KU-043-083

TEXTBOOK OF
RHEUMATOLOGY

VOLUME 1

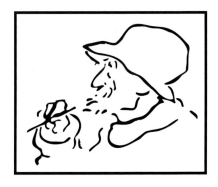

TEXTBOOK OF
RHEUMATOLOGY

FIFTH EDITION

WILLIAM N. KELLEY, M.D.
Chief Executive Officer
University of Pennsylvania Medical Center and
    Health System
Executive Vice President, University of
    Pennsylvania
Dean, University of Pennsylvania School of
    Medicine
Robert G. Dunlop Professor of Medicine and
    Biochemistry and Biophysics, University of
    Pennsylvania
Philadelphia, Pennsylvania

SHAUN RUDDY, M.D.
Elam Toone Professor of Internal Medicine,
    Microbiology, and Immunology
Chairman, Division of Rheumatology, Allergy, and
    Immunology
Department of Internal Medicine
Medical College of Virginia
Virginia Commonwealth University
Richmond, Virginia

EDWARD D. HARRIS, Jr., M.D.
George DeForest Barnett Professor
Department of Medicine
Stanford University School of Medicine
Palo Alto, California

CLEMENT B. SLEDGE, M.D.
John B. and Buckminster Brown Professor of
    Orthopedic Surgery
Harvard Medical School
Chairman, Department of Orthopedic Surgery
Brigham and Women's Hospital
Boston, Massachusetts

W.B. SAUNDERS COMPANY
A Division of Harcourt Brace & Company
Philadelphia   London   Toronto   Montreal   Sydney   Tokyo

W.B. SAUNDERS COMPANY
A Division of Harcourt Brace & Company

The Curtis Center
Independence Square West
Philadelphia, Pennsylvania 19106

Library of Congress Cataloging-in-Publication Data

Textbook of rheumatology / William N. Kelley . . . [et al.]. —5th ed.

    p.   cm.

Includes bibliographical references and index.

ISBN 0–7216–5692–7 (set)

1. Rheumatology.   I. Kelley, William N. [DNLM: 1. Rheumatic
   Diseases.   2. Arthritis.   WE 544 T355 1997]

RC927.T49 1997   616.7'23—dc20

DNLM/DLC   96–4866

SBRLSMP	
CLAS	WE540 TEX V.1
CIR(	OWK.
SUPPLIER	BMBC 11/97 £147.00 (2 vol)
BINDING	

TEXTBOOK OF RHEUMATOLOGY, Fifth Edition   ISBN 0–7216–5692–7

Copyright © 1997, 1993, 1989, 1985, 1981 by W.B. Saunders Company

All rights reserved.   No part of this publication may be reproduced or transmitted in any form or by any means, electronic or mechanical, including photocopy, recording, or any information storage and retrieval system, without permission in writing from the publisher.

Printed in the United States of America

Last digit is the print number: 9   8   7   6   5   4   3   2   1

This edition of the
Textbook of Rheumatology
is dedicated to our families.

Lois Kelley, Paige Kelley Nath, Ginger Kelley Yost, Lori Kelley, and Mark Kelley.

Joan Lonergan, Ned Harris, Tom Harris, and Chandler Harris.

Millicent Ruddy, Christi Ruddy Hulcher, and Candace Ruddy Lau-Hansen.

*Georgia Sledge, Margaret Sledge Tracy, John Sledge, Matthew Sledge,
and Claire Sledge Smith.*

Contributors

ROY ALTMAN, M.D.
Professor of Medicine, University of Miami School of
Medicine. Director, Clinical Research, Geriatric Research,
Education, and Clinical Center (GRECC), Miami Veterans
Affairs Medical Center, Miami, Florida.
Hypertrophic Osteoarthropathy

WILLIAM P. AREND, M.D.
Professor, Departments of Medicine and Immunology, and
Head, Division of Rheumatology, University of Colorado
School of Medicine, Denver, Colorado.
Cytokines and Growth Factors

M. AMIN ARNAOUT, M.D.
Professor of Medicine, Harvard Medical School, Boston.
Director, Leukocyte Biology and Inflammation Program,
Massachusetts General Hospital, Charlestown,
Massachusetts.
*Structural Diversity of Cell Adhesion Molecules and Their Role
in Inflammation*

RONALD A. ASHERSON, M.D., F.A.C.R., F.R.C.P.,
F.C.A.
Principal Scientific Officer, Department of Medicine,
University of Cape Town. Honorary Consultant Physician,
Rheumatic Disease Unit, Department of Medicine, Groote
Schuur Hospital, Cape Town, South Africa.
Antiphospholipid Syndrome

K. FRANK AUSTEN, M.D.
Theodore Bevier Bayles Professor of Medicine, Harvard
Medical School. Director, Inflammation and Allergic
Diseases Research Section, Division of Rheumatology and
Immunology, Brigham and Women's Hospital, Boston,
Massachusetts.
Prostaglandins, Leukotrienes, and Related Compounds

STANLEY P. BALLOU, M.D.
Associate Professor of Medicine, Case Western Reserve
University School of Medicine. Director, Arthritis and
Lupus Clinics, MetroHealth Medical Center, Cleveland,
Ohio.
Laboratory Evaluation of Inflammation

N. NICHOLE BARRY, M.D.
Clinical Fellow, Department of Immunology/Rheuma-
tology, Stanford University Medical Center, Palo Alto,
California.
Hip and Knee Pain

ROBERT M. BENNETT, M.D., F.R.C.P.
Professor, Department of Medicine, and Chairman,
Division of Arthritis and Rheumatic Diseases, Oregon
Health Sciences University, Portland, Oregon.
*The Fibromyalgia Syndrome; Mixed Connective Tissue Disease
and Other Overlap Syndromes*

HÅKAN BERGSTRAND, Ph.D.
Scientific Advisor and Associate Director, Department
of Cell and Molecular Biology, Astra Draco, Lund,
Sweden.
Neutrophils and Eosinophils

ALAN L. BISNO, M.D.
Professor and Vice-Chairman, Department of Medicine,
University of Miami School of Medicine. Chief, Medical
Service, Miami Veterans Affairs Medical Center, Miami,
Florida.
Rheumatic Fever

JOSEPH J. BIUNDO, Jr., M.D.
Professor of Medicine and Chief of Physical Medicine and
Rehabilitation, Louisiana State University Medical Center,
New Orleans, Louisiana.
Rehabilitation of Patients with Rheumatic Diseases

DAVID R. BLAKE, M.B., Ch.B., F.R.C.P.
Professor of Rheumatology, St. Bartholomew's and
The Royal London Hospital School of Medicine and
Dentistry. Honorary Consultation Rheumatologist,
Royal Hospitals NHS Trust, Mile End Hospital,
London, England.
Biology of the Normal Joint

MAARTEN BOERS, M.D., Ph.D., M.Sc.
Associate Professor, Department of Internal Medicine/
Rheumatology, University of Maastricht, Maastricht, The
Netherlands.
Clinical Epidemiology of the Rheumatic Diseases

ARTHUR L. BOLAND, M.D.
Assistant Clinical Professor, Orthopaedic Surgery, Harvard
Medical School. Visiting Orthopaedic Surgeon,
Massachusetts General Hospital and Brigham and
Women's Hospital, Boston, Massachusetts.
Sports Medicine

KENNETH D. BRANDT, M.D.
Professor of Medicine, Indiana University School of
Medicine. Head, Rheumatology Division, and Director,
Multipurpose Arthritis and Musculoskeletal Diseases
Center, Indiana University Medical Center, Indianapolis,
Indiana.
Pathogenesis of Osteoarthritis; Management of Osteoarthritis

DOREEN B. BRETTLER, M.D.
Professor of Medicine, University of Massachusetts
Medical School. Director, New England Hemophilia
Center, Medical Center of Central Massachusetts,
Worcester, Massachusetts.
Hemophilic Arthropathy

DAVID M. BRISCOE, M.D.
Assistant Professor in Pediatrics, Harvard Medical School. Assistant in Medicine, Children's Hospital, Boston, Massachussets.
Endothelial Cells in Inflammation

REBECCA H. BUCKLEY, M.D.
J. Buren Sidbury Professor of Pediatrics and Professor of Immunology, Duke University School of Medicine. Chief, Division of Allergy and Immunology, Department of Pediatrics, Duke University Medical Center, Durham, North Carolina.
Specific Immunodeficiency Diseases, Excluding Acquired Immunodeficiency Syndrome

DAVID S. CALDWELL, M.D.
Associate Professor, Duke University School of Medicine, Durham, North Carolina.
Musculoskeletal Syndromes Associated with Malignancy

EVAN CALKINS, M.D.
Emeritus Professor of Medicine and Family Medicine, School of Medicine and Biomedical Sciences, State University of New York at Buffalo. Senior Physician and Coordinator, Geriatric Programs, Health Care Plan. Partner, Medical Partners of Western New York, Buffalo, New York.
Some Aspects of Rheumatic Disease in the Older Patient

MARCUS E. CARR, Jr., M.D., Ph.D.
Associate Professor, Departments of Internal Medicine and Pathology, Medical College of Virginia, Virginia Commonwealth University. Staff Physician, Hunter Holmes McGuire Veterans Affairs Medical Center. President and Founder of Hemodyne, Inc., Virginia BioTech Park, Richmond, Virginia.
Platelets

DENNIS A. CARSON, M.D.
Professor of Medicine and Director, The Sam and Rose Stein Institute for Research on Aging, University of California–San Diego School of Medicine, La Jolla, California.
Rheumatoid Factors

JAMES T. CASSIDY, M.D.
Professor of Child Health, University of Missouri–Columbia School of Medicine. Attending Physician, Department of Child Health, University of Missouri Health Sciences Center, Columbia, Missouri.
Juvenile Rheumatoid Arthritis; Systemic Lupus Erythematosus, Juvenile Dermatomyositis, Scleroderma, and Vasculitis

RICARD CERVERA, M.D., Ph.D.
Specialist Internist, Systemic Autoimmune Diseases Unit, Hospital Clinic, Villarroel, Barcelona, Catalonia, Spain.
Antiphospholipid Syndrome

MICHAEL J. CHMELL, M.D.
Clinical Instructor, Department of Surgery, University of Illinois College of Medicine. Staff Orthopedic Surgeon, Rockford Memorial Hospital, Swedish American Hospital, and St. Anthony Medical Center, Rockford, Illinois.
Surgical Management of Juvenile Rheumatoid Arthritis

PHILIP J. CLEMENTS, M.D.
Professor, Department of Medicine, University of California–Los Angeles School of Medicine, Los Angeles, California.
Nonsteroidal Antirheumatic Drugs

ROBERT H. COFIELD, M.D.
Professor, Mayo Medical School. Consultant in Orthopedics, Mayo Clinic, and Dean, Mayo Graduate School of Medicine, Rochester, Minnesota.
The Shoulder

DOYT L. CONN, M.D.
Clinical Professor of Medicine, Emory University School of Medicine. Senior Vice President for Medical Affairs, Arthritis Foundation, National Office, Atlanta, Georgia.
Vasculitis and Related Disorders

PHILIP G. COOGAN, M.D.
Instructor in Orthopaedics, Duke University School of Medicine. Hand and Microsurgery Fellow, Duke University Medical Center, Durham, North Carolina.
Osteonecrosis

RAMZI S. COTRAN, M.D.
F.B. Mallory Professor of Pathology, Harvard Medical School. Chairman, Department of Pathology, Brigham and Women's Hospital and Children's Hospital, Boston, Massachusetts.
Endothelial Cells in Inflammation

JOE CRAFT, M.D.
Associate Professor, Department of Medicine, and Chief, Section of Rheumatology, Yale University School of Medicine. Attending Physician, Yale–New Haven Hospital, New Haven, Connecticut.
Antinuclear Antibodies

JODY A. DANTZIG, Ph.D.
Research Associate, Department of Physiology, University of Pennsylvania School of Medicine/Pennsylvania Muscle Institute, Philadelphia, Pennsylvania.
Skeletal Muscle

LAURIE S. DAVIS, Ph.D.
Assistant Professor of Internal Medicine, Southwestern Medical School, University of Texas Health Science Center at Dallas, Dallas, Texas.
T Cells and B Cells

RICHARD O. DAY, M.B.B.S., M.D.
Professor, Clinical Pharmacology, School of Physiology and Pharmacology, University of New South Wales. Director, Clinical Pharmacology and Therapeutics, St. Vincent's Hospital, Sydney, New South Wales, Australia.
Sulfasalazine

JEAN-MICHEL DAYER, M.D.
Associate Professor of Immunology, Geneva University Medical School. Head, Division of Immunology and Allergy, University Hospital, Geneva, Switzerland.
Cytokines and Growth Factors

MICHAEL F. DILLINGHAM, M.D.
Clinical Professor, Division of Orthopedic Surgery,
Stanford University School of Medicine. Director,
Orthopedics, and Team Physician, Stanford University,
Stanford. Team Physician, San Francisco Forty-Niners, San
Francisco. Team Physician, Santa Clara University, Santa
Clara, California.
Hip and Knee Pain

MICHAEL J. DUVAL, M.D.
Assistant Professor, Department of Orthopaedic Surgery,
Louisiana State University School of Medicine, Lafayette,
Louisiana.
Arthroscopy and Synovectomy

PENG THIM FAN, M.D.
Clinical Professor of Medicine, University of
California–Los Angeles School of Medicine, Los Angeles,
California.
Reiter's Syndrome

ANTHONY S. FAUCI, M.D.
Director, National Institute of Allergy and Infectious
Diseases, National Institutes of Health, Bethesda,
Maryland.
Immunoregulatory Agents

JOHN A. FEAGIN, Jr., M.D.
Associate Professor, Biomedical Engineering, Department
of Surgery, Division of Orthopaedics, Duke University
School of Medicine, Durham, North Carolina.
Sports Medicine

ANTHONY S. FELSOVANYI, M.D.
Emeritus Clinical Professor of Medicine (Active), Stanford
University School of Medicine. Attending Physician,
Stanford University Medical Center, Palo Alto, California.
Weakness

GARY S. FIRESTEIN, M.D.
Professor of Medicine, University of California–San Diego
School of Medicine, La Jolla, California.
Etiology and Pathogenesis of Rheumatoid Arthritis

IRVING H. FOX, B.Sc., M.D., C.M.
Clinical Professor of Medicine, Harvard Medical School.
Vice-President of Medical Affairs, Biogen, Inc. Clinical
Associate, Massachusetts General Hospital, Boston,
Massachusetts.
Antihyperuricemic Drugs

ROBERT I. FOX, M.D., Ph.D.
Member, Division of Rheumatology, Scripps Clinic and
Research Foundation, La Jolla, California.
Sjögren's Syndrome

ANDREW G. FRANKS, Jr., M.D.
Clinical Associate Professor, Department of Dermatology,
New York University School of Medicine. Chief,
Connective Tissue Disease, Skin and Cancer Clinic, New
York University. Senior Rheumatologist, Lenox Hill
Hospital, New York, New York.
Cutaneous Manifestations of Rheumatic Diseases

HOWARD FUCHS, M.D.
Associate Professor of Medicine, Vanderbilt University
School of Medicine, Division of Rheumatology. Chief,
Section of Rheumatology Medical Service, Nashville
Department of Veterans Affairs Medical Center, Nashville,
Tennessee.
Silicone Breast Implants and Rheumatic Diseases

THOMAS D. GEPPERT, M.D.
Assistant Professor, Department of Internal Medicine,
Southwestern Medical School, University of Texas Health
Science Center at Dallas, Dallas, Texas.
T Cells and B Cells

WILLIAM W. GINSBURG, M.D.
Associate Professor, Mayo Medical School, Rochester,
Minnesota. Consultant in Rheumatology, Mayo Clinic
Jacksonville, Jacksonville, Florida.
Multicentric Reticulohistiocytosis

DAFNA D. GLADMAN, M.D., F.R.C.P.C.
Professor of Medicine, University of Toronto Faculty of
Medicine. Deputy Director, Center for Prognosis Studies in
the Rheumatic Diseases, The Toronto Hospital, Toronto,
Ontario, Canada.
Psoriatic Arthritis

JOSEPH GOLBUS, M.D.
Associate Professor of Medicine, Section of
Arthritis–Connective Tissue Diseases, Northwestern
University Medical School, Chicago. Head, Division of
Rheumatology, Evanston Hospital, Evanston, Illinois.
Monarticular Arthritis

DON L. GOLDENBERG, M.D.
Professor of Medicine, Tufts University School of
Medicine, Boston. Chief of Rheumatology, Newton-
Wellesley Hospital, Newton, Massachusetts.
Bacterial Arthritis

YALE E. GOLDMAN, E.E., M.D., Ph.D.
Professor, Department of Physiology, University of
Pennsylvania School of Medicine. Director, Pennsylvania
Muscle Institute, Philadelphia, Pennsylvania.
Skeletal Muscle

DUNCAN A. GORDON, M.D., F.R.C.P.C., F.A.C.P.
Professor of Medicine, University of Toronto Faculty of
Medicine. Editor, *Journal of Rheumatology*. Senior
Rheumatologist, The Toronto Hospital Arthritis Centre,
Ontario, Canada.
Gold Compounds and Penicillamine in the Rheumatic Diseases

PETER K. GREGERSEN, M.D.
Associate Professor of Medicine, Cornell University
Medical College, New York. Chief, Division of Biology
and Human Genetics, Department of Medicine, North
Shore University Hospital, Manhasset, New York.
Genetic Analysis of Rheumatic Diseases

BEVRA HANNAHS HAHN, M.D., F.A.C.R.
Professor of Medicine and Chief of Rheumatology,
University of California–Los Angeles School of Medicine,
Los Angeles, California.
*Pathogenesis of Systemic Lupus Erythematosus; Management of
Systemic Lupus Erythematosus*

LENA HÅKANSSON, Ph.D.
Associate Professor, Department of Clinical Chemistry, Uppsala University. Research Engineer, University Hospital, Uppsala, Sweden.
Neutrophils and Eosinophils

STEPHEN HALL, M.B.B.S., F.R.A.C.P.
Clinical Associate Professor of Medicine, Monash University. Head, Rheumatology Unit, Box Hill Hospital, Melbourne, Australia.
Vasculitis and Related Disorders

SIGVARD T. HANSEN, Jr., M.D.
Professor and Chairman Emeritus, Department of Orthopaedics, University of Washington School of Medicine. Chief, Section of Foot/Ankle/Amputee Care, Harborview Medical Center, Seattle, Washington.
The Ankle and Foot

JOHN A. HARDIN, M.D.
Professor and Chairman, Department of Medicine, Medical College of Georgia, Augusta, Georgia.
Antinuclear Antibodies

J. TIMOTHY HARRINGTON, Jr., M.D.
Clinical Associate Professor, University of Wisconsin Medical School. Chair, Department of Rheumatology, Physicians Plus Medical Group, Madison, Wisconsin.
Mycobacterial and Fungal Infections

EDWARD D. HARRIS, Jr., M.D.
George DeForest Barnett Professor, Department of Medicine, Stanford University School of Medicine, Palo Alto, California.
Clinical Features of Rheumatoid Arthritis; Treatment of Rheumatoid Arthritis

MARC C. HOCHBERG, M.D., M.P.H.
Professor of Medicine and Epidemiology and Preventive Medicine, and Head, Division of Rheumatology and Clinical Immunology, University of Maryland School of Medicine, Baltimore, Maryland.
Polychondritis

GENE G. HUNDER, M.D., M.S.
Professor of Medicine, Mayo Medical School. Chairman, Division of Rheumatology, Mayo Clinic, Rochester, Minnesota.
Examination of the Joints; Giant Cell Arteritis and Polymyalgia Rheumatica

JOHN N. INSALL, M.D.
Attending Physician, Beth Israel Medical Center, North Division, New York, New York.
The Knee

SILVIU ITESCU, M.D., F.R.A.C.P.
Assistant Professor of Pediatrics, and Director, Transplantation Immunology, Department of Surgery, Columbia University, College of Physicians and Surgeons. Attending Physician, Presbyterian Hospital, New York, New York.
Rheumatologic Manifestations of Human Immunodeficiency Virus Infection

JOHN S. JOHNSON, M.D.
Associate Professor of Medicine, Vanderbilt University School of Medicine. Chairman, Department of Medicine, St. Thomas Hospital, Nashville, Tennessee.
Silicone Breast Implants and Rheumatic Diseases

WILLIAM N. KELLEY, M.D.
Chief Executive Officer, University of Pennsylvania Medical Center and Health System. Executive Vice President; Dean, School of Medicine; and Robert G. Dunlop Professor of Medicine and Biochemistry and Biophysics, University of Pennsylvania, Philadelphia, Pennsylvania.
Gout and Hyperuricemia

EDWARD C. KEYSTONE, M.D., F.R.C.P.(C)
Professor of Medicine, University of Toronto Faculty of Medicine. Director, Division of Rheumatology, The Wellesley Hospital, Toronto, Ontario, Canada.
Biologic Agents in the Treatment of Rheumatoid Arthritis

JOSEPH H. KORN, M.D.
Professor of Medicine and Biochemistry, and Director, Arthritis Center, Boston University School of Medicine. Chief, Rheumatology Section, Department of Medicine, Boston University Medical Center and Boston Veterans Affairs Medical Center, Boston, Massachusetts.
Fibroblast Function and Fibrosis

JOEL M. KREMER, M.D.
Professor of Medicine, and Head, Division of Rheumatology, The Albany Medical College. Attending Physician, Albany Medical Center Hospital, Albany, New York.
Nutrition and Rheumatic Diseases

IRVING KUSHNER, M.D.
Professor of Medicine and Pathology, Case Western Reserve University School of Medicine. Acting Director, Division of Rheumatology, MetroHealth Medical Center, Cleveland, Ohio.
Laboratory Evaluation of Inflammation

ROBERT G. LAHITA, M.D., Ph.D.
Associate Professor, Columbia University College of Physicians and Surgeons. Chief of Rheumatology and Connective Tissue Disease, Saint Lukes Roosevelt Hospital, New York, New York.
Clinical Presentation of Systemic Lupus Erythematosus

R. ELAINE LAMBERT, M.D.
Assistant Professor, Division of Immunology and Rheumatology, Department of Internal Medicine, Stanford University School of Medicine, Stanford, California.
Arthropathies Associated with Endocrine Disorders; Iron Storage Disease

JOHN V. LANNIN, M.D.
Orthopaedic Surgeon, Palo Alto Medical Foundation, Palo Alto, California.
Hip and Knee Pain

MERYL S. LeBOFF, M.D.
Associate Professor, Harvard Medical School. Director, Skeletal Health and Osteoporosis Program, and Associate

Physician, Brigham and Women's Hospital, Boston, Massachusetts.
Metabolic Bone Disease

MATTHEW H. LIANG, M.D., M.P.H.
Professor of Medicine, Harvard Medical School. Professor of Health Policy and Management, Harvard School of Public Health. Director, Rehabilitation Services, and Robert B. Brigham Multipurpose Arthritis and Musculoskeletal Diseases Center, Brigham and Women's Hospital, Boston, Massachusetts.
Psychosocial Management of Rheumatic Diseases

SCOTT A. LINTNER, M.D.
Staff Orthopaedic Surgeon, Orthopaedics Indianapolis, Indianapolis, Indiana.
Sports Medicine

PETER E. LIPSKY, M.D.
Professor, Departments of Internal Medicine and Microbiology, Southwestern Medical School, University of Texas Health Science Center at Dallas, Dallas, Texas.
T Cells and B Cells; Monocytes and Macrophages

STEPHEN J. LIPSON, M.D.
Associate Professor, Department of Orthopedic Surgery, Harvard Medical School. Orthopedic Surgeon-in-Chief, Beth Israel Hospital, Boston, Massachusetts.
Low Back Pain; The Cervical Spine

CARLO L. MAINARDI, M.D.
Professor of Medicine, University of Maryland School of Medicine. President and Chief Executive Officer, University Health Care, Baltimore, Maryland.
Localized Fibrotic Diseases

HENRY J. MANKIN, M.D.
Edith M. Ashley Professor of Orthopaedic Surgery, Harvard Medical School. Chief of the Orthopaedic Service, Massachusetts General Hospital, Boston, Massachusetts.
Pathogenesis of Osteoarthritis

W. JOSEPH McCUNE, M.D.
Associate Professor, Department of Internal Medicine, Division of Rheumatology, University of Michigan Medical School, Ann Arbor, Michigan.
Monarticular Arthritis

JAMES L. McGUIRE, M.D.
Chairman, Department of Medicine, Mount Auburn Hospital. Executive Vice President, Medical Director, and Chief Operating Officer, Mount Auburn Professional Services, Inc., Mount Auburn Hospital, Cambridge, Massachusetts.
Iron Storage Disease; Arthropathies Associated with Endocrine Disorders

KATHERYN MEEK, D.V.M.
Assistant Professor, Departments of Internal Medicine and Microbiology, Southwestern Medical School, University of Texas at Dallas, Dallas, Texas.
T Cells and B Cells

KENJI C. MIYASAKA, M.D.
Surgical Arthritis Fellow, Center for Total Joint Replacement, Department of Orthopaedic Surgery, Lenox Hill Hospital, New York, New York.
The Hip

KEVIN G. MODER, M.D.
Assistant Professor, Division of Rheumatology, Department of Internal Medicine, Mayo Graduate School of Medicine.
Senior Associate Consultant, Mayo Clinic, Rochester, Minnesota.
Examination of the Joints

B. F. MORREY, M.D.
Professor of Orthopedics, Mayo Medical School. Chair, Department of Orthopedics, Mayo Clinic, Rochester, Minnesota.
The Elbow

GEORGE MOXLEY, M.D.
Associate Professor, Department of Internal Medicine, Medical College of Virginia, Virginia Commonwealth University. Chief, Rheumatology Section, Hunter Holmes McGuire Veterans Affairs Medical Center, Richmond, Virginia.
Immune Complexes and Complement

HIDEAKI NAGASE, Ph.D.
Professor, Department of Biochemistry and Molecular Biology, University of Kansas School of Medicine, Kansas City, Kansas.
Proteinases and Matrix Degradation

KENNETH K. NAKANO, M.D., M.P.H., M.S., F.R.C.P.(C)
Neurologist, Straub Clinic, Honolulu, Hawaii.
Neck Pain; Entrapment Neuropathies and Related Disorders

J. DESMOND O'DUFFY, M.B.
Professor of Medicine, Mayo Medical School. Consultant, Division of Rheumatology, Mayo Clinic, Rochester, Minnesota.
Vasculitis and Related Disorders; Multicentric Reticulohistiocytosis

YASUNORI OKADA, M.D., Ph.D.
Professor, Department of Molecular Immunology and Pathology, Cancer Research Institute, Kanazawa University, Kanazawa, Ishikawa, Japan.
Proteinases and Matrix Degradation

NANCY OPPENHEIMER-MARKS, Ph.D.
Assistant Professor, Department of Internal Medicine, Southwestern Medical School, University of Texas Health Science Center at Dallas, Dallas, Texas.
T Cells and B Cells

DUNCAN S. OWEN, Jr., M.D.
Taliaferro/Scott Professor of Internal Medicine, Medical College of Virginia, Virginia Commonwealth University. Attending Physician, Medical College of Virginia Hospitals. Consultant, Hunter Holmes McGuire Department of Veterans Affairs Medical Center, Richmond, Virginia.
Aspiration and Injection of Joints and Soft Tissues

HAROLD E. PAULUS, M.D.
Professor, Department of Medicine, University of
California–Los Angeles, School of Medicine, Los Angeles,
California.
Nonsteroidal Antirheumatic Drugs

STANFORD L. PENG, B.A., B.S.
Fellow, Medical Scientist Training Program, Department of
Biology, and Section of Rheumatology, Department of
Internal Medicine, Yale University School of Medicine,
New Haven, Connecticut.
Antinuclear Antibodies

JOHN F. PENROSE, M.D.
Assistant Professor, Harvard Medical School. Associate
Rheumatologist/Pediatric Rheumatologist, Division of
Rheumatology/Immunology, Brigham and Women's
Hospital, Boston, Massachusetts.
Prostaglandins, Leukotrienes, and Related Compounds

ROBERT S. PINALS, M.D.
Professor of Medicine, University of Medicine and
Dentistry of New Jersey–The Robert Wood Johnson
Medical School, New Brunswick. Chairman, Department
of Medicine, The Medical Center at Princeton, Princeton,
New Jersey.
Felty's Syndrome

THEODORE PINCUS, M.D.
Professor of Medicine, Division of Rheumatology–
Immunology, Vanderbilt University School of Medicine,
Nashville, Tennessee.
Glucocorticoids

DARWIN J. PROCKOP, M.D., Ph.D.
Professor and Chairman, Department of Biochemistry and
Molecular Biology, Jefferson Medical College, Thomas
Jefferson University. Director, Jefferson Institute of
Molecular Medicine, Philadelphia, Pennsylvania.
Collagen and Elastin

ERIC L. RADIN, M.D.
Clinical Professor of Orthopedic Surgery, University of
Michigan, Ann Arbor, Michigan. Professor of Orthopedic
Surgery, Case Western Reserve University School of
Medicine, Cleveland, Ohio. The Breech Chair, Bone and
Joint Center, Henry Ford Hospital, Detroit, Michigan.
Biomechanics of Joints

CHITRANJAN S. RANAWAT, M.D.
Professor of Orthopaedic Surgery, Cornell University
Medical College. Director, Department of Orthopaedic
Surgery and Center for Total Joint Replacement, Lenox
Hill Hospital, New York, New York.
The Hip

ANTHONY M. REGINATO, Ph.D., M.D.
Resident-Internal Medicine, Yale–New Haven Hospital,
Yale University School of Medicine, New Haven,
Connecticut.
*Diseases Associated with Deposition of Calcium Pyrophosphate
or Hydroxyapatite*

ANTONIO J. REGINATO, M.D.
Professor of Medicine and Head, Division of
Rheumatology, University of Medicine and Dentistry of
New Jersey–Robert Wood Johnson Medical School,
Camden, New Jersey. Associate Clinical Professor,
University of Pennsylvania. Recipient of the American
College of Physicians International Professorship,
American College of Physicians, Philadelphia,
Pennsylvania.
*Diseases Associated with Deposition of Calcium Pyrophosphate
or Hydroxyapatite*

DONALD RESNICK, M.D.
Professor, Department of Radiology, University of
California–San Diego School of Medicine, La Jolla. Chief,
Osteoradiology Section, Veterans Affairs Medical Center,
San Diego, California.
Imaging

JOSE A. RODRIGUEZ, M.D.
Instructor of Orthopaedic Surgery, Cornell University
Medical College. Assistant Adjunct Attending Orthopaedic
Surgeon, Lenox Hill Hospital, New York, New York.
The Hip

ANDREW E. ROSENBERG, M.D.
Associate Professor, Harvard Medical School. Assistant
Pathologist, Massachusetts General Hospital, Boston,
Massachusetts.
*Tumors and Tumor-Like Lessons of Joints and Related
Structures*

DAVID W. ROWE, M.D.
Professor of Pediatrics, Division of Endocrinology/
Diabetes, University of Connecticut School of Medicine,
Farmington, Connecticut.
Heritable Disorders of Structural Proteins

CLINTON T. RUBIN, Ph.D.
Professor, Department of Orthopaedics, and Director,
Program in Biomedical Engineering, School of Medicine,
State University of New York at Stony Brook, Stony Brook,
New York.
The Biology, Physiology, and Morphology of Bone

JANET E. RUBIN, M.D.
Associate Professor, Department of Medicine, Emory
University School of Medicine. Attending Physician,
Veterans Affairs Medical Center, Decatur, Georgia.
The Biology, Physiology, and Morphology of Bone

SHAUN RUDDY, M.D.
Elam Toone Professor of Internal Medicine, Microbiology,
and Immunology, and Chairman, Division of
Rheumatology, Allergy, and Immunology, Department of
Internal Medicine, Medical College of Virginia, Virginia
Commonwealth University, Richmond, Virginia.
*Immune Complexes and Complement; Complement Deficiencies
and Rheumatic Diseases*

PERRY J. RUSH, M.D.
Assistant Professor, University of Toronto Faculty of
Medicine. Associate Physician, Mt. Sinai Hospital, and
Consultant, Baycrest Hospital, Toronto, Ontario, Canada.
Rehabilitation of Patients with Rheumatic Diseases

RICHARD I. RYNES, M.D.
Clinical Professor of Medicine, Albany Medical College, Albany. Rheumatologist, Community Health Program, Latham, New York.
Antimalarial Drugs

DAVID SARTORIS, M.D.
Professor, Department of Radiology, University of California–San Diego School of Medicine, La Jolla. Chief, Quantitative Bone Densitometry, University Medical Center, San Diego, California.
Imaging

ROBERT J. SCARDINA, D.P.M.
Clinical Instructor in Orthopaedics, Harvard Medical School. Chief, Podiatric Unit, Massachusetts General Hospital, and Director, Podiatric Division, Brigham and Women's Hospital, Boston, Massachusetts.
Ankle and Foot Pain

ALAN L. SCHILLER, M.D.
Irene Heinz Given and John LaPorte Given Professor and Chairman of Pathology, Mt. Sinai School of Medicine. Chairman of Pathology, The Mt. Sinai Hospital, New York, New York.
Tumors and Tumor-Like Lesions of Joints and Related Structures

THOMAS J. SCHNITZER, M.D., Ph.D.
Willard L. Wood, M.D., Professor of Medicine, and Director, Section of Rheumatology and Geriatric Medicine, Rush Medical College. Medical Director, Johnston R. Bowman Health Center for the Elderly, Rush-Presbyterian–St. Luke's Medical Center, Chicago, Illinois.
Viral Arthritis

H. RALPH SCHUMACHER, Jr., M.D.
Professor of Medicine, University of Pennsylvania School of Medicine. Director, Arthritis Immunology Center, Veterans Affairs Medical Center. Rheumatologist, Hospital of the University of Pennsylvania, Philadelphia, Pennsylvania.
Hemoglobinopathies and Arthritis; Synovial Fluid Analysis and Synovial Biopsy; Antihyperuricemic Drugs

LAWRENCE B. SCHWARTZ, M.D., Ph.D.
Charles and Evelyn Thomas Professor of Medicine, Department of Internal Medicine, Medical College of Virginia, Virginia Commonwealth University, Richmond, Virginia.
The Mast Cell

RICHARD D. SCOTT, M.D.
Associate Clinical Professor, Department of Orthopaedic Surgery, Harvard Medical School. Attending Surgeon, Brigham and Women's Hospital and New England Baptist Hospital, Boston, Massachusetts.
Surgical Management of Juvenile Rheumatoid Arthritis

JAMES R. SEIBOLD, M.D.
Director, Scleroderma Program, University of Medicine and Dentistry of New Jersey–Robert Wood Johnson Medical School. Attending Physician, Medicine and Rheumatology, Robert Wood Johnson University Hospital, New Brunswick, New Jersey.
Scleroderma

WINSTON SEQUEIRA, M.D., F.A.C.P.
Associate Professor, Rush Medical College. Chairman, Division of Rheumatology, Cook County Hospital, Chicago, Illinois.
Rheumatic Manifestations of Sarcoidosis

JOHN S. SERGENT, M.D.
Chief Medical Officer, Vanderbilt University Medical Center, Nashville, Tennessee.
Approach to the Patient with Pain in More Than One Joint; Silicone Breast Implants and Rheumatic Diseases

JAY R. SHAPIRO, M.D.
Professor of Medicine, Johns Hopkins University School of Medicine, Division of Geriatric Medicine and Gerontology. Program Director, General Clinical Research Center, Johns Hopkins Bayview Medical Center, Baltimore, Maryland.
Heritable Disorders of Structural Proteins

NIGEL E. SHARROCK, M.B., Ch.B.
Assistant Clinical Professor in Anesthesiology, Cornell University Medical College. Senior Scientist and Attending Physician in Anesthesia, Hospital for Special Surgery, New York, New York.
Anesthetic Considerations

BARRY P. SIMMONS, M.D.
Associate Clinical Professor of Orthopedic Surgery, Harvard Medical School. Chief, Department of Orthopedics, Division of Hand and Upper Extremity Service, Brigham and Women's Hospital, Boston, Massachusetts.
The Hand and Wrist

SHELDON R. SIMON, M.D.
Judson Wilson Professor of Orthopaedics, Ohio State University School of Medicine. Chief, Division of Orthopaedics, Department of Surgery, Ohio State University Hospitals, Columbus, Ohio.
Biomechanics of Joints

MARTHA SKINNER, M.D.
Professor of Medicine, Boston University School of Medicine. Director, Amyloid Clinical and Research Program, Boston University Medical Center, Boston, Massachusetts.
Amyloidosis

CLEMENT B. SLEDGE, M.D.
John B. and Buckminster Brown Professor of Orthopedic Surgery, Harvard Medical School. Chairman, Department of Orthopedic Surgery, Brigham and Women's Hospital, Boston, Massachusetts.
Biology of the Normal Joint; Introduction to Surgical Management of the Patient with Arthritis

LIV MARIT SMEDSTAD, M.D.
Research Fellow, Department of Behavioral Sciences in Medicine, University of Oslo, Oslo, Norway.
Psychosocial Management of Rheumatic Diseases

GARTH R. SMITH, M.D.
Clinical Fellow in Orthopedic Surgery, Harvard Medical School. Clinical Fellow, Department of Orthopedics,

Division of Hand and Upper Extremity Service, Brigham and Women's Hospital, Boston, Massachusetts.
The Hand and Wrist

LOUIS SOLOMON, M.D., F.R.C.S.
Emeritus Professor of Orthopaedic Surgery, University of Bristol. Consultant Orthopaedic Surgeon, Bristol Royal Infirmary, Bristol, United Kingdom.
Clinical Features of Osteoarthritis

NICHOLAS A. SOTER, M.D.
Professor, The Ronald O. Perelman Department of Dermatology, New York University School of Medicine. Medical Director, Charles C. Harris Skin and Cancer Pavilion. Attending Physician, Tisch Hospital (University Hospital), New York, New York.
Cutaneous Manifestations of Rheumatic Diseases

ALLEN C. STEERE, M.D.
Professor of Medicine, Tufts University School of Medicine. Chief, Rheumatology/Immunology, New England Medical Center, Boston, Massachusetts.
Lyme Disease

C. MICHAEL STEIN, M.B., Ch.B., M.R.C.P.(UK)
Assistant Professor of Medicine and Pharmacology, Vanderbilt University School of Medicine, Nashville, Tennessee.
Glucocorticoids

VIBEKE STRAND, M.D., F.A.C.P.
Clinical Associate Professor, Division of Immunology, Stanford University School of Medicine. Biopharmaceutical Consultant, Stanford, California.
Biologic Agents in the Treatment of Rheumatoid Arthritis

JERRY TENENBAUM, M.D., F.R.C.P.(C), F.A.C.P.
Associate Dean of Continuing Medical Education and Associate Professor of Medicine, University of Toronto Faculty of Medicine. Staff Physician, Mt. Sinai Hospital. Staff Consultant (Rheumatology), Baycrest Geriatric Center, and Toronto Hospital, Toronto, Ontario, Canada.
Hypertrophic Osteoarthropathy

RANJENY THOMAS, M.B.B.S., M.D.
Senior Lecturer in Rheumatology, University of Queensland. Rheumatologist, Princess Alexandra Hospital, Brisbane, Queensland, Australia.
Monocytes and Macrophages

THOMAS S. THORNHILL, M.D.
Associate Clinical Professor of Orthopedic Surgery, Harvard Medical School. Chief of Orthopedic Surgery, New England Baptist Hospital, and Orthopedic Surgeon, Brigham and Women's Hospital, Boston, Massachusetts.
Shoulder Pain

HELEN TIGHE, Ph.D.
Assistant Adjunct Professor, University of California–San Diego School of Medicine, La Jolla, California.
Rheumatoid Factors

ROBERT L. TRELSTAD, M.D.
Professor and Chair, Department of Pathology and Laboratory Medicine, University of Medicine and

Dentistry of New Jersey–Robert Wood Johnson Medical School. Attending Physician, Robert Wood Johnson University Hospital, New Brunswick, New Jersey.
Matrix Glycoproteins and Proteoglycans

PETER TUGWELL, M.D., M.Sc., F.R.C.P.C.
Professor and Chairman, Department of Medicine, and Professor, Department of Epidemiology and Community Medicine, University of Ottawa School of Medicine. Physician-in-Chief, Department of Medicine, Ottawa General Hospital, Ottawa, Ontario, Canada.
Clinical Epidemiology of the Rheumatic Diseases

MARC E. UMLAS, M.D.
Attending Orthopaedic Surgeon, Mt. Sinai Medical Center, Miami Beach, Florida.
The Hip

KATHERINE S. UPCHURCH, M.D.
Assistant Professor of Medicine, University of Massachusetts Medical School. Chief, Department of Rheumatology, Medical Center of Central Massachusetts, Worcester, Massachusetts.
Hemophilic Arthropathy

JAMES R. URBANIAK, M.D.
Virginia Flowers Baker Professor of Orthopaedic Surgery, Duke University School of Medicine. Chief, Division of Orthopaedic Surgery, and Vice Chairman, Department of Surgery, Duke University Medical Center, Durham, North Carolina.
Osteonecrosis

ROBERT M. VALENTE, M.D.
Assistant Professor, Department of Internal Medicine, Division of Rheumatology, Mayo Medical School. Consultant in Rheumatology, Mayo Clinic, Rochester, Minnesota.
Vasculitis and Related Disorders

PHILIPP VANDENBERG, M.D., Ph.D.
Senior Staff Scientist, Origen Biotechnology AG, Berlin, Germany.
Collagen and Elastin

SJEF van der LINDEN, M.D.
Professor of Rheumatology, University of Limburg, Department of Medicine, Division of Rheumatology, Maastricht, The Netherlands.
Ankylosing Spondylitis

PER VENGE, M.D., Ph.D.
Professor, Department of Clinical Chemistry, University of Uppsala. Head, Department of Clinical Chemistry, University Hospital, Uppsala, Sweden.
Neutrophils and Eosinophils

DAVID A. WALSH, Ph.D., M.R.C.P.
Lecturer, Inflammation Research Group, London Hospital Medical College, London, England.
Biology of the Normal Joint

ROBERT S. WEINBERG, M.D.
Ophthalmologist, Richmond Eye Associates, Glen Allen, Virginia. Staff Ophthalmologist, Richmond Eye and Ear

Hospital, and Medical Director, Old Dominion Eye Bank, Richmond, Virginia.
The Eye and Rheumatic Disease

MICHAEL E. WEINBLATT, M.D.
Associate Professor of Medicine, Harvard Medical School. Director of Clinical Rheumatology, Brigham and Women's Hospital, Boston, Massachusetts.
Methotrexate

BARBARA N. WEISSMAN, M.D.
Professor of Radiology, Harvard Medical School. Chief, Musculoskeletal Radiology, and Vice-Chair, Radiology Ambulatory Services, Brigham and Women's Hospital, Boston, Massachusetts.
Radiographic Evaluation of Total Joint Replacement

TERRY L. WHIPPLE, M.D.
Clinical Professor of Orthopaedic Surgery, Bowman Gray School of Medicine, Wake Forest University, Winston-Salem, North Carolina. Clinical Associate Professor in Orthopaedic Surgery, Department of Surgery, Medical College of Virginia, Virginia Commonwealth University, Richmond, Virginia. Clinical Associate Professor of Orthopaedics and Rehabilitation, University of Virginia School of Medicine, Charlottesville, Virginia. Director, Orthopaedic Research of Virginia, Richmond, Virginia.
Arthroscopy and Synovectomy

CHARLENE J. WILLIAMS, Ph.D.
Research Associate Professor, Department of Biochemistry and Molecular Biology, Jefferson Institute of Molecular Medicine, Jefferson Medical College, Thomas Jefferson University, Philadelphia, Pennsylvania.
Collagen and Elastin

ROBERT J. WINCHESTER, M.D.
Professor of Pediatrics and Pathology, Columbia University College of Physicians and Surgeons, New York, New York.
Rheumatologic Manifestations of Human Immunodeficiency Virus Infection

RUSSELL E. WINDSOR, M.D.
Associate Professor of Orthopedic Surgery, Cornell University Medical College. Associate Attending Orthopaedic Surgeon, Hospital for Special Surgery and New York Hospital. Chief of the Knee Service, Hospital for Special Surgery, New York, New York.
The Knee

FRANK A. WOLLHEIM, M.D., Ph.D.
Professor of Rheumatology, Lund University School of Medicine. Chairman, Department of Rheumatology, Lund University Hospital, Lund, Sweden.
Enteropathic Arthritis

RICHARD WONG, M.B., Ch.B.
Registrar in Rheumatology, Princess Alexandra Hospital, Brisbane, Queensland, Australia.
Monocytes and Macrophages

BRUCE T. WOOD, D.P.M.
Formerly, Associate in Orthopedics/Podiatry Harvard Medical School. Formerly, Attending Physician, Brigham and Women's Hospital, Boston, Massachusetts. Formerly, Staff Podiatrist, MIT Medical Department, Cambridge, Massachusetts.
Ankle and Foot Pain

ROBERT L. WORTMANN, M.D.
Professor and Chairman, Department of Medicine, East Carolina University School of Medicine. Chief of Medical Service, University Medical Center of Eastern North Carolina and Pitt County Memorial Hospital, Greenville, North Carolina.
Inflammatory Diseases of Muscle and Other Myopathies; Gout and Hyperuricemia

K. RANDALL YOUNG, Jr., M.D.
Director, Division of Pulmonary and Critical Care Medicine, Department of Medicine, University of Alabama at Birmingham. Staff Physician, University of Alabama Hospital, Birmingham, Alabama.
Immunoregulatory Agents

DAVID TAK YAN YU, M.D.
Professor of Medicine, University of California–Los Angeles, Los Angeles, California.
Reiter's Syndrome

JOSEPH S. YU, M.D.
Assistant Professor, Department of Radiology, Ohio State University College of Medicine. Director of Musculo-skeletal Division, Department of Radiology, Ohio State University Medical Center, Columbus, Ohio.
Imaging

NOTICE

Medicine is an ever-changing field. Standard safety precautions must be followed, but as new research and clinical experience broaden our knowledge, changes in treatment and drug therapy become necessary or appropriate. The editors of this work have carefully checked the generic and trade drug names and verified drug dosages to ensure that the dosage information in this work is accurate and in accord with the standards accepted at the time of publication. Readers are advised, however, to check the product information currently provided by the manufacturer of each drug to be administered to be certain that changes have not been made in the recommended dose or in the contraindications for administration. This is of particular importance in regard to new or infrequently used drugs. It is the responsibility of the treating physician, relying on experience and knowledge of the patient, to determine dosages and the best treatment for the patient. The editors cannot be responsible for misuse or misapplication of the material in this work.

THE PUBLISHER

Exciting fields in clinical medicine are sparked by basic science. When advances in the laboratory lead to new understandings of pathophysiology and promising leads for therapy, the modern paradigm of "bench to bedside" turns from an ideal to a reality. Rheumatology is now at that place. This fact makes production of the fifth edition of the *Textbook of Rheumatology* both a challenge and an opportunity.

The format that led to establishment of the *Textbook of Rheumatology* as the best of its genre through the first four editions has again served us well. The first few sections present new concepts of immunogenetics and immunology in clear and succinct fashion that lead logically into sections on diagnosis and pharmacology. The subsequent sections include individual diseases and blend all the previously presented concepts on basic mechanisms of disease into a background for comprehending the broad range of illnesses that rheumatologists, clinical immunologists, and orthopedic surgeons see in their offices and clinics.

New authors provide vigor and energy to a revision of a textbook. As before, for this edition of *Textbook of Rheumatology*, we have brought in writers from the stock of talent in clinical and basic fields. Authors who have written distinguished chapters in earlier editions have been invited to return, and some of the best investigator/authors have written yet another outstanding chapter on the subject that they know so well.

Reading this textbook from start to finish is not practicable. A problem should be defined, and then the basic, diagnostic, and clinical chapters searched for, found, and appreciated. On the topic of rheumatoid arthritis, for example Chapter 14, "Genetic Analysis of Rheumatic Diseases," describes the HLA-DR haplotypes that lend predisposition to the disease. Chapter 7, "T Cells and B Cells," and Chapter 8, "Monocytes and Macrophages," explain how T cells are activated by antigen-presenting cells and costimulatory factors and how activated monocytes become "angry" macrophages. Chapter 18, "Cytokines," clarifies the soluble substances that act in autocrine and paracrine fashion to change phenotypic expression of lymphocytes, endothelial cells, synovial cells, mast cells, and macrophages in the developing synovitis. Activated B cells generate rheumatoid factor, and Chapter 16, "Rheumatoid Factor," describes the somatic mutations of germline genes that lead to production of high-affinity antibodies against immunoglobulin G. In the several years since publication of

the fourth edition of the *Textbook of Rheumatology*, one field, detailed in Chapter 20 on cell adhesion molecules, has made enormous advances. This chapter presents clear information on the proteins that are responsible for the binding of circulating leukocytes to endothelial cells and, after translocating to the synovium, fixing the inflammatory cells in the activated joint lining.

The immune reactions may initiate the process, but many other inflammatory and proliferative pathways enter the sequence, including those presented in Chapter 19, "Prostaglandins, Leukotrienes, and Related Compounds"; Chapter 21, "Proteinases and Matrix Degradation"; and Chapter 9, "Neutrophils and Eosinophils." An entire section of the book, Clinical Pharmacology for Rheumatic Diseases (Section VI), presents the drugs used in treating rheumatoid arthritis. Beginning with NSAIDs, then sulfasalazine and antimalarial drugs, the chapters cover details of pharmacokinetics, dosing, and side effects of the many compounds used alone and in combination in treatment of inflammatory arthritis as well as the diffuse connective tissue diseases, crystal synovitis, and osteoarthritis. Methotrexate is the second-line drug of choice now used for rheumatoid arthritis; Chapter 49, "Methotrexate," completely revised, describes why. A new chapter, "Biologic Agents in the Treatment of Rheumatoid Arthritis" (Chapter 53), contains a well-organized, concise, and up-to-date review of the monoclonal antibodies and recombinant proteins that may have focused targets in the inflammatory diseases that comprise rheumatology.

With these early chapters providing the scientific basis of immunopathology, diagnostic techniques, and therapy, the student is well prepared to appreciate the presentations of specific rheumatologic diseases and syndromes that follow, again, with a focus on rheumatoid arthritis. Chapters 54 to 56 bring the disease mechanisms and the clinical features of rheumatoid arthritis together and lead naturally to the treatment algorithms that have evolved from evidence-based clinical trials in this disease.

Similar approaches are used in Section VIII, Spondyloarthropathies; Section IX, Systemic Lupus Erythematosus and Related Syndromes; Section X, Vasculitic Syndromes; Section XI, Connective Tissue Diseases Characterized by Fibrosis; Section XII, Inflammatory Diseases of Muscle; Section XV, Crystal-Associated Synovitis; and Section XVI, Osteoarthritis and Polychondritis. The expanding breadth of rheumatology, however, does not allow for simplistic inclusion of all the relevant syndromes in standard groups. For instance, a new section (Section XIV, Syndromes of Impaired Immune Function) has been prepared, with three chapters devoted to rheumatologic manifestations of HIV infection, specific immunodeficiency diseases excluding AIDS, and complement deficiencies and rheumatic diseases. Similarly, a special series of chapters is clustered under the heading Special Issues of the Rheumatic Diseases (Section IV). Syndromes and focused special problems are addressed in chapters such as "The Fibromyalgia Syndrome," "Nutrition and Rheumatic Diseases," "Psychosocial Management of Rheumatic Diseases," "Some Aspects of Rheumatic Diseases in the Older Patient," "Sports Medicine," and "Entrapment Neuropathies and Related Disorders."

The editors have recognized that, increasingly, primary care physicians are turning to the *Textbook of Rheumatology* for help in diagnosis and treatment of patients with many diverse syndromes involving the musculoskeletal system. Accordingly, Section III, Evaluation of the Patient, describes in detail the efficient and effective examination of the joints; this is followed by chapters that facilitate differential diagnosis of monarticular arthritis, polyarticular arthritis, weakness, neck pain, shoulder pain, low back pain, hip and knee pain, and ankle and foot pain. In Section V, Diagnostic Tests and Procedures for Rheumatic Diseases, the techniques of joint aspiration and injection and synovial biopsy as well as the cost-effective, focused approach to laboratory evaluations of connective tissue diseases and imaging are outlined. In Chapter 12, "Imaging," the student and the physician are led to algorithms that direct them to the most useful imaging technique for every type of problem involving each joint.

One of the most interesting attractions of rheumatology is the association of musculoskeletal complaints with illnesses not primarily involving muscles, bones, and joints. The Editors have expanded Section XVII, Infiltrative Disorders Associated with Rheumatic Diseases, to include chapters on amyloidosis, sarcoidosis, iron storage diseases, and multicentric reticulohistiocytosis. Also expanded is Section XIX, Arthritis as a Manifestation of Other Systemic Diseases, which focuses on the musculoskeletal aspects of hemophilia, hemoglobinopathies, endocrine disorders, and malignancy. This is followed by a section of increasing importance in this time of emerging pathogens, Infectious Arthritis (Section XVIII), which includes a completely revised and relevant chapter on Lyme disease.

More and more, rheumatologists and primary care physicians are developing capabilities in evaluation and treatment of bone disease. Section XX, Disorders of Bone and Structural Proteins, includes a new chapter, "Metabolic Bone Disease" (Chapter 100), that coordinates the new appreciation of bone physiology, receptors on bone cells for hormones, and effective compounds that modulate bone metabolism and are useful therapeutic agents for osteoporosis. Similarly, primary care physicians and rheumatologists who care for patients with arthritis increasingly need guidance about what to expect and ask for in consultation from orthopedic surgeons. The expanded Section XXIII, Reconstructive Surgery for Rheumatic Disease, comprising 11 chapters by orthopedic surgeons specializing in arthritis, provides an overview on anesthesia of the arthritic patient, and then presents evidence-based information on the surgical management of each joint, including the spine. This section should be read in conjunction with Section XXII, Rehabilitation, which provides a rationale for the physician in prescribing modality therapy and orthotics for patients with pain and disability from joint disease.

Like a universe, rheumatology is expanding in all directions. With expansion comes excitement and comprehension, as the multiple disciplines of immunology, biochemistry, cell biology, pharmacology, clinical medicine, and surgery converge to help physicians and students understand and treat the traditional as well as newly recognized rheumatic diseases. This fifth edition of the *Textbook of Rheumatology* is a worthy companion for the journey toward comprehending and being confident in treating rheumatic diseases.

WILLIAM N. KELLEY
EDWARD D. HARRIS, JR.
SHAUN RUDDY
CLEMENT B. SLEDGE

Contents

Color Plates Follow Table of Contents

SECTION *I*

Structure and Function of Joints, Connective Tissue, and Muscle, 1

CHAPTER **1**

Biology of the Normal Joint 1
David A. Walsh, Clement B. Sledge,
and David R. Blake

CHAPTER **2**

Collagen and Elastin 23
Charlene J. Williams, Philipp Vandenberg,
and Darwin J. Prockop

CHAPTER **3**

Matrix Glycoproteins and
Proteoglycans 37
Robert L. Trelstad

CHAPTER **4**

The Biology, Physiology, and
Morphology of Bone 55
Clinton T. Rubin and Janet E. Rubin

CHAPTER **5**

Skeletal Muscle 76
Jody A. Dantzig and Yale E. Goldman

CHAPTER **6**

Biomechanics of Joints 86
Sheldon R. Simon and Eric L. Radin

SECTION **II**

Immune and Inflammatory Responses, 95

CHAPTER **7**

T Cells and B Cells 95
Laurie S. Davis, Thomas D. Geppert,
Katheryn Meek, Nancy Oppenheimer-Marks,
and Peter E. Lipsky

CHAPTER **8**

Monocytes and Macrophages 128
Ranjeny Thomas, Richard Wong, and Peter E. Lipsky

CHAPTER **9**

Neutrophils and Eosinophils 146
Per Venge, Håkan Bergstrand, and Lena Håkansson

CHAPTER **10**

The Mast Cell 161
Lawrence B. Schwartz

CHAPTER **11**

Platelets 176
Marcus E. Carr, Jr.

CHAPTER **12**

Endothelial Cells in Inflammation 183
Ramzi S. Cotran and David M. Briscoe

xix

CHAPTER **13**

Fibroblast Function and Fibrosis 199
Joseph H. Korn

CHAPTER **14**

Genetic Analysis of Rheumatic Diseases ... 209
Peter K. Gregersen

CHAPTER **15**

Immune Complexes and Complement 228
George Moxley and Shaun Ruddy

CHAPTER **16**

Rheumatoid Factors 241
Helen Tighe and Dennis A. Carson

CHAPTER **17**

Antinuclear Antibodies 250
Stanford L. Peng, John A. Hardin, and Joe Craft

CHAPTER **18**

Cytokines and Growth Factors 267
Jean-Michel Dayer and William P. Arend

CHAPTER **19**

Prostaglandins, Leukotrienes, and
Related Compounds 287
John F. Penrose and K. Frank Austen

CHAPTER **20**

Structural Diversity of Cell
Adhesion Molecules and
Their Role in Inflammation 303
M. Amin Arnaout

CHAPTER **21**

Proteinases and Matrix Degradation 323
Hideaki Nagase and Yasunori Okada

SECTION **III**
Evaluation of the Patient, 343

CHAPTER **22**

Clinical Epidemiology of the
Rheumatic Diseases 343
Peter Tugwell and Maarten Boers

CHAPTER **23**

Examination of the Joints 353
Kevin G. Moder and Gene G. Hunder

CHAPTER **24**

Monarticular Arthritis 371
W. Joseph McCune and Joseph Golbus

CHAPTER **25**

Approach to the Patient with Pain
in More Than One Joint 381
John S. Sergent

CHAPTER **26**

Weakness 388
Anthony S. Felsovanyi

CHAPTER **27**

Neck Pain 394
Kenneth K. Nakano

CHAPTER **28**

Shoulder Pain 413
Thomas S. Thornhill

CHAPTER **29**

Low Back Pain 439
Stephen J. Lipson

CHAPTER **30**

Hip and Knee Pain 457
Michael F. Dillingham, N. Nichole Barry,
and John V. Lannin

CHAPTER **31**

Ankle and Foot Pain 479
Robert J. Scardina and Bruce T. Wood

CHAPTER **32**

The Eye and Rheumatic Disease 488
Robert S. Weinberg

CHAPTER **33**

Cutaneous Manifestations of
Rheumatic Diseases 497
Nicholas A. Soter and Andrew G. Franks, Jr.

SECTION **IV**

Special Issues of the Rheumatic Diseases, 511

CHAPTER **34**

The Fibromyalgia Syndrome 511
Robert M. Bennett

CHAPTER **35**

Nutrition and Rheumatic Diseases 521
Joel M. Kremer

CHAPTER **36**

Psychosocial Management of
Rheumatic Diseases 534
Liv Marit Smedstad and Matthew H. Liang

CHAPTER **37**

Some Aspects of Rheumatic Disease
in the Older Patient 541
Evan Calkins

CHAPTER **38**

Sports Medicine 546
Scott A. Lintner, John A. Feagin, Jr.,
and Arthur L. Boland

CHAPTER **39**

Entrapment Neuropathies and
Related Disorders 564
Kenneth K. Nakano

SECTION **V**

Diagnostic Tests and Procedures in Rheumatic Diseases, 591

CHAPTER **40**

Aspiration and Injection of
Joints and Soft Tissues 591
Duncan S. Owen, Jr.

CHAPTER **41**

Synovial Fluid Analysis and
Synovial Biopsy 609
H. Ralph Schumacher, Jr.

CHAPTER **42**

Imaging 626
Donald Resnick, Joseph S. Yu, and David Sartoris

CHAPTER **43**

Arthroscopy and Synovectomy 687
Terry L. Whipple and Michael J. Duval

CHAPTER **44**

Laboratory Evaluation of Inflammation 699
Stanley P. Ballou and Irving Kushner

SECTION **VI**

Clinical Pharmacology for Rheumatic Diseases, 707

CHAPTER **45**

Nonsteroidal Antirheumatic Drugs 707
Philip J. Clements and Harold E. Paulus

CHAPTER **46**

Sulfasalazine 741
Richard O. Day

CHAPTER **47**

Antimalarial Drugs 747
Richard I. Rynes

CHAPTER **48**

*Gold Compounds and Penicillamine
in the Rheumatic Diseases* 759
Duncan A. Gordon

CHAPTER **49**

Methotrexate 771
Michael E. Weinblatt

CHAPTER **50**

Glucocorticoids 787
C. Michael Stein and Theodore Pincus

CHAPTER **51**

Immunoregulatory Agents 805
Anthony S. Fauci and K. Randall Young, Jr.

CHAPTER **52**

Antihyperuricemic Drugs 829
H. Ralph Schumacher, Jr., and Irving H. Fox

CHAPTER **53**

*Biologic Agents in the Treatment
of Rheumatoid Arthritis* 839
Vibeke Strand and Edward C. Keystone

SECTION **VII**

Rheumatoid Arthritis, 851

CHAPTER **54**

*Etiology and Pathogenesis of
Rheumatoid Arthritis* 851
Gary S. Firestein

CHAPTER **55**

*Clinical Features of
Rheumatoid Arthritis* 898
Edward D. Harris, Jr.

CHAPTER **56**

Treatment of Rheumatoid Arthritis 933
Edward D. Harris, Jr.

CHAPTER **57**

Felty's Syndrome 951
Robert S. Pinals

CHAPTER **58**

Sjögren's Syndrome 955
Robert I. Fox

SECTION **VIII**
Spondyloarthropathies, 969

CHAPTER **59**

Ankylosing Spondylitis 969
Sjef van der Linden

CHAPTER **60**

Reiter's Syndrome 983
Peng Thim Fan and David Tak Yan Yu

CHAPTER **61**

Psoriatic Arthritis 999
Dafna D. Gladman

CHAPTER **62**

Enteropathic Arthritis 1006
Frank A. Wollheim

SECTION **IX**
Systemic Lupus Erythematosus and Related Syndromes, 1015

CHAPTER **63**

Pathogenesis of Systemic
Lupus Erythematosus 1015
Bevra Hannahs Hahn

CHAPTER **64**

Clinical Presentation of Systemic
Lupus Erythematosus 1028
Robert G. Lahita

CHAPTER **65**

Management of Systemic
Lupus Erythematosus 1040
Bevra Hannahs Hahn

CHAPTER **66**

Antiphospholipid Syndrome 1057
Ronald A. Asherson and Ricard Cervera

CHAPTER **67**

Mixed Connective Tissue Disease
and Other Overlap Syndromes 1065
Robert M. Bennett

SECTION **X**
Vasculitic Syndromes, 1079

CHAPTER **68**

Vasculitis and Related Disorders 1079
Robert M. Valente, Stephen Hall,
J. Desmond O'Duffy, and Doyt L. Conn

CHAPTER **69**

Giant Cell Arteritis and
Polymyalgia Rheumatica 1123
Gene G. Hunder

SECTION **XI**

Connective Tissue Diseases Characterized by Fibrosis, 1133

CHAPTER **70**

Scleroderma 1133
James R. Seibold

CHAPTER **71**

Localized Fibrotic Diseases 1163
Carlo L. Mainardi

CHAPTER **72**

Silicone Breast Implants and
Rheumatic Diseases 1169
John S. Sergent, Howard Fuchs, and John S. Johnson

SECTION **XII**

Inflammatory Diseases of Muscle, 1177

CHAPTER **73**

Inflammatory Diseases of Muscle
and Other Myopathies 1177
Robert L. Wortmann

SECTION **XIII**

Rheumatic Diseases of Childhood, 1207

CHAPTER **74**

Juvenile Rheumatoid Arthritis 1207
James T. Cassidy

CHAPTER **75**

Rheumatic Fever 1225
Alan L. Bisno

CHAPTER **76**

Systemic Lupus Erythematosus,
Juvenile Dermatomyositis,
Scleroderma, and Vasculitis 1241
James T. Cassidy

SECTION **XIV**

Syndromes of Impaired Immune Function, 1265

CHAPTER **77**

Rheumatologic Manifestations of Human
Immunodeficiency Virus Infection 1265
Silviu Itescu and Robert J. Winchester

CHAPTER **78**

Specific Immunodeficiency
Diseases, Excluding Acquired
Immunodeficiency Syndrome 1282
Rebecca H. Buckley

CHAPTER **79**

Complement Deficiencies and
Rheumatic Diseases 1305
Shaun Ruddy

SECTION **XV**

Crystal-Associated Synovitis, 1313

CHAPTER **80**

Gout and Hyperuricemia 1313
William N. Kelley and Robert L. Wortmann

CHAPTER **81**

Diseases Associated with Deposition
of Calcium Pyrophosphate
or Hydroxyapatite 1352
Antonio J. Reginato and Anthony M. Reginato

SECTION **XVI**

Osteoarthritis and Polychondritis, 1369

CHAPTER **82**

Pathogenesis of Osteoarthritis 1369
Henry J. Mankin and Kenneth D. Brandt

CHAPTER **84**

Management of Osteoarthritis 1394
Kenneth D. Brandt

CHAPTER **83**

Clinical Features of Osteoarthritis 1383
Louis Solomon

CHAPTER **85**

Relapsing Polychondritis 1404
Marc C. Hochberg

SECTION **XVII**

Infiltrative Disorders Associated with Rheumatic Diseases, 1409

CHAPTER **86**

Amyloidosis 1409
Martha Skinner

CHAPTER **88**

Iron Storage Disease 1423
R. Elaine Lambert and James L. McGuire

CHAPTER **87**

Rheumatic Manifestations
of Sarcoidosis 1418
Winston Sequeira

CHAPTER **89**

Multicentric Reticulohistiocytosis 1430
William W. Ginsburg and J. Desmond O'Duffy

SECTION **XVIII**

Infectious Arthritis, 1435

CHAPTER **90**

Bacterial Arthritis 1435
Don L. Goldenberg

CHAPTER **92**

Lyme Disease 1462
Allen C. Steere

CHAPTER **91**

Mycobacterial and Fungal Infections 1450
J. Timothy Harrington, Jr.

CHAPTER **93**

Viral Arthritis 1473
Thomas J. Schnitzer

SECTION *XIX*

Arthritis as a Manifestation of Other Systemic Diseases, 1485

CHAPTER **94**

Hemophilic Arthropathy 1485
Katherine S. Upchurch and Doreen B. Brettler

CHAPTER **95**

Hemoglobinopathies and Arthritis 1493
H. Ralph Schumacher, Jr.

CHAPTER **96**

Arthropathies Associated with
Endocrine Disorders 1499
James L. McGuire and R. Elaine Lambert

CHAPTER **97**

Hypertrophic Osteoarthropathy 1514
Roy D. Altman and Jerry Tenenbaum

CHAPTER **98**

Musculoskeletal Syndromes
Associated with Malignancy 1521
David S. Caldwell

SECTION *XX*

Disorders of Bone and Structural Proteins, 1535

CHAPTER **99**

Heritable Disorders of
Structural Proteins 1535
David W. Rowe and Jay R. Shapiro

CHAPTER **100**

Metabolic Bone Disease 1563
Meryl S. LeBoff

CHAPTER **101**

Osteonecrosis 1581
Philip G. Coogan and James R. Urbaniak

SECTION *XXI*

Tumors Involving Joints, 1593

CHAPTER **102**

Tumors and Tumor-Like Lesions of
Joints and Related Structures 1593
Andrew E. Rosenberg and Alan L. Schiller

SECTION **XXII**
Rehabilitation, 1619

CHAPTER **103**

Rehabilitation of Patients with
Rheumatic Diseases 1619
Joseph J. Biundo, Jr., and Perry J. Rush

SECTION **XXIII**
Reconstructive Surgery for Rheumatic Disease, 1633

CHAPTER **104**

Introduction to Surgical Management
of the Patient with Arthritis 1633
Clement B. Sledge

CHAPTER **105**

Anesthetic Considerations 1640
Nigel E. Sharrock

CHAPTER **106**

The Hand and Wrist 1647
Barry P. Simmons and Garth R. Smith

CHAPTER **107**

The Elbow 1675
B. F. Morrey

CHAPTER **108**

The Shoulder 1696
Robert H. Cofield

CHAPTER **109**

The Cervical Spine 1713
Stephen J. Lipson

CHAPTER **110**

The Hip 1723
Chitranjan S. Ranawat, Kenji C. Miyasaka,
Marc E. Umlas, and Jose A. Rodriguez

CHAPTER **111**

The Knee 1739
Russell E. Windsor and John N. Insall

CHAPTER **112**

The Ankle and Foot 1759
Sigvard T. Hansen, Jr.

CHAPTER **113**

Surgical Management of Juvenile
Rheumatoid Arthritis 1773
Michael J. Chmell and Richard D. Scott

CHAPTER **114**

Radiographic Evaluation of Total
Joint Replacement 1782
Barbara N. Weissman

Appendices, 1849

APPENDIX **1**

Guidelines for the Medical
Management of Osteoarthritis:
Part I, Osteoarthritis of the Hip 1850

APPENDIX **2**

Guidelines for the Medical
Management of Osteoarthritis:
Part II, Osteoarthritis of the Knee 1855

APPENDIX 3

Methotrexate for Rheumatoid Arthritis:
Suggested Guidelines for Monitoring
Liver Toxicity 1860

APPENDIX 4

Empiric Parenteral Antibiotic Treatment
of Patients with Fibromyalgia and Fatigue
and a Positive Serologic Result for Lyme
Disease: A Cost-Effectiveness Analysis 1872

APPENDIX 5

Guidelines for the Initial Evaluation
of the Adult Patient with Acute
Musculoskeletal Symptoms 1880

APPENDIX 6

Guidelines for the Management
of Rheumatoid Arthritis 1888

APPENDIX 7

Guidelines for Monitoring Drug Therapy
in Rheumatoid Arthritis 1897

Index, i

TEXTBOOK OF
RHEUMATOLOGY

Color Plates

PLATE 1

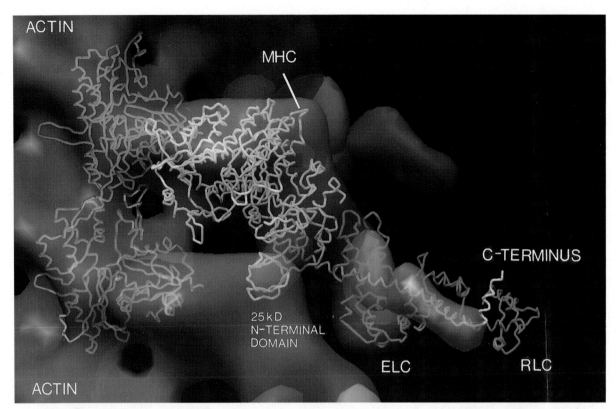

FIGURE 5–4. The atomic structure of actin and myosin (colored "ribbons"), determined by x-ray crystallography, superimposed on a three-dimensional reconstruction (shaded) of the thin filament decorated with S1, from cryoelectron microscopy and Fourier image analysis. The myosin heavy chain (MHC, yellow) binds with two actin monomers (orange and gray) to form a tight complex in the absence of nucleotide. Bound to an unusually long α-helix of the MHC are the essential light chain (ELC, green) and the regulatory light chain (RLC, red). A small extension (pink shading) of the 25 kD, NH_2-terminal region of S1 appears to contact an adjacent S1. The x-ray crystal structures fit uniquely within the electron microscopic image reconstruction, verifying the three-dimensional relationship between actin and S1. The C terminus of S1, shown here, ends just beyond the light chain binding region, but in whole myosin the heavy chain extends further to become the coiled-coil rod portion of the molecule. A putative hinge between the nucleotide-binding and light chain-binding regions is implicated in the conformational changes associated with force production and filament sliding. (Courtesy of Dr. Ron Milligan and Dr. Michael Whittaker, Scripps Research Institute, La Jolla, Calif.)

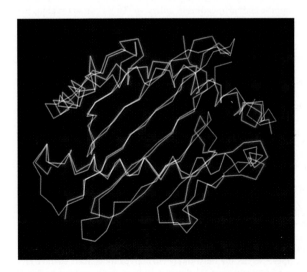

FIGURE 14–4. The superimposed peptide binding clefts of HLA class I and class II molecules. The alpha carbon backbone of class I is shown in red; that of HLA class II is shown in blue. Areas of complete overlap are white. The two clefts are very similar in size and shape. The major difference relates to the absence of α-helical structure in class II at the upper left hand "wall" of the cleft. Note the more extended conformation of the blue alpha carbon backbone of class II in this region. The major consequence of this and other differences is that class II molecules can bind peptides that are longer and more variable in size. (From Brown JH, Jardetzky TS, Gorga JC, et al. Three-dimensional structure of the human class II histocompatibility antigen HLA-DR1. Nature 364:33, 1993. © 1993, Macmillan Magazines Limited.)

PLATE 2

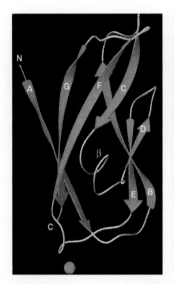
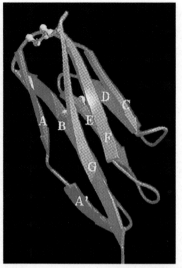

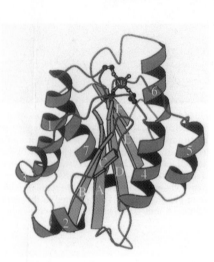
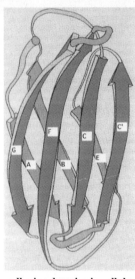
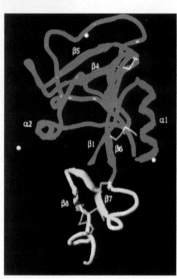

FIGURE 20–2. Ribbon diagrams of the structure of known adhesion domains in cellular adhesion molecule (CAM) families.

A, The overall structure of the N-terminal cadherin domain from N-cadherin. The seven β-strands are arranged as two β-sheets connected by a quasi β-helix region. Residues from strands C, D, F, G, and β mediate homophilic cadherin-cadherin adhesion. These contact regions are far from the metal-binding site (green sphere) located near the carboxy terminus. The metal is coordinated by residues from two adjacent domains within each cadherin. Residues from β-strand A mediate dimerization of cadherins expressed on the same cell surface. The cadherin structure bears considerable similarity to the immunoglobulin (Ig) domain (see Fig. 2–2B), despite lack of any amino acid homology. (From Shapiro L, Fannon AM, Kwong PD, et al: Structural basis of cell-cell adhesion by cadherins. Nature 374:327–337, 1995. © 1995, Macmillan Magazines Limited.)

B, Structure of the immunoglobulin domain 1 of CD106. Mutational analysis has confirmed that the CD49d/CD29 ($\alpha 4\beta 1$) binding site is composed of residues clustered on the CFG face, with a key asparate (Asp 40 in CD106) projecting from the distinctive CD loop. (From Jones EL, Harlos K, Bottomley MJ, et al: Crystal structure of an intern-binding fragment of vascular cell adhesion molecule-1 at 1.8 Å resolution. Nature 373:539–544, 1995. © 1995, Macmillan Magazines Limited.)

C, Structure of the A-domain from integrin CD11b. The structure reveals a well-coordinated metal ion exposed on the surface of the domain. In the generated crystals, the sixth metal coordination site is provided by an acidic residue from a neighboring domain. Under physiologic conditions, the acidic residue from an integrin ligand probably completes metal coordination. (From Lee J-O, Rieu P, Arnaout MA, Liddington R: Crystal structure of the A-domain from the α-subunit of β_2 integrin complement receptor type 3 (CR3, CD11b/CD18). Cell 80:631–638, 1995. Courtesy of Cell Press.)

D, Structure of the third FN-III domain of tenascin. The structure consists of seven β-strands arranged into two β-sheets (ABE and C'CFG). The Arg-Gly-Asp sequence is located in the flexible FG loop, which projects from the protein surface. The homology of the FN-III fold to that of Ig (see Fig. 2–2B) is apparent. (From Graves BJ, Crowther RL, Chandran C: Insight into E-selectin/ligand interaction from the crystal structure and mutagenesis of the lec/EGF domains. Nature 367:532–538, 1994. © 1994, Macmillan Magazines Limited.)

E, Structure of the C-type lectin-EGF domains from E-selectin shown in red and yellow, respectively. The three Ca²⁺ positions are shown as white spheres, and the five disulfide bridges as green sticks. The left and right Ca²⁺ (neighboring α_2 and α_1 helices, respectively) are weakly coordinated. Mutagenesis studies identified a finite region in the vicinity of the upper Ca²⁺ as the most likely carbohydrate contact surface (see text). (From Leahy DJ, Hendrickson WA, Aukhil I, Erickson HP: Structure of a fibronectin type III domain from tenascin phased by MAD analysis of the selenomethionyl protein. Nature 258:987–991, 1992. © 1992, Macmillan Magazines Limited.)

PLATE 3

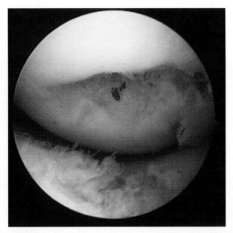

FIGURE 30–15. Osteochondritis dissecans of the femoral condyle, as seen by arthroscopy.

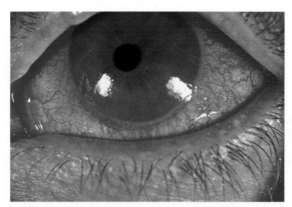

FIGURE 32–1. Keratoconjunctivitis sicca. Intense hyperemia of the conjunctival vessels accounts for the prominent redness. Dryness of the corneal epithelium causes the reflection from the photographic flash to be dull and irregular rather than normally sharp and highly polished.

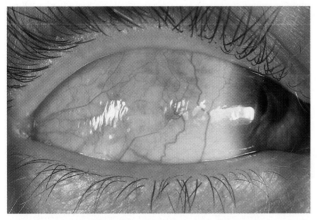

FIGURE 32–2. Episcleritis. Localized episcleral injection with overlying conjunctival injection adjacent to areas with no vascular congestion.

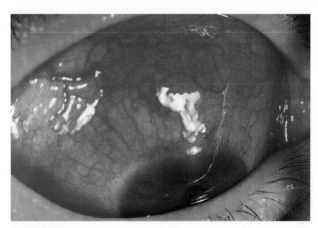

FIGURE 32–3. Diffuse scleritis. Diffuse scleritis in a patient with rheumatoid arthritis. There is intense vascular engorgement, overlying conjunctival injection, but no discharge.

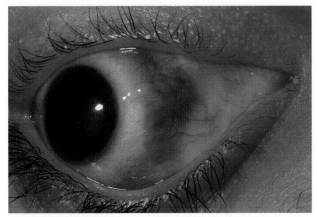

FIGURE 32–5. Scleromalacia. Therapy for scleritis can decrease scleral inflammation. Once active inflammation has decreased, the sclera may be thin and translucent, appearing bluish-gray.

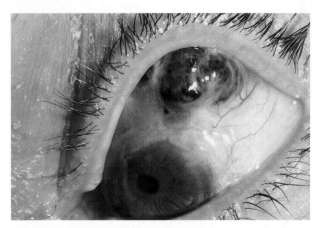

FIGURE 32–6. Scleromalacia perforans. Severe scleral thinning and translucency with bulging of underlying uveal tissue in a patient with severe rheumatoid arthritis.

PLATE 4

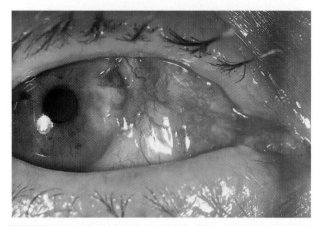

FIGURE 32–9. Scleritis and keratitis in Wegener's granulomatosis. Localized keratitis at the limbus, adjacent to an area of localized scleritis in Wegener's granulomatosis. The corneal thinning is approximately 90 percent, with a high risk of corneal perforation.

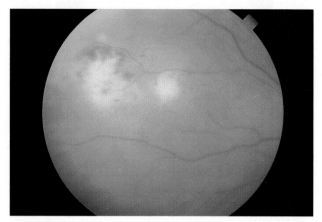

FIGURE 32–11. Retinal ischemia in Behçet's disease. Areas of white retinal ischemia in the mid-periphery of the retina in a patient with Behçet's disease. Ischemic areas are partially surrounded by retinal hemorrhages.

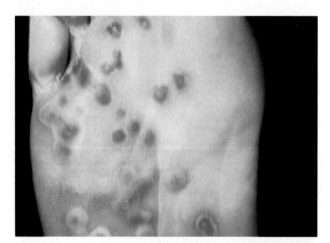

FIGURE 33–1. Keratoderma blennorrhagica. Vesicles and pustules of the sole in a patient with Reiter's syndrome. (From Soter NA, Franks AG Jr: Cutaneous manifestations of rheumatic diseases: An update. *In* Kelley WN, et al: Textbook of Rheumatology, 4th ed. Philadelphia, WB Saunders. Update No. 15, pp 1–24, 1995.)

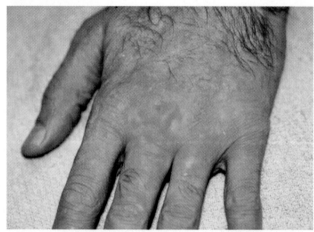

FIGURE 33–5. Systemic lupus erythematosus. Note bulla over the dorsum of the hand. (From Soter NA, Franks AG Jr: Cutaneous manifestations of rheumatic diseases: An update. *In* Kelley WN, et al: Textbook of Rheumatology, 4th ed. Philadelphia, WB Saunders. Update No. 15, pp 1–24, 1995.)

PLATE 5

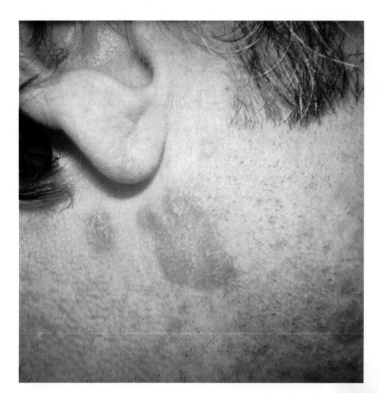

FIGURE 33–6. Tumid lupus erythematosus. Erythematous, indurated plaques. (From Soter NA, Franks AG Jr: Cutaneous manifestations of rheumatic diseases: An update. *In* Kelley WN, et al: Textbook of Rheumatology, 4th ed. Philadelphia, WB Saunders. Update No. 15, pp 1–24, 1995.)

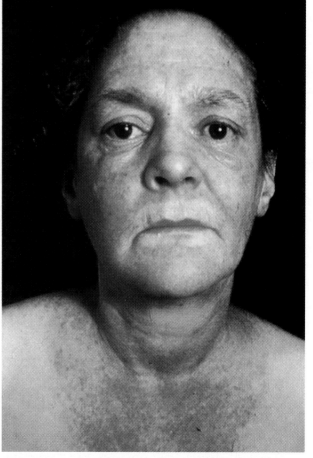

FIGURE 33–9. Dermatomyositis. Photosensitivity. (From Soter NA, Franks AG Jr: Cutaneous manifestations of rheumatic diseases: An update. *In* Kelley WN, et al: Textbook of Rheumatology, 4th ed. Philadelphia, WB Saunders. Update No. 15, pp 1–24, 1995.)

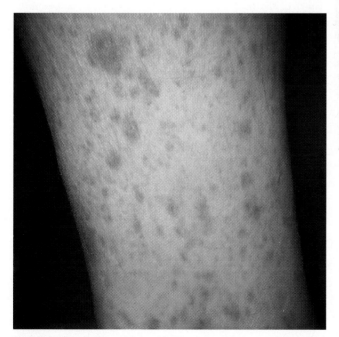

FIGURE 33–8. Necrotizing venulitis. Palpable purpura distributed over the lower extremities.

PLATE 6

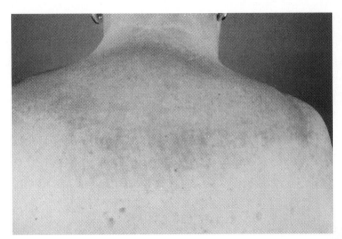

FIGURE 33–11. Dermatomyositis. Shawl pattern of erythema on the upper back. (From Soter NA, Franks AG Jr: Cutaneous manifestations of rheumatic diseases: An update. *In* Kelley WN, et al: Textbook of Rheumatology, 4th ed. Philadelphia, WB Saunders. Update No. 15, pp 1–24, 1995.)

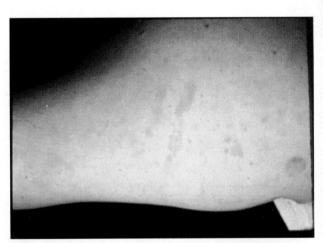

FIGURE 33–14. Juvenile rheumatoid arthritis. Salmon-colored lesions on the arm. (From Soter NA, Franks AG Jr: Cutaneous manifestations of rheumatic diseases: An update. *In* Kelley WN, et al: Textbook of Rheumatology, 4th ed. Philadelphia, WB Saunders. Update No. 15, pp 1–24, 1995.)

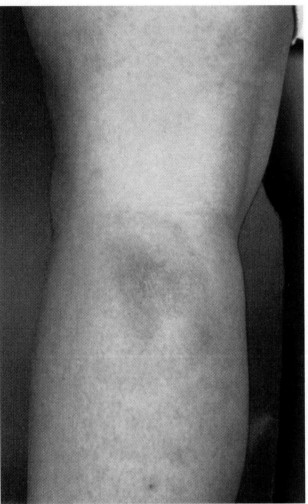

FIGURE 33–15. Lyme borreliosis. Erythema migrans. (From Soter NA, Franks AG Jr: Cutaneous manifestations of rheumatic diseases: An update. *In* Kelley WN, et al: Textbook of Rheumatology, 4th ed. Philadelphia, WB Saunders. Update No. 15, pp 1–24, 1995.)

PLATE 7

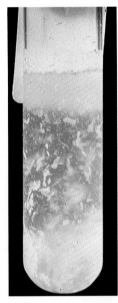

Figure 41–2

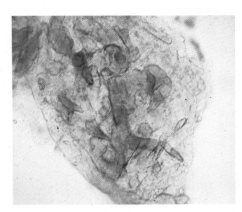

Figure 41–3

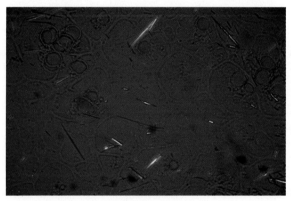

Figure 41–4

FIGURE 41–2. Synovial fluid rice bodies containing fibrin and debris from degenerated villi are especially common in rheumatoid arthritis but can also be seen in other conditions such as tuberculous arthritis.

FIGURE 41–3. Any fragments floating in fluid should be examined. They may be cartilage or synovium and contain crystals or other diagnostic clues. Shards of golden or ochre cartilage fragments here are embedded in detached synovium found in synovial fluid in a patient with ochronotic arthropathy.

FIGURE 41–4. Monosodium urate crystals from a gouty synovial fluid as viewed with compensated polarized light. The crystals are yellow parallel to the axis of slow vibration marked on the compensator (negative birefringence). Do not expect to see so many crystals, as even a few can cause acute gout.

FIGURE 41–5. Calcium pyrophosphate dihydrate (CPPD) crystals can be needle, rod, or rhomboid shaped but usually have blunt ends *(A)*. They often have fainter birefringence than is seen with urates *(B)*. CPPD are blue when aligned longitudinally with the axis of slow vibration of the compensator (positive birefringence).

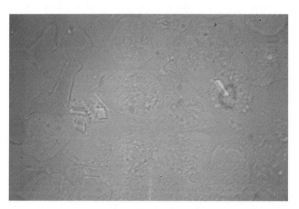

Figure 41–5A

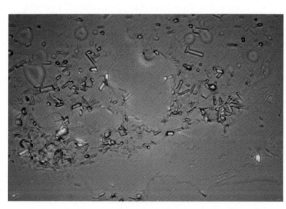

Figure 41–5B

PLATE 8

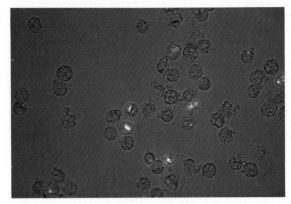

Figure 41–6

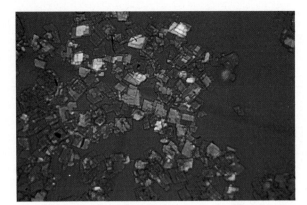

Figure 41–7

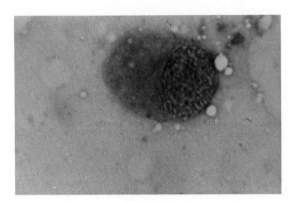

Figure 41–8

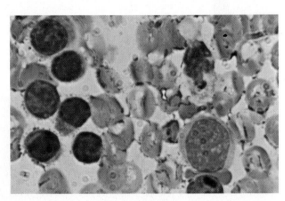

Figure 41–9

FIGURE 41–6. Triamcinolone acetonide (Aristospan) crystals phagocytized by synovial fluid cells after intra-articular injection.

FIGURE 41–7. Cholesterol crystals from a chronic rheumatoid olecranon bursal effusion. These are most often flat plates with notched corners.

FIGURE 41–8. Synovial lining cell. The prominent homogeneous blue cytoplasm is typical of type B or synthetic cells. Other large cells with a nucleus:cytoplasm ratio of less than 50 percent have vacuolated cytoplasm and are either phagocytic lining cells or large monocytes (macrophages).

FIGURE 41–9. Synovial fluid small lymphocytes with one activated lymphocyte, the larger cell with nucleus filling most of the cytoplasm.

PLATE 9

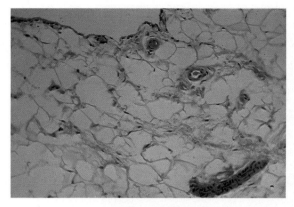

Figure 41–14

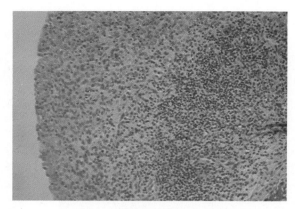

Figure 41–15

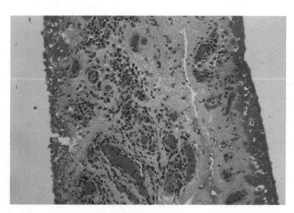

Figure 41–16

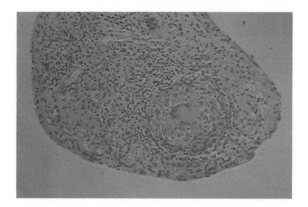

Figure 41–18

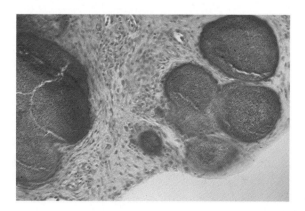

Figure 41–19

FIGURE 41–14. Normal synovial membrane of the knee. There is a single layer of flattened synovial cells overlying areolar connective tissue. Note the small synovial vessels immediately under the lining layer and the larger vessel in the lower right corner. (× 100, Hematoxylin & eosin stain.)

FIGURE 41–15. Rheumatoid arthritis synovium showing many layers of synovial lining cells on the left and infiltration of lymphocytes and plasma cells on the right. (× 100, Hematoxylin & eosin stain.)

FIGURE 41–16. Synovial membrane in early scleroderma shows massive superficial fibrin, loss of lining cells, and infiltration with lymphocytes and plasma cells. (× 100, Hematoxylin & eosin stain.)

FIGURE 41–18. Granuloma in superficial synovium in tuberculous arthritis. Some superficial granulomas, such as this one, do not show caseation. There is also scattered chronic inflammatory cell infiltration. (× 100, Hematoxylin & eosin stain.)

FIGURE 41–19. Tophus-like deposits in synovium containing positively birefringent crystals in pseudogout. (× 100, Hematoxylin & eosin stain.)

PLATE 10

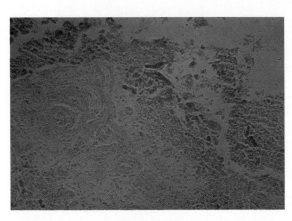

Figure 41–20

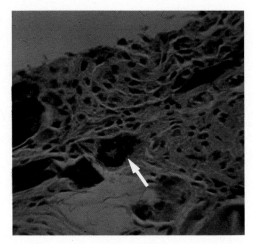

Figure 41–21

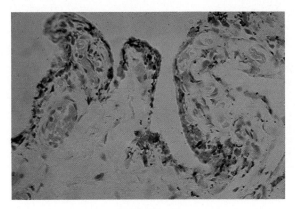

Figure 41–22

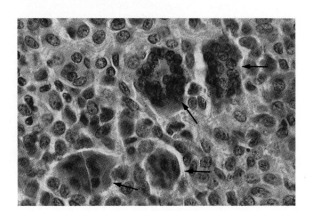

Figure 41–23

FIGURE 41–20. Amyloid arthritis as seen here in a patient with multiple myeloma is characterized by Congo red staining on the surface and sparing of the synovial vessels (V). (×100, Congo red stain.)

FIGURE 41–21. Dark, angular cartilage shards pigmented brown with homogentisic acid polymer are embedded in ochronotic synovium. Note also a giant cell *(arrow)* and mild proliferation of synovial lining cells. (×400, Hematoxylin & eosin stain.)

FIGURE 41–22. Iron stain of synovial membrane in idiopathic hemochromatosis shows blue (dark) staining predominantly in the lining cells. (×100, Prussian blue stain.)

FIGURE 41–23. Pigmented villonodular synovitis is characterized by golden brown hemosiderin in deep macrophages, giant cells *(arrows),* monotonous proliferation of deep cells with pale nuclei, and, not illustrated here, foam cells, lining cell hyperplasia (dark), and villous proliferation. (×400, Hematoxylin & eosin stain.) (Courtesy of Schumacher HR: Semin Arthritis Rheum 12:32, 1982.)

Structure and Function of Joints, Connective Tissue, and Muscle

David A. Walsh
Clement B. Sledge
David R. Blake

Biology of the Normal Joint

The joint is a specialized structure whose design allows for both stability and movement. During activity, the normal joint cartilage may be exposed to severe shearing forces and to compression forces equivalent to several times the body weight. In the inflamed joint, movement generates repeated hypoxic-reperfusion cycles. Joint structure is well adapted to resisting such insults but includes many unique features that may help explain the particular predisposition of articular tissues to chronic inflammation. Constituents of articular cartilage, synovium, and its vasculature and innervation and of synovial fluid have all been implicated in the pathogenesis of arthritis, and deviations from normal may provide useful markers of articular disease. Furthermore, differentiation of articular tissues during embryogenesis dictates their capacity to respond to insults in later life. Angiogenesis, macrophage recruitment, and fibroblast proliferation, all normal processes in the development of joints, occur again during the development of arthritis. An understanding of the embryogenesis, structure, and function of the normal joint is therefore essential in unraveling the dominant mechanisms of human arthritis.

It is useful to recognize two basic types of articulation: *synovial* or *diarthrodial* joints (Fig. 1–1), which are articulations with free movement and synovial lining cells bordering the joint cavity; and *synarthroses*, at which very little movement occurs. There are four subclassifications of synarthroses:

- *Symphyses:* A fibrocartilaginous disc separates bone ends that are joined by firm ligaments (e.g., symphysis pubis and intervertebral joints).
- *Synchondroses:* Bone ends are covered with articular cartilage, but there is no synovium or significant joint cavity (e.g., sternomanubrial joint).
- *Syndesmoses:* Bones are joined directly by fibrous ligaments without a cartilaginous interface (the dis-

tal tibiofibular articulation is the only joint of this type outside the cranial vault).
- *Synostoses:* Bone bridges between bones, producing ankylosis.

This chapter concentrates on the developmental biology and relationship between structure and function of a "typical" normal human diarthrodial joint, the joint that is most likely to develop arthritis. Most

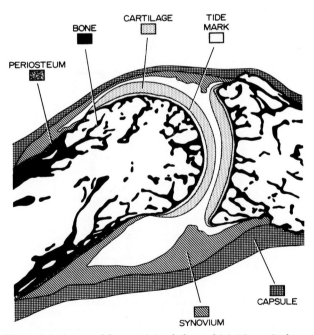

Figure 1–1. A normal human interphalangeal joint in sagittal section, as an example of a synovial or diarthrodial joint. The "tidemark" represents the calcified cartilage that bonds articular cartilage to the subchondral bone plate. (With permission from Sokoloff L, Bland JH: The Musculoskeletal System. Baltimore, Williams & Wilkins, 1975. © 1975, the Williams & Wilkins Co, Baltimore.)

research has been performed on the knee because of its accessibility, but other joints are described when appropriate.

DEVELOPMENTAL BIOLOGY OF DIARTHRODIAL JOINTS

The appendicular skeleton develops in the human embryo from limb buds, first visible at around 4 weeks of gestation. Structures resembling adult joints are generated between about 4½ and 7 weeks of gestation,[1] preceding many other crucial phases of musculoskeletal development, including vascularization of epiphyseal cartilage (8 to 12 weeks), appearance of villous folds in synovium (10 to 12 weeks), evolution of bursae (3 to 4 months), and appearance of fat pads (4 to 5 months). The upper limbs develop approximately 24 hours earlier than the homologous portions of the lower limb, and proximal structures, such as the glenohumeral joint, develop before more distal ones, such as the wrist and hand. As a consequence, insults to embryonic development during the period of limb formation affect a more distal portion of the upper limb than of the lower limb.

The normal sequences of limb bud formation are well described by O'Rahilly and Gardner.[2] A summary follows in Figure 1–2. Long bones differentiate by the sequential processes of condensation, chondrification, and endochondral ossification; the first two are necessary precursors of joint development and are discussed here.

The cellular accumulation first identifiable as the precursor of a part of an organ is called an *anlage.* Common precursor mesenchyme cells divide into both myogenic and chondrogenic lineages, and it remains unclear as to what determines the differentiation of cartilage centrally and muscle peripherally. Zwilling and coworkers proposed that positional information was imparted by diffusible agents generated at the tip of the limb bud and along its posterior margin, promoting the development of a cartilaginous anlage along proximodistal and anteroposterior axes, respectively.[3] Signals from the apical ectoderm of the limb bud probably initiate formation of the anlage by activating homeobox gene expression in the undifferentiated mesenchyme.[4]

Condensation

Shortly after limb buds appear, cellular aggregation generates a *blastema,* a condensed, growing mass of embryonic mesenchyme in which definitive tissues, such as a cartilaginous matrix, cannot yet be distinguished.[5] The precise stimulus for condensation remains unclear, although transforming growth factor-β has been implicated.[6] Initiation of condensation depends on expression of the adhesion molecule N-cadherin, and stabilization of the blastema requires the development of intercellular gap junctions and expression of neural cell adhesion molecules (NCAMs).[7, 8]

Chondrification

In the human, chondrification (Fig. 1–3) can be detected when the embryo is as small as 11.7 mm (stage 17 of embryologic development). Chondrification effectively divides the blastema into cartilaginous precursors of individual limb bones. Differentiation of chondrocytes is associated with the switching of gene expression from mesenchymal matrix proteins, such as type I collagen, to cartilage-specific proteins, such as collagen types II and IX, and cartilage proteoglycan core protein.[9, 10] (See Chapters 2 and 3 for a discussion of cartilage matrix.)

Chondrification is under both positive and negative regulatory control. Hyaluronate, retinoic acid, platelet-derived growth factor (PDGF), and activators of protein kinase C inhibit chondrification,[11–14] whereas bone morphogenetic protein-2 (BMP-2) and fragmentation of hyaluronate by hyaluronidase may stimulate chondrocyte differentiation.[6, 15] Hyaluronate can be demonstrated at the tip of the developing limb bud, before chondrification, and hyaluronidase is localized to the base of the limb bud. This provides a mechanism to remove the inhibitory hyaluronate and to allow chondrogenesis to proceed from the proximal to the distal end of the limb.[15]

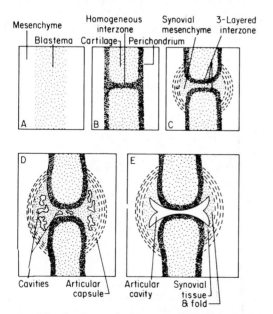

Figure 1–2. The development of a synovial joint. *A, Condensation.* Joints develop from the blastema, not the surrounding mesenchyme. *B, Chondrification and formation of the interzone.* The interzone remains avascular and highly cellular. *C, Formation of synovial mesenchyme.* Synovial mesenchyme forms from the periphery of the interzone and is invaded by blood vessels. *D, Cavitation.* Cavities are formed in the central and peripheral interzone and merge to form the joint cavity. *E, The mature joint.* (From O'Rahilly R, Gardner E: The embryology of movable joints. *In* Sokoloff L [ed]: The Joints and Synovial Fluid. Vol 1. New York, Academic Press, 1978.)

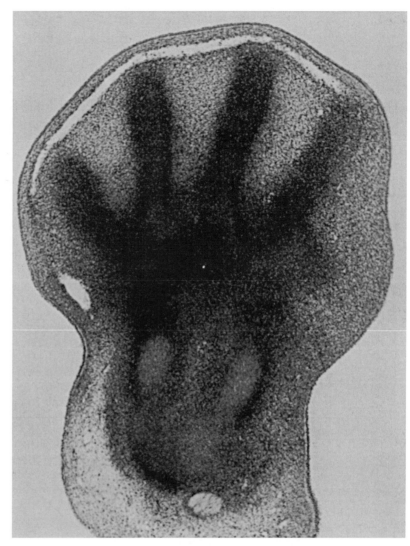

Figure 1–3. Coronal section of the hand at 11.7 mm (stage 17). The blastema with its increased cellularity serves to outline the form of the hand. Faint lightening in the region of the third and fourth metacarpals indicates very early chondrification. Chondrification in the radius and ulna is more advanced. (From O'Rahilly R: The development of joints. Ir J Med Sci 6:456, 1957.)

Interzones, the Future Joints

Interzones (Fig. 1–4) first appear as avascular, homogeneous, densely cellular areas between segments undergoing chondrification. Vascular infiltration precedes the recruitment of macrophages from the fetal circulation into the periphery of the interzone. At the same time, mesenchymal cells throughout the interzone proliferate and develop fibroblastoid characteristics, such as expression of the collagen-synthesizing enzyme prolyl hydroxylase.[16, 17] Hyaluronan synthase, hyaluronan, and the CD44 hyaluronan receptor are present in the interzone, and the hyaluronan precursor synthetic enzyme uridine diphosphoglucose dehydrogenase (UDPGD) localizes to a narrow band of fibroblastoid cells at the presumptive joint line.[16] It is proposed that loss of cellular adhesion in response to increased hyaluronan concentration may determine synovial cavitation, perhaps signaled or facilitated by vascular invasion of the interzone.

Synovial Mesenchyme

The joint capsule evolves as a dense layer of collagen deposited by fibroblasts surrounding the interzone, enclosing into the future joint some of the vascularized mesoderm. This mesoderm will give rise eventually to the synovial lining, intracapsular ligaments, menisci, and tendons. In common usage, the term "synovium" refers to both the true synovial lining and the subjacent vascular and areolar tissue, up to but excluding the capsule.

Synovial lining cells can be distinguished as soon as the multiple cavities within the interzone begin to coalesce. At first, these are exclusively fibroblast-like (type B) cells. As the joint cavity increases in size, synovial lining cell layers expand by proliferation of fibroblast-like cells and recruitment of macrophage-like (type A) cells from the circulation.[17] Further synovial expansion results in the appearance of synovial villi at the end of the second month, early in the fetal period, which greatly increases the surface area

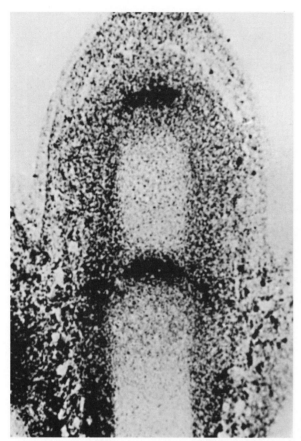

Figure 1–4. Histochemical preparation demonstrating intense localization of acid phosphatase (representing lysosomal activity) in the zone of presumptive joint formation in a mouse embryo. This enzymatic removal of matrix allows cavitation to occur, separating the limb elements. (From Milaire J: *In* Frantz CH [ed]: Normal and Abnormal Embryological Development. Washington, DC, National Research Council, 1947, p 61.)

pletely defined, but extracellular matrix destruction by enzymes, apoptosis of interzone cells, and secretion of hyaluronate by synovial fibroblasts may all play a role.[16, 19] In chick embryos, it has been shown that movement of the limb is essential for normal cavitation,[20] but equivalent data from human embryonic joints are difficult to obtain.[21] In all large joints in the human, complete joint cavities are apparent at the beginning of the fetal period.

Articular Cartilage

The peripheral interzone is absorbed into each adjacent chondrogenous zone, evolving into the articular surface. The articular surface is a specialized, permanently cartilaginous structure that does not normally undergo vascularization and ossification. In these respects, it differs from the cartilaginous anlage of the bone but resembles other permanent cartilages, such as the costal cartilages. Articular chondrocytes continue to express cartilage-specific type II collagen rather than switching to express type I collagen present in bone matrix.[22] They also express tenascin, a glycoprotein that is characteristic of nonossifying cartilage.[23]

Thus, a potential space in the body has developed, lined on all surfaces either by cartilage or by synovial lining cells. These two very different tissues merge at the "enthesis" (the region at the periphery of the joint where the cartilage melds into bone and where ligaments are attached).

In contrast to other joints, the temporomandibular joint develops slowly, with cavitation at a crown-

available for exchange between the joint cavity and the vascular space.

A dense capillary network develops in the subsynovial tissue with numerous capillary loops into the true synovial lining layer. The human synovial microvasculature is already innervated by 8 weeks of gestation, as demonstrated by immunoreactivity for the neuronal "housekeeping" enzyme ubiquitin C-terminal hydrolase (PGP 9.5).[18] However, evidence of neurotransmitter function is not found until much later, with the appearance of the sensory neuropeptide substance P at 11 weeks. The putative sympathetic neurotransmitter, neuropeptide Y, appears at 13 weeks of gestation together with the catecholamine synthesizing enzyme tyrosine hydroxylase.[18]

The Joint Cavity

Cavitation begins in the central interzone at about the time the synovial mesenchyme differentiates into a pseudomembrane (Figs. 1–5 and 1–6). The precise mechanisms causing cavitation have not been com-

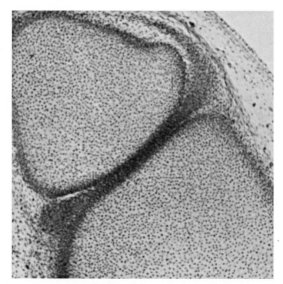

Figure 1–5. The embryonic joint developing between the femur and tibia at 31 mm (stage 23). The lateral meniscus is outlined by cavitation on the femoral side. Cavitation will subsequently spread in a medial direction as well as developing spontaneously at other foci. (From Gardner E, O'Rahilly R: The early development of the knee joint in staged human embryos. J Anat 102:289, 1968. Used by permission of Cambridge University Press.)

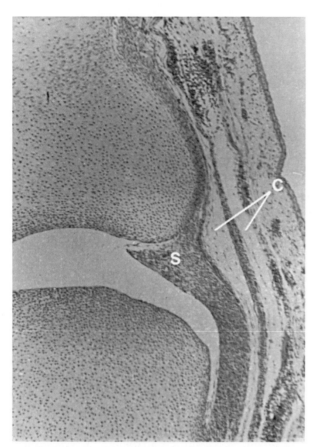

Figure 1–6. Adjacent phalanges in a human embryo hand are separated by a clearly demarcated joint space containing early synovial tissue. The densely collagenous joint capsule lying exterior to the synovium is clearly demonstrated. S, synovium; C, capsule. (From Sledge CB: *In* Resnick D, Niwayana G [eds]: Diagnosis of Bone and Joint Disorders, 2nd ed. Philadelphia, WB Saunders, 1988, p 618.)

rump length of 57 to 75 mm (i.e., well into the fetal stage).[24] This may be because this joint develops in the absence of a continuous blastema and involves the insertion between bone ends of a fibrocartilaginous disc that arises from muscular and mesenchymal derivatives of the first pharyngeal arch.

The development of synostoses (cartilaginous and fibrous joints) is similar to that of diarthrodial joints, except that cavitation does not occur and synovial mesenchyme is not formed. In these respects, synostoses resemble the "fused" peripheral joints induced by paralyzing chicken embryos,[25] and symphyses may develop as they do because there is relatively little motion during their formation.

Human vertebrae and intervertebral discs develop as units, each derived from a homogeneous blastema arising from a somite.[26] Each embryonic intervertebral disc serves as a rostral and a caudal chondrogenous zone for the two adjacent evolving vertebral bodies. The periphery of the embryonic "disc" is replaced by the annulus fibrosus.[27] The intervertebral disc bears many similarities to the joint; the annulus is the joint capsule, the nucleus pulposus is the joint cavity, and

the vertebral end-plates are the cartilage-covered bone ends composing the articulation. Because the nucleus pulposus contains proteoglycans as well as type II (cartilaginous) collagen,[28–30] it is thought to represent segmented inclusions of the original embryonic disc still active in chondrification.

ORGANIZATION OF THE MATURE JOINT

The mature diarthrodial joint is a complex structure. Understanding it demands consideration of biomechanics (see Chapter 6), and structural differences between joints are determined by their different functions. Components of the "typical" synovial joint are described next.

Muscles

The physiology of muscle is described in detail in Chapter 5. Muscles generate forces required for both joint movement and stabilization. Ligaments and the conforming anatomy of apposing articular surfaces also impart stability but at the same time limit the joint's range of movement. Joints such as the shoulder and hip, which have wide ranges of movement, are stabilized by large muscle masses, whereas the ankle moves only in one plane through limited arcs and is stabilized by its hinge-like anatomy and dense ligaments. Inter-individual variability in passive joint motion has a broad range—from the muscular athlete who is often at risk for muscle "pulls and strains," to the "loose-jointed" asthenic person who suffers frequent joint sprains and who may have a predisposition for the development of osteoarthritis.[31] A person at the most loose-jointed end of the normal range may resemble the patient with Ehlers-Danlos type III syndrome (see Chapter 99).

Most joints have their muscle insertions close to the fulcrum (articular surface) so that small muscle contractions produce an extensive arc of motion of the terminal member (hand or foot). However, this means that the muscle is at a mechanical disadvantage and must generate large forces in order to move the limb. These forces are transmitted through the articular cartilage.

Tendons[32]

Tendons are functional and anatomic bridges between muscle and bone. They focus the force of a large mass of muscle into a localized area on bone and, by splitting to form numerous insertions, may distribute the force of a single muscle to different bones.[33]

Tendons are formed of longitudinally arranged type I collagen bundles interlaced by a delicate reticular network of type III collagen, blood vessels, lymphatics, and fibroblasts.[34] Tendon fibroblasts synthesize and secrete matrix components, such as type I collagen and proteoglycans, as well as metalloproteinases and their inhibitors that have implications in the breakdown and repair of tendon components.

Many tendons, particularly those with a large range of motion, run through vascularized, discontinuous sheaths of collagen lined with mesenchymal cells resembling synovium. Gliding of tendons through their sheaths is enhanced by hyaluronic acid, produced by the lining cells.[35] Tendon movement is essential for the embryogenesis and maintenance of tendons and their sheaths.[36, 37] Degenerative changes appear in tendons and fibrous adhesions form between tendons and sheaths when inflammation or surgical incision is followed by long periods of immobilization.[37]

At the myotendinous junction, recesses between muscle cell processes are filled with collagen fibrils, which blend into the tendon. At its other end, collagen fibers of the tendon typically blend into fibrocartilage, mineralize, then merge into bone.[36] At some tendon insertions, such as the insertion of the pectoralis major tendon into the humerus, there are no intervening tiers of fibrocartilage.[38] Instead, tendon fibrils run through the periosteum and become continuous with outer bone lamellae ("Sharpey's perforating fibers").

It is unusual for the muscle-tendon apparatus to fail, but when it does, it is secondary to enormous, quickly generated forces across a joint and usually occurs near the tendon insertion into bone. Factors that may predispose to tendon failure include the following:

- Aging processes, including loss of extracellular water and an increase in intermolecular cross-links of collagen
- Tendon ischemia
- Iatrogenic factors, including intratendon injection of glucocorticoids
- Deposition of calcium hydroxyapatite crystals

Ligaments[39]

Ligaments provide a stabilizing bridge between bones, permitting a limited range of movements. Often the ligaments are recognized only as hypertrophied components of the fibrous joint capsule. Ligaments are structurally similar to tendons, although some have a much higher ratio of elastin to collagen (1:4) than do tendons (1:50),[33] which permits a greater degree of stretch. For example, the high elastin content of the ligamentum flavum, between adjacent vertebral laminae, allows it to stretch during spinal flexion.

Ligaments play a major role in the passive stabilization of joints, aided by the capsule and, when present, menisci. In the knee (the most studied of all joints), the collateral ligaments and cruciate ligaments provide stability when there is little or no load upon the joint. As compressive load increases, there is an increasing contribution to stability from the joint surfaces themselves.

Bursae

The many bursae in the human body facilitate gliding of one tissue over another, much as a tendon sheath facilitates movement of its tendon. Bursae are closed sacs, lined sparsely with mesenchymal cells similar to synovial cells, but are generally less well vascularized than synovium. Most bursae differentiate concurrently with synovial joints during embryogenesis. During life, however, trauma or inflammation may lead to the development of new bursae, hypertrophy of previously existing ones,[40] and communication between deep bursae and joints.[33] In patients with rheumatoid arthritis, for example, communications may exist between subacromial bursae and the glenohumeral joint, between gastrocnemius or semimembranous bursae and knee joint, and between the iliopsoas bursa and hip joint. It is unusual, however, for subcutaneous bursae (e.g., the prepatellar bursa or olecranon bursa) to develop communication with the underlying joint.

Menisci[41]

The meniscus, a fibrocartilaginous, wedge-shaped structure, is best developed in the knee but is also found in the acromioclavicular and sternoclavicular joints, the ulnocarpal joint, and the temporomandibular joint. Until recently, menisci were felt to have little function and an indolent metabolism with no capability of repair. However, it has been observed that removal of menisci from the knee may lead to premature arthritic changes in the joint,[42] and thus there has been increased attention directed toward preserving the meniscus by repair of tears.

The microanatomy of the meniscus is complex and age-dependent. The characteristic shape of both the lateral and medial meniscus is obtained early in prenatal development. At that time, the menisci are very cellular and highly vascularized throughout their substance; with maturation, however, vascularity decreases progressively from the central margin to the peripheral margin. After skeletal maturity, the peripheral 10 to 30 percent of the meniscus remains highly vascularized by a circumferential capillary plexus and is well innervated. Tears in this vascularized peripheral zone undergo repair and remodeling.[43] The central portion of the mature meniscus, however, is an avascular, aneural, and alymphatic fibrocartilage consisting of cells surrounded by an abundant extracellular matrix of collagens, chondroitin sulfates, dermatan sulfates, and hyaluronic acid. Tears in this central zone are repaired poorly.

Collagen constitutes 60 to 70 percent of the dry weight of the meniscus and is mostly type I collagen, with lesser amounts of types III, V, and VI (see Chapter 2). A small quantity of cartilage-specific type II collagen is localized to the inner, avascular portion of the meniscus. Collagen fibers in the periphery are mostly circumferentially oriented, with radial fibers extending toward the central portion.[44]

ARTICULAR CARTILAGE

Articular cartilage enables low-friction, high-velocity movement between bones; absorbs transmitted forces, thereby protecting the underlying bone end; and contributes to joint stability. Its unique structure is exquisitely adapted to the high compressional and shearing stresses that inevitably accompany such functions. A brief synthesis of the structure and function of articular cartilage follows; details of its structural components can be found in Chapters 2 and 3.

Organization

Cartilage can be identified as hyaline cartilage, white or yellow fibrocartilage, and cellular cartilage according to its macroscopic appearance. Normal articular cartilage is hyaline, with a glassy appearance when cut. It is composed predominantly of water, collagen, and proteoglycans, respectively, accounting for 65 to 80 percent, 10 to 30 percent, and 5 to 10 percent of wet weight. Although chondrocytes occupy only 0.4 to 2 percent of articular cartilage volume, they are responsible for synthesis and maintenance of cartilage matrix and are the source of nonstructural proteins, such as metalloproteases and their inhibitors localized within cartilage.[45]

Figure 1–7 is a diagrammatic representation of the various zones and regions of cartilage.

The *superficial zone* (5 to 10 percent of total thickness) is called the lamina splendens. It differs in biochemical composition and structure from the middle and deep zones, reflecting its subjection to high shearing forces and resistance to invasion by synovial cells.[46] Its collagen fibrils are oriented tangentially to the articular surface at an angle to the usual direction of motion of the joint, much like the reinforcing fibers in a radial tire. It has a high water content (80 percent of wet weight), and some glycoproteins, such as fibronectin and tenascin, are localized preferentially to the superficial zone.[47, 48]

Collagen

Collagen fibrils impart tensile strength to articular cartilage and provide a framework in which proteoglycans and chondrocytes are embedded. Tangential collagen fibers in the superficial zone blend with radial fibers, which form plates sweeping vertically through the middle zone. Type II collagen composes 90 percent of this fibrillar network, with further contributions from collagen types III, V, VI, IX, and XI. Type X collagen is restricted to the deep, calcified zone of mature articular cartilage. Collagen types II, IX, and XI are cartilage specific, and products of their degradation may be useful markers of cartilage turnover. The matrix immediately surrounding chondrocytes forms a specialized subcompartment of articular cartilage containing small-diameter collagen fibrils and the minor collagen types III, V, and VI.[49–51]

Proteoglycans

Proteoglycans impart elasticity to articular cartilage. They make up core protein with covalently attached glycosaminoglycans and form massive, polyanionic aggregates with hyaluronate and link protein; total molecular weights are about 10^{11}. These aggregates attract water, but swelling is restricted to about 20 percent of the potential maximum swelling by the surrounding collagen network. Compression causes water to be forced out of the aggregates but is opposed by repellent forces between electronegative charges within the proteoglycan molecules. After compression is released, mutual repulsion of negative charges forces the proteoglycans back to their fully extended state, and water and nutrients are pulled back into the aggregates until expansion is restricted again by the collagen network.[52] Aggrecan is the major proteoglycan imparting elasticity to articular cartilage. Smaller proteoglycans, such as decorin, may additionally affect the formation of collagen fibrils, and others may inhibit cartilage calcification.[53, 54]

Glycoproteins

Articular cartilage contains a diverse range of glycoproteins synthesized and secreted by chondrocytes. These include proteases and their inhibitors, important in matrix turnover (see Chapter 14). Some of these glycoproteins can retard the development of osteoclasts[55] and inhibit neovascularization.[56, 57] Inhibitors of angiogenesis may help to maintain the avascular nature of articular cartilage and may contribute to its resistance against neoplastic infiltration. Fibronectin is important for adhesion of articular chondrocytes via cell surface integrins and may also contribute to the organization of a stable collagen network.[58]

Chondrocytes

Chondrocytes exist in relative isolation, living singly or in small clusters. They are highly specialized to synthesize matrix components as well as enzymes capable of breaking them down, such as collagenase, neutral proteinases, and cathepsins. The chondrocyte is subjected to repeated and abrupt pressure changes and deformations and modifies its synthetic function in response to such mechanical stimuli. For example, proteoglycan synthesis may be stimulated by compression in a frequency-dependent manner.[59] Such mechanoreceptor activity may contribute to the degenerative changes observed in cartilage after forced immobilization.

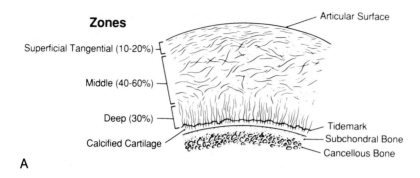

A

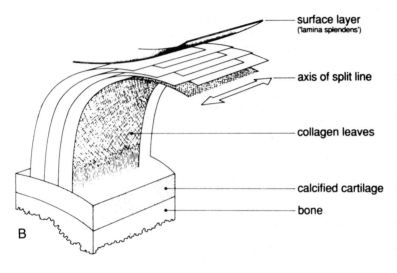

B

Figure 1–7. *A,* Zones of articular cartilage showing organization of collagen fibrils. *B,* Three-dimensional view of collagen plates in articular cartilage illustrating how the appearance of the collagen changes from "arcades" to random to plates, depending on the orientation of the section. *C,* Diagrammatic representation of the zones and regions of bovine articular cartilage. (*A,* From Mow VC, et al: *In* Nordin M, Frankel VH [eds]: Basic Biomechanics of the Musculoskeletal System, 2nd ed. Philadelphia, Lea & Febiger, 1989. *B,* From Jeffery AK, et al: Three-dimensional collagen architecture in bovine articular cartilage. J Bone Joint Surg [Br] 73B:795, 1991. *C,* From Poole AR, et al: An immuno-electron microscope study of the organization of proteoglycan monomer, link protein and collagen in the matrix of articular cartilage. J Cell Biol 93:921, 1982. By copyright permission of the Rockefeller University Press.)

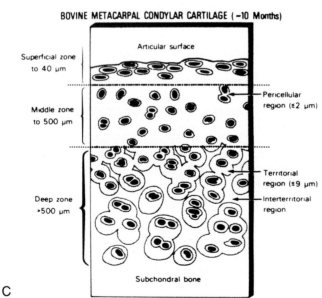

C

In addition to responding to mechanical stimuli, articular chondrocyte synthetic functions and proliferation may be regulated by a variety of cytokines and growth factors. Chondrocytes bear receptors for, among others, interleukin-1 (IL-1), insulin-like growth factor-I (IGF-I), transforming growth factor-β (TGF-β), and basic fibroblast growth factor (bFGF).[60, 61] Some growth factors, such as IGF-I and TGF-β, can be synthesized by chondrocytes themselves, possibly serving an autocrine role.[62, 63] TGF-β and bFGF are localized to cartilage extracellular matrix, bound to proteoglycans, and may be released during cartilage remodeling.[64] IL-1β stimulates the generation of other proinflammatory factors by chondrocytes, including monocyte chemoattractants, nitric oxide, and metalloproteases[65, 66] and together with bFGF stimulates articular chondrocyte proliferation.[67, 68] TGF-β and IGF-I stimulate chrondrocyte differentiation and the synthesis of cartilage matrix components, such as proteoglycans and type II collagen.[67–69] These factors may be important not only in embryogenesis and cartilage remodeling during development but also in cartilage maintenance and repair in response to traumatic and inflammatory insults.

Nutrition

As demonstrated by William Hunter in 1743, normal adult articular cartilage contains no blood vessels.[70] Vascularization of cartilage would inevitably alter its mechanical properties. Furthermore, blood flow would be repeatedly occluded during weight bearing and exercise, with reactive oxygen species generated during reperfusion, resulting in repeated damage to both cartilage matrix and to chondrocytes. In order to maintain articular cartilage as an avascular structure, chondrocytes synthesize specific inhibitors of angiogenesis.[56, 57]

As a result of the lack of adjacent blood vessels, the chondrocyte normally lives in a hypoxic and acidotic environment, with extracellular fluid pH values around 7.1 to 7.2,[71] principally utilizing anaerobic glycolysis for energy production.[72] High lactate levels in normal synovial fluid compared with paired plasma may partly reflect this anaerobic metabolism.[73] There are two potential sources of nutrients for articular cartilage: (1) subchondral blood vessels and (2) the synovial fluid.

In the growing child, the deeper layers of articular cartilage are vascularized. Here in the hypertrophic zone, as in the growth plate, blood vessels penetrate between columns of chondrocytes and active endochondral ossification occurs. It is likely that nutrients diffuse from these tiny end capillaries through matrix to chondrocytes. Diffusion from subchondral blood vessels has been thought unlikely to be a major route for the nutrition of normal adult articular cartilage because of the barrier provided by its densely calcified lower layer, the "tidemark."[74] Nonetheless, partial defects may normally exist in the osteocartilaginous barrier,[75] and, in pathologic states, such as rheumatoid arthritis, neovascularization of the deeper layers of articular cartilage may contribute to cartilage nutrition.[76] Furthermore, experimental studies have indicated that cartilage lesions of chondromalacia may develop if the subchondral blood supply of the patella is compromised.[77]

Much evidence indicates that synovial fluid and, indirectly, the synovial lining region, through which synovial fluid is generated, are major sources of nutri-ents for articular cartilage. The extracellular fluid of articular cartilage is continuous with synovial fluid, with no intervening basement membrane, and solutes pass easily from the synovial fluid into cartilage. Articular cartilage cannot survive without contact with synovial fluid in vivo; indeed, loose bodies of cartilage in joints actually grow in size.[78] In experimental systems, sufficient agitation of synovial fluid results in nourishment of even the deepest layers of articular cartilage.[79]

Nutrients may enter cartilage from synovial fluid either by diffusion or by mass transport of fluid during compression-relaxation cycles. Molecules as large as hemoglobin (MW, 65 kD) can diffuse through normal articular cartilage,[79] and solutes needed for cellular metabolism are much smaller. It is of interest that diffusion of uncharged small solutes, such as glucose, is not impaired in matrices containing large amounts of glycosaminoglycans, and diffusivity of small molecules through hyaluronate is actually enhanced.[80, 81]

The concept that intermittent compression may serve as a pump mechanism for solute exchange in cartilage has arisen from observations that joint immobilization[82] or dislocation,[83] which interferes with normal movement of one articular surface on its counterpart, leads to degenerative changes. Exercise, in contrast, increases solute penetration into cartilage in experimental systems.[79] Pressing filter paper against cartilage squeezes out liquid that has the ionic composition of extracellular fluid.[84] McCutchen suggested that during weight bearing, fluid escapes from the load-bearing region by flow to other cartilage sites.[85] When the load is removed, cartilage reexpands and draws back fluid, thereby exchanging nutrients with waste materials.

Mechanical Properties of Cartilage

Articular cartilage remains healthy despite being subjected to substantial compressive forces during normal activity. However, conditions that lead to small increases in those forces are associated with premature osteoarthritis, as seen in the longer limb's knee in individuals with leg length disparity and in the uneven articular surface following intra-articular fracture. Joints are protected from excessive unit load (force per unit area) by four mechanisms, one active (muscle contraction) and three passive:

• Transfer of forces into surrounding soft tissue, ligaments, and muscles
• Joint incongruity, which allows increasing contact area with increasing load
• Compliance of the cartilage/cancellous bone unit

Unit load is further minimized by the ends of the bones being flared, thereby providing a large articular surface for joint contact. Indeed, dissipation of forces from weight-bearing joints to surrounding structures is normally so effective that repetitive, unaccustomed exercise will lead to stress fracture through the bony diaphysis several centimeters from the joint rather than to damage to the joint itself.

The demands placed on each joint dictate the precise relationships among the three mechanisms of force dissipation. The shoulder, having an extensive range of motion, must have a small area of contact and minimal constraint. Stress overload is prevented by dissipation of forces into surrounding soft tissues and by the high compliance conferred by having one side of the articulation (the scapula) "floating" in a mass of muscle. The ankle, which provides limited and essentially uniaxial motion, experiences enormous forces. This joint must, however, remain small, with limited contact areas, because a large articular surface would exacerbate the inertia against the acceleration of a large, heavy body segment around a distant fulcrum. Forces are dissipated to the fibula and, to a lesser extent, by incongruity and expansion of the articulation with increasing force.

An essential function of cartilage—its ability to be compressed by a load and recover from this deformity—has been an object of research since Bar's studies in 1926 (Fig. 1–8).[86] When a load is applied to cartilage, there is a rapid ("instantaneous") indentation, followed by a time-dependent "creep" phase during which indentation increases while load remains constant. On removal of the load, there is an initial immediate recovery, followed by a long, sustained recovery to normal volume. The initial rapid deformation results from a bulk movement of water and compression of collagen fibers. In the creep phase, water flows through the matrix.

Studies of bone-bone contact in the absence of cartilage have demonstrated that a function of cartilage is to absorb some of the energy of impact loading by deforming, thereby spreading the load over a broad area. Both collagen and proteoglycans contribute to load carriage in normal cartilage.[87] The tensile strength of collagen resists deformation, maintaining the structural framework in which proteoglycans remain in place. The proteoglycans, through strong charge interactions with water, control solute flow and, therefore, both instantaneous and creep phases of deformation. Studies of matrix-depleted cartilage, using specific digestion with enzymes such as collagenase, trypsin, and cathepsin D, have helped to clarify the relative contributions of collagen and proteoglycans in the mechanical properties of cartilage. Collagen-depleted articular cartilage becomes filmy, flimsy, and transparent, devoid of tensile strength.[88] Proteoglycan-depleted cartilage has low compressive stiffness, losing its ability to rebound from a deforming load.[89] Changes in matrix composition of osteoarthritic cartilage may perpetuate joint damage by compromising resistance to normal compressive forces.

Repair of Articular Cartilage[90]

Articular cartilage has a poor capacity for repair, and pharmacologic enhancement of cartilage repair would have considerable potential in the treatment of arthritides and intra-articular fractures. Cartilage defects may be either superficial or deep, according to whether they penetrate the subchondral bone plate. Repair of superficial defects depends on chondrocyte proliferation and matrix remodeling and may be enhanced by mitogens for chondrocytes, such as bFGF.[91] Deep cartilage defects through the subchondral plate are filled by granulation tissue, which is eventually replaced by fibrocartilage but rarely by true hyaline cartilage.[92, 93] Transplantation of cultured autologous chondrocytes in humans, however, has resulted in the filling of full-thickness defects by hyaline cartilage.[94]

Aging of Articular Cartilage

The biochemical composition, structure, and mechanical properties of articular cartilage all change with age, and it is important, but often difficult, to distinguish between aging itself and diseases, such as osteoarthritis, that become more common with increasing age.

Proteoglycans in aged cartilage have a wide range of sizes, with small forms resulting from low substitution of glycosaminoglycan residues and their short length compared with glycosaminoglycan in young articular cartilage.[95] The unsubstituted proteoglycan core proteins—aggrecan and biglycan—are detectable in articular cartilage from elderly subjects.[96, 97] Hyaluronan content increases in aged cartilage but with a reduced mean chain length, and link protein appears also to be fragmented.[98, 99] Collagen fibrils become

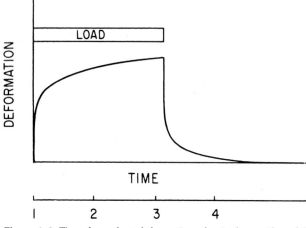

Figure 1–8. Time-dependent deformation of articular cartilage following application of a load. Four phases of deformation can be discerned as a function of time: 1, instantaneous deformation coincident with application of the load; 2, slow deformation that reaches a plateau with sustained loading; 3, instantaneous recovery following removal of load; 4, slow recovery to normal cartilage thickness. (After Bär E: Elasticitätsprufungen der Gelenkkorpel. Arch J Entwicklungsmech Organ 108:739, 1926; and Kempson GE: Mechanical properties of articular cartilage. *In* Freeman MAR [ed]: Adult Articular Cartilage. New York, Grune & Stratton, 1974, p 196.)

thinner with age, are less densely packed, and have an increased proportion of pentosidine cross-links.[87, 100, 101] Such biochemical changes may result in part from changes in chondrocyte synthetic function with age and also from changes in matrix degradation.

Biochemical changes are reflected by changes in cartilage structure. The thickness of articular cartilage, as demonstrated by magnetic resonance imaging (MRI), decreases with increasing age.[102] Fatigue fracture of superficial collagen bundles and a heterogeneous depletion of glycosaminoglycans at the periphery of joint surfaces may contribute to the mild splitting and fraying of superficial cartilage; this is referred to as "fibrillation."[103, 104] If fibrillation progresses into deeper layers of cartilage, an abnormal multicellular cluster of chondrocytes that stain intensely for glycosaminoglycans is found at the base of clefts.[105] Fibrillation, by itself, need not necessarily lead to osteoarthritis and may best be considered a "regressive change."

Together with these biochemical and structural changes, stiffness of cartilage decreases with increasing age, with fibrillated areas becoming soft or malacic. Furthermore, the tensile strength of articular cartilage decreases considerably with age, particularly in the femoral head.[106] The relevance of age-related changes in the predisposition to osteoarthritis requires further research. (See Chapter 82 for a detailed discussion of the changes in osteoarthritis.)

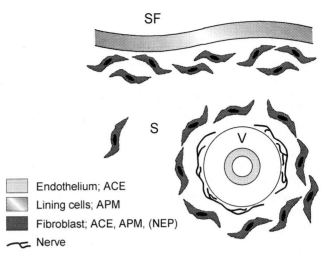

Figure 1–9. Schematic diagram showing functional compartmentalization of human synovium with respect to the regulatory neuropeptide substance P. Vascular (V), stromal (S) and synovial fluid (SF) compartments are not divided by basement membranes or tight junctions, but, instead, are segregated by condensations of cells bearing membrane peptidases capable of degrading substance P. Substance P is released from perivascular nerve terminals and acts on specific receptors on the microvascular endothelium. Microvessels are surrounded by fibroblast-like cells bearing angiotensin converting enzyme (ACE), aminopeptidase M (APM) and, in inflamed synovium, neutral endopeptidase (NEP). Synovial stroma is further separated from the synovial cavity by the lining cell layers, richly endowed with APM, underlined by a condensation of fibroblast-like cells bearing ACE, APM, and NEP. Other enzymes, such as dipeptidyl peptidase IV and matrix metalloproteases, may also contribute to synovial compartmentalization.

Subchondral Bone

The plate of bone beneath the calcified base of articular cartilage may have many effects on the cartilage above it. Its stiffness modifies the compressive forces to which articular cartilage is subjected, its blood supply may be important in cartilage nutrition (see earlier), and its cells may produce peptides that regulate chondrocyte function.[107, 108] An increase in subchondral bone density is an early feature of osteoarthritis, and ischemia of the subchondral bone leads to a rapidly destructive arthropathy, as seen in avascular necrosis of the femoral head. Furthermore, subchondral bone contains follicular lymphoid aggregates, at least in established rheumatoid arthritis, and therefore may be a site of immune-mediated disease activity.[109]

SYNOVIUM

The synovium, the tissue between the fibrous joint capsule and fluid-filled synovial cavity, is divided into functional compartments comprising the lining region (synovial intima), the subintimal stroma, and the vasculature (Fig. 1–9). These compartments are not circumscribed by basement membranes but nonetheless have distinct functions; they are separated from each other by chemical barriers, such as membrane peptidases, which limit the diffusion of regulatory factors between compartments.[110] Furthermore, synovial compartments are unevenly distributed within a single joint; vascularity, for example, is high at the enthesis where synovium, ligament, and cartilage coalesce. Far from being a homogeneous tissue in continuity with the synovial cavity, synovium is highly heterogeneous, and synovial fluid may poorly represent the tissue fluid composition of any synovial compartment.

Synovial Lining

The synovial lining comprises a specialized condensation of cells and extracellular matrix, which is localized between the synovial cavity and stroma. In normal synovium, the lining layer is three to four cells deep, although intra-articular fat pads are usually covered by only a single layer of synovial cells, and ligaments and tendons are covered by synovial cells, which are widely separated. At some sites, lining cells are absent and the extracellular connective tissue constitutes the lining layer.[111] Such bare areas become increasingly frequent with increasing age.[112]

The region containing synovial lining cells is often referred to as the *synovial membrane*. The term *membrane*, however, is more correctly reserved for epithelia that have basement membranes, intercellular tight junctions, and desmosomes. Instead, synovial lining cells lie loosely in a bed of hyaluronate interspersed with collagen fibrils. This is the macromolecular sieve that imparts the semipermeable nature of the synovium. This absence of any true epithelial tissue is a major determinant of joint physiology.

Lining cells can be categorized as (1) bone marrow, (2) macrophage-derived type A synoviocytes, and (3) mesenchymal, fibroblast-derived type B synoviocytes (Fig. 1–10).[113] Normal synovium is lined predominantly by fibroblast-like cells, whereas macrophage-like cells compose only 10 to 20 percent of lining cells.

Fibroblast-like cells are particularly concentrated in

A

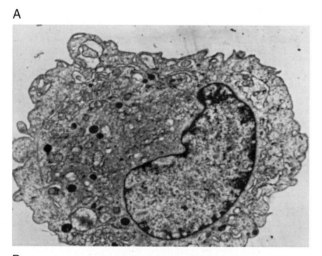

B

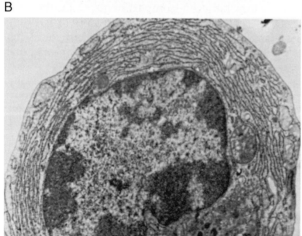

Figure 1–10. *A,* Type A human synovial cell with many undulations, a prominent Golgi complex and many microvesicles, various and heterogeneous inclusions (residual bodies), and lysosomes. The nucleus contains dense chromatin. Microfilaments are abundant, lying in the long axis of the cell. This cell type has phagocytic capabilities and antigenically resembles mature macrophages. (×11,200.) *B,* Type B human synovial cell with a very-well-developed rough endoplasmic reticulum with few cell processes and vacuoles. Nuclear chromatin is less dense, and nucleoli are more developed. Cytoplasmic vacuoles and vesicles are rare. These features are consistent with a synthetic function. Type B synovial cells contain the enzyme prolyl hydroxylase, important in collagen synthesis, and so resemble mature fibroblasts. (×17,500.) (*A, B,* Courtesy of Donald Gates.)

the deeper parts of the lining region and have fine cytoplasmic processes that extend toward the synovial surface. Like other fibroblasts, they express the collagen-synthesis enzyme prolyl hydroxylase, synthesize extracellular matrix, and have the potential to proliferate, although proliferation markers are rarely seen in normal synovium.[114] Unlike stromal fibroblasts, however, type B synoviocytes express UDPGD and synthesize hyaluronan, an important constituent of synovial fluid.[115] Furthermore, they express CD44, the principal receptor for hyaluronan and the vascular cell adhesion molecule-1 (VCAM-1).[116, 117]

The extent to which these specific features of type B synoviocytes contribute to the predisposition of synovium to chronic inflammation awaits further investigation. Hyaluronan, in particular, has many biologic functions, including roles in joint cavitation in the embryo (see earlier), regulation of cell-cell and cell-matrix interactions, and lubrication (see below) in the mature joint. Hyaluronan is structurally modified in rheumatoid synovial fluids and may be directly involved in the pathogenesis of synovitis through its angiogenic potential.[118]

Type A synoviocytes can express most of the antigens characteristic of fully differentiated, mature macrophages. They are certainly phagocytic and, like other tissue macrophages, have little capacity to proliferate; however, they are recruited from the circulation during synovial inflammation.

Although these two types of synoviocytes can be broadly defined morphologically and appear to have distinct ontogenies, some overlap may exist between their respective functions and it would be oversimplistic to regard type A and type B synoviocytes as purely phagocytic and synthetic, respectively. Type B cells may display phagocytic activity,[119] whereas type A cells synthesize a wide variety of regulatory factors and even matrix components.[120]

Despite not being a true epithelium, and despite being boundary to a cavity with no communication to the exterior, synovial lining cells bear abundant membrane peptidases on their surface, capable of degrading a wide range of regulatory peptides, such as substance P and angiotensin II.[110] These enzymes may be important in limiting the diffusion of these potent peptide mediators away from the immediate vicinity of their release and action. Synovial cells also synthesize non–membrane-bound proteases and their inhibitors and may regulate matrix turnover, not only in the synovium but also, via the synovial fluid, in articular cartilage.

Components of the intercellular matrix of the synovial lining region distinguish it from the underlying stroma, reflecting the specific synthetic activity of lining cells. Hyaluronan, type VI collagen, and chondroitin-6-sulfate are localized to the lining region, with tenascin localized immediately beneath the lining cells.[121–124] Normal synovial lining cells also express a rich array of adhesion molecules.[117, 125, 126] These are probably essential for cellular attachment to specific matrix components in the synovial lining region, preventing loss into the synovial cavity of cells subjected to deformation and shear stresses during joint movement. Adhesion molecules potentially are also involved in the recruitment of inflammatory cells during the evolution of arthritis.

Synovial Stroma

A variable depth of heterogeneous mesenchymal tissue is interposed between the synovial lining region and joint capsule. At the lateral joint margin of the knee, this synovial stroma is well vascularized and cellular but becomes increasingly fibrous with increasing depth until it blends with the joint capsule. The synovial lining of cruciate ligaments is in direct continuity with the underlying hypocellular collagenous fibers; in the suprapatellar pouch, the synovial stroma predominantly composes adipose tissue. This synovial heterogeneity can make assessment by synovial biopsy difficult.

Stromal cells in normal synovium are predominantly fibroblasts. Fibroblasts accumulate immediately beneath the lining region and around blood vessels; they bear surface peptidases, such as angiotensin converting enzyme (ACE), dipeptidyl peptidase IV, aminopeptidase M, and, in inflamed synovium, neutral endopeptidase. These enzymes contribute to the functional compartmentalization of peptide regulatory systems within the tissue.[110, 127] The synovial stroma plays an important role in the response of synovium to arthritis, being host to inflammatory cell infiltrates and lymphoid follicles.

Synovial Vasculature

Normal synovium is richly vascularized,[128] providing the high blood flow required for solute and gas exchange, not only for the synovium itself but also for meeting the needs of the avascular articular cartilage. In addition, the synovial vasculature is essential in generating synovial fluid; it behaves as an endocrine organ, generating factors that regulate synoviocyte function, and it is a selective gateway, recruiting inflammatory cells in times of need. Finally, synovial blood flow regulates intra-articular temperature. The following text details the structure and function of blood vessels in normal synovium.

Arterial and venous networks of the joint are complex and are characterized by arteriovenous anastomoses that communicate freely with blood vessels in periosteum and periarticular bone.[129] As large synovial arteries enter the deep layers of the synovium near the capsule, they give off branches, which branch again to form "microvascular units" in the subsynovial layers. The synovial lining region, the surfaces of intra-articular ligaments, and the entheses (in the angle of ligamentous insertions into bone) are particularly well vascularized. The distribution of synovial vessels displays considerable plasticity. Angiogenesis is characteristic of inflammatory arthritis; immobilization in experimental animals, however, actually decreases the number of capillary plexuses as well as blood flow in joints.[130]

The synovial vasculature can be divided on morphologic and functional grounds into arterioles, capillaries, and venules. In addition, lymphatics accompany arterioles and larger venules.[131]

Arterioles regulate regional blood flow; capillaries and postcapillary venules are sites of fluid and cellular exchange. Correspondingly, regulatory systems are differentially distributed along the vascular axis. For example, ACE, which generates the vasoconstrictor/growth factor angiotensin II, is localized predominantly to arteriolar and capillary endothelia.[110] Specific receptors for angiotensin II and for the neuropeptide substance P are abundant on synovial capillaries, with lower densities on adjacent arterioles.[132, 133] Dipeptidyl peptidase IV, a peptide-degrading enzyme, is specifically localized to the cell membranes of venular endothelium.[110] The synovial vasculature, therefore, is not only functionally compartmentalized from the surrounding stroma but also highly specialized along its arteriovenous axis.

Synovial blood flow is regulated by both *intrinsic* (autocrine and paracrine) and *extrinsic* (neural and humoral) systems (Fig. 1–11). Locally generated factors, such as the peptide vasoconstrictors angiotensin II and endothelin-1 and the endothelium-derived relaxing factor (EDRF) nitric oxide, act on adjacent arteriolar smooth muscle to regulate regional vascular tone.[132, 134, 135] Normal synovial arterioles are richly innervated by sympathetic nerves containing vasoconstrictors, such as norepinephrine and neuropeptide Y, and by "sensory" nerves, which also play an efferent vasodilatory role by releasing the neuropeptides substance P and calcitonin gene-related peptide.[136]

Complex regulatory systems are no doubt essential for responding to the repeated mechanical stresses that can interrupt synovial perfusion during joint movement, particularly in the presence of a synovial effusion. In normal joints, intra-articular pressures are slightly subatmospheric at rest (0 to −5 mm Hg).[137, 138] During exercise, hydrostatic pressure in the normal joint may decrease further.[139] Chronic arthritis leads to increased intra-articular pressures because of the increased volume of synovial fluid and decreased compliance of the joint capsule.[140] Resting intra-articular pressures in rheumatoid joints are around 20 mm Hg; during isometric exercise, they may rise above 100 mm Hg, well above capillary perfusion pressure and, at times, above arterial pressure.[138]

Elevation of intra-articular pressure interrupts not only synovial blood flow but also blood flow in the subchondral bone plate.[141] High resting intra-articular pressures contribute to resting synovial hypoxia in rheumatoid arthritis and, therefore, may be damaging to the joint. The potential volume, and thus the pressure of the synovial cavity, varies according to the degree to which the joint is flexed.[142, 143] During exer-

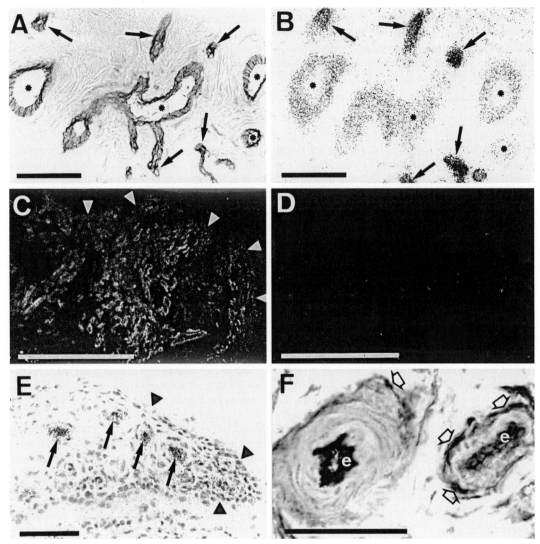

Figure 1–11. Microvascular regulatory systems in human synovium. *A,* Microvascular endothelium immunoreactive for platelet-endothelial cell adhesion molecule (CD31). *B,* Receptors for the vasoconstrictor/growth factor angiotensin II in a consecutive section to *A.* In *A* and *B,* silver grains represent dense specific binding of [^{125}I](Sar^1, Ile^8)-angiotensin II to microvessels *(arrows),* and less dense binding to the media of larger arterioles *(asterisks).* *C, D,* Microvascular localization of nitric oxide synthase (NOS) to human synovium. *C,* Annular and punctate binding of the NOS ligand [^{3}H]nitro-L-arginine (100 nM) to synovial microvessels. *D,* Abolition of [^{3}H]nitro-L-arginine binding by an excess of the specific NOS inhibitor N-nitro-L-arginine methyl ester (200 μM). Nitro-L-arginine binds with high affinity to constitutive NOS on microvessels in noninflamed as well as in inflamed human synovium. (Further details in Walsh DA, et al: Inducible nitric oxide synthase in human synovium. Br J Rheumatol 33[S1], 175, 1994.) *E,* Receptors for the vasodilator/growth factor substance P. Silver grains represent specific binding of [^{125}I]Bolton Hunter-labeled substance P to synovial microvessels *(arrows).* *F,* Angiotensin-converting enzyme localized to vascular endothelium (e) and perivascular fibroblast-like cells *(open arrows).* *C, E,* Arrowheads indicate the synovial surface. *A, F,* Immunoperoxidase method. *B, E,* Emulsion-dipped in vitro receptor autoradiography preparations with hematoxylin and eosin counterstain. *C, D,* Reversal prints of film autoradiograms. *A, B, E, F,* Calibration bar = 100 μm. *C, D,* Calibration bar = 3 mm.

cise, such as walking, synovial blood flow in the chronically inflamed knee is cyclically occluded, with intermittent reperfusion. Reactive oxygen species generated during these hypoxic-reperfusion cycles may further injure the synovium.[144] The coordinated interplay of vasodilator and vasoconstrictor regulatory systems may normally be designed to relieve synovial hypoxia while limiting transient reperfusion.

Massive elevation of intra-articular pressure during exercise is a feature of the chronic synovial inflammation of rheumatoid arthritis but not of acute traumatic effusions.[137] Reflex muscle inhibition may normally protect against elevated joint pressures in acute synovitis, and failure of such mechanisms may underlie the persistence of rheumatoid joint disease.[137]

Regulation of synoviocyte function by the synovial vasculature extends beyond nutrition and excretion. Regulatory peptides, such as angiotensin II and endothelin-1, generated by microvascular endothelium may induce nonvascular cells to proliferate and synthesize other regulatory factors and matrix.[132, 134] Expression of adhesion molecules on the venular endothelium of normal synovium is important in type A synoviocyte recruitment from the circulation and in the initiation of synovial inflammation; other adhesion molecules are expressed or up-regulated during the evolution of the inflammatory response (see Chapter 12).

The synovial microvasculature is essential for the generation of synovial fluid, formed by admixture of a protein-rich filtrate of blood with synoviocyte-derived hyaluronate. Capillary depth is proposed as the major factor governing fluid exchange in joints.[145] Synovial capillaries are fenestrated; they contain small pores covered by a thin membrane (Fig. 1–12).[146] These fenestrations may facilitate rapid exchange of small molecules, such as glucose and lactate.

The vascular system of the extremities acts as a countercurrent distribution system for tissue temperature, and peripheral joints normally function with intra-articular temperatures well below the core body temperature of 37°C. Non–weight-bearing active movements increase intra-articular temperature by as much as 1°C, probably by increasing subsynovial tissue blood flow, although normal intra-articular temperatures in the knee are always below 36°C (at ambient temperatures of around 20°C). Low intra-articular temperatures are important because enzymatic reactions observed in vitro at 37°C may proceed only slowly in the normal joint but may be enhanced during synovial inflammation. At 37°C, for instance, destruction of articular cartilage collagen fibers by synovial collagenase is substantial; at 32°C, it is imperceptible.[147]

Intra-articular temperatures may vary widely according to ambient room temperature. In small, peripheral joints with very little overlying insulation of fat or muscle (e.g., the metacarpophalangeal joint), intra-articular temperatures closely parallel those of skin between resting temperatures and 40°C.[148] By contrast, in larger joints (e.g., the knee), there are wide variations between joint and skin temperature.[149] In the knee, cold or hot packs applied to the skin reflexly change intra-articular temperatures in the opposite direction.[150] Similarly, a painful stimulus (e.g., apprehension, alarm, or smoking) lowers the skin temperature and elevates intra-articular temperature. Possible disparities between skin and intra-articular temperatures complicate the interpretation of thermographic data derived from large joints.

INNERVATION OF THE JOINT

Normal joints have both *afferent* (sensory) and *efferent* (motor) innervations. Fast-conducting, myelinated A-fibers innervating the joint capsule are important for proprioception and detection of joint movement; slow-conducting, unmyelinated C-fibers transmit diffuse pain sensation and regulate synovial microvascular function. Abnormalities of articular innervation are associated with inflammatory arthritis,[136, 151] and

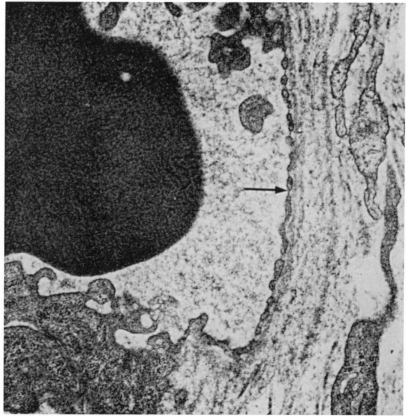

Figure 1–12. Fenestrated blood capillary in human synovium. The capillary is situated just beneath the lining layer. Pores in the endothelium are indicated by the arrow. A red blood cell lies in the lumen of the capillary. ($\times$11,000.) (From Bassleer R, et al: *In* Franchimont P [ed]: Articular Synovium: Anatomy, Physiology, Pathology, Pharmacology, and Therapy. Basel, Karger, 1982, pp 1–26.)

neurogenic mechanisms may underlie symmetric joint involvement in rheumatoid arthritis.[152]

Afferent Innervation

Dissection studies have shown that each joint has a dual nerve supply, composing specific articular nerves that penetrate the capsule as independent branches of adjacent peripheral nerves, and articular branches that arise from related muscle nerves. The definition of joint position and the detection of joint motion are monitored separately and by a combination of multiple inputs from different receptors in varied systems. Nerve endings in muscle and skin as well as in the joint capsule mediate sensation of joint position[153] and movement.[154] Patients who have had capsulectomy along with total hip replacement[155] or surgical removal of proximal interphalangeal or metacarpophalangeal joints of the hand[156] still retain good awareness of joint position. Indeed, joint replacement may partially reverse the impairment of joint position sense that results from articular inflammation.[157, 158] It has been suggested that impaired proprioception may contribute to the propensity of early osteoarthritis to develop in hypermobile subjects.[159]

Normal synovium is richly innervated by fine, unmyelinated nerve fibers that follow the courses of blood vessels and extend into the synovial lining layers.[136] Many of these contain markers of sensory nerves, such as the neuropeptide substance P. They do not have specialized endings, are slow-conducting, and may transmit diffuse, burning, or aching pain sensation.

Mechanisms of joint pain have been reviewed by Schaible and Grubb.[160] In the noninflamed joint, most sensory nerve fibers do not respond to movement within the normal range; these are referred to as "silent nociceptors." In the acutely inflamed joint, however, these nerve fibers become sensitized by mediators, such as bradykinin and prostaglandins ("peripheral sensitization"), such that normal movements induce pain. Pain sensation is further up-regulated or down-regulated in the central nervous system, both at the level of the spinal cord and in the brain, by central sensitization and "gating" of nociceptive input. Thus, although the normal joint may respond predictably to painful stimuli, there is often a poor correlation between apparent joint disease and perceived pain in chronic arthritis. Pain on joint movements within the normal range is a characteristic symptom described by the patient with chronically inflamed joints caused by rheumatoid arthritis. Despite this, however, chronically inflamed joints may not be painful at rest, although they become so with super-added acute inflammation, such as infection.

Afferent nerve fibers from the joint play an important role in the reflex inhibition of muscle contraction. Reflex muscle inhibition comprises complex phenomena ranging from the abrupt "giving way" and "dropping" described by patients with painful knees and hands, to the rapid quadriceps wasting observed in patients with an acutely swollen knee. Fast-conducting, myelinated and slow-conducting, unmyelinated afferent nerve fibers as well as descending inputs from the central nervous system may each contribute to these phenomena. Trophic factors generated by motor neurons, such as the neuropeptide calcitonin gene-related peptide, are important in maintaining muscle bulk and a functional neuromuscular junction.[161] Decreases in motor neuron trophic support during articular inflammation probably contribute to muscle wasting.

Acute synovial effusion in the knee reflexly inhibits quadriceps contraction even in the absence of pain.[161] Such inhibition limits the peak intra-articular pressure during attempted exercise and should be seen as a normal protective mechanism in knees with acute traumatic effusions. Suppression of these reflexes in the chronically inflamed joint may exacerbate arthritis and contribute to its persistence. (See Synovial Vasculature earlier.)

Efferent Innervation

Sympathetic nerve fibers surround blood vessels, particularly in the deeper regions of normal synovium.[136] They contain (and release) both classic neurotransmitters (norepinephrine) and neuropeptides (neuropeptide Y), which constrict synovial blood vessels. In addition, sympathetic neurotransmitters may facilitate transmission of nociceptive information by sensory fibers and enhance synovial inflammation.[163, 164] Sympathetic nervous activity is increased in a range of both inflammatory and noninflammatory conditions associated with peripheral pain, and sympathetic blockade may improve symptoms in rheumatoid arthritis.[165]

"Afferent" nerves containing substance P also have an efferent role in the synovium. Substance P is released from peripheral nerve terminals into the joint, and specific, G protein–coupled receptors for substance P are localized to microvascular endothelium in normal synovium.[133, 166] Substance P is a vasodilator, enhances plasma extravasation, and stimulates angiogenesis.[167, 168] Furthermore, in vitro studies have implicated substance P in the stimulation of synoviocyte proliferation and collagenase production, lymphocyte activation, and inflammatory cell chemotaxis.[169–171] These apparently proinflammatory actions of neuropeptides may contribute to synovial inflammation. Sensory neuropeptides are, however, also important in wound healing[172] and maintenance of tissue integrity, and the partial denervation of synovium observed in rheumatoid arthritis may contribute to the failure of synovial inflammation to resolve.[136]

SYNOVIAL FLUID

Fluid in normal joints is present in small quantities (2.5 ml in the normal knee), sufficient to coat the synovial surface but not to separate one surface from another. Tendon sheath fluid and synovial fluid are biochemically similar[173]; both are essential for the nutrition and lubrication of adjacent avascular structures (tendon and articular cartilage) and may help to limit adhesion formation and, therefore, maintain movement. Measurement of synovial fluid constituents has, appropriately, proved popular in attempts to identify locally generated regulatory factors, markers of cartilage turnover, and the metabolic status of the joint and in assessing access of pharmaceutical agents to the joint. However, interpretation of such data requires an understanding of the generation and clearance of synovial fluid and its various components.

Generation and Clearance of Synovial Fluid

Synovial fluid is an ultrafiltrate of plasma to which locally generated factors have been added. Generation of this ultrafiltrate depends on the difference between intracapillary and intra-articular hydrostatic pressures and between colloid osmotic pressures of capillary plasma and synovial tissue fluid. Fenestrations in synovial endothelium (see Fig. 1–12) and the macromolecular sieve of hyaluronic acid[174] permit the selective entry of water and low-molecular-weight solutes into the synovium, assisted, in the case of glucose, by an active transport system.[175] Proteins are present in synovial fluid in concentrations inversely proportional to molecular size, with synovial fluid albumin concentrations being about 45 percent of those in plasma (Fig. 1–13).[176]

Hyaluronic acid is synthesized by fibroblast-like synovial lining cells, and it appears in high concentra-

tions in synovial fluid (≈ 3 g/L) compared with plasma (≈ 30 μg/L). Lubricin, a glycoprotein that assists articular lubrication, is another constituent of synovial fluid which is generated by the lining cells. In addition, a wide range of regulatory factors may be generated locally within the joint, as are products of synoviocyte metabolism and cartilage breakdown, resulting in marked differences between the composition of synovial fluid and plasma ultrafiltrate.

Synovial fluid is cleared through lymphatics in the synovium, assisted by joint movement. Unlike ultrafiltration, lymphatic clearance of solutes is independent of molecular size. In addition, constituents of synovial fluid, such as regulatory peptides, may be locally degraded by enzymes, and low-molecular-weight metabolites may diffuse along concentration gradients into plasma. Clearance of synovial fluid and its constituents, therefore, may be increased in inflamed joints as a result of increased lymphatic drainage,[177] up-regulation of membrane peptidases,[110, 127] or increased synovial blood flow. Lymphatics, however, appear damaged or depleted in rheumatoid synovium,[131] and there is indirect evidence to suggest that clearance of some synovial fluid components is inadequate in severe inflammation. For instance, complement components and leukocyte-derived proteinases accumulate in synovial fluid in rheumatoid arthritis and may contribute to joint damage.[178, 179]

Synovial Fluid As an Indicator of Joint Function

In the absence of a basement membrane separating synovium or cartilage from synovial fluid, measurements made on synovial fluid may reflect the activity of these structures. Furthermore, because there is little capacity for the selective concentration of solutes in synovial fluid, those present at higher concentration than in plasma probably are synthesized locally. However, such assumptions must be treated with caution. Furthermore, solutes present in synovial fluid at lower concentrations than in plasma can be assumed to be locally generated only if the local clearance rate is known.

Despite the absence of a basement membrane, synovial fluid does not mix freely with synovial tissue fluid. Hyaluronan may trap molecules within the synovial cavity by acting as a "filtercake" on the surface of the synovial lining and thereby resisting the movement of synovial fluid out from the joint space.[180] Membrane peptidases may limit the diffusion of regulatory peptides from their sites of release into synovial fluid.

Synovial fluid and its constituent proteins have a rapid turnover time (around 1 hour in normal knees), and equilibrium is not usually reached between all parts of the joint. Tissue fluid around fenestrated endothelium, therefore, is likely to reflect plasma ultrafiltrate most closely, with a low content of hyaluronate compared with synovial fluid, whereas locally gener-

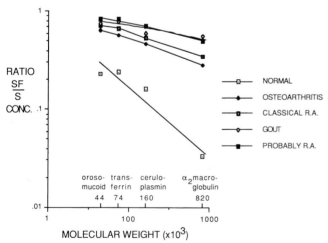

Figure 1–13. Ratio of the concentration of proteins in synovial fluid to that found in serum, plotted as a function of molecular weight. Larger proteins are selectively excluded from normal synovial fluid, but this macromolecular sieve is less effective in diseased synovium. Conc., concentration; R.A., rheumatoid arthritis; SF, synovial fluid; S, serum. (From Kushner I, Somerville JA: Permeability of human synovial membrane to plasma proteins. Arthritis Rheum 14:560, 1971. Reprinted with permission of the American College of Rheumatology.)

ated or released peptides, such as endothelin and substance P, may attain much higher perivascular concentrations than those measured in synovial fluid.

Solutes detected in synovial fluid at higher concentrations than in plasma are likely to have been locally generated. However, clearance rates from synovial fluid may be slower than those from plasma, and synovial fluid levels of drugs or urate, for example, may remain elevated after plasma levels have declined.[181] Furthermore, the turnover time for hyaluronan in the normal joint (≈13 hours) is an order of magnitude slower than that of small solutes and proteins. Association with hyaluronan may thus result in trapping of solutes within synovial fluid.[182]

Comparisons of synovial fluid constituents between disease groups are often limited by the sparsity of data on normal synovial fluid[183] as a result of difficulties in its collection. Extrapolation from synovial fluid concentrations to local synthetic rates is further complicated because of variations in clearance rates and in synovial fluid volume. Plasma proteins are less effectively filtered in inflamed synovium, perhaps because of increased size of endothelial cell fenestrations or because interstitial hyaluronate-protein complexes are fragmented by enzymes associated with the inflammatory process.[176] Concentrations of proteins, such as α_2-macroglobulin (the principal proteinase inhibitor of plasma), fibrinogen, and immunoglobulin M (IgM), therefore, are elevated in inflammatory synovial fluids (see Fig. 1–13), as are associated, protein-bound cations.

Despite these reservations, however, cautious interpretation of synovial fluid analysis will, no doubt, continue to provide useful information about synovial function.

LUBRICATION

The complicated subject of joint lubrication has been extensively reviewed.[184] Lubrication is essential for the protection of joint structures from friction and shear stresses associated with movement under loading. Multiple mechanisms contribute to joint lubrication, falling into two basic categories:

1. *Fluid-film lubrication*, in which cartilage surfaces are separated by an incompressible fluid film.
2. *Boundary lubrication*, in which surface-to-surface contact exists, with special molecules attached to cartilage surfaces offering protection by decreasing its coefficient of friction.

In addition, the articular cartilage is deformable by compression and by tangential stretching, and this further reduces frictional stresses at the articular surface (elastohydrodynamic lubrication).[185] Fluid-film lubrication is possibly the major mechanism in moving normal joints, but boundary lubrication becomes more important during static loading and in disease. During loading, a film of fluid is trapped between opposing cartilage surfaces and, because the fluid film is noncompressible, prevents the surfaces from touching, resulting in so-called "squeeze film" lubrication.[186] Irregularities in the cartilage surface and its deformation during compression may augment this trapping of fluid. During loading, fluid and low-molecular-weight solutes are forced into articular cartilage from the synovial cavity, thereby concentrating a hyaluronic acid–protein macromolecular gel between cartilage surfaces, preventing cartilage-cartilage contact and "boosting" lubrication.[187] This stable gel layer is approximately 0.1 μm thick in the normal human hip joint, but it can be much thinner in the presence of inflammatory synovial fluids or with increased cartilage porosity.[188, 189]

Lubricin is a major boundary lubricant in the human joint.[35, 190] A glycoprotein synthesized by synovial cells, it has a molecular weight of 225,000 daltons, is 200 nm in length, and is 1 to 2 nm in diameter; it is analogous to bovine synovial lubricating factor.[191, 192] The lubricating mechanism of these glycoproteins is uncertain, but sugar digestions indicate that terminal galactose residues may be important. Dipalmitoyl phosphatidylcholine, which constitutes 45 percent of lipid in normal synovial fluid, may also act as a boundary lubricant.[193] Lipid composes 1 to 2 percent of dry weight of cartilage,[194] and experimental treatment of cartilage surfaces with fat solvents impairs lubrication qualities.[195] Hyaluronate appears to be less important than glycoproteins in boundary lubrication,[196] but the two may act synergistically.[197]

Articular surfaces are also protected by other mechanisms not involving lubrication. During impact loading, muscles and bone absorb the great majority of force and energy, leaving only a small amount to be absorbed by cartilage itself.[198] Finely tuned neuromuscular reflexes are essential for this system to work effectively.[199] Small failures in these reflex arcs may lead to insufficient attenuation of impact loading, resulting in degenerative changes in joints and subchondral bone.

CONCLUSIONS

The normal human synovial joint is a complicated structure, well adapted to provide nutrition and lubrication to an avascular cartilage. It maintains this function despite the repeated stresses inherent in joint movement, providing sufficient stability to permit normal function. Cartilage and synovium are heterogeneous and very different structures in almost all aspects of their cellular and matrix composition, nutrition, and mechanical properties. Synovium is essential for normal cartilage nutrition; synovial folds are normally applied to the cartilage surface and the two structures meld together at the joint margin. However, normal cartilage is resistant to synovial invasion, a resistance that breaks down in inflammatory arthritis, leading to pannus formation, erosions, and joint destruction. The regulation of cellular activity and matrix composition and the maintenance of functionally distinct compartments within articular structures appear to be essential in sustaining the normal joint, whose physiology is dramatically altered in acute and chronic inflammatory states.

References

1. Sledge CB, Zaleske DJ: Developmental anatomy of joints. In Resnick D, Niwayama G (ed): Diagnosis of Bone and Joint Disorders: Philadelphia, WB Saunders, 1988.
2. O'Rahilly R, Gardner E: The embryology of movable joints. In Sokoloff L(ed): The Joints and Synovial Fluid. New York, Academic Press, 1978, p 49.
3. Zwilling E, Saunders JW Jr, Gasseling JT: Involvement of the apical ectodermal ridge in chick limb development. Anat Rec 136:307, 1960.
4. Davidson DR, Crawley A, Hill RE, Tickle C: Position-dependent expression of two related homeobox genes in developing vertebrate limbs. Nature 352:429, 1991.
5. Rahilly R: The development of joints. Ir J Med Sci 6:456, 1957.
6. Roark EF, Greer K: Transforming growth factor-β and bone morphogenetic protein-2 act by distinct mechanisms to promote chick limb cartilage differentiation in vitro. Dev Dyn 200:103, 1994.
7. Tavella S, Raffo P, Tacchetti C, Cancedda R, Castagnola P: N-CAM and N-cadherin expression during in vitro chondrogenesis. Exp Cell Res 215:354, 1994.
8. Coelho CN, Kosher RA: Gap junctional communication during limb cartilage differentiation. Dev Biol 144:47, 1991.
9. Sasano Y, Mizoguchi I, Kagayama M, et al: Distribution of type I collagen, type II collagen and PNA binding glycoconjugates during chondrogenesis of three distinct embryonic cartilages. Anat Embryol 186:205, 1992.
10. Kulyk WM, Coelho CN, Kosher RA: Type IX collagen gene expression during limb cartilage differentiation. Matrix 11:282, 1991.
11. Toole BP, Jackson G, Gross J: Hyaluronate in morphogenesis: Inhibition of chondrogenesis in vitro. Proc Natl Acad Sci USA 69:1384, 1972.
12. Motoyama J, Eto K: Antisense retinoic acid receptor γ-1 oligonucleotide enhances chondrogenesis of mouse limb mesenchymal cells in vitro. FEBS Lett 338:319, 1994.
13. Chen P, Carrington JL, Paralkar VM, Pierce GF, Reddi, AH: Chick limb bud mesodermal cell chondrogenesis: Inhibition by isoforms of platelet-derived growth factor and reversal by recombinant bone morphogenetic protein. Exp Cell Res 200:110, 1992.
14. Kulyk WM: Promotion of embryonic limb cartilage differentiation in vitro by staurosporine, a protein kinase C inhibitor. Develop Biol 146:38, 1991.
15. Toole BP: Hyaluronate turnover during chondrogenesis in the developing chick limb and axial skeleton. Dev Biol 29:321, 1972.
16. Edwards JC, Wilkinson LS, Jones HM, et al: The formation of human synovial cavities: A possible role for hyaluronan and CD44 in altered interzone cohesion. J Anat 185:355, 1994.
17. Izumi S, Takeya M, Takagi K, Takahashi K: Ontogenetic development of synovial A cells in fetal and neonatal rat knee joints. Cell Tissue Res 262:1, 1990.
18. Hukkanen MV, Mapp PI, Moscoso G, et al: Innervation of the human knee joint: A study in foetal material. Br J Rheumatol 29(S2):32, 1990.
19. Mitrovic D: Development of the diarthrodial joints in the rat embryo. Am J Anat 151:475, 1978.
20. Drachman DB, Sokoloff L: The role of movement in embryonic joint development. Dev Biol 14:401, 1966.
21. Yasuda Y: Differentiation of human limb buds in vitro. Anat Rec 175:561, 1973.
22. Mundlos S, Zabel B: Developmental expression of human cartilage matrix protein. Dev Dyn 199:241, 1994.
23. Pacifici M, Iwamoto M, Golden EB, et al: Tenascin is associated with articular cartilage development. Dev Dyn 198:123, 1993.
24. Symons NBB: The development of the human mandibular joint. J Anat 86:326, 1952.
25. Bradley SJ: An analysis of self-differentiation of chick limb buds in chorio-allantoic grafts. J Anat 107:479, 1970.
26. Bauer R: Zur Problem der Neugliederung der Wurbelsaule. Acta Anat 72:321, 1969.
27. Walmsley R: The development and growth of the intervertebral disc. Edinburgh Med J 60:341, 1983.
28. Linsenmeyer TF, Trelstad RL, Gross J: The collagen of chick embryonic notochord. Biochem Biophys Res Commun 3:39, 1973.
29. Eyre DR, Muir H: Collagen polymorphism: Two molecular species in pig intervertebral discs. FEBS Lett 42:192, 1974.
30. Herbert CM, Lindberg KA, Jayson MIV, et al: Changes in the collagen of human intervertebral discs during ageing and degenerative joint disease. J Mol Med 1:79, 1975.
31. Bird HA, Tribe DR, Bacon PA: Joint hypermobility leading to osteoarthritis and chondrocalcinosis. Ann Rheum Dis 37:203, 1978.
32. Gelberman R, Goldberg V, An K-N, et al: Tendon. In Woo SL-Y, Buckwalter JA (eds): Injury and Repair of the Musculoskeletal Soft Tissues: Park Ridge, Ill, American Academy of Orthopaedic Surgeons, 1988.
33. Canoso JJ: Bursae, tendons and ligaments. Clin Rheum Dis 7:189, 1981.
34. Gay S, Miller EJ: Collagen in the Physiology and Pathology of Connective Tissue. Stuttgart, Gustav Fisher, 1978.
35. Swann DA: Macromolecules of synovial fluid. In Sokoloff L (ed.): The Joints and Synovial Fluid. New York, Academic Press, 1978, pp 407–435.
36. Kieny M, Chevallier A: Autonomy of tendon development in the embryonic duck wing. J Embryol Exp Morphol 49:153, 1979.
37. Kannus P, Jozsa L, Dvist M, Lehto M, Jarvinen M: The effect of immobilization on myotendinous junction: An ultrastructural, histochemical and immunohistochemical study. Acta Physiol Scand 144:387, 1992.
38. Cooper RR, Misol S: Tendon and ligament insertion: A light and electron microscopic study. J Bone Joint Surg 82A:1, 1970.
39. Frank C, Woo S, Andriacchi T, et al: Normal ligament: Structure, function, and composition. In Woo SL-Y, Buckwalter JA (eds): Injury and Repair of the Musculoskeletal Soft Tissues: Park Ridge, Ill, American Academy of Orthopaedic Surgeons, 1988, p 45.
40. Kuhns JG: Adventitious bursa. Arch Surg 46:687, 1943.
41. Arnoczky S, Adams M, DeHaven K, et al: Meniscus. In Woo SL-Y, Buckwalter JA (eds): Injury and Repair of the Musculoskeletal Soft Tissues: Park Ridge, Ill, American Academy of Orthopaedic Surgeons, 1988, p 487.
42. Fairbank TJ: Knee joint changes after meniscetomy. J Bone Joint Surg 30B:664, 1948.
43. Arnoczky SP, Warren RF: The microvasculature of the meniscus and its response to injury: An experimental study in the dog. Am J Sports Med 11:131, 1983.
44. McDevitt CA, Webber RJ: The ultrastructure and biochemistry of meniscal cartilage. Clin Orthop 252:8, 1990.
45. Stockwell RA, Meachim G: The chondrocytes. In Freeman MAR (ed): Adult Articular Cartilage. London, Pitman Medical, 1979, pp 69–145.
46. Siozawa S, Yoshihara R, Kuroki Y, et al: Pathogenic importance of fibronectin in the superficial region of articular cartilage as a local factor for the induction of pannus extension on rheumatoid articular cartilage. Ann Rheum Dis 51:869, 1992.
47. Salter DM: Tenascin is increased in cartilage and synovium from arthritic knees. Br J Rheumatol 32:780, 1993.
48. Chevalier X, Groult N, Labat-Robert J: Biosynthesis and distribution of fibronectin in normal and osteoarthritic cartilage. Clin Phys Biochem 9:1, 1992.
49. Poole AR, Pidoux I, Reiner A, et al: Localization of proteoglycan monomer and link protein in the matrix of bovine articular cartilage: An immunohistochemical study. J Histochem Cytochem 28:621, 1980.
50. Wotton SF, Duance VC: Type II collagen in normal human articular cartilage. Histochem J 26:412, 1994.
51. Poole CA, Ayad S, Schofield JR: Chondrons from articular cartilage: I. Immunolocalization of type VI collagen in the pericellular capsule of isolated canine tibial chondrons. J Cell Sci 90:635, 1988.
52. Mow V, Rosenwasser M: Articular cartilage: Biomechanics. In Woo SL-Y, Buckwalter JA (eds): Injury and Repair of the Musculoskeletal Soft Tissues: Park Ridge, Ill, American Academy of Orthopaedic Surgeons, 1988, p 427.
53. Poole BP, Lowther DA: The effect of chondroitin sulfate protein on the formation of collagen fibrils in vitro. Biochem J 109:857, 1968.
54. DiSalvo J, Schubert M: Specific interaction of some cartilage protein polysaccharides with freshly precipitating calcium phosphate. J Biol Chem 242:705, 1967.
55. Horton JE, Wezeman FH, Kuettner KE: Inhibition of bone resorption in vitro by a cartilage-derived anticollagenase factor. Science 199:1342, 1978.
56. Langer R, Brem H, Flaterman K, et al: Isolation of a cartilage factor that inhibits tumor neo-vascularization. Science 193:70, 1976.
57. Moses MA, Sudhalter J, Langer R: Identification of an inhibitor of neovascularization from cartilage. Science 248:1408, 1990.
58. Loeser RF: Integrin-mediated attachment of articular chondrocytes to extracellular matrix proteins. Arthritis Rheum 36:1103, 1993.
59. Urban JP: The chondrocyte: A cell under pressure. Br J Rheumatol 33:901, 1994.
60. Martel-Pelletier J, McCollum R, DiBattista J, et al: The interleukin-1 receptor in normal and osteoarthritic human articular chondrocytes: Identification as the type-I receptor and analysis of binding kinetics and biologic function. Arthritis Rheum 35:530, 1992.
61. Dore S, Pelletier JP, DiBattista JA, et al: Human osteoarthritic chondrocytes possess an increased number of insulin-like growth factor 1 binding sites but are unresponsive to its stimulation: Possible role of IGF-1-binding proteins. Arthritis Rheum 37:253, 1994.
62. Middleton JFS, Tyler JA: Upregulation of insulin-like growth factor I gene expression in the lesions of osteoarthritic human articular cartilage. Ann Rheum Dis 51:440, 1992.

63. Frazer A, Seid JM, Hart KA, et al: Detection of mRNA for the transforming growth factor β family in human articular chondrocytes by the polymerase chain reaction. Biochem Biophys Res Commun 180:602, 1991.

64. Ruoslahti E, Yamaguchi Y: Proteoglycans as modulators of growth factor activities. Cell 64:867, 1991.

65. Villiger PM, Terkeltaub R, Lotz M: Monocyte chemoattractant protein-1 (MCP-1) expression in human articular cartilage: Induction by peptide regulatory factors and differential effects of dexamethasone and retinoic acid. J Clin Invest 90:488, 1992.

66. Murrell GA, Jang D, Williams RJ: Nitric oxide activates metalloprotease enzymes in articular cartilage. Biochem Biophys Res Commun 206:15, 1995.

67. Peracchia F, Ferrari G, Poggi A, et al: IL-1β-induced expression of PGDF-AA isoform in rabbit articular chondrocytes is modulated by TGF-β₁. Exp Cell Res 193:208, 1991.

68. Osborne KD, Trippel SB, Mankin HJ: Growth factor stimulation of adult articular cartilage. J Orthop Res 7:35, 1989.

69. Centrella M, McCarthy TL, Canalis E: Skeletal tissue and transforming growth factor β. FASEB J 2:3066, 1988.

70. Hunter W: On the structure and diseases of articulating cartilage. Philos Trans R Soc Lond [Biol] 42:514, 1743.

71. Pita JC, Howell DS: Micro-biochemical studies of cartilage. The Joints and Synovial Fluid. New York, Academic Press, 1978, p 273.

72. Bywaters EGL: The metabolism of joint tissues. J Pathol Bacteriol 44:247, 1937.

73. Naughton DP, Haywood R, Blake DR, et al: A comparative evaluation of the metabolic profiles of normal and inflammatory knee-joint synovial fluids by high resolution proton NMR spectroscopy. FEBS Lett 317:221, 1993.

74. Collins, D.H. The Pathology of Articular and Spinal Disease. London, Arnold, 1949.

75. Mitul MA, Millington PF: Osseous pathway of nutrition to articular cartilage of the human femoral head. Lancet 1:842, 1970.

76. Bromley M, Bertfield H, Evanson JM, Wooley DE: Bidirectional erosion of cartilage in the rheumatoid knee joint. Ann Rheum Dis 44:676, 1985.

77. Graf J, Neusel E, Freese U, Simank HG, Niethard FU: Subchondral vascularisation and osteoarthritis. Int Orthop 16:113, 1992.

78. Strangeways TSP: The nutrition of articular cartilage. Br Med J. 1:661, 1920.

79. Maroudas A, Bullough P, Swanson SAV, et al: The permeability of articular cartilage. J Bone Joint Surg 50B:166, 1968.

80. Hadler NM: The biology of the extracellular space. Clin Rheum Dis 7:71, 1981.

81. O'Hara BP, Urban JP, Maroudas A: Influence of cyclic loading on the nutrition of articular cartilage. Ann Rheum Dis 49:536, 1990.

82. Sood SC: A study of the effects of experimental immobilization on rabbit articular cartilage. J Anat 108:497, 1971.

83. Bennett G, Bauer W: Joint changes resulting from patellar displacement and their relation to degenerative hip disease. J Bone Joint Surg 19A:667, 1937.

84. Lewis PR, McCutchen CW: Experimental evidence for weeping lubrication in mammalian joints. Nature 184:1285, 1959.

85. McCutchen CW: An approximate equation for weeping lubrication, solved with an electrical analogue. Ann Rheum Dis 34:85, 1975.

86. Bar E: Elasticitatsprufungen der Gelenkkorpel. Arch J Entwicklungsmech Organ 108:1926.

87. Freeman MAR, Kempson GE: Load carriage. In Freeman MAR (ed): Adult Cartilage. New York, Grune & Stratton, 1974, pp 228–246.

88. Harris ED, DiBona DR, Krane SM: A mechanism for cartilage destruction in rheumatoid arthritis. Trans Assoc Am Physicians 83:267, 1970.

89. Harris ED Jr, Parker HG, Radin EL et al: Effects of proteolytic enzymes on structural and mechanical properties of cartilage. Arthritis Rheum 15:497, 1972.

90. Buckwalter J, Rosenberg L, Coutts R, et al: Articular cartilage: Injury and repair. In Woo SL-Y, Buckwalter JA (eds): Injury and Repair of the Musculoskeletal Soft Tissues: Park Ridge, Ill, American Academy of Orthopaedic Surgeons, 1988, p 465.

91. Cuevas P, Burgos J, Baird A: Basic fibroblast growth factor (FGF) promotes cartilage repair in vivo. Biochem Biophys Res Commun 156:611, 1988.

92. Landells JW: The reactions of injured human articular cartilage. J Bone Joint Surg 39B:548, 1957.

93. Meachim G, Osborne GV: Repair at the femoral articular cartilage surface in osteoarthritis of the hip. J Pathol 102:1, 1970.

94. Brittberg M, Lindahl A, Nilsson A, et al: Treatment of deep cartilage defects in the knee with autologous chondrocyte transplantation. N Engl J Med 331:889, 1994.

95. Buckwalter JA, Roughley PJ, Rosenberg LC: Age-related changes in cartilage proteoglycans: Quantitative electron microscopic studies. Micros Res Tech 28:398, 1994.

96. Roughley PJ, White RJ, Magny MC, et al: Non-proteoglycan forms of biglycan increase with age in human articular cartilage. Biochem J 295:421, 1993.

97. Vilim V, Fosang AJ: Proteoglycans isolated from dissociative extracts of differently aged human articular cartilage: Characterization of naturally occurring hyaluronan-binding fragments of aggrecan. Biochem J 304:887, 1994.

98. Holmes MW, Bayliss MT, Muir H: Hyaluronic acid in human articular cartilage. Age-related changes in content and size. Biochem J 250:435, 1988.

99. Mort JS, Caterson B, Poole AR, Roughley PJ: The origin of human cartilage proteoglycan link-protein heterogeneity and fragmentation during ageing. Biochem J 232:805, 1985.

100. Wachtel E, Maroudas A, Schneiderman R: Age-related changes in collagen packing of human articular cartilage. Biochim Biophys Acta 1243:239, 1995.

101. Uchiyama A, Ohishi T, Takahashi M: Fluorophores from ageing human articular cartilage. J Biochem 110:714, 1991.

102. Karvonen RL, Negendank WG, Teitge RA, et al: Factors affecting articular cartilage thickness in osteoarthritis and ageing. J Rheumatol 21:1310, 1994.

103. Bollet AJ, Nance JL: Biochemical findings in normal and osteoarthritic articular cartilage: II. Chondroitin sulfate concentration and chain length, water and ash content. J Clin Invest 4:1170, 1966.

104. Mankin HJ, Lippiello L: Biochemical and metabolic abnormalities in articular cartilage from osteoarthritic human hips. J Bone Joint Surg 52A:424, 1970.

105. Collins DH, Meachim G: Sulphate (³⁵SO₄) fixation by human articular cartilage compared in the knee and shoulder joints. Ann Rheum Dis 20:117, 1961.

106. Kempson GE: Age-related changes in the tensile properties of human articular cartilage: A comparative study between the femoral head of the hip joint and the talus of the ankle joint. Biochim Biophys Acta 1075:223, 1991.

107. Burr DB, Radin EL: Trauma as a factor in the initiation of osteoarthritis. In Brandt KD(ed): Cartilage Changes in Osteoarthritis. Indianapolis, Indiana University School of Medicine, 1990, p 73.

108. Oegema TR, Thompson RCJ: Cartilage-bone interface (tidemark). In Brandt KD (ed): Cartilage Changes in Osteoarthritis. Indianapolis, Indiana University School of Medicine, 1990, p 43.

109. Watson WC, Tooms RE, Carnesale PG, Dutkowsky JP: A case of germinal center formation by CD45RO T and CD20 B lymphocytes in rheumatoid arthritic subchondral bone: Proposal for a two-compartment model of immune-mediated disease with implications for immunotherapeutic strategies. Clin Immunol Immunopathol 73:27, 1994.

110. Walsh DA, Mapp PI, Wharton J, Polak JM, Blake DR: Neuropeptide degrading enzymes in normal and inflamed human synovium. Am J Pathol 142:1610–1621, 1993.

111. Bassleer R, Lhoest-Ganthier M-P, Renard A-M, et al: Histological structure and functions of synovium. In Franchimont P (ed): Articular Synovium: Basel, Karger, 1982, pp 1–26.

112. Pasquali-Ronchetti I, Frizziero L, Guerra D, et al: Ageing of the human synovium: An in vivo and ex vivo morphological study. Semin Arthritis Rheum 21:400, 1992.

113. Ghadially FN, Roy S: Ultrastructure of Synovial Joints in Health and Disease. London, Butterworth, 1969.

114. Qu Z, Garcia CH, O'Rourke LM, et al: Local proliferation of fibroblast-like synoviocytes contributes to synovial hyperplasia. Arthritis Rheum 37:212, 1994.

115. Wilkinson LS, Pitsillides AA, Worrall JG, Edwards JC: Light microscopic characterization of the fibroblast-like synovial intimal cell (synoviocyte). Arthritis Rheum 35:1179, 1992.

116. Henderson KJ, Edwards JC, Worrall JG: Expression of CD44 in normal and rheumatoid synovium and cultured synovial fibroblasts. Ann Rheum Dis 53:729, 1994.

117. Morales-Ducret J, Wayner E, Elices MJ, et al: Alpha 4/beta 1 integrin (VLA-4) ligands in arthritis: Vascular cell adhesion molecule-1 expression in synovium and on fibroblast-like synoviocytes. J Immunol 149:1424, 1992.

118. Henderson EB, Grootveld M, Farrell A, et al: A pathological role for damaged hyaluronan in synovitis. Ann Rheum Dis 50:196, 1991.

119. Norton WL, Lewis DC, Ziff M: Electron-dense deposits following injection of gold sodium thiomalate and thiomalic acid. Arthritis Rheum 11:436, 1968.

120. Roy S, Ghadially FN: Synthesis of hyaluronic acid by synovial cells. J Pathol Bacteriol 93:555, 1967.

121. Okada Y, Naka K, Minamoto T, et al: Localization of type VI collagen in the lining cell layer of normal and rheumatoid synovium. Lab Invest 63:647, 1990.

122. Worrall JG, Bayliss MT, Edwards JCW: Morphological localization of hyaluronan in normal and diseased synovium. J Rheumatol 18:1466, 1991.

123. Cutolo M, Picasso M, Ponassi M, Sun MZ, Balza E: Tenascin and fibronectin distribution in human normal and pathological synovium. J Rheumatol 19:1439, 1992.

124. Worrall JG, Wilkinson LS, Bayliss MT, Edwards JC: Zonal distribution

of chondroitin-4-sulphate/dermatan sulphate and chondroitin-6-sulphate in normal and diseased human synovium. Ann Rheum Dis 53:35, 1994.

125. Demazier A, Athanasou NA: Adhesion receptors of intimal and subintimal cells of the normal synovial membrane. J Pathol 168:209, 1992.

126. Johnson BA, Haines GK, Harlow LA, Koch AE: Adhesion molecule expression in human synovial tissue. Arthritis Rheum 36:137, 1993.

127. Mapp PI, Walsh DA, Kidd BL, et al: Localisation of the enzyme neutral endopeptidase to the human synovium. J Rheumatol 19:1838, 1992.

128. Stevens CR, Blake DR, Merry P, Revell PA, Levick JR: A comparative study by morphometry of the microvasculature in normal and rheumatoid synovium. Arthritis Rheum 34:1508, 1991.

129. Liew M, Dick C: The anatomy and physiology of blood flow in a diarthrodial joint. Clin Rheum Dis 7:131, 1981.

130. Lindstrom J: Microvascular anatomy of synovial tissue. Acta Rheum Scand 7:1, 1963.

131. Wilkinson LS, Edwards JCW: Demonstration of lymphatics in human synovial tissue. Rheumatol Int 11:151, 1991.

132. Walsh DA, Suzuki T, Knock G, et al: AT$_1$ receptor characteristics of angiotensin analogue binding in human synovium. Br J Pharmacol 112:435, 1994.

133. Walsh DA, Mapp PI, Wharton J, et al: Localisation and characterisation of substance P binding to human synovium in rheumatoid arthritis. Ann Rheum Dis 51:313, 1992.

134. Wharton J, Rutherford RAD, Walsh DA, et al: Autoradiographic localisation and analysis of endothelin-1 binding sites in rheumatoid synovial tissue. Arthritis Rheum 35:894, 1992.

135. Farrell AJ, Blake DR, Palmer RM, Moncada, S: Increased concentrations of nitrite in synovial fluid and serum samples suggest increased nitric oxide synthesis in rheumatic diseases. Ann Rheum Dis 51:1219, 1992.

136. Mapp PI, Kidd BL, Gibson SJ, et al: Substance P-, calcitonin gene-related peptide- and C-flanking peptide of neuropeptide Y-immunoreactive fibres are present in normal synovium but depleted in patients with rheumatoid arthritis. Neuroscience 37:143, 1990.

137. Merry P, Williams R, Cox N, King JB, Blake DR: Comparative study of intra-articular pressure dynamics in joints with acute traumatic and chronic inflammatory effusions: Potential implications for hypoxic-reperfusion injury. Ann Rheum Dis 50:917, 1991.

138. Gaffney K, Williams RB, Jolliffe VA, Blake DR: Intra-articular pressure changes in rheumatoid and normal peripheral joints. Ann Rheum Dis 54:670, 1995.

139. Jayson MIV, Dixon A St J: Intra-articular pressure in rheumatoid arthritis of the knee: III. Pressure changes during joint use. Ann Rheum Dis 29:401, 1970.

140. Myers DB, Palmer DG: Capsular compliance and pressure-volume relationships in normal and arthritic knees. J Bone Joint Surg 54B:710, 1972.

141. Gronlund J, Kofoed H, Svalastoga E: Effect of increased knee joint pressure on oxygen tension and blood flow in subchondral bone. Acta Physiol Scand 121:127, 1984.

142. Jayson MIV, Rubenstein D, Dixon ASJ: Intra-articular pressure and rheumatoid geodes (bone "cysts"). Ann Rheum Dis 29:496, 1970.

143. Jayson MIV, Dixon ASJ: Valvular mechanisms in juxta-articular cysts. Ann Rheum Dis 29:415, 1970.

144. Blake DR, Merry P, Unsworth J, et al: Hypoxic-reperfusion injury in the inflamed human joint. Lancet 1:289, 1989.

145. McDonald JN, Levick JR: Pressure induced deformation of the interstitial route across synovium and its relation to hydraulic conductance. J Rheum 17:341, 1990.

146. Schumacher HR: The microvasculature of the synovial membrane of the monkey: Ultrastructural studies. Arthritis Rheum 112:387, 1969.

147. Harris ED Jr, McCroskery PA: The influence of temperature and fibril stability on degradation of cartilage collagen by rheumatoid synovial collagenase. N Engl J Med 290:1, 1974.

148. Mainardi CL, Walter JM, Spiegel PK, et al: The lack of effect of daily heat therapy on the progression of rheumatoid arthritis. Arch Phys Med Rehabil 60:390, 1979.

149. Horvath SM, Hollander JL: Intra-articular temperature as a measure of joint reaction. J Clin Invest 28:469, 1949.

150. Hollander JL, Horvath SM: The influence of physical therapy procedures on the intra-articular temperature of normal and arthritic subjects. Am J Med Sci 218:543, 1949.

151. Bruckner FE, Howell A: Neuropathic joints. Semin Arthritis Rheum 2:47, 1972.

152. Kidd BL, Gibson SJ, O'Higgens F, et al: A neurogenic mechanism for symmetrical arthritis. Lancet ii:1128, 1989.

153. Ferrell WR, Craske B: Contribution of joint and muscle afferents to position sense at the human proximal interphalangeal joint. Exp Physiol 77:331, 1992.

154. Dee R: Structure and function of hip joint innervation. Ann R Coll Surg Engl 45:357, 1969.

155. Griff P, Finerman GA, Riley LHR: Joint position sense after total hip replacement. J Bone Joint Surg 55:1016, 1973.

156. Cross MJ, McCloskey D: Position sense following surgical removal of joints in man. Brain Res 55:443, 1973.

157. Barrett DS, Cobb AG, Bentley G: Joint proprioception in normal, osteoarthritic and replaced knees. J Bone Joint Surg 73A:53, 1991.

158. Ferrell WR, Crighton A, Sturrock RD: Position sense at the proximal interphalangeal joint is distorted in patients with rheumatoid arthritis of finger joints. Exp Physiol 77:675, 1992.

159. Hall MG, Ferrell WR, Sturrock RD, Hamblen DL, Baxendale RH: The effect of the hypermobility syndrome on knee joint proprioception. Br J Rheumatol 34:121, 1995.

160. Shaible HG, Grubb BD: Afferent and spinal mechanisms of joint pain. Pain 55:5, 1993.

161. New HV, Mudge AW: Calcitonin gene-related peptide regulates muscle acetylcholine receptor synthesis. Nature 323:809, 1986.

162. Spencer JD, Hayes KC, Alexander IJ: Knee joint effusion and quadriceps reflex inhibition in man. Arch Phys Med Rehabil 65:171, 1984.

163. Coderre TJ, Abbott FV, Melzack R: Effects of peripheral antisympathetic treatments in the tail-flick, formalin and autonomy tests. Pain 18:13, 1984.

164. Levine JD, Coderre TJ, Helms C, Basbaum AI: β_2-Adrenergic mechanisms in experimental arthritis. Proc Natl Acad Sci USA 85:4553, 1988.

165. Levine JD, Fye K, Heller P, Basbaum AI, Whiting-O'Keefe Q: Clinical response to regional intravenous guanethidine in patients with rheumatoid arthritis. J Rheumatol 13:1040, 1986.

166. Yaksh TL: Substance P release from knee joint afferent terminals: Modulation by opioids. Brain Res 458:319, 1988.

167. Green PG, Basbaum AI, Levine JD: Sensory neuropeptide interactions in the production of plasma extravasation in the rat. Neuroscience 50:745, 1992.

168. Lam FY, Ferrell WR: Effects of interactions of naturally-occurring neuropeptides on blood flow in the rat knee joint. Br J Pharmacol 108:694, 1993.

169. Lotz M, Carson DA, Vaughan JH: Substance P activation of rheumatoid synoviocytes: Neural pathway in pathogenesis of arthritis. Science 235:893, 1987.

170. Payan DG, Brewster DR, Goetzl EJ: Specific stimulation of human T-lymphocytes by substance P. J Immunol 131:1613, 1983.

171. Wiedermann CJ, Wiedermann FJ, Apperl A, et al: In vitro human polymorphonuclear leukocyte chemokinesis and human monocyte chemotaxis are different activities of aminoterminal and carboxyterminal substance P. Naunyn-Schmiedeberg's Arch Pharmacol 340:185, 1989.

172. Kjartansson J, Dalsgaard C-J, Jonsson CE: Decreased survival of experimental critical flaps in rats after sensory denervation with capsaicin. Plast Reconstr Surg 79:218, 1987.

173. Hagberg L, Heinegard D, Ohlsson K: The contents of macromolecular solutes in the flexor tendon sheath fluid and their relation to synovial fluid: A quantitative analysis. J Hand Surg 17:167, 1992.

174. Nettelbladt E, Sundblad L, Jonsson E: Permeability of the synovial membrane to proteins. Acta Rheum Scand 9:28, 1963.

175. Simkin PA, Pizzoro JE: Transsynovial exchange of small molecules in normal human subjects. J Appl Physiol 36:581, 1974.

176. Kushner I, Somerville JA: Permeability of human synovial membrane to plasma proteins. Arthritis Rheum 14:560, 1971.

177. Wallis WJ, Simkin PA, Nelp WB: Protein traffic in human synovial effusions. Arthritis Rheum 30:57, 1987.

178. Ruddy S, Austen KF: Activation of the complement and properdin systems in rheumatoid arthritis. Ann N Y Acad Sci 256:96, 1975.

179. Opdenakker G, Masure S, Grillet B, van Damme J: Cytokine-mediated regulation of human leukocyte gelatinases and role in arthritis. Lymphokine Cytokine Res 10:317, 1991.

180. Levick JR, McDonald JN: Fluid movement across synovium in healthy joints: Role of synovial fluid macromolecules. Ann Rheum Dis 54:417, 1995.

181. Simkin PA: Synovial perfusion and synovial fluid solutes. Ann Rheum Dis 54:424, 1995.

182. Myers SL: Effect of synovial fluid hyaluronan on the clearance of albumin from the canine knee. Ann Rheum Dis 54:433, 1995.

183. Ropes MW, Bauer W: Synovial Fluid Changes in Joint Diseases. Cambridge, Harvard University Press, 1953.

184. McCutchen CW: Lubrication of joints. In Sokoloff L (ed): The Joints and Synovial Fluid. New York, Academic Press, 1978, p 437.

185. Dintenfass L: Lubrication in synovial joints. Nature 197:496, 1963.

186. Fein RS: Are synovial joints squeeze-film lubricated? Proc Inst Mech Eng 181:125, 1967.

187. Walker PS, Dowson D, Longfield MD, et al: "Boosted lubrication" in synovial joints by fluid entrapment and enrichment. Ann Rheum Dis 27:512, 1968.

188. Hlavecek M: The role of synovial fluid filtration by cartilage in lubrication of synovial joints: II. Squeeze-film lubrication: Homogeneous filtration. J Biomech 26:1151, 1993.

189. Jin ZM, Dowson D, Fisher J: The effect of porosity of articular cartilage on the lubrication of a normal human hip joint. J Eng Med 206:117, 1992.

190. Swann DA, Silver FH, Slayter HS, et al: The molecular structure and lubricating activity of lubricin isolated from bovine and human synovial fluids. Biochem J 225:195, 1985.

191. Swann DA: Structure and function of lubricin, the glycoprotein responsible for the boundary lubrication of articular cartilage. *In* Franchimont P(ed): Articular Synovium. Basel, Karger, 1982, pp 45–58.
192. Jay GD: Charcterization of a bovine synovial fluid lubricating factor: I. Chemical, surface activity and lubricating properties. Connect Tissue Res 28:71, 1992.
193. Williams PF, Powell GL, LaBerge M: Sliding friction analysis of phosphatidylcholine as a boundary lubricant for articular cartilage. J Eng Med 207:59, 1993.
194. Stockwell RA: Lipid content of human costal and articular cartilage. Ann Rheum Dis 26:481, 1967.
195. Little T, Freeman MAR, Swanson SAV: Experiments on friction in the human hip joint. *In* Wright V (ed): Lubrication and Wear in Joints. London, Sector, 1969, p 110.
196. Radin EL, Swann DA, Weisser PA: Separation of hyaluronate-free lubricating fraction from synovial fluid. Nature 288:377, 1970.
197. Jay GD, Lane BP, Sokoloff L: Characterization of a bovine synovial fluid lubricating factor: III. The interaction with hyaluronic acid. Connect Tissue Res 28:245, 1992.
198. Radin EL, Paul IL: A consolidated concept of joint lubrication. J Bone Joint Surg 54A:607, 1972.
199. Ito H, Nagasaki H, Hashizume K, et al: Time-course of force production by fast isometric contraction of the knee extensor in young and elderly subjects. J Hum Ergol (Tokyo) 19:23, 1990.

Charlene J. Williams
Philipp Vandenberg
Darwin J. Prockop

Collagen and Elastin

Connective tissue and extracellular matrix are loosely defined as the compartments and components that provide the structural support of the body and bind together its cells, organs, and tissues. The major connective tissues are bone, skin, tendons, ligaments, and cartilage. The term connective tissue is also applied to blood vessels and to synovial spaces and fluids. In effect, however, all organs and tissues contain connective tissue in the form of membranes and septa.

All connective tissues contain large amounts of water, salt, albumin, and other components of plasma. The characteristic feature of connective tissues, how-ever, is that they contain a series of specific macromol-ecules that are assembled into large and complex structures that define the size and shape of most organs. Two of the most characteristic macromole-cules of connective tissue are the fibrous proteins *collagen* and *elastin*. Connective tissues also contain a series of proteoglycans and related molecules.

The differences among connective tissues such as bone, skin, and cartilage are, in part, attributable to differences in their contents of specific macromole-cules (Table 2–1). Tendons and ligaments, for exam-ple, consist primarily of fibrils of type I collagen bound together into large fibers. They also contain

Table 2–1. CONSTITUENTS OF CONNECTIVE TISSUE IN VARIOUS TISSUES

Connective Tissue	Known Constituents	Approximate Amounts (% dry weight)	Characteristics
Skin (dermis), ligaments, tendons	Type I collagen	80	Bundles of fibers of high tensile strength
	Type III collagen	5 to 15	Thin fibrils
	Type IV collagen, laminin, nidogen	<5	In basal laminae under epithelium and in blood
	Types V to VII	<5	Distributions and functions unclear
	Fibronectin	<5	Associated with collagen fibers and cell surfaces
	Proteoglycans*	0.5	Provide resiliency
	Hyaluronate	0.5	Provides resiliency
Bones (demineralized)	Type I collagen	90	Complex organization of fibrils
	Type V collagen	1 to 2	Function unclear
	Proteoglycans	1	Function unclear
	Sialoproteins	1	Function unclear
	Osteonectin	2 to 3	Role in ossification
	Osteocalcin	1	Probable role in ossification
	α_2-Glycoprotein	1	Possible role in ossification
Aorta	Type I collagen	20 to 40	Thick fibrils
	Type III collagen	20 to 40	Thin fibrils
	Elastin, microfibrillar protein	20 to 40	Amorphous, elastic fibrils
	Type IV collagen, laminin, nidogen	<5	In basal lamina / Functions unclear
	Types V and VI collagens	<2	Mucopolysaccharides, mainly chondroitin sulfate and dermatan sulfate; heparan sulfate in basal lamina
	Proteoglycans	<3	
Cartilage	Type II collagen	40 to 50	Thin fibrils
	Types IX and XI collagen	5 to 25	Possible flexible spacers
	Type X collagen	5	Undefined role in hypertrophic region
	Proteoglycans	15 to 50	Provides resiliency
	Hyaluronate	0.5 to 2	Provides resiliency

*Proteoglycan structures are incompletely defined. About five different protein cores have been identified, and each has one or more kinds of mucopolysac-charides attached. Major mucopolysaccharides of skin and tendon are dermatan sulfate and chondroitin-4-sulfate; of aorta, chondroitin-4-sulfate and dermatan sulfate; of cartilage; chondroitin-4-sulfate, chondroitin-6-sulfate, and keratan sulfate. Basal lamina contains a heparan sulfate.

small amounts of other types of collagen that bind to and probably help organize the fibrils of type I collagen. Cartilage contains large amounts of type II collagen, a protein very similar to type I collagen. The fibrils of type II collagen in cartilage form an arcade-like network that is distended by the presence of highly charged proteoglycans that trap large amounts of water and salts. Blood vessels such as the aorta contain large amounts of another fibrillar collagen known as type III and large amounts of elastin. The differences among connective tissues also depend on variations in the size, orientation, and packing of collagen fibrils. Fibrils and fibers of type I collagen in tendon are in a parallel orientation. Whereas the type I collagen fibrils of skin are randomly oriented in the plane of the skin, the type I collagen fibrils in cortical bone are deposited in complex helical rays around haversian canals. Accordingly, the differences in the morphology and function of connective tissues are based in part on their content of specific macromolecules and in part on the organization of the macromolecules in the extracellular spaces.

Collagen and elastin, the subjects of this chapter, are similar, in that they are tough fibrous proteins. At the same time, they are dramatically different, in that the monomers of most collagens spontaneously self-assemble into highly ordered structures, whereas elastin forms amorphous fibrils in which it is difficult to find any evidence of an ordered structure.

COLLAGENS

More than 15 different kinds of collagens have now been identified in different tissues of vertebrates.[1–3] This family of collagens can be divided into four subclasses (Table 2–2):

Table 2–2. MAJOR TYPES OF COLLAGEN AND THEIR α-CHAIN COMPOSITIONS*

Classes	α-Chain Composition
Fibrillar	
Type I	Two α1(I) and one α2(I)
Type II	Three α1(II)
Type III	Three α1(III)
Type V	α1(V), α2(V), and α3(V)
Type XI	α1(XI), α2(XI), and α3(XI)
Basement Membrane– Associated	
Type IV†	α1(IV), α2(IV), ± α3(IV), ± α4(IV), and ± α5(IV)
Type VII	α1(VII)
Fiber-Associated†	
Type IX	α1(IX), α2(IX), and α3(IX)
Type XII	α1(XII)
Short-Chain	
Type VIII	α1(VIII)
Type X	α1(X)

*For more complete descriptions, see references 1 to 3.
†Chain composition apparently varies in different tissues, with α3(IV), α4(IV), and α5(IV) prominent in kidney.

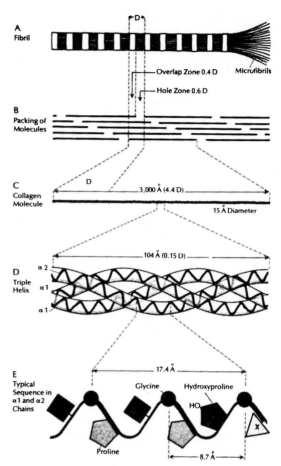

Figure 2–1. *A–E,* Schematic representation of the structure of a fibril of type I collagen. (From Prockop DJ, Guzman NA: Collagen diseases and the biosynthesis of collagen. Hosp Pract 12:61–68, 1977. © 1977, The McGraw-Hill Companies, Inc. Illustration by Bunji Tagawa.)

- Fibrillar collagens
- Basement membrane–associated collagens
- Fibril-associated collagens
- Short-chain collagens

All the fibrillar collagens form fibrils that appear similar by electron microscopy. They vary in diameter and probably length, but they have a characteristic cross-striated pattern that reflects the gaps between the ends of the molecules found on the surface of the fibrils (Fig. 2–1, *Panel A*).[4] The major fibrillar proteins (types I, II, and III) are among the most abundant proteins in the body. Fibrils and fibril bundles or fibers of type I collagen account for 60 to 90 percent of the dry weight of skin, ligaments, and bone (demineralized).

Type I collagen is also found in many thin tissues, including the lungs and dentin and the sclerae of the eyes. In addition, it is the major constituent of mature scars.

Type II collagen accounts for more than half the dry weight of cartilage, and it is found in the vitreous gel of the eye. It is also transiently present in many tissues during embryonic development.

Type III collagen is abundant in large blood vessels and is found in small amounts in most tissues that contain type I collagen, but it is not present in bone. Of special interest is a large fraction of the type III collagen found in some tissues, particularly skin; it is found as a partially processed precursor form that retains the N-propeptides (see later). The partially processed form, defined as type III pNcollagen, binds to the surface of type I collagen fibrils and thereby limits their lateral growth.[5] The less abundant fibrillar collagen, known as type V collagen, is found as thin fibrils in synovial membranes, lung, skin, and a few other tissues.

Type XI collagen is uniformly distributed in articular cartilage, where it can account for 5 to 20 percent of the total collagen. The fibrils formed by type V and type XI collagens appear to be similar to those of the major fibrillar collagens, but they have not been studied as extensively.[3]

Type IV collagen is a major constituent of all basement membranes. Monomers of the protein bind to one another through globular extensions found at both ends of the molecules to form large structures resembling a wire network (Fig. 2–2). The network-like structures serve as filtration barriers and as a scaffolding for the binding of other basement membrane constituents, such as laminin, nidogen, and a large heparan sulfate proteoglycan. The decorated scaffold then serves as an important barrier for fluids and solutes and as an important surface for the attachment and movement of cells. Type VII collagen is found in the upper layers of the dermis, where it forms thin and short structures that serve as "anchoring fibrils" between the basement membrane of the skin and the dermis.

The fiber-associated collagens (types VIII, IX, and XIV) are found on the surface of fibrils of type I and type II collagens, where they probably serve as flexible spacers among the fibrils. The structures assembled from the short-chain collagens (types VIII and X) and a number of other recently identified collagens are poorly defined, but they may form specialized networks among specific cell types.[1–3]

Structure of Collagen Fibrils

The fibrils formed by the fibrillar collagens consist almost entirely of monomers of the protein tightly packed in a quarter-stagger array (see Fig. 2–1). The molecular structure of type I collagen is composed of two identical polypeptide chains called $\alpha1(I)$ and one slightly different polypeptide chain called $\alpha2(I)$ (see Table 2–2). Type II collagen is a homotrimer made up of three identical $\alpha1(II)$-chains, and type III collagen is a homotrimer composed of three $\alpha1(III)$-chains. The structure of each α-chain of the fibrillar collagens is highly repetitive. Glycine is every third amino acid, and each α-chain has about 1000 amino acids. Therefore the sequence of each α-chain can be defined as $(Gly-X-Y)_{333}$. The X-position in the sequence is frequently occupied by proline, and the Y-position is frequently occupied by hydroxyproline, an unusual amino acid that is abundant in collagen but rare in any other protein. An important feature of the triple helix of collagen is that the glycine residues are packed into a restricted space near the center of the triple helix that can accommodate only glycine, the smallest amino acid residue.[1] Because proline and hydroxyproline are saturated ring amino acids, they keep the α-chains in an extended configuration that stabilizes the structure of the triple helix. Some of the X- and Y-positions in each α-chain contain hydrophobic or charged amino acids that appear in clusters.

Figure 2–2. Schematic representation of the network-like structures formed by the assembly of type IV collagen in basement membranes. The NC1 domains are the globular extensions at the C terminus of the molecule. The 7S domains are noncollagenous domains at the N terminus of the protein.

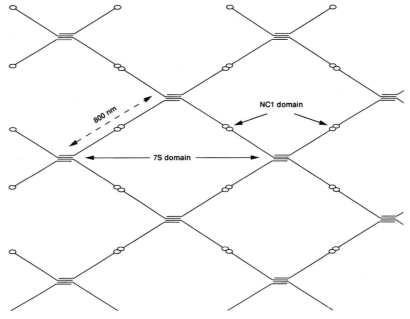

The clusters of hydrophobic and charged amino acids on the surface of the triple helix direct binding of one molecule to another so that each is quarter-staggered relative to a nearest neighbor in a fibril (see Fig. 2-1). Each of the α-chains of a fibrillar collagen also contains short sequences of about 25 amino acids at each end (telopeptides) that do not have a triple-helical structure and that play an important but incompletely defined role in assembly of the proteins into fibrils.

All collagens have at least one triple-helical domain similar to the large triple-helical domain that accounts for most of the structure of a fibrillar collagen. In the nonfibrillar collagens, however, the repetitive Gly-X-Y sequences are frequently interrupted by short regions of other amino acid sequences that introduce more flexible hinge regions into the proteins.[17] Type IV collagen, for example, has numerous short interruptions of its large triple-helical domain that are probably important for its assembly into network-like structures (see Fig. 2–2) or binding of other basement membrane constituents. One of the hinge regions of type IX collagen is an attachment site for a mucopolysaccharide chain (chondroitin sulfate).

Structure of Collagen Genes

The genes for collagens have several unusual features. Each of the genes for the major fibrillar collagens (types I, II, and III) has 52 to 54 exons that code for the large triple-helical domain of the protein.[1–3, 6] The most common exon size is 54 base pairs (bp); some exons are 108 bp (twice 54), and one is 162 (three times 54). Still other exons are variations on the 54-bp theme in that they are 99 bp (54 plus 45). With one exception, the sizes of specific exons are identical in the two genes for type I procollagen (COL1A1 and COL1A2), the gene for type II procollagen (COL2A1), and the gene for type III procollagen (COL3A1). In addition, the same exons have the same sizes in the genes from humans, rodents, and chickens. The unusual 54-bp motif of the genes for fibrillar collagens may indicate either that the genes arose by duplication of a 54-bp exon or that the molecular mechanisms for replication of the genes specifically perpetuate a 54-bp motif.

The same 54-bp motif is seen in parts of the structures for nonfibrillar collagens. However, some of the exons of the genes for these other collagens have varying structures, and many of the exons begin with the second base for a glycine codon rather than a complete codon for glycine, as seen in the exons for fibrillar collagens.

Biosynthesis

The biosynthesis of collagen involves a large number of post-translational processing steps.[1]

The major fibrillar collagens (types I, II, and III) are first assembled as large precursor procollagens that have additional N-terminal and C-terminal propeptides not found in the nonfibrillar collagens (Fig. 2–3). The three proα-chains of a procollagen are initially synthesized with N-terminal signal sequences that direct their binding to the ribosomes of the cisternae of the rough endoplasmic reticulum. As the proα-chains pass into the cisternae, the signal peptides are cleaved and the proα-chains undergo a series of hydroxylations and glycosylations. About 100 prolyl residues in the Y-positions are hydroxylated to hydroxy-4-proline, and about 10 lysyl residues in the Y-positions are hydroxylated to hydroxylysine. Some of the hydroxylysyl residues are subsequently modified by the addition of galactose or both galactose and glucose to the epsilon-hydroxyl (ε-hydroxyl) group. Both the hydroxylation of proline and that of lysine require ascorbic acid. Of the two hydroxylations, the hydroxylation of proline to hydroxyproline is more critical, since a stable collagen triple helix cannot be formed at body temperature unless each α-chain contains about 100 hydroxyprolyl residues. The requirement for ascorbic acid in the enzymatic hydroxylation of proline probably explains the failure of wounds to heal in scurvy. In addition to the modifications of the prolyl and lysyl residues, a mannose-rich carbohydrate is added to the C-terminal propeptide of each proα-chain. As these modifications of the proα-chains are occurring, the three chains come together through their globular C-propeptides and become disulfide linked. After the three chains associate and acquire the necessary content of hydroxyproline, a nucleus of triple helix forms near the C terminal of the α-chain domains. The triple-helical conformation is then propagated from the C to the N terminus of the molecule.

An unusual relationship exists between the folding of procollagen into a triple-helical conformation and the post-translational modifications that introduce hydroxyproline, hydroxylysine, and glycosylated hydroxylysine.[1–3] The two hydroxylases and the two glycosyl transferases involved in the reactions can modify only proα-chains or α-chains that are in a random coil conformation. As soon as the protein folds into a triple helix, the enzymes no longer interact with the proα-chains. Since the protein cannot fold into a triple helix until most of the Y-position prolyl residues are hydroxylated to hydroxyproline, the content of hydroxyproline in most fibrillar collagens is essentially the same. The contents of hydroxylysine and glycosylated hydroxylysine vary, however, and depend on several poorly controlled factors, such as the relative concentrations of the proα-chain substrates, the enzymes, and the cofactors for the enzymes in the cisternae of the rough endoplasmic reticulum. The lack of precise control of these factors probably explains why the contents of hydroxylysine and glycosylated hydroxylysine are higher in embryonic tissues than in adult tissues. The content of glycosylated hydroxylysine in collagen affects its biologic function, since the glycosylated hydroxylysyl residues project from the surface of the triple helix and interfere with lateral packing of the molecule into fibrils.

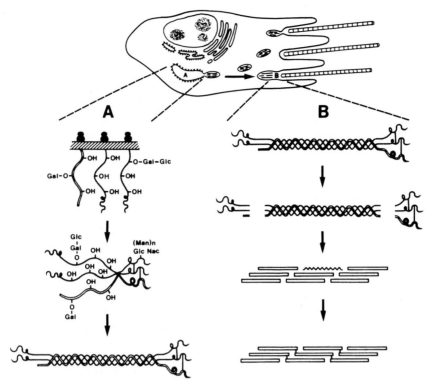

Figure 2–3. *A, B,* Schematic representation of how a fibroblast assembles collagen fibrils. *A,* Intracellular post-translational modifications of proα-chains, association of C-propeptide domains, and folding into the triple-helical conformation. *B,* Enzymatic cleavage of procollagen to collagen, self-assembly of collagen monomers into fibrils, and cross-linking of fibrils into fibers. (From Prockop DJ, Kivirikko KI: Heritable diseases of collagen. N Engl J Med 311:376–386, 1984. Reprinted with permission from the New England Journal of Medicine.)

Therefore, an increase in glycosylated hydroxylysine decreases the diameter of the fibrils formed. Any condition that delays folding of the proα-chains into a triple helix increases the contents of hydroxylysine and glycosylated hydroxylysine. As a result, most mutations that change the amino acid sequences of proα-chains increase the content of hydroxylysine and glycosylated hydroxylysine in procollagen and collagen (see later).

The folding of procollagen into a triple-helical conformation is also intimately related to its secretion from cells. Under normal conditions, secretion begins only after the protein is correctly folded. In a condition such as ascorbate deficiency, the rate of hydroxylation of prolyl residues, and hence the rate of protein folding, is decreased. Consequently, there is an accumulation of nonhelical proα-chains in the rough endoplasmic reticulum and an overall decrease in the secretion of helical procollagen molecules. Accumulation of nonhelical proα-chains is also seen with agents that inhibit prolyl hydroxylase and with mutations in the structure of the proα-chains that delay folding (see later).

As soon as the protein folds into a triple-helical conformation, it is transported from the rough endoplasmic reticulum to Golgi vesicles, from which it is secreted. The protein is then further processed extracellularly by a specific procollagen N-proteinase that cleaves the N-propeptides and a separate procollagen C-proteinase that cleaves the C-propeptides. After the propeptides are cleaved, the solubility of the protein decreases over 1000-fold to less than 1 μg/ml at 37°C, and it spontaneously self-assembles into fibrils.[1, 7, 8] The fibers initially assembled have the same morphology as mature fibers of collagen, but they do not achieve their optimal tensile strength until some of the lysyl and glycosylated hydroxylysyl residues are enzymatically deaminated by the enzyme lysyl oxidase to generate aldehydes that project from the surfaces of the molecules. The aldehydes then spontaneously form covalent cross-links among adjacent molecules in the fibril. The formation of the cross-links stabilizes the fibril structure so that it acquires a tensile strength approximating that of a steel wire.

Two recent observations about procollagen C-proteinase have illuminated unexpected features of the collagen biosynthetic pathway. One is that enzyme can process an inactive precursor form of lysyl oxidase to the active enzyme in vitro.[9] Therefore, it may play a role in the synthesis of the covalent cross-links that are essential for the normal tensile strength of fibers of both collagen and elastin (see below). The second observation is that the C-proteinase is a product of the same gene that synthesizes bone morphogenic protein-1.[10, 11] Bone morphogenic protein-1, in turn, was shown to be similar in structure to a large family of proteins that play critical roles in the development of organisms that include *Drosophila*, hydra, sea urchin, frogs, fish, and mammals. Therefore, the enzyme that is essential to assemble the collagen fibrils that largely define the size, shape, and strength of most complex organisms may play additional roles in embryonic development.

The biosynthetic pathways for nonfibrillar collagens are similar to those for the fibrillar collagens, but they have not been as extensively studied. Most of the nonfibrillar collagens have globular extensions at both ends, but there is no evidence that the globular ends of the proteins are cleaved in a manner comparable to that of the globular ends of fibrillar procollagens. Instead, the globular ends persist in tissues and appear to be involved in the assembly of matrix structures (see Fig. 2–2).

Metabolic Turnover

The collagens in adult tissues are highly stable structures. However, dramatic degradation and resynthesis of collagen fibrils occur during embryonic development as tissues change their shape and increase in size.[1] Considerable metabolic turnover of collagens continues throughout the growth of the organism. After maturity of the skeleton, the collagen fibrils and fibers in most tissues become stable metabolically so that they have half-lives of many weeks or months. In bone, however, collagen continues to be degraded and resynthesized as remodeling continues throughout life. In addition, large amounts of collagen can be lost from the skin and other connective tissues during periods of malnutrition or starvation.

The collagen in many tissues, therefore, is a replenishable source of amino acids for gluconeogenesis. Also, diseases of connective tissue produce marked increases in collagen turnover. For example, there are marked increases in the metabolic turnover of collagen in bone in Paget's disease, hyperparathyroidism, and metastatic diseases. There are large increases in the turnover of collagen as well as most other proteins in hyperthyroidism. Increases in collagen turnover are accompanied by increases in the excretion in urine of peptide-bound hydroxyproline and hydroxylysine that arise from incomplete degradation of collagen polypeptides. Assays of the urinary excretion of hydroxyproline and glycosylated hydroxylysine have therefore been used clinically to measure turnover of collagen. Immunoassays of serum levels of procollagen propeptides have been used to follow changes in rates of collagen biosynthesis. The most widely used have been assays of the serum levels of the N-propeptide of type III procollagen and the 7S fragment of type IV, which have been particularly useful in following liver fibrosis.[12, 13]

The degradation of the collagen in tissues is initiated by cleavage of the molecule by one of several specific collagenases. The collagenases cleave the molecule at a site that is about three quarters of the distance from the N to the C terminal. The resulting three-quarter and one-quarter fragments then partially unfold so that they are further degraded by nonspecific proteases such as gelatinases and stromelysin. In addition to the extracellular degradation of collagen fibrils, part of the newly synthesized proα-chains in cells appears to be degraded before they are incorporated into functional procollagen or collagen molecules. The intracellular degradation of the newly synthesized chains may represent a mechanism for correcting errors in biosynthesis.

Principle of Nucleated Growth in Collagen Biosynthesis

One of the unusual features of collagen biosynthesis is that it extensively employs a principle of nucleated growth whereby a few molecules first assemble into a structure defined as a nucleus, and the structure of the nucleus is then propagated by the orderly and rapid addition of thousands of the same molecules.[7, 8] The principle of nucleated growth is used extensively in nature in the formation of crystals by many inorganic materials, including the formation of snowflakes by water. In collagen biosynthesis, the principle of nucleated growth is used in folding of the protein in that a nucleus of triple helix is formed near the C terminus of the procollagen molecule and is then rapidly propagated to the N terminus (see Fig. 2–3). In addition, the principle of nucleated growth is employed in the assembly of fibrils in that a few molecules of the protein first form a nucleus of a fibril, and then the nucleus grows by the orderly and rapid addition of many collagen molecules.

Nucleated growth is a highly efficient mechanism for assembly of large structures with a precisely defined architecture; however, it requires that all the molecules or subunits in the system have the same structure. As illustrated by the growth of inorganic crystals, a few molecules with a defective structure prevent propagation of the nucleus and "poison" the system. Because collagen biosynthesis extensively employs the principle of nucleated growth, it is markedly disturbed by mutations that change the amino acid sequence of the protein. In particular, single-base mutations that convert a glycine codon to a codon for an amino acid with a bulkier side residue can prevent propagation of the triple helix so that the molecule cannot form a functional protein. The presence of one proα-chain with a single glycine substitution can prevent folding and cause degradation of both the abnormal proα-chain and two normal proα-chains in a process referred to as "procollagen suicide" (Fig. 2–4). Surprisingly, however, some mutations substituting bulkier amino acids for glycine residues have little effect on the folding of the protein but produce subtle changes in conformation such as a flexible "kink" in the triple helix that is visible by electron microscopy (Fig. 2–5). The presence of conformational kinks in the molecule can poison fibril assembly so as to generate fibrils with highly distorted morphology

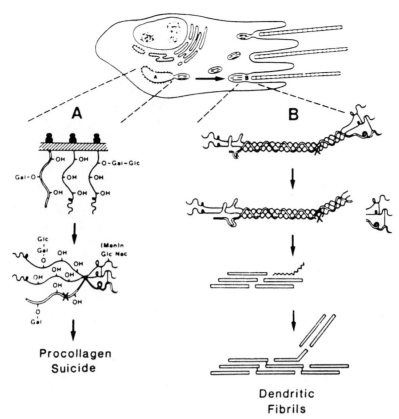

Figure 2–4. *A, B,* Schematic representation of how mutations that change the structure of type I collagen can interfere with either the intracellular assembly of the protein or the subsequent assembly of collagen fibrils. As discussed in the text, a mutation that converts a codon for a glycine residue to a codon for a bulkier amino acid can prevent the folding of the protein into a triple-helical conformation. If folding is prevented, both the normal proα-chains and the mutated proα-chains are degraded through a process referred to as "procollagen suicide." Alternatively, a glycine substitution or other mutation can allow folding into a triple-helical conformation but introduces a subtle change in conformation of the protein, such as a "kink." Monomers with an altered conformation can interfere with fibril assembly so that highly abnormal fibrils are generated. (From Prockop DJ, Kivirikko KI: Heritable diseases of collagen. N Engl J Med 311:376–386, 1984. Reprinted with permission from the New England Journal of Medicine.)

(Fig. 2–6) or markedly decrease the amount of collagen incorporated in the fibrils.

Mutations in Collagen Genes That Produce Human Diseases

Mutations in collagen genes were first encountered in studies on osteogenesis imperfecta, a heritable disorder characterized by brittleness of bones that is frequently associated with changes in other tissues rich in collagen. More than 90 percent of patients with osteogenesis imperfecta have a mutation in the gene for the proα1(I)-chain *(COL1A1)* or the gene for the proα2(I)-chain *(COL1A2)* of type I procollagen.[3, 16, 17] As yet, no patient with osteogenesis imperfecta has been shown to have a mutation in any other gene-protein system. Mild forms of osteogenesis imperfecta are caused primarily by mutations that decrease the synthesis of proα1(I)-chains. More severe variants of osteogenesis imperfecta, however, are caused by mutations that produce synthesis of abnormal but partially functional proα1(I)- or proα2(I)-chains of type I procollagen. Unrelated patients and families rarely

have the same mutation, and more than 150 different mutations have now been defined.

The devastating effects of mutations that change the structure of a proα1(I)-chain or proα2(I)-chain are explained by the extensive use of nucleated growth in collagen biosynthesis.[7, 8] Of special interest has been a large number of single-base mutations that convert a codon for glycine to a codon for a bulkier amino acid. The glycine substitutions are highly position-specific, in that a substitution of one glycine position can produce procollagen suicide, whereas a substitution of the same or a similar amino acid for a nearby glycine position has essentially no effect on the folding of the triple helix but can markedly alter fibril assembly (Fig. 2–7 and Table 2–3). Also, the glycine substitutions are position-specific, in the sense that substitutions for some glycine residues produce severe osteogenesis imperfecta that is lethal in utero or shortly after birth, whereas others cause only mild forms of the disease. The results suggest that some regions of the α-chains may be more critical to the stability of triple helix than others. Also, some regions of the molecule may be important for its normal function in tissues such as bone, whereas other re-

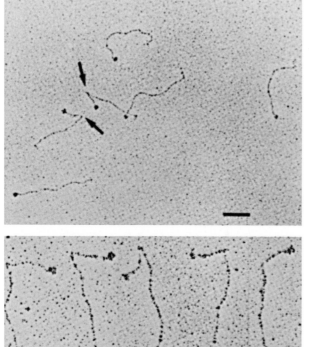

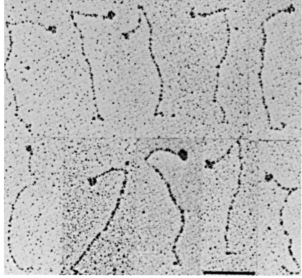

Figure 2–5. Rotary shadowing electron microscopy of mutated type I procollagen molecules. A panel of individual molecules is presented. The C terminus of the protein can be identified because the globular C-propeptide is larger than the globular N-propeptide. The molecules demonstrate the presence of a flexible kink at the site of a mutation that has converted the codon for glycine at position α1-748 to a codon for cysteine. (From Vogel BE, et al: A substitution of cysteine for glycine 748 of the α1 chain produces a kink at this site in the procollagen I molecule and an altered N-proteinase cleavage site over 225 nm away. J Biol Chem 263:19249–19255, 1988.)

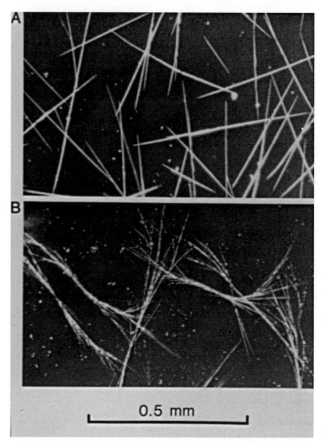

Figure 2–6. Collagen fibrils assembled from normal human type I collagen *(A)* and collagen from a proband with a heterozygous mutation that converted the codon for glycine at position α1-748 to a codon for cysteine *(B)*. About 10 percent of the protein in the fibrils is the mutated type I collagen, and 90 percent is normal type I collagen. As indicated, the presence of the mutated protein generates fibrils that are abnormally branched. (From Kadler KE, Torre-Blanco A, et al: A type I collagen with substitution of a cysteine for glycine-748 in the α1(I) chain copolymerizes with normal type I collagen and can generate fractal-like structures. Biochemistry 30:5081–5088, 1991. Reproduced by permission from Biochemistry. Copyright 1991, American Chemical Society.)

gions are more important for its function elsewhere. Such generalizations probably explain why some patients with moderately severe osteogenesis imperfecta have fragile bones together with evidence of decreased collagen in other tissues, such as blue sclerae, severe dentinogenesis imperfecta, and strikingly thin skin, whereas other patients with equally fragile bones have apparently normal sclerae, teeth, and skin.

The large number of mutations in the type I procollagen genes causing osteogenesis imperfecta prompted a search for mutations in other procollagen genes that might cause other heritable disorders of connective tissue. A series of mutations in the gene

for type II procollagen have been found to cause severe chondrodysplasias.[17] Similarly, mutations in the gene for type III procollagen have been shown to cause the potentially lethal form of Ehlers-Danlos

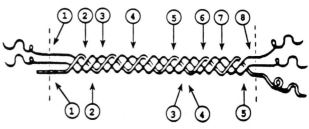

Figure 2–7. Approximate sites of mutations that alter the primary structure of type I procollagen. *Numbers above the molecule:* approximate sites of mutations in the proα1(I)-chain. *Numbers below the molecule:* approximate sites of mutations in the proα2(I)-chain. Effects of the mutations are summarized in Table 2–3.

Table 2–3. MUTATIONS IN TYPE 1 PROCOLLAGENS, THEIR EFFECTS ON THE PROTEIN, AND THE PHENOTYPES THEY PRODUCE*

| | Molecular Mechanism | | |
Mutation	Procollagen Suicide	Abnormal Fibrils	Disease Phenotype
Proα1-Chain			
(1) Splicing of exon 6		+	Loose joints (EDS VIIA)†
(2) Gly^{175}→Cys	±	+	Moderate OI
(3) Gly^{244}→Cys	0	(+)	Lethal OI
(4) Gly^{391}→Arg	±	(+)	Lethal OI
(5) Gly^{598}→Ser	+		Lethal OI
(6) Gly^{748}→Cys	+	+	Lethal OI
(7) Gly^{832}→Cys	±	(+)	Moderate OI
(8) Gly^{988}→Cys	+	+	Lethal OI
Proα2-Chain			
(1) Splicing of exon 6		+	Loose joints (EDS VIIA)†
(2) Partial deletion of IVS10/exon 11	+	+	Loose joints or fragile bones
(3) Gly^{646}→Cys	±	(+)	Mild OI
(4) Gly^{661}→Ser	0	(+)	Osteoporosis
(5) Gly^{907}→Asp	+	(?)	Lethal OI

*For recent summaries of mutations and their effects, see Kuivaniemi et al[17] and Byers.[16]
†Mutations that prevent cleavage of the N-propeptide.
Key: +, proven mechanism; ±, secondary mechanism; (+), probable mechanism. Superscript numbers indicate amino acid position in the α1(I)- or α2(I)-chains.
Abbreviations: EDS, Ehlers-Danlos syndrome; OI, osteogenesis imperfecta.

syndrome known as type IV, a disease that produces marked changes in tissues rich in type III collagen, such as thinness and scarring of skin and rupture of large arteries and other whole organs. Mutations in the gene for the α5(IV)-chain of type IV collagen are known to cause X-linked forms of Alport's syndrome,[18] a hereditary disorder characterized by hematuria and nephritis frequently associated with deafness. Mutations in the gene for type VII collagen may cause the dystrophic form of epidermolysis bullosa, in which blistering occurs below the basement membrane of the skin associated with a decrease in the anchoring fibrils[19, 20] formed by type VII collagen.

In addition, it is possible that mutations in collagen genes may be a cause of more common diseases of connective tissues. A glycine substitution in type III procollagen was shown to cause aortic aneurysms in a family without any of the characteristic features of Ehlers-Danlos syndrome type IV or Marfan's syndrome.[21] Linkage studies suggested that a mutation in the gene for type II procollagen was the cause of osteoarthritis in two large Finnish families.[22] In addition, a mutation that converted an arginine codon to a codon for cysteine[23] was shown to cause osteoarthritis associated with a mild chondrodysplasia in one family (Figs. 2–8 to 2–10).

Subsequently, three additional families with similar syndromes were found to have the same mutation that converted the codon for Arg-519 to a codon for Cys.[24] Also, three families with similar syndromes had similar mutations that converted the codon for Arg-75 to a codon for Cys and two families with similar mutations that converted the codon for Arg-789 to Cys.[25, 26] All of the families appeared to be unrelated. Therefore, these sites may be "hot spots" for mutations in the gene for type II procollagen.

Similarly, several reports indicate that mutations in the genes for type I procollagen may be the cause of some forms of postmenopausal osteoporosis.[27–29] The results demonstrate that mutations in genes for fibrillar collagens are the cause of at least subsets of these common diseases (Table 2–4). The data suggest that such mutations account for 1 to 2 per cent of the common forms of postmenopausal osteoporosis, aortic aneurysms, or primary generalized osteoarthritis.

ELASTIN

The elastic properties of tissues such as skin, large blood vessels, lung, and large ligaments depend largely on the presence of rubber-like elastic fibers.[30–33] In contrast with collagen fibrils and fibers, elastic fibers are amorphous structures, in the sense that their molecular components are not assembled in a regular pattern that can be detected by electron microscopy or x-ray diffraction. The major constituent of elastic fibers is elastin, an unusual protein composed of a single polypeptide chain of 72 kD. The protein has large domains of hydrophobic amino acids joined by shorter sequences that are rich in alanine and lysine. The amino acid sequences of the hydrophobic domains are similar to the α-chains of collagen in that they frequently have sequences of Gly-X-Y. A few of the prolines in the Y-position of the sequences are hydroxylated to hydroxyproline, but the presence of hydroxyproline in elastin appears to have no functional significance. The regions rich in alanine and lysine are sites for covalent cross-links among different regions of the same chain and among

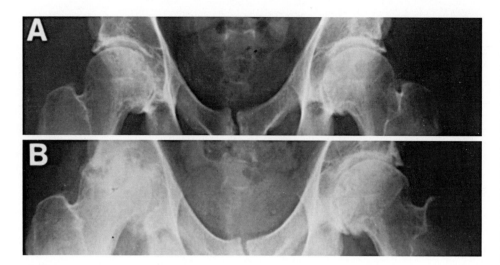

Figure 2–8. Radiographs from an affected member of the family with primary generalized osteoarthritis associated with mild chondrodysplasia. *A,* Radiograph showing osteoarthritis in both hips, but no apparent dysplasia. *B,* Radiograph of same patient 3 years later. There is a progressive increase in osteoarthritis-induced changes that are more pronounced on the right. (From Knowlton RG, et al: Genetic linkage of a polymorphism in the type II procollagen gene (COL2A1) to primary osteoarthritis associated with mild chondrodysplasia. N Engl J Med 322:526, 1990. Reprinted with permission from the New England Journal of Medicine.)

different chains of the protein. The elastic properties of the protein derive from the marked tendency of the hydrophobic domains to fold in on themselves and from coil-like compartments within the fibers.[30] Stretching the fibers unfolds the hydrophobic domains and extends the polypeptide chains so that they are held together primarily by the cross-links. As soon as the stretching force is released, the hydrophobic domains spontaneously refold. Detailed studies on elastin, however, are hampered by the fact that the protein is among the most insoluble proteins in nature and cannot be extracted from tissues with solvents as harsh as 8 M urea or hot alkali.

In addition to elastin, the elastic fibers in tissues contain poorly defined microfibrillar structures. The microfibrillar structures are seen early in embryonic development as elastic fibers are first formed. They are also seen at the edges of elastic fibrils in mature tissues. The composition of the microfibrillar structures has not been fully defined, but a major component has been identified as *fibrillin,* a large glycoprotein of about 300 kD that appears to be associated with most elastin fibrils.[34]

The Gene for Elastin and Fibrillin

The human gene for elastin contains 34 exons that range in size from 27 to 186 bp and code for a polypeptide chain of 786 amino acids.[35] The hydrophobic and the cross-linking domains of the protein are coded by separate exons. The introns of the gene are

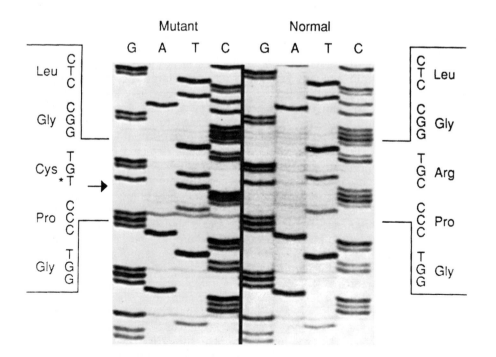

Figure 2–9. DNA sequencing film of an appropriate region of the cosmid clone containing the mutation from an affected member of the family with osteoarthritis and mild chondrodysplasia. An asterisk marks the single-base change that converts the codon CGT for arginine at position 519 of the α1(II)-chain to TGT, a codon for cysteine. The sequences are from the appropriate allele of the patient shown in Figure 2–8. (From Ala-Kokko L, et al: Single base mutation in the type II procollagen gene (COL2A1) as a cause of primary osteoarthritis associated with a mild chondrodysplasia. Proc Natl Acad Sci USA 87:6565–6568, 1990.)

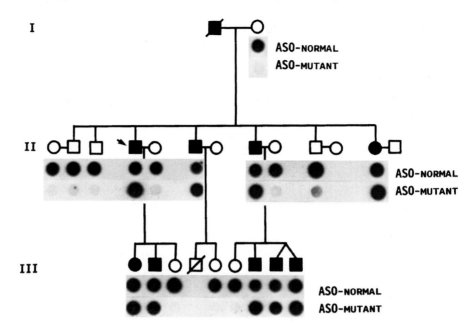

Figure 2–10. Hybridization assays for the presence of the normal allele for type II collagen and the mutated allele for type II collagen containing cysteine at position 519 of the α1(II)-chain. Genomic DNA from members of the family was amplified with a polymerase chain reaction. Products of the polymerase chain reaction were blotted on nitrocellulose filters and hybridized with ^{32}P-labeled DNA probes specific for either the normal base sequence (ASO-normal) or the mutated sequence (ASO-mutant). Black squares and circles in the pedigree indicate affected members of the family. (From Ala-Kokko L, et al: Single base mutation in the type II procollagen gene (COL2A1) as a cause of primary osteoarthritis associated with a mild chondrodysplasia. Proc Natl Acad Sci USA 87:6565–6568, 1990.)

relatively large compared with genes for collagens and other proteins, and they contain a large number of Alu repetitive sequences, particularly at the 3' end of the gene.

One of the most interesting features of the elastin gene is that RNA transcripts are spliced by a large number of alternative pathways to generate a large series of messenger RNAs (mRNAs) that differ because they lack the codons from one or more exons of the gene.[35, 36] As a result, cells synthesizing elastin produce a variety of polypeptide chains of different sizes and amino acid composition. The reasons for these variations are not known.

The elastin found in tissues is usually associated with a complex mixture of other proteins and glycoproteins that frequently form microfibrils with diameters of 10 to 12 nm.[31, 34] The best characterized of the microfibrillar components are two similar 350-kD

glycoproteins known as fibrillin-1 and fibrillin-2.[34, 37, 38] Both have complex repetitive structures that include 43 domains, similar to the precursor of epidermal growth factor that has a consensus sequence for calcium binding. The isolated proteins are found as long strands of globular structures joined by thin fibrils.[37] The proteins are encoded by multi-exonic genes with the gene for fibrillin-1 on chromosome 15 and the similar gene for fibrillin-2 on chromosome 5.[38]

Biosynthesis and Metabolic Turnover

Elastin is synthesized by smooth muscle cells and, to a lesser extent, by fibroblasts. Initial studies suggested that the protein was first synthesized as a larger and more soluble precursor protein, but this possibility was subsequently excluded by more detailed biosynthetic studies.[39] Therefore, it is not apparent how this highly insoluble protein is synthesized without premature aggregation in cells. Also, little information is available about the biosynthesis of fibrillin, the best-defined of the several proteins associated with elastin in elastic fibers.

After elastin is secreted, it undergoes extensive cross-linking reactions.[33] The cross-linking reactions (Fig. 2–11) begin with removal of the ε-amino group of lysine by lysyl oxidase, the same enzyme involved in collagen cross-linking. About 40 lysine residues in elastin are deaminated to generate aldehydes that undergo a series of apparently spontaneous interactions to form complex aromatic structures. The parent compound is desmosine, but a number of variations on the structure are also found, including reduced aldehyde condensation products.

Elastases that degrade elastin are present in polymorphonuclear leukocytes and in the pancreas.[40, 41] Because desmosine is metabolized poorly, if at all, the

Table 2–4. TYPES OF COLLAGENS AND DISEASES CAUSED BY MUTATIONS IN COLLAGEN GENES

Collagen	Human Disorder	
	Most Severe	*Mildest*
Fibrillar		
Type I	Lethal osteogenesis imperfecta	A subset of osteoporosis
Type II	Lethal chondrodysplasia	A subset of osteoarthritis
Type III	Ehlers-Danlos syndrome IV (lethal)	A subset of aortic aneurysm
Basement Membrane–Associated		
Type IV	Alport's syndrome	
Type VII	Epidermolysis bullosa (dystrophic form)	

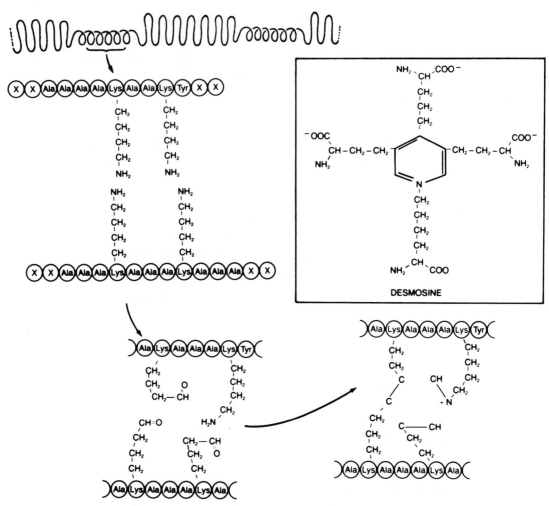

Figure 2–11. Formation of peptidyl cross-links in the conversion of soluble elastin to insoluble elastin. The large loop of the tropoelastin structure represents hydrophilic stretchable areas composed primarily of the amino acids, glycine, proline, valine, phenylalanine, isoleucine, and leucine. The small coiled areas represent the alanine-rich areas that surround the lysine residues involved in cross-link formation. This is an α-helical region containing two lysine residues separated by two and three alanine residues. Two peptide chains are parallel such that the side chains of lysine or allysine after oxidative deamidation can spontaneously condense to form the stable peritoneum ring structure with three double bonds (as depicted). The desmosine molecule, therefore, is composed of three allysine residues and one lysine residue in a peritoneum ring structure to form the tetrafunctional amino acid that participates in both inter- and intrachain cross-linking.

urinary excretion of desmosine has been used to assay metabolic turnover of elastin. The results suggest that only about 1 percent of total body elastin is degraded per year in a normal adult.[42]

Diseases Related to Elastin and Fibrillin

Genetic defects in elastin that cause human disease have long been suspected, but no such diseases have been definitively identified.

The extreme looseness of skin seen in cutis laxa is probably caused by a genetic defect in elastin.[43] Decreased levels of mRNA for elastin were found in fibroblasts from a few patients with the disease. However, no gene defect has yet been defined, and some forms of the disease may be explained by an increase in elastase activity. Similarly, defects in elastin may well be the cause of pseudoxanthoma elasticum, which is characterized by abnormal accumulations of calcified elastic fibers in the mid-dermis.[43] Also, defects in the elastin gene may explain the skin tumors rich in elastic fibers and the osteopoikilotic bone lesions of Buschke-Ollendorff syndrome.[43] Studies with cultured fibroblasts from patients with the syndrome suggest that there is an unexplained increase in elastin biosynthesis.

Deficiencies in serum α_1-antitrypsin cause a heritable form of emphysema that is sometimes associated with hepatitis and cirrhosis.[44] Serum α_1-antitrypsin is the major inhibitor of neutrophil elastase in the lower respiratory tract, and deficiencies of the inhibitor apparently cause destruction of lung tissue because of increased elastase activity. The causal relationship between deficiency of the inhibitor and the disease is strongly supported by the observation that similar emphysematous changes are seen in experimental animals in which elastase is introduced into the lungs. The hepatic injury seen in some forms of the disease is related to mutations that change the structure of α_1-antitrypsin so that it is not secreted by hepatocytes, in which it is normally synthesized. Several different defects in the gene for α_1-antitrypsin have now been identified.[45]

Recently, mutations in the gene for fibrillin-1 have been shown to be a primary cause of the Marfan syndrome. The mutations include premature termination codons, partial gene deletions, and single base substitutions, including single base substitutions that probably alter the binding of calcium to the epidermal growth factor-like (EGF) domains.[37, 38] Mutations in the fibrillin-2 gene cause a rarer form of the Marfan syndrome, which is characterized by contractual arachnodactyly.

References

1. Prockop DJ, Kivirikko KI: Heritable diseases of collagen. N Engl J Med 311:376, 1984.
2. van der Rest M, Garrone R: Collagen family of proteins. FASEB J 5:2814–2823, 1991.
3. Prockop DJ, Kivirikko KI: Collagen: Molecular biology, diseases and potentials for therapy. Annu Rev Biochem 64:403–434, 1995.
4. Prockop DJ, Guzman NA: Collagen diseases and the biosynthesis of collagen. Hosp Pract 12:61, 1977.
5. Romanic AM, Adachi E, Kadler KE, Hojima Y, Prockop DJ: Copolymerization of pNcollagen III and collagen I: pNcollagen III decreases the rate of incorporation of collagen I into fibrils, the amount of collagen incorporated, and the diameter of fibrils formed. J Biol Chem 266:12703, 1991.
6. Chu ML, Prockop DJ: Collagen: Gene structure. In Royce PM, Steinmann B (eds): Connective Tissue and Its Heritable Disorders. New York, Wiley-Liss, 1993, pp 149–165.
7. Prockop DJ: Mutations that alter the primary structure of type I collagen: The perils of a system for generating large structures by the principle of nucleated growth. J Biol Chem 265:15349, 1990.
8. Engel J, Prockop DJ: The zipper-like folding of collagen triple helices and the effects of mutations that disrupt the zipper. Annu Rev Biophys Biophys Chem 20:137, 1991.
9. Panchenko MV, Stetler-Stevenson WG, Trubetskoy OV, Gacheru SN, Kagan HM: Metalloproteinase activity secreted by fibrogenic cells in the processing of prolysyl oxidase: Potential role of procollagen C-proteinase. J Biol Chem. In press.
10. Li SW, Sieron AL, Fertala A, Hojima Y, Arnold WV, Prockop DJ: The C-proteinase that processes procollagens to fibrillar collagens is identical to the protein previously identified as bone morphogenic protein-1. Proc Natl Acad Sci USA. In press.
11. Kessler E, Takahara K, Biniaminov L, Brusel M, Greenspan DS: Bone morphogenetic protein-1: The type I procollagen C-proteinase. Science 271:360, 1996.
12. Rohde H, Vargas L, Hahn E, Kalbfleisch H, Bruguera M, Timpl R: Radioimmunoassay for type III procollagen peptide and its application to human liver disease. Eur J Clin Invest 9:451, 1979.
13. Ala-Kokko L, Günzler V, Hoek JB, Rubin E, Prockop DJ: Hepatic fibrosis in rats produced by carbon tetrachloride and dimethyl-nitrosamine: Observations suggesting immunoassays of serum for the 7S fragment of type IV collagen are a more sensitive index of liver damage than immunoassays for the NH$_2$-terminal propeptide of type III procollagen. Hepatology 16:167, 1992.
14. Vogel BE, Doelz R, Kadler KE, Hojima Y, Engel J, Prockop DJ: A substitution of cysteine for glycine-748 of the α1 chain produces a kink at this site in the procollagen I molecule and an altered N-proteinase cleavage site over 225 nm away. J Biol Chem 263:19249, 1988.
15. Kadler KE, Torre-Blanco A, Adachi E, Vogel BE, Hojima Y, Prockop DJ: A type I collagen with substitution of a cysteine for glycine-748 in the α1(I) chain copolymerizes with normal type I collagen and can generate fractal-like structures. Biochemistry 30:5081, 1991.
16. Byers PH: Osteogenesis imperfecta. In Royce PM, Steinmann B (eds): Connective Tissue and Its Heritable Disorders. New York, Wiley-Liss, 1993, pp 317–350.
17. Kuivaniemi H, Tromp G, Prockop DJ: Mutations in collagens type I, II, III, X and XI cause a spectrum of diseases of bone, cartilage and blood vessels. Hum Mutation. In press.
18. Barker DF, Hostikka SL, Zhou J, Chow LT, Oliphant AR, Gerken SC, Gregory MC, Skolnick MH, Atkin CL, Tryggvason K: Identification of mutations in the COL4A5 collagen gene in Alport syndrome. Science 248:1224, 1990.
19. Ryynänen, N, Knowlton, RG, Parente MG, Chung LC, Chu M-L, Uitto J: Human type VII collagen: Genetic linkage of the gene (COL7A1) on chromosome 3 to dominant dystrophic epidermolysis bullosa. Am J Hum Genet 49:797, 1991.
20. Bachinger HP, Morris NP, Lunstrum GP, Keene DR, Rosenbaum LM, Compton LA, Burgeson RE: The relationship of the biophysical and biochemical characteristics of type VII collagen to the function of anchoring fibrils. J Biol Chem 265:10095, 1990.
21. Kontusaari S, Tromp G, Kuivaniemi H, Romanic A, Prockop DJ: A mutation in the gene for type III procollagen (COL3A1) in a family with aortic aneurysms. J Clin Invest 86:1465, 1990.
22. Palotie A, Vaisanen P, Ott J, Ryhanen L, Ilma K, Vikkula M, Cheah K, Vuorio E, Peltonen L: Predisposition to familial osteoarthrosis linked to type II collagen gene. Lancet 1:924, 1989.
23. Ala-Kokko L, Baldwin CT, Moskowitz RW, Prockop DJ: Single base mutation in the type II procollagen gene (COL2A1) as a cause of primary osteoarthritis associated with a mild chondrodysplasia. Proc Natl Acad Sci USA 87:6565, 1990.
24. Bleasel JF, Holderbaum D, Haqqi TM, Moskowitz RW: Clinical correlations of osteoarthritis associated with single base mutations in the type II procollagen gene. J Rheumatol 43:34–36, 1995.
25. Williams CJ, Rock M, Considine E, McCarron S, Gow P, Ladda R, McLain D, Michels VM, Murphy W, Prockop DJ, Ganguly A: Three new point mutations in type II procollagen (COL2A1) and identification of a fourth family with the COL2A1 ARG519 → CYS base substitution using conformation sensitive gel electrophoresis. Hum Molec Genet 4:309–312, 1995.
26. Bleasel JR, Bisagni-Faure A, Holderbaum D, Vacher-Lavenu MC, Haqqi TM, Moskowitz RW, Menkes CJ: Type II procollagen gene (COL2A1) mutation in exon 11 associated with spondyloepiphyseal dysplasia, tall stature and precocious osteoarthritis. J Rheumatol 22:255–261, 1995.
27. Spotila LD, Constantinou CD, Sereda L, Ganguly A, Riggs BL, Prockop DJ: Mutation in a gene for type I procollagen (COL1A2) in a woman with post-menopausal osteoporosis: Evidence for phenotypic and genotypic overlap with mild OI. Proc Natl Acad Sci USA 88:6624, 1991.
28. Constantinou CD, Pack M, Prockop DJ: A mutation in the type I procollagen gene on chromosome 17q21.31-q22.05 or 7q21.3-q22.1 that decreases the thermal stability of the protein in a woman with ankylosing spondylitis and osteopenia. Cytogenet Cell Genet 51:979, 1990.
29. Shapiro JR, Burn VE, Chipman SD, Velis KP, Bansal M: Osteoporosis and familial idiopathic scoliosis: Association with an abnormal α2(I) collagen. Connect Tissue Res 21:117, 1989.
30. Urry DW: Molecular prospectives of vascular wall structure and disease—elastin component. Perspect Biol Med 21:265, 1978.
31. Sandberg LB, Soskel NJ, Solt MS: Structure of the elastin fiber: An overview. J Invest Dermatol 79:128, 1982.
32. Rucker RB, Dubick MA: Elastin metabolism and chemistry: Potential roles in lung development and structure. Environ Health Perspect 55:179, 1984.
33. Siegel RC: Lysyl oxidase. Int Rev Connect Tissue Res 8:73, 1979.
34. Sakai LY, Keene DR, Glanville RW, Bachinger HP: Purification and partial characterization of fibrillin, a cysteine-rich structural component of connective tissue microfibrils. J Biol Chem 266:14763, 1991.
35. Rosenbloom J, Bashir M, Yeh H, Rosenbloom J, Ornstein-Goldstein N, Fazio M, Kahari F-M, Uitto J: Regulation of elastin gene expression. Ann NY Acad Sci 624:116, 1991.
36. Indik Z, Yeh H, Ornstein-Goldstein N, Sheppard P, Anderson N, Rosenbloom JC, Peltinen L, Rosenbloom J: Alternate splicing of human elastin mRNA indicated by sequence analysis of cloned genomic and complementary DNA. Proc Natl Acad Sci USA 84:5680, 1987.
37. Raghunath M, Kielty CM, Kainulainen K, Child A, Peltonen L, Steinmann B: Analyses of truncated fibrillin caused by a 336 bp deletion in the FBN1 gene resulting in Marfan syndrome. Biochem J 302:889–896, 1994.
38. Dietz HC, Ramirez F, Sakai LY: Marfan's syndrome and other microfibrillar diseases. Adv Hum Genet 22:153–186, 1994.
39. Bressan GM, Prockop DJ: Synthesis of elastic in aortas from chick embryos: Conversion of newly secreted elastin to cross-linked elastin without apparent proteolysis of the molecule. Biochemistry 16:1406, 1977.
40. Shapiro SD, Campbell EJ, Welgus HG, Senior RM: Elastin degradation by mononuclear phagocytes. Ann NY Acad Sci 624:69, 1991.
41. Snider GL, Ciccolella DE, Morris SM, Stone PJ, Lucey EC: Putative role of neutrophil elastase in the pathogenesis of emphysema. Ann NY Acad Sci 624:45, 1991.

42. Partridge SM, Elsden DF, Thomas J: Biosynthesis of the desmosine and isodesmosine cross-bridges in elastin. Biochem J 93:30, 1964.
43. Uitto J, Christiano AM, Veli-Matti K, Bashir MM, Rosenbloom J: Molecular biology and pathology of human elastin. Biochem Soc Trans 19:824, 1991.
44. Cox DW: α1-Antitrypsin deficiency. *In* Scriber CR, Beaudet AL, Sly WS, Valle D (eds): The Metabolic Basis of Inherited Disease, 6th ed. New York, McGraw-Hill, 1989, pp 2409–2437.
45. Okayama H, Brantly M, Holmes M, Crystal RG: Characterization of the molecular basis of the α1-antitrypsin F allele. Am J Hum Genet 48:1154, 1991.

CHAPTER 3

Robert L. Trelstad

Matrix Glycoproteins and Proteoglycans

Improved understanding of the roles of the extracellular matrix in biology and medicine can be expected based on new information about the dynamics of cell-matrix relationships. Principal among these dynamics is the extracellular matrix as a ligand, reversibly binding biologically active agents that affect cells in an autocrine, paracrine, and endocrine manner. Second among these is the matrix as an agonist in both the *solid phase* (transmitting information to contiguous cells) and the *fluid phase* (transmitting information through the pericellular space and the circulation). These matrix attributes of receptor and agonist add to the better-known matrix functions as adhesives, biomaterials, and filters and, as a text, recording events in the history of the organism.

This chapter emphasizes the dynamic nature of the matrix and its multiple relationships with cells. Details of matrix chemistry and its macroscopic structures are available in other reviews.[1-4] The major matrix components described cover terminology, chemistry, intermolecular relationships, and overall organization as a three-phase system (Fig. 3–1):

- A solid phase
- A fluid phase
- A cell surface phase

All three phases are composed of matrix components commonly known as collagens, proteoglycans, structural glycoproteins, and elastins.[5-11]

MATRIX PHASES

Solid Phase Matrix

The solid phase extracellular matrix is well known and functions at a macroscopic level as a supporting structure. At the cellular level, it serves as (1) a substrate for cell migration; (2) an adhesive for cell anchorage; (3) a ligand for ions, growth factors, and other bioactive agents; (4) signals to contacting cells; and (5) a recording device.[12-14] The cells that produce, store, and excrete these matrices include nearly all cell types, ranging from circulating mast cells to neurons. The principal sources of the solid phase matrices are fibroblasts, chondrocytes, osteoblasts, smooth muscle cells, and various epithelia.[15]

Fluid Phase Matrix

Derivatives of most components of the solid phase matrix can also be found in fluid forms in the extracellular fluids, lymph, or blood. Secreted matrix components are transiently in a fluid phase prior to polymerization. The fluid phase forms may be derived from solid phase components by some form of cleavage, whereas others are unique isoforms.[16] Hyaluronan, aggrecan, fibronectin, vitronectin, thrombospondin, cartilage matrix protein, and laminin are found intact or as fragments in blood, lymph, synovial fluid, and bronchoalveolar lavage fluid.[17, 18] Following injury, matrix components are found in fluid phases in sites ranging from joints to the peritoneum.[19, 20]

Cell Surface Matrix

The location of matrix components at the cell's surface is affected as follows:

- In part, by membrane receptors that bind matrix components (e.g., the integrins)[21]
- In part, as integral components of the plasma membrane (e.g., the syndecans)[22]
- In part, as covalently linked elements to membrane glycolipids (e.g., betaglycan)[23]
- In part, through biosynthetic steps that result in direct transmembrane penetration of product bypassing the Golgi apparatus (e.g., hyaluronan)[24]

By whichever of these means, the cell surface matrix consists of polyvalent molecules that can bind other ligands and amplify and extend the surface of the cell into the pericellular space (Fig. 3–2). The cell surface matrix can be indirectly or directly visualized on living cells and is several micrometers in thickness and in constant motion.[25]

The *basement membrane* is an extracellular matrix that is noncovalently associated with the plasma membranes of most animal cells (see Fig. 3–1). The term basement membrane is well ingrained, even though it is neither on the "bottom" of cells nor a membrane in the traditional sense. It coats nearly the entire surface of smooth, cardiac, and skeletal muscle cells; fat cells; and Schwann cells and the basal surface of most epithelia.[26]

In essence, the basement membrane, or *basal lam-*

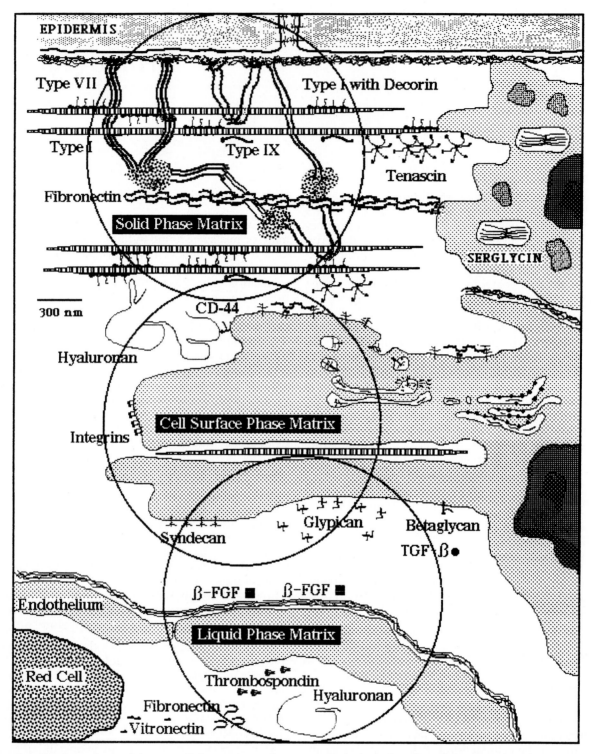

Figure 3–1. The three phases of the extracellular matrix are drawn to scale for both the cells and the matrix components. *Top*, Basal portion of an epidermal cell, covered on its basal surface by basement membrane. Type VII collagen aggregates are linked to the basement membrane to form anchoring fibrils, which create "loops," entrapping collagen fibrils and other matrix components. Taken together, the elements in the upper circle constitute a solid phase of the matrix. *Middle*, The fibroblast shows a convoluted topography with cell surface receptors and matrix components associated with the cell surface. Hyaluronan, bound to the cell surface by the CD44 receptor or penetrating the cell during biosynthesis, forms an extended pericellular coat. Syndecan, glypican, and betaglycan, three membrane-associated proteoglycans, are important components of the cell surface phase matrix. In that glypican is not a transmembrane protein, but rather linked by phosphoinositol, it can readily be released from the cell surface phase to enter the liquid phase matrix. *Lower left*, A capillary is carrying soluble forms of fibronectin, vitronectin, hyaluronan, and thrombospondin. Fluid phase elements from the circulation and from the interstitial fluids surrounding the cells move throughout the liquid phase matrix.

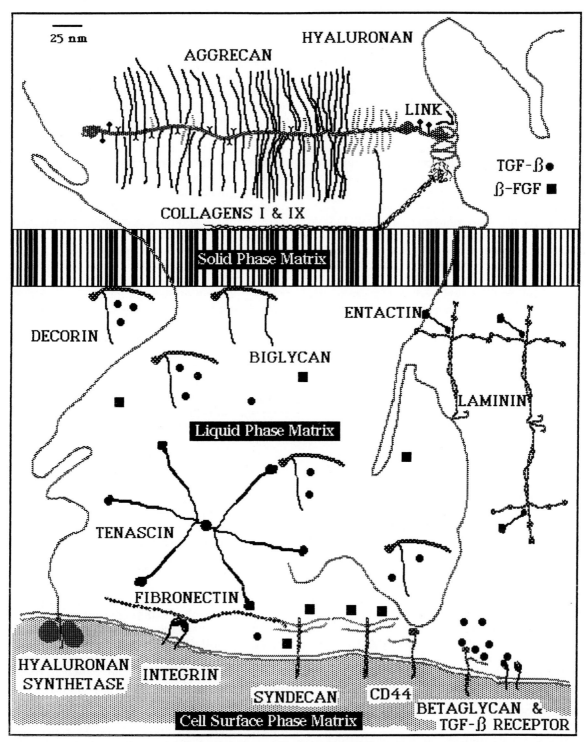

Figure 3–2. A detailed view of the cell surface and the pericellular matrix drawn to scale. The type I collagen fibril is present as a 67-nm striated structure with associated components: decorin, biglycan, and a type IX molecule. The type IX molecule is covalently cross-linked to the type I. Both decorin and biglycan interact with the fibril, and both influence fibril formation. The upper portion of the diagram illustrates the solid phase matrix. The external surface of the cell in the lower half shows fibronectin bound to an integrin receptor with syndecan interacting with one end of the same fibronectin molecule. Syndecan is also shown interacting with basic fibroblast growth factor (bFGF). Hyaluronan bound to the cell via CD44 as well as anchored through the membrane during synthesis leads to the formation of an extension of the cell and contributes significantly to the cell surface phase of the matrix. The binding of transforming growth factor–beta (TGF-β) to decorin, betaglycan, and its receptors occurs in all three phases of the matrix.

ina,[27] is a cell surface matrix, filtering and protecting the cell surface; reversibly binding regulators and growth factors; partitioning tissues during morphogenesis and repair; and all the while being traversed by components involved in nutrition, respiration, and metabolic waste. The basal lamina is a heteropolymeric mixture of molecules, including type IV collagen, laminin, perlecan, and entactin.[27–30] These relatively constant molecular constituents undergo a variety of self-assembly reactions of both a homopolymeric and a heteropolymeric nature to produce a cell surface matrix that ranges from 50 to 200 nm in thickness.[31] The linkages to the cell surface are noncovalent, calcium-dependent, and mediated via a variety of its constituents acting individually or together with receptors or through unknown means.[27]

Although its filtration functions are well known, particularly in the glomerulus, the basement membrane plays additional important binding and storage roles for drugs, ions, enzymes, and growth factors.[28, 32, 33] Transforming growth factor-β (TGF-β), a potent regulator of cell proliferation and matrix production and degradation, is down-regulated when cells are cultured on a reconstituted basement membrane. Because of their ubiquity and the polyvalency of their constituents, basement membranes play a central role in cell-matrix interactions ranging from cell anchorage to regulation of cytokines and growth factors.[34]

MATRIX NOMENCLATURE

The nomenclature and classification of matrix components have simultaneously blurred and come more into focus as details of their overlapping chemistries have developed. The triple helical structure of collagen, once thought to be a unique attribute, is shared with a variety of molecules, including surfactant, macrophage scavenger receptor, C1q, and acetylcholinesterase.[35–38] In that proteins are modular structures, often shared with unrelated molecules, the possession of a particular module, such as a growth factor sequence, does not help to define a clear nosology.[39, 40] Further, because proteins often have extensive postsynthetic modifications ranging from oxidations to glycosylation, these attributes do not assist in providing clarity of definitions.

Most matrix proteins have attached one or more of four classes of carbohydrate polymers:

• Simple hexoses
• Branched N-linked oligosaccharides
• Branched O-linked (mucinous) oligosaccharides
• Unbranched O-linked glycosaminoglycans (GAGs)

The hexose chains on collagen are simple monosaccharides and disaccharides linked to hydroxylysine. The oligosaccharides are branched structures, often rich in mannose and sialic acid, which undergo extensive alterations during synthesis and postsynthetic modifications. Such oligosaccharides are an essential feature of a glycoprotein. The glycosaminoglycans are unbranched, long chains that are highly sulfated and that have a motif of a disaccharide repeat.[41] Glycosaminoglycans are an essential feature of a proteoglycan.

The examples of types IX and XII collagens underscores the above-mentioned naming problem. Type IX collagen has covalently bound oligosaccharides and glycosaminoglycans and should be classified as a collagen, a glycoprotein, and a proteoglycan.[42] Type XII collagen presents a similar ambiguity, in that it is a chimeric molecule with reiterated fibronectin type III motifs, von Willebrand factor A motifs, a domain homologous to a noncollagenous region of type IX collagen, and short collagenous domains with an Arg-Gly-Asp (RGD) site, the classic integrin-binding sequence.[43] Proteins to which glycosaminoglycans are inconstantly linked have been called part-time proteoglycans (see betaglycan, brevican, CD44, and thrombomodulin later in this chapter).

Thus, although the initial logic of earlier taxonomies of matrix components was chemistry or function, it is now clear that overlapping chemistries and functions do not lend themselves to simple classifications. The current tendency is to "name" each matrix macromolecule with a new term, number, or both (e.g., syndecan-1[44] or the α_1 chain of type XIX collagen[45]). Although this tendency is bound to lead to some confusion, the need to expand beyond the intellectual constraints of the prior nomenclature is clear because proteoglycans, glycoproteins, and collagens are polymorphic, polyfunctional, and widely distributed.

MATRIX CHEMICAL STRUCTURES

Proteins, Aggregated or Cross-Linked, with Attached Carbohydrates

The principal chemistry of the matrix is that of proteins with covalently attached carbohydrates. Post-translation modifications include hydroxylation of prolyl, lysyl, and asparagine residues[46]; glycosylation to form the various N-linked or O-linked oligosaccharides or glycosaminoglycans; acylation by the long-chain fatty acids myristate and palmitate; and tyrosine-O-sulfation.[47] The proteins may also be oxidized to create covalent cross-linkages among proteins of the same group and between proteins of different groups.[48] The carbohydrate polymers are covalently linked at one of four amino acids: asparagine, threonine, serine, and hydroxylysine. The linkage at the asparagine residues occurs through a nitrogen atom (*N-linked*); linkages through threonine, serine, and hydroxylysine are through an oxygen atom (*O-linked*) (Fig. 3–3).

The protein cores of matrix glycoproteins and proteoglycans vary in molecular weight from approximately 40 to 600 kD and in physical size from less than 30 nm to greater than 300 nm in greatest dimension (Fig. 3–4). The core protein of perlecan, for example, is 50 percent greater than type IV collagen in

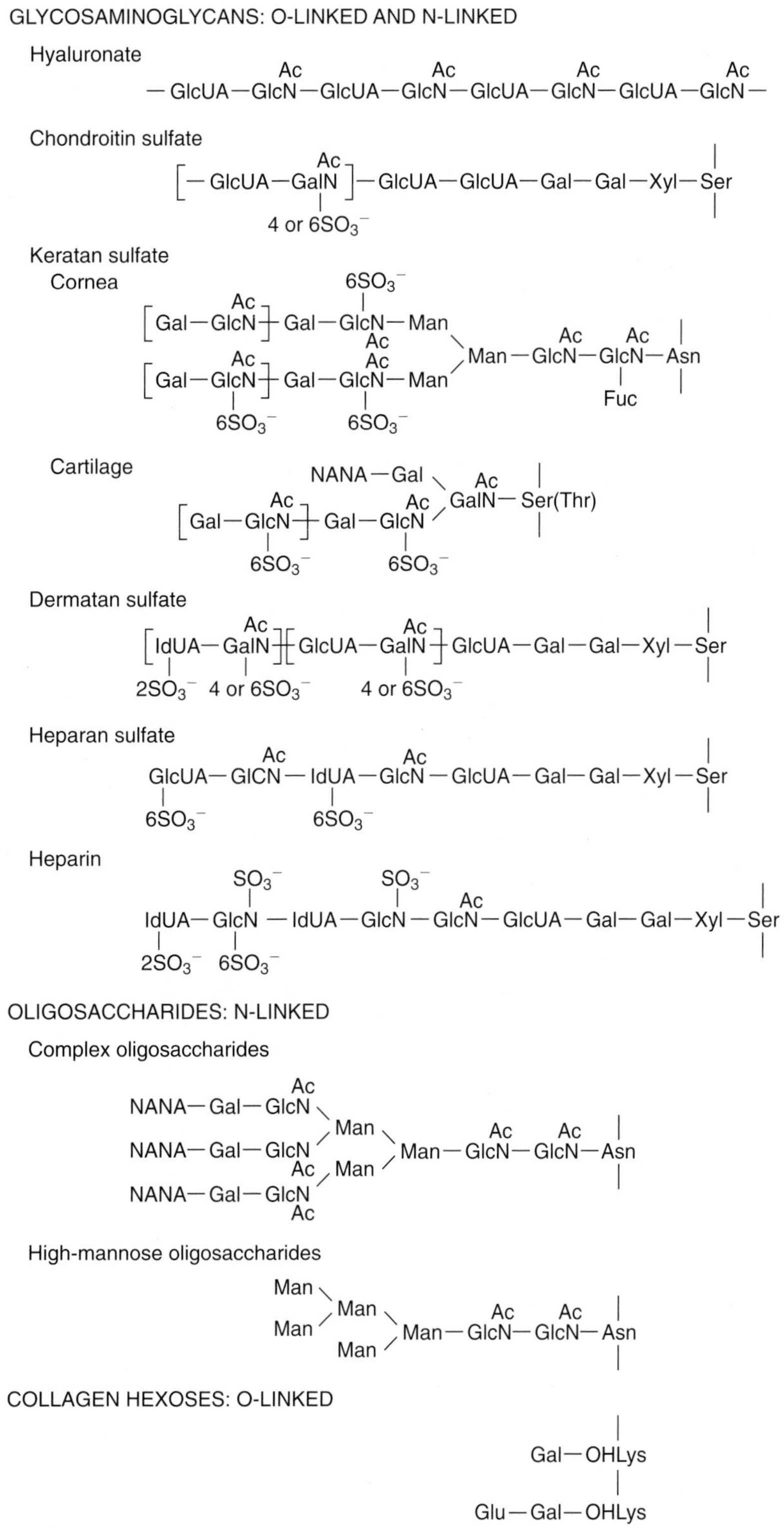

GLYCOSAMINOGLYCANS: O-LINKED AND N-LINKED

Hyaluronate

$$\begin{array}{ccccccc} & Ac & & Ac & & Ac & & Ac \\ & | & & | & & | & & | \\ -\,GlcUA-GlcN-GlcUA-GlcN-GlcUA-GlcN-GlcUA-GlcN- \end{array}$$

Chondroitin sulfate

$$\left[-\,GlcUA-\overset{\overset{\displaystyle Ac}{|}}{\underset{\underset{\displaystyle 4\ \text{or}\ 6SO_3^-}{|}}{GalN}}\right]-GlcUA-GlcUA-Gal-Gal-Xyl-Ser$$

Keratan sulfate

Cornea

Cartilage

Dermatan sulfate

$$\left[\,IdUA-\overset{\overset{\displaystyle Ac}{|}}{\underset{\underset{\displaystyle 2SO_3^-}{|}}{GalN}}\right]\!\!\left[\,GlcUA-\overset{\overset{\displaystyle Ac}{|}}{\underset{\underset{\displaystyle 4\ \text{or}\ 6SO_3^-}{|}}{GalN}}\right]-GlcUA-Gal-Gal-Xyl-Ser$$

4 or 6SO₃⁻

Heparan sulfate

$$\underset{\underset{\displaystyle 6SO_3^-}{|}}{GlcUA}-\overset{\overset{\displaystyle Ac}{|}}{GlcN}-\underset{\underset{\displaystyle 6SO_3^-}{|}}{IdUA}-\overset{\overset{\displaystyle Ac}{|}}{GlcN}-GlcUA-Gal-Gal-Xyl-Ser$$

Heparin

$$\underset{\underset{\displaystyle 2SO_3^-}{|}}{IdUA}-\overset{\overset{\displaystyle SO_3^-}{|}}{\underset{\underset{\displaystyle 6SO_3^-}{|}}{GlcN}}-IdUA-\overset{\overset{\displaystyle SO_3^-}{|}}{GlcN}-GlcN-GlcUA-\overset{\overset{\displaystyle Ac}{|}}{Gal}-Gal-Xyl-Ser$$

OLIGOSACCHARIDES: N-LINKED

Complex oligosaccharides

High-mannose oligosaccharides

COLLAGEN HEXOSES: O-LINKED

$$Gal-OHLys$$
$$Glu-Gal-OHLys$$

Figure 3–3. Linkage patterns in N-linked and O-linked oligosaccharides, in O-linked hexoses in the collagens, and O-linked and N-linked (keratan sulfate) patterns in the glycosaminoglycans. The vertical lines attached to the amino acids indicate the protein chain. IdUA, iduronic acid; GlcUA, glucuronic acid; GlCN, glucosamine; GalN, galactosamine; Gal, galactose; Glu, glucose; Man, mannose; Fuc, fucose; Xyl, xylose; Ser, serine; Thr, threonine; Asn, asparagine; OHLys, hydroxylysine; 2SO₃, O-sulfation at position 2; 6SO₃, O-sulfation at position 6; SO₃, N-sulfation; Ac, N-acetylation.

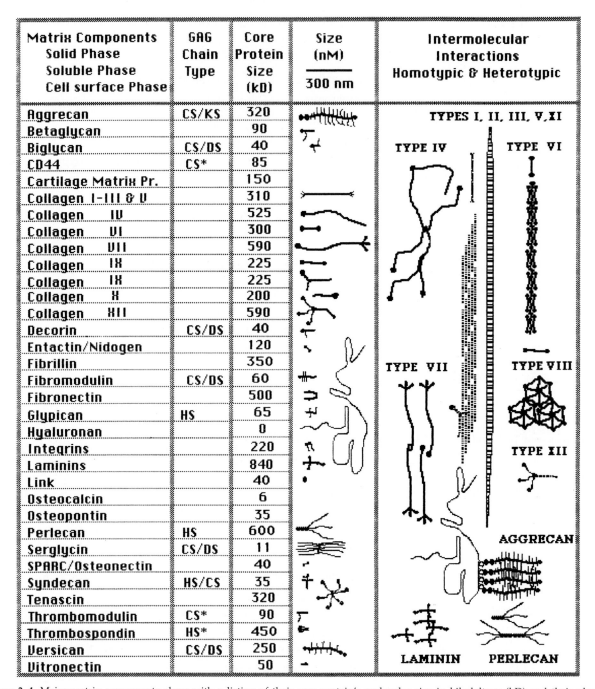

Matrix Components Solid Phase Soluble Phase Cell surface Phase	GAG Chain Type	Core Protein Size (kD)
Aggrecan	CS/KS	320
Betaglycan		90
Biglycan	CS/DS	40
CD44	CS*	85
Cartilage Matrix Pr.		150
Collagen I-III & V		310
Collagen IV		525
Collagen VI		300
Collagen VII		590
Collagen IX		225
Collagen IX		225
Collagen X		200
Collagen XII		590
Decorin	CS/DS	40
Entactin/Nidogen		120
Fibrillin		350
Fibromodulin	CS/DS	60
Fibronectin		500
Glypican	HS	65
Hyaluronan		0
Integrins		220
Laminins		840
Link		40
Osteocalcin		6
Osteopontin		35
Perlecan	HS	600
Serglycin	CS/DS	11
SPARC/Osteonectin		40
Syndecan	HS/CS	35
Tenascin		320
Thrombomodulin	CS*	90
Thrombospondin	HS*	450
Versican	CS/DS	250
Vitronectin		50

Figure 3–4. Major matrix components along with a listing of their core protein's molecular size in kilodaltons (kD) and their physical size in nanometers (nm). The mass of the core protein and the size of the natural configuration are not closely related. CS, chondroitin sulfate; HS, heparan sulfate; DS, dermatan sulfate. Asterisk indicates a variably glycosylated status of the protein.

mass (600 kD versus 400 kD) but is about ¼ its size (100 nm versus 400 nm) in linear dimension. Such size and mass differences result from globular packing and indicate that the three-dimensional size of components cannot be predicted from simple mass. Because aggregates of matrix components establish and maintain form in most tissues in the animal kingdom, the manner of component folding, interacting, and aggregating is of considerable importance.[48–50]

Most matrix proteins are modular when the modular unit is based on sequence similarities or homologies among polypeptide stretches of 45 to 90 amino acids and frequently contain intra-module disulfide cross-links. Modules presumably arise within one protein by exon duplication and among unrelated proteins by exons that have shuffled from one gene to another. Matrix proteins have an extensive modular character.[51]

Carbohydrate Structures

The characters of the carbohydrate chains of both the oligosaccharides of the glycoproteins and the glycosaminoglycans of the proteoglycans[41, 52, 53] are dictated by:

1. The intrinsic properties of the individual sugars.
2. The specific sites and stereochemistry of the linkages between adjacent sugars.
3. The order in which they are added or removed during biosynthesis.
4. Postsynthetic modifications, which include epimerization and sulfation.

Chondroitin sulfate (CS) and dermatan sulfate (DS) glycosaminoglycan (GAG) chains are similar because of the epimerization of glucuronic acid in CS to iduronic acid in DS, a conversion that occurs after the oligosaccharide is synthesized. The biologic and pharmacologic importance of the epimerizations that occur in the iduronic acid to glucuronic acid shift should not be underestimated. A variety of agents, from sulfate to vitamin A deficiency, cause reduction of GAG incorporation into the decorin class of proteoglycans and also to a decreased epimerization of D-glucuronic to L-iduronic acid.[54]

MATRIX FUNCTIONS

From the preceding discussion, it is apparent that the extracellular matrix is broadly involved in functions ranging from roles as adhesives, biomaterials, filters, receptors, signals, and archives. Each of these functions is described next.

Adhesives

In and of themselves, matrix components are adhesives, historically acting as glues and binding to each other in both native and denatured forms in homotypic and heterotypic combinations. These important practical, clinical, and commercial uses of matrix continue to develop[55]; however, it is the cell receptor–matrix interactions or the cell surface–matrix interactions that are new to adhesive considerations. Adhesion molecules and adhesive phenomena have generally excluded cell-matrix interactions. In the past, traditional adhesion molecules dealt with homotypic cell-cell adhesions, as with the calcium-independent cell adhesion molecules (CAMs); the calcium-dependent cadherens; the selectins; desmosomes; and a variety of receptors on lymphocytes. That cell-matrix interactions overlap with traditional adhesive interactions can be inferred from the modular chemistry of the components. In the mouse, for example, perlecan has five distinct domains: a heparan sulfate attachment domain, a low-density-lipoprotein (LDL) receptor-like domain, two different laminin-like domains, and a neural cell adhesion molecule (NCAM)–like domain. This polyvalency leads to molecular interactions of considerable complexity and suggests endless variations of cell-cell and cell-matrix adhesion.[14, 56]

A compelling argument for cell-matrix interactions as an adhesive process is the extensive involvement of integrins in biologic adhesivity.[57–59] The regulation of integrin expression by pharmacologic means, using natural as well as synthesized agents, and the altered regulation of integrin expression in human disease suggest new avenues for study and modulation of cell-matrix adhesion.[60–64]

Microorganisms use the matrix as an adhesive substrate to establish infections. Organisms from various species express cell-surface molecules called *adhesins*, which bind to the matrix. Typical organisms and an example of their matrix ligands[65] include:

- *Pneumocystis carinii* (fibronectin)
- *Trypanosoma cruzi* (collagen)
- *Aspergillus* (fibrinogen)
- *Staphylococcus aureus* (vitronectin)
- *Plasmodium falciparum* (heparan sulfate)

Biomaterials

The biomaterials properties of natural and reconstituted matrices are well understood at macroscopic levels. Matrix components can be reassembled in a theoretically limitless number of combinations, in differing sizes and shapes, to form implantable devices or substrates for cells at sites of injury. It is reasonable to predict that biomaterials, composed of extracellular matrix components and their cells, will increasingly be available for clinical use.[66–68]

Filters

All nutrients, gases, cytokines, hormones, and drugs must pass through the extracellular matrix in moving from one tissue or tissue compartment to another. In particular, most agents must traverse the basement membrane at least twice: when the agent exits the vasculature and before it enters the cell, or vice versa. Both the matrix and the basement membranes bind, select, inhibit, facilitate, release, or reversibly remove components with which they come in contact, acting as a filter with physiologic consequences.[69, 70] In addition to these filtration functions, the glomerular basement membrane plays a major role in homeostasis and is central to a number of disease processes.[71]

Ligands

Solid phase matrix components are ligands that bind, store, protect, and release growth factors and other regulatory agents.[72–75] The release of such ligands bound to the matrix may occur through (1) matrix degradation, (2) specific intermediary binding factors,[76] (3) competitive interactions with other ligands, or (4) some change in the ligand itself. This "storage/receptor" activity in the matrix shows considerable specificity and is a major matrix function.[77]

At the same time that the solid phase matrix is a storage/receptor, cell surface matrix molecules, such as the syndecans,[78] CD44,[79] betaglycan,[23] and glypican,[80] are probably signal-transducing receptors,[81] although the transduction mechanisms need to be clarified.

Signals

In early studies of developing embryos and in cell culture studies in which collagen was shown to support and promote differentiation in vitro, the roles of the matrix in signaling and mediating cell-cell interactions were apparent.[82, 83] Studies of hyaluronic acid and fibronectin opened a new view of the broad biologic effects of matrix components as signals.[12, 84] The signaling functions of matrix macromolecules may be detected by cells when the molecules are in a complex macroaggregate and as small polypeptides or oligosaccharides, released from the parent molecule by hydrolysis.[81] The solid phase signals operate in a variety of biologic situations, for example, during cell migrations in development,[85] in neutrophil reactions in injury,[86] in allergic reactions,[87] in malignant transformations of epithelia,[58] and in endometrial changes associated with menstruation or pregnancy.[88] The Arg-Gly-Asp (RGD) peptide in solid phase in intact fibronectin or released from fibronectin can effectively inhibit cell binding to a number of serum and matrix components.[89]

As with peptides, short sequences of carbohydrates or oligosaccharides have similar regulatory effects. The replication of smooth muscle cells is significantly inhibited by oligosaccharides derived from heparin, and this effect is dependent on both the size and the charge of the oligosaccharide. The inhibition involves a competition between basic fibroblast growth factor (bFGF) binding to cell-associated heparin sulfate proteoglycans and the released oligosaccharides with the consequent inhibition of a protein kinase C–dependent pathway.[90] The matrix also has "positional information" sufficient to influence the homing and orientation of cells, as shown by the effects of matrix on neural crest cell migration or the polarizing influence of the COOH terminus of the α chain of laminin on nephrogenic mesenchyme.[83, 91, 92]

Archives

Finally, the matrix is a text, a record of events that have taken place around a cell and within a tissue. It is a repository of information and a historical document, recording local events from the time of synthe-

sis to later events, such as cell migrations, inflammation, transformation, and matrix cross-linking. These postdepositional events involve deliberate or accidental glycosylation,[93] cross-linking,[48] oxidation,[94] phosphorylation, and epimerization, to name but a few. Some of the history of an organism is written in this text, and its epigenetic character will make it a challenge to read. For the physical anthropologist, reading this text gives insight to matters from the cultural to the medical.

MATRIX REGULATORS

The regulatory factors that affect matrix synthesis, degradation, and function are many and include "growth factors," cytokines, hormones, vitamins, matrix metalloproteinases (MMPs), and tissue inhibitors of metalloproteinases (TIMPs). The logistics of matrix regulation differs from the logistics of intracellular proteins, in that the matrix is more distant from the genetic and biosynthetic machinery inside the cell. Nonetheless, the matrix is directly and indirectly involved in feedback on its production, polymerization, and degradation.[95] These important topics are covered in other chapters.

MATRIX COMPONENTS

Next is a brief overview of the various macromolecules; they are presented individually or as families, primarily in alphabetical order of the best known member.

Agrin, Dystroglycan

Agrin

Agrin and related isoforms are secreted molecules produced by nerves and muscle that induce the aggregation of acetylcholine receptors (AChRs).[96] Acetylcholine receptor genes are specifically transcribed by synaptic nuclei in response to signals from the synaptic basement membrane.[97] Various isoforms of agrin are generated by alternative splicing, and these isoforms have differing interactive properties with proteoglycans and other components of the basement membrane.[98]

The C terminus of agrin that is responsible for causing AChRs of muscle to aggregate contains three laminin modules separated by epidermal growth factor (EGF)–like modules. Alternative splicing in the laminin modules leads to the formation of isoforms that are devoid of AChR-aggregating activity.

In the N terminus, all isoforms contain follistatin-related modules that, like those in follistatin and osteonectin, may bind the TGF-β or platelet-derived growth factor (PDGF) families.[99]

Dystroglycan

Structural similarities of agrin and laminin allow both to bind to the laminin receptor dystroglycan-α and dystrophin-related protein (DRP/utrophin) in a calcium-dependent manner inhibitable by heparin and laminin, but not by fibronectin.[100] α-Dystroglycan is the major agrin-binding protein in Torpedo and myotube membranes.[101]

Aggrecan, Versican

Aggrecan is the major proteoglycan derived from a variety of cartilages. It consists of a long core protein (350 nm) with three distinct globular domains: two near the NH_2 terminus and one at the COOH terminus. It contains an extensive array of keratan sulfate and chondroitin sulfate GAG chains, which give it its classic bottle-brush appearance (see Fig. 3–2). The amino terminal globular domain shows sequence similarity to link protein and the carboxy terminal globule to lectin-binding proteins. The amino terminal globule binds to hyaluronan and forms a macroaggregate that contributes to the three-dimensional organization of most cartilages.

Aggrecan provides cartilage with osmotic properties that give articular cartilages resistance to compression.[102] In the mouse, an autosomal recessive deficiency (cmd), characterized by cleft palate, short limbs, tail, and snout, results from a 7 base pair (bp) deletion in exon 5 of aggrecan and consequent truncation of the molecule.[103] The GAG chains and the core protein undergo shortening in the tissues long after synthesis and deposition, which possibly accounts for some of the changes that occur in cartilages with aging.[104, 105]

Versican is a large chondroitin sulfate proteoglycan (also known as PG-M) that inhibits cell-substratum adhesion. In fibroblast cultures, versican is abundant in the subcellular space but is selectively absent from focal contacts where vinculin, integrins, and fibronectin have been localized. Hyaluronan, CD44, and tenascin have a similar distribution.[14]

Betaglycan

Betaglycan is an integral membrane protein and part-time proteoglycan as well as a soluble matrix element. Betaglycan directly regulates the access of TGF-β to its signaling receptors. In its membrane phase, betaglycan is the type III receptor for TGF-β, where it functions to present TGF-β directly to the kinase subunit of the signaling receptor, forming a high-affinity complex.[106] By itself TGF-β binds with low affinity to the heteromeric serine-threonine protein kinase receptor. Betaglycan thereby enhances cell responsiveness to TGF-β and its isoforms. Soluble betaglycan binds TGF-β but does not enhance binding to membrane receptors, and recombinant betaglycans act as potent inhibitors of TGF-β. In the solid matrix phase, betaglycan is an enhancer of TGF-β action; in its soluble matrix phase, it is a TGF-β antagonist.[23]

Biglycan, Decorin, Fibromodulin, Lumican

The small proteoglycans—biglycan, decorin, fibromodulin, and lumican—are a family of structurally similar but distinct molecules found in a diverse array of connective tissues.[107] Fibromodulin and decorin interact with collagens I and II at different sites on the striated fibrils. Fibromodulin has an average of one binding site per type I collagen molecule, whereas decorin has several, some possibly mediated by the dermatan sulfate chain.[108] Fibromodulin is functionally similar to decorin, in that it binds to collagen types I and II during fibrillogenesis. The fibromodulin isolated from cartilage contains at least one keratan sulfate chain, which suggests that this group of molecules may show structural heterogeneities from tissue to tissue on the basis of their GAG adducts.

When decorin is present during collagen fibril assembly, fibrils of smaller diameter are formed. Such fibrils have less biomechanical strength because tensile properties of woven polymers (e.g., collagen) are dependent, in part, on the fibril diameter.

Although the "solid-phase" functions of these small proteoglycans are important as a structural element, their binding of TGF-β in a regulatory manner is likely to be of equal or greater importance. TGF-β binding presumably involves both the "solid phase" and "fluid phase" forms in vivo, in that the decorin-type proteoglycans all bind to similar sites on TGF-β as betaglycan and do so in a competitive manner.[109] In addition to their interactions with TGF-β, biglycan and decorin accelerate heparin cofactor II inhibition of thrombin, an effect mediated by the GAG chains.

Biglycan and decorin are also bound to type V collagen in a saturable manner and in the bound state accelerate the heparin cofactor II/thrombin inhibition reaction as efficiently as the proteoglycans in solution.[110]

Brevican, Neurocan, Phosphacan

The extracellular matrix in the central nervous system (CNS) is modest in its interstitial distribution but is present nonetheless. The structural roles of the matrix in the CNS are likely to be less prominent than the roles of signal, receptor, and text. The following recently described proteoglycans in the CNS, in conjunction with hyaluronan, are serving new roles in morphogenesis and eventually should be involved in signaling.[53]

Brevican

Brevican, a part-time proteoglycan, contains chondroitin sulfate chains when glycanated and, within its short protein core (relative to aggrecan, versican, or neurocan), a hyaluronan-binding domain at the N terminus, an EGF-like repeat, a lectin-like domain, and a complement regulatory protein-like domain in the C terminus. Brevican is present predominantly in the brain and is expressed in primary cerebellar astrocytes but not in neurons.[111]

Neurocan

Neurocan is a multidomain proteoglycan synthesized by neurons and binds to hyaluronic acid. Neurocan interacts with the neuronal-glial and neural-cell adhesion molecules NgCAM and NCAM, and it competes with the effects of these two adhesion molecules. In that neurocan, NgCAM, and NCAM colocalize in the developing cerebellum, it is likely that their interactions affect neuronal adhesion and neurite growth during morphogenesis.[112]

Phosphacan

Phosphacan is synthesized by glia and represents an extracellular variant of the receptor-type protein tyrosine phosphatase.[113, 114] Tenascin binds phosphacan and neurocan, which suggests that interactions among chondroitin sulfate proteoglycans and tenascin are involved in neurogenesis, possibly by modulating signal transduction across the plasma membrane.[115]

CD44, RHAMM

CD44

CD44 is a transmembrane family of proteins with various isoforms generated by alternative splicing and/or post-translational modification. CD44 is a major hyaluronan receptor, a part-time proteoglycan, and a lymphocyte homing receptor.[116] The interactions of the CD44 with hyaluronan are inhibited by low concentrations of hyaluronan and high concentrations of chondroitin sulfate, which suggests that the receptor ligand interaction may mimic the interactions of aggrecan, link protein, and hyaluronan in the matrix, a suggestion supported by sequence homologies among the hyaluronan-binding domains in aggrecan and versican with the protein core of CD44.

CD44 on lymphocytes is responsible for their homing to high endothelium during physiologic and pathologic extravasation and for the ability of macrophages to internalize hyaluronan during lung development.[117] In addition to these binding and receptor functions, CD44 plays a role in matrix assembly, where it acts to organize the immediate pericellular zone.[25, 118]

Receptor for Hyaluronan-Mediated Motility (RHAMM)

RHAMM is a family of proteins that act at the cell surface to bind hyaluronan, particularly during cell migration. RHAMM is not an integral membrane protein but is dependent on binding to the cell surface by undefined means. RHAMM contains two hyaluronan-binding sites, each in a sequence of nine amino acids. The RHAMM-binding domains lack cysteines and operate under reducing conditions; in contrast, the binding domains in CD44 and link protein contain disulfides, and their binding to hyaluronan is sensitive to reduction.[119]

Cartilage Matrix Protein

Cartilage matrix protein is a 148-kD protein composed of three identical units and is present in non-articular cartilages. It can be extracted with EDTA-containing buffers indicating a divalent cation-dependent anchorage in the matrix. Although its functions are not well understood, cartilage matrix protein is released into the serum in some, but not all, rheumatoid conditions. The subunits have a modular organization with one EGF-like domain and two domains having homologies with the type A repeats of von Willebrand factor, complement factors B and C2, α chains of the integrins, and a globular domain on type VI collagen. Three ellipsoid subunits, connected at the carboxy terminus by a coiled-coil α-helical assembly domain, have been observed by electron microscopy.[120] In the developing chick limb, the expressions of the genes for cartilage matrix protein, type II collagen, link protein, and aggrecan are all independent.

Fibrillin

Elastin is a hydrophobic molecule that, following secretion, assembles with other elastin monomers and forms covalent cross-links with other elastin monomers to create an extended, insoluble fabric that provides tissues with elastic properties.[121] In tissues, elastin is found in close association with another structural glycoprotein, fibrillin. The fibrillins are a family of structural glycoproteins initially identified in association with the amorphous core of elastin but also found as isolated bundles of 10-nm-diameter microfibrils in most connective tissues.[122]

Marfan's syndrome is associated with mutations in fibrillin-1 that are located primarily in the calcium-binding domain. Fibrillin-1 contains 43 precursor epidermal growth factor (pEGF)–like domains that have a consensus sequence for calcium binding and a separate domain for an unusual β-hydroxylation of Asp/Asn.[46] In the heart, fibrillin is distributed at the interface of the cardiac muscle cell surface and matrix, transferring tension from the contracting myocardial cells to the cardiac matrix. At the dermal-epidermal junction, fibrillin penetrates into the lamina densa of the basement membrane. In bone, fibrillin is found in conjunction with type III collagen, and at the bone-periosteum interface it is associated with linking the mineralized bone cortex to ligaments and tendons.

Entactin (Nidogen)

Entactin, also known as nidogen, is a major constituent of the basement membrane. It is a dumbbell-shaped molecule with three domains, a NH_2 terminal globular domain linked by a relatively rigid rod to a COOH terminal globular domain. The rod-like domain consists of EGF modules and a thyroglobulin module; it has an overall mass of 150 kD. Entactin is a structural element that binds laminin to type IV collagen. The COOH terminal domain of entactin has a high affinity for laminin near the intersection of the laminin arms, and the NH_2 terminal domain of entactin has a high affinity for calcium. Entactin contains the RGD, -Arg-Gly-Asp-, sequence, and potential tyrosine O-sulfation and N-glycosylation sites.[123]

Fibronectin

Fibronectin is an adhesive, a solid phase element; a cell surface–matrix protein bound to receptors; and a fluid phase element in the blood serving as an opsonin and chemoattractant. It is a polyvalent molecule with affinities for fibrin, collagen, heparin, thrombospondin, integrins, components in bacterial cell coats, and itself. Fibronectin is produced early in embryogenesis and is important in guiding migratory cells during early morphogenesis. In wound healing, fibronectin, as an intact molecule and as peptide fragments, is chemotactic. It also forms a substrate to which the cells involved in the repair reaction can adhere.[124] Microorganisms have cell surface adhesive molecules–adhesins–that bind to fibronectin and participate in infectivity.[125] Elevated levels of fibronectin occur in the joint fluid of patients with arthritis.

The polyfunctional binding of fibronectin is accomplished by the presence of unique domains along the axis of the two polypeptide chains (~p200 kD). Three types of such repeating sequences are present in fibronectin: types I, II, and III. More than 30 of these three repeats are arranged along one fibronectin chain. The absence of a single type III repeat near the carboxy terminus, by way of alternative splicing, determines the differences between the serum and cell-associated forms. Three exons in fibronectin are candidates for alternative splicing, thus making it possible to construct more than 20 different proteins from one gene. The repeating domains are grouped into larger functional domains that have binding affinities for heparin, fibrin, collagen, and cell surfaces. The binding of fibronectin to the cell is mediated by the sequence -Arg-Gly-Asp- (RGD). The major cell receptor for the fibronectins is the *integrins*.

The multiplicities of interactions that are possible because of the domain structure of matrix monomers and their multimers are well illustrated by the contra-dictory effects of fibronectin and its proteolytic fragments on cell migration and anchorage, sometimes promoting, sometimes inhibiting. Add to this elegant complexity the competitive binding of fibronectin by other matrix components, and a pattern emerges of matrix molecules as an "orchestra" with an unlimited repertoire.[126, 127]

Free Glycosaminoglycans

The idea of free GAGs, while somewhat at odds with the paradigm of the proteoglycans, is just another example of the constrained thinking that occurs when paradigms become platitudes. Matrix biologists have struggled with the taxonomy of hyaluronan for just this reason—it is a GAG without a protein. Free GAG, of a sulfated character, can be found in tissues, on the cell surface, and inside the cell. The production of free GAGs does not necessarily involve degradation of proteoglycans.[128] Free heparan sulfate GAG chains produced in the environment of the developing kidney have profound effects on nephron formation.[129]

Glypican, Cerebroglycan

Glypican

Glypican is a cell surface heparan sulfate proteoglycan, with a core protein linked to the cell surface by a glycosyl-phosphatidylinositol (GPI) linkage. The core protein has both N-linked carbohydrate and four potential sites for O-linked heparan sulfate. The anchorage of the core protein to the cell surface via a phosphoinositol linkage renders it susceptible to cleavage by phospholipases, and glypican is readily shed from the cell surface.

Cerebroglycan

Additional GPI-anchored heparan sulfate proteoglycans have been identified in neuronal tissues and intestinal epithelial cells, with the former named cerebroglycan. Cerebroglycan appears in neurons only during their migratory phase through areas containing laminin[130] and fibronectin,[131] which suggests an important role in the development of the nervous system.[132]

Hyaluronan

Hyaluronan is found in all three phases of the matrix (see Figs. 3–1 and 3–2):

1. As a solid phase matrix element, it occurs in association with aggrecan and link proteins, forming the compressible structure of cartilage.

2. As a fluid phase matrix element, it circulates in

the plasma and flows in the synovial space under normal and abnormal conditions.

3. As a cell surface matrix element, it is present on the cell surface in both a receptor-bound form and as an integral membrane component.

Hyaluronan is not covalently bound to protein. It is the only GAG that is not sulfated and consists of a repeating disaccharide of glucuronic acid and N-acetyl-glucosamine. Hyaluronan is involved in biologic processes as varied as embryonic development, wound healing, and tumor invasion, and it is an important constituent of many tissues. Hyaluronan is present in human serum and is cleared by the liver. The serum levels are elevated in various clinical disorders, including liver disease and arthritis. Patients with rheumatoid arthritis show elevated plasma levels, particularly early in the day in association with morning stiffness. Because of its extended conformation, hyaluronan is highly hydrated and is usually associated with edematous, loosely organized matrices (see Figs. 3–1 and 3–2).

Hyaluronan is synthesized in the cytosol and extrudes directly through the cell membrane, thus providing the cell with an extended "whisker" or "antenna."[25, 118] After synthesis and extension into the extracellular space, non–surface-bound hyaluronan is released by an unknown mechanism.[24] In the matrix, hyaluronan plays a central role in tissue structure through interactions with other matrix molecules, including aggrecan, link protein, and type VI collagen.[133]

Integrins

Integrins constitute a family of membrane-spanning, heterodimeric proteins that mediate adhesive interactions between cells and surrounding extracellular matrices (or other cells) and participate in signal transduction.[21, 134]

Each integrin consists of a noncovalently associated $\alpha\beta$ subunit. The integrins are involved in both cell-cell and cell-matrix interactions. There are nearly a dozen α subunits and half as many β subunits that can associate in a variety of combinations, leading to various binding affinities. A full review of the integrins is beyond the scope of this chapter.

Laminins

The laminins are a family of polyvalent structural glycoproteins, first isolated from the Englebreth-Holm-Swarm (EHS) sarcoma and shown to be a prominent component of most basement membranes. The monomer is composed of three polypeptide chains, originally named A, B1, and B2, but recently renamed alpha, beta, and gamma.[135] At present, three isoforms of the $\alpha\beta$ chains and two of the gamma have been described in seven different arrangements:

- Laminin-1: α_1, β_1, γ_1
- Laminin-2: α_2, β_1, γ_1, previously called merosin
- Laminin-3: α_1, β_2, γ_1, previously called s-laminin
- Laminin-4: α_2, β_2, γ_1, previously called s-merosin
- Laminin-5: α_3, β_3, γ_2, previously called kalinin, nicein, or epiligrin
- Laminin-6: α_3, β_1, γ_1
- Laminin-7: α_3, β_2, γ_1, called κ-laminin and κs-laminin, respectively[10]

The three chains are entwined to form a cross-shaped structure composed of both globular and nonglobular regions. Receptor-mediated cell attachment promotion of neurite outgrowth and heparin binding reside in the terminal region of the long arm; a separate cell attachment site, a solid phase signaling site with mitogenic capacity, binding sites for entactin, and the calcium-dependent sites involved in aggregation are in the short arms.[136] These various sites are composed mainly of cysteine-rich regions with EGF and perlecan homologies.[26]

The list of laminin functions grows rapidly, ranging from the structural to the regulatory.

As a structural element, laminin is a major constituent of the basement membrane; the neuromuscular junction, where its structural functions are matched by its solid phase signaling; and the glomerulus, where its structural functions are closely related to its being a filter and, perhaps, an incidental antigen and ligand of DNA-histone complexes.

As a regulatory element, laminin is a major promoter of neurite outgrowth; it is significantly increased on the surfaces of transformed cells and is a stimulant of metastasis.[137] Proteolytic fragments of the laminin α chain are strongly chemotactic for mast cells that, having been attracted to a site of laminin α chain degradation, are able to produce laminin β chains, type IV collagen, and heparan sulfate proteoglycan.[87]

Laminin and its complex with entactin play an important modulatory role in angiogenesis in a dose-dependent manner, with low concentrations stimulating and high concentrations inhibiting. These effects suggest that the basement membrane is a dynamic regulator of angiogenesis whose function varies according to the concentration of its molecular components and on the presence of additional factors, such as bFGF.[138]

Link

Link is a protein isolated from cartilage that stabilizes the interactions of the NH_2 terminus of aggrecan with hyaluronan. The structure of link shows similarities to CD44. Link is not restricted to cartilaginous structures but has also been found in the embryonic chick mesonephros.[139]

Osteocalcin

The proteins in the organic matrix of bone are many, including those made by bone (type I collagen, alkaline phosphatase, SPARC, biglycan, decorin, osteocalcin, and osteopontin) and others (α_2–heparan sulfate–glycoprotein, TGF-β, PDGF, insulin-like growth factor [IGF-1], FGF-α, FGF-β, and interleukin-1 [IL-1]), which are synthesized elsewhere and which bind secondarily to the bone matrix. Osteocalcin is seemingly a specific bone cell product and is one of the few matrix proteins that contains a high content of gamma-carboxyglutamic acid (GLA). Osteocalcin can be detected in the circulation and is associated with an increased risk for osteoporosis and hip fracture.[140, 141]

Interestingly, although osteocalcin is relatively restricted to bone, its release from bone fragments does not stimulate mononuclear cells to release IL-1 and is likely not to play a role in the increased IL-1 secretion by circulating monocytes in patients with high turnover osteoporosis. Rather, it appears that the collagen from bone fragments, detected by integrin receptors on the monocytes, is responsible for IL-1 release.[142]

Osteopontin

Osteopontin, originally called *bone sialoprotein*, is an acidic glycoprotein that is prominent in bone and teeth, but it is also found in other connective tissues.[143] It binds to both an integrin receptor and the inorganic hydroxyapatite in the mineral phase of bone. Its synthesis is increased by both TGF-β and 1,25-dihydroxyvitamin D_3. Osteoclast adherence to bone and its subsequent resorption of bone stem from interactions between osteopontin or bone sialoprotein and an integrin receptor.[144] The tartrate-resistant acid phosphatase (TRAP) of osteoclasts dephosphorylates osteopontin and bone sialoprotein, reducing osteoclast binding.[145] An interesting feature of osteopontin is the presence of a thrombin-cleavage site close to its integrin-binding site. Cell attachment and spreading are increased on thrombin-cleaved osteopontin, possibly through exposure of the integrin-binding site.[146]

Perlecan

Perlecan is the major heparan sulfate proteoglycan of basement membranes. It has a modular structure with domains homologous to the LDL receptor, laminin, EGF, and NCAM. At the carboxy terminus are three glycosaminoglycan (GAG) chains of the heparan sulfate type.[147] Perlecan plays an integral role in the structure of basement membranes.[27] As a structural element, it plays a major charge-dependent sieving function in the basement membrane. It interacts with itself, through its protein core and GAG chains, and with type IV collagen, laminin, basic FGF (bFGF), and extracellular superoxide dismutase C.

The glycosaminoglycan chains of heparin and heparan sulfate can serve as potent signals if released by endoglycosidases. In addition to known effects on hemostasis, the fragments of these GAG chains can dampen the stimulus to replication of smooth muscle cells that have been subjected to stimulation by PDGF. Regulation of bFGF-stimulated vascular smooth muscle cell proliferation, by vascular cell-secreted heparin-like compounds, correlates with inhibition of bFGF binding to cell-associated heparin sulfate proteoglycans.[90] Endothelial cells bind to perlecan via the core protein, but in a manner influenced by the GAG chains[148]; hematopoeitic cells in the bone marrow do not adhere to perlecan but are possibly dependent on its ligand functions for granulocyte-macrophage colony-stimulating factor (GM-CSF).[149]

Direct relationships between perlecan production, amyloid formation, and Alzheimer's disease have been demonstrated.[150] Perlecan, laminin, and type IV collagen are synthesized at sites of amyloid deposition before amyloid fibrils form. The polymerized perlecan induces serum amyloid A (SAA) protein to assume a beta-pleated sheet structure. Administration of low-molecular-weight anionic sulfate or sulfonate compounds apparently competes with the perlecan-SAA interactions with reduction of splenic AA amyloid progression in a murine model.[151]

Serglycin

All types of hematopoeitic cells produce a secretory form of proteoglycans. The best known of these is serglycin, so named because of the frequent sequences Ser-Gly, consensus sequences for O-linkage of GAG chains. Serglycin is produced by all types of hematopoeitic cells in both a regulated and a constitutive fashion, including mast cells, basophils, T lymphocytes, and natural killer cells.

Serglycin is a proteinase-resistant proteoglycan that stores and protects a variety of agonists with which it is copackaged. The serglycin protein core is highly glycosylated by a variety of GAG chains, and this secretory, fluid phase matrix component has been implicated in the regulation of inflammation, immune responses, and coagulation of blood. In circulating cells, such as mast cells, platelets, and natural killer cells, there is evidence that serglycin is complexed with cationic proteins and pharmacologic amines, such as histamine, complexes that show variable sensitivities to environmental conditions (e.g., pH and counter ions). Presumably, the interactions of serglycin with these agonists, both within the cell and after discharge into the matrix, represent a means for regulating the release and rates of degradation of bioactive reagents.

SPARC

SPARC, a *s*ecreted *p*rotein *a*cidic *r*ich in *c*ysteine, is also called *osteonectin* and BM-40. It is a solid phase, fluid phase, and cell surface phase matrix glycoprotein found in bone, serum, and basement membrane. It is present in platelets and is released by collagen or thrombin from platelets in a dose-dependent manner. SPARC is also present on the platelet cell surface. The platelet form of SPARC appears to be larger than that found in bone.

In vitro, SPARC induces cell rounding, as do thrombospondin and tenascin, and all three thus can act to inhibit cell spreading. SPARC interacts with collagen types III and V and with thrombospondin. The affinities of SPARC for the matrix are calcium-dependent and act in concert with other regions of the molecule to inhibit cellular spreading. Endothelial cells, for example, do not adhere to type III collagen gels that contain SPARC. Cell shape influences might also be operating in the Leydig and Sertoli cells in the testis. SPARC is released from endothelial cells during injury, which results in a rounded cell morphologic appearance and in gaps between the cells. If the cell's F-actin is stabilized with phallicidin prior to injury, this effect is not apparent, which suggests that SPARC regulates endothelial barrier function through F-actin–dependent changes in cell shape.[152]

When SPARC is added to cells in culture, the effects on cell anchorage and migration are not inhibited by the RGD peptide. The biologic effects of SPARC depend on calcium binding at both NH_2 and COOH terminal "E-F" hand modules. The 90-kD protein contains a high percentage of cysteine, and there is high homology among SPARC proteins obtained from various species.

Syndecan

The syndecans are a family of integral membrane cell surface proteoglycans that are found primarily on epithelial cells but also transiently on mesenchyme at sites of epithelial-mesenchymal interactions. At present, four different syndecans have been described, and the nomenclature (as syndecan-1 to syndecan-4) should presumably replace a variety of names that have emerged (e.g., ryudocan, amphiglycan) for various members. The syndecans associate extracellularly through their ectodomain with various matrix molecules and growth factors and intracellularly through their cytoplasmic domain with the actin cytoskeleton.[153]

The principal glycosaminoglycan chain linked to the syndecans is heparan sulfate. Syndecan-1 on mouse mammary epithelial cells shows preferential increase in chondroitin sulfate when treated with TGF-β, and syndecan-1 on the vaginal epithelium of the mouse is significantly modulated by either endogenous or exogenous estrogens and progesterones.[154]

Syndecans act as matrix receptors binding to most components of the interstitial matrix, including collagen types I, III, and V; fibronectin; thrombospondin; and tenascin in a calcium-independent manner. Syndecan is shed from the cell surface when the cells round up; conversely, epithelial cells made syndecan-deficient assume a mesenchymal morphologic ap-

pearance. In the adult mouse, syndecan is distributed predominantly on the surface of epithelial cells in various patterns, depending on the tissue of origin. Syndecan is not present on stromal cells in the adult mouse except for plasma cells and Leydig cells; however, it is transiently expressed on mesenchyme in embryonic tissues during epithelial-mesenchymal interactions in the tooth and limb. Syndecan is expressed on the surface of plasma cells, initially when present as pre-B cells in the marrow but not when circulating in the blood, and then again when present in such tissues as the lymph nodes and spleen.[22]

A major function of the syndecans is as a co-receptor; the syndecan presents bound ligands to adjacent receptors that possess higher ligand specificity or signaling capacities. This seems to be the case with bFGF, fibronectin, and antithrombin III in their interactions with the syndecans, which is analogous to the case for the interactions of TGF-β with betaglycan. A precedent for this kind of function exists in the multiple steps in antigen presentation and processing that occur in the immune system and in the various binding steps and effectors of the cytokines.

Tenascin

Tenascin is a large matrix glycoprotein that is prominent in states of high tissue remodeling and morphogenesis. Tenascin was originally described at the myotendinous junction, where it appears to play an important biomechanical function linking the muscle cell surface to the tendon. The binding of tenascin to fibronectin has been questioned, but recent studies indicate a weak affinity, which is sufficient to block cell binding and migration on fibronectin. This effect of tenascin is probably based on its capacity to block or mask either the fibronectin or its receptors.

A review of Figure 3–2 demonstrates that the large extended configuration of tenascin may have significant, nonspecific effects, not only on fibronectin-cell surface interactions but also on other ligand-receptor interactions. In the developing chick limb, a tenascin-rich sheet that extends from the ectodermal basement membrane to the proximally located muscle anlage has been identified. This sheet lies in the position where tendons form, and it may represent a template that influences the spatial organization of the tendons during their development.[155]

Thrombomodulin

Thrombomodulin is an integral membrane protein on the endothelial cell surface and a part-time proteoglycan. Thrombomodulin influences coagulation by acting as a cofactor for thrombin-induced protein C activation; by altering the procoagulant activity of thrombin; and by accelerating antithrombin III inhibition of thrombin. These activities are significantly influenced by the presence or absence of the solitary chondroitin sulfate chain.[156] Transcriptional down-regulation of thrombomodulin occurs when cultured endothelial cells are exposed to cytokines; up-regulation occurs after exposure to retinoic acid and dibutyryl cyclic adenosine monophosphate (cAMP).[157]

Thrombospondin

Thrombospondin is a family of glycoproteins of three identical disulfide-bonded subunits, a constituent of platelet α-granules and the product of a variety of cells. Thrombospondin binds to cell surfaces and becomes incorporated into the extracellular matrix, where it exerts a broad spectrum of activities ranging from activation of TGF-β[158] to inhibition of enzymes, such as plasmin and neutrophil elastase.[52] It forms specific complexes with active TGF-β in platelet releasate and activates endogenous latent TGF-β secreted by endothelial cells; this indicates that thrombospondin is a regulatory factor in the control of TGF-β activity.[159] Thrombospondin influences platelet aggregation, fibrin formation and lysis, cell adhesion and migration, and cell proliferation.[160] It specifically promotes neutrophil adhesion and migration and monocyte recruitment at sites of injury.[161] Thrombospondin is also an antiadhesive, in that it can cause a loss of focal adhesion plaques from spread endothelial cells and fibroblasts.[162]

Vitronectin

Vitronectin (VN), also known as serum spreading factor, complement S protein, or epibolin, is an adhesive glycoprotein that interacts with complement, coagulation, fibrinolytic and immunologic components as well as cells and platelets.[18] The non-plasma form of vitronectin, abundant in platelets and subendothelium, assumes the conformation of the heparin binding form. By assuming different conformations, vitronectin exposes unique multivalent properties and unique functions.[163] Many of the interactions of vitronectin with complement derivatives C7, C8, and C9 occur via this heparin-binding domain near the COOH terminus. Vitronectin also binds to collagens and elastins, but it does not bind to laminin or fibronectin. Vitronectin interacts with the integrin class receptors through an RGD consensus sequence, and vitronectin receptor also has specificity for osteopontin.[164] Cross-linked multimers of vitronectin can be generated by a transgluaminase, and the alignment of the vitronectin monomers during this cross-linking is facilitated by their interaction with GAG. The cross-linked forms of vitronectin retain binding affinities to heparin, platelets, and plasminogen activator inhibitor type-1 (PAI-1).[165]

References

1. Carey DJ: Control of growth and differentiation of vascular cells by extracellular matrix proteins. Annu Rev Physiol 53:161, 1991.
2. Jackson RL, Busch SJ, Cardin AD: Glycosaminoglycans: Molecular properties, protein interactions and role in physiological processes. Physiol Rev 71:481, 1991.
3. Martini R: Expression and functional roles of neural cell surface molecules and extracellular matrix components during development and regeneration of peripheral nerves. J Neurocytol 23:1, 1994.
4. Ruoslahti E: Control of cell motility and tumour invasion by extracellular matrix interactions. Br J Cancer 66:239, 1992.
5. Burgeson RE, Nimni ME: Collagen types: Molecular structure and tissue distribution: Clin Orthop 282:250, 1992.
6. David G: Integral membrane heparan sulfate proteoglycans. FASEB J 7:1023, 1993.
7. Erickson HP: Tenascin-C, tenascin-R and tenascin-X: a family of talented proteins in search of functions. Curr Opin Cell Biol 5:869, 1993.
8. Mayne R, Brewton RG: New members of the collagen superfamily. Curr Opin Cell Biol 5:883, 1993.
9. Rosenbloom J, Abrams WR, Mecham R: Extracellular matrix 4: The elastic fiber. FASEB J 7:1208, 1993.
10. Timpl R, Brown JC: The laminins. Matrix Biol 14:275, 1994.
11. Van der Rest M, Garrone R: Collagen family of proteins. FASEB J 5:2814, 1991.
12. Juliano RL, Haskill S: Signal transduction from the extracellular matrix. J Cell Biol 120:577, 1993.
13. Tanaka Y, Adams DH, Shaw S: Proteoglycans on endothelial cells present adhesion-inducing cytokines to leukocytes. Immunol Today 14:111, 1993.
14. Yamagata M, Saga S, Kato M, Bernfield M, Kimata K: Selective distributions of proteoglycans and their ligands in pericellular matrix of cultured fibroblasts: Implications for their roles in cell-substratum adhesion. J Cell Sci 106:55, 1993.
15. Yurchenco PD, Birk DE, Mecham RP (eds): Extracellular Matrix Assembly and Structure. San Diego, Academic Press, 1994.
16. Hynes RO: Fibronectins. New York, Springer-Verlag, 1990.
17. Poole AR, Ionescu M, Swan A, Dieppe PA: Changes in cartilage metabolism in arthritis are reflected by altered serum and synovial fluid levels of the cartilage proteoglycan aggrecan: Implications for pathogenesis. J Clin Invest 94:25, 1994.
18. Teschler H, Pohl WR, Thompson AB, Konietzko N, Mosher DF, Costabel U, Rennard SI: Elevated levels of bronchoalveolar lavage vitronectin in hypersensitivity pneumonitis. Am Rev Respir Dis 147:332, 1993.
19. Berg S, Hesselvik JF, Laurent TC: Influence of surgery on serum concentrations of hyaluronan. Crit Care Med 22:810, 1994.
20. Edelstam GA, Lundkvist O, Venge P, Laurent TC: Hyaluronan and myeloperoxidase in human peritoneal fluid during genital inflammation. Inflammation 18:141, 1994.
21. Hynes RO: Integrins: Versatility, modulation, and signaling in cell adhesion. Cell 69:11, 1992.
22. Bernfield M, Kokenyesi R, Kato M, Hinkes MT, Spring J, Gallo RL, Lose EJ: Biology of the syndecans: A family of transmembrane heparan sulfate proteoglycans. Annu Rev Cell Biol 8:365, 1992.
23. Lopez CF, Payne HM, Andres JL, Massague J: Betaglycan can act as a dual modulator of TGF-β access to signaling receptors: Mapping of ligand binding and GAG attachment sites. J Cell Biol 124:557, 1994.
24. Calabro A, Hascall VC: Differential effects of brefeldin A on chondroitin sulfate and hyaluronan synthesis in rat chondrosarcoma cells. J Biol Chem 269:22764, 1994.
25. Lee GM, Johnstone B, Jacobson K, Caterson B: The dynamic structure of the pericellular matrix on living cells. J Cell Biol 123:1899, 1993.
26. Yurchenco PD: Assembly of laminin and type iv collagen into basement membrane networks. In Yurchenco PD, Birk DE, Mecham RP (eds): Extracellular Matrix Assembly and Structure. San Diego, Academic Press, 1994, p 351.
27. Yurchenco PD, O'Rear JJ: Basal lamina assembly. Curr Opin Cell Biol 5:674, 1994.
28. Aumailley M, Battaglia C, Mayer U, Reinhardt D, Nischt R, Timpl R, Fox JW: Nidogen mediates the formation of ternary complexes of basement membrane components. Kidney Int 43:7, 1993.
29. Hagen SG, Michael AF, Butkowski RJ: Immunochemical and biochemical evidence for distinct basement membrane heparan sulfate proteoglycans. J Biol Chem 268:7261, 1993.
30. Noonan DM, Hassell JR: Perlecan, the large low-density proteoglycan of basement membranes: Structure and variant forms. Kidney Int 43:53, 1993.
31. Chan FL, Inoue S, Leblond CP: The basement membranes of cryofixed or aldehyde-fixed, freeze-substituted tissues are composed of a lamina densa and do not contain a lamina lucida. Cell Tissue Res 273:41, 1993.
32. Reinhardt D, Mann K, Nischt R, Fox JW, Chu ML, Krieg T, Timpl R: Mapping of nidogen binding sites for collagen type IV, heparan sulfate proteoglycan, and zinc. J Biol Chem 268:10881, 1993.
33. Vettel U, Brunner G, Bar SR, Vlodavsky I, Kramer MD: Charge-dependent binding of granzyme A (MTSP-1) to basement membranes. Eur J Immunol 23:279, 1993.
34. Streuli CH, Schmidhauser C, Kobrin M, Bissell MJ, Derynck R: Extracel-

lular matrix regulates expression of the TGF-β 1 gene. J Cell Biol 120:253, 1993.

35. Acton S, Resnick D, Freeman M, Ekkel Y, Ashkenas J, Krieger M: The collagenous domains of macrophage scavenger receptors and complement component C1q mediate their similar, but not identical, binding specificities for polyanionic ligands. J Biol Chem 268:3530, 1993.

36. el Khoury J, Thomas CA, Loike JD, Hickman SE, Cao L, Silverstein SC: Macrophages adhere to glucose-modified basement membrane collagen IV via their scavenger receptors. J Biol Chem 269:10197, 1994.

37. Petry F, Reid KB, Loos M: Isolation, sequence analysis and characterization of cDNA clones coding for the C chain of mouse C1q: Sequence similarity of complement subcomponent C1q, collagen type VIII and type X and precerebellin. Eur J Biochem 209:129, 1992.

38. Sastry K, Ezekowitz RA: Collectins: Pattern recognition molecules involved in first line host defense. Curr Opin Immunol 5:59, 1993

39. Colombatti A, Bonaldo P, Doliana R: Type A modules: Interacting domains found in several non-fibrillar collagens and in other extracellular matrix proteins. Matrix 13:297, 1993.

40. Engel J: Common structural motifs in proteins of the extracellular matrix. Curr Opin Cell Biol 3:779, 1991.

41. Hardingham TE, Fosang AJ: Proteoglycans: Many forms and many functions. FASEB J 6:861, 1992.

42. Brewton RG, Wright DW, Mayne R: Structural and functional comparison of type IX collagen-proteoglycan from chicken cartilage and vitreous humor. J Biol Chem 266:4752, 1991.

43. Yamagata M, Yamada KM, Yamada SS, Shinomura T, Tanaka H, Nishida Y, Obara M, Kimata K: The complete primary structure of type XII collagen shows a chimeric molecule with reiterated fibronectin type III motifs, von Willebrand factor A motifs, a domain homologous to a noncollagenous region of type IX collagen, and short collagenous domains with an Arg-Gly-Asp site. J Cell Biol 115:209, 1991.

44. Liebersbach BF, Sanderson RD: Expression of syndecan-1 inhibits cell invasion into type I collagen. J Biol Chem 269:20013, 1994.

45. Myers JC, Yang H, D'Ippolito JA, Presente A, Miller MK, Dion AS: The triple-helical region of human type XIX collagen consists of multiple collagenous subdomains and exhibits limited sequence homology to alpha 1(XVI). J Biol Chem 269:18549, 1994.

46. Glanville RW, Qian RQ, McClure DW, Maslen CL: Calcium binding, hydroxylation, and glycosylation of the precursor epidermal growth factor-like domains of fibrillin-1, the Marfan gene protein. J Biol Chem 269:26630, 1994.

47. Iozzo RV, Kovalszky I, Hacobian N, Schick PK, Ellingson JS, Dodge GR: Fatty acylation of heparan sulfate proteoglycan from human colon carcinoma cells. J Biol Chem 265:19980, 1990.

48. Wu JJ, Woods PE, Eyre DR: Identification of cross-linking sites in bovine cartilage type IX collagen reveals an antiparallel type II–type IX molecular relationship and type IX to type IX bonding. J Biol Chem 267:23007, 1992.

49. Birk DE, Silver FH, Trelstad RL: Matrix assembly. In Hay ED (ed): Cell Biology of Extracellular Matrix. New York, Plenum Press, 1991, p 221.

50. Iwata M, Wight TN, Carlson SS: A brain extracellular matrix proteoglycan forms aggregates with hyaluronan. J Biol Chem 268:15061, 1993.

51. Goetinck P, Winterbottom N: Proteoglycans: Modular macromolecules of the extracellular matrix. In Goldstein L (ed.): Biochemistry and Physiology of the Skin. Oxford, Oxford University Press, 1991.

52. Hogg PJ, Owensby DA, Mosher DF, Misenheimer TM, Chesterman CN: Thrombospondin is a tight-binding competitive inhibitor of neutrophil elastase. J Biol Chem 268:7139, 1993.

53. Lander AD: Proteoglycans in the nervous system. Curr Opin Neurobiol 3:716, 1993.

54. Silbert CK, Humphries DE, Palmer ME, Silbert JE: Effects of sulfate deprivation on the production of chondroitin/dermatan sulfate by cultures of skin fibroblasts from normal and diabetic individuals. Arch Biochem Biophys 285:137, 1991.

55. Ennker IC, Ennker J, Schoon D, Schoon HA, Rimpler M, Hetzer R: Formaldehyde-free collagen glue in experimental lung gluing. Ann Thorac Surg 57:1622, 1994.

56. Morris JE: Proteoglycans and the modulation of cell adhesion by steric exclusion. Dev Dyn 196:246, 1993.

57. Klein S, Giancotti FG, Presta M, Albelda SM, Buck CA, Rifkin DB: Basic fibroblast growth factor modulates integrin expression in microvascular endothelial cells. Mol Biol Cell 4:973, 1993.

58. Mette SA, Pilewski J, Buck CA, Albelda SM: Distribution of integrin cell adhesion receptors on normal bronchial epithelial cells and lung cancer cells in vitro and in vivo. Am J Respir Cell Mol Biol 8:562, 1993.

59. Sutherland AE, Calarco PG, Damsky CH: Developmental regulation of integrin expression at the time of implantation in the mouse embryo. Development 119:1175, 1993.

60. Chen D, Magnuson V, Hill S, Arnaud C, Steffensen B, Klebe RJ: Regulation of integrin gene expression by substrate adherence. J Biol Chem 267:23502, 1992.

61. Handagama P, Bainton DF, Jacques Y, Conn MT, Lazarus RA, Shuman MA: Kistrin, an integrin antagonist, blocks endocytosis of fibrinogen into guinea pig megakaryocyte and platelet alpha-granules. J Clin Invest 91:193, 1993.

62. Sheppard D, Cohen DS, Wang A, Busk M: Transforming growth factor-β differentially regulates expression of integrin subunits in guinea pig airway epithelial cells. J Biol Chem 267:17409, 1992.

63. Zhang Z, Tarone G, Turner DC: Expression of integrin alpha-1 beta-1 is regulated by nerve growth factor and dexamethasone in PC12 cells: Functional consequences for adhesion and neurite outgrowth. J Biol Chem 268:5557, 1993.

64. Zhou Y, Damsky CH, Chiu K, Roberts JM, Fisher SJ: Preeclampsia is associated with abnormal expression of adhesion molecules by invasive cytotrophoblasts. J Clin Invest 91:950, 1993.

65. Patti JM, Allen BL, McGavin M, Hook M: MSCRAMM-mediated adherence of microorganisms to host tissues. Ann Rev Microbiol 48:585, 1994.

66. Huang LL, Wu JH, Nimni ME: Effects of hyaluronan on collagen fibrillar matrix contraction by fibroblasts. J Biomed Mater Res 28:123, 1994.

67. Petite H, Frei V, Huc A, Herbage D: Use of diphenylphosphorylazide for cross-linking collagen-based biomaterials. J Biomed Mater Res 28:159, 1994.

68. Rao JK, Ramesh DV, Rao KP: Implantable controlled delivery systems for proteins based on collagen—pHEMA hydrogels. Biomaterials 15:383, 1994.

69. Nettelbladt O, Bergh J, Schenholm M, Tengblad A, Hallgren R: Accumulation of hyaluronic acid in the alveolar interstitial tissue in bleomycin-induced alveolitis. Am Rev Respir Dis 139:759, 1989.

70. Valeyre D, Soler P, Basset G, Loiseau P, Pre J, Turbie P, Battesti JP, Georges R: Glucose, K⁺, and albumin concentrations in the alveolar milieu of normal humans and pulmonary sarcoidosis patients. Am Rev Respir Dis 143:1096, 1991.

71. Koide H, Hayashi T(eds): Extracellular Matrix in the Kidney. Basel, Karger, 1994.

72. Benezra M, Vlodavsky I, Ishai MR, Neufeld G, Bar SR: Thrombin-induced release of active basic fibroblast growth factor-heparan sulfate complexes from subendothelial extracellular matrix. Blood 81:3324, 1993.

73. Kato S, Ishii T, Hara H, Sugiura N, Kimata K, Akamatsu N: Hepatocyte growth factor immobilized onto culture substrates through heparin and matrigel enhances DNA synthesis in primary rat hepatocytes. Exp Cell Res 211:53, 1994.

74. Upchurch HF, Conway E, Patterson MJ, Maxwell MD: Localization of cellular transglutaminase on the extracellular matrix after wounding: Characteristics of the matrix bound enzyme. J Cell Physiol 149:375, 1991.

75. Witt DP, Lander AD: Differential binding of chemokines to glycosaminoglcyan subpopulations. Curr Biol 4:394, 1994.

76. Taipale J, Miyazona K, Heldin C-H, Keski-Oja J: Latent transforming growth factor-β1 associates to fibroblast extracellular matrix via latent TGF-β binding protein. J Cell Biol 124:171, 1994.

77. Aviezer D, Levy E, Safran M, Svahn C, Buddecke E, Schmidt A, David G, Vlodavsky I, Yayon A: Differential structural requirements of heparin and heparan sulfate proteoglycans that promote binding of basic fibroblast growth factor to its receptor. J Biol Chem 269:114, 1994.

78. Kato M, Wang H, Bernfield M, Gallagher JT, Turnbull JE: Cell surface syndecan-1 on distinct cell types differs in fine structure and ligand binding of its heparan sulfate chains. J Biol Chem 269:18881, 1994.

79. Bourguignon LY, Lokeshwar VB, He J, Chen X, Bourguignon GJ: A CD44-like endothelial cell transmembrane glycoprotein (GP116) interacts with extracellular matrix and ankyrin. Mol Cell Biol 12:4464, 1992.

80. Carey DJ, Stahl RC, Asundi VK, Tucker B: Processing and subcellular distribution of the Schwann cell lipid-anchored heparan sulfate proteoglycan and identification as glypican. Exp Cell Res 208:10, 1993.

81. Brunner G, Metz CN, Nguyen H, Gabrilove J, Patel SR, Davitz MA, Rifkin DB, Wilson EL: An endogenous glycosylphosphatidylinositol-specific phospholipase D releases basic fibroblast growth factor–heparan sulfate proteoglycan complexes from human bone marrow cultures. Blood 83:2115, 1994.

82. Hay ED: Extracellular matrix alters epithelial differentiation. Curr Opin Cell Biol 5:1029, 1993.

83. Howlett AR, Bissell MJ: The influence of tissue microenvironment (stroma and extracellular matrix) on the development and function of mammary epithelium. Epithelial Cell Biol 2:79, 1993.

84. Hershkoviz R, Gilat D, Miron S, Mekori YA, Aderka D, Wallach D, Vlodavsky I, Cohen IR, Lider O: Extracellular matrix induces tumour necrosis factor-α secretion by an interaction between resting rat CD4⁺ T cells and macrophages. Immunology 78:50, 1993.

85. Jones PL, Schmidhauser C, Bissell MJ: Regulation of gene expression and cell function by extracellular matrix. Crit Rev Eukaryot Gene Expr 3:137, 1993.

86. Hermann M, Jaconi ME, Dahlgren C, Waldvogel FA, Stendahl O, Lew DP: Neutrophil bactericidal activity against Staphylococcus aureus adherent on biological surfaces: Surface-bound extracellular matrix proteins activate intracellular killing by oxygen-dependent and -independent mechanisms. J Clin Invest 86:942, 1990.

87. Thompson HL, Thomas L, Metcalfe DD: Murine mast cells attach to and migrate on laminin-, fibronectin-, and matrigel-coated surfaces in response to Fc-ε RI-mediated signals. Clin Exp Allergy 23:270, 1993.

88. Lessey BA, Castelbaum AJ, Buck CA, Lei Y, Yowell CW, Sun J: Further characterization of endometrial integrins during the menstrual cycle and in pregnancy. Fertil Steril 62:497, 1994.

89. Pfaff M, Aumailley M, Specks U, Knolle J, Zerwes HG, Timpl R: Integrin and Arg-Gly-Asp dependence of cell adhesion to the native and unfolded triple helix of collagen type VI. Exp Cell Res 206:167, 1993.

90. Nugent MA, Karnovsky MJ, Edelman ER: Vascular cell-derived heparan sulfate shows coupled inhibition of basic fibroblast growth factor binding and mitogenesis in vascular smooth muscle cells. Circ Res 73:1051, 1993.

91. Ekblom P, Ekblom M, Fecker L, Klein G, Zhang HY, Kadoya Y, Chu ML, Mayer U, Timpl R: Role of mesenchymal nidogen for epithelial morphogenesis in vitro. Development 120:2003, 1994.

92. Zhang HY, Kluge M, Timpl R, Chu ML, Ekblom P: The extracellular matrix glycoproteins BM-90 and tenascin are expressed in the mesenchyme at sites of endothelial-mesenchymal conversion in the embryonic mouse heart. Differentiation 52:211, 1993.

93. Reiser KM, Amigable MA, Last JA: Nonenzymatic glycation of type I collagen: The effects of aging on preferential glycation sites. J Biol Chem 267:24207, 1992.

94. Kato Y, Uchida K, Kawakishi S: Oxidative fragmentation of collagen and prolyl peptide by Cu(II)/H2O2: Conversion of proline residue to 2-pyrrolidone. J Biol Chem 267:23646, 1992.

95. Hausser H, Witt O, Kresse H: Influence of membrane-associated heparan sulfate on the internalization of the small proteoglycan decorin. Exp Cell Res 208:398, 1993.

96. McMahan UJ, Horton SE, Werle MJ, Honig LS, Kroger S, Ruegg MA, Escher G: Agrin isoforms and their role in synaptogenesis. Curr Opin Cell Biol 4:869, 1992.

97. Jennings CG, Burden SJ: Development of the neuromuscular synapse. Curr Opin Neurobiol 3:75, 1993.

98. Ferns M, Hoch W, Campanelli JT, Rupp F, Hall ZW, Scheller RH: RNA splicing regulates agrin-mediated acetylcholine receptor clustering activity on cultured myotubes. Neuron 8:1079, 1992.

99. Patthy L, Nikolics K: Functions of agrin and agrin-related proteins. Trends Neurosci 16:76, 1993.

100. Gee SH, Montanaro F, Lindenbaum MH, Carbonetto S: Dystroglycan-alpha, a dystrophin-associated glycoprotein, is a functional agrin receptor. Cell 77:675, 1994.

101. Sugiyama J, Bowen DC, Hall ZW: Dystroglycan binds nerve and muscle agrin. Neuron 13:103, 1994.

102. Roughley PJ, Lee ER: Cartilage proteoglycans: Structure and potential functions. Microsc Res Techn 28:385, 1994.

103. Watanabe H, Kimata K, Line S, Strong D, Gao LY, Kozak CA, Yamada Y: Mouse cartilage matrix deficiency (cmd) caused by a 7 bp deletion in the aggrecan gene. Nature Genet 7:154, 1994.

104. Buckwalter JA, Roughley PJ, Rosenberg LC: Age-related changes in cartilage proteoglycans: Quantitative electron microscopic studies. Microsc Res Tech 28:398, 1994.

105. Hardingham TE, Fosang AJ, Dudhia J: The structure, function and turnover of aggrecan, the large aggregating proteoglycan from cartilage. Eur J Clin Chem Clin Biochem 32:249, 1994.

106. Fukushima D, Butzow R, Hildebrand A, Ruoslahti E: Localization of transforming growth factor-β binding site in betaglycan: Comparison with small extracellular matrix proteoglycans. J Biol Chem 268:22710, 1993.

107. Funderburgh JL, Funderburgh ML, Brown SJ, Vergnes JP, Hassell JR, Mann MM, Conrad GW: Sequence and structural implications of a bovine corneal keratan sulfate proteoglycan core protein: Protein 37B represents bovine lumican and proteins 37A and 25 are unique. J Biol Chem 268:11874, 1993.

108. Walker A, Turnbull JE, Gallagher JT: Binding of fibromodulin and decorin to separate sites on fibrillar collagens. J Biol Chem 268:27307, 1993.

109. Hildebrand A, Romaris M, Rasmussen LM, Heinegard D, Twardzik DR, Border WA, Ruoslahti E: Interaction of the small interstitial proteoglycans biglycan, decorin and fibromodulin with transforming growth factor beta. Biochem 302:527, 1994.

110. Whinna HC, Choi HU, Rosenberg LC, Church FC: Interaction of heparin cofactor II with biglycan and decorin. J Biol Chem 268:3920, 1993.

111. Yamada H, Watanabe K, Shimonaka M, Yamaguchi Y: Molecular cloning of brevican, a novel brain proteoglycan of the aggrecan/versican family. J Biol Chem 269:10119, 1994.

112. Friedlander DR, Milev P, Karthikeyan L, Margolis RK, Margolis RU, Grumet M: The neuronal chondroitin sulfate proteoglycan neurocan binds to the neural cell adhesion molecules Ng-CAM/L1/NILE and N-CAM, and inhibits neuronal adhesion and neurite outgrowth. J Cell Biol 125:669, 1994.

113. Maurel P, Rauch U, Flad M, Margolis RK, Margolis RU: Phosphacan, a chondroitin sulfate proteoglycan of brain that interacts with neurons and neural cell adhesion molecules, is an extracellular variant of a receptor-type protein tyrosine phosphatase. Proc Natl Acad Sci USA 91:2512, 1994.

114. Milev P, Friedlander DR, Sakurai T, Karthikeyan L, Flad M, Margolis RK, Grumet M, Margolis RU: Interactions of the chondroitin sulfate proteoglycan phosphacan, the extracellular domain of a receptor-type tyrosine phosphatase with neurons, glia and neural cell adhesion molecules. J Cell Biol 127:1703, 1994.

115. Grumet M, Milev P, Sakurai T, Karthikeyan L, Bourdon M, Margolis RK, Margolis RU: Interactions with tenascin and differential effects on cell adhesion of neurocan and phosphacan, two major chondroitin sulfate proteoglycans of nervous tissue. J Biol Chem 269:12142, 1994.

116. Lesley J, Hyman R, Kincade PW: CD44 and its interaction with the cellular matrix. Adv Immunol 54:271, 1993.

117. Underhill CB, Nguyen HA, Shizari M, Culty M: CD44 positive macrophages take up hyaluronan during lung development. Dev Biol 155:324, 1993.

118. Knudson W, Bartnik E, Knudson CB: Assembly of pericellular matrices by COS-7 cells transfected with CD44 lymphocyte-homing receptor genes. Proc Natl Acad Sci USA 90:4003, 1993.

119. Sherman L, Sleeman J, Herrlich P, Ponta H: Hyaluronate receptors: Key players in growth, differentiation, migration and tumor progression. Curr Opin Cell Biol 6:726, 1994.

120. Hauser N, Paulsson M: Native cartilage matrix protein (CMP): A compact trimer of subunits assembled via a coiled-coil alpha-helix. J Biol Chem 269:25747, 1994.

121. Mecham RP, Davis EC: Elastic fiber structure and assembly. In Yurchenco PD, Birk DE, Mecham RP (eds): Extracellular Matrix Assembly and Structure. San Diego, Academic Press, 1994, p 281.

122. Zhang H, Apfelroth SD, Hu W, Davis EC, Sanguineti C, Bonadio J, Mecham RP, Ramirez F: Structure and expression of fibrillin-2, a novel microfibrillar component preferentially located in elastic matrices. J Cell Biol 124:855, 1994.

123. Mayer U, Timpl R: Nidogen: A versatile binding protein of basement membranes. In Yurchenco PD, Birk DE, Mecham RP (eds): Extracellular Matrix Assembly and Structure. San Diego, Academic Press, 1994, p 389.

124. Anwar AR, Walsh GM, Cromwell O, Kay AB, Wardlaw AJ: Adhesion to fibronectin primes eosinophils via alpha-4 beta-1 (VLA-4). Immunology 82:222, 1994.

125. Klotz SA, Hein RC, Smith RL, Rouse JB: The fibronectin adhesin of Candida albicans. Infect Immun 62:4679, 1994.

126. Sipes JM, Guo N, Negre E, Vogel T, Krutzsch HC, Roberts DD: Inhibition of fibronectin binding and fibronectin-mediated cell adhesion to collagen by a peptide from the second type I repeat of thrombospondin. J Cell Biol 121:469, 1993.

127. Barkalow FJ, Schwarzbauer JE: Interactions between fibronectin and chondroitin sulfate are modulated by molecular context. J Biol Chem 269:3957, 1994.

128. Piepkorn M, Lo C, Plowman G: Amphiregulin-dependent proliferation of cultured human keratinocytes: Autocrine growth, the effects of exogenous recombinant cytokine, and apparent requirement for heparin-like glycosaminoglycans. J Cell Physiol 159:114, 1994.

129. Platt JL, Trescony P, Lindman B, Oegema TR: Heparin and heparan sulfate delimit nephron formation in fetal metanephric kidneys. Dev Biol 139:338, 1990.

130. Hunter DD, Llinas R, Ard M, Merlie JP, Sanes JR: Expression of S-laminin and laminin in developing rat central nervous system. J Comp Neurol 323:238, 1992.

131. Sheppard AM, Hamilton SK, Pearlman AL: Changes to the distribution of extracellular matrix components accompany early morphogeneic events of mammalian cortical development. J Neurosci 11:3928, 1991.

132. Stipp CS, Litwack ED, Lander AD: Cerebroglycan: An integral membrane heparan sulfate proteoglycan that is unique to the developing nervous system and expressed specifically during neuronal differentiation. J Cell Biol 124:149, 1994.

133. Kielty CM, Whittaker SP, Grant ME, Shuttleworth CA: Type VI collagen microfibrils: Evidence for a structural association with hyaluronan. J Cell Biol 118:979, 1992.

134. Grinblat Y, Zusman S, Yee G, Hynes RO, Kafatos FC: Functions of the cytoplasmic domain of the beta PS integrin subunit during Drosophila development. Development 120:91, 1994.

135. Burgeson RE, Chiquet M, Deutzmann R, Ekblom R, Engel J, Kleinman H, Martin GR, Meneguzzi G, Paulsson M, Sanes J, Timpl R, Tryggvason K, Yurchenco PD: A new nomenclature for laminins. Matrix Biol 5:209, 1994.

136. Sung U, O'Rear JJ, Yurchenco PD: Cell and heparin binding in the distal long arm of laminin: Identification of active and cryptic sites with recombinant and hybrid glycoprotein. J Cell Biol 123:1255, 1993.

137. De Rosa G, Barra E, Guarino M, Staibano S, Donofrio V, Boscaino A: Fibronectin, laminin, type IV collagen distribution, and myofibroblastic stromal reaction in aggressive and nonaggressive basal cell carcinoma. Am J Dermatopathol 16:258, 1994.

138. Nicosia RF, Bonanno E, Smith M, Yurchenco P: Modulation of angiogenesis in vitro by laminin-entactin complex. Dev Biol 164:197, 1994.

139. Binette F, Cravens J, Kahoussi B, Haudenschild DR, Goetinck PF: Link protein is ubiquitously expressed in non-cartilaginous tissues where it enhances and stabilizes the interaction of proteoglycans with hyaluronic acid. J Biol Chem 269:19116, 1994.

140. Ingram RT, Park YK, Clarke BL, Fitzpatrick LA: Age- and gender-related changes in the distribution of osteocalcin in the extracellular matrix of normal male and female bone: Possible involvement of osteocalcin in bone remodeling. J Clin Invest 93:989, 1994.

141. Szulc P, Chapuy MC, Meunier PJ, Delmas PD: Serum undercarboxylated osteocalcin is a marker of the risk of hip fracture in elderly women. J Clin Invest 91:1769, 1993.

142. Pacifici R, Carano A, Santoro SA, Rifas L, Jeffrey JJ, Malone JD, McCracken R, Avioli LV: Bone matrix constituents stimulate interleukin-1 release from human blood mononuclear cells. J Clin Invest 87:221, 1991.

143. Denhardt DT, Guo X: Osteopontin: A protein with diverse functions. FASEB J 7:1475, 1993.

144. Kato M, Wang H, Bernfield M, Gallagher JT, Turnbull JE: Interactions between the bone matrix proteins osteopontin and bone sialoprotein and the osteoclast integrin $\alpha_5\beta_3$ potentiate bone resorption. J Biol Chem 268:9901, 1993.

145. Binette F, Cravens J, Kahoussi B, Haudenschild DR, Goetinck PF: Dephosphorylation of osteopontin and bone sialoprotein by osteoclastic tartrate-resistant acid phosphatase: Modulation of osteoclast adhesion in vitro. J Biol Chem 269:14853, 1994.

146. Senger DR, Perruzzi CA, Papadopoulos SA, Van de Water L: Adhesive properties of osteopontin: Regulation by a naturally occurring thrombin-cleavage in close proximity to the GRGDS cell-binding domain. Mol Biol Cell 5:565, 1994.

147. Iozzo RV: Perlecan: A gem of a proteoglycan. Matrix Biol 14:203, 1994.

148. Hayashi K, Madri JA, Yurchenco PD: Endothelial cells interact with the core protein of basement membrane perlecan through b1 and b3 integrins: An adhesion modulated by glycosaminoglycan. J Cell Biol 119:945, 1992.

149. Klein G, Conzelmann S, Beck S, Timpl R, Muller CA: Perlecan in human bone marrow: A growth-factor-presenting, but anti-adhesive, extracellular matrix component for hematopoietic cells. Matrix Biol 14:457, 1995.

150. Jucker M, Ingram DK: Age-related fibrillar material in mouse brain: Assessing its potential as a biomarker of aging and as a model of human neurodegenerative disease. Ann N Y Acad Sci 719:238, 1994.

151. Kisilevsky R, Lemieux LJ, Fraser PF, Kong X, Hultin PG, Szarek WA: Arresting amyloidosis in vivo using small-molecule anionic sulphonates or sulphates: Implications for Alzheimer's disease. Nature Med 1:143, 1995.

152. Goldblum SE, Ding X, Funk SE, Sage EH: SPARC (secreted protein acidic and rich in cysteine) regulates endothelial cell shape and barrier function. Proc Natl Acad Sci USA 91:3448, 1994.

153. Hinkes MT, Goldberger OA, Neumann PE, Kokenyesi R, Bernfield M: Organization and promoter activity of the mouse syndecan-1 gene. J Biol Chem 268:11440, 1993.

154. Hayashi K, Hayashi M, Boutin E, Cunha GR, Bernfield M, Trelstad RL: Hormonal modification of epithelial differentiation and expression of cell surface heparan sulfate proteoglycan in the mouse vaginal epithelium: An immunohistochemical and electron microscopic study. Lab Invest 58:68, 1988.

155. Hurle JM, Ros MA, Ganan Y, Macias D, Critchlow M, Hinchliffe JR: Experimental analysis of the role of ECM in the patterning of the distal tendons of the developing limb bud. Cell Differ Dev 30:97, 1990.

156. Liu LW, Rezaie AR, Carson CW, Esmon NL, Esmon CT: Occupancy of anion binding exosite 2 on thrombin determines Ca^{2+} dependence of protein C activation. J Biol Chem 269:11807, 1994.

157. Conway EM, Liu L, Nowakowski B, Steiner MM, Jackman RW: Heat shock of vascular endothelial cells induces an up-regulatory transcriptional response of the thrombomodulin gene that is delayed in onset and does not attenuate. J Biol Chem 269:22804, 1994.

158. Schultz CS, Murphy UJ: Thrombospondin causes activation of latent transforming growth factor-β secreted by endothelial cells by a novel mechanism. J Cell Biol 122:923, 1993.

159. Schultz CS, Ribeiro S, Gentry L, Murphy UJ: Thrombospondin binds and activates the small and large forms of latent transforming growth factor-β in a chemically defined system. J Biol Chem 269:26775, 1994.

160. Iruela AM, Liska DJ, Sage EH, Bornstein P: Differential expression of thrombospondin 1, 2, and 3 during murine development. Dev Dyn 197:40, 1993.

161. Mansfield PJ, Suchard SJ: Thrombospondin promotes chemotaxis and haptotaxis of human peripheral blood monocytes. J Immunol 153:4219, 1994.

162. Murphy UJ, Gurusiddappa S, Frazier WA, Hook M: Heparin-binding peptides from thrombospondins 1 and 2 contain focal adhesion-labilizing activity. J Biol Chem 268:26784, 1993.

163. Stockmann A, Hess S, Declerck P, Timpl R, Preissner KT: Multimeric vitronectin. Identification and characterization of conformation-dependent self-association of the adhesive protein. J Biol Chem 268:22874, 1993.

164. Seiffert D, Crain K, Wagner NV, Loskutoff DJ: Vitronectin gene expression in vivo: Evidence for extrahepatic synthesis and acute phase regulation. J Biol Chem 269:19836, 1994.

165. Lawrence DA, Berkenpas MB, Palaniappan S, Ginsburg D: Localization of vitronectin binding domain in plasminogen activator inhibitor-1. J Biol Chem 269:15223, 1994.

CHAPTER 4

Clinton T. Rubin
Janet E. Rubin

The Biology, Physiology, and Morphology of Bone

Bone is an extremely complex tissue that regulates its mass and architecture to meet two critical and competing responsibilities: one structural and the other metabolic. In the first case, the skeleton provides a sophisticated framework for the body; it protects vital organs and facilitates locomotion. Second, it serves as a mineral reservoir that contains 99 percent of the body's total calcium, 85 percent of its phosphorus, and 66 percent of its magnesium. It is this dual responsibility that creates conflicting goals and competing stimuli in the regulation of skeletal tissues. Metabolic aberrations, such as hypocalcemia, hyperparathyroidism, endocrinopathy, and aging, put the skeleton's structural integrity at risk to ensure calcium homeostasis. On the other hand, altered functional responsibilities, such as exercise and bed rest, stimulate the skeleton to adapt (i.e., add or remove tissue) to these new mechanical demands. The adaptation presumably occurs to retain a structurally optimized skeleton, yet ignores the potential consequences of rapid fluctuations in serum calcium (e.g. renal lithiasis) or the metabolic burden of producing, retaining, and transporting mineralized tissue. Although metabolic processes may occur independently of the skeleton's structural functions and vice versa, the viability of the organism is critically dependent on an intricate balance between them.

The balance between structural and metabolic responsibilities is achieved via the complex and tightly regulated processes of formation and resorption of bone tissue. Beginning at the level of the cell, this chapter covers local and systemic factors that influence bone turnover, the composition and mineralization of the matrix, the architecture and material properties of the tissue, and the adaptive capacity of the skeleton. This multilevel, multidisciplinary overview is intended to provide the reader with an appreciation of not only the complexity of bone but also its success in meeting its wide-ranging responsibilities. Ultimately, as more is known of the normal biology, physiology, and morphology of bone, an understanding of the pathogenesis and etiology of metabolic bone disease will follow.

THE CELLULAR BASIS OF BONE REMODELING

Bone tissue is a highly specialized, mineralized connective tissue, metabolically active and intrinsically capable of adapting to subtle changes in its functional (i.e., mechanical) environment. Bone's toughness, hardness, and resilience to fatigue belie its appearance as an inert, structural material. The constant modeling and remodeling of the tissue are necessary for repair of scars left by fracture and infection, for the rapid mobilization of mineral as required for metabolic homeostasis, and for the fine adjustment of skeletal mass and morphology to achieve the optimal supporting structure. Indeed, far from inert, bone tissue is the ultimate "smart material."

The skeleton's capacity to adapt to changes in both its functional and metabolic milieu is achieved through its sophisticated network of osteoregulatory cells. The cells of this network—the osteoblasts, osteoclasts, and osteocytes—mediate the remodeling balance of the skeleton as well as provide the cellular machinery necessary for maintenance of calcium homeostasis in the extracellular fluid.

Although it was once believed that a common stem cell ancestry existed for osteoblasts and osteoclasts, it is now understood that these cells derive from distinct precursors. The osteoblast arises from an osteogenic mesenchymal cell[1] that, when surrounded by calcified matrix, terminally differentiates into an osteocyte.[2] The multinucleated osteoclast arises from the fusion of mononuclear precursors of hematopoietic origin.[3] The recruitment and differentiated function of these bone cells are carefully orchestrated systemically by humoral factors and locally by cytokines and physical factors.

Osteoblasts

The primary function of the osteoblasts, which are plump, cuboidal cells, is to synthesize and mineralize the extracellular matrix. Osteoblasts are connected to one another via extended cell processes that are interconnected via gap junctions,[4] establishing a single, continuous blanket of cells on the bone surface (Fig. 4-1). These features help to distinguish osteoblasts from the mesenchymal precursors (pre-osteoblasts), which are also found on bone surfaces, but they are thin and flat rather than plump and cuboidal. Together, these two cell types are known as "bone-lining" cells. Morphologically, the tight canopy of the lining cells enables the selective isolation of the min-

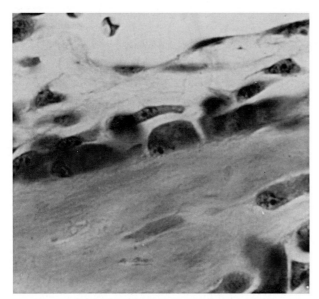

Figure 4–1. Polyhedral osteoblasts lying on the surface of newly formed bone matrix. (Courtesy of Dr. B. Boothroyd.)

formative part of the bone remodeling unit, the "coupling" of formation to resorption.[12]

The osteoblast's principal function is to form bone, first with secretion of the osteoid and then with subsequent nucleation and mineralization of the osteoid matrix. The osteoblast can thus be functionally described by a panel of secretory proteins consisting of type I collagen and several noncollagenous proteins and proteoglycans that are critical to the appropriate orchestration of the remodeling response (Table 4–1). The formation of protocollagen and its processing by the osteoblast, which requires vitamin C,[13] is typified by cross-linking of lysine and proline residues to form procollagen trimers.[14] The processed collagen is organized into parallel fiber sheets of tropocollagen.[15] Within each sheet, or lamellae, the fibers lie parallel to each other[16] whereas the fibril orientation on adjacent lamellae runs in directions distinct from this axis (Fig. 4–2), contributing to the strength of bone, as in the structure of plywood. This structure also facilitates the seeding of hydroxyapatite crystals from a supersaturated extracellular fluid.

eralized surface from the extracellular milieu, which is critical for the site-specific control of mineralization or resorption.[5] The cytoplasmic elements of the osteoblast include abundant endoplasmic reticulum with cisternae, a well-developed Golgi body, and numerous free ribosomes that are responsible for the basophilia seen in sections stained with hematoxylin and eosin.

Induction of osteoblast differentiation is influenced by a number of cell-secreted factors. Urist's identification of a factor in demineralized bone powder which initiated bone formation has led to the cloning and sequencing of at least seven bone morphogenetic proteins (BMPs) belonging to the transforming growth factor-β (TGF-β) family of growth potentiators.[6] These polypeptide factors appear to be important regulators of bone growth and repair through their ability to activate migration of mesenchymal cells and induce osteoblastic differentiation followed by proliferation.[7] BMP-4, for instance, initiates the sequential gene expression of osteopontin and osteocalcin in chondrocytes and osteoblasts.[8] Interestingly, BMP-2 is homologous to *Drosophila* decapentaplegic protein, which directs segmental development of the adult fly[9]; it is likely that several BMPs have primary roles in mammalian skeletal embryogenesis as well. The differential effects of the various BMPs to induce cartilage and bone formation in vivo are currently being examined to determine their potential to accelerate the healing of complex fractures and to improve the rate of allograft and autograft successes.[10]

TGF-β itself is abundant in bone matrix. In vitro cell work has shown that TGF-β has both positive and negative effects on osteoblast proliferation, differentiation, and matrix synthesis.[11] A matrix-bound protein, TGF-β is released during the process of osteoclastic bone resorption, and may serve to initiate the

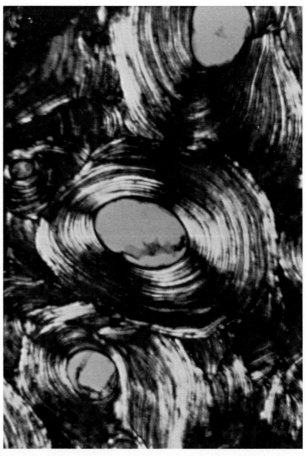

Figure 4–2. Ground section of bone photographed with polarized light showing the concentric lamellar structure of the basic unit of mature bone, the osteon. The central vascular canal (empty in this preparation) is surrounded by multiple lamellae of bone. The adjacent lamellae are composed of collagen bundles with differing orientations, giving rise to alternating light and dark bands in polarized light.

Table 4–1. COMPOSITION OF BONE OSTEOID

Collagen
  Type I, some III, V, XI, XIII
Proteoglycans
  Biglycan, decorin, hyaluronan
Glycoproteins
  Osteonectin, bone sialoprotein, osteopontin, thombospondin,
    fibronectin, gamma carboxyglutamic acid containing
    proteins: osteocalcin, matrix gla protein
Enzymes
  Alkaline phosphatase, collagenase, cysteine proteinases,
    plasminogen activator, tissue inhibitor of
    metalloproteinase
Growth factors
  Fibroblast growth factor, insulin-like growth factor,
    transforming growth factor, bone morphogenetic protein,
    α_2–human serum–glycoprotein
Proteolipids

The noncollagenous proteins entrapped in the bone matrix space, which make up 10 to 15 percent of total bone content, serve several critical roles in the mineralization and maintenance of bone tissue. Many of these proteins are secreted by the osteoblasts and have signaling roles in bone remodeling, such as the suggested role of osteocalcin to recruit osteoclasts,[17] or the plasminogen activator, which initiates the cascade of collagen breakdown.[18] Others, such as osteopontin and bone sialoprotein, strongly bind ionic calcium and may serve as cell attachment factors.[19]

Perhaps the most important humoral factor for maintaining extracellular calcium homeostasis is parathyroid hormone (PTH), which is secreted when the serum calcium level falls below normal. The effects of PTH in bone are complex but are certainly initiated at the level of the osteoblast, which has a membrane receptor for PTH. Continuous treatment with PTH causes inhibition of bone formation, largely through a direct inhibition of bone collagen synthesis. In contrast, intermittent exposure to PTH is anabolic, probably through stimulation of osteoblast proliferation and differentiation, and is being studied as a potential prophylaxis for osteoporosis.[20]

The functional life of the osteoblast varies, depending on the host, from 3 days in young rabbits[21] to reports of the human osteoblast surviving up to 8 weeks.[22] A typical active osteoblast in humans produces a seam of osteoid about 15 mm thick, at a rate of 0.5 to 1.5 μm/day,[23] suggesting the average osteoblast life in humans to be 15 days. Although seams can exceed 70 mm,[24] such a seam width can also indicate a disruption or flaw in the mineralization process (e.g., rickets or osteomalacia).

As mineralization proceeds, the osteoblast may become engulfed in its own calcifying osteoid matrix.[25] Osteoblasts remaining behind in small lacunae retain connections with other similarly disposed cells, creating the osteocyte network.

Osteocytes

Osteocytes, once considered irrelevant by-products of the mineralization process, are now recognized as essential to the metabolic regulation of bone tissue. Although the sequestered osteoblast has lost size and organelles, in its new phenotype it is connected to other osteocytes and bone-lining cells through cytoplasmic extensions that pass through a network of catacombs radiating outward from the central vascular canal (Fig. 4–3). These interconnecting canaliculi are ideal pathways for chemical, electrical, and stress-generated fluid communication through the dense bone matrix.[26] Importantly, the processes themselves

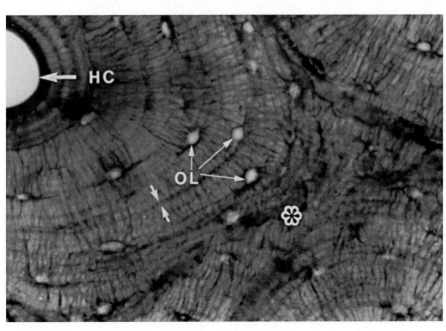

Figure 4–3. Ground section of bone photographed in normal light showing empty osteocyte lacunae (OL) connected by fine darkly stained canaliculi. The central haversian canal (HC) is seen in the upper left hand corner; the reversal line (*) marking the junction between two adjacent osteons and the cement line (→ ←) separating adjacent lamellae are seen.

are interconnected by gap junctions composed of connexin 43, facilitating integration of many of these regulatory messages.[27] Indeed, the three-dimensional nature of this osteocyte syncytium is ideally configured to perceive biophysical stimuli, not unlike the function of an antenna. That these cells are interconnected potentiates their role in orchestrating site-specific formation and resorption in response to such signals.

The volume of bone occupied by this syncytium is approximately 5 percent for the canalicular network and 2 percent for the lacunar spaces.[28] Interestingly, this cell syncytium deteriorates markedly with increasing age[29] and may well contribute to the increasing insensitivity of bone tissue to chemical and physical signals. The surface area of the lacunar and canalicular system is at least 250 m²/L of calcified bone matrix and communicates with a submicroscopic, interfibrillar space representing 35,000 mm²/mm³. Thus, exchange of mineral, nutrients, and chemical and physical stimuli through this enormous network may be both rapid and substantial and certainly

may be essential to the homeostatic control of the skeleton.

Osteoclasts

The osteoclast, functioning as the bone macrophage, is found wherever existing bone tissue is being removed. This large, multinucleated cell migrates over the bone surface, creating irregular, scalloped cavities, or Howship's lacunae (Fig. 4–4). Activated osteoclasts can travel up to 100 μm/day, resorbing a cavity 300 μm in diameter, excavating 200,000 μm³ of bone. The reclamation of this volume of bone requires seven to ten generations of osteoblasts to follow and fill the resorption space.[30] Absence of osteoclasts, or a population of dysfunctional osteoclasts, leads to osteopetrosis, or *marble bone disease*, which can be fatal in childhood secondary to pancytopenias resulting from the absent marrow space.[31]

Osteoclast precursors arise from hematopoeitic stem cells in the bone marrow, as was first suggested

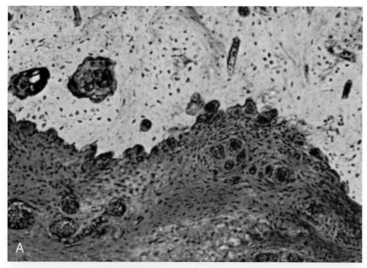

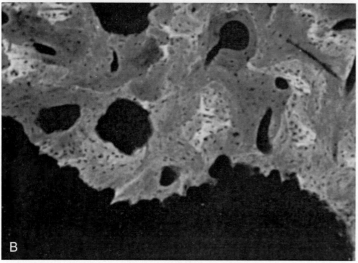

Figure 4–4. *A,* Paragon-stained mineralized section with large multinucleate osteoclasts lying along the pale staining bone surface. *B,* Microradiograph of the same area showing Howship's lacunae in the areas of osteoclastic resorption. (From Jowsey J, Gordan G: *In* Bourne GH [ed]: The Biochemistry and Physiology of Bone, 2nd ed. Vol III. New York, Academic Press, 1972, pp 201–238.)

by Kahn and Simmons.[32] The processes controlling osteoclast differentiation have been the subject of intense scrutiny over the past several years, and the number of cytokines and growth factors along with hormones known to affect this process continues to grow.

Several hematopoeitic growth factors, such as interleukin-3 (IL-3) and granulocyte-macrophage colony-stimulating factor (GM-CSF), are important for establishing the colony-forming unit for granulocytes and macrophages. At that point, the single most important factor promoting entry into the monocytic lineage, from whence the osteoclast ultimately derives, is macrophage colony-stimulating factor (MCSF). Loss of MCSF action engenders deficiencies of both osteoclasts and macrophages; the osteopetrotic op/op mouse, which secretes an ineffective MCSF, is cured by infusions of recombinant MCSF.[33] MCSF alone, however, is unable to generate osteoclasts in in vitro culture systems; further progression into the osteoclast lineage (appearance of functional osteoclast characteristics, such as calcitonin receptor and carbonic anhydrase II expression) requires other local stimuli. For example, an absence of the tyrosine kinase c-fos has been shown to be associated with inhibition of the divergence of osteoclasts from the macrophage pathway.[34] The systemic factors $1,25(OH)_2D_3$, PTH, and tumor necrosis factor (TNF) can enhance the development of osteoclasts from hematopoietic progenitor cells in the presence of stromal elements from bone.[35] Cytokines, such as IL-6 and IL-11, also influence osteoclast development and may have particular significance in some pathogenic states, such as postmenopausal osteoporosis[36] and Paget's disease.[37]

Mature osteoclasts possess several unique ultrastructural characteristics that allow their very active functional phenotype. These characteristics include abundant pleomorphic mitochondria, vacuoles, and lysosomes, which store the multiple secretory products necessary for digestion of bone substance.[38] The apical membrane of the osteoclast is tightly sealed to the calcified matrix, creating a clear zone that has no cellular organelles but is rich in contractile proteins. Toward the center of the cell, the membrane becomes deeply folded, creating the characteristic ruffled border.[39] Under this ruffled border is the resorption pit, where the osteoclast creates an acid environment by secretion of protons through a vacuolar proton pump[40] and several lysosomal enzymes. One of these, tartrate-resistant acid phosphatase (TRAP), can be used to identify these cells in bone sections. Osteoclasts also can be identified by their unique possession of a receptor for calcitonin, which, on exposure to this hormone, causes the osteoclast to retract and loosen from the bone surface.

Osteoclast function is specialized for bone resorption (Fig. 4–5). The highly polarized nature of the cell allows unidirectional secretion of protons from the proton pump into the resorption bay. The protons accumulate within this confined subosteoclastic space, lowering the pH of this micromilieu to a level sufficient to dissolve the mineral phase of the matrix (pH of 2 to 4) and activate osteoclastic hydrolytic enzymes. The organic matrix that remains is subsequently dissolved by lysosomal enzymes (e.g., cathepsin B) released across the ruffled border, leaving the osteoclasts's signature scalloped resorption cavities.[41] As the excavation proceeds, the ionized calcium levels just beyond the clear zone rise from a basal level of 1 to 2 mM to as high as 20 mM.[42] Protons are generated for the pump through the actions of carbonic anhydrase II, an enzyme subtype also associated with vacuolar proton pumps in the renal cortex and the gastric parietal cell.

Deficiencies in carbonic anhydrase II lead to a mild form of osteopetrosis.[43] The bicarbonate resulting from this activity is transported via a chloride bicarbonate exchanger on the marrow-facing side of the osteoclast. The motility of the osteoclast is under con-

Figure 4–5. The osteoclast is a polarized cell that adheres to bone, generating a subosteoclastic space where bone resorption occurs. Into this space, the osteoclast pumps hydrogen ions and lysosomal enzymes. The protons that create the acid pH in the resorption space derive from the action of carbonic anhydrase II on bicarbonate, which has entered the cell via a chloride bicarbonate exchanger on the marrow side of the cell. Calcitonin receptors distinguish this cell, as does the characteristic ruffled border seen on electron micrographs.

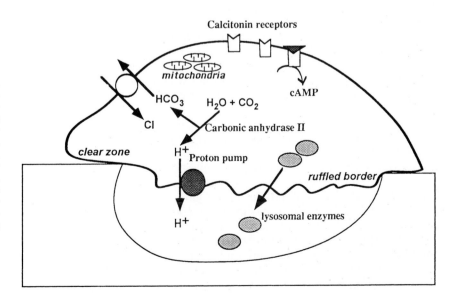

trol of many factors, including the recognition of substances in the bone matrix by integrin receptors, such as vitronectin.

Specific deficiency of another ubiquitous tyrosine kinase, c-src, has been associated with diminished osteoclast function. Targeted disruption of the murine src gene results in offspring with osteopetrosis as a result of dysfunctional osteoclasts.[44] Also notable is the ability to control osteoclast acid secretion through inhibition of the calmodulin kinase through non–estrogen receptor–mediated actions of estrogen agonists.[45] Although our understanding of the complex controls by which osteoclasts are recruited and regulated has advanced rapidly over the last several years, much remains to be learned before therapeutic tools are developed to finely manipulate osteoclastic bone resorption.

SYSTEMIC REGULATION OF BONE CELL METABOLISM

Regulation of bone formation and resorption not only occurs at the local level but also is controlled by systemic factors. For example, osteoclasts are incapable of independently resorbing bone unless the osteoid lining is first removed. This denuding is typically accomplished via proteases such as collagenase, an enzyme that osteoclasts do not produce. In the presence of the parathyroid hormone, however, osteoblasts produce collagenase and may actually secrete it complexed with a peptide inhibitor of collagen formation,[46] further facilitating the *resorptive* process.

Parathyroid Hormone

Many systemic factors play a critical role in the regulation of bone metabolism, even though it could easily be argued that the principal responsibility of these peptide or steroid hormones is to regulate mineral homeostasis rather than focally control skeletal morphology. For example, a primary function of PTH is to maintain serum ionized calcium levels within a narrow physiologic range. PTH secretion is stimulated as calcium levels drop below 8 mg/dl, but a calcium level above 10 mg/dl is identified with high levels of serum PTH; thus, a diagnosis of hyperparathyroidism can be made.[47]

Parathyroid hormone regulates serum calcium in part by influencing the formation and resorption of bone. By stimulating osteoclast activity and in turn bone resorption, PTH provides calcium and phosphate for mineral homeostasis. Membrane receptors for PTH on osteoblasts stimulate substantial morphologic and metabolic changes in these cells and subsequently in osteoclasts[48] through intracellular increases in cyclic adenosine monophosphate (cAMP) and by mobilization of cytosolic calcium ion,[49] both of which serve as second messengers. Although PTH receptors do not exist on osteoclasts,[50] these cells are activated

within minutes of osteoblast exposure to PTH. PTH also targets renal 1α-hydroxylase, which generates the active metabolite, 1,25-dihydroxyvitamin D, from vitamin D. 1,25-Dihydroxyvitamin D has direct effects on osteoclast recruitment[35] and also stimulates intestinal calcium absorption. Thereby, PTH contributes to maintaining serum calcium via both direct and indirect interactions with the skeleton.

Vitamin D

Vitamin D is another systemic factor that plays a critical role in both bone remodeling and calcium homeostasis. Brief exposure of the skin (10 to 20 minutes) to ultraviolet light (sun) endogenously produces sufficient quantities of vitamin D_3 from 7-dehydrocholestrol. Diet is the principal source of its isomer, vitamin D_2. In a series of steps, these fat-soluble vitamins are first hydroxylated to 25-hydroxyvitamin D. In the kidney, 25-hydroxyvitamin D is further hydroxylated to 1,25-dihydroxyvitamin D. Often referred to as calcitriol, 1,25-dihydroxyvitamin D stimulates intestinal absorption of calcium, thereby elevating serum calcium concentrations and establishing a positive milieu for the mineralization of new bone. Even though the mineral mobilizing effects of 1,25-dihydroxyvitamin D are necessary to provide calcium and phosphorus for bone formation, high levels induce bone resorption by stimulating differentiation of osteoclast precursors.[51] Clearly, by influencing both the calcium levels and resident bone cell population, vitamin D has a complex but important role in both the formation and resorption of bone.[52]

Estrogens and Androgens

The rapid decline of skeletal mass following the menopause underscores the critical regulatory role of sex steroids in bone cell metabolism. The expression of estrogen receptors by osteoblasts[53, 54] designates these cells as targets of this sex steroid. Elevated estrogen levels both increase osteoblast proliferation[55] and attenuate the osteoblast response to PTH.[50] In addition, estrogens increase both osteoblastic collagen gene expression[55] and insulin-like growth factor (IGF-2) production[56] and may even directly affect osteoclasts to regulate the production of lysosomal enzymes.[57] It has also been recognized that IL-6 is a potent stimulator of osteoclastic bone resorption in the estrogen-deficient state.[36]

Estrogen may also be important in the male skeleton; a unique patient shown to be unresponsive to estrogen through an abnormal estrogen receptor never experienced fusion of the epiphyses despite an intact androgen axis.[58] Androgen receptors have been identified within the osteoblast of the male,[59] and androgens affect these cells in a manner similar to that of estrogens.[60] Considering the ever-escalating percentage of our population that is elderly and the severe social, clinical, and economic burden caused by osteoporosis,[61] it is clear that an improved understanding of estrogen and androgen interactions on formation and resorption of bone will ultimately improve the treatment of these skeletal disorders.

Prostaglandins

In response to hormonal stimuli, osteoblasts also secrete prostaglandin E_2 (PGE_2), a stimulator of both bone formation and resorption, and serve as an osteoclast-tactic factor.[62] Although PGE_2 and PTH stimulate the same second messengers in osteoblasts, PGE_2 can also influence osteoclasts directly. PGE_2 stimulates several second messenger responses in bone cells, including an increase in cytosolic calcium, elevated cAMP production, and activation of the phosphatidyl inositol pathway.[63] Therefore, variable levels of PGE_2 directly modulate the response of forming and resorbing cells both locally and systemically.

Calcitonin

Calcitonin is a calcium regulatory hormone that works independently of either PTH or vitamin D and possesses a potent capacity to modulate serum calcium and phosphate levels.[64] Similar to the regulation of PTH secretion from parathyroid cells, serum calcium levels regulate the secretion of calcitonin from parafollicular or "C" cells of the thyroid. In contrast to PTH secretion, which is inversely proportional to serum calcium levels, calcitonin secretion is directly related to serum calcium; as serum calcium values go up, calcitonin secretion follows.[65] Through binding to its receptor on osteoclasts,[66] calcitonin causes a marked decrease in osteoclast metabolic activity and cell retraction[67, 68] through the effects of at least two second messengers, cAMP and release of intracellular calcium.[69] For these reasons, calcitonin has been used successfully in the acute treatment of the humoral hypercalcemia of malignancy and in Paget's disease;

the use of calcitonin in the treatment of hyperresorptive osteoporosis is also effective.[70]

Growth Factors

Osteoblasts also produce a number of growth factors and cytokines that are critical to the process of bone formation, remodeling, and repair (Fig. 4–6). Many of these soluble products are also released by circulating macrophages and lymphocytes. For example, insulin-like growth factor I (somatomedin C) directly stimulates osteoblast replication and function.[71] Another osteoblast stimulator, TGF-β, is released by the matrix during the process of bone resorption,[72] establishing a protective feedback loop, or coupled response, for osteoblast and osteoclast activity. This growth factor not only increases levels of osteoblast activity[73] but also appears to inhibit differentiation and maturation of osteoclast precursors.[74]

Bone morphogenetic proteins are also osteoblast products that can, under the correct conditions, set off a cascade of bone formation, whereas MCSF is necessary for osteoclast precursors to enter the monocytic lineage and proliferate.[33] Cells of monocyte-macrophage lineage release other factors that enhance osteoclastic bone resorption, such as IL-1 and IL-6, and tumor necrosis factor-α (TNF-α).[75] Although our understanding of growth factors is only embryonic, considering their potency in the remodeling process and the possibility of using recombinant techniques to produce them, these peptides are certain to make a major contribution to the treatment of skeletal disorders.

Biophysical Stimuli

Working systemically, vitamin D, PGE_2, steroids, and other "chemical" factors play vital roles in the determination of the modulation of cell types and skeletal modeling and remodeling. Although their role as "stimuli" is clear, depending on the circum-

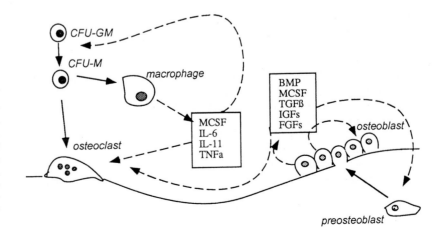

Figure 4–6. Osteoclasts and osteoblasts interact through cytokines released into the bone micromilieu. Macrophages secrete M-CSF, various interleukins (IL), and tumor necrosis factor, all of which promote osteoclast differentiation from hematopoeitic stem cells, from the colony-forming unit for granulocyte-macrophages (CFU-GM) and the CFU-M (CFU for macrophage) to terminal osteoclast phenotype. Osteoblasts interact by secreting factors that affect osteoclasts, including MCSF and transforming growth factor-β (TGF-β) as well as factors affecting bone mineralization and progression of their own phenotype, such as insulin-like growth factors (IGFs) and basic fibroblast growth factors (FGFs). TNF, tumor necrosis factor.

stances these factors can elevate either resorption or formation. There is increasing evidence that the ultimate role that these "mediators of change" play is orchestrated by local factors that are not chemical in origin. One of the most potent influences of the development and maintenance of the skeleton is a by-product of function and is referred to as a physical (mechanical-electrical) factor. Indeed, it is essential to keep the role of chemical mediators in perspective and to acknowledge physical factors as critical control mechanisms in tissue differentiation regulation, growth, repair, and remodeling.[76] Physical stimuli as potent determinants of skeletal morphology have even been postulated as primary regulators of chondro-osseous morphogenesis.[77] The influence of physical stimuli in the formation and resorption of bone is detailed later in this chapter.

In summary, through the interactions of systemic and local factors, a cellular symbiosis exists in which an integrated "activation, resorption, reversal, formation" (ARRF) occurs, reflecting an intricate control of both osteoblasts and osteoclasts.[78] To initiate this sequence, osteoclasts are activated by chemical or physical signals that recruit them to specific remodeling areas. Once activated and attached to the matrix, they begin the resorption cycle and create the Howship's lacunae. When resorption is completed, new bone formation begins within the cavity, a process that leaves a boundary that is visible in histologic sections as a "reversal line."[79] This "pocket" of new bone is known as a *bone structural unit.*[80] A similar line, called a *cement line,* is seen between the adjacent lamellae of bone (see Fig. 4–3).

COMPOSITION OF BONE MATRIX

Bone is composed of inorganic mineral (70 percent of weight), organic matrix and cells (25 percent), and water (5 percent). Before its calcification, newly synthesized bone matrix is essentially completely organic and is called *osteoid. Collagen* is the predominant organic component in bone, accounting for approximately 94 percent of the unmineralized matrix (see Table 4–1). Other noncollagenous proteins unique to bone are found in osteoid, accounting for approximately 4 percent of its weight. These include glycoproteins and phosphoproteins, such as osteonectin[81]; sialoproteins, which are predominantly osteopontin[82]; bone Gla protein, also called BGP, or osteocalcin[83]; and bone morphogenetic protein.[84] Extracts of bone also include enzymes, hormones, growth factors, and other metabolites essential for bone metabolism.[85] Bone cells, for all their responsibility to mineral and structural homeostasis, make up only 2 percent of the organic tissue's constituents. While beyond the scope of this chapter, an extensive review by Robey on the biochemistry of bone provides an excellent discussion of the function and interrelatedness of these matrix components.[86]

Collagen

Bone collagen is primarily type I and resembles other type I collagens found in skin and tendon. The basic unit of bone collagen, the tropocollagen molecules, is a triple helix of three polypeptide (α) chains, each of approximately 1000 amino acids.[87] By stabilizing these soluble molecules with cross-links of hydroxylysine and lysine, the bone collagen fibrils become essentially insoluble.[88] Type I collagen differs from the type II collagen of cartilage in several salient aspects. Each of the three α chains of type II collagen is identical, yet their amino acid composition is different from any of the three (one pair, one unique) α chains of the type I tropocollagen of bone.[89] Compared with type I, the chains of type II contain much more glycosylated hydroxylysine, making cartilage more resistant to degradation by collagenase.

The triple helix of type I collagen forms a linear molecule approximately 300 nm long.[90] Each molecule is aligned parallel to the next, producing a collagen fibril. Within the collagen fibril, gaps called "hole zones" exist between the end of one molecule and the beginning of the next. It is thought that noncollagenous proteins reside in these spaces, which chemotactically attract and initiate the mineralization process.[85] The fibrils are further grouped in bundles to form the collagen fiber.

Proteoglycans

Proteoglycans constitute the principal noncollagenous protein in the mineralized matrix. They form the major macromolecule of the ground substance, consisting of approximately 95 percent polysaccharide (glycosaminoglycans) and 5 percent protein. This bone proteoglycan, similar in structure to the cartilage proteoglycan, consists of a thin protein core with multiple covalently bound glycosaminoglycan chains[91] composed of repeating disaccharide units of the amino sugars chondroitin sulfate and keratan sulfate.[92]

Although the role of these proteins in bone has not been determined, it has been proposed that they may actually store load information following functional activity, serving as a form of strain memory.[93] Proteoglycans protrude into canalicular spaces and even touch osteocyte membranes. These molecules deform rapidly in response to load, yet reestablish their original orientation relatively slowly. Although somewhat speculative, this matrix cell interaction may well serve as a signal transduction mechanism to transfer mechanical information from the matrix to the entombed osteocytes.

Osteonectin

Glycoprotein matrix molecules, such as osteonectin, serve as binding catalysts between the extracellular matrix and cell processes.[94] The acidic PO_4 complexes on these glycoproteins bind to collagen and have a high affinity for calcium and hydroxyapatite,[95] suggesting their direct role in mineral formation. It is thought that the acidic phospholipids of osteonectin first form on matrix vesicles to facilitate collagen-mediated nucleation and perhaps serve as seeding sites for mineralization at the collagen fibril "hole zones."[96]

Osteocalcin

Also present in the matrix are substantial quantities of osteocalcin, a protein found almost exclusively in bone, composing 1 to 2 percent of the total bone protein. Osteocalcin synthesis, which can be stimulated by 1,25-dihydroxyvitamin D, takes place in the osteoblasts during the carboxylation of glutamate, a vitamin K–dependent reaction.[97] 1,25-Dihydroxyvitamin D enhances the synthesis of this noncollagenous protein, further evidence that vitamin D has a direct stimulatory effect on osteoblasts.[98] The function of this protein remains unclear, but it may play a role in osteoclast recruitment and bone formation.[99] Along with bone alkaline phosphatase measurements, serum osteocalcin levels can be used clinically as a reflection of bone formation activity.[100]

Hydroxyapatite

Bone mineral is generically referred to as hydroxyapatite [$Ca_{10}(PO_4)_6(OH)_2$], a plate-like crystal 20 to 80 nm long and 2 to 5 nm thick. Bone hydroxyapatite is quite different from naturally occurring apatite, containing a number of impurities, including sodium, fluorine, strontium, lead, and radium. It is smaller in size than natural apatites (100 versus 400 Å) and more reactive and soluble because of its less perfect atomic arrangement.[101] The nucleation sites of bone mineral may not be the plates of hydroxyapatite but more energetically favorable crystal spicules, such as amorphous calcium phosphate and octacalcium phosphate.[102] It is believed these unstable precursors are formed first and gradually transformed to the more crystalline hydroxyapatite.[103] Mineral exchange is facilitated by the enormous surface area of amorphous calcium phosphate, including its hydration shell. This is reflected in the greater avidity of new bone for "bone-seeking" isotopes (technetium, fluorine, strontium). The bone mineral continues to mature through an individual's lifetime,[104] becoming more and more "perfect" and thus exposing less surface area for a given volume of mineral. Indeed, the process of crystal maturity may contribute to the etiology of osteopenia[105]; not only would greater levels of systemic factors be needed to liberate calcium from the more stable crystal, but stress-generated zeta potentials would attenuate as a function of the diminished surface area of the mineral constituents. The magnitude of these stress-generated potentials, produced by the ionic constituents of the fluid flowing by the charged phase of the mineral, drops proportionally as less mineral is exposed at the microboundary layer. In the elderly, therefore, the same degree of functional strain would generate a weaker regulatory signal.

DEVELOPMENT OF THE SKELETON

Most of the bones of the skeleton are first formed in the embryo as cartilaginous models, which are later resorbed and replaced by bone tissue. This cartilage template, or *anlage,* is formed by the condensation of mesenchymal cells in the developing limb bud. While the shape of the anlage resembles that of the adult bone and appears to be genetically determined, the bone that replaces the cartilage template is greatly influenced by physical factors (e.g., weight bearing, muscle pull) and is constantly modeled and remodeled as these forces change according to the dictums of *Wolff's law.*[106]

The cartilage anlage expands and elongates by interstitial growth in which chondrocytes divide, enlarge, and surround themselves by the new matrix. At about the same time, cells in the connective tissues surrounding the anlage (perichondrium) begin to lay down bone tissue and form a collar of bone around the center of the cartilage model. At the time it is formed, the anlage is pierced by a capillary that invades the calcified cartilage matrix and begins to hollow out its center, replacing the excavated cartilage with bone and creating the primitive marrow space. This process of vascular invasion of the cartilage model, followed by bone deposition, is referred to as *enchondral ossification.* The process continues until the entire shaft of the anlage is replaced by marrow and bone, confining the growth process of chondrocyte multiplication to the epiphyseal ends of the bone, away from the primary center of ossification. As the epiphysis swells, the central chondrocytes find themselves too remote from the blood supply to survive solely by means of diffusion. Cartilage canals facilitate diffusion of nutrients and provide conduits for subsequent capillary ingrowth. The hypertrophic chondrocytes survive and elaborate angiotrophic substances.

Rosenberg and coworkers[107] characterized the changes that occur in the lower hypertrophic bone, demonstrating the deposition of a 35,000-molecular-weight protein (probably osteocalcin) and the modification of existing proteoglycans. Mineral deposition begins in the matrix vesicles located in the columns between the last hypertrophic chondrocytes on the extreme metaphyseal end of the physis.[108] Invasion by osteoblasts and osteoclasts results in the resorption of this woven bone and its replacement by mature lamellar bone.[109] The hydroxyapatite formed during primary ossification is a rather rough crystal whose imperfections may render it more vulnerable to resorption,[110] which also implies the facility with which woven bone is removed.

The controlling mechanism for the mineralization and morphogenesis of the cartilage anlage is unknown, but this process is typically considered templated by genetic determinants. Alternative regulatory mechanisms include that first proposed by Roux,[111] in which he hypothesized that the differentiation of connective tissues was controlled by mechanical stresses. More recently, this general "stress" postulation has been refined by Carter and coworkers,[112] who proposed that intermittently applied shear stresses promote enchondral ossification and that intermittent hydrostatic compression inhibits cartilage degeneration and ossification. Therefore, the mechanical stress environment to which the anlage is exposed would contribute heavily to the bone's ultimate shape.

Although growth in length occurs at the growth plate, growth in diameter occurs by the centrifugal proliferation of cartilage cells along the groove of Ranvier,[113] an anatomic structure bordered outwardly by a continuation of the fibrous periosteum and inwardly by the physeal cartilage. When swelling of the cartilaginous anlage first begins, a condensed layer of mesenchyme develops around it as a membrane of cells and collagen, called *perichondrium*. As the cartilage is replaced by bone, this membrane is renamed *periosteum*. In the growing skeleton, this periosteum is clearly divided into an inner cellular layer and an outer fibrous layer that merge gradually into the surrounding muscle. Muscles take origin from the periosteum; collagen bundles can be traced from tendon and ligament, through the periosteum, to anchor directly into the bone via Sharpey's fibers.[114]

MINERALIZATION OF BONE TISSUE

The mineralization of bone begins 10 to 15 days after the organic osteoid matrix has been laid down.[115] At this point, mineral increases almost immediately to 70 percent of the ultimate content, whereas deposition of the final 30 percent takes several months.[116] The process of mineralization is extremely complex and temporally dynamic.[117] There is emerging evidence that hydroxyapatite deposition and seeding of mineralization are strongly interdependent on both cartilage and bone-derived macromolecules, such as osteonectin, phosphoproteins, and proteolipids. Surprisingly, the initial sites of calcium-phosphate nucleation in growing bone, fracture callus, and calcifying cartilage appear to be not at the bone surface but on the processes of matrix vesicles.[118] Matrix vesicles are small, round, extracellular lipid-bilaminar bound organelles, which bud from hypertrophic chondrocytes or osteoblasts undergoing the process of apoptosis[119] as well as from cell processes originating from the plasma membrane.[120] There is a definite polarity to the vesicles, with mineralization occurring in a predictable and organized way adjacent to the requisite

phosphatases on the inner leaflet of the membrane.[121] The matrix vesicles contain alkaline phosphatase, AT-Pase, inorganic pyrophosphatase, 5'-nucleotidase, and ATP-pyrophosphohydrolase[122] in addition to phospholipids (especially phosphatidyl serine), which have a strong affinity for calcium ions.[123] It is believed that these ions accumulate in the matrix vesicle because of their affinity for the phospholipids and a membrane-bound calcium pump. At a point of supersaturation, nucleation of the mineral begins.[124]

Nucleation

Alkaline phosphatase, a biosynthetic product of osteoblasts, is present in very high concentrations during development and osteoid production.[125] The regulatory role of this disulfide-linked dimer is not known, but its presence may increase local concentrations of P and thereby facilitate hydroxyapatite deposition.[126] Increasing the concentration of P in the micromilieu exceeds the local solubility product and catalyzes deposition along the inner leaflet of the vesicle.

Following this accretion, the destruction of the membrane has been attributed to an increasing concentration of lysophospholipids within the matrix vesicles, which suggests that they are programmed to self-destruct.[127] Following dissolution of the matrix vesicle membrane, the hydroxyapatite crystals are exposed to the extravesicular environment, where additional mineral accretes to the newly formed crystal.[128] The crystal is then believed to chemotactically move toward and preferentially bind at the hole zones between collagen fibrils, precipitated by the nesting osteonectin[129] and fibronectin.[130] Mineralization proceeds and extends over the collagen matrix, with the long axis of the hydroxyapatite crystal parallel to the collagen fiber. The arrangement of the collagen matrix that is synthesized during osteoblast activity ultimately determines the orientation of the bone mineral crystals.[89]

In the extravesicular milieu, glycosaminoglycans inhibit the calcification process by modulating the advancing mineral front.[131] Indeed, it may be just these proteoglycan macromolecules, found in high concentrations in noncalcifying collagenous structures, such as ligament, tendon, and skin, that may prevent mineral deposition.[132] Other theories for the noncalcification of dense connective tissues include the tighter packing of their collagen fibrils, impeding the access of phosphate ions to the interfibrillar nucleation sites, and the existence of crystallization inhibitors such as pyrophosphate, present in synovial fluid, plasma, and urine at concentrations sufficient to prevent deposition of calcium carbonates.[133] Once the concentration of these inhibitors reaches a threshold, mineralization is halted, leaving a thin layer of osteoid between the lining cells and the mineralization front. This establishes the *syncytium*, or cellular canopy, that must be retracted to expose the mineral and reinitiate the remodeling cycle.

Turnover

In undecalcified ground sections, microradiography demonstrates subtle differences in the calcium content of the bone tissue, thus allowing separation into "old" and "new" bone on the basis of contrast intensity (Fig. 4–7). For example, young osteons, in the process of formation, have large central vascular canals that narrow with infilling, showing progressively less mineralization toward the center. This contrasts sharply with the active tunneling process of *resorption*, in which case the inside rim of the osteon appears equally mineralized as with the outer rings. Static remodeling parameters, such as osteoid seam width, number of resorptive events, and number of formative events, can thus be inferred from these morphologic characteristics. By using double fluorescent labels (e.g., tetracyclines), administered at known intervals, one can determine dynamic parameters of bone remodeling (i.e., rates of turnover, infilling, and

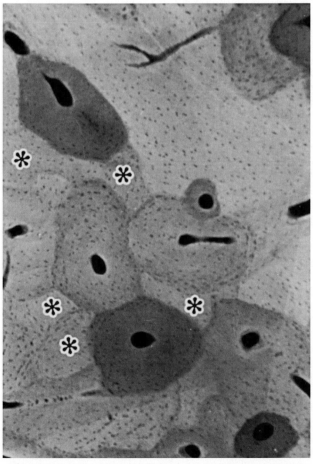

Figure 4–7. Microradiograph of cortical bone showing osteons in varying degrees of mineralization with numerous interstitial fragments (*).

formation). Static and dynamic histomorphometric studies, quantified via biopsy specimens harvested from such areas as the iliac crest, are extremely powerful means of evaluating the systemic state of the skeleton.[134]

The complex, composite nature of bone achieved through the secretion of the collagen matrix and its subsequent mineralization is a product of the synergistic interrelationships of the cell types, the systemic regulators of calcium metabolism, and the matrix-bound proteins that locally control bone remodeling. The product of this sophisticated and interdependent process is an extremely successful tissue that serves both as a structural organ and as a mineral reservoir.

ARCHITECTURE OF BONE

Bones are remarkably well suited for their structural role. At the gross level, as hollow tubes they derive maximal strength from minimal weight.[135] Descending to the next structural level, cortical and cancellous morphology is strategically arranged to evenly distribute functional stresses.[136] Lower still, the arrangement of the collagen within the cancellous or cortical bone, combined with the two-phase composite matrix of the collagen and mineral, provides both tensile and compressive strength.[137] The ultimate tensile strength of bone approaches that of cast iron, and its capacity to absorb and release energy is twice that of oak, yet the weight of bone is only one-third that of steel. And while proving a resilient and resistant material, this tissue's capacity to remodel, adapt, and repair itself is what identifies bone as the ultimate biomaterial. An excellent review of the architecture of bone can be found in the monograph by Martin and Burr.[138]

The structural success of skeletal morphology can be examined at a series of levels:

1. By its gross anatomy and functional responsibility.
2. By its ultrastructural morphology (cortical or cancellous).
3. By its microscopic organization (lamellar or woven).
4. On the basis of its mineralization process (enchondral or intramembranous).

Macroscopic Organization

At the gross, structural level, each bone has diverse and distinct morphologic features. Regardless of function, each bone is composed of dense cortical tissue (e.g., diaphyseal shaft) and cancellous tissue, such as the trabecular cascades found in the neck of the femur or the metaphysis of the proximal tibia (Fig. 4–8). At the microscopic level, two types of bone are identified: the disorganized, hypercellular woven bone, and the highly organized, relatively hypocellular lamellar

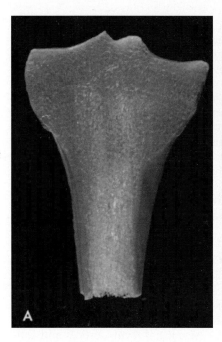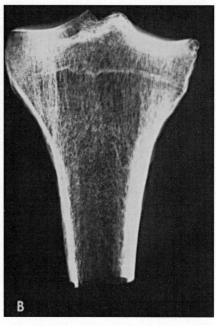

Figure 4–8. *A,* Macerated preparation of the human knee showing the trabecular structure that supports the flared articular surface. *B,* Radiograph of the specimen shown in *A.*

bone. Essentially, all bone tissue can be described by either of these two morphologic patterns, whether mature, growing, pathologic, or healing.

Woven bone is a product of rapid bone formation. Architecturally, it has an irregular, disorganized pattern of collagen orientation and osteocyte distribution (Fig. 4–9). While woven bone is characteristic of embryonic and fetal development, it is also found in the healthy adult skeleton at ligament and tendon

insertions as well as in specific disease states, such as Paget's, osteogenic sarcoma, and metastases. Under less severe pathologic conditions (fracture callus, inflammatory responses, stress fractures), woven bone is usually reabsorbed and replaced by lamellar bone within a few weeks of its deposition.[139] Mechanical stimulation, if potent enough, can even cause a rapid production of woven bone, which ultimately remodels into dense lamellar bone.[140] Many consider woven bone an aberrant response. That it is laid down so quickly and is so readily remodeled, however, distinguishes this type of bone to be a wise strategy in accommodating new, intense structural challenges.

Lamellar, or *mature, bone* can be packed tightly to form the dense cortex of a bone, or it can be organized as the trabecular struts in cancellous bone. In contrast to the random and disorganized structure of woven bone, the lamellar appearance of this mature bone is the product of highly organized mineralized plates. In cancellous bone, the lamellae run parallel to the trabeculae. In cortical bone, several patterns occur. The predominant one is that found in *osteons,* which are composed of small concentric lamellar cylinders surrounding a central vascular channel, not unlike the rings in a tree trunk (Fig. 4–10). Osteons are typically 200 to 300 μm in diameter, consisting of up to six or seven concentric osteocyte rings composed of up to 20 lamellar plates.[141] Canaliculi in lamellar bone are consistent in diameter and orientation and in toto contain less osteocytes per unit volume than woven bone (20,000 cells/μm^3 versus 80,000 cells/μm^3).

During growth in diameter, new bone must be added appositionally. Following formation of the periosteal cuff about the primary center of ossification, bone increases its diameter by one of two methods. During rapid growth, spicules of new woven bone are formed perpendicular to the surface, which

Figure 4–9. Outer cortex of bone showing the results of rapid periosteal bone formation producing woven bone *(arrows),* followed by the slower formation of primary osteons surrounding blood vessels.

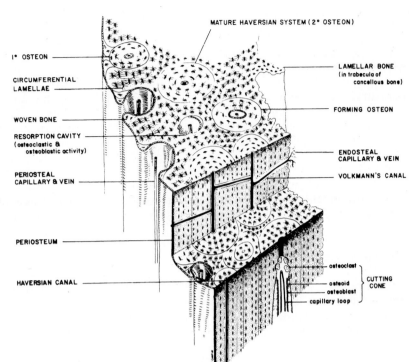

MATURE HAVERSIAN SYSTEM (2° OSTEON)

1° OSTEON

CIRCUMFERENTIAL
LAMELLAE

WOVEN BONE

RESORPTION CAVITY
(osteoclastic &
osteoblastic activity)

PERIOSTEAL
CAPILLARY & VEIN

PERIOSTEUM

HAVERSIAN CANAL

LAMELLAR BONE
(in trabecula of
cancellous bone)

FORMING OSTEON

ENDOSTEAL
CAPILLARY & VEIN

VOLKMANN'S CANAL

osteoclast
osteoid   CUTTING
osteoblast   CONE
capillary loop

Figure 4–10. Diagrammatic representation of the architectural organization of cortical bone.

allows maximal radial expansion with minimal material. The gaps between the spicules are subsequently filled in and consolidated by the formation of lamellar bone. In this process, individual periosteal blood vessels that lie in the valley of the spicules are surrounded by the encroaching new lamellar formation, creating *primary osteons* parallel to the long axis of the bone. An osteon that has formed de novo, as in the woven bone consolidation process just described, is known as a primary osteon. If this occurs intracortically via a resorptive process to replace preexisting bone tissue, it is referred to as a *secondary osteon*, or haversian system, and constitutes the bulk of adult human bone.[142]

When slow diametric growth occurs, seams of new bone are laid appositionally on the existing surface. As discussed previously, the birefringent pattern of both circumferential lamellae and single osteons is believed to be produced by the altering of collagen bundle direction from one layer to the next, therefore maximizing strength in a number of different planes. Although the collagen bundles within each of these lamellar plates are highly oriented, individual fibers often traverse interlamellar spaces. Such a composite integration increases both the individual osteon's resistance to external loads and the effective strength of the bone structure.[143]

An alternative theory for the polarized light birefringence of an osteon is based on fiber-rich, fiber-poor lamellar rings, in which the thinner (1 to 2 μm) plates contain a greater degree of glycosaminoglycans (ground substance) than the adjacent 5 to 7 μm collagen-rich layers.[144] These glycosaminoglycans are thought to be continuous from the "thin" lamellar plate, through the cement line, to interdigitate with the ground substance of the "thick" plate. This architecture, with a true continuity between plates, would produce an increase in the stiffness of each osteon or each circumferential plate. Perhaps the morphology of lamellar bone will prove to be some combination of these two postulations, thus maximizing both the stiffness of the material (continuity of ground substance) and its toughness (integration of collagen layers).

Cortical Drifts

If periosteal surface modeling were to occur in the absence of endosteal resorption, the overall thickness of the cortex would increase with increasing age, leaving too much bone and too little marrow space. This is avoided by coordinating the increasing periosteal diameter with a concomitant increase in the diameter of the endosteal envelope, achieved through resorption at this inner surface.[145] Although these rapid surface drifts diminish in the mature skeleton, they rise again in the elderly. In the aged skeleton, the rate of surface erosion of the endosteal surface exceeds the formation rate of the periosteum, resulting in a net decrease in total bone mass. However, this age-related expansion of the cortex establishes a biomechanical compensatory mechanism via the concurrent increase in the cross-sectional moments of inertia, which results in an increased capacity of the bone to resist bending loads.[146]

Metaphyseal Reshaping

During growth in length, the inverse to periosteal expansion with endosteal resorption can occur. As the metaphysis and diaphysis elongate, resorption at the periosteal surface must be closely coordinated with deposition at the endosteum, a process known as metaphyseal reshaping.[147] Under these circumstances, some of the cortical bone within the epiphyseal shell is spared and subsequently becomes a component of the cancellous structure within the metaphysis. Where fragments of osteons as well as new lamellae and abundant cement lines are seen, the ultrastructural organization of trabeculae reflects their cortical origin.

Haversian Remodeling

Bone remodeling is a process of "real time" tissue replacement. In places, trabeculae are covered with osteoblasts making new bone; in others, osteoclasts are eroding the surface. By this process of resorption and formation, orientation of the trabeculae can be rapidly altered to accommodate changes in manner or loading or shifts in alignment secondary to disease or fracture.[148] To remodel cortical bone so that intracortical damage or dead tissue can be replaced, the cortex must first be resorbed from within, thus creating a surface for apposition. When haversian systems replace or remodel existing bone, it is not necessarily achieved through the identical pathway of the original osteon. Indeed, these secondary osteons can persist directly through an existing arrangement of osteons and circumferential lamellae, leaving only remnants of these preexisting structures. These fragments of lamellar or woven bone are called *interstitial lamellae.* Because the structural integrity of the bone must be preserved during this remodeling, this replacement process must be undertaken with close integration between resorption and formation. For the strength of each skeletal element to be retained, the cutting cone of the osteoclast must be followed rapidly by a capillary and the simultaneous intrusion of a population of osteoblasts infilling the lamellar rings of the secondary osteon. As discussed previously, matrix-bound proteins, such as TGF-β, which are released via the resorption process, are critical to the retention of the close integration of this coupling process.

Although levels of intracortical remodeling may be elevated by changes in the organism's nutritional status (e.g., calcium deficiency),[149] endocrine imbalance (hyperparathyroidism, menopause),[150] or even aging (osteopenia),[105] one of the most potent stimuli for remodeling is a change in the level of physical activity.[151] If physical demands are altered (e.g., an increased or decreased level of activity), or if the manner in which the bone is loaded is changed (e.g., distribution of strain or loading rate), the bone remodels internally to adapt to the new demands.[152] Evidence of this osteonal turnover has been demon-strated in rabbits, in which a 150 percent increase in the number of labeled secondary osteons arose in the subchondral plate of the proximal tibia subjected to repetitive impulsive loads.[153]

Not only does loading activate modeling and remodeling; by-products of loading are also believed to influence morphology. For example, one of the strongest correlates to elevated intracortical turnover is increased strain rate.[154] Another alternative to strain magnitude, strain frequency is a potent determinant of bone morphology.[155] This sensitivity to discrete components of the biophysical milieu opens several distinct avenues for the treatment of musculoskeletal disorders, including induced electric fields,[156] ultrasound,[157] and low-magnitude, high-frequency mechanical stimulation.[158]

Blood Supply of Bone

Bone is extremely vascular and requires approximately 10 percent of the cardiac output.[159] Blood supply to the cortical diaphysis is derived from the *nutrient artery* and the periosteal vessels. In the metaphyseal ends of the bone, where metabolism is most active, the periosteal vessels are large and abundant and are also referred to as *metaphyseal arteries,* although they are entirely analogous to the periosteal capillaries. The third set of vessels, the *epiphyseal arteries,* supplies the subarticular ends of the bones and assumes special importance because of the growth process in this area and the vulnerability of these vessels to injury.

During infancy and adolescence, the epiphyseal plate serves as a barrier separating the epiphysis from the metaphysis. Although a few vessels crossing the plate have been described, it is widely accepted that there is no effective circulation across the plate. Essentially, therefore, the epiphyses have an isolated blood supply via the epiphyseal arteries, but those few vessels do present a potential route for spread of infection or tumor from metaphysis into the epiphysis. In most joints, there are abundant soft tissue attachments to the epiphyses (muscles, ligaments, capsule), so that numerous vessels supply the bone through these attachments (Fig. 4–11). In a few locations, such as the proximal femur, the entire epiphysis may be intra-articular and therefore may be covered by articular cartilage. Since neither the articular nor growth cartilage is penetrated by vessels, the few epiphyseal arteries must pass alongside the growth plate, covered by a thin layer of periosteum, to perforate the epiphysis.[160] This route of blood supply is extremely vulnerable to trauma (fractures through the growth plate), increased intra-articular pressure (joint infections or bleeding into the joint), or idiopathic interruption (Legg-Perthes disease in children, avascular necrosis in adults).

Epiphyseal vessels arborize within the bony nucleus to supply the marrow, cancellous bone, and the dividing chondrocytes in the microepiphyseal plates

A

Articular Cartilage

Growth Plate

B

Periosteum

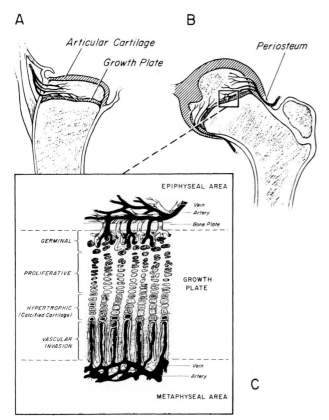

EPIPHYSEAL AREA

Vein
Artery
Bone Plate

GERMINAL

PROLIFERATIVE

GROWTH
PLATE

HYPERTROPHIC
(Calcified Cartilage)

VASCULAR
INVASION

Vein

Artery

C

METAPHYSEAL AREA

Figure 4–11. Epiphyseal blood supply of growing bone. *A,* The blood supply of most secondary centers of ossification is abundant by virtue of the numerous soft tissue attachments. *B,* Certain secondary centers, such as the proximal femur, are devoid of soft tissue attachments, and the blood supply therefore follows a tenuous route through the joint, where it is liable to injury. *C,* Diagrammatic representation of the blood supply to the growth plate showing the contribution of the epiphyseal artery to the germinal portion of the growth plate. (From Sledge CB: *In* Cave EF [ed]: Trauma Management. Chicago, Year Book Medical Publishers, 1974.)

in the depths of the articular cartilage and the growth plate itself. Because of this, interruption of the vessels leads to cessation of longitudinal growth and diametric growth of the epiphysis and joint surface.

Within the cortex of bone, capillaries travel primarily in the longitudinal direction within haversian canals. Occasional branching is seen, and lateral communications with the periosteal vessels through Volkmann's canals provide collateral circulation. The usual haversian system is 100 mm or less in diameter; thus, individual osteocytes are not more than 50 mm from their blood supply. The rich system of canaliculi radiating out from the central canal enhances microcirculation to the most distant osteocytes.

MECHANICAL PROPERTIES OF BONE

Even considering the elaborate cell kinetics, mineralization process, and morphology of bone, its success as a structure is, in large part, a product of bone's

mechanical properties; how stiff it is, how resilient to fatigue, and how effectively it withstands the extremes of physical activity. An excellent review of this subject is addressed in a monograph edited by Cowin.[161]

The mechanical strength of fully mature osteonal bone is greater than that of immature bone composed of circumferential lamellae and a few osteons that may only be partially mineralized.[162] Values for the mechanical properties of individual osteons range from tensile elastic modulus of 12 gigapascals (GPa) and 114 megapascals (MPa) ultimate tensile strength for a fully mature, mineralized osteon, to less than half that modulus and only 75 percent the ultimate tensile strength for a younger, less mineralized osteon. For normal tensile or compressive loading, the stiffness of the material, or elastic modulus, shows human haversian bone to be about 17.0 GPa in the longitudinal direction, 11.5 GPa in the transverse direction, and 3.3 GPa in shear.[163] The degree of mineralization (young bone) or porosity (old bone) compromises the stiffness of the bone and thereby lowers the elastic modulus. However, the "effective" modulus of the bone can compensate for decreased stiffness by changes in morphology (e.g., periosteal expansion).

Strength

A major contributor to the strength of bone is derived through its composite nature of haversian, circumferential, and interstitial lamellae that works synergistically to avoid *yield*, or *ultimate strain*. *Strain*, a dimensionless unit of change in length divided by its original length, is used in bone physiology as 10^{-6} strain, or *microstrain*. The yield strain of bone, or that degree of deformation reached at which the bone does not elastically recover, is approximately 7000 microstrain; that is, a 0.7 percent change in length causes irreversible damage to the tissue. Ultimate strain in bone, or that degree of deformation where the material actually fractures, is 15,000 microstrain.[164]

An analogy of a bundle of straws versus a solid stick illustrates how such a composite structure, such as bone, can prove more successful in resisting loads by avoiding yield and ultimate strain of the material. The solid stick breaks with relatively little bending, because relatively high strains are generated within the periphery of the material; however, the bundle of straws composed of the same mass and subjected to the same bending conditions continue to deform (strain) rather than break, as each independent element slips relative to adjacent bundles. By dissipating the strains generated by identical forces, the chance of exceeding yield strains or ultimate failure is greatly diminished.

This analogy is often put into practice with the use of multistranded wire chosen over the use of single-strand wire. During flexion, each individual strand slips relative to its neighbor rather than strain, thus minimizing the generation of potentially damaging levels of strain. In the same manner, individual lamellae "slip" relative to adjacent lamellae, dissipating energy and minimizing strain levels within the material, thus allowing the entire system to react in a more elastic manner rather than to sustain brittle failure or ultimate fracture.

Toughness

Bone, as an organ, needs to be both stiff (to resist deformation) and tough (to prevent crack propagation). However, there is a compromise between these two objectives, as they are attained through a balance of the composite between the resiliency to crack propagation provided by collagen and the resiliency to deformation provided by mineral. Comparatively small changes in the mineral content of bone tissue can have substantial effects on its properties as a material, as demonstrated by Curry in his determination of the mechanical properties of diverse types of bone.[165] By comparing the bovine femur, the deer antler, and the whale tympanic bulla, he illustrated that as the morphologic responsibility of the skeletal element changed, so did its mineral content. In the extreme, the mineral content ranged from 86 percent in the bulla, which requires a high acoustic impedance, to 59 percent in the antler, which must be resilient to high-impact loads. The consequence of this high mineral content is revealed by comparing the relative work to fracture of these bones; the bulla is only 3 percent that of the antler.

The material properties of the appendicular skeleton, however, remain remarkably consistent through a wide range of animals.[166] Over an animal mass range of 0.09 to 700 kg the bending strength of those bones relegated to traditional load-bearing responsibilities remains approximately 200 to 250 MPa with an elastic modulus consistently approaching 20 GPa. To adapt to changes in the physical demands placed on it, it appears that the appendicular skeleton responds not by changing its material properties but by altering its shape and morphology.[167] This is achieved by functionally regulated alterations in bone mass and architecture.

STRUCTURAL ADAPTATION IN BONE

Bone tissue has the capacity to adapt to its functional environment such that its morphology is "optimized" for its mechanical demand. Indeed, the concept proposed in 1892—that the course and balance of bone remodeling can be affected by mechanical function—is one of the oldest in modern medicine and is widely referred to as *Wolff's law*.[106] But what component of the functional environment is osteoregulating, and what is the structural objective of bone morphology? Strains measured during functional activity should indicate what the architecture of the skeleton is trying to amplify or suppress. Loads can be sustained with the smallest strains if they are applied axially. However, the axial component of functional activity is responsible for only a small percentage of the total strain measured at the bone surface; the femur, humerus, radius, ulna, and tibia all show that well over 80 percent of the measured strain is caused by bending moments.[168] As the neutral axis of strain typically passes across the marrow cavity, a significant portion of the tissue is in fact subjected to tension.[169] Although bending moments cannot be extinguished, their effect would be minimized if the bone's longitudinal curvature were oriented such that the moment created by curvature counteracted those externally imposed by activity. Surprisingly, long bone curvature does not appear directed toward the neutralization of bending, and in some cases this curvature is oriented such that bending is increased.[170] Perhaps bone curvature, a morphologic modification attributable to functional loading,[171] acts to accentuate bone strain rather than cancel it.

Dynamic Strain Similarity

Contrary to our normal interpretation of Wolff's law, it appears that minimizing strain is not the ultimate goal of adaptation; instead, skeletal morphology strives to generate a certain type of strain. But what kind of strain is morphology trying to achieve? Although vertebrate design and function are diverse, at the level of small volumes of tissue all loads and bending moments resolve into strain. Peak strain magnitudes measured in adult species, including horse, human, lizard, sheep, goat, goose, pig, macaque, turkey, sunfish, and dog, are remarkably similar, ranging from 2000 to 3500 microstrain. This relationship has been called "dynamic strain similarity" and suggests that skeletal morphology and locomotion character combine to elicit a very specific and perhaps beneficial level of strain.[172]

This limited range of strain has implications beyond the maintenance of a twofold safety factor within the bone material. Although the structural benefit of a safety factor cannot be denied, it is difficult to imagine a cellular process that could monitor how close to deleterious strain levels the skeleton came during activity and then adjust the tissue's mass simply to avoid them. It seems reasonable that the cell population responsible for adjusting skeletal mass can respond only to the strains to which it is subjected, not the potential strain it might see should an aberrant loading incident occur. Instead, perhaps the safety factors within bone are simply a valuable by-product of a tissue that strives for some cytologic benefit generated by this common strain milieu. The interspecies similarity in strain magnitudes is strong evidence for the existence of a common strain-sensitive cellular population within the skeletal tissues of each of these animals. Further, it suggests the existence of a generic cellular mechanism that strives toward a common, strain-determined structural goal that is desired by and beneficial to the bone cell population.

Strain-Regulated Adaptation

Although the nature of this structure-function relationship is only poorly understood, it has been proposed that bone remodeling is continually influenced by the level and distribution of the functional strains within the bone.[173] One striking example of the skeleton's capacity to adapt to its functional environment has been demonstrated in professional tennis players; by comparing the humeral mass of the racquet arm to the side that simply throws the ball into the air, Jones and colleagues[174] observed a 35 percent increase in men and a 28 percent increase in women in the cortical thickness of the more active humerus.

The converse can also be demonstrated, as immobilization and bed rest can cause negatively balanced bone remodeling either locally or within the entire skeleton. Healthy adult males restricted to complete bed rest for up to 36 weeks showed a total body calcium loss during that period averaging 4.2 percent; however, bone mineral content measurements of the calcaneus showed a mean decrease of 34 percent; in one case, 45 percent bone mineral was lost,[175] demonstrating that at specific weight-bearing sites the negatively balanced bone remodeling stimulated by diminished demand can be severe.

Optimal Strain Stimulus

Attempts to identify those aspects of the skeleton's functional milieu that are responsible for generating and controlling this adaptive response have demonstrated that alterations in bone mass, turnover, and internal replacement are sensitive to changes in the magnitude,[176] distribution,[177] and rate of strain[154] generated within the bone tissue. A loading regimen must be dynamic in nature; static loads do not influence bone morphology,[178] yet its full osteogenic potential is achieved after only an extremely short exposure to this stimulus.[179] The potency of the stimulus is proportional to the magnitude of the strain.[176] As strain levels that are acceptable in one location induce adaptive remodeling in others, each region of each bone may be genetically programmed to accept a particular amount and pattern of intermittent strain as normal. Deviation from this optimal strain environment stimulates changes in the bone's remodeling balance, resulting in adaptive increases or decreases in its mass.

It is not clear whether a discrepancy in strain is picked up at the level of each individual osteocyte, that the cell has the ability to manipulate the structural milieu of its adjacent space, or whether the osteocyte network somehow spatially integrates the load information across the cortex.[180] However, bone mass is substantially influenced by strain situations engendered by short periods of particularly osteogenic activity (e.g. vigorous and diverse exercise) rather than by the strain situation experienced during a predominant activity (e.g. walking) or by the fatigue damage that this might produce.

Isolating specific components of the physical milieu that regulate skeletal morphology has been difficult; no single parameter of the mechanical environment has been shown to reliably predict bone remodeling in all naturally observed or experimentally created conditions.[152] Perhaps our limited success in identifying these elusive stimuli has in part been due to our presumption that structural efficiency (minimal strain with minimal mass) is an essential goal of skeletal morphology. That the skeleton has "optimized" its structure is supported by the similarity in peak strains generated in the cortex regardless of animal or activity (2000 to 3000 microstrain), indicating a common, peak-strain determined goal. Contrasting with this perspective, however, is the nonuniform, but consistent distribution of normal and shear strains that exist throughout the stance phase, leaving large areas of the diaphyseal shaft subjected only to extremely low levels of strain energy density.[155] Further, rather than a signal to repair accumulated damage, a new strain milieu need be applied for only a very short time to maximize the tissue response.[172] Perhaps the engineering perspective that strain is harmful to bone and that remodeling is a repair drive process needs to be reconsidered. Instead, there may be some by-product of strain, such as stress-generated potentials, piezoelectric currents, or increased perifusion, which enhances the cell population's vitality.

Perhaps a principal objective of tissue adaptation is to promote and regulate some specific aspect of the functional milieu such that the matrix or cells within the tissue enjoy some direct or indirect benefit of strain.[181] Indeed, it may not even be the predominant components of the physical milieu that regulate these processes. Very-low-intensity electric fields (<1 mV/cm[182]) as well as low-magnitude strains (<100 microstrain[158]), when induced within a specific, hyperphysiologic (10- to 50-Hz) frequency band, influence bone mass as effectively as stimuli of greater intensity induced at more "physiologic" frequencies. Importantly, strains at this frequency and magnitude are induced as by-products of muscle contractions, which resonate between 20 and 50 Hz.[183] Perhaps we should be more hesitant to presume skeletal morphology to be a product of dominant strain parameters with the structural goal of minimizing strain and instead consider the matrix and cellular advantages of a tissue exposed to a dynamic functional milieu.

Bioelectric Stimuli

Although these data demonstrate some relationship of function to form, they do not suggest the means by which the physical signal is transduced by the cell and extracellular matrix into the adaptive process. A potential mechanism for the coupling of mechanical deformation and control of cellular metabolic activity may be the stress-generated electric potential (SGP). A change in the bone's level or type of activity in turn alters the magnitude of this potential charge at the bone-fluid interface. Vascular channels within haversian systems, combined with the lacunae and cannaliculi occupied by cells and the microporosity of the matrix, may consume as much as 10 percent of the bone tissue's volume and are filled with fluids and/or cellular components. The deformation, or straining of the skeleton caused by functional activity, initiates this fluid to flow, similar to the way in which water flows through a sponge that is stretched or compressed. While at one level this fluid behavior may contribute to increased perifusion and nutrient delivery, the ionic constituents of the fluid interact with the charged nature of the mineral to generate electrokinetic potentials.[184] In 1962, Bassett and Becker hypothesized that a primary step in translating functional load-bearing to an adaptive cellular response was linked to the electrical potential generated by the mechanical deformation of the bone tissue.[185] This postulation has been strongly supported by many subsequent investigators showing the relationship between electric potential and regulation of bone cell activity. Several excellent reviews are available.[156, 186]

Because fluid pressure gradients and the resultant streaming potentials affect primarily those cells confined within the cortices of the extracellular matrix (osteocytes) and changes in the "normal" electrokinetic signal would be generated by alterations in the type and/or amplitude of function, this intracortical syncytium might be a key regulator of osteoblast or osteoclast activity. This potential in turn may act to effect proliferation of osteoprogenitor cells.[187] or catalyze the production[188] or mineralization[189] of the extracellular matrix. Indeed, electric fields of extremely low magnitude can affect both differentiation of osteoblasts[190] and recruitment of osteoclasts.[191]

Whatever the signal transduction pathway of transforming physical information to something the cell population can perceive and respond to, it is clear that the capacity of bone tissue to adapt to its functional demands is critical to the skeleton's structural success. Indeed, as we attempt to evaluate the cellular mechanisms responsible for the positive control of bone mass, the osteogenic potential of physical stimuli cannot be ignored.

SUMMARY

This chapter has provided a brief overview of the cells responsible for the regulation of bone mass as well as the local and systemic factors that influence their activity. Clearly, these cells and matrix that make up the tissue of bone reflect a sophisticated interaction of organic and inorganic constituents that contribute to the skeleton's admirable capacity to serve both as mineral reservoir and structural entity. The process of cell proliferation and differentiation, matrix synthesis and mineralization, growth, and adaptation all contribute to this elaborate balance of modeling and remodeling. It is hoped that this chapter has diminished the skeleton's rather blasé reputation as a static entity and has demonstrated its critical role in the dynamic process of mineral homeostasis and its unparalled capacity to facilitate locomotion. It is neither solely a reservoir of mineral nor uniquely a structure. The skeleton represents an extremely complex and successful combination of these responsibilities.

References

1. Raisz LG, Kream BE: Regulation of bone formation. N Engl J Med 309:29–35, 1983.
2. Rodan G, Rodan S: Expression of the osteoblastic phenotype. In Peck W (ed): Bone and Mineral Research Annual. II. Amsterdam, Excerpta Medica, 1984, pp 244–285.
3. Roodman GD, Ibbotson KJ, MacDonald BR, Kuehl TJ, Mundy GR: 1,25(OH)2-vitamin D₃ causes formation of multinucleated cells with osteoclast characteristics in cultures of primate marrow. Proc Natl Acad Sci USA 82:8213–8217, 1985.
4. Doty S: Morphological evidence of gap junctions between bone cells. Calcif Tiss Int 33:509–512, 1981.
5. Rodan GA, Martin TJ: Role of osteoblasts in hormonal control of bone resorption: A hypothesis. Calcif Tissue Int 33:349–351, 1981.
6. Urist MF, Mikulski A, Lietze A: Solubilized and insolubilized bone morphogenetic protein. Proc Nat Acad Sci USA 76:1828–1832, 1979.
7. Wozney JM: Bone morphogenetic protein family and osteogenesis. Molec Reprod Dev 32:160–167, 1992.
8. Hirota S, Takaoka K, Hashimoto J, Takemura T, Morii E, Fukuyama A, Morihana K, Kitamura Y, Nomura S: Expression of mRNA of murine bone-related proteins in ectopic bone induced by murine bone morphogenetic protein 4. Cell Tissue Res 277:27–32, 1994.
9. Iimura T, Oida S, Takda K, Maruoka T, Sasaki S: Changes in homeobox-containing gene expression during ectopic bone formation induced by bone morphogenetic protein. Biochem Biophys Res Commun 201:980–987, 1994.
10. Stevenson S, Cunningham N, Toth J, Davy D, Reddi A: The effect of osteogenin (a bone morphogenetic protein) on the formation of bone in orthotopic segmental defects in rats. J Bone Joint Surg 76A:1676–1687, 1994.
11. Elima K: Osteoinductive proteins. Ann Med 24:395–402, 1993.
12. Takaishi T, Matsui T, Tsukamoto T, Ito M, Taniguchi T, Fukase M, Chihara K: TGF-β induced macrophage colony-stimulating factor gene expression in various mesenchymal cell lines. Am J Physiol 267:C25–C31, 1994.
13. Rhodas RE, Volenfriend S: Decarboxylation of X-hetoglutarate coupled to collagen prolin hydroxylate. Proc Natl Acad Sci USA 60:1473, 1968.
14. Rosenbloom J, Prockop DJ: Biochemical aspects of collagen biosynthesis. Repair and regeneration. In Dunphy JS, Van Winkle W (eds): Scientific Basis of Surgical Practice. New York, McGraw-Hill, 1969, pp 117–135.
15. Pritchard JJ: General histology of bone. In Bourne GH (ed): The Biochemistry and Physiology of Bone, 2nd ed. Vol I. New York, Academic Press, 1972, p 15.
16. Ascenzi A, Bonucci E: Relationship between ultrastructure and "pin test" in osteons. Clin Orthop 121:275, 1976.
17. Owen TA, Aronow M, Shalhoub V, Barone LM, Wilming L, Tasinari MS, Kennedy MB, Pockwsinse S, Lian JB, Stein GS: Progressive development of the rat osteoblast phenotype in vitro: Reciprocal relationships in expression of genes associated with osteoblast proliferation and differentiation during formation of the bone extracellular matrix. J Cell Physiol 143:420–430, 1990.
18. Martin TJ, Allan EH, Fukumoto S: The plasminogen activator and inhibitor system in bone remodeling. Growth Reg 3:209–214, 1993.
19. Reinholt FP, Hultenby K, Oldberg A, Heinegard D: Osteopontin—a possible anchor of osteoclasts to bone. Proc Natl Acad Sci USA 87:4473–4475, 1990.
20. Canalis E, Centrella M, Burch W, McCarthy TL: Insulin-like growth factor I mediates selective anabolic effects of parathyroid hormone in bone cultures. J Clin Invest 83:60–65, 1989.
21. Owen M: Cellular dynamics of bone. In Bourne GH (ed): The Biochem-

istry and Physiology of Bone, 2nd ed. Vol III. New York, Academic Press, 1972, p 271.

22. Jaworski ZFG: Lamellar bone turnover system and its effector organ. Calcif Tissue Int 36S:46, 1984.

23. Jowsey J: Metabolic Diseases of Bone. Philadelphia, WB Saunders, 1977, p 61.

24. Parfitt AM: Osteomalacia and related disorders. In Avioli LV, Krane SM (eds): Metabolic Bone Disease and Clinically Related Disorders. Philadelphia, WB Saunders, 1990, p 329.

25. Menton DN, Simmons DJ, Chang SL, Orr BY: From bone lining cell to osteocyte: An SEM study. Anat Rec 209:29–39, 1984.

26. Curtis TA, Ashrafi SH, Weber DF: Canalicular communication in the cortices of human long bones. Anat Rec 212:336–344, 1985.

27. VanderMolen M, Rubin C, Donahue H: Decreased hormonal responsiveness in gap junction deficient osteoblasts. Trans 41st Orthop Res Soc 20:295, 1995.

28. Robinson RA: Observations regarding compartments for tracer calcium in the body. In Frost HM (ed): Bone Biodynamics. Boston, Little, Brown, 1964.

29. Atkinson PJ, Hallsworth B: The changing pore structure of aging human mandibular bone. Gerontology 2:57–63, 1983.

30. Albright JA, Skinner C: Bone: Structural organization and remodeling dynamics. In Albright JA, Brand RA (eds): The Scientific Basis of Orthopaedics, 2nd ed. East Norwalk, Conn, Appleton & Lange, 1987, pp 161–198.

31. Boyce BF, Chen H, Soriano P, Mundy G: Histomorphometric and immunocytochemical studies of src-related osteopetrosis. Bone 14:335–340, 1993.

32. Kahn AJ, Simmons DJ: Investigation of cell lineage in bone using a chimaera of chick and quail embryonic tissue. Nature 258:325, 1975.

33. Felix R, Cecchini M, Fleisch H: MCSF restores in vivo bone resorption in the op/op osteopetrotic mouse. Endocrinology 127:2592, 1990.

34. Grigoradis AE, Wang A, Cecchini MG, Hofstetter W, Felix R, Fleisch HA, Wagner EF: c-Fos: A key regulator of osteoclast-macrophage lineage determination and bone remodeling. Science 266:443–448, 1994.

35. Suda T, Takahashi N, Martin TJ: Modulation of osteoclast differentiation. Endocr Rev 13:66–80, 1992.

36. Jilka RL, Hangoc G, Girasole G, Passeri G, Williams D, Abrams JS, Boyce B, Broxmeier H, Manolagas SC: Increased osteoclast development after estrogen loss: Mediation by interleukin-6. Science 257:88–91, 1992.

37. Roodman G, Kurihara N, Ohsaki Y, Kukita A, Hosking D, Demulder A, Smith JF, Singer FR: Interleukin 6: A potential autocrine/paracrine factor in Paget's disease of bone. J Clin Invest 98:46–52, 1992.

38. Walker DG: Enzymatic and electron microscopic analysis of isolated osteoclasts. Calcif Tissue Res 9:296, 1972.

39. Baron R: Polarity and membrane transport in osteoclasts. Conn Tissue Res 20:109–120, 1989.

40. Blair HC, Teitelbaum SL, Chiselli R, Gluck S: Osteoclastic bone resorption by a polarized vacuolar proton pump. Science 245:855–857, 1989.

41. Jones SJ, Boyde A, Ali NN, Maconnachie E: A review of bone cell substratum interactions. Scanning 7:5–24, 1985.

42. Silver A, Murrills RJ, Etherington DJ: Microelectrode studies on the acid microenvironment beneath adherent macrophages and osteoclasts. Exp Cell Res 175:266–276, 1988.

43. Biskobing D, Nanes M, Rubin J: 1,25(OH)₂D is required for protein kinase C upregulation of carbonic anhydrase 11 in a mono-myelocytic cell line. Endocrinology 139:1493–1498, 1994.

44. Soriano P, Montgomery C, Geske R, Bradley A: Targeted disruption of the c-src protoncogene leads to osteopetrosis in mice. Cell 64:693, 1991.

45. Williams JP, Blair H, Jordan S, McDonald JM: Tamoxifen inhibits osteoclastic bone resorption and H⁺-ATPase activity by an estrogen receptor independent mechanism. J Bone Min Res 9:62, 1994.

46. Partridge NC, Jeffrey JJ, Ehlich LL, Teitelbaum SL, Fliszar C, Welgus HG, Kahn AJ: Hormonal regulation of the production of collagenase and a collagenase inhibitor activity by rat osteogenic sarcoma cells. Endocrinology 120:1956–1962, 1987.

47. Diagnosis and management of asymptomatic primary hyperparathyroidism: Consensus Development Conference Statement. Ann Intern Med 1145:593–597, 1991.

48. McSheehy PMJ, Chambers TJ: Osteoblast-like cells in the presence of parathyroid hormone release soluble factor that stimulates osteoclastic bone resorption. Endocrinology 119:1654–1659, 1986.

49. Donahue HJ, Fryer MJ, Eriksen EF, Heath H III: Differential effects of parathyroid hormone and its analogues on cytosolic calcium ion and cAMP levels in cultured rat osteoblast-like cells. J Biol Chem 263:13522–13527, 1988.

50. Rouleau MF, Warshawsky H, Goltzman D: Parathyroid hormone binding in vivo to renal, hepatic, and skeletal tissues of the rat using a radioautographic approach. Endocrinology 118:919–931, 1986.

51. Pharoah MJ, Heersche JNM: 1,25-Dihydroxyvitamin D₃ causes an increase in the number of osteoclast-like cells in cat bone marrow cultures. Calcif Tissue Int 37:276–281, 1985.

52. Stern PH: Vitamin D and bone. Kidney Int 38:S17–S21, 1990.

53. Eriksen EF, Colvard DS, Berg NJ, Graham ML, Mann KG, Spelsberg TC, Riggs L: Evidence of estrogen receptors in normal human osteoblast-like cells. Science 241:84–86, 1988.

54. Komm B, Terpening C, Benz D, Graeme K, Gallegos A, Korc M, Gree G, O'Malley B, Haussler M: Estrogen binding, receptor mRNA, and biologic response in osteoblast-like osteosarcoma cells. Science 241:81–84, 1988.

55. Ernst M, Schmid CH, Froesch ER: Enhanced osteoblast proliferation and collagen gene expression by estradiol. Proc Natl Acad Sci USA 85:2307–2310, 1988.

56. Gray TK, Mohan S, Linkhart TA, Baylink DJ: Estradiol stimulates in vitro the secretion of insulin-like growth factors by the clonal osteoblastic cell line, UMR 106. Biochem Biophys Res Commun 158:407–412, 1989.

57. Oursler MJ, Landers JP, Riggs BL, Spelsberg TC: Oestrogen effects on osteoblasts and osteoclasts. Ann Med 25:361–371, 1993.

58. Smith EP, et al: Estrogen resistance caused by a mutation in the estrogen-receptor gene in a man. N Engl J Med 16:1056–1061, 1994.

59. Colvard DS, Eriksen EF, Keeting PE, Wilson EM, Lubahn DB, French FS, Riggs BL, Spelsberg TC: Identification of androgen receptors in normal human osteoblast-like cells. Proc Natl Acad Sci USA 86:854–857, 1989.

60. Fukayama S, Tashjian AH: Direct modulation by androgens of the response of human bone cells (SaOS-2) to human parathyroid hormone (PTH) and PTH-related protein. Endocrinology 125:1789–1790, 1989.

61. NIH Consensus Development Conference on Osteoporosis. JAMA 252:799–802, 1984.

62. Raisz LG, Niemann I: Effect of phosphate, calcium and magnesium on bone resorption and hormonal responses in tissue culture. Endocrinology 85:446–452, 1969.

63. Yamaguchi DT, Hahn TJ, Beeker TG, Kleeman CR, Muallem S: Relationship of cAMP and calcium messenger systems in prostaglandin-stimulated UMR-106 cells. J Biol Chem 263:10745–10753, 1988.

64. Austin LA, Heath H III: Calcitonin: Physiology and pathophysiology. N Engl J Med 304:269–278, 1981.

65. Arnaud CD, Kolb FO: The calciotropic hormones and metabolic bone disease. In Greenspan FS, Forsham PH (eds): Basic and Clinical Endocrinology. Los Altos, Calif, Lange Medical Publications, 1983, pp 187–250.

66. Nicholson GC, Moseley JM, Sexton PM, Mendelsohn FAO, Martin TJ: Abundant calcitonin receptors in isolated rat osteoclasts: Biochemical and autoradiographic characterization. J Clin Invest 78:355–360, 1986.

67. Chambers TJ, Athanasou NA, Fuller K: Effect of parathyroid hormone and calcitonin on the cytoplasmic spreading of isolated osteoclasts. J Endocrinol 102:281, 1984.

68. Murrills RJ, Dempster DW: The effects of stimulators of intracellular cyclic AMP on rat and chick osteoclasts in vitro: Validation of a simplified light microscope assay of bone resorption. Bone 11:333–344, 1990.

69. Deftos LJ, Roos B: Medullary thyroid carcinoma and calcitonin gene expression. In Peck WA (ed): Bone and Mineral Research. II. Excerpta Medica, Amsterdam, 1989, pp 267–316.

70. Raisz LG: Local and systemic factors in the pathogenesis of osteoporosis. N Engl J Med 318:818–828, 1988.

71. Canalis E, McCarthy T, Centrella M: Growth factors and the regulation of bone remodeling. J Clin Invest 81:277–281, 1988.

72. Pfeilschifter JP, Seyedin S, Mundy GR: Transformed growth factor-β inhibits bone resorption in fetal rat long bone cultures. J Clin Invest 82:680–685, 1988.

73. Noda M, Camilliere JJ: In vivo stimulation of bone formation by transforming growth factor-β. Endocrinology 124:2991–2994, 1989.

74. Chenu C, Pfeilschifter J, Mundy GR, Roodman GD: Transforming growth factor-β inhibits formation of osteoclast-like cells in long-term human marrow cultures. Proc Natl Acad Sci USA 85:5683–5687, 1988.

75. Goldring MJ, Goldring SR: Skeletal tissue response to cytokines. Clin Orthop 258:245–278, 1990.

76. Rubin CT, Hausman MR: The cellular basis of Wolff's law: Transduction of physical stimuli to skeletal adaptation. Rheum Dis Clin North Am 14:503–517, 1988.

77. Carter D, Wong A: Mechanical stresses and endochondral ossification in chondroepiphysis. J Orthop Res 6:148, 1988.

78. Parfitt AM: The coupling of bone resorption to bone formation: A critical analysis of the concept and of its relevance to the pathogenesis of osteoporosis. Metab Bone Dis Relat Res 4:1–6, 1982.

79. Bain SD, Impeduglia TM, Rubin CT: Cement line staining in undecalcified thin sections of cortical bone. Stain Tech 65:159–163, 1990.

80. Parfitt AM: The cellular basis of bone remodeling: The quantum concept re-examined in light of recent advances in cell biology of bone. Calcif Tissue Int 36(Suppl):S37–S45, 1984.

81. Fisher LW, Gehron RP, Tuross N, et al: The Mr 24,000 phosphoprotein from developing bone is the NH2-terminal propeptide of the α chain of type I collagen. J Biol Chem 262:13457, 1987.

82. Noda M, Yoon, Prince CW, et al: Transcriptional regulation of osteopontin production in rat osteosarcoma cells by type β transforming growth factor. J Biol Chem 263:13916, 1988.

83. Price PA, Otsuka AS, Poser JW, et al: Characterization of gamma-carboxyglutamic acid containing protein from bone. Proc Natl Acad Sci USA 73:1447, 1976.

84. Urist MR, Juo YK, Brownell AG, et al: Purification of bovine bone morphogenetic protein by hydroxyapatite chromatography. Proc Natl Acad Sci USA 81:371, 1984.

85. Termine JD, Belcourt AB, Conn KM, et al: Mineral and collagen-binding proteins of fetal calf bone. J Biol Chem 256:10403, 1981.

86. Robey PG: The biochemistry of bone. Endocrinol Metab Clin North Am 18:859–902, 1989.

87. Eyre DR: Collagen: Molecular diversity in the body's protein scaffold. Science 207:1315, 1980.

88. Boskey AL, Posner AS: Bone structure, composition and mineralization. Orthop Clin North Am 15:597, 1984.

89. Veis A, Sharkey M, Dickson I: Non-collagenous proteins of bone and dentin extracellular matrix and their role in organized mineral deposition. In Wasserman RH (ed): Calcium Binding Proteins and Calcium Function. New York, Elsevier, 1977, pp 409–418.

90. Glimcher MJ: Studies of the structure, organization and reactivity of bone collagen. In Gibson T (ed): Proceedings of the International Symposium on Wound Healing. Montreaux Foundation of International Cooperative Medical Science, 1975, p 253.

91. Herring GM: The chemical structure of tendon cartilage, dentin and bone matrix. Clin Orthop 60:261, 1968.

92. Boskey AL: Mineral-matrix interactions in bone and cartilage. Clin Orthop 281:244, 1992.

93. Skerry TM, Suswillo R, ElHaj AJ, Ali NN, Dodds RA, Lanyon LE: Load-induced proteoglycan orientation in bone tissue in vivo and in vitro. Calcif Tissue Int 46:318–326, 1990.

94. Termine JD, Kleinman HK, Whitson SW, et al: Osteonectin, a bone-specific protein linking mineral to collagen. Cell 26:99, 1981.

95. Romberg RW, Werness PG, Lollar P, et al: Isolation and characterization of native adult osteonectin. J Biol Chem 260:2728, 1985a.

96. Termine JD, Eanes ED, Conn KM: Phosphoprotein modulation of apatite crystallization. Calcif Tissue Int 31:247–251, 1980.

97. Hauschka PV, Lian JB, Cole DEC, Gundberg CM: Osteocalcin and matrix Gla protein: Vitamin K–dependent protein in bone. Phys Rev 69:990–1047, 1988.

98. Lian JB, Coutts M, Canalis E: Studies of hormonal regulation of osteocalcin synthesis in cultured fetal rat calvariae. J Biol Chem 260:8706–8710, 1985.

99. Canalis E, McCarthy T, Centrella M: Growth factors and the regulation of bone remodeling. J Clin Invest 81:277–281, 1988.

100. Lian JB, Gundberg CM: Osteocalcin: Biochemical considerations and clinical applications. Clin Orthop 262:267–291, 1988.

101. Weiner S, Traub W: Bone structure: From angstroms to microns. FASEB J 6:879–885, 1992.

102. Posner AS: Crystal chemistry of bone mineral. Physiol Rev 49:760, 1969.

103. Moradian-Oldak J, Weiner S, Addadi L, Landis WJ, Traub W: Electron imaging and diffraction study of individual crystals of bone, mineralized tendon and synthetics carbonate apatite. Connect Tissue Res 25:219–228, 1991.

104. Bonar LC, Roufosse AH, Sabine WK, Grynpas MD, Glimcher MJ: X-ray diffraction studies of the crystallinity of bone mineral in newly synthesized and density fractioned bone. Calcif Tissue Int 35:202–209, 1983.

105. Rubin CT, Bain S, McLeod KJ: Suppression of the osteogenic response in the aging skeleton. Calcif Tissue Int 50:306–313, 1992.

106. Wolff J: The Law of Remodeling. Berlin, Springer Verlag, 1986 (original manuscript 1892). Translated by P. Maquet, R. Furlong.

107. Rosenberg LC, Choi HU, Poole AR: Biological processes involved in endochondral ossification. In Rubin RT, Weiss GB, Putney JB (eds): Calcium in Biological Systems. New York, Plenum Publishing, 1985, pp 617–624.

108. Eggli PS, Herrmann W, Hunziker EB, Schenk RK: Matrix compartments in the growth plate of the proximal tibia of rats. Anat Rec 211:246, 1985.

109. Floyd WE, Zaleske DJ, Schiller AL, Trahan C, Mankin HJ: Vascular events associated with the appearance of the secondary center of ossification in the murine distal femoral epiphysis. J Bone Joint Surg 69A:185, 1987.

110. Trelstad RL, Silver FH: Matrix assembly. In Hay ED (ed): Cell Biology of Extracellular Matrix. New York, Plenum Publishing, 1981, pp 179–215.

111. Roux W: Gesammelte Abhandlungen uber Entwicklungsmechanik der Organismen. Vol I and II. Leipzig, Wilhelm Engelmann, 1895. Terminologie der Entwicklungsmechanik der Tiere und Pflanzen. Leipzig, Wilhelm Engelmann, 1912. Virchows Arch (A):209:168, 1912.

112. Carter DR, Orr TE, Fyhrie DP, Schurman DJ: Influences of mechanical stress on prenatal and postnatal skeletal development. Clin Orthop 219:237, 1987.

113. Shapiro F, Holtrop ME, Glimcher MJ: Organization and cellular biology of the perichondrial ossification groove of Ranvier. J Bone Joint Surg 59A:703, 1977.

114. Cooper RR, Misol S: Tendon and ligament insertion: A light and electron microscopic study. J Bone Joint Surg 52A:1, 1970.

115. Christoffersen J, Landis WJ: A contribution with review to the description of bone and other calcified tissues in vivo. Anat Rec 230:435–450, 1991.

116. Jowsey J: Microradiography: A morphologic approach to quantitating bone turnover. Excerpta Medica International Congress Series No. 270. Amsterdam, Excerpta MedicaFoundation, 1972, p 114.

117. Glimcher MJ, Lian JB: The Chemistry and Biology of Mineralized Tissues. Proceedings of the Third International Conference on the Chemistry and Biology of Mineralized Tissues. New York, Gordon and Breach Science Publishers, 1988.

118. Wuthier RE, Jajeska RJ, Collins GM: Biosynthesis of matrix vesicles in epiphyseal cartilage. 1. In vivo incorporation of 32P-orthophosphate into phospholipid of chondrocyte, membrane and matrix vesicle fractions. Calcif Tissue Res 23:135–139, 1977.

119. Kerr JFR, Wyllie AH, Currie AR: Apoptosis: A basic biological phenomenon with wide ranging implications in tissue kinetics. Br J Cancer 26:239, 1972.

120. Russell RGG, Caswell AM, Hearn PR, Sharrard RM: Calcium in mineralized tissues and pathological calcification. Br Med Bull 42:435, 1986.

121. Anderson HC: Electron microscopic studies of induced cartilage development and calcification. J Cell Biol 35:81, 1967.

122. Anderson HC: Matrix vesicle calcification: Review and update. In Peck WA (ed): Bone and Mineral Research. Vol 3. New York, Elsevier, 1985.

123. Wuthier RE: Lipid composition of isolated cartilage cells, membranes and matrix vesicles. Biochim Biophys Acta 409:128, 1975.

124. Endo A, Glimcher MJ: The potential role of phosphoproteins in the in vitro calcification of bone collagen. In Goldberg VM (ed): Transactions of the 32nd Meeting of Orthopaedic Research Society. Chicago, Adept Printing, 1986, pp 221.

125. Puzas JE: Phosphotyrosine phosphatase activity in bone cells: An old enzyme with a new function. Adv Protein Phosphatases 3:237–256, 1986.

126. Anderson HC: Biology of disease: Mechanism of mineral formation in bone. Lab Invest 60:320, 1989.

127. Wuthier RE: The role of phospholipids in biological calcification: Distribution of phospholipase activity in calcifying epiphyseal cartilage. Clin Orthop 90:191, 1973.

128. Peress NS, Anderson HC, Sajdera SW: The lipids of matrix vesicles from bovine fetal epiphyseal cartilage. Calcif Tissue Res 14:275, 1974.

129. Termine JD, Belcourt AB, Conn KM, et al: Mineral and collagen-binding proteins of fetal calf bone. J Biol Chem 256:10403, 1981.

130. Hynes RO: The molecular biology of fibronectin. Ann Rev Cell Biol 1:67, 1985.

131. Glimcher MJ, Krane SM: The organization and structure of bone and the mechanism of calcification. In Ramachandran GN, Gould BS (eds): Treatise on Collagen. Vol 11B. Biology of Collagen. New York, Academic Press, 1968, p 68.

132. Baylink D, Wengedal J, Thompson E: Loss of protein polysaccharides at sites where bone mineralization is initiated. J Histochem Cytochem 20:279, 1972.

133. Glimcher MJ: Composition, structure and organization of bone and other mineralized tissues and the mechanism of calcification. In Handbook of Physiology: Endocrinology. Vol VII. Baltimore, Williams & Wilkins, 1976, p 25.

134. Parfitt AL: Bone histomorphometry: Proposed system for standardization of nomenclature, symbols and units. Calcif Tissue Int 42:284–286, 1988.

135. Hayes WC, Gerhart TN: Biomechanics of bone: Applications for assessment of bone strength. In Peck WA (ed): Bone and Mineral Research, 3rd ed. New York, Elsevier, 1985, p 259.

136. Lanyon LE: Analysis of surface bone strain in the calcaneus of sheep during normal locomotion: Strain analysis of the calcaneus. J Biomech 6:41–49, 1973.

137. Ascenzi A: The micromechanics versus the macromechanics of cortical bone: A comprehensive presentation. J Biomech Eng 110:357–363, 1988.

138. Martin RB, Burr DB: Structure, Function, and Adaptation of Compact Bone. New York, Raven Press, 1989, pp 1–275.

139. Jones BH, Harris J McA, Vinh TN, Rubin CT: Exercise-induced stress fractures and stress reactions of bone: Epidemiology, etiology, and classification. In Pandolf KB (ed): Exerc Sport Sci Rev 17:379–422, 1989.

140. Rubin CT, Gross T, McLeod K, Bain SD: Morphologic stages in lamellar bone formation stimulated by a potent mechanical stimulus. J Bone Miner Res 10:488–495, 1995.

141. Albright JA, Skinner HCW: Bone: structural organization and remodeling dynamics. In Albright JA, Brand RA (eds): The Scientific Basis of Orthopaedics, 2nd ed. East Norwalk, Conn, Appleton & Lange, 1987, pp 161–198.

142. Frost HM: Secondary osteon population densities: An algorithm for estimating the missing osteons; Yearbook of Physical Anthropology 30:221–238, 1987.

143. Ascenzi A, Benvenuti A: Orientation of collagen fibers at the boundary between two successive osteonic lamellae and its mechanical interpretation. J Biomech 19:455–463, 1986.

144. Schaffler MB, Burr DB, Fredrickson RG: Morphology of the osteonal cement line in human bone. Anat Rec 217:223–228, 1987.

145. Garn SM: The course of bone gain and the phases of bone loss. Orthop Clin North Am 3:503, 1972.

146. Ruff CV, Hayes WC: Subperiosteal expansion and cortical remodeling of the human femur and tibia with aging. Science 217:945, 1982.

147. Enlow DH: Principles of Bone Remodeling. Springfield, Ill, Charles C Thomas, 1963.

148. Koch JC: The laws of bone architecture. Am J Anat 21:177, 1917.

149. Lanyon LE, Rubin CT, Baust G: Modulation of bone loss during calcium insufficiency by controlled dynamic loading. Calcif Tissue Int 38:209–216, 1986.

150. Bain SD, Rubin CT: Metabolic modulation of disuse osteopenia: Endocrine-dependent site specificity of bone remodeling. J Bone Miner Res 5:1069–1075, 1990.

151. Rubin CT: The benefits and consequences of structural adaptation in bone. *In* Fitzgerald R (ed): Non-Cemented Total Hip Arthroplasty. New York, Raven Press, 1988, pp 41–48.

152. Brown TD, Pedersen DR, Gray ML, Brand RA, Rubin CT: Toward an identification of mechanical parameters initiating periosteal remodeling: A combined experimental and analytic approach. J Biomech 23:893–905, 1990.

153. Radin EL, Martin RB, Burr DB, Caterson B, Boyd RD, Goodwin C: Effects of mechanical loading on the tissues of the rabbit knee. J Orthop Res 2:221–234, 1984.

154. O'Connor JA, Lanyon LE, MacFie H: The influence of strain rate on adaptive bone remodeling. J Biomech 15:767–781, 1982.

155. Rubin C, Gross T, Donahue H, Guilak F, McLeod K: Physical and environmental influences on bone formation. *In* Brighton CT, Friedlaender GE, Lane JM (eds): Bone Formation and Repair. Rosemont, Ill, American Academy of Orthopaedic Surgeons, 1994.

156. Bassett CA: Fundamental and practical aspects of therapeutic uses of pulsed electromagnetic fields (PEMFs). Crit Rev Biomed Eng 17:451–529, 1989.

157. Heckman J, Ryaby J, McCabe J, Frey J, Kilcoyne R: Acceleration of tibial fracture healing by noninvasive low intensity ultrasound. J Bone Joint Surg 76A:165–174, 1994.

158. Rubin CT, McLeod KJ: Promotion of bony ingrowth by frequency specific, low-amplitude mechanical strain. Clin Orthop 298:165–174, 1994.

159. Shim SS: Physiology of blood circulation of bone. J Bone Joint Surg 50A:812, 1968.

160. Sledge CB: Epiphyseal injuries. *In* Cave EF, Burke JF, Boyd RJ (eds): Trauma Management. Chicago, Year Book Medical Publishers, 1974.

161. Cowin SC: Bone mechanics. Boca Raton, Fla, CRC Press, p 313, 1989.

162. Ascenzi A, Bell GH: Bone as a mechanical engineering problem. *In* Bourne GH (ed): The Biochemistry and Physiology of Bone. Vol 1. Structure. New York, Academic Press, 1972, p 311.

163. Reilly DT, Burstein AH: The elastic and ultimate properties of compact bone tissue. J Biomech 8:393–405, 1975.

164. Carter DR, Harris WH, Caler WE: The mechanical and biological response of cortical bone to in vivo strain histories. *In* Cowin SC (ed): Mechanical Properties of Bone, AMD. Vol 45. New York, American Society of Mechanical Engineers, 1981, pp 81–92.

165. Curry JD: Mechanical properties of bone with greatly differing functions. J Biomech 12:313, 1979.

166. Lanyon LE, Rubin CT: Functional adaptation in skeletal structures. *In* Hildebrand M, Bramble DM, Leim KF, Wake DB (eds): Functional Vertebrate Morphology. Cambridge, Harvard University Press, 1985, pp 1–25.

167. Woo SLY: The relationships of changes in stress levels on long bone remodeling. *In* Cowen S (ed): Mechanical Properties of Bone, AMD. Vol 45. New York, American Society of Mechanical Engineers, 1981, p 107.

168. Rubin CT, Lanyon LE: Limb mechanics as a function of speed and gait: A study of functional strains in the radius and tibia of horse and dog. J Exp Biol 101:187–211, 1982.

169. Gross T, McLeod K, Rubin C: Characterizing the bone strain distributions in vivo using three triple rosette strain gages. J Biomech 25:1081–1087, 1992.

170. Rubin CT: Skeletal strain and the functional strain significance of bone architecture. Calcif Tissue Int 36:S11–S18, 1984.

171. Lanyon LE: The influence of function on the development of bone curvature: An experimental study on the rat tibia. J Zool Lond 192:457–466, 1980.

172. Rubin CT, Lanyon LE: Dynamic strain similarity in vertebrates: An alternative to allometric limb bone scaling. J Theor Biol 107:321–327, 1984.

173. Rubin CT, Lanyon LE: Osteoregulatory nature of mechanical stimuli: Function as a determinant for adaptive remodeling in bone. J Orthop Res 5:300–310, 1987.

174. Jones HH, Pries JD, Hayes WC, Tichenor CC, Nagel DA: Humeral hypertrophy in response to exercise. J Bone Joint Surg 59A:204–208, 1977.

175. Donaldson CL, Hulley SB, Vogel JM, Hattner RS, Bayers JH, McMillan DE: Effect of prolonged bed rest on bone mineral. Metabolism 19:1071, 1970.

176. Rubin CT, Lanyon LE: Regulation of bone mass by mechanical loading: Ether effect of peak strain magnitude. Calcif Tissue Int 37:411, 1985.

177. Lanyon LE, Goodship AE, Pye C, MacFie H: Mechanically adaptive bone remodeling: A quantitative study on function adaptation in the radius following ulna osteotomy in sheep. J Biomech 15:141–154, 1982.

178. Lanyon LE, Rubin CT: Static versus dynamic loads as an influence on bone remodeling. J Biomech 17:897, 1984.

179. Rubin CT, Lanyon LE: Regulation of bone formation by applied dynamic loads. J Bone Joint Surg 66A:397–402, 1984.

180. Sun Y, McLeod K, Rubin C: Upregulation of collage type 1 mRNA following mechanical loading as measured by in situ RT PCR. Trans 41st Orthop Res Soc 20:290, 1995.

181. Rubin CT, McLeod KJ: Biologic modulation of mechanical influence sin bone remodeling. *In* Mow VC, Ratcliffe A, Woo SLY (eds): Biomechanics of Diarthrodial Joints. Vol II. New York, Springer-Verlag, 1990, pp 97–118.

182. McLeod KJ, Rubin CT: The effect of low frequency electric fields on osteogenesis. J Bone Joint Surg 74A:920–929, 1992.

183. McLeod K, Rubin C: Strain frequency spectra in the appendicular skeleton during normal activity. J Biomech (in press).

184. Berretta D, Pollack SR: Ion concentration effects on the zeta potential of bone. J Orthop Res 4:337–345, 1986.

185. Bassett CA: Biophysical principles affecting bone structure. *In* The Biochemistry and Physiology of Bone. Vol 3. New York, Academic Press, 1971, pp 1–76.

186. Brighton CT, McCluskey WP: Cellular response and mechanism of action of electrically induced osteogenesis. *In* Peck WA (ed): Bone and Mineral Research, 4th ed. Elsevier, 1986.

187. Ashihara T, Kagawa K, Kamich M, et al: 3H-Thymidine autoradiographic studies of the cell proliferation and differentiation in electrically stimulated osteogenesis. *In* Brighton CT, Black J, Pollack SR (eds): Electrical Properties of Bone and Cartilage. New York, Grune & Stratton, 1979.

188. McLeod KJ, Lee RD, Ehrlich HP: Frequency dependence of electric field modulation of fibroblast protein synthesis. Science 236:1465–1469, 1987.

189. Bassett CAL, Chokshi HR, Hernandez E, et al: The effect of pulsing electromagnetic fields on cellular calcium and calcification of nonunions. *In* Brighton CT, Black J, Pollack SR (eds): Electrical Properties of Bone and Cartilage. New York, Grune & Stratton, 1979.

190. McLeod K, Fontaine MA, Donahue HJ, Rubin CT: Electric fields modulate bone cell function in a density dependent manner. J Bone Miner Res 8:977–983, 1993.

191. Rubin J, McLeod K, Titus L, Nanes MS, Catherwood BD, Rubin CT: Formation of osteoclast-like cells is suppressed by low frequency, low intensity electric fields. J Orthop Res 14:7–15, 1996.

CHAPTER 5

Skeletal Muscle

Jody A. Dantzig
Yale E. Goldman

The approximately 640 skeletal muscles that support and move the body, under control of the central nervous system (CNS), constitute up to 40 percent of the adult human body mass. Skeletal muscles are positioned across joints and are fastened to two or more bones by *tendons* composed mainly of type I and type XII collagen and fibroblasts. Movement of the skeleton is accomplished when the muscles shorten by transduction of chemical energy into mechanical work. The specialization of muscle cells for this task is evident from the intricate architecture and kinetics of both the contractile proteins and the intracellular membrane systems. Muscle cells are normally subjected to wide variations in their levels of activity and are able to adapt in size, isoenzyme composition, and membrane organization. This *plasticity* can be surprisingly swift and extensive. This chapter outlines the development, structure, and function of muscle and introduces the basis for its highly adaptive response to altered demands. These processes affect the course of many diseases.

MUSCLE DEVELOPMENT

During embryogenesis, mesodermal stem cells differentiate into connective tissue, bone, and skeletal muscle. The events that control the expression of skeletal muscle–specific (SMS) genes and regulate skeletal muscle cell differentiation and maturation are emerging from molecular biologic studies.[1-6] Sequentially expressed regulators, such as the myocyte enhancer factors (e.g., MEF2A, MEF2B)[6] and the myogenic basic helix-loop-helix (bHLH) proteins (MyoD, myf5, mrf4, and myogenin),[1-5] initiate the transcription of SMS genes in *presumptive myoblasts* (precursors of muscle cells). These transcription factors can also switch SMS genes on when expressed in non-muscle cells.[7] Myogenic bHLH proteins and MEF2 bind cooperatively to neighboring sites on the DNA and coordinate the developmental program of the muscle cell lineage.[6, 8] The detailed relationships of these control proteins with other ubiquitous regulatory factors[9, 10] and the "master switch" for myogenesis remain to be determined.

When the mesenchymal cells commit to the myogenic cell line, the presumptive myoblasts proliferate and migrate to sites of muscle development within the embryo. They withdraw from the cell cycle and differentiate into spindle-shaped *myoblasts* containing the initial framework for the contractile apparatus. They align and fuse to produce multinucleated *primary myotubes* (Fig. 5–1), which continue to synthesize embryonic isoforms of the muscle-specific proteins.[11] Myofibrils are assembled near the periphery of the myotubes and move in toward the center of the cell, now termed *muscle fiber.* Myofibrillogenesis continues until the cytoplasm is filled with parallel and laterally aligned myofibrils. The nuclei then migrate from the center to the periphery of the cell, where they remain in the mature muscle fiber.

An extracellular matrix of type IV collagen, proteoglycans, fibronectin, and laminin is secreted by the myotubes to form the *basal lamina,* which ensheaths the cell completely except at the neuromuscular junction.[12] Secondary generations of myoblasts elongate, fuse, and differentiate within the basal laminae of the primary myotubes, forming independent, secondary myotubes.[13] The myotubes develop into phenotypically distinct types of muscle fibers by sequentially expressing a series of embryonic, neonatal, and mature isoforms of the contractile proteins. The developmental and mature isoforms of the contractile proteins (*myosin, actin, tropomyosin,* and *troponin*) expressed in fast, slow, and cardiac muscle are either encoded by multigene families or determined by alternative splicing of messenger RNA (mRNA).

Under normal conditions, the number of muscle fibers within a skeletal muscle remains constant throughout life. However, a pool of myogenic stem cells (*satellite cells*) remains in the mature muscles, providing a reservoir of myoblasts for muscle repair and growth.[14] Satellite cells are situated between the cell membrane (*sarcolemma*) and basal laminae of the muscle fibers. When a cell is structurally damaged or necrosed, the basal lamina provides a scaffold for migration of the satellite cells into the affected area. The myoblasts fuse to form a new muscle fiber. This process is initiated by mitogenic factors and peptide regulators released from the damaged cells.[15]

STRUCTURE

Muscle fibers make up 85 percent of muscle tissue; the remainder is innervation and blood supply as well as connective tissue structures that provide support, elasticity, and force transmission to the skeleton. The fibers are 10 to 150 μm in diameter and a few millimeters to a few centimeters long. Some of the mechanical

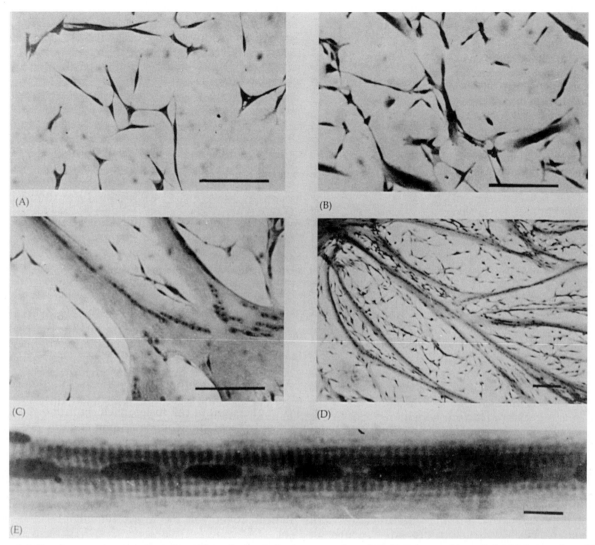

Figure 5–1. Developmental progression of myoblasts during fusion into myotubes. *A,* Unicellular myoblasts. *B,* Initial fusion of myoblasts. *C,* Multinucleated myotubes. *D,* Lower-magnification micrograph of multinucleated myotubes showing the extent of cell fusion. *E,* Multinucleated myotube with cross-striations. *A–D,* Calibration bar = 0.1 mm. *E,* Calibration bar = 0.01 mm. (From Buckley PA, Konigsberg IR: Dev Biol 37:198, 1974.)

properties of the muscle arise from variations in the geometric arrangement of the fibers: parallel, fan-shaped, fusiform (spindle-like), or pennate (feather-like). The slant of the fibers in a pennate muscle increases the magnitude of force generation at the expense of speed and range of movement compared with a muscle of similar size that has fibers aligned parallel to the tendons.[16] Typically, muscles designed for strength (e.g., gastrocnemius) are pennate, whereas those designed for speed (e.g., biceps) are parallel. Muscles are commonly arranged around joints as antagonistic pairs facilitating bidirectional motion. When one (*agonist*) set of muscles contracts, another (*antagonist*) is passively extended.

Each muscle cell is innervated at one or two sites along its length by axonal branches of an α-motoneuron. At the *neuromuscular junction* (NMJ), the axon tapers and loses its myelin sheath and the postsynaptic membrane is indented in folds that increase the

surface area. Mitochondria and nuclei are concentrated beneath these folds and form the *motor end plate*. The *synaptic cleft* is a 500 Å wide space between the axon and the muscle cell membranes. An α-motoneuron arising from the ventral horn of the spinal column and the 5 to 1600 homogeneous muscle fibers it innervates constitute a *motor unit*. Although the spatial domains of different units are intermingled, when an α-motoneuron is excited, all fibers in the motor unit are triggered to contract together. Functional properties of a motor unit, such as speed and susceptibility to fatigue, vary with the dynamic requirements set by the neuronal firing pattern and the mechanical load.

Invaginations of the sarcolemma at regular intervals constitute the transverse tubule (*T tubule*) network, which pervades the fiber and surrounds the contractile apparatus with connected longitudinal and lateral segments (Fig. 5–2). Because the lumen of

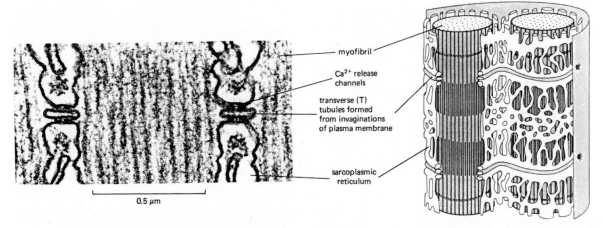

myofibril

Ca²⁺ release channels

transverse (T) tubules formed from invaginations of plasma membrane

sarcoplasmic reticulum

0.5 μm

Figure 5–2. Membrane systems that relay the excitation signal from the sarcolemma to the cell interior. In the electron micrograph, two T tubules are cut in cross-section. The electron densities spanning the gap between the T tubules and sarcoplasmic reticulum membranes are the ryanodine receptors, channels that release calcium into the myoplasm. (From Alberts B, et al: Molecular Biology of the Cell, 2nd ed. New York, Garland Publishers, 1989, p 622. Micrograph courtesy of Dr. Clara Franzini-Armstrong, University of Pennsylvania, Philadelphia.)

this network is open to the extracellular space, it contains the high Na⁺ and low K⁺ concentrations of interstitial fluid.[17] A specialized type of endoplasmic reticulum forms an entirely intracellular membrane system termed the *sarcoplasmic reticulum* (SR). The *triad* is a prevalent structure containing a T tubule flanked by two *terminal cisternae* of the sarcoplasmic reticulum. These sacs contain the Ca²⁺-binding protein, *calsequestrin*, providing the fiber with a reservoir of calcium ions. *Dihydropyridine receptors* (DHPR, homologous to plasma membrane Ca²⁺ channels) are localized in the T tubule membranes of skeletal muscle[18] juxtaposed to the cytoplasmic domain of the *ryanodine receptor* (RyR or foot protein, sarcoplasmic reticulum Ca²⁺-release channels) in the terminal cisternae membranes.[19] Although no direct association between the RyR and DHPR proteins has been demonstrated in skeletal muscle to date, glyceraldehyde-3-phosphate dehydrogenase[20] (170 kD) and triadin[21–23] (95 kD) have been implicated as possible links between these signaling molecules. The membrane proteins are further characterized in Table 5–1.

The *myofibrils* (Fig. 5–3) are the organelles that contain the contractile machinery responsible for work production, force generation, and shortening. They are 1-μm-diameter cylindrical arrays of contractile proteins that extend the whole length of the fiber. Each myofibril is a chain of *sarcomeres*, the basic contractile units, 2.5 μm in length between densely packed *Z lines* containing α-actinin (see Fig. 5–3, diagrams 4 and 5). The contractile and structural proteins are arranged within each sarcomere in a highly ordered, nearly crystalline lattice of interdigitating thick and thin *myofilaments*[24] (see Fig. 5–3, diagrams 5, 11, and 12). The myofilaments are remarkably uniform in both length and lateral registration even during contraction,[25] giving rise to the cross-striated histologic appearance of skeletal and cardiac muscles. This orderly and highly periodic organization has facili-

tated biophysical studies of muscle by sophisticated structural[24] and spectroscopic techniques.[26] The specific locations and putative functions of the contractile proteins are listed in Table 5–1.

Thick filaments (1.6 μm long), containing *myosin*, are located in the center of the sarcomere in the optically anisotropic *A band* (see Fig. 5–3, diagram 4). The thick filaments are arranged laterally in a hexagonal lattice stabilized by M filaments[27] and muscle-specific creatine phosphokinase[28] (MM-CK) in the M line (see Fig. 5–3, diagrams 4 and 5). Myosin is an asymmetric molecule (see Fig. 5–3, diagram 13) with a long α-helical, coiled-coil rod and a globular head (termed the *cross-bridge* or *subfragment 1,* S1). Each myosin molecule contains two 220-kD heavy chains making up the rod and two S1 heads. Two *light chains, essential* and *regulatory,* ranging from 15 to 22 kD, are associated with each S1. The rod portions of approximately 300 myosin molecules polymerize to form the backbone of the thick filament in a three-stranded helix with a 14.3-nm subunit spacing and a 42.9-nm axial repeat. The cross-bridges, protruding from the filament backbone (Fig. 5–3, diagram 12), contain a site for adenosine triphosphate (ATP) binding and an actin-binding region responsible for the conversion of chemical energy into mechanical work.

Thin filaments extend 1.1 μm from each side of the Z line and form the optically isotropic *I band* (see Fig. 5–3, diagrams 4 and 5). They are double-stranded helical polymers of *actin* (see Fig. 5–3, diagram 11) with 5.1-, 5.9-, and 72-nm helical pitches. A regulatory complex containing one tropomyosin and three troponin molecules (TnC, TnT, and TnI) is associated with each successive group of seven actin monomers along the thin filament.[24] In the region where the thick and thin filaments overlap, the thin filaments are positioned within the hexagonal lattice of the A band, equidistant from three thick filaments (in the *trigonal position*) (see Fig. 5–3, diagram 9). Both sets of fila-

Table 5–1. SIGNALING AND CONTRACTILE PROTEINS OF SKELETAL MUSCLE

Protein	Molecular Weight	Subunits	Location	Function
Acetylcholine receptor	~250 kD	5 × ~50 kD	Post-synaptic membrane of neuromuscular junction	Neuromuscular signal transmission
Dihydropyridine receptor	~380 kD	1 × ~160 kD 1 × ~130 kD 1 × ~60 kD 1 × ~30 kD	T-tubule membrane	Voltage sensor
Ryanodine receptor or foot protein	1800 kD	4 × 450 kD	Terminal cisternae of SR	SR Ca^{2+} release channel
Ca^{2+} ATPase	110 kD	—	Longitudinal SR	Uptake of Ca^{2+} into the SR
Triadin	95 kD	—	T-tubule membrane	Potential connector for DHPR and RyR
Troponin	78 kD	1 × 18 kD 1 × 21 kD 1 × 31 kD	Thin filament	Regulation of contraction
Tropomyosin	64 kD	2 × 33 kD	Thin filament	Regulation of contraction
Myosin	500 kD	2 × 220 kD 2 × 15 kD 2 × 20 kD	Thick filament	Chemomechanical energy transduction
Actin	42 kD	—	Thin filament	Chemomechanical energy transduction
MM creatine phosphokinase	40 kD	—	M line	ATP buffer, structural protein
α-Actinin	190 kD	2 × 95 kD	Z line	Structural protein
Titin	3000 kD	—	From Z line to M line	Structural protein
Nebulin	600 kD	—	Thin filaments, in the I-band	Structural protein
Dystrophin	400 kD	—	Subsarcolemma	Structural integrity of sarcolemma

Abbreviations: SR, sarcoplasmic reticulum; ATP, adenosine triphosphate; DHPR, dihydropyridine receptor; RyR, ryanodine receptor.

ments are polarized so that their interactions in an active muscle cause a concerted translation of the thin filaments toward the M line that shortens the sarcomere.

A major advance in the structural biology of the contractile proteins came in the early 1990s with the determination of the three-dimensional atomic structure of actin[29] and the myosin head[30, 31] and (to 2 and 2.8 Å resolution, respectively) by x-ray crystallography. Diagrams of the actin and myosin peptide backbones in the crystal structures are superimposed on an electron density map of the thin filament, decorated with S1 heads (Fig. 5–4). (See also Color Plate.) In this image, the thin filament axis is vertical, with S1 bound to two adjacent actin monomers. The crystal structures fit precisely into the electron density map and show a unique, three-dimensional macromolecular arrangement.[32] Specific ionic and hydrophobic interactions between actin and myosin have been identified in this myosin-decorated thin filament as well as the nucleotide-binding pocket and several important domains and clefts. Both of the light chains bind to and stabilize an unusually long (11 nm) single α-helix of the myosin heavy chain that extends radially away from actin.

Two giant proteins appear to function in assembling and maintaining the structural integrity of the sarcomere. Individual *titin* molecules are associated with the thick filament and extend from the M line to the Z line.[33] *Nebulin* is associated with the thin filaments.[34] The cytoskeleton of muscle fibers is composed of cytoplasmic actin, microtubules, intermediate filaments,[35] and membrane-associated proteins such as *dystrophin*.[36] Duchenne muscular dystrophy results from mutations in the dystrophin gene,[37] which emphasizes the importance of cytoskeletal elements to the structural integrity of the cell.

EVENTS DURING MUSCLE CONTRACTION

Normally, a skeletal muscle fiber is activated briefly and then relaxes. This *twitch*, which is 5 to 40 msec long, is initiated by an action potential propagated from the CNS along an α-motoneuron to the motor end plate at the neuromuscular junction. The level of muscle activity is controlled by varying the rate of firing twitches and the number of active motor units. As activity increases, more and larger units are recruited. Afferent feedback pathways from *Golgi tendon organs* and *spindle receptors* modulate activity to control the desired movement. The same feedback system generates the stretch reflex.

When the nerve action potential reaches the presynaptic terminal of the neuromuscular junction, the membrane depolarization gates local Ca^{2+} channels open allowing influx of extracellular Ca^{2+}. The Ca^{2+} triggers fusion of acetylcholine (ACh)-loaded mem-

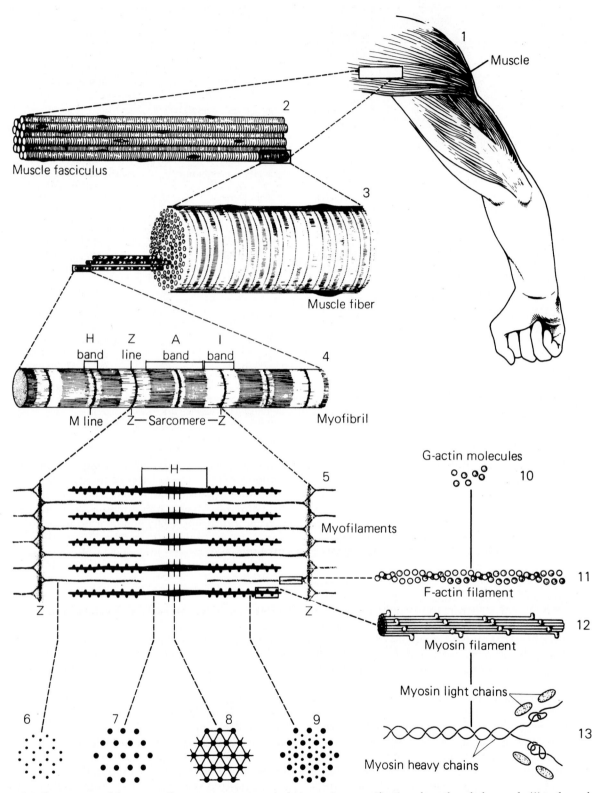

Figure 5–3. Components of the contractile apparatus at successively increasing magnifications from the whole muscle *(1)* to the molecular level *(10–13)*. The myofibril *(4)* shows the banding pattern created by the lateral alignment of the myofilaments *(11, 12)* in the sarcomeres *(4, 5)*. Diagrams *6* to *9* show the cross-sectional structure of the filament lattice at various points within the sarcomere. (From Junqueira LC, et al: Basic Histology, 5th ed. Norwalk, Conn, Appleton-Lange, 1986, p 238. Modified from Bloom W, Fawcett DW: A Textbook of Histology, 10th ed. Philadelphia, WB Saunders, 1975.)

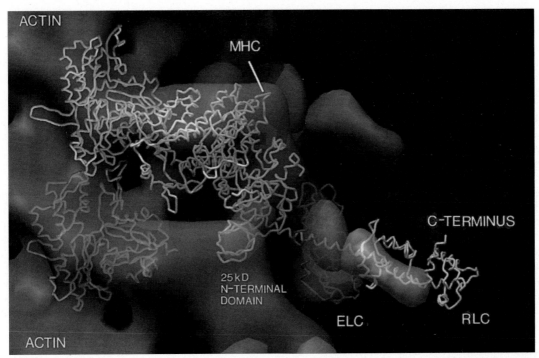

Figure 5–4. The atomic structure of actin and myosin (colored α-carbon chains), determined by x-ray crystallography, superimposed on a three-dimensional reconstruction (shaded) of the thin filament decorated with S1, from cryoelectron microscopy and Fourier image analysis. The myosin heavy chain (MHC, yellow) binds with two actin monomers (orange and gray) to form a tight complex in the absence of nucleotide. Bound to an unusually long α-helix of the MHC are the essential light chain (ELC, green) and the regulatory light chain (RLC, red). A small extension (pink shading) of the 25 kD, NH_2-terminal region of S1 appears to contact an adjacent S1. The x-ray crystal structures fit uniquely within the electron microscopic image reconstruction, verifying the three-dimensional relationship between actin and S1. The C terminus of S1, shown here, ends just beyond the light chain–binding region, but in whole myosin the heavy chain extends further to become the coiled-coil rod portion of the molecule. A putative hinge between the nucleotide-binding and light chain–binding regions is implicated in the conformational changes associated with force production and filament sliding. (See also Color Plate.) (Courtesy of Dr. Ron Milligan and Dr. Michael Whittaker, Scripps Research Institute, La Jolla, Calif.)

brane vesicles with the presynaptic membrane of the neuron, releasing ACh into the junctional cleft.[38] *Synapsin I,* a phosphoprotein associated with these vesicles,[39] as well as a family of vesicle-associated membrane proteins called *synaptobrevins*[40] participate with the cytoplasmic actin in transporting the vesicles to the terminal membrane for exocytosis. Release of the neurotransmitter probably involves docking and fusion proteins analogous to the N-ethylmaleimide-sensitive factor (NSF),[41] soluble NSF-attachment proteins (SNAPs), and SNAP receptors (SNAREs) recently discovered in brain neurons.[42] Following exocytosis, ACh rapidly diffuses across the junctional cleft to the postsynaptic membrane and binds to nicotinic, ACh-gated ion channels in the sarcolemma. Cloning and sequencing of the ACh receptor[43] and resolution of the molecular structure from two-dimensional crystals[44] launched a productive era in structure-function studies of membrane proteins.

ACh binding to sarcolemmal receptors causes an increase in cation permeability that initiates an action potential, mediated by voltage-gated Na^+ and K^+ channels. The action potential propagates at velocities up to 5 meters/second from the motor end plate throughout the sarcolemma and T-tubule network to uniformly activate a twitch. In skeletal muscle, the DHPR, primarily a voltage sensor, detects the consequent membrane depolarization during the action potential and transmits the signal from the T tubule directly to the RyR. Ca^{2+} is then released from the sarcoplasmic reticulum into the myoplasm, where it activates the contractile machinery.[45] This sequence of events is termed *excitation-contraction* (E-C) coupling. The twitch ends when Ca^{2+} is transported back into the sarcoplasmic reticulum by Ca^{2+}-ATPase pumps located in longitudinal regions of the sarcoplasmic reticulum membranes. During cardiac muscle action potentials, the DHPR serves as both a voltage sensor and an ionic channel that transports extracellular Ca^{2+} into the myoplasm[46] to signal the RyRs to release the Ca^{2+} from the sarcoplasmic reticulum. Thus extracellular Ca^{2+} is required for cardiac, but not skeletal, E-C coupling.

Some strains of dysgenic mice are paralyzed because membrane depolarization of skeletal muscle does not initiate the release of Ca^{2+} from the sarcoplasmic reticulum. E-C coupling can be restored in cultured cells from these mice by transfection with the complementary DNA (cDNA) encoding for the α-subunit of the DHPR.[47] Expression of chimeras of skeletal and cardiac DHPRs[48] have pinpointed the cytoplasmic domain of the DHPR that specifies skeletal or cardiac type E-C coupling. Human malignant hyperthermia occurs in individuals with mutant RyRs that become trapped in the open state after exposure to halothane anesthetic agents.[49]

At rest, the thin filament regulatory proteins—troponin and tropomyosin—inhibit contraction. During a twitch, Ca^{2+} released from the sarcoplasmic reticulum binds to troponin C, relieving this inhibition and thus allowing cross-bridges to attach to actin. A contraction results from a cyclic interaction between actin and myosin (the *cross-bridge cycle*) that produces a relative sliding force between the thin and the thick filaments. The energy for this work is derived from the hydrolysis of ATP to adenosine diphosphate (ADP) and orthophosphate (P_i).

A simplified model of the chemomechanical events in the cross-bridge cycle is illustrated in Figure 5–5. When Ca^{2+} is present, a complex of myosin, ADP, and P_i attaches to the thin filament (step *a*) and a structural change associated with P_i release (*b*) generates the sliding force.[50, 51] The conformational change in the cross-bridge that leads to force generation is apparently a tilting motion of the light chain region of S1[52, 53] (see Fig. 5–5). After ADP is released (*c*), ATP binds to the active site and dissociates myosin from actin (*d*). Myosin then hydrolyzes ATP (*e*) to form the ternary myosin-ADP-P_i complex, which can reattach to actin for the next cycle.

If the mechanical load on the muscle is high, the contractile apparatus produces a matching force (*isometric contraction*). If the load is moderate, the thin filaments slide toward the M line of the sarcomere, resulting in shortening of the muscle. Skeletal muscles maintain a constant volume; they broaden when they shorten. Work production (force and sliding) is associated with an increase of the ATPase rate. The thermodynamic efficiency (mechanical power/ATPase activity) approaches 50 percent, a remarkable figure considering that manmade machines seldom achieve efficiencies greater than 2 percent. The ATP concentration in skeletal muscle is buffered by MM-CK, which catalyzes the transfer of P_i from creatine phosphate to ADP, re-forming ATP. Glycolysis and mitochondrial oxidative phosphorylation reestablish and maintain metabolic conditions on a slower time scale.

During intense or prolonged activity, muscle *fatigue* is caused by alterations of metabolite levels that suppress force generation at the contractile apparatus[54] and/or in E-C coupling.[55] Marked increases in myoplasmic P_i and H^+ concentrations have been detected by magnetic resonance spectroscopy.[56] The chemomechanical linkage between P_i release and force generation (see Fig. 5–5) implies that the increase of myoplasmic P_i in fatigued muscle reduces the magnitude of force simply by mass action.[51]

PLASTICITY

Muscles are remarkably adaptable. Motor units and their muscle fibers can be classified according to their size, twitch duration, speed of contraction, balance between aerobic and glycolytic metabolism, and resistance to fatigue (Table 5–2). In addition, isoenzymes of the signaling, regulatory, and contractile proteins and the surface area of the sarcoplasmic reticulum

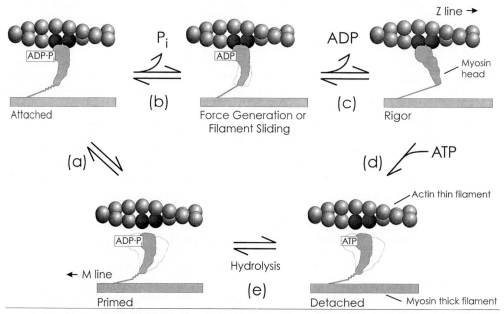

Figure 5–5. The actomyosin cross-bridge cycle. Myosin molecules normally have two globular head regions (cross-bridges), but for clarity only one is shown. Each head binds with two actins (shown as darkened monomers). The sequence of reactions is attachment (*a*), P_i release and the force generating transition (*b*), ADP release (*c*), ATP binding and detachment (*d*), and ATP hydrolysis (*e*). The *dashed lines* near the detached and force generating myosin heads indicate high mobility of the cross-bridges in these states. ADP, adenosine diphosphate; ATP, adenosine triphosphate.

Table 5–2. CLASSIFICATION OF MUSCLE FIBER TYPES

Fiber Type	I	IIA	IIB	IIC
		General Features		
Size	Moderate	Small	Large	Small
Mitochondria	Many	Intermediate	Few	Intermediate
Capillary blood supply	Extensive	Sparse	Sparse	Sparse
SR membrane	Sparse	Extensive	Extensive	Extensive
Z line	Wide	Wide	Narrow	Narrow
		Protein Isoforms		
Myosin heavy chain	MHCI	MHCIIA	MHCIIB	MHCI and MHCIIA
Myosin essential light chain	MLC1s	MLC1f, MLC3f	MLC1f, MLC3f	MLC1f, MLC3f and MLC1s
Myosin regulatory light chain	MPLC2s	MPLC2f	MPLC2f	MPLC2f and MPLC2s
Regulatory proteins	Slow	Fast	Fast	Fast
		Mechanical Properties		
Contraction time	Slow and sustained	Fast twitch	Fast twitch	Moderate twitch
SR calcium ATPase rate	Low	High	High	High
Actomyosin ATPase rate	Low	High	High	Moderate
Shortening velocity	Slow	Fast	Fast	Moderate
Resistance to fatigue	High	Moderate	Low	Moderate
		Metabolic Profile		
Oxidative capacity	High	Intermediate	Low	High
Glycolytic capacity	Moderate	High	High	High
NADH-TR/SDH/MDH	High	Moderate	Low	Moderate
LDH and phosphorylase	Low	Medium	High	NA
Glycogen	Low	High	High	Variable
Myoglobin	High	Medium	Low	NA

Abbreviations: s, slow; f, fast; MHC, myosin heavy chain; MLC, myosin alkali light chain; MPLC, myosin phosphorylatable light chain (regulatory); NADH-TR, nicotinamide adenine dinucleotide tetrazolium reductase; SDH, succinate dehydrogenase; MDH, malate dehydrogenase; LDH, lactate dehydrogenase; NA, not available from the literature; SR, sarcoplasmic reticulum; ATP, adenosine triphosphate.

membranes are key features that distinguish functional properties of fiber types. For instance, the duration of the twitch is influenced by the rates of the sarcoplasmic reticulum Ca^{2+} release and reuptake. The velocity of shortening is determined by myosin isoenzyme composition. Classification schemes are not, however, absolute because some motor units have composite or intermediate functional, ultrastructural, and histochemical characteristics.

During development, fiber type specificity may be partly determined prior to innervation.[57] Although the biologic events and signals responsible for designating functional specialization in motor units are not fully understood, classic cross-innervation experiments demonstrate that the innervation can dynamically specify and modify the muscle fiber type.[58] Following cross-innervation, the functional and histologic properties listed in Table 5–2 shift toward the target fiber type over a few weeks, indicating the ability of muscles to adapt and remodel in accordance with the pattern of neuronal activity. This type of plasticity is observed in many physiologic and clinical situations.

Exercise leads to adaptations in the muscle fibers that include alterations in specific contractile, regulatory, structural, and metabolic proteins. The frequency, intensity, and duration of a training stimulus mediate the adaptive response.[59] Specifically, strength training causes hypertrophy of fast type IIB fibers (Table 5–2), whereas endurance training enhances metabolism in type I and IIA fibers. Long-term hyperplasia does not usually occur following training in humans. There is also little evidence that voluntary training regimens can switch fibers between the major categories. When physical activity is reduced, for instance in limb immobilization, the cross-section of the fibers decreases and endurance is reduced as a result of a decreased metabolic reserve. Acute exercise hypertrophy and disuse atrophy are both reversible, but after extensive alterations the reversion may be incomplete.[60] The roles of neural trophic and growth factors in plasticity are still being identified.

The endocrine system also participates in adaptation. For example, normal circulating levels of thyroid hormones are required during muscle development and differentiation.[61] Experimental alterations of thyroid hormone concentrations promote changes in the relative levels of myosin and regulatory protein isoforms as well as changes in the activity of some metabolic enzymes.[62] An intact nerve supply is required for these effects, but involvement of growth factors has not been excluded.

SUMMARY

The complex functional capacity of muscle to produce finely tuned and coordinated movements is ultimately expressed as transduction of chemical to mechanical energy by actomyosin. A twitch is initiated via an action potential propagated from the CNS along an α-motoneuron, neuromuscular chemical transmission, direct protein-protein communication at the T tubule/sarcoplasmic reticulum junction, Ca^{2+} diffusion in the myoplasm, and Ca^{2+} binding to thin filament regulatory proteins. Since the CNS controls activity through recruitment of motor units, gradation and coordination of movement depend critically on the pattern of connections between the α-motoneurons and the muscle fibers and on variations of properties among motor units. Development and maintenance of the muscular system involve a complex series of genetic programs and cellular interactions that are just beginning to be understood at the molecular level. Adaptation of motor unit properties is evident not only in training regimens but also in reduced activity caused by pain or joint immobilization and in compromised metabolic, hormonal, or nutritional conditions. Hence, the plasticity of muscle impacts on the clinical course of many diseases. In addition to its importance in pathophysiology, muscle serves as an excellent substrate for understanding the molecular basis of cell development, protein structure-function relationships, cell signaling, and energy transduction processes.

References

1. Weintraub H, Davis R, Tapscott S, Thayer M, Krause M, Benezra R, Blackwell TK, Turner D, Rupp R, Hollenberg S, Zhuang Y, Lassar A: The *myoD* gene family: Nodal point during specification of the muscle cell lineage. Science 251:761, 1991.
2. Olson EN: MyoD family: A paradigm for development? Genes Dev 4:1454, 1990.
3. Edmondson DG, Olson EN: Helix-loop-helix proteins as regulators of muscle-specific transcription. J Biol Chem 268:755, 1993.
4. Emerson CP: Myogenesis and developmental control genes. Curr Opin Cell Biol 2:1065, 1990.
5. Olson EN: Signal transduction pathways that regulate skeletal muscle gene expression. Mol Endocrinol 7:1369, 1993.
6. Kaushal S, Schneider JW, Nadal-Ginard B, Mahdavi V: Activation of the myogenic lineage by MEF2A, a factor that induces and cooperates with MyoD. Science 266:1236, 1994.
7. Tapscott SJ, Davis RL, Thayer MJ, Cheng P-F, Weintraub H, Lassar AB: MyoD1: A nuclear phosphoprotein requiring a myc homology region to convert fibroblasts to myoblasts. Science 242:405, 1988.
8. Leibham D, Wong MW, Cheng T-C, Schroeder S, Weil PA, Olson EN, Perry M: Binding of TFIID and MEF2 to the TATA element activates transcription of the *Xenopus MyoDa* promoter. Mol Cell Biol 14:686, 1994.
9. Lassar AB, Davis RL, Wright WE, Kadesch T, Murre C, Voronova A, Baltimore D, Weintraub H: Functional activity of myogenic HLH proteins requires hetero-oligomerization with E12/E47-like proteins in vivo. Cell 66:305, 1991.
10. Blackwell TK, Weintraub H: Differences and similarities in DNA-binding preferences of MyoD and E2A protein complexes revealed by binding site selection. Science 250:1104, 1990.
11. Buckley PA, Konigsberg IR: Myogenic fusion and the duration of the post-mitotic gap (G_1). Dev Biol 37:193, 1974.
12. Kühl U, Öcalan M, Timpl R, Mayne R, Hay E, von der Mark K: Role of muscle fibroblasts in the deposition of type-IV collagen in the basal lamina of myotubes. Differentiation 28:164, 1984.
13. Kelly AM, Rubinstein NA: Development of neuromuscular specialization. Med Sci Sports Exerc 18:292, 1986.
14. Bischoff R: Interaction between satellite cells and skeletal muscle fibers. Development 109:943, 1990.
15. Florini JR: Hormonal control of muscle growth. Muscle Nerve 10:577, 1987.
16. Gowitzke BA, Milner M: Scientific Bases of Human Movement, 3rd ed. Baltimore, Williams & Wilkins, 1988, pp 144–145.
17. Somlyo AV, Gonzalez-Serratos H, Shuman H, McClellan G, Somlyo AP: Calcium release and ionic changes in the sarcoplasmic reticulum of tetanized muscle: An electron-probe study. J Cell Biol 90:577, 1981.
18. Schwartz LM, McCleskey EW, Almers W: Dihydropyridine receptors in muscle are voltage-dependent but most are not functional calcium channels. Nature 314:747, 1985.
19. Block BA, Imagawa T, Campbell KP, Franzini-Armstrong C: Structural evidence for direct interaction between the molecular components of the transverse tubule/sarcoplasmic reticulum junction in skeletal muscle. J Cell Biol 107:2587, 1988.
20. Brandt NR, Caswell AH, Wen S-R, Talvenheimo JA: Molecular interactions of the junctional foot protein and dihydropyridine receptor in skeletal muscle triads. J Membrane Biol 113:237, 1990.
21. Kim KC, Caswell AH, Talvenheimo JA, Brandt NR: Isolation of a terminal cisterna protein which may link the dihydropyridine receptor to the junctional foot protein in skeletal muscle. Biochemistry 29:9281, 1990.
22. Caswell AH, Brandt NR, Brunschwig J-P, Purkerson S: Localization and partial characterization of the oligomeric disulfide-linked molecular weight 95 000 protein (triadin) which binds the ryanodine and dihydropyridine receptors in skeletal muscle triadic vesicles. Biochemistry 30:7507, 1991.
23. Flucher BE, Andrews SB, Fleischer S, Marks AR, Caswell A, Powell JA: Triad formation: Organization and function of the sarcoplasmic reticulum calcium release channel and triadin in normal and dysgenic muscle in vitro. J Cell Biol 123:1161, 1993.
24. Squire J: The Structural Basis of Muscular Contraction. New York, Plenum Press, 1981.
25. Sosa H, Popp D, Ouyang G, Huxley HE: Ultrastructure of skeletal muscle fibers studied by a plunge quick freezing method: Myofilament lengths. Biophys J 67:283, 1994.
26. Thomas DD: Spectroscopic probes of muscle cross-bridge rotation. Annu Rev Physiol 49:691, 1987.
27. Chowrashi PK, Pepe FA: M-band proteins: Evidence for more than one component. *In* Pepe FA, Sanger JW, Nachmias VT (eds): Motility in Cell Function. New York, Academic Press, 1979.
28. Walliman T, Pelloni G, Turner DC, Eppenberger HM: Removal of the M-line by treatment with Fab' fragments of antibodies against MM-creatine kinase. *In* Pepe FA, Sanger JW, Nachmias VT (eds): Motility in Cell Function. New York, Academic Press, 1979.
29. Kabsch W, Mannherz HG, Suck D, Pai EF, Holmes KC: Atomic structure of the actin: DNase I complex. Nature 347:37, 1990.
30. Rayment I, Rypniewski WR, Schmidt-Base K, Smith R, Tomchick DR, Benning MM, Winkelmann DA, Wesenberg G, Holden HM: Three-dimensional structure of myosin subfragment-1: A molecular motor. Science 261:50, 1993.
31. Xie X, Harrison DH, Schlichting I, Sweet RM, Kalabokis VN, Szent-Györgyi AG, Cohen C: Structure of the regulatory domain of scallop myosin at 2.8 Å resolution. Nature 368:306, 1994.
32. Rayment I, Holden HM, Whittaker M, Yohn CB, Lorenz M, Holmes KC, Milligan RA: Structure of the actin-myosin complex and its implications for muscle contraction. Science 261:58, 1993.
33. Higuchi H, Suzuki T, Kimura S, Yoshioka T, Maruyama K, Umazume Y: Localization and elasticity of connectin (titin) filaments in skinned frog muscle fibres subjected to partial depolymerization of thick filaments. J Musc Res Cell Motil 13:285, 1992.
34. Wang K: Sarcomere-associated cytoskeletal lattices in striated muscle. *In* Shay JW (ed): Cell and Muscle Motility. Vol 6. New York, Plenum Press, 1985.
35. Toyama Y, Forry-Schaudies S, Hoffman B, Holtzer H: Effects of taxol and colcemid on myofibrillogenesis. Proc Natl Acad Sci USA 79:6556, 1982.
36. Ibraghimov-Beskrovnaya O, Ervasti JM, Leveille CJ, Slaughter CA, Sernett SW, Campbell KP: Primary structure of dystrophin-associated glycoproteins linking dystrophin to the extracellular matrix. Nature 355:696, 1992.
37. Hoffman EP, Brown RH Jr, Kunkel LM: Dystrophin: The protein product of the Duchenne muscular dystrophy locus. Cell 51:919, 1987.
38. Südhof TC: The synaptic vesicle cycle: a cascade of protein-protein interactions. Nature 375:645, 1995.
39. Greengard P, Valtorta F, Czernik AJ, Benfenati F: Synaptic vesicle phosphoproteins and regulation of synaptic function. Science 259:780, 1993.
40. Bennett MK, Scheller RH: The molecular machinery for secretion is conserved from yeast to neurons. Proc Natl Acad Sci USA 90:2559, 1993.
41. Balch WE, Dunphy WG, Braell WA, Rothman JE: Reconstitution of the transport of protein between successive compartments of the Golgi measured by the coupled incorporation of N-acetylglucosamine. Cell 39:405, 1984.
42. Söllner T, Whiteheart SW, Brunner M, Erdjument-Bromage H, Geromanos S, Tempst P, Rothman JE: SNAP receptors implicated in vesicle targeting and fusion. Nature 362:318, 1993.
43. Mishina M, Takai T, Imoto K, Noda M, Takahashi T, Numa S, Methfessel C, Sakmann B: Molecular distinction between fetal and adult forms of muscle acetylcholine receptor. Nature 321:406, 1986.
44. Brisson A, Unwin PNT: Quaternary structure of the acetylcholine receptor. Nature 315:474, 1985.

45. Rios E, Brum G: Involvement of dihydropyridine receptors in excitation-contraction coupling in skeletal muscle. Nature 325:717, 1987.
46. Fabiato A: Time and calcium dependence of activation and inactivation of calcium-induced release of calcium from the sarcoplasmic reticulum of a skinned canine cardiac Purkinje cell. J Gen Physiol 85:247, 1985.
47. Tanabe T, Beam KG, Powell JA, Numa S: Restoration of excitation-contraction coupling and slow calcium current in dysgenic muscle by dihydropyridine receptor complementary DNA. Nature 336:134, 1988.
48. Tanabe T, Beam KG, Adams BA, Niidome T, Numa S: Regions of the skeletal muscle dihydropyridine receptor critical for excitation-contraction coupling. Nature 346:567, 1990.
49. Gillard EF, Otsu K, Fujii J, Khanna VK, De Leon S, Derdemezi J, Britt BA, Duff CL, Worton RG, MacLennan DH: A substitution of cysteine for arginine 614 in the ryanodine receptor is potentially causative of human malignant hyperthermia. Genomics 11:751, 1991.
50. Goldman YE: Kinetics of the actomyosin ATPase in muscle fibers. Annu Rev Physiol 49:637, 1987.
51. Dantzig JA, Goldman YE, Millar NC, Lacktis J, Homsher E: Reversal of the cross-bridge force-generating transition by photogeneration of phosphate in rabbit psoas muscle fibres. J Physiol 451:247, 1992.
52. Hirose K, Franzini-Armstrong C, Goldman YE, Murray JM: Structural changes in muscle crossbridges accompanying force generation. J Cell Biol 127:763, 1994.
53. Irving M, Allen TStC, Sabido-David C, Craik JS, Brandmeier B, Kendrick-Jones J, Corrie JET, Trentham DR, Goldman YE: Tilting of the light-chain region of myosin during step length changes and active force generation in skeletal muscle. Nature 375:688, 1995.
54. Dawson MJ, Gadian DG, Wilkie DR: Muscular fatigue investigated by phosphorus nuclear magnetic resonance. Nature 274:861, 1978.
55. Lännergren J, Westerblad H: Force and membrane potential during and after fatiguing, continuous high-frequency stimulation of single Xenopus muscle fibres. Acta Physiol Scand 128:359, 1986.
56. Meyer RA, Brown TR, Kushmerick MJ: Phosphorus nuclear magnetic resonance of fast- and slow-twitch muscle. Am J Physiol 248:C279, 1985.
57. Miller JB, Stockdale FE: What muscle cells know that nerves don't tell them. Trends Neurosci 10:325, 1987.
58. Buller AJ, Eccles JC, Eccles RM: Differentiation of fast and slow muscles in the cat hind limb. J Physiol 150:399, 1960.
59. Faulkner JA, White TP: Adaptations of skeletal muscle to physical activity. In Bouchard C, Shephard RJ, Stephens T, Sutton JR, McPherson BD (eds): Exercise, Fitness, and Health. Champaign, Ill, Human Kinetics Publishers, 1990.
60. Appell HJ: Muscular atrophy following immobilisation: A review. Sports Med 10:42, 1990.
61. Rubinstein NA, Lyons GE, Kelly AM: Hormonal control of myosin heavy chain genes during development of skeletal muscles. Ciba Found Symp 138:35, 1988.
62. Nwoye L, Mommaerts WFHM: The effects of thyroid status on some properties of rat fast-twitch muscle. J Musc Res Cell Motil 2:307, 1981.

CHAPTER 6

Biomechanics of Joints

Sheldon R. Simon
Eric L. Radin

NORMAL JOINTS

Joint Stability

In general, joint motion is minimally translational and primarily rotational (Fig. 6–1).[1] Joint stability is created by bony configurations, ligaments, and muscles, with different joints using different combinations of these constructs.[2] Although each joint is characterized by its own unique contour, one side is usually concave and the other is convex.[3] Since bone is the most rigid anatomic structure, the greater the arc of motion enclosed by the bone, the greater the amount of inherent stability that exists. By contrast, the shoulder, with a flatter radius of curvature and a less enclosed humeral head, is easier to dislocate or sublux than the hip, whose femoral spherical head is almost enclosed by a hemispherical arc of bony acetabulum (Fig. 6–2). In such circumstances, ligaments may provide some stability; however, they provide stability only in circumstances of modest loading, because they can tear.

In resisting displacement, ligaments have some stretch.[4] Muscle-tendon complexes are similar to ligaments in the way they stabilize joints. Muscles have the added advantage of active shortening. Because ligaments are only passive stabilizers, the advantage of muscles, which are active, in controlling joint motion is obvious. Muscle action, in fact, protects ligaments from tearing.[5]

The spine illustrates the intricate balance between the three structural stabilizers. To protect the spinal cord while allowing rotatory motions of the trunk, a sophisticated stabilizing arrangement has evolved.

The intervertebral "unit" (vertebra–intervertebral disc–vertebra) is composed of the following (Fig. 6–3):

1. One amphiarthrodial joint (the intervertebral disc) and two diarthrodial intervertebral facet joints.
2. Multiple ligaments (anterior and posterior longitudinal, ligamentum flavum, and interspinous).
3. Paraspinal muscles.

The disc is the major supporting unit between the vertebral bony units and helps to maintain the vertical rigidity of the system.[6] Although the disc stabilizes vertical loads and prevents vertical translation, it does not stabilize horizontal translation.[7] Bending to tie a shoelace puts the body's weight anterior to the spine. This configuration compresses the disc and tends to topple the spine by creating forces that tilt and slide one vertebral unit over the one below it. The posterolateral intervertebral facet joints prevent sliding and direct rotation. The ligaments and muscles limit the extent of motion, control the degree of and speed with which motions occur, and act as the major source of stability in rotation (Fig. 6–4). When all is said and done, control of the position of the loaded spine ultimately depends on the paraspinal muscles.[8]

Joint Motions

The types of motions and the degree to which each motion is allowed are distinct in each joint.[9] In the human, the primary function of the upper extremities is to carry and manipulate objects; the primary function of the lower extremities is locomotion. To provide for the wide sphere of function that an extremity can encompass, the most proximal joint must have the widest range of motion.

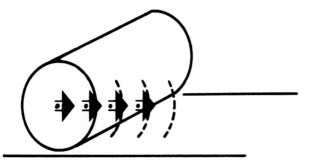

Figure 6–1. If a body rotates in place, the center of its rotation does not move. If the body translates as it rotates, movement of the center of rotation reflects this motion.

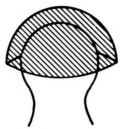
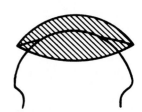

Figure 6–2. Neither the hip nor the shoulder joints have no rotational restrictions and each has a similar ball-in-socket shape. The glenoid socket does not stabilize the humeral head as well as the acetabulum stabilizes the femoral head.

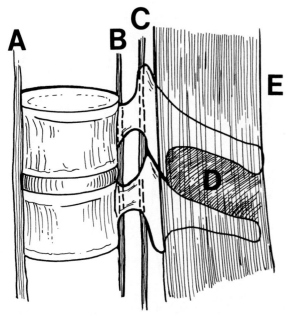

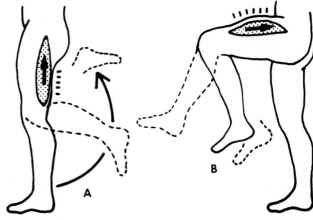

Figure 6–5. *A,* If the femur is stationary, knee motions alone are not an effective means of producing limb shortening. Under such circumstances, the foot can move only in a single prescribed 180-degree arc behind the knee. *B,* However, if at the same time the thigh is allowed to move by rotatory motions produced about the hip, the limb can be shortened or placed within a wide spherical volume.

Figure 6–3. Schematic representation of the motion segment. The vertebral bodies are separated by the intervertebral disc. Each vertebral body is connected to its posterior elements and spinous process. The anterior-longitudinal ligament (A) and posterior-longitudinal ligament (B) run up the front and back of the vertebral bodies. The ligamentum flavum (C) runs behind the spinal canal, which is the space between B and C. The interspinous ligament (D) joins the spinous processes. Muscles are applied to the posterior surfaces of the bones and vertical surfaces of the spinous processes (E).

The joint configuration established to suit these demands at the shoulder is a ball on a relatively flat surface, requiring significant muscular and ligamentous stability, with minimal bony constraint.[10] The hip, which functions to balance body mass, needs greater stability to prevent translational motions and a smaller range of rotational motion. It derives much of its stability from encapsulating bony contours; it is a ball and socket, with muscles playing an important role. Paralyzed individuals are more likely to dislocate their hips than people with functional hip musculature.[11]

In order for an extremity to function at all points within its range, a means is provided to alter the length of the limb. Rotational motion of the elbow and knee joints allows length changes as adjacent limb segments move (Fig. 6–5). It is most efficient to provide such control with a single muscle that spans two joints. One joint moves in a direction to stretch the muscle, and the other rotates in an opposite direction, lessening the degree of active contraction necessary (Fig. 6–6). Of necessity, muscle-tendon systems must span the periphery of rotational joints to control their actions and stabilize them in all directions.

Joint Forces

The force causing joint rotation about an axis is not merely the contractile or stretching force produced in the muscle; it is the product of this force multiplied by the distance between the joint's center of rotation and the tendon (Fig. 6–7). The tendon, placed at the periphery of the joint, gives the muscle a mechanical advantage—leverage—which creates the greatest torque with the least effort.[12] Because most external forces on the extremity are exerted at some distance

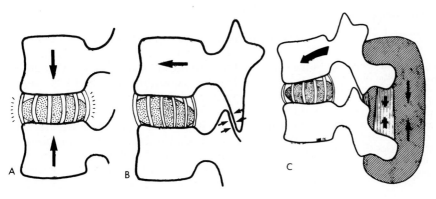

Figure 6–4. The intervertebral unit of the spine has multiple structures contributing to its stability. *A,* The disc prevents vertical translational motions, like a balloon placed in a coffee can. *B,* The facet joints prevent forward translation, permitting the more proximal vertebrae only to rotate about the more distal one in a prescribed arc. *C,* Multiple ligaments and paraspinal muscles control the speed and extent of motion within this arc of movement through their "clamping" effect on the posterior elements.

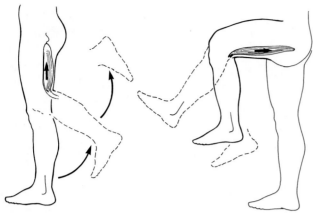

Figure 6–6. The hamstring muscles originate above the hip and insert below the knee. With the hip straight, considerable contraction of the hamstrings is necessary to bend the knee. With the hip flexed, however, the hamstrings are stretched behind the hip, and a relatively modest contraction is all that is necessary to bend the knee in that circumstance.

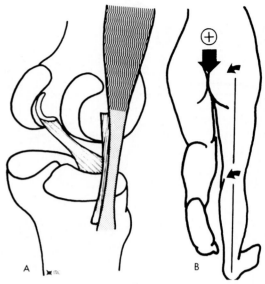

Figure 6–8. Being eccentrically placed, a muscle will produce compressive force that will prevent a joint from pivoting open. At the knee the vastus lateralis assists knee ligaments (A), preventing body weight medially placed from opening up the lateral side of the joint during one-legged support (B).

from the joint, stabilizing forces around the most proximal joint are high.[13]

Muscle contraction produces compressive forces across the joint, tending to squeeze the joint together. This force also maintains stability against forces that might pivot a joint open (Fig. 6–8). The joint surfaces

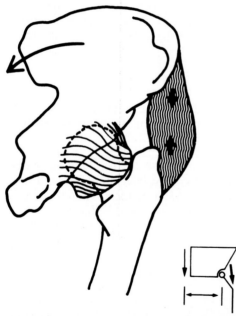

Figure 6–7. When one-legged support is required, the abductor muscles contract to produce a rotational force about the hip joint opposite to that produced by body weight. The farther away the muscle-tendon complex is from the center of the joint, the lower the muscle force needs to be to create the same rotational force. In most cases the distance of the muscle-tendon complex from the center of the joint is less than that of the weight it is trying to counteract. This produces a larger force in the muscles than the weight it balances. As a consequence, during the functional activities of daily living the major muscles about the hip typically produce forces two to four times body weight.

sustain substantial forces created by highly leveraged muscles. In some movements, if the joint is rotated into certain positions, the muscles become more parallel to the joint surface. The muscles then lose their mechanical advantage and must increase the force applied to maintain the applied torque. In most of the weight-bearing joints in the lower extremities, the intra-articular forces are in the range of three to four times body weight.[14]

In some cases, the shear force or rotational torque parallel to the joint line is helpful in stabilizing the joint against inertial or weight-bearing forces that tend to translate the two sides of the joint. In other cases, they work in concert with ligaments to minimize the strain on these soft tissues (i.e., muscles about the knee versus the anterior or posterior cruciate ligaments). Sometimes, as in the flexor tendons of the fingers, pulleys are provided to maintain a constant direction of pull across the joint (Fig. 6–9). In some cases, shear forces can be detrimental.[15]

Joint Structure

It is estimated that each year the joints of a person's lower extremities undergo at least 2 million oscillatory cycles in the activities of daily living. Even under this extreme loading condition, for up to 80 years, most of our joints do not wear out.[16] The joint lubricant (synovial fluid), the bearing surfaces, and articular cartilage are built to withstand the intra-articular frictional forces created. The biochemical composition and geometric distribution of water and organic matrix within the articular cartilage provide conformational load bearing. The subchondral trabecular bony

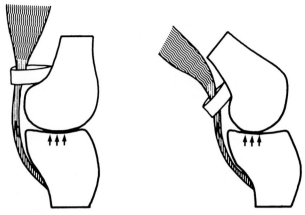

Figure 6–9. At certain joints, pulleys located proximal to the joint maintain flexor tendons at fixed distances and orientation to the joint's surface.

bed on which the cartilage sits absorbs some of the shock of impulsive loading.[17] Each aspect of the joint structure is optimized to allow joint movement to occur, reduce the mechanical forces that it must withstand, and provide nourishment and protection.

Minimization of Frictional Forces

Rotational movements of a joint create a sliding motion of one articular surface on another. Such motion could create shear or frictional forces between the two surfaces, causing joint breakdown; yet joints do not wear down by pure rubbing—their lubrication is too good.[18]

Frictional force is defined as the resistance one moving surface exerts on the other to impede its progress. Such resistance depends on compressional load, the composition of the materials, and the characteristics of the lubricant interposed between the two surfaces (Fig. 6–10). The resistance to movement may be quantified by a dimensionless number called the "coefficient of friction." The lower this number, the more slippery is the movement of the two surfaces, and the lower the shear forces created between them. Good manmade joints, such as steel-on-steel lubricated by oil, operate at coefficients of friction between 0.1 and 0.5. Biologic diarthrodial joints operate at coefficients of friction of approximately 0.002, nearly one-hundredth that of what humans can at present design.[19] Thus, if a walking man weighing 70 kg creates a 200-kg compressive force across the lower extremity joint, the shear, or frictional, force at the joint would be less than 0.4 kg. The low frictional forces that minimize surface wear appear to be related to a number of biologic constructs of the joint. The porous deformable collagen surface is arranged with its surface fibers parallel to the surface of the joint. This orientation is ideal for preserving surface integrity because it strongly resists shear forces that tend to disrupt the surface by pulling the fibers apart.[20]

Articular cartilage, with an intact surface layer but

without any fluid imbibed within it, has a coefficient of friction of 0.3.[21] If saline is added, the cartilage imbibes the fluid like a sponge; and when the wet cartilage surfaces slide against each other, the coefficient of friction is reduced to as much as 0.010.[19] If glycoprotein molecules ("lubricin"), which naturally occur in synovial fluid, are added to the saline, the coefficient of friction is further reduced to 0.002.[22] The self-pressurized fluid that is squeezed out of the fluid-soaked cartilage[23] and the lubricin in the synovial fluid are the major features that reduce the frictional forces so effectively that the articular surface sees little shear stress at its surface.

How the various lubricating mechanisms interact to produce low levels of frictional resistance is still a matter of controversy. Many theories have been proposed[1, 24, 25]; common to all is the movement of fluid in and out of the porous cartilage. McCutchen[23] postulated that as the cartilage is compressed, the fluid from within seeps out and forms a self-pressurized layer separating the two surfaces. Theoretical evidence and in vitro tests[26] suggest that in the trailing area of compression, fluid is imbibed into articular surfaces, whereas at the leading edge where compression is developing, fluid is expressed (Fig. 6–11).

The lubrication mechanisms in joints are so efficient that the joint's frictional forces do not appear to be a cause of articular cartilage breakdown.

Maximization of Contact Area

The breakdown of any mechanical structure depends on the total force and the area over which it is loaded. For example, if a tack is pressed into a person's finger, the person's reaction will depend on whether the point or the flat part of the tack is being pushed into the skin. Joint structures are designed to

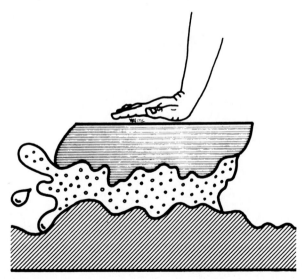

Figure 6–10. The ease with which one surface may be slid over another is dependent on the compressive load, the characteristics of the two opposing materials and their surfaces, and the nature of the material interposed between the two surfaces.

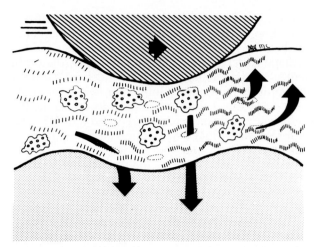

Figure 6–11. To minimize the resistance of moving one cartilage surface over another, the porous cartilaginous surface is layered with viscous macromolecules but primarily weeps synovial fluid dialysate at the leading edge, absorbs this fluid in the trailing area, and deforms in the "area of contact," allowing the two cartilaginous surfaces to be kept apart.

provide an increasing contact surface with increasing forces to keep articular compressive stress minimal.

Joints provide this contact area in different ways. In all joints, under load the articular cartilage under contact is squeezed down (i.e., it compresses). The load-bearing contact area of the knee becomes greater with increasing loads because the menisci come into play and increase the contact area.[27] The acetabulum spreads and the femoral head flattens to increase the hip contact area.[28] The contact area of the tibiotalar joint increases with load-sharing of the fibulotalar joint.[29] Articular cartilage and subchondral bone can withstand only so much pressure. Physiologic joint pressure approximates 5.0 meganewtons (MN)/m²,[30]

and pressures in all joints are equivalent. Even though the joints in the upper extremities are smaller than those in the lower extremities, so are their loads.

Resistance to Compressive Stresses

Cartilage is constructed in an ideal way to withstand compressive stresses.[31] It has two components: a liquid and a solid. The liquid is a dialysate of synovial fluid and is incompressible but can flow.[32, 33] However, for this fluid to withstand the compressive loads that joints sustain, it must be contained. The cartilage matrix resembles a sponge with directional pores. The small diameter[34] of these functional pores and their arrangement in circuitous "tunnels," created by the hydrophilic collagen and proteoglycan matrix components, prevent large molecules from entering the cartilage and offer considerable resistance to interstitial fluid flow (Fig. 6–12).[35] These characteristics provide adequate containment for the fluid to support the load.

At any instant, only a part of the joint is load-bearing or compressed. If one part is in compression, the adjacent area is being stretched and pulled apart. This places high compressive and tensile stresses on the organic matrix of cartilage.

Although there is agreement about the tangential parallel arrangement of the collagen fibers on the surface of the articular cartilage and the perpendicular ones at its base, controversy about the arrangement of the collagen in the middle zone of articular cartilage persists.[36–38] Some believe that the midzone fibers alter their alignment under compression to provide maximal resistance against load. Such changes allow the matrix to accommodate the imposed loads, decrease the pore size, and increase resistance to fluid flow through the cartilage, with permeability of the

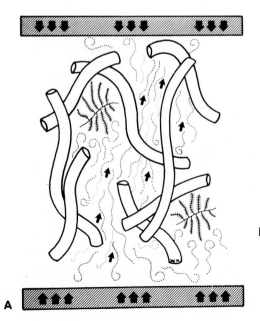

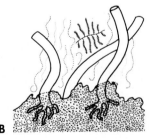

Figure 6–12. Cartilage is composed of a liquid and a multicomponent solid consisting of collagen and hydrophilic proteoglycan molecules. In the middle layer *(A)*, the mechanical and electrical properties and architectural design of the solid "contain" the fluid, preventing it from being compressed while still allowing fluid flow, providing nourishment for cartilage cells. In the deepest zone *(B)*, although the content of proteoglycans decreases, the collagen is secured tightly to subchondral bone similar to liquid-solid properties.

tissue (ease of flow) decreasing exponentially.[39] The mechanical strength of cartilage increases as greater loads are imposed.[40] The greater the depth of the cartilage layer examined, the larger the importance of these relationships.[28]

The electrical properties of proteoglycans and their interaction with the surrounding substances contribute to the material properties of the articular cartilage. The carboxyl and sulfate groups of the glycosaminoglycans are endowed with highly polyionic charge characteristics.[41] The charge correlates with the fixed negative charge density found in the surface. The large, fixed proteoglycan molecules are highly charged and attract a large volume of water, which tends to neutralize the fixed negative charge. Under compressive loads, water is pushed out of the zone of highest pressure, allowing the cartilage to compress and increasing its fixed charge density. This increases the resistance to the flow of such fluid away from it, increasing the mechanical strength of the cartilage. When the pressure is removed, the fixed negative charge osmotically attracts water and the cartilage regains its precompressed thickness. Under most circumstances, this fluid flow, under pressure, allows articular cartilage to compress under load without permanent damage to its matrix.[40]

In light of the preceding discussion, it is easy to understand how enzymatic destruction of cartilage matrix in arthritic (primarily inflammatory) joint conditions can lead to cartilage destruction.[42] In osteoarthrotic (primarily mechanical) joint deterioration, it is believed that repetitive, impulsive loading damages the matrix.[43] In this circumstance, the compressive load is applied too rapidly for the interstitial cartilage water to have the time to flow and the cartilage matrix is then subjected to compression and fails in fatigue.[44]

Additional Resistance to Compressive Loads

The articular cartilage rests on a layer of calcified cartilage, supported by a subchondral bone plate. This plate is supported by subchondral trabecular bone whose lattice arrangement follows the major stress trajectories of the transmitted load.[45] The trabecular bone density is related to the quantity of the habitually transmitted load. The articular ends of the joints are expanded to increase their potential contact area and thus diminish the articular stress. Trabecular bone is ten times more compliant than cortical bone,[46] and micromotion of the subchondral trabecular bone and subchondral plate aids in joint conformation under load[47] and can probably help absorb impulsive loads if they are not applied too quickly.[48]

As an example, at the hip (Fig. 6–13) the concave acetabulum, under low loads, contacts the head of the femur about its periphery. As the load increases, the surface tends to flare out for maximum joint confinement under load.[49] Movement of the marrow and slight bending of the acetabular and femoral head trabeculae allow subchondral deformation without

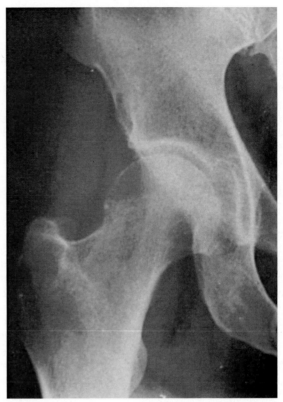

Figure 6–13. At the hip, trabecular bone in the femoral head is concentrated along an axis 160 degrees to the vertical, where the greatest concentration of forces occurs. In contrast, the trabecular bone on the acetabular side flares out to occupy an area greater than the joint's contacting surface, distributing the same forces over a wide area and thereby reducing the stresses and allowing some of the stresses to be absorbed by bone deformation.

matrix damage.[50] At very high rates of loading, however, there is insufficient time for marrow flow and the trabecular bone can be subjected to microdamage. This microdamage, from repetitive impulsive loading, can accumulate and lead to fatigue failure.[44] The repair of the subchondral bone damage stiffens the trabecular structure. This process also turns on once dormant endochondral ossification, which duplicates the tidemark base on which the articular cartilage rests. As the ossification front advances, the articular cartilage is thinned. This thinning increases the shear stress on the articular cartilage, particularly in its depth, which can lead to fragmentation.[51]

The ability of the subchondral bone to absorb compressive loads provides added protection for the cartilage under most circumstances. Although cartilage is very compliant, even in its normal state it is not thick enough to deform adequately to absorb impulsive loads.[52] It is thought that chronic mechanically induced progressive cartilage loss requires subchondral plate thickening and cartilage thinning as a prerequisite[51] (see Chapter 82).

Joint Control

The magnitude of the intra-articular forces depends on what the functional activity is, how the activity is performed, and how fast it is performed.[53-56] For example, during walking, the knee flexes 15 to 20 degrees during the early stance phase. The quadriceps muscle attempts to prevent collapse of the leg under the body's weight as the leg is decelerating. Most of the force exerted is compressive. If an individual walks faster, greater muscle activity is needed for deceleration, creating higher compressive loads across the joint (Fig. 6–14). Quadriceps activity increases even further during running, when muscle action is needed for acceleration.[57] In contrast, during the swing phase of walking, most of the forces are internal, no significant muscle activity is needed, and knee joint forces are minimal.[56]

Quadriceps and other muscle activity at all joints during common activities appears to be dictated by fixed, preprogrammed neurologic responses, so-called locomotion or pattern generators, located in the brainstem. There are separate generators for the upper and lower extremities.[58] Activities requiring involvement of the low back require the participation of one or more joints of the upper and lower extremities.

The speed at which an activity is carried out can be controlled voluntarily by the higher cortical centers. The locomotion generators and cerebellum coordinate these motions and such common activities of daily living as walking and writing. This may have important implications in regard to the progression of osteoarthrosis. Both bone (see Chapter 4) and articular cartilage (see Chapter 1) are viscoelastic; that is, when they are compressed slowly, their interstitial water flows and protects the matrix. Rapidly compressed interstitial water has no time to flow, and matrix can be damaged. It is thus advantageous to avoid impulsive loading of joints during activities of daily living. One can accomplish this primarily by decelerating the limb just before it is about to hit an object. This momentary deceleration may be very important in avoiding the matrix microdamage that is found in significant amounts in osteoarthrotic tissues.[59]

About one third of normal adults lack protective timely limb deceleration; as a result, people impulsively load their joints during activities of daily living. Such individuals have been referred to as "microklutzes."[60] Such repetitive impulsive loading can be deleterious to joints over time.[61]

The ability of an individual to perform a task in a chosen manner depends on the strength of various relevant muscle groups. For example, if a person has strong enough back muscles, he or she may pick something up by keeping the legs straight and bending only the spine (Fig. 6–15A, diagram A), or the person may bend at the hips, knees, and ankles, keeping the back straight, and lift the object mainly with the leg muscles (Fig. 6–15A, diagram B) if there is sufficient strength in the leg muscles.[62] A person might choose to use a combination of these two methods, employing both back and lower extremity muscles (Fig. 6–15A, diagram C).[63] Using a combination of upper and lower extremity efforts plus the paraspinal muscles places less stress on the lumbar region.

BIOMECHANICS OF JOINT DEGENERATION

Under normal conditions, joints last. Nature's marvelous mechanical architecture allows most individuals years of good service from their joints. Yet, under certain circumstances, joints can wear out. This loss is remarkably disabling. Proper restoration requires therapeutic modalities that consider the joint as an organ and that respect the physiologic interrelationships of its tissue.

Normal function of any joint requires that all structures (cartilage, bone, ligaments, synovium, capsule, muscle, nerves, and higher control centers) act in combination to allow smooth steady motion while maintaining stability. Alteration of any individual component affects the delicate balance and can lead to mechanical breakdown of the joint. Although many factors may initiate cartilage damage, by definition it is mechanical factors that lead to the progressive joint dysfunction known as *osteoarthrosis* (see Chapter 82). If the condition is primarily inflammatory, it should not be considered an arthrosis but, rather, an arthritis.

CONCLUSION

Joint physiology and pathophysiology depend on interactions of tissue biology and biomechanics. Osteoarthrosis—mechanically induced joint failure—can be fully understood and treated only if the mechanics of

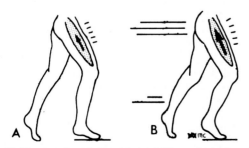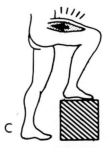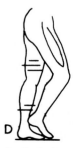

Figure 6–14. The muscle activity of the quadriceps depends on the type of activity that is being performed, that is, the early stance phase of walking *(A)*, running *(B)*, and going up stairs *(C)* and the early swing phase of walking or running *(D)*.

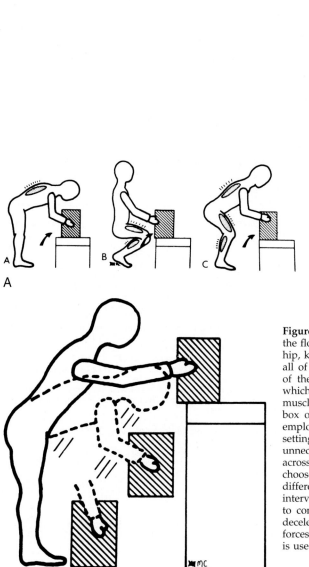

Figure 6–15. *A,* A person attempting to lift a box off the floor may utilize hip, trunk, and arm motions (A); hip, knee, and ankle motions (B); or a combination of all of these (C). Muscles needed, and the magnitude of the force from each that is required, depend on which method the individual chooses. *B,* Whatever muscles a person chooses to utilize when lifting a box off the floor, nonpurposeful movement may be employed, such as overshooting the table and then setting the box back down. Muscles needed for such unnecessary movements create forces and stresses across respective joints. *C,* Whatever method a person chooses to utilize when lifting a box off the floor, different speeds may be employed during different intervals of the act. Changes in speeds require muscles to control both weight and inertial acceleration and deceleration, creating additional, often unnecessary forces and stresses across the joints if "improper form" is used.

the joints and their compensating mechanisms are appreciated.

References

1. MacConaill MA: The movements of bones and joints. J Bone Joint Surg 31B:100,1949.
2. O'Connor M, Shercliff T, Goodfellow J: The mechanics of the knee in the sagittal plane: Mechanical interactions between muscles, ligaments, and articular surfaces. *In* Muller W, Hackenbruch W (eds): Surgery and Arthroscopy of the Knee. New York, Springer-Verlag, 1988.
3. Simkin PA, Graney DO, Fiechtner JJ: Roman arches, human joint, and disease: Differences between convex and concave sides of joints. Arthritis Rheum 23:1308, 1980.
4. Benedict JV, Walker LB, Harris EH: Stress-strain characteristics and tensile strength of unembalmed human tendon. J Biomech 1:53, 1968.
5. Marshall JL, Girgis FG, Zelko RR: The biceps femoris tendon and its functional significance. J Bone Joint Surg 54A:1444, 1972.
6. Parke WW, Schiff DCM: The applied anatomy of the intervertebral disc. Orthop Clin North Am 2:309, 1971.
7. MacNab I: The traction spur: An indicator of segmental instability. J Bone Joint Surg 53A:663, 1971.
8. Morris JM: Biomechanics of the spine. Arch Surg 107:418, 1973.
9. Kapandji IA: The Physiology of Joints, 2nd ed. Edinburgh, ERS Livingstone, 1970.
10. Saha AK: Theory of Shoulder Mechanism. Springfield, Ill, Charles C Thomas, 1961.
11. Somerville EW: Paralytic dislocation of the hip. J Bone Joint Surg 41B:279, 1959.
12. Dec JB, Inman VT, Eberhart MS: The major determinants in normal and pathological gait. J Bone Joint Surg 35A:543, 1953.
13. Cleland J: The shoulder-girdle and its movements. Lancet 1:293, 1881
14. Denham RA: Hip mechanics. J Bone Joint Surg 41B:550, 1959.
15. Flatt AE: The pathomechanics of ulnar drift. Social and Rehabilitation Services Final Report, Grant No. RD, 225m, 1971.
16. Sokoloff L: The Biology of Degenerative Joint Disease. Chicago, University of Chicago Press, 1969.
17. Radin EL, Paul IL: Importance of bone in sparing articular cartilage from impact. Clin Orthop 78:342, 1971.
18. Radin EL, Paul IL: Response of joints to impact loading: I. In vitro wear. Arthritis Rheum 14:356, 1971.

19. Linn FC, Radin EL: Lubrication of animal joints: III. The effect of certain chemical alterations of the cartilage and lubricant. Arthritis Rheum 2:674, 1968.

20. Kempson GE, Freeman MAR, Swanson SAV: Tensile properties of articular cartilage. Nature 220:1127, 1968.

21. Jones ES: Joint lubrication. Lancet 226:1426, 1934.

22. Radin EL, Swann DA, Weisser PA: Separation of a hyaluronate-free lubricating fraction from synovial fluid. Nature 228:377, 1970.

23. McCutchen CW: Mechanism of animal joints: Sponge-hydrostatic and weeping bearings. Nature 184:1284, 1959.

24. Walker PS, Dowson D, Longfield MD, et al: Boosted lubrication in synovial joints by fluid entrapment. Ann Rheum Dis 27:512, 1968.

25. Mansour JM, Mow VC: On the natural lubrication of synovial joints: Normal and degenerate. J Lubrication Technol 99:163, 1977.

26. Torzilli PA, Mow VC: On the fundamental fluid transport mechanisms through normal and pathological articular cartilage during function: II. The analysis, solution and conclusions. J Biomech 9:587, 1976.

27. Kettelkamp DB, Jacobs AW: Tibiofemoral contact area: Determination and implications. J Bone Joint Surg 54A:348, 1972.

28. Bullough PG, Goodfellow JB, Greenwald AS, et al: Incongruent surfaces in the human joint. Nature 217:1290, 1968.

29. Greenwald AS, Matejczyk M-B: A contact area study of the human ankle joint. Orthop Rev 6:85, 1967.

30. Walker PS: Human Joints and Their Artificial Replacements. Springfield, Ill, Charles C Thomas, 1977.

31. Freeman MAR: Articular Cartilage. New York, Grune & Stratton, 1974.

32. MacConaill MA: The movement of bones and joints: IV. The mechanical structure of articulating cartilage. J Bone Joint Surg 33B:251, 1951.

33. Linn FC, Sokoloff L: Movement and composition of interstitial fluid of cartilage. Arthritis Rheum 8:481, 1965.

34. McCutchen CW: The frictional properties of animal joints. Wear 5:1, 1962.

35. Hayes WC, Mockros LF: Viscoelastic properties of human articular cartilage. J Appl Physiol 31:562, 1971.

36. McCall J: Load deformation response of the microstructure of articular cartilage. In Wright V (ed): Lubrication and Wear in Joints. London, Sector Publishing Limited, 1969.

37. Benninghoff A: Form und Bau der gelenkknorpel in ihren Beziehungen zur funktion: I. Die modellierenden und formerhaltenden faktoren des knorpelreliefs. Z Gesammelte Anat 76:43, 1925.

38. Clark JR: Variation of collagen fiber alignment in a joint surface: A scanning electron microscope study of total plateau in dog, rabbit, and man. J Orthop Res 9:246, 1991.

39. Mansour JM, Mow VC: The permeability of articular cartilage under compressive strain and at high pressures. J Bone Joint Surg 58A:509, 1976.

40. Maroudas A: Physico-chemical properties of articular cartilage. In Freeman, MAR (ed): Adult Articular Cartilage. New York, Grune & Stratton, 1974.

41. Rosenberg L: Cartilage proteoglycans. Fed Proc 32:1467, 1973.

42. Smith RL: Soluble mediators of articular cartilage degradation in juvenile rheumatoid arthritis. Clin Orthop 259:21, 1990.

43. Simon LR, Radin EL, Paul IL, Rose RM: Response of joints to impact loading: II. In vivo behavior of subchondral bone. J Biomech 5:267, 1972.

44. Radin EL, Parker HG, Pugh JW, Steinberg RS, Paul IL, Rose RM: Response of joints to impact loading: III. Relationship between trabecular microfractures and cartilage degeneration. J Biomech 6:61, 1973.

45. Wolff J: The How of Bone Remodeling, 1892. [Translation by P. Maquet and R. Furlong.] New York, Springer-Verlag, 1986.

46. Radin EL, Paul IL, Lowy M: A comparison of the dynamic force-transmitting properties of subchondral bone and articular cartilage. J Bone Joint Surg 52A:444, 1970.

47. Radin EL, Paul IL: The biomechanics of congenital dislocated hips and their treatment. Clin Orthop 98:32, 1974.

48. Pugh JW, Rose RM, Radin EL: Elastic and viscoelastic properties of trabecular bone: Dependence on structure. J Biomech 6:475, 1973.

49. Bullough PG, Goodfellow J: The significance of the fine structure of articular cartilage. J Bone Joint Surg 50B:852, 1968.

50. Ochoa JA, Heck DA, Brandt KD, Hillberry BM: The effect of intertrabecular fluid on femoral head mechanics. J Rheumatol 18:580, 1991.

51. Radin EL, Fyhrie D: Joint physiology and biomechanics. In Mow VC, Woo SYL, Ratcliffe T (eds): Symposium on Biomechanics of Diarthrodial Joints. Vol II. New York, Springer-Verlag, 1990.

52. Radin EL, Paul IL: Importance of bone in sparing articular cartilage from impact. Clin Orthop 78:342, 1971.

53. Johns RJ, Draper IT: The control of movement in normal subjects. Bull Johns Hopkins Hosp 115:447, 1964.

54. Basmajian JV, Latif A: Integrated actions and functions of the chief flexors of the elbow. J Bone Joint Surg 39A:1106, 1957.

55. Barnett CH, Harding D: The activity of antagonist muscles during voluntary movement. Ann Phys Med 2:290, 1955.

56. Elftman H: Biomechanics of muscle with particular application to studies of gait. J Bone Joint Surg 48A:363, 1966.

57. Bigland B, Lippold OJC: The relation between force, velocity, and integrated activity in human muscles. J Physiol 123:214, 1954.

58. Grillner S: Locomotion in vertebrates: Central mechanisms and reflex interactions. Physiol Rev 55:247–304. 1975

59. Radin EL, Fulkerson JP, Hungerford DS: Symposium: Anterior knee pain. Contemp Orthop 22:453–482, 1991.

60. Radin EL, Yang KH, O'Connor JJ, Reigger C, Kish VL: Relationship between lower limb dynamics and knee joint pain. J Orthop Res 9:398–405, 1991.

61. Radin EL, Burr DB, Fyhrie D, Brown TD, Boyd RD: Characteristics of joint loading as it applies to osteoarthrosis. In Mow VC, Woo SYL, Ratcliffe T (eds): Symposium on Biomechanics of Diarthrodial Joints. Vol I. New York, Springer-Verlag, 1990, p 437.

62. Davis PR: Posture of the trunk during the lifting of weights. Br Med J 5114:87, 1959.

63. Davis PR, Troup JD, Barnard JH: Movements of the thoracic and lumbar spine when lifting: A chondrocyclophotographic study. J Anat 99:13, 1965.

Immune and Inflammatory Responses

CHAPTER 7

Laurie S. Davis
Thomas D. Geppert
Katheryn Meek
Nancy Oppenheimer-Marks
Peter E. Lipsky

T Cells and B Cells

The salient features of the immune system are:

1. The capacity to respond specifically to the universe of foreign antigens.

2. The capacity to develop enhanced responsiveness to encountered antigens during the first exposure (*priming*).

3. The capacity to retain specific memory of an encountered antigen and respond more vigorously and quickly to a second exposure.

4. The capacity to discern self from non-self.

All of these characteristic features can be accounted for by the activities of thymus-derived lymphocytes (T cells) and bone marrow–derived lymphocytes (B cells), the antigen-specific cellular elements of the immune system.

Both T cells and B cells express clonally distributed antigen receptors, which endow these cells with the ability to respond to all the antigens that an organism will encounter during its lifetime. T cells differ from B cells in (1) the nature of their antigen receptors, (2) the nature of the antigens they recognize, (3) the mechanisms by which they recognize antigens, and (4) their responses to such antigens.

B cells utilize a membrane form of immunoglobulin (Ig) as their receptors to recognize soluble antigens. After stimulation, they respond by clonal expansion and differentiation into Ig-secreting cells. In contrast, T cells express one of two types of antigen receptor that recognizes cell-associated antigenic peptides bound to polymorphic determinants of either class I or class II major histocompatibility complex (MHC) molecules. After stimulation, T cells proliferate and acquire a number of effector functions, such as the capacity to kill specific target cells, as well as regulatory activities, many of which are accomplished by a variety of secreted, antigen-nonspecific molecules, or *cytokines*. In concert, the actions of antigen-specific T and B cells and their various secreted effector molecules account for the exquisite specificity, acquired reactivity, memory, and self/non-self discrimination that are hallmarks of the immune system.

CELLS OF THE IMMUNE SYSTEM

B Lymphocytes

B lymphocytes are the cells in the body that are specialized to produce immunoglobulin. Their name denotes their origin in the bone marrow in mammals and the bursa of Fabricius in birds.[1] The most characteristic feature of B lymphocytes is the capacity to synthesize Ig and both to express it as an integral membrane protein and to secrete it. Developmentally, B lymphocytes constitute a distinct lineage of cells, whose various members differ in degree of maturation and activation, and extent of differentiation.[2, 3] Distinct stages of B cell maturation and development can be recognized, including early B lineage precursors (pro-B cells, pre–pre-B cells), pre-B cells, immature and mature B cells, and plasma cells. In general, these can be distinguished by the status of Ig gene rearrangements and the production of Ig gene products as well as the expression of other B lineage markers.[4]

Most mature peripheral B lymphocytes express two immunoglobulins on their surface (IgM and IgD), each with identical light chains and antigen-binding capabilities.[5] More immature B cells express only surface membrane IgM, whereas pre-B cells express cytoplasmic mu (μ) heavy chains, but neither kappa (κ) nor lambda (λ) light chains and no surface Ig. After activation, B cells rapidly lose surface IgD expression and, if they undergo switch recombination, IgM expression as well. Post-switch memory B cells, therefore, can be identified by the expression of membrane-associated IgG, IgA, or IgE. When B lineage cells undergo terminal differentiation to high rate Ig-secreting plasma cells, they cease to express all surface membrane–associated Ig.

B Cell Surface Markers

Besides immunoglobulin, B cells express a number of non-Ig surface proteins, some of which are B lin-

Table 7–1. HUMAN B CELL DIFFERENTIATION MOLECULES

Molecule	Other Designation	Molecular Weight (kD)	Function	Distribution	Comments
CD5	T1, Leu-1, Ly-1	67	Signaling molecule	B cell subset, T cells	Possibly identifies autoantibody-producing cells
CD9	—	24	Unknown	Pre-B cells, monocytes, platelets	Induction of homotypic adhesion
CD19	B4	90	Signaling molecule	B cells	Modulation of B cell proliferation
CD20	B1	35–37	Signaling molecule	B cells	Activation or inhibition of B cell function
CD21	B2	140	C3d receptor (CR2) EBV receptor	B cell subset	Stimulation of B cell proliferation
CD22	—	135	Signaling molecule	B cells	Augmentation of B cell activation
CD23	Blast-2	45–50	Low-affinity IgE receptor	B cell subset, activated monocytes, eosinophils	Induced by IL-4, shed as 33-kD B cell growth factor
CD24	—	38–41	Signaling function	B cells, granulocytes	Costimulates B cell proliferation, inhibits differentiation
CD40	—	45–50	Signaling molecule, receptor for CD40 ligand on activated T cells	B cells, some carcinomas, activated T cells, dendritic cells	Facilitates B cell activation and Ig class switch
CD72	Lyb-2	45	Signaling molecule	B cells	Receptor for CD5
CD80	BB-1, B7	46	Facilitates T-B cell collaboration	Activated B cells	Receptor for CD28
CD86	B70, B7-2		Facilitates T-B cell collaboration	Activated B cells	Receptor for CD28

Abbreviations: CD, cluster of differentiation; EBV, Epstein-Barr virus; kD, kilodalton; IL, interleukin; Ig, immunoglobulin.

eage–specific or uniquely expressed by B cell subsets. Many of these markers are expressed in a developmentally regulated way or are altered as a result of activation stimuli (Table 7–1).[6]

CD19 is the first of the B cell–specific differentiation markers to be expressed. It is found on pro-B cells, the earliest committed precursors of the B cell lineage. Its expression is up-regulated after activation and is lost only at the terminal stages of B cell maturation. CD19 is a 90-kD heavily glycosylated transmembrane glycoprotein that is a member of the Ig supergene family.

CD20 is a 33-kD transmembrane glycoprotein that has several transmembrane spanning regions. CD20 is expressed exclusively on B cells. It is expressed by pre–pre-B cells, after CD19 can first be detected but before the appearance of cytoplasmic μ chains. CD20 expression is lost after B cells differentiate into Ig-secreting cells.

CD21 is a 140-kD B cell–specific glycoprotein. It is the receptor for the C3d subunit of complement as well as a receptor for Epstein-Barr virus. The expression of CD21 can first be found on pre-B cells, after CD19 and CD20.

CD22 is a B cell–specific 135-kD member of the Ig supergene family, whose expression parallels that of CD21.

CD72 is a 43-kD transmembrane protein that is expressed at all stages of B cell maturation, except by plasma cells when it is lost. It belongs to a family of genes that contain a lectin-homology domain in its external C-terminal domain.[7] CD72 is the human equivalent of the murine Lyb-2 molecule.

Ligation of each of the preceding molecules provides unique activation signals to B cells.

B cells express a number of other molecules that are not B lineage–specific but that can be useful in identifying the stage of B cell differentiation and that may play a role in regulating B cell activation. Among these is CD23, the low-affinity receptor for IgE, which is distinct from the high-affinity IgE receptor on mast cells and basophils. Expression of CD23 on B cells is limited to IgM- and IgD-bearing B cells and is increased by activation and regulated by the action of cytokines. CD23 belongs to the same gene superfamily of lectin-containing molecules as CD72.

CD40 is a 45- to 50-kD integral membrane protein whose expression is largely, but not completely, limited to B lineage cells. CD40 is a member of a family of cell surface receptors, including the tumor necrosis factor (TNF) receptors. Engagement of CD40 by its ligand expressed by activated T cells plays an important role in stimulating initial activation and subsequent Ig class switching during B cell:T cell collaboration.[8, 9]

B Cell Subsets

A subpopulation of B cells expresses the pan–T cell marker, CD5.[10] These cells constitute 10 to 20 percent of the total circulating B cells in healthy adults. Larger numbers of CD5+ B cells are present in fetal spleen, neonatal blood, and in the blood of patients following bone marrow transplantation. The CD5 marker is also expressed on most chronic lymphocytic leukemia B cells. In the mouse, CD5+ B cells and their progenitors constitute a major fraction of peritoneal B cells. That CD5+ B cells represent a distinct population is suggested by the findings that levels of CD5+ B cells are genetically regulated in the mouse and humans. It has been suggested that the CD5+ B cell subpopulation is a distinct B cell lineage.

A role for these cells in the pathogenesis of autoimmune disease has been suggested because elevated levels of CD5+ B cells are found in autoimmune mice, in which they produce IgM autoantibodies constitutively. Studies in humans indicate that CD5+ B cell levels are elevated in patients with rheumatoid arthritis and Sjögren's syndrome and that these cells produce autoantibodies.[11] In humans, however, CD5+ B cells do not preferentially produce autoantibodies.[12] Moreover, CD5 may not identify a unique lineage of B cells in humans, as this marker is induced by activation of CD5+ B cells.[13] Therefore, the role of CD5+ B cells in the pathogenesis of autoimmunity in humans is unclear.

T Lymphocytes

T Cell Surface Markers

A number of cell surface molecules are uniquely expressed by T lineage cells (Table 7–2).[6] The earliest of these is CD7, a 40-kD transmembrane glycoprotein with an extracellular portion composed of a single Ig

variable (V) region–like domain. CD7 is expressed by all T cells, including prethymic precursor T cells in the bone marrow, although it may be transiently modulated after stimulation. It is also expressed at diminished density on memory T cells.

The most characteristic T cell surface molecule is the T cell antigen receptor (TCR) heterodimer.[14] The TCR is an 80- to 90-kD disulfide-linked heterodimer that is noncovalently associated with as many as five invariant chains of the CD3 complex.[15] The TCR is composed of a 48- to 54-kD acidic α-chain and a 37- to 42-kD more basic β-chain. Each chain is an integral membrane protein with both constant (C) and variable domains. Both chains are members of the Ig gene superfamily. A small subpopulation of T cells expresses a similar, but distinct TCR composed of gamma (γ)- and delta (δ)-chains, also associated with the CD3 molecular complex. The γ-chains range in size from 35 to 55 kD and are disulfide bonded to the 45- to 52-kD δ-chain. T cells expressing the γδ TCR usually fail to express either CD4 or CD8, whereas most of the αβ TCR-expressing T cells are either CD4+ or CD8+.[16] The structural variability and antigenic specificity of the TCR are explained by the organization, recombination, and expression of the genes encoding these chains.

In contrast to Ig molecules, TCRs occur only as membrane-bound molecules. Each T cell expresses only a single TCR consisting of either an αβ or γδ heterodimer. All four TCR polypeptides consist of two Ig domains, one variable, and one constant. The one exception is the Cγ2 molecule, which has undergone gene duplication.[17] Each polypeptide has transmembrane and cytoplasmic domains encoded by separate exons. The αβ and γδ heterodimers are covalently

Table 7–2. HUMAN T CELL DIFFERENTIATION MOLECULES

Molecule	Other Designation	Molecular Weight (kD)	Function	Distribution	Comments
CD1a,b,c	T6	43–46	Unknown	Thymocytes, dendritic cells, some B cells	Associated with β_2-microglobulin
CD2	T11	50	Receptor for LFA-3	T cells, some NK cells	Triggers alternative activation pathway
CD3	T3	5 chains of 16–25	Components of TCR	Thymocytes, T cells	Generates activation signals from TCR
TCR	Ti	Heterodimer of 42 and 45	Antigen recognition	Thymocytes, T cells	Polymorphic receptor for antigen-MHC complex
CD4	T4	59	Binds MHC class II	Thymocytes, helper/inducer T cells, monocytes	Receptor for HIV, associated with p56[lck]
CD5	T1, Leu-1, Ly-1	67	Signaling molecule	Thymocytes, T cells, B cell subset	Receptor for CD72
CD7	—	40	Unknown	Prethymocytes, thymocytes, T cells	Earliest T cell marker
CD8	T8	Heterodimer of 32	Binds MHC class I	Thymocytes, suppressor/cytotoxic T cells, some natural killer cells	Associated with p56[lck]

Abbreviations: TCR, T cell antigen receptor; HIV, human immunodeficiency virus; kD, kilodalton; MHC, major histocompatibility complex; CD, cluster of differentiation; LFA, leukocyte function-associated antigen.

bound via disulfide bonds C terminal to the constant region domains. As with Ig, TCRs are glycosylated proteins. The function of the TCR is to recognize cell-associated antigenic fragments bound to molecules of the MHC on the surface of specialized antigen-presenting cells (APCs). Both $\alpha\beta$ and $\gamma\delta$ TCRs are expressed on the cell surface in association with the CD3 complex. CD3 is a multichain complex of 16- to 28-kD subunits, consisting of γ, δ, epsilon (ϵ), zeta (ζ), and eta (η) chains.[14, 18] Each chain is the product of an individual gene, except for ζ and η, which are alternatively spliced forms of the same gene.[18] γ, δ, and ϵ are present as single chains, whereas ζ and η form dimers. Zeta (ζ) is found primarily as a disulfide-linked homodimer, but it may also form a heterodimer with the η chain. The exact organization of the CD3 complex has not been determined, although it appears that separate complexes may contain γ or δ associated with one or more ϵ chains.[19]

CD3 and the TCR appear to be physically associated on the surface of T cells. Moreover, both the TCR and the components of the CD3 complex are necessary for surface expression of both structures. Association of the TCR with the CD3 complex appears to relate to the presence of charged amino acids in the transmembrane domains of the molecules.[20] CD3 is thought to play a central role in T cell activation after engagement of the TCR. Because CD3 components are not polymorphic, the role of CD3 does not involve antigen recognition, rather, CD3 transmits signals from the TCR to the interior of the cell.

CD2 is another transmembrane protein that identifies T cells and may play a role in signal transduction. Originally recognized as a receptor for sheep erythrocytes, CD2 is a 50-kD glycoprotein that binds predominantly to leukocyte function-associated molecule-3 (LFA-3, CD58), expressed by a variety of cell types, but also to CD48 and CD59.[6] CD2 is expressed by the vast majority of thymocytes and all peripheral T cells as well as by some natural killer (NK) cells. It has been suggested that CD2 may provide an alternative activation pathway, which might be important during ontogeny before the TCR/CD3 complex is expressed. Alternatively, interactions between CD2 and LFA-3, expressed by a variety of accessory cells, may serve to costimulate T cell activation after antigen recognition.

CD4 is a 59-kD member of the Ig gene superfamily[16, 21] expressed by specific subsets of thymocytes, one of the two major subsets of $\alpha\beta$ expressing peripheral T cells, some monocyte/macrophages, and dendritic cells.[22] CD4 was originally thought to denote T cells with the capacity to function as helper cells for B cell responses or as inducer cells for the maturation of other T cell subsets, but more recent information indicates that CD4 is expressed by T cells whose capacity to recognize antigen is restricted by class II molecules of the MHC.[23]

CD4 plays at least two roles in this process. First, it directly binds to nonpolymorphic determinants on class II MHC molecules, increasing the avidity of the interaction between the TCR and the antigenic pep-tide bound to the antigen-binding groove of class II MHC molecules displayed on the surface of an APC. Second, engagement of CD4 provides a costimulatory signal that amplifies T cell activation induced by recognition of antigen. For many T cells, the binding and costimulatory roles of CD4 are critical to allow antigen recognition to result in T cell activation. Interactions with CD4 molecules are not necessary for activation of some T cells with very-high-avidity TCRs. CD4 is also the receptor for the envelope glycoprotein gp120 of the human immunodeficiency virus (HIV).[24, 25] The signaling capacity of CD4 molecules relates to the fact that its cytoplasmic domain associates with a lymphocyte-specific tyrosine kinase, p56[lck].[26] Aggregation of CD4 with the TCR/CD3 molecular complex brings this kinase into association with new substrates, whose phosphorylation appears to be important in the cascade of biochemical events involved in T cell activation.

CD8 is expressed by specific subsets of thymocytes (a subpopulation of peripheral T cells that generally does not express CD4) and by many NK cells.[16, 21] Whereas the human CD4 molecule is present on the cell surface as a monomer, the CD8 molecule is expressed on the T cell surface as a dimer consisting of 32- to 34-kD monomers.

Two forms of CD8 may be expressed on T cells; either CD8α/α homodimers or CD8α/β heterodimers. Both the α- and β-chains are similar in size and are members of the Ig gene superfamily. They are encoded by two closely linked genes. T cells expressing $\alpha\beta$ TCRs may express both CD8α/α and CD8α/β on the same cell, although coexpression of the two forms varies between individuals. CD8$^+$ T cells expressing the $\gamma\delta$ TCR and CD8$^+$ NK cells express only the CD8α/α homodimer. Although the expression of CD8 was originally thought to denote T cells with suppressor or cytotoxic activity, more recent information indicates that CD8 is expressed by T cells whose capacity to recognize antigen is restricted by class I MHC molecules. CD8 binds to nonpolymorphic amino acids of the $\alpha3$ domain of class I MHC molecules.[27] Such binding not only increases the avidity of interactions between CD8$^+$ T cells and APCs expressing antigenic peptides bound into the antigen-binding cleft of class I MHC molecules but also delivers a costimulatory signal to the T cell. Associations between the cytoplasmic domain of CD8 and p56[lck] appear to play an important role in the capacity of CD8 to costimulate T cell activation.[26]

Many other molecules are expressed by T cells, some of which play a role in modulating the function of these cells (Table 7–3).[6] One of these is CD28, a homodimeric transmembrane glycoprotein consisting of two 44-kD polypeptide chains.[28, 29] This member of the Ig gene superfamily is expressed on nearly all CD4$^+$ and about 50 percent of CD8$^+$ T cells. The natural ligands for CD28 are CD80 and CD86 expressed by B cells and other APCs.[30, 31] Engagement of CD28 provides an activation signal to T cells that is unique, in that it is not dependent on the expression of the TCR/CD3 complex.[29] Blocking this interaction during

Table 7–3. T CELL SURFACE MOLECULES THAT PLAY A ROLE IN SIGNAL TRANSDUCTION

Surface Antigens	Early Activation Events	Comments
CD1	$[Ca^{2+}]_i$	Costimulates with PMA; CD3-independent
CD2	$[Ca^{2+}]_i$, PI, Tyr P	APC ligand—LFA-3 (CD58); surface CD3 required
CD3-TCR	$[Ca^{2+}]_i$, PI, Tyr P, PKC	APC ligand—polymorphic MHC
CD4/CD8	$[Ca^{2+}]_i$, Tyr P via p56^{lck}	APC ligand—nonpolymorphic class II/I MHC; costimulates with CD3
CD5	$[Ca^{2+}]_i$, PI	B cell ligand—CD72; surface CD3 required; costimulates with CD3
CD6	Modest $[Ca^{2+}]_i$	Costimulates with CD3
CD7	Modest $[Ca^{2+}]_i$	Absence is associated with immunodeficiency
CD11a/CD18 (LFA-1)	Augment $[Ca^{2+}]_i$	APC ligand—ICAM-1 (CD54), ICAM-2; costimulates with CD3
CD26	Unknown	Costimulates with CD2, CD3
CD28	Tyr P	Ligand on APC—CD80, CD86; costimulates with PMA, CD3; CD3-independent
VLA-4 (CD49d/CD29)	Unknown	Ligand is fibronectin and VCAM-1; costimulates with CD3
CD43 (sialophorin)	$[Ca^{2+}]_i$, PI, PKC	Costimulates with CD3, PMA; absence is associated with immunodeficiency; ligand—ICAM-1
CD44	Unknown	Ligand—hyaluronic acid; costimulates with CD2 or CD3
CD45	Tyrosine phosphatase	Various isoforms expressed by cells at different maturation stages
CD55 (DAF)	Augment $[Ca^{2+}]_i$	Ligand—complement components; costimulates with CD3, AC + PMA
CDw60	Unknown	Costimulates with AC or PMA
CD69	$[Ca^{2+}]_i$	Costimulates with PMA
CD73	Unknown	Costimulates with PMA
MHC class I	$[Ca^{2+}]_i$	Ligand—CD8; requires cross-linking and CD3 expression

Abbreviations: PI, phosphatidylinositol; PKC, protein kinase C; PMA, phorbol myristate acetate; APC, antigen-presenting cell; AC, accessory cell; MHC, major histocompatibility complex; Tyr P, tyrosine kinase activity; CD, cluster of differentiation; ICAM, intercellular adhesion molecule.

antigen recognition can lead to T cell nonresponsiveness, or *anergy*.[32]

T Cell Subsets

A wide variety of activities have been attributed to T cells. Early studies suggested that CD4+ cells represented helper/inducer cells and that CD8+ cells represented cytolytic/suppressor cells. Subsequent studies documented that these activities were not strictly related to the expression of CD4 and CD8; rather, the CD4+ or CD8+ phenotype of the T cell related more closely to its capacity to recognize antigen in the context of either class II or class I MHC antigens, respectively.[16, 21, 33]

It is clear that recognition of antigen by T cells is fundamentally distinct from antigen recognition by B cells. Cell-bound antigen, rather than soluble antigen, is the form recognized by T cells. Cell-bound antigenic peptides are recognized by T cells after association with molecules of the MHC. A direct physical interaction between antigenic peptides and class I and class II MHC molecules has been demonstrated.[34, 35] Class I MHC molecules play the major role as restricting elements for peptides derived endogenously within antigen presenting cells, whereas class II MHC molecules largely restrict T cell responses to exogenous proteins that are taken up and degraded in the lysosomes of APCs to reveal antigenic peptides.[33] The strong association between class I and class II MHC restriction and the CD8+ and CD4+ subsets of T cells, respectively, is likely to reflect a fundamental role of the CD4 and CD8 molecules during T cell activation and also during the selection of the T cell repertoire in the thymus.

CD4+ T cells make up approximately 60 percent of the circulating T cell population. These cells seem to be the most effective—but not the only cells—that can provide help for B cell differentiation and that mediate delayed type hypersensitivity (DTH) reactions. In addition, these cells appear to play a major role in mediating graft-versus-host disease and allograft rejection when class II MHC molecules are the major alloantigenic stimulus. Of importance, these cells appear to play a major immunopathogenic role in a number of autoimmune diseases in experimental animals.[36–40] Much of the functional activity of these cells appears to relate to their capacity to produce a variety of cytokines that affect the function of a myriad of other cell types. In addition, CD4+ T cells can exert several effector functions, including the capacity to kill targets expressing appropriate class II MHC molecules and the ability to down-modulate the function of B lymphocytes.

Recent studies in the mouse have suggested that CD4+ T cell clones can be generated that express specific functional activities (Table 7–4) although differences in the expression of differentiation markers have not been appreciated.[41] T helper-1 (Th1) cells are effective mediators of DTH and are the primary producers of interleukin-2 (IL-2) and gamma interferon (IFN-γ), whereas Th2 cells produce IL-4, IL-5, and IL-6 and are effective helper cells for B cell differentiation and especially the secretion of IgE. Th1 cells appear to regulate the activities of Th2 cells by producing IFN-γ, whereas Th2 cells interfere with the function of Th1 cells by secreting IL-10, which limits the capacity of APCs to activate Th1 cells. The unique actions of Th1 and Th2 cells may bias the immune response toward DTH or humoral immunity and especially IgE production, respectively. It has been difficult to identify Th1 and Th2 type helper cells in

Table 7–4. FUNCTIONAL PROPERTIES OF MURINE CD4 SUBSETS

Function	T Helper-1 Cell	T Helper-2 Cell
Lymphokine secretion		
IL-2	+	±
IFN-γ	+	−
IL-3	+	+
GM-CSF	+	+
IL-4	−	+
IL-5	−	+
IL-6	−	+
IL-9	−	+
IL-10	−	+
IL-15	+	+
Help for B cells		
IgM, IgG	+	+
IgE	−	+
Delayed type hypersensitivity	+	−

Abbreviations: IL, interleukin; Ig, immunoglobulin; GM-CSF, granulocyte-monophage colony-stimulating factor; IFN, interferon.

humans, although specific subpopulations that produce IL-4 and not IFN-γ have been found.[42]

In both humans and mice, as well as other species, CD4+ T cells have been separated into "memory" and "naive" subsets based on the expression of a variety of markers (Table 7–5).[43–46] Although these subsets differ in the level of expression of several cell surface molecules, the most useful ones to separate them have proved to be the isoforms of CD45, with the higher-molecular-weight form, CD45RA, expressed by naive T cells and the lower-molecular-weight form, CD45RO, by memory T cells. These isoforms differ only in the extracellular portion of the molecule and are generated by alternative splicing. Monoclonal antibodies against CD45RA or CD45RO recognize reciprocal populations of resting T cells. After activation, there is a predominantly unidirectional transition from expression of CD45RA to CD45RO, which is thought to parallel the differentiation from naive to memory T cells.

A number of other observations support the conclusion that CD45RA and CD45RO are expressed on naive and memory T cells, respectively. First, neonatal T cells are largely CD45RA+, with the percentage of CD45RO+ cells progressively increasing with age. Moreover, in vitro responses to recall antigens are exhibited by CD45RO+ cells, whereas both populations respond to mitogenic stimulation and allogeneic stimulator cells. The capacity of CD45RO+ memory cells to produce certain cytokines is also enhanced compared with that of CD45RA+ naive cells. Thus, memory cells produce IL-4, IFN-γ, and IL-6, whereas both populations can secrete IL-2 after appropriate stimulation. Within the memory population, smaller subsets of more differentiated cells with unique functional activities can be identified by the diminished expression of another CD45 isoform, CD45RB, or the lack of expression of CD27.[47, 48]

The CD8+ T cell subset comprises approximately 35 percent of peripheral T cells. These cells recognize antigenic peptides that are bound to class I MHC molecules. Because this pathway of peptide presentation is most important in the recognition of endogenously synthesized proteins, CD8+ T cells are particularly involved in host defense to intracellular pathogens, such as viruses and other intracellular microorganisms. In some situations, the response of CD8+ T cells to microbial peptides may be sufficiently vigorous, not only to eradicate the organism but also to cause tissue pathology.[49] Prominent among the activities of CD8+ T cells is the capacity to differentiate into cytolytic effector cells.[50] This activity is not unique to CD8+ T cells, in that CD4+ T cells can also differentiate into killer cells. However, the specificity of CD4+ cytolytic cells is different, with the activity directed toward class II MHC molecules or peptides presented by class II MHC molecules. Moreover, CD8+ T cells are not limited in their effector functions; they can also produce a variety of cytokines, including IL-2, TNF-α, and IFN-γ. Under certain circumstances, CD8+ T cells can also support B cell differentiation. Although it was previously believed that the differen-

Table 7–5. SURFACE MARKERS ON NAIVE AND MEMORY T CELLS

Molecule	Other Designation	Molecular Weight (kD)	Characteristic	Expression	
				Memory	*Naive*
CD58	LFA-3	45–66	Ligand for CD2	+ +	+
CD2	T11	50	Alternative activation pathway	+ + +	+ +
CD11a/CD18	LFA-1	180–195	Receptor for ICAM-1, ICAM-2, ICAM-3	+ + +	+ +
CD29	—	130	β-chain of β₁ (VLA) integrins	+ + + +	+
CD45RO	—	220	Isoform of CD45	+ + + +	−
CD45RA	—	80–95	Isoform of CD45	−	+ + + +
CD44	Pgp-1	90	Receptor for hyaluronic acid	+ +	+ +
CD54	ICAM-1	120	Counter-receptor for LFA-1	+	−
CD26	—	40	Dipeptidyl peptidase IV	+	−
CD7	—	Multichain complex	T cell lineage marker	+ / −	+ +
CD3	—		Part of TCR complex	+	+

Abbreviations: VLA, very late activation antigen; LFA, leukocyte function-associated antigen; ICAM, intercellular adhesion molecule; TCR, T cell antigen receptor; CD, cluster of differentiation.

tiation of cytolytic effector cells from CD8+ T cell precursors required an interaction with CD4+ T cells, more recent evidence indicates that in many circumstances this is not necessary.

The mechanism by which cytolytic effector cells kill their targets involves a complex series of steps. Initially, there is TCR-mediated recognition of the target, which is facilitated by adhesion molecules on the killer cell, such as LFA-1 (CD11a/CD18) and CD2, which recognize intercellular adhesion molecule-1 (ICAM-1, CD54) and CD58 (LFA-3), respectively, on the target cell. Subsequently, the lytic mechanism is activated. This involves the action of a number of preformed granule-associated proteins, including several serine esterases (granzymes) and a membrane pore–forming protein, perforin. The action of these various secreted granule components leads to direct lysis of non-nucleated targets and a more complex form of death of nucleated targets that involves deoxyribonucleic acid (DNA) fragmentation similar to that noted with apoptosis or programmed cell death. In certain circumstances, secreted cytokines, such as TNF-α and lymphotoxin, may contribute to target cell death.

T cells expressing the γδ TCR represent a distinct set of peripheral T cells.[51] Most of these cells express neither CD4 nor CD8. They represent a minor percentage of T cells in the peripheral blood (2 to 5 percent) but appear to be enriched at epithelial surfaces including the skin, reproductive tract, respiratory system, and gastrointestinal tract. In general, their capacity to recognize antigens appears to be more limited than that of αβ T cells, recognizing bacterial antigens, heat shock proteins, and MHC or MHC-related proteins. Unlike the situation with αβ T cells, recognition of some antigens by γδ T cells does not appear to be restricted by class I or class II MHC molecules. Functionally, γδ cells can act as cytolytic effector cells and also secrete a variety of cytokines.[52]

The function of γδ cells has not been completely delineated. However, their capacity to migrate through endothelial cells, their ability to respond to specific bacterial antigens, their tissue distribution at epithelial surfaces, and their cytolytic potential suggest that they may play a unique role as the first line of defense against invasion by certain bacterial pathogens. A potential role for γδ cells in perpetuating certain autoimmune diseases,[53] including rheumatoid arthritis,[54] Behçet's syndrome,[55] polymyositis,[56] and lupus nephritis[57] has also been proposed.

EFFECTOR MOLECULES OF THE IMMUNE SYSTEM

Cytokines

Cytokines are soluble protein or glycoprotein molecules secreted by a variety of cells in response to a challenge by a foreign antigen or other stimulus. Cytokines regulate the growth, differentiation, and function of cells in an autocrine, paracrine, and endocrine manner. They are involved primarily in regulating immune and inflammatory responses. Whereas cytokines are involved primarily in immune surveillance, they can also be responsible for tissue injury and even death that occurs in response to some infections and autoimmune diseases.[58]

Because cytokines were thought to be the products of leukocytes and to function to communicate regulatory signals to other leukocytes, the name *interleukin* (IL) was coined to simplify the categorization of these molecules.[59] Other cytokines are grouped into functional families, such as the interferons, growth factors, and colony-stimulating factors (CSFs).[60, 61] Despite their original designations, many of the cytokines exhibit a number of additional activities, including the ability to regulate the growth and differentiation of lymphocytes, to regulate hematopoiesis, and to participate in promoting inflammation and destruction of infected cells or tissue.

Some of the cytokines that are produced by T cells and that contribute to the inflammatory response are listed in Table 7–6. The cytokines that regulate the growth and differentiation of mature leukocytes include IL-1, IL-2, IL-4, IL-5, IL-11, IL-12, IL-13, IL-14, IL-15, TNF-α, lymphotoxin, and transforming growth factor-β (TGF-β).[41, 42, 62] Cytokines that promote hematopoiesis include IL-3, IL-7, IL-9, granulocyte-macrophage-CSF (GM-CSF), monocyte-CSF (M-CSF), and granulocyte-CSF (G-CSF). Some cytokines affect many different cell types and participate in regulating inflammatory responses. These include IL-1, IL-5, IL-6, IL-8, IFN-γ, TNF-α, and lymphotoxin. Other cytokines function to down-regulate immune responses, such as TGF-β, and IL-10. In addition, a number of other nonimmune mediators, such as hormones and prostaglandins, can up-regulate or dampen systemic or local development of an immune response by altering or disrupting cytokine production. T cells produce some cytokines exclusively and along with other cells produce several other cytokines.

Cytokine Function

Cytokines that are produced in the rheumatoid synovium, including IL-1, IL-2, IL-6, IFN-γ, TNF-α, TGF-β, and GM-CSF, are discussed in more detail in Chapter 13. Some of the cytokines that are the most important for the growth and differentiation of peripheral blood T cells and B cells are discussed next.

Specific Cytokines

Interleukin-2. IL-2 was first named "T cell growth factor" and is produced exclusively by activated T cells.[63] IL-2 has been cloned and sequenced.[64–66] In the mouse, only some CD4+ T cell clones produce IL-2 (Th1 cells), whereas other clones produce IL-4, IL-5, and IL-6 (Th2 cells).[41] In humans, almost all freshly isolated peripheral blood T cells have the capacity to produce IL-2 and thus resemble the murine Th0 cell

Table 7-6. T CELL–DERIVED CYTOKINES

Cytokine	Abbreviation	Other Names	Mr of Natural Protein (kD)	Amino Acids of Mature Protein	Chromosome	Receptor	Activity
Interleukin-1α	IL-1α	Lymphocyte-activating factor (LAF) Endogenous pyrogen (EP); catabolin Osteoclast activating factor (OAF) Epidermal cell-derived thymocyte-activating factor (ETAF)	17.5	159	2	Single chain; CDw121a; type I receptor; 80 kD or p80; binds IL-1α, IL-1β, and IL-1R antagonist	Costimulates T and B cell activation and the secretion of cytokines (IL-2, IFN-γ) and antibody; increases killing by NK cells; myriad of effects on non-lymphoid cells
Interleukin-2	IL-2	T cell growth factor (TCGF)	15–20	133	4	Low-affinity, CD25, IL-2Rα, p55; CD122, IL-2Rβ, p75; non–IL-2 binding p64 IL-2γ; intermediate affinity IL-2R, IL-2Rα/γ or IL-2Rβ/γ; high affinity is IL-2Rα/β/γ. γ-chain associated with IL-4R, IL-7R, IL-15R (? IL-13R and IL-9R)	Promotes growth and differentiation of activated T and B cells; activates NK cells, macrophages
Interleukin-3	IL-3	Multipotential colony-stimulating factor (multi-CSF) Mast cell growth factor (MCGF) Erythroid colony-stimulating factor (ECSF) Megakaryocyte colony-stimulating factor (Meg-CSF) Eosinophil colony-stimulating factor (Eo-CSF)	14–30	133	5	α-chain, p70; β-chain, p120; IL-3R associated with a tyrosine kinase activity	Stimulates proliferation and differentiation of precursors of all hematopoietic cell lineages
Interleukin-4	IL-4	B cell stimulatory factor I (BSF-1) B cell differentiation factor-γ (BCDF-γ) T cell growth factor-2 (TCGF-2) Mast cell growth factor-2 (MCGF-2)	15–20	129	5	High-affinity, IL-4Rα + IL-2R γ-chain or "common γ-chain," γc; CD124 is IL-4R α-chain, p140; low-affinity IL-4R reported; soluble IL-4Rα is potent IL-4 antagonist	Promotes growth and differentiation of T cells, B cells; enhances tumoricidal activity of macrophages, but inhibits IL-1 and TNF-α production
Interleukin-5	IL-5	B cell growth factor II (BCGF-II) T cell replacing factor (TRF) Eosinophil differentiation factor (EDF) IgA-enhancing factor (IgA-EF)	45	115	5	Low-affinity, CD125, IL-5α, p60; IL-5R β-chain is nonbinding and shared with IL-3R and GM-CSFR	Promotes growth of cytotoxic cells and differentiation of B cells
Interleukin-6	IL-6	Interferon-β2 (IFN-β2) B cell stimulatory factor-2 (BSF-2) Hepatocyte stimulatory factor II (HSF-II) Hybridoma plasmacytoma growth factor (HPGF, IL-HP1) Myeloma cell growth factor (MCGF)	26	183	7	High-affinity, IL-6R α-chain (p80) + gp130; gp130 is nonbinding and forms homodimer when complexed with IL-6Rα, acts to transduce signal	Enhances IL-2 production from T cells and Ig production by B cells; myriad of effects on non-lymphoid cells
Interleukin-8	IL-8	Neutrophil-activating protein (NAP-1) Granulocyte chemotactic protein (GCP)	6–8	77	4	High-affinity IL-8R, CDw128, p58–67; low affinity IL-8R also binds GRO/MGSA, NAP-2	Produced by many cell types, mainly acts as neutrophil and lymphocyte chemoattractant and activation factor

Cytokine	Abbreviation	Other names	Size (kDa)	Amino acids	Chromosome	Receptor	Functions
Interleukin-9	IL-9	P40, mast cell growth-enhancing activity; T cell growth factor III	32–39	126	5	IL-9R is single chain, p64	Produced by activated Th2 cells; enhances T cell proliferation, mast cell lines and erythroid precursors
Interleukin-10	IL-10	Cytokine synthesis inhibition factor (CSIF) B cell-derived T cell growth factor (B-TCGF)	35–40	160	1	IL-10R is single chain, p90–110	Stimulates Th2 cell and thymocyte growth; inhibits Th1 cell proliferation, IL-2 and IFN-γ production; inhibits macrophage cytokine production
Interleukin-12	IL-12	Natural killer cell stimulatory factor (NKSF) Cytotoxic lymphocyte maturation factor (CLMF)	30–33 / 35–44	196/306	?	High-affinity, IL-12R, type I receptor, p180	Induces Th1 cell differentiation; enhances IFN-γ production by T cells and NK cells; stimulates proliferation of T cells
Interleukin-13	IL-13	Murine P600	10–17	112	5	Unknown; may share non-binding chain with IL-4	Produced by activated T cells; inhibits production of inflammatory cytokines (IL-1β, IL-6, TNFα, IL-8); induces CD23 on B cells, promotes human B cell proliferation and Ig secretion
Interleukin-14	IL-14	High-molecular-weight B cell growth factor (HMW-BCGF)	60	483	?	Unknown; also binds Bb component of complement	Produced by activated T cells; promotes B cell proliferation, inhibits Ig secretion; shares homology with complement factor Bb
Interleukin-15	IL-15	None	14–15	114	?	IL15R binding chain unknown; shares IL-2Rβ and γ-chains (not IL-2Rα)	Produced by many cells; enhances T cell proliferation, cytotoxic activity and LAK activity
Granulocyte-macrophage colony-stimulating factor	GM-CSF	Colony-stimulating factor-α Pluripoietin Colony-stimulating factor 2	22	127	5	Low-affinity, CDw116, α-chain, p80; β-chain, p130, shared with IL-3R and IL-5R; high affinity α- + β-chains	Activates macrophages
Interferon-γ	IFN-γ	Macrophage-activating factor (MAF)	20–25	143	12	High-affinity, CDw119, binding chain; second chain transduces signal	Enhances differentiation of T and B cells; counteracts effects of IL-4; enhances killing by NK cells; activates macrophages; induces class II MHC molecules on many non-immune cells
Lymphotoxin	LT	Tumor necrosis factor-β (TNF-β)	25	171	6	Type I receptor, CD120a, p55; second receptor is type II receptor, CD120b, p75; both members of NGFR/TNFR superfamily	LT and TNF-α have the same activities; enhance T and B cell proliferation; enhance B cell differentiation; increase killing by NK cells
Tumor necrosis factor-α	TNF-α	Cachectin	52	157	6	Same as LT	Same as LT
Transforming growth factor-β	TGF-β	None	25	2×112	19/14	Three receptors; high-affinity type I and II, p55 and p80; low-affinity type III, p250–300	Inhibits T cell growth and cytokine secretion; inhibits B cell growth and differentiation; counteracts effects of IFN-γ on non-immune cells

phenotype. IL-2 appears to be the most important growth factor for human T and B cells. Studies have suggested that a lack of sufficient IL-2 to drive a proliferative response may cause activated T cells to enter an anergic state and therefore may be unable to respond to subsequent antigenic challenge (anergy).[67, 68] Both CD4[+] and CD8[+] T cells can produce IL-2.[69] However, only a small subset of cells in a T cell population may produce IL-2 in response to a given stimulus, whereas almost all stimulated T cells will become activated and express high-avidity IL-2 receptors (IL-2R).

IL-2R expression is limited to a few types of cells of hematopoietic origin compared with receptors for many other cytokines.[70, 71] IL-2Rs are expressed by activated T cells, activated B cells, activated monocytes, and NK cells. As is shown in Table 7–6, the IL-2R is composed of three chains, which together make up the high-affinity receptor for IL-2.[70] The α-chain (p55), originally named Tac and now designated CD25, binds IL-2 with low avidity but does not transmit an activation signal; the β-chain (p70 or CD122) binds IL-2 with higher avidity and conveys an activation signal after being engaged via the third chain, which does not bind IL-2, called the γ-chain (p64). Together the molecules form the high-avidity IL-2R, with the capacity to transmit growth signals to the cells. The γ-chain also acts as a component for IL-4R, IL-7R, IL-9R, and IL-15R.

Engagement of IL-2Rs on activated T cells, B cells, and NK cells causes proliferation, whereas IL-2Rs on monocytes, which are up-regulated by stimulation with IFN-γ, leads to enhanced functional activation. Some studies indicate that the IL-2R is associated with the lymphocyte tyrosine kinase, p56[lck], which also plays an important role in TCR-mediated signaling. A soluble form of CD25, probably produced by proteolytic cleavage of the membrane-bound form, is found in the serum and synovial fluid of patients with rheumatoid arthritis and other inflammatory diseases.[72] Although inhibitors for IL-2 have been reported, it is doubtful that the soluble form of the IL-2R can compete with cell-bound high-avidity and intermediate-avidity IL-2Rs. It has also been suggested that antibodies might act as IL-2 inhibitors.

Interleukin-4. IL-4 is a 14-kD growth factor that is produced by activated T cells and mast cells.[73–76] In mice, IL-4 is produced by a distinct subset of CD4[+] cells that also produce IL-5 and IL-6 in response to antigen stimulation.[41] In humans, IL-4 production appears to be restricted to a subpopulation of CD4[+] memory T cells.[42, 77] A wide variety of cells bear receptors for IL-4 (CD124), including cells in brain and muscle.[78, 79] However, most of the work with IL-4 has focused on the effects of IL-4 on bone marrow–derived cells. IL-4 was first described as a growth factor for B cells and is the only factor to date that can induce murine B cells to switch to IgE production.[80] IL-4 can also increase production of IgE from human B cells, but it does not appear to be unique in this capacity. IL-4 stimulates a subset of T cells to

grow and promotes the generation of cytotoxic T cells. IL-4 up-regulates macrophage function and is a growth factor for murine mast cells.

Interleukin-5. IL-5 is a 45- to 50-kD molecule produced by a subset of T cells and mast cells.[80, 81] IL-5 was originally described as a B cell growth factor and appears to facilitate B cell growth and differentiation in combination with other cytokines.[80–83] IL-5 enhances Ig production by murine B cells and especially appears to induce enhanced production of IgA by facilitating the growth of post-switch IgA expressing B cells.[82] IL-5 promotes the generation of murine cytotoxic T cells and promotes the growth, differentiation, and activation of eosinophils.[80–85] Thus, in murine models IL-5 is important in limiting parasitic infection. The role of IL-5 in human immune responses is much less well delineated.

Interleukin-10. IL-10, originally called "cytokine synthesis inhibitory factor," is produced by both murine and human T cells and human monocytes.[86–88] It is produced by the Th2 subset of murine T cells and promotes the growth of these cells. IL-10 inhibits IL-2 and IFN-γ production by the Th1 subset of T cells, resulting in inhibition of the growth of these cells. IL-10 also inhibits the production of cytokines by macrophages.

Interleukin-12. IL-12 is a heterodimeric molecule produced by B cells, monocytes, and other accessory cells.[89, 90] IL-12 induces CD4[+] T helper cells to develop into Th1 cells. IL-12 augments the cytotoxic activity of T cells and regulates γ-IFN production. IL-12 downregulates the ability of T cells to produce IL-4 and can be the deciding factor in disease resistance, as has been shown in a number of experimental models of infectious diseases.[90] In addition, IL-12 is able to limit some parasitic and viral infections and has antitumor activity. Because IL-12 is relatively nontoxic compared with IL-2, it is considered a potential candidate in therapeutic regimens for infectious diseases and possibly for tumors.

Cytokine Regulation

Most T cell–derived cytokines are secreted only after T cells have been stimulated via a TCR-specific mechanism. Monocytes and other cells secrete cytokines in response to microbial products or other cytokines. Several features of cytokines contribute to the complexity of an immune response. For example, the same stimulus may induce different cytokines from T cells, depending on the state of differentiation of the T cells. Thus, when T cells are activated with monoclonal antibodies to the TCR/CD3 complex or potent mitogens, human memory T cells produce more IFN-γ and IL-4 than naive T cells and murine Th1 cells secrete IL-2, lymphotoxin, and IFN-γ, whereas Th2 cells secrete IL-4, IL-5, IL-6, and IL-10.[41] Moreover, the presence of additional cytokines or other immunomodulatory molecules also influences cytokine production. For example, monocyte-derived IL-1 augments T cell IL-2 production[91]; however, IL-1 can also induce monocytes to produce prostaglandins that inhibit both IL-1 and IL-2 production.[91, 92] By contrast, prostaglandins have no effect on IL-4 production and have been reported to enhance IL-5 and GM-CSF production.[92, 93]

Several other general principles appear to apply to the understanding of most cytokines. Cytokine production is highly regulated and self-limited. The production of each cytokine is under the control of several regulatory elements in the 5′ promoter region of the gene.[94] These elements bind specific proteins that either up-regulate or down-regulate transcription of the gene. For example, glucocorticoid response elements have been identified in the 5′ promoter region of several cytokine genes.[94] The immunosuppressive agents cyclosporine and FK-506 prevent IL-2, IL-3, IL-4, and GM-CSF production by interacting with distinct cytosolic proteins, cyclophilin, and FK-binding protein, respectively, each of which is a *cis-trans* prolyl isomerase and binds calcineurin inhibiting its activity.[95, 96] Calcineurin is a calmodulin-dependent phosphatase that activates the cytoplasmic half (NFAT$_c$) of the NFAT heterodimer, causing it to translocate to the nucleus and activate IL-2 gene transcription.[97–99] Even after stimulation, cytokine gene transcription is tightly regulated and is usually limited to a brief period. Moreover, the messenger ribonucleic acid (mRNA) produced is usually very unstable. For example, the half-life of IL-2 mRNA is approximately 30 minutes.[100]

Once the cytokines are secreted, they usually have a short half-life in vivo. The activity of each cytokine is determined by the presence of specific receptors on the responding cells. There is little or no cross-reactivity of cytokines, such that each cytokine is recognized by its specific receptor. For example, although IL-1 and TNF-α have many similar activities, the receptors for each cytokine are specific and cells bearing only IL-1Rs do not respond to TNF-α and vice versa.[91]

In general, activated cells bear increased numbers of cytokine receptors and different cytokines may up-regulate or down-regulate their own or each other's receptors. In addition, different cytokines may affect the same cell in similar ways. For example, several cytokines (IL-4, IL-6, IFN-γ) all promote B cell growth.[62] Alternatively, the same cytokine may affect different cells in different ways, although the intracellular signaling is induced through the same receptor. Thus, IL-1 promotes the growth of many cells, including lymphocytes and fibroblasts, but is cytotoxic for other cells such as β cells of the human pancreatic islets and thyrocytes.[91]

Finally, new T cell cytokines continue to be discovered and tested for function.

Immunoglobulin

Antibody molecules were the first members of the Ig gene superfamily described[101] and now often serve as prototypes in regard to molecules of this multigene

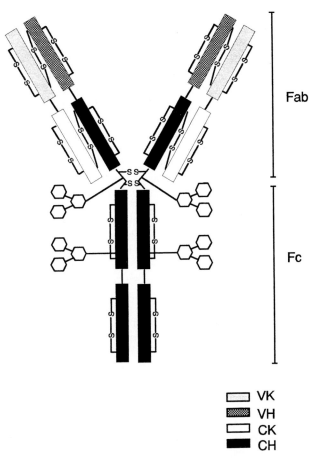

Figure 7–1. Schematic representation of a prototypic immunoglobulin monomer. Individual Ig domains (intrachain disulfide bonded) are represented by rectangles. Interchain disulfide bonds (between heavy and light and between the two heavy chains) have also been demonstrated. Carbohydrate moieties are depicted attached in C_H2 and C_H3, although carbohydrate can be found attached at other locations.

family. Characteristically, these proteins share amino acid sequence homology encompassing a fundamental structure, the Ig "domain." The Ig domain is a compact globular structure made up of seven antiparallel β-pleated sheets ("immunoglobulin fold" or "β-barrel").[102]

A prototypic Ig molecule is depicted in Figure 7–1.[103] Ig molecules consist of two identical heavy chains disulfide bonded to two identical light chains. In general, heavy chains contain four domains. Each heavy chain contains a variable domain (V_H), encoded by the variable region exon, which is derived by bringing together three separate genetic elements during ontogeny: V_H, or variable segment, the D_H, (diversity) segment, and the J_H (joining) region.

Heavy chains contain three constant region domains: C_H1, C_H2, and C_H3. Light chains (either κ or λ) have two domains: variable (Vκ or Vλ) and constant (Cκ or Cλ). Each domain is made up of approximately 110 amino acids.[104]

Early studies using various proteolytic enzymes demonstrated that Ig monomers could be cleaved into two functional units, termed *Fab* and *Fc*, for *fraction antigen binding* and *fraction crystallizable*.[105] The Fab consists of V_L and C_L paired with V_H and C_H1; Fc is composed of dimers of C_H2 and C_H3. The Fc portion of the molecule is the site of all known effector functions, whereas the Fab gives an antibody molecule its capacity to recognize a specific antigen. Because immunoglobulins have two Fab fragments per Fc, each antibody molecule can bind two identical antigenic moieties simultaneously and thus are bivalent.

Crystal structures of antigen-specific antibody molecules demonstrate that the portions of the molecule that are involved in antigen recognition are the loops between the β-pleated sheets.[106] These portions of the molecule are more variable than the parts which encode the β-pleated sheets.[107] There are three of these regions in both Ig heavy and light chains, and they have been termed the *hypervariable regions* (HVR1-3) or *complementarity-determining regions* (CDR1 to CDR3). The third hypervariable region of both heavy and light chains is encoded by the portion of the variable region exon that was generated by V(D)J joining. Generally, the most variable portion of any of the immune receptor molecules is the CDR3, and variations in this region engender different antigenic specificities.

In the heavy chain, there is an additional exon between the exons encoding C_H1 and C_H2, which encodes the hinge region. This relatively short protein sequence connects the two Fab fragments to the Fc portion of the molecule and allows for considerable flexibility between the antigen-binding part of the molecule and the effector region.[104] The IgM and IgE constant regions do not have hinge regions but, instead, have four constant domains (C_H1 to C_H4).

Certain constant region isotypes allow for the formation of Ig multimers. Specifically, secreted IgM usually occurs as a pentamer, whereas secreted IgA is usually a dimer. In both instances, an accessory molecule, the J (joining) chain is involved in multimer formation.[108] Multimeric Ig molecules have higher valences than their monomeric counterparts and potentially can bind more antigenic copies of specific antigen. Another accessory molecule secreted by epithelial cells (*secretory component*) now known as the *poly-Ig receptor* and also a member of the Ig supergene family, associates with IgA and facilitates transport of IgA across epithelial cells.[109]

Ig molecules all have numerous specific effector functions, and the capacity of each heavy chain isotype for each effector function differs.[104]

IgM is produced in primary immune responses, and as the antigen receptor, monomeric IgM is an important signaling molecule. Secreted IgM can form antigen/antibody complexes with high avidity, and IgM is a potent activator of complement.

IgG antibodies are the predominant antibodies formed in secondary immune responses and are important in many functions, including phagocytosis and antibody-dependent cellular cytotoxicity (ADCC). These functions are mediated by a variety of different cells, such as macrophages, mast cells, and polymorphonuclear cells, which bind IgG via Fc receptors.

IgA is found predominantly in mucosal secretions, including tears, saliva, nasal mucus, and milk.

Finally, IgE is the primary defense against parasitic infections. Dysregulation of IgE synthesis results in allergic disease.

Table 7–7 summarizes the characteristics of the different heavy chain isotypes.

Antigen-Specific Recognition: The Origin of Diversity

The efficiency with which higher organisms can defend themselves from pathogens is, in large part, a consequence of the ability to generate an enormous variety of antigen receptor molecules.

B Lymphocytes

The number of different antibody molecules in an individual at any given time is approximately 10^7. The origin of such enormous antibody diversity was not understood, because it was thought that each protein must be encoded by a separate gene. Since it was known that the approximate total number of

Table 7–7. PROPERTIES OF HUMAN IMMUNOGLOBULIN (Ig)

Property	IgG	IgA	IgM	IgD	IgE
Molecular form (usual)	Monomer	Monomer, dimer	Pentamer	Monomer	Monomer
Subclasses	IgG1, IgG2, IgG3, IgG4	IgA1, IgA2	–	–	–
Molecular weight	150,000	160,000	950,000	175,000	190,000
Serum level, approximate (mg/dl, adult)	1250	210	125	4	0.03
Half-life (days)	23	5.8	5.1	2.8	2.5
Valence	2	2	5 or 10	?	?
Complement fixation Classic	+ (IgG1/IgG2/IgG3)	–	+	–	–
Alternative	+ (IgG4)	+ (IgA1/IgA2)	–	+	–
Binding to cells	Macrophages; neutrophils	–	–	–	–
Biologic properties	Secondary response; placental transfer	Secretions	Primary response	Surface molecule	Mast cells Anaphylaxis; allergy

genes in the human genome is only about 10^6, this presented a puzzle. The mechanism by which this enormous diversity is generated from a limited number of genes has now been delineated. The genes of the immune receptor molecules are not encoded within the germline as functional genes but, rather, as gene segments, which must be juxtaposed by a somatic recombination event to create a functional gene.

Thus, different combinations of germline gene segments can generate many different antigen receptors from a limited amount of germline information.[110, 111] Furthermore, because imprecisions exist in the recombination process, significant additional differences can be generated at the sites at which the genetic elements are joined. This results in the generation of antigen receptor molecules that can differ in their antigen specificity even though they derive from the same genetic information. Whereas recombination generates antigen receptor diversity in both T cell receptors and Ig, B cells also generate their effector function diversity via an additional somatic recombination event called *switch recombination,* in which the same set of genes encoding antigenic binding is used to encode antibody molecules of different heavy chain classes and, therefore, different functional activities.[112]

There are seven immune receptor loci: TCR α, β, γ, and δ, the Ig heavy chains (IgH), Igκ, and Ig-λ. T cells express TCRs for antigen composed of either $\alpha\beta$ heterodimers or $\gamma\delta$ heterodimers in conjunction with the CD3 complex.[113, 114] B cells express Ig heterodimers consisting of a heavy chain and a light chain. These molecules are expressed in association with a complex of nonpolymorphic proteins, Ig-α and Ig-β, that appear to play analogous roles to CD3 in T cells.[115] Ig not only serves as the B cell antigen receptor (membrane bound Ig) but also is itself an immune mediator as a secreted molecule. There are nine Ig heavy chain isotypes (IgM, IgD, IgG1 to IgG4, IgA1, IgA2, and IgE), all encoded at the IgH locus on chromosome 14, and two light chain isotypes (κ and λ) encoded at distinct loci on chromosome 2 and 22, respectively. The TCRs are encoded by separate genes on chromosome 14 (α,δ) and 7 (β,γ) with the δ locus residing within the α-chain locus.

In general, the organization of the immune receptor loci is analogous. At the Ig heavy chain, TCR β, and TCR δ, the general order of the gene segments is V (variable), D (diversity), and J (joining), although there are exceptions. The Ig-κ, Ig-λ, TCR α, and TCR γ are similar, except that there are no D segments. In B and T cells, somatic recombination events juxtapose two or three gene segments, V(D)J, to create a functional gene, which generates a single exon encoding the "variable" region of the mature immune receptor molecule. This is illustrated in Figure 7–2. The functional variable region exon is expressed in conjunction with downstream exons, which encode the "constant" region of the immune receptor molecule. A schematic of the gene organization at each locus is depicted in Figure 7–3. For the purpose of describing V(D)J

recombination, the IgH locus is used as an example. Analogous events occur during recombination of the light chain and TCR loci.

There are about 50 different functional V_H gene segments in humans, 30 different D_H gene segments, and six different J_H gene segments. Because any J_H gene segment can recombine with any of the D_H gene segments, which in turn can rearrange with any of the V_H gene segments, the number of possible VDJ combinations to generate a heavy chain variable region exon is about $50 \times 30 \times 6$, or 9000. In addition, it is thought that heavy chains can pair with various light chains (κ or λ), although preferential pairing occurs. Light chains are also derived by somatic recombination of distinct gene segments. Finally, additional diversity is generated during DNA rearrangement, because the recombination event is not precise, in that there is the deletion or addition of non-germline encoded nucleotides at the joining sites of recombination.

Specific DNA elements are involved in the rearrangement process.[116] Immune receptor genes have palindromic heptamer and nonamer sequences immediately adjacent to their coding sequences. The heptamer is separated from the nonamer by a nonconserved spacer of either 12 (± 1) or 23 (± 1) base pairs, approximately one or two turns of the DNA helix. This highly conserved sequence motif is found flanking the rearranging elements in the immune receptor genes of all species that have been studied. These sequences are evidently the binding, or recognition site of the enzyme or enzymes involved in the rearrangement process.

At each receptor locus, the organization of the genes is such that a recombination signal sequence with a 12 base-pair spacer rearranges to a recombination signal sequence with a 23 base-pair spacer. This 12/23 base-pair recombination rule has been maintained at all seven of the immune receptor loci (IgH, Ig-κ, Ig-λ, TCR α, TCR β, TCR γ, TCR δ), although less common rearrangements (e.g., D_H-D_H rearrangements) that violate the "12 of 23 rule" do occur but at a lower frequency.[117] Even these less common rearrangements can contribute to the generation of additional diversity.

The recombination reaction involves two double-stranded DNA (dsDNA) cuts and subsequent religations. This results in the formation of two new DNA joints: *coding* joints, which contain the coding information, and *reciprocal* joints, which contain the two recombination signal sequences. The DNA between the two rearranging gene segments can either be deleted from the chromosome, or it can be inverted and thus maintained on the chromosome but in opposite orientation (see Fig. 7–2).[118] The orientation of the two recombination signal sequences dictates whether rearrangement will be by deletion or inversion.

A number of mechanisms permit modification of rearrangements. These include deletion of nucleotides by exonuclease activity and addition of nucleotides including palindromes to overhanging breakpoints[119]

1. Germline Configuration

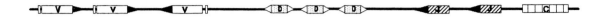

2. D-J Rearrangement (Deletion)

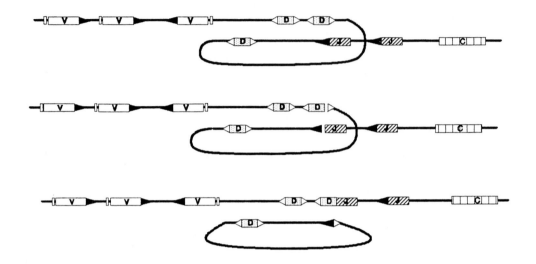

3. V-DJ Rearrangement (Inversion)

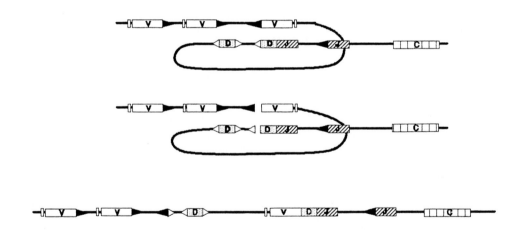

4. Transcription and processing

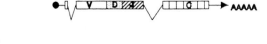

Figure 7–2. Schematic representation of VDJ rearrangement. In this example, so that both direct and inverted rearrangements could be demonstrated, D to J rearrangement is demonstrated as deletional rearrangement, whereas V to DJ rearrangement is via inversion. Whether or not rearrangement occurs by either of these mechanisms is entirely dependent on the relative transcriptional orientation of the two rearranging gene segments. The constant region in this example is depicted as a single exon, although in most situations the constant regions of the immune receptor molecules are encoded by multiple exons.

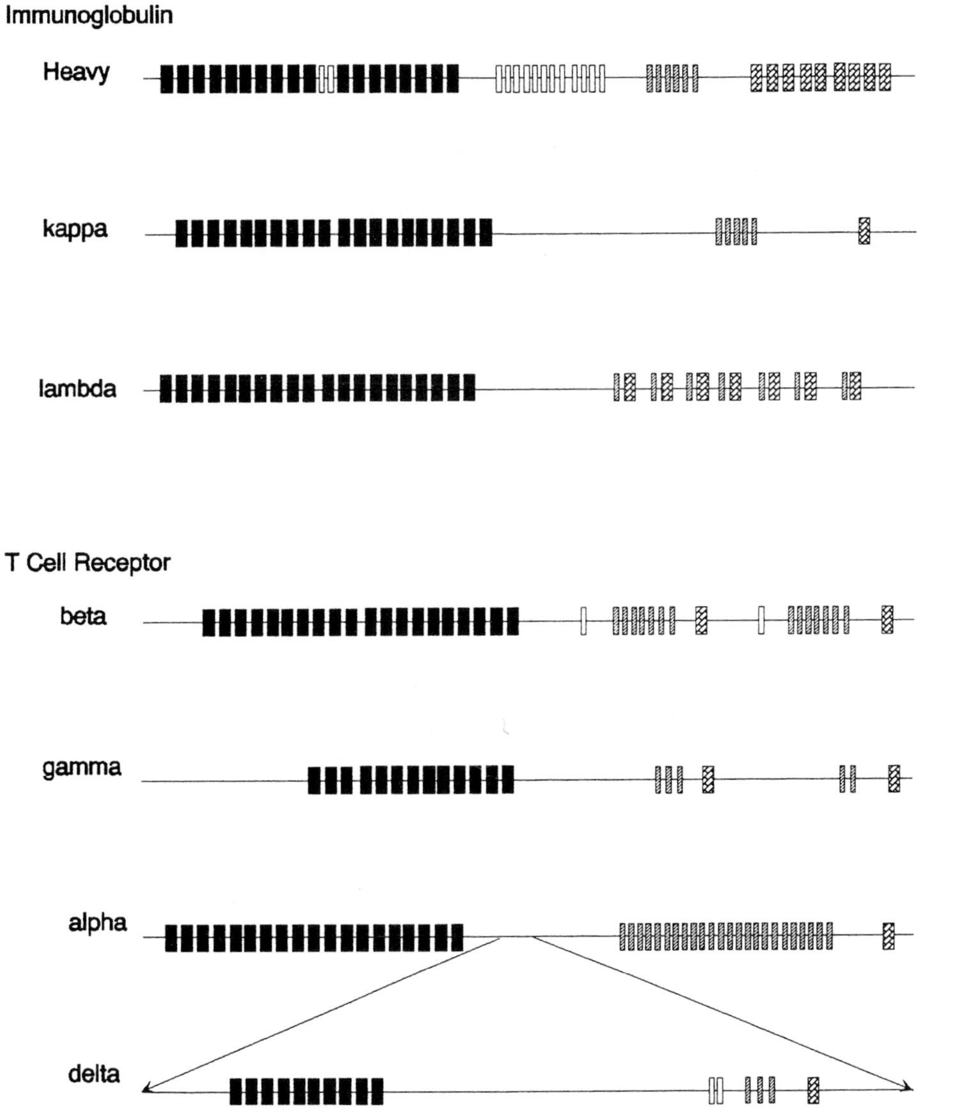
Immunoglobulin
Heavy
kappa
lambda
T Cell Receptor
beta
gamma
alpha
delta
V (variable) Gene Segment
D (diversity) Gene Segment
J (joining) Gene Segment
Constant Region Gene

	Chromosome	#V	#D	#J	#C
heavy	14	~150	~30	6	9
kappa	2	~110	-	5	1
lambda	22	~40	-	~7	~7
beta	7	~60	2	13	2
gamma	7	~10	-	2	2
alpha	14	~100	-	~60	1
delta	14	~10	2	3	1

Figure 7–3. Schematic representation of the seven immune receptor loci. Chromosomal location and approximate number of each type of gene segment are listed below.

and those resulting from the activity of terminal deoxyribonucleotidyl transferase (TdT), termed *N segments*.[120] Signal joints are precise ligations, whereas coding joints usually have small deletions.

Expression of TdT is not uniform in all lymphocytes undergoing immune receptor rearrangements. Because expression of TdT in developing B cells diminishes drastically from the time of heavy chain rearrangement to the time of light chain rearrangement (see later), κ and λ chains, unlike the other immune receptor molecules, lack N segments.[107] TdT is also differentially regulated during development. This results in a relative lack of N segment additions in fetal Ig molecules and TCRs.[121] The rearrangement process itself is an ordered one, in which different receptor genes are rearranged in a defined sequence during lymphocyte development.[114] In B cells, first D_H to J_H rearrangements occur, usually on both alleles, followed by V_H to D_HJ_H rearrangements. V_H to D_H rearrangements are not found. V_H to D_HJ_H

rearrangements continue until a functional product is generated on one allele. If nonfunctional $V_H D_H J_H$ rearrangements are generated on both alleles, the B cell dies.

Once a functional variable region exon is generated, μ chain is expressed. Experimental evidence indicates that the presence of μ chain signals both termination of rearrangement at the heavy chain locus and initiation of κ rearrangement. Two surrogate proteins that resemble Ig light chains (V pre-B, λ5), but that do not undergo somatic recombination, pair with the membrane but not the secreted form of μ chain; they are expressed on the surface of pre-B cells before κ and λ rearrangement.[122]

If initial κ rearrangement on both alleles does not result in a functional light chain exon, rearrangement can continue at both κ alleles by Vκ genes rearranging to other more downstream Jκ gene segments. Alternatively, much of the κ locus can be deleted by rearrangement to a heptamer sequence, termed the κ deleting element, found 3' of the Cκ gene.[123] In most but not all situations, rearrangement at the λ locus begins only after Cκ is deleted. As is the case with μ chain, expression of a functional light chain signals termination of light chain rearrangement. This provides the mechanism of allelic exclusion that dictates expression of only a single Ig molecule from any one B cell.

An accessibility model for the ordering of rearrangement has been proposed.[123] This model is largely based on the observation that transcription of unrearranged genes ("germline transcription") often precedes rearrangement. In this model, B cell–specific factors are proposed to act on the promoters of specific variable regions resulting in transcription of these unrearranged genes. Chromatin is in an open configuration during transcription. The openness of the chromatin may also allow the recombinase enzymes access to their substrate and therefore may explain the correlation between transcription and recombination. Alternatively, the actual transcription process, or even the germline transcripts themselves, may have some role in recombination. The factors that initiate germline variable region transcription by either T cells or B cells are only beginning to be understood.

B cells have an additional mechanism to generate diversity. Somatic mutation allows for the generation of very-high-affinity antigen recognition. There is a large body of experimental evidence demonstrating hypermutation of expressed Ig genes during the maturation of an antibody response.[124] Although mutations appear to occur randomly, B cells expressing mutated antibodies, which have a higher antigen-binding avidity, are selectively expanded by a process that appears to be mediated by T cells or T cell factors (*antigen selection*). B cells expressing higher avidity surface Ig antigen receptors are preferentially expanded in the microenvironment of the germinal center. Mutations found in the high-avidity antibodies have a higher than random rate of mutations in coding rather than silent nucleotides. Moreover, these mutations are most apparent in the portion of the molecule that is directly involved in antigen binding—the CDRs. The estimated rate of somatic hypermutation in B cells is approximately 10^{-3}/base-pair/cell division. The molecular mechanism of hypermutation is still obscure. T cells have a much more limited degree of somatic mutation of TCR genes, although somatic mutation of TCR α-chain genes by germinal center T cells has been reported.[125]

Although the process of rearrangement has been intensely studied for the last decade, relatively little is known about the enzymes or recombinases that mediate V-D-J rearrangement. Recently, two highly conserved genes were isolated, recombinase activating genes 1 and 2 (RAG-1 and RAG-2), which are encoded within the same genetic locus and appear to be necessary for recombination of antigen receptors.[126] Thus, deletion of RAG-1 or RAG-2 prevents the development of B cells and T cells. Although RAG-1 and RAG-2 are essential for recombinase activity, several ubiquitously expressed DNA repair factors are also involved in VDJ recombination.

In summary, unique T and B cell antigen receptors are generated by several mechanisms:

1. Selection of particular V, D, and J segments to form a complete antigen-combining site.
2. Junctional diversity generated at the joints of V-D-J or V-J rearrangement.
3. The addition of nucleotides at the junctions of rearranged gene segments.
4. Pairing of heavy/β/δ chains with κ or λ/α/γ chains to form heterodimeric molecules.
5. Somatic hypermutation of rearranged gene segments in B cells.

These various processes generate an enormous number of immune receptors that give the organism the potential to respond to an almost limitless number of encountered antigens. Except for somatic hypermutation, each of these events is intrinsically controlled and regulated and occurs in the absence of antigenic exposure.

Expression of the immune receptor genes is regulated at two levels. First, since productive rearrangement of these genes is limited to the appropriate cell lineage, this represents a major mechanism for regulation of gene expression. In addition, numerous *cis*- and *trans*- acting genetic elements regulate the tissue specific expression of the immune receptor genes.[127–129]

The rate-limiting step in Ig production is at the level of transcription. Two major DNA regulatory sequence elements are responsible. There are the *promoter elements*, found before all Ig V regions, and the *enhancer elements*, found between the J regions and the constant region genes. VDJ rearrangement brings these two sequence elements into proximity, which appears to facilitate Ig expression.

The two most well characterized sequence motifs of the Ig promoters are the TATA box and the octamer motif. TATA boxes are found in most eukaryotic promoters; the octamer motif is more specific, although not completely unique to Ig promoters. The octamer motif is essential for B cell–specific expression of Ig as well as for optimal levels of Ig gene transcription.[130]

Immunoglobulin enhancer regions are complex DNA sequences composed of numerous different sequence motifs that affect transcription of the Ig genes. Both the IgH and Ig-κ enhancers have relatively well characterized sequence motifs (E *boxes*). In addition, the IgH enhancer includes an octamer motif, whereas the κ enhancer has a binding site termed *nuclear factor, κ binding* (NFκB). Two *trans-* acting factors that bind to the octamer site have been isolated (OTF1 and OTF2, octamer transcription factors 1 and 2) as well as the *trans-* acting element, NFκB.[131–133] Ig gene transcription involves not only these elements but also numerous other DNA binding sites in both the promoters and enhancers of the Ig genes and *trans-* acting factors that interact with these sequences.

Transcription of fully rearranged Ig genes initiates upstream of the promoter regions, proceeding through the leader exon, VDJ exon, through the downstream unrearranged J regions and enhancer element, and finally through the constant region exons. Generation of a mature transcript is accomplished via messenger RNA (mRNA) splicing (see Fig. 7–2). In the case of Ig molecules, either secreted or membrane bound forms of the mRNA can be generated by differential use of polyadenylation signals and splicing.

Ig switch recombination is the molecular mechanism by which functional diversity is generated. Class switching provides a mode for a variety of different biologic functions to be associated with any particular set of rearranged Ig variable regions (VλJλ or VκJκ and $V_H D_H J_H$). Class switch involves the molecular association of a $V_H D_H J_H$ rearrangement with one of the different Ig constant region genes.

The human Ig constant region locus is composed of nine functional and two nonfunctional constant region genes. The μ and δ genes are the most J_H proximal constant regions; the remaining genes are located on two duplication units (Cγ-Cγ-Cε-Cα) centromeric of Cμ. The epsilon (ε) gene in the more Cμ proximal unit is a pseudogene, and the two units are separated by an additional gamma pseudogene. Thus, the organization of the locus is as follows: Cμ-Cδ-Cγ3-Cγ1-ψCε-Cα1-ψCγ-Cγ2-Cγ4-Cε-Cα2.

The ability of a single $V_H D_H J_H$ to be expressed with different constant regions is accomplished predominantly via a DNA recombination between tandemly repeated sequences (*switch regions*) located 5′ of each CH gene (except Cδ). The result of this somatic recombination event is that downstream constant regions are juxtaposed in the same relative position that the μ constant region occupies in germline configuration. For example, when a B cell switches from IgM to IgG production, the following events transpire: (1) a double-stranded DNA break occurs in the Cμ switch region, (2) a second break occurs in the Cγ switch region, and (3) the J_H proximal portion of Sμ and the

J_H distal portion of Sγ are ligated. Thus, the original $V_H D_H J_H$ is juxtaposed to the Cγ1 gene.

The genomic structure of the nine human Ig constant region genes are analogous. The IgG, IgD, and IgA constant regions have three constant region exons (C_H1 to C_H3) that encode Ig domains and a hinge exon; IgE and IgM have four constant region exons that encode Ig domains (C_H1 to C_H4). Each isotype can be expressed as either a membrane or a secreted form.[134] There are generally two additional exons downstream of C_H3 (or C_H4 for μ and ε) that encode a short transmembrane segment usually 26 amino acids and a cytoplasmic tail that is variable in length, depending on the isotype. The secreted or membrane form of each mRNA can be differentially expressed by using one of two cleavage/polyadenylation sites, one before the transmembrane exon and one after the cytoplasmic exon and differential mRNA splicing. Resting B cells express the membrane form of the mRNA, whereas activation and differentiation generally results in expression of the secreted form of the mRNA.

Unlike the other constant region genes, the δ constant region lacks a switch region. IgD and IgM are coexpressed in developing B cells via cotranscription of a single, long transcript beginning 5′ of the variable exon and continuing through the δ membrane exon.[135]

Whereas VDJ recombination is directed by recombination signal sequences that are rigidly conserved, the specific DNA sequences that direct switch recombination are very large (up to 10 kb) and are characterized by short tandem repeats that are not strictly conserved.[136] The human switch regions are composed of pentameric sequences similar to those found in murine switch regions.

Antibody responses to specific antigens are tailored in response to the eliciting antigen.[137] For example, the responses to polysaccharide antigens are generally IgG2 in humans and IgG3 in mice, whereas the responses to parasitic antigens are generally IgE antibodies. This bias during immune responses to particular types of antigens for particular constant region utilization appears to be independent of the particular $V_H D_H J_H$ rearrangement employed. These observations suggest that isotype expression is precisely regulated and not random during immune responses. More recent experimental evidence demonstrates that switch recombination is, in fact, a directed and regulated process, not a random one.

Switch specificity is accomplished by controlling the ability of the recombinase to interact with specific switch regions. The "accessibility" of the gene segments may be regulated by transcription factors. Thus, as with VDJ rearrangement, switch recombination is preceded by germline transcription of the gene segments involved.[138]

The validity of the accessibility model has been supported by a large body of data demonstrating germline transcription of unrearranged constant region genes is required for switch recombination. These germline transcripts initiate 5′ of the various switch regions and proceed through the constant region exons. No protein product is generated. Thus, T cell factors, by inducing sterile transcription, direct switch recombination and the expression of the different Ig isotypes.

T Lymphocytes

The genes of the TCR undergo a similar rearrangement process to generate functional genes.[139] The TCR α-chain consists of a single C region gene, approximately 60 J region genes, and approximately 100 Vα genes.[140] For α-chains, the mechanism of recombination appears to be deletion of the DNA between Vα and Jα. Allelic exclusion of α-chain genes is not as precise as for β-chain genes or Ig genes, but the mechanism has not been delineated.

There are two tandemly arranged β-chain constant region genes. There are no known functional differences between the two, and they are used interchangeably by T cells. Upstream of each Cβ region are seven J regions and one D segment. The order of rearrangement of the β chain locus is analogous to that of the immunoglobulin heavy chain locus.[141]

The γ-chain locus consists of at least 14 V region genes, of which six are pseudogenes, each capable of rearranging to any of five J region genes.[17] In humans, there are two C region genes that are significantly different, in that Cγ2 contains reduplicated second exons that lack the cysteine residues involved in the interchain disulfide bond, thereby giving rise to larger γ-chains that are not disulfide bonded to δ-chains. Assembly of the γ-chain gene is analogous to the TCR α-chain and λ and κ, resulting from a single V to J rearrangement. The δ-chain genes are located within the α-chain gene between Vα and Jα.[142] There is a single C region gene and at least two J and two D regions. Rearrangement is comparable to that of TCR β and V_H.

Expression of TCRs during ontogeny also occurs in a very ordered fashion with respect to the use of αβ versus γδ type receptors and with respect to the use of specific V region gene segments.[143–147] Transcription of rearranged γδ genes begins first, increasing through days 15 to 17 of fetal life in the mouse and then decreasing so as to be barely detectable in adult thymocytes. TCR β transcription can be detected on day 14 of fetal life in the mouse, but mRNA is truncated and incomplete (D-J only). Complete V-D-J rearrangements are first seen on day 16 and correspond to the appearance of full-length mRNA. TCR β-chains can be expressed on the surface of T cells in combination with a surrogate α-chain that is analogous to the surrogate light chains associated with Ig heavy chain gene products.[148] TCR α gene transcription is the last to begin, with full-length mRNA first detectable on day 17 of fetal life in the mouse. The level of α and β gene transcription increases from this time through birth.

Consistent with the pattern of TCR gene transcription, cell surface expression of γδ receptors occurs before that of αβ receptors. TCR γδ+ cells are detectable on day 14 of fetal life in the mouse and increase in number through day 17. The absolute number of γδ cells remains at a plateau from day 17 until birth. After day 17, γδ cells rapidly decrease as a percentage of total TCR+ thymocytes. This results from a sudden expansion of αβ cells. TCR αβ+ thymocytes are occasionally detectable on day 16, rapidly expand in number on days 17 and 18, and outnumber γδ cells after day 18. In the murine adult thymus, δγ cells account for only 0.3 to 0.5 percent of all TCR+ cells.[149]

In addition to the order of appearance of γδ TCRs before αβ TCRs, there is also ordered expression of γ and δ V region genes. Thus, during ontogeny, particular Vγ and Vδ genes are preferentially rearranged and expressed at certain times during thymic ontogeny.[150] The physiologic explanation for this phenomenon remains to be delineated.

Based on the order of appearance of γδ TCRs before αβ TCRs in ontogeny and on the observation that many αβ T cells also have γ gene rearrangements, it has been suggested that γδ and αβ cells belonged to the same lineage. According to this model, precursor cells attempt to rearrange γ and δ genes and, if successful, become γδ T cells. If the attempt is unsuccessful, these same cells would go on to rearrange their α and β genes. Because the δ genes are found within the α locus, rearrangements of Vα to Jα would result in deletion of δ. If the above model is correct, the DNA deleted during V-Jα rearrangement would be expected to contain rearranged δ genes. In most cases, however, the δ gene of αβ cells genes remain in a germline configuration,[151] making this an unlikely alternative.

More recently, information obtained through the use of γδ transgenic mice has led to the conclusion that γδ and αβ T cells develop along independent lines.[152, 153] In γδ transgenic mice, the extent to which αβ T cells develop depends on the presence or absence of a cis-acting DNA element, called a "silencer," in the flanking regions of γ.[153] When the γ transgene included the silencer, αβ T cells developed normally. When the silencer was eliminated from the γ transgene, αβ T cell development was blocked. It appears that activation of the γ silencer occurs in a portion of T cell precursors and the αβ lineage develops from these cells. In contrast, multiple cis-acting elements that silence the TCR α enhancer are active in γδ cells and a variety of non–T cell lines but not in αβ cells.[154] Entry into the αβ T cell lineage may involve inhibition of these elements.

ONTOGENY AND SELF/NON-SELF DISCRIMINATION

T Lymphocytes

Immunocompetent T cells develop in the thymus from bone marrow–derived or fetal liver-derived precursors.[155, 156] During this complex maturational process, deletion of autoreactive T cells (negative selection) and expansion of T cells whose antigen reactivity is restricted by self MHC antigens (positive selection) occur. During the development of T cells in the thymus, more than 90 percent of immature thymocytes are eliminated and the remainder exit the thymus to constitute the T cell arm of the immune system. Distinct stages of thymic ontogeny have been identified by surface phenotype, rearrangement and expression of T cell receptors, and functional capability.

The ultimate thymocyte precursors are derived from multipotent precursors in the fetal liver and later in life in the bone marrow.[155, 156] The CD7 molecule is the earliest T cell–specific cell surface molecule and can be identified in human fetal liver, yolk sac, and upper thorax as early as 7 to 8½ weeks of human embryonic development.[155–157] CD7 is expressed by prethymocytes as well as by all thymocytes and most peripheral T cells. Prethymocytes may contain cytoplasmic CD3 but have not rearranged their TCR genes and, hence, do not express the TCR/CD3 complex on their surface. In addition, they express neither CD4 nor CD8. CD7⁺ precursors of T cells colonize the thymus very early in fetal life (day 11 in mice, weeks 7 and 8 in humans) and continue to migrate into the thymus from the bone marrow during postnatal and adult life. Under the influence of thymic epithelium-derived chemotactic factors, thymocyte precursors localize initially to the subcapsular portion of the thymic cortex.[158]

During the process of thymic maturation, thymocytes migrate from the cortex to the medulla as they mature. After entry of cells into the thymus and the initiation of maturation, they begin to express a variety of differentiation markers, such as CD2 and CD1.[155, 157] Although mature T cells continue to express CD2, CD1 expression is lost as T cells mature in the thymus. By contrast, mature, functionally differentiated thymocytes acquire expression of CD5.[159]

A host of other changes in the phenotype of T cells occur in a programmed manner as they mature in the thymus. The most characteristic changes involve expression of the TCR/CD3 complex and CD4 and CD8.[156] The induction of TCR gene rearrangement and expression occurs in the subcapsule of the thymus under the influence of the thymic epithelium. For αβ T cells, this is the exclusive site of TCR rearrangements, whereas γδ T cells may also mature in extrathymic sites.[155, 160] In the subcapsule of the thymus, TCR gene rearrangement begins as a result of direct interactions with thymic epithelium and perhaps macrophages.[161, 162] This process appears to be mediated by a number of adhesive interactions, including those involving CD2 and LFA-1 on the thymocytes and their counterreceptors on thymic stromal cells, LFA-3 and ICAM-1, respectively. These cells remain CD4-, CD8-, and CD3-negative and are the likely precursors of the next stage of thymic maturation.

In the thymic cortex, the CD4⁻ CD8⁻ thymocytes begin to express both CD4 and CD8 as well as CD3 and the TCR. Among the CD4⁺ CD8⁺ CD3⁺ TCR⁺ thymocytes, there is positive selection of those recognizing self-MHC molecules expressed primarily on cortical epithelium.[163] The exact nature of the thymic epithelial cells involved in positive selection remains to be completely delineated, but thymic nurse cells probably play a role. In the absence of positive selection, there is an accumulation of CD4⁺ CD8⁺ cells followed by their elimination by means of programmed cell death or apoptosis.[164] CD4⁺ CD8⁺ cells that have undergone positive selection up-regulate expression of CD3. Negative selection of autoreactive T cells with high-avidity receptors for self-peptides follows.[163] The populations inducing negative selection include bone marrow–derived macrophages, dendritic cells, and B cells, which leads to apoptosis of self-reactive T cells. Thymocytes that progress beyond negative selection continue to up-regulate CD3 and lose either CD4 or CD8, becoming mature single positive thymocytes in the medulla. Afterward, these cells exit the thymic medulla and populate peripheral lymphoid organs. As a result of positive and negative selection in the thymus, mature CD4⁺ and CD8⁺ T cells are generated that are restricted in their capacity to recognize antigenic peptides bound to class II and class I MHC molecules, respectively, and that have been purged of cells expressing TCRs for self antigens.

Some autoreactive T cells escape deletion in the thymus. These T cells are maintained in a state of nonresponsiveness by a process known as *peripheral anergy*.[165] In this process, potentially autoreactive T cells are rendered nonresponsive by encountering antigen displayed on the surface of an inappropriate APCs. These cells differ from classic or "professional" APCs, such as macrophages, dendritic cells, and B cells, in that they lack the capacity to provide costimulatory signals necessary for antigen recognition to lead to T cell activation.[31] The exact nature of these costimulatory signals and the surface receptors involved have not been delineated. It is clear, however, that when potentially autoreactive T cells encounter antigen displayed by an APC that is unable to deliver these signals, anergy, not activation, results. Such induced nonresponsiveness appears to be a major mechanism in preventing autoreactive T cells that escape the thymus from causing autoimmune disease.

B Lymphocytes

B cells develop from precursors initially found in the placenta and fetal liver and subsequently in the bone marrow.[2, 3, 166, 167] During adult life, B cell precursors reside in the bone marrow. The development of B cells involves the commitment of hematopoietic stem cells to the B cell lineage, with subsequent rearrangement of Ig genes and expression of membrane-associated Ig and other specific B cell lineage markers (see Table 7–1).

In prenatal and adult life, the decision to enter the B cell lineage occurs in the fetal liver and bone marrow, respectively. Adherent bone marrow stromal cells play a critical role in the commitment of precursors to the B cell lineage.[167] Stromal cells secrete growth factors for pre-B cells that appear to play a critical role in this process. Bone marrow macrophages and other stromal cells also contribute to the induction of stem cell commitment to the B cell lineage.

The maturation of stem cell precursors into functional human B lymphocytes represents a multistep process of programmed development that involves both Ig gene rearrangements and the induction of expression of a number of B lineage differentiation molecules. CD19 appears to be the earliest B lineage differentiation molecule expressed by developing B cells.[2, 3] These pro-B cells also express HLA-DR, CD10 (enkephalinase), CD34, and TdT. These early B cell precursors evolve through a complex series of maturation changes into pre–pre B cells and then pre-B cells and immature B cells, eventually giving rise to mature B cells, which exit the bone marrow. Ig rearrangement begins in CD19 positive pre–pre B cells before they have begun to express CD20 or CD21.[3] Pre-B cells first express cytoplasmic μ chains but do not express membrane IgM; immature B cells express surface IgM but not IgD. Mature B cells express both IgD and IgM.

During the maturation of B cells, specific cytokines appear to facilitate the growth and differentiation of precursors at different stages. Thus, for example, low-molecular-weight B cell growth factor and IL-3, but not IL-1, IL-4, IL-5, or IL-6, induce proliferation of pro-B cells.[3, 167] Similarly, a subpopulation of fetal liver pro-B cells proliferate in response to IL-7, a 15-kD stromal cell–derived cytokine.[168, 169] As B cell precursors mature, the expression of cytokine receptors changes in a programmed manner. IL-7 receptors are lost during the pre-B cell stage, whereas IL-3 receptors are lost as cells become immature B cells.[3] Immature membrane IgM$^+$IgD$^-$ B cells first express receptors for IL-4, whereas receptors for IL-1, IL-2, IL-5, and IL-6 are first expressed by mature IgM$^+$IgD$^+$ B cells.

Peripheral B cells can be classified as either *naive* or *memory* cells, depending on their antigenic experience. Naive B cells that have not yet encountered antigen account for the majority of mature, peripheral B cells. These cells express both membrane IgM and IgD and are continuously replenished from the maturational process in the bone marrow. Memory B cells, which have been selected for expansion in T cell–dependent immune responses for high-avidity binding to their target antigen, frequently express somatically mutated Ig VDJ region genes and persist in the immune system for a long time.[170] They usually do not express IgD, may express IgM, but generally express IgG, IgA, or IgE on their surface membranes.

The repertoire of Ig receptors expressed by peripheral B lymphocytes is influenced by positive and negative selection in a manner that is analogous to the shaping of the T cell repertoire during ontogeny.

Thus, newly generated B cells appear to undergo a process of positive selection as they differentiate from pre-B cells into the mature peripheral B cell pool.[171] The nature of the cells and molecules responsible for this positive selection process is unknown. B cells expressing membrane Ig receptors that recognize autoantigens are deleted during B cell ontogeny.[172–174] This is particularly effective for B cells that recognize cell-bound antigens. Autoreactive B cells that escape into the periphery become unresponsive to the autoantigen by a process that involves down-regulation of their surface Ig receptors as well as functional anergy, which is similar to that observed with autoreactive T cells that escape the thymus.

LYMPHOCYTE ACTIVATION

T Lymphocytes

Activation is the series of steps that begin with antigen recognition and includes the biochemical events that will initiate cell cycle entry and sustain cell cycle progression to mitosis and the production of daughter cells. An important result of T cell activation is the production of a number of cytokines, since T cell activation results in the up-regulation of cytokine gene transcription. Cytokines not only are required for T cell cycle progression but also have important regulatory effects on B cells, monocytes, and other cells of the immune system.

T cell activation can be conveniently separated into three series of events:

1. The required cellular interactions.
2. Generation of the initial transmembrane signals.
3. The subsequent gene activation events that occur in orderly progression to induce the production of cytokines and other proteins or cell products needed to sustain cell cycle progression and to stimulate cellular division and growth.

Cellular Interactions

Under normal circumstances, T cells recognize antigen bound to MHC molecules on the surface of specialized APCs. Cell surface molecules have evolved on both the T cell and the APC to mediate antigen presentation and recognition. The T cell expresses the clonally distributed TCR, which recognizes antigen complexed with an MHC molecule present on the surface of the APC (Fig. 7–4). The TCR is a heterodimer whose ligand-binding domain is unique to each clone of T cells.[175] Both of these chains belong to the Ig superfamily, have a single membrane spanning region and short cytoplasmic tails (4 to 12 amino acids), and are linked by a single disulfide bond.[175] The TCR is always noncovalently associated on the cell surface with the CD3 complex. The CD3 complex is composed of five different polypeptide chains that are invariant in structure in all T cells. The association of CD3 with the TCR appears to involve interactions

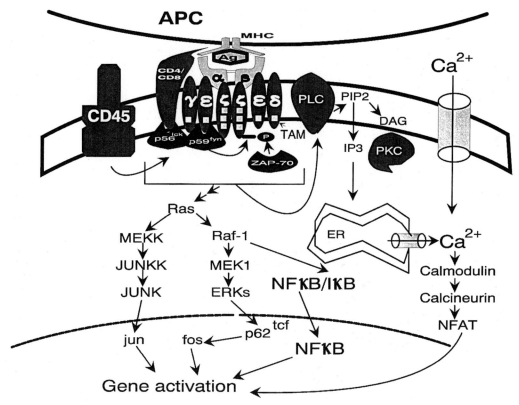

Figure 7–4. Signaling events involved in T cell activation resulting from recognition of an antigenic peptide–MHC molecule complex. APC, antigen-presenting cell; MHC, major histocompatibility complex.

between charged amino acids of their cytoplasmic domains. The TCR structure determines the specificity of antigen recognition. The CD3 complex mediates transduction of activation signals to the T cell.

Three of the proteins found in the CD3 complex—γ, δ, and ϵ—are coded for on human chromosome 11, are highly homologous in structure, and probably have arisen by gene duplication. Only γ (28 kD) and δ (20 kD) are glycosylated.[175] The other two TCR associated proteins are ζ-ζ homodimers, or ζ-η or ζ-Fcϵ-γ heterodimers that have no structural homology to γ, δ, or ϵ and are independently associated with the TCR.[175]

CD3-ζ is not glycosylated. It maps to human chromosome 1, and has a short extracellular domain, but a cytoplasmic domain of 113 amino acids. Approximately 90 percent of ζ is found as a homodimer. CD3-η is derived by alternative splicing from the same gene locus on chromosome 1 as CD3-ζ.[176] Fcϵ-γ is homolgous to CD3-ζ, which is associated with the Fcϵ receptor and is found on NK cells. Each TCR unit consists of four relatively independent dimers: $\alpha\alpha$, $\epsilon\delta$, $\epsilon\gamma$, and $\zeta\zeta$.

ζ, η, and all of the CD3 molecules contain a sequence motif of approximately 26 amino acids found in the cytoplasmic domain of various molecules that associate with receptors, called the *antigen receptor homology motif* (ARH1) or *tyrosine activation motif* (TAM).[177] The sequence is characterized by six con-

served amino acids in the sequence D/E-X$_7$-D/E-X$_2$-Y-X$_2$-L/I-X$_7$-Y-X$_2$-L/I. ζ and η contain three ARH1 regions; the other CD3 molecules contain one. The tyrosine residues within these regions are phosphorylated on antigen recognition and are required for signal transduction to occur.[178] Each of the molecules can tranduce signals leading to T cell activation.[179]

T cell–APC recognition requires not only that an appropriate antigen be presented to be recognized by a unique TCR but also that the antigen be bound to the correct class I or class II MHC molecule on the APC. This further restriction occurs because CD4$^+$ T cells recognize antigenic peptides bound to class II MHC molecules on the APC, whereas CD8$^+$ T cells recognize peptide presented on APC class I MHC molecules.[16] CD4 can directly bind nonpolymorphic regions of class II MHC molecules, whereas CD8 can bind the nonpolymorphic regions of the α3 domain of class I MHC proteins. The restriction of the T cell–APC interaction on the basis of CD4 or CD8 phenotype in part relates to the signaling function of these molecules. CD4 and CD8 physically associate with the TCR when antigen is recognized, thus forming a complex in which antigen recognition and CD4 or CD8 association occurs on the same MHC molecule (see Fig. 7–4).[180] As CD4 and CD8 are associated with the lymphocyte-specific intracellular tyrosine kinase, p56^{lck}, one result of formation of this complex is to bring p56^{lck} into association with the TCR complex.[181]

An important advance in the understanding of the role of the MHC encoded molecules has occurred as a result of determination of the three-dimensional structure of the heterodimeric class I MHC.[34] The larger α-chain (44 kD), coded for by the MHC, is organized into three extracellular domains: an α_1 and α_2 domain, which forms the antigen-binding region, and an α_3 Ig-like domain. In addition, the polypeptide has a transmembrane sequence and a cytoplasmic tail. There is one peptide-binding site per molecule, and the cleft that is formed to bind antigen is large enough to bind a peptide fragment of about nine amino acids. Most of the polymorphic amino acid residues of the heavy chain are found in the α-helical sides or the β-pleated sheet floor of the peptide-binding cleft. These allelic differences in the peptide-binding cleft contribute to the ability of the molecule to bind different peptides.[182] The heavy chain is noncovalently associated with a smaller peptide (12 kD), β_2-microglobulin, which is not MHC-encoded and is entirely extracellular. β_2-microglobulin is folded in an Ig-like conformation and associates with the α_3 domain of the heavy chain. This association seems to be critical in maintaining the tertiary structure of the complex and in stabilizing peptide binding and expression on the cell surface.

The crystallographic structure of class II MHC molecules has also been determined.[35, 183] The molecule is unlike the class I MHC molecule, in that it is composed of two noncovalently associated chains: a nonpolymorphic α-chain and a polymorphic β-chain, both of which are similar in structure. The class II MHC molecule has antigen-binding cleft with α-helical sides and a β-pleated sheet forming the floor. The polymorphic amino acid residues of the β-chain point toward the groove where the antigenic peptide is proposed to reside. Unlike the class I MHC molecule, however, the antigen-binding site is formed by both chains.[183]

Although the interactions of TCR–MHC are critical for stimulation of specific T cells, these ligand receptor interactions may not be sufficient to activate the T cell; in fact, in isolation, subsequent T cell unresponsiveness, a form of anergy, can result.[31, 165] A number of additional interactions with other molecules expressed on the T cell surface are important in providing a sufficient stimulus to activate the resting T cell (see Table 7–3). APCs are known to express ligands for some of these T cell antigens, including CD2, CD4/CD8, CD28, and LFA-1. Many of these molecules function to increase adhesive interactions between T cells and APCs, and they also can generate activation signals. Therefore, it is likely that T cells receive multiple signals from engagement of these various receptors during interactions with APCs that can summate and thus facilitate T cell activation.[31] Some studies have suggested that the interaction between CD28 on T cells and B7-1 (CD86) and B7-2 (CD87) on accessory cells may be critical in providing costimulatory signals to T cells.[30, 31, 165]

Transmembrane Signaling

Once an appropriate T cell–antigen APC couple has been formed, information must be transmitted to the T cell to initiate the cascade of biochemical events that will eventually result in cytokine receptor expression, cytokine gene expression, cell cycle progression, and clonal expansion. Phosphorylation or dephosphorylation of proteins is one of the central biochemical mechanisms used to regulate intracellular events in response to extracellular signals. In fact, the earliest detectable event that occurs after TCR/CD3 ligation is phosphorylation of a variety of polypeptides on their tyrosine residues.[184] The critical role of tyrosine kinase phosphorylation is indicated by the observation that inhibition of tyrosine kinase–mediated phosphorylation prevents T cell activation and IL-2 production.[185] Tyrosine phosphorylation of some proteins has been detected as early as 5 seconds after ligation of the TCR/CD3 complex, and tyrosine phosphorylation of the ζ chain of the TCR occurs within minutes.[186] Such tyrosine phosphorylation occurs before detectable phospholipase C activation.[186]

Although tyrosine phosphorylation is initiated by ligation of the TCR/CD3 complex, the T cell receptor is not itself a tyrosine kinase. It is thought that tyrosine phosphorylation is catalyzed by tyrosine kinases that associate with the TCR and/or CD4/CD8 molecules. As mentioned earlier, the *src* family tyrosine kinase *lck* is physically associated with CD4 or CD8.[181] Another src family kinase, *fyn*, is physically associated with the CD3 molecules.[187] In both cases, the association can be detected in the resting state. A third tyrosine kinase, ZAP-70, is not associated with the TCR in resting cells but associates with the TCR complex on activation.[188] ZAP-70 is not a member of the src family of tyrosine kinases. The mechanism whereby these kinases cooperate to bring about T cell activation is not yet clear, but it appears that all of them must be present for optimal activation to occur.[181, 188–191] The activity of *src* family tyrosine kinases are themselves regulated by tyrosine phosphorylation. The tyrosine kinase *csk* constitutively phosphorylates a C-terminal tyrosine residue that inactivates both *lck* and *fyn*.[191] Activation requires dephosphorylation of this residue and autophosphorylation at an internal site. Autophosphorylation is favored by aggregation, which occurs on antigen recognition.

An important mediator of dephosphorylation is the CD45 molecule, which is expressed as different isoforms on T cell subsets, B cells, and other bone marrow–derived cells. The cytoplasmic domain of CD45 has tyrosine phosphatase activity,[192] and cells that do not express CD45 cannot be activated appropriately.[193] CD45 can remove the inhibitory phosphate from *src* family kinases, thus allowing activation to take place.[194] CD45 can physically associate with CD3 and with CD2.[195] Thus, one result of ligation of the TCR/CD3 is to bring CD45 into aggregates containing *lck*, *fyn*, and ZAP-70, where it presumably allows activation to occur.

Physiologically, other pathways appear to be linked to surface receptors by the action of the tyrosine kinases described above. Tyrosine phosphorylation is required for activation of phospholipase C (PLC), following CD3 ligation resulting in tyrosine phosphorylation of the PLC-γ1 isoform.[196] Inhibition of tyrosine phosphorylation inhibits the activation of phospholipase C and generation of the increase in $[Ca^{2+}]_i$ observed in response to ligation of the TCR/CD3 complex.[197] Membrane-bound phospholipase C hydrolyzes phosphatidylinositol-4,5-bisphosphate, a minor membrane lipid, to produce intracellular inositol trisphosphate (IP_3) and diacylglycerol (DAG) in response to engagement of TCR/CD3.[198] IP_3 mobilizes an intracellular store of calcium that, when released, contributes to the initial increase in intracellular calcium ($[Ca^{2+}]_i$) that is observed after mitogen activation of T cells. DAG is believed to be the physiologic activator of protein kinase C, a serine-threonine kinase.

The increase in $[Ca^{2+}]_i$ observed after mitogen stimulation is not entirely a result of mobilization of intracellular stores by IP_3, as movement of calcium from the extracellular medium into the cell is necessary both for T cell activation and for the maintenance of the sustained increase in $[Ca^{2+}]_i$ associated with T cell activation.[199] How calcium moves across the T cell membrane is not yet clear, although a cation movement that is stimulated by mitogens has been detected.[200] This cation entry is not voltage-gated, and thus it is unlike the classic voltage-gated calcium channels found in most other cells. Activation of T cells requires concomitant increases in $[Ca^{2+}]_i$ and the activation of protein kinase C. Moreover, several hours of a sustained increase in $[Ca^{2+}]_i$ and PKC activation is required to maximize the T cell proliferative response.[201] The importance of this pathway is underscored by the observation that it can be mimicked pharmacologically by the addition of a calcium ionophore to raise $[Ca^{2+}]_i$ and a phorbol ester to activate protein kinase C, a combination which activates the vast majority of T cells. This is the minimal stimulus required to activate T cells to produce cytokines and to proliferate.[201, 202]

The tyrosine kinase activity stimulated by antigen recognition triggers a series of events that increase the percentage of Ras, a low-molecular weight G protein, that is bound to GTP.[203] GTP-bound Ras then binds to the serine threonine kinase Raf-1, bringing it to the membrane where it becomes activated.[204] Both Ras and Raf-1 are required for optimal T cell IL-2 production.[205, 206] Downstream of Raf-1, a number of mitogen-activated protein (MAP) kinase or extracellular signal-regulated kinase (ERK) kinases (MEKs) are activated; these, in turn, activate a variety of MAP kinases. MAP kinases are thought to control the transcriptional activity of a nuclear binding factor p62[tfc], which promotes c-*fos* transcription.[207] Studies have described a *jun* kinase (JNK) that is homologous to ERKs. Phosphorylation of c-*jun* by JNK increases its transcriptional activity. The activity of this kinase is controlled at least in part by a recently described JNK

kinase that functions downstream of a MEK kinase (MEKK). Optimal activation of this pathway appears to depend on signals derived from an increase in intracellular free calcium and the activation of protein kinase C, which suggests that two or more signaling pathways may converge on JNK to regulate its activity.[208] It activity controls the transcriptional activity of c-*jun*. Both c-*jun* and c-*fos* play critical roles in T cell IL-2 production.[209]

In the physiologic T cell–APC interaction, multiple different surface molecules are engaged in addition to the TCR/CD3. Ligation of these additional T cell surface molecules is required for T cell activation, cytokine gene expression, and progression to mitosis after T cell recognition of antigen (see Table 7–3). Such binding of multiple surface molecules may increase the avidity of the cellular interaction. However, it is probably more important that ligation of different surface molecules stimulates transmembrane signaling events required to move the G_0 resting T cell into the cell cycle.

The importance of these interactions has been inferred in several ways. First, monoclonal antibodies that recognize the specific surface antigen can either stimulate or inhibit the T cell response, usually when another surface molecule, such as CD3 or CD2, is simultaneously engaged. In some cases, monoclonal antibodies to a specific determinant can partially block the accessory cell–dependent stimulation, which demonstrates the importance of that interaction in T cell activation. More importantly, known ligands exist for many of these receptors on T cells. In addition, ligation of certain surface antigens can be directly shown to provide signaling information to the T cell, such as inducing an increase in $[Ca^{2+}]_i$ (see Table 7–3). Finally, deletion of these gene products by homologous recombination or antisense approaches has directly documented their roles as T cell costimulatory molecules.[210]

The CD2 surface antigen was the first antigen-independent activation pathway to be described.[6, 211] The major ligand for CD2 is LFA-3 (CD58), which is expressed on a variety of cell types. Ligation of CD2 can stimulate a rise in $[Ca^{2+}]_i$ and phosphatidylinositol turnover and can costimulate phosphorylation of CD3-γ or tyrosine phosphorylation of CD3 ζ.[31, 211] Although CD2-stimulated cell activation does not require additional signals delivered via CD3, surface CD3 expression does seem to be required for this pathway to be active, which suggests cross-talk between CD3 and CD2.[31]

The CD28 molecule mediates a distinct signaling pathway. CD28 is a 90-kD glycoprotein homodimer expressed on 80 percent of human T cells. Ligation of CD28 costimulates T cell activation; however, unlike many other T cell surface molecules that transduce signals, CD3 surface expression is not required and the resultant induction of IL-2 secretion is resistant to cyclosporine.[29, 212] Some studies have demonstrated that ligation of CD28 results in tyrosine phosphorylation of several substrates[213] and that the cytoplasmic domain of CD28 binds to PI-3 kinase.[214] Moreover, mutants of CD28, which do not bind PI-3 kinase, do not costimulate T cell activation.[214] The mechanism by which PI-3 kinase regulates T cell activation is not yet known. However, CD28 stimulation results in stabilization of several lymphokine mRNAs, including IL-2 mRNA, and can augment IL-2 gene transcription.[214] Two known ligands for CD28 are CD86 and CD80 molecules expressed by a variety of APCs, including dendritic cells, activated B cells, and monocytes.[30, 31]

Not all of the ligands for these T cell surface antigens (see Table 7–2) are yet known, and it is not yet clear which of these interactions are critical to T cell activation. It is interesting that the absence of expression of certain of these T cell molecules, including CD7 and CD43, is associated with immunodeficiency states. Moreover, inhibition of the CD28 interaction with its ligands blocks immune responses in vivo and may induce tolerance to specific antigen.

Gene Activation and DNA Synthesis

Although the subsequent sequence of events after generation of second messengers that lead to gene activation are not completely known, a large number of genes that are activated in an orderly sequence have been identified. Immediate genes are expressed within minutes and do not require protein synthesis, whereas early and late genes require protein synthesis.[215] Immediate and early genes are expressed before cell division, late genes after mitosis.

IL-2 is produced specifically by T cells and is critical in maintaining the progression of events that lead to mitosis.[70, 71] The location of the IL-2 gene transcriptional enhancer has been determined and contains four regions critical to regulation by the TCR.[215] The gene most proximal region is designated NFIL-2A and binds a complex that consists of the constitutively expressed nuclear binding factor, Oct-1, and the induced nuclear binding factor, c-jun.[216–218] Adjacent to NFIL-2A is NFIL-2B, which binds to AP-1 complexes and unknown factors regulated by CD28 binding.[216–218] AP-1 is the product of the c-jun proto-oncogene, and its binding affinity to DNA is enhanced when it forms a complex with protein products of the c-fos proto-oncogene, resulting in a "leucine zipper" structure.[216, 218] NFIL-2D contains an Oct-1 binding site that differs from that found in NFIL-2A and may bind Oct-1 without c-jun. Finally, NFIL-2E binds a complex consisting of the nuclear factor of activated T cells (NFAT-1), c-jun, and c-fos.[217, 218] NFAT-1 is synthesized approximately 20 minutes after T cell activation and precedes appearance of IL-2 mRNA.[215, 218] Like JNK, NFAT-1 is modified by agents that increase intracellular free calcium or protein kinase C independently, which indicates that distinct signaling pathways may also converge on NFAT-1 to regulate its function.[209, 215, 218] NFIL-2C contains an NFκB binding site that is not significantly induced upon antigen recognition.[209] The receptor for IL-2 (IL-2R) is not detected on resting T cells but is rapidly expressed after stimulation by mitogen or antigen.[71] The IL-2R is composed of a 55 kD (α), a 70-kD (β) and a 64-kD (γ) proteins.[71, 218] The α- and β-chains bind IL-2 with low (α) or intermediate (β) affinity, but the physical interaction of α and β forms the tertiary structure, which binds IL-2 with high affinity. The γ- and β-chains are both required for signal transduction.[218]

Investigation of second messenger signals, which result from IL-2 binding to the IL-2R, has shown that binding of IL-2 to its receptor does not increase $[Ca^{2+}]_i$ or phosphatidylinositol turnover.[219] Although translocation of protein kinase C has been reported, it is not necessary for the effects of IL-2.[220] IL-2 binding is known to trigger tyrosine phosphorylation, and the receptor is known to bind the src family kinase p56[lck].[218, 221] Tyrosine kinase inhibitors or mutations in the receptor that block the capacity of the receptor to interact with tyrosine kinases block its ability to promote cell growth.[221] Like antigen recognition, IL-2 binding stimulates the association of Ras with GTP and activates the MAP kinase pathway leading to c-fos transcription and an increase in the transcriptional activity of AP-1.[209, 218] IL-2 binding also stimulates c-myc transcription.[209, 218] IL-2 mRNA and IL-2 secretion are detected much sooner than IL-2R. IL-2 itself stimulates an up-regulation of IL-2R transcription and cell surface expression. A binding site for the phorbol ester–sensitive factor NFκB has been defined in the IL-2R gene transcription initiation region.[215] Mutations in one of the IL-2R chains are responsible for X-linked severe combined immunodeficiency (X-SCID) in humans.[222]

B Lymphocytes

Many of the initial signaling events that have been defined in B cells are triggered in response to ligation of surface Ig. Mature B cells express surface IgM or IgD. Membrane Ig has a very short 3–amino acid cytoplasmic tail and no known enzymatic activity or binding domains for kinases or G proteins. Therefore, the Ig heavy chain is unlikely to mediate signal transduction directly, although the cytoplasmic tail is important in some functions, as deletion eliminates calcium signaling and antigen presentation in response to ligation of surface Ig.[223] Surface IgM and IgD are nonconvalently associated with additional proteins. In most of cases, surface Ig associates with a heterodimer consisting of Ig-α (CD79a), a 43-kD protein coded for by the mb-1 gene, and Ig-β (CD79b), a 39-kD peptide coded for by the B29 gene.[224] In low-density B cells and bone marrow cells, surface Ig associates with a heterodimer of Ig-α and Ig-γ, which is a truncated form of Ig-β.[224] The transmembrane sequences of surface Ig are important for its association with the Ig-α/Ig-β heterodimer. The cytoplasmic tails of both Ig-β and IgM-α contain ARH1 regions.[224] The Ig-α chain also contains sequences with the ARH1 that bind src-family kinases.[225] This interaction occurs in the absence of tyrosine phosphorylation and occurs constitutively in resting cells.[225]

As in T cells, tyrosine phosphorylation may be critical to integrating different pathways of signal transduction. The tyrosine kinase *syk*, which is homologous to ZAP-70, is physically associated with the transmembrane or cytoplasmic domain of IgM, whereas *src*-family kinases, such as *blk, fyn, lck,* and *lyn,* are associated with Ig-α.[224] Ligation of surface Ig stimulates an increase in tyrosine phosphate and stimulates the phosphorylation of tyrosine residues with the ARH1 regions of Ig-α and Ig-β.[224–226] Additional *src*-family kinases and *syk* are recruited to the receptor complex via interactions between phosphotyrosine in the ARH1 region of Ig-α and Ig-β and the SH2 domains of the tyrosine kinase.[224] One of the proteins that is tyrosine-phosphorylated is the γ1 form of B cell phospholipase C. The activation of phospholipase C results in the production of IP_3 and DAG, with the resultant increase in $[Ca^{2+}]_i$ and the translocation of protein kinase.[226] These events depend on CD45 expression. Consistent with the importance of this pathway in B cell activation, treatment of B cells with phorbol ester and a calcium ionophore will trigger B cell proliferation.

Signal transduction in physiologic B cell activation stimulated by interaction with T cells may involve many B cell surface molecules other than surface Ig. B cells express a number of surface molecules that have signaling capacity (see Table 7–1).[4, 62] Of the B cell–specific molecules, CD19, CD20, CD21, and CD23 either increase $[Ca^{2+}]_i$ when cross-linked or augment anti-IgM calcium signaling. CD40 appears to play a major role in inducing responses of B cells during T cell–B cell collaboration. CD40 is a 50-kD glycoprotein that is expressed predominantly by B cells during most stages of B cell differentiation. It is a member of a family of signaling molecules that includes the TNF receptor, CD27, and CD30. Engagement of CD40 by its ligand expressed by activated T cells induces activation, promotes proliferation and Ig class switching, and presents apoptosis by germinal center B cells.[9, 227, 228] The central role of CD40–CD40 ligand interactions in T cell–B cell collaboration is emphasized by the clinical features of the X-linked hyper-IgM immunodeficiency syndrome, which is characterized by mutations in the external domain of the CD40 ligand such that binding CD40 is eliminated.[229] As a result, children with this syndrome do not produce antibody encoded by downstream heavy chain isotype genes and do not form germinal centers in lymph nodes.[229] The signaling pathways activated by ligation of CD40 have not been completely delineated, although there is rapid activation of protein tyrosine kinases, including *lyn,* and activation of a variety of serine-threonine kinases.[230–232] At a nuclear level, ligation of CD40 induces activation of both B cell NFAT and NFκB.

The role of the class II MHC molecule on B cells may also be important, because it can interact with CD4 on the T cell helper population. Ligation of class II MHC molecules on B cells leads to an increase in B cell $[Ca^{2+}]_i$, phosphatidylinositol turnover, protein phosphorylation, and B cell proliferation.[233–234] Other B cell ligands are known to bind T cell surface molecules, including CD72, which is the ligand for CD5,[7, 10] and LFA-1 on B cells, which interacts with ICAM-1 (CD54) on CD4$^+$ T cells.[235] It is likely that these B cell surface molecules transduce intracellular signals to B cells, as anti-CD72 monoclonal antibodies induce proliferation in B cells[236] and ligating LFA-1 can increase $[Ca^{2+}]_i$ in T cells.[237] Thus, the T cell–B cell cognate interaction may result in summation of multiple signals generated by mutual interaction of cell surface ligands to lead to the initial activation of the resting B cell (Fig. 7–5).

CELL-CELL INTERACTIONS

Lymphocyte Trafficking

Newly generated lymphocytes leave their site of production, which under usual circumstances is the bone marrow or thymus, and migrate via the blood stream through essentially all tissues and organs. Continuous recirculation through tissues provides a perpetual surveillance function, which is of critical importance for the generation of immune responses.[238] The resultant distribution of lymphocytes is not random, inasmuch as lymphocytes possess specific homing mechanisms that facilitate their trafficking into distinct tissues. Lymphocytes recirculate through tissues by two main routes:

1. Entry into lymphoid tissue via specialized postcapillary venules, called *high endothelial venules* (HEVs). HEVs are morphologically distinguishable on the basis of the cuboidal shape of the cells.

2. Crossing of postcapillary venules that are lined by flat endothelium and thus lack specialized HEV.[239]

Entry via HEVs is important for the high-volume movement of lymphocytes through lymphoid tissue.

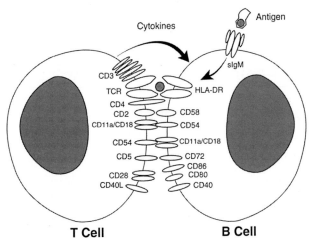

Figure 7–5. Schematic representation of T cell–B cell collaboration.

The less frequent movement into other tissues, such as gut or skin, occurs by lymphocyte recognition of counterreceptors on flat endothelium.

Endothelium with morphology similar to that of HEVs is observed in inflamed synovium and other inflammatory sites.[240, 241] It is not clear whether the appearance of HEV-like endothelial cells in inflamed tissue is caused by the differentiation of flat endothelial cells already present in the tissue or results from the emergence of endothelial cells of a new phenotype as part of the neovascularization occurring in the inflamed tissue. Endothelial cells possess the ability to alter their morphologic and biologic phenotypes in response to environmental stimuli. The microenvironment of the endothelium appears to be an important determinant of its functional capacity. Activated T cells play a role in the development and maintenance of HEV and lymphocyte recirculation into tissue, as evidenced by the findings that morphologic changes in endothelium can be induced in response to the cytokines TNF-α and IFN-γ and that flattening of HEVs occurs following T cell depletion.[242] HEV morphology is not necessary for lymphocyte extravasation, however, inasmuch as transendothelial migration occurs through flat endothelium as well, although the transit time is considerably longer.[238] Thus, HEVs may offer a biologic advantage over flat endothelial cells by presentation of the optimum architecture for the organization of cell surface adhesion receptors necessary for the efficient transendothelial migration of lymphocytes, but do not appear to be absolutely necessary for lymphocyte entry into tissue.

Table 7–8 lists currently known receptors and counterreceptors that mediate the specific interactions of lymphocytes with endothelial cells of different lymphoid tissues. Lymphocytes also can home to organs such as spleen, bone marrow, lung, and liver in which HEVs are not prominent, but little is known about specific receptor-ligand interactions in these tissues.[243]

T lymphocytes have different migration patterns, depending on whether they have encountered antigen. "Naive" (CD45RA⁺) T cells, which have not encountered antigen since their development in the thymus, express the adhesion receptor CD62L (L-selectin, Leu-8, leukocyte-endothelial cell adhesion molecule-1 [LECAM-1], leukocyte adhesion molecule-1 [LAM-1]), which is essential for lymphocyte binding to peripheral lymph node HEV. CD62L is a member of the selectin family of adhesion molecules. It is constitutively expressed by lymphocytes and can bind specific glycoproteins expressed by endothelial cells.[238] Thus, naive T cells, which are the predominant population in peripheral lymph nodes, enter lymph nodes as a result of receptor-mediated interactions between CD62L on lymphocytes with its counterreceptor, peripheral node addressin (PNAd). PNAd consists of at least two separate heavily glycosylated proteins, a smaller-molecular-weight glycosylated cell adhesion molecule (GlyCAM-1) and a larger CD34.[244] The unique glycosylation of CD34 on lymph node HEV allows it to be recognized as a specific homing receptor.

B cells also utilize CD62L to bind the endothelium of peripheral lymph node. Lymphocytes utilize a different set of adhesion receptors, including CD44 and the integrin α4β7, during their extravasation into Peyer's patch. The precise counterreceptor on the HEV of Peyer's patch that binds CD44 has not been completely delineated. CD44 is an adhesion molecule that shares homology with proteoglycan link protein, and which binds hyaluronic acid as well as other extracellular matrix molecules.[245] Trafficking of lymphocytes into Peyer's patch also involves the lymphocyte adhesion receptor, α4β7, which binds to mucosal addressin cell adhesion molecule-1 (MAdCAM-1), an adhesion molecule of the Ig family expressed by endothelial cells of Peyer's patch and other mucosal tissues.[246] α4β7 is a heterodimer of noncovalently associated α and β chains and is a member of the integrin family of adhesion receptors.

A number of other adhesion receptors also facilitate lymphocyte entry into lymphoid tissue. These include the β2 integrin, CD11a/CD18 (LFA-1), which binds to CD54 (ICAM-1), which is expressed by endothelium.[247]

Whereas naive T cells seem to migrate through HEV into lymphoid tissue, "memory" T cells (CD45RO⁺) enter lymph nodes from the afferent lymphatics.[248] By contrast, CD45RO⁺ "memory" T cells

Table 7–8. ADHESION RECEPTORS MEDIATING LYMPHOCYTE HOMING INTO LYMPHOID TISSUE

Lymphocyte Receptor	Common Name	Adhesion Receptor Family	Endothelial Counterreceptor	Tissue Expressing Counterreceptor
CD62L	L-selectin, LAM-1, leu-8, LECAM-1	Selectin	PNAd (GlyCAM-1, CD34); charged oligosaccharides	Lymphoid (peripheral, mesenteric)
CD44	Homing-CAM	H-CAM	Mucosal vascular addressin	Lymphoid (Peyer's patch, mesenteric)
CD49d/β7	α4β7	Integrin	MAdCAM-1	Mucosal
CD11a/CD18	LFA-1	Integrin	CD54 (ICAM-1), CD102 (ICAM-2)	Widespread

Abbreviations: LAM, leukocyte adhesion molecule; LECAM, leukocyte-endothelial cellular adhesion molecule; ICAM, intercellular adhesion module; GlyCAM, glycosylated cell adhesion molecule; PNAd, peripheral node addressin; MAdCAM, mucosal addressin cell adhesion molecule; CD, cluster of differentiation; H-CAM, homing cell adhesion molecule.

Table 7–9. ADHESION RECEPTORS MEDIATING ENTRY OF T CELLS INTO INFLAMMATORY SITES

Lymphocyte Receptor	Common Name	Endothelial Cell Counterreceptor	Regulation of Endothelial Cell Counterreceptor
CD11a/CD18	LFA-1	CD54 (ICAM-1), CD102 (ICAM-2)	CD54 (constitutive, increased with cytokines, endotoxin); CD102 (constitutive)
CD49d/CD29	VLA-4, α4β1	CD106 (VCAM-1)	Induced by cytokines
CLA		CD62E (E-selectin)	Induced by cytokines
CD49d/β7	α4β7	MAdCAM-1	Induced by cytokines

Abbreviations: LFA, leukocyte function-associated antigen; VLA, very late (activation) antigen; VCAM, vascular cell adhesion molecule; ICAM, intercellular adhesion molecule; MAdCAM, mucosal addressin cell adhesion molecule; CD, cluster of differentiation; CLA, cutaneous lymphocyte-associated antigen.

are recruited from the blood into nonlymphoid tissues by migration through flat endothelium. This process is greatly amplified by local inflammation. Memory T cells leave tissue sites via the lymphatics, from which they can reenter the circulation or can enter lymph nodes. Memory T cells are believed to have encountered antigen since their development in the thymus, and are the primary T cell population in inflammatory sites.

A number of specific adhesive interactions mediate the extravasation of T cells into sites of inflammation (Table 7–9). The cutaneous lymphocyte-associated (CLA) antigen is expressed by 80 to 90 percent of the memory T cells in chronically inflamed skin lesions, and it mediates the binding of these memory T cells to the endothelium of inflamed skin by binding CD62E (E-selectin, endothelial-leukocyte adhesion molecule-1 [ELAM-1], another member of the selectin family of adhesion molecules.[238] Other adhesion receptor pairs, including CD49d/CD29 (α4β1; VLA-4)-CD106 (VCAM-1), and CD11a/CD18-CD54 are also important during the binding and transendothelial migration, respectively, of T cells into sites of inflammation.[249]

Vascular adhesion protein-1 (VAP-1) is a recently described endothelial cell adhesion receptor that binds lymphocytes. It is expressed by endothelial cells in different tissues, including rheumatoid synovium.[250] Whether it is important during the trafficking of lymphocytes into rheumatoid synovium has not yet been determined. Thus, mechanisms involving specific adhesion receptors (e.g., CD62L-PNAd, α4β7-MAdCAM-1, CLA-CD62E) are involved in the arrest of specific lymphocyte populations on the endothelium of distinct tissues, whereas other receptors (e.g., CD11a/CD18-CD54) play a more global role in facilitating the transendothelial migration of various bound T cells out of the blood stream and into the tissue. It is likely that there are as yet unidentified adhesion receptors that also play important roles in the extravasation of T cells into sites of inflammation.

The expression of endothelial cell adhesion receptors is modulated by inflammatory cytokines. Thus, CD54 is increased on endothelium at sites of inflammation and when endothelial cells are activated by cytokines in culture.[251] CD54, together with its T cell ligand CD11a/CD18, plays a prominent role in the migration of bound T cells through the intercellular

junctions of endothelial cells by a process that appears to involve progressive interactions between CD54 and CD11a/CD18.[252] CD54 is also the counterreceptor for CD11b/CD18 (Mac-1, CR3), which appears to play a more important role in the migration of neutrophils rather than lymphocytes. The endothelial cell adhesion receptors CD62E and CD106 are found at sites of inflammation and are both induced by cytokines such as IL-1 and TNF-α.[251]

Soluble mediators emerging from the tissue are also involved in controlling the adhesiveness of lymphocytes and their transendothelial migration. Thus, aside from cytokines influencing adhesion receptor expression by endothelial cells, cytokines known as *chemokines* may play an important role in recruiting lymphocyte populations out of the blood as well as directing their movements within the tissue. Chemokines are structurally and functionally related proteins that have affinity for heparan sulfate proteoglycan, and they share a common ability to stimulate the chemotactic migration of distinct sets of cells.[252] The chemokines RANTES, MIP-1α, MIP-1β, MCP-1, and IL-8 are produced by a number of cell types (including endothelial cells, activated T cells, and monocytes), are present at inflammatory sites (including rheumatoid synovium), and may stimulate the directed migration of distinct subsets of lymphocytes.[253] Thus, a complicated interplay of regulatory factors derived from the endothelium and the inflamed tissue governs the entry of lymphocytes into tissue.

T Cell–B Cell Collaboration

For many antigens, the induction of antibody production requires collaboration between antigen-specific T cells and B cells. Recent experimental results have provided an explanation for the observation that this interaction is restricted by class II molecules of the MHC, although the T cell and B cell respond to different aspects of the stimulating antigen. A variety of cells that express class II MHC molecules can function as APCs, but during T cell–B cell collaboration, it appears that the B cell acts as the APC (see Fig. 7–5). Expression of membrane Ig allows B cells to recognize specific antigen effectively. B cell Ig receptors recognize native intact antigen without the need for initial enzymatic degradation. After binding, antigen is internalized and degraded within an acid compartment. Particular antigenic peptides bind to class II MHC molecules within this compartment, and the complexes are subsequently expressed on the surface of the B cell, where they can be recognized by CD4⁺ helper T cells. Engaging surface Ig with antigen may also activate the B cell to become a more effective APC.

After the antigen bound into the peptide-binding cleft of the class II MHC molecules is displayed on the surface of the B cell, it can be recognized by helper T cells. The requirement for helper T cells to recognize peptides bound to self class II MHC molecules accounts for the genetic restriction of T cell–B cell collaboration. A number of receptors on B cells and counterreceptors on T cells appear to be capable of facilitating the activation of T cells during this interaction. These include LFA-1, ICAM-1, LFA-3, MHC II, CD80/CD86, and CD72 on the B cell interacting with ICAM-1, LFA-1, CD2, CD4, CD28, and CD5 on the T cell.[6, 30, 31] As a result of these various costimulatory interactions, antigen-specific T cells are activated in an antigen-specific manner restricted by class II MHC molecules.

The activated T cell develops the capacity to stimulate the antigen-presenting B cell.[8, 62] This involves both a contact-dependent event and the action of a variety of cytokines. One of the major B cell stimulatory molecules expressed by activated T cells is the 33-kD ligand for CD40 (CD40L). Genetic abnormalities in the CD40L results in the X-linked hyper-IgM immunodeficiency syndrome, characterized by elevated levels of IgM, but absent IgG, IgA, or IgE and the absence of lymph node germinal centers.[226–230] Once the T cells have been stimulated, their capacity to activate the antigen-presenting B cells is restricted not by class II MHC molecules but, rather, by the CD40–CD40L interactions and various other receptor/counterreceptor interactions described.

Stimulation of B cells is a complex process in which resting B cells are activated to enter the cell cycle, undergo several rounds of proliferation, and finally undergo differentiation into high-rate Ig-secreting cells.[62] This sequence of events is tightly modulated by activating signals provided by the interaction with stimulated T cells and a series of cytokines. The cytokines regulating B cell responsiveness originate from a variety of cell types, including cells that are not members of the immune system, such as fibroblasts and endothelial cells. However, T cells or their products are necessary for the production of antibody to many antigens and polyclonal B cell activators, emphasizing the central role for T cell–derived cytokines in regulating B cell responses. A number of these cytokines play distinct roles in the regulation of B cell responses.

Because resting B cells express few receptors for cytokines, activation signals that promote the expression of cytokine receptors are necessary for the development of B cell cytokine responsiveness. Clonal expansion of the responding B lymphocyte is an inte-

gral component of the immune response. Beyond this, it has been demonstrated that proliferation is an essential event in the subsequent differentiation of Ig-secreting cells. After initial activation, proliferation, and differentiation, individual B cells may cease secreting Ig of one antibody isotype and commence producing antibody encoded for by the same VDJ gene segments but a different, more 3′, heavy chain constant region gene segment. The usual mechanism for this isotype switch appears to be deletional recombination induced or selected for by T cell–derived cytokines.[254]

A number of cytokines influence human B cell responses, of which IL-2 appears to play a central role. After resting B cells are activated, they express high-avidity receptors for IL-2. As a result, IL-2 can sustain ongoing proliferation of activated human B cells.[255, 256] In humans, IL-2 also appears to play a central role in stimulating proliferating B cells to secrete Ig.[256] The effect of IL-2 on human B cell differentiation is not Ig heavy chain isotype-specific.[256] Several cytokines that cannot induce differentiation of Ig-secreting cells alone can augment the Ig production induced by IL-2. These include the interferons, IL-1, IL-6, TNF-α, and TNF-β.

IL-4 plays a central role in regulating murine B cell function, with effects on activation, proliferation, and differentiation.[257] IL-4 alone stimulates small resting murine B cells to increase their volume and expression of class II MHC molecules and CD23. In addition, IL-4 cofacilitates entry into the S phase by activated B cells.

Finally, IL-4 exerts a major influence on murine B cell differentiation, promoting the production of IgG1 and IgE by appropriately costimulated B cells.[71, 72] In humans, IL-4 can promote growth and Ig production by B cells stimulated by ligation of CD40. Although most Ig heavy chain isotypes are produced, the response is biased toward production of IgG4 and IgE.[62]

References

1. Roitt IM, Torrigiani G, Greaves MF, Brostoff J, Playfair JH: The cellular basis of immunological responses. Lancet 2:367, 1969.
2. Loken M, Shah V, Dattilio K, Civin C: Flow cytometric analysis of human bone marrow: II. Normal B cell development. Blood 70:1316, 1987.
3. Uckun FM: Regulation of human B-cell ontogeny. Blood 76:1908, 1990.
4. Clark EA, Ledbetter JA: Structure, function and genetics of human B cell associated surface molecules. Adv Cancer Res 52:81, 1989.
5. Abney ER, Cooper MD, Kearney JF, Lawton AR, Parkhouse RME: Sequential expression of immunoglobulin on developing B lymphocytes: A systematic survey that suggests a model for the generation of immunoglobulin isotype diversity. J Immunol 120:2041, 1978.
6. Schlossman SF, Boumsell L, Gilks W, Harlan JM, Kishimoto T, Morimoto C, Ritz J, Shaw S, Silverstein RL, Springer TA, Tedder TF, Todd RF (eds): Leucocyte typing V: White cell differentiation antigens. Proceedings of the Fifth International Workshop and Conference, Boston, November 3–7, 1993. New York, Oxford University Press, 1995.
7. Nakayama E, Von Hoegen I, Parnes JR: Sequence of the Lyb-2 B cell differentiation antigen defines a gene superfamily of receptors with inverted membrane orientation. Proc Natl Acad Sci USA 86:1352, 1989.
8. Noelle RJ, Ledbetter JA, Aruffo A: CD40 and its ligand, an essential ligand receptor pair for thymus dependent B-cell activation. Immunol Today 13:431, 1992.
9. Spriggs MK, Fanslow WC, Armitage RJ, Belmont J: The biology of the human ligand for CD40. J Clin Immunol 13:373, 1993.

10. Kipps TJ: The CD5 B cell. Adv Immunol 47:117, 1989.
11. Hardy RR, Hayakawa K, Shimizu M, Yamasaki K, Kishimoto T: Rheumatoid factor secretion from human Leu-1⁺ B cells. Science 236:81, 1987.
12. Suzuki N, Sakane T, Engelman EG: Anti-DNA antibody production by CD5⁺ and CD5⁻ B cells of patients with systemic lupus erythematosus. J Clin Invest 85:238, 1990.
13. Vernino LA, Pisetsky DS, Lipsky PE: Analysis of the expression of CD5 by human B cells and correlation with functional activity. Cell Immunol 139:185, 1992.
14. Allison JP, Lanier LL: Structure, function and serology of the T-cell antigen receptor complex. Annu Rev Immunol 5:503, 1987.
15. Ashwell JD, Klausner RD: Genetic and mutational analysis of the T-cell antigen receptor. Annu Rev Immunol 8:139, 1990.
16. Parnes JR: Molecular analysis and function of CD4 and CD8. Adv Immunol 44:265, 1989.
17. LeFranc MP, Forster A, Rabbitts TH: Genetic polymorphism and exon changes of the constant regions of the human T-cell rearranging gene gamma. Proc Natl Acad Sci USA 83:9596, 1986.
18. Baniyash M, Garcia-Morales P, Bonifacino JS, Samelson LE, Klausner RD: Disulfide linkage of the ζ and η chains of the T cell receptor: Possible identification of two structural classes of receptors. J Biol Chem 263:9874, 1988.
19. Alarcon B, Ley SC, Sanchez-Madrid F, Blumberg RS, Lee ST, Fresno M, Terhorst C: The CD3-γ and CD3-δ subunit of the T cell antigen receptor can be expressed within distinct functional TCR/CD3 complexes. EMBO J 10:903, 1991.
20. Manolios N, Bonifacino JS, Klausner RD: Transmembrane helical interactions and the assembly of the T cell antigen receptor complex. Science 249:274, 1990.
21. Littman DR: The structure of the CD4 and CD8 genes. Annu Rev Immunol 5:561, 1987.
22. Szabo G, Miller CL, Kodys K: Antigen presentation by the CD4 positive monocyte subset. J Leukocyte Biol 47:111, 1990.
23. Swain SL: T cell subsets and the recognition of MHC class. Immunol Rev 74:129, 1983.
24. Dalgleish AG, Beverly PCL, Clapham PR, Crawford DH, Greaves MF, Weiss RA: The CD4 (T4) antigen is an essential component of the receptor for the AIDS retrovirus. Nature 312:763, 1984.
25. Maddon PJ, Dalgleish AG, McDougal JS, Clapham PR, Weiss RA, Axel R: The T4 gene encodes the AIDS virus receptor and is expressed in the immune system and the brain. Cell 47:333, 1986.
26. Turner JM, Brodsky MH, Irving BA, Levin SD, Perlmutter RM, Littman DR: Interaction of the unique N-terminal region of tyrosine kinase p56ˡᶜᵏ with cytoplasmic domains of CD4 and CD8 is mediated by cysteine motifs. Cell 60:755, 1990.
27. Norment AM, Salter RD, Parham P, Engelhard VH, Littman DR: Cell-cell adhesion mediated by CD8 and MHC class I molecules. Nature 336:79, 1988.
28. Aruffo A, Seed B: Molecular cloning of a CD28 cDNA by a high efficiency COS cell expression system. Proc Natl Acad Sci USA 84:8573, 1987.
29. Linsley PS, Clark EA, Ledbetter JA: T-cell antigen CD28 mediates adhesion with B cells by interacting with activation antigen B7/BB1. Proc Natl Acad Sci USA 87:5031, 1990.
30. Caux C, Vanbervliet B, Massacrier C, Azuma M, Okumura K, Lanier LL, Banchereau J: B70/B7-2 is identical to CD86 and is the major functional ligand for CD28 expressed on human dendritic cells. J Exp Med 180:1841, 1994.
31. Geppert TD, Davis LS, Gur H, Wacholtz MC, Lipsky PE: Accessory cell signals involved in T cell activation. Immunol Rev 117:5, 1990.
32. Tan P, Anasetti C, Hansen JA, Melrose J, Brunvand M, Bradshaw J, Ledbetter JA, Linsley PS: Induction of alloantigen-specific hyporesponsiveness in human T lymphocytes by blocking interaction of CD28 with its natural ligand B7/BB1. J Exp Med 177:165, 1993.
33. Morrison LA, Lukacher AE, Braciale VL, Fan DP, Braciale TJ: Differences in antigen presentation to MHC class I and class II restricted influenza virus-specific cytolytic T lymphocyte clones. J Exp Med 163:903, 1986.
34. Young ACM, Nathenson SG, Sacchettini JC: Structural studies of class I major histocompatibility complex proteins: Insights into antigen presentation. FASEB J 9:26, 1995.
35. Engelhard VH: Structure of peptides associated with class I and class II MHC molecules. Ann Rev Immunol 12:181, 1994.
36. Waldor MK, Sriram S, Hardy R, Herzenberg LA, Herzenberg LA, Lanier L, Lim M, Steinman L: Reversal of experimental allergic encephalomyelitis with monoclonal antibody to a T-cell subset marker. Science 227:415, 1985.
37. Shizuru JA, Taylor-Edwards C, Banks BA, Gregory AK, Fathman G: Immunotherapy of the nonobese diabetic mouse: Treatment with an antibody to T-helper lymphocytes. Science 240:659, 1988.
38. Wofsy D, Seaman WE: Successful treatment of autoimmunity in NZB/NZW F₁ mice with monoclonal antibody to L3T4. J Exp Med 161:378, 1985.
39. Ranges GE, Sriram S, Cooper SM: Prevention of type II collagen-induced arthritis by in vivo treatment with anti-L3T4. J Exp Med 162:1105, 1985.
40. Kong YM, Waldmann H, Cobbold SP, Giraldo AA, Fuller BE: Altered pathogenic mechanisms in murine autoimmune thyroiditis after depletion in vivo of L3T4⁺ and Lyt2⁺ cells. Immunobiology (Suppl) 3:30, 1987.
41. Street NE, Mosmann TR: Functional diversity of T lymphocytes due to secretion of different cytokine patterns. FASEB J 5:171, 1991.
42. Romagnani S: Lymphokine production by human T cells in disease states. Annu Rev Immunol 12:227, 1994.
43. Akbar AN, Salmon M, Janossy G: The synergy between naive and memory T cells during activation. Immunol Today 12:184, 1991.
44. Seder RA, Paul WE: Acquisition of lymphokine-producing phenotype by CD4⁺ T cells. Annu Rev Immunol 12:635, 1994.
45. Sanders ME, Makgoba MW, Shaw S: Human naive and memory T cells: Reinterpretation of helper-inducer and suppressor-inducer subsets. Immunol Today 9:195, 1988.
46. Cerotini JC, MacDonald HR: The cellular basis of T-cell memory. Annu Rev Immunol 7:77, 1989.
47. Hintzen RQ, de Jong R, Lens SMA, Brouwer M, Baars P, van Lier RAW: Regulation of CD27 expression on subsets of mature T-lymphocytes. J Immunol 151:2426, 1993.
48. Thomas R, McIlraith M, Davis LS, Lipsky PE: Rheumatoid synovium is enriched in CD45RBᵈⁱᵐ mature memory T cells that are potent helpers for B cell differentiation. Arthritis Rheum 35:1455, 1992.
49. Oldstone MBA, Nerenberg M, Southern P, Price J, Lewicki H: Virus infection triggers insulin-dependent diabetes mellitus in a transgenic model: Role of anti-self (virus) immune response. Cell 65:319, 1991.
50. Nabholz M, MacDonald HR: Cytolytic T lymphocytes. Annu Rev Immunol 1:273, 1983.
51. Janeway CA, Jones B, Hayday A: Specificity and function of T cells bearing γδ receptors. Immunol Today 9:73, 1988.
52. Patel SS, Wacholtz MC, Duby AD, Thiele DL, Lipsky PE: Analysis of the functional capabilities of CD3⁺CD4⁻CD8⁻ and CD3⁺CD4⁺CD8⁺ human T cell clones. J Immunol 143:1108, 1989.
53. Haregewoin A, Singh B, Gupta RS, Finberg RW: A mycobacterial heat-shock protein-responsive gamma delta T cell clone also responds to the homologous human heat-shock protein: A possible link between infection and autoimmunity. J Infect Dis 163:156, 1991.
54. Soderstrom K, Halapi E, Nilsson E, Gronberg A, van Emdben J, Klareskog L, Kiessling R: Synovial cells responding to a 65-kDa mycobacterial heat shock protein have a high proportion of a TcR gamma delta subtype uncommon in peripheral blood. Scand J Immunol 32:503, 1990.
55. Fortune F, Walker J, Lehner T: The expression of gamma delta T cell receptor and the prevalence of primed, activated and IgA-bound T cells in Behçet's syndrome. Clin Exp Immunol 82:326, 1990.
56. Hohlfeld R, Engel AG, Ii K, Harper MC: Polymyositis mediated by T lymphocytes that express the gamma/delta receptor. N Engl J Med 324:877, 1991.
57. Rajagopalan S, Zordan T, Tsokos GC, Datta SK: Pathogenic anti-DNA autoantibody-inducing T helper cell lines from patients with active lupus nephritis: Isolation of CD4-8⁻ T helper cell lines that express the gamma delta T-cell antigen receptor. Proc Natl Acad Sci USA 87:7020, 1990.
58. Lipsky PE, Davis LS, Cush JJ, Oppenheimer-Marks N: The role of cytokines in the pathogenesis of rheumatoid arthritis. Springer Semin Immunopathol 11:123, 1989.
59. Aarden LA, Brunner TK, Cerottini JC, Dayer JM, deWeck AL, Dinarello CA, Disabato G, Farrar JJ, Gery I, Gillis S, Handschumacher RE, Henney CS, Hoffman MK, Koopman WJ, Krane SM, Lachman LB, Lefkowits I, Mishell RI, Mizel SB, Oppenheim JJ, Paetkau V, Plate J, Rollinghoff M, Rosenstreich D, Rosenthal AS, Rosenwasser LJ, Schimpl A, Shin HS, Simon PL, Smith KA, Wagner H, Watson JD, Wecker E, Wood DD: Revised nomenclature for antigen-nonspecific T cell proliferation and helper factors. J Immunol 123:2928, 1979.
60. Lopez AF, Elliott MJ, Woodcock J, Vadas MA: GM-CSF, IL-3, and IL-5: Cross-competition on human haemopoietic cells. Immunol Today 13:495, 1992.
61. Hamilton JA: Colony stimulating factors, cytokines and monocyte-macrophages—some controversies. Immunol Today 14:18, 1993.
62. Splawski JB, Lipsky PE: Human B-cell regulation by growth and differentiation factors. In Cambier JC (ed): Ligands, Receptors, and Signal Transduction in Regulation of Lymphocyte Function. Washington, DC, American Society for Microbiology, 1990, p 149.
63. Smith KA: T cell growth factor. Immunol Rev 51:337, 1980.
64. Devos R, Plaetinck G, Cheroutre H, Simons G, Degrave W, Tavernier J, Remaut E, Fiero W: Molecular cloning of human interleukin 2 cDNA and its expression in E. coli. Nucleic Acids Res 11:4307, 1983.
65. Taniguchi T, Matsui H, Fujita T, Takaoka C, Kashiman N, Yoshimoto R, Hamuro J: Structure and expression of a cloned cDNA for human interleukin-2. Nature 302:305, 1983.
66. Fujita T, Takaoka C, Matsui H, Taniguchi T: Structure of the human interleukin 2 gene. Proc Natl Acad Sci USA 80:7437, 1983.

67. Norton SD, Havinen DE, Jenkins MK: IL-2 secretion and T cell clonal anergy are induced by distinct biochemical pathways. J Immunol 146:1125, 1991.

68. Jenkins MK: The role of cell division in the induction of clonal anergy. Immunol Today 13:69, 1992.

69. Robb RJ: Interleukin-2: The molecule and its function. Immunol Today 5:203, 1984.

70. Waldmann TA: The IL-2/IL-2 receptor system: A target for rational immune intervention. Immunol Today 14:264, 1993.

71. Waldmann TA: The interleukin-2 receptor. J Biol Chem 266:2681, 1991.

72. Symons JA, Wood NC, DiGiovine FS, Duff GW: Soluble IL-2 receptor in rheumatoid arthritis: Correlation with disease activity, IL-1 and IL-2 inhibition. J Immunol 141:2612, 1988.

73. Arai N, Nomura D, Villaret D, Malefijt RD, Yoshida M, Minoshima S, Fukuyama R, Maekawa M, Kudoh J, Shimizu N, Yokota K, Abe E, Yokota T, Takeabe Y, Arai K: Complete nucleotide sequence of the chromosomal gene for human IL-4 and its expression. J Immunol 142:274, 1989.

74. Kishimoto T: B-cell stimulatory factors (BSFs): Molecular structure, biological function, and regulation of expression. J Clin Immunol 7:343, 1987.

75. Paul WE: Interleukin 4/B cell stimulatory factor 1: One lymphokine, many functions. FASEB J 1:456, 1987.

76. Yokota T, Otsuka T, Mosmann T, Bancherau J, DeFrance T, Blanchard D, DeVries JE, Lee F, Arai K-I: Isolation and characterization of a human interleukin cDNA clone, homologous to mouse B-cell stimulatory factor 1, that expresses B-cell–and T-cell–stimulating activities. Proc Natl Acad Sci USA 83:5894, 1986.

77. Bettens F, Walker C, Gauchat JF, Gauchar D, Wyss T, Pichler WJ: Lymphokine gene expression related to CD4 T cell subset (CD45R/CDw29) phenotype conversion. Eur J Immunol 19:1569, 1989.

78. Lowenthal JW, Castle BE, Christiansen J, Schreurs J, Rennick D, Arai N, Hoy P, Takebe Y, Howard M: Expression of the high affinity receptors for murine interleukin-4 (BSF-1) on hemopoietic and nonhemopoietic cells. J Immunol 140:456, 1988.

79. Mosley B, Beckmann MP, March CJ, Idzerda RL, Gimpel SD, VandenBos T, Friend D, Alpert A, Anderson D, Jackson J, Wignall JM, Smith C, Gallis B, Sims JE, Urdal D, Widmer MB, Cosman D, Park LS: The murine interleukin-4 receptor: Molecular cloning and characterization of secreted and membrane bound forms. Cell 59:335, 1989.

80. Street NE, Mosmann TR: IL4 and IL5: The role of two multifunctional cytokines and their place in the network of cytokine interactions. Biotherapy 2:347, 1990.

81. Campbell HD, Tucker WQJ, Hort Y, Martinson ME, Mayo G, Clutterbuck EJ, Sanderson CJ, Young IG: Molecular cloning, nucleotide sequence, and expression of the gene encoding human eosinophil differentiation factor (interleukin-5). Proc Natl Acad Sci USA 84:6629, 1987.

82. Yokota T, Coffman RL, Hagiward H, Rennick DM, Takebe Y, Yokota K, Gemmell L, Shrader B, Yang G, Meyerson P, Luh J, Hoy P, Pene J, Briere F, Spits H, Bancherau J, deVries J, Lee FD, Arai N, Arai K-I: Isolation and characterization of lymphokine cDNA clones encoding mouse and human IgA-enhancing factor and eosinophil colony-stimulating factor activities: Relationship to interleukin-5. Proc Natl Acad Sci USA 84:7388, 1987.

83. Rasmussen R, Takatsu K, Harada N, Takahashi T, Bottomly K: T cell-dependent hapten-specific and polyclonal B cell responses require release of interleukin-5. J Immunol 140:705, 1988.

84. Takatsu K, Kikuchi Y, Takahashi T, Honjo T, Matsumoto M, Harada N, Yamaguchi N, Tominaga A: Interleukin-5, a T-cell–derived B-cell differentiation factor also induces cytotoxic T lymphocytes. Proc Natl Acad Sci USA 84:4234, 1987.

85. Waren DJ, Moore MAS: Synergism among interleukin-1, interleukin-3, and interleukin-5 in the production of eosinophils from primitive hemopoietic stem cells. J Immunol 140:94, 1988.

86. Fiorentino DF, Bond MW, Mosmann TR: Two types of mouse T helper cell. IV: T_H2 clones secrete a factor that inhibits cytokine production by T_H1 clones. J Exp Med 170:2081, 1989.

87. Moore KW, Vieira P, Fiorentino DF, Trounstine ML, Khan TA, Mosmann TR: Homology of cytokine synthesis inhibitory factor (IL-10) to the Epstein-Barr virus gene BCRFI. Science 248:1230, 1990.

88. MacNeil IA, Suda T, Moore KW, Mosmann TR, Zlotnik A: IL-10, a novel growth cofactor for mature and immature T cells. J Immunol 145:4167, 1990.

89. Trinchieri G: Interleukin-12 and its role in the generation of T_H1 cells. Immunol Today 14:335, 1993.

90. Trinchieri G, Scott P: The role of interleukin-12 in the immune response, disease and therapy. Immunol Today 15:460, 1994.

91. Dinarello CA: Modalities for reducing interleukin-1 activity in disease. Immunol Today 14:260, 1993.

92. Betz M, Fox BS: Prostaglandin E_2 inhibits production of T_H1 lymphokines but not of T_H2 lymphokines. J Immunol 146:18, 1991.

93. Quill H, Gaur A, Phipps RP: Prostaglandin E_2-dependent induction of granulocyte-macrophage colony-stimulating factor secretion by cloned murine helper T cells. J Immunol 142:813, 1989.

94. Masuda ES, Naito Y, Arai K-I, Arai N: Expression of lymphokine genes in T cells. The Immunologist 1:198, 1993.

95. Fruman DA, Burakoff SJ, Bierer BE: Immunophilins in protein folding and immunosuppression. FASEB J 8:391, 1994.

96. Liu J: FK506 and cyclosporin, molecular probes for studying intracellular signal transduction. Immunol Today 14:290, 1993.

97. Jain J, McCaffrey PG, Valge AV, Rao A: Nuclear factor of activated T cells contains Fos and Jun. Nature 356:801, 1992.

98. Jain J, McCaffrey PG, Miner Z, Kerppola TK, Lambert JN, Verdine GL, Curran T, Rao A: The T-cell transcription factor NFATp is a substrate for calcineurin and interacts with Fos and Jun. Nature 365:352, 1993.

99. Rao A: NFATp: A transcription factor required for the coordinate induction of several cytokine genes. Immunol Today 15:274, 1994.

100. Shaw JP, Meerovitch JK, Cleackley RC, V Paetkau: Mechanisms regulating the level of IL-2 mRNA in T lymphocytes. J Immunol 140:2243, 1988.

101. Hunkapillar T, Hood L: Diversity of the immunoglobulin gene superfamily. Adv Immunol 44:1, 1989.

102. Edmundson AB, Ely KR, Abola EE, Schiffer M, Panagiotopoulos N: Rotational allomerism and divergent evolution of domains in immunoglobulin light chains. Biochemistry 14:3953, 1975.

103. Saul FA, Amzel LM, Poljak RJ: Preliminary refinement and structural analysis of the Fab fragment of human immunoglobulin new at 2.09 A resolution. J Biol Chem 253:585, 1977.

104. Hasemann CA, Capra JD: Immunoglobulins: Structure and Function. In Paul WE (ed): Fundamental Immunology, 2nd ed. New York, Raven Press, 1989, p 209.

105. Fleischman JB, Pain RH, Porter RR: Reduction of gammaglobulins. Arch Biochem Biophys Suppl 1:174, 1962.

106. Amit AG, Mariuzza RA, Phillips SEV, Poljak RJ: Three-dimensional structure of an antigen antibody complex at 2.8 A resolution. Science 233:747, 1986.

107. Kabat EA, Wu TT, Reid-Miller M, Perry HM, Gottesman KS: Sequences of Proteins of Immunologic Interest, 4th ed. Bethesda, Md, U.S. Department of Health and Human Services, 1987.

108. Mole JE, Bhown AS, Bennett J: Primary structure of human J chain: Alignment of peptides from chemical and enzymatic hydrolyses. Biochemistry 16:3507, 1977.

109. Mostov KE, Friedlander M, Blobel G: The receptor for transepithelial transport of IgA and IgM contains multiple immunoglobulin-like domains. Nature 308:37, 1984.

110. Honjo T: Immunoglobulin genes. Annu Rev Immunol 1:499, 1983.

111. Tonegawa S: Somatic generation of antibody diversity. Nature 302:575, 1983.

112. Lutzker S, Alt FW: Immunoglobulin heavy-chain class switching. In Berg DE, Howe MM (eds): Mobile DNA. Washington, DC, American Society for Microbiology, 1988, pp 691–714.

113. Hedrick SM: T Lymphocyte Receptors. In Paul WE (ed): Fundamental Immunology, 2nd ed. New York, Raven Press, 1989.

114. Max E: Immunoglobulins: Molecular Genetics. In Paul WE (ed): Fundamental Immunology, 2nd ed. New York, Raven Press, 1989, p 235.

115. Reth M, Hombach J, Wienards J, Campbell KS, Chien N, Justement LB, Cambier KS: The B-cell antigen receptor complex. Immunol Today 12:196, 1991.

116. Rathbun GA, Tucker PW: Conservation of sequences necessary for V gene recombination. In Kelsoe G, Shultz D (eds): Evolution of the Immune Response. San Francisco, Academic Press, 1986, p 75.

117. Meek KD, Hasemann CA, Capra JD: Novel rearrangements at the immunoglobulin D locus: Inversions and fusions add to somatic diversity. J Exp Med 170:39, 1989.

118. Lewis S, Gifford A, Baltimore D: DNA elements are asymmetrically joined during the site specific recombination of Kappa immunoglobulin genes. Science 228:677, 1985.

119. Lafaille JJ, DeCloux A, Bonneville M, Takagake Y, Tonegawa S: Junctional sequences of T cell receptor γδ genes: Implications for γδ T cell lineages and for a novel intermediate of V-(D)-J joining. Cell 59:859, 1989.

120. Alt FW, Baltimore D: Joining of immunoglobulin heavy chain gene segments. Implications from a chromosome with evidence of three D-JH fusions. Proc Natl Acad Sci USA 79:4118, 1982.

121. Meek K: Analysis of junctional diversity during B lymphocyte development. Science 250:820, 1990.

122. Kudo A, Melchers F: A second gene, V preB in the lambda 5 locus of the mouse, which appears to be selectively expressed in pre-B lymphocytes. EMBO J 6:103, 1987.

123. Siminovitch KA, Bakhski A, Goldman P, Korsmeyer SJ: A uniform deleting element mediates the loss of K genes in human B cells. Nature 316:260, 1985.

124. Clarke SH, Huppi K, Ruezinsky D, Staudt L, Gerhard W, Weigert M: Inter- and intraclonal diversity in the antibody response to influenza hemagglutinin. J Exp Med 161:687, 1985.

125. Zheng B, Xue W, Kelsoe G: Locus-specific somatic hypermutation in germinal centre T cells. Nature 372:556, 1994.

126. Schatz DG, Oettinger MA, Baltimore D: The V(D)J recombination activating gene, RAG-1. Cell 59:1035, 1989.

127. Bergman Y, Rice D, Grosschedl R, Baltimore D: Two regulatory elements for immunoglobulin kappa light chain gene expression. Proc Natl Acad Sci USA 81:7041, 1984.

128. Ballard DW, Bothwell A: Mutational analysis of the immunoglobulin heavy chain promoter region. Proc Natl Acad Sci USA 83:9626, 1986.

129. Mizushima-Sugano J, Roeder RG: Cell-type specific transcription of an immunoglobulin kappa light chain gene in vitro. Proc Natl Acad Sci USA 83:8511.

130. Wirth T, Staudt L, Baltimore D: An octamer oligonucleotide upstream of a TATA motif is sufficient for lymphoid-specific promoter activity. Nature 329:174, 1987.

131. Scheidereit C, Heguy A, Roeder RG: Purification and characterization of a human lymphoid-specific octamer-binding protein (OTF-2) that activates transcription of an immunoglobulin promoter in vitro. Cell 51:783, 1987.

132. Fletcher C, Heintz N, Roeder RG: Purification and characterization of OTF-1, a transcription factor regulating cell cycle expression of a human histone H2b gene. Cell 51:773, 1987.

133. Sen R, Baltimore D: Inducibility of kappa immunoglobulin enhancer-binding protein NF-kappa B by a post-translational mechanism. Cell 47:921, 1986.

134. Early P, Rogers J, Davis M, Calame K, Bond M, Wall R, Hood L: Two mRNAs can be produced from a single immunoglobulin mu gene by alternative RNA processing pathways. Cell 20:313, 1980.

135. Knapp MR, Liu CP, Newell N, Ward RB, Tucker PW, Strober S, Blattner F: Simultaneous expression of immunoglobulin mu and delta heavy chains by a clones B-cell lymphoma: A single copy of the VH gene is shared by two adjacent CH genes. Proc Natl Acad Sci USA 79:2996, 1982.

136. Kenter A, Birshtein B: Chi, a promoter of generalized recombination of λ phage, is present in immunoglobulin genes. Nature 293:402, 1983.

137. Perlmutter R, Hansburg D, Briles D, Nicolotti R, Davie J: Subclass restriction of murine anticarbohydrate antibodies. J Immunol 121:566, 1978.

138. Lutzker S, Rothman P, Pollock R, Coffman R, Alt FW: Mitogen and IL4 regulated expression of germline Ig γ2b transcripts: Evidence for directed heavy chain class switching. Cell 53:177, 1988.

139. Kronenberg M, Siu G, Hood LE, Shastri N: The molecular genetics of the T cell receptor and T cell antigen recognition. Annu Rev Immunol 4:529, 1986.

140. Yoshikai Y, Clark SP, Taylor S, Sohn U, Wilson BI, Mindon MD, Mak TW: Organization and sequences of the variable, joining and constant region genes of the human T cell receptor alpha chain. Nature 316:837, 1985.

141. Lai E, Concannon P, Hood L: Conserved organization of the human and murine T cell receptor beta gene families. Nature 331:5436, 1985.

142. Chien YH, Isashima M, Kaplan KB, Elliot JF, Davis MM: A new T cell receptor gene located within the alpha locus and expressed early in T cell differentiation. Nature 327:677, 1987.

143. Raulet DH, Garman RD, Saito H, Tonegawa S: Developmental regulation of T-cell receptor gene expression. Nature 314:103, 1985.

144. Snodgrass HR, Dembic Z, Steinmetz M, von Boehmer H: Expression of T-cell antigen receptor genes during fetal development in the thymus. Nature 315:232, 1985.

145. Haars R, Kronenberg M, Gallatin WM, Weissman IL, Owen FL, Hood L: Rearrangement and expression of T cell antigen receptor and γ genes during thymic development. J Exp Med 164:1, 1986.

146. Chien Y-H, Iwashima M, Wettstein DA, Kaplan KB, Elliott JF, Born W, Davis MM: T-cell receptor δ gene rearrangements in early thymocytes. Nature 330:722, 1987.

147. Born W, Rathbun G, Tucker P, Marrack P, Kappler J: Synchronized rearrangement of T-cell γ and β chain genes in fetal thymocyte development. Science 234:479, 1986.

148. Saint-Ruf C, Ungewiss K, Groettrup M, Bruno L, Fehling HJ, von Boehmer H: Analysis and expression of a cloned pre-T cell receptor gene. Science 266:1208, 1994.

149. Havran WL, Allison JP: Developmentally ordered appearance of thymocytes expressing different T-cell antigen receptors. Nature 335:443, 1988.

150. Houlden BA, Cron RQ, Coligan JE, Bluestone JA: Systematic development of distinct T cell receptor-γδ T cell subsets during fetal ontogeny. J Immunol 141:3753, 1988.

151. Winoto A, Baltimore D: Separate lineages of T cells expressing the αβ and γδ receptors. Nature 338:430, 1989.

152. Bonneville M, Janeway CA Jr, Ito K, Haser W, Ishida I, Nakanishi N, Tonegawa S: Intestinal intraepithelial lymphocytes are a distinct set of γδ T cells. Nature 336:479, 1988.

153. Ishida I, Verbeek S, Bonneville M, Itohara S, Berns A, Tonegawa S: T-cell receptor γδ and γ transgenic mice suggest a role of a γ gene silencer in the generation of αβ T cells. Proc Natl Acad Sci USA 87:3067, 1990.

154. Winoto A, Baltimore D: αβ lineage-specific expression of the α T cell receptor gene by nearby silencers. Cell 59:649, 1989.

155. Haynes BF: The human thymic microenvironment. Adv Immunol 36:87, 1984.

156. Fowlkes BJ, Pardoll DM: Molecular and cellular events of T cell development. Adv Immunol 44:207, 1989.

157. Haynes BF, Martin ME, Kay HH, Kurtzberg J: Early events in human T cell ontogeny. Phenotypic characterization and immunologic localization of T cell precursors in early human fetal tissues. J Exp Med 168:1061, 1988.

158. Deugnier MA, Imhof BA, Bauvois B, Dunon D, Denoyelle M, Thiery J-P: Characterization of rat T cell precursors sorted by chemotactic migration toward Thymotaxin. Cell 56:1073, 1989.

159. Reinherz EL, Kung PC, Goldstein G, Schlossman SF: A monoclonal antibody with selective reactivity with functionally mature human thymocytes and all peripheral human T cells. J Immunol 123:1312, 1979.

160. Poussier P, Julius M: Thymus-independent T cell development and selection in the intestinal epithelium. Annu Rev Immunol 12:521, 1994.

161. Boyd RL, Hugo P: Toward an integrated view of thymopoiesis. Immunol Today 12:71, 1991.

162. Nikolic-Zugic J: Phenotypic and functional stages in the intrathymic development of αβ T cells. Immunol Today 12:65, 1991.

163. Sprent J, Lo D, Gao K-K, Ron Y: T cell selection in the thymus. Immunol Rev 101:173, 1988.

164. Zacharchuk CM, Mercep M, Chakraborti PK, Simons SS Jr, Ashwell JD: Programmed T lymphocyte death: Cell activation- and steroid-induced pathways are mutually antagonistic. J Immunol 145:4037, 1990.

165. Mueller DL, Jenkins MK, Schwartz RH: Clonal expansion versus functional inactivation: A costimulatory signaling pathway determines the outcome of T cell antigen receptor occupancy. Annu Rev Immunol 7:445, 1989.

166. Kincade PW: Formation of B lymphocytes in fetal and adult life. Adv Immunol 31:177, 1981.

167. Kincade PW, Lee G, Pietrangeli CE, Hayashi S-I, Gimble JM: Cells and molecules that regulate B lymphopoiesis in bone marrow. Annu Rev Immunol 7:111, 1989.

168. Namen AE, Lupton S, Njerrild K, Wignall J, Mochizuki DY, Schmierer A, Mosley B, March CJ, Urdal D, Gillis S, Cosman D, Goodwin RG: Stimulation of B cell precursors by cloned murine interleukin 7. Nature 333:571, 1988.

169. Takeda S, Gillis S, Palacio S: In vitro effects of recombinant interleukin 7 on growth and differentiation of bone marrow pro-B and pro-T lymphocyte clones and fetal thymocyte clones. Proc Natl Acad Sci USA 86:1634, 1989.

170. Kocks C, Rojewsky K: Stable expression somatic hypermutation of antibody V regions in B cell development pathways. Annu Rev Immunol 7:537, 1989.

171. Gu H, Tarlinton D, Muller W, Rajewsky K, Forster I: Most peripheral B cells in mice are ligand selected. J Exp Med 173:1357, 1991.

172. Goodnow CC, Adelstein S, Basten A: The need for central and peripheral tolerance in the B cell repertoire. Science 248:1373, 1990.

173. Erikson J, Radic MZ, Camper SA, Hardy RR, Carmack C, Weigert M: Expression of anti-DNA immunoglobulin trans genes in non-autoimmune mice. Nature 349:331, 1991.

174. Nemazee DA, Burki K: Clonal deletion of B lymphocytes in a transgenic mouse bearing anti-MHC class I antibody genes. Nature 337:562, 1989.

175. Rudd CE, Janssen O, Cai Y-C, Da Silva AJ, Raab M, Prasad KVS: Two-step TCRzeta/CD3-CD4 and CD28 signaling in T cells: SH2/SH3 domains, protein-tyrosine and lipid kinases. Immunol Today 15:225, 1994.

176. Yin YJ, Clayton LK, Howard FD: Molecular cloning of the CD3eta subunit identifies a CD3zeta-related product in thymus derived cells. Proc Natl Acad Sci USA 87:3319, 1990.

177. Klausner RD, Samelson LE: T cell antigen receptor activation pathways: The tyrosine kinase connection. Cell 64:875, 1991.

178. Weissman AM: The T-cell antigen receptor: A multisubunit signaling complex. Chem Immunol 59:1, 1994.

179. Wegener AM, Letourneur F, Hoeveler A, Brocker T, Luton F, Malissen B: The T cell receptor/CD3 complex is composed of at least two autonomous transduction molecules. Cell 68:83, 1992.

180. Janeway CA Jr, Rojo J, Saizawa K, Dianzani U, Portoles P, Tite J, Haque S, Jones B: The co-receptor function of murine CD4. Immunol Rev 109:77, 1989.

181. Barber EK, Dasgupta JD, Schlossman SF, Trevillyan JM, Rudd CE: The CD4 and CD8 antigens are coupled to a protein-tyrosine kinase (p56lck) that phosphorylates the CD3 complex. Proc Natl Acad Sci USA 86:3277, 1989.

182. Bjorkman PJ, Saper MA, Samraoui B, Bennett WS, Strominger JL, Wiley DC: The foreign antigen binding site and T cell recognition regions of class I histocompatibility antigens. Nature 329:512, 1987.

183. Stern LJ, Brown JH, Jardetzky TS, Gorga JC, Urban RG, Strominger JL, Wiley DC: Crystal structure of the human class II MHC protein HLA-DR1 complexed with an influenza virus peptide. Nature 368:215, 1994.

184. Hsi ED, Siegel JN, Minami Y, Luong ET, Klausner RD, Samelson LE: T cell activation induces rapid tyrosine phosphorylation of a limited number of cellular substrates. J Biol Chem 264:10836, 1989.

185. June CH, Fletcher MC, Ledbetter JA, Schieven GL, Siegel JN, Phillips

AF, Samelson LE: Inhibition of tyrosine phosphorylation prevents T-cell receptor-mediated signal transduction. Proc Natl Acad Sci USA 87:7722, 1990.

186. June CH, Fletcher MC, Ledbetter JA, Samelson LE: Increases in tyrosine phosphorylation are detectable before phospholipase C activation after T cell receptor stimulation. J Immunol 144:1599, 1990.

187. Samelson LE, Phillips AF, Luong ET, Klausner RD: Association of the fyn protein-tyrosine kinase with the T-cell antigen receptor. Proc Natl Acad Sci USA 87:4358, 1990.

188. Straus DB, Weiss A: The CD3 chains of the T cell antigen receptor associate with the ZAP-70 tyrosine kinase and are tyrosine phosphorylated after receptor stimulation. J Exp Med 178:1523, 1993.

189. Elder ME, Lin D, Clever J, Chan AC, Hope TJ, Weiss A, Parslow TG: Human severe combined immunodeficiency due to a defect in ZAP-70, a T cell tyrosine kinase. Science 264:1596, 1994.

190. Appleby MW, Gross JA, Cooke MP, Levin SD, Qian XA, Perlmutter RM: Defective T cell receptor signaling in mice lacking the thymic isoform of p59^{fyn}. Cell 70:751, 1992.

191. Chow LML, Fournel M, Davidson D, Veillette A: Negative regulation of T-cell receptor signalling by tyrosine protein kinase p50^{csk}. Nature 365:156, 1993.

192. Tonks NK, Diltz CD, Fischer EH: CD45, an integral membrane protein tyrosine phosphatase. J Biol Chem 265:10674, 1990.

193. Pingel JT, Thomas ML: Evidence that the leukocyte-common antigen is required for antigen-induced T lymphocyte proliferation. Cell 58:1055, 1989.

194. Mustelin T, Coggeshall KM, Altman A: Rapid activation of the T-cell tyrosine protein kinase pp56^{lck} by the CD45 phosphotyrosine phosphatase. Proc Natl Acad Sci USA 86:6302, 1989.

195. Volarevic S, Burns CM, Sussman JJ: Intimate association of thy-1 and the T-cell receptor with the CD45 tyrosine phosphatase. Proc Natl Acad Sci USA 87:7085, 1990.

196. Mustelin T, Coggeshall KM, Isakov N, Altman A: T cell antigen receptor–mediated activation of phospholipase C requires tyrosine phosphorylation. Science 247:1584, 1990.

197. June CH, Fletcher MC, Ledbetter JA, Schieven GL, Siegel JN, Phillips AF, Samelson LE: Inhibition of tyrosine phosphorylation prevents T-cell receptor–mediated signal transduction. Proc Natl Acad Sci USA 87:7722, 1990.

198. Weiss A, Imboden J, Hardy K, Stobo J: The role of the antigen receptor/T3 complex in T-cell activation. Adv Exp Med Biol 213:45, 1987.

199. Imboden JB, Weiss A: The T-cell antigen receptor regulates sustained increases in cytoplasmic free Ca^{2+} through extracellular Ca^{2+} influx and ongoing intracellular Ca^{2+} mobilization. Biochem J 247:695, 1987.

200. Gardner P: Patch clamp studies of lymphocyte activation. Annu Rev Immunol 8:231, 1990.

201. Davis LS, Lipsky PE: T cell activation induced by anti-CD3 antibodies requires prolonged stimulation of protein kinase C. Cell Immunol 118:208, 1989.

202. Kumagal N, Benedict SH, Mills GB: Induction of competence and progression signals in human T lymphocytes by phorbol esters and calcium ionophores. J Cell Physiol 137:329, 1988.

203. Downward J, Graves JD, Warne PH, Rayter S, Cantrell DA: Stimulation of p21ras upon T-cell activation. Nature 346:719, 1990.

204. Warne PH, Viciana PR, Downward J: Direct interaction of Ras and the amino-terminal region of Raf-1 in vitro. Nature 364:352, 1993.

205. Rayter SI, Woodrow M, Lucas SC, Cantrell DA, Downward J: p21^{ras} mediates control of IL-2 gene promoter function in T cell activation. EMBO J 11:4549, 1992.

206. Owaki H, Varma R, Gillis B, Bruder JT, Rapp UR, Davis LS, Geppert TD: Raf-1 is required for T cell IL2 production. EMBO J 12:4367, 1993.

207. Gille H, Sharrocks AD, Shaw PE: Phosphorylation of transcription factor p62^{TCF} by MAP kinase stimulates ternary complex formation at c-fos promoter. Nature 358:414, 1992.

208. Su B, Jacinto E, Hibi M, Kallunki T, Karin M, Ben-Neriah Y: JNK is involved in signal integration during costimulation of T lymphocytes. Cell 77:727, 1994.

209. Riegel JS, Corthesy B, Flanagan WM, Crabtree GR: Regulation of the interleukin 2 gene. In Kishimoto T (ed): Chemical Immunology: Interleukins, Molecular Biology and Immunology. Vol 51. Basel, Karger, 1992, p 266.

210. Pfeffer K, Mak TW: Lymphocyte ontogeny and activation in gene targeted mutant mice. Annu Rev Immunol 12:367, 1994.

211. Monostori E, Desai D, Brown MH: Activation of human T lymphocytes via the CD2 antigen results in tyrosine phosphorylation of T cell antigen receptor ζ chains. J Immunol 144:1010, 1990.

212. June CH, Ledbetter JA, Linsley PS: Role of the CD28 receptor in T-cell activation. Immunol Today 11:211, 1990.

213. Prasad KVS, Cai Y-C, Raab M, Duckworth B, Cantley L, Shoelson SE, Rudd CE: T-cell antigen CD28 interacts with the lipid kinase phosphatidylinositol 3-kinase by a cytoplasmic Tyr(P)-Met-Xaa-Met motif. Proc Natl Acad Sci USA 91:2834, 1994.

214. Fraser JD, Irving BA, Crabtree GR, Weiss A: Regulation of interleukin-2 gene enhancer activity by the T cell accessory molecule CD28. Science 251:313, 1991.

215. Crabtree GR: Contingent genetic regulatory events in T lymphocyte activation. Science 243:355, 1989.

216. Schuermann M, Neuberg M, Hunter JB: The leucine repeat motif in fos protein mediates complex formation with jun/AP-1 and is required for transformation. Cell 56:507, 1989.

217. Northrop JP, Ho SN, Chen L, Thomas DJ, Timmerman LA, Nolan GP, Admon A, Crabtree GR: NF-AT components define a family of transcription factors targeted in T-cell activation. Nature 369:497, 1994.

218. Gaulton GN, Williamson P: Interleukin-2 and the interleukin-2 receptor complex. In Samelson LE (ed): Chemical Immunology. Lymphocyte Activation. Vol 59. Basel, Karger, 1994, pp 91–114.

219. Mills GB, Stewart DJ, Mellors A: Interleukin-2 does not induce phosphatidylinositol hydrolysis in activated T cells. J Immunol 136:3019, 1986.

220. Mills GB, Girard P, Grinstein S: Interleukin-2 induces proliferation of T lymphocyte mutants lacking protein kinase C. Cell 55:91, 1988.

221. Horak ID, Gress RE, Lucas PJ, Horak EM, Waldmann TA, Bolen JB: T-lymphocyte interleukin 2-dependent tyrosine protein kinase signal transduction involves the activation of p56^{lck}. Proc Natl Acad Sci USA 88:1996, 1991.

222. Puck JM: Molecular and genetic basis of X-linked immunodeficiency disorders. J Clin Immunol 14:81, 1994.

223. Shaw AC, Mitchell RN, Weaver YK, Campos-Torres J, Abbas AK, Leder P: Mutations of immunoglobulin transmembrane and cytoplasmic domains: Effects on intracellular signaling and antigen presentation. Cell 63:381, 1990.

224. Pleiman CM, D'Ambrosio D, Cambier JC: The B cell receptor complex: Structure and signal transduction. Immunol Today 15:393, 1994.

225. Clark MR, Johnson SA, Cambier JC: Analysis of Ig-α-tyrosine kinase interaction reveals two levels of binding specificity and tyrosine phosphorylated Ig-α stimulation of Fyn activity. EMBO J 13:1911, 1994.

226. Campbell KS, Justement LB, Cambier JC: Murine B-cell antigen receptor–mediated signal transduction. In Cambier JC (ed): Ligands, Receptors, and Signal Transduction in Regulation of Lymphocyte Function. Washington DC, American Society for Microbiology, 1990, pp 1–50.

227. Tsubata T, Wu J, Honjo T: B-cell apoptosis induced by antigen receptor crosslinking is blocked by a T-cell signal through CD40. Nature 364:645, 1993.

228. Jumper MD, Splawski JB, Lipsky PE, Meek K: Ligation of CD40 induces sterile transcripts of multiple Ig H chain isotypes in human B cells. J Immunol 152:438, 1994.

229. Callard RE, Armitage RJ, Fanslow WC, Spriggs MK: CD40 ligand and its role in X-linked hyper-IgM syndrome. Immunol Today 14:559, 1993.

230. Uckun FM, Schieven GL, Dibirdik I, Chandan-Langlie M, Tuel-Ahlgren L, Ledbetter JA: Stimulation of protein tyrosine phosphorylation, phosphoinositide turnover, and multiple previously unidentified serine/threonine-specific protein kinases by the pan–B-cell receptor CD40/Bp50 at discrete developmental stages of human B-cell ontogeny. J Biol Chem 266:17478, 1991.

231. Knox KA, Gordon J: Protein tyrosine phosphorylation is mandatory for CD40-mediated rescue of germinal center B cells from apoptosis. Eur J Immunol 23:2578, 1993.

232. Ren CL, Morio T, Fu SM, Geha RS: Signal transduction via CD40 involves activation of lyn kinase and phosphatidylinositol-3-kinase, and phosphorylation of phospholipase Cγ2. J Exp Med 179:673, 1994.

233. Lane PJL, McConnell FM, Schieven GL: The role of class II molecules in human B cell activation: Association with phosphatidyl inositol turnover, protein tyrosine phosphorylation and proliferation. J Immunol 144:3684, 1990.

234. Cambier JC, Morrison DC, Chein MM: Modeling of T cell contact dependent B cell activation. IL-4 and antigen receptor ligation primes quiescent B cell to mobilize calcium in response to Ia cross-linking. J Immunol 146:2075, 1991.

235. Tohma S, Hirohata S, Lipsky PE: The role of CD11a/CD18-CD54 interactions in human T cell dependent B cell activation. J Immunol 146:492, 1991.

236. Subbarao B, Mosier DE: Induction of B lymphocyte proliferation by monoclonal anti-Lyb 2 antibody. J Immunol 130:2033, 1983.

237. Wacholtz MC, Patel SS, Lipsky PE: Leukocyte function-associated antigen 1 is an activation molecule for human T cells. J Exp Med 170:431, 1989.

238. Picker LJ, Butcher EC: Physiological and molecular mechanisms of lymphocyte homing. Annu Rev Immunol 10:561, 1992.

239. Mackay CR: T cell memory: The connection between function, phenotype, and migration pathways. Immunol Today 12:189, 1991.

240. Jalkanen S, Steere AC, Fox RI: A distinct endothelial cell recognition system that controls lymphocyte traffic into inflamed synovium. Science 233:557, 1986.

241. Oppenheimer-Marks N, Ziff M: Binding of normal human mononuclear cells to blood vessel in rheumatoid arthritis synovial membrane. Arth Rheum 29:789, 1986.

242. Manolios N, Geczy C, Schrieber L: Lymphocyte migration in health and inflammatory rheumatic disease. Semin Arth Rheum 20:339, 1991.

243. Munro JM, Pober JS, Cotran RS: Tumor necrosis factor and interferon-γ induce distinct patterns of endothelial activation and associated leukocyte accumulation in skin of *Papio anubis*. Am J Pathol 135:121, 1989.

244. Butcher EC: Cellular and molecular mechanisms that direct leukocyte traffic. Am J Pathol 136:3, 1990.

245. Baumhueter S, Singer MS, Henzel W, Hemmerich S, Renz M, Rosen SD, Lasky LA: Binding of L-selectin to the vascular sialomucin CD34. Science 262:436, 1993.

246. Haynes BF, Telen MJ, Hale LP, Denning SM: CD44: A molecule involved in leukocyte adherence and T cell activation. Immunol Today 10:423, 1989.

247. Berlin C, Berg EL, Briskin MJ, Andrew DP, Kilshaw PJ, Holzmann B, Weissman IL, Hamann A, Butcher EC: α4β7 Integrin medicates lymphocyte binding to the mucosal vascular addressin MAdCAM-1. Cell 74:185, 1993.

248. Springer TA: Adhesion receptors of the immune system. Nature 346:425, 1990.

249. Oppenheimer-Marks N, Lipsky PE: Transendothelial migration of T cells in chronic inflammation. The Immunologist 2:58, 1994.

250. Salmi M, Kalimo K, Jalkanen S: Induction of vascular adhesion protein-1 at sites of inflammation. J Exp Med 178:2255, 1993.

251. Pober JS, Cotran RS: The role of endothelial cells in inflammation. Transplantation 50:537, 1990.

252. Miller MD, Krangel MS: Biology and biochemistry of the chemokines: A family of chemotactic and inflammatory cytokines. Crit Rev Immunol 12:17, 1992.

253. Oppenheimer-Marks N, Lipsky PE: The role of cell adhesion in the evolution of inflammatory arthritis. *In* Wegner CD (ed): Handbook of Immunopharmacology: Adhesion Molecules. San Diego, Academic Press, 1994, p 141.

254. Calame K: Mechanisms that regulate immunoglobulin gene expression. Annu Rev Immunol 3:159, 1985.

255. Nakagawa T, Hirano T, Nakagawa N, Yoshizaki K, Kishimoto T: Effect of recombinant IL-2 and γ-IFN on proliferation and differentiation of human B cells. J Immunol 134:959, 1985.

256. Jelinek D, Splawski J, Lipsky P: The roles of interleukin-2 and interferon-gamma in human B cell activation, growth and differentiation. Eur J Immunol 16:925, 1986.

257. Splawski J, Jelinek D, Lipsky P: Immunomodulatory role of interleukin-4 on the secretion of immunoglobulin by human B cells. J Immunol 142:1569, 1989.

CHAPTER 8

Monocytes and Macrophages

Ranjeny Thomas
Richard Wong
Peter E. Lipsky

Mononuclear phagocytes reside in every organ and tissue in the body and carry out a number of diverse functions that are essential for host defense and normal homeostasis. Members of this family of cells play a critical role in the induction and regulation of both humoral and cellular immune responses[1]; act as the main protection against a number of microorganisms; are involved in the removal of senescent or dying cells from the circulation; participate in bone remodeling and resorption[2]; aid in tissue repair and scar formation following injury; and may help to prevent the spread and development of neoplastic cells.[3] Finally, mononuclear phagocytes play an important role as effector cells at sites of chronic inflammation. Their migratory, pinocytic, phagocytic, intracellular digestive, and secretory activities as well as the capacity to respond to a number of environmental stimuli enable them to carry out these varied activities. Thus, the mononuclear phagocytes constitute a family of lineally related but diverse cells scattered throughout the body that can respond to environmental stimuli and differentiate to achieve their various functions.

HISTORICAL PERSPECTIVE

In 1883, the Russian biologist Elie Metchnikoff first described the function and distribution of phagocytes in invertebrates and then in the liver, spleen, lymph nodes, and central nervous system (CNS) of vertebrates, including humans.[4] He distinguished mononuclear phagocytes, or *macrophages*, from the smaller leukocytes of the circulating blood, which he called *microphages*.

Aschoff subsequently introduced the term *reticuloendothelial system* (RES) to cover the entire range of cells with the endocytic capacity to take up vital dyes. These cells were thought to be involved in the formation of the reticulum of the lymph nodes and spleen or were those cells lining blood or lymph sinusoids. The concept of the reticuloendothelial system has been largely abandoned because it defines a system of cells linked only by their ability to take up vital dyes in vivo.[5] Certain cells, such as blood monocytes, which do not take up vital dyes efficiently in vivo, are excluded inappropriately from this system. Moreover, the reticuloendothelial system includes such cells as reticulum cells and endothelial cells, which are not lineally related to other cells of the system.

Evolving knowledge indicated that macrophages were a family of cells with unique features, especially those of phagocytosis, derived from a common bone marrow precursor. This morphologically, functionally, and lineally related family of cells[6] is now known as the *mononuclear phagocyte system* (Table 8–1).

CHARACTERISTICS OF MATURE MONONUCLEAR PHAGOCYTES

Morphology of Peripheral Blood Monocytes

Peripheral blood monocytes and tissue and organ macrophages are mature mononuclear phagocytes. The peripheral blood monocyte is a large round cell with a diameter of 10 to 18 μm. Its cytoplasm contains a well-developed Golgi apparatus, numerous lysosomal granules, and mitochondria. The nucleus is eccentric and kidney-shaped, with moderately condensed chromatin. Pseudopodia extend from the cell surface, and there is evidence of endocytic activity (Fig. 8–1).

Monocytes circulate in the peripheral blood, and the half-life in humans is estimated from 8 to 71 hours. Monocytes subsequently penetrate tissues in a random fashion independent of age[7] and in numbers proportional to the size of the organ. Once monocytes leave the circulation, they do not return. The total blood monocyte pool is composed of circulating and marginated components. The marginated pool, which

Table 8–1. THE MONONUCLEAR PHAGOCYTE SYSTEM

Cell Type	Location
Monoblast	Bone marrow
Promonocyte	Bone marrow
Monocyte	Bone marrow and peripheral blood
Macrophage	Tissue and organs
	Connective tissue (histiocytes)
	Liver (Kupffer cells)
	Lung (alveolar macrophages)
	Lymph nodes (free and fixed macrophages)
	Spleen (macrophages)
	Bone marrow (macrophages)
	Serous cavities (pleural and peritoneal macrophages)
	Bone (osteoclasts)
	Nervous system (microglial cells)
	Synovium (type A and C cells)
	Inflammatory sites (macrophages, epithelioid and giant cells)

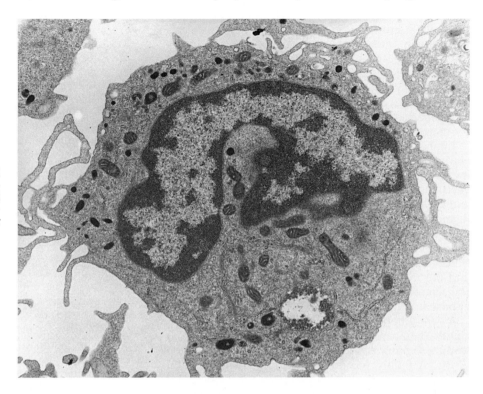

Figure 8–1. A human peripheral blood monocyte. The reniform nucleus, numerous mitochondria, and endocytic vacuoles are typical morphologic features of mononuclear phagocytes.

constitutes up to 75 percent of the total, consists of monocytes adhering to or rolling along the endothelial cells of blood vessels.

Entry of Peripheral Blood Monocytes into the Tissues

Monocytes are adherent to the endothelial cells of all the postcapillary venules and can migrate between them, through the basement membrane to enter tissues.[8] Because monocytes leaving the circulation acquire the characteristics of macrophages within a few hours, vascular endothelium may be an important substrate with which monocytes interact in order to differentiate further. Several leukocyte cell surface glycoprotein families known as the *integrins* (see Chapter 20) have been demonstrated to be involved in both monocyte and neutrophil/endothelial cell interactions.[9]

The most important integrins involved in monocyte adhesion to endothelial cells are known as the CD18 family, or β_2-*integrins*, as they share a common β-subunit.[9] There are three adhesion receptors:

- Leukocyte functional antigen-1 (LFA-1), also known as CD11a/CD18
- Mac-1 (CD 11b/CD18)
- Protein 150,95 (CD 11c/CD18)

LFA-1 is found on all leukocytes; Mac-1 is found on monocytes, macrophages, granulocytes, natural killer (NK) cells, and some lymphocytes; and GP 150/95 is found on monocytes, granulocytes, and some cytotoxic lymphocytes.

LFA-1 binds to three transmembrane glycoprotein counterreceptors—intercellular adhesion molecules-1 (CD54), -2 (CD102), and -3 (CDw50) (ICAM-1, ICAM-2, and ICAM-3), all of which are members of the immunoglobulin supergene family.[10] Whereas ICAM-1 and ICAM-2 are inducible molecules expressed on leukocytes, endothelial cells, and epithelial cells in response to cytokines, endotoxin, and phorbol esters, ICAM-3 is constitutively expressed on endothelial as well as other cells and is not enhanced by inflammatory stimuli.

CD11b/CD18 has been identified as the receptor (CR3) for the complement component C3bi (CR3bi), but it also can recognize and bind to ICAM-1.[9]

p150,95, which is a receptor for the complement component C3bi, can also function as an adhesion molecule, mediating the binding of monocytes to stimulated human endothelial cells independent of other receptor-ligand interactions.[11] Its ligand on endothelial cells has not been characterized.

After cell activation, up-regulation of surface CD11b/CD18 and CD11c/CD18 occurs by the translocation of receptors stored in intracellular vesicles to the cell surface.[12] Conformational changes or phosphorylation of the receptors also appear to be required for regulating adhesive interactions.

Additional adhesion receptors used to bind various connective tissue molecules are expressed by monocytes, including receptors for hyaluronic acid (probably CD44), and B_1 integrin receptors for laminin, elastin, collagen, and fibronectin. Adherence of monocytes to exposed vascular substratum, especially following injury, may be another mechanism of migration from blood vessels.

Finally, a group of lymphoid tissue homing receptors, known as the *selectins*, may be involved in monocyte and neutrophil migration into inflammatory sites. L-selectin (CD62-L) is expressed by neutrophils and monocytes. During inflammation, CD62-L is down-regulated or lost by neutrophils.[13] In contrast, inflammation increases the binding of monocytes to counterreceptors of CD62-L.[13]

Transendothelial leukocyte migration involves several stages.[14] The initial interaction of leukocyte rolling on the endothelial surface of the postcapillary venule is mediated by the selectins (CD62-E, CD62-L, and CD62-P) and their corresponding carbohydrate ligands (see later).[14, 15] Before migration, the rolling cells become tightly adherent to the endothelium by up-regulation and activation of β_2-integrins. CD31 (PECAM-1), expressed by monocytes, neutrophils, and the interendothelial cell junction, is involved in transendothelial leukocyte migration between tightly apposed endothelial cells.[14, 15]

A rare inherited abnormality in the gene encoding CD18 (leukocyte adhesion deficiency-1 [LAD-1]), leading to diminished expression of all three members of the β2 family, has enhanced understanding of the role of these molecules.[12] Defects in adhesion-related functions of phagocytes occur, including chemotaxis, aggregation, endothelial cell and complement (C3bi) binding, and cell-mediated cytotoxicity (ADCC). Affected children experience recurrent and often fatal bacterial infections. Studies of these patients indicate that all three of the CD11/CD18 antigens are crucial in adhesion-dependent functions of monocytes and granulocytes.[12]

A second form of leukocyte adhesion deficiency, LAD-2, is characterized by the inability to add fucose to carbohydrate structures, including the selectin ligands sialyl-Lewis a (sLe^a) and sialyl-Lewis x (SLe^x), resulting in disordered selectin/ligand interactions and thus impaired phagocyte adhesion/motility but normal phagocytic function, and recurrent bacterial infections.[16]

The accumulation of monocytes at inflammatory sites is also governed by local elaboration of chemoattractants, which influence the direction and speed of their movement. Monocytes move in the direction of increasing concentrations of chemoattractant. A number of factors are known to be chemotactic for monocytes, including bacterial products such as N-formylated oligopeptides, cleavage products generated as a result of complement activation, and connective tissue components. In addition, several monocyte- and lymphocyte-derived cytokines and factors produced by erythrocytes, tumor cells, and platelets, such as platelet-derived growth factor (PDGF) and transforming growth factor-β (TGF-β), are chemoattractants.

Members of a family of chemoattractant cytokines, known as *chemokines*, are important in monocyte chemoattraction.[17, 18] The β subfamily includes:

• Monocyte chemotactic and activating factor (MCAF)
• Monocyte chemoattractant protein-1 (MCP-1)

• RANTES (regulated *a*ctivation, *n*ormal *T* cell expressed and *s*ecreted)

In addition to being chemotactic for monocytes, MCAF induces the release of lysosomal enzymes and the production of reactive oxygen intermediates (ROIs) by monocytes. MCP-1 is secreted by activated fibroblasts and endothelial cells, and RANTES is secreted by T cells. Activated lymphocytes also produce a cytokine, migration inhibition factor (MIF), that inhibits macrophage migration and may contribute to the localization of recently arrived monocytes.[19] Finally, macrophage-stimulating protein (MSP) is an unrelated protein that can transiently activate and chemoattract mature macrophages.[20]

Besides stimulating directional cell movement, chemoattractants induce random motility (*chemokinesis*), cell-to-substrate adhesiveness, and cell-to-cell aggregation. Alternate cycles of hyperadherence to (through enhanced expression of leukocyte adhesion molecules) and detachment from tissue substrates may be the basis of directional cell movement in response to chemoattractants. Higher concentrations of chemoattractants also induce exocytosis of lysosomal enzymes and production of ROIs and reactive nitrogen intermediates (RNIs).

Cellular movement is initiated by a rapidly regulated remodeling of the branching network of actin filaments found in the macrophage cytoplasm. Chemoattractants exert their concentration-dependent effects on mononuclear phagocytes through a series of membrane chemoattractant receptor-mediated biochemical and cellular events, leading to regulation of the cytoskeleton and cell movement. Thus, exposure of monocytes to a chemoattractant, such as f-methionine-leucine-phenylalanine (f-MLP), leads to phosphorylation of CD18 within seconds.[21] In evidence of this, cells from patients with leukocyte adhesion deficiency cannot polymerize actin filaments in response to chemoattractants.

Peripheral Blood Monocyte Differentiation into Tissue Macrophages

Once in the tissues, the monocyte matures into a functionally more active cell, the *tissue macrophage*. This cell varies in diameter from 10 to 80 μm. Tissue macrophages contain one or more oval or indented, often eccentrically located, nuclei and may have prominent nucleoli. Their cytoplasm is more abundant than that of the monocyte and contains numerous lysosomes, endocytic vacuoles, and mitochondria. Lysosomes are membrane-bound structures that contain a variety of hydrolytic enzymes. A membrane-associated proton pump maintains an acid environment. Primary lysosomes bud from the Golgi apparatus and may fuse with phagocytic vacuoles to form digestive bodies or secondary lysosomes. Ruffles, pseudopodia, and flaps can be seen on the surface of macrophages.

Macrophages have a very long life span in the tissues, often surviving for months or even years. It has generally been held that tissue macrophages are the direct descendants of blood monocytes. Although this may be true for alveolar macrophages,[22] some resident macrophage populations, such as Kupffer cells and peritoneal macrophages, may renew themselves by local proliferation.[23] In this case, an influx of monocytes may be important only during inflammation.[22]

In chronic inflammation, macrophages may form tight clusters or *granulomas* and take on the characteristics of epithelioid cells (i.e., large macrophage-like cells with abundant cytoplasm and round or oval nuclei that contain numerous mitochondria, lysosomes, and large vacuoles). In some cases, newly emigrated monocytes fuse to form multinucleated giant cells. The resulting syncytia have a life span of only a few days. Both IL-4 and interferon (IFN) may be involved. Many giant cells express class II MHC antigens and may function as antigen-presenting cells (APCs).[24] Giant cells appear to represent highly stimulated cells of the mononuclear phagocytic lineage at a terminal stage of differentiation.[25]

Macrophages are found outlining blood vessels in the connective tissue and are particularly prominent in the lung, liver, spleen, and bone marrow (see Table 8–1). The synovial lining layer also contains cells of macrophage lineage. Primarily on the basis of light and electron microscopic studies, these cells have been classified as macrophage-like types A and C cells, as distinct from fibroblast-like type B cells. Synovial lining type A cells are phagocytic, express monocyte/macrophage-associated antigens detected by a variety of monoclonal antibodies and receptors for the Fc region of the IgG molecule and the third component of complement (C3), and are likely to be derived from bone marrow. The deeper type B cells react only with monoclonal antibodies that identify fibroblasts and are probably derived locally.[26] Finally, mature dendritic cells (see later), expressing abundant major histocompatibility complex (MHC) class II antigen and adhesion molecules are enriched in rheumatoid synovial fluid and tissue.[27]

Macrophage Heterogeneity

As might be expected from their widespread tissue distribution, macrophages are heterogeneous with respect to morphology and functions, such as antigen-presenting capacity, tumor-cell killing, and cytokine secretion. Mononuclear phagocyte heterogeneity probably results from the differences in their stage of differentiation, as well as the local environment during normal and altered homeostasis. For instance, resident tissue macrophages overall are a more functionally quiescent population of cells than are peripheral blood monocytes. In contrast, macrophages activated at inflammatory sites exhibit enhancement in phagocytosis, pinocytosis, and microbicidal and tumoricidal activities.[28]

MATURATION OF THE MONONUCLEAR PHAGOCYTES IN BONE MARROW

Five regulatory glycoproteins, referred to as the *colony-stimulatory factors* (CSFs), are essential for the survival and proliferation of myeloid cells (Table 8–2).[29] Colony-stimulatory factors can be considered in two groups:

- Group 1 stimulates the growth and differentiation of pluripotent stem cells and progenitor cells.
- Group 2 directs mature progenitor cells toward specific cell lineages.

Granulocyte-macrophage CSF (GM-CSF) and multi-CSF (interleukin-3 [IL-3]) stimulate the formation of granulocytes and macrophages.[30] Granulocyte CSF (G-CSF) stimulates only granulocyte formation, and macrophage CSF (M-CSF) stimulates only monocyte formation. Restricted development of cells of monocyte or granulocyte lineage from the bipotential stem cell depends on the relative concentrations of these CSFs. Thus, low concentrations of GM-CSF produce few colonies that are predominantly monocytic, and high concentrations result in predominantly granulocyte colonies.[30] The protein sequence shows a distinct similarity to that of G-CSF.[31] Recombinant human IL-

Table 8–2. COLONY-STIMULATING FACTORS (CSFs)

Human CSF	Other Names	Cellular Sources
Group 1		
Multi-CSF	IL-3	T cells
		Keratinocytes
GM-CSF	CSF-α	T cells
	CSF2	Macrophages
	Pluriprotein-α	Endothelial cells
		Fibroblasts
		Osteoblasts
		Smooth muscle cells
		Epithelial cells
		Mesangial cells
IL-6		T cells
		B cells
		Monocytes/macrophages
		Endothelial cells
		Fibroblasts
		Epithelial cells
		Mesangial cells
Group 2		
G-CSF	CSF-β	Macrophages
	Pluriprotein	Endothelial cells
		Fibroblasts
M-CSF	CSF1	Macrophages
		Endothelial cells
		Fibroblasts
		Epithelial cells
		Embryonic yolk sac
Erythropoietin		Renal cells
		Liver cells

Based on data from Ruef C, Coleman DL: Granulocyte-macrophage colony-stimulating factor: Pleiotropic cytokine with potential clinical usefulness. Rev Infect Dis 12:41, 1990.

Abbreviations: IL, interleukin; M-CSF, macrophage colony-stimulating factor; GM-CSF, granulocyte-macrophage colony-stimulating factor; G-CSF, granulocyte colony-stimulating factor.

6 synergizes with IL-3 in the proliferation of stem cell colonies but does not induce colony formation by itself at the bipotential cell stage. However, IL-6 suppresses colony formation induced by G-CSF but not M-CSF.[32] This may occur either by competitive inhibition or down-regulation of G-CSF receptors by IL-6.

Stem cell factor (SCF, Steel factor, *kit* ligand), produced by bone marrow stromal cells, shows modest effects on pluripotent stem cells by itself, but it synergizes dramatically with other factors, such as erythropoietin, IL-1, IL-6, IL-7, IL-13, and the CSFs.[33, 34] The importance of stem cell factor is evidenced by the severe deficiency of hematopoiesis in animals with defects in its production. IL-13 enhances SCF-induced proliferation of mouse bone marrow stem cells. Whereas the combination of SCF and G-CSF results in the formation of 90 percent granulocytes, addition of IL-13 results in production of macrophages exclusively.[34]

Unique membrane receptors exist for each CSF and are found on stem cells and their progeny. Most cells simultaneously exhibit receptors for more than one type of CSF (Table 8–3). Progenitor cells can respond to any of the four CSFs. One CSF may modulate the capacity of myelomonocytic precursors to respond to other CSFs and thereby regulate their capacity to differentiate down specific pathways.[35] Thus, binding of GM-CSF to its receptor down-modulates receptors for G-CSF and M-CSF.[35] In addition, receptor binding of G-CSF down-modulates receptors for M-CSF, whereas receptor binding of M-CSF down-modulates binding for GM-CSF. The M-CSF and SCF receptors have been identified as the proto-oncogene products *c-fms* and *c-kit*, respectively. Both of these contain intracellular tyrosine kinase domains.[33, 36]

There is marked synergy between CSFs and IL-1. IL-1 may regulate hematopoiesis by inducing alterations of progenitor responsiveness or by enhancing CSF production by auxiliary stromal cells (especially T cells, but also monocytes, endothelial cells, and fibroblasts). IL-1 allows IL-3 to act on multipotent stem cells that are more primitive than those normally responsive to IL-3 alone.[37] This action is mediated in part by the enhancement of CSF receptors on primi-tive multipotent hematopoietic precursors. In cells of hemopoietic stroma, IL-1 can increase translation of IL-6, GM-CSF, and G-CSF genes by stabilizing their messenger ribonucleic acid (mRNA) transcripts.[38] Thus IL-1 provides another mechanism by which immature cells may be directed to the monocytic lineage. Although it is not clear whether the factors produced by inflammatory tissue macrophages reach the bone marrow to stimulate the earliest monocyte/macrophage progenitors, it is likely that their ontogeny is regulated by cells of the mononuclear phagocyte lineage as well as other cell types (Fig. 8–2). Resting peripheral monocytes have no detectable mRNA for G-CSF or M-CSF, but gene expression and protein secretion are inducible by activation with IFN-γ, GM-CSF, and IL-3.[39] GM-CSF and IL-3 appear to induce monocyte M-CSF secretion selectively, whereas endotoxin induces G-CSF. Both endothelial cells and fibroblasts produce M-CSF, G-CSF, and GM-CSF, although production of M-CSF by human endothelial cells requires activation by IL-1 and tumor necrosis factor (TNF).[40]

Growth hormone may also influence myelopoiesis by increasing the number of granulocyte colonies in the presence of GM-CSF. Bone marrow stromal cells thus appear to respond to growth hormone by synthesizing somatomedin-C in a paracrine fashion.[41]

Besides the proliferative actions of the CSFs, each is capable of maintaining membrane integrity, inducing cellular maturation, and stimulating the functional activity of mature cells.[30] The CSF receptors, therefore, mediate diverse biologic responses, depending on the differentiation status of the myeloid cell. M-CSF primes mature monocytes to secrete IL-1, TNF-α, and colony-stimulating activity, and it enhances cell-mediated cytotoxicity. GM-CSF and IL-3 stimulate macrophage cytotoxicity. Both GM-CSF and IL-3 stimulated monocytes kill more effectively when exposed to a second activating signal provided by endotoxin.[40] It is likely that TNF-α secretion is responsible for these effects. Because both GM-CSF and IL-3 are secreted by activated T lymphocytes, these factors may serve to enhance endotoxin-induced macrophage killing in an area of local inflammation. GM-CSF also stimu-

Table 8–3. DIFFERENTIATION MARKERS OF MYELOID CELLS

Designation	Characteristics/Function of Molecule	Pluripotent Cell	Bipotential Cell	Blood Monocyte	Granulocyte	Dendritic Cell
CD34	Glycoprotein (phosphorylated by protein kinase C)	+ +	+ +	−	−	−
CD33	Glycoprotein	+	+	+ +	+ +	+ +
CD13	Aminopeptidase N (a membrane-anchored metalloprotease)	−	+	+ +	+ +	+ +
CD15	LNF-III "X hapten" polysaccharide	−	−	+ +	+ +	−
CD14	Receptor for endotoxin-endotoxin-binding protein complex	−	−	+ +	+	−
CD115	M-CSF receptor (c-fms oncoprotein)	−	+	+ +	−	−
CDw116	GM-CSF receptor	−	+	+ +	+ +	+ +

Abbreviations: LNF-III, lacto-N-fucopentanose III; M-CSF, macrophage colony-stimulating factor; GM-CSF, granulocyte-macrophage colony-stimulating factor; CD, cluster of differentiation.

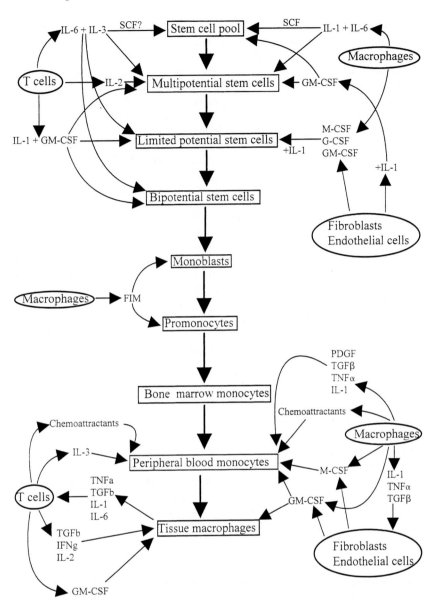

Figure 8–2. Regulation of mononuclear phagocyte development. Factors produced by mononuclear phagocytes as well as by other cell types, such as T cells, fibroblasts, and endothelial cells, control mononuclear phagocyte ontogeny and differentiation. SCF, stem cell factor; IL, interleukin; IFN, interferon; PDGF, platelet-derived growth factor; CSF, colony-stimulating factor; GM, granulocyte-macrophage; TGF, transforming growth factor; TNF, tumor necrosis factor.

lates the expression of class II MHC molecules by monocytes and thereby may allow them to be more effective APCs at sites of inflammation.[42]

Recombinant deoxyribonucleic acid (DNA) technology has enabled the production of CSFs for clinical use.[43] Administration of recombinant GM-CSF leads to a significant increase in nadir white blood cell count following cycles of chemotherapy, with only mild side effects, including cutaneous reactions at injection sites, low-grade fever, bone discomfort, myalgia, and headache.[44] In vitro, continuous exposure of cells to GM-CSF is required to stimulate proliferation and functional activity.[30] Likewise, clinically, subcutaneous and continuous intravenous (IV) routes of administration are more effective than IV pulse or bolus doses of GM-CSF. In a study of adjunctive treatment with GM-CSF for induction therapy of non-Hodgkin's lymphoma, the number of days of neutro-

penia, fever, IV antibiotics, and hospitalization for infection, was significantly reduced.[44]

Factor increasing monocytopoiesis (FIM), a thermolabile protein with a molecular weight of about 20 kD, is secreted by macrophages at the site of inflammation and then transported to the bone marrow.[45] In the marrow, it stimulates monocyte production by increasing the proliferative activity of monoblasts and promonocytes and enhancing the transit of monocytes from bone marrow to blood. This may lead to the appearance in the circulation of immature monocytes normally retained in the bone marrow. FIM has no chemotactic activity, but it stimulates bone marrow monocyte production at times of acute demand for monocytes or macrophages.[46]

Monocyte maturation is accompanied by alterations in cellular morphology and histochemistry. Monoblasts contain cytoplasmic enzymes, including peroxidase, nonspecific esterase, and lysozyme; are phago-cytically active; and possesses receptors for both the Fc region of immunoglobulin G (IgG) and C3.[47] Pro-monocytes constitute about 0.25 percent of all nucle-ated bone marrow cells.[7] They are adherent to glass, contain cytoplasmic esterase and peroxidase activity, but have few Fc and C3 receptors.[7, 47] Although capa-ble of endocytosis, these cells are poorly phagocytic compared with monocytes.[47]

Table 8–3 depicts the differentiation markers of my-eloid cells, demonstrating similarities and differences between the developing cells and their mature prog-eny. Table 8–4 shows the surface markers of mature cells divided into functional groups. The function of some of these cell surface molecules is not yet known. Mature monocytes, macrophages, and activated mac-rophages bear different constellations of cell surface markers. Furthermore, functional subsets of macro-phages can be defined by their expression of different cell surface markers.[48]

ACTIVITIES OF MATURE MONONUCLEAR PHAGOCYTES

The various activities of mononuclear phagocytes can be considered in terms of simple and complex functions (Table 8–5). A simple function is a single ability or activity; a complex function involves the coordination of a variety of simple functions. For example, phagocytosis, pinocytosis, and intracellular digestion are simple functions that are part of micro-bial digestion, a complex function.

Mononuclear phagocytes possess a number of physiologic characteristics that permit them to accom-plish their varied functions. Among these features is the display of a variety of cell surface molecules. Mononuclear phagocytes express more than 30 dis-tinct receptors that enable them to recognize and in-teract with various molecules in their external envi-ronment (see Table 8–4). Another feature is the capacity to synthesize and secrete some 100 defined substances that act both intracellularly and extracellu-larly.

Cell Surface Molecules

Immunoglobulin Fc Receptors

Mononuclear phagocytes possess surface receptors that specifically recognize the Fc region of the IgG and IgE antibody molecules. The human Fc receptors (FcR) can be divided into three classes on the basis of ligand affinity and reactivity with class-specific monoclonal antibodies and genetic structure.

- FcRI (CD64) has high affinity for monomeric IgG and is found only on cells of monocytic origin.
- FcRII (CD32) binds aggregated or polyvalent IgG (IgG1 or IgG3) and is found on monocytes, lympho-cytes, and granulocytes.

- FcRIII (CD16) has a low affinity for aggregated IgG and is found mainly on granulocytes and natural killer cells and, to a lesser extent, on monocytes and macrophages.[49]

The major biologic role for Fc receptors is the facili-tation of phagocytosis. Although antibody is not an obligatory requirement for endocytosis of many parti-cles, its presence greatly enhances phagocytosis. Al-though interaction with FcR initiates fairly weak binding of particles to mononuclear phagocytes, such interactions are potent stimulators of phagocytosis.[50] The FcR is also likely to play a central role in a number of other functions of macrophages, including cell-mediated cytotoxicity, "arming" in tumor immu-nity, and triggering of the secretion of biologically active molecules (prostaglandins, lysosomal acid hy-drolases, and reactive oxygen metabolites).[50] In addi-tion, cytophilic antibody bound to Fc receptors can enhance the amount of foreign antigen taken up by a macrophage and subsequently presented to antigen-specific T cells.[51]

Complement Receptors

Mononuclear phagocytes bear at least three cell surface receptors that recognize activation fragments of the third component of complement (C3a, C3b, and C3bi) and one for an activation fragment of the fifth component of complement, anaphylotoxin (C5a)[52]. Two distinct C3 receptors (CR1 and CR3) appear to recognize different portions of the C3 molecule (C3 and C3bi, respectively.[52] In addition, CD11c/CD18 recognizes C3bi (CR4). Whereas binding of particles is effectively induced by interaction with C3 recep-tors, such interactions are ineffective triggers of phagocytosis by resting macrophages.[53, 54] There is marked synergy between C3 and Fc receptors in facili-tation of phagocytosis, with C3 mediating binding and Fc receptors mediating internalization. Engage-ment of C3 receptors can also lead to release of prosta-glandin.[54] The interaction of C5a with its macrophage receptor induces secretion of IL-1 and initiates chemo-taxis.

Fibronectin Receptors

Fibronectin and laminin are found in the substra-tum of blood vessels and in connective tissue. The fibronectin and laminin receptors are members of the very-late-antigen (VLA) family of integrins, which share a common β_1-subunit (CD29). $\alpha1\beta1$ (VLA-1,CD49a/CD29) and $\alpha2\beta1$ (VLA-2, CD49b/CD29) bind collagen and $\alpha4\beta1$ (VLA-4, CD49d/CD29), $\alpha5\beta1$ (VLA-5, CD49e/CD29) and $\alpha_v\beta1$ (CD51) bind fibro-nectin. $\alpha3\beta1$ (VLA-3, CD49c/CD29) acts as a receptor for epiligrin, collagen, laminin, and fibronectin, and $\alpha6\beta1$ (VLA-6, CD49f/CD29) is a laminin receptor.[9] $\alpha4\beta1$ also mediates adhesion of leukocytes to an in-ducible endothelial cell surface protein, called vascu-lar cell adhesion molecule (VCAM-1, CD106),[55] while

Table 8–4. SURFACE MARKERS ON MYELOID CELLS

Designation	Characteristics/Function of Molecule	Blood Monocyte	Granulocyte	Macrophage
Adhesion Molecules				
CD11a	LFA-1 α chain; p180	+ +	+ +	+
CD11c	p150,95 α chain (CR4)	+ +	+ +	+
CD18	95-kD glycoprotein chain, linked to CD11a, b, and c	+ +	+ +	+ +
CD49d	VLA-α4 chain. Binds VCAM (α4β1), MAdCAM (α4β7), and fibronectin	+ +	−	
CD49f	VLA-α6 chain; laminin receptor	+ +	−	
CD29	Common β chain of VLA protein family	+ +	+ +	+ +
CD44	LECAM-III hyaluronic acid receptor	+ +	+ +	+ +
CD58	LFA-3; binds CD2 molecule on T cells	+ +	+ +	+ +
CD36	85-kD glycoprotein; thrombospondin receptor	−	−	+ +
CD54	ICAM-1	+	+	+ +
CD102	ICAM-2	+	−	+ +
CD31	PECAM	+ +	+ +	+
	Heterophilic and homophilic adhesive interactions			
Complement Receptors				
CD11b	α subunit of complement receptor C3bi (CR3); fibrinogen receptor	+ +	+ +	
CD35	CR1. Binds C3b, C3bi, C3c, C4b	+ +	+ +	−
Immunoglobulin Receptors				
CD64	FcγRI. High-affinity IgG receptor	+ +	+	+ +
CD32	FcγRII. Low-affinity IgG receptor	+ +	+ +	+ +
CD16	FcγRIII. Low-affinity IgG receptor	+ +	+ +	+ +
CD23	FcεRIIa, b; low-affinity IgE receptor	−	+ +	−
Other Receptors				
CD74	Invariant chain	+ +	−	+ +
CD45,	Transmembrane glycoprotein (tyrosine phosphatase) with 4 isoforms, resulting	+ +	+ +	+ +
CD45RA,	from differential splicing	+ +	−	−
CD45RB		+ +	−	+ +
CD45RO		+ +	+ +	+ +
CD25	α-chain of IL-2 receptor complex; low-affinity IL-2 receptor	−	−	−
CD9	24-kD single-chain protein	+ +	−	−
CD46	Doublet glycoprotein of 56-66 kD. Membrane co-factor protein (MCP)	+ +	+ +	+ +
CD47	47 to 52-kD glycoprotein	+ +	+ +	+ +
CD48	41 kD PI-linked glycoprotein, receptor for CD2	+ +	+ +	+ +
CD43	95-kD highly sialated integral membrane protein	+ +	+ +	+ +
CD53	35-kD transmembrane glycoprotein	+ +	+ +	+ +
CD55	70 kD PI-linked membrane glycoprotein. Decay accelerating factor	+ +	+ +	+ +
CD59	18- to 20-kD glycoprotein. Mediates inhibition of the membrane attack complex	+ +	+ +	+ +
CD63	53-kD glycoprotein	+ +	+ +	+ +
CD68	110-kD glycoprotein	+ +	−	+ +
CD71	Transferrin receptor	+ +	+ +	+ +
CDw17	Lactosyl ceramide	+ +	+ +	−
CDw50	ICAM-3; binds LFA-1	+ +	+ +	+ +
CDw52	21- to 29-kD glycoprotein; campath antigen	+ +	+ +	+ +
CDw65	Fucoganglioside; ceramide dodecasaccharide 4c	+	+ +	−
CD40	gp50; ligation leads to monocyte activation	+	−	−
CD80	B7-BB1; CD28 counterreceptor	−	−	+
CD86	B-70, B7-2; CD28 counterreceptor	−	−	+
CD91	α₂-macroglobulin receptor (α-subunit)	+ +	−	+

Data from The CD system of human leukocyte surface molecules. *In* Coligan JE, Kruisbeek AM, Margulies DH, et al: Current Protocols in Immunology. Vol 1, Appendix 4. New York, Greene Publishing Associates, Wiley Interscience, 1991; and Singer NG, Todd RF, Fox DA: Structures on the cell surface. Update from the Fifth International Workshop on Human Leukocyte Differentiation Antigens. Arthritis Rheum 37:1245, 1994.
Abbreviations: CD, cluster of designation; LFA, leukocyte-function associated antigen; kD, kilodalton; VLA, very-late-antigen; VCAM, vascular cellular adhesion molecule; LECAM, leukocyte endothelial cellular adhesion molecule; ICAM, intercellular adhesion molecule; PI, protease inhibitor; CR, complement receptor; Ig, immunoglobulin; MAdCAM, mucosal addressin cell adhesion molecule; PECAM, platelet endothelial cell adhesion molecule.

α4β7 binds the mucosal addressin cell adhesion molecule (MAdCAM-1). The sites on VLA-4 involved in VCAM-1 binding are distinct from those involved in fibronectin binding.

Interaction of these matrix molecules with their specific mononuclear phagocyte receptors may be involved in migration of macrophages to sites of exposed interstitium, as in damaged tissue. In addition,

Table 8–5. PANOPLY OF MONONUCLEAR PHAGOCYTE ACTIVITIES

Simple Functions	Complex Functions
Migration	Tissue remodeling
Pinocytosis	Senescent or dead cell removal
Phagocytosis	Antimicrobial activity
Intracellular digestion	Antiviral activity
	Antineoplastic activity
	Antibody-dependent cell-mediated cytotoxicity
	Immunoregulation
	Lipid and lipoprotein metabolism
	Wound healing

engagement of fibronectin receptors in vitro results in enhanced functional expression of Fc and C3 receptors and consequently augmented phagocytosis and secretion of neutral proteases. CD11b/CD18, fibronectin, vitronectin, and laminin receptors are stored in vesicles in monocytes and neutrophils, and activation of the cell leads to their rapid expression on the cell surface.

Cytokine Receptors

Mononuclear phagocytes have receptors for many cytokines that modify their behavior. These include receptors for chemoattractants, CSFs, IL-1, IL-2, IL-4, IL-6, IL-13, IFN-α and IFN-γ, TGF-β, and PDGF.[30, 56] The IL-1 receptor on monocytes is immunologically distinct from that on T lymphocytes and is up-regulated in a synergistic fashion by dexamethasone and prostaglandin E_2.[57] Monocytes respond to IL-1 by up-regulating endogenous IL-1 production and by producing cyclooxygenase metabolites of arachidonic acid. The IL-6 receptor is conserved between monocytes, T cells, and B cells. IL-1 and IL-6 down-regulate IL-6 receptor mRNA levels in monocytes.[58] Low-affinity and high-affinity IL-2 receptors are found on stimulated but not resting macrophages.[59] They are up-regulated by lipopolysaccharide and IFN-γ. Stimulation of IL-2 leads to a respiratory burst by activated macrophages.[59]

The effects of TGF-β illustrate that the state of monocyte activation often determines its response to cytokines. Thus, TGF-β up-regulates the expression of FcRIII in monocytes, thereby modulating phagocytosis, and stimulates production of IL-1, TNF-α, IL-6, and additional TGF-β by resting monocytes. In contrast, TGF-β inhibits the release of these cytokines by activated monocytes.[60] Furthermore, autoregulation of TGF-β production may provide a negative feedback loop by which monocytes are able to limit their own activity and, therefore, host damage. TGF-β_1 and TGF-β_2 also inhibit production of reactive oxygen and reactive nitrogen intermediates (ROIs and RNIs) by macrophages.

G-CSF and M-CSF, but not other cytokines, are up-regulated by IL-4 in resting human monocytes.[60] In contrast, IL-4 suppresses cytokine production by activated monocytes. IL-4 also down-regulates the expression of CD14 on human monocytes.[61] Similarly, IL-4 exhibits suppressive activity on RNI and ROI production.[60]

In contrast, IL-10, which is secreted by a variety of cells, including macrophages and T cells, down-regulates macrophage cytokine production at the mRNA level in a much more uniform manner compared with TGF-β and IL-4.[60] Furthermore, the production of IL-10 is autoregulated by macrophages.[60, 62] Production of ROIs and RNIs is markedly suppressed by IL-10 in human monocytes. Much higher concentrations of IL-10 are required for suppression of ROI and RNI production than for inhibition of TNF-α or IL-1 expression.[60, 63] Thus, depending on the prevailing IL-10 concentration, macrophages can be influenced either to limit T cell responses (low levels of IL-10) or to become permissive to the growth of microbial pathogens and tumor cells (high levels of IL-10).

IL-13, synthesized by activated T cells, prolongs human monocyte survival in culture and alters their morphology and phenotype.[64] Like IL-4, IL-13 suppresses the production of proinflammatory cytokines and hematopoietic growth factors by activated monocytes.[64, 65]

Hormone and Other Biologic Messenger Receptors

Mononuclear phagocytes express receptors for polypeptide hormones, bioactive lipids, and other biologically active substances.[56] Many of these have the capacity to regulate the function of mononuclear phagocytes. Insulin suppresses expression of Fc receptors. Glucocorticoids may exert their anti-inflammatory effects by inhibition of phospholipase A_2 activity and thus the synthesis of prostaglandins. In addition, they may inhibit IL-1 secretion, proteinase secretion, and the response to IFN-γ. Calcitriol facilitates monocyte maturation. It thus exerts a paracrine effect on differentiated monocytes and macrophages, which are present at the sites of granulomata, where calcitriol is produced by macrophage 1α-hydroxylase activity. Phorbol esters augment many macrophage functions by directly activating protein kinase C. Prostaglandins of the E series diminish phagocytic potential, decrease MHC class II expression, and decrease the secretion of IL-1 and TNF-α.[66]

Secretory Products

Mononuclear phagocytes secrete a variety of substances either constitutively or after a specific stimulus, such as a cell surface receptor-ligand interaction. The array of products secreted by macrophages is determined by their stage of differentiation, local environmental influences, and state of activation. Substances released by macrophages are shown in Table 8–6. It is clear that macrophages produce diverse sub-

Table 8–6. SECRETORY PRODUCTS OF MACROPHAGES

Polypeptide Hormones

Interleukin-1α and β (IL-1)
Interleukin-1 receptor antagonist (IL-1ra)
Interleukin-6 (IL-6)
Interleukin-10 (IL-10)
Interleukin-12 (IL-12)
Interleukin-15 (IL-15)
Tumor necrosis factor-α (TNF-α)
Interferon-α
Neutrophil activating factor
Transforming growth factor-β (TGF-β)
Transforming growth factor α
Platelet-derived growth factor (PDGF)
Fibroblast growth factor (FGF)
Fibroblast activating factor
Plasmacytoma growth factor
Thymosin B4
Insulin-like growth factor-1 (somatomedin-C)
Somatotropin
Erythropoietin
Colony-stimulating factor for granulocytes and macrophages (GM-CSF)
Colony stimulating factor for macrophages (M-CSF, CSF-1)
Colony stimulating factor for granulocytes (G-CSF)
Factor increasing monocytopoiesis (FIM)
Macrophage inflammatory proteins (MIP): 1α, 1β, 2
Monocyte chemotactic and activating factor (MCAF)/monocyte chemoattractant protein-1 (MCP-1)
Erythroid colony-potentiating factor/tissue inhibitor of metalloproteinases (TIMP)
Adrenocorticotrophic hormone (ACTH)
β-Endorphin
Bombesin
Substance P

Complement (C) Components

Classical pathway: C1, C2, C3, C4, C5, C6, C7, C8, C9; active component fragments generated by macrophage proteinases: C3a, C3b, C5a, Bb
Alternative pathway: factor B, factor D, properdin
Inhibitors: factor I (of C3b), factor H (β-1H)

Coagulation Factors

Intrinsic pathway: IX, X, V, prothrombin
Extrinsic pathway: VII
Surface activities: tissue factor, prothrombinase
Antithrombolytic: plasminogen activator, inhibitor-2, plasmin inhibitors

Proteolytic Enzymes

Metalloproteases: macrophage elastase, collagenase, stromelysin, 92-kD and 68-kD gelatinase, angiotensin convertase
Serine proteases: urokinase-type plasminogen activator (UPA), cytolytic proteinase
Aspartyl proteases: cathepsin D
Cystein protease: cathepsin L, cathepsin B

Other Enzymes

Lipases: lipoprotein lipase, phospholipase
Glucosaminidase: lysozyme
Lysosomal acid hydrolases: proteases, lipases, (deoxy)ribonucleases, phosphatases, glycosidases, sulfatases (~40)
Deaminase: arginase

Inhibitors of Enzymes

Protease inhibitors: α₂-macroglobulin, α₁-protease inhibitor (α₁-PI)/α₁-antitrypsin, plasminogen activator inhibitor-2 (PAI-2), plasmin inhibitors, TIMP/collagenase inhibitor
Phospholipase inhibitor: lipomodulin (macrocortin)

Proteins of Extracellular Matrix or Cell Adhesion

Fibronectin
Gelatin binding protein/92-kD gelatinase
Thrombospondin
Chondroitin sulfate proteoglycans
Heparin sulfate proteoglycans

Other Binding Proteins

For metals: transferrin, acidic isoferrins
For vitamins: transcobalamin II
For lipids: apolipoprotein E, lipid transfer protein
For growth factors: α₂-macroglobulin, IL-1
For inhibitors: TGF-β–binding protein
For biotin: avidin

Bioactive Lipids

Cyclooxygenase products: prostaglandin E₂ (PGE₂)
Prostaglandin F₂α, prostacyclin (PGI₂), thromboxane
Lipoxygenase products: monohydroxyeicosatetraenoic acids (HETE), leukotrienes (LT), B4, C, D, E
Platelet-activating factors (PAF):1-O alkyl-2-acetyl-sn-glyceryl-3-phosphocholine

Other Bioactive Low-Molecular-Weight Substances

Oligopeptides: glutathione
Steroid hormones: 1α25-dihydroxyvitamin D₃
Purine and pyrimidine products: thymidine, uracil, uric acid, deoxycytidine, cyclic adenosine monophosphate (cAMP), neopterin
Reactive oxygen intermediates (ROIs): superoxide, hydrogen peroxide, hydroxyl radical, singlet oxygen, hypohalous acids
Reactive nitrogen intermediates (RNIs): nitric oxide (NO), nitrites, nitrates

Adapted from Rappolee DA, Werb Z: Secretory products of phagocytes. Curr Opin Immunol 1:47,1988.

stances with potentially opposing or complementary effects on the organism.

Enzymes

The lysosomal acid hydrolases of macrophages are involved primarily in intracellular digestion; however, macrophages may also be stimulated to release these enzymes selectively into the environmental milieu. Phagocytosis of particles, such as latex particles or erythrocytes, induces the release of about 10 to 25 percent of the macrophage's lysosomal granules, whereas ingested streptococcal cell walls, zymosan, or asbestos induces the release of up to 80 percent of the lysosomal enzymes into the extracellular environment. Lysosomal release may also be induced by interaction of macrophages with immune complexes or IFN-γ.[67]

Lysozyme is the major secretory product of the macrophage. It is a cationic protein that hydrolyzes N-acetyl muramic beta-1,4-N-acetyl glucosamine linkages in bacterial cell walls, leading to lysis of susceptible organisms. The synthesis and secretion of a number of neutral proteinases (see Table 8–6) are inducible in activated macrophages and are markedly stimulated by phagocytosis.[68] Up to 75 percent of the newly synthesized enzymes are secreted into the extracellular fluid.

Enzyme and Cytokine Inhibitors

Cultured human monocytes secrete products that are inhibitory to enzymes and cytokines and that play a role in autocrine regulation. Enzyme inhibitors include α_2-macroglobulin, a protease inhibitor of lysosomal hydrolases, plasminogen activator, elastase, and collagenase. When α_2-macroglobulin-protease complexes bind to the α_2-macroglobulin receptor, secretion of neutral proteases is shut off.[69] The regulation of this reciprocal secretion of active enzymes and enzyme inhibitors remains to be delineated.

Activated human monocytes secrete an inhibitor of IL-1, known as *IL-1 receptor antagonist* (IL-1ra).[70, 71] It is a 22-kD secreted protein with some homology to IL-1 that acts by competitively inhibiting IL-1 binding to the type I IL-1 receptor. IL-1ra may have utility as an anti-inflammatory agent. The production of IL-1ra by lipopolysaccharide (LPS)–stimulated monocytes is increased by the cytokines IL-4, IL-10, and IL-13 and may partially explain their anti-inflammatory effects.[60, 65] TGF-β and prostaglandin E_2 also inhibit the effects of IL-1. Of note, both IL-1 and tumor necrosis factor (TNF) induce prostaglandin synthesis by macrophages and other cell types.[72] Macrophages are capable of synthesizing the whole spectrum of lipoxygenase (leukotriene) and cyclooxygenase (prostaglandin) products. This differs from other cells, which tend to be more specialized. The specific spectrum synthesized by a macrophage population at any one time depends on the following[73]:

• The nature of the stimulus
• The tissue of origin of the cells
• Their stage of cellular activity

Simple Functions

Phagocytosis

Phagocytosis is an essential component of many complex functions, such as tissue remodeling, wound healing, microbial destruction, and clearance of senescent or dead cells, particulate debris, and biologically active molecules. The most critical step in phagocytosis is the cell's ability to discriminate between normal self and damaged self or foreign particles. This recog-

nition and attachment process is mediated primarily through cell surface receptors. In the case of bacteria, opsonins function by binding specifically to bacterial surface molecules as well as to the macrophage receptors.

There are two types of opsonin:[74]

• The C3b and C3bi fragments of C3
• Antimicrobial IgG (and other immunoglobulins)

Receptors for immunoglobulin, complement, and fibronectin bind particles complexed with these opsonins. Marked synergy exists between the opsonins, in that particle-bound C3 can markedly reduce the amount of IgG necessary to induce phagocytosis. Only activated macrophages can ingest particles opsonized by C3 alone.[54] Other receptors, such as those for mannose or fucose-terminal glycoproteins and acetylated proteins, bind ligands directly. A nonspecific particle receptor has also been defined on the surface of macrophages.

Binding of a particle to the macrophage membrane leads to initiation of ingestion. The cytoplasm extends to form pseudopodia, which spread to surround the particle. The pseudopodia fuse on the distal side of the particle, resulting in the formation of a phagocytic vesicle or phagosome. The lining of this vacuole is composed of inverted plasma membrane. The vesicle buds off from the cell periphery and migrates to the cytoplasm. Initial binding of a particle to the macrophage surface, even after opsonization with IgG antibody, does not always trigger ingestion. Rather, for IgG-opsonized particles, a "zipper-like" mechanism seems to be involved. Phagocytosis of a particle requires initial attachment of the particle to the Fc receptor, followed by sequential attachment of sites on the particle to adjacent macrophage Fc receptors. In this way, the macrophage membrane is guided around the particle. Phagocytosis of one particle does not trigger ingestion of other particles attached to the macrophage surface.

Pinocytosis

Materials not specifically bound to the plasma membrane are taken up as simple solutes, in a process called *fluid phase pinocytosis*.[75] Compounds bound to the membrane are concentrated at that site and are interiorized to a greater extent. The clathrin-coated pit is the main port of entry of pinocytosed ligands.[75] Both occupied and unoccupied receptors are internalized by clathrin-coated pits. Very rapidly, the internalized vesicles lose their coats (referred to as *early endosomes*) and are capable of fusing with one another. Within minutes, these are converted into a *sorting endosome*, where the fate of receptors and ligands is decided. Some molecules recycle back to the surface in recycling endosomes, whereas others are directed to the lysosome in *late endosomes*. The late endosome fuses with the lysosome.[76]

Fluid-phase pinocytosis and hormone-stimulated endocytosis can also occur in the absence of coated pits. The uptake of soluble immune complexes provides an example of such pinocytosis. These are bound by macrophage FcR and thus are interiorized at a markedly accentuated rate compared with that of soluble protein alone.

Intracellular Digestion

Fusion of endocytic vacuoles with primary or secondary lysosomes initiates the process of intracellular digestion, which results in the degradation of internalized microorganisms or other ingested materials. Intracellular vacuoles are able to exchange their contents by means of membrane fusion. This leads to a constant exchange of digestive enzymes and materials from the extracellular environment.

Intracellular digestion is an enzymatic process that uses preformed lysosomal hydrolases. Acid hydrolases are synthesized in the endoplasmic reticulum and stored within the cell in primary and secondary lysosomes. Endocytosis of a number of materials leads to an increase in the level of intracellular macrophage lysosomal hydrolases and other enzymes.[77]

Materials that are endocytosed by macrophages usually do not regain access to the external environment in an undigested form unless the macrophage is killed.[78] Following uptake, nondigestible materials, such as colloidal gold and certain bacterial constituents, are stored within secondary lysosomes of the macrophages, where they remain for long periods.

Complex Functions

Complex functions of mononuclear phagocytes include the following:

- Selective removal of senescent autologous cells
- Resistance to bacterial and viral infections
- Protection against the development and spread of neoplastic cells
- Initiation and regulation of immune responses

Antimicrobial Function

Several lines of evidence suggest that one of the major antimicrobial mechanisms by mononuclear phagocytes is the production of reactive nitrogen intermediates (RNIs). Nitric oxide (NO) is a particularly important mediator of the antimicrobial activity in at least murine macrophages.[79, 80] Nitric oxide synthase (NOS) exists in *constitutive* and *inducible* forms. The constitutive form leads to production of brief pulses of low to intermediate amounts of nitric oxide that mediate physiologic functions via an increase in cyclic guanosine monophosphate (cGMP) levels in target cells. In contrast, when induced by immunologic stimuli (e.g., LPS, IFN-γ, and TNF-α), inducible nitric oxide synthase produces large amounts of nitric oxide over longer phases. High levels of nitric oxide increase cGMP levels but also inactivate various iron-sulfur (Fe-S)–containing enzymes, leading to metabolic failure and thus cell death.[81] Although nitric oxide produced by murine macrophages is an important cytotoxic defense molecule, controversy remains as to the importance of nitric oxide in human macrophage microbicidal activity.[81]

Reactive oxygen intermediates (ROIs) are also an important antimicrobial effector system.[82] The susceptibility of an organism to killing is directly related to its ability to trigger the secretion of oxygen metabolites during its ingestion and is inversely related to its level of antioxidant defense pathways. Oxygen metabolites mediate cell injury by disrupting the structure of proteins, lipids, and nucleic acids and by activating thiol groups in enzymes. Oxygen-independent antimicrobial mechanisms include[82–84]:

- Growth inhibition by acidification of the phagosome
- Iron removal by iron-binding proteins
- Action of cationic proteins, IFN, and complement components
- Digestion by lysozyme and lysosomal hydrolases

Macrophage Activation

Monocytes or macrophages recruited in response to injury or infection are less mature than resident macrophages but are able to generate a respiratory burst, produce ROIs, release secretory products, and exhibit enhancement in phagocytosis and microbicidal and tumoricidal activities.[85] This is as a result of activation by cytokines produced at the inflammatory site and by microbial products, such as LPS and muramyl dipeptide. The most important macrophage-activating cytokine is IFN-γ, secreted by T cells. Other cytokines, including GM-CSF and TNF-α, induce generation of ROI and RNI by macrophages. TNF-α and IL-4 independently synergize with IFN-γ for macrophage activation in parasitic killing.[86] Concomitant with the development of the activated state, other functions, such as the ability to multiply, may be lost. Some resident macrophages are selectively refractory to the actions of IFN-γ. Thus, Kupffer cells fail to generate a respiratory burst after IFN-γ, although class II MHC antigen expression is enhanced.

The term "macrophage activation" refers to the development by macrophages of enhanced microbicidal function.[4] Although this phenomenon is induced primarily by IFN-γ,[87] this cytokine can either up-regulate or down-regulate many functional, metabolic, and morphologic properties of macrophages, only some of which are involved in enhanced antimicrobial function. Thus, some investigators consider macrophage activation to encompass all the cellular effects of IFN-γ. The concept of macrophage activation is further complicated by the finding that factors other than IFN-γ, such as IL-2, IL-4, IL-13, and GM-CSF, can mimic or enhance its action on macrophages. Consequently, there is no current consensus on the definition of macrophage activation, except that it is a differentiation stage of heightened functional competence.

Three murine macrophage inflammatory proteins (MIP-1α, MIP-1β, and MIP-2) are secreted by LPS-stimulated macrophages.[18] All cause a localized inflammatory reaction, are chemotactic for and activate human neutrophils in vitro, and synergize with GM-CSF or M-CSF (but not G-CSF) to stimulate hemopoietic colony formation. MIP-1α/β can act as endogenous pyrogens.[18, 88] Both MIP-1α and MIP-1β are also members of the chemokine β subfamily. MIP-2 is a member of the chemokine subfamily, which also includes platelet factor 4 and IL-8, and is chemotactic for monocytes.[17, 18, 65] IL-8 is produced by LPS-stimulated macrophages. Both IL-8 and platelet factor 4 are chemotactic for neutrophils.[18, 88, 89] Thus, these chemokines, secreted by stimulated macrophages and other cells at the site of inflammation, are important attractors of activated macrophages and neutrophils to these sites.

Antiviral Function

Mononuclear phagocytes are important in host defense against viral infection. Host susceptibility to a number of viruses is related to its ability to replicate within the mononuclear phagocytes. Newborn mice, for example, are highly susceptible to herpes simplex infection, which can replicate in the macrophages of newborn mice.[90] On the other hand, pathogens that resist intracellular killing can use macrophage Fc and C3 receptors to gain entry into the macrophage and then commence replication unchecked. In the presence of subneutralizing amounts of antiviral antibodies, this phenomenon is known as *antibody-dependent enhancement* (ADE) of viral infectivity.[91]

An important example is the entry of human immunodeficiency virus (HIV) I into macrophages via human FcRII and FcRIII.[92] Macrophages may also become infected with HIV via the CD4 receptor, as in T cells.[93] Infected macrophages and dendritic cells are crucial in the pathogenesis of acquired immunodeficiency syndrome (AIDS).[94] Infected macrophages may act as major, persistent, fixed reservoirs of HIV, infecting CD4+ T cells as they recirculate by attracting and presenting viral proteins to them. IL-13 in vitro inhibits HIV replication in human monocytes but not in T cells.[64, 95] In contrast, IL-4, TGF-β, and IFN paradoxically both suppress and enhance HIV replication in monocytes and macrophages.[95]

Antineoplastic Function

Large numbers of macrophages are commonly found within tumors. The number can be influenced by the nature of the tumor; that is, some tumors produce chemotactic factors or CSFs, whereas others secrete substances preventing macrophage activation,

chemotaxis-inhibiting factors, lymphokines, or complement.[96]

Young mononuclear phagocytes, such as inflammatory macrophages, but not resident tissue macrophages, acquire competence to lyse neoplastic cells in a contact-dependent, nonphagocytic manner. In the first stage of this process, macrophages interact with IFN-γ and thereby gain responsiveness to a second signal, such as the lipid A component of bacterial endotoxin or maleylated proteins.[69] Interferon-γ renders macrophages capable of selectively binding tumor cells but not lysing them. Cytolytic competence is acquired only after full activation by the triggering stimuli.

Other factors, which may or may not be secreted by mononuclear phagocytes themselves, can prime the macrophage for cytolytic competence. Interferon-γ and TNF-α are synergistic in their induction of tumoricidal activity in macrophages. Prostaglandin E_2 stimulates tumoricidal activity in activated macrophages but depresses antitumor effects in resident macrophages.[97] TGF-β also suppresses the tumoricidal activity of macrophages.[60] Somatotropin is as effective as IFN-γ in priming macrophages for superoxide production. Finally, the macrophage products hydrogen peroxide,[82] nitric oxide,[98] and the complement components[99] are important in tumoricidal killing.

Another antineoplastic mechanism involves antibody coating ("arming") of tumor cells. Antibody-coated tumor cells can interact with Fc receptors on activated macrophages and thereby trigger the release of RNIs, ROIs, hydrogen peroxide, and lysosomal enzymes, which either kill tumor cells or limit their growth.[100]

DENDRITIC CELLS

A number of characteristic features distinguish the specialized (or professional) antigen-presenting cells (APCs) known as dendritic cells (DCs) from monocytes and macrophages. These include long dendritic processes, exceptional motility, lack of macrophage-specific cell surface markers, limited phagocytic capacity, and the ability to present antigen to T cells in the primary immune response.[101]

The dendritic cell is one of the most potent APCs to be described. Dendritic cells have therefore been defined functionally as APCs with the ability to activate resting T cells.[102] Although first identified in lymphoid organs, cells with these features have since been isolated from many nonlymphoid tissues in both rodents and humans. These include skin (Langerhans cells), lung, circulating blood, and rheumatoid synovium.[103–105] Dendritic cells constitute 1 to 2 percent of the mononuclear cells in most fluids and tissues in which they have been identified.[101]

Despite the differences between dendritic cells and mononuclear phagocytes, accumulating evidence demonstrates that dendritic cells belong to the myeloid lineage and dendritic cells and monocytes derive from a common myeloid precursor. Although dendritic cell differentiation from CD34$^+$ multipotential stem cells in bone marrow is enhanced by GM-CSF and TNF in humans,[106] other factors also appear to lead to dendritic cell differentiation. Thus, dendritic cells have been cultured from adherent human blood mononuclear cells in the presence of GM-CSF and IL-4.[107] Furthermore, mice that have had the GM-CSF gene inactivated have normal numbers of monocytes, granulocytes, and dendritic cells in peripheral tissues, which suggests that GM-CSF is not essential for the development of myeloid lineage cells.[108] Blood and skin dendritic cells and precursors express myeloid lineage markers, including CD13 and CD33.[105] Thus, dendritic cells can be identified among circulating human non–T cells as CD13$^+$ CD33$^+$ CD14$^-$ cells.[105]

After maturation in the bone marrow, dendritic cells circulate in blood as precursors that, when isolated by cell sorting, are round in shape and express relatively modest amounts of MHC and adhesion molecules. However, they differentiate in culture into cells with the typical morphologic, functional, and phenotypic features of mature dendritic cells.[105] Circulating mature dendritic cells make up just 0.1 percent of mononuclear cells and can be identified by their expression of CD11c as well as a greater expression of CD33, MHC, and adhesion molecules than by dendritic cell precursors.[109, 110]

GM-CSF in vitro is essential for the maturation and development of potent APC function of Langerhans cells, and it up-regulates the APC function of other dendritic cells.[103, 111] In vivo antigen administration or exposure, likely in the context of local inflammation and cytokine secretion, leads to the differentiation of Langerhans cells similar to that noted after in vitro culture with GM-CSF.

IMMUNOREGULATION

Antigens enter macrophages and dendritic cells by fluid phase pinocytosis (Fig. 8–3). In contrast to macrophages, mature dendritic cells show little or no phagocytic capacity.[101] However, mouse bone marrow dendritic cell precursors and freshly isolated Langerhans cells are phagocytically active before their differentiation into functional APCs.[112] Particularly in the case of macrophages, antigen may be taken up by absorptive endocytosis following the interaction of antigen with receptors on the surface of the cell, and antigen uptake is augmented by IgG Fc receptor binding in the presence of IgG.[113] Autologous, homologous, and heterologous proteins are taken up in a similar manner, indicating that foreignness per se is not recognized by APCs.[114] In some cases, soluble antigen may be derived from macrophages regurgitating particulate matter. Endocytosed antigens meet newly synthesized class II MHC molecules in an acidic endosomal compartment and are transported to the plasma membrane via the Golgi apparatus and its vesicles.[115] Expression of the peptide MHC complex is associated with dendritic cell differentiation and migration. Thus, after taking up antigen applied topically, Langerhans cells migrate from the epidermis to local lymph nodes via the afferent lymphatics and there prime antigen-specific proliferative and cytotoxic responses in naive T cells.[116–118]

An alternative, cytosolic processing pathway exists for proteins that are endogenously synthesized or penetrate plasma or endosomal membranes. Endogenous synthesis of viral proteins within the target cell and the fusion of a virus with cell membranes are examples of this process. These determinants typically associate with class I MHC molecules.[115]

Class I molecules consist of a highly polymorphic glycoprotein chain noncovalently bound to β_2-microglobulin. Class II molecules consist of two noncovalently bound membrane glycoproteins (α and β), at least one of which is polymorphic. Crystallographic analysis of the structure of class I and II molecules reveals a groove at the surface of the molecule formed by the two amino terminal domains to which antigenic peptide binds.[119, 120]

The expression of class II MHC molecules can be up-regulated by macrophages in response to IFN-γ as well as IL-4, IL-13, and GM-CSF.[60, 65, 121] In contrast, prostaglandins of the E series, IFN-α, TGF-β_1, IL-6, IL-10, LPS, glucocorticoids, and maleylated proteins in the α_2-macroglobulin protease complex are known inhibitors of MHC class II expression.[121, 122] TNF-α down-regulates macrophage class II expression to a moderate degree, mostly by suppression of transcription.

Of the other tissue macrophages, Kupffer cells constitutively express class I and class II MHC molecules and can function as APCs.[123] Microglial cells can also express class II MHC molecules and function as APCs after exposure to IFN-γ.[124] In contrast, alveolar macrophages have poor antigen-presenting ability. Some resident tissue (e.g., lung and liver) macrophages that express class II antigens are inadequate APCs for resting T cells.[125, 126] T cell activation requires physical interaction between the T cell receptor (TCR) and processed antigen presented by the MHC molecule of the APC. Signals thus generated may be transduced to T cells via CD3—a molecular complex of at least five components that is noncovalently linked to the TCR.[127] In addition to the interaction between the processed antigen–class II complex on the macrophage and the antigen receptor on the T cell, other accessory activation signals to resting T cells are required.[128] These involve a variety of T cell surface molecules and their macrophage ligands, including CD28/CD80, CD86, CD4/class II, LFA-1/ICAM-1, -2, -3, and CD2/LFA-3.[128]

Other molecules may also act as accessory molecules (Fig. 8–3). For example, monocyte-derived cytokines, including IL-1, IL-6, and TNF-α, costimulate by enhancing responses of T cells.[129] Macrophages that possess all or even some of the properties of a

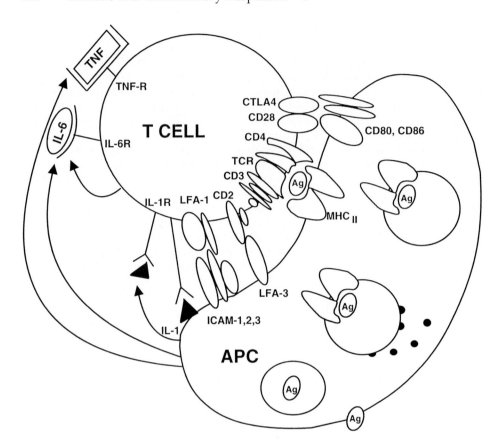

Figure 8–3. Mononuclear phagocytes as antigen-presenting cells (APCs). Mononuclear phagocytes endocytose and then process foreign antigen (Ag), which associates with class II major histocompatibility complex (MHC) molecules (MHC$_{II}$) in the endosome. T cell stimulation requires physical interaction between the class II–Ag complex and the T cell receptor (TCR). During this interaction, a variety of receptor ligand interactions transmit costimulatory signals that enhance T cell activation. In addition, cytokines produced by mononuclear phagocytes enhance T cell responses. ICAM, intercellular adhesion molecule; TNF, tumor necrosis factor; IL, interleukin; LFA, leukocyte function–associated molecule.

complete APC are capable of facilitating the function for such incomplete APCs.[130] Macrophages can also play an auxiliary role in antigen presentation to resting T cells through their roles as accessory cells and in the secretion of cytokines that stimulate dendritic cell differentiation and activation.

The potent APC function of dendritic cells derives in part from their dense expression of MHC class I and II molecules, integrins, and adhesion molecules.[101, 131–133] Expression of the B7 family of molecules (CD80, CD86), the costimulatory ligands for CD28 on T cells, increases after in vitro maturation of human and mouse dendritic cells.[131, 134] CD28 ligands, although not expressed by dendritic cell precursors, plays an important role in the accessory function of differentiated dendritic cells and monocytes.[111, 131, 135] However, the expression of MHC molecules or their bound peptides is likely to be of major importance in the markedly enhanced capacity of dendritic cells to act as APCs for resting T cells.[131]

Several secretory products of macrophages are involved in immunoregulation. This can occur by interaction of macrophage secretory products with either dendritic cell or T cells. Thus, secretory products of macrophage subsets may either enhance or downregulate dendritic cell function. GM-CSF and IL-1 upregulate the APC function of dendritic cells,[136] whereas IL-10 down-regulates dendritic cell MHC molecule and B7 expression as well as their APC function. In the mouse, nitric oxide derived from a subset of alveolar macrophages may serve to prevent dendritic cell activation under normal physiologic conditions.[137] IL-1 was the first example of a macrophage-derived cytokine involved in the initiation and propagation of immune responses by its effects on T cells.[138] IL-1 enhances IL-2 and IFN-γ production, induces IL-2 receptors on T cells, and augments cytotoxic T cell activity. TNF-α may augment T cell responsiveness to antigen directly or via stimulation of other cytokines, such as IL-6.[139, 140] TNF-α may also enhance or diminish the capacity of macrophages to initiate T cell responses by stimulating them to produce IL-1 or prostaglandin E$_2$, respectively.[72] Thus, macrophage products that suppress T cell activation directly or indirectly include prostaglandin, hydrogen peroxide, arginase, ROIs, nitric oxide, and IL-1ra.[70, 71, 82, 83] IL-10 is a potent inhibitor of T cell IL-2 production by a direct effect as well as indirectly through the inhibition of antigen presentation and accessory cell functions of macrophages and dendritic cells and, thereby, T cell stimulation.[62]

Finally, macrophages may be important in the control of T helper (Th1) cell subtype differentiation. In the mouse, IL-12 secreted by macrophages may direct the development of uncommitted, naive T cells toward the T$_H$1 subtype, thus contributing to cell-mediated immunity.[141] This occurs both as a direct action of IL-12, as well as by increasing the production of IFN-γ, which promotes Th1 subtype differentiation. The Th2 products IL-4, IL-10, and IL-13 all inhibit the generation of IL-12 by human monocytes, thus suppressing Th1 and enhancing Th2 development.[64, 65, 142]

CONCLUSIONS

The mononuclear phagocyte system is a dynamic collection of lineally related cells whose functions are extremely varied and critical to normal homeostasis and host defense. Mononuclear phagocytes participate in a variety of physiologic and pathologic events. This ability relies on their capacity to respond to environmental stimuli with an increase in maturation of effector cells, enhancement of tissue migration, and functional modulation of individual cells to meet the immediate needs of the organism.

References

1. Unanue ER, Allen PM: The basis for the immunoregulatory role of macrophages and other accessory cells. Science 236:551, 1987.
2. Stashenko P, Dewhirst FE, Peros WJ, et al: Synergistic interactions between interleukin 1, tumor necrosis factor, and lymphotoxin in bone resorption. J Immunol 138:1464, 1987.
3. Varesio L: Induction and expression of tumoricidal activity by macrophages. In Dean RT, Jessup W (eds): Mononuclear Phagocytes: Physiology and Pathology. Amsterdam, Elsevier, 1985.
4. Metchnikoff E: Lectures on the comparative pathology of inflammation. In Starling FA, Starling EH (eds): London, Kegan, Paul, Trench, Treubner and Company, 1883.
5. van-Furth R, Langevoort HL, Schaberg A: Mononuclear phagocytes in human pathology: Proposal for an approach to improved classification. In van-Furth R (ed): Mononuclear Phagocytes in Immunity, Infection and Pathology. Oxford, Blackwell Scientific Publications, 1975.
6. van-Furth R, Cohn ZA, Hirsch JG, et al: The mononuclear phagocyte system: A new classification of macrophages, monocytes, and their precursor cells. Bull WHO 46:845, 1972.
7. van-Furth R: Macrophage activity and clinical immunology: Origin and kinetics of mononuclear phagocytes. Ann N Y Acad Sci 278:161, 1976.
8. Harlan JM: Leukocyte-endothelial interactions. Blood 65:513, 1985.
9. Albelda SM, Buck CA: Integrins and other cell adhesion molecules. FASEB J 4:2868, 1990.
10. Wawryk SO, Novotny JR, Wicks IP, et al: The role of the LFA-1/ICAM-1 interaction in human leukocyte homing and adhesion. Immunol Rev 108:135, 1989.
11. Stacker SA, Springer TA: Leukocyte integrin p150,95 (CD11c/CD18) functions as an adhesion molecule binding to a counter-receptor on stimulated endothelium. J Immunol 146:648, 1991.
12. Dana N, Arnaout MA: Leukocyte adhesion molecular (CD11/CD18) deficiency. In Kazatchine M (ed): Balliere's Clinical Immunology and Allergy. Philadelphia, WB Saunders, 1988.
13. Kishimoto TK, Jutila MA, Berg EL, et al: Neutrophil Mac-1 and MEL-14 adhesion proteins inversely regulated by chemotactic factors. Science 245:1238, 1989.
14. Muller WA, Weigl SA, Deng X, et al: PECAM-1 is required for transendothelial migration of leukocytes. J Exp Med 178:449, 1993.
15. Bevilacqua MP, Nelson RM: Selectins. J Clin Invest 91:379, 1993.
16. Etzioni A, Frydman M, Pollack S, et al: Brief report: Recurrent severe infections caused by a novel leukocyte deficiency. N Engl J Med 327:1789, 1992.
17. Miller MD, Krangel MS: Biology and biochemistry of the chemokines: A family of chemotactic and inflammatory cytokines. Crit Rev Immunol 12:17, 1992.
18. Oppenheim JJ, Zachariae CO, Mukaida N, et al: Properties of the novel proinflammatory supergene "intercrine" cytokine family. Annu Rev Immunol 9:617, 1991.
19. Weiser WY, Temple PA, Witek-Giannotti JS, et al: Molecular cloning of a cDNA encoding a human macrophage migration inhibitory factor. Proc Natl Acad Sci USA 86:7522, 1989.
20. Skeel A, Leonard EJ: Action and target cell specificity of human macrophage stimulating protein (MSP). J Immunol 152:4618, 1994.
21. Chatila TA, Geha RS, Arnaout MA: Constitutive and stimulus-induced phosphorylation of CD11/CD18 leukocyte adhesion molecules. J Cell Biol 109:3435, 1989.
22. van-Furth R, Diesselhoff-Den Dulk MMC, Sluiter W, et al: New perspectives on the kinetics of mononuclear phagocytes. In van-Furth R (ed): Mononuclear Phagocytes: Characteristics, Physiology and Function. Dordrecht, The Netherlands, Martinus Nijhoff, 1985.
23. Bouwens L, Baekeland M, Wisse E: A balanced view on the origin of Kupffer cells. In Kirn A, Knook DL, Wisse E (eds): Cells of the Hepatic Sinusoid. Rijswijk, The Netherlands, Kupffer Cell Foundation, 1986.
24. Papadimitriou JM, van Bruggen I: Evidence that multi-nucleate giant cells are examples of mononuclear phagocytic differentiation. J Pathol 148:149, 1986.
25. Kreipe H, Radzun HJ, Rudolph P, et al: Multinucleated giant cells generated in vitro: Terminally differentiated macrophages with down-regulated c-fms expression. Am J Pathol 130:232, 1988.
26. Burmester GR, Dimitriu-Bona A, Waters SJ, et al: Identification of three major synovial lining cell populations by monoclonal antibodies directed to Ia antigens and antigens associated with monocytes/macrophages and fibroblasts. Scand J Immunol 17:69, 1983.
27. Thomas R, Davis LS, Lipsky PE: Rheumatoid synovium is enriched in mature antigen-presenting dendritic cells. J Immunol 152:2613, 1994.
28. Todd RF, Schlossman S: Utilization of monoclonal antibodies in the characterization of monocyte-macrophage differentiation antigens. In Bellanti JA, Herscowitz HB (eds): Immunology of the Reticuloendothelial System: A Comprehensive Treatise. New York, Plenum Press, 1984.
29. Ruef C, Coleman DL: Granulocyte-macrophage colony-stimulating factor: Pleiotropic cytokine with potential clinical usefulness. Rev Infect Dis 12:41, 1990.
30. Metcalf D: The molecular control of cell division, differentiation commitment and maturation in hemopoietic cells. Nature 339:27, 1989.
31. Ikebuchi K, Wong GG, Clark SC, et al: Interleukin-6 enhancement of interleukin-3–dependent proliferation of multipotential hemopoietic progenitors. Proc Natl Acad Sci USA 84:9035, 1987.
32. Katayama K, Koizumi S, Ueno Y, et al: Antagonistic effects of interleukin 6 and G-CSF in the later stage of human granulopoiesis in vitro. Exp Hematol 18:390, 1990.
33. Zsebo KM, Williams DA, Geissler EN, et al: Stem cell factor is encoded at the SI locus of the mouse and is the ligand for the c-kit tyrosine kinase receptor. Cell 63:213, 1990.
34. Jacobsen SEW, Okkenhaug C, Veiby OP, et al: Interleukin 13: Novel role in direct regulation of proliferation and differentiation of primitive hematopoietic progenitors. J Exp Med 180:75, 1994.
35. Walker F, Nicola NA, Metcalf D, et al: Hierarchical down-modulation of hemopoietic growth factor receptors. Cell 43:269, 1985.
36. Sherr CJ, Rettenmier CW, Sacca R, et al: The c-fms proto-oncogene product is related to the receptor for the mononuclear phagocyte growth factor, CSF-1. Cell 41:665, 1985.
37. Stanley ER: Action of the colony-stimulating factor, CSF-1. In Evered D, Nugent J, O'Connor M (eds): Biochemistry of Macrophages. London, Pitman, 1986.
38. Bagby GC, Shaw G, Segal GM: Human vascular endothelial cells, granulopoiesis, and the inflammatory response. J Invest Dermatol 93:48S, 1989.
39. Horiguchi J, Warren MK, Kufe D: Expression of the macrophage-specific colony-stimulating factor in human monocytes treated with granulocyte-macrophage colony-stimulating factor. Blood 69:1259, 1987.
40. Cannistra SA, Griffin JD: Regulation of the production and function of granulocytes and monocytes. Semin Hematol 15:173, 1988.
41. Kelley KW: The role of growth hormone in modulation of the immune response. Ann N Y Acad Sci 594:95, 1990.
42. Alvaro-Gracia JM, Zvaifler NJ, Firestein GS: Cytokines in chronic inflammatory arthritis: IV. Granulocyte/macrophage colony-stimulating factor–mediated induction of class II MHC antigen on human monocytes: A possible role in rheumatoid arthritis. J Exp Med 170:865, 1989.
43. Jones TC: The effects of rhGM-CSF on macrophage function. Eur J Cancer 29A(Suppl 3):S10, 1993.
44. Gerhartz HH, Englehard M, Meusers P, et al: Randomized, double-blind, placebo-controlled phase III trial of recombinant human granulocyte-macrophage colony-stimulating factor as adjunct to induction treatment of high-grade malignant non-Hodgkin's lymphomas. Blood 82:2329, 1993.
45. Sluiter W, Nibbering PH, van-Furth R, et al: Increased activity of FIM in serum of mice during a Mycobacterium bovis (BCG) infection. Immunology 70:327, 1990.
46. Annema A, Sluiter W, van-Furth R: Effect of interleukin 1, macrophage colony-stimulating factor, and factor increasing monocytopoiesis on the production of leukocytes in mice. Exp Hematol 20:69, 1992.
47. Tomida M: Regulation of differentiation of normal and leukemic precursors. In Dean RT, Jessup W (eds): Mononuclear Phagocytes: Physiology and Pathology. Amsterdam, Elsevier, 1985.
48. Thiele DL, Lipsky PE: Mononuclear phagocytes: Phenotype and function. Surv Immunol Res 3:142, 1984.
49. Mellman IS: Relationships between structure and function in the Fc receptor family. Curr Opin Immunol 1:16, 1988.
50. Unkeless JC, Fleit H, Mellman IS: Structural aspects and heterogeneity of immunoglobulin Fc receptors. Adv Immunol 31:247, 1981.

51. Grey HM, Chesnut R: Antigen processing and presentation to T cells. Immunol Today 6:101, 1985.

52. Dierich MP: Complement-dependent ligand receptor interactions in inflammatory respones. *In* Russo F, Mencia-Huerta MJM, Chignard M (eds): Advances in Inflammation Research. New York, Raven Press, 1986.

53. Bodmer JL: Membrane receptors for particles and opsonins. *In* Dean RT, Jessup W (eds): Mononuclear Phagocytes: Physiology and Pathology. Amsterdam, Elsevier, 1985.

54. Griffin FM Jr: Activation of macrophage complement receptors for phagocytosis. Contemp Top Immunobiol 13:57, 1984.

55. Elices MJ, Osborn L, Takada Y, et al: VCAM-1 on activated endothelium interacts with the leukocyte integrin VLA-4 at a site distinct from the VLA-4/fibronectin binding site. Cell 60:577, 1990.

56. Adams DO, Hamilton TA: Phagocytic cells: Cytotoxic activities of macrophages. *In* Gallin JI, Goldstein R, Snyderman R (eds): Inflammation: Basic Principles and Clinical Correlates. New York, Raven Press, 1988.

57. Spriggs MK, Lioubin PJ, Slack J, et al: Induction of an interleukin-1 receptor (IL-1R) on monocytic cells: Evidence that the receptor is not encoded by a T cell-type IL-1R mRNA. J Biol Chem 265:22499, 1990.

58. Bauer J, Bauer TM, Kalb T, et al: Regulation of interleukin 6 receptor expression in human monocytes and monocyte-derived macrophages: Comparison with the expression in human hepatocytes. J Exp Med 170:1537, 1989.

59. Holter W, Goldman CK, Casabo L, et al: Expression of functional IL-2 receptors by lipopolysaccharide and interferon-gamma stimulated human monocytes. J Immunol 138:2917, 1987.

60. Bogdan C, Nathan C: Modulation of macrophage function by transforming growth factor-β, interleukin-4, and interleukin-10. Ann N Y Acad Sci 685:713, 1993.

61. Lauener RP, Goyert SM, Geha RS, et al: Interleukin 4 down-regulates the expression of CD14 in normal human monocytes. Eur J Immunol 20:2375, 1990.

62. Moore KW, O'Garra A, de Waal Malefyt R, et al: Interleukin-10. Annu Rev Immunol 11:165, 1993.

63. Bogdan C, Vodovotz Y, Nathan C: Macrophage deactivation by interleukin 10. J Exp Med 174:1549, 1991.

64. Zurawski G, De Vries JE: Interleukin 13, an interleukin 4-like cytokine that acts on monocytes and B cells, but not on T cells. Immunol Today 15:19, 1994.

65. de Waal Malefyt R, Figdor CG, Huijbens R, et al: Effects of IL-13 on phenotype, cytokine production, and cytotoxic function of human monocytes: Comparison with IL-4 and modulation by IFN-gamma or IL-10. J Immunol 151:6370, 1993.

66. Knudsen PJ, Dinarello CA, Strom TB: Prostaglandins posttranscriptionally inhibit monocyte expression of interleukin 1 activity by increasing intracellular cyclic adenosine monophosphate. J Immunol 137:3189, 1986.

67. Pantalone RM, Page RC: Lymphokine-induced production and release of lysosomal enzymes by macrophages. Proc Natl Acad Sci USA 72:2091, 1975.

68. Gordon S: Regulation of enzyme secretion by mononuclear phagocytes: Studies with macrophage plasminogen activator and lysozyme. Fed Proc 37:2754, 1978.

69. Johnson WJ, Pizzo SV, Imber MJ, et al: Receptors for maleylated proteins regulate secretion of neutral proteases by murine macrophages. Science 218:574, 1982.

70. Arend WP, Joslin FG, Massoni RJ: Effects of immune complexes on production by human monocytes of interleukin 1 or an interleukin 1 inhibitor. J Immunol 134:3868, 1985.

71. Arend WP: Interleukin-1 receptor antagonist. Adv Immunol 54:167, 1993.

72. Bachwich PR, Chensue SW, Larrick JW, et al: Tumor necrosis factor stimulates interleukin-1 and prostaglandin E2 production in resting macrophages. Biochem Biophys Res Commun 136:94, 1986.

73. Schade UF, Burmeister I, Elekes E, et al: Mononuclear phagocytes and eicosanoids: Aspects of their synthesis and biological activities. Blut 59:475, 1989.

74. Ofek I, Sharon N: Lectinophagocytosis: A molecular mechanism of recognition between cell surface sugars and lectins in the phagocytosis of bacteria. Infect Immun 56:539, 1988.

75. Duncan R, Pratten MK: Pinocytosis: Mechanism and regulation. *In* Dean RT, Jessup W (eds): Mononuclear Phagocytes: Physiology and Pathology. Amsterdam, Elsevier, 1985.

76. Kaplan J, Ward DM: Movement of receptors and ligands through the endocytic apparatus in alveolar macrophages. Am J Physiol 258:L263, 1990.

77. Axline SG: Functional biochemistry of the macrophage. Semin Hematol 7:142, 1970.

78. Andrews PW, Jackett PS, Lowrie DB: Killing and degradation of microorganisms by macrophages. *In* Dean RT, Jessup W (eds): Mononuclear Phagocytes: Physiology and Pathology. Amsterdam, Elsevier, 1985.

79. Kolb H, Kolb-Bachofen V: Nitric oxide: A pathogenic factor in autoimmunity. Immunol Today 13:157, 1992.

80. Nathan CF, Hibbs JB: Role of nitric oxide synthesis in macrophage antimicrobial activity. Curr Opin Immunol 3:65, 1991.

81. James SL, Nacy C: Effector functions of activated macrophages against parasites. Curr Opin Immunol 5:518, 1993.

82. Nathan CF: Secretion of toxic oxygen products by macrophages: Regulatory cytokines and their effect on the oxidase. *In* Evered D, Nugent J, O'Connor M (eds): Biochemistry of Macrophages. London, Pitman, 1986.

83. Nathan CF: Secretion of oxygen intermediates: Role in effector functions of activated macrophages. Fed Proc 41:2206, 1982.

84. Rothermel CD, Rubin BY, Jaffe EA, et al: Oxygen-independent inhibition of intracellular *Chlamydia psittaci* growth by human monocytes and interferon-gamma–activated macrophages. J Immunol 137:689, 1986.

85. Nathan CF: Mechanisms of macrophage antimicrobial activity. Trans R Soc Trop Med Hyg 77:620, 1983.

86. Bogdan C, Mol H, Solbach W, et al: Tumor necrosis factor-alpha in combination with interferon-gamma, but not with interleukin-4 activates murine macrophages for elimination of *Leishmania major* amastigotes. Eur J Immunol 20:1131, 1990.

87. Nathan CF: Interferon-gamma and macrophage activation in cell-mediated immunity. *In* Steinman RM, North RJ (eds): Mechanisms of Host Resistance to Infectious Agents, Tumors and Allografts. New York, Rockefeller University Press, 1986.

88. Wolpe SD, Cerami A: Macrophage inflammatory proteins 1 and 2: Members of a novel superfamily of cytokines. FASEB J 3:2565, 1989.

89. Djeu JT, Matsushima K, Oppenheim JJ, et al: Functional activation of human neutrophils by recombinant monocyte-derived neutropil chemotactic factor/IL-8. J Immunol 144:2205, 1990.

90. Hirsch MS, Zisman B, Allison AC: Macrophages and age-dependent resistance to herpes simplex virus in mice. J Immunol 104:1160, 1970.

91. Kauffmann SH, Reddehase MJ: Infection of phagocytic cells. Curr Opin Immunol 2:43, 1989.

92. Homsy J, Meyer M, Tateno M, et al: The Fc and not CD4 receptor mediates antibody enhancement of HIV infection in human cells. Science 244:1357, 1989.

93. Weiss RA: How does HIV cause AIDS? Science 260:1273, 1993.

94. Mosier D, Seiburg H: Macrophage-tropic HIV: Critical for AIDS pathogenesis? Immunol Today 15:332, 1994.

95. Montaner LJ, Doyle AG, Collin M, et al: Interleukin 13 inhibits human immunodeficiency virus type 1 production in primary blood-derived human monocytes in vitro. J Exp Med 178:743, 1993.

96. Lipton JH, Sachs L: Characterization of macrophage- and granulocyte-inducing proteins for normal and leukemic myeloid cells produced by the Krebs ascites tumor. Biochim Biophys Acta 673:552, 1981.

97. Taffet SM, Russell SW: Macrophage-mediated tumor cell killing: Regulation of expression of cytolytic activity by prostaglandin E₂. J Immunol 126:424, 1981.

98. Martin HJJ, Edwards SW: Changes in mechanisms of monocyte/macrophage-mediated cytotoxicity during culture: Reactive oxygen intermediates are involved in monocyte-mediated cytotoxicity, whereas reactive nitrogen intermediates are employed by macrophages in tumor cell killing. J Immunol 150:3478, 1993.

99. Pettersen HB, Johnson E, Hetland G: Human alveolar macrophages synthesize active complement components C6, C7, and C8 in vitro. Scand J Immunol 25:567, 1987.

100. Adams DO, Johnson WJ, Fiorito E, et al: Hydrogen peroxide and cytolytic factor can interact synergistically in effecting cytolysis of neoplastic targets. J Immunol 127:1973, 1981.

101. Steinman RM: The dendritic cell system and its role in immunogenicity. Annu Rev Immunol 9:271, 1991.

102. MacPherson GG: What don't we know about dendritic cells? Res Immunol 140:877, 1989.

103. Schuler G, Steinman RM: Murine epidermal Langerhans cells mature into potent immunostimulatory dendritic cells in vitro. J Exp Med 161:526, 1985.

104. Holt PG, Schon-Hegrad MA, McMenamin PG: Dendritic cells in the respiratory tract. Int Rev Immunol 6:139, 1990.

105. Thomas R, Davis LS, Lipsky PE: Isolation and characterization of human peripheral blood dendritic cells. J Immunol 150:821, 1993.

106. Caux C, Dezutter-Dambuyant C, Schmitt D, et al: GM-CSF and TNF-α cooperate in the generation of dendritic Langerhans cells. Nature 360:258, 1992.

107. Sallusto F, Lanzavecchia A: Efficient presentation of soluble antigen by cultured human dendritic cells is maintained by granulocyte/macrophage colony-stimulating factor plus interleukin 4 and downregulated by tumor necrosis factor-alpha. J Exp Med 179:1109, 1994.

108. Dranoff G, Crawford AD, Sadelain M, et al: Involvement of granulocyte-macrophage colony-stimulating factor in pulmonary homeostasis. Science 264:713, 1994.

109. Thomas R, Lipsky PE: Human peripheral blood dendritic cell subsets: Isolation and characterization of precursor and mature antigen-presenting cells. J Immunol 153:4016, 1994.

110. O'Doherty U, Peng M, Gezelter S, et al: Human peripheral blood con-

tains two dendritic cell subsets: One mature and one immature. Immunology 82:487, 1994.

111. Thomas R, Davis LS, Lipsky PE: Comparative accessory function of human peripheral blood dendritic cells and monocytes. J Immunol 151:6840, 1993.

112. Inaba K, Inaba M, Naito M, et al: Dendritic cell progenitors phagocytose particulates, including Bacillus Calmette-Guérin organisms, and sensitize mice to mycobacterial antigens in vivo. J Exp Med 178:479, 1993.

113. Cohn ZA: Biochemistry of macrophages: The first line of defence—Chairman's introduction. Ciba Found Symp 118:1, 1986.

114. Babbitt BP, Matsueda G, Haber E, et al: Antigenic competition at the level of peptide-Ia binding. Proc Natl Acad Sci USA 83:4509, 1986.

115. Yewdell JW, Bennink JR: The binary logic of antigen processing and presentation to T cells. Cell 62:203, 1990.

116. Cumberbatch M, Illingworth I, Kimber I: Antigen-bearing dendritic cells in the draining lymph nodes of contact sensitized mice: Cluster formation with lymphocytes. Immunology 74:139, 1991.

117. Macatonia SE, Knight SC, Edwards AJ, et al: Localization of antigen on lymph node dendritic cells after exposure to the contact sensitizer fluorescein isothiocyanate. Functional and morphological studies. J Exp Med 166:1654, 1987.

118. Larsen CP, Steinman RM, Witmer-Pack M, et al: Migration and maturation of Langerhans cells in skin transplants and explants. J Exp Med 172:1483, 1990.

119. Bjorkman PJ, Saper MA, Samraoui B, et al: The foreign antigen binding site and T cell recognition regions of class I histocompatibility antigens. Nature 329:512, 1987.

120. Brown JH, Jardetzky TS, Gorga JC, et al: Three-dimensional structure of the human class II histocompatibility antigen HLA-DR1. Nature 364:33, 1993.

121. Stuart PM, Zlotnik A, Woodward JG: Induction of class I and class II MHC antigen expression on murine bone marrow-derived macrophages by IL-4 (B cell stimulatory factor 1). J Immunol 140:1542, 1988.

122. Fertsch D, Schoenberg DR, Germain RN, et al: Induction of macrophage Ia antigen expression by rIFN-gamma and down-regulation by IFN-alpha/beta and dexamethasone are mediated by changes in steady-state levels of Ia mRNA. J Immunol 139:244, 1987.

123. Rogoff TM, Lipsky PE: Role of the Kupffer cells in local and systemic immune responses. Gastroenterology 80:854, 1981.

124. Frei K, Siepl C, Groscurth P, et al: Immunobiology of microglial cells. Ann N Y Acad Sci 540:218, 1988.

125. Mayernik DG, Ul-Haq A, Rinehart JJ: Differentiation-associated alteration in human monocyte-macrophage accessory cell function. J Immunol S130:21, 1983.

126. Toews GB, Vial WC, Dunn MM, et al: The accessory cell function of human alveolar macrophages in specific T cell proliferation. J Immunol 132:181, 1984.

127. Brenner MB, Trowbridge IS, Strominger JL: Cross-linking of human T cell receptor proteins: Association between the T cell idiotype beta subunit and the T3 glycoprotein heavy subunit. Cell 40:183, 1985.

128. Geppert TD, Lipsky PE: Antigen presentation at the inflammatory site. Crit Rev Immunol 9:313, 1989.

129. Ruppert J, Peters JH: IL-6 and IL-1 enhance the accessory activity of human blood monocytes during differentiation to macrophages. J Immunol 146:144, 1991.

130. Rubinstein D, Roska AK, Lipsky PE: Antigen presentation by liver sinusoidal lining cells after antigen exposure in vivo. J Immunol 138:1377, 1987.

131. Symington FW, Brady W, Linsley PS: Expression and function of B7 on human epidermal Langerhans cells. J Immunol 150:1286, 1993.

132. Freudenthal PS, Steinman RM: The distinct surface of human blood dendritic cells, as observed after an improved isolation method. Proc Natl Acad Sci USA 87:7698, 1990.

133. Pure E, Inaba K, Crowley MT, et al: Antigen processing by epidermal Langerhans cells correlates with the level of biosynthesis of major histocompatibility complex class II molecules and expression of invariant chain. J Exp Med 172:1459, 1990.

134. Larsen CP, Ritchie SC, Pearson TC, et al: Functional expression of the costimulatory molecule B7/BB1 on murine dendritic cell populations. J Exp Med 176:1215, 1992.

135. Young JW, Koulova L, Soergel SA, et al: The B7/BB1 antigen provides one of several costimulatory signals for the activation of CD4+ T lymphocytes by human blood dendritic cells in vitro. J Clin Invest 90:229, 1992.

136. Koide S, Steinman RM: Induction of interleukin 1a mRNA during the antigen-dependent interaction of sensitized T lymphoblasts with macrophages. J Exp Med 168:409, 1988.

137. Holt PG, Oliver J, Bilyk N, et al: Downregulation of the antigen presenting cell function(s) of pulmonary dendritic cells in vivo by resident alveolar macrophages. J Exp Med 177:397, 1993.

138. Oppenheim JJ, Kovacs EJ, Matsushima K, et al: There is more than one interleukin-1. Immunol Today 1986.

139. Lotz M, Jirik F, Kabouridis P, et al: B cell stimulating factor 2/interleukin 6 is a costimulant for human thymocytes and T lymphocytes. J Exp Med 167:1253, 1988.

140. Yokota S, Geppert TD, Lipsky PE: Enhancement of antigen- and mitogen-induced human T lymphocyte proliferation by tumor necrosis factor-alpha. J Immunol 140:531, 1988.

141. Scott P: IL-12: Initiation cytokine for cell-mediated immunity. Science 260:496, 1993.

142. Trinchieri G, Wysocka M, D'Andrea A, et al: Natural killer cell stimulatory factor (NKSF) or interleukin-12 is a key regulator of immune response and inflammation. Prog Growth Factor Res 4:355, 1992.

CHAPTER 9

Neutrophils and Eosinophils

Per Venge
Håkan Bergstrand
Lena Håkansson

The vital importance of the neutrophil granulocyte in the defense against bacteria is easily demonstrated by the life-threatening infections experienced by patients who lack these cells in their peripheral blood or who have a major defect in the function of the cell.[1, 2] It is assumed, and even probable, that the neutrophil plays a major pathophysiologic role in a number of various diseases, including rheumatic disorders, as a result of the destructive power of this cell.

On the other hand, although the eosinophil granulocyte was discovered more than 100 years ago, its physiologic role is still enigmatic. Currently, the most popular hypothesis is that the eosinophil plays a role in the defense against invading parasites. Indeed, the eosinophil and eosinophil products are capable of killing various parasites in vitro. Eosinophils have been seen accumulating around invading parasites in tissue, but the few individuals who seem to lack eosinophils are surprisingly healthy. A very interesting possibility is a major role of the eosinophil in cancer cell killing. That the eosinophil has a role in disease, however, has become increasingly clear during the last decade. Thus, activated eosinophils are found in most inflammatory diseases adjacent to sites of tissue destruction, and patients who have hypereosinophilia in their blood generally experience severe and often life-threatening symptoms directly related to the number of eosinophils present in tissues and in the peripheral blood.

THE NEUTROPHIL

The neutrophil granulocyte matures from a common stem cell for erythrocytes, thrombocytes, macrophages, eosinophils, basophils, and mast cells (i.e., the hematopoietic stem cell).[1] Thus, the neutrophil is remotely related to all other blood cells with only one major exception—the lymphocytes.

The first identifiable neutrophil precursor cell in the bone marrow in myelopoiesis is the *myeloblast*. This precursor further matures into the promyelocyte. These two precursor cells contain a rather homogeneous population of primary, or azurophil, granules.

The next maturation stage is the *myelocyte*, which contains another population of granules (i.e., the specific, or secondary, granules). The mature neutrophil granulocyte has an abundance of small heterogeneous granules that may be separated into several different subpopulations based on their densities and their con-

tent of specific proteins (Table 9–1). The marrow transit time (the time it takes for a myeloblast to become a mature neutrophil) is about 14 days in normal healthy individuals. After this time, the neutrophil survives for 2 more days, with a blood transit time (half-life) of about 6 to 7 hours. The graveyard of the neutrophil is mainly the spleen and liver, but a number of neutrophils also die in the lungs and intestine. It has been estimated that the turnover of neutrophils is about 10^{11} cells/day. In various diseases, such as in acute and chronic inflammatory conditions, the turnover of neutrophils may be dramatically increased.

The principles that regulate myelopoiesis and differentiation to the mature neutrophil include a number of growth and differentiation factors collectively called *cytokines* (see later). With respect to myelopoiesis, the best known are the granulocyte-macrophage colony-stimulating factor (GM-CSF) and granulocyte colony-stimulating factor (G-CSF), which are now used clinically to stimulate myelopoiesis in neutropenic patients.

Biochemistry

Azurophil (Primary) Granules

The azurophil granules contain as their main constituents several proteolytic enzymes and a wide array of bactericidal proteins (see Table 9–1).[3–5]

Table 9–1. NEUTROPHIL GRANULE POPULATIONS AND SOME OF THEIR PROTEIN CONTENTS

Primary (Azurophil) Granules	Secondary (Specific) Granules	Tertiary Granules
Cathepsin G	Lactoferrin	Gelatinase
Elastase	Lysozyme	
Proteinase 3	Plasminogen activator	
Myeloperoxidase (MPO)	B_{12}-binding protein	
Lysozyme	C5a-cleaving enzyme	
Defensins	Cytochrome b_{558}	
Azurocidin	NADPH-oxidase	
Bactericidal/permeability-increasing protein (BPI)	Human neutrophil lipocalin (HNL)	
Acid hydrolases	β_2-Microglobulin	
	Guanosine triphosphate (GTP)–binding protein	

146

Proteases

Cathepsin G. Cathepsin G is one of the most basic proteins in the human organism, with an isoelectric point (pI) above pH 11. It is a chymotrypsin-like protease with optimal protease activity at near neutral pH. In addition to the enzymatic activity, cathepsin G is also capable of killing certain bacteria. The proteolytic activity is neutralized by several plasma protease inhibitors, among which α_1-antichymotrypsin is the most specific. However, α_1-antitrypsin (α_1-proteinase inhibitor) and α_2-macroglobulin are also efficient inhibitors of cathepsin G.

The major biologic activities of cathepsin G are probably related to its proteolytic activity and comprise the cleavage of a number of proteins, including complement factors, coagulation factors, angiotensin, bradykinin, and basement membrane laminin. In many instances, these cleavages give rise to active products; in other cases, active products are inactivated. Examples are the generation of chemotactic products after cleavage of the complement factor C5 and the activation of latent neutrophil collagenase or matrix metalloproteinases and the inactivation of chemotactic peptides. The activities of cathepsin G may also be directed against various cells, such as platelets and neutrophils, and may induce functional changes of biologic importance. One such activity is the induction of platelet aggregation.

Elastase. Elastase is a basic serine protease with an elastolytic enzyme activity. The major inhibitor of elastase in plasma is α_1-antitrypsin (α_1-proteinase inhibitor), but α_2-macroglobulin is also an effective inhibitor. In addition, elastase is inhibited by a locally produced inhibitor, the so-called secretory leukocyte-protease inhibitor (SLPI). The proteolytic activity of elastase provides it with a role in tissue injury. Subjects deficient in the major elastase inhibitor α_1-antitrypsin have an increased propensity for the development of emphysema. Other studies have suggested that elastase is involved in the glomerular injury in glomerulonephritis. Digestion of several clotting factors by elastase released to the extracellular plasma environment may account for the coagulation abnormalities seen in patients with septicemia. Basement membrane structures, such as laminin, are also degraded by elastase, and endothelial cells are injured. Degradation of fibronectin by elastase gives rise to several biologically active products, some having cell-adhesive properties and others having gelatin-binding properties.

Proteinase 3. Proteinase 3 has a broad serine protease activity and the capacity to degrade collagen. The amino acid sequence shows a high degree of homology with the other serine-proteases in the azurophil granules and with azurocidin (see later). The enzyme specificity of proteinase 3 is very similar to that of elastase, and like elastase, proteinase 3 produces emphysema when it is given intratracheally to hamsters. The proteolytic activity of proteinase 3 is inhibited by α_1-antitrypsin and α_2-macroglobulin. Proteinase 3 enhances platelet aggregation induced by cathepsin G. Autoantibodies specific for proteinase 3 (c-ANCA) are found in patients with Wegener's granulomatosis.

Antibiotic Proteins

Myeloperoxidase. Myeloperoxidase (MPO) is a basic heme-containing protein. It is a strong peroxidase and takes part in the production of short-lived and reactive oxygen-derived radicals, such as OCl^- (hypochlorite), and long-lived radicals, such as chloramines. Biologic activities related to this property of MPO include microbicidal activities, tumor cell killing, the inactivation of a_1-proteinase inhibitor and chemotactic peptides, induction of platelet release, transformation of prostaglandins, reduction of the opsonizing activity of immunoglobulin G (IgG) and complement factor C3b, down-regulation of natural killer (NK) cells activity against tumors, damage to fibronectin, and the potential involvement in degradation of articular cartilage proteoglycan and hyaluronic acid. In spite of these demonstrations, the precise role of MPO in vivo is still enigmatic. Thus, the deficiency of MPO, which in certain areas is relatively common, is rarely related to any specific problems of the individual. Immunoassays have been developed for MPO and used to measure MPO in blood and in various tissue fluids.[6] MPO measurements in blood may be used to quantitatively estimate bone marrow activity in leukemic patients.[7] Autoantibodies against MPO (p-ANCA) may be found in blood in some inflammatory diseases, such as systemic vasculitis.

Lysozyme. Lysozyme is located in both primary (azurophil) and secondary (specific) granules and is detailed later; see Specific (Secondary) Granules.

Defensins. Defensins comprise a group of four peptides with molecular weights of less than 4 kD. The defensins are the most abundant of all granule proteins in the neutrophil, making up about 50 percent of all proteins in the granules. Defensins are active in the killing of both bacteria and viruses but are less potent than the other antibiotic proteins of the neutrophil. Defensins are also found in intestinal and respiratory cells. Defensins are chemotactic to monocytes and may have other hormonal effects.

Azurocidin. Azurocidin is an antibiotic protein, which is a member of the serine-protease family of proteins of the neutrophil. Azurocidin, however, has no protease activity due to an amino-acid replacement in the catalytic site of the sequence. Azurocidin is also a potent chemotactic principle for monocytes.

Bactericidal/Permeability-Increasing Protein (BPI). BPI is probably the same protein as the more recently described protein, cationic antimicrobial protein (CAP57) (Mr 57,000). BPI/CAP57 is a potent killer of gram-negative bacteria, such as *Escherichia coli*. BPI also binds to lipopolysaccharides (LPS) and may neutralize some of the effects of endotoxin on neutrophils, such as receptor up-regulation.

Specific (Secondary) Granules

Most prominent among the components of the secondary granules are lactoferrin, lysozyme, and human neutrophil lipocalin (HNL). Other proteins in the secondary granules include a B_{12}-binding protein, β_2-microglobulin, a guanosine triphosphate (GTP)–binding protein, a specific collagenase. In addition, the secondary granules seem to function as a reservoir of components of the (reduced) nicotinamide-adenine dinucleotide phosphate (NADPH) oxidase and of plasma membrane receptors.[3-5]

Lactoferrin. Lactoferrin is an iron-binding protein with a high degree of homology with transferrin. Lactoferrin is produced by several exocrine glands, such as the mammary gland, and is believed to take part in the first-line defense against microorganisms by interfering with the iron metabolism of the microbes. The role of lactoferrin in the neutrophil is not clear, but the few children described with a lactoferrin deficiency are all highly susceptible to life-threatening infections. Lactoferrin takes part in the feedback regulation of myelopoiesis, possibly by regulating cytokine release from mononuclear cells. A role for lactoferrin in the negative feedback mechanism of the prevention of recruitment and activation of neutrophils at sites of inflammation has been suggested. Furthermore, by virtue of its iron-binding capacity, lactoferrin may interfere with the oxygen-derived molecules produced by the neutrophil, although there is no real consensus as to the biologic consequence of this interaction. Sensitive immunoassays have been developed for lactoferrin and are used to measure the lactoferrin level in the circulation as a sensitive and quantitative marker of the turnover and activity of neutrophils in patients with leukemia and in patients with inflammatory disease.

Lysozyme. Lysozyme is found both in the specific and in the azurophil granules of human neutrophils. As with lactoferrin, lysozyme is also produced by a number of other cells, including monocytes/macrophages and glandular cells. Lysozyme probably has a role as a first-line defense molecule, because it has some bactericidal properties and is ubiquitously distributed on all mucus membranes. Lysozyme may be measured in the circulation as a marker of macrophage activity, since approximately 90 percent of all lysozyme in the circulation derives from the monocyte/macrophage pool of cells. Thus, the classical use of serum/plasma measurements of lysozyme is in the diagnosis of monocytic leukemia. Lysozyme has also been used to a certain extent in the monitoring of sarcoidosis and lately in the management of patients with human immunodeficiency virus (HIV) infection.

Human Neutrophil Lipocalin. HNL is a recently discovered protein of the secondary granules.[8] It is highly homologous to proteins of the lipocalin family, which bind hydrophobic molecules, such as vitamins and other lipids. HNL may bind to gelatinase and is therefore also named neutrophil gelatinase-associated lipocalin (NGAL).[9] HNL also interacts with the chemotactic tripeptide f-MLP (formyl-methionyl-leucyl-phenylalanine) and may take part in the regulation of f-MLP–induced chemotaxis of the neutrophil. HNL may be measured in body fluids as a specific marker of neutrophil turnover and activity. Serum measurements of HNL can accurately distinguish between acute infections caused by bacteria or viruses.[10]

Other Secretory Organelles

In addition to the just described primary and secondary secretory granules, the neutrophil contains some other organelles from which various components are secreted when the neutrophil is stimulated. These organelles include the so-called tertiary or gelatinase granules, which contain as one major component gelatinase and also cytochrome b and ubiquinone. Other secretory organelles are the secretory vesicles, which among other things contain alkaline phosphatase and the complement factor 3 receptors, CR1 and CR3.[3]

Stimulus-Response Coupling

The processes that transmit the message of a stimulus into a functional phagocyte response are complex and not fully clarified (Fig. 9–1). Although basically similar, stimulus-response couplings for degranulation, oxidative metabolism, and motility/chemotaxis may differ. Within response, they may also differ with the stimulus examined. Thus, soluble and insoluble immune complexes (IC) utilize partly separate signal transduction pathways; the phorbol ester PMA (phorbol myristate acetate) induces an oxidative response with little degranulation, whereas f-MLP triggers granule exocytosis with transient and restricted H_2O_2 generation. Even exocytosis of different granules may be distinctly regulated.[11-13] In many respects, these pathways are also valid for the eosinophil.

PLC-PKC Pathway. Chemoattractants bind to specific seven-transmembrane-domain receptors[14, 15] and trigger, via GTP-binding proteins, phospholipase C (PLC) to generate two second messengers: inositol 1,4,5-trisphosphate (IP_3) and diacylglycerol (DAG).

IP_3 induces calcium release from intracellular stores; oscillations in calcium levels may generate the signal. Possibly, inositol 1,3,4,5-tetrakisphosphate (IP_4) complements IP_3 in regulating cytosolic Ca^{2+} levels.[14, 16-18] Moreover, a role for phosphatidylinositol 3,4,5-trisphosphate (PI) in the chemotactic response is a possibility.[15]

DAG, like the phorbol ester PMA, activates protein kinase C (PKC). The PKC family consists of at least 12 different isozymes that probably play specific roles in signal transduction pathways.

Ras-Raf Kinase-Mitogen Activated Protein (MAP) Kinase Pathway. An ubiquitous signal transduction pathway involving tyrosine kinase activities, a Ras-like G-protein and Raf kinase, MAP kinase kinase (MEK), and MAP kinase (Erk) transduces signals in neutrophils triggered by f-MLP or C5a (but not platelet-activating factor [PAF]), by GM-CSF, by soluble

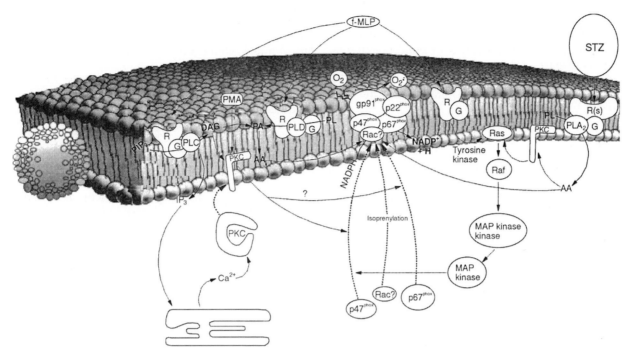

Figure 9–1. Schematic representation of the concepts of the phagocyte oxidative burst and signal transduction pathways. AA, arachidonic acid; DAG, 1,2-sn-diacylglycerol; f-MLP, formyl-methionyl-leucyl-phenylalanine; G, GTP-binding protein; IP$_3$, inositol 1,4,5-trisphosphate; IP$_4$, inositol 1,3,4,5-tetrakisphosphate; MAP kinase, mitogen-activated protein kinase; MEK, MAP kinase/*ex*tracellular receptor kinase *k*inase; PA, phosphatidic acid; PKC, protein kinase C; PLC, phospholipase C; PLD, phospholipase D; PMA, phorbol myristate acetate; STZ, serum-treated zymosan.

immune complex, or even by PMA.[13, 19, 20] Studies with tyrosine kinase inhibitors suggest that this pathway may be involved in chemoattractant-induced oxidative burst rather than in degranulation. Specificity prevails because the phosphotyrosine protein pattern may differ with stimuli employed.[20] Moreover, cross-linking of FcγRI or FcγRII may lead to activation of the Src-like tyrosine kinases Syk and Fgr. Ras-related G-proteins are carboxyl methylated during f-MLP–induced stimulus-response coupling. Inhibitors of this reaction block neutrophil responses to f-MLP, including generation of superoxide O$_2^-$.[21]

Crosstalk. Protein kinase C isozymes may modulate other signal transduction pathways. One example is the PKC-mediated inhibition of agonist-induced rises in polymorphonuclear neutrophil (PMN) cytosolic Ca^{2+}. Also activation of cyclic adenosine monophosphate (cAMP)–dependent kinase may lead to a reduced cellular response. Increased cAMP blocks f-MLP–induced MAP kinase activation and superoxide O$_2^-$ generation.[19] There is also a cross-talk between protein kinase C and MAP kinase pathways.

Phospholipases. G-Protein–regulated phospholipases A$_2$ (PLA$_2$) and D, generating arachidonic acid (AA) and phosphatidic acid (PA) as putative second messengers, respectively, play important but less clearly defined roles in signal transduction.[16, 22] Some effects of arachidonic acid may occur via inhibition of a GTPase-activating protein (GAP), others possibly via direct activation of protein kinase C or, more likely, the NADPH oxidase.[14, 23] Insoluble immune complex and

serum-treated zymosan (STZ), interacting with the C3b, C3bi, and FcRII and FcRIII receptors, trigger production of PLA$_2$-generated arachidonic acid and generation of IP$_3$ and DAG, and trigger the tyrosine kinase/Ras-Raf-MAP kinase pathway.

Adenosine. Two receptors for adenosine exist on human neutrophils—the adenosine receptors A1 and A2.[24] The interaction with these receptors promotes chemotaxis but inhibits the generation of reactive oxygen molecules, such as hydrogen peroxide (H$_2$O$_2$) and O$_2^-$. Adenosine also affects adherence of neutrophils to endothelial cells and protects the endothelial cells from neutrophil-mediated injury. These different effects of adenosine are mediated differentially by the interaction with the two adenosine receptors with the occupancy of the A1 receptor promoting adherence and chemotaxis but with the occupancy of the A2 receptor inhibiting adherence and the generation of oxygen radicals. Adenosine may therefore act both as a proinflammatory and as an anti-inflammatory agent. The interaction with the A2 receptor and the inhibition of neutrophil activities may be a novel approach in the development of anti-inflammatory drugs, and indeed the anti-inflammatory effect of methotrexate may be mediated by the increase of adenosine production at sites of inflammation.

Neutrophil Functions

Adherence

Adherence of neutrophils to the vascular endothelial cells is the initial key event leading to the accumulation of neutrophils at an inflammatory site. The increased adherence of neutrophils to endothelial cells and the increased adhesiveness of endothelial cells, which is a part of the inflammatory response, are regulated by a series of events involving adhesion molecules expressed on neutrophils and endothelial cells (see Chapters 12 and 20).

Migration

Migration of neutrophils out into the tissue after adhesion to the endothelial cells is the second crucial mechanism behind the accumulation of neutrophils at an inflammatory focus. To accomplish the migration of neutrophils to an inflammatory site, the cells are subjected to substances that regulate their direction and speed of migration.[25]

Chemotactic and Chemokinetic Factors. Chemotactic agents govern the direction of cell migration. When exposed to a gradient of a chemotactic agent, neutrophils migrate toward the increasing concentration of the agent. Chemokinetic factors enhance the speed of directed as well as undirected migration. As a result of the lack of adequate methods, the relative importance of chemotactic and chemokinetic factors has not been studied in vivo. Based on results obtained in vitro, however, it is hypothesized that chemotactic factors govern the final step of migration to the inflammatory foci, whereas chemokinetic factors—by enhancing the speed of migration—increase the possibility of the neutrophils to detect the gradient of a chemotactic factor.

Neutrophils respond to a number of chemotactic factors in vitro (Table 9–2). The complement-derived C5a, the arachidonic acid metabolite leukotriene B4 (LTB4), PAF, the tripeptide f-MLP, and IL-8 are the most potent of these chemotactic factors, active at nanomolar concentrations.[26–31] The chemokinetic factors are less well characterized. Apart from the fact that some of the chemotactic factors, such as C5a and

Table 9–2. CHEMOTACTIC AND CHEMOKINETIC FACTORS FOR NEUTROPHILS AND EOSINOPHILS

Chemotactic factors

C5a (complement-derived)
f-MLP (formyl-leucyl-phenylanaline) (bacterial origin)
HETEs (metabolite of arachidonic acid)
LTB4 (leukotriene B4, metabolite of arachidonic acid)
PAF (platelet-activating factor, 1-O-alkyl-2-acetyl-sn-glycero-3 phosphocholine)
LCF (lymphocyte chemotactic factor)
IL-2 (interleukin-2)
IL-5 (interleukin-5)
IL-8 (interleukin-8)
RANTES (regulated on activation, normal T cell expressed, and secreted)

Chemokinetic factors

C3-related products
α_1-Antiproteinase inhibitor, α_2-macroglobulin, orosomucoid
Albumin (ethanol-treated)

PAF, also possess chemokinetic effects, the plasma proteins α_1-antiproteinase and α_2-macroglobulin and orosomucoid have been identified as chemokinetic factors.[32]

The Motile Apparatus of Neutrophils. Migration as well as phagocytosis and degranulation requires changes of the shape and consistency of the cell's peripheral cytoplasm and pseudopods, which are the regions involved in these movements. The extension of the cytoplasm is maintained by a network of actin microfilaments.[33] Actin exists in two forms: as a monomer (*G-actin*) and as filaments (*F-actin*). The three-dimensional network formed by actin is based on actin-binding protein and α-actinin. Actin-binding protein is a cross-linking protein that forms the right angles of the network. α_1-Actinin, the other cross-linking agent, joins the actin filaments side to side as bundles. The length and maintenance of actin filaments are regulated by the proteins acumentin, gelsolin, and profilin. Strong evidence suggests that the extensive action of actin is counteracted by the contractile action of myosin.

Phagocytosis

Phagocytosis is the process by which particles recognized by neutrophils are internalized. Recognition depends on the presence of opsonins, such as immunoglobulins and complement components (C3b) on the particles, and is mediated by receptors for immunoglobulins and complement components on the surface membrane of neutrophils. Binding of opsonins to the cell surface receptor activates the motile apparatus of the cell via gelation and contraction of actin filaments, and pseudopods are formed around the particle, which is eventually engulfed.

Fc- and C3b-Receptors on the Surface Membrane of the Neutrophil (Table 9–3). The receptors that recognize the Fc- part of IgG and C3b/iC3b are the most important receptors involved in phagocytosis. Under normal conditions, the neutrophils express the low-affinity receptors FcγRII (CD32) and FcγRIII (CD16).[34, 35] FcγRII interacts with IgG complexes consisting of two or more IgG molecules and thereby induces phagocytosis, respiratory burst, and degranulation. FcγRIII interacts with dimeric complexes of IgG and can induce granule secretion but not phagocytosis or respiratory burst. The FcγRIII, however, possesses the unique ability to induce opsonin-independent phagocytosis of bacteria that possesses lectin-like substances on their surface. The FcγRIII is coupled to a phospholipase C–sensitive glycosyl-phosphatidylinositol anchor.

Two forms of neutrophil FcγRIII have been identified that correspond to the previously described biallelic NA1/NA2 neutrophil antigen system. The expression of FcγRIII depends on up-regulation and release of the receptor. Expression of the high-affinity FcγRI is induced on neutrophils by IFN-γ. FcγRI mediates phagocytosis of monomeric IgG and IgG complexes.

Table 9–3. IMMUNOGLOBULIN AND COMPLEMENT RECEPTORS ON NEUTROPHILS AND EOSINOPHILS

Receptor	Cell	Cellular Function
FcαR	Neutrophil Eosinophil	Phagocytosis Secretion Respiratory burst
FcγRI (CD64)	Neutrophil	Cytokine- activated phagocytosis Respiratory burst Secretion
FcγRII (CD32)	Neutrophil Eosinophil	Phagocytosis Respiratory burst Secretion
FcγRIII (CD16)	Neutrophil	Secretion
FcεRII (CD23-rel)	Eosinophil	Secretion Respiratory burst
CR1 (CD35)	Neutrophil Eosinophil	Phagocytosis Secretion
CR3 (CD11b/CD18)	Neutrophil Eosinophil	Phagocytosis Secretion

Neutrophils express two kinds of C3b-receptors[36]:

• CR1, which interacts with C3b and C4b
• CR3, which interacts with iC3b

CR1 interacts with the actin filaments of the cytoskeleton of neutrophils. Expression of CR1 is increased by TNF-α and f-MLP, probably by recruitment of receptors from the secretory vesicles.

CR3 is present both in the plasma membrane and in the specific granule fraction. Tumor necrosis factor (TNF-α) and f-MLP up-regulate CR3 by recruitment from the specific granule fraction. It has long been recognized that coating of particles with both C3b and IgG enhances the rate of phagocytosis compared with that of particles coated with IgG only. The demonstration of an association between the CR3-receptor and the FcγR, by a subset of CD11b/CD18 receptors, is probably one explanation for the synergistic effect of C3b on IgG-mediated phagocytosis.

The FcαRs on neutrophils, under normal conditions, exist in a low-affinity state, but activation of granulocytes with GM-CSF and G-CSF induces a change to a high-affinity state and an acquisition of IgA-mediated phagocytic capability, superoxide generation, and killing of various microorganisms.[37]

Secretion

The extracellular release of granule constituents may be brought about by active mobilization of the granule material to the exterior of the cell and the passive diffusion out of the cell because of loss of cellular integrity. The latter may take place at cell death but is also believed to take place during phagocytosis because of the imperfect closure of the phagocytic vacuole.[3, 4] Thus, when the neutrophil ingests a particle such as a bacterium, the granules are mobilized to the vacuolar membrane in order to release their material into the vacuole. At a very early stage of this process, part of the granule material is released into the vacuole before the ingestion phase is completed and the phagocytic vacuole properly closed. This phenomenon is sometimes referred to as "regurgitation while feeding." Active secretion of granule material may take place during the chemotactic migration of the neutrophil. The actual meaning of this secretion is not well understood but may be of importance for the capacity of the neutrophil to penetrate certain tissue structures, such as basal membranes during the migration from blood to tissues.

The kinetics of secretion from the various secretory organelles is very different, which implies that the mechanisms that govern secretion from these compartments are fundamentally different. With most stimuli, the kinetics of mobilization of the various compartments has the following rank order: secretory vesicles are mobilized first, followed by the tertiary granules, secondary granules, and primary granules. The primary granules, with their contents of very potent and potentially destructive material, seem to release their content mainly into the phagocytic vacuole; the constituents of the other secretory organelles are mobilized to the plasma membrane and released to the exterior of the cell. Secretion of the constituents of all secretory organelles may be achieved with C5a, PMA, or other soluble stimuli, but it requires, in the case of primary granules, concentrations that are 10 to 100 times higher than those needed to induce secondary, tertiary granule, or secretory vesicle secretion. Even with these high concentrations, hardly more than 15 to 25 percent of the primary granule constituents are released in contrast to the other compartments, which release 50 to 100 percent of their material with the lower secretagogue concentrations.

Induction of neutrophil degranulation is brought about by a variety of soluble stimuli, such as the chemotactic agents C5a, IL-8, LTB₄, f-MLP, the phorbol ester PMA, Ca-ionophores, or the exposure to particles opsonized with immunoglobulins and complement products (e.g., C3b). As shown in Table 9–3, secretion is induced by the interaction with either IgA and IgG and the IgG signal for secretion is mediated primarily through the FcγRII and RIII receptors. Some cytokines, such as GM-CSF, enhance the secretion of primary and secondary granule proteins from human neutrophils partly by up-regulation of receptors in the plasma membrane (compare with Table 9–4) but probably also by changing intracellular Ca^{2+} levels.

The cytosol of neutrophils contains the fusogenic protein annexin I. In the presence of Ca^{2+}, annexin I has been shown in vitro to attach to the secondary granules and to promote aggregation of these granules and fusion with plasma membranes.[38] Annexin I may be one of the major intracellular principles operative in the fusion of secondary granules with the plasma membrane when the neutrophil is exposed to secretagogues.

Table 9–4. PRIMING OF NEUTROPHILS AND EOSINOPHILS BY CYTOKINES

Cytokine	Affected Cell	Effect on
IL-3	Neutrophil Eosinophil	Adherence CR3 expression Cytotoxicity
IL-4	Neutrophil	Phagocytosis
IL-5	Eosinophil	Adherence CR3 expression Cytotoxicity Secretion
IL-6	Neutrophil	Secretion
IL-8	Neutrophil	Adherence CR1, CR3 expression Chemotaxis Respiratory burst Secretion
GM-CSF	Neutrophil Eosinophil	Adherence CR1, CR3 expression FcγRIII expression Phagocytosis Cytotoxicity
IFN-γ	Neutrophil Eosinophil	FcγRII and RIII expression Cytotoxicity
IFN-α	Eosinophil	Cytotoxicity
IFN-β	Eosinophil	Cytotoxicity
TNF-α	Neutrophil Eosinophil	Adherence CR1, CR3 expression Respiratory burst Phagocytosis
EAF	Eosinophil	Respiratory burst CR3 expression Secretion
ECEF	Eosinophil	Cytotoxicity

Abbreviations: IL, interleukin; GM-CSF, granulocyte-macrophage colony-stimulating factor; IFN, interferon; TNF, tumor necrosis factor; EAF, eosinophil-enhancing factor; ECEF, eosinophil cytotoxicity-enhancing factor.

Priming

Priming denotes an increased responsiveness of granulocytes to stimuli of, for instance, chemotactic responses, adherence responses, and secretion responses. Several interleukins (ILs) are capable of priming the function of neutrophils (see Table 9–4). IL-4 facilitates the killing of opsonized bacteria by an increased phagocytosis and IL-6 enhances the cytotoxicity of neutrophils.[39, 40] IL-8, also called *neutrophil-activating peptide* (NAP), is a potent primer of most aspects of neutrophil function, such as chemotaxis, respiratory burst, secretion, and cytotoxicity.[31] An increased expression of CD11b/CD18 (CR3) and CR1 might be one explanation behind its priming activity. Apart from its effect on neutrophil proliferation and differentiation, GM-CSF also affects the function of mature neutrophils, such as adherence, phagocytosis, and degranulation.[41] GM-CSF also induces an increased FcγRIII expression as a result of de novo protein synthesis. TNF-α enhances neutrophil respiratory burst, phagocytosis, and adherence to endothelium.[42, 43]

Oxidative Metabolism

Appropriately triggered neutrophils respond with a marked increase in oxygen consumption (see Fig. 9–1). This respiratory burst is due to the activation of an oxidase catalyzing the one-electron reduction of oxygen to superoxide radicals at the expense of NADPH generated in the hexose monophosphate (HMP) shunt according to the reaction $2O_2 + NADPH \rightarrow 2O_2^- + NADP^+ + H^+$. The O_2^- radicals formed are dismutated to H_2O_2; further conversion to hydroxyl radicals and other reactive oxygen species (ROS) involves MPO. This respiratory or oxidative burst is part of the phagocyte's armament for microbicidal purposes. However, if inappropriately released from the cell, the reactive oxygen species formed are potentially harmful to the tissue. The oxidative burst may be induced and modulated independently from other neutrophil functions. A monograph[44] and several comprehensive reviews detail this process.[45–51]

The NADPH Oxidase. In vitro, the respiratory burst is usually assayed as O_2^--induced ferricytochrome C reduction, as chemiluminescence enhanced by lucigenin (O_2^--dependent) or luminol (H_2O_2 and MPO-dependent), or by the reduction of nitroblue tetrazolium (NBT). It is technically more difficult to demonstrate generation of reactive oxygen species in vivo; principles that have been used in this respect are electron spin resonance measurements and spin trapping.

The NADPH oxidase is dormant in phagocytes. It is composed of at least four subunits (see Fig. 9–1): a membrane-associated cytochrome consisting of two chains, gp91-*phox* (phagocyte *ox*idase) and p22-*phox*, two cytosolic proteins (p47-*phox* and p67-*phox*), and a Ras-like G-protein, p21-*rac*. Upon activation of the cell, p47-*phox* and p67-*phox* are translocated to the membrane and assembled with the cytochrome.[52] The G-protein *Rac2* is also required for oxidase activation but does not participate in the early interaction between p47-*phox* and cytochrome b_{558}; p21-*rac*2 is also translocated after stimulation of the cells.[21] Association of the NADPH complex with the cytoskeleton may be of vital importance for its activation.

The *cytochrome* is a 1:1 complex of gp91-*phox* and p22-*phox* containing two hemes, FAD and probably an NADPH-binding site. Its redox potential, -245 mV, facilitates a single electron reduction of oxygen to O_2^- and an a band of absorption at 558 nm. It is referred to as cytochrome b_{-245} or cytochrome b_{558}. Both p47-*phox* and p67-*phox* contain two SH3 regions through which they may interact with proline-rich domains in other proteins[50]; p47-*phox* also possesses multiple phosphorylation sites in its C-terminal region.[53] Evidence also favors participation in the oxidase of the following:

• Another G-protein, *Rap1A*, evidently linked to the cytochrome

- A 40-kD protein with some homology to p47-*phox*
- A 45-kD *flavoprotein* of unknown function
- A 32-kD *NADPH-binding component*

Priming enables a low-responsive cell to respond optimally to a stimulus. Priming of PMNs for an oxidative burst often results from treating cells with low concentrations of chemoattractants or lipopolysaccharide, or with appropriate cytokines, such as GM-CSF and TNF-α, or even with PMA at concentrations that per se do not induce the response. The mechanisms for the priming are not clarified, but primers do not necessarily use pathways, which trigger a response. Physiologic agents prime cells by mechanisms that differ from those of the frequently used *cytochalasin B* (an inhibitor of actin polymerization). Physiologic primers exert their effects at or distal to G-protein activation but proximal to protein kinase C activation; changes in intracellular levels of calcium and/or DAG/PA may contribute to the priming effect. TNF-α–primed cells express a lower cAMP increase in response to IL-8 compared with non-primed cells. A normal down-regulatory function may thus be reduced at priming. Neutrophils in *suspension* respond to chemoattractant challenge with a transient oxidative burst, whereas *adherent* cells may respond according to a more protracted time course, which implies differences in the control of the burst or in priming in these situations.[45, 54]

The oxidative burst is activated by chemoattractants or soluble immune complexes or by particulate stimuli, such as serum-treated zymosan and insoluble immune complexes. More artificial secretagogues, such as PMA and calcium ionophores, are often used to trigger a vigorous, longstanding burst in vitro. The stimulus-secretion coupling involved differs with the stimulus. Most stimuli induce generation of DAG and IP_3 with the ensuing stimulation of protein kinase C and increase of cytosolic Ca^{2+}. However, a proposed obligate role for Ca^{2+} is under debate. A rise in cytosolic free Ca^{2+} or oscillations in Ca^{2+} levels is neither sufficient nor required for O_2^- generation. Moreover, most stimuli, including PMA, induce activation of tyrosine kinase and the Ras-Raf kinase-MAP kinase pathway. Figure 9–1 represents an attempt to schematically integrate different pathways reportedly involved in triggering of the granulocyte respiratory burst. Main prerequisites for NADPH oxidase activation include phosphorylations of p47-*phox*, and possibly p67-*phox*, and translocation of these proteins from the cytosol to the membrane-localized cytochrome b_{558}.

Phosphorylations of p47-*phox* are mediated by protein kinase C and probably by MAP kinase.[53, 55, 56] Moreover, neutrophils contain four f-MLP-stimulated, wortmannin-sensitive kinases that may be involved in O_2^- release.[57] Phosphorylation of 47-*phox* is needed for activation of the oxidase. Continuous PKC-mediated phosphorylations of p47-*phox*, and possibly also p67-*phox*, are suggested to maintain the oxidase in the activated state.[56] Moreover, inhibitors of phosphoserine phosphatase activity, such as okadaic acid, normally enhance superoxide generation induced by f-MLP. Inhibition of a vigorous phosphatase activity possibly leads to activation of the respiratory burst[14, 56]; however, phosphatase inhibition may paradoxically block PMA-triggered O_2^- release. Both chains of cytochrome b_{558} are also phosphorylated during O_2^- generation. These phosphorylations may be involved in cessation of the activity.

Tyrosine Kinase. Tyrosine kinase–mediated phosphorylations of selected proteins are also implicated in NADPH oxidase activation induced by f-MLP, C5a, and concanavalin A (ConA).[13, 20, 58] Such responses are not necessarily dependent on increase in intracellular levels of Ca^{2+}; second messengers generated by phospholipase A_2, C, or D; or on protein kinase C. f-MLP induces the phosphorylation of p43 MAP kinase (ERK-1), whereas ConA induces phosphorylation of p45 MAP kinase and PMA triggers both MAP kinases. With f-MLP and ConA, tyrosine phosphorylations of MAP kinases and of p75 (Raf-1 kinase?) can be involved in NADPH oxidase activation. PMA can induce the oxidative burst independently of these phosphorylations.[20] Inhibitors of tyrosine kinase activity block O_2^- generation triggered by f-MLP but not that triggered by PMA.[13, 20, 58] Moreover, exposure of PMNs to culture fluid from *Fusobacterium nucleatum* induces increased activity of a CD45-associated phosphotyrosine phosphatase activity; such cells are incapable of mounting a respiratory burst at challenge with f-MLP but do respond to PMA.[58]

Phospholipase D. The early f-MLP–induced respiratory burst is largely unaffected when protein kinase C and phospholipase D (PLD) are inhibited.[59] Conceivably, activation of the NADPH oxidase occurs at cytochrome b_{558} molecules already present on the plasma membrane. However, although protein kinase C and phospholipase D are not required for the initiation or maximal rate of oxidant generation, they are needed to sustain oxidase activity. Inhibitor studies show that protein kinase C is not involved in f-MLP–induced phospholipase D activation, whereas tyrosine kinase may be.[13] However, protein kinase C may be essential for concomitant NADPH oxidase activation. f-MLP–stimulated oxidase activity is more dependent on phospholipase D activity in the presence of cytochalasin B than in its absence. In this situation, NADPH oxidase may be inactivated more quickly and new cytochrome b_{558} molecules may have to be recruited from the cytosol. The translocation and activation of these molecules may be PLD-dependent.[59] A possible second messenger is phosphatidic acid; DAG may *enhance* such responses and ceramide modulate them.[13, 14, 16, 54, 55, 60]

Arachidonic Acid and Additional Pathways. Another possible messenger is arachidonic acid. O_2^- generation induced by PMA is blocked by inhibitors of phospholipase A_2, and there is, *besides* phosphorylation and translocation of p47-*phox* and p67-*phox*, a co-requirement for phospholipase A_2 activation for superoxide generation to occur in PMA- or STZ-triggered neutrophils.[23] In f-MLP–triggered cells, activation of the respiratory burst occurs in the absence of phospholipase A_2 activation if both p43 and p45 MAK kinases are tyrosine phosphorylated.[20] Triggering of an oxidative response by serum-treated zymosan or ConA can utilize pathways that do not involve Ca^{2+} increase and protein kinase C activation and differ from those utilized at stimulation by f-MLP.[12] A novel post-translational incorporation of tyrosine into multiple proteins in activated human neutrophils, which is correlated with phagocytosis and activation of the respiratory burst, may be functionally relevant to physiologic host-defense responses of human neutrophils.[61]

Translocations. To become active, the NADPH oxidase subunits have to assemble. Although the continuous translocations to the membrane of p47-*phox* and p67-*phox* are essential for the activation as well as for its maintenance,[55] and although phosphorylations of p47-*phox* and p67-*phox* are conceivable prerequisites for these translocations,[56] the latter can be quantitatively dissociated from the translocations.[20, 46] More recent data implicate the SH3 domains of these subunits in the translocations, which apparently involves a "docking" of the p47-*phox* protein to the C-terminal tail of the 91-kD cytochrome b_{558} subunit.[50]

Cellular Acidification and Alkalinization. The respiratory burst is accompanied by metabolic acid production. A lowering of intracellular pH is counteracted by at least three H^+ extrusion mechanisms: (1) an electroneutral Na^+/H^+ antiport, (2) an adenosine triphosphate (ATP)–driven vacuolar type H^+ pump, and (3) a passive H^+ conductance. The latter, but not the two former, requires assembly of the NADPH oxidase but not its redox function.[62] Various agonists also induce Cl^- efflux, a common phenomenon related to an intracellular alkalinization induced by agonists.

The NADPH oxidase can be activated in suitably composed subcellular systems by arachidonic acid or detergents, such as sodium dodecyl sulfate (SDS). In such a system, protein kinase C is not necessary.[46] Arachidonic acid, and not phosphorylation, is possibly the immediate activator of the NADPH oxidase in cytoplasts.[63] Arachidonic acid is reported to increase the activity of the assembled NADPH oxidase in cytoplasmic membranes by elevating the number of its active complexes and increasing its affinity to the substrate.[23] One mode of action of arachidonic acid is possible disruption of the binding of Rac to its modulator GDP dissociation inhibitor (GDI) protein.[64] Reconstitution of full NADPH oxidase activity in a cell-free system can be accomplished with four components: the cytochrome b_{558}, the p47-*phox*, the p67-*phox*, and p22-*rac*.[65]

Physiologic and Pharmacologic Modulation of the Oxidative Burst. A number of endogenous and experimental modulators of the oxidative burst have been identified.[66] Some of these are listed in Table 9–5. With respect to clinically used drugs, it is noteworthy that most reports do not record substantial

Table 9–5. SOME INHIBITORS OF NADPH OXIDASE-MEDIATED REACTIVE OXYGEN SPECIES (ROS) GENERATION

Agents	Proposed Target/Mode of Action
Endogenous agents	
Adenosine	Via seven transmembrane domain receptor, increase in cAMP
1-O-alkyl-L-acyl-sn-glycerol	Protein kinase C?
Sphingoid bases/sphingosine	Protein kinase C, phospholipase C, and others
Ceramides	? (Not protein kinase C)
α_1-antichymotrypsin	Assembled NADPH oxidase
Lipid thiobisester	NADPH oxidase
Nitric oxide	Prevention of oxidase assembly
Polyamines	?
Clinically available drugs	
Azelastine	?
Xanthine derivatives	Cyclic nucleotide phosphodiesterase inhibition → increased cAMP

Abbreviations: NADPH, reduced nicotinamide-adenine dinucleotide phosphate; cAMP, cyclic adenosine monophosphate.

inhibition of phagocyte oxygen radical generation by glucocorticoid treatment either in vitro or in vivo.

Chronic Granulomatous Disease (CGD). CGD is a rare but severe clinical syndrome characterized by serious infections associated with granuloma formation. It is due to lack of phagocyte NADPH oxidase activity. Genetically distinct forms of CGD exist. Approximately 50 percent of all cases of CGD are a result of X-linked defects in gp91-*phox*, and about one third are due to autosomal recessive defects in the p47-*phox* (the protein cannot be phosphorylated). In a few cases, patients with CGD lack functional p67-*phox* or p22-*phox*.[67]

Tissue Injury Induced by Reactive Oxygen Species. It is not clear to which extent reactive oxygen species (ROS) induce injury in various pathologic conditions. One reason for this is the lack of drugs specifically reducing the oxidative burst. In joints, the role of reactive oxygen species may be a primary one; oxidant attack on proteins may transform them to autoantigens or may increase their susceptibility to degradation by proteolytic agents. Reactive oxygen species may play an important role in the pathogenesis of Crohn's disease and ulcerative colitis and may also contribute to the induction of acute lung injury, to neutrophil-induced tissue damage at vascular sites of immune complex deposition, and to hyperreactivity in asthma.

The NADPH Oxidase as a Signal Transducer. Cells of the immune system often react to oxidants with changes in reactivity. Early reports that trace such changes into oxidant-induced effects on signal transduction pathways include H_2O_2-induced activation of transmembrane tyrosine kinases and modulation of transcription factor activity.[49] A signaling function of the reactive oxygen species, analogous to that of nitric

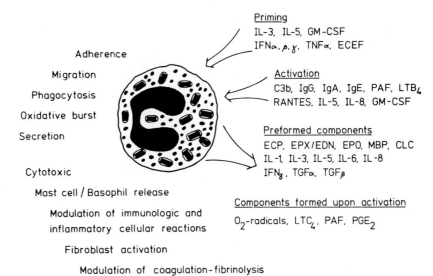

Figure 9–2. The human eosinophil. C, complement; CLC, Charcot-Leyden crystal; ECEF, eosinophil cytotoxicity-enhancing factor; ECP, eosinophil cationic protein; EPO, eosinophil peroxidase; EPX/EDN, eosinophil protein X, eosin-derived neurotoxin; GM-CSF, granulocyte-macrophage colony-stimulating factor; IFN, interferon; Ig, immunoglobulin; IL, interleukin; LTB, LTC, leukotrienes; MBP, major basic protein; PAF, platelet-activating factor; PGE$_2$, prostaglandin E$_2$; RANTES, regulated on activation, normal T cell expressed, and secreted; TGF, transforming growth factor; TNF, tumor necrosis factor.

oxide, might be a reason why an NADPH oxidase-like system is also expressed in B cells and why an NADPH oxidase-like system exists in fibroblasts and glomerular mesangial cells.

Neutrophils and Nitric Oxide. In recent years, nitric oxide has been defined as a product of many mammalian cells with critical functions in homeostasis and host defense. The characteristics of various nitric oxide synthase isoforms have been schematically compared with the NADPH oxidase.[48] However, although a well-characterized murine phagocyte inducible nitric oxide synthase (iNOS) exists, there is still controversy whether human neutrophils produce nitric oxide.[68]

THE EOSINOPHIL

The human eosinophil granulocyte derives from a common hematopoietic stem cell and is remotely related to neutrophils, basophils, mast cells, and monocytes/macrophages. Important growth factors involved in eosinophil maturation are GM-CSF and IL-3 at an early stage and IL-5 at a later stage.[69] The most immature and identifiable eosinophil precursor cell is the *promyelocytic eosinophil*, which is characterized by its content of large crystalloid-containing granules in which eosinophil-specific proteins are found. These granules are also abundant in mature human eosinophil granulocytes and help to identify these cells under the electron microscope.

Normally, only 1 to 4 percent of all leukocytes in the blood are eosinophil granulocytes. The tissue contains 100 to 300 times as many eosinophils, which indicates that the eosinophil is to be regarded predominantly as a tissue cell. The half-life of the eosinophil in the blood is 13 to 18 hours, whereas the half-life in tissues is considerably longer, probably several days and perhaps even weeks.

Like the neutrophil, the eosinophil may express its activity by the production and extracellular release of the granule proteins and other newly formed mediators, such as oxygen-derived metabolites and some lipids (Fig. 9–2).[70–72]

Biochemistry

Granules and Granule Proteins

The granules of human eosinophils are separated into two major populations: peroxidase-positive and peroxidase-negative. The peroxidase-positive granules contain as one feature characteristic crystalloids. These crystalloids are made up by one of the four major proteins of the human eosinophil, i.e., the *major basic protein* (MBP). The three other major proteins, contained in the matrix, are:

- Eosinophil cationic protein (ECP)
- Eosinophil peroxidase (EPO)
- Eosinophil protein X, or eosinophil-derived neurotoxin (EPX/EDN)

All four proteins appear to be present in the heavy, peroxidase-positive granules, but only ECP and EPX/EDN are present in the other lighter population.

A fifth major protein of the eosinophil is the Charcot-Leyden crystal (CLC) protein, which presumably is a plasma membrane protein. It is shed from the eosinophil and forms typical extracellular needle-like crystals in tissues with heavy eosinophil infiltration.

Both major basic protein and the Charcot-Leyden crystal protein are also found in basophils, whereas ECP, EPO, and presumably EPX/EDN are specific to the eosinophil. These specificities have important implications when these proteins are to be used as specific markers of eosinophil activity in vivo.

Characteristic of the four granule proteins are their high isoelectric points, about pH 11 for ECP and EPO. They are also fairly small, ranging from about 14 kD for major basic protein to 67 kD for EPO. All four proteins have been cloned, and their primary structures have revealed large contents of the basic amino acid arginine. The amino acid sequence of ECP and EPX/EDN shows a large degree of homology, about 70 percent, with each other. Also a homology to pancreatic ribonuclease has been shown, and both proteins have ribonuclease activities, with EPX/EDN being the most active. The close relationship between ECP and EPX/EDN is also demonstrated by the monoclonal antibody EG2, which recognizes a common epitope on the two proteins.

The relative content of these four major proteins in normal human eosinophil granules is roughly the same, ranging from 10 to 15 µg/10⁶ eosinophils; however, the content in eosinophils obtained from patients with eosinophilia may vary considerably.

Eosinophil Cationic Protein (ECP). ECP is a one-chain, zinc-containing protein with a molecular weight varying from 18 to 21 kD. The heterogeneity is due to differences in glycosylation of the protein molecule. Besides being a ribonuclease, ECP is a potent cytotoxic molecule with the capacity to kill mammalian cells as well as nonmammalian cells, such as parasites. The noncytotoxic properties of ECP include the alteration of glycosaminoglycan production by human fibroblasts and stimulation of airway mucus secretion. The former finding may point to a role in tissue repair processes and may have a bearing on the findings of the eosinophil presence in fibrotic processes. The latter may be very important for the understanding of the role of the eosinophil in diseases such as asthma, which among other things is characterized by hypersecretion of the airways. ECP increases microvascular transport of macromolecules, which may point to a role of ECP in causing increased vascular permeability.

Another finding of potential interest is the capacity of ECP to inhibit T-lymphocyte proliferation and immunoglobulin synthesis by B cells. ECP also shortens the coagulation time of plasma by mechanisms related to the enhancement of the activity of factor XII. These findings may be relevant in the *hypereosinophilic syndrome*, in which thromboembolic phenomena are very common, and in allergic reactions, in which activation of factor XII has been demonstrated concomitant to the activation of the eosinophil.

Another study has shown an effect on fibrinolysis with preactivation of plasminogen with consequent enhancement of plasminogen activator activation of plasminogen. Most of the described effects of ECP in vitro take place at concentrations that are comparable to those found in vivo (10^{-9} to 10^{-6} mol/L). Locally, these concentrations may even be exceeded. Thus, in sputum of asthmatic patients and in synovial fluid of patients with rheumatoid arthritis, concentrations as high as 10^{-5} mol/L have been found.

One important question, therefore, is how the cytotoxic activity of these proteins is regulated extracellularly. So far, two potential mechanisms have been described. Thus, by virtue of its acidic nature, heparin binds and neutralizes the activity of ECP; however, no data exist in vivo to support this potential mechanism.

Another potential mechanism is the binding of ECP to α_2-macroglobulin, probably at the site of the binding of proteolytic enzymes. The binding of ECP to α_2-macroglobulin in vivo is indicated by the existence of high-molecular-weight forms of ECP in serum of patients with eosinophilia and with very high levels of ECP in serum. This interaction with α_2-macroglobulin may be an important mechanism in neutralizing the actions of ECP, since it is the only obvious interaction of ECP with any plasma component.

Sensitive immunoassays for ECP serve as an indicator of eosinophil activation and turnover not only in asthma and allergic diseases but also in inflammatory diseases of the gut, skin, joints, and brain.[6, 73]

Eosinophil Protein X and Eosinophil-Derived Neurotoxin (EPX/EDN). EPX and EDN are the same protein. EPX/EDN is a one-chain protein; it is slightly less basic than ECP of a similar size (molecular weight, 18 kD). EPX/EDN is a potent ribonuclease and about 100 times more active than ECP. EPX/EDN also has some cytotoxic properties, as the name EDN implies. Thus, when injected into the brains of experimental animals, EPX/EDN produces damage to the tissues; this is reminiscent of the so-called *Gordon phenomenon*, with destruction of Purkinje cells of the cerebellum and the development of ataxia of the animals. The neurotoxic activity of EPX/EDN, however, is not restricted to this protein, because ECP produces the Gordon phenomenon at concentrations about 100 times lower compared with EPX/EDN.

In analogy with ECP, EPX/EDN inhibits T lymphocyte proliferation in a noncytotoxic fashion and at concentrations similar to those of ECP. EPX/EDN does not seem to kill parasites as efficiently as ECP does. The effect of EPX/EDN on parasites, such as the larvae of *Schistosoma mansoni*, is characteristic and differs from the effect of ECP. Thus, when the parasite is exposed to EPX/EDN, it is reversibly paralyzed. This phenomenon may be an important defense mechanism and may facilitate eradication of the parasite.

Eosinophil Peroxidase (EPO). EPO is a two-chain protein with a total molecular weight of 67 kD. Its main function is that of a peroxidase. Together with a halide and H_2O_2, EPO constitutes a potent cytotoxic mechanism but may also increase microvascular permeability. EPO damages nasal sinus mucosa and also exerts a number of noncytotoxic effects on mammalian cells. Thus, EPO induces degranulation of mast cells and causes platelet aggregation.

In addition, EPO may be involved in the inactivation of lipid mediators, such as the leukotrienes. EPO also acts as an allosteric antagonist of the muscarinic M2 receptor, which may have a bearing on the role of eosinophils in diseases such as asthma.[74] EPO is taken up by the neutrophils by a specific and probably a receptor-related mechanism. This uptake may be an important regulatory mechanism, which actively neutralizes the toxic effects of EPO, but it also increases the adhesiveness of the neutrophil. EPO can be measured in several body fluids, including plasma by sensitive immunoassays.

Major Basic Protein (MBP). The name *major basic protein* derives from the fact that in guinea pig eosinophils this protein seems to dominate, making up about 50 percent of the protein content of the granule proteins. As mentioned previously, MBP (molecular weight, 13.9 kD) is stored in the granules in the peculiar and typical crystalloids. Major basic protein is not unique to the eosinophil; it is also found in other cells, such as basophils and some placenta cells. Its main biologic function is related to its cytotoxic activities and involves the killing and damage of parasites and mammalian cells, such as pneumocytes and nasal mucosa. In analogy to the other eosinophil granule proteins, MBP also produces a number of noncytotoxic effects on various cells. These include degranulation of basophils and mast cells, platelet aggregation, induction of neutrophil superoxide production and enhancement of the expression of the neutrophil receptors CR3 and p150,95 (CR4), contraction of airway smooth muscle, and inhibition of airway mucus production. Interesting functions of major basic protein are the effects on respiratory epithelium, which partly may explain the development of the hyperresponsiveness of the airways of asthmatics.

Similar to ECP, major basic protein also causes increased microvascular transport of macromolecules, and similar to EPO, it acts as an allosteric antagonist of the muscarinic M2 receptor. Major basic protein and, to some extent, the other eosinophil granule proteins, impair thrombomodulin function, which may play a role in the thromboembolism seen in patients with hypereosinophilia.

The physiologic control of MBP activities is not well understood. Two potential mechanisms have been discovered. One includes the binding and neutralization of the activities by heparin. Another interesting observation is that mast cells can sequester major basic protein. Major basic protein may also be measured in various body fluids by means of a sensitive immunoassay. These data indicate that measurement of major basic protein in serum or plasma is less suitable as marker of eosinophil turnover and activity in the body than the above-mentioned proteins, since very high levels of major basic protein are also found in conditions unrelated to eosinophil involvement, such as pregnancy.

In addition to the four major proteins, the human eosinophil contains in its granules several other enzymatic activities, including those of gelatinase,[75] arylsulfatase B, histaminase, and phospholipase. These activities may indicate a regulatory role of eosinophils in allergy, since the eosinophil, by means of these activities, acquires the potential to inactivate a number of the putative mediators of the allergic inflammation, such as histamine, PAF, and leukotrienes. One study has also shown that eosinophils produce several different cytokines, such as IL-3, IL-5, IL-6, trans-

forming growth factors (TGF-α and TGF-β), and GM-CSF, which emphasizes the substantial potential of the eosinophil to interfere with many central processes of inflammation.[76]

Newly Formed Mediators

The eosinophil is a very capable producer of oxygen-derived toxic metabolites, such as O_2^-, H_2O_2, and $OH\cdot$. In this respect, the eosinophil is fully comparable to the neutrophil. The eosinophil also produces a number of lipid mediators, including prostaglandins (PGE_2), LTC_4, and PAF. Both LTC_4 and PAF are potent spasmogenic lipids.

Eosinophil Functions

Adherence

Eosinophil adherence to vascular endothelium is essentially governed by the same mechanisms that affect neutrophil adherence. The important difference between eosinophil and neutrophil adherence is that eosinophils can adhere to vascular cell adhesion molecule-1 (VCAM-1) as a result of their expression of very late antigen-4 (VLA-4).[77]

Migration

Eosinophils respond to the chemotactic factors C5a, LTB_4, PAF, and f-MLP.[77] PAF is claimed to be the most potent chemotactic factor for eosinophils, and their response to f-MLP is weaker than that of neutrophils. To explain the selective accumulation of eosinophils observed, for instance, in connection with allergic disorders, many investigators have been searching for eosinophil chemotactic factors that do not attract neutrophils, such as the common chemotactic factors just mentioned. The cytokines IL-2, IL-5, RANTES, and LCF, act as selective chemotactic factors for eosinophils.[78]

Another possible mechanism behind eosinophil accumulation (i.e., an increased responsiveness of the cells) has also been described. Eosinophils from patients with asthma demonstrated enhanced chemotactic and chemokinetic responses compared with normal eosinophils.[79]

Secretion

Secretion of granule proteins from eosinophils may be induced by a receptor-coupled mechanism. The receptors most commonly involved are probably IgG, IgA, IgE, and C3b-receptors (see Table 9–3), but lipid mediators, such as PAF, may also induce eosinophil degranulation.[70–72, 76]

Secretion of granule proteins may be brought about by several mechanisms. One is by granule fusion with the plasma membrane; another is by vesicular transport. These mechanisms are important in our understanding of the selective release of granule proteins, which may occur in response to certain stimuli. Thus, release of peroxidase and MBP (but not of ECP) was demonstrated after exposure of hypodense cells to IgE complexes in contrast to the release of ECP only, after exposure to IgG complexes.

A common method for studying secretion from human eosinophils is the use of C3b-coated particles. This model emphasizes the importance of a large surface in addition to a specific ligand in order to induce degranulation of the eosinophil and probably to involve the interaction with the cell surface receptors CD18/CD11b. This phenomenon is reminiscent of the putative mechanism of parasite killing. The rate and extent of secretion are greatly enhanced by several cytokines, of which IL-3, IL-5, and GM-CSF seem to be of particular interest.

Priming

Interleukin-5 is a potent primer of most aspects of eosinophil function (see Table 9–4).[79–81] IL-5 increases the adherence of eosinophils to endothelial cells via the CD11/CD18 adhesion molecules by an up-regulation of the expression of CD11/CD18. The observed enhanced cytotoxicity induced by IL-5 is probably partly related to increased adherence. IL-3 increases the cytotoxicity of eosinophils and GM-CSF induces increased survival, adherence, and cytotoxicity of eosinophils.[82–84] IFN-α, IFN-β, and IFN-γ are all inducers of increased eosinophil cytotoxicity, although IFN-γ is reported to be the most potent of all cytokines.[85] The two cytokines called eosinophil enhancing factor (EAF) and eosinophil cytotoxicity-enhancing factor (ECEF), which are derived from supernatants of cultured monocytes (and, in the case of ECEF, from T lymphocytes), both induce increased cytotoxicity of eosinophils.[86, 87] EAF and ECEF, which are now molecularly characterized, are distinct from all other hitherto described cytokines. ECEF, which shows molecular heterogeneity, however, may include EAF.

Eosinophilia and the Hypereosinophilic Syndrome

Eosinophilia, a common finding in humans, is generally defined as more than 400×10^6 eosinophils/L

Table 9–6. SOME CAUSES OF BLOOD EOSINOPHILIA

Allergic disease
Asthma
Parasite disease
Chronic inflammatory diseases (e.g., rheumatoid disorders, skin conditions)
Cancer (e.g., Hodgkin's disease, colon and urogenital cancer, lung cancer)
Postinfectious and post-acute inflammation (e.g., after acute myocardial infarction)
Hematological (e.g., chronic myeloid leukemia, eosinophil leukemia)
Hypereosinophilic syndrome
Others

Table 9–7. FREQUENT SYMPTOMS IN PATIENTS WITH THE HYPEREOSINOPHILIC SYMDROME*

80–100 Percent:
  Retinal lesions
  Endomyocardial disease
  Thromboembolic disease

50–80 Percent:
  Skin involvement
  Lymphatic and spleen involvement
  Anorexia, weight loss
  Fever, sweating
  Central nervous system involvement

20–50 Percent:
  Lung involvement
  Renal disease
  Gastrointestinal involvement, including diarrhoea
  Joint disease

Adapted from Spry CJF: Eosinophils: A Comprehensive Review and Guide to the Scientific and Medical Literature, New York, Oxford University Press, 1988.
*Symptoms are ordered in the relative frequency of occurrence.

of blood. In nonatopic, healthy individuals, this number is seldom above 250×10^6/L. The most common causes of blood eosinophilia (Table 9–6) can roughly be categorized into asthma, allergy, chronic inflammatory disease, postinfectious eosinophilia, parasite infestation, cancer, hematologic disease, and a group of unknown causes. It is wise to regard eosinophilia as a signal of disease until proven otherwise. To take full advantage of eosinophil counts, one must ensure that the eosinophils are counted either in a chamber or in one of the modern machines. Calculation of eosinophils based on differential counts under the microscope is of little value.

Although eosinophilia usually signals an underlying disease and generally disappears when the disease has been cured, sometimes eosinophilia by itself may give rise to disease. This is the case in the hypereosinophilic syndrome of unknown cause and in tropical eosinophilia.[70, 88] In patients with these diseases, most of the symptoms can be directly related to the activity of the eosinophils; consequently, the therapeutic strategy is to reduce the number of eosinophils (e.g., by corticosteroids or, in severe cases, by cytostatics). The most common symptoms of patients with the hypereosinophilic syndrome (Table 9–7) clearly reflect the potential of the eosinophil. The recognition and definition of the hypereosinophilic syndrome during the 1970s constituted a very important component in the recognition of the eosinophil as a proinflammatory and potentially harmful cell.

References

1. Bainton DF: Developmental biology of neutrophil and eosinophils. *In* Gallin JI, Goldstein IM, Snyderman R (eds): Inflammation. Basic Principles and Clinical Correlates, 2nd ed. New York, Raven Press, 1992, pp 303–324.
2. Gallin JI: Disorders of phagocytic cells. *In* Gallin JI, Goldstein IM, Sny-

derman R (eds): Inflammation. Basic Principles and Clinical Correlates, 2nd ed. New York, Raven Press, 1992, pp 859–874.

3. Borregaard N, Lollike K, Kjeldsen L, Sengelov H, Bastholm L, Nielsen MH, Bainton DF: Human neutrophil granules and secretory vesicles. Eur J Haematol 51:187, 1993.

4. Henson PM, Henson JE, Fittschen C, Bratton DL, Riches DWH: Degranulation and secretion by phagocytic cells. In Gallin JI, Goldstein IM, Snyderman R (eds): Inflammation: Basic Principles and Clinical Correlates, 2nd ed. New York, Raven Press, 1992, pp 511–540.

5. Weiss SJ: Tissue destruction by neutrophils. N Engl J Med 320:365, 1989.

6. Venge P: Soluble markers of allergic inflammation. Allergy 5:128, 1994.

7. Höglund M, Simonsson B, Smedmyr B, Öberg G, Venge P: The effect of rGM-CSF on neutrophil and eosinophil regeneration after ABMT as monitored by circulating levels of granule proteins. Br J Haematol 86:709, 1994.

8. Xu SY, Carlson M, Engström ÅA, Garcia R, Peterson CGB, Venge P: Purification and characterization of a human neutrophil lipocalin (HNL) from the secondary granules of human neutrophils. Scand J Clin Lab Invest 54:365 1994.

9. Kjeldsen L, Johnsen AH, Sengelov H, Borregaard N: Isolation and primary structure of NGAL, a novel protein associated with human neutrophil gelatinase. J Biol Chem 268:10425, 1993.

10. Xu SY, Petersson CGB, Carlson M, Venge P: The development of an assay for human neutrophil lipocalin (HNL)—to be used as a specific marker of neutrophil activity in vivo and vitro. J Immunol Methods 171:245, 1994.

11. Downey GP: Mechanisms of leukocyte motility and chemotaxis. Curr Opin Immunol 6:113, 1994.

12. Robinson JJ, Watson F, Buchnall RC, Edwards SW: Stimulation of reactive oxidant production in neutrophils by soluble and insoluble immune complexes occurs via different receptor/signal transduction systems. FEMS Immunol Med Microbiol 8:249, 1994.

13. Yasui K, Yamazaki M, Miyabayashi M, Tsuno T, Komiyama A. Signal transduction pathway in human polymorphonuclear leukocytes for chemotaxis induced by a chemotactic factor. Distinct from the pathway for superoxide generation. J Immunol 152:5922, 1994.

14. Baggiolini M, Boulay F, Badwey JA, Curnutte JT: Activation of neutrophil leukocytes: Chemoattractant receptors and respiratory burst. FASEB J 7:1004, 1993.

15. Gerard C, Gerard NP: The pro-inflammatory seven-transmembrane segment receptors of the leukocyte. Curr Opin Immunol 6:140, 1994.

16. Cockcroft S: G-protein–regulated phospholipases C, D and A₂-mediated signalling in neutrophils. Biochim Biophys Acta 1113:135, 1992.

17. Taylor CW, Marshall ICB: Calcium and inositol 1,4,5-trisphosphate receptors: A complex relationship. Trends Biochem Sci 17:403, 1992.

18. Balla T, Catt KJ: Phosphoinositides and calcium signaling: New aspects and diverse functions in cell regulation. Trends Endocrinol Metab 5:250, 1994.

19. Buhl AM, Avdi N, Worthen GS, Johnson GL: Mapping of the C5a receptor signal transduction network in human neutrophils. Proc Natl Acad Sci USA 91:9190, 1994.

20. Dusi S, Donini M, Rossi F: Tyrosine phosphorylation and activation of NADPH oxidase in human neutrophils: A possible role for MAP kinases and for a 75 kDa protein. Biochem J 304:243, 1994.

21. Philips MR, Pillinger MH, Staud R, Volker C, Rosenfeld MG, Weissmann G, Stock JB: Carboxyl methylation of Ras-related proteins during signal transduction in neutrophils. Science 259:977, 1993.

22. Thelen M, Wirthmueller U: Phospholipases and protein kinases during phagocyte activation. Curr Opin Immunol 6:106, 1994.

23. Dana R, Malech HL, Levy R: The requirement for phospholipase A₂ for activation of the assembled NADPH oxidase in human neutrophils. Biochem J 297:217, 1994.

24. Cronstein BN: Adenosine, an endogenous anti-inflammatory agent. J Appl Physiol 76: 5, 1994.

25. Keller HU, Wilkinson PC, Abercombie M, Becker EL, Hirsch JG, Miller ME, Ramsey WS, Zigmond SH: A proposal for the definition of terms related to locomotion of leukocytes and other cells. Clin Exp Immunol 27:377, 1977.

26. Gerard NP, Gerard C: The chemotactic receptor for human C5a anaphylatoxin. Nature 349:614, 1991.

27. Palmblad J, Malmsten CL, Uden A-M, Rådmark O, Engstedt L, Samuelsson B: Leukotriene B4 is a potent and stereospecific stimulator of neutrophil chemotaxis and adherence. Blood 58:658, 1981.

28. Valone FH, Goetzl EJ: Specific binding by human polymorphonuclear leukocytes of the immunological mediator 1-O-hexadecyl/octadecyl-2-acetyl-sn-glycero-3-phophorylcholine. Immunology 48:141, 1983.

29. Ingraham LM, Coates TD, Allen JM, Higgins CP, Baehner RL, Boxer LA: Metabolic, membrane, and functional responses of human polymorphonuclear leukocytes to platelet-activating factor. Blood 59:1259, 1982.

30. Showell HJ, Freer RJ, Zigmond SH, Schiffmann E, Aswanikumar S, Corcoran B, Becker EL: The structure-activity relations of synthetic peptides as chemotactic factors and inducers of lysosomal enzyme secretion for neutrophils. J Exp Med 143:1154, 1976.

31. Baggiolini M, Imboden P, Detmers P: Neutrophil activation and the effects of interleukin-8/neutrophil-activating peptide 1 (IL-8/NAP-1). Cytokines 4:1, 1992.

32. Håkansson L, Venge P: Partial characterization and identification of chemokinetic factors in serum. Scand J Immunol 18:531, 1983.

33. Stossel TP: The mechanical responses of white blood cells. In Gallin JI, Goldstein IM, Snyderman R (eds): Inflammation: Basic Principles and Clinical Correlates. New York, Raven Press, 1992, pp 459–475.

34. Lin C-T, Shen Z, Boros P, Unkeless JC: Fc receptor-mediated signal transduction. J Clin Immunol 14:1, 1994.

35. Van de Winkel JGJ, Capel PJA: Human IgG Fc receptor heterogeneity: Molecular aspects and clinical implications. Immunol Today 14:215, 1993.

36. Wright SD: Receptors for complement and the biology of phagocytosis. In Gallin JI, Goldstein IM, Snyderman R (eds): Inflammation: Basic Principles and Clinical Correlates. New York, Raven Press, 1992, pp 477–495.

37. Shen L: Receptors for IgA on phagocytic cells. Immunol Res 11:273, 1992.

38. Meers P, Mealy T, Tauber AI: Annexin I interactions with human neutrophil-specific granules: Fusogenicity and coaggregation with plasma membrane vesicles. Biochim Biophys Acta 1147:177, 1993.

39. Boey H, Rosenbaum R, Castracane J, Borish L: Interleukin 4 is a neutrophil activator. J Allergy Clin Immunol 83:978, 1989.

40. Borish L, Rosenbaum R, Albury L, Clark S: Activation of neutrophils by recombinant interleukin 6. Cell Immunol 121:280, 1989.

41. Steinbeck MJ, Roth JA: Neutrophil activation by recombinant cytokines. Rev Infect Dis 11:549, 1989.

42. Berger M, Wetzler EM, Wallis RS: Tumor necrosis factor is the major monocyte product that increases complement receptor expression on mature human neutrophils. Blood 71:151, 1988.

43. Capsoni F, Bonara P, Minonzio F, Ongari AM, Colombo G, Rizzardi GP, Zanussi C: The effect of cytokines on human neutrophil Fc receptor-mediated phagocytosis. J Clin Lab Immunol 34:115, 1991.

44. Sbarra AJ, Strauss RR (ed): The Respiratory Burst and Its Physiological Significance. New York, Plenum Press, 1988.

45. Morel F, Doussiere J, Vignais PV: Review: The superoxide-generating oxidase of phagocytic cells: Physiological, molecular and pathological aspects. Eur J Biochem 201:523, 1991.

46. Nauseef WM: Cytosolic oxidase factors in the NADPH-dependent oxidase of human neutrophils. Eur J Haematol 51:301, 1993.

47. Segal AW, Abo A: The biochemical basis of the NADPH oxidase of phagocytes. Trends Biochem Sci 18:43, 1993.

48. Bastian NR, Hibbs JB: Assembly and regulation of NADPH oxidase and nitric oxide synthase. Curr Opin Immunol 6:131, 1994.

49. Chanock SJ, El Benna J, Smith RM, Babior BM: The respiratory burst oxidase. J Biol Chem 269:24519, 1994.

50. McPhail LC: SH3-dependent assembly of the phagocyte NADPH oxidase. J Exp Med 180:2011, 1994.

51. Umeki S: Minireview: Activation factors of neutrophil NADPH oxidase. Life Sci 55:1, 1994.

52. Uhlinger DJ, Taylor KL, Lambeth DJ: p67-phox enhances binding of p47-phox to the human neutrophil respiratory burst oxidase complex. J Biol Chem 269:22095, 1994.

53. El Benna J, Faust LRP, Babior B: The phosphorylation of the respiratory burst oxidase component p47phox during neutrophil activation. Phosphorylation of sites recognized by protein kinase C and by proline-directed kinases. J Biol Chem 269:23431, 1994.

54. Nakamura T, Abe A, Balazovich KJ, Wu D, Suchard SJ, Boxer LA, Shayman JA: Ceramide regulates oxidant release in adherent human neutrophils. J Biol Chem 269:18384, 1994.

55. Dusi S, Della Bianca V, Grzeskowiak M, Rossi F: Relationship betwen phosphorylation and translocation to plasma membrane of p47phox and p67phox and activation of the NADPH oxidase in normal and Ca²⁺-depleted human neutrophils. Biochem J 290:173, 1993.

56. Curnutte JT, Erickson RW, Ding J, Badwey JA: Reciprocal interactions between protein kinase C and components of the NADPH oxidase complex may regulate superoxide production by neutrophils stimulated with a phorbol ester. J Biol Chem 269:10813, 1994.

57. Ding J, Badwey JA: Wortmannin and 1-butanol block activation of a novel family of protein kinases in neutrophils. FEBS Lett 348:149, 1994.

58. Cui Y, Harvey K, Akard L, Jansen J, Hughes C, Siddiqui RA, English D: Regulation of neutrophil responses by phosphotyrosine phosphatase. J Immunol 152:5420, 1994.

59. Watson F, Lowe GM, Robinsson JJ, Galvani DW, Edwards SW: Phospholipase D-dependent and -independent activation of the neutrophil NADPH oxidase. Biosci Rep 14:91, 1994.

60. McPhail LC, Qualliotine-Mann D, Agwu DE, McCall CE: Phospholipases and activation of the NADPH oxidase. Eur J Haematol 51:294, 1993.

61. Nath J, Ohno Y, Gallin JI, Wright DG: A novel post-translational incorporation of tyrosine into multiple proteins in activated human neutrophils: Correlation with phagocytosis and activation of the NADPH oxidase-mediated respiratory burst. J Immunol 149:3360, 1992.

62. Nanda A, Curnutte JT, Grinstein S: Activation of H⁺ conductance in neutrophils requires assembly of components of the respiratory burst oxidase but not its redox function. J Clin Invest 93:1770, 1994.

63. Henderson LM, Moule SK, Chappel JB: The immediate activator of the NADPH oxidase is arachidonate not phosphorylation. Eur J Biochem 211:157, 1993.

64. Bokoch GM, Knaus UG: The role of small GTP-binding proteins in leukocyte function. Curr Opin Immunol 6:98, 1994.

65. Rotrosen D, Yeung CL, Katkin JP: Production of recombinant cytochrome b_{558} allows reconstitution of phagocyte NADPH oxidase solely from recombinant proteins. J Biol Chem 268:14256, 1993.

66. Cross AR: Inhibitors of the leukocyte superoxide generating oxidase: Mechanisms of action and methods for their elucidation. Free Radical Biol Med 8:71, 1990.

67. Curnutte JT: Molecular basis of the autosomal recessive forms of chronic granulomatous disease. Immunodeficiency Rev 3:149, 1992.

68. Yan L, Vandivier RW, Suffredini AF, Danner RL: Human polymorphonuclear leukocytes lack detectable nitric oxide synthase activity. J Immunol 153:1825, 1994.

69. Clutterbuck EJ, Sanderson CJ: Regulation of human eosinophil precursor production by cytokines: A comparison of recombinant human interleukin-1 (rhIL-1), rhIL-3, rhIL-5, rhIL-6, and rh granulocyte-macrophage colony-stimulating factor. Blood 75:1774, 1990.

70. Spry CJF: Eosinophils: A Comprehensive Review and Guide to the Scientific and Medical Literature. New York, Oxford University Press, 1988.

71. Gleich GJ, Adolphson CR, Leiferman KM: The biology of the eosinophilic leukocyte. Annu Rev Med 44:85, 1993.

72. Venge P: Human eosinophil granule proteins: Structure function and release. In Smith H, Cook RM (eds): Immunopharmacology of Eosinophils. San Diego, Academic Press, 1993, p 43.

73. Hällgren R, Venge P: The eosinophil in inflammation. In Matsson P, Ahlstedt S, Venge P, Thorell J (eds): Clinical Impact of the Monitoring of Allergic Inflammation. San Diego, Academic Press, 1991, pp 119–140.

74. Jacoby DB, Gleich GJ, Fryer AD: Human eosinophil major basic protein is an endogenous allosteric antagonist at the inhibitory muscarinic M2 receptor. J Clin Invest 91:1314, 1993.

75. Ståhle-Bäckdahl M, Parks WC: 92-kd Gelatinase is actively expressed by eosinophils and stored by neutrophils in squamous cell carcinoma. Am J Pathol 142:995, 1993.

76. Wardlaw AJ: Eosinophils in the 1990s: New perspectives on their role in health and disease. Postgrad Med J 70:536, 1994.

77. Resnick MB, Weller PF: Mechanisms of eosinophil recruitment. Am J Respir Cell Mol Biol 8:349, 1993.

78. Rand TH, Cruikshank WW, Center DM, Weller PF: CD4-mediated stimulation of human eosinophils: Lymphocyte chemoattractant factor and other CD4-binding ligands elicit eosinophil migration. J Exp Med 173:1521, 1991.

79. Håkansson L, Carlson M, Ståalenheim G, Venge P: Migratory responses of eosinophil and neutrophil granulocytes from asthmatic patients. J Allergy Clin Immunol 85:743, 1990.

80. Sanderson CJ: Interleukin-5: An eosinophil growth and activation factor. Dev Biol Stand 69:23, 1988.

81. Harriman GR, Strober W: The immunobiology of interleukin-5. In Cruse JM, Lewis E Jr (eds): The Year in Immunology 1988. Immunoregulatory Cytokines and Cell Growth. Basel, Karger, 1989, pp 160–177.

82. Silberstein DS, David JR: The regulation of human eosinophil function by cytokines. Immunol Today 8:380, 1987.

83. Lopez AF, To LB, Yang Y-C, Gamble JR, Shannon MF, Burns GF, Dyson PG, Juttner CA, Clark S, Vadas MA: Stimulation of proliferation, differentiation, and function of human cells by primate interleukin 3. Proc Natl Acad Sci USA 84:2761, 1987.

84. Silberstein DS, Owen WF, Gasson JC, DiPersio JF, Golde DW, Bina JC, Soberman R, Austen KF, David JR: Enhancement of human eosinophil cytotoxicity and leukotriene synthesis by biosynthetic (recombinant) granulocyte-macrophage colony-stimulating factor. J Immunol 137:3290, 1986.

85. Valerius T, Repp R, Kalden JR, Platzer E: Effects of IFN on human eosinophils in comparison with other cytokines: A novel class of eosinophil activators with delayed onset of action. J Immunol 145:2950, 1990.

86. Silberstein DS, Ali MH, Baker SL, David JR: Human eosinophil cytotoxicity-enhancing factor: Purification, physical characteristics, and partial amino acid sequence of an active polypeptide. J Immunol 143:979, 1989.

87. Elsas PX, Elsas MICG, Dessein AJ: Eosinophil cytotoxicity enhancing factor: Purification, characterization and immunocytochemical localization on the monocyte surface. Eur J Immunol 20:1143, 1990.

88. Liesveld JL, Abboud CN: State of the art: The hypereosinophilic syndromes. Blood Rev 5:29, 1991.

CHAPTER 10

Lawrence B. Schwartz

The Mast Cell

The mast cell is the principal cell type that initiates the humoral and cellular inflammatory response characteristic of immediate type hypersensitivity reactions (type I). The early phase of these reactions (5 to 30 minutes, depending on the target tissue), involves local edema, smooth muscle contraction, vasodilation, and increased permeability of postcapillary venules. The late phase of immediate type hypersensitivity involves the recruitment and activation of basophils, eosinophils, and other cell types. Mediators of mast cells stored preformed inside secretory granules (Table 10–1) are released with cell activation. Other mediators not present preformed are synthesized and secreted directly. In humans, the principal preformed mediators include histamine, proteoglycans (heparin, chondroitin sulfates), and neutral proteases (tryptase, chymase, cathepsin G, and carboxypeptidase). Basic fibroblast growth factor (bFGF) also may reside preformed in at least some mast cells. The primary newly generated mediators include the arachidonic acid metabolites, prostaglandin D_2 (PGD_2), and leukotriene C_4 (LTC_4). Also, Th2-like cytokines, such as interleukin-4 (IL)-4, IL-5, IL-6, and IL-13, and tumor necrosis factor-α (TNF-α), are produced by activated mast cells (see Table 10–1). Together, these products of mast cells account for much of the host response.

Mast cells occupy a sentinel position in tissues where noxious substances might attempt entry and immediate type hypersensitivity reactions typically begin. Basophils normally reside in the circulation but enter tissues at sites of inflammation, particularly during the late phase of allergic reactions and during the early phase of delayed type hypersensitivity reactions. These are the two cell types that constitutively express substantial quantities of the high-affinity receptor for IgE (FcϵRI) in an active form and store histamine in their secretory granules. Two mast cell phenotypes have been observed in human tissues, suggesting a purposeful presence for each and a higher level of complexity concerning the pathobiologic mechanisms and pharmacologic control of mast cell–mediated reactions than previously appreciated. The selected participation of basophils and different types of mast cells in various clinical conditions—as well as the duration, intensity, and tissue distribution of a particular response—depends on various characteristics of the agonist, the immunologic sensitivity of the host, the target tissue involved, and any underlying pathology. Because of their obvious relevance to human disease, this chapter focuses on the different types of human mast cells and on human basophils.

DIFFERENT TYPES OF MAST CELLS

Histochemistry, Composition, Distribution, and Morphology

Two distinct types of human mast cells have been described based on different protease compositions of the secretory granules. MC_{TC} cells contain chymase, mast cell carboxypeptidase, cathepsin G, and tryptase; MC_T cells contain only tryptase (see Table 10–1).[1] These proteases are the most discriminating markers of different mast cell types in humans. In histologically normal tissues (Table 10–2), mast cell concentrations are particularly high in the human alveolar wall, bowel mucosa, dermis, and nasal and conjunctival mucosa and around blood vessels, consistent with the clinical alterations known to occur in allergic diseases at these sites. Only modest numbers of mast cells reside in normal human synovium. MC_T cells are the predominant, but not exclusive, type of mast cell found in the lung, particularly alveoli, and the small intestinal mucosa, whereas MC_{TC} cells are the predominant type found in the skin, gastrointestinal submucosa,[2] and normal synovium. The relative abundance of MC_{TC} and MC_T cells may change with tissue inflammation or fibrosis, making it impossible to base a subtype designation on location alone.

As shown in Figure 10–1, mature mast cells of all types have a nucleus without deeply divided lobes, numerous cytoplasmic granules, and thin, elongated folds of the plasma membrane.[3] Human basophils are polymorphonuclear, contain larger and less numerous granules, and have a comparatively smooth plasma membrane contour. Among mature, unstimulated MC_{TC} and MC_T cells, differences in granule morphology correspond to differences in protease composition[4, 5]; MC_T granules often are scroll-rich, whereas MC_{TC} granules have gratings and lattices and are scroll-poor. All granules in both cell types contain tryptase and heparin; all granules in MC_{TC} cells also contain chymase.

Functional and Pharmacologic Differences

Although immunologic stimulation (IgE and allergen) as well as calcium ionophores activate all tissue-derived mast cells, nonimmunologic agonists of biologic importance show selectivity for mast cells from different tissue sites, independent of the protease phe-

Table 10–1. MEDIATORS OF HUMAN MAST CELLS AND BASOPHILS

Mediator	MC$_{TC}$ Cell	MC$_T$ Cell	Basophil
Preformed (granules)			
Histamine	+ +	+ +	+ +
Tryptase	+ +	+ +	±
Chymase	+ +	–	–
Carboxypeptidase	+ +	–	–
Cathepsin G	+ +	–	–
Heparin	+	+	–
Chondroitin sulfate E	+	+	–
Chondroitin sulfate A			+
Newly generated			
Lipoxygenase metabolite			
LTC$_4$	+ +	+ +	+ +
LTB$_4$	+	+	+
Cyclooxygenase metabolite			
PGD$_2$	+ +	+ +	–
Cytokines			
TNF-α	+ +	+ +	+ +
IL-4, -5, -6, -13	+ +	+ +	+ +

Abbreviations: LTC, leukotriene; PGD$_2$, prostaglandin D$_2$; TNF-α, tumor necrosis factor-α; IL, interleukin.

Table 10–2. CHARACTERISTICS OF HUMAN MC$_{TC}$ AND MC$_T$ TYPES OF MAST CELLS

Characteristic	MC$_{TC}$ Cell	MC$_T$ Cell
Normal tissue distribution		
Skin	+ +	–
Intestinal submucosa	+ +	+
Intestinal mucosa	+	+ +
Alveolar wall	–	+ +
Bronchi and bronchioles	+	+ +
Nasal mucosa	+ +	+ +
Conjunctiva	+ +	+
Synovium	+ +	+
Combined immunodeficiency or acquired immunodeficiency syndrome (small intestine)	Amounts unchanged	Amounts decreased
Granule morphology	Grating or lattice; complete scroll-poor	Complete scroll-rich

notype of the mast cell. Mast cells derived from human skin release histamine in response to morphine sulfate, substance P, vasoactive intestinal peptide (VIP), somatostatin, calcitonin gene-related protein (CGRP), and the anaphylatoxins C5a and C3a, whereas mast cells from rheumatoid synovial fluid,

lung, tonsils, adenoids, and colon do not.[6–10] Mast cells from heart uniquely respond to C5a but not to substance P.[11, 12] In contrast, basophils respond to C5a and C3a but not to substance P. Unlike all mast cells, basophils respond to f-Met-Leu-Phe; also, basophils do not respond to morphine or codeine. The desArg derivatives of C3a and C5a are inactive on skin mast cells but still show limited agonist activity against basophils.[10, 13] Whether these basic peptides activate mast cells and basophils by stereospecific receptor

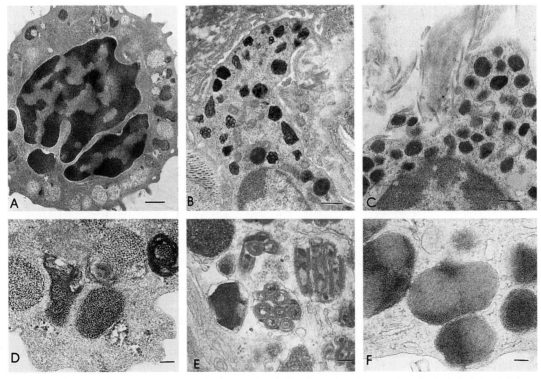

Figure 10–1. Ultrastructural features of human mast cells and basophils. Electron micrographs of a human basophil from peripheral blood (A), MC$_T$ cell from lung (B), MC$_{TC}$ cell from skin (C), and their corresponding secretory granules at a higher magnification (D–F) are shown. Bars in A–C = 0.5 μm; in D–F = 0.1 μm. (Courtesy of Dr. Shirley S. Craig, Virginia Commonwealth University, Richmond.)

interactions or by ionic perturbations of membrane components is unclear.[14] Complement anaphylatoxin activation of rodent mast cells is abolished if sialic acid is removed from the membrane surface and thus may act as a direct stimulator of pertussis-sensitive G-proteins,[15] whereas substance P activity is blocked by a receptor antagonist. Differences in the secretory response between mast cells isolated from different tissues may relate to microenvironmental influences rather than to lineage. For example, the rat mucosal mast cell line, called RBL, acquires responsiveness to substance P when co-cultured with 3T3 fibroblasts without otherwise changing its phenotype.[16]

Histamine-releasing factors also have received considerable attention as alternatives to FcεRI-mediated activation of basophils and possibly mast cells.[17] Mononuclear-derived proteins of the chemokine family, initially discovered because of their abilities to attract predominantly monocytes or neutrophils, include potent basophil histamine-releasing agents. Active chemokines include monocyte chemotactic protein (MCP)-1, -2 and -3; RANTES; monocyte inflammatory peptide (MIP)-1α and -1β; human inflammatory proteins 1α and 1β; connective tissue activating peptide (CTAP)-III; neutrophil-activating peptide (NAP)-2; and fibroblast-induced cytokine (FIC).[18–21] Other nonactivating chemokines may inhibit the activating chemokines by competing for the same binding sites on the basophil cell surface.[22] Although the activities of these cytokines on human mast cells have not been reported in as much detail, basophil-activating chemokines tend to cause chemotaxis of mast cells without causing histamine release in human[23] and rodent[24] studies. Whether MC$_T$ and MC$_{TC}$ or mast cells from different tissue sites exhibit different response patterns remains to be determined.

The pharmacologic responsiveness of mast cells also varies depending on the tissue source. At high concentrations, disodium cromoglycate and nedocromil (used for the treatment of allergic asthma, rhinitis, and conjunctivitis) are weak inhibitors of lung-derived mast cells, but not those from skin and intestine.[25] β-Adrenoreceptor agonists, at concentrations theoretically achievable on the airway surface with inhaled medication, produce 10 to 50 percent inhibition of IgE-dependent histamine release in vitro from dispersed human lung mast cells,[26, 27] whereas generation of LTC$_4$ and PGD$_2$ is inhibited to a greater extent.[28]

Cyclosporine and FK-506 produce rapid and long-lasting inhibition of IgE-dependent histamine release from human basophils and skin-derived and lung-derived mast cells.[29–33] Rapamycin interferes with the inhibitory activity of FK-506 by competing for the same FK-506 binding protein but by itself does not inhibit mast cell or basophil activation. In rodents, cyclosporine and FK-506 prevent induction of cytokine messenger ribonucleic acid (mRNA) and TNF-α protein production by inhibiting calcineurin phosphatase activity.[34–36] Adenosine added to antigen or calcium ionophore–stimulated human mast cells at low concentrations augments ongoing release of both histamine and LTC$_4$, but has no effect on mediator release from unstimulated mast cells.[37] In contrast, release of these mediators from human basophils is inhibited by adenosine. Dexamethasone in vitro inhibits activation and secretion by human basophils,[38] but not by human lung–derived mast cells.[39] In vivo, local instillation of nasal glucocorticosteroids diminished mediator release during the immediate response to nasal allergen challenge,[40] perhaps because of the capacity for local steroids to diminish mast cell concentrations, as demonstrated in the synovium,[41] skin,[42] and rectal mucosa,[43] or to prevent the superficial migration of mast cells, which apparently occurs in atopic subjects during the allergy season.[44, 45]

Mast Cell Types and Human Rheumatic Disease

Alterations in the numbers or distribution of mast cells may occur in human disease. For example, mast cell hyperplasia (near sites of cartilage erosion) has been observed in rheumatoid synovium (Fig. 10–2).[46]

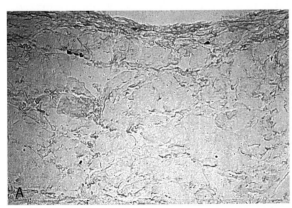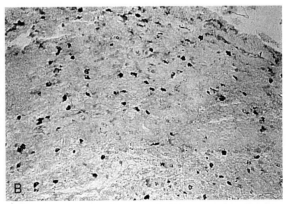

Figure 10–2. Mast cells in human synovium. Tissues were fixed in Carnoy's fluid, embedded in paraffin, and stained sequentially with antitryptase and antichymase antibodies (see Irani et al., 1989).[171] MC$_{TC}$ cells stain brown; MC$_T$ cells stain blue. *A*, Normal synovium. *B*, Rheumatoid synovium. (Courtesy of Dr. Anne-Marie A. Irani, Virginia Commonwealth University, Richmond.)

MC$_{TC}$ cells appear to be associated with areas of dense fibrosis in the rheumatoid synovium, whereas variable ratios of both MC$_T$ and MC$_{TC}$ cells were found at sites of active inflammation.[47]

Involvement of mast cells in other disorders of inflammation and fibrosis has been suggested based on the observation of increased numbers and activation of mast cells in fibrotic lung diseases[48-51] and keloids.[52] In sclerodermatous lung, mast cell numbers or activation may correlate with the level of pulmonary impairment as judged by the chest radiograph.[53] Although mast cell numbers in scleroderma skin are not elevated, the cells often appear fragmented, perhaps reflecting a cytotoxic factor.[54] Studies of the tight skin (Tsk) mouse model of human scleroderma suggest that mast cell hyperplasia may correlate to the severity of the fibrosis but not to its initiation.[55]

Experimentally, bidirectional effects have been reported between mast cells and fibroblasts. Mouse skin–derived 3T3 fibroblasts prolong the survival of human lung mast cells[56] and rodent mast cells. The maturational effect is consistent with previous findings in mice,[57] which suggest that mast cell differentiation from noncommitted cells depends on factors secreted by T lymphocytes whereas maturation of granules depends on fibroblast factors. As discussed later, the production of stem cell factor (SCF) by fibroblasts accounts for a substantial portion of the fibroblast effect on mast cell growth and differentiation. Also, cultured rat embryonic skin fibroblasts phagocytose granules released from co-cultured rat mast cells.[58] Degranulation of lymph node–derived murine mast cells co-cultured with murine embryonic skin fibroblasts results in structural alterations in the fibroblast monolayer.[59] Mouse 3T3 fibroblasts co-cultured with mouse bone marrow–derived mast cells lose their contact inhibition.[60] Tryptase also enhances proliferation of fibroblasts, although contact inhibition is maintained.[61] The ability of purified tryptase to activate latent collagenase derived from rheumatoid synovium[62] and of tryptase[61, 63] and bFGF[64] to stimulate fibroblasts may be relevant to these observations. In mice, production of transforming growth factor-β (TGF-β) and TNF-α by mast cells is associated with increased collagen production by neighboring fibroblasts.[65]

Growth and Differentiation of Mast Cells

Although both mast cells and basophils originate from hematopoietic stem cells, like most myeloid cells, basophils complete their differentiation in the bone marrow whereas mast cells complete their differentiation in peripheral tissues (Fig. 10–3). Basophils develop largely under the influence of IL-3,[66, 67] a process that is augmented by TGF-β.[68] Mast cells differentiate under the influence of stem cell factor,[69–71] the ligand for Kit, a product of the c-*kit* proto-oncogene. IL-3 has little if any influence on the differentiation of human mast cells other than to expand the

pool of hematopoietic progenitor cells; this is in contrast to rodent mast cells, in which IL-3 is an important growth and differentiation factor. Mast cell progenitors identified in peripheral blood have been clearly distinguished from basophils, monocytes, and other leukocytes,[72, 73] and thus represent a distinct myeloid lineage. Conditions that influence the selective development or recruitment of MC$_{TC}$ and MC$_T$ cells are not yet understood. However, commitment to a particular mast cell phenotype appears to have occurred by the time granules begin to form.[74] Unlike other myelocytes that stop expressing Kit as they mature, mast cells express increasing amounts of Kit as they develop. Thus, stem cell factor exerts various effects on mast cells throughout their development, including differentiation, survival,[75–77] chemotaxis,[23, 78] activation,[79, 80] and priming.[80, 81] The effects of differentiation and survival are particularly evident in certain strains of mice with defects in either Kit or stem cell factor in which a profound mast cell deficiency results. Removal of stem cell factor from mast cells in mice[75, 76] and presumably humans[77] results in apoptosis. Of potential interest is the observation that TGF-β inhibits the ability of stem cell factor to rescue murine mast cells from apoptosis.[82] Why mast cells fail to develop in the bone marrow, where stem cell factor clearly exerts an effect on other lineages, is an enigma. Either the bone marrow microenvironment lacks an accessory factor present in peripheral sites or the microenvironment contains additional factors that do not permit mast cell development. The latter seems in part to be the case, because IL-4 appears to prevent the stem cell factor–dependent development of mast cells from progenitors in vitro[77, 83] but has little effect on more mature mast cells. The capacity for IL-4 to down-regulate expression of Kit may explain this observation.[84] Glucocorticosteroids have a similar inhibitory effect on mast cell development, whereas mature mast cells are relatively resistant.[85]

Two experiments suggest that MC$_{TC}$ and MC$_T$ cells develop along distinct pathways. First, in humans with inherited combined immunodeficiency disease and/or acquired immunodeficiency syndrome (AIDS), marked and selective decreases in MC$_T$ cell concentrations occur in the bowel, whereas the concentration and distribution of MC$_{TC}$ cells are unaffected.[86] This suggests that the appearance in tissues of MC$_T$ cells depends on functional T lymphocytes and that MC$_{TC}$ cell development proceeds independently. Second, immature MC$_T$ cells contain granules with complete scrolls and tryptase alone, whereas MC$_{TC}$ cells have granules with electron-dense cores surrounded by a less electron-dense matrix and tryptase together with chymase.[74] Thus, commitment to a particular mast cell type occurs by the time granules begin to form.

MEDIATORS OF MAST CELLS AND BASOPHILS
Preformed Granule-Associated Mediators
Biogenic Amines

Derived from histidine, *histamine* (β-imidazolylethylamine) is the sole biogenic amine in human mast

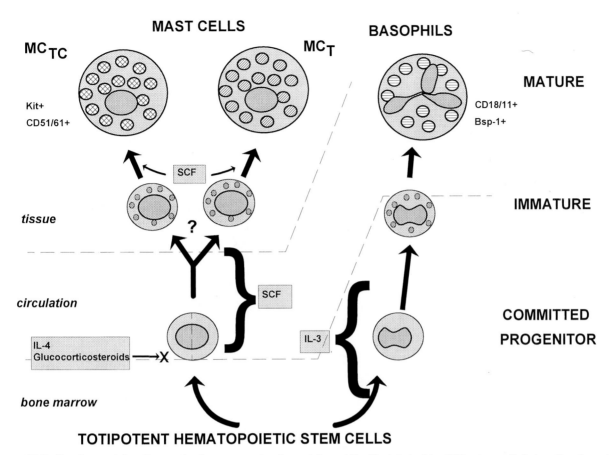

Figure 10–3. Developmental pathways for human mast cells and basophils. IL, interleukin; SCF, stem cell factor. Bsp, basophil-specific protein.

cells and basophils. It is formed from histidine[87] by histidine decarboxylase (Fig. 10–4)[88, 89] and is then stored in secretory granules. Histamine is the only preformed mediator of human mast cells with direct potent vasoactive and smooth muscle spasmogenic effects. With degranulation, histamine is released and diffuses rapidly. Extracellular histamine is metabolized within minutes of release, which suggests that it is destined to act quickly and locally. Human mast cells and basophils contain 1 to 3 picograms (pg) of histamine per cell. Histamine concentrations of about 0.1 mol/L and 2 nmol/L are estimated to exist inside secretory granules and in plasma, respectively. Intermediate levels in samples obtained from other sites reflect rates of local production and removal. Elevated levels of histamine in plasma or urine are detected after anaphylactic reactions to allergens or radiocontrast dyes and in a portion of patients with mastocytosis, a consistent finding with mast cell involvement. Histamine levels are not elevated, however, in patients in septic shock or those with hereditary angioneurotic edema during attacks, consistent with a lack of mast cell involvement.

Histamine exerts its biologic and pathobiologic effects through its interaction with cell-specific receptors designated H1, H2, and H3,[90–92] which initially were defined with the recognition of specific agonists

and antagonists. H1 receptors are blocked by chlorpheniramine; H2 receptors are blocked by cimetidine; and H3 receptors are blocked by thioperamide. Many of the previously described H2 effects were based on using burimamide or impromidine, which shows H3 cross-antagonism. Examples of receptor-specific agonists include 2-methylhistamine at H1 receptors, dimaprit at H2 receptors, and α-methylhistamine at H3 receptors.

Effects of histamine (see Fig. 10–4) mediated by H1 receptors include enhanced permeability of postcapillary venules, vasodilation, contraction of bronchial and gastrointestinal smooth muscle, and increased mucus secretion at mucosal sites. Increased vasopermeability facilitates the tissue deposition of factors from plasma that may be important for tissue growth and repair and of foreign material or immune complexes that result in tissue inflammation. H2 receptor agonists stimulate gastric acid secretion by parietal cells. H2 agonists also inhibit secretion by cytotoxic lymphocytes and granulocytes, augment suppression by T lymphocytes,[93] enhance epithelial permeability across human airways,[94] stimulate chemokinesis of neutrophils and eosinophils and expression of eosinophil C3b receptors, and activate endothelial cells to release a potent inhibitor of platelet aggregation, prostacyclin. Stimulation of H3 receptors affects neu-

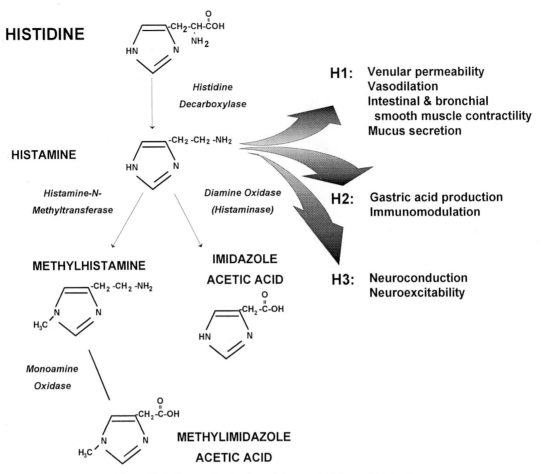

Figure 10–4. The synthesis, degradation, and biology of histamine.

rotransmitter release and histamine formation in the central and peripheral nervous system.[95] H3 receptors are postulated but not proven to be involved in cross-talk between mast cells and peripheral nerves. Bronchial hyperreactivity in atopic patients with asthma to irritant stimuli may be mediated in part by histamine-mediated neurogenic hyperexcitability.

The combined effects of H1 receptor and H2 receptor–mediated activities of histamine are required for the full expression of vasoactivity. For example, the triple response caused by an intradermal injection of histamine—namely, a central erythema within seconds (histamine arteriolar vasodilation), followed by circumferential erythema (axon reflex vasodilation mediated by neuropeptides) and a central wheal (histamine vasopermeability, edema), peaking at about 15 minutes—is mostly blocked by H1 receptor antagonists but is completely blocked only with a combination of H1 and H2 receptor antagonists.[96] Analogous results have been observed for the tachycardia, widened pulse pressure, diastolic hypotension, flushing, and headaches that result from intravenous infusion of histamine.[97]

Neutral Proteases of Human Mast Cells

Neutral proteases cleave peptide bonds near neutral pH. Such enzymes are the dominant protein com-

ponents of secretory granules in human and rodent mast cells.[98] In addition, neutral proteases serve as selective markers that distinguish mast cells from other cell types, including basophils, and different mast cell subpopulations from one another.

Tryptase. Tryptase is the principal enzyme accounting for the trypsin-like activity first detected in human mast cells by histochemical techniques.[99, 100] Substantial amounts of tryptase are present in MC_{TC} cells derived from foreskin (35 pg/cell) and in MC_T cells derived from lung (10 pg/cell), where it is located in secretory granules and is released in parallel with histamine during degranulation.[101] Negligible amounts have been measured in human basophils (0.04 pg/cell), where tryptase mRNA levels approximately 10^5-fold lower than levels in tissue mast cells have been measured.[102] Other cell types have no detectable tryptase protein or mRNA. Thus, the enzyme is a discriminating marker of human mast cells.

Tryptase is a tetrameric serine endoprotease of 134 kD with N-glycosylated subunits of 31 to 34 kD, each with an active enzymatic site.[99] Although at least two homologous tryptase complementary DNA (cDNA) molecules (α and β) and corresponding genes have been identified on human chromosome 16,[103–105] β-tryptase appears to account for all of the enzymatically active tryptase.[105a] A mutation in the leader sequence of α-tryptase prevents processing to a mature form, causing it to be constitutively secreted without being stored in secretory granules. Thus, when tryptase activity for mast cell–derived material is being discussed, β-tryptase is the species actually being measured.

Tryptase activity is measured by hydrolysis of synthetic trypsin-like substrates, and the absence of inhibition by the biologic inhibitors of serine esterases present in plasma, lung, and urine clearly distinguishes tryptase from pancreatic trypsin and from most other serine esterases. Tryptase stored in secretory granules is fully active, uniquely stabilized in its active tetrameric form by binding to heparin.[106] When free in solution, tryptase subunits rapidly dissociate from one another into inactive monomers without any evidence for autodegradation.[107]

Several tryptase-mediated activities of potential biologic interest have been examined in vitro (Table 10–3). Tryptase rapidly inactivates fibrinogen as a coagulable substrate for thrombin[108]; the lack of fibrin deposition and rapid resolution of urticarial and angioedematous reactions may, in part, reflect this same activity in vivo. Tryptase activates latent collagenase derived from rheumatoid synovial cells, apparently by first activating prostromelysin (metalloproteinase III),[62] which then activates latent collagenase. The increased numbers of mast cells found in rheumatoid synovium[41] and in inflammatory cutaneous lesions of scleroderma,[109] together with the increased tissue turnover that occurs in each condition, suggest a related role for tryptase. Also of interest are the abilities of tryptase to stimulate smooth muscle cells[110] and fibroblasts.[61] The recent availability of tryptase inhibitors as potential therapeutics should provide better information on the biologic and pathobiologic roles of this enzyme in humans.

Chymase. Chymase is the enzyme that accounts for most of the chymotrypsin-like activity in human cutaneous mast cells. The enzyme was purified from human skin,[111] and the corresponding gene was cloned and localized to human chromosome 14.[112] Chymase was selectively localized to a subpopulation of mast cells by enzymatic and immunohistochemical techniques.[2] Dispersed MC_{TC} cells obtained from skin contain 4.5 pg of chymase per mast cell.

Human chymase is a monomer of 30 kD with chymotryptic activity on synthetic substrates. Like tryptase, chymase is a serine esterase that is stored fully active in mast cell secretory granules, presumably bound to heparin, chondroitin sulfate E, or both. Unlike tryptase, chymase stability is not substantially affected by heparin,[113] and its activity is inhibited by classic biologic inhibitors of serine proteinases, such as $α_1$-antichymotrypsin, $α_1$-proteinase inhibitor, and $α_2$-macroglobulin.[114] Neither chymotrypsin-like enzymatic activity nor chymase mRNA is detected in MC_T cells.[102]

Potential biologic activities of chymase, like those of tryptase, are based on in vitro observations (see Table 10–3). Chymase is a potent activator of angiotensin I,[115] inactivates bradykinin,[116] and attacks the lamina lucida of the basement membrane at the dermal-epidermal junction of human skin.[117] The physiologic importance of angiotensin II generation by mast cell chymase is supported by a study in marmosets showing that administration of an angiotensin II derivative, capable of being activated by chymase but not by angiotensin-converting enzyme, raised arterial blood pressure. Dog chymase stimulates mucus production from glandular cells in vitro,[118] which suggests a similar role in asthma and allergic rhinitis, in which release of chymase in proximity to glandular tissue might be involved in the state of hypersecretion.

Human Mast Cell Cathepsin G. This is a serine-class neutral protease found in mast cells as well as in neutrophils and monocytes. The enzyme resides with chymase in MC_{TC} cells[119, 120] and has a molecular weight of 30 kD.

Human Mast Cell Carboxypeptidase. This protease resides with chymase and cathepsin G in secretory granules of MC_{TC} cells.[121] Stored fully active, when released it cleaves the carboxy terminal His^9–Leu^{10} bond of angiotensin I and behaves like a zinc metalloexopeptidase.[122] Human mast cells dispersed from skin contain 5 to 16 pg of carboxypeptidase per cell.[123] Human mast cell carboxypeptidase is a monomer with a molecular weight of 34.5 kD.[123] Based on analysis of the cDNA-derived amino acid sequence and gene structure,[124] the human enzyme is more homologous to human pancreatic carboxypeptidase B than A, but the catalytic site is more homologous to human pancreatic carboxypeptidase A, as are its substrate specificities for carboxy terminal Phe and Leu residues.

Proteoglycans

The presence of highly sulfated proteoglycans in secretory granules of mast cells and basophils results in metachromasia when these cells are stained with basic dyes. Proteoglycans are composed of glycosaminoglycan side chains (repeating unbranched disaccha-

Table 10–3. POTENTIAL BIOLOGIC PROPERTIES OF HUMAN TRYPTASE AND CHYMASE

Protease	Property
Tryptase	Fibrinogenolysis
	High-molecular-weight kininogen destruction
	Neuropeptide degradation
	Prostromelysin activation
	Cellular activation
	Fibroblast proliferation
	Pulmonary smooth muscle hyperreactivity to histamine
Chymase	Generation of angiotensin II
	Procollagenase activation
	Basement membrane degradation
	Glandular mucus secretion
	Neuropeptide degradation

ride units of a uronic acid and hexosamine moieties that are variably sulfated) covalently linked to a single-chain protein core by means of a specific trisaccharide-protein linkage region consisting of -Gal-Gal-Xyl-Ser. The intracellular proteoglycans of concern to mast cells are *heparin* and *chondroitin sulfate E*.[125, 126] *Chondroitin sulfate A* is the predominant type in human basophils.[127] Heparin is selectively concentrated only in mast cells but is present in all mature mast cells[128]; chondroitin sulfates A and E are also found in other cell types.

The characteristic disaccharide units of heparin and chondroitin sulfates E and A are shown in Figure 10–5. The average number of sulfate residues per disaccharide is 2.5, 1.5, and 1.0, respectively. The characteristic susceptibility of heparin to nitrous acid is due to attack at the N-sulfate residue; chondroitin sulfates lack this residue and are resistant to nitrous acid.

The same peptide core is associated with heparin and chondroitin sulfate proteoglycans, and both proteoglycan types may reside in the same cell, even on the same peptide core. In humans, the 17.6-kD core protein contains a glycosaminoglycan attachment region of 18 amino acids,[129] where two or three glycosaminoglycans of about 20 kD are attached.[130, 131] The attachment region is rich in alternating Ser-Gly residues, and the gene is located on chromosome 10.

The biologic functions of endogenous mast cell proteoglycans are somewhat speculative. These proteoglycans bind to histamine, neutral proteases, and acid hydrolases at the acidic pH inside mast cell secretory granules and may facilitate processing of the enzymes as well as uptake and packaging of these mediators into the secretory granules. The stabilizing effect of heparin and, to a lesser degree, chondroitin sulfate E on human tryptase activity[106, 107] may be crucial for the full expression of mast cell–mediated events. Heparin and, to a lesser extent, chondroitin sulfate E express anticoagulant, anticomplement, antikallikrein, and Hageman factor autoactivation activities. Heparin neutralizes the ability of eosinophil-derived major basic protein to kill schistosomula and enhances the binding of fibronectin to collagen. Heparin protects and facilitates bFGF activity,[132] which appears to reside in cutaneous mast cells,[64] and modulates the cell adhesion properties of matrix proteins such as vitronectin, fibronectin, and laminin. Binding of heparin to L- and P-selectins inhibits inflammation,[133] perhaps by blocking leukocyte rolling. The anticoagulant activities of human and commercial porcine heparin are similar and depend on a specific pentasaccharide

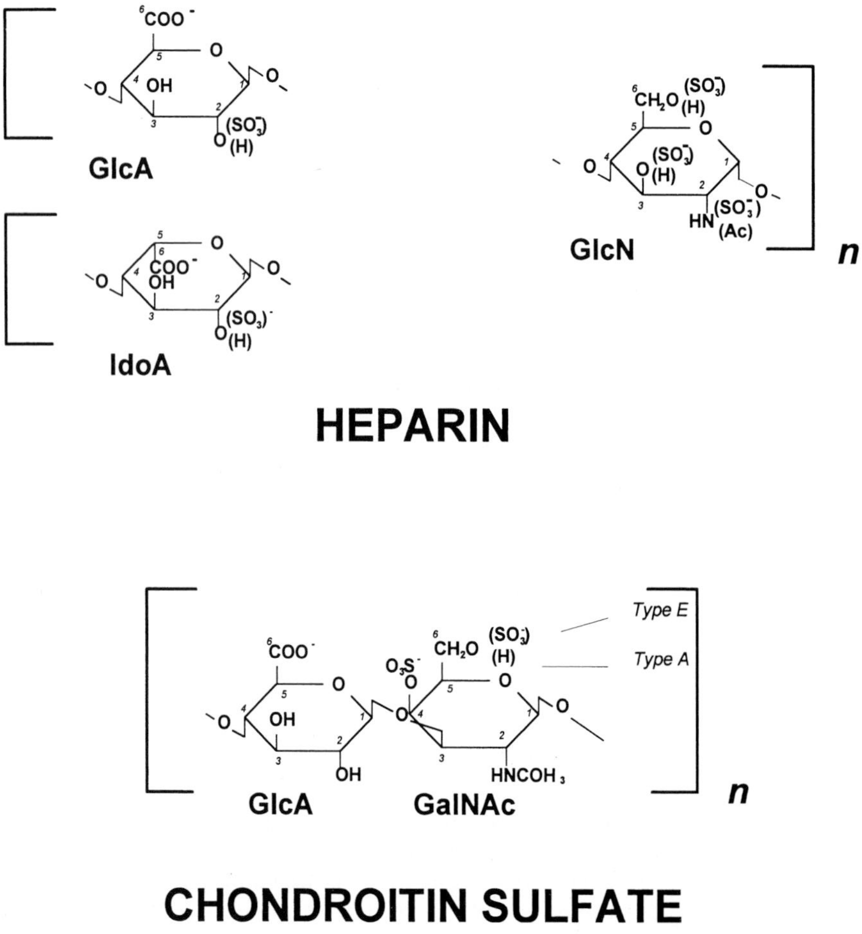

HEPARIN

Figure 10–5. Structural characteristics of mast cell and basophil proteoglycans. GlcA, glucuronic acid; IdoA, iduronic acid; GlcN, glucosamine; GalNAc, N-acetylgalactosamine.

CHONDROITIN SULFATE

sequence.[134] When heparin is saturated with tryptase and other mast cell proteases, however, these activities may be attenuated.

Newly Generated Lipid Mediators

Liberation of the 20-carbon polyunsaturated fatty acid called *arachidonic acid* from cellular lipid stores by phospholipase A occurs with mast cell activation, whereupon it is reincorporated into lipids, released, or oxidatively metabolized. Unstimulated human mast cells derived from lung incorporate exogenous arachidonic acid into neutral lipids and phospholipids in a ratio of about 7:2[135] and store these lipids in membranes and cytoplasmic lipid bodies.[136] Arachidonate released by hydrolysis of these lipids is then metabolized along either the cyclooxygenase pathway to prostaglandins and thromboxanes, or the 5-, 12-, or 15-lipoxygenase pathway to monohydroxyl fatty acids, leukotrienes—which include both LTB_4 and the sulfidopeptides LTC_4, LTD_4, and LTE_4 (slow-reacting substances of anaphylaxis [SRS-A]—and lipoxins. Platelet activating factor (PAF), made by acetylating the lysophospholipid remaining after arachidonic

acid departs, has not been shown to be a major secretory product of human mast cells and basophils. The major eicosanoid products of mast cells and selected properties are shown in Figure 10–6.

On activation, dispersed and purified preparations of human mast cells obtained from lung, skin, and intestine produce PGD_2 and LTC_4 in weight ratios of approximately 5:1.[137] Smaller amounts of LTB_4 isomers are also produced. Ratios of these metabolites cannot be used to distinguish MC_T from MC_{TC} cell activation. In contrast, peripheral blood basophils obtained from normal humans, when activated, synthesize LTC_4 but not PGD_2.[138] Cells other than mast cells and basophils, however, produce PGD_2 and LTC_4. Thus, when these products are detected in a complex biologic milieu, their cell source may be ambiguous.

The biologic importance of mast cell–derived products of arachidonic acid has gained support with the advent of 5-lipoxygenase inhibitors and LTD_4 inhibitors, both of which are helpful in atopic and aspirin-induced asthma, each condition also involving activation of mast cells.[139] A metabolite of PGD_2 has been detected in the urine of patients with active systemic mastocytosis but not in normal subjects.[140] The importance of PGD_2 production in the subgroup of these

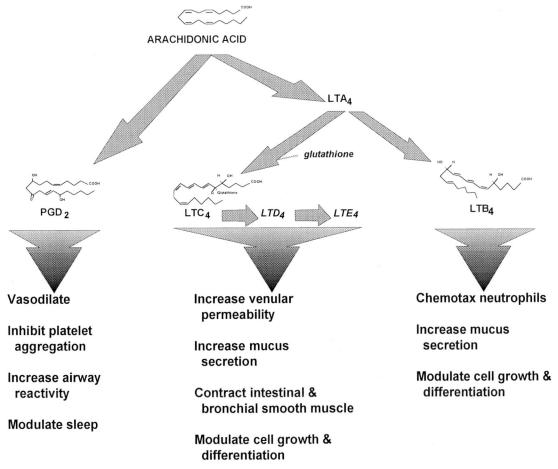

Figure 10–6. Major leukotriene and prostaglandin products of mast cells and basophils. LT, leukotriene; PG, prostaglandin.

patients with recurrent hypotensive episodes was suggested when administration of aspirin inhibited generation of the PGD$_2$ metabolite and led to clinical improvement.

Cytokines (see Table 10–1)

Human mast cells and basophils, when activated, produce a diverse array of cytokines, including TNF-α and IL-4, IL-5, IL-6, and IL-13.[141–143] Cytokine production occurs minutes to hours after mast cells or basophils are activated, in marked variance to the unloading of granule mediators within minutes and the generation of arachidonic acid metabolites beginning within minutes and lasting up to about 30 minutes. These cytokines serve to activate endothelial cells to recruit eosinophils and other cell types during the late-phase response of immediate type hypersensitivity reactions. They provide a mechanism for mast cell involvement in sustaining allergic inflammation hours after release of granule mediators may have finished.

ACTIVATION AND REGULATED SECRETION

Immunologic activation of mast cells and basophils typically begins by cross-linkage of IgE bound to the high-affinity Fcε receptor (FcεR1, $K_a = 10^9$ M^{-1}) with multivalent allergen. The FcεR1 receptor is composed of four subunits,[144] αβγ$_2$, shown schematically in Figure 10–7. The α-chain contains the IgE-binding domain. The β-chain and two disulfide-linked γ-chains are not accessible on the surface. The γ-chains are involved in signal transduction and also are present in the CD16 FcγRIII receptors of natural killer cells and may substitute for the T cell receptor (TCR) ζ-chain. In vivo, autoantibodies against FcεRIα[145] and against IgE[146] in patients with idiopathic urticaria have been detected, suggesting an autoimmune cause in some patients with this disorder.

Regulated secretion by mast cells and basophils also may be induced by nonimmunologic agonists. Multivalent lectins, like bivalent concanavalin A (Con A), cross-link membrane FcεRI or IgE. Calcium ionophores activate by translocating calcium. Basic biomolecules, such as compound 48/80, C3a, C5a, mor-

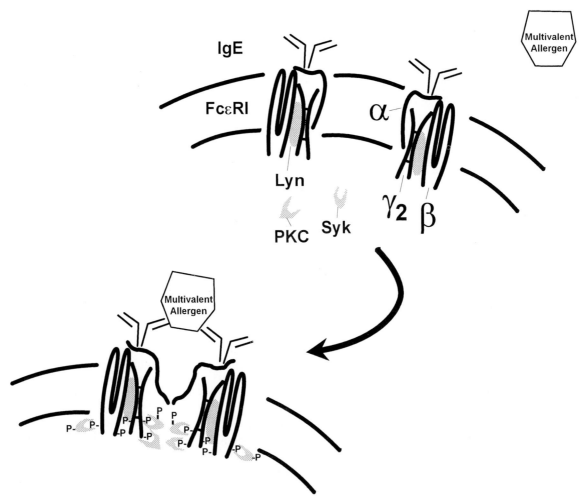

Figure 10–7. Early biochemical steps involved in the activation of mast cells. IgE, immunoglobin E. PKC, protein kinase C.

phine, mellitin, and eosinophil-derived major basic protein, and various neuropeptides, such as substance P, directly perturb the plasma membrane of human mast cells derived from skin but are inactive against mast cells derived from most other tissues or against basophils. The peptide f-Met-Leu-Phe activates human basophils but not mast cells. Various histamine-releasing factors derived from monocytes, lymphocytes, platelets, and neutrophils also have been described that are of potential clinical significance.

Mast cells undergo regulated exocytosis when FcεRI (α, β, γ₂) receptors are dimerized by multivalent antigen or anti–receptor antibody. The earliest biochemical events involved in signal transduction after FcεR1 aggregation involve phosphorylation of the β- and γ-chains of the high-affinity receptor (see Fig. 10–7). Phosphorylation of tyrosines in membrane proteins often occurs on a special motif consisting of six conserved amino acids (two Tyr residues) distributed over a 26–amino acid stretch called ITAM (immunoreceptor tyrosine activation motif), previously called ARH1 (antigen receptor homology 1), ARAM (antigen receptor activation motif), and TAM (tyrosine activation motif). These ITAMs associate with Src-family protein tyrosine kinases (PTKs). Activation of these PTKs lead to the phosphorylation of Tyr residues in the ITAMs and the phosphorylation and activation of downstream effector molecules such as phospholipase Cγ, Ras, and phosphatidylinositol-3 kinase (PI3-k). ITAMs are found on both γ and β, and these two subunits are phosphorylated within seconds after receptor cross-linking and are dephosphorylated almost immediately on disruption of the receptor aggregates. The PTK Lyn associates with the β- and γ-chains when the cells are at rest and initiates phosphorylation of these chains after receptor aggregation.[147] Also, a calcium-independent isoform of protein kinase C appears to associate with and phosphorylate the γ-chain.

Phosphorylation of these sites increases the affinity of cytoplasmic PTK Syk for these chains. Syk is then phosphorylated by Lyn and possibly by itself and is required for mast cell activation.[148–150] These early events also are regulated by CD45, a protein tyrosine phosphatase, because mast cells from mice that are deficient in this enzyme do not exhibit IgE-dependent activation.[151] The hematopoietic cytoplasmic phosphatase also is thought to down-regulate Lyn-dependent events. Phosphorylated Syk then carries the activation signal to pathways involving phospholipase Cγ, MAP kinase,[152] and PI-3 kinase.

Degranulation is associated with activation of small G-proteins that cause actin polymerization and actin relocalization. Metabolism of phospholipids, which reside mostly in secretory granules,[153] occurs early during the secretory response, is necessary for the later secretion of lipid mediators, and may be important for regulated secretion to ensue. Generation of inositol 1,4,5-triphosphate (IP₃) and diacylglycerol (DAG) after FcεRI receptor aggregation occurs and results in release of calcium from the endoplasmic reticulum. This in turn stimulates calcium-dependent isoforms of protein kinase C[154] and may directly facilitate fusion of lipid bilayers as exocytosis proceeds.

BIOLOGY AND PATHOBIOLOGY OF HUMAN MAST CELLS

A precise assessment of mast cell involvement in various diseases has been facilitated by use of monoclonal antibodies that selectively recognize the proteases specific to this cell type. The finding of a secretory granule marker for human basophils[155] holds promise that similar tests for basophil involvement will become available.

Specific immunoassays for tryptase have been developed to quantify total amounts of the enzyme in complex biologic fluids as a reflection of mast cell activation and mast cell number. One immunoassay,[156] termed *G5 capture*, detects primarily β-tryptase[157] and therefore reflects mast cell activation. Baseline levels of tryptase with the G5 capture assay are less than 1 ng/ml but rise during systemic anaphylaxis if clinical severity is sufficient to cause hypotension.[158, 159] In fact, peak levels of tryptase correlate closely with the drop in mean arterial pressure seen with systemic anaphylaxis to insect stings.[160] The other immunoassay,[161] termed *B12 capture*, detects both α- and β-tryptase.[157] Baseline levels of tryptase with the B12 assay are about 5 ng/ml, indicating that the predominant form of tryptase in baseline serum is α-tryptase. This form is markedly elevated in people with systemic mastocytosis.[157] Elevated levels of tryptase by the G5 assay in postmortem serum have been used to suggest premortem anaphylaxis as a cause of death[162] and have implicated anaphylaxis as a cause of death in a substantial number of victims of sudden infant death syndrome.[163]

Arthritis

Possible roles for mast cell involvement in arthritis are well documented.[164] Increased concentrations and depth of mast cells in synovial tissue are found in patients with rheumatoid arthritis.[165, 166] Increased numbers of the MC_T type of mast cells are seen in regions with mononuclear infiltrates; MC_TC cells are seen in regions with fibrosis.[47] Mast cells free in synovial fluid are occasionally observed.[167] Suppression of mast cell hyperplasia occurs after intrasynovial injection of glucocorticosteroid but not after treatment with low-dose methotrexate.[41] IgE rheumatoid factors have been observed in synovial fluid capable of activating mast cells in vitro.[168] One study, however, found no effect of astemizole on the clinical course of rheumatoid arthritis; this suggests that if mast cells are involved, released histamine has little impact on the disease.[169] Released tryptase may affect cartilage and bone turnover and synovial fibrosis. In synovial fluid taken from patients with various arthritides, including osteoarthritis, rheumatoid arthritis, and acute gout, levels of tryptase did not correlate with a particular pathogenic cause or with the degree of complement activation, although lower levels of tryptase were found more often in fluids with higher levels of C3a.[170]

Whether tryptase levels in synovial fluid accurately reflect levels of mast cell activation in synovial tissue is unclear. Larger volumes of synovial fluid, faster rates of exchange of soluble proteins across vascular surfaces, and higher turnover rates in inflamed tissue may obscure higher production rates of tryptase at such sites. Thus, a better understanding of the mechanism of mast cell involvement in synovial inflammation is needed.

References

1. Irani AA: Tissue and developmental variation of protease expression in human mast cells. In Caughey GH (ed): Mast Cell Proteases in Immunology and Biology. New York, Marcel Dekker, 1995, pp 127–144.
2. Irani AA, Schechter NM, Craig SS, et al: Two types of human mast cells that have distinct neutral protease compositions. Proc Natl Acad Sci USA 83:4464, 1986.
3. Dvorak AM: The fine structure of human basophils and mast cells. In Holgate ST (ed): Mast Cells, Mediators and Disease. London, Kluwer Academic Publishers, 1988, pp 29–97.
4. Craig SS, Schechter NM, Schwartz LB: Ultrastructural analysis of human T and TC mast cells identified by immunoelectron microscopy. Lab Invest 58:682, 1988.
5. Craig SS, Schwartz LB: Human MC$_{TC}$ type of mast cell granule: The uncommon occurrence of discrete scrolls associated with focal absence of chymase. Lab Invest 63:581, 1990.
6. Church MK, Pao GJK, Holgate ST: Characterization of histamine secretion from mechanically dispersed human lung mast cells: Effects of anti-IgE, calcium ionophore A 23187, compound 48/80, and basic polypeptides. J Immunol 129:2116, 1982.
7. Fox CC, Dvorak AM, Peters SP, et al: Isolation and characterization of human intestinal mucosal mast cells. J Immunol 135:483, 1985.
8. Schmutzler W, Delmich K, Eichelberg D, et al: The human adenoidal mast cell: Susceptibility to different secretagogues and secretion inhibitors. Int Arch Allergy Appl Immunol 77:177, 1985.
9. Bloch JG, Asch L, Landry Y, et al: Effects of different secretagogues on synovial fluid mast cells from patients with rheumatoid arthritis. Agents Actions 36 (Suppl C):C290, 1992.
10. El-Lati SG, Dahinden CA, Church MK: Complement peptides C3a- and C5a-induced mediator release from dissociated human skin mast cells. J Invest Dermatol 102:803, 1994.
11. Patella V, Marinò I, Lampärter B, et al: Human heart mast cells: Isolation, purification, ultrastructure, and immunologic characterization. J Immunol 154:2855, 1995.
12. Sperr WR, Bankl HC, Mundigler G, et al: The human cardiac mast cell: Localization, isolation, phenotype, and functional characterization. Blood 84:3876, 1994.
13. Bürgi B, Brunner T, Dahinden CA: The degradation product of the C5a anaphylatoxin C5a$_{desarg}$ retains basophil-activating properties. Eur J Immunol 24:1583, 1994.
14. Mousli M, Hugli TE, Landry Y, et al: Peptidergic pathway in human skin and rat peritoneal mast cell activation. Immunopharmacology 27:1, 1994.
15. Mousli M, Hugli TE, Landry Y, et al: A mechanism of action for anaphylatoxin C3a stimulation of mast cells. J Immunol 148:2456, 1992.
16. Swieter M, Midura RJ, Nishikata H, et al: Mouse 3T3 fibroblasts induce rat basophilic leukemia (RBL-2H3) cells to acquire responsiveness to compound 48/80. J Immunol 150:617, 1993.
17. Baggiolini M, Dahinden CA: CC chemokines in allergic inflammation. Immunol Today 15:127, 1994.
18. Kuna P, Reddigari SR, Schall TJ, et al: Characterization of the human basophil response to cytokines, growth factors, and histamine releasing factors of the intercrine/chemokine family. J Immunol 150:1932, 1993.
19. Alam R, Kumar D, Anderson-Walters D, et al: Macrophage inflammatory protein-1α and monocyte chemoattractant peptide-1 elicit immediate and late cutaneous reactions and activate murine mast cells in vivo. J Immunol 152:1298, 1994.
20. Dahinden CA, Geiser T, Brunner T, et al: Monocyte chemotactic protein 3 is a most effective basophil- and eosinophil-activating chemokine. J Exp Med 179:751, 1994.
21. Alam R, Forsythe P, Stafford S, et al: Monocyte chemotactic protein-2, monocyte chemotactic protein-3, and fibroblast-induced cytokine: Three new chemokines induce chemotaxis and activation of basophils. J Immunol 153:3155, 1994.
22. Kuna P, Reddigari SR, Rucinski D, et al: Chemokines of the α, β-subclass inhibit human basophils' responsiveness to monocyte chemotactic and activating factor/monocyte chemoattractant protein-1. J Allergy Clin Immunol 95:574, 1995.
23. Nilsson G, Butterfield JH, Nilsson K, et al: Stem cell factor is a chemotactic factor for human mast cells. J Immunol 153:3717, 1994.
24. Harris RB, You JL, Milton CF, et al: The role of propeptide hormone protein conformation in limited endoproteolysis: Processing mammalian hypothalamic progonadotropin-releasing hormone (GnRH) precursor protein. In Hedin PA, Menn JJ, Hollingworth RM (eds): Natural and Engineered Pest Management Agents. Washington, DC, American Chemical Society, 1994, pp 230–248.
25. Okayama Y, Benyon RC, Rees PH, et al: Inhibition profiles of sodium cromoglycate and nedocromil sodium on mediator release from mast cells of human skin, lung, tonsil, adenoid and intestine. Clin Exp Allergy 22:401, 1992.
26. Church MK, Hiroi J: Inhibition of IgE-dependent histamine release from human dispersed lung mast cells by anti-allergic drugs and salbutamol. Br J Pharmacol 90:421, 1987.
27. Peters SP, Schulman ES, Schleimer RP, et al: Dispersed human lung mast cells: Pharmacologic aspects and comparison with human lung tissue fragments. Am Rev Respir Dis 126:1034, 1982.
28. Undem BJ, Peachell PT, Lichtenstein LM: Isoproterenol-induced inhibition of immunoglobulin E–mediated release of histamine and arachidonic acid metabolites from the human lung mast cell. J Pharmacol Exp Ther 247:209, 1988.
29. Marone G, Triggiani M, Cirillo R, et al: Cyclosporin A inhibits the release of histamine and peptide leukotriene C4 from human lung mast cells. Ric Clin Lab 18:53, 1988.
30. Stellato C, De Paulis A, Ciccarelli A, et al: Anti-inflammatory effect of cyclosporin A on human skin mast cells. J Invest Dermatol 98:800, 1992.
31. Casolaro V, Spadaro G, Patella V, et al: In vivo characterization of the anti-inflammatory effect of cyclosporin A on human basophils. J Immunol 151:5563, 1993.
32. De Paulis A, Stellato C, Cirillo R, et al: Anti-inflammatory effect of FK-506 on human skin mast cells. J Invest Dermatol 99:723, 1992.
33. Cirillo R, Triggiani M, Siri L, et al: Cyclosporin A rapidly inhibits mediator release from human basophils presumably by interacting with cyclophilin. J Immunol 144:3891, 1990.
34. Kaye RE, Fruman DA, Bierer BE, et al: Effects of cyclosporin A and FK506 on Fc$_ε$ receptor type I-initiated increases in cytokine mRNA in mouse bone marrow-derived progenitor mast cells: Resistance to FK506 is associated with a deficiency in FK506-binding protein FKBP12. Proc Natl Acad Sci USA 89:8542, 1992.
35. Wershil BK, Furuta GT, Lavigne JA, et al: Dexamethasone or cyclosporin A suppress mast cell–leukocyte cytokine cascades: Multiple mechanisms of inhibition of IgE- and mast cell–dependent cutaneous inflammation in the mouse. J Immunol 154:1391, 1995.
36. Fruman DA, Bierer BE, Benes JE, et al: The complex of FK506-binding protein 12 and FK506 inhibits calcineurin phosphatase activity and IgE activation-induced cytokine transcripts, but not exocytosis, in mouse mast cells. J Immunol 154:1846, 1995.
37. Peachell PT, Lichtenstein LM, Schleimer RP: Differential regulation of human basophil and lung mast cell function by adenosine. J Pharmacol Exp Ther 256:717, 1991.
38. Schleimer RP, Lichtenstein LM, Gillespie E: Inhibition of basophil histamine release by anti-inflammatory steroids. Nature (Lond) 292:454, 1981.
39. Schleimer RP, Schulman ES, MacGlash DW, et al: Effects of dexamethasone on mediator release from human lung fragments and purified human lung mast cells. J Clin Invest 71:1830, 1983.
40. Pipkorn U, Proud D, Lichtenstein LM, et al: Inhibition of mediator release in allergic rhinitis by pretreatment with topical glucocorticosteroids. N Engl J Med 316:1506, 1987.
41. Malone DG, Wilder RL, Saavedra-Delgado AM, et al: Mast cell numbers in rheumatoid synovial tissues: Correlations with quantitative measures of lymphatic infiltration and modulation by anti-inflammatory therapy. Arthritis Rheum 30:130, 1987.
42. Lavker RM, Schechter NM: Cutaneous mast cell depletion results from topical corticosteroid usage. J Immunol 135:2368, 1985.
43. Goldsmith P, McGarity B, Walls AF, et al: Corticosteroid treatment reduces mast cell numbers in inflammatory bowel disease. Digest Dis Sci 35:1409, 1990.
44. Enerbäck L, Pipkorn U, Granerus G: Intraepithelial migration of nasal mucosal mast cells in hay fever. Int Arch Allergy Appl Immunol 80:44, 1986.
45. Bentley AM, Jacobson MR, Cumberworth V, et al: Immunohistology of

the nasal mucosa in seasonal allergic rhinitis: Increases in activated eosinophils and epithelial mast cells. J Allergy Clin Immunol 89:877, 1992.

46. Wasserman SI: The mast cell and synovial inflammation: Or, what's a nice cell like you doing in a joint like this? Arthritis Rheum 27:841, 1984.

47. Irani AA, Golzar N, DeBlois G, et al: Distribution of mast cell subsets in rheumatoid arthritis and osteoarthritis synovia (abstr). Arthritis Rheum 30:66, 1987.

48. Kawanami O, Ferrans V, Fulmer JD, et al: Ultrastructure of pulmonary mast cells in patients with fibrotic lung disorders. Lab Invest 40:717, 1979.

49. Goto T, Befus D, Low R, et al: Mast cell heterogeneity and hyperplasia in bleomycin-induced pulmonary fibrosis in rats. Am Rev Respir Dis 130:797, 1984.

50. Hunt LW, Colby TV, Weiler DA, et al: Immunofluorescent staining for mast cells in idiopathic pulmonary fibrosis: Quantification and evidence for extracellular release of mast cell tryptase. Mayo Clin Proc 67:941, 1992.

51. Pesci A, Bertorelli G, Gabrielli M, et al: Mast cells in fibrotic lung disorders. Chest 103:989, 1993.

52. Smith CJ, Smith JC, Finn MC: The possible role of mast cells (allergy) in the production of keloid and hypertrophic scarring. J Burn Care Rehabil 8:126, 1987.

53. Chanez P, Lacoste J-Y, Guillot B, et al: Mast cells' contribution to the fibrosing alveolitis of the scleroderma lung. Am Rev Respir Dis 147:1497, 1993.

54. Irani A-MA, Gruber BL, Kaufman LD, et al: Mast cell changes in scleroderma: Presence of MC$_T$ cells in the skin and evidence of mast cell activation. Arthritis Rheum 35:933, 1992.

55. Everett ET, Pablos JL, Harley RA, et al: The role of mast cells in the development of skin fibrosis in tight-skin mutant mice. Comp Biochem Physiol [A] 110A:159, 1995.

56. Levi-Schaffer F, Austen KF, Caulfield JP, et al: Co-culture of human lung-derived mast cells with mouse 3T3 fibroblasts: Morphology and IgE-mediated release of histamine, prostaglandin D2, and leukotrienes. J Immunol 139:494, 1987.

57. Davidson SMA, Mansour A, Gallily R, et al: Mast cell differentiation depends on T cells and granule synthesis on fibroblasts. Immunology 48:439, 1983.

58. Subba Rao PV, Friedman MM, Atkins FM, et al: Phagocytosis of mast cell granules by cultured fibroblasts. J Immunol 130:341, 1983.

59. Ginsburg H, Amira M, Padawer J, et al: Structural alterations in fibroblast monolayers caused by mast cell degranulation. J Leukocyte Biol 45:491, 1989.

60. Dayton ET, Caulfield JP, Hein A, et al: Regulation of the growth rate of mouse fibroblasts by IL-3–activated mouse bone marrow–derived mast cells. J Immunol 142:4307, 1989.

61. Hartmann T, Ruoss SJ, Raymond WW, et al: Human tryptase as a potent, cell-specific mitogen: Role of signaling pathways in synergistic responses. Am J Physiol Lung Cell Mol Physiol 262:L528, 1992.

62. Gruber BL, Marchese MJ, Suzuki K, et al: Synovial procollagenase activation by human mast cell tryptase dependence upon matrix metalloproteinase 3 activation. J Clin Invest 84:1657, 1989.

63. Ruoss SJ, Hartmann T, Caughey GH: Mast cell tryptase is a mitogen for cultured fibroblasts. J Clin Invest 88:493, 1991.

64. Reed JA, Albino AP, McNutt NS: Human cutaneous mast cells express basic fibroblast growth factor. Lab Invest 72:215, 1995.

65. Gordon JR, Galli SJ: Promotion of mouse fibroblast collagen gene expression by mast cells stimulated via the FcεRI. Role for mast cell–derived transforming growth factor β and tumor necrosis factor α. J Exp Med 180:2027, 1994.

66. Valent P, Schmidt G, Besemer J, et al: Interleukin-3 is a differentiation factor for human basophils. Blood 73:1763, 1989.

67. Dvorak AM, Saito H, Estrella P, et al: Ultrastructure of eosinophils and basophils stimulated to develop in human cord blood mononuclear cell cultures containing recombinant human interleukin-5 or interleukin-3. Lab Invest 61:116, 1989.

68. Sillaber C, Geissler K, Scherrer R, et al: Type β transforming growth factors promote interleukin-3 (IL-3)–dependent differentiation of human basophils but inhibit IL-3–dependent differentiation of human eosinophils. Blood 80:634, 1992.

69. Irani AA, Nilsson G, Miettinen U, et al: Recombinant human stem cell factor stimulates differentiation of mast cells from dispersed human fetal liver cells. Blood 80:3009, 1992.

70. Mitsui H, Furitsu T, Dvorak AM, et al: Development of human mast cells from umbilical cord blood cells by recombinant human and murine C-kit ligand. Proc Natl Acad Sci USA 90:735, 1993.

71. Valent P, Spanblöchl E, Sperr WR, et al: Induction of differentiation of human mast cells from bone marrow and peripheral blood mononuclear cells by recombinant human stem cell factor/kit-ligand in long-term culture. Blood 80:2237, 1992.

72. Valent P: The phenotype of human eosinophils, basophils, and mast cells. J Allergy Clin Immunol 94 (Suppl):1177, 1994.

73. Agis H, Willheim M, Sperr WR, et al: Monocytes do not make mast cells when cultured in the presence of SCF: Characterization of the circulating mast cell progenitor as a c-kit$^+$, CD34$^+$, Ly$^-$, CD14$^-$, CD17$^-$, colony-forming cell. J Immunol 151:4221, 1993.

74. Craig SS, Schechter NM, Schwartz LB. Ultrastructural analysis of maturing human T and TC mast cells in situ. Lab Invest 60:147, 1989.

75. Iemura A, Tsai M, Ando A, et al: The c-kit ligand, stem cell factor, promotes mast cell survival by suppressing apoptosis. Am J Pathol 144:321, 1994.

76. Yee NS, Paek I, Besmer P: Role of kit-ligand in proliferation and suppression of apoptosis in mast cells: Basis for radiosensitivity of white spotting and Steel mutant mice. J Exp Med 179:1777, 1994.

77. Nilsson G, Miettinen U, Ishizaka T, et al: Interleukin-4 inhibits the expression of Kit and tryptase during stem cell factor–dependent development of human mast cells from fetal liver cells. Blood 84:1519, 1994.

78. Meininger CJ, Yano H, Rottapel R, et al: The c-kit receptor ligand functions as a mast cell chemoattractant. Blood 79:958, 1992.

79. Sperr WR, Czerwenka K, Mundigler G, et al: Specific activation of human mast cells by the ligand for c-kit: Comparison between lung, uterus and heart mast cells. Int Arch Allergy Immunol 102:170, 1993.

80. Columbo M, Horowitz EM, Botana LM, et al: The human recombinant c-kit receptor ligand, rhSCF, induces mediator release from human cutaneous mast cells and enhances IgE-dependent mediator release from both skin mast cells and peripheral blood basophils. J Immunol 149:599, 1992.

81. Bischoff SC, Dahinden CA: c-kit Ligand: A unique potentiator of mediator release by human lung mast cells. J Exp Med 175:237, 1992.

82. Mekori YA, Metcalfe DD: Transforming growth factor-β prevents stem cell factor–mediated rescue of mast cells from apoptosis after IL-3 deprivation. J Immunol 153:2194, 1994.

83. Sillaber C, Sperr WR, Agis H, et al: Inhibition of stem cell factor dependent formation of human mast cells by interleukin-3 and interleukin-4. Int Arch Allergy Immunol 105:264, 1994.

84. Sillaber C, Strobl H, Bevec D, et al: IL-4 regulates c-kit proto-oncogene product expression in human mast and myeloid progenitor cells. J Immunol 147:4224, 1991.

85. Irani AA, Nilsson G, Ashman LK, et al: Dexamethasone inhibits the development of mast cells from dispersed human fetal liver cells cultured in the presence of recombinant human stem cell factor. Immunology 84:72, 1995.

86. Irani AA, Craig SS, DeBlois G, et al: Deficiency of the tryptase-positive, chymase-negative mast cell type in gastrointestinal mucosa of patients with defective T lymphocyte function. J Immunol 138:4381, 1987.

87. Bauza MT, Lagunoff D: Histidine transport by isolated rat peritoneal mast cells. Biochem Pharmacol 30:1271, 1981.

88. Schayer RW: Histidine decarboxylase in mast cells. Ann N Y Acad Sci 103:164, 1963.

89. Yamauchi K, Sato R, Tanno Y, et al: Nucleotide sequence of the cDNA encoding L-histidine decarboxylase derived from human basophilic leukemia cell line, KU-812-F. Nucleic Acids Res 18:5891, 1990.

90. Polk RE, Healy DP, Schwartz LB, et al: Vancomycin and the red-man syndrome: Pharmacodynamics of histamine release. J Infect Dis 157:502, 1988.

91. Arrang JM, Garbarg M, Lancelot JC, et al: Highly potent and selective ligands for histamine H3-receptors. Nature 327:117, 1987.

92. Black JW, Duncan WAM, Durant CJ, et al: Definition and antagonism of histamine H2-receptors. Nature 236:385, 1972.

93. Melmon KL, Rocklin RE, Rosenkranz RP: Autacoids as modulators of the inflammatory and immune response. Am J Med 71:100, 1981.

94. Braude S, Coe C, Royston D, et al: Histamine increases lung permeability by an H2-receptor mechanism. Lancet 2:372, 1984.

95. Arrang JM, Devaux B, Chodkiewicz JP, et al: H3-receptors control histamine release in human brain. J Neurochem 51:105, 1988.

96. Robertson I, Greaves MW: Responses of human skin blood vessels to synthetic histamine analogues. Br J Clin Pharmacol 5:319, 1978.

97. Kaliner M, Shelhamer JH, Ottesen EA: Effects of infused histamine: Correlation of plasma histamine levels and symptoms. J Allergy Clin Immunol 69:283, 1982.

98. Schwartz LB (ed): Monographs in Allergy: Neutral Proteases of Mast Cells. Basel, Karger, 1990.

99. Schwartz LB, Lewis RA, Austen KF: Tryptase from human pulmonary mast cells: Purification and characterization. J Biol Chem 256:11939, 1981.

100. Hopsu VK, Glenner GG: A histochemical enzyme kinetic system applied to the trypsin-like amidase and esterase activity in human mast cells. J Cell Biol 17:503, 1963.

101. Schwartz LB, Lewis RA, Seldin D, et al: Acid hydrolases and tryptase from secretory granules of dispersed human lung mast cells. J Immunol 126:1290, 1981.

102. Xia H-Z, Kepley CL, Sakai K, et al: Quantitation of tryptase, chymase, FcεRI-α and FcεRI-gamma mRNAs in human mast cells and basophils by competitive RT-PCR. J Immunol 154:5472, 1995.

103. Miller JS, Westin EH, Schwartz LB: Cloning and characterization of complementary DNA for human tryptase. J Clin Invest 84:1188, 1989.

104. Vanderslice P, Ballinger SM, Tam EK, et al: Human mast cell tryptase: Multiple cDNAs and genes reveal a multigene serine protease family. Proc Natl Acad Sci USA 87:3811, 1990.

105. Miller JS, Moxley G, Schwartz LB: Cloning and characterization of a second complementary DNA for human tryptase. J Clin Invest 86:864, 1990.

105a. Sakai K, Ren S, Schwartz LB: A novel heparin-dependent processing pathway for human tryptase: Autcatalysis followed by activation with dipeptidyl peptidase I. J Clin Invest 97:988, 1996.

106. Schwartz LB, Bradford TR: Regulation of tryptase from human lung mast cells by heparin: Stabilization of the active tetramer. J Biol Chem 261:7372, 1986.

107. Alter SC, Metcalfe DD, Bradford TR, et al: Regulation of human mast cell tryptase: Effects of enzyme concentration, ionic strength and the structure and negative charge density of polysaccharides. Biochem J 248:821, 1987.

108. Schwartz LB, Bradford TR, Littman BH, et al: The fibrinogenolytic activity of purified tryptase from human lung mast cells. J Immunol 135:2762, 1985.

109. Hawkins RA, Claman HN, Clark RA, et al: Increased dermal mast cell populations in progressive systemic sclerosis: A link in chronic fibrosis. Ann Intern Med 102:182, 1985.

110. Brown JK, Jones CA, Tyler CL, et al: Tryptase-induced mitogenesis in airway smooth muscle cells: Potency, mechanisms, and interactions with other mast cell mediators. Chest 107 (Suppl):95S, 1995.

111. Schechter NM, Fraki JE, Geesin JC, et al: Human skin chymotryptic protease: Isolation and relation to cathepsin G and rat mast cell protein-ase. J Biol Chem 258:2973, 1983.

112. Caughey GH, Zerweck EH, Vanderslice P: Structure, chromosomal as-signment, and deduced amino acid sequence of a human gene for mast cell chymase. J Biol Chem 266:12956, 1991.

113. Sayama S, Iozzo RV, Lazarus GS, et al: Human skin chymotrypsin-like proteinase chymase: Subcellular localization to mast cell granules and interaction with heparin and other glycosaminoglycans. J Biol Chem 262:6808, 1987.

114. Schechter NM, Sprows JL, Schoenberger OL, et al: Reaction of human skin chymotrypsin-like proteinase chymase with plasma proteinase in-hibitors. J Biol Chem 264:21308, 1989.

115. Wintroub BU, Schechter NB, Lazarus GS, et al: Angiotensin I conversion by human and rat chymotryptic proteinases. J Invest Dermatol 83:336, 1984.

116. Reilly CF, Tewksbury DA, Schechter NM, et al: Rapid conversion of angiotensin I to angiotensin II by neutrophil and mast cell proteinases. J Biol Chem 257:8619, 1982.

117. Briggaman RA, Schechter NM, Fraki J, et al: Degradation of the epider-mal–dermal junction by a proteolytic enzyme from human skin and human polymorphonuclear leukocytes. J Exp Med 160:1027, 1984.

118. Sommerhoff CP, Caughey GH, Finkbeiner WE, et al: Mast cell chymase: A potent secretagogue for airway gland serous cells. J Immunol 142:2450, 1989.

119. Schechter NM, Irani A-MA, Sprows JL, et al: Identification of a cathep-sin G–like proteinase in the MC_TC type of human mast cell. J Immunol 145:2652, 1990.

120. Schechter NM, Mei Wang Z, Blacher RW, et al: Determination of the primary structures of human skin chymase and cathepsin G from cuta-neous mast cells of urticaria pigmentosa lesions. J Immunol 152:4062, 1994.

121. Irani A-MA, Goldstein SM, Wintroub BU, et al: Human mast cell car-boxypeptidase: Selective localization to MC_TC cells. J Immunol 147:247, 1991.

122. Goldstein SM, Kaempfer CE, Proud D, et al: Detection and partial characterization of a human mast cell carboxypeptidase. J Immunol 139:2724, 1987.

123. Goldstein SM, Kaempfer CE, Kealey JT, et al: Human mast cell carboxy-peptidase: Purification and characterization. J Clin Invest 83:1630, 1989.

124. Reynolds DS, Gurley DS, Stevens RL, et al: Cloning of cDNAs that encode human mast cell carboxypeptidase A, and comparison of the protein with mouse mast cell carboxypeptidase A and rat pancreatic carboxypeptidases. Proc Natl Acad Sci USA 86:9480, 1989.

125. Thompson HL, Schulman ES, Metcalfe DD: Identification of chondroitin sulfate E in human lung mast cells. J Immunol 140:2708, 1988.

126. Stevens RL, Fox CC, Lichtenstein LM, et al: Identification of chondroitin sulfate E proteoglycans and heparin proteoglycans in the secretory granules of human lung mast cells. Proc Natl Acad Sci USA 85:2284, 1988.

127. Metcalfe DD, Bland CE, Wasserman SI: Biochemical and functional characterization of proteoglycans isolated from basophils of patients with chronic myelogenous leukemia. J Immunol 132:1943, 1984.

128. Craig SS, Irani A-MA, Metcalfe DD, et al: Ultrastructural localization of heparin to human mast cells of the MC_TC and MC_T types by labeling with antithrombin III-gold. Lab Invest 69:552, 1993.

129. Stevens RL, Avraham S, Gartner MC, et al: Isolation and characteriza-tion of a cDNA that encodes the peptide core of the secretory granule

130. Metcalfe DD, Soter NA, Wasserman SI, et al: Identification of sulfated mucopolysaccharides including heparin in the lesional skin of a patient with mastocytosis. J Invest Dermatol 74:210, 1980.

131. Metcalfe DD, Lewis RA, Silbert JE, et al: Isolation and characterization of heparin from human lung. J Clin Invest 64:1537, 1979.

132. Spivak-Kroizman T, Lemmon MA, Dikic I, et al: Heparin-induced oligo-merization of FGF molecules is responsible for FGF receptor dimeriza-tion, activation, and cell proliferation. Cell 79:1015, 1994.

133. Nelson RM, Cecconi O, Roberts WG, et al: Heparin oligosaccharides bind L- and P-selectin and inhibit acute inflammation. Blood 82:3253, 1993.

134. Oscarsson LG, Pejler G, Lindahl U: Location of the antithrombin-bind-ing sequence in the heparin chain. J Biol Chem 264:296, 1989.

135. Peters SP, MacGlashan DW, Schulman ES, et al: Arachidonic acid metab-olism in purified human lung mast cells. J Immunol 132:1972, 1984.

136. Dvorak AM, Dvorak HF, Peters SP, et al: Lipid bodies: Cytoplasmic organelles important to arachidonate metabolism in macrophages and basophils. J Immunol 131:2965, 1983.

137. Robinson C: Mast cells and newly-generated lipid mediators. In Holgate ST (ed): Immunology and Medicine: Mast Cells, Mediators and Disease. London, Kluwer Academic Publishers, 1988, pp 149–174.

138. MacGlashan DW Jr, Peters SP, Warner J, et al: Characteristics of human basophil sulfidopeptide leukotreine release: Releasability defined as the ability of basophils to respond to dimeric cross-links. J Immunol 136:2231, 1986.

139. Israel E, Rubin P, Kemp JP, et al: The effect of inhibition of 5-lipoxygen-ase by Zileuton in mild-to-moderate asthma. Ann Intern Med 119:1059, 1993.

140. Roberts LJ II, Sweetman BJ, Lewis RA, et al: Increased production of prostaglandin D2 in patients with systemic mastocytosis. N Engl J Med 303:1400, 1980.

141. Walsh LJ, Trinchieri G, Waldorf HA, et al: Human dermal mast cells contain and release tumor necrosis factor α, which induces endothelial leukocyte adhesion molecule 1. Proc Natl Acad Sci USA 88:4220, 1991.

142. Bradding P, Feather IH, Wilson S, et al: Immunolocalization of cytokines in the nasal mucosa of normal and perennial rhinitic subjects: The mast cell as a source of IL-4, IL-5, and IL-6 in human allergic mucosal inflammation. J Immunol 151:3853, 1993.

143. Burd PR, Thompson WC, Max EE, et al: Activated mast cells produce interleukin 13. J Exp Med 181:1373, 1995.

144. Metzger H, Alcarez G, Hohman R, et al: The receptor with high affinity for immunoglobulin E. Annu Rev Immunol 4:419, 1986.

145. Hide M, Francis DM, Grattan CE, et al: Autoantibodies against the high-affinity IgE receptor as a cause of histamine release in chronic urticaria. N Engl J Med 328:1599, 1993.

146. Gruber BL, Baeza ML, Marchese MJ, et al: Prevalence and functional role of anti-IgE autoantibodies in urticarial syndromes. J Invest Derma-tol 90:213, 1988.

147. Wilson BS, Kapp N, Lee RJ, et al: Distinct functions of the FcεR1 gamma and β subunits in the control of FcεR1-mediated tyrosine kinase activation and signaling responses in RBL-2H3 mast cells. J Biol Chem 270:4013, 1995.

148. Oliver JM, Burg DL, Wilson BS, et al: Inhibition of mast cell FcεR1-mediated signaling and effector function by the Syk-selective inhibitor, piceatannol. J Biol Chem 269:29697, 1994.

149. Vallé A, Kinet J-P: N-acetyl-L-cysteine inhibits antigen-mediated Syk, but not Lyn tyrosine kinase activation in mast cells. FEBS Lett 357:41, 1995.

150. Rivera VM, Brugge JS: Clustering of Syk is sufficient to induce tyrosine phosphorylation and release of allergic mediators from rat basophilic leukemia cells. Mol Cell Biol 15:1582, 1995.

151. Berger SA, Mak TW, Paige CJ: Leukocyte common antigen (CD45) is required for immunoglobulin E–mediated degranulation of mast cells. J Exp Med 180:471, 1994.

152. Tsai M, Chen R-H, Tam S-Y, et al: Activation of MAP kinases, pp90^rsk and pp70-S6 kinases in mouse mast cells by signaling through the c-kit receptor tyrosine kinase or FcεRI: Rapamycin inhibits activation of pp70-S6 kinase and proliferation in mouse mast cells. Eur J Immunol 23:3286, 1993.

153. Chock SP, Schmauder-Chock EA: Phospholipid storage in the secretory granule of the mast cell. J Biol Chem 264:2862, 1989.

154. Buccione R, Di Tullio G, Caretta M, et al: Analysis of protein kinase C requirement for exocytosis in permeabilized rat basophilic leukaemia RBL-2H3 cells: A GTP-binding protein(s) as a potential target for pro-tein kinase C. Biochem J 298:149, 1994.

155. Kepley CL, Craig SS, Schwartz LB: The identification and partial charac-terization of a unique marker for human basophils. J Immunol 154:6548, 1995.

156. Enander I, Matsson P, Nystrand J, et al: A new radioimmunoassay for human mast cell tryptase using monoclonal antibodies. J Immunol Methods 138:39, 1991.

proteoglycan of human promyelocytic leukemia HL-60 cells. J Biol Chem 263:7287, 1988.

157. Schwartz LB, Sakai K, Bradford TR, et al: The α form of human tryptase is the predominant type present in blood at baseline in normal subjects, and is elevated in those with systemic mastocytosis. J Clin Invest 96:2702, 1995.

158. Schwartz LB, Yunginger JW, Miller JS, et al: The time course of appearance and disappearance of human mast cell tryptase in the circulation after anaphylaxis. J Clin Invest 83:1551, 1989.

159. Schwartz LB, Metcalfe DD, Miller JS, et al: Tryptase levels as an indicator of mast-cell activation in systemic anaphylaxis and mastocytosis. N Engl J Med 316:1622, 1987.

160. Van der Linden PG, Hack CE, Poortman J, et al: Insect-sting challenge in 138 patients: Relation between clinical severity of anaphylaxis and mast cell activation. J Allergy Clin Immunol 90:110, 1992.

161. Schwartz LB, Bradford TR, Rouse C, et al: Development of a new, more sensitive immunoassay for human tryptase: Use in systemic anaphylaxis. J Clin Immunol 14:190, 1994.

162. Yunginger JW, Nelson DR, Squillace DL, et al: Laboratory investigation of deaths due to anaphylaxis. J Forensic Sci 36:857, 1991.

163. Platt MS, Yunginger JW, Sekula-Perlman A, et al: Involvement of mast cells in sudden infant death syndrome. J Allergy Clin Immunol 94:250, 1994.

164. Mican JM, Metcalfe DD: Arthritis and mast cell activation. J Allergy Clin Immunol 86(Suppl):677, 1990.

165. Crisp AJ, Chapman CM, Kirkham SE, et al: Articular mastocytosis in rheumatoid arthritis. Arthritis Rheum 27:845, 1984.

166. Godfrey HP, Ilardi C, Engber W, et al: Quantitation of human synovial mast cells in rheumatoid arthritis and other rheumatic diseases. Arthritis Rheum 27:852, 1984.

167. Malone DG, Irani AM, Schwartz LB, et al: Mast cell numbers and histamine levels in synovial fluids from patients with arthritides of various etiologies. Arthritis Rheum 29:956, 1986.

168. Gruber B, Ballan D, Gorevic PD: IgE rheumatoid factors: quantification in synovial fluid and ability to induce synovial mast cell histamine release. Clin Exp Immunol 71:289, 1988.

169. Chard MD, Crisp AJ: Astemizole, an H_1 antagonist, has no additional therapeutic effect in rheumatoid arthritis. J Rheumatol 18:203, 1991.

170. Brodeur JP, Ruddy S, Schwartz LB, Moxley G: Synovial fluid levels of complement SC5b-9 and fragment Bb are elevated in patients with rheumatoid arthritis. Arthritis Rheum 34:1531, 1991.

171. Irani A-MA, Bradford TR, Kepley CL, et al: Detection of MC_T and MC_{TC} types of human mast cells by immunohistochemistry using new monoclonal anti-tryptase and anti-chymase antibodies. J Histochem Cytochem 37:1509, 1989.

CHAPTER 11

Platelets

Marcus E. Carr, Jr.

Recognized primarily for their critical role in blood coagulation, platelets are thought to play pivotal roles in early inflammatory processes and wound repair. This chapter briefly reviews platelet structure and platelet function in hemostasis and summarizes the role of platelets in inflammation.

Platelets, the smallest of the constituent blood elements, are derived from megakaryocytes found in the bone marrow and pulmonary vasculature.[1, 2] Platelet production is stimulated by thrombopoietin. Thrombopoietin, which has been cloned, is the ligand for the c-Mpl proto-oncogene.[3] Produced as an enucleate cell fragment, platelets are surrounded by a complex, multifunctional membrane. Glycoprotein receptors, such as GPIIb/IIIa and GPIb, mediate adhesion of platelets to other platelets and subendothelium.[4] Other receptors initiate platelet activation in response to external stimuli.[5] Signal transduction involves G-protein activation, phosphorylation reactions, and intracytoplasmic calcium shifts.[5] With the membrane serving as the primary source of arachidonic acid, platelet activation is amplified via eicosanoid synthesis.[6] Finally, membrane phospholipid augments clotting by concentrating coagulation factors on the platelet surface. Factor Xa activation and prothrombinase complex formation are thus facilitated.[7] These multifactor complexes are the primary determinants of the rate of clot formation.

Beneath the membrane, a collection of fibrous microtubules and filaments form a dynamic cytoskeleton, which preserves the resting discoid platelet shape but facilitates rapid shape change on platelet activation.[8] Within the cytoskeleton, platelets contain an array of organelles and membrane-bound granules. Mitochondria produce the energy required for platelet function, and platelet lysosomes exhibit digestive activity similar to that found in other cells capable of phagocytosis (Table 11–1).

Platelets contain two types of unique storage granules. *Dense* granules contain potent, low-molecular-weight chemical mediators such as serotonin, calcium, and adenine nucleotides.[9] *Alpha*-granules (α-granules) are larger and more numerous and contain an impressive array of soluble proteins.[10] Proteins found in α-granules include:

- Coagulation factors (fibrinogen, plasminogen, factor V)
- Adhesion molecules (fibronectin, von Willebrand factor)
- Plasma proteins (albumin, immunoglobulin G [IgG])
- Platelet-specific proteins (platelet factor-4 [PF-4], β-thromboglobulin)
- Mitogenic proteins (platelet-derived growth factor [PDGF], transforming growth factor-β [TGF-β])

Proteins contained within the α-granule are derived from the plasma or synthesized by the megakaryocyte. The α-granule membrane also contains glycoprotein receptors, which can be exposed to the platelet exterior by fusion of the α-granules with the external platelet membrane.

The *dense tubular system* (DTS) and *open canalicular system* (OCS) are platelet structures that are critical to platelet activation and function. The dense tubular system pumps Ca^{2+} from the cytoplasm into itself. The resulting lower cytoplasmic Ca^{2+} concentration stabilizes the microtubular apparatus and preserves platelet shape. Enzymes contained within the dense tubular system are essential for eicosanoid production.[11]

The open canalicular system directly connects the deep cytoplasm to the external cell surface. Movement of proteins through this system allows transfer of plasma proteins into the platelet via endocytosis, and rapid secretion of granule contents via fusion of granules with the open canalicular system.[12]

PLATELET-NEUTROPHIL INTERACTIONS

Tissue damage exposes procoagulant materials, which leads to rapid platelet adhesion and activation (Fig. 11–1). Platelet activation is followed by granule secretion and exposure of P-selectin on the platelet surface.[13] P-selectin is normally hidden as a granule membrane protein. Release of PF-4, PDGF, and arachidonic acid metabolites recruits leukocytes to the site via chemotaxis.[14, 15] P-selectin mediates adhesion of recruited leukocytes to activated platelets.[13, 16] PDGF further augments neutrophil function by inducing degranulation, enhancing phagocytosis,[17] and increasing cellular respiratory burst. The close apposition of platelets and neutrophils allows sharing of secreted metabolites. Via combined metabolism, platelets increase production of the leukotriene B_4 (LTB$_4$) by neutrophils and cause the conversion of LTA$_4$ into the potent vasoconstrictor LTC$_4$.[18] In turn, activated neutrophils enhance platelet calcium mobilization and

Table 11–1. PLATELET STRUCTURAL CONSTITUENTS

Structure	Component	Function
Cell membrane	Glycoprotein receptors Phospholipid Arachidonic acid	Activation, adhesion Facilitation of hemostasis Synthesis of eicosanoids
Cytoskeleton	Microtubules, filaments	Maintenance of resting discoid shape; control of shape change during activation
Dense tubular system	Calcium pumps Synthetic enzymes	Maintenance of low cytoplasmic Ca^{2+} Eicosanoid synthesis
Open canalicular system	Membrane connecting deep cytoplasm to external membrane	Secretion, endocytosis
Secretory granules α-Granules	Coagulation factors (fibrinogen, factor V) Adhesion molecules (vWF, fibronectin) Platelet-specific proteins (PF-4, β-thromboglobulin) Mitogenic proteins (PDGF, TGF-β) Plasma proteins (albumin, IgG)	Augmentation of coagulation Adhesion to injury site Multiple functions Stimulation of cell growth Multiple activities
Dense granules	Serotonin, calcium, adenine nucleotides	Platelet activation

Abbreviations: vWF, von Willebrand factor; PF, platelet factor; PDGF, platelet-derived growth factor; TGF-β, transforming growth factor-β; Ig, immunoglobulin.

thromboxane B_2 production in response to platelet-activating factor (PAF).[19]

Actin polymerization is a critical early step in neutrophil activation. In vitro studies demonstrate that co-incubation of neutrophils and platelets increases neutrophil F-actin content.[20] Platelets also potentiate agonist-induced actin polymerization and intracellular calcium increases within neutrophils.[20] Because G-protein activation is known to increase actin polymerization, one possible mechanism for these events may be platelet-mediated enhancement of neutrophil G-protein expression.[21]

In vivo evidence of the biologic significance of platelet-neutrophil interactions comes from several sources. Platelet activation is known to occur during cardiopulmonary bypass, and circulating platelet-neutrophil-monocyte aggregates have been documented during this procedure.[22] In addition, postischemic myocardial dysfunction is greater in the presence of platelets and neutrophils than in the presence of either alone.[23] In patients with asthma, IgE-sensitized leukocytes produce PAF, which leads to bronchospasm via a platelet-dependent mechanism.[24] Finally, platelets amplify neutrophil-dependent damage in immune complex glomerulonephritis.[25] This is demonstrated by the protective effect of induced thrombocytopenia.

Although platelets and neutrophils tend to mutually enhance their activation, there is evidence that platelets can dampen neutrophil responses. These negative influences include inhibition of oxygen radical production[26] and reduction, via TGF-β release, of neutrophil binding to endothelial cells.[27]

TRANSFORMING GROWTH FACTOR-β

The multiple properties of TGF-β and its potential functions in inflammation and wound healing have been reviewed.[28–30] Whereas most cells can produce TGF-β and all cells express TGF-β receptors, TGF-β is a major platelet product.[31] Released by platelets during the earliest stages of wound repair, TGF-β is a potent chemoattractant for leukocytes (Fig. 11–2).[32] Once they have been recruited, adhesion of leukocytes is augmented by TGF-β induction of adhesion molecule receptors.[33] Stimulated neutrophils, monocytes, and lymphocytes produce additional TGF-β, which leads to high levels at the inflammatory site.[28] These higher TGF-β levels induce monocyte expression of CD16 (FcγRIII receptors for the Fc portion of IgG), leading to enhanced immunophagocytosis.[34] TGF-β also induces monocyte production of interleu-

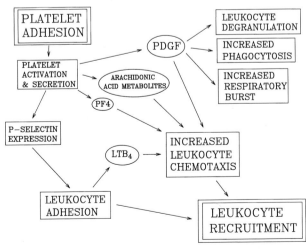

Figure 11–1. Platelet participation in early inflammatory events. PDGF, platelet-derived growth factor; PF4, platelet factor-4; LTB₄, leukotriene B₄.

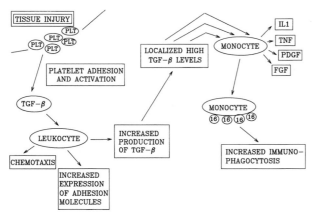

Figure 11–2. Platelet-leukocyte interactions mediated by transforming growth factor-β (TGF-β). PLT, platelet; IL1, interleukin-1; TNF, tumor necrosis factor; PDGF, platelet-derived growth factor; FGF, fibroblast growth factor; 16, CD16.

kin-1 (IL-1), tumor necrosis factor (TNF), PDGF, and fibroblast growth factor (FGF).[35]

Control of TGF-β is multifactorial, involving regulation of TGF-β activation and TGF-β receptor expression and antagonism of TGF-β functions. TGF-β is produced as a latent molecule that is activated by stimulated macrophages.[36] Activation is sensitive to microenvironmental influences, such as pH, and is enhanced in the acidic conditions found at inflammatory sites. Although exposure to TGF-β induces monocytes to produce additional TGF-β, exposure to lipopolysaccharides or γ-interferon (IFN-γ) leads to 90 percent loss of TGF-β receptors.[37] Specific activities of TGF-β are also antagonized (e.g., IL-4 blockade of TGF-β induction of CD16 expression).

While primarily a stimulant of granulocytes, TGF-β inhibits T and B lymphocyte growth.[38, 39] A potent immunosuppressor,[38] TGF-β suppresses B cell immunoglobulin production[39] and inhibits the effects of IL-1, IL-2, and IL-3.[38] Thus, TGF-β expresses both proinflammatory and immunosuppressive effects.

As a result of its pleiotropic functions, the global effects of TGF-β may be categorically opposed if the mode of administration is altered. If TGF-β is injected into a joint cavity of a nonarthritic animal, a pronounced monocytic infiltrate will occur, with associated swelling, erythema, and deformity peaking at 48 to 72 hours.[40] If administered systemically, TGF-β suppresses both the acute and chronic phases of streptococcal cell wall–induced erosive polyarthritis in the same animal model.[41] Thus, although TGF-β is almost certainly involved locally in the pathogenesis of inflammatory disease, systemic application of TGF-β or related molecules may eventually provide therapeutic benefits via its anti-inflammatory effects. In animal models, benefit is apparently accomplished with limited toxicity.

PLATELET-ACTIVATING FACTOR

Platelet-activating factor is a potent inducer of platelet aggregation and was first isolated from IgE-stimulated basophils.[42] Identified as 1-0-alkyl-2-acetyl-sn-glycero-3-phosphocholine, PAF is also produced by macrophages, mast cells, platelets, neutrophils, eosinophils, monocytes, and endothelial cells.[43] PAF is not stored but is rapidly generated upon cell activation. PAF synthesis can be initiated by an influx of Ca^{2+} [44] and involves processing of membrane phospholipids by phospholipase A_2 to form the intermediate molecule lyso-PAF (Fig. 11–3). Further processing, mediated by acetyl transferase, involves the addition of acetate. PAF may be converted back to inactive lyso-PAF by acetylhydrolase. Thus, lyso-PAF is both an intermediate synthetic product and a primary degradation product.

PAF activity is markedly dependent on its chemical structure.[43] The ether linkage at sn-1 is critical for activity, and only the natural (R-form) stereoisomer is active. The length of the alkyl side chain at sn-1 is also important, with 16:0 being more active than 18:0. Acetate at sn-2 produces the highest activity, and hydrolysis of this acetate results in the inactive lyso-PAF form.

High-affinity receptors for PAF are found on platelets, neutrophils, macrophages, and monocytes and in tissues such as brain and lung.[45] Binding of PAF to its receptors results in G-protein activation (see Fig. 11–3). Activated G-protein activates a phosphoinositide-specific phospholipase C, which results in mobilization of intracellular Ca^{2+} and activation of protein kinase C. Adenylate cyclase is inhibited. The end result is prostaglandin, leukotriene, and cytokine release.[46]

The proinflammatory effects of PAF have been studied in animal models and are known to depend on the mode of PAF administration. If administered systemically, PAF produces hypotension and shock.[47] If injected into the pleural space of rats, PAF causes a rapid decline in pleural leukocytes and marked exudation of fluid.[48] Intradermal PAF injection in rats

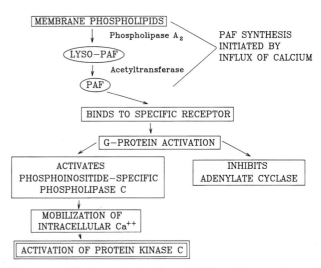

Figure 11–3. Platelet-activating factor (PAF) synthesis and signal transduction pathways.

causes increased vascular permeability, vascular lesions, thrombosis, and edema formation.[49] Intradermal injection in humans causes acute accumulation of neutrophils and monocytes with enhanced chemotaxis and degranulation.[50]

The role of PAF in chronic inflammatory diseases, such as rheumatoid arthritis, is postulated but not proven. PAF is present in high concentrations in synovial fluid of a rat model of adjuvant-induced arthritis,[51] but PAF concentrations have not been elevated in synovial fluid of arthritic joints. PAF is detected in psoriatic skin sites and appears to play a role in the persistence of these lesions.[52]

PLATELET-COMPLEMENT INTERACTIONS

Although normal complement function is required for adequate vascular hemostasis in some mammalian systems,[53] coagulation and platelet function appear to be normal in humans with inherited deficiencies of C3, C5, C6, or C7.[54] There is considerable evidence, however, that complement components and activation can alter platelet function. C1q can induce platelet aggregation and release, whereas the membrane attack complex (C5b-9) produces non–receptor-mediated phospholipase C activation with subsequent platelet secretion and enhanced platelet procoagulant activity.[55]

Platelet Interactions with Early Complement Components

Although free C1q inhibits collagen-induced platelet aggregation, clustered or aggregated C1q can initiate platelet aggregation and release.[56, 57] Both of these effects may be mediated by C1q binding to the platelet collagen receptor. Although platelets do not have receptors for C3a, C4a, or C5a,[58] they express membrane cofactor protein, which is necessary for inactivation of C3b,[59] and decay-accelerating factor (DAF), which accelerates dissociation of C3/C5 convertase.[60]

Platelet/C5b-9 Interactions

Zymosan induces platelet aggregation and secretion in normal platelet-rich plasma. If plasma deficient in C3, C5, C6, or C7 is used, zymosan-mediated aggregation is abolished.[61] In similar fashion, 5-hydroxytryptamine (5-HT) release from anti-I antibody–exposed platelets is blocked in plasma deficient of C6.[62] IgG antibodies to platelet Pl^{A1} antigen fail to produce platelet release in heparinized plasma-deficient in terminal complement components.[63] In nonplasma systems, C5b-9 complex potentiates platelet responses to thrombin and arachidonate and increases thromboxane synthesis.

The mechanism by which C5b-9 complex assembly activates platelets is incompletely understood, but it is known to involve an increase in Na^+ conductance and rapid membrane depolarization. Platelet lysis occurs if greater than 10^3 complexes accumulate on the platelet surface. Lysis is prevented by platelet membrane vesiculation.[64] C5b-9 complexes are caught up in the membrane vesicles and are shed from the membrane surface.[65] Transient permeabilization of the membrane leads to inward Ca^{2+} flux, an increase in cytosolic Ca^{2+}, and phosphorylation of protein kinase C substrates.[66] As a result, platelet granules fuse with the surface membrane and secretion is initiated. This activation appears not to require receptor-mediated phospholipase C activation.

Vascular thrombosis is frequently associated with complement activation. Complement-mediated platelet activation increases platelet uptake of factor Xa and acceleration of plasma clotting. Membrane vesiculation that occurs in response to C5b-9 complex formation results in expression of high-affinity binding sites for factor Va[67, 68] and factor VIII.[69] These membrane structures support formation of both the tenase and prothrombinase enzyme complexes. Combined complement and platelet activation have been documented in paroxysmal nocturnal hemoglobinuria,[70] immune complex disease, chronic immune thrombocytopenic purpura (ITP), and some cases of thrombotic thrombocytopenic purpura.

SCLERODERMA

Platelet function may be enhanced in scleroderma.[71] In a study of 29 patients with scleroderma, 19 patients with Raynaud's disease, and 19 patients with systemic lupus erythematosus (SLE), the only consistent abnormalities in platelet function were noted in patients with scleroderma. Platelets from these patients exhibited enhanced collagen-induced platelet aggregation. Adenosine diphosphate (ADP) and epinephrine-induced aggregation were normal. Elevations in plasma fibrinogen and von Willebrand factor (vWF) levels were also noted, and vWF levels appeared to correlate with disease severity.

Antiplatelet autoantibodies are apparently common in patients with scleroderma and may be detected in asymptomatic, nonthrombocytopenic patients.[72] In a study of 16 patients with scleroderma, 15 had normal platelet counts. Twelve of these patients had platelet-associated IgG, and four patients had platelet-bindable IgG in their serum.

SYSTEMIC LUPUS ERYTHEMATOSUS

The association between SLE, antiplatelet antibodies, and ITP is well established.[73, 74] There is increasing evidence, however, that although most patients with chronic ITP have antibodies directed against GPIIIa, GPIIb/IIIa, or GPIb-Ix,[75, 76] many patients with SLE or primary antiphospholipid syndrome have antibodies directed against a 50- to 70-kD internal platelet protein.[77] It is also increasingly apparent that autoimmune hemolytic anemia and ITP are on a continuum of autoimmune processes that overlap and include SLE.[78] Patients with ITP who are also positive for antinuclear antibodies but who never develop SLE are well described.[79] Interestingly, ITP in SLE is not protective against antiphospholipid-associated thrombotic events.[80] Concurrent steroid therapy also does not appear to reduce the thrombotic risk.

In vitro investigations indicate that circulating immune complexes in patients with SLE may alter GPIIb/IIIa binding to fibrinogen.[81] In 12 of 29 patients with nonthrombocytopenic SLE, serum-inhibited GPIIb/IIIa binding of fibrinogen by 5 to 60 percent. Polyethylene glycol extraction reduced the inhibitory activity, whereas the redissolved precipitates exhibited substantial inhibitory properties. The clinical significance of this finding has not been demonstrated.

Neuropsychiatric symptoms occur in up to 75 percent of patients with SLE, and pathologically documented central nervous system (CNS) involvement is noted in 50 percent.[82, 83] CNS lesions are known to involve vasculopathies and microinfarctions. Potential involvement of platelets in the pathogenesis of these lesions has been raised with the demonstration of platelet membrane fragments in the walls of involved cortical and meningeal vessels.[84]

References

1. Wright JH: The histogenesis of the blood platelets. J Morphol 21:263–278, 1910.
2. Handagama PJ, Feldman BF, Janin NC, et al: Circulating proplatelets: Isolation and quantitation in healthy rats and in rats with induced acute blood loss. Am J Vet Res 48:1142–1146, 1987.
3. Lok S, Kaushansky K, Holly RD, et al: Cloning and expression of murine thrombopoietin cDNA and stimulation of platelet production in vivo. Nature 369:565–568, 1994.
4. Phillips DR, Charo IF, Parise LV, et al: The platelet membrane glycoprotein IIb-IIIa complex. Blood 71:831–843, 1988.
5. Hourani SMO, Cusack NJ: Pharmacological receptors on blood platelets. Pharmacol Rev 43:243–298, 1991.
6. Lagarde M: Metabolism of fatty acids by platelets and the functions of various metabolites in mediating platelet function. Prog Lipid Res 27:135–152, 1988.
7. Davie EW, Fujikawa K, Kisiel W: The coagulation cascade: Initiation, maintenance, and regulation. Biochemistry 30:10363–10370, 1991.
8. White JG: Ultrastructural modifications in platelet membranes and cytoskeleton following activation. Blood Cells 9:237–261, 1983.
9. Fukami MH, Salganicoff L: Human platelet storage organelles: A review. Thromb Haemost 38:963–970, 1977.
10. Harrison P, Cramer EM: Platelet alpha-granules. Blood Rev 7:52–62, 1993.
11. Carey F, Menashi S, Crawford N: Localization of cyclo-oxygenase and thromboxane synthetase in human platelet intracellular membranes. Biochem J 204:847–851, 1982.
12. White JG, Escolar G: The blood platelet open canalicular system: A two-way street. Eur J Cell Biol 56:233–242, 1991.
13. McEver RP: GMP-140: A receptor for neutrophils and monocytes on activated platelets and endothelium. J Cell Biochem 45:156–161, 1991.
14. Deuel TF, Senior RM, Chang D, et al: Platelet factor 4 is chemotactic for neutrophils and monocytes. Proc Natl Acad Sci USA 78:4584–4587, 1981.
15. Deuel TF, Senior RM, Huang JS, et al: Chemotaxis of monocytes and neutrophils to platelet-elevated growth factor. J Clin Invest 69:1046–1049, 1982.
16. Nash GB: Adhesion between neutrophils and platelets: A modulator of thrombotic and inflammatory events. Thromb Res 74(Suppl 1):S3–S11, 1994.
17. Sakamoto H, Yokoya Y: Purification and characterization of macromolecular phagocytosis activators released from platelets. J Leukoc Biol 50:356–363, 1991.
18. Maclouf AJ, Murphy RC: Transcellular metabolism of neutrophil-derived leukotriene A4 by human platelets. J Biol Chem 263:174–181, 1988.
19. Del Maschio A, Evangelista V, Ratjar G, et al: Platelet activation by polymorphonuclear leukocytes exposed to chemotactic agents. Am J Physiol 258:870–879, 1990.
20. Bengtsson T, Grenegard M: Platelets amplify chemotactic peptide-induced changes in F-actin and calcium in human neutrophils. Eur J Cell Biol 63:345–349, 1994.
21. Brom C, Brom J, König W: GTPases and low molecular weight G proteins during cell-cell interaction between neutrophils and platelets. Int Arch Allergy Appl Immunol 99:397–399, 1992.
22. Rinder CS, Bonan JL, Rinder HM, et al: Cardiopulmonary bypass induces leukocyte-platelet adhesion. Blood 79:1201–1205, 1992.
23. Alloatti G, Montrucchio G, Emanuelli G, et al: Platelet-activating factor (PAF) induces platelet/neutrophil co-operation during myocardial reperfusion. J Mol Cell Cardiol 24:163–171, 1992.
24. Vargaftig BB, Lefort J, Chignard M, et al: Platelet-activating factor induces a platelet-dependent bronchoconstriction unrelated to the formation of prostaglandin derivatives. Eur J Pharmacol 65:185–192, 1980.
25. Johnson RJ, Alpers CE, Pritzl P, et al: Platelets mediate neutrophil-dependent immune complex nephritis in the rat. J Clin Invest 82:1225–1235, 1988.
26. Moon DG, van Der Zee H, Weston LK, et al: Platelet modulation of neutrophil superoxide anion production. Thromb Haemost 63:91–96, 1990.
27. Gamble JR, Vadas MA: Endothelial adhesiveness for blood neutrophils is inhibited by transforming growth factor-β. Science 242:97–99, 1988.
28. Wahl SM: The role of transforming growth factor-beta in inflammatory processes. Immunol Res 10:249–254, 1991.
29. Wahl SM: Transforming growth factor beta (TGF-β) in inflammation: A cause and a cure. J Clin Immunol 12:61–74, 1992.
30. Ruscetti F, Varesio L, Ochoa A, et al: Pleiotropic effects of transforming growth factor-β on cells of the immune system. Ann NY Acad Sci 685:488–500, 1993.
31. Assoian RK, Sporn MB: Type-beta transforming growth factor in human platelets: Release during platelet degranulation and action on vascular smooth muscle cells. J Cell Biol 102:1217–1223, 1986.
32. Wahl SM, Hunt DA, Wakefield LM, et al: Transforming growth factor-beta (TGF-β) induces monocyte chemotaxis and growth factor production. Proc Natl Acad Sci USA 84:5788–5792, 1987.
33. Ignotz RA, Heino J, Massague J: Regulation of cell adhesion receptors by transforming growth factor-β: Regulation of vitronectin receptor and LFA-1. J Biol Chem 264:389–393, 1989.
34. Welch G, Wong H, Wahl SM: Selective induction of FcRIII on human monocytes by transforming growth factor-β. J Immunol 144:3444–3448, 1990.
35. McCartney-Francis N, Mizel D, Wong H, et al: TGF-β regulates production of growth factors and TGF-β by human peripheral blood monocytes. Growth Factors 4:27–35, 1990.
36. Wakefield LM, Smith DM, Masui T, et al: Distribution and modulation of the cellular receptor for transforming growth factor-beta. J Cell Biol 105:965–975, 1987.
37. Brandes ME, Wakefield LM, Wahl SM: Modulation of monocyte type I TGF-β receptors by inflammatory stimuli. J Biol Chem 266:19697–19703, 1991.
38. Kehrl JH, Wakefield LM, Roberts AB, et al: Production of transforming growth factor β by human T lymphocytes and its potential role in the regulation of T cell growth. J Exp Med 163:1037–1050, 1986.
39. Kehrl JH, Roberts AB, Wakefield LM, et al: Transforming growth factor β is an important immunomodulatory protein for human B lymphocytes. J Immunol 137:3855–3860, 1986.
40. Allen JB, Manthey CL, Hand AR, et al: Rapid onset synovial inflammation and hyperplasia induced by TGF-β. J Exp Med 171:231–247, 1990.
41. Brandes ME, Allen JB, Ogawa Y, et al: TGF-β1 suppresses leukocyte recruitment and synovial inflammation in experimental arthritis. J Clin Invest 87:1108–1113, 1991.
42. Benveniste J, Henson PM, Cochrane CG: Leukocyte-dependent histamine release from rabbit platelets: The role of IgE basophils and a platelet activating factor. J Exp Med 136:1356–1377, 1972.
43. Braquet P, Touqui L, Shen TY, et al: Perspectives in platelet-activating factor research. Pharmacol Rev 39:97–145, 1987.
44. Yue TL, Rabinovici R, Feuerstein G: Platelet-activating factor (PAF)—a putative mediator in inflammatory tissue injury. Adv Exp Med Biol 314:223–233, 1991.
45. Hwang SB: Specific receptors of platelet-activating factor, receptor heterogeneity, and signal transduction mechanisms. J Lipid Mediat 2:123–158, 1990.
46. Peplow PV, Mikhailidis DP: Platelet-activating factor (PAF) and its relation to prostaglandins and leukotrienes and other aspects of arachidonate metabolism. Prostaglandins Leukot Essent Fatty Acids 41:71–82, 1990.
47. Watanabe M, Ohuchi K, Sugidachi A, et al: Platelet-activating factor in the inflammatory exudate in the anaphylactic phase of allergic inflammation in rats. Int Arch Allergy Appl Immunol 84:396–403, 1987.

48. Martins MA, Silva PMR, Neto HCCF, et al: Pharmacological modulation of Paf-induced rat pleurisy and its role in inflammation by zymosan. Br J Pharmacol 96:363–371, 1989.

49. Pirotzky E, Page CP, Roubin RA, et al: PAF-acether–induced plasma exudation in rat skin is independent of platelets and neutrophils. Microcirc Endothelium Lymphatics 1:107–122, 1984.

50. Archer CB, Morley J, MacDonald DM: Accumulation of inflammatory cells in response to intracutaneous platelet activating factor (PAF-acether) in man. Br J Dermatol 112:285–290, 1985.

51. Pettipher ER, Higgs GA, Henderson B: PAF-acether in chronic arthritis. Agents Actions 21:98–103, 1987.

52. Ramesha CS, Soter N, Pickett WC: Identification and quantitation of PAF from psoriatic scales. Agents Actions 21:382–383, 1987.

53. Zimmerman TS, Arroyove CM, Müller-Eberhard HJ: A blood coagulation abnormality in rabbits deficient in the sixth component of complement (C6) and its correction by purified C6. J Exp Med 134:1591–1600, 1971.

54. Blajchman MA, Ozge-Anwar AH: The role of the complement system in hemostasis. Prog Hematol 14:149–182, 1986.

55. Sims PJ, Wiedmer T: The response of human platelets to activated components of the complement system. Immunol Today 12:338–342, 1991.

56. Cazenave JP, Assimeh SN, Painter RH, et al: C1q inhibition of the interaction of collagen with human platelets. J Immunol 116:162–163, 1976.

57. Peerschke EIB, Ghebrehiwet B: Human blood platelets possess specific binding sites for C1q. J Immunol 138:1537–1541, 1987.

58. Meuer S, Hugli TE, Andreatta RH, et al: Comparative study on biological activities of various anaphylatoxins (C4a, C3a, C5a). Investigations on their ability to induce platelet secretion. Inflammation 5:263–273, 1981.

59. Yu GH, Holers VM, Seya T, et al: Identification of a third component of complement-binding glycoprotein of human platelets. J Clin Invest 78:494–501, 1986.

60. Nicholson-Weller A, March JP, Rosen CE, et al: Surface membrane expression by human blood leukocytes and platelets of decay-accelerating factor, a regulatory protein of the complement system. Blood 65:1237–1244, 1985.

61. Breckenridge RT, Rosenfeld SI, Graff KS, et al: Hereditary C5 deficiency in man: III. Studies on hemostasis and platelet responses to zymosan. J Immunol 118:12–16, 1977.

62. Dixon RH, Rosse WF: Mechanism of complement-mediated activation of human blood platelets in vitro: Comparison of normal and paroxysmal nocturnal hemoglobinuria platelets. J Clin Invest 59:360–368, 1977.

63. Cines DB, Schreiber AD: Effect of anti-P1A1 antibody on human platelets: I. The role of complement. Blood 53:567–577, 1979.

64. Sims PJ, Wiedmer T: Repolarization of the membrane potential of blood platelets after complement damage: Evidence for a Ca⁺⁺-dependent exocytotic elimination of C5b-9 pores. Blood 68:556–561, 1986.

65. Wiedmer T, Sims PJ: Participation of protein kinases in complement C5b-9–induced shedding of platelet plasma membrane vesicles. Blood 78:2880–2886, 1991.

66. Wiedmer T, Ando B, Sims PJ: Complement C5b-9–stimulated platelet secretion is associated with a Ca²⁺-initiated activation of cellular protein kinases. J Biol Chem 262:13674–13681, 1987.

67. Wiedmer T, Shattil SJ, Cunningham M, et al: Role of calcium and calpain in complement-induced vesiculation of the platelet plasma membrane

68. and in the exposure of the platelet factor Va receptor. Biochemistry 29:623–632, 1990.

68. Sims PJ, Faioni EM, Wiedmer T, et al: Complement proteins C5b-9 cause release of membrane vesicles from the platelet surface that are enriched in the membrane receptor for coagulation factor Va and express prothrombinase activity. J Biol Chem 263:18205–18212, 1988.

69. Gilbert GE, Sims PJ, Wiedmer T, et al: Platelet-derived microparticles express high affinity receptors for factor VIII. J Biol Chem 266:17261–17268, 1991.

70. Wiedmer T, Hall SE, Ortel TL, et al: Complement-induced vesiculation and exposure of membrane prothrombinase sites in platelets of paroxysmal nocturnal hemoglobinuria. Blood 82:1192–1196, 1993.

71. Goodfield MJ, Orchard MA, Rowell NR: Whole blood platelet aggregation and coagulation factors in patients with systemic sclerosis. Br J Haematol 84:675–680, 1993.

72. Girelli G, Sorgi ML, Conti L, et al: Red blood cell and platelet autoantibodies in scleroderma. Clin Exp Rheumatol 11:347–348, 1993.

73. Rabinowitz Y, Dameshek W: Systemic lupus erythematosus after 'idiopathic' thrombocytopenic purpura, a review: A study of systemic lupus erythematosus occurring after 78 splenectomies for "idiopathic' thrombocytopenic purpura, with a review of the pertinent literature. Ann Intern Med 52:1–28, 1960.

74. Kaplan C: Antiplatelet antibodies in systemic lupus erythematosus: An overview. Curr Stud Hematol Blood Transfus 55:90–93, 1988.

75. Berchtold P, Harris JP, Tani P, et al: Autoantibodies to platelet glycoproteins in patients with disease-related immune thrombocytopenia. Br J Haematol 73:365–368, 1989.

76. Waters AH: Autoimmune thrombocytopenia: Clinical aspects. Semin Hematol 29:18–25, 1992.

77. Fabris F, Steffan A, Cordiano I, et al: Specific antiplatelet autoantibodies in patients with antiphospholipid antibodies and thrombocytopenia. Eur J Haematol 53:232–236, 1994.

78. Miescher PA, Tucci A, Beris P, et al: Autoimmune hemolytic anemia and/or thrombocytopenia associated with lupus parameters. Semin Hematol 29:13–17, 1992.

79. Panzer S, Penner E, Graninger W, et al: Antinuclear antibodies in patients with chronic idiopathic autoimmune thrombocytopenia followed 2–30 years. Am J Hematol 32:100–103, 1989.

80. Rosove MH, Brewer PMC: Antiphospholipid thrombosis: Clinical course after the first thrombotic event in 70 patients. Ann Intern Med 117:303–308, 1992.

81. Kamiyama M, Arkel YS, Chen K, et al: Inhibition of platelet GPIIb/IIIa binding to fibrinogen by serum factors: Studies of circulating immune complexes and platelet antibodies in patients with hemophilia, immune thrombocytopenic purpura, human immunodeficiency virus–related immune thrombocytopenia purpura, and systemic lupus erythematosus. J Lab Clin Med 117:209–217, 1991.

82. Lim L, Ron MA, Ormerod IE, et al: Psychiatric and neurological manifestations in systemic lupus erythematosus. Q J Med 66:27–38, 1988.

83. Ellis SG, Verity MA: Central nervous system involvement in systemic lupus erythematosus: A review of neuropathological findings in 57 cases, 1955–1977. Semin Arthritis Rheum 8:212–221, 1979.

84. Ellison D, Gatter K, Heryet A, et al: Intramural platelet deposition in cerebral vasculopathy of systemic lupus erythematosus. J Clin Pathol 46:37–40, 1993.

CHAPTER 12

Ramzi S. Cotran
David M. Briscoe

Endothelial Cells in Inflammation

Endothelial cells line the lumina of all blood vessels and, in this unique position, form the interface between the blood and tissues. They perform a wide variety of critical physiologic functions and interact in an active way with cellular and soluble components of the blood and with other cells in the vascular wall.[1-4] Endothelial cells respond to various pathologic stimuli by undergoing alterations in function and structure that directly influence the initiation and evolution of the inflammatory reaction. Many of these responses are due to alterations in gene expression leading to modulation of synthesis or release of biologically active molecules. This chapter briefly reviews the roles of endothelium in inflammation that may be particularly relevant to rheumatic diseases. The numerous metabolic functions of the endothelium are not discussed but have been the subject of recent comprehensive studies.[5]

Endothelial cells contribute to all phases of acute and chronic inflammation: from the initial vascular events characterized by vasodilatation and increased vascular permeability; to the acute cellular events manifested by leukocyte adhesion, transmigration, and activation; to the chronic cellular response, dominated by lymphocytic infiltration; and, finally, to the healing and fibrotic reactions, highlighted by neovascularization (*angiogenesis*) and fibroplasia. Endothelial cells are also involved in the thrombotic phenomena of inflammation.

ENDOTHELIAL CELL RESPONSES IN INFLAMMATION

Before we present the role of endothelium in these events, certain terms that are being used increasingly to define these endothelial responses operationally should be introduced.

Necrosis and *lysis* are endothelial reactions that have long been appreciated from ultrastructural studies and that have been ascribed to direct effects of exogenous injurious agents, such as burns, chemicals, and bacterial toxins[6]; however, they also might potentially be caused by endogenous chemical mediators, such as oxygen-derived free radicals released from leukocytes. This type of injury results in increased vascular permeability and, frequently, in local thrombus formation. It often results in *desquamation* of the endothelium, but desquamation can in principle occur without the endothelial cells necessarily undergoing necrosis or lysis. It is possible, for example, that activation of certain proteolytic enzymes in the subendothelial space may cause a disruption of the cell-matrix adhesive proteins, followed by endothelial detachment.[7] Such an event may also cause increased vascular permeability.

Apoptosis also occurs in endothelial cells.[8] A variety of stimuli, such as ionizing radiation, peroxide oxidants, bacterial lipopolysaccharide (LPS),[9] tumor necrosis factor (TNF-α),[10] certain lysophospholipids,[11] hemorrhagic snake venom,[12] and deprivation of growth factors induce apoptosis in cultured endothelial cells.[13] Genes known to regulate apoptosis (e.g., BCl_2 and BCl_x) in other cells are also found in endothelium.

Recent studies suggest two pathways for apoptotic cell death in cultured endothelium. The first involves the intracellular generation of oxidants, particularly hydroxyl radicals.[14] Apoptosis caused by peroxides, LPS, and TNF-α is induced by this mechanism and can be prevented by antioxidants that cross cell membranes. In other cell types, BCl_2 and BCl_x overexpression prevents this oxidant-associated apoptotic cell death. The second pathway results from deprivation of growth factors, allowing the death program to be activated, and in cultured endothelial cells it is age-dependent.[8] This type of apoptosis is not inhibited by antioxidant treatment but is reduced by factors that activate protein kinase C. The expression of A20, a novel zinc-finger protein, first identified as one of the earliest genes induced in cultured endothelial cells with TNF-α, correlates with protection from cell death after both growth factor deprivation and TNF-α, and thus may act along both pathways of apoptosis.[8, 15, 16]

Endothelial apoptosis may also play a role in the regression of new blood vessels during angiogenesis. In cultured endothelial cells, inhibition of anchorage-dependent cell spreading triggers apoptosis,[17] a phenomenon that may be related to intracellular signaling by integrins.[18] During tumor angiogenesis in vivo, inhibition of endothelial cell adhesion by antagonists of integrin $\alpha_V\beta 3$ induces apoptosis in angiogenic blood vessels and promotes tumor regression.[19] Similarly, certain endothelial growth factors, such as *vascular endothelial growth factor* (VEGF), act as survival factors in newly formed vessels; down-regulation of

VEGF, induced by hyperoxia, results in foci of endothelial apoptosis and regression of newly formed retinal vessels in experimental animals.[20]

Endothelial stimulation here denotes a rapid (in minutes), reversible response of the endothelium that is independent of new protein synthesis.[2] The best example of endothelial stimulation is the endothelial cell contraction, which occurs immediately after injection of histamine, serotonin, and other vasoactive mediators and that results in the formation of the classic intracellular gaps in venules.[21] Another is the rapid redistribution of the adhesive glycoprotein P-selectin (also called GMP-140, PADGEM, and CD62)[22, 23] when endothelial cells are stimulated with thrombin or histamine (see later).

In contrast to stimulation, *endothelial activation* is a response that depends on new or altered protein synthesis; it is induced by inflammatory cytokines, such as interleukin-1 (IL-1), TNF-α, and interferon-γ (IFN-γ).[1–3] Classic examples of endothelial activation are the induction of the endothelial adhesion molecule E-selectin (also called ELAM-1 or CD62E)[24, 25] by IL-1 and induction of class II major histocompatibility complex (MHC) molecules by IFN-γ.[26] Recent work indicates that a variety of nonimmune stimuli, such as hypoxia, disturbed shear stress, and lipid products, also cause endothelial activation (discussed later).

Endothelial dysfunction is a relatively nonspecific term, first used in the context of the role of endothelial injury in atherogenesis, to describe endothelial cells undergoing potentially irreversible alterations in functional state without losing their structural integrity.[27] Increased pinocytosis, changes in membrane fluidity, and altered growth characteristics are some examples of such dysfunctions. Although such sublethal injury to the endothelium may be of importance, most of the examples initially described as representing endothelial dysfunction are now known to be examples of either endothelial activation or what was defined earlier as endothelial stimulation.

Finally, *neovascularization* (angiogenesis) is a process that represents an integrated series of endothelial responses, endothelial migration, proliferation, and maturation. It is characteristic of the healing phase of inflammation and chronic inflammatory responses. This topic is discussed later in this chapter.

There is a great deal of overlap among these responses, in terms of mediators and mechanisms involved as well as final effects. For example, cytokines, such as TNF-α that are classic inducers of endothelial activation, render endothelial cells more susceptible to endothelial lysis by leukocyte products[28] and may also cause angiogenesis.[29]

THE ROLE OF ENDOTHELIUM IN THE VASCULAR EVENTS OF ACUTE INFLAMMATION

Vasodilatation

The first hallmark of acute inflammation is local vasodilation. Vasodilatation serves to enhance the subsequent increases in vascular permeability and neutrophil exudation that characterize the inflammatory response. Although vasodilatory mediators may originate from plasma, leukocytes (e.g., monocytes, macrophages), or platelets, vascular endothelium is a known regulator of vascular tone and can contribute to the vasodilation.

Endothelial cells regulate basal vascular tone through the release of both endothelium-derived contracting and relaxing factors.[30] The most important contracting factors are endothelin-1, angiotensin-II, and certain eicosanoids (thromboxane A_2 and prostaglandin H_2). The principal relaxing factors are prostacyclin (PGI_2) and nitric oxide (NO). A variety of agonists, such as thrombin, histamine, leukotriene C, acetylcholine, and cytokines (IL-1, TNF-α), as well as endotoxin, hypoxia, and mechanical shear[30, 31] stimulate endothelial production of these vasodilators in vitro. Thus, vascular endothelium can contribute to the vasodilation by elaborating these potential vasodilators. The effects of PGI_2 are described fully in Chapter 19.

Nitric oxide is a soluble free radical gas that is produced by endothelial cells, macrophages, specific neurons in the brain, and a variety of other cell types.[32–34] It is synthesized from L-arginine, molecular oxygen, NADPH, and other cofactors by the enzyme nitric oxide synthase (NOS). There are several isoforms of NOS. Constitutive NOS forms, found in endothelium (eNOS) and certain neurons (nNOS) produce small amounts of nitric oxide, which can be activated rapidly by an increase in cytoplasmic calcium ions in the presence of calmodulin. In contrast, inducible NOS (iNOS), originally identified in macrophages, is not calcium-dependent and is highly regulated by cytokines; iNOS can also be induced in smooth muscle cells, hepatocytes, and other cells. Some cytokines (IFN-γ, IL-1, TNF-α) promote but others (TGF-β) inhibit the induction of the enzymes.

Particularly high levels of nitric oxide can be generated by iNOS. Nitric oxide has a half-life of 6 to 30 seconds and is inactivated by superoxide and oxygen. In addition to its effect on smooth muscle, causing vasodilatation, nitric oxide has other effects in inflammation. It inhibits platelet adhesion and aggregation, suppresses leukocyte adhesion[34, 35] and aggregation, and inhibits proliferation of vascular smooth muscle and other cells. High levels of nitric oxide and its free radical derivatives are also cytotoxic and may be responsible for tissue damage.

Although endothelial NOS is constitutive, this isoform can actually be induced by such stimuli as shear stress, chronic exercise, and high oxygen concentrations. Hyperoxia up-regulates and hypoxia down-regulates eNOS expression through both transcriptional and post-transcriptional mechanisms.[36]

Most of the NOS inhibitors now in use (L-arginine analogs) inhibit both constitutive and inducible NOS. In various experimental animal models, such inhibitors protect against the profound vasodilation in septic shock and reduce the severity of inflammation and tissue damage in acute inflammation,[37] arthritis,[38] autoimmune, glomerulonephritis,[39] and immune complex lung injury.[40] Although it is thought that iNOS, rather than eNOS, is a more likely target of these agents, as discussed earlier, eNOS plays a more important role in regulation of vascular tone. Thus, the relative contributions of eNOS, and iNOS to the vasodilatory response in vivo are unclear and may depend on the precise pathologic condition.

On the other hand, failure of the vascular endothelium to elicit nitric oxide–mediated vasodilation as a result of decreased formation, increased degradation, or decreased sensitivity to nitric oxide may contribute to vasoconstriction in systemic and pulmonary hypertension, atherosclerosis, and diabetic vasculopathy.

Increased Vascular Permeability

Much more is known of the role of endothelium in the *increased vascular permeability* characteristic of acute inflammation. The ultrastructural studies of the 1960s and more recent studies in vitro and in vivo have established several fundamental types of endothelial responses that result in increased vascular permeability. Although certain stimuli specifically cause only one type of response, most natural inflammatory reactions are associated with combinations of such events.

Endothelial Contraction

In most experimental models of inflammation studied—from the simple injection of vasoactive amines (histamine, serotonin) to the complex permeability changes induced by physical, chemical, thermal, toxic, or immunogenic injury—the principal morphologic basis for vascular leakage is the formation of intercellular gaps in the endothelium that allow the passage of plasma across the vascular wall. Except in some experimental models, this histamine type of vascular injury occurs almost exclusively in small and medium-sized venules.[41, 42] Persuasive evidence suggests that the gaps form as a result of contraction of endothelial cells mediated by the vasoactive agents, a classic example of endothelial stimulation. This sort of mediated injury is relatively short-lived and is seen with all the permeability-increasing chemical mediators thus far studied, including histamine, serotonin, bradykinin, C3a, C5a, platelet-activating factor (PAF), and the vasoactive leukotrienes.[43] Although the precise cause of the venular localization of such increased permeability is still uncertain, Simionescu and colleagues found a greater density of surface histamine receptors in venular endothelium than in capillary endothelium.[44] In vitro studies have confirmed that histamine causes endothelial cell contraction and that the process is mediated by an intracellular pathway involving calmodulin myosin light chain phosphorylation[45] and changes in peripheral actin.

Endothelial Retraction, Cytoskeletal Reorganization, and Sublethal Injury

An apparently different mechanism of reversible endothelial intracellular leakage has been reported in cultured endothelial cells in vitro. When exposed to cytokines such as IL-1, TNF-α, and IFN-γ for 4 to 6 hours, endothelial cells in confluent monolayers begin to undergo a structural reorganization of their cytoskeleton in such a way that they retract from each other at the junctions, causing intercellular discontinuities that lead to long-lived (24 hours or more) increases in permeability.[46, 47] The retraction is reversible and requires protein synthesis. Its genesis is thus altogether different from that of endothelial contraction induced by histamine and is an example of cytokine-induced endothelial activation. Whether there are in vivo correlates to this type of increased permeability is unclear, but cytokine-induced retraction is an attractive explanation for the vascular leakage caused in immunologically mediated delayed hypersensitivity or by toxins, which cause a delayed or prolonged type of vascular leakage.

Endothelial retraction with cytoskeletal reorganization can also be induced by sublethal doses of agents that in higher concentrations may be cytotoxic. Sublethal concentrations of hydrogen peroxide, for example, produce reversible endothelial cell retraction accompanied by loss of normal cytoskeletal spatial organization of endothelial cell adhesion molecules.[48] In addition, the increased permeability induced in vitro by hypoxia[49] and by engagement of advanced glycation end-products by their endothelial receptor[50] may reflect such cytoskeletal reorganization and endothelial cell retraction.

Direct Endothelial Injury

This type of vascular leakage, originally described after necrotizing thermal and chemical injury, is characterized ultrastructurally by degenerative changes in the endothelium with vacuolization, fragmentation, membrane blebbing, and frequently outright denudation with local thrombus formation. This diffuse microvascular injury involves capillaries, venules, and arterioles and results in immediate and sustained increases in local vascular permeability.[6]

Leukocyte-Mediated Vascular Leakage

A variety of in vitro and in vivo studies indicate that leukocytes, in the process of adhesion and transmigration across the vascular wall, may injure endothelial cells, which results in increased vascular permeability. The mechanism of such injury involves oxygen-derived free radicals and proteolytic enzymes[51] (detailed elsewhere). The occurrence and severity of the endothelial injury that accompanies leukocyte-endothelial interactions are variable and appear to depend on the state of activation of neutrophils. For example, during the process of neutrophil extravasation induced by serum in the rat, closed junctions are maintained and no vascular leakage occurs. In contrast, the leukocytic exudation, which accompanies immune complex–mediated injury, or injections of chemotactic complement fragments, which also cause leukocyte activation, result in a considerable increase in vascular permeability and ultrastructural evidence of endothelial injury and denudation. The process has been most extensively studied in pulmonary-induced inflammation in which increases in vascular permeability can be measured. In some of these models, interventions that prevent leukocyte adhesion[52] or protect against toxic oxygen leukocyte products[53] inhibit edema formation.

Regenerating Endothelium

This mechanism of leakage accounts for the increased permeability of new regenerating capillaries in healing inflammation during the process of endothelial proliferation. Leakage in this setting occurs as a result of open intercellular junctions and is enhanced by the relatively incomplete basement membranes in immature endothelial cells.[54] In addition, proliferation of endothelium in the microcirculation may cause endothelial regeneration without the formation of new blood vessels but with the occurrence of distinct increases in vascular permeability that mostly involve capillaries.[55]

Increased Transcytosis

Although the role of caveolae (noncoated endocytic vesicles) in transendothelial transport of macromolecules has been a matter of controversy, studies by Schnitzer and associates have shown specific proteins and binding sites on the surface of endothelial cells, which interact with such circulating molecules as albumin, transferrin, and insulin.[56, 57] For example, a cell surface protein, called *albondin*, mediates albumin transport across endothelium in vitro and in situ, and the alkylating agent *N*-ethylmaleimide, which interferes with intervesicular locking and fusion, significantly inhibits such transport.[58] That increased transcytosis by a *vesicovacuolar* transcellular pathway causes increased permeability has been recently shown convincingly in blood vessels within tumors by Dvorak and colleagues.[55a]

LEUKOCYTE-ENDOTHELIAL INTERACTIONS AND ENDOTHELIAL ACTIVATION

Leukocyte-Endothelial Adhesion

A critical function of inflammation is the delivery of leukocytes to the site of injury. The process involves leukocyte adhesion to endothelium, followed by transmigration across the endothelium through intercellular junctions, and emigration toward chemoattractants emanating from the source of injury. Although the roles of leukocytes are to ingest offending agents, kill bacteria and other microbes, and degrade necrotic tissue and foreign antigens, they can also induce tissue damage by releasing enzymes, chemical mediators, and toxic oxygen free radicals.

Leukocyte-induced injury contributes to many acute and chronic inflammatory diseases, including arthritis, and may be subject to therapeutic intervention. There has been an explosion of research on the mechanisms of leukocyte-endothelial adhesion and transmigration in the past decade.[59–61] This work has shown that both adhesion and transmigration are determined, in large part, by the interaction of complementary adhesion molecules on the leukocytes and endothelium and that the expression, adhesion avidity, and surface modulation of these molecules are governed by a variety of factors, principally chemical

Table 12–1. MAJOR FAMILIES OF LEUKOCYTE-ENDOTHELIAL ADHESION PROTEINS

Family	Members	Distribution
Selectins	E-selectin	Activated endothelium
	P-selectin	Platelets; endothelium
	L-selectin	Leukocytes
Immunoglobulins	ICAM-1/2	Endothelium; leukocytes
	VCAM-1	Endothelium; leukocytes
	MAdCAM-1	HEV; gut endothelium
	PECAM-1	Endothelium; leukocytes
Integrins	VLA-4 ($\alpha4\beta_1$)	Lymphocytes; monocytes; eosinophils
	LPAM-1 ($\alpha4\beta7$)	B and T cells
	LFA-1($\alpha L\beta2$)	Lymphocytes; monocytes; neutrophils
	Mac-1 ($\alpha M\beta2$)	Monocytes; neutrophils
	P-250 ($\alpha X\beta2$)	Monocytes; neutrophils; eosinophils
Mucin-like proteins	GlyCAM-1	High endothelial venules
(linked to sialyl-	P-selectin glycoprotein ligand-1	Leukocytes
Lewis[x,a])	E-selectin ligand-1	Leukocytes
	CD34	Leukocytes

Abbreviations: ICAM, intercellular adhesion molecules; VCAM, vascular cell adhesion molecules; MAdCAM, mucosal addressin cell adhesion molecules; PECAM-1, platelet-endothelial adhesion molecule-1; VLA, very late antigen; LPAM-1, lymphocyte Peyer's patch adhesion molecule; LFA, leukocyte function-associated antigen; GlyCAM, glycosylated cell adhesion molecule; HEV, high endothelial venule.

mediators. The molecular characteristics of adhesion molecules are detailed in Chapter 20. Here we describe only the role of endothelium in these events, and particularly, with the process of endothelial activation.

The adhesion receptors involved in leukocyte-endothelial interactions belong to five molecular families (Table 12–1):

• Selectins
• Immunoglobulins
• Integrins
• Mucins
• Certain proteoglycans

The principal adhesion molecules and their possible role in inflammation are shown in Table 12–2. Several mechanisms modulate these molecules so that endothelial adhesion is induced.

Redistribution of Adhesion Molecules to the Cell Surface

This mechanism has been most well studied for P-selectin. Originally described in the α-granule of platelets, P-selectin is present constitutively on the membrane of Weibel-Palade granules and can be rapidly translocated to the plasma membrane on exposure of endothelium to thrombin, histamine, and PAF.[22, 23] This process occurs within minutes, does not require protein synthesis, depends on increased concentrations of cytosolic calcium, and serves to deliver preformed adhesion molecules in short order to the surface. P-selectin mediates neutrophil, monocyte, and lymphocyte binding to endothelium by interacting with carbohydrate ligands (sialyl-Lewis^x) O-linked to the glycoprotein mucin *P-selectin glycoprotein ligand-1* (PSGL-1).[62] In addition to cytokines, oxidants[63] and hypoxia[64] may also cause P-selectin surface expression.

Another endothelial cell adhesion molecule, *intercellular adhesion molecule-1* (ICAM-1), may also be increased slightly by mobilization of intracellular stores.[65, 66]

Increased Avidity of Binding

Increased avidity of binding is most relevant to the binding of leukocyte integrins, including the $\beta 2$-integrin molecule *lymphocyte function-associated antigen-1* (LFA-1, CD11aCD18) and the $\alpha 4\beta 1$-integrin molecule *very late antigen-4* (VLA-4, CD49dCD29). LFA-1, normally present on leukocytes—neutrophils, monocytes, and lymphocytes—has a low affinity for its ligand ICAM-1 on endothelium.[65] When leukocytes are activated by chemoattractants, such as chemotactic peptides and chemokines (e.g., macrophage inflammatory protein [MIP]-1α and β, IL-8, MCP-1 and Rantes), LFA-1 is converted to a high-affinity binding state, probably as a result of a conformational change, that increases its affinity for endothelial ICAM-1, as

Table 12–2. LEUKOCYTE-ENDOTHELIAL CELL ADHESION MOLECULES IN INFLAMMATION

Endothelial Molecule	Leukocyte Ligand	Main Function
E-selectin (CD62E, ELAM-1)	Sialyl-Lewis^x, SSEA-1, ESL-1, PSGL-1, CLA GlyCAM-1, (?) L-selectin	Neutrophil, eosinophil, basophil, macrophage, and memory T cell rolling/early adhesion, (?) Angiogenesis
P-selectin (CD62P, GMP-140)	Sialyl-Lewis^x, PSGL-1, (?) L-selectin, ?others	Neutrophil, monocyte, and lymphocyte rolling/early adhesion, (?) platelet–leukocyte–endothelial cell interaction
Peripheral L-selectin ligand (?)	L-selectin (CD62L)	Neutrophil, monocyte, and lymphocyte rolling/early adhesion
GlyCAM-1	L-selectin, $\alpha 4\beta 7$	Lymphocyte homing
MadCAM-1	L-selectin, $\alpha 4\beta 7$, $\alpha 4\beta 1$	Lymphocyte homing
CD34	L-selectin	Lymphocyte homing
ICAM-1	LFA-1 (CD11aCD18) Mac-1 (CD11bCD18)	All leukocyte subsets. Adhesion/stable arrest and transmigration, costimulation of CD4$^+$ T cell activation
ICAM-2	LFA-1 (CD11aCD18)	Neutrophils and lymphocytes, other leukocyte subsets trafficking/low-affinity adhesion, (?) transmigration, (?) costimulation of T cell activation
VCAM-1 (INCAM-110)	$\alpha 4\beta 1$ (VLA-4, CD49dCD29) $\alpha 4\beta 7$ (LPAM-1)	Lymphocyte, monocyte, eosinophil, and basophil adhesion, transmigration
LFA-3	CD2	Lymphocyte adhesion and costimulation
CD31 (PECAM-1)	CD31 (homophillic)	Neutrophil, monocyte, lymphocyte subset transmigration, platelet-endothelial cell adhesion, integrin activation
CD44 (Hermes)	Hyaluronic acid, collagen, fibronectin, laminin, extracellular matrix	Leukocyte adhesion, lymphocyte homing, endothelial cell binding of chemokines (e.g., MIP-1β)
CD40	CD40 ligand (gp39, TRAP)	Leukocyte adhesion, stimulation of endothelial cell activation, induction of adhesion molecule expression
VAP-1	(?) Lymphocyte ligand	Lymphocyte adhesion, (?) trafficking, (?) synovial addressin
L-VAP-2	(?) Lymphocyte ligand	Lymphocyte adhesion, (?) trafficking
$\alpha 6\beta 1$	(?) Extracellular matrix laminin	Lymphocyte homing to thymus

well as an altered interaction with the cytoskeleton.[59, 60, 60a]

Induction of Adhesion Molecules on Endothelium

A number of agents, and particularly cytokines, cause profound and often selective increases in the synthesis and surface expression of endothelial cell adhesion molecules, including E-selectin,[24, 25, 67] ICAM-1,[65] and *vascular cell adhesion molecule-1* (VCAM-1)[68, 69] as part of the process of endothelial activation (also see Chapter 20). TNF-α and IL-1 induce de novo E-selectin expression and increased expression of ICAM-1, VCAM-1, and L-selectin ligand on peripheral endothelial cells.[2, 60] For E-selectin, expression is maximal 4 to 6 hours after cytokine treatment. Expression then declines even in the presence of cytokine. In cell culture, E-selectin promotes the adhesion of neutrophils, eosinophils, basophils, monocytes, and a subpopulation of memory T cells.[70, 71] Its major ligand is the carbohydrate sialyl-Lewis[x] linked to several mucins,[72] including ESL-1[73] and PSGL-1,[74] the ligand for P-selectin (see Table 12–2). The time sequence of ICAM-1 induction differs from that of E-selectin. ICAM-1, present basally, is increased by 4 hours and is maximal 12 to 24 hours after cytokine treatment; it may remain elevated for days.[75] ICAM-1 mediates both neutrophil and lymphocyte adhesion to cytokine-activated endothelial cells in vitro through the leukocyte integrin receptors LFA-1 (CD11aCD18)[65] and Mac-1 (CD11bCD18).[76] VCAM-1 is also induced slowly, reaching peak expression at about 12 to 24 hours after cytokine treatment, but it declines in expression over several days following stimulation.[69, 77]

Induction of these endothelial cell adhesion molecules can be regulated by combinations of cytokines.[2, 4] For instance, IFN-γ accelerates and prolongs and IL-4 decreases TNF-α–mediated induction of E-selectin and ICAM-1.[75, 78] In contrast, there is synergism between IL-4 and TNF-α in the induction of VCAM-1.[79, 80] VCAM-1 mediates adhesion of lymphocytes, monocytes, eosinophils, and basophils but not neutrophils, via the β1-integrin α4β1 and α4β7 (also known as α4βp and LPAM-1).[60, 61, 68]

The molecular mechanism underlying adhesion and the precise roles of the adhesion molecules are being dissected in numerous in vitro and in vivo models of inflammation.[59, 81–83] Several points should be made with regard to the role of endothelial cell adhesion molecules in inflammation.

First, hemodynamic conditions, such as altered shear stress, clearly influence both adhesion and transmigration.[84] For example, LFA-1 contributes to the adhesion of neutrophils to endothelium under static conditions but not under flow with shear stresses at levels estimated to exist in postcapillary venules.[85] In contrast, P-selectin mediates neutrophil binding under flow but is only minimally functional under static conditions.

The second factor is the state of activation of the leukocyte itself.[86] The resting neutrophil readily adheres to cytokine-activated endothelial cells bearing E-selectin. Activated neutrophils shed L-selectin and therefore do not adhere to the putative L-selectin ligand on endothelium. In addition, activated neutrophils are less adhesive to E- and P-selectin,[87] but they bind ICAM-1 more avidly as a result of the high-avidity binding state of LFA-1 and Mac-1. The loss of L-selectin– and E-selectin–dependent binding, associated with neutrophil activation, coupled with the increased avidity for ICAM-1 favors LFA-1–dependent transmigration events.[88, 89]

A third influence on leukocyte adhesion and transmigration is the potential role of endogenous endothelial mediators—induced pari passu with the initial stimulant or activator of endothelium—on subsequent endothelial interactions. As will be discussed later, activated endothelial cells synthesize and secrete a variety of endogenous cytokines with potential biologic activities, including IL-1,[90] IL-8 family molecules,[91, 92] and MCP-1,[93] which have the potential of priming or activating leukocytes and causing chemokinesis and chemotaxis.

Fourth, the actual topographic distribution of adhesion molecules on leukocytes governs contact initiation under flow. L-selectin, for example, which is involved in *rolling* and is an efficient initiator of adhesion, is clustered on the tips of leukocyte microvilli.[94] Cells transfected with mutants of L-selectin that lack the ability to localize to the microvillus have markedly decreased binding to their ligand. Thus, microvillus presentation of adhesion molecules is important in increasing binding under flow conditions.

Fifth, a number of adhesion inhibitors have been described. These include nitric oxide,[95] transforming growth factor (TGF-β),[96, 97] and the lipoxins.[98] The relative contributions of these molecules in inflammatory responses have been described in detail elsewhere.

A current model (Fig. 12–1) postulates three or more steps for signaling leukocyte trafficking across the endothelium in inflammation.[59, 83, 84, 94, 99] These steps are postulated to occur in sequence and include:

1. *Rolling.* An initial primary rapid and relatively loose adhesion pathway that involves L- and P-selectins as well as E-selectin on cytokine-activated endothelium. This step is reflected by the tethering of leukocytes to the vessel wall, followed by rolling, which can be readily seen in vivo by intravital microscopy to precede adhesion.[82, 100]

2a. *Arrest and adhesion strengthening.* This step is dependent on the presence of chemoattractants or leukocyte-activating factors, produced by endothelium, and other cells. This process may be stimulated by initial interactions with selectin molecules.

2b. *Stable arrest.* Loosely adherent leukocytes increase their ability to bind stably to endothelium, largely through the integrin-immunoglobulin receptor-ligand pairs.

3. *Transmigration.* This step necessitates directional

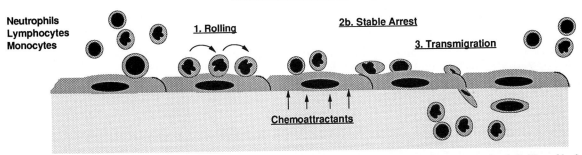

Figure 12–1. Illustration of the proposed events leading to the recruitment of leukocytes into an inflammatory site. *1, Rolling* of leukocytes (e.g., neutrophils, monocytes, lymphocytes) involving low-affinity interactions with endothelial cells and the selectin family of molecules. *2a, Arrest and adhesion strengthening,* mediated by leukocyte-activating factors, including peptides, chemoattractants, and chemokines. *2b, Stable arrest,* mediated by high-affinity binding involving integrin-immunoglobulin family interactions. *3, Transmigration,* mediated by the integrins and immunoglobulin family of molecules, including CD31-CD31 interactions. (Adapted from Springer TA: Traffic signals on endothelium for lymphocyte recirculation and leukocyte emigration. Annu Rev Physiol 57:827, 1995. Adapted, with permission by Annual Reviews Inc. © 1995.)

cues from chemoattractants as well as specific adhesion molecules. The integrin/immunoglobulin pairs as well as homotypic PECAM-1 (CD31) interactions are important in such transmigration.[101]

The existence of numbers of receptor-ligand pairs as well as the proposed requirement for several sequential events in recruitment of leukocytes provides likely mechanisms for the diversity and specificity of endothelial-leukocyte adhesion in different forms of inflammation.

Persuasive evidence for the relevance of adhesion molecules in inflammation comes from several sources. First is the existence in humans of *leukocyte adhesion deficiency syndromes* (LAD-1 and LAD-2).[102-105] LAD-1 is caused by a congenital defect in the biosynthesis of the β2-chain (CD18) of the leukocyte integrins LFA-1, Mac-1, and p150,95. Patients with LAD-1 have a profound defect in adhesion and emigration of neutrophils and monocytes, leading to recurrent bacterial infections[102, 103] (see Chapter 20). LAD-2 is a congenital defect that results from generalized fucose deficiency, thus the expression of sialyl-Lewis[x], the carbohydrate ligand for the selectins. Neutrophils from patients with LAD-2 have normal levels of L-selectin and the β2-integrin complexes but bind minimally or not at all to E-selectin or P-selectin.[104, 105] These patients also exhibit marked impairment in neutrophil emigration to skin windows, but have a relatively mild clinical course compared with patients with LAD-1. This is probably due to the ability of LAD-2 neutrophils to adhere and transmigrate via the β2-integrins under conditions of reduced shear stress.

Second, adhesion molecules can be demonstrated in experimentally induced reactions or natural disease processes by immunohistochemical techniques. E-selectin, ICAM-1, VCAM-1, and P-selectin have been localized in a variety of human diseased tissues, including delayed hypersensitivity reactions,[106] the late-phase reaction of immediate hypersensitivity,[107] septic shock,[108] the vasculature of tumors characterized by

excessive cytokine production,[42] allograft rejection,[109] atherosclerosis,[110, 111] arthritis,[112-114] and other inflammatory conditions of the skin and viscera.[115] Similarly, injection of cytokines in animals mimic some of the in vitro effects.[80, 116] Thus, TNF-α causes rapid rises in E-selectin, beginning 2 hours after TNF-α injection, that correlates with neutrophil adhesion and extravasation; later it causes rises in ICAM-1 and VCAM-1, which correlate with lymphocytic influx. Further, IL-4, as it does in vitro, enhances VCAM-1 expression induced by TNF-α. IFN-γ induces emigration of monocytes and lymphocytes but not neutrophils.

Third, numerous studies[61] have shown that antibodies to adhesion molecules inhibit leukocyte accumulation and tissue injury in models of inflammation. For example, the neutrophil accumulation that occurs in ischemia-reperfusion injury is partially inhibited by antibodies to P-selectin, L-selectin, and ICAM-1; and neutrophil recruitment in immune-mediated lung injury, inflamed skin, and peritonitis is inhibited by antibodies to, E-, P-, and L-selectin; ICAM-1; and PECAM-1 (CD31).[61] Similarly, lymphocytic and monocytic infiltration is partially prevented with antibodies to ICAM-1, VCAM-1, and VLA-4 in allografts and in a variety of chronic inflammatory disorders, including collagen or adjuvant-induced arthritis, anti–glomerular basement membrane (GBM) nephritis, allergic encephalomyelitis, and delayed hypersensitivity reactions.[4, 61] Antibodies to the β2-integrins have also been effective in reducing leukocyte influx in models of acute inflammation. In certain instances, combinations of antibodies are even more protective. For example, in a model of anti-GBM crescentic glomerulonephritis in the rat, a combination of anti–ICAM-1 and anti–LFA-1 antibodies cause marked inhibition of proteinuria, leukocyte infiltration, and crescent formation.[117]

Finally, studies of genetically engineered mice lacking one or combinations of adhesion molecules ("knockout" mice) lend great credence to the role of adhesion molecules in vivo. P-selectin–deficient mice exhibit virtually no leukocyte rolling in vessels in the mesentery, and the emigration of neutrophils into the peritoneum is markedly delayed after thioglycollate injections.[118] P-selectin deficiency also inhibits leukocyte influx in mouse ears subjected to delayed hypersensitivity reactions. L-selectin deficiency induces defects in lymphocyte homing and reduced leukocyte rolling, and delays thioglycolate-induced peritonitis.[119] E-selectin–deficient mice develop a defect in thioglycolate-induced peritonitis and delayed hypersensitivity but only if anti–P-selectin antibodies are also infused.[120] Mice lacking both P- and E-selectin exhibit minimal leukocyte rolling, even in inflamed vessels, and neutrophil emigration is severely reduced. These animals exhibit extreme leukocytosis, elevated cytokine levels, alterations in hematopoiesis, and bacterial infections characterized by ulcerative dermatitis, a phenotype that resembles human LAD-2.[121] ICAM-1 deficiency induces leukocytosis, reduced mixed lymphocyte reactions, and reduced leukocyte influx in delayed hypersensitivity lesions and affords significant protection from lethality in septic shock.[122]

Mechanisms of Endothelial Activation

Induction of endothelial adhesion molecules is but one of the repertoire of induced endothelial gene expression in endothelial activation (Table 12–3). Cytokine-activation of endothelial cells results in the synthesis and secretion of a variety of other endothelial cell-derived cytokines,[1, 123] including:

- IL-1, IL-6, IL-8, and MCP-1
- Growth factors, such as platelet-derived growth factor (PDGF), colony-stimulating factor (CSF), granulocyte-monophage CSF (GM-CSF), and TGF-β
- MHC class I and II molecules
- A variety of vasoactive mediators, including nitric oxide, prostacyclin, and other eicosanoids
- A number of coagulation proteins, including tissue factor, tissue plasminogen activator (tPA), and plasminogen activator inhibitor (PAI)

These mediators may themselves influence the further evolution of inflammation, as in the case of IL-8.[124–126] Similarly, as discussed earlier, a number of

Table 12–3. INDUCED ENDOTHELIAL GENE EXPRESSION

Adhesion molecules
Cytokines (interleukin-1, -6, -8; macrophage inflammatory
   protein-1)
Growth factors (platelet-derived growth factor, colony-
   stimulating factor, transforming growth factor-β,
   epidermal growth factor)
Major histocompatibility complex molecules (class I, II)
Vasoactive molecules (eicosanoids, nitric oxide)
Coagulation proteins (tissue plasminogen activator,
   plasminogen activator inhibitor, tissue factor)

Table 12–4. INDUCERS OF ENDOTHELIAL ACTIVATION

Cytokines
Bacterial products (endotoxin)
Hemodynamic stresses (altered shear)
Viruses
Lipid products (oxidized low-density lipoproteins;
   lysophophatidylcholine)
Advanced glycosylation end-products
Hypoxia

stimuli other than cytokines can activate endothelial cells (Table 12–4). These include endotoxin, viruses, hemodynamic stresses (e.g., altered shear stress), lipid products, including oxidized low-density lipoprotein (LDL) and lysophosphatidylcholine, and advanced glycosylation end-products. Hypoxia, for example, induces increased synthesis of endothelin and basic fibroblast growth factor (bFGF); up-regulation of expression of IL-1, IL-6, and IL-8; PAF; and ICAM-1.[127–132] Bacterial LPS mimics most of the effects of IL-1 and TNF-α. Alterations in shear stress induce eicosanoids, adhesion molecules, and nitric oxide. Lysophosphatidylcholine induces VCAM-1, ICAM-1, PDGF-α, PDGF-β, epidermal growth factor (EGF), nitric oxide, and PGI$_2$.

The molecular mechanisms underlying the pleiotropic effects of these disparate agents are now the subject of intense investigation and are beyond the scope of this chapter. A growing body of evidence, however, suggests that the NF-kB/IkB system of transcription factors may regulate endothelial cell gene activation[133–136] (Fig. 12–2). Many genes induced during endothelial activation, in particular E-selectin, ICAM-1, and VCAM-1, have NF-kB binding sites in their 5' flanking sequences. NF-kB is present in resting endothelial cells in an inactive cytosolic form, complexed to members of inhibitory proteins known as IkB. NF-kB can be activated by a variety of agents, including oxidants, cytokines (IL-1 and TNF-α), endotoxin, viral products, advanced glycosylation end-products, and physical forces. On activation, the inhibitor IkB is phosphorylated and subsequently degraded, releasing NF-kB from IkB, thus allowing NF-kB to translocate to the nucleus, bind to its recognition DNA elements, and participate in the activation of transcription. The NF-kB system is autoregulatory, in that NF-kB also induces activation of IkB gene. This results in a negative feedback loop to inhibit transcription of the target gene and to ensure that the activated endothelial cell returns to a quiescent state within a relatively short period following activation. All the components of this system are present in endothelial cells. The proteasome pathway is required for these events.[137]

Collins and associates have hypothesized that activation of NF-kB could coordinate the expression of numerous endothelial products that are important in endothelial activation, including adhesion molecules,

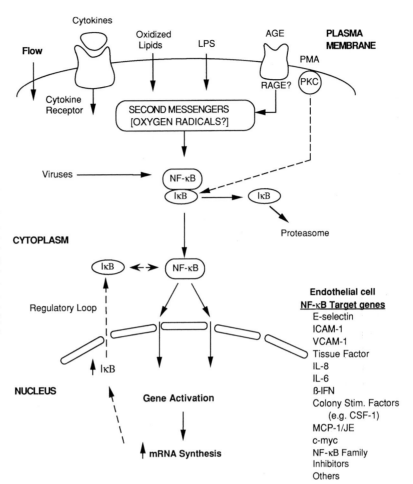

Figure 12–2. The NF-kB/IkB family of transcription factors in endothelial cell gene regulation. NF-kB is present in the cytoplasm of resting endothelial cells bound to its inhibitor IkB. Upon endothelial activation, NF-kB is released from IkB and translocates into the nucleus. NF-kB may then bind to specific DNA recognition sites and participate in the transcriptional activation of specific genes including E-selectin, ICAM-1, and VCAM-1. Nuclear translocation of NF-kB is also associated with IkB production, to regulate this process. (Modified from Collins T: Biology of disease: Endothelial nuclear factor-KB and the initiation of the atherosclerotic lesion. Lab Invest 68:499, 1993.)

growth factors, and components of the coagulation system[133, 136] (see Fig. 12–2). However, NF-kB sites, although necessary, are not sufficient for full transcription. The requirement for other transcription factor gene families, possibly targeted by second environmental signals, would potentially increase diversity and potential specificity of the endothelial responses.

ROLE OF ENDOTHELIAL CELLS IN CHRONIC INFLAMMATORY AND IMMUNOLOGIC REACTIONS

We conclude by examining the role of endothelial cells in chronic inflammatory and immunologic reactions, since these may be particularly relevant to chronic inflammatory arthritis. A wide body of literature, reviewed in detail elsewhere,[1, 3, 65] has shown important interactions among cytokines, endothelial cell surface molecules, and lymphocytes in lymphocyte homing, infiltration, and proliferation at sites of acute and chronic inflammation. In addition, angiogenesis, a characteristic component of the healing phase of inflammation, is of particular relevance to the pathophysiology of chronic arthritis.

Lymphocyte Trafficking

The trafficking of lymphocytes into lymphoid tissues and from lymph nodes into peripheral tissues is an extremely complex and highly regulated process that involves multiple molecular interactions.[86, 138, 139] One of the governing principles for "normal" selective recirculation of lymphocytes is that lymphocytes tend to preferentially recirculate to the organ where they initially encountered a specific antigen. However, several factors govern the homing of lymphocytes into inflamed tissues. These include (1) the different cell surface phenotype of naive and memory lymphocytes, (2) the tissue distribution of vascular addressins on inflamed endothelium, and (3) the different abilities of naive and memory lymphocytes to respond to a diversity of molecular signals. These are described in Chapter 20 and are only briefly discussed here.

Lymphocyte homing to peripheral lymph nodes is governed by complementary adhesion molecules on lymphocytes and endothelial cells[60, 86] (see Table 12–2). Because of the selectivity of tissues to which lymphocyte populations home, there are thought to be specific endothelial ligands for the homing receptors.[139] These are called *addressins*.[140] Naive and memory lymphocytes as well as activated T cells use different sets of molecules in their journey through the vascular system.[138, 141] The cell surface phenotype of naive lymphocytes promotes their recirculation through specialized blood vessels called *high endothelial venules* (HEVs) in peripheral lymph nodes.[142] Antigen-specific activation of naive lymphocytes in a peripheral lymph node results in proliferation and clonal expansion of cells (now called *memory T cells*) that have a new repertoire of cell surface receptors. The best-known marker for naive and memory T cells is the expression of CD45, naive cells expressing the high-molecular-weight form of the molecule (CD45RA) and memory cell expressing the low molecular isoform (CD45RO). These two populations of cells also express different cell surface adhesion molecules. Varying expression of these adhesion molecules on each T cell subset governs its trafficking pattern via different interactions with complementary molecules on endothelial cells.

The best studied of the homing receptors is L-selectin.[119, 143, 144] L-selectin is predominantly, but not exclusively, expressed by naive lymphocytes. Initially defined as the Mel-14 antigen in the mouse, it was found to be expressed on lymphocytes that recognize peripheral lymph node HEVs, but not Peyer's patch HEV. Antibody MECA-79, which blocked L-selectin–directed adhesion of lymphocytes, recognized the MECA-79 carbohydrate antigen, also called *peripheral node addressin* (PNAd).[145] This molecule was subsequently found to be a carbohydrate determinant expressed by multiple molecules on HEVs, including *glycosylated cell adhesion molecule-1* (GlyCAM-1) and CD34.[144, 146–148] GlyCAM-1 is present on, and is secreted by, HEVs; CD34 is a cell surface–associated molecule. Similarly, the endothelial addressin in Peyer's patch HEV, recognized by antibody MECA-367, is now called *mucosal addressin cell adhesion molecule-1* (MAdCAM-1).[149] MAdCAM-1 is expressed on endothelial cells in mucosal tissues, Peyer's patch HEVs, and endothelial cells in intestinal lamina propria. MAdCAM-1 binds lymphocyte L-selectin as well as the integrin molecule $\alpha 4\beta 7$ (also called LPAM). Antibodies to L-selectin, MAdCAM-1, or $\alpha 4\beta 7$ block the binding of lymphoid cells to Peyer's patch.[150] Thus, the increased expression of L-selectin and $\alpha 4\beta 7$ on naive cells might govern trafficking to lymph node HEV. In addition, other molecules involved in the migration of lymphoid cells to HEV are lymphocyte LFA-1,[151] L-VAP-2,[152] a G-protein–coupled receptor of the $\alpha 1$ class,[153] and endothelial VAP-1.[154] VAP-1 is worthy of special note because it is defined by a monoclonal antibody that was generated by immunizing mice with human synovium. It is expressed constitutively on endothelium in a variety of tissues, including peripheral lymph node and synovial HEV. It is not yet known whether VAP-1 is the specific synovial vascular addressin.

Lymphocyte Recruitment

As originally described for neutrophils, a series of sequential steps have been proposed to govern the recruitment of lymphocytes into sites of immune inflammation[59, 60, 99] (see Fig. 12–1). First, lymphocytes roll on endothelial cells, and second, they become firmly adherent to endothelial cells. This involves "triggering" of the lymphocyte, in which there is activation of lymphocyte cell surface receptors. Third, lymphocytes flatten on the endothelial cell surface, and quickly transmigrate across endothelial cells into the tissue.

E- and P-selectins, which mediate low-affinity adhesive events and rolling,[155] preferentially bind lymphocytes of the memory (CD45RO) phenotype, even under flow conditions in vitro.[156] Subsequent higher-affinity binding and stable arrest are mediated by the integrins. The chemokine MIP-1β mediates activation of lymphocyte cell surface integrin molecules, including LFA-1 and VLA-4, which results in an enhanced avidity for endothelial cell ICAM-1 and VCAM-1, respectively. Triggering by chemokines involves association of the chemokine with endothelial cell surface molecules, including proteoglycans such as CD44.[60, 60a, 139]

Integrin-immunoglobulin interactions for lymphocyte adhesion include the pairs LFA-1/ICAM-1 or ICAM-2, Mac-1/ICAM-1, $\alpha 4\beta 1$ (VLA-4) or $\alpha 4\beta 7$/VCAM-1, and $\alpha 4\beta 7$/MAdCAM-1 (see Table 12–2). Endothelial cell CD31 (PECAM-1), $\alpha 4\beta 1$, $\alpha 5\beta 1$, LFA-1, CD44, and extracellular matrix mediate the subsequent transmigration events.[60, 61, 139]

In addition to the steps described above, an immune inflammatory response may be amplified by cell surface proteins expressed on activated T cells, which directly impart activation signals to the endothelial cell. Recent studies have shown that the cell surface molecule CD40 is induced in vitro and in vivo on endothelial cells.[157, 158] CD40 was initially described on B cells, where it mediates B cell proliferation, secretion of immunoglobulins, and rescue of germinal center B cells from undergoing apoptosis. Interaction between the CD40 ligand gp39 and endothelial CD40 results in endothelial cell activation, leukocyte adhesion, and the expression of E-selectin, ICAM-1, and VCAM-1. Thus, recently activated T cells can impart a direct signal to endothelial cells to up-regulate adhesion molecules and augment immune inflammatory reactions.

Endothelium in Immunologic Interactions with T Cells

In addition to its role in lymphocyte recruitment, the endothelium responds to its interaction with lymphocytes by directly activating T cells. The bidirectionality of these interactions enables endothelial cells to act as active components in the evolution of a cell-mediated immune reaction.

Antigen-specific CD4$^+$ T cells migrate from lymph nodes into the periphery, where they may reencounter specific antigen. Following antigen-specific activation,

T-helper type 1 (Th1) cells secrete IL-2, IFN-γ, and TNF-β, and T-helper type 2 (Th2) cells secrete IL-4, IL-5, IL-6, and IL-10.[159, 160] Th1 cells are thought to be effective stimulators of cell-mediated immune reactions, whereas Th2 cells are more potent helpers for humoral responses and may play a role down-regulating the immune response. In vitro studies using cultured human and mouse endothelial cells have shown that endothelial cells can effectively present antigen to CD4+ T cells in both antigen-specific and alloimmune inflammatory reactions. This indicates that endothelial cells can initiate an antigen-specific signal (called "signal 1") and a costimulatory signal (called "signal 2") to T cells.[161–163] Signal 1 is initiated by specific engagement of the T cell receptor–CD3 complex of molecules with antigenic peptides in association with MHC class I or class II molecules on an *antigen-presenting cell* (APC), such as an endothelial cell. Signal 2 is initiated via additional accessory cell surface receptor-ligand interactions that alone cannot activate T cells. Cell surface receptors that mediate such costimulatory signals include T cell CD2, LFA-1, VLA-4, and CD28 interacting with LFA-3, ICAM-1, VCAM-1, and the B7 family molecules, respectively, on the APC.[162, 164, 165] Endothelial cells express a variety of costimulatory molecules, including LFA-3, ICAM-1, and VCAM-1. In addition, although human endothelial cells have not been shown to express the B7 family of molecules as yet, they are expressed on endothelium of other species.[166]

Different populations of helper T cells have different requirements for accessory molecules, such that the level of expression of endothelial-specific costimulators might be an important regulator of specific immune responses.[3, 167] For instance, endothelial LFA-3, ICAM-1, and VCAM-1 can costimulate cytokine gene activation. Endothelial LFA-3 directly costimulates T cell IL-2 production, and ICAM-1 and VCAM-1 can costimulate both IL-2 and IL-4 production. Thus, the tissue-specific phenotype of microvascular endothelial cell or the expression of costimulators in inflammation may determine the local T cell activation response. Indeed, endothelial cells undergo phenotypic changes during the course of an acute and chronic inflammatory reaction.

While activated endothelial cells mediate the recruitment and binding of lymphocytes, they also have profound effects on T cell activation. Endothelial cells costimulate IL-2 and IFN-γ cytokine gene production in an antigen-independent but costimulator-dependent manner.[3, 168] IL-2 is the predominant T cell growth factor and may thus enhance the local T cell proliferation. Costimulation of IFN-γ may result in further direct effects on endothelial cells to induce the expression of MHC class I and II molecules as well as to up-regulate the expression of ICAM-1.[78] Once endothelial cells express MHC class II molecules, they may now activate T cells entering the inflammatory site in an antigen-specific manner. Endothelial cell expression of MHC class II occurs in vivo in many models of immune inflammation, including classic

delayed type hypersensitivity reactions,[116] experimental allergic encephalomyelitis,[169] and acute and chronic allograft rejection.[4, 170] Whether such MHC class II expression plays a role in vivo is still uncertain.

Finally, activated endothelial cells elaborate a variety of cytokines, some of which can act as costimulators of T cell activation.[90, 171] For example, IL-1 enhances T cell activation and T cell–B cell interactions and, in some circumstances, may be important in overcoming T cell anergy. IL-6 has pleiotropic effects relevant to immune reactions and may in part account for the augmented B cell responses ascribed to endothelial cells. Other endothelium-derived cytokines that may be involved in the various phases of chronic inflammation include the IL-8 family of chemokines and the growth factors GM-CSF, TGF-β, PGDF-α, and PDGF-β, and *endothelium-derived growth factor* (EDGF).

Angiogenesis

The formation of new blood vessels—angiogenesis or neovascularization—is an important component of wound repair and all chronic inflammatory reactions.[172, 173] A fundamental process in the growth and development of tissues, it is one of the most intensively studied processes in biology today because of its critical role in the growth of tumors and in such poorly understood conditions as retrolental fibroplasia, macular degeneration, and psoriasis.[174] In addition, therapeutic strategies that may interfere with angiogenesis offer the hope of causing reduced tumor growth or progression of chronic inflammatory actions. Angiogenesis is a constant feature of many chronic arthritides, including rheumatoid arthritis, and experimental studies have shown that angiogenic factors are involved in the progression of arthritic lesions and that inhibition of angiogenesis may suppress arthritis.[175, 176]

Endothelial cells and their extracellular matrix are central to angiogenesis. New blood vessels arise by budding or sprouting from preexisting vessels, a process involving proteolytic degradation of the basement membrane of the parent vessel to allow, followed by migration of endothelial cells toward the angiogenic stimulus, proliferation of endothelial cells just behind the leading front of migrating cells, and finally, maturation of cells and their organization into capillary tubes, vascular loops, and networks. These events are modulated by a variety of endogenous growth promoters (angiogenic factors), negative regulators of vessel growth (angiogenesis inhibitors), and the extracellular matrix (ECM). The extracellular matrix interacts with the soluble molecules and endothelial cells in formation of the resultant three-dimensional vascular structure and also in regression.[177, 178]

The major angiogenic factors, listed in Table 12–5, can be induced by a variety of cell types, including endothelium.[172, 179, 180] Angiogenic factors are considered to be *direct* when they cause neovascularization

Table 12–5. ANGIOGENIC FACTORS*

Angiogenesis Factors	Angiogenesis Inhibitors
Fibroblast growth factor (FGF)	α-Interferon
Basic and acidic	Tissue inhibitors
Vascular endothelial growth factor (VEGF)	Metalloproteinases (TIMPs)
Tumor necrosis factor-α	Prolactin
Transforming growth factor-α (TGF-α)	Thrombospondin-1
Transforming growth factor-β*	Platelet factor-4
Interleukin-8	Angiostatin
Hepatocyte growth factor	Transforming growth factor-β
Angiogenin*	
Granulocyte colony-stimulating factor	

*In vivo only.
For more detail, see Folkman J: N Engl J Med 333:1757, 1995.

in vivo and also stimulate endothelial cell proliferation or migration in vitro. Indirect angiogenic factors do not have in vitro effects but can produce neovascularization in vivo, either by promoting the synthesis and release of endogenous growth factors by other cells or by other unknown mechanisms. The two factors currently thought to be most likely candidates for neovascularization in vivo are bFGF and VEGF.[181] Basic FGF can mediate all the steps of neovascularization in vitro.[182] It stimulates the synthesis of proteases that may degrade basement membranes and connective tissue matrix, migration and proliferation of endothelial cells, and the development of capillary tubes under appropriate conditions. It is synthesized by endothelial cells, macrophages, and a variety of tumor cells, and it has strong affinity for heparan and heparan sulfate proteoglycans. It thus binds to basement membranes and extracellular matrix. One class of FGF receptor includes the low-affinity cell surface heparan sulfate proteoglycans, the other, high-affinity receptors with tyrosine kinase activity. The process by which bFGF is released from the cell is unclear because it lacks a signal peptide, but the protein is present in body fluids. Indeed, quantitative assays of bFGF show increased concentrations in the sera of 10 percent of patients with cancer, in the cerebrospinal fluid of children with brain tumors, and in the urine of infants with hemangiomas.[172, 174, 183] VEGF (~45 kD), also a heparan-binding protein, causes endothelial cell proliferation in vitro, angiogenesis in vivo, and increased vascular permeability to proteins.[55] It also stimulates synthesis and release of proteases. It thus recapitulates all the components of angiogenesis, and there is increasing evidence that it is a central mediator of tumor angiogenesis, of blood vessel growth in normal development. VEGF may also be involved in chronic inflammation and wound healing. It is produced by tumor cells, macrophages, and several other cell types, including activated T cells.[184, 185] Its synthesis is markedly enhanced in the hypoxic conditions that are present in necrotic tumors or foci of inflammation.[186] Further, VEGF and bFGF act syner-

gistically in vitro to induce endothelial growth and capillary formation.[187] Both VEGF and FGF also act as survival factors for endothelium. Their withdrawal in culture causes apoptosis, as described earlier. Soluble E-selectin and VCAM-1 also cause angiogenesis,[188] and antibodies to E-selectin may inhibit tube formation in vitro.[189, 189a]

Acting to down-regulate new vessel growth are a group of endogenous inhibitors of endothelial cell proliferation or chemotaxis in vitro and of neovascularization in vivo. These include such cytokines as IFN-α and TGF-β. TGF-β inhibits endothelial cell proliferation in vitro but causes induced angiogenesis when injected in vivo. Platelet factor IV, tissue inhibitors of metalloproteinases (TIMPs), connective tissue adhesive proteins (e.g. thrombospondin-1) and tumor-derived factors, such as angiostatin, a 38-kD fragment of plasminogen, are other angiogenesis inhibitors. These endogenous negative influences may also be involved in regression of new blood vessels.

Extracellular matrix proteins and the organization of the extracellular matrix also play important roles in angiogenesis.[177, 178, 190] For example, secretion of type I collagen in bovine aortic endothelial cells in vitro is necessary for the formation of networks, possibly because of physical interactions among cells and matrix.[191, 192] Additionally, proteolysis of extracellular matrix through the release of proteases facilitates angiogenesis, whereas inhibition of endogenous metalloproteinases by TIMPs blocks angiogenesis.[193]

Finally, the various adhesive integrins are also involved in angiogenesis.[194–197] Antibodies against $\alpha_V\beta3$-integrin, for example, inhibit angiogenesis in the chick chorioallantoic membrane.[197] This integrin interacts with type I collagen, fibrinogen, and vitronectin and is expressed during angiogenesis. Inhibitors of $\alpha_V\beta3$-integrin not only inhibit angiogenesis but also cause regression of newly formed blood vessels by inducing apoptosis in such vessels.[19]

SUMMARY

Endothelial cells contribute to all phases of acute and chronic inflammation by undergoing specific alterations in structure and function and by elaborating adhesion molecules, cytokines, growth factors, and other mediators. Endothelial cells participate in the acute events of inflammation by producing vasodilatory mediators, including prostacyclin and nitric oxide-EDRF, and by the expression of cell surface adhesion molecules that mediate a series of selective leukocyte-endothelial adhesion and transmigration events. A number of stimuli, including cytokines, chemoattractants, and chemokines, cause activation of the leukocytes or endothelium or both. Rheologic factors, such as shear stress and the precise localization of molecules on leukocyte microvilli, also affect adhesion. Stimuli other than cytokines may also cause endothelial activation, including endotoxin, physical factors, advanced glycosylation end-products, certain lipids, and hypoxia. All of these stimuli induce gene expression of a number of molecules in endothelium, including adhesion molecules, cytokines, growth factors, MHC molecules, and coagulation proteins. The molecular mechanisms regulating activation are complex, but recent studies suggest that the NF-kB/IkB system of transcription factors may be one of the pathways that play a common regulatory role. Endothelial cells also contribute to lymphocyte trafficking, T cell activation, and the process of angiogenesis by a number of mechanisms.

Therapeutic interventions that interfere with the endothelium to dysregulate endothelial-leukocyte interactions and angiogenesis may suppress acute and chronic inflammation.

References

1. Pober JS, Cotran RS: Cytokines and endothelial cell biology. Physiol Rev 70:427, 1990.
2. Pober JS, Cotran RS: The role of endothelial cells in inflammation. Transplantation 50:537, 1990.
3. Briscoe DM, Cotran RS: Endothelial cells in immune inflammation. In Austen KF, Bruakoff SJ, Rosen FS, Strom TB (eds): Therapeutic Immunology. Cambridge, Mass, Blackwell Science, 1996, pp 12–20.
4. Briscoe DM, Cotran RS: Role of leukocyte-endothelial cell adhesion molecules in renal inflammation: In vitro and in vivo studies. Kidney Int 44(Suppl 42):S27, 1993.
5. Silverman ES, Gerritson ME, Collins T: Metabolic functions of the pulmonary endothelium. In Crystal RG, West JB, Weibel E, Barnes P (eds): The Lung: Scientific Foundations, 1996. In press.
6. Cotran RS, Majno G: A light and electron microscopic analysis of vascular injury. Ann N Y Acad Sci 116:750, 1964.
7. Weiss SJ: Tissue destruction by neutrophils. N Engl J Med 320:365, 1989.
8. Varani J, Dame MK, Taylor CG, et al: Age-dependent injury in human umbilical vein endothelial cells: Relationship to apoptosis and correlation with a lack of A20 expression. Lab Invest 73:851, 1995.
9. Buchman TG, Abello PA, Smith EH, Bukley GB: Induction of heat shock response leads to apoptosis in endothelial cells previously exposed to endotoxin. Am J Physiol 265:H165, 1993.
10. Robaye B, Mosselmans R, Fiers W, Dumont JE, Galand P: Tumor necrosis factor induces apoptosis (programmed cell death) in normal endothelial cells in vitro. Am J Pathol 138:447, 1991.
11. Araki S, Tsuna I, Kaji K, Hayashi H: Programmed cell death in response to alkyllysophospholipids in endothelial cells. J Biochem 115:245, 1994.
12. Araki S, Ishida T, Yamamoto T, Kaji K, Hayashi H: Induction of apoptosis by hemorrhagic snake venom in vascular endothelial cells. Biochem Biophys Res Commun 190:148, 1993.
13. Araki S, Shimada Y, Kaji K, Hayashi H: Apoptosis of vascular endothelial cells by fibroblast growth factor deprivation. Biochem Biophys Res Commun 169:1248, 1990.
14. Abello PA, Fidler SA, Bukley GB, Buchman TG: Antioxidants modulate induction of programmed endothelial cell death (apoptosis) by endotoxin. Arch Surg 129:134, 1994.
15. Opipari AW, Boguski MS, Dixit VM: The A20 cDNA induced by tumor necrosis factor alpa encodes a novel type of zinc finger protein. J Biol Chem 265:14705, 1990.
16. Opipari AW, Hu HM, Yabkowitz R, Dixit VM: The A20 zinc finger protein protects cells from tumor necrosis factor cytotoxicity. J Biol Chem 267:12424, 1992.
17. Re F, Zanetti A, Sironi M, et al: Inhibition of anchorage-dependent cell spreading triggers apoptosis in cultured human endothelial cells. J Cell Biol 127:537, 1994.
18. Ruoslahti E, Reed JC: Anchorage dependence, integrins, and apoptosis. Cell 77:477, 1994.
19. Brooks PC, Montgomery AMP, Rosenfeld M, et al: Integrin $\alpha_v\beta_3$ antagonists promote tumor regression by inducing apoptosis of angiogenic blood vessels. Cell 79:1157, 1994.
20. Alon T, Hemo I, Itin A, Pe'er J, Stone J, Keshet E: Vascular endothelial growth factor acts as a survival factor for newly formed retinal vessels and has implications for retinopathy of prematurity. Nature Med 1:1024, 1995.
21. Majno G, Shea SM, Leventhal M: Endothelial contraction induced by histamine-type mediators: An electron microscopic study. J Cell Biol 42:647, 1969.
22. Hattori R, Hamilton KK, Fugate RD, McEver RD, Sims PJ: Stimulated secretion of endothelial von Willebrand factor is accompanied by rapid redistribution to the cell surface of the intercellular granule membrane associated protein GMP-140. J Biol Chem 264:7768, 1989.
23. Johnston GI, Cook RG, McEver RP: Cloning of GMP-140, a granule membrane protein of platelets and endothelium: sequence similarity to proteins involved in cell adhesion and inflammation. Cell 56:1033, 1989.
24. Bevilacqua M, Pober JS, Mendrick DL, Cotran RS, Gimbrone MA Jr: Identification of an inducible endothelial-leukocyte adhesion molecule. Proc Natl Acad Sci USA 84:9238, 1987.
25. Bevilacqua MP, Stengelin S, Gimbrone MA Jr, Seed B: Endothelial leukocyte adhesion molecule 1: An inducible receptor for neutrophils related to complement regulatory proteins and lectins. Science 243:1160, 1989.
26. Pober JS, Gimbrone MA Jr, Cotran RS, et al: Ia expression by vascular endothelium is inducible by activated T cells and by human γ-interferon. J Exp Med 157:1339, 1983.
27. Gimbrone MA: Endothelial dysfunction and the pathogenesis of atherosclerosis. In Gotto AM Jr, Smith LC (eds): Atherosclerosis. New York, Springer-Verlag, 1980, pp 415–425.
28. Varani J, Bendelow MJ, Sealey DE: Tumor necrosis factor enhances susceptibility of vascular endothelial cells to neutrophil-mediated killing. Lab Invest 59:292, 1988.
29. Leibovich SJ, Polverini PJ, Shepard HM, Wiseman DM, Shively V, Nuseir N: Macrophage-induced angiogenesis is mediated by tumour necrosis factor-α. Nature 329:630, 1987.
30. Conger JD: Endothelial regulation of vascular tone. Hosp Pract 117–126, 1994.
31. Awolesi MA, Sessa WC, Sumpio BE: Cyclic strain upregulates nitric oxide synthase in cultured bovine aortic endothelial cells. J Clin Invest 96:1449, 1995.
32. Schmidt HW, Walker U: NO at work. Cell 78:919, 1994.
33. Moncada S, Higgs EA: Molecular mechanisms and therapeutic strategies related to nitric oxide. FASEB J 9:1319, 1995.
34. Hunley TE, Iwasaki S, Homma T, Kon V: Nitric oxide and endothelin in pathophysiological settings. Pediatr Nephrol 9:235, 1995.
35. Salvemini D, Manning PT, Zweifel BS, et al: Dual inhibition of nitric oxide and prostaglandin production contributes to the antiinflammatory properties of nitric oxide synthase inhibitors. J Clin Invest 96:301, 1995.
36. Liao JK, Zulueta JJ, Yu FS, Peng HB, Cote CG, Hassoun PM: Regulation of bovine endothelial constitutive nitric oxide synthase by oxygen. J Clin Invest 96:2661, 1995.
37. Ialenti A, Ianaro A, Moncada S, DiRosa M: Modulation of acute inflammation by endogenous nitric oxide. Eur J Pharmacol 211:177, 1992.
38. McCartney-Francis N, Allen JB, Mizel DE, et al: Suppression of arthritis by an inhibitor of nitric oxide synthase. J Exp Med 178:749, 1993.
39. Weinberg JB, Granger DL, Pisetsky DS, et al: The role of nitric oxide in the pathogenesis of spontaneous murine anutoimmune disease: Increased nitric oxide production and nitric oxide synthase expression in MRL-lpr/lpr mice, and reduction of spontaneous glomerulonephritis and arthritis by orally administered NG-monomethyl-L-arginine. J Exp Med 179:651, 1994.
40. Mulligan MS, Hevel JM, Marletta MA, Ward PA: Tissue injury caused by deposition of immune complexes is L-arginine dependent. Proc Natl Acad Sci USA 88:6338, 1991.
41. Majno G, Palade GE, Schoefl GI: Studies on inflammation. II. The site of action of histamine and seratonin along the vascular tree: A topographic study. J Biophys Biochem Cytol 11:607, 1961.
42. Cotran RS, Pober JS: Endothelial activation: Its role in inflammatory and immune reactions. In Simionescu N, Simionescu M (eds): Endothelial Cell Biology. Plenum Publishing, 1988, pp 335–347.
43. Joris I, Majno G, Corey EJ, Lewis RA: The mechanism of vascular leakage induced by leukotriene E4: Endothelial contraction. Am J Pathol 126:19, 1987.
44. Simionescu N, Heltianu C, Autohe F, Simionescu M: Endothelial cell receptors for histamine. Ann N Y Acad Sci 401:132, 1982.
45. Wysolmerski RB, Lagunoff D: Involvement of myosin light chain kinase in endothelial cell retraction. Proc Natl Acad Sci USA 87:16, 1990.
46. Stolpen AH, Guinen EC, Fiers W, Pober JS: Recombinant tumor necrosis factor and immune interferon act singly and in combination to reorganize human vascular endothelial cell monolayers. Am J Pathol 123:16, 1986.
47. Brett J, Gerlach H, Nawroth P, Steinberg S, Godman G, Stern D: Tumor necrosis factor/cachectin increases permeability of endothelial cell monolayers by a mechanism involving regulatory G proteins. J Exp Med 169:1977, 1989.
48. Bradley JR, Thiru S, Pober JS: Hydrogen peroxide-induced endothelial retraction is accompanied by a loss of the normal spatial organization of endothelial cell adhesion molecules. Am J Pathol 147:627, 1995.
49. Shreeniwas R, Ogawa S, Cozzolino F, et al: Macrovascular and microvascular endothelium during long-term exposure to hypoxia: alterations in cell growth, monolayer permeability, and cell surface anticoagulant properties. J Cell Physiol 146:8, 1991.

50. Schmidt AM, Hori O, Chen JX, et al: Advanced glycation endproducts interacting with their endothelial receptor induce expression of vascular cell adhesion molecule-1 (VCAM-1) in cultured human endothelial cells and in mice: A potential mechanism for the accelerated vasculopathy of diabetes. J Clin Invest 96:1395, 1995.

51. Varani J, Ginsburg I, Schuger L: Endothelial cell killing by neutrophils: Synergistic interaction of oxygen products and proteases. Am J Pathol 135:435, 1989.

52. Mulligan MS, Varani J, Dame MK, et al: Role of endothelial-leukocyte adhesion molecule-1 (ELAM-1) in neutrophil-mediated lung injury in rats. J Clin Invest 88:1396, 1991.

53. Johnson KJ, Ward PA: Role of oxygen metabolites in immune complex injury of the lung. J Immunol 126:2365, 1981.

54. Schoefl G: Studies on inflammation. III. Growing capillaries: Their structure and permeability. Virchows Arch A337:97, 1963.

55. Dvorak HF, Brown LF, Detmar M, Dvorak AM: Vascular permeability factor/vascular endothelial growth factor, microvascular hyperpermeability, and angiogenesis. Am J Pathol 146:1029, 1995.

55a. Dvorak AM, Kohn S, Morgan ES, Fox P, Nagy JA, Dvorak HF: The vesiculo-vacuolar organelle (VVO): A distinct endothelial cell structure that provides a transcellular pathway for macromolecular extravasation. J Leukocyte Biol 58:100, 1996.

56. Schnitzer JE: Update on the cellular and molecular basis of capillary permeability. Trends Cardiovasc Med 3:124, 1993.

57. Schnitzer JE, Oh P: Albondin-mediated capillary permeability to albumin: Differential role of receptors in endothelial transcytosis and endocytosis of native and modified albumins. J Biol Chem 269:6072, 1994.

58. Schnitzer JE, Allard J, Oh P: NEM inhibits transcytosis, endocytosis, and capillary permeability: Implication of caveolae fusion in endothelia. Am J Physiol 268:H48, 1995.

59. Springer TA: Traffic signals on endothelium for lymphocyte recirculation and leukocyte emigration. Annu Rev Physiol 57:827, 1995.

60. Imhof BA, Dunin D: Leukocyte migration and adhesion. Adv Immunol 58:345, 1995.

60a. Angel del Pozo M, Sánches-Mateos P, Sánches-Madrid F: Cellular polarization induced by chemokines: A mechanism for leukocyte recruitment. Immunol Today 17:127, 1996.

61. Carlos TM, Harlan JM: Leukocyte-endothelial adhesion molecules. Blood 84:2068, 1994.

62. Sako D, Comess KM, Barone KM, Camphausen RT, Cumming DA, Shaw GD: A sulfated peptide segment at the amino terminus of PSGL-1 is critical for P-selectin binding. Cell 83:323, 1995.

63. Patel KD, Prescott SM, McEver RP: Oxygen radicals induce human endothelial cells to express GMP-140 and bind neutrophils. J Cell Biol 112:749, 1991.

64. Pinsky DJ, Naka Y, Liao H, et al: Hypoxia-induced exocytosis of endothelial cell Weibel-Palade bodies: A mechanism for rapid neutrophil recruitment after cardiac preservation. J Clin Invest 97:493, 1996.

65. Marlin SD, Springer TA: Purified intercellular adhesion molecule-1 (ICAM-1) is a ligand for lymphocyte function-associated antigen 1 (LFA-1). Cell 51:813, 1987.

66. Sugama Y, Tiruppathi C, Janakidevi K, Anderson TT, Fenton JW II, Malik AB: Thrombin-induced expression of endothelial P-selectin and intercellular adhesion molecule-1: A mechanism for stabilizating neutrophil adhesion. J Cell Biol 119:935, 1992.

67. Bevilacqua M, Butcher E, Furie B, et al: Selectins: A family of adhesion receptors. Cell 67:233, 1991.

68. Osborn L, Hession C, Tizard R, et al: Direct expression cloning of vascular cell adhesion molecule-1, a cytokine-induced endothelial protein that binds to lymphocytes. Cell 59:1203, 1989.

69. Rice EG, Bevilacqua MP: An inducible cell surface glycoprotein mediates melanoma cell adhesion. Science 246:1303, 1989.

70. Shimizu Y, Shaw S, Graber N, et al: Activation-independent binding of human memory T cells to adhesion molecule ELAM-1. Nature 349:799, 1991.

71. Picker LJ, Kishimoto TK, Smith CW, Warnock RA, Butcher EC: ELAM-1 is an adhesion molecule for skin-homing T cells. Nature 349:796, 1991.

72. Walz G, Aruffo A, Kolanus W, Bevilacqua MP, Seed B: Recognition by ELAM-1 of the sialyl-Lex determinant on myeloid and tumor cells. Science 23:1132, 1990.

73. Steegmaler M, Levinovitz A, Isenmann S, et al: The E-selectin ligand ESL-1 is a variant of a receptor for fibroblast growth factor. Nature 373:615, 1995.

74. Asa D, Raycroft L, Ma L, et al: The P-selectin glycoprotein ligand function as a common human leukocyte ligand for P- and E-selectin. J Biol Chem 270:11662, 1995.

75. Pober JS, Gimbrone MA Jr, Lapierre LA, et al: Overlapping patterns of activation of human endothelial cells by interleukin-1, tumor necrosis factor, and immune interferon. J Immunol 137:1893, 1986.

76. Diamond MS, Staunton DE, de Fougerolles AR, et al: ICAM-1 (CD54): A counter-receptor for MAC-1 (CD11b/CD18). J Cell Biol 111:3129, 1990.

77. Rice EG, Munro JM, Bevilacqua MP: Inducible cell adhesion molecule-110 (INCAM-110) is an endothelial receptor for lymphocytes. J Exp Med 171:1369, 1990.

78. Doukas J, Pober JS: IFN-γ enhances endothelial activation induced by tumor necrosis factor but not IL-1. J Immunol 145:1727, 1990.

79. Thornhill MH, Haskard DO: IL-4 regulates endothelial cell activation by IL-1, tumor necrosis factor, or IFN-γ. J Immunol 145:865, 1990.

80. Briscoe DM, Cotran RS, Pober JS: Effects of tumor necrosis factor, lipopolysaccharide, and IL-4 on the expression of vascular cell adhesion molecule-1 in vivo: Correlation with CD3+ T cell infiltration. J Immunol 149:2954, 1992.

81. Ley K, Gaehtgens P, Fennie C, Singer MS, Lasky LA, Rosen SD: Lectin-like cell adhesion molecule 1 mediates leukocyte rolling in mesenteric venules in vivo. Blood 77:2553, 1991.

82. Ley K, Tedder TF: Leukocyte interactions with vascular endothelium: New insights into selectin-mediated attachment and rolling. J Immunol 155:525, 1995.

83. Lawrence MB, Springer TA: Leukocytes roll on a selectin at physiologic flow rates: Distinction from and prerequisite for adhesion through integrins. Cell 65:859, 1991.

84. Tozeren A, Ley K: How do selectins mediate leukocyte rolling in venules? Biophys J 63:700, 1992.

85. Patel KD, Moore KL, Nollert MU, McEver RP: Neutrophils use both shared and distinct mechanisms to adhere to selectins under static and flow conditions. J Clin Invest 96:1887, 1995.

86. Springer TA: Traffic signals for lymphocyte recirculation and leukocyte emigration: The multistep paradigm. Cell 76:1, 1994.

87. Lorant DE, McEver RP, McIntyre TM, Moore KL, Prescott SM, Zimmerman GA: Activation of polymorphonuclear leukocytes reduces their adhesion to P-selectin and causes redistribution of ligands for P-selectin on their surfaces. J Clin Invest 96:171, 1995.

88. Smith CW, Rothlein R, Hughes BJ, et al: Recognition of an endothelial determinant of CD18-dependent human neutrophil adherence and transendothelial migration. J Clin Invest 82:1746, 1988.

89. Oppenheimer-Marks N, Davis LS, Bogue DT, Ramberg J, Lipsky PE: Differential utilization of ICAM-1 and VCAM-1 during the adhesion and transendothelial migration of human T cells. J Immunol 147:2913, 1991.

90. Kurt-Jones EA, Fiers W, Pober JS: Membrane IL-1 induction on human endothelial cells and dermal fibroblasts. J Immunol 139:2317, 1987.

91. Matsushima K, Oppenheim JJ: Interleukin 8 and MCAF: Novel inflammatory cytokines inducible by IL 1 and TNF. Cytokine 1:2, 1989.

92. Kaplanski G, Teysseire N, Farnarier C, et al: IL-6 and IL-8 production from cultured human endothelial cells stimulated by infection with Rickettsia conorii via a cell-associated IL-1a–dependent pathway. J Clin Invest 96:2839, 1995.

93. Rollins BJ, Yoshimura T, Leonard EJ, Pober JS: Cytokine-activated human endothelial cells synthesize a monocyte chemoattractant, MCP-1/JE. Am J Pathol 136:1229, 1990.

94. von Andrian UH, Hassien SR, Nelson RD, Erlandsen SL, Butcher EC: A central role for microvillous receptor presentation in leukocyte adhesion under flow. Cell 82:989, 1995.

95. De Caterina R, Libby P, Peng HB, et al: Nitric oxide decreases cytokine-induced endothelial activation: Nitric oxide selectively reduces endothelial expression of adhesion molecules and proinflammatory cytokines. J Clin Invest 96:60, 1995.

96. Gamble JR, Vadas MA: Endothelial cell adhesiveness for human T lymphocytes is inhibited by transforming growth factor-β 1. J Immunol 146:1149, 1991.

97. Gamble JR, Khew-Goodall Y, Vadas MA: Transforming growth factor-β inhibits E-selectin expression on human endothelial cells. J Immunol 150:4494, 1993.

98. Brady HR, Serhan CN: Adhesion promotes transcellular leukotriene biosynthesis during neutrophil-glomerular endothelial cell interactions: Inhibition by antibodies against CD18 and L-selectin. Biochem Biophys Res Comm 186:1307, 1992.

99. Butcher EC: Leukocyte-endothelial cell recognition: Three (or more) steps to specificity and diversity. Cell 67:1033, 1991.

100. Olofsson M, Arfors KE, Ramezani L, Wolitzky BA, Butcher EC, von Andrian U: E-selectin mediates leukocyte rolling in interleukin-1-treated rabbit mesentery venules. Blood 84:2749, 1994.

101. Muller WA, Weigl SA, Deng X, Phillips DM: PECAM-1 is required for transendothelial migration of leukocytes. J Exp Med 178:449, 1993.

102. Anderson DC, Springer TA: Leukocyte adhesion deficiency: An inherited defect in the Mac1, LFA-1 and p150.95 glycoproteins. Annu Rev Med 38:175, 1987.

103. Anderson DC, Schmalsteig FC, Feingold MJ, et al: The severe and moderate phenotypes of heritable Mac-1, LFA-1 deficiency: Their quantitative definition and relation to leukocyte dysfunction and clinical features. J Infect Dis 152:668, 1985.

104. Etzioni A, Frydman M, Pollack S, Avidor I, Phillips ML, Gershoni-Baruch R: Recurrent severe infections caused by a novel leukocyte adhesion deficiency. N Engl J Med 327:1789, 1992.

105. Price TH, Ochs HD, Gershoni-Baruch R, Harlan JM, Etzioni A: In vivo neutrophil and lymphocyte function studies in a patient with leukocyte adhesion deficiency type II. Blood 84:1635, 1994.

106. Cotran RS, Gimbrone MA Jr, Bevilacqua MP, Mendrick DL, Pober JS: Induction and detection of a human endothelial activation antigen in vivo. J Exp Med 164:661, 1986.

107. Leung DC, Pober JS, Cotran RS: Expression of endothelial-leukocyte adhesion molecule-1 in elicited late phase reactions. J Clin Invest 87:1805, 1991.

108. Redl H, Dinges HP, Buurman WA, et al: Expression of endothelial leukocyte adhesion molecule-1 in septic but not traumatic/hypovolemic shock in the baboon. Am J Pathol 139:461, 1991.

109. Briscoe DM, Yeung AC, Schoen FJ, et al: Predictive value of inducible endothelial cell adhesion molecule expression for acute rejection of human cardiac allografts. Transplantation 59:204, 1995.

110. Cybulsky MI, Gimbrone MA Jr: Endothelial expression of a mononuclear leukocyte adhesion molecule during atherogenesis. Science 251:788, 1991.

111. Li H, Cybulsky MI, Gimbrone MA Jr, Libby P: An atherogenic diet rapidly induces VCAM-1, a cytokine-regulatable mononuclear leukocyte adhesion molecule, in rabbit aortic endothelium. Arterioscler Thromb 13:197, 1993.

112. van Dinther-Janssen AC, Horst E, Koopman G, Newmann W, Meijer CJ, Pals ST: The VLA-4/VCAM-1 pathway is involved in lymphocyte adhesion to endothelium in rheumatoid synovium. J Immunol 147:4207, 1991.

113. Iigo Y, Takashi T, Tamatani T, et al: ICAM-1–dependent pathway is critically involved in the pathogenesis of adjuvant arthritis in rats. J Immunol 147:4167, 1991.

114. Gerritson ME, Carley WW, Ranges GE, et al: Flavinoids inhibit cytokine-induced endothelial cell adhesion protein gene expression. Am J Pathol 147:278, 1995.

115. Pober JS, Cotran RS: What can be learned from the expression of endothelial adhesion molecules in tissues? Lab Invest 64:301, 1991.

116. Munro JM, Pober JS, Cotran RS: Tumor necrosis factor and interferon-γ induce distinct patterns of endothelial activation and associated leukocyte accumulation in skin of Papio anubis. Am J Pathol 135:121, 1989.

117. Kawasaki K, Yaoita E, Yamamoto T, Tamatani T, Miyasaka M, Kihara I: Antibodies against intercellular adhesion molecule-1 and lymphocyte function-associated antigen-1 prevent glomerular injury in rat experimental crescentic glomerulonephritis. J Immunol 150:1074, 1993.

118. Mayadas TN, Johnson RC, Rayburn H, Hynes RO, Wagner DD: Leukocyte rolling and extravasation are severely compromised in P-selectin-deficient mice. Cell 74:541, 1993.

119. Arbones ML, Ord DC, Ley K, et al: Lymphocyte homing and leukocyte rolling and migration are impaired in L-selectin–deficient mice. Immunity 1:247, 1994.

120. Labow MA, Norton CR, Rumberger JM, et al: Characterization of E-selectin–deficient mice: Demonstration of overlapping function of the endothelial selectins. Immunity 1:709, 1994.

121. Frenett PS, Mayadas TN, Rayburn H, Hynes RO, Wagner DD: Leukocyte adhesion defects, altered hematopoiesis and susceptibility to infection in P- and E-selectin–deficient mice. Cell 84:563–574, 1996.

122. Xu H, Gonzalo JA, St Pierre Y, et al: Leukocytosis and resistance to septic shock in intercellular adhesion molecule 1–deficient mice. J Exp Med 180:95, 1994.

123. Mantovani A, Bussolino F, DeJana E: Cytokine regulation of endothelial cell function. FASEB J 6:2591, 1992.

124. Shuster DE, Kehrli ME, Ackermann MR: Neutrophilia in mice that lack the murine IL-8 receptor homolog. Science 269:1590, 1995.

125. Simonet WS, Hughes TM, Nguyen HQ, Trebasky LD, Danilenko DM, Medlock ES: Long-term impaired neutrophil migration in mice overexpressing human interleukin-8. J Clin Invest 94:1310, 1994.

126. Hechtman DH, Cybulsky MI, Fuchs HJ, Baker JB, Gimbrone MA Jr: Intravascular IL-8: Inhibitor of polymorphonuclear leukocyte accumulation at sites of acute inflammation. J Immunol 147:883, 1991.

127. Korembanas S, Marsden PA, McQuillan LP, Faller DV: Hypoxia induces endothelin ene expression and secretion in cultured human endothelium. J Clin Invest 88:1054, 1991.

128. Kuwabara K, Ogawa S, Matsumoto M, et al: Hypoxia-mediated induction of acidic/basic FGF and PDGF in mononuclear phagocytes stimulates growth of hypoxic endothelial cells. Proc Natl Acad Sci USA 92:4606, 1995.

129. Shreeniwas R, Koga S, Karakurum M, et al: Hypoxia mediated induction of endothelial cell interleukin 1α: An autocrine mechanism promoting expression of leukocyte adhesion molecules on the vessel surface. J Clin Invest 90:2333, 1992.

130. Yan SF, Tritto I, Pinsky DJ, et al: Induction of interleukin 6 (IL-6) by hypoxia in vascular cells: Central role of the binding site for nuclear factor IL-6. J Biol Chem 370:11463, 1995.

131. Karakurum M, Shreeniwas R, Chen J, et al: Hypoxic induction of interleukin-8 gene expression in human endothelial cells. J Clin Invest 93:1564, 1994.

132. Arnould T, Michiels C, Remacle J: Increased PMN adherence on endothelial cells after hypoxia: Involvement PAF, CD18/CD11b, and ICAM-1. Am J Physiol 264:C1102, 1993.

133. Collins T, Read MA, Neish AS, Whitley MZ, Thanos D, Maniatis T: Transcriptional regulation of endothelial cell adhesion molecules: NF-KB and cytokine-inducible enhancers. FASEB J 9:899, 1995.

134. Collins T, Palmer HJ, Whitley MZ, Neish AS: A common theme in endothelial activation: Insights from the structural analysis of the genes for E-selectin and VCAM-1. Trends Cardiovasc Med 3:16, 1993.

135. Collins T: Biology of disease: Endothelial nuclear factor-KB and the initiation of the atherosclerotic lesion. Lab Invest 68:499, 1993.

136. Read MA, Whitley MZ, Williams AJ, Collins T: NF-KB and IKBa: An inducible regulatory system in endothelial activation. J Exp Med 179:503, 1994.

137. Read MA, Neish AS, Luscinskas FW, Palombella VJ, Maniatis T, Collins T: The proteasome pathway is required for cytokine-induced endothelial-leukocyte adhesion molecule expression. Immunity 2:493, 1995.

138. Shimizu Y, Newman W, Tanaka Y, Shaw S: Lymphocyte interactions with endothelial cells. Immunol Today 13:106, 1992.

139. Mackay CR, Imhof BA: Cell adhesion in the immune system. Immunol Today 14:99, 1993.

140. Butcher EC: Cellular and molecular mechanisms that direct leukocyte trafficking. Am J Pathol 136:3, 1990.

141. Stoolman LM: Adhesion molecules controlling lymphocyte migration. Cell 56:907, 1989.

142. Mackay CR, Marston WL, Dudler L: Naive and memory T cells show distinct pathways of lymphocyte recirculation. J Exp Med 171:801, 1990.

143. Gallatin WM, Weissman IL, Butcher EC: A cell surface molecule involved in organ-specific homing of lymphocytes. Nature 303:30, 1983.

144. Lasky LA, Singer MS, Dowbenko D, et al: An endothelial ligand for L-selectin is a novel mucin-like molecule. Cell 69:927, 1992.

145. Streeter PR, Rouse BT, Butcher EC: Immunohistologic and functional characterization of a vascular addressin involved in lymphocyte homing into peripheral lymph nodes. J Cell Biol 107:1853, 1988.

146. Imai Y, Lasky LA, Rosen SD: Sulphation requirement for GlyCAM-1, an endothelial ligand for L-selectin. Nature 361:555, 1993.

147. Hoke D, Mebius RE, Dybdal N, et al: Selective modulation of the expression of L-selectin ligands by an immune response. Curr Biol 5:670, 1995.

148. Baumhueter S, Singer MS, Henzel W, et al: Binding of L-selectin to the vascular sialomucin, CD34. Science 262:436, 1993.

149. Berg EL, McEvoy LM, Berlin C, Bargatze RF, Butcher EC: L-selectin–mediated lymphocyte rolling on MAdCAM-1. Nature 366:695, 1993.

150. Hamann A, Andrew DP, Jablonski-Westrich D, Holzmann B, Butcher EC: Role of alpha 4-integrins in lymphocyte homing to mucosal tissues in vivo. J Immunol 152:3282, 1994.

151. Springer TA, Dustin ML, Kishimoto TK, Marlin SD: The lymphocyte function associated LFA-1, CD2, and LFA-3 molecules: Cell adhesion receptors of the immune system. Annu Rev Immunol 5:223, 1987.

152. Airas L, Salmi M, Jalkanen S: Lymphocyte-vascular adhesion protein-2 is a novel 70-kDa molecule involved in lymphocyte adhesion to vascular endothelium. J Immunol 151:4228, 1993.

153. Bargatze RF, Butcher EC: Rapid G protein regulated activation event involved in lymphocyte binding to high endothelial venules. J Exp Med 178:367, 1993.

154. Salmi M, Jalkanen S: A 90-kilodalton endothelial cell molecule mediating lymphocyte binding in humans. Science 257:1407, 1992.

155. Luscinskas FW, Ding H, Lichtman AH: P-selectin and vascular cell adhesion molecule-1 mediate rolling and arrest, respectively, of CD4 + T lymphocytes on tumor necrosis factor α–activated vascular endothelium under flow. J Exp Med 181:1179, 1995.

156. Lichtman AH, Ding H, DesRoches LE, Luscinskas FW: E- and P-selectins mediate preferential rolling of CD4+ memory cells compared to naive T cells. FASEB J 9:A34, 1995.

157. Hollenbaugh D, Mischel-Petty N, Edwards CP, et al: Expression of functional CD40 by vascular endothelial cells. J Exp Med 182:33, 1995.

158. Karmann K, Hughes CCW, Schechner J, Fanslow WC, Pober JS: CD40 on human endothelial cells: Inducibility by cytokines and functional regulation of adhesion molecule expression. Proc Natl Acad Sci USA 92:4342, 1995.

159. Abbas AK, Williams ME, Burstein HJ, Chang T, Bossu P, Lichtman AH: Activation and functions of CD4+ T cell subsets. Immunol Rev 123:5, 1991.

160. Paul WE, Seder RA: Lymphocyte responses and cytokines. Cell 76:241, 1994.

161. Germain RN: MHC-dependent antigen processing and peptide presentation: Providing ligands for T lymphocyte activation. Cell 76:287, 1994.

162. Janeway CA Jr, Bottomly K: Signals and signs for lymphocyte responses. Cell 76:275, 1994.

163. Jenkins MK: The ups and downs of T cell costimulation. Immunity 1:443, 1994.

164. Schwartz RH: Costimulation of T lymphocytes: The role of CD28, CTLA-4, and B7/BB1 in interleukin-2 production and immunotherapy. Cell 71:1065, 1992.

165. Damle NK, Klussman K, Linsley PS, Aruffo A: Differential costimulatory effects of adhesion molecules B7, ICAM-1, LFA-3, and VCAM-1 on

resting and antigen-primed CD4⁺ T lymphocytes. J Immunol 148:1985, 1992.

166. Murray AG, Khodadoust MM, Pober JS, Bothwell AL: Porcine aortic endothelial cells activate human T cells: Direct presentation of MHC antigens and costimulation by ligands for human CD2 and CD28. Immunity 1:57, 1994.

167. Briscoe DM, DesRoches LE, Kiely JM, Lederer JA, Lichtman AH: Antigen-dependent activation of T helper cell subsets by endothelium. Transplantation 59:1638, 1995.

168. Pober JS, Doukas J, Hughes CCW, Savage COS, Munro JM, Cotran RS: The potential roles of vascular endothelium in immune reactions. Human Immunol 28:258, 1990.

169. Sobel RA, Blanchette BW, Bhan AK, Colvin RB: The immunopathology of experimental allergic encephalomyelitis. II. Endothelial cell Ia increases prior to inflammatory cell infiltration. J Immunol 132:2402, 1984.

170. Libby P, Hansson GK: Involvement of the immune system in human atherogenesis: Current knowledge and unanswered questions. Lab Invest 64:5, 1991.

171. Leeuwenberg JF, von Asmuth EJ, Jeunhomme TM, Buurman WA: IFN-γ regulates the expression of the adhesion molecules ELAM-1 and IL-6 production by human endothelial cells in vitro. J Immunol 145:2110, 1990.

172. Folkman J: Tumor angiogenesis. In Mendelsohn J, Howley PM, Israel MA, Liotta LA (eds): The Molecular Basis of Cancer. Philadelphia, WB Saunders, 1995, pp 206–232.

173. Folkman J: Clinical applications of research on angiogenesis. N Engl J Med 333:1757, 1995.

174. Nguyen M, Watanabe H, Budson AE, Richie JP, Hayes DF, Folkman J: Elevated levels of an angiogenic peptide, basic fibroblast growth factor, in the urine of patients with a wide spectrum of cancers. J Natl Cancer Inst 86:356, 1994.

175. Peacock DJ, Banquerigo ML, Brahn E: Angiogenesis inhibition suppresses collagen arthritis. J Exp Med 175:1135, 1992.

176. Paulus HE: Minocycline treatment of rheumatoid arthritis. Ann Intern Med 122:147, 1995.

177. Vernon RB, Sage EH: Between molecules and morphology: Extracellular matrix and creation of vascular form. Am J Pathol 147:873, 1995.

178. Ingber DE, Folkman J: Mechanochemical switching between growth and differentiation during fibroblast growth factor-stimulated angiogenesis in vitro: Role of extracellular matrix. J Cell Biol 109:317, 1989.

179. Zagzag D: Angiogenic growth factors in neural embryogenesis and neoplasia. Am J Pathol 146:293, 1995.

180. Folkman J, Klagsburn M: Angiogenic factors. Science 235:442, 1987.

181. Potgens AJG, Westphal HR, de Waal RMW, Ruiter DJ: The role of vascular permeability factor and basic fibroblast growth factor in tumor angiogenesis. Biol Chem Hoppe-Seyler 376:57, 1995.

182. Montesano R, Vassalli JD, Baird A, Gullemin R, Orci L: Basic fibroblast growth factor induces angiogenesis in vitro. Proc Natl Acad Sci USA 83:7297, 1986.

183. Folkman J: Angiogenesis in cancer, vascular, rheumatoid, and other disease. Natl Med 1:27, 1995.

184. Freeman MR, Schneck FX, Gagnon ML, et al: Peripheral blood T lymphocytes and lymphocytes infiltrating human cancers express vascular endothelial growth factor: A potential role for T cells in angiogenesis. Cancer Res 55:4140, 1995.

185. Peoples GE, Blotnick S, Takahashi K, Freeman MR, Klagsbrun M, Eberlein TJ: T lymphocytes that infiltrate tumors and atherosclerotic plaques produce heparin-binding epidermal growth factor–like growth factor and basic fibroblast growth factor: A potential pathologic role. Proc Natl Acad Sci USA 92:6547, 1995.

186. Mukhopadhyay D, Tsiokas L, Zhou XM, Foster D, Brugge JS, Sukhatme VP: Hypoxic induction of human vascular endothelial growth factor expression through c-Src activation. Nature 375:577, 1995.

187. Pepper MS, Ferrara N, Orci L, Montesano R: Potent synergism between vascular endothelial growth factor and basic fibroblast growth factor in the induction of angiogenesis in vitro. Biochem Biophys Res Commun 189:824, 1992.

188. Koch AE, Halloran MM, Haskell CJ, Shah MR, Polverini PJ: Angiogenesis mediated by soluble forms of E-selectin and vascular cell adhesion molecule-1. Nature 376:517, 1995.

189. Nguyen M, Strubel NA, Bischoff J: A role for sialyl Lewis-X/A glycoconjugates in capillary morphogenesis. Nature 365:267, 1993.

189a. Polverini PJ: Cellular adhesion molecules: Newly identified mediators of angiogenesis. Am J Pathol 148:1023, 1996.

190. Ingber DE, Dike L, Hansen L, et al: Cellular tensegrity: Exploring how mechanical changes in the cytoskeleton regulate cell growth, migration, and tissue pattern during morphogenesis. Int Rev Cytol 150:173, 1994.

191. Vernon RB, Lara SL, Drake CJ, et al: Organized type I collagen influences endothelial patterns during "spontaneous angiogenesis in vitro": Planar cultures as models of vascular development. In Vitro Cell Dev Biol Animal 31:120, 1995.

192. Jackson CJ, Jenkins KL: Type I collagen fibrils promote rapid vascular tube formation upon contact with the apical side of cultured endothelium. Exp Cell Res 192:319, 1991.

193. Fisher C, Gilbertson-Beadling S, Powers EA, Petzold G, Poorman R, Mitchel MA: Interstitial collagenase is required for angiogenesis in vitro. Dev Biol 162:499, 1994.

194. Gamble JR, Matthias LJ, Meyer G, et al: Regulation of in vitro capillary tube formation by anti-integrin antibodies. J Cell Biol 121:931, 1993.

195. Vernon RB, Angello JC, Iruela-arispe ML, Lane TF, Sage EH: Reorganization of basement membrane matrices by cellular traction promotes the formation of cellular networks in vitro. Lab Invest 66:536, 1992.

196. Klein S, Giancotti FG, Presta M, Albelda ST, Buck CA, Rifkin DB: Basic fibroblast growth factor modulates integrin expression in microvascular endothelial cells. Mol Biol Cell 4:973, 1993.

197. Brooks PC, Clark RAF, Cheresh DA: Requirement of vascular integrin αᵥβ3 for angiogenesis. Science 264:569, 1994.

CHAPTER 13

Joseph H. Korn

Fibroblast Function and Fibrosis

The fibroblast plays a critical role in tissue repair, i.e., in laying down collagen and other matrix proteins in response to injury. This reparative function may be a response to physical injury (e.g., a surgical incision) or to tissue destruction from other causes. In each instance, the fibroblast responds to sets of signals from its microenvironment (Fig. 13–1). These signals include mediators, cytokines and growth factors, released by immune and inflammatory cells, platelets, endothelial cells, and smooth muscle cells as well as signals from the noncellular environment. The noncellular environment includes plasma and serum factors, oxygen tension, pH, and matrix proteins.

Cytokines were originally described as products of immune cells that affected metabolism or activation of other immune cells. It soon became clear that some cytokines affected nonimmune cells as well, in particular fibroblasts and hematopoietic cell precursors; in some cases, these were identical to cytokines previously identified for their effects on immune cells. Growth factors were identified by their effects on proliferation of mesenchymal and epithelial cells. These factors also affect cell activities other than proliferation and may be products of both immune cells and other cells. The distinction between growth factors and cytokines is thus historical and artificial.

Excessive stimulation of the fibroblast may lead to persistent activation, with resulting fibrosis.[1, 2] This can result from increased matrix, especially collagen, deposition with or without an increase in fibroblast numbers. The process of repair also involves tissue remodeling that necessitates degradation of matrix proteins. Fibroblasts release a variety of enzymes that can degrade collagen, proteoglycans, and other matrix components. In some instances, such as in rheumatoid synovitis, net matrix destruction, rather than fibrosis, may result; the fibrosis is due to activation of synovial fibroblasts with release of matrix-degrading enzymes (Fig. 13–2).

Several areas of fibroblast biology have received increasing attention in recent years and have significant bearing on the processes of inflammation and repair. A large repertoire of cytokines have been defined that influence fibroblast function.[3–5] The delineation of these and their mechanisms of action has shed considerable light on the fibrotic process. It has also become clear that the fibroblast is a cell involved in inflammation by actions other than synthesis and degradation of matrix. The original concept was that the fibroblast was only a responder to environmental signals that governed its level of metabolic activity. However, the fibroblast is capable of interacting with the immune system, hematopoietic cell precursors, and other cell types in more complex and interdependent ways (Fig. 13–3). This capability can occur through release from the fibroblast of soluble mediators, including cytokines thought originally to derive only from immune cells (and originally called *lymphokines*), or through direct cell-cell interactions mediated by adhesion ligands. These interactions can result in profound alterations of immune cell localization and function that, in turn, may alter fibroblast metabolism.

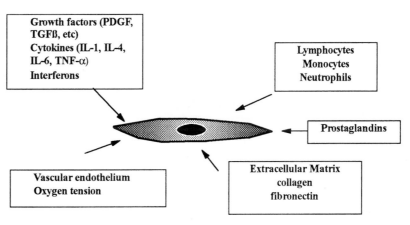

Figure 13–1. Features of the microenvironment that influence fibroblast growth and metabolism. Cells, matrix, nutritive factors, and spatial orientation provide signals that regulate fibroblast activity. Theses factors may individually or in combination relay signals through intracellular messengers and initiating or inhibiting gene transcription. PDGF, platelet-derived growth factor; TGF, transforming growth factor; IL, interleukin; TNF, tumor necrosis factor.

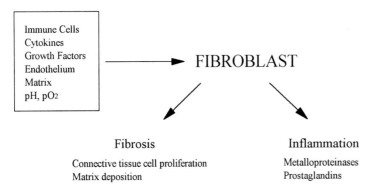

Immune Cells
Cytokines
Growth Factors
Endothelium
Matrix
pH, pO2

→ FIBROBLAST

Fibrosis

Connective tissue cell proliferation
Matrix deposition

Inflammation

Metalloproteinases
Prostaglandins

Figure 13–2. Alternative pathways of fibroblast activation. The mix of signals to which the fibroblast is exposed and the type of responding fibroblast determine whether responses are primarily fibrotic/reparative or degradative/inflammatory in nature. Both types of processes coexist in most situations, and inflammation followed by repair is a common and "normal" sequence.

Another area in which the view of fibroblast biology has expanded is in the appreciation of differences among and within fibroblast populations. Fibroblasts are mesenchyme-derived cells that have a widespread tissue distribution. Morphologically, fibroblasts from a variety of sites can be quite similar; indeed, fibroblasts have been "identified" by their spindle-shaped morphology in culture. In special instances, subtypes of fibroblasts have been identified either by histology or electron microscopy, such as myofibroblasts and type A and type B synovial cells. It is clear, however, that differences exist among fibroblasts from the skin, lung, synovium, periosteum, gingiva, cornea, bone marrow, and interstitium of various organs. Furthermore, it is evident that even among fibroblasts derived from a single site, there are substantial differences in proliferation and in biosynthetic activity.[6]

This chapter reviews the manifold aspects of fibroblast metabolism, including the role of cytokines in regulating fibroblast function, the synthesis of cytokines by fibroblasts, the adhesive interactions important in localization of immune cells to connective tissue, and the alterations of fibroblast functions in disease states. Finally, differences among fibroblasts from various tissues, fibroblast heterogeneity within a given tissue, and ways in which alterations in heterogeneity might play a role in disease are presented.

FIBROBLAST RESPONSE TO INJURY

In the unperturbed state, fibroblasts in vivo are relatively quiescent with little cell turnover and low levels of matrix synthesis. In response to injury, an increase in fibroblast number and in metabolic activity occurs. Fibroblasts synthesize collagens, fibronectin, proteoglycans, elastin, and a variety of glycoproteins. In addition to types I and III collagen (the predominant types synthesized by skin and interstitial fibroblasts), several other collagens that are important in collagen fibril organization are synthesized by fibroblasts; these include types V, VI, and VII (see Chapter 2).

In the most straightforward type of injury, a surgical wound either of the skin or another site, it is clear that platelet-derived growth factor (PDGF) plays an important role in the reparative response.[7] With the vascular damage associated with the surgical wound, a platelet plug forms and PDGF is released from platelet α-granules. PDGF is also released by other cell types, including endothelial cells, smooth muscle cells, macrophages, renal mesangial cells, and Langerhans cells. PDGF thus can play a role in fibroproliferative events not only following mechanical injury to the skin but also following damage at other sites.

PDGF may exist as either a homodimer or a heterodimer of PDGF-A and PDGF-B chains.[8] Some cells release one isoform of PDGF preferentially; others, such as platelets, release both isoforms. The PDGF receptor also functions optimally as a dimer, constituted as either a homodimer or heterodimer of α- and β-chains, with different cells having different receptor forms.[9] The BB PDGF isoform binds to all possible receptor dimers (αα, αβ, and ββ) with high affinity;

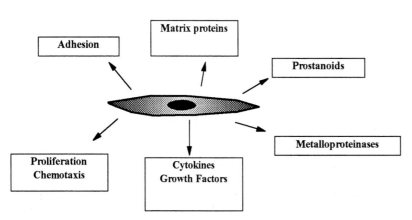

Adhesion

Matrix proteins

Prostanoids

Metalloproteinases

Proliferation
Chemotaxis

Cytokines
Growth Factors

Figure 13–3. Fibroblast products that alter the microenvironment. Fibroblast responses to signals in the microenvironment include not only proliferation but also expression of new surface proteins, matrix proteins, matrix degrading enzymes, and soluble molecules that can influence the metabolic activity of other cells.

PDGF-AA binds with high affinity only to the αα-receptor.[10] The binding of PDGF to specific fibroblast cell surface αα-receptors is followed by receptor activation, autophosphorylation, and initiation of fibroblast proliferation.[11]

In addition to increased fibroblast proliferation, there may be directed migration of fibroblasts from adjacent sites. Migration occurs in response to chemotactic stimuli, including PDGF and transforming growth factor-β (TGF-β) from platelets, thrombin, and peptides of collagen, fibronectin, and elastin, which may be released in the course of injury.[12–17] In addition, the accompanying vascular injury and endothelial cell perturbation can lead to release of TGF-β and PDGF from endothelial cells.[18, 19] The accumulated fibroblasts are activated by these and other stimuli to initiate local fibrosis. TGF-β and PDGF stimulate increased synthesis of matrix proteins, which form the scar tissue of the wound.[20] Interleukin-1 (IL-1) and tumor necrosis factor-α (TNF-α) may be released by both activated endothelial cells and Langerhans cells in the skin.[21–23] IL-1 and TNF-α stimulate fibroblast proliferation, and IL-1 stimulates fibroblast collagen synthesis.[24–26] IL-1 and TNF-α also can stimulate the release of additional regulatory cytokines from other cells, including fibroblasts (see later). Endothelial cells also release endothelin, known primarily for its vasoconstrictive properties and also as a stimulus for fibroblast chemotaxis, proliferation, and collagen synthesis.[27–29] Thus, "simple" mechanical injury initiates a sequence of events that rapidly lead to fibroblast recruitment and activation.

The fibroblast reparative response following or accompanying inflammation, in the pulmonary fibrosis of scleroderma, for example, obviously depends much more on immune cells than on platelet activation. Immune cell cytokines modulate proliferation, connective tissue biosynthesis, and other functions of fibroblasts. The role of these cytokines is discussed more fully below. Less well appreciated is the critical role of the immune system in normal wound healing. Surgical wounds of animals depleted of monocytes do not heal normally, presumably as a result of absence of monocyte factors that stimulate proliferation, chemotaxis, and matrix biosynthesis of fibroblasts.[30] Immune cells thus provide important activation signals to the fibroblast in settings that are not obviously inflammatory.

Cell Signaling

The availability of purified or recombinant cytokines and growth factors has allowed the precise definition of action of some of the signals regulating fibroblast metabolism.[31] Growth factors act both independently and, more often, in synergy with or by stimulating other growth factors. In the body, of course, cells are not exposed to single growth factors. Interactions among the many growth factors and between growth factors and other features of the fibroblast milieu play an important role in determining the ultimate fibroblast response. Some growth factors, such as PDGF and basic fibroblast growth factor (bFGF), stimulate quiescent cells to enter the cell cycle.[32, 33] At that point, other factors, termed *progression factors*, are needed for completion of cell replication. Some factors may act as both competence and progression factors, either by their direct effects or by induction of synthesis of competence and progression factors (Table 13–1).

Growth factors and cytokines activate intracellular signaling pathways, which affect a variety of metabolic processes. These "second messengers" include cyclic nucleotides (cyclic adenosine monophosphate [cAMP]), changes in intracellular Ca^{2+} concentration, and G-proteins. Receptor-associated and other kinases can phosphorylate and activate inositol phosphates, important second messengers that regulate intracellular calcium[34] and affect fibroblast proliferation.[35–37] The mitogenic effect of several fibroblast growth factors, including PDGF, IL-1, endothelin, and TGF-β, is dependent on stimulation of inositol phosphate turnover.[35–38] Activation of phospholipase (e.g., by IL-1) and generation of arachidonic acid metabolites, including PGE_2, lead to cAMP generation with suppression of cellular proliferation.[39–41]

In addition to generation of second messengers, cytokines and growth factors directly activate transcription of a series of genes. The products of these genes include transcription factors (i.e., proteins that then activate transcription of other genes), factors that regulate cell cycle, factors that regulate or are involved in metabolic pathways, and end-products, such as matrix macromolecules and fibroblast-derived cytokines (Table 13–2).[31] Thus, the initial stimulation of a fibroblast by a single stimulus, such as PDGF or IL-1 or another cytokine, leads to receptor activation, initiation of signaling through intracellular messen-

Table 13–1. FUNCTIONAL CLASSIFICATION OF CYTOKINES THAT AFFECT CELLULAR PROLIFERATION

Competence Factors	Progression Factors	Unclassified
Platelet-derived growth factor	Insulin-like growth factor-1	Interleukin-1
Fibroblast growth factor	Insulin	Tumor necrosis factor
α-Thrombin	Epidermal growth factor	Transforming growth factor-β
Bombesin		

Adapted with permission from Goldring MB, Goldring SR: Cytokines and cell growth control. Crit Rev Eukaryotic Gene Expression 1:302, 1991. Copyright CRC Press, Boca Raton, Florida.

Table 13–2. GENES INVOLVED IN REGULATION OF FIBROBLAST PROLIFERATION

Immediate Early (Transiently 15–120 min)	Progression (1–2 hr)	Intermediate (2–8 hr)	Late Response (2–8 hr, Stable mRNA Expression)
c-*fos*	Thymidine kinase	JE	Metalloproteinases
c-*jun*	Dihydrofolate reductase	KC	Plasminogen activator
Jun B	Thymidylate kinase	gro	Proteinase inhibitors
c-*myc*	Histones	IL-8	Fibronectin
Egr-1/Zif-268/Krox-24/NGF1-B	Maturation proliferation factor	IL-6	Collagens I and III
Egr-2/Krox-20	MAP kinase	M-CSF	Actin
ets-1/PEA3	Focal adhesion kinase (FAK)	Cyclooxygenase	

Adapted with permission from Goldring MB, Goldring SR: Cytokines and cell growth control. Crit Rev Eukaryotic Gene Expression 1:303, 1991. Copyright CRC Press, Boca Raton, Florida.

Abbreviations: mRNA, messenger ribonucleic acid; MAP, microtuble-associated protein; IL, interleukin; M-CSF, macrophage colony-stimulating factor.

gers, activation of a multitude of other regulatory gene products, and, ultimately, cellular proliferation and matrix biosynthesis.

The Fibroblast Environment

Fibroblasts in vivo exist under environmental conditions markedly different from those used to study growth factors in vitro. Such conditions, including the presence of a surrounding extracellular matrix and different oxygen tension, profoundly influence fibroblast behavior in general as well as responses to growth factors. For example, in vitro responses to PDGF, as well as to epidermal growth factor (EGF), are altered by the presence of an extracellular matrix[42–44]; PDGF signaling, which occurs via receptor autophosphorylation, is decreased when cells are grown in an in vitro matrix.[45] There is evidence that other cytokines and growth factors that stimulate fibroblast proliferation may mediate their effect via PDGF action. IL-1 and TNF stimulate synthesis and release of endogenous fibroblast PDGF-AA.[46] TGF-β1 appears to increase expression of fibroblast PDGF-αα receptors.[47] Some growth factors, for example, insulin-like growth factor (IGF),[48] are not mitogenic by themselves but potentiate the mitogenic action of other substances. At low oxygen tension, which may occur following vascular injury, binding of TGF-β and EGF[47] is decreased whereas proliferative responses to EGF may be augmented.[49]

The low level of fibroblast proliferation in undisturbed skin and other tissues may be due not only to the absence of "on" signals (e.g., growth factors) but also to the presence of "off" signals.[44, 50] The fibroblast interacts with its matrix environment via discrete receptors to regulate cell function.[51–53] *Integrins* are heterodimers involved in cell-cell and cell-matrix interactions. The β1-integrin family are involved largely in cell-matrix interactions, whereas β2-integrins are involved in cell-cell adhesion (e.g., lymphocyte-endothelial and lymphocyte-fibroblast binding). Fibroblasts express α1β1-, α2β1-, and α5β1-integrins that interact with specific ligands on collagen and fibronectin.[54, 55] The amino acid sequence RGDS (argi-nine-glycine-aspartate-serine) on fibronectin acts as a ligand or counterreceptor for integrins expressed on the fibroblast.[56]

In the unperturbed state, the spatial orientation of the fibroblast and its interaction with matrix proteins provides an "off" signal.[50] Disruption of the extracellular matrix from injury changes this relationship. Signals from cytokines and growth factors may lead to fibroblast proliferation, migration, or new matrix biosynthesis. Structural focal adhesions form between the fibroblast and connective tissue proteins or cells. The binding of fibroblasts to fibronectin and collagen can lead to activation of a variety of cellular signals. Both disengagement and engagement of integrin receptors occur, which leads to activation of protein kinases, including the focal adhesion kinase (FAK) pp125FAK, present at the site of focal fibroblast adhesions and microtubule-associated kinases.[57–60] FAK, in turn, can transduce intracellular signals via inositol triphosphate (IP$_3$).[61] Focal adhesions also lead to changes in the organization of cytoskeletal proteins, such as actin, talin, and vinculin, cytoskeletal proteins that are linked to intracellular signaling pathways.[62] Thus, matrix reorganization can have profound effects on fibroblast intracellular processes.

IMMUNE MODULATION OF FIBROBLAST METABOLISM

Lymphocyte Recruitment and Localization

Lymphocytes normally reside in specialized lymphoid tissues (i.e., lymph nodes and spleen) and in the circulation. Lymphocytes may gain entry to the circulation from lymphoid organs or other tissues, and they may leave to recirculate through the lymphatic system. Establishment of a chronic inflammatory focus is characterized by increased lymphocyte and monocyte emigration from the vasculature and localization of these cells to tissue (Fig. 13–4). Recirculation as well as homing and localization of immune cells are rigorously controlled by the expression and engagement of cell surface receptors.[63]

Lymphocytes and monocytes express cell surface

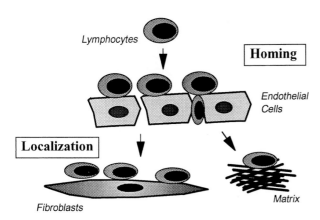

Figure 13–4. Homing and localization of mononuclear cells to connective tissue. The localization of lymphocytes and monocytes requires cellular activation, egress from the vasculature, and binding to cellular and matrix elements of the connective tissue. These processes are tightly regulated by the expression of specific adhesion ligands.

molecules that interact with ligands on endothelial cells, fibroblasts, and extracellular matrix to promote cell adhesion (see Chapter 20). As an initial event, activation of immune cells leads to increased expression and function of adhesion ligands. Endothelial cells at sites of inflammation are activated by immune cell cytokines, particularly IL-1 and TNF-α from monocytes, or by other stimuli (e.g., endotoxin) to increase expression of counterreceptors, or ligands, for lymphocyte and monocyte receptors. The endothelial cell ligands (see Chapters 12 and 20) include:

- Vascular cell adhesion molecule (VCAM-1)
- Endothelial-leukocyte adhesion molecule (ELAM-1; E-selectin)
- Mucosal addressin cell adhesion molecule (Mad-CAM-1)
- CD34 (CD, or cell determinant, designations are catalog numbers for identified proteins)
- P-selectin
- Intercellular adhesion molecule-1 (ICAM-1)

Lymphocyte and monocyte ligands, including L-selectin; sialated glycoproteins; the β2-integrin lymphocyte function-associated antigen-1/LFA-1 (CD11a, CD18, or α1β2); very late activation antigen VLA-4 (CD49d, CD29, or α4β1); and MAC-1 (α1β2 or CD11b, CD18), bind to these endothelial cell receptors and modulate the egress of lymphocytes and monocytes from the vasculature. The egress can be facilitated by chemotactic stimuli, such as the chemokines IL-8, RANTES, macrophage inflammatory protein-1α (MIP-1α), and monocyte chemotactic protein-1 (MCP-1), as well as by other chemotactic stimuli, including collagen peptides.[64–67]

Lymphocyte localization requires activation of fibroblasts and expression of functional ICAM-1, which mediates lymphocyte-fibroblast attachment (Fig. 13–5).[68, 69] ICAM-1 on fibroblasts is induced by gamma interferon (IFN-γ), TFN-α, IL-1, and IL-4.[69–71] In addi-

tion, lymphocytes may bind to noncellular ligands expressed on collagen and fibronectin via surface integrins, which include VLA-1 (α1β1) and VLA-4 (α4β1).[55, 72, 73] Lymphocytes initially leaving the vasculature and binding to connective tissue are presumably activated; however, there is further recruitment of monocytes and lymphocytes in response to immune cell and connective tissue signals, including the chemotactic factors noted above. Cellular binding per se may result in activation of immune cells and connective tissue cells as a consequence of receptor activation.[74]

Fibroblast Proliferation and Matrix Biosynthesis

Although direct cell contact between fibroblasts and immune cells may have reciprocal effects on cell metabolism, the preponderant regulation of fibroblast metabolism occurs via release from immune cells of soluble cytokines and growth factors (Table 13–3). These are often active at nanomolar (10^{-9} molar) concentrations, a range readily achieved in the confines of the interstitial space. Cytokines and growth factors released by lymphocytes and monocytes that regulate fibroblast metabolism include IL-1, IL-4, IL-6, IL-10, TNF-α, IFN-γ, TGF-β, and PDGF. As already noted, IL-1, TGF-β, and PDGF stimulate both proliferation and collagen synthesis by fibroblasts, whereas IL-4 stimulates fibroblast chemotaxis, proliferation, and matrix synthesis.[75–77] IL-6 stimulates synthesis of collagen and glycosaminoglycans.[78] TNF-α increases fibroblast proliferation, such as IL-1, by stimulating endogenous fibroblast PDGF-AA. TNF-α has variable effects on collagen synthesis, stimulates proteoglycans, and suppresses fibronectin production.[79–81] IFN-γ, TNF-α, and IL-10 suppress collagen synthesis.[82] The

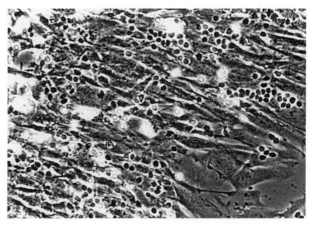

Figure 13–5. Photomicrograph of T lymphocytes bound to fibroblasts. Purified human T lymphocytes are bound to human dermal fibroblasts grown in culture. Fibroblasts were activated by γ-interferon prior to binding process. Fibroblasts appear as spindle-shaped cells. Lymphocytes are small, round dark cells that are tightly adherent and flattened or bright round cells that are more loosely adherent and rounded. (Viewed under phase contrast microscopy; original magnification, ×400.)

Table 13–3. CYTOKINES MODULATING FIBROBLAST FUNCTION*

	Proliferation	Matrix Biosynthesis	Metalloproteinases	Adhesion Molecule Expression	Chemotaxis
Stimulation	PDGF	TGF-β	TNF-α	IFN-γ	TGF-β
	FGF	IL-1	IL-1	TNF-α	PDGF
	IL-1 via PDGF	IL-4	IL-10	IL-1	IL-4
	IL-4	IL-6 (proteoglycan)		IL-4	IFN-γ
	CTAPs	PDGF			TNF-α
	Endothelin	FGF			Fibronectin
	TNF-α	Endothelin			Collagen peptides
					EGF
					C5a/C5
					Endothelin
					Leukotriene B4
					Thrombin
Suppression	IL-1 via PGE	IFN-γ	TGF-β		IFN-γ
	IFN-γ	TNF-α	IFN-γ		IFN-α
	TGF-β	IL-8			
		IL-10			

*Predominant effects of cytokines and growth factors on fibroblast metabolism are shown. Effects are often concentration dependent and may vary with particular types of fibroblasts. In some instances, as noted in text, effects of a single cytokine may not be concordant for different matrix components or different proteinases. Connective tissue activating peptides (CTAPs) include platelet factor 3. C5a is the activation fragment of the fifth complement component.

Abbreviations: PDGF, platelet-derived growth factor; FGF, fibroblast growth factor; IL, interleukin; TNF, tumor necrosis factor; IFN, interferon; TGF, transforming growth factor; EGF, epidermal growth factor.

overall effect on collagen synthesis thus depends on the balance of cytokines and growth factors, the type of responding fibroblast, and other environmental factors.

The net amount of accumulated collagen and other matrix components depends not only on synthesis but also on degradation. Fibroblasts as well as other cell types elaborate connective tissue matrix degrading enzymes, termed *matrix metalloproteinases* (MMPs) because of their dependence of metal ions for activity. Seven of these enzymes are related structurally and genetically, the prototype being interstitial collagenase[83] (see Chapter 21). These enzymes are secreted as latent enzymes and are activated extracellularly.

Fibroblast (interstitial) collagenase (MMP-1) and neutrophil collagenase (MMP-8) can cleave native (non-denatured) collagen.[84] Once cleaved, collagen becomes denatured (gelatin = denatured collagen) and is susceptible to further degradation by gelatinases.

MMP-2 (also called 72-kD gelatinase because of its molecular weight) and MMP-3 (stromelysin) are gelatinases produced constitutively by fibroblasts. MMP-9, stromelysin-2, and pump-1 (uterine MMP) are inducible gelatinases. MMP-3 also degrades proteoglycans, fibronectin, laminin, and cartilage link protein and activates latent procollagenase. Fibroblasts also make elastases, cathepsins, and other enzymes, some of which are membrane-bound enzymes.[85, 86] Elastases not only are important in degradation of vascular, skin, and lung elastin but also can degrade matrix proteins and cause significant tissue injury.

Cytokines may have concordant or discordant effects on synthesis of collagen and of the enzymes that degrade collagen and other matrix macromolecules. IL-1, which stimulates production of collagen, also stimulates production of collagenase (MMP-1) and stromelysin.[87–89] TNF-α is a potent stimulator of MMP-9 and also stimulates production of collagenase and stromelysin.[90] Both IL-1 and TNF-α induce c-*jun* in fibroblasts and the increase in c-*jun* likely plays a direct role in activating collagenase gene transcription.[91, 92] IL-1 and TNF-α also individually and synergistically stimulate fibroblast prostaglandin E₂ (PGE₂) synthesis, and PGE₂ suppresses collagenase production.[93–96] In direct contrast to IL-1, IFN-γ suppresses both collagen synthesis and synthesis of collagenase and stromelysin.[97, 98] TGF-β, perhaps the most potent stimulus for collagen synthesis, suppresses synthesis of collagenase and stromelysin.[99, 100] Glucocorticoids, in general, suppress production of MMPs. Finally, fibroblasts synthesize *autokines* (self-stimulating cytokines), which augment collagenase production.[101]

In addition to elaborating matrix and matrix-degrading enzymes, fibroblasts synthesize inhibitors of metalloproteinases. Tissue inhibitor of metalloproteinases (TIMP or TIMP-1) inhibits the action of the entire family of mammalian MMPs.[83] TIMP is induced in fibroblasts by IL-1, IL-6, and IL-11.[102–104] Both IL-6 and IL-11 are fibroblast products, or autokines, whose production in fibroblasts is, in turn, stimulated by IL-1 and TNF-α.[21, 105] IL-11 production can also be stimulated by TGF-β.[106] Thus, TGF-β has an overall matrix-promoting effect, augmenting production of collagen and collagenase inhibitor, suppressing collagenase production, and potentially playing a critical role in the development of fibrotic disease.

The balance of forces on the fibroblast, as well as the particular tissue involved, determine whether inflammatory stimuli will lead to net proliferation and repair or to tissue degradation and destruction. The skin fibroblast is normally a relatively quiescent cell that divides slowly and, in the absence of injury, elaborates little matrix. Inflammation in the skin tends to lead to net increases in matrix (e.g., wound healing). In contrast, synovial tissue responds to inflammation predominantly with increased MMP production and destruction of subadjacent cartilage and bone. Within the synovium per se, however, synovial fibroblast proliferation and matrix deposition are increased. A similar situation exists for the gingival fibroblast, in which proliferation and matrix deposition in the gingiva are accompanied by destruction and resorption of adjacent bony tissues.

FIBROBLAST CYTOKINES

As just noted, the stimulation of fibroblasts by IL-1, TNF-α, and other cytokines leads to fibroblast proinflammatory activities by stimulation of matrix degradation. Peptides of degraded collagen and fibronectin may further stimulate lymphocyte and monocyte recruitment by their chemotactic properties. Fibroblasts may also have more direct effects on leukocyte recruitment and activation. Stimulation of fibroblasts by TNF-α leads to synthesis of the chemotaxin IL-8 and leukemia inhibition factor (LIF), which is chemotactic for and activates leukocytes.[74, 107] Fibroblasts also elaborate the lymphocyte chemotactic factors MCP-1 and MIP-1a.[67, 108] TNF-α also stimulates production of membrane-associated IL-1α in fibroblasts; IL-1 has multiple stimulatory influences on lymphocytes and monocytes. Both IL-1 and TNF-α stimulate production of IL-6 by fibroblasts[21, 105]; IL-6 is a major inducer of acute phase proteins in hepatocytes and is an important promoter of plasma cell proliferation.[109–112]

Fibroblasts also are an important source of cytokines, which regulate development of hematopoietic precursors. In this respect, bone marrow fibroblasts serve key nutritive and differentiating functions; fibroblasts make granulocyte colony-stimulating factor (G-CSF), granulocyte-monocyte colony-stimulating factor (GM-CSF), and IL-11 augmented in response to IL-1, TNF-α, and/or TGF-β.[106, 113, 114] Finally, fibroblasts make growth factors, including TGF-β and PDGF, which not only can serve as autokines but also act on other cells.[46, 115] Thus, fibroblast-derived cytokines affect a variety of cells, including immune cells, mesenchymal cells, and bone marrow stem cells.

FIBROBLAST HETEROGENEITY

In addition to the obvious differences in functional expression among dermal, synovial, lung, and other fibroblast populations, it has become apparent that even fibroblasts derived from a single source are heterogeneous. Thus, among fibroblasts derived from human skin, there are marked differences in proliferation and in synthesis of collagen, glycosaminoglycans, prostaglandins, and metalloproteinases.[116–119] Furthermore, there are differences in responses to growth regulatory cytokines and in adhesion molecule expression.[120, 121] Finally, monoclonal antibodies have identified surface membrane molecules that are differentially expressed among fibroblasts. This heterogeneity among fibroblasts has been ascertained in studies of cloned fibroblast populations and of whole populations by flow cytometry, immunohistochemistry, and in situ hybridization. Similar heterogeneity has been seen in populations of fibroblasts derived from lung and other tissues.[122]

The iportance of this heterogeneity is difficult to assess. One possibility is that it represents a continuum of states of fibroblast differentiation. Alternatively, there may be discrete subtypes of fibroblast lineage, each with somewhat different metabolic capabilities. Because subtypes may have differential responses to environmental factors, including growth modulatory cytokines, it is possible that subpopulations of fibroblast may become selectively increased. This process of "clonal selection" may explain some abnormalities of fibroblast metabolism seen in fibrotic states. Scleroderma fibroblasts, for example, maintain increased collagen synthesis in vitro in the absence of continued stimulation by immune-derived cytokines, which might have stimulated collagen synthesis in vivo.[123]

One possibility that could explain this finding is that in vivo processes have "selected" for high-collagen-producing cells or clones. Indeed, the fibroblast subpopulation with high levels of receptors for C1q (first complement component) also maintains high levels of collagen synthesis.[124] Similarly, the persistent abnormalities displayed by rheumatoid synovial cells in vitro may reflect overgrowth of particular synovial cell subpopulations.

SUMMARY

The fibroblast is the foremost cell involved in reparative functions in both skin and visceral tissues. Reparative processes are initiated in response to injury or inflammatory stimuli. The fibroblast responds to cytokines and growth factors, which are released in these circumstances, by initiating cellular proliferation and matrix biosynthesis. In addition, the fibroblast is capable of matrix degradation and remodeling, a process that normally accompanies repair. With excessive activity of the immune system, reparative processes may not cease, either because of persistent stimulatory signals or because of the failure of inhibitory signals to retard fibroblast activity. In the latter instance, excessive and pathologic fibrosis may result. In addition, the fibroblast elaborates a variety of regulatory cytokines that modulate the proliferation and biosynthetic activity of other cell types.

References

1. Agelli M, Wahl SM: Cytokines and fibrosis. Clin Exp Rheumatol 4:379, 1986.
2. Kovacs EJ: Fibrogenic cytokines: The role of immune mediators in the development of scar tissue. Immunol Today 12:17, 1991.
3. Postlethwaite AE: Dermal fibroblast function. In Nickoloff BJ (ed): Dermal Immune System. Boca Raton, Fla, CRC Press, 1993, pp 163–184.
4. Korn JH, Piela-Smith T: Interaction of immune and connective tissue cells. In Nickoloff BJ (ed): Dermal Immune System. Boca Raton, Fla, CRC Press, 1993, pp 185–208.
5. Piela TH, Korn JH: Lymphokines and cytokines in the reparative process. In Cohen S Z(ed): The Role of Lymphokines in the Immune Response. Boca Raton, Fla, CRC Press, 1990, pp 255–273.
6. Fries KM, Blieden T, Looney RJ, et al: Evidence of fibroblast heterogeneity and the role of fibroblast subpopulations in fibrosis. Clin Immunol Immunopathol 72:283, 1995.
7. Pierce GF, Mustoe TA, Altrock BW, et al: Role of platelet-derived growth factor in wound healing. J Cell Biochem 45:319, 1991.
8. Beckmann MP, Betsholtz C, Heldin C-H, et al: Comparison of biological properties and transforming potential of human PDGF-A and PDGF-B chains. Science 241:1346, 1988.
9. Seifert RA, Hart CE, Phillips PE, et al: Two different subunits associate to create isoform-specific platelet-derived growth factor receptors. J Biol Chem 264:8771, 1989.
10. Hart CE, Forstrom JW, Kelly JD, et al: Two classes of PDGF receptor recognize different isoforms of PDGF. Science 240:1529, 1988.
11. Heldin C-H, Ernlund A, Rorsman C, et al: Dimerization of B-type platelet-derived growth factor receptors occurs after ligand binding and is closely associated with receptor kinase activation. J Biol Chem 264:8905, 1989.
12. Gu X-F, Raynaud F, Evain-Brion D: Increased chemotactic and mitogenic response of psoriatic fibroblasts to platelet-derived growth factor. J Invest Dermatol 91:599, 1988.
13. Postlethwaite AE, Keski-Oja J, Moses HL, et al: Stimulation of the chemotactic migration of human fibroblasts by transforming growth factor β. J Exp Med 165:251, 1987.
14. Dawes KE, Gray AJ, Laurent GJ: Thrombin stimulates fibroblast chemotaxis and replication. Eur J Cell Biol 61:126, 1993.
15. Postlethwaite AE, Seyer JM, Kang AH: Chemotactic attraction of human fibroblasts to type I, II, and III collagens and collagen-derived peptides. Proc Natl Acad Sci USA 75:871, 1978.
16. Fukai F, Suzuki H, Suzuki K, et al: Rat plasma fibronectin contains two distinct chemotactic domains for fibroblastic cells. J Biol Chem 266:8807, 1991.
17. Senior RM, Griffin GL, Mecham RP: Chemotactic responses of fibroblasts to tropoelastin and elastin-derived peptides. J Clin Invest 70:614, 1982.
18. Antonelli-Orlidge A, Saunders KB, Smith SR, et al: An activated form of transforming growth factor β is produced by cocultures of endothelial cells and pericytes. Proc Natl Acad Sci USA 86:4544, 1989.
19. Kavanaugh WM, Harsh GR IV, Starksen NF, et al: Transcriptional regulation of the A and B chain genes of platelet-derived growth factor in microvascular endothelial cells. J Biol Chem 263:8470, 1988.
20. Pierce GF, Vande Berg J, Rudolph R, et al: Platelet-derived growth factor-BB and transforming growth factor beta-1 selectively modulate glycosaminoglycans, collagen, and myofibroblasts in excisional wounds. Am J Pathol 138:629, 1991.
21. Zilberstein A, Ruggieri R, Korn JH, et al: Structure and expression of cDNA and genes for human interferon-beta-2, a distinct species inducible by growth-stimulatory cytokines. EMBO J 5:2529, 1986.
22. Nawroth PP, Bank I, Handley D, et al: Tumor necrosis factor/cachectin interacts with endothelial cell receptors to induce release of interleukin 1. J Exp Med 163:1363, 1986.
23. Shanahan WR, Hancock WW, Korn JH: Expression of IL-1 and tumor necrosis factor by endothelial cells: Role in stimulating fibroblast PGE$_2$ synthesis. J Exp Pathol 4:17, 1989.
24. Schmidt JA, Mizel SB, Cohen D, et al: Interleukin 1, a potential regulator of fibroblast proliferation. J Immunol 128:2177, 1982.
25. Sugarman BJ, Aggarwal BB, Hass PE, et al: Recombinant human tumor necrosis factor-α: Effects on proliferation of normal and transformed cells in vitro. Science 230:943, 1985.
26. Postlethwaite AE, Raghow R, Stricklin GP, et al: Modulation of fibroblast functions by interleukin 1: Increased steady-state accumulation of type I procollagen messenger RNAs and stimulation of other functions but not chemotaxis by human recombinant interleukin 1α and β. J Cell Biol 106:311, 1988.
27. Takuwa N, Takuwa Y, Yanagisawa M, et al: A novel vasoactive peptide endothelin stimulates mitogenesis through inositol lipid turnover in Swiss 3T3 fibroblasts. J Biol Chem 264:7856, 1989.
28. Peacock AJ, Dawes KE, Shock A, et al: Endothelin-1 and endothelin-3 induce chemotaxis and replication of pulmonary artery fibroblasts. Am J Respir Cell Mol Biol 7:492, 1992.
29. Kahaleh MB: Endothelin, an endothelial-dependent vasoconstrictor in scleroderma: Enhanced production and profibrotic action. Arthritis Rheum 34:978, 1991.
30. Leibovich SJ, Ross R: The role of the macrophage in wound repair: A study with hydrocortisone and an antimacrophage serum. Am J Pathol 78:71, 1975.
31. Goldring MB, Goldring SR: Cytokines and cell growth control. Crit Rev Eukaryotic Gene Expression 1:301, 1991.
32. Paris S, Pouyssegur J: Mitogenic effects of fibroblast growth factors in cultured fibroblasts: Interaction with G-protein-mediated signaling pathways. Ann N Y Acad Sci 638:139, 1991.
33. Pledger WJ, Stiles CD, Antoniades HN, et al: An ordered sequence of events is required before BALB/c-3T3 cells become committed to DNA synthesis. Proc Natl Acad Sci USA 75:2839, 1978.
34. Huang C-L, Takenawa T, Ives HE: Platelet-derived growth factor-mediated Ca^{2+} entry is blocked by antibodies to phosphatidylinositol 4,5-bisphosphate but does not involve heparin-sensitive inositol 1,4,5-tris-phosphate receptors. J Biol Chem 266:4045, 1991.
35. Matuoka K, Fukami K, Nakanishi O, et al: Mitogenesis in response to PDGF and bombesin abolished by microinjection of antibody to PIP$_2$. Science 239:640, 1988.
36. Ballou LR, Barker SC, Postlethwaite AE, et al: Interleukin 1 stimulates phosphatidylinositol kinase activity in human fibroblasts. J Clin Invest 87:299, 1991.
37. Muldoon LL, Rodland KD, Forsythe ML, et al: Stimulation of phosphatidylinositol hydrolysis, diacylglycerol release, and gene expression in response to endothelin, a potent new agonist for fibroblasts and smooth muscle cells. J Biol Chem 264:8529, 1989.
38. Muldoon LL, Rodland KD, Magun BE: Transforming growth factor β and epidermal growth factor alter calcium influx and phosphatidylinositol turnover in Rat-1 fibroblasts. J Biol Chem 263:18834, 1988.
39. Dayer J-M, Goldring SR, Robinson DR, et al: Effects of human mononuclear cell factor on cultured rheumatoid synovial cells. Interactions of prostaglandin E$_2$ and cyclic adenosine-3′,5′-monophosphate. Biochim Biophys Acta 586:87, 1979.
40. Magnaldo I, Pouysségur J, Paris S: Cyclic AMP inhibits mitogen-induced DNA synthesis in hamster fibroblasts, regardless of the signalling pathway involved. FEBS Lett 245:65, 1989.
41. Korn JH, Halushka PV, LeRoy EC: Mononuclear cell modulation of connective tissue function: Suppression of fibroblast growth by stimulation of endogenous prostaglandin production. J Clin Invest 65:543, 1980.
42. Rhudy RW, McPherson JM: Influence of the extracellular matrix on the proliferative response of human skin fibroblasts to serum and purified platelet-derived growth factor. J Cell Physiol 137:185, 1988.
43. Nakagawa S, Pawelek P, Grinnell F: Extracellular matrix organization modulates fibroblast growth and growth factor responsiveness. Exp Cell Res 182:572, 1989.
44. Nishiyama T, Akutsu N, Horii I, et al: Response to growth factors of human dermal fibroblasts in a quiescent state owing to cell-matrix contact inhibition. Matrix 11:71, 1991.
45. Lin YC, Grinnell F: Decreased level of PDGF-stimulated receptor autophosphorylation by fibroblasts in mechanically relaxed collagen matrices. J Cell Biol 122:663, 1993.
46. Raines EW, Dower SK, Ross R: Interleukin 1 mitogenic activity for fibroblasts and smooth muscle cells is due to PDGF-AA. Science 243:393, 1989.
47. Ishikawa O, LeRoy EC, Trojanowska M: Mitogenic effect of transforming growth factor beta 1 on human fibroblasts involves the induction of platelet-derived growth factor alpha receptors. J Cell Physiol 145:181, 1990.
48. Phillips PD, Pignolo RJ, Cristofalo VJ: Insulin-like growth factor-I: Specific binding to high and low affinity sites and mitogenic action throughout the life span of WI-38 cells. J Cell Physiol 133:135, 1987.
49. Storch TG, Talley GD: Oxygen concentration regulates the proliferative response of human fibroblasts to serum and growth factors. Exp Cell Res 175:317, 1988.
50. Grinnell F, Nakagawa S: Spatial regulation of fibroblast proliferation: An explanation for cell regression at the end of the wound repair. Prog Clin Biol Res 365:155, 1991.
51. Juliano RL, Haskill S: Signal transduction from the extracellular matrix. J Cell Biol 120:577, 1993.
52. Hynes RO: Integrins: versatility, modulation, and signaling in cell adhesion. Cell 69:11, 1992.
53. Mauch C, Kreig T: Fibroblast-matrix interactions and their role in the pathogenesis of fibrosis. Rheum Dis Clin North Am 16:93, 1990.
54. Klein CE, Dressel D, Steinmayer T, et al: Integrin alpha 2 beta 1 is upregulated in fibroblasts and highly aggressive melanoma cells in

three-dimensional collagen lattices and mediates the reorganization of collagen I fibrils. J Cell Biol 115:1427, 1991.

55. Gullberg D, Gehlsen KR, Turner DC, et al: Analysis of alpha 1 beta 1, alpha 2 beta 1 and alpha 3 beta 1 integrins in cell-collagen interactions: Identification of conformation dependent alpha 1 beta 1 binding sites in collagen type I. EMBO J 11:3865, 1992.

56. D'Souza SE, Ginsberg MH, Burke TA, et al: Localization of an Arg-Gly-Asp recognition site within an integrin adhesion receptor. Science 242:91, 1988.

57. Chen Q, Kinch MS, Lin TH, et al: Integrin-mediated cell adhesion activates mitogen-activated protein kinases. J Biol Chem 269:26602, 1994.

58. Lin TH, Yurochko A, Kornberg L, et al: The role of protein tyrosine phosphorylation in integrin-mediated gene induction in monocytes. J Cell Biol 126:1585, 1994.

59. Morino N, Mimura T, Hamasaki K, et al: Matrix/integrin interaction activates the mitogen-activated protein kinase, p44erk-1 and p42erk-2. J Biol Chem 270:269, 1995.

60. Kornberg L, Juliano RL: Signal transduction from the extracellular matrix: The integrin-tyrosine kinase connection. Trends Pharmacol Sci 13:93, 1992.

61. Chen HC, Guan JL: Association of focal adhesion kinase with its potential substrate phosphatidylinositol 3-kinase. Proc Natl Acad Sci USA 91:10148, 1994.

62. Sanchez-Mateos P, Campanero MR, Balboa MA, et al: Co-clustering of beta 1 integrins, cytoskeletal proteins, and tyrosine-phosphorylated substrates during integrin-mediated leukocyte aggregation. J Immunol 151:3817, 1993.

63. Springer TA: Traffic signals for lymphocyte recirculation and leukocyte emigration: The multistep paradigm [review]. Cell 76:301, 1994.

64. Korn JH, Downie E: Clonal interactions in fibroblast proliferation: Recognition of self vs. non-self. J Cell Physiol 141:437, 1989.

65. Cruikshank WW, Center DM, Nisar N, et al: Molecular and functional analysis of a lymphocyte chemoattractant factor: Association of biologic function with CD4 expression. Proc Natl Acad Sci USA 91:5109, 1994.

66. Taub DD, Lloyd AR, Wang JM, et al: The effects of human recombinant MIP-1 alpha, MIP-1 beta, and RANTES on the chemotaxis and adhesion of T cell subsets. Adv Exp Med Biol 351:139, 1993.

67. Carr MW, Roth SJ, Luther E, et al: Monocyte chemoattractant protein 1 acts as a T-lymphocyte chemoattractant. Proc Natl Acad Sci USA 91:3652, 1994.

68. Piela TH, Korn JH: Lymphocyte-fibroblast adhesion induced by interferon-γ. Cell Immunol 114:149, 1988.

69. Rothlein R, Czajkowski M, O'Neill MM, et al: Induction of intercellular adhesion molecule 1 on primary and continuous cell lines by pro-inflammatory cytokines: Regulation by pharmacologic agents and neutralizing antibodies. J Immunol 141:1665, 1988.

70. Piela-Smith TH, Broketa G, Hand A, et al: Regulation of ICAM-1 expression and function in human dermal fibroblasts by IL-4. J Immunol 148:1375, 1992.

71. Piela TH, Korn JH: ICAM-1 dependent fibroblast-lymphocyte adhesion: Discordance between expression and function of ICAM-1. Cell Immunol 129:125, 1990.

72. Liao N-S, St. John J, McCarthy JB, et al: Adhesion of lymphoid cells to the carboxyl-terminal heparin-binding domains of fibronectin. Exp Cell Res 181:348, 1989.

73. Takada Y, Elices MJ, Crouse C, et al: The primary structure of the α4 subunit of VLA-4: Homology to other integrins and a possible cell-cell adhesion function. EMBO J 8:1361, 1989.

74. Lorenzo JA, Jastrzebski SL, Kalinowski JF, et al: Tumor necrosis factor alpha stimulates production of leukemia inhibitory factor in human dermal fibroblast cultures. Clin Immunol Immunopathol 70:260, 1994.

75. Postlethwaite AE, Seyer JM: Fibroblast chemotaxis induction by human recombinant interleukin-4: Identification by synthetic peptide analysis of two chemotactic domains residing in amino acid sequences 70–88 and 89–122. J Clin Invest 87:2147, 1991.

76. Monroe JG, Haldar S, Prystowsky MB, et al: Lymphokine regulation of inflammatory processes: Interleukin-4 stimulates fibroblast proliferation. Clin Immunol Immunopathol 49:292, 1988.

77. Postlethwaite AE, Katai H, Raghow R: Stimulation of extracellular matrix biosynthesis in fibroblasts by interleukin-4 (abstr). Arthritis Rheum 32:S78, 1989.

78. Duncan MR, Berman B: Stimulation of collagen and glycosaminoglycan production in cultured human adult dermal fibroblasts by recombinant human interleukin 6. J Invest Dermatol 97:686, 1991.

79. Paulsson Y, Austgulen R, Hofsli E, et al: Tumor necrosis factor–induced expression of platelet-derived growth factor A-chain messenger RNA in fibroblasts. Exp Cell Res 180:490, 1989.

80. Mauviel A, Daireaux M, Rédini F, et al: Tumor necrosis factor inhibits collagen and fibronectin synthesis in human dermal fibroblasts. FEBS Lett 236:47, 1988.

81. Duncan MR, Berman B: Differential regulation of collagen, glycosaminoglycan, fibronectin, and collagenase activity production in cultured

82. human adult dermal fibroblasts by interleukin 1-alpha and beta and tumor necrosis factor-alpha and beta. J Invest Dermatol 92:699, 1989.

82. Reitamo S, Remitz A, Tamai K, et al: Interleukin-10 modulates type I collagen and matrix metalloprotease gene expression in cultured human skin fibroblasts. J Clin Invest 94:2489, 1994.

83. Woessner JF Jr: Matrix metalloproteinases and their inhibitors in connective tissue remodeling. FASEB J 5:2145, 1991.

84. Harris ED Jr, DiBona DR, Krane SM: Collagenase in human synovial fluid. J Clin Invest 48:2104, 1969.

85. Piela-Smith TH, Korn JH: Aminopeptidase N: A constitutive cell surface protein on human fibroblasts. Cell Immunol 162:42, 1995.

86. Rédini F, Lafuma C, Pujol J-P, et al: Effect of cytokines and growth factors on the expression of elastase activity by human synoviocytes, dermal fibroblasts and rabbit articular chondrocytes. Biochem Biophys Res Commun 155:786, 1988.

87. Dayer JM, Russell RGG, Krane SM: Collagenase production by rheumatoid synovial cells: Stimulation by a human lymphocyte factor. Science 195:181, 1977.

88. Postlethwaite AE, Lachman LB, Mainardi CL, et al: Interleukin 1 stimulation of collagenase production of cultured fibroblasts. J Exp Med 157:801, 1983.

89. Sirum-Connolly K, Brinckerhoff CE: Interleukin-1 or phorbol induction of the stromelysin promoter requires an element that cooperates with AP-1. Nucleic Acids Res 19:335, 1991.

90. Dayer JM, Beutler B, Cerami A: Cachectin/tumor necrosis factor stimulates collagenase and prostaglandin E2 production by human synovial cells and dermal fibroblasts. J Exp Med 162:2163, 1985.

91. Brenner DA, O'Hara M, Angel P, et al: Prolonged activation of jun and collagenase genes by tumour necrosis factor-α. Nature 337:661, 1989.

92. Conca W, Kaplan PB, Krane SM: Increases in levels of procollagenase messenger RNA in cultured fibroblasts induced by human recombinant interleukin 1β or serum follow c-jun expression and are dependent on new protein synthesis. J Clin Invest 83:1753, 1989.

93. Krane SM, Dayer J-M, Simon LS, et al: Mononuclear cell-conditioned medium containing mononuclear cell factor (MCF), homologous with interleukin 1, stimulates collagen and fibronectin synthesis by adherent rheumatoid synovial cells: Effects of prostaglandin E$_2$ and indomethacin. Collagen Relat Res 5:99, 1985.

94. Mizel SB, Dayer JM, Krane SM, et al: Stimulation of rheumatoid synovial cell collagenase and prostaglandin by partially purified lymphocyte-activating factor (interleukin-1). Proc Natl Acad Sci USA 78:2474, 1981

95. Dayer J-M, Breard J, Chess L, et al: Participation of monocytes-macrophages and lymphocytes in the production of a factor that stimulates collagenase and prostaglandin release by rheumatoid synovial cells. J Clin Invest 64:1386, 1979.

96. Elias JA, Gustilo K, Baeder W, et al: Synergistic stimulation of fibroblast prostaglandin production by recombinant interleukin-1 and tumor necrosis factor. J Immunol 138:3812, 1987.

97. Shapiro SD, Campbell EJ, Kobayashi DK, et al: Immune modulation of metalloproteinase production in human macrophages: Selective pre-translational suppression of interstitial collagenase and stromelysin biosynthesis by interferon-gamma. J Clin Invest 86:1204, 1990.

98. Unemori EN, Bair MJ, Bauer EA, et al: Stromelysin expression regulates collagenase activation in human fibroblasts: Dissociable control of two metalloproteinases by interferon-gamma. J Biol Chem 266:23477, 1991.

99. Varga J, Jimenez SA: Stimulation of normal human fibroblast collagen production and processing by transforming growth factor-beta. Biochem Biophys Res Commun 138:974, 1986.

100. Overall CM, Wrana JL, Sodek J: Independent regulation of collagenase, 72-kDa progelatinase, and metalloendoproteinase inhibitor expression in human fibroblasts by transforming growth factor-β. J Biol Chem 264:1860, 1989.

101. Brinckerhoff CE, Mitchell TI, Karmilowicz MJ, et al: Autocrine induction of collagenase by serum amyloid A-like and β$_2$-microglobulin-like proteins. Science 243:655, 1989.

102. Murphy G, Reynolds JJ, Werb Z: Biosynthesis of tissue inhibitor of metalloproteinases by human fibroblast cultures: Stimulation by 12-0-tetradecanoylphorbol 13-acetate and interleukin-1 in parallel with collagenases. J Biol Chem 260:3079, 1985.

103. Lotz M, Guerne P-A: Interleukin-6 induces the synthesis of tissue inhibitor of metalloproteinases-1/erythroid potentiating activity (TIMP-1/EPA). J Biol Chem 266:2017, 1991.

104. Maier R, Ganu V, Lotz M: Interleukin-11, an inducible cytokine in human articular chondrocytes and synoviocytes, stimulates the production of the tissue inhibitor of metalloproteinases. J Biol Chem 268:21527, 1993.

105. Walther Z, May LT, Sehgal PB: Transcriptional regulation of the interferon-β2/B cell differentiation factor BSF-2/hepatocyte-stimulating factor gene in human fibroblasts by other cytokines. J Immunol 140:974, 1988.

106. Elias JA, Zheng T, Whiting NL, et al: IL-1 and transforming growth factor-beta regulation of fibroblast-derived IL-11. J Immunology 152:2421, 1994.

107. DeMarco D, Kunkel SL, Strieter RM, et al: Interleukin-1 induced gene expression of neutrophil activating protein (interleukin-8) and monocyte chemotactic peptide in human synovial cells. Biochem Biophys Res Commun 174:411, 1991.

108. Taub DD, Conlon K, Lloyd AR, et al: Preferential migration of activated CD4+ and CD8+ T cells in response to MIP-1α and MIP-1β. Science 260:355, 1993.

109. Gauldie J, Richards C, Harnish D, et al: Interferon β₂/B-cell stimulatory factor type 2 shares identity with monocyte-derived hepatocyte-stimulating factor and regulates the major acute phase protein response in liver cells. Proc Natl Acad Sci USA 84:7251, 1987.

110. Vink A, Coulie PG, Wauters P, et al: B cell growth and differentiation activity of interleukin-HP1 and related murine plasmacytoma growth factors: Synergy with interleukin 1. Eur J Immunol 18:607, 1988.

111. Geiger T, Andus T, Bauer J, et al: Cell-free-synthesized interleukin-6 (BSF-2/IFN-β2) exhibits hepatocyte-stimulating activity. Eur J Biochem 175:181, 1988.

112. Marinkovic S, Jahreis GP, Wong GG, et al: IL-6 modulates the synthesis of a specific set of acute phase plasma proteins in vivo. J Immunol 142:808, 1989.

113. Fibbe WE, Van Damme J, Billiau A, et al: Human fibroblasts produce granulocyte-CSF, macrophage-CSF, and granulocyte-macrophage-CSF following stimulation by interleukin-1 and poly(rI)·poly(rC). Blood 72:860, 1988.

114. Mantovani L, Henschler R, Brach MA, et al: Regulation of gene expression of macrophage-colony stimulating factor in human fibroblasts by the acute phase response mediators interleukin (IL)-1β, tumor necrosis factor-α and IL-6. FEBS Lett 280:97, 1991.

115. Needleman BW, Choi J, Burrows-Mezu A, et al: Secretion and binding of transforming growth factor beta by scleroderma and normal dermal fibroblasts. Arthritis Rheum 33:650, 1990.

116. Goldring SR, Stephenson ML, Downie E, et al: Heterogeneity in hormone responses and patterns of collagen synthesis in cloned dermal fibroblasts. J Clin Invest 85:798, 1990.

117. Whiteside TL, Ferrarini M, Hebda P, et al: Heterogeneous synthetic phenotype of cloned scleroderma fibroblasts may be due to aberrant regulation in the synthesis of connective tissues. Arthritis Rheum 31:1221, 1988.

118. Korn JH: Substrain heterogeneity in prostaglandin E₂ synthesis of human dermal fibroblasts: differences in prostaglandin E₂ synthetic capacity of substrains are not stimulus restricted. Arthritis Rheum 28:315, 1985.

119. Korn JH, Brinckerhoff CE, Edwards RL: Synthesis of PGE₂, collagenase and tissue factor by fibroblast substrains: Substrains are differentially activated for different metabolic products. Coll Relat Res 5:437, 1985

120. Korn JH, Torres D, Downie E: Clonal heterogeneity in the fibroblast response to mononuclear cell derived mediators. Arthritis Rheum 27:174, 1984.

121. Needleman BW: Increased expression of intercellular adhesion molecule 1 on the fibroblasts of scleroderma patients. Arthritis Rheum 33:1847, 1990.

122. Jordana M, Schulman J, McSharry C, et al: Heterogeneous proliferative characteristics of human adult lung fibroblast lines and clonally derived fibroblasts from control and fibrotic tissue. Am Rev Respir Dis 137:579, 1988.

123. LeRoy EC: Increased collagen synthesis by scleroderma skin fibroblasts in vitro. J Clin Invest 54:880, 1974.

124. Bordin S, Page RC, Narayanan AS: Heterogeneity of normal human diploid fibroblasts: Isolation and characterization of one phenotype. Science 223:171, 1984.

CHAPTER 14

Peter K. Gregersen

Genetic Analysis of Rheumatic Diseases

The genetic factors that underlie susceptibility to the rheumatic diseases primarily involve gene families that control the immune response. By far, the best studied of these is the cluster of genes contained within the major histocompatibility complex (MHC) and encoding the human leukocyte antigens (HLAs). Not only are there a large number of HLA genes within the MHC, but a hallmark of these genes is the enormous degree of structural variability (polymorphism) in these molecules between different individuals in the population. The delineation of these HLA polymorphisms has provoked a major effort to relate these genetic differences to alterations in immune function, including the propensity to develop autoimmunity. A major portion of this chapter, therefore, is devoted to a description of the advances that have been made in this area during the past decade.

A major challenge for the late 1990s concerns the identification of additional genes outside the MHC (i.e., non-HLA genes) that may predispose to rheumatic diseases. This aspect of the field is still in the early stages of development but is progressing rapidly, fueled in part by the information being gathered by the Human Genome Project.[1] To evaluate future advances in this area, it will be important for rheumatologists to understand the concepts underlying the various approaches to the genetic analysis of rheumatic diseases, a group of illnesses that are multifactorial and likely to be genetically heterogeneous. Therefore, the second part of this chapter discusses basic genetic concepts and methods employed for the analysis of genetically complex traits.

CONCEPT OF GENETIC SUSCEPTIBILITY

In the case of simple dominant or recessive mendelian inheritance, a straightforward correlation usually exists between the inheritance of the relevant disease genes and the presence of the disease phenotype in an affected individual. For example, homozygosity for the sickle hemoglobin allele is nearly always associated with the clinical syndrome of sickle cell anemia. In contrast, inheritance of genes that predispose to autoimmunity does *not* give rise to the clinical syndrome of autoimmunity in most cases. This is demonstrated most directly by the data on disease concordance rates in monozygotic twins with autoimmune diseases.

When one monozygotic twin is affected with an autoimmune disease, the probability that the same illness will develop in other twin of the pair is approximately one in four, although the exact concordance rates vary somewhat for different rheumatic diseases. The concordance rate for clinical lupus in identical twins has been reported as 24 percent.[2] Similar concordance rates have been observed in other autoimmune diseases, such as multiple sclerosis and type I (juvenile) diabetes.[3, 4] Early studies of twin concordance for rheumatoid arthritis have also suggested that about 30 percent of monozygotic twin pairs were concordant for rheumatoid arthritis.[5] Large studies of twins in the Finnish and British populations, however, have reported concordance rates in the range of 12 to 15 percent.[6, 7] Thus, in most cases, only one member of a monozygotic twin pair is affected with these rheumatic diseases, despite their identical genetic inheritance. Clearly, other factors must come into play in causing the development of autoimmunity. These factors can be attributed to two other general sources of variation among individuals: (1) differences in exposure to disease-related environmental factors[8] and (2) differences arising out of developmental processes.[9] Thus, when one is searching for genetic factors that may predispose to autoimmunity in the general population, it must be kept in mind that these effects will be obscured by the multifactorial nature of autoimmune diseases.

The genetic influences on rheumatic diseases are usually described in terms of conferring susceptibility to, or risk for, the disease. The degree of risk conferred by a given genetic polymorphism can be calculated as the estimated relative risk, described later. This pattern of conferring genetic susceptibility for disease is typical of the associations between HLA genes and rheumatic disease and is revealed by a higher frequency of such genes in certain populations of patients compared with normal subjects. Nevertheless, the relatively low concordance rate in monozygotic twins suggests that even genes directly involved in causing autoimmunity are found in a substantial number of normal individuals in whom the disease never develops.

At first consideration, this relatively weak relationship between inheritance and autoimmunity may appear to have limited utility. However, the analysis of HLA associations with autoimmune disease has revealed the power of detailed genetic studies to suggest new hypotheses about the causes of autoimmunity. Thus, even if particular genetic factors play a role only in a subset of patients or only in certain environmental settings, they may nevertheless provide important insights into disease pathogenesis. This is a major rationale for continuing to search for additional genetic factors underlying autoimmunity.

MAJOR HISTOCOMPATIBILITY COMPLEX

The chromosomal region containing the MHC was originally identified because of the ability of genes in this region to regulate transplant rejection,[10] as well as to control the immune response of mice and guinea pigs to simple antigens,[11] a series of observations that led to the 1980 Nobel Prize. The analogous genetic region in humans was subsequently shown to encode the HLAs. The HLA molecules themselves, and their counterparts in rodents, have now been shown to be directly responsible for immune response differences between individuals as well as for determining the likelihood of graft rejection.[10–13] In addition, a large number of studies since the mid-1970s have shown that genetic variants of HLA molecules predispose to a wide variety of disorders.[14]

Function of HLA Molecules in T Cell Recognition

The proximate function of the HLA molecules encoded within the MHC is the presentation of antigenic peptides to T cells.[11–13] With some exceptions,[15] most antigen-specific T cell recognition events involve the formation of a trimolecular complex consisting of an HLA molecule and its bound peptide antigen interacting with the T cell receptor at the cell surface[16] (Fig. 14–1). The functional result of this interaction is the cross-linking of the T cell receptor and associated signal transduction into the T cell. The exact geometry of this trimolecular complex has not been established, but it is likely that the T cell receptor contacts both the bound peptide and the HLA molecule directly.[16] This requirement for MHC molecules to present antigen to T cells is frequently referred to as *MHC-restricted* T cell recognition. In each person, T cell recognition of antigen is restricted to one's own MHC molecules. Thus, allelic differences in HLA structure may result in subtle differences between individuals in the types of antigenic peptides presented or in the types of T cells used to respond to these antigens.

The model for T cell recognition shown in Figure 14–1 is highly simplified and does not reflect the participation of a large number of accessory molecules that are also involved in the activation of antigen-specific T cells. These accessory molecules include the CD3 complex and a variety of adhesion

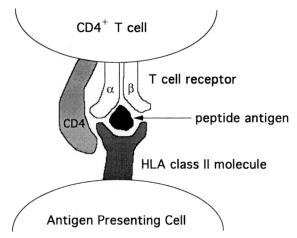

Figure 14–1. Schematic representation of major histocompatibility complex (MHC)–restricted CD4+ T cell recognition. A trimolecular complex of a T cell receptor, a peptide antigen, and an HLA molecule is formed during antigen-specific T cell recognition. The topographic details of this interaction are unknown, but it is probable that the T cell receptor makes direct contact with both the HLA molecule and its bound peptide antigen (Davis and Bjorkman: Nature 334:395, 1988).[16] In addition, accessory molecules, such as CD4, make direct contact with the HLA class II molecule. In the case of CD8+ T cells, HLA class I molecules present the bound peptide antigen for T cell receptor recognition in an analogous interaction to the one shown here.

molecules and other co-ligands (see Chapters 7 and 20). In addition, CD4+ and CD8+ T cells use different isotypes of HLA molecules for immune recognition. As shown in Figure 14–1, CD4+ T cells are generally restricted to HLA class II molecules, whereas CD8+ T cells recognize peptide antigens bound to HLA class I molecules (see later). The fact that HLA molecules are directly involved in the specificity of T cell responses has provided a rationale for the detailed investigation of their structure and diversity in the human population.

Structure of HLA Molecules

The HLA molecules encoded within the human MHC are of two basic isotypes—HLA class I and HLA class II. Their features are summarized in Figure 14–2. HLA class I molecules consist of a 45-kD α-chain encoded within the MHC, noncovalently associated with β2-microglobulin (12 kD). In contrast, HLA class II molecules consist of noncovalently associated α- (32-kD) and β- (28-kD) chains, both of which are encoded within the MHC. Both HLA class I and class II molecules are cell surface glycoproteins, anchored to the membrane by hydrophobic transmembrane segments. HLA class I molecules are distributed widely among most somatic cells of the body, with the major exception of red blood cells. In contrast, HLA class II molecules have a much more restricted tissue distribution, generally limited to cells of the immune system, such as B cells, macrophages, den-

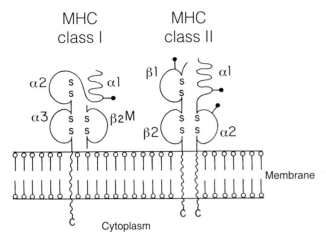

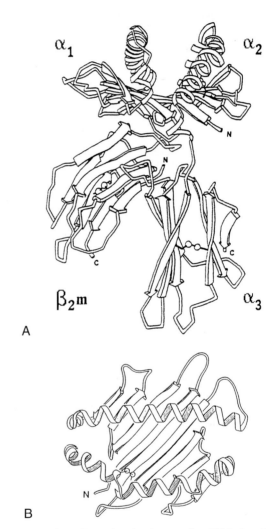

Figure 14–2. A schematic comparison of the structural features of major histocompatibility complex (MHC) class I and class II molecules. MHC class I molecules are anchored in the membrane by a single transmembrane segment contained in the 45-kD α-chain. The MHC class I α-chain is noncovalently associated with β_2-microglobulin. There are four external domains, three of which contain intramolecular disulfide bonds, as indicated. In contrast, MHC class II molecules consist of noncovalently associated α- (32-kD) and β- (28-kD) chains, both of which are anchored within the membrane. The overall domain organization of the two molecules is highly similar, however. Glycosylation sites on both molecules are indicated by a *solid circle*.

dritic cells, and some subsets of T cells. This is consistent with the fact that HLA class II molecules are primarily involved in presenting foreign antigens to CD4+ T cells during the initiation and propagation of the immune response. The expression of HLA class II molecules can also be induced on a variety of other cell types, however, by inflammatory cytokines such as γ-interferon.

A major breakthrough in the understanding of HLA molecules came in 1987, when Bjorkman and colleagues reported on the crystal structure of an HLA class I molecule.[17, 18] More recently, the structures of an HLA class II molecule[19] and of several different HLA class I alleles[20, 21] have been determined by x-ray crystallography. The similarities and differences between these homologous structures can be appreciated by examining Figures 14–3 and 14–4. In the side view of the class I molecule shown in Figure 14–3*A*, the base of the molecule (directly adjacent to the cell membrane) is formed by β_2-microglobulin and the immunoglobulin-like α3 domain. The α1 and α2 domains form a distinct cleft or groove at the top of the molecule. The function of this cleft is to bind antigenic peptides for presentation to T cells, as discussed earlier. A top view of this cleft is shown in Figure 14–3*B*. The "floor" of the peptide binding cleft consists of β-sheets, whereas the "walls" of the cleft are bounded by extended regions of α-helical structure. The cleft in HLA class I molecules is approximately 10 × 20 angstroms and generally accommodates antigenic peptides nine amino acids long.[21–25]

The structure of HLA class II molecules is analogous to class I, in that a peptide binding cleft sits on

top of a base formed by the α2 and β2 immunoglobulin-like domains. The geometry of the cleft itself is also highly similar, but not identical, to that found in the HLA class I molecule.[19] Figure 14–4 shows a comparison of the α carbon backbone of the two proteins in this region. In terms of the overall size and shape of the cleft, the two HLA molecules can almost be superimposed (see Color Plate). Subtle differences exist, however, particularly at the ends of the cleft. The α-chain of the class II molecule (shown in blue in Fig. 14–4) (see Color Plate) assumes an extended conformation instead of an α-helical structure

Figure 14–3. Three-dimensional structure of an HLA class I molecule, based on the x-ray crystallographic analysis of Bjorkman et al. (Nature 329:506, 512, 1987).[17, 18] *A*, Side view. A peptide binding cleft is formed by the α1 and α2 domains at the top of the molecule. The α3- and β_2-microglobulin domains are similar in structure to immunoglobulin domains; essentially, they act as a platform on which the peptide binding cleft rests and provide contact sites for the CD8+ molecule during CD8+ T cell recognition. *B*, Top view of the empty peptide binding cleft. This "T cell view" of the MHC molecule would normally include a peptide bound within the cleft. The disulfide bond connects the α-helix of the α2 domain with the floor of the cleft. (From Bjorkman SJ, Saper MA, Samraoui B, et al: Structure of the human class I histocompatibility antigen HLA-A2. Reprinted with permission from Nature 329:506, 1987. Copyright 1987 Macmillan Magazines Limited.)

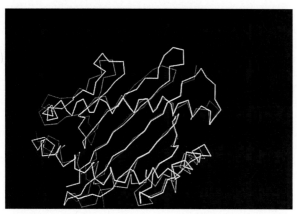

Figure 14–4. The superimposed peptide binding clefts of HLA class I and class II molecules. The alpha carbon backbone of class I is shown in red; that of HLA class II is shown in blue. Areas of complete overlap are white. The two clefts are very similar in size and shape. The major difference relates to the absence of α-helical structure in class II at the upper left hand "wall" of the cleft. Note the more extended conformation of the blue alpha carbon backbone of class II in this region. The major consequence of this and other differences is that class II molecules can bind peptides that are longer and more variable in size. (See also Color Plate.) (From Brown JH, Jardetzky TS, Gorga JC, et al. Three-dimensional structure of the human class II histocompatibility antigen HLA-DR1. Reprinted with permission from Nature 364:33, 1993. Copyright 1993 Macmillan Magazines Limited.)

at the upper left-hand section of the cleft. This results in a less rigid "wall" in this region and potentially allows an opening to form at this end of the cleft. Not shown on the diagram is the fact that the amino acid R groups at the other end of the cleft (the right-hand end in the figure) differ in size between class I and class II. A relatively bulky tyrosine is located here in class I, whereas an arginine is at this position in class II and is slightly lower in the cleft.

Several other structural features appear to distinguish class I and class II molecules, including the possibility that class II molecules may form dimers at the cell surface.[19] The most obvious consequence of these differences is an alteration in the size of the peptides accommodated by class I and class II molecules. Direct analysis of peptides bound to HLA class II molecules has shown that their size commonly varies from 12 to 19 amino acids.[24] Thus, relatively longer peptides lie in the cleft of class II molecules, possibly extending beyond the ends of the cleft, whereas class I molecules contain peptides that are much shorter and are buried down within the cleft at either end.

Intracellular Trafficking and Peptide Loading of HLA Molecules

In addition to the size difference in the peptides bound by class I and class II molecules, a fundamental difference exists in the source of these peptide antigens. In general, class I molecules present and process

peptide antigens derived from proteins that are actively synthesized within the endoplasmic reticulum of antigen-presenting cells, whereas HLA class II molecules present and process antigens taken up from outside the cell by endocytosis. These differences are reflected in the antigen-processing machinery and trafficking patterns of HLA class I and class II molecules within the cell. The cellular and molecular biology of this process are complex and have been recently reviewed.[25]

At the time of synthesis in the endoplasmic reticulum, the MHC class II α- and β-chains associate with a third polypeptide, designated the *invariant chain* (Ii; actually a group of related molecules[25]). Several functions have been ascribed to the invariant chains, including the prevention of peptide binding to the newly synthesized class II molecule and transport to endosomal compartments. When class II molecules arrive in the endosomes, the invariant chain is removed and peptides derived from external antigens are loaded onto the class II molecule. This complex is then transported to the cell surface for recognition by T cells. An important consequence of this pathway is that loading with peptides synthesized by the cell in the endoplasmic reticulum (potential autoantigens) is avoided.

In contrast, HLA class I molecules undergo peptide loading close to the time of synthesis in the endoplasmic reticulum. Indeed, a number of molecular complexes have been identified that are specifically engaged in processing and transporting peptides from the cytoplasm to the endoplasmic reticulum for loading onto class I molecules.[26] Some of the genes encoding these transporter molecules are encoded within the MHC region itself, such as the TAP1 and TAP2 genes discussed later. Thus, like class II molecules, the HLA class I molecules present at the cell surface have peptides bound in the cleft; in a normal cell, most of these peptides are derived from self proteins.[22, 23, 25]

Genetic Organization of the Human Major Histocompatibility Complex

The human MHC extends over some 4 million base pairs on the short arm of chromosome 6 (6p21.3). The HLA class I and class II gene clusters are found in distinct locations (Fig. 14–5). In addition to the HLA genes themselves, a number of other genes are dispersed throughout this genetic region, some of which are obviously related to immune function and antigen presentation, and others of which are not.

The HLA class I α-chain genes are found on the telomeric side of the cluster. HLA-A, HLA-B, and HLA-C are among the most polymorphic of these genes and are often referred to as the "classic" transplantation antigens. (As discussed earlier, HLA class I molecules consist of an α-chain noncovalently associated with β2-microglobulin. The invariant β2-microglobulin is not encoded within the MHC but, rather,

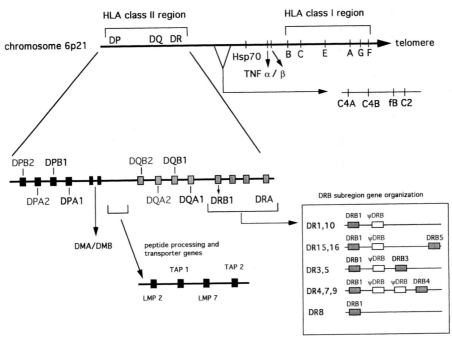

Figure 14–5. Map of the human major histocompatibility complex (MHC). The HLA class I and class II molecules are encoded in distinct regions of the MHC. In between are encoded complement components (C4A, C4B, C2, and factor B), tumor necrosis factor (TNF)-α and -β, and the heat shock protein Hsp70. The HLA class II region itself contains three subregions: DR, DQ, and DP. Each of these contains a variable number of α- and β-chain genes. HLA class II loci with known functional protein products are labeled in bold. In the case of DR, different numbers of DRB genes are present in different haplotypes. A summary of the most common of these is shown in the box. (The DR3, DR5, and DR6 group includes haplotypes carrying the DR11, DR12, DR13, and DR14 allelic families; most of these carry a functional DRB3 gene.) The DQ and DP subregions each contain one pair of functional α- and β-chain genes. A number of genes involved in antigen processing and presentation by class I molecules are situated between the DP and DQ subregions (see Germain and Margulies, Ann Rev Immunol 11:403, 1993). In addition, the DMA and DMB genes are required for normal antigen presentation by HLA class II molecules.[29, 30] (See Campbell and Trowsdale, Immunol Today 14:349, 1993, for a detailed map.[100])

on chromosome 15.) Additional ("nonclassic") class I genes have been defined more recently. These include HLA-G, whose expression appears to be limited to placental trophoblasts.[27] The HLA-E and HLA-F loci encode relatively nonpolymorphic molecules that are expressed in most tissues.

The HLA class II genes are situated centromeric to the class I genes and have a more complicated organization. There are three major subregions of the class II cluster, designated DR, DQ, and DP. Each of these subregions contains a variable number of both α- and β-chain genes. Particularly in the case of the DR subregion, this variability has led to confusion over the nomenclature to describe these genes. An international standard for this nomenclature has now been established.[28]

The DR subregion contains a single α-chain gene, designated DRA, that does not exhibit significant allelic variation. In contrast, the genes encoding the DR β-chains are highly polymorphic and vary in number among different individuals in the population. This is shown in the box at the lower right of Figure 14–5, in which several examples of common DR haplotypes are displayed. (*Haplotype* refers to a group of alleles at closely linked loci that are commonly inherited together.) Many of these DRB genes are nonfunctional pseudogenes, indicated by the symbol psi (Ψ), al-

though all haplotypes contain at least one functional DRB1 gene and many haplotypes contain a second functional DRB gene (DRB3, DRB4, or DRB5).

The DQ subregion contains one pair of functional α- and β-chain genes, designated DQA1 and DQB1. These two genes encode all the known HLA-DQ molecules. Protein products of the DQA2 and DQB2 loci have not been reported. A similar situation exists in the DP subregion, where only the DPA1 and DPB1 genes give rise to known protein products, the HLA-DP molecules.

Between the class I and class II loci are found several genes with potential relevance to immune function. These include tumor necrosis factors-α and -β (TNF-α and TNF-β) and the complement components C4A, C4B, C2, and factor B. In addition, a number of genes distributed within the class II region itself are involved in antigen processing and loading of peptides onto HLA molecules. The TAP1 and TAP2 genes have been of particular interest because they exhibit a modest degree of polymorphism and are involved in delivering peptides for loading onto HLA class I molecules.[26] More recently, genes involved in antigen presentation by HLA class II molecules have been mapped to the class II region.[29, 30] These genes have been designated DMA and DMB; their exact function is still unknown.

High Polymorphism of HLA Molecules

One of the most dramatic aspects of the HLA system is the extreme degree of polymorphism at most of the loci. The formal definition of polymorphism usually requires that the most common allele at the locus does not exceed a frequency of 98 percent. By contrast, at many HLA loci, it is uncommon for a single HLA allele to exceed a frequency of 50 percent in the population. Furthermore, the number of different alleles present in the population is much larger than in any other known polymorphic locus encoding functional genes. For example, at the HLA-A locus, 50 different alleles have been reported; at HLA-B, the number of reported alleles approaches 100. A similar degree of allelic diversity is seen at the DRB1 locus and to a lesser degree at DQA and DQB. These alleles are listed in Tables 14–1 and 14–2.

The naming of the various HLA alleles has been a major source of confusion in the literature. The difficulty with the nomenclature stems in part from the different methods used to define HLA polymorphisms. Originally, HLA class I alleles were detected through the use of alloantisera. (The prefix *allo-* refers to the genetic differences that exist between individuals of the same species. Thus, *alloantisera* are sera that detect antigenic differences between individuals in the population.) Alloantisera directed toward HLA molecules are commonly found in the context of pregnancy, in which the mother mounts an immune response against the "foreign" HLA molecules carried by the fetus (derived from the father). Anti-HLA responses are also seen after blood transfusion, because the HLA molecules on the donor cells are highly immunogenic. In the case of HLA class II alleles, differences were originally detected using mixed lymphocyte responses. When T cells from a responder are mixed with lymphocytes from another person, differences in HLA class II alleles cause the responder's T cells to proliferate. Data on mixed lymphocyte culture typing dominated this early HLA literature, and such typing was the method first used to detect the HLA class II associations with rheumatoid arthritis.[31] Subsequently, serologic methods were also used to detect class II polymorphisms.

In contrast to the early nomenclature, the current names of the HLA class I and class II alleles are attached to the specific DNA sequence and locus for each allele and thus are definitive.[28] Many older publications, however, used the previous serologic definitions of alleles, and these are also given in Tables 14–1 and 14–2. In practice, the old serologic names are often used in oral discussion because they are less cumbersome. For example, the DRB1*03011 allele is common in whites (frequency of 10 to 15 percent in many populations) and is often referred to as simply "DR3," after its original serologic designation. It should be clear from Table 14–2 that there are at least five distinct alleles that are detected by such DR3 alloantisera; therefore, the term *DR3* is imprecise; when used in the context of a discussion about white populations, however, "DR3" is often used to refer to the DRB1*03011 allele that is overwhelmingly predominant.

Linkage Disequilibrium of HLA Alleles

In addition to their highly polymorphic nature, a characteristic feature of HLA genes is the tendency for certain HLA alleles to be found together on the same haplotype. This phenomenon, referred to as *linkage disequilibrium,* is central to understanding the significance of HLA associations with disease. Linkage disequilibrium is present when the frequency of two alleles occurring together on the same haplotype exceeds that predicted by chance. For example, a common haplotype that exhibits linkage disequilibrium in the white population carries the following combination of alleles: A*0101–B*0801–DRB1*03011, commonly referred to as the A1–B8–DR3 haplotype. This haplotype is present in about 9 percent of the Danish population, a typical Northern European white group. To understand why this reflects the presence of linkage disequilibrium, consider the fact that the A1 allele is present in 17 percent of Danes and the B8 allele is present in 12.7 percent of Danes. Thus, one would expect to find them together only $12.7 \times 17 = 2.1$ percent of the time, much less than what is observed (9 percent). The extent of linkage disequilibrium is measured as the Δ value, as follows:

$$\Delta = \underset{\text{(observed)}}{0.09} - \underset{\text{(expected)}}{0.021} = 0.069$$

In general, there are two likely explanations for linkage disequilibrium:

1. The population may have originated from a mixture of two populations, one of which had a high frequency of a particular haplotype (in this case A1–B8–DR3). If this happened recently, there would not have been time (i.e., a sufficient number of generations) to randomize alleles at closely linked loci by recombination at meiosis. Inasmuch as human history is marked by large population migrations, it is probable that population admixture explains many examples of linkage disequilibrium.

2. The alleles in linkage disequilibrium may be maintained together because of a selective advantage. For example, one could argue that A1 and B8 confer an advantage for immune defense when they are present together in the same person. While this hypothesis is plausible, it is difficult to prove it for any particular haplotype, and there is no direct evidence for it.

HLA ASSOCIATIONS WITH RHEUMATIC DISEASES

Population Association Studies and Calculation of the Odds Ratio

The most straightforward way to establish whether a gene confers risk for a disease is by performing a

Table 14–1. HLA CLASS I ALLELES DEFINED AT THE HLA-A AND HLA-B LOCI

HLA-A Allele Name	HLA Specificity†	HLA-B Allele Name	HLA Specificity†	HLA-B Allele Name	HLA Specificity†
A*0101	A1	B*0701	B7	B*3801	B38(16)
A*0102	A1	B*0702	B7	B*3802	B38(16)
A*0201	A2	B*0703	B703	B*39011	B3901
A*0202	A2	B*0704	B7	B*39013	B3901
A*0203	A203	B*0801	B8	B*39021	B3902
A*0204	A2	B*0802	B8	B*39022	B3902
A*0205	A2	B*1301	B13	B*3903	B39(16)
A*0206	A2	B*1302	B13	B*3904	B39(16)
A*0207	A2	B*1401	B64(14)	B*40011	B60(40)
A*0208	A2	B*1402	B65(14)	B*40012	B60(40)
A*0209	A2	B*1501	B62(15)	B*4002	B61(40)
A*0210	A210	B*1502	B75(15)	B*4003	B40
A*0211	A2	B*1503	B72(70)	B*4004	B40
A*0212	A2	B*1504	B62(15)	B*4005	B4005
A*0213	A2	B*1505	B62(15)	B*4006	B61(40)
A*0301	A3	B*1506	B62(15)	B*4101	B41
A*0302	A3	B*1507	B62(15)	B*4201	B42
A*1101	A11	B*1508	B62(15)	B*4402	B44(12)
A*1102	A11	B*1509	B70	B*4403	B44(12)
A*2301	A23(9)	B*1510	B71(70)	B*4404	B44(12)
A*2401	A24(9)	B*1511	B15	B*4501	B45(12)
A*2402	A24(9)	B*1512	B76(15)	B*4601	B46
A*2403	A2403	B*1513	B77(15)	B*4701	B47
A*2501	A25(10)	B*1514	B76(15)	B*4801	B48
A*2601	A26(10)	B*1515	B62(15)	B*4802	B48
A*2602	A26(10)	B*1516	B63(15)	B*4901	B49(21)
A*2603	A26(10)	B*1517	B63(15)	B*5001	B50(21)
A*2604	A26(10)	B*1518	—	B*5101	B51(5)
A*2901	A29(19)	B*1519	B76(15)	B*5102	B5102
A*2902	A29(19)	B*1520	B62(15)	B*5103	B5103
A*3001	A30(19)	B*1801	B18	B*5104	B51(5)
A*3002	A30(19)	B*1802	B18	B*5105	B51(5)
A*3003	A30(19)	B*2701	B27	B*52011	B52(5)
A*31011	A31(19)	B*2702	B27	B*52012	B52(5)
A*31012	A21(19)	B*2703	B27	B*5301	B53
A*3201	A32(19)	B*2704	B27	B*5401	B54(22)
A*3301	A33(19)	B*27051	B27	B*5501	B55(22)
A*3302	A33(19)	B*27052	B27	B*5502	B55(22)
A*3401	A34(10)	B*2706	B27	B*5601	B56(22)
A*3402	A34(10)	B*2707	B27	B*5602	B56(22)
A*3601	A35	B*2708	—	B*5701	B57(17)
A*4301	A43	B*3501	B35	B*5702	B57(17)
A*6601	A66(10)	B*3502	B35	B*5801	B58(17)
A*6602	A66(10)	B*3503	B35	B*5901	B59
A*68011	A68(28)	B*3504	B35	B*6701	B67
A*68012	A68(28)	B*3505	B35	B*7301	B73
A*6802	A68(28)	B*3506	B35	B*7801	B7801
A*6901	A69(28)	B*3507	B35		
A*7401	A74(19)	B*3508	B35		
A*8001		B*3701	B37		

†The numbers in parentheses indicate the original specificities from which the current ones are derived (e.g., A23 and A24 are "splits" of A9).

Table 14–2. HLA CLASS II ALLELES DEFINED AT THE HLA-DR AND HLA-DQ LOCI

HLA-DR Allele Name	HLA-DR Specificities†	HLA-DR Allele Name	HLA-DR Specificities†	HLA-DR Allele Name	HLA-DR Specificities†	HLA-DQ Allele Name	HLA-DQ Specificities†
DRA1*0101	—	DRB1*11012	R11(5)	DRB1*1412	—	DQA1*0101	—
DRA1*0102	—	DRB1*1102	DR11(5)	DRB1*1413	—	DQA1*0102	—
DRB1*0101	DR1	DRB1*1103	DR11(5)	DRB1*1414	—	DQA1*0103	—
DRB1*0102	DR1	DRB1*11041	DR11(5)	DRB1*1415	—	DQA1*0104	—
DRB1*0103	DR103	DRB1*11042	DR11(5)	DRB1*1416	—	DQA1*0201	—
DRB1*0104	DR1	DRB1*1105	DR11(5)	DRB1*1417	—	DQA1*03011	—
DRB1*1501	DR15(2)	DRB1*1106	DR11(5)	DRB1*0701	DR7	DQA1*03012	—
DRB1*15021	DR15(2)	DRB1*1107	—	DRB1*0801	DR8	DQA1*0302	—
DRB1*15022	DR15(2)	DRB1*11081	DR11(5)	DRB1*08021	DR8	DQA1*0401	—
DRB1*1503	DR15(2)	DRB1*11082	DR11(5)	DRB1*08022	DR8	DQA1*0501	—
DRB1*1504	DR15(2)	DRB1*1109	DR11(5)	DRB1*08031	DR8	DQA1*05011	—
DRB1*1601	DR16(2)	DRB1*1110	—	DRB1*08032	DR8	DQA1*05012	—
DRB1*1602	DR16(2)	DRB1*1111	—	DRB1*08041	DR8	DQA1*05013	—
DRB1*1603	—	DRB1*1112	—	DRB1*08042	DR8	DQA1*0502	—
DRB1*1604	DR16(2)	DRB1*1113	—	DRB1*0805	DR8	DQA1*0601	—
DRB1*1605	—	DRB1*1201	DR12(5)	DRB1*0807	DR8	DQB1*0501	DQ5(1)
DRB1*1606	DR2	DRB1*1202	DR12(5)	DRB1*0806	DR8	DQB1*0502	DQ5(1)
DRB1*03011	DR17(3)	DRB1*1203	DR12(5)	DRB1*0808	DR8	DQB1*05031	DQ5(1)
DRB1*03012	DR17(3)	DRB1*1301	DR13(6)	DRB1*0809	DR8	DQB1*05032	DQ5(1)
DRB1*0302	DR18(3)	DRB1*1302	DR13(6)	DRB1*0810	DR8	DQB1*0504	—
DRB1*0303	DR18(3)	DRB1*1303	DR13(6)	DRB1*0811	DR8	DQB1*06011	DQ6(1)
DRB1*0304	DR3	DRB1*1304	DR13(6)	DRB1*09011	DR9	DQB1*06012	DQ6(1)
DRB1*0401	DR4	DRB1*1305	DR13(6)	DRB1*09012	DR9	DQB1*0602	DQ6(1)
DRB1*0402	DR4	DRB1*1306	DR13(6)	DRB1*1001	DR10	DQB1*0603	DQ6(1)
DRB1*0403	DR4	DRB1*1307	—	DRB3*0101	DR52	DQB1*0604	DQ6(1)
DRB1*0404	DR4	DRB1*1308	DR13(6)	DRB3*0201	DR52	DQB1*06051	DQ6(1)
DRB1*0405	DR4	DRB1*1309	—	DRB3*0301	DR52	DQB1*06052	DQ6(1)
DRB1*0406	DR4	DRB1*1310	DR13(6)	DRB4*01	DR53	DQB1*0606	—
DRB1*0407	DR4	DRB1*1311	DR13(6)	DRB4*01011	DR53	DQB1*0607	—
DRB1*0408	DR4	DRB1*1312	—	DRB4*01012N	DR53	DQB1*0608	—
DRB1*0409	DR4	DRB1*1313	—	DRB4*0102	DR53	DQB1*0609	—
DRB1*0410	DR4	DRB1*1401	DR14(6)	DRB4*0103	DR53	DQB1*0201	DQ2
DRB1*0411	DR4	DRB1*1402	DR14(6)	DRB5*0101	DR51	DQB1*0202	DQ2
DRB1*0412	DR4	DRB1*1403	DR14(6)	DRB5*0102	DR51	DQB1*0301	DQ7(3)
DRB1*0413	DR4	DRB1*1404	DR14(6)	DRB5*0201	DR51	DQB1*0302	DQ8(3)
DRB1*0414	DR4	DRB1*1405	DR14(6)	DRB5*0202	DR51	DQB1*03031	DQ9(3)
DRB1*0415	DR4	DRB1*1406	DR14(6)	DRB5*0203	DR51	DQB1*03032	DQ9(3)
DRB1*0416	DR4	DRB1*1407	DR14(6)	DRB6*0101	—	DQB1*0304	DQ7(3)
DRB1*0417	DR4	DRB1*1408	DR14(6)	DRB6*0201	—	DQB1*0305	—
DRB1*0418	DR4	DRB1*1409	DR14(6)	DRB6*0202	—	DQB1*0401	DQ4
DRB1*0419	DR4	DRB1*1410	DR14(6)	DRB7*01011	—	DQB1*0402	DQ4
DRB1*11011	DR11(5)	DRB1*1411	—	DRB7*01012	—		

†The numbers in parentheses indicate the original specificities from which the current ones are derived (e.g., DR15 and DR16 are "splits" of DR2).

prospective cohort study. The disease outcome in a group of individuals carrying (exposed to) the gene is compared with the outcome in a control group that does not carry the gene. The results can be displayed in a contingency table (Table 14–3A). On examination of Table 14–3A, it is apparent that the fraction of exposed individuals who contract the disease is a/(a + b), whereas the fraction of unexposed individuals who acquire the disease is c/(c + d). The ratio of these two fractions is known as the *relative risk* (RR) and is equal to a/(a + b) ÷ c/(c + d) = (ac + ad)/ (ac + bc). If the disease is rare in the population, ac is very small, and the RR is approximated by (a × d)/(b × c), also referred to as the cross-product.

In reality, such prospective cohort studies often are impractical and a retrospective case-control design is thus used. In this type of study, subjects are initially identified who have the disease, and individuals without the disease are controls. The data can be tabulated as in Table 14–3B. In this case, the cross-product (a × d)/(b × c) is known as the *odds ratio* (OR). In practice, this quantity is often reported as the estimated relative risk, since the cross-product is close to the relative risk when the disease is rare. An odds ratio of 1 indicates that the genetic factor confers no risk for the disease. An odds ratio below 1 suggests that the genetic factor under study may be negatively associated with the disease and is frequently reported as negative inverse value. Thus, an odds ratio of +0.5 may be reported as −2.0. With the exception of HLA-B27–associated diseases, most HLA associations with rheumatic diseases have odds ratios less than 10. Some of the most common of these associations are shown in Table 14–4.

Table 14–3. CONTINGENCY TABLES FOR A PROSPECTIVE COHORT STUDY AND FOR A CASE-CONTROL STUDY*

A. Prospective Cohort Study		
	Disease	*No Disease*
Exposed	a	b
Not exposed	c	d

B. Case-Control Study		
	Exposed	*Not Exposed*
Disease	a	b
No disease	c	d

*The letters a, b, c, and d stand for number of individuals observed in each category.

HLA Class I Associations: HLA-B27 and Spondyloarthropathies

One of the strongest and earliest[32] reported HLA associations with the rheumatic diseases is the association of HLA-B27 with ankylosing spondylitis. In whites, more than 90 percent of patients with ankylosing spondylitis carry HLA-B27, in contrast to approximately 8 percent of normal individuals, giving estimated relative risks of 50 to 100 in many studies.[33] This association with HLA-B27 has held up in many different population groups around the world, although the strength of the association varies with ethnicity.[33] The consistency of this finding lends support to the contention that the HLA-B27 alleles themselves are directly involved in the pathogenesis of ankylosing spondylitis. HLA-B27 is also associated with reactive arthritis, including Reiter's syndrome and the arthritis seen in the context of inflammatory bowel disease. As shown in Table 14–4, the strength of the association of HLA-B27 with these diseases is lower, in terms of estimated relative risk, than for ankylosing spondylitis.

The serologic specificity of HLA-B27 actually encompasses nine distinct HLA class I alleles. These differ from one another at a number of amino acid positions; examples are shown in Table 14–5. In white populations, B*2705 is the most common allele and is present in nearly 90 percent of the HLA-B27–positive individuals in the population. In contrast, fewer than 50 percent of HLA-B27–positive Asians carry this particular allele. The fact that these different HLA-B27 alleles are associated with disease in the various ethnic groups suggests that the differences between them are not relevant to disease. A possible exception to this is the B*2703 allele, which does not appear to be associated with risk for ankylosing spondylitis.[33] An examination of the sequences in Table 14–5 reveals that B*2703 differs from B*2705 by virtue of one substitution at position 59 (histidine for tyrosine). The presence of histidine at this position is unique among all known class I MHC molecules and thus may radically alter the function of B*2703 with respect to peptide binding, T cell recognition, or both.

Some hypotheses can be derived by combining the sequence information on the various B27 alleles with recent structural information about the HLA-B27 molecule and the peptides bound to it.[21] The structure of the B*2705 allele has been solved by x-ray crystallography, which revealed the presence of a characteristic "pocket" in the floor of the peptide binding cleft. This has been referred to as the "45 pocket," because amino acid position 45 is situated at the base of this pocket and, in the case of the B27 alleles, contains a negatively charged glutamic acid.[21] Furthermore, the peptides that bind to B27 alleles are all nine amino acids long and invariably contain a positively charged arginine at the second position from the N terminal.[21] This arginine appears to be situated within the 45 pocket when a peptide is bound to the HLA-B27 molecule. This sequence motif is distinct from peptides that are bound to other HLA class I alleles, such as HLA-A2, which lacks a glutamic acid in the 45 pocket.

A number of other sequence motifs of B27-associated peptides have also been described. These data suggest that the reason for the HLA-B27 association with spondylitic disease may relate to the specific

Table 14–4. SOME COMMON HLA ASSOCIATIONS WITH RHEUMATIC AND AUTOIMMUNE DISEASES

Disease	HLA Allele (Serologically Defined)	Approximate Allele Frequency in White Patients (%)	Approximate Allele Frequency in White Controls (%)	Approximate Relative Risk
Ankylosing spondylitis	B27	90	8	90
Reiter's syndrome	B27	70	8	40
Spondylitis or inflammatory bowel disease	B27	50	8	10
Rheumatoid arthritis	DR4	70	30	6
Systemic lupus erythematosus	DR2	45	20	3.5
	DR3	50	25	3
Multiple sclerosis	DR2	60	20	4
Juvenile diabetes	DR3	55	25	3
	DR4	75	30	6

Table 14–5. AMINO ACID DIFFERENCES IN VARIOUS SUBTYPES OF HLA-B27

Allele	Amino Acid Position										
	59	74	77	80	81	97	113	114	116	131	152
B*2701	Tyr	Tyr	Asn	Thr	Ala	Asn	Tyr	His	Asp	Ser	Val
B*2702	—	Asp	—	Ile	—	—	—	—	—	—	—
B*2703	His	Asp	Asp	—	Leu	—	—	—	—	—	—
B*2704	—	Asp	Ser	—	Leu	—	—	—	—	—	Glu
B*2705	—	Asp	Asp	—	Leu	—	—	—	—	—	—
B*2706	—	Asp	Ser	—	Leu	—	—	Asp	Tyr	—	Glu
B*2707	—	Asp	Asp	—	Leu	Ser	His	Asn	Tyr	Arg	—

peptides that are bound and presented to CD8+ T cells by these molecules. As discussed later, a number of alternative hypotheses are also plausible. In this regard, a negatively charged 45 pocket is not uniquely present in B27 alleles but is also found in class I molecules that are not associated with spondyloarthropathies.

HLA Class II Associations with Autoimmune Diseases

A large number of HLA class II associations with autoimmune diseases have been described.[14] Generally, the disease associations with HLA class II alleles are weaker and more complex than those seen with HLA-B27. Rheumatoid arthritis has received particularly intense scrutiny, but the reasons for the HLA associations with this disease are still unclear. Although HLA class II associations with rheumatoid arthritis are observed in almost every ethnic group, the particular alleles involved may differ. In addition, the relationship of HLA to disease severity is still under study. By contrast, in the case of systemic lupus and related illnesses, the HLA class II associations appear to relate primarily to the presence of specific autoantibodies or clinical phenotypes. These differences suggest that different mechanisms may be involved in the HLA associations with these diseases.

Rheumatoid Arthritis

The initial descriptions of an association between MHC genes and rheumatoid arthritis were made by Stastny in the mid-1970s.[31, 34] This was followed by a large number of studies showing that rheumatoid arthritis is associated with HLA-DR4 in many populations, with estimated relative risks between 3 and 10.[35] During the 1980s, many different HLA-DR4 alleles were defined by mixed lymphocyte culture typing[36] and subsequently by DNA sequence analysis[37] (see Table 14–2 for a list of DR4-associated DRB1 alleles). In addition, in some ethnic groups, rheumatoid arthritis is not associated with HLA-DR4 but, rather, with HLA-DR1,[38] HLA-DR10,[39] or HLA-DR14.[40] In an attempt to explain these findings, the

shared epitope hypothesis was proposed.[41] It rests on the observation that HLA-DR alleles that are associated with rheumatoid arthritis share a common amino acid sequence motif (Q K/R R A A) from residues 70 to 74 of the DR β-chain. A summary of these sequences is shown in Table 14–6. The utility of the shared epitope hypothesis to explain the HLA associations with rheumatoid arthritis has been extensively discussed and reviewed.[35, 42, 43] Nevertheless, the significance of the Q K/R R A A sequence motif for disease risk remains a topic of debate, for the following reasons.

Although the Q K/R R A A sequence (the shared epitope) on the DRB1 chain has been associated with rheumatoid arthritis in many different population groups, there are some exceptions. For example, in the American black population, a specific association with the shared epitope is not observed[44]; HLA-DR4 itself is associated weakly with rheumatoid arthritis in this ethnic group. A similar pattern of DR4 association has been reported in a New York Hispanic population.[45] In addition, the DR10 (DRB1*1001) allele, which is associated with rheumatoid arthritis in Spanish[39] and Israeli[46] populations, contains a slightly different sequence at positions 70 to 74: R R R A A. Furthermore, in some reports, the degree of risk for rheumatoid arthritis is weaker for DR1- than for DR4-associated alleles.[35, 47] These data suggest that the shared epitope may not be entirely equivalent when present in the context of different HLA-DR molecules or in the setting of different genetic backgrounds, and

Table 14–6. AMINO ACID SUBSTITUTIONS AT POSITIONS 70 TO 74 (THE "SHARED EPITOPE") OF DRB1 ALLELES ASSOCIATED WITH RHEUMATOID ARTHRITIS

DRB1 Alleles	Amino Acid Position				
	70	71	72	73	74
0101	Gln	Arg	Arg	Ala	Ala
0401	—	Lys	—	—	—
0404	—	—	—	—	—
0405	—	—	—	—	—
0408	—	—	—	—	—
1402	—	—	—	—	—
1001	Arg	—	—	—	—

therefore is not a complete explanation for the HLA associations with rheumatoid arthritis.[48]

The role of specific combinations of HLA alleles and their relation to disease severity have also been investigated. An early study of adult-type seropositive juvenile rheumatoid arthritis indicated that heterozygosity for DRB1*0401/0404 had the strongest association with disease.[49] These observations suggested that the "dosage" of DR susceptibility alleles might influence disease risk or severity. Indeed, the role of various DR4 alleles in disease severity remains under active investigation.[35, 50–56] A number of studies have reported a higher frequency of DR4 in patients with erosions[52] or extra-articular disease, such as Felty's syndrome and vasculitis.[53, 54] More recently, homozygosity for the shared epitope has been strongly associated with severe disease in a population of North American whites.[55] Early results from a 5-year prospective study in Great Britain support the view that DR1 is primarily associated with early inflammatory arthritis but that DR4 may be more specifically associated with progression to true rheumatoid arthritis.[35, 56] These long-term prospective studies, performed in different ethnic groups, will be important for sorting out the subtle differences between the various HLA alleles that share the Q K/R R A A sequence.

Systemic Lupus Erythematosus and Related Disorders

Phenotypically, systemic lupus erythematosus (SLE) is a much more heterogeneous disorder than rheumatoid arthritis, and it is therefore perhaps not surprising that the HLA associations with the disease are similarly more complicated. HLA-B8 was the first HLA allele to be associated with lupus.[57] This association was subsequently shown to be due to linkage disequilibrium (see earlier) between the serologically defined HLA-B8 and HLA-DR3 alleles; both DR3 and DR2 give higher estimated relative risks for SLE than any class I allele. It is now apparent that these HLA associations are more directly related to the presence of particular autoantibodies than to SLE itself.[58] In contrast to the findings in rheumatoid arthritis, the strongest associations involve the HLA-DQ loci, rather than HLA-DR. Furthermore, it has been proposed that an autosomal dominant "autoimmunity" gene may be involved in SLE,[59] in the setting of which particular HLA alleles may control autoantibody status or clinical phenotype. The identification of such non-HLA genes is obviously crucial to fully understanding the role of HLA in this group of diseases.

The DQ subregion presents special challenges for the newcomer to HLA, because the old serologic nomenclature does not generally have a simple correlation with a group of alleles at a single locus. Because most of the HLA correlations with autoantibodies in lupus involve the DQ loci, it is important to understand this at the outset. The problem arises because both the α- and β-chains are polymorphic in DQ molecules. This is different from HLA-DR molecules, in which the DR α-chain is essentially invariant in the population. For example, the serologic specificity of DQ2 may detect either of two related DQB1 alleles, DQB1*0201 or DQB1*0202 (see Table 14–2). In addition, the DQ2 serologic specificity also detects these alleles on several different haplotypes, which may encode quite different DQ α-chains. Thus, in white populations, the DQB1*0201 allele is commonly found on both DR3 haplotypes (in association with DQA1*0501) and DR7 haplotypes (in association with DQA1*0201), yet both these haplotypes would type serologically as DQ2. When reviewing the literature and discussing DQ polymorphisms, the reader should distinguish serologically defined polymorphisms, which may vary within the group of alleles on both the α- and β-chains, from polymorphisms defined at a specific locus (either DQA1 or DQB1).

The HLA associations with the Ro (SS-A) and La (SS-B) autoantibody systems have been the most thoroughly studied. The anti-Ro response is present in 25 to 50 percent of patients with lupus[60] and even more frequently in the setting of primary Sjögren's syndrome.[61] Although early serologic studies indicated an association with HLA-DR3 and -DR2, a detailed molecular analysis of these HLA haplotypes has provided evidence that HLA-DQ alleles in linkage disequilibrium with DR2 and DR3 are responsible for controlling this autoantibody response.[62] In addition, heterozygous individuals who inherit both a DR2–DQ1 haplotype and a DR3–DQ2 haplotype tend to have very high anti-Ro antibody titers in the setting of lupus or Sjögren's syndrome.[62] The strongest associations involve a DQA1*0501–DQB1*0201 haplotype (frequently found in linkage disequilibrium with DR3) and a DQA1*06–DQB1*06 haplotype (frequently found in linkage disequilibrium with DR2).[58]

Arnette and colleagues have attempted to further refine these associations by looking in detail at DQ alleles in Ro antibody–positive patients who do not inherit one of these two associated haplotypes. These data have led to the hypothesis that particular amino acid substitutions in the DQ α-chain (glutamine at position 34) and DQ β-chain (leucine at position 26) may contribute to the risk for development of a Ro antibody response.[58] Proof of this hypothesis is unlikely to come solely from additional genetic studies and is more likely to come from experiments that directly test the influence of these DQ polymorphisms on the immune response to specific autoantigens.[63, 64]

HLA-DQ associations have also been reported for other autoantibody systems, including antiphospholipid antibodies,[65, 66] anti-Sm responses,[67] and anti–DNA antibodies.[58] The overall pattern of HLA-DQ associations with these antibody responses is similar to patterns seen for anti-Ro responses, although the alleles involved are quite different. For some of these autoantibodies, specific amino acid substitutions have also been proposed as being of predominant importance.[58]

Population Association Studies: What Do They Mean?

Almost all of the studies on HLA and disease involve population associations that are detected by means of retrospective case-control studies. It is essential to understand the strengths and weaknesses of this approach to genetic analysis to judge the significance of these HLA associations. In general, there are three possible reasons for detecting an association between a particular allele and a disease:

1. The allele under investigation is directly involved in the pathogenesis of the disease. This assumption actually underlies most of the foregoing discussion on HLA and rheumatic disease. The studies described reflect the search for evermore precise definition of particular amino acid substitutions or structural characteristics of disease-associated alleles. This effort derives from the belief that HLA alleles themselves directly predispose to disease by virtue of their ability to control the immune response.[12] This may involve a number of mechanisms, which are discussed in the next section.

2. A gene in linkage disequilibrium with HLA may be the disease gene. As mentioned, linkage disequilibrium is a characteristic feature of the HLA region. This applies to non-HLA genes within the complex, which may themselves be directly involved in predisposing to autoimmunity. As shown in Figure 14–5, genes involved in antigen processing (TAP1 and TAP2) and complement activation (C4, C2, and factor B) and cytokines such as TNF are all encoded in this region and could potentially be responsible for disease risk. Indeed, lupus-like disease is frequently seen in the context of a variety of complement deficiencies,[68] and this may explain at least some of the HLA associations with lupus. Polymorphisms of TAP genes have been specifically investigated for their role in disease, but the results have been negative.[69, 70] Nevertheless, the possibility that these or other genes involved in antigen processing predispose to some forms of autoimmunity cannot be ruled out. Likewise, the involvement of TNF in modulating autoimmunity in animals[71] and its utility as a target for immunotherapy in humans[72] suggest that it may also be involved in genetic predisposition to autoimmune disease. As additional non-MHC genes are discovered in HLA regions, new candidate genes will emerge for testing this hypothesis.

3. The HLA associations may be artifactual as a result of population stratification of patients and controls. The potential for population stratification is a major problem in genetic epidemiology and one that is particularly relevant to population association studies. The concern is that the control group may not be genetically matched to the disease group at loci that are unrelated to disease. An extreme example of such a problem would result from the failure to study a control group that is ethnically matched to the disease group. Thus, when studying the frequency of the DRB1*0401 allele in Scandinavian patients with rheumatoid arthritis, one should not use Ashkenazi Jews as a control population, since the rarity of DRB1*0401 in the latter population would lead to false-positive results. Indeed, any number of genetically determined characteristics might vary between these two ethnic groups. For example, in doing such a study, one might also conclude that the genes controlling blue eye color also predispose to rheumatoid arthritis.

Because of this problem, retrospective use of published control frequencies for HLA alleles is not acceptable methodology, and all good HLA association studies go to great efforts to match patients and controls with regard to ethnicity. Nevertheless, it is difficult to be certain that the two populations are not stratified in some subtle way, particularly in the United States, where ethnic admixture in the population is common. The usual solutions to this difficulty are to rely on repeated studies in a new set of patients and controls and to look at HLA associations in a variety of different ethnic groups. However, a number of approaches have been described that can circumvent the problem of population stratification. These have not yet been used widely by workers in the field.

Consider the family shown in Figure 14–6. The affected child carries DR4 and DR3, each of which is inherited from one parent. The laws of mendelian inheritance require that one DR haplotype from each parent is not inherited by any given offspring—DR2 in the father and DR5 in the mother in this example. These two noninherited haplotypes can be thought of as forming a genotype for a "control" individual. In this manner, issues of population stratification are eliminated because both patients and "controls" are sampled from the identical (parental) gene pool.

This approach to disease association has been termed the *haplotype relative risk method.*[73, 74] Its validity depends on a number of assumptions; one is that the genetic marker under study does not influence mating preference or the production of gametes. Because of the potential for recombination between the marker locus and the disease locus, the haplotype relative

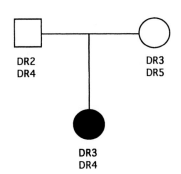

Figure 14–6. Family structure for determination of haplotype relative risk. The affected child carries the DR3 and DR4 alleles. A fictitious "control" individual can be constructed from the noninherited DR2 and DR5 alleles and used for a relative risk calculation. This method avoids potential artifacts, which result from population stratification (see text).

risk may underestimate the true relative risk. Nevertheless, this disadvantage (the need for a somewhat larger study population to achieve statistical significance) is minor compared with the elimination of artifactual results due to population stratification. Obviously, the haplotype relative risk requires the availability of parents, which may not always be possible for late-onset diseases, and requires additional expense in that two control individuals (the parents) have to be typed, instead of one. This method of analysis has been used successfully to detect HLA associations in juvenile diabetes[75] and SLE.[76]

HLA Allele Association with Autoimmune Diseases

While it is important to keep in mind these different interpretations of HLA and disease association studies, it appears likely that particular HLA alleles are directly involved in disease pathogenesis in at least some cases. In general, there are three possible mechanisms by which HLA alleles may confer disease susceptibility.

The first relates to the specific peptides that are bound by different HLA alleles. For example, as mentioned for the HLA-B27 alleles, consistent sequence motifs are present in the peptide antigens bound by these HLA molecules.[21] Thus, B27 may be biased in its ability to present particular autoantigens, or cross-reactive foreign antigens, to T cells. A similar argument can be made for HLA class II alleles associated with disease, although the sequence motifs found in peptides bound to class II molecules are generally more diverse than for class I–associated peptides.[76]

A second possibility is that the HLA molecule *itself* is an autoantigen. For example, peptides derived from HLA molecules can be found in the cleft of other HLA molecules and in some cases are recognized by T cells.[78] An interesting corollary to this idea is that molecular mimicry may occur between foreign antigens and portions of disease-associated HLA molecules.[79] Both of these models predict that peripheral T cell responses restricted to, or specific for, the disease-associated HLA allele initiate or maintain the disease process.

The hypothesis that HLA-B27 is directly involved in disease pathogenesis has led to a series of experiments with dramatic results. Taurog and colleagues have constructed transgenic rats using the human B27 gene.[80] These animals experience an illness strikingly similar to human spondyloarthropathies, particularly Reiter's syndrome. This illness appears to be mediated by bone marrow–derived cells[81] and to be specific to rats that receive the B27 allele compared with other human class I alleles. Furthermore, a germ-free environment markedly reduces the incidence of disease in the rats,[82] directly implicating a role for microbes, as in the human illness. This animal model provides an exciting opportunity to investigate disease mechanisms in detail as well as test candidate

therapies. Similar approaches to the study of rheumatoid arthritis–associated HLA alleles are being pursued.

A third mechanism by which HLA alleles may predispose to autoimmune disease relates to the role of HLA molecules in guiding the process of T cell development in the thymus. During differentiation in the thymus, thymocytes undergo a process of selection in which autoreactive T cells are deleted by programmed cell death.[83] In addition, certain T cells are positively selected, by mechanisms that are unclear.[83] Both of these selective processes are influenced by the MHC molecules present in the person.[84] Thus, the repertoire of T cell receptors (and hence the recognition capabilities) of an individual's peripheral T cell population is a direct result of this process. A series of experiments in a collagen-induced arthritis model in mice has provided evidence that thymic selection events can influence susceptibility to disease.[85]

ALTERNATIVE APPROACHES TO THE ANALYSIS OF GENETICALLY COMPLEX DISEASE

The previous discussion has focused on population association studies as the primary means of detecting the involvement of HLA or other genetic loci in rheumatic diseases. Two other methods of genetic analysis offer powerful alternatives to this approach: (1) linkage analysis of multiplex families and (2) analysis of allele sharing between affected individuals (usually siblings) within a family. Both methods are beginning to be applied to autoimmune diseases. Therefore, it is important for the rheumatologist to have some understanding of the concepts underlying these methods, since they are likely to be used extensively for the genetic analysis of rheumatic diseases in the future.

Linkage Analysis

Linkage analysis is the classic genetic approach to studying the segregation of genetic markers with disease in families. It has been used successfully in humans to map a number of single-gene disorders, which follow simple mendelian inheritance patterns. The statistical computations involved in carrying out a project in linkage analysis are formidable and are the subject of a classic textbook.[86] This section considers the principles underlying linkage analysis.

The basic purpose of linkage analysis is to determine whether a particular genetic marker and a disease (or phenotype) tend to be inherited together in families. The experimental approach to this question rests on the occurrence of recombination during the first meiotic division. This leads to the production of gametes that contain different combinations of the disease gene and any given marker gene. As discussed later, the frequency of these combinations depends on the relative locations of the disease gene and the genetic marker being examined.

Figure 14–7 illustrates the possible outcome of meiosis for two genes situated in different regions of the genome. One of the genes may carry a disease allele, D, or the corresponding wild-type (normal) allele, d, at the disease gene locus, designated *D*. A second marker gene can also carry one of two alleles, M and m, at locus *M*. In Figure 14–7A, the possible meiotic products are given when the *D* and *M* loci are on different chromosomes and the parent is heterozygous at both loci (genotypes D/d and M/m). Because

the two chromosomes segregate independently, the four meiotic products occur with equal frequency (25 percent each for D/M, D/m, d/M, and d/m). In Figure 14–7B, the two loci are on the same chromosome but are widely separated. In this case, the four possible meiotic products also occur with equal frequency, because the likelihood of a crossover (recombination) event occurring between the two loci is high, effectively producing random combinations of marker and disease alleles in the meiotic products. (At least one recombination event occurs in every chromosome at every meiosis. On average, about 66

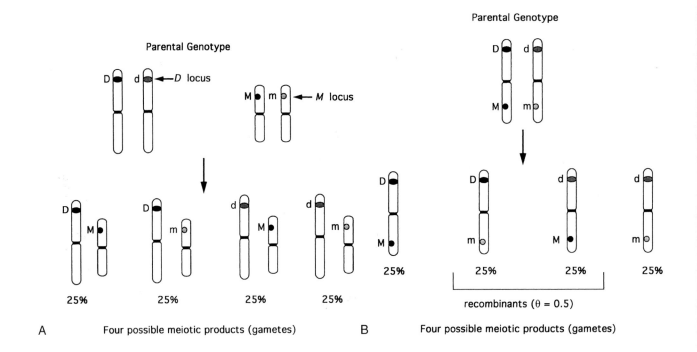

Figure 14–7. Segregation of alleles at the *M* and *D* loci depends on their relative locations. *A,* These loci are on different chromosomes, and thus the four combinations of alleles occur with equal frequency in the meiotic products. *B,* The *M* and *D* loci are far apart on the same chromosome, and thus recombination during the first meiotic division again results in an equal distribution of the four meiotic products. *C,* The *M* and *D* loci are close to one another in the same chromosomal region, which makes recombination between them an uncommon event during meiosis. The frequency of recombination, in this case 10 percent, is expressed as the recombination fraction, $\theta = 0.1$.

recombination events at each meiosis are spread over the 23 chromosomes. This number is slightly higher for females and slightly lower for males.)

The situation in Figure 14–7C is slightly different. In this case, the D and M loci are close together on the same chromosome. Therefore, the likelihood that recombination will occur between them is low but not zero. The same four meiotic products can occur but at different frequencies. Two of the meiotic products are recombinants and in this case constitute 10 percent of the total. This quantity is called the *recombination fraction*, θ. When 10 percent of the meiotic products are recombinants, θ = 0.1. If the marker gene is extremely close to or identical with the disease gene, θ = 0; no recombinants would be observed in the meiotic products.

Now let us apply these principles to the two families with an autosomal dominant disease shown in Figure 14–8. In family "A," two of the four children with the disease inherit the marker allele M from their affected father (through the grandmother), whereas the unaffected children do not inherit the M allele. In this family, marker M segregates with the disease. Can we conclude that marker M is linked to the disease locus? Remember, we do not know at the outset whether the M locus is near to the disease

locus. It could be that D and M are far apart (θ = 0.5). If this is the case, what is the probability that the co-segregation of disease with marker M happened by chance in family "A"? Going back to Figure 14–7A and B, it can be seen that half of the father's meiotic products that carry the disease allele (D) are expected to also carry M, if D and M are unlinked (θ = 0.5). Therefore, the probability that D will always segregate with M (and d with m) in four of four offspring is $(1/2)^4$ = 1 in 16, even if the M and D loci are on different chromosomes. Obviously, we cannot conclude anything with certainty on the basis of family "A" alone. If 10 offspring were available for analysis, however, as shown in family "B," with the same pattern of complete co-segregation between the disease and the marker allele M, chance alone would be unlikely to explain this pattern. In this case, the probability would be $(1/2)^{10}$ = 1 in 1024, and linkage between M and the disease would be highly likely, although not certain.

In practice, the calculation of a likelihood ratio is used to derive conclusions from such family data. In the case of family "B" (see Fig. 14–8), the best fit for the data is that the disease locus and marker M are close to or identical to one another (θ = 0). If this is the case, the probability of observing the outcome

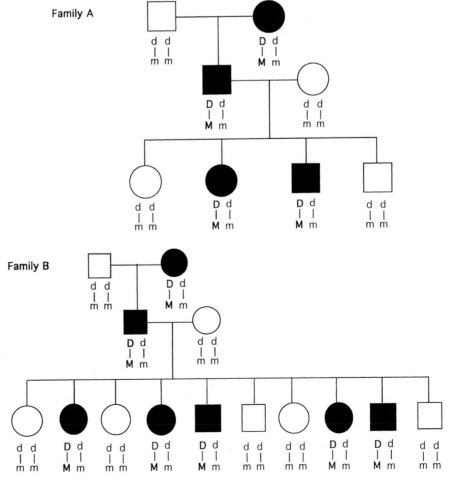

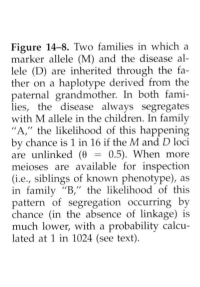

Figure 14–8. Two families in which a marker allele (M) and the disease allele (D) are inherited through the father on a haplotype derived from the paternal grandmother. In both families, the disease always segregates with M allele in the children. In family "A," the likelihood of this happening by chance is 1 in 16 if the M and D loci are unlinked (θ = 0.5). When more meioses are available for inspection (i.e., siblings of known phenotype), as in family "B," the likelihood of this pattern of segregation occurring by chance (in the absence of linkage) is much lower, with a probability calculated at 1 in 1024 (see text).

shown in family "B" is 1. On the other hand, if the disease gene and the marker allele M are nowhere near each other (θ = 0.5), the likelihood of observing the pattern of segregation in family "B" is 1 in 1024, as discussed earlier. The ratio of these two probabilities is termed the *likelihood ratio*, Z(θ).

$$Z(\theta) = \frac{L(\theta)}{L_{(1/2)}} = \frac{\text{likelihood of the data if } \theta = 0}{\text{likehood of the data if } \theta = 0.5} = \frac{1}{1/1024} = 1024$$

The $\log_{10}$ of this ratio is referred to as the *LOD score*. In this case, the LOD score is slightly greater than 3. For the purpose of linkage analysis, an LOD score of 3 is considered a statistically significant result and is used as a cutoff. Thus, family "B" provides enough information to conclude that the marker locus is very near the disease locus.

In linkage studies, a candidate genetic marker is often near, but not immediately adjacent to, the disease gene (0 < θ < 0.5). Suppose, for example, that one of the ten offspring in family "B" is affected in the absence of the marker allele M. Assuming that the *M* and *D* loci are linked, this would imply that recombination between the marker locus and the disease locus occurs 10 percent of the time. In this case, the LOD score would be calculated on the basis of using the probability of the data if θ = 0.1 in the numerator of the likelihood ratio, Z(θ). In practice, the calculations for a large amount of family data are done with various values of θ to determine which θ gives the best fit for the data and therefore the highest LOD score. For example, Table 14–7 is taken from recently published data on linkage between the HLA region and ankylosing spondylitis.[87] In this analysis, LOD scores of 3 or higher are obtained at many different values of θ, with the maximum at θ = 0.05. Of course, a maximum LOD score at θ = 0.05 does not necessarily imply that the actual recombination frequency between the disease locus and the HLA locus is 5 percent. Indeed, the data in Table 14–7 show a significant LOD score at θ = 0. Thus, it is highly likely that a gene in the HLA region, presumably the HLA-B gene itself, is involved in ankylosing spondylitis.

Perhaps the best example of the successful use of linkage methods in mapping a rheumatic disease is familial Mediterranean fever (FMF). FMF is known to be transmitted as an autosomal recessive trait and thus is well suited to linkage analysis. A study of 27 families (involving about 120 meioses) led to the localization of the FMF gene to chromosome 16.[88] The relevant genetic region has been narrowed down to a relatively small area (less than 10^6 base-pairs) at 16p13.3.[89] It is likely that the specific genetic defects or defects in FMF will be identified in the near future as a direct consequence of this mapping effort.

Allele-Sharing Methods

One of the drawbacks to classic linkage analysis is that, to be most useful, it requires some knowledge about the genetic model underlying the disease (e.g., dominant versus recessive, penetrance values, genetic homogeneity of the disease). In contrast, allele-sharing methods require no knowledge about the underlying genetic model, a feature that is particularly attractive for the study of autoimmune diseases, which have a complex genetic basis.[90]

The most common approach to allele sharing is the *affected sibling pair method*. This method is based on a simple question: when two siblings are both affected with a disease, do they share particular genetic markers more frequently than would be expected by chance? By the laws of mendelian inheritance, both parental alleles should be shared by two siblings 25 percent of the time, one allele should be shared 50 percent of the time, and there should be no sharing of parental alleles in the remaining 25 percent of sibling pairs. A significant deviation from this 25:50:25 distribution toward sharing of particular alleles in affected sibling pairs implies a role for that genetic region in the disease. The closer the marker is to the disease locus (θ close to 0), the greater the deviation will be from a 25:50:25 distribution, the fewer sibling pairs will be required to detect a significant difference, or both.

These relationships can be appreciated by examining Figure 14–9. The segregation of a disease gene with a marker locus (with alleles i, j, k, and l in the parents) is shown for a sample mating. If the marker locus is distant from the disease locus, free recombination occurs between the two loci, and eight possible genotypes occur in the offspring. If one randomly selects twice from the offspring who carry the disease allele, D (i.e., affected sibling pairs), there is a 25:50:25 probability of sharing two, one, or no markers in common. If the marker locus is very near or identical to the disease locus (θ = 0), however, the probability that two affected sibs will share two, one, or no marker alleles is 50:50:0.

This method is most powerful when the parental origin of all the markers is known and when sibling "identity by descent" can be unequivocally established. In some cases, the parents are not available and one can establish only "identity by state." In this case, corrections have to be made for the possibility that a shared allele may have been present in and transmitted from different parents. One important feature of affected sibling pair analysis is that if par-

Table 14–7. LOD SCORES BETWEEN ANKYLOSING SPONDYLITIS AND THE HLA REGION AT VARIOUS RECOMBINATION FRACTIONS

Number of Pedigrees	Recombination Fraction (θ)					
	0.0	*0.01*	*0.05*	*0.1*	*0.2*	*0.3*
13	3.27	3.36	3.48	3.29	2.47	1.40

Adapted from Rubin LA, Amos CI, Wade JA, et al: Investigating the genetic basis for ankylosing spondylitis. Arthritic Rheum 37:1212, 1994.

Parental Haplotypes

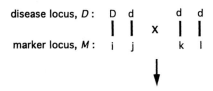

disease locus, *D* :   D   d   d   d

marker locus, *M* :   i   j   k   l

possible genotypes of offspring:

Free recombination (θ = 0.5) between *D* and *M* loci	Di/dk Di/dl Dj/dk Dj/dl di/dk di/dl dj/dk dj/dl
No recombination (θ = 0) between *D* and *M* loci	Di/dk Di/dl dj/dk dj/dl

Figure 14–9. The possible genotypes of offspring of a mating in which both parents are heterozygous at a marker locus: i, j, k, and l signify alleles at locus *M*. If the marker locus is not near to the disease locus, *D*, eight possible genotypes can be found in the children, four of which contain the disease allele, D. If the marker locus and the disease locus are close or identical (θ = 0), only four genotypes will be observed in the offspring, two of which carry the disease allele, D. Conceptually, affected sibling pair analysis involves picking consecutively from these possibilities at random and determining whether the frequency at which marker alleles are shared differs from that predicted under free recombination. Under free recombination, it would be expected that 25 percent of the time, two affected siblings would not share any marker allele in common (e.g., for two siblings with the genotypes Di/dk and Dj/dl). In contrast, if there is no recombination between the marker locus and the disease gene (θ = 0), there would always be sharing of at least one marker allele (e.g., allele i). At intermediate values of θ, the absence of allele sharing would occur but significantly less frequently than 25 percent.

ents are available, the unaffected siblings are not used for the calculations, so false-negative assignment of phenotypes will not affect the results. This is vastly different from classic linkage analysis, in which false assignment of a family member as unaffected can confound the results. This aspect of sibling pair analysis is particularly appealing for a disease such as rheumatoid arthritis, which may not manifest itself until late in life, and therefore the assignment of unaffected status is never certain.

The affected sibling pair method has been used to study a variety of autoimmune diseases.[91, 92] The most dramatic results have been obtained in juvenile onset diabetes, in which up to 18 different chromosomal regions have been tentatively identified as relevant to disease.[91] It is doubtful that all of these regions will turn out to be significant, but this result does emphasize the complexity of the genetic background involved in these diseases. Recently, affected sibling pair analysis has also been used to investigate the role of T cell receptor β genes in rheumatoid arthritis.[93] One marker within the T cell receptor β gene cluster yielded a result of borderline significance (P = .005). (An LOD score of 3 [equivalent to P = .001] is generally required to establish linkage. Indeed, even lower P values may be appropriate for reaching significance in sibling pair analysis.[90])

Future of Genetics in the Rheumatic Diseases

Until now, the search for additional, non-HLA genes involved in autoimmunity have focused primarily on candidate gene families such as T cell receptor, immunoglobulin, and cytokine genes. The results so far have been conflicting and inconclusive.[93–98] Efforts to define the genetic basis of rheumatic diseases are certain to expand in the near future, however, and will probably use a combination of population association studies, linkage analysis, and allele-sharing methods.

These approaches will be strengthened by the large number of informative genetic markers, designated *microsatellites*, that are being identified throughout the human genome. Microsatellite markers consist of unique genetic regions that contain repeated elements, most often dinucleotide repeats; the number of these repeats commonly varies greatly between individuals. Several thousand microsatellites have been identified and assigned to specific chromosomal regions.[1, 90] For the study of human disease, the remaining problem is to gather large numbers of multiplex families and affected sibling pairs. This task is beginning to be taken on by a number of groups for various diseases.[91, 99] In addition, microsatellite-based methods are being used to clarify the genetic basis of animal models of autoimmunity, and this may lead to the identification of candidate genes relevant to human disease.[98] It is reasonable to expect that when additional genes involved in autoimmunity are identified, it will result in a much better understanding of the pathogenesis of these diseases, with attendant benefits for diagnosis and therapy.

References

1. Cox DR, Green ER, Lander ES, et al: Assessing mapping progress in the Human Genome Project. Science 265:2031, 1994.
2. Deapen D, Escalante A, Weinrib L, et al: A revised estimate of twin concordance in systemic lupus erythematosus. Arthritis Rheum 35:311, 1992.
3. Olmos P, Hern RA, Heaton DA, et al: The significance of the concordance rate for type I (insulin-dependent) diabetes in identical twins. Diabetologia 31:747, 1988.
4. Ebers GC, Bulman DE, Sadovnick AD, et al: A population-based study of multiple sclerosis in twins. N Engl J Med 315:1638, 1986.
5. Lawrence JS: Rheumatoid arthritis: Nature or nurture? Ann Rheum Dis 28:257, 1970.
6. Aho K, Koskenvuo M, Tuominen J, et al: Occurrence of rheumatoid arthritis in a nationwide series of twins. J Rheumatol 13:899, 1986.
7. Silman AJ, MacGregor AJ, Thomson W, et al: Twin concordance rates for rheumatoid arthritis: Results from a nationwide study. Br J Rheumatol 32:903, 1993.
8. Jarvinen P, Aho K: Twin studies in rheumatic diseases. Semin Arthritis Rheum 24:19, 1995.
9. Gregersen PK: Discordance for autoimmunity in monozygotic twins: Are "identical" twins really identical? Arthritis Rheum 36:1185, 1993.
10. Snell GD, Dausset J, Nathenson SG: Histocompatibility. New York, Academic Press, 1976.
11. Benacerraf B: Role of MHC gene products in immune regulation. Science 212:1229, 1981.
12. McDevitt HL, Benacerraf B: Genetic control of specific immune responses. Adv Immunol 11:31, 1969.
13. Schwartz RH: T lymphocyte recognition of antigen association with gene products of the major histocompatibility complex. Annu Rev Immunol 3:237, 1985.
14. Tiwari JL, Terasaki PI: HLA and Disease Associations. Berlin, Springer-Verlag, 1985.

15. Beckman EM, Porcellii SM, Morita CT, et al: Recognition of a lipid antigen by CD1 restricted α/β + T cells. Nature 372:691, 1994.
16. Davis MM, Bjorkman PJ: T cell antigen receptor genes and T cell recognition. Nature 334:395, 1988.
17. Bjorkman PJ, Saper MA, Samraoui B, et al: Structure of the human class I histocompatibility antigen, HLA-A2. Nature 329:506, 1987.
18. Bjorkman PJ, Saper MA, Samraoui B, et al: The foreign antigen binding site and T cell recognition regions of class I histocompatibility antigens. Nature 329:512, 1987.
19. Brown JH, Jardetzky TS, Gorga JC, et al: Three dimensional structure of the human class II histocompatibility antigen HLA-DR1. Nature 364:33, 1993.
20. Garrett TPJ, Saper MA, Bjorkman PJ, et al: Specificity pockets for the side chains of peptide antigens in HLA-Aw68. Nature 342:692, 1989.
21. Madden DR, Gorga JC, Strominger JL, et al: The structure of HLA-B27 reveals nonamer self-peptides bound in an extended conformation. Nature 353:321, 1991.
22. Hunt DF, Henderson RA, Shabanowitz J, et al: Characterization of peptides bound to the class I MHC molecule HLA-A2.1 by mass spectrometry. Science 255:1261, 1992.
23. Rammensee H-G, Falk K, Rotzschke O: Peptides naturally presented by MHC class I molecules. Annu Rev Immunol 11:213, 1993.
24. Engelhard VH: Structure of peptides associated with class I and class II MHC molecules. Annu Rev Immunol 12:181, 1994.
25. Germain RG, Margulies DH: The biochemistry and cell biology of antigen processing and presentation. Annu Rev Immunol 11:403, 1993.
26. Neefjes JJ, Momburg F, Hammerling GJ: Selective and ATP-dependent translocation of peptides by the MHC-encoded transporter. Science 261:769, 1993.
27. Kovats S, Main EK, Librach C: A class I antigen, HLA-G, expressed in human trophoblasts. Science 248:220, 1990.
28. Bodmer JG, Marsh SGE, Albert ED, et al: Nomenclature for factors of the HLA system, 1994. Tissue Antigens 44:1, 1994.
29. Morris P, Shaman J, Ataya M, et al: An essential role for HLA-DM in antigen presentation by class II major histocompatibility molecules. Nature 368:551, 1994.
30. Fling SP, Arp B, Pious D: HLA-DMA and -DMB genes are both required for MHC class II/peptide complex formation in antigen presenting cells. Nature 368:554, 1994.
31. Stastny P: Mixed lymphocyte culture typing cells from patients with rheumatoid arthritis. Tissue Antigens 4:571, 1974.
32. Brewerton DA, Caffrey M, Hart FD, et al: Ankylosing spondylitis and HLA-B27. Lancet 1:904, 1973.
33. Khan MA, Kellner H: Immunogenetics of spondyloarthropathies. Rheum Dis Clin North Am 18:837, 1992.
34. Stastny P: Association of the B-cell alloantigen DRw4 with rheumatoid arthritis. N Engl J Med 298:869, 1978.
35. Ollier W, Thompson W: Population genetics of rheumatoid arthritis. Rheum Dis Clin North Am 18:741, 1992.
36. Reinsmoen NL, Bach F: Five HLA-D clusters associated with HLA-DR4. Hum Immunol 4:249, 1982.
37. Gregersen PK, Shen M, Song Q, et al: Molecular diversity of HLA-DR4 haplotypes. Proc Natl Acad Sci USA 83:2642, 1986.
38. Nichol RE, Woodrow J: HLA-DR antigens in Indian patients with rheumatoid arthritis. Lancet 1:220, 1981.
39. Sanchez B, Moreno I, Jagarino R, et al: HLA-DRw10 confers the highest susceptibility to rheumatoid arthritis in a Spanish population. Tissue Antigens 36:174, 1990.
40. Wilkens RF, Nepom GT, Marks CR, et al: Associations of HLA-Dw16 with rheumatoid arthritis in Yakima Indians. Arthritis Rheum 34:43, 1991.
41. Gregersen PK, Silver J, Winchester RJ: The shared epitope hypothesis: An approach to understanding the molecular genetics of susceptibility to rheumatoid arthritis. Arthritis Rheum 30:1205, 1987.
42. Winchester R, Dwyer E, Rose S: The genetic basis of rheumatoid arthritis: The shared epitope hypothesis. Rheum Dis Clin North Am 18:761, 1992.
43. Nepom GT, Nepom BS: Prediction of susceptibility to rheumatoid arthritis by human leukocyte typing. Rheum Dis Clin North Am 18:785, 1992.
44. McDaniel O, Reveille JD, Pratt PW, et al: The large majority of African-American patients with seropositive RA do not possess the "rheumatoid epitope" (abstr). Arthritis Rheum 37:S169, 1994.
45. Teller K, Budhai L, Davidson A: Non-Caucasian populations with RA: The shared epitope hypothesis may not apply (abstr). Arthritis Rheum 37:S373, 1994.
46. Gao X, Gazit E, Livneh A, et al: Rheumatoid arthritis in Israeli Jews: Shared sequences in the third hypervariable region of DRB1 alleles are associated with susceptibility. J Rheumatol 18:801, 1991.
47. Ploski R, Mellbye OJ, Roinningen KS, et al: Seronegative and weakly seropositive rheumatoid arthritis differ from clearly seropositive rheumatoid arthritis. J Rheumatol 21:1397, 1994.
48. Dizier M-H, Eliaou J-F, Babron M-C, et al: Investigation of the HLA component involved in rheumatoid arthritis (RA) by using the marker association segregation X^2 (MASC) method: Rejection of the unifying shared epitope hypothesis. Am J Hum Genet 53:715, 1993.
49. Nepom B, Nepom GT, Schaller J, et al: Characterization of specific HLA-DR4 associated histocompatibility molecules in patients with juvenile rheumatoid arthritis. J Clin Invest 74:287, 1984.
50. Salmon M, Wordsworth P, Emery P, et al: The association of HLA-DR beta alleles with self-limiting and persistent forms of early symmetrical polyarthritis. Br J Rheum 32:628, 1993.
51. Walker DJ, Griffiths M, Dewar P, et al: Association of MHC antigens with susceptibility to and severity of rheumatoid arthritis in multicase families. Ann Rheum Dis 44:519, 1985.
52. Young A, Jaraquemada D, Awad J, et al: Association of HLA-DR4/Dw4 and DR2/Dw2 with radiologic changes in a prospective study of patients with rheumatoid arthritis: Preferential relationship with HLA-Dw rather than HLA-DR specificities. Arthritis Rheum 27:20, 1984.
53. Klouda PT, Corbin SA, Bidwelll JL, et al: Felty's syndrome and HLA-DR antigens. Tissue Antigens 27:112, 1986.
54. Hillarby MC, Hopkins J, Grennan DM: A re-analysis of the association between rheumatoid arthritis with and without extra-articular features, HLA-DR4 and DR4 subtypes. Tissue Antigens 37:39, 1991.
55. Weyand CM, Hicok KC, Conn DL, et al: The influence of HLA-DRB1 genes on disease severity in rheumatoid arthritis. Ann Intern Med 117:801, 1992.
56. Thompson W, Pepper L, Payton A, et al: Absence of an association between HLA-DRB1*04 and rheumatoid arthritis in newly diagnosed cases from the community. Ann Rheum Dis 52:539, 1993.
57. Grumet FC, Coukell A, Bodmer JG, et al: Histocompatibility HLA antigens associated with systemic lupus erythematosus: A possible genetic predisposition to disease. N Engl J Med 285:193, 1971.
58. Arnett FC, Reveille JD: Genetics of systemic lupus erythematosus. Rheum Dis Clin North Am 18:865, 1992.
59. Bias WB, Beatty TLH, Meyers DA, et al: Evidence that autoimmunity in man is a mendelian dominant trait. Am J Hum Genet 39:584, 1986.
60. Hamilton RG, Harley JB, Bias WB, et al: Two Ro(SS-A) autoantibody responses in systemic lupus erythematosus: Correlation of HLA-DR/DQ specificities with quantitative expression of Ro(SS-A) autoantibody. Arthritis Rheum 31:496, 1988.
61. Harley JB, Alexander EL, Arnett FC, et al: Anti-Ro/SSA and anti-La/SSB in patients with Sjögren's syndrome. Arthritis Rheum 29:196, 1986.
62. Harley JB, Reichlin M, Arnett FC, et al: Gene interaction at HLA-DQ enhances autoantibody production in primary Sjögren's syndrome. Science 232:1145, 1986.
63. Hoffman RW, Takeda Y, Sharp GC, et al: Human T cell clones reactive against U-small nuclear ribonucleoprotein autoantigens from connective tissue disease patients and healthy individuals. J Immunol 151:6460, 1993.
64. Mamula MJ, Fatenejad S, Craft J: B cells process and present lupus autoantigens that initiate autoimmune T cell responses. J Immunol 152:1453, 1994.
65. Arnett FC, Olsen ML, Anderson KL, et al: Molecular analysis of major histocompatibility complex alleles associated with the lupus anticoagulant. J Clin Invest 87:1490, 1991.
66. Gulko PS, Reveille JD, Koopman WJ, et al: Anticardiolipin antibodies in systemic lupus erythematosus: Clinical correlates, HLA associations, and impact on survival. J Rheumatol 20:1684, 1993.
67. Olsen ML, Arnett FC, Reveille JD: Contrasting molecular patterns of MHC class II alleles associated with the anti-Sm and anti-RNP precipitin autoantibodies in systemic lupus erythematosus. Arthritis Rheum 36:94, 1993.
68. Moulds JM, Drych M, Holers VM, et al: Genetics of the complement system and rheumatic diseases. Rheum Dis Clin North Am 18:893, 1992.
69. Wordsworth BP, Pile KD, Gibson K, et al: Analysis of the MHC-encoded transporters TAP1 and TAP2 in rheumatoid arthritis: Linkage with DR4 accounts for the association with a minor TAP2 allele. Tissue Antigens 42:153, 1993.
70. Burney RO, Bile KED, Gibson K, et al: Analysis of the MHCV class II encoded components of the HLA class I antigen processing pathway in ankylosing spondylitis. Ann Rheum Dis 53:58, 1994.
71. Keffer J, Probert L, Cazlaris H, et al: Transgenic mice expressing human tumour necrosis factor: A predictive genetic model of arthritis. EMBO J 10:4015, 1991.
72. Elliott MJ, Maini RN, Feldman M, et al: Randomized double blind comparison of chimeric monoclonal antibody to tumour necrosis factor-alpha (cA2) versus placebo in rheumatoid arthritis. Lancet 344:1105, 1994.
73. Falk CR, Rubinstein P: Haplotype relative risks: An easy, reliable way to construct a proper control sample for risk calculations. Ann Hum Genet 51:227, 1987.
74. Knapp M, Seuchter SA, Baur MP: The haplotype relative risk (HRR) method for analysis of association in nuclear families. Am J Hum Genet 52:1085, 1993.
75. Rubinstein P, Walker M, Carpenter C, et al: Genetics of HLA disease

associations: The use of the haplotype relative risk (HRR) and the "haplo-delta" (Dh) estimates in juvenile diabetes from three racial groups. Hum Immunol 3:384, 1981.

76. Seuchter SA, Knapp M, Hartung K, et al: Testing for associations in SLE families. Genet Epidemiol 8:409, 1991.

77. Hill CM, Liu A, Marshall KW, et al: Exploration of requirements for peptide binding to HLA DRB1*0101 and DRB1*0401. J Immunol 152:2890, 1994.

78. Liu Z, Sun YK, Xi YP, et al: Contribution of direct and indirect recognition pathways to T cell alloreactivity. J Exp Med 177:1643, 1993.

79. Roudier J, Petersen J, Rhodes G, et al: Susceptibility to rheumatoid arthritis maps to a T cell epitope shared by the HLA-Dw4 DR beta 1 chain and the Epstein-Barr virus glycoprotein gp 110. Proc Natl Acad Sci USA 86:5104, 1989.

80. Hammer RE, Maika SD, Richardson JA, et al: Spontaneous inflammatory disease in transgenic rats expressing HLA-B27 and human β2m: An animal model of HLA-B27 associated human disorders. Cell 63:1099, 1990.

81. Breban M, Hammer RE, Richardson JA, et al: Transfer of the inflammatory disease of HLA-B27 transgenic rats by bone marrow engraftment. J Exp Med 178:1607, 1993.

82. Taurog JD, Richardson JA, Croft JT, et al: The germfree state prevents development of gout and joint inflammatory disease in HLA-B27 transgenic rats. J Exp Med 180:2359, 1994.

83. Blackman M, Kappler J, Marrack P: The role of the T cell receptor in positive and negative selection of developing T cells. Science 248:1335, 1990.

84. Sprent J, Gao E-K, Webb SR: T cell reactivity to MHC molecules: Immunity versus tolerance. Science 248:1357, 1990.

85. David CS: Genes for MHC, TCR and Mls determine susceptibility to collagen-induced arthritis. APMIS 98:575, 1990.

86. Ott J: Analysis of Human Genetic Linkage. Baltimore, Johns Hopkins University Press, 1992.

87. Rubin LA, Amos CI, Wade JA, et al: Investigating the genetic basis for ankylosing spondylitis. Arthritis Rheum 37:1212, 1994.

88. Pras E, Aksentijevich I, Gruberg L, et al: Mapping of a gene causing familial Mediterranean fever to the short arm of chromosome 16. N Engl J Med 326:1509, 1992.

89. Ajksentijevich I, Chen X, Levy E, et al: Genetic and physical localization of the gene causing familial Mediterranean fever (abstr). Am J Hum Genet 55:A253, 1994.

90. Lander ES, Schork NJ: Genetic dissection of complex traits. Science 265:2037, 1994.

91. Davies JL, Kawaguchi Y, Bennett ST, et al: A genome-wide search for human type 1 diabetes susceptibility genes. Nature 371:130, 1994.

92. Seboun E, Robinson MA, Doolittle TH, et al: A susceptibility locus for multiple sclerosis is linked to the T cell receptor β chain complex. Cell 57:1095, 1989.

93. McDermott M, Kastner DL, Holloman JD, et al: The role of T cell receptor β chain genes in susceptibility to rheumatoid arthritis. Arthritis Rheum 38:91, 1995.

94. Scofield RH, Frank MB, Neas BR, et al: Cooperative association of T cell beta receptor and HLA-DQ alleles in the production of anti-Ro in systemic lupus erythematosus. Clin Immunol Immunopathol 72:335, 1994.

95. Charmley P, Nepom BS, Concannon P: HLA and T cell receptor beta chain DNA polymorphisms identify a distinct subset of patients with pauciarticular onset juvenile rheumatoid arthritis. Arthritis Rheum 37:695, 1994.

96. Moxley G: Variable-constant segment genotype of immunoglobulin kappa is associated with increased risk for rheumatoid arthritis. Arthritis Rheum 35:19, 1992.

97. Singh R, Mullinax PF, Moxley G: Systemic lupus erythematosus is not associated with allotypic markers of immunoglobulin kappa in Caucasians. J Rheumatol 21:839, 1994.

98. Theofilopoulos AN: The basis of autoimmunity: Part II. Genetic predisposition. Immunol Today 16:150, 1995.

99. Hay EM, Ollier WE, Silman AJ: The Arthritis and Rheumatism Council's national family material repository. Br J Rheumatol 32:443, 1993.

100. Campbell RD, Trowsdale J: Map of the human MHC. Immunol Today 14:349, 1993.

CHAPTER 15

Immune Complexes and Complement*

George Moxley
Shaun Ruddy

When antibodies bind to antigens to form immune complexes, immune recognition is linked to protective biologic consequences by means of receptors for the immunoglobulin Fc portions and for complement cleavage fragments. Combining viral protein and antibody, for example, influences the immune response to that protein[1, 2] and starts the complement cascade. Portions of the C1q, C4, and C3 complement components modify the immune complex structure and thereby inhibit precipitation in tissues or solubilize already deposited complexes. Complement fragments coating the immune complex interact with complement receptors on various cell surfaces, modifying immune complex processing and enhancing delivery to phagocytic cells.[3]

Secondary antibody responses directed toward T cell–dependent antigens and generation of memory B cells and plasma cells are highly dependent on immune complexes. Germinal centers of lymphoid tissues contain a network of follicular dendritic cells. The follicular dendritic cell surface displays immune complexes that contain intact antigens and fixed complement for extended periods, even longer than a year. Each germinal center attracts three B cell precursors on average, and these precursors undergo clonal expansion and hypermutation of the rearranged immunoglobulin variable (V) region genes (somatic mutation). If the B cell surface immunoglobulin binds tightly to complexed antigen on the follicular dendritic cell, such B cells may then take antigen from the follicular dendritic cell, process it, and present it to T cells. Under T cell influence, germinal center B cells may undergo apoptosis, may emerge as memory B cells undergoing isotype switching, or may further differentiate into plasma cells.[4, 5] The presence of immune complexes on follicular dendritic cells, therefore, is essential to secondary antibody responses and B cell memory.[6, 7]

Fcγ receptors (FcγR) also link immune complexes with cellular effects. The three closely related FcγR families are FcγRI (CD64), FcγRII (CD32), and FcγRIII (CD16).

The high-affinity immunoglobulin G (IgG) receptor, FcγRI, binds monomeric IgG, occurs constitutively on monocytes and macrophages, and may be induced on neutrophils and eosinophils. The low-affinity IgG receptor, FcγRII, is widely expressed on immune and inflammatory cells and binds immune complexes. FcγRIII has either medium or low affinity and binds monomeric IgG and immune complexes. FcγRIII is expressed constitutively on macrophages, natural killer cells, mast cells, some T cells, and some monocytes, and occurs inducibly on monocytes and eosinophils. Immune complexes cause cellular effects by cross-linking Fcγ receptors.[8]

These FcγR-mediated effects include phagocytosis; superoxide generation; cytotoxicity (FcγRIII); mediator release (lysosomal enzymes, tumor necrosis factor-α [TNF-α], IL-1, and IL-6); enhancement of antigen presentation (FcγRIIb2, FcγRIII, and the IgE receptor FcεRII); and regulation of immunoglobulin production (FcγRIIb1).[9–11] Allelic variations of certain Fcγ receptors exist and may have pathogenetic importance. One FcγRII allotype (the LR allotypic form of FcγRIIa receptor) is the only Fcγ receptor that binds the IgG2 subclass; the lack of this allotype may confer risk for infections with bacteria such as *Haemophilus influenzae* and *Streptococcus pneumoniae*. Similarly, allotypic forms of FcγRIII may also make one susceptible to bacterial infections.[10]

Immune complexes can be cleared from the circulation by interaction with complement and Fc receptors.[12] Because individuals with inherited complement deficiencies frequently experience diseases associated with immune complex–mediated injury,[13, 14] complement-related interactions are important to immune complex clearance. Following immune complex formation, complement may be activated with resulting C3b deposition on the immune complex. The C3b-opsonized immune complex then may bind to a nearby erythrocyte through clustered CR1 (C3b) receptors.

Platelets also have complement receptors, such as CR2 (C3d receptor), CR3 (C3bi receptor), and membrane cofactor protein, but they do not have CR1. Platelets are less important than erythrocytes in immune complex clearance. After passing through the hepatic or splenic circulation, the fixed mononuclear cells remove the immune complexes from the erythrocyte.[14] The immune complexes engage the fixed mononuclear cell system in liver and spleen primarily through surface Fc receptors and not complement

---

*Supported by National Institutes of Health Grant Nos. AR38478, AR07079, and AI28532; the Arthritis Foundation; and the Alpha Omicron Pi Foundation.

receptors. Some disease states, such as systemic lupus erythematosus (SLE), show impaired immune complex clearance.[12]

The venerated idea that immune complexes cause disease began with von Pirquet's observations on serum sickness. Eight to 12 days after an initial injection of horse serum, patients experienced urticaria, fever, edema, and arthralgias; the reaction to a second injection was more rapid and more severe. Von Pirquet suggested that when the immunogens interacted with host antibodies, resulting toxic substances caused clinically apparent illness.[15] Germuth[16] and Dixon and colleagues[17] supported this proposed mechanism with evidence from an animal model of serum sickness. Cardiovascular and renal manifestations due to tissue deposition of immune complexes occurred at the same time that both antigen and specific antibody occurred in the circulation. They proposed that the antigen and antibody had interacted in the circulation, deposited locally, and resulted in anaphylactic and inflammatory responses.

That immune complexes cause disease has been central to the notion that rheumatoid arthritis, SLE, and other illnesses are autoimmune diseases. This theory also helps to explain such diverse diseases as glomerulonephritis and vasculitis, as well as certain manifestations of subacute bacterial endocarditis and other infectious diseases.[1, 2] Chapters on immune complexes in previous editions of this book have analyzed evidence of pathogenetic mechanisms in immune complex diseases. In some conditions, immune complexes form in the circulation and then localize in various tissues to cause inflammation; a prime example is serum sickness. In others, immune complexes form in interstitial fluids and cause local inflammation. A classic example is the *Arthus reaction*, in which antigens injected intradermally combine with antibody found in the interstitial fluid to trigger inflammation at the site of injection. Because animals deficient in Fc receptors have an attenuated Arthus reaction, immune complex–mediated tissue injury is started by cell surface Fc receptors and then amplified through mediator release and local complement activation.[18]

Not all immune complexes are alike in their capacity to induce tissue damage. Antigens differ in size, charge, and ability to bind to macromolecules. For example, multivalent antigens such as polysaccharides and proteins favor lattice formation and precipitation. Positively charged antigens can bind to anionic tissue sites. This may relate to histone deposition in lupus nephritis or antigenic localization in reactive arthritis.[19] Similarly, antibodies may differ in isotype, valence, affinity, relative charge, and ability to activate complement. IgM, particularly pentameric IgM, fixes complement well, but IgA does not. IgG subclasses vary in complement fixation. IgG1 and IgG3 are quite effective, IgG2 is moderately effective, and IgG4 does not bind complement. The structural basis of this subclass variation includes a single amino acid differ-

ence in the second heavy chain domain (C_H2), namely *proline* in IgG1 versus *serine* in IgG4 at position 331.[20]

IgG subclasses also vary in binding Fcγ receptors. IgG1 and IgG3 bind tightly to FcγRI, IgG4 binds less well, and IgG2 does not bind at all. The structural basis is a short stretch of amino acids in the C_H2 domain (positions 234 to 236). For the FcγRII family, IgG3 and IgG1 bind best, and IgG2 binding shows an allotypic difference.[10] The FcγRIII family binds IgG2 and IgG4 poorly. The structural variation responsible for FcγRII binding pattern appears to reside in the IgG C_H2 domain, and that for FcγRIII pattern in the C_H3 domain.[20] The proportions of antigen and antibody contained in the complex vary, and, depending on the antibody isotype, rheumatoid factors may bind.

Other important pathogenetic factors in immune complex disease include local blood flow patterns, changes in vascular permeability, altered phagocytic function, and the effects of released complement fragments. In addition, the bound complement fragments modify the immune complexes and route them to complement receptors on cell surfaces for further modification and ultimate disposition.[3] Large complexes (favored by antibody excess) activate complement well and are rapidly cleared through binding to cell surface receptors. Small complexes (favored by antigen excess), which do not activate complement as well, are not very inflammatory. Complexes of intermediate size, which escape clearance mechanisms and activate complement well, are the most effective in inducing tissue damage. In any patient, when one samples immune complex levels in the circulation, there is likely to be various sizes and compositions of immune complexes. Therefore, immune complex diseases reflect the sum of various immune complex effects.

METHODS THAT DEMONSTRATE CIRCULATING IMMUNE COMPLEXES

In tissues, immune complexes are identified by indirect immunofluorescence methods, which detect granular deposits of immunoglobulin and complement. In biologic fluids, one can easily detect immune complexes if the antigen is known; for example, a virus or viral product in a complex may be precipitated with antibodies directed toward immunoglobulin or complement, or may be sedimented rapidly together with immunoglobulin in the ultracentrifuge.

Detecting specific antigens in circulating immune complexes can be helpful in linking etiologic agents to specific illnesses. For example, the vasculitic illness type II cryoglobulinemia occurs with complexed polyclonal IgG plus monoclonal IgM rheumatoid factor. With availability of hepatitis C tests, not only was there frequent evidence of hepatitis C infection in the circulation,[21, 22] but there also was antibody directed toward hepatitis C and hepatitis C RNA concentrated in the cryoglobulin.[22] Similarly, in persons suspected of having Lyme disease but seronegative for anti–Lyme antibody, antibody to *Borrelia burgdorferi* in immune complexes provides an explanation of the seronegative illness.[23, 24] In some disorders of unknown etiology, however, including many rheumatic diseases, nonspecific methods detect materials with attributes of immune complexes, such as bound complement fragments or high molecular weight.

There are more than 40 different antigen-nonspecific methods. Seven of the most commonly used are described in Table 15–1. Most methods detect aggregated γ-globulin, not just immune complexes, and therefore are subject to interference by heating of sera or freeze–thaw effects. There are substantial biases in the kinds of immune complexes detected.

Some methods react more with large immune complexes. Some ignore materials between the size of monomeric IgG and pentameric IgM (200 to 900 kD).[25] Some see only certain immunoglobulin isotypes. Variation within and between assays may exceed 50 percent and is highest for the Raji cell assay.[25] The use of heat-aggregated γ-globulin as the standard accounts for part of this variation. In one collaborative survey, the range of values obtained by the various laboratories for an unknown, namely tetanus-antitetanus at 40 μg/ml, was 35 to 1420.[26] Because of this variation among laboratories, some have proposed international standards for immune complexes,[26] but this idea has not gained wide acceptance. *Therefore, the technical characteristics of the assays do not favor uniform*

Table 15–1. COMMONLY USED ANTIGEN-NONSPECIFIC ASSAYS FOR CIRCULATING IMMUNE COMPLEXES

Assay	Properties Allowing Detection	Complex Size Bias[25]	Isotypes Detected	Confounding Factors
Fluid phase C1q binding[94]	Binding of radiolabeled C1q to complex Insolubility in 2.5% PEG	Large	IgG1, IgG2, IgG3, pentameric IgM	Heparin, C-reactive protein, rheumatoid factor
Solid phase C1q[95]	Binding of complex to C1q adsorbed on microtiter well		Monomeric IgG1, IgG2, IgG3	Rheumatoid factor; often reflects anti-C1q antibody[41, 42]
	Detection by radiolabeled antibody		Monomeric and pentameric IgM	
Raji cell[96]	Display of C3bi or C3dg on complex Binding to CR2 on Raji cell Detection by radiolabeled anti-IgG	Large	IgG, IgM	EDTA, heat inactivation, rheumatoid factor, anti-lymphocyte antibody[97]
Monoclonal rheumatoid factor (RF)[98]	Competition with IgG immunosorbent for binding to radiolabeled rheumatoid factor Competition with radiolabeled aggregated γ-globulin for binding to solid phase rheumatoid factor	Large	IgG1, IgG2, IgG4	DNA, rheumatoid factor
Staphylococcal binding[99]	Binding to protein A of *Staphylococcus aureus* Removal of monomeric IgG by competition with rabbit IgG Detection by radiolabeled anti-human IgG	Minimal	IgG1-4, IgA1, IgM	Rheumatoid factor, endotoxin, heparin
Conglutinin[100]	Display of C3bi on complex Binding via C3bi on conglutinin coated on microtiter well Developed with labeled anti-IgG or staphylococcal protein A	Large	IgG, IgM	Endotoxin, heparin, EDTA, heat inactivation
Anti-C3[101]	Display of C3 on complex Binding to C3-specific monoclonal antibody coated on microtiter well Detection by labeled anti-human immunoglobulin	Not addressed		Not addressed

Abbreviations: CR2, complement receptor 2; EDTA, ethylenediamine tetraacetic acid; Ig, immunoglobulin; PEG, polyethylene glycol.

detection of all sizes and kinds of immune complexes or following levels except in serially obtained specimens compared in the same assay.

USE OF IMMUNE COMPLEX ASSAYS IN RHEUMATIC DISEASES

The various immune complex assays may distinguish patients with certain rheumatic diseases from normal persons. The accuracy in rheumatoid arthritis, SLE, or vasculitis is illustrated in Table 15–2. Even studies using the same published assay method show a wide range of values, such as the fluid-phase C1q binding assay for SLE. Despite the variation among studies, the positive and negative predictive values tell the empirical usefulness in distinguishing diseased from normal individuals.

The most useful positive test for distinguishing patients with rheumatoid arthritis from normal persons is the staphylococcal binding assay, followed closely by the Raji cell assay; the most useful negative test in excluding rheumatoid arthritis is the fluid phase C1q binding assay. For distinguishing SLE from normal, the most useful test, if positive, is the staphylococcal binding test followed closely by the Raji cell assay; the diagnostic accuracy of the Raji cell assay for SLE partly reflects anti-lymphocyte assay. In contrast, the most useful test in excluding SLE, if negative, is the monoclonal rheumatoid factor test, followed by the solid phase C1q binding assay.

For the diseases characterized by vasculitis, the most useful positive tests are the monoclonal rheumatoid factor and staphylococcal binding assays, and the most useful negative tests are the Raji cell and staphylococcal binding assays. Antigen-nonspecific immune complex assays may be positive in any of the diseases listed in Table 15–3. Although positive immune complex assays have no differential diagnostic value, they often reflect certain clinical subsets of disease. When compared with the immune complex levels in patients with rheumatoid arthritis restricted to the joints, levels from patients with extra-articular forms of rheumatoid arthritis (such as rheumatoid nodules and Sjögren's syndrome) were higher in several studies.[27] Patients with rheumatoid vasculitis also have positive test results more frequently[28] and typically have higher levels of immune complexes.[29] Overall, these levels are higher in the more complicated forms of rheumatoid arthritis, but the difference in positive frequency is not enough to allow reliable identification of the clinical subset.

In patients with SLE, no particular clinical manifestations correlate with the presence of antigen-nonspecific immune complexes as detected by the solid phase C1q binding assay, but patients with skin disease alone do not have positive immune complex test results.[30] This is similar to demonstrating tissue-associated immunoglobulin and complement in clinically normal skin by the lupus band test: In discoid lupus, the results are negative; in SLE, about half the patients have positive results.[31] In a study of patients with lupus nephritis, the levels of reactivity detected by the solid phase C1q binding assay were twice as high in diffuse proliferative as in membranous lupus glomerulonephritis, and this was due to material the size of monomeric IgG.[32] One study of SLE patients using the Raji cell assay showed a positive correlation with the numbers of organ systems involved,[33] and a second correlated with central nervous system involvement.[34]

In patients with cutaneous vasculitis of either the necrotizing or the lymphocytic type, the presence of fluid phase C1q binding activity was found to a far greater extent in the group with necrotizing vasculitis.[35] In one study of patients with scleroderma, those with positive Raji cell test results more frequently had diffuse disease, tendon friction rubs, and positive results for antinuclear antibodies, and those with positive fluid phase C1q binding assays had more pulmonary involvement and were positive for rheumatoid factors.[36] A second scleroderma study showed that results for fluid phase C1q binding, solid phase C1q binding, and conglutinin binding assays were only infrequently positive.[37]

Immune complex assays have sometimes been used as indices of disease activity. An analysis of immune complex assays in rheumatic disease activity is included in a previous edition of this book.[38] To summa-

Table 15–2. PREDICTIVE VALUE OF IMMUNE COMPLEX ASSAYS*

Assay	Positive Predictive Value			Negative Predictive Value		
	RA	*SLE*	*Vasculitis*	*RA*	*SLE*	*Vasculitis*
Fluid phase C1q	88	91	67	81	50	76
Solid phase C1q	82	95	70	73	64	73
Raji cell	96	97	74	57	56	87
Monoclonal rheumatoid factor	92	85	90	54	66	58
Staphylococcal binding	98	99	92	63	42	90
Conglutinin	86	94	71	51	50	87

*This table represents accuracy in comparison between each clinical group and normal individuals. The figures reflect the mean, weighted for number of subjects, of all studies identified by use of Grateful Med with search terms for disease and prognosis or activity and antigen–antibody complex or immune complex.
Abbreviations: RA, rheumatoid arthritis; SLE, systemic lupus erythematosus.

Table 15–3. DISEASES ASSOCIATED WITH POSITIVE RESULTS FOR IMMUNE COMPLEXES

Rheumatic Diseases

Rheumatoid arthritis and Felty's syndrome
Primary Sjögren's syndrome
Juvenile rheumatoid arthritis
Systemic lupus erythematosus
Scleroderma
Mixed connective tissue disease
Seronegative spondyloarthropathies
 Reiter's syndrome
 Ankylosing spondylitis[102]
 Psoriasis
Behçet's syndrome, idiopathic inflammatory bowel disease
Vasculitis
 Mixed cryoglobulinemia
 Polyarteritis nodosa
 Wegener's granulomatosis
 Serum sickness
 Henoch-Schönlein purpura
 Hypocomplementemic cutaneous vasculitis
Infectious arthritides
 Lyme disease
 Viral arthritides
Sarcoidosis

Neoplastic Disease (including but not limited to):

Solid tumors (e.g., melanomas)
Lymphoproliferative disorders

Glomerulonephritides

Bacterial Infections (including but not limited to):

Endocarditis
Meningococcal infection
Gonococcemia
Streptococcal infections
Syphilis
Chronic infections, such as in patients with underlying cystic fibrosis
Recurrent infections in children
Otitis media

Viral Infections (including but not limited to):

Cytomegalovirus
Hepatitis B
Infectious mononucleosis
Acquired immunodeficiency syndrome (AIDS)
AIDS-related complex[103]

Various Parasitic Infections (such as toxoplasmosis and quartan malaria)

Many Other Disorders (including inflammatory bowel disease, myocardial infarction, sickle cell anemia, atopic conditions, and other less common diseases)

Data from Williams RC: Immune Complexes in Clinical and Experimental Medicine. Cambridge, Harvard University Press, 1980; and Theofilopoulos AN, Dixon FJ: The biology and detection of immune complexes. Adv Immunol 28:89, 1979.

rize, except for the solid phase C1q binding assay in SLE, no assay for circulating immune complexes uniformly assesses or predicts rheumatic disease activity. The solid phase C1q binding assay has generally correlated strongly with various measures of lupus disease activity, including arthritis and nephritis; the exception is that skin disease alone was not associated with positive test results.[30] Correlation of disease severity with solid phase C1q binding has been confirmed,[39] and positive test results are found with most

flares of lupus.[40] Despite the empirical value, the positive assay result may reflect an artifactual reactivity from anti-C1q antibody rather than true immune complexes.[41, 42]

Summary of Clinical Uses

Circulating immune complex assays may be useful in *categorization*. Specifically, a disease state typically characterized by immune complexes, such as early rheumatoid arthritis, might be distinguished from a condition in which there are typically no immune complexes, such as arthralgia.[43] Preliminary indications are that a positive result would be likely to suggest rheumatoid arthritis with 75 percent accuracy, and a negative result would be likely to suggest arthralgia with slightly over 80 percent accuracy[43]; this has not been confirmed by other published reports. One can probably sharpen this distinction by the judicious repetition of the assay; if the results are again positive, it is more likely that the true underlying cause of the joint pain is related to a disease associated with immune complexes. The optimal clinical use of these assays requires careful consideration of disease likelihood before obtaining the study.

The second clinical setting is the assessment of *disease activity*. However, other tests for disease activity not only reflect the actual clinical state better but are cheaper, such as the Westergren erythrocyte sedimentation rate (ESR) for rheumatoid arthritis or temporal arteritis. For SLE, however, there may continue to be a role for some immune complex assays. Specifically, the solid phase C1q binding together with anti-DNA antibodies[44, 45] and levels of C3 and C4 may be used to assess and predict disease activity. To avoid the considerable assay-to-assay variation, side-by-side comparison of serially obtained specimens should be performed.

COMPLEMENT ACTIVATION

The complement system includes 14 plasma proteins that interact in a cascade sequence to mediate a variety of inflammatory effects, including the opsonization of particles for phagocytosis, activation of leukocytes, and assembly of the membrane attack complex (MAC).[46–48] Six plasma proteins and five integral membrane proteins regulate this cascade (Table 15–4).[49] Recognition of activating agents by either of two proteolytic pathways (Fig. 15–1) leads to a final common sequence that assembles the MAC (Fig. 15–2). The *classical activation pathway*—so called because it was discovered first—is triggered primarily by immune complexes formed from the union of IgG or IgM antibodies with their antigens. The *alternative pathway*—phylogenetically the more primitive—is activated principally by repeating polysaccharides and similar polymeric structures.[50, 51] Activation by either pathway generates enzymes with identical specificity:

Table 15-4. PROTEINS OF THE COMPLEMENT SYSTEM

Complement System and Components	Molecular Weight (kD)	Mean Serum Concentration (µg/ml)	Cleavage Fragments
Classical Activation Pathway			
C1q	410	70	—
C1r	83	35	—
C1s	83	35	—
C4	209	430	C4a, C4b, C4c, C4d
C2	110	25	C2a, C2b
Alternative Activation Pathway			
Properdin	220	25	—
D	23.5	2	—
B	93	250	Bb, Ba
C3	195	1300	C3a, C3b, C3c, C3d, C3g
Terminal Sequence			
C5	190	75	C5a, C5b
C6	128	60	—
C7	121	55	—
C8	153	80	—
C9	79	160	—
Plasma Control Proteins			
C1 inhibitor	105	200	—
C4 binding protein	550	250	—
Factor H	150	360	—
Factor I	88	35	—
Anaphylatoxin inactivator	310	40	—
S-protein (vitronectin)	83	500	—
Membrane Control Proteins			
Complement receptor 1 (CD35)	190–280	—	—
Membrane cofactor protein (MCP)	45–70	—	—
Decay-accelerating factor (DAF)	70	—	—
Homologous restriction factor	65	—	—
Membrane inhibitor of reactive lysis (CD59)	18	—	—

Both pathways cleave the third complement component, C3, releasing the 8000-kD activation peptide C3a and generating nascent C3b that has a metastable thioester bond capable of reacting with amino or hydroxyl groups on the activating agent or adjacent cell membranes, linking C3b to them covalently.[52, 53] Both pathways also lead to cleavage of C5 and assembly of the membrane attack complex from the terminal sequence (C5b-9).[54, 55]

Classical Activation Pathway

C1 is a calcium-dependent pentamolecular complex of one molecule of C1q with two molecules of C1r and C1s. The C1q molecule bears six globular heads that are recognition units for sites on the Fc portions of immunoglobulins and probably for other activators of the classical pathway, including lipopolysaccharide and porins from gram-negative bacteria and ligand-bound C-reactive protein.[56–58] The binding of two or more recognition heads of C1q to an activator induces a rearrangement in C1r, converting it to a protease that cleaves and activates both itself and C1s. The natural substrates of the active C$\overline{1s}$ protease are C4 and C2. Both are cleaved, releasing activation pep-

tides. The major fragments join in a magnesium-dependent enzyme complex, C$\overline{4b2b}$, the classical pathway C3 convertase. C4 resembles C3 in that it also contains a labile thioester bond. Cleavage to C4b generates a nascent binding site capable of forming covalent amide or ester linkages with nearby proteins or carbohydrates. Normal serum contains an α_2-neuraminoglycoprotein member of the serpin family, the C1 inhibitor, which complexes with both C$\overline{1s}$ and C$\overline{1r}$, irreversibly blocking the activities of these proteases and thereby preventing the activation of C1s and the cleavage of C4 and C2. Formation of the classical pathway convertase is also inhibited by proteins that bind to C4b and inhibit its complexing with C2b. These include C4 binding protein (C4BP), complement receptor 1 (CR1), and decay-accelerating factor (DAF).[59] C4BP and CR1 also act as cofactors for factor I, which further cleaves C4b into two inactive fragments, C4c and C4d.

Alternative Activation Pathway

Activation of the alternative pathway does not require antibody and is triggered by polysaccharides such as those found in the coats of yeasts, pneumo-

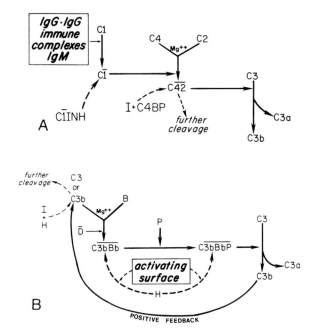

Figure 15–1. Pathways for complement activation. *A,* Classical pathway. *B,* Alternative pathway.

cocci, and many gram-negative bacteria.[50, 51] In a reaction strikingly similar to that of the classical pathway, four factors participate in the formation of the alternative pathway convertase. Factor $\overline{D}$, C3, and factor B are the homologous proteins for C1s, C4, and C2, respectively. An extra protein, *properdin,* serves to stabilize the magnesium-dependent complex enzyme C3 convertase, $\overline{C3bBb}$, which is identical to $\overline{C4b2b}$ in its capacity to cleave C3 and C5 and to initiate the terminal sequence. Just as cleavage of C4 to C4b reveals a site for interaction with C2, cleavage of C3 to C3b permits its participation in a complex with factor B. Cleavage of C3b-bound B by $\overline{D}$ yields $\overline{C3bBb}$. Unlike C1, factor $\overline{D}$ already exists in plasma in its active form. Control of proteolysis is limited by the availability of substrate: $\overline{D}$ acts only on B that has complexed with C3b, and not on free or unbound B.

A positive feedback or amplification loop is built into the alternative pathway. C3b, the product of the cleavage reaction catalyzed by $\overline{C3bBb}$, is itself capable of complexing with additional B, making it susceptible to cleavage by $\overline{D}$, thereby producing additional $\overline{C3bBb}$. Uncontrolled cycling of this loop is prevented by the following reactions: (1) CR1, DAF, and factor H dissociate the $\overline{C3bBb}$ complex, rendering it inactive; and (2) factor I further degrades C3b in the presence of CR1, MCP, or factor H, yielding C3c and C3dg.[60, 61]

Agents that trigger the alternate pathway do so by protecting newly formed $\overline{C3bBb}$ from dissociation and degradation by the control proteins. These agents increase the formation of the alternative pathway convertase by transforming an inefficient fluid phase reaction into effective assembly of the C3bBb complex on a surface. In the fluid phase, a small amount of C3 is continuously being hydrolyzed at its internal

thioester bond,[62] inducing a conformational change in C3 that permits B to complex with it and become susceptible to cleavage by $\overline{D}$. This reaction generates small amounts of C3 convertase and produces small amounts of C3b equivalents. If C3b binds to the surface of host cells, regulatory mechanisms involving factor H, CR1, and MCP prevent further activation. Binding of C3b to foreign activators provides a haven on which the small amount of C3b produced by the fluid phase reactions can be deposited and protected from the action of control proteins.

Terminal Sequence

Assembly of the MAC from the terminal components (C5 to C9) leads to membrane damage.[63] Binding of C3b to $\overline{C4b2b}$ forms a trimolecular complex that efficiently cleaves C5; binding of a second C3b molecule to $\overline{C3bBb}$ has the same effect. The C5 convertases of both the classical and alternative pathways cleave C5 at the same site, yielding the 11-kD activation peptide, C5a, and the remainder of the molecule, C5b. Activated C5b has a specific metastable binding site for C6 and combines with it to form $\overline{C5b6}$, which reacts with C7. Attachment of the nascent hydrophobic $\overline{C5b67}$ complex to cell membranes is the first step in assembling the MAC. Addition of C8 to the complex induces some membrane damage, but formation of a stable transmembrane channel requires the binding of up to 14 molecules of C9, which polymerize to form the mature MAC. The C5b-9 complex is inserted through the lipid bilayer of the cell membrane, with hydrophobic residues on the exterior in contact with the lipid bilayer, and leads to osmotic lysis of the cell. C9 is homologous, both in amino acid sequence and function, to perforins, the pore-forming proteins found in cytotoxic T lymphocytes and the granules of eosinophils.

Action of the membrane attack complex is regulated by the glycolipid-anchored membrane proteins homologous restriction factor and membrane inhibitor of reactive lysis (CD59).[49, 64] Both of these proteins

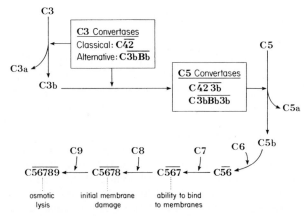

Figure 15–2. Assembly of the membrane attack complex.

prevent membrane damage by MACs formed from plasma proteins of the same species as the cells on which they are located, thereby protecting host cells from lysis as innocent bystanders during complement activation.[65] Vitronectin, or S-protein, which prevents the insertion of the $C\overline{5b67}$ complex into the lipid bilayer of cell membranes, probably also protects host cells from lysis.[66, 67]

BIOLOGIC CONSEQUENCES OF COMPLEMENT ACTIVATION (Table 15–5)

Although assembly of the C5b-9 complex and membrane damage is the most notorious effect of complement activation, a variety of other inflammatory events also ensue. These include changes in vascular permeability that have been associated with the cleavage of C4 and C2 by C1 and that may explain the pathogenesis of the angioedema associated with C1 inhibitor deficiency in hereditary angioedema.[68] The active enzyme $C\overline{3bBb}$ is chemotactic for polymorphonuclear neutrophils (PMNs). The Bb fragment of factor B induces peritoneal macrophages to spread and increase their surface area. The activation peptides C3a and C5a are anaphylatoxins capable of inducing the secretion of histamine by mast cells and basophils. The degranulating effects on skin mast cells are observable at concentrations of 10^{-12} and 10^{-15} M for C3a and C5a, respectively. Both peptides also possess smooth muscle contractile activity that is independent of histamine release. The anaphylatoxic activities are blocked by cleavage of the terminal arginine from either C3a or C5a by carboxypeptidase N, a magnesium-dependent enzyme, which also has been termed the *anaphylatoxin inactivator*. C5a activates neutrophils and monocytes by means of a specific receptor, leading to increases in intracellular calcium, mobilization of membrane arachidonate, degranulation, production of oxygen free radicals, increased expression of adhesion molecules, chemokinesis, and chemotaxis.

Table 15–5. BIOLOGIC ACTIVITIES OF COMPLEMENT ACTIVATION

Product	Activity
C4, C2 kinin	Increase in vascular permeability; putative mediator of edema in hereditary angioedema
C3bBb	Chemotaxis of polymorphonuclear leukocytes
Bb	Spreading of monocytes
C3a	Anaphylatoxin: release of histamine from basophils and mast cells, serotonin from platelets, contracts smooth muscle
C5a	Anaphylatoxin: same activities as C3a on mast cells; activation and chemotaxis of monocytes and polymorphonuclear leukocytes
C5b-9	Membrane attack complex: formation of transmembrane channels leading to cytolysis

The biologic activities of C3b and its degradation products iC3b and C3dg are governed by the types of cells bearing the receptors to which they bind (Table 15–6).[69] In addition to its function as a regulator of complement activation, CR1 on the membranes of erythrocytes promotes the clearance of immune complexes by binding and transporting them to the liver and spleen, where they are removed from the circulation by sinusoidal macrophages.[70] CR1 on PMNs and monocytes enhances the phagocytosis of C3b-coated particles by these cells.

CR2, the receptor for C3d and C3dg, is present on B lymphocytes in a membrane complex that also contains CD19, a member of the immunoglobulin superfamily, as well as three other proteins of 130, 50, and 20 kD.[71, 72] Interaction of this complex with polymeric C3dg lowers the threshold for signaling B lymphocytes by means of antigen-specific membrane IgM. The Epstein-Barr virus binds to the same domains of CR2, as do C3d and C3dg, and achieves infection of cells by this route.[73] CR3 and CR4 are members of the integrin family of adhesion molecules, heterodimers sharing a common β-chain (CD18) and different α-chains (CD11b or CD11c) (see Chapter 20). CR3 specifically binds iC3b to PMNs and monocytes and promotes the phagocytosis of iC3b-coated particles by these cells. CR3 also promotes the attachment of PMNs and monocytes to endothelium through direct interaction that does not involve complement proteins. The function of CR4 is less well characterized, but it also binds iC3b, fibrinogen, and endotoxic lipopolysaccharide.[74, 75]

COMPLEMENT SYNTHESIS AND METABOLISM

Although in vitro culture studies have detected synthesis of many complement proteins by monocytes and macrophages,[76] the liver is the primary source of synthesis in vivo. Patients with severe hepatic failure have marked depressions of the levels of C4 and C3 in sera, and impaired synthesis of C3 has been measured directly in metabolic turnover studies.

Measurements of the fractional catabolic rates of C4, C3, C5, and B indicate that complement proteins are among the most rapidly metabolized of all plasma proteins.[77] The mean fractional catabolic rates in normal individuals are in the range of 50 percent of the plasma pool per 24 hours. Synthetic rates are significantly correlated with levels in serum, indicating that the rate of synthesis is the major determinant of concentration in plasma in normal persons. Levels in plasma reflect the balance between catabolism and synthesis. Increased synthetic rates induced by an inflammatory condition may produce elevated levels of complement proteins. When the disease progresses to a state in which increased utilization of complement proteins is occurring, levels may then fall into the normal range. For this reason, serial determinations of levels in an individual patient are often much

Table 15–6. C3 AND C4 RECEPTORS

Receptor	Molecular Structure	Ligand	Cell Type	Function
CR1 (CD35)	190–280 kD Variable number of tandem SCRs	C3b > iC3b C4b	Erythrocytes Neutrophils Monocytes B lymphocytes T lymphocytes Follicular dendritic cells Glomerular epithelial cells	Immune complex clearance Enhanced phagocytosis Immune complex binding Antigen localization
CR2 (CD21)	145 kD; 15 SCRs	iC3b C3dg C3d Epstein-Barr virus Interferon-α	B lymphocytes Follicular dendritic cells	B cell activation (part of CD19 complex) Antigen localization Lymphocyte memory Mediation of viral infection
CR3 (CD11b/CD18)	α: 150 kD β: 95 kD Heterodimer member of integrin family	iC3b Zymosan ICAM-1 Fibrinogen Factor X	Neutrophils Monocytes Macrophages	Enhanced phagocytosis Adhesion to endothelium
CR4 (CD11c/CD18)	α: 150 kD β: 95 kD Heterodimer member of integrin family	iC3b Fibrinogen Lipopolysaccharide	Neutrophils Monocytes Macrophages	Enhanced phagocytosis Adhesion to endothelium

Abbreviations: ICAM-1, intercellular adhesion molecule-1; SCRs, short consensus repeats.

more informative than measurements at isolated times.

With the exception of properdin, which is X-linked, the synthesis of complement proteins is encoded by genes inherited in an autosomal codominant fashion (see Chapter 79).[78] Congenital deficiency is the consequence of inheritance of a null gene, which codes for nonsynthesis of the protein and which is allelic with the normal structural gene. Inheritance of C4 is complicated by the existence of two adjacent loci, C4A and C4B.[79] At both of these loci, null (Q0) alleles are common and levels in serum roughly correspond to the number of expressed C4 genes. Individuals homozygous for null alleles in both loci (C4AQ0,BQ0/C4AQ0,BQ0) are rare, but those with one, two, or three null alleles and levels in serum equal to three fourths, one half, or one fourth of the normal mean occur more frequently. The relatively high frequency of null alleles coding for nonsynthesis of complement proteins leads to wide variations in normal levels. C4 levels in individuals who inherit a null allele at one of the two C4 loci, and who would be expected to have a level in plasma that was about 75 percent of the normal mean, overlap broadly with levels in those who have four fully functional C4 genes. Even those who are heterozygous for null alleles at both loci and who would be expected to have a level in plasma 50 percent of normal are often difficult to identify.

The result is a broad range of normal in the population. For most complement proteins, the normal range is within about 50% either way of the normal mean. The very large normal range probably also reflects the fact that most complement proteins are acute-phase reactants, members of a class of proteins whose plasma levels rise in response to IL-1, IL-6, and TNF (see Chapter 44).

COMPLEMENT MEASUREMENT

Hemolytic Complement Assays

The total hemolytic complement assay (also called the CH50 assay) is the traditional method for the determination of complement in serum or other body fluid.[80] It measures the ability of the test sample to lyse 50 percent of a standard suspension of sheep erythrocytes coated with optimal amounts of rabbit antibody in a reaction that includes the entire classical activation pathway and the terminal sequence. The CH50 assay is a useful screening procedure for detecting homozygous deficiency of a complement protein, but it does not reliably detect heterozygous deficiency states. Because complement *activity* is heat labile, considerable care is required in collecting and handling specimens to preserve this activity.

Immunoassays

The concentrations of individual complement proteins can be measured by radial immunodiffusion or nephelometry using specific antibody. Most widely available clinically are assays for C4 and C3. Immunoassays measure the complement protein as antigen, without regard to whether it is active, so that special handling or processing of plasma samples is not required.

With the exception of certain kindreds with C1 inhibitor deficiency, in which the synthesis of nonfunctional but antigenically intact C1 inhibitor is inherited, the difference between the results of functional and immunochemical determinations in plasma is not clinically important. Functionally inactive products of the component sequence are cleared rapidly from the plasma, so that participation of a component in an in vivo reaction is usually reflected by depressed levels in serum as measured by either functional or antigenic assays. In the case of closed body spaces, such as the synovial, pleural, pericardial, and subarachnoid spaces, clearance of spent complement protein proceeds at a much slower rate, so that considerable divergence between the results of functional assays and immunoassays may occur.

Detection of Activation or Cleavage Products

Measurement of cleavage fragments, the concentrations of which are normally close to zero in plasma or interstitial fluids, may be a more sensitive index of complement activation during disease than a fall in the plasma concentration of a complement protein.[81]

Sensitive and reproducible methods for the detection of nanogram quantities of the anaphylatoxin peptides (C3a, C4a, and C5a) have been developed. The plasma of patients undergoing extracorporeal circulation transiently contains elevated levels of C5a, which are temporally associated with the leukopenia and depressed PO_2 observed during the initiation of this procedure.[82] Synovial fluid from patients with rheumatoid arthritis or gout has markedly increased levels of C3a, whereas the level of C5a is within normal limits.[83] Measurement of C3a is a more sensitive index of in vivo complement activation than C5a, because the latter peptide is rapidly cleared from the circulation.

Antibodies to neoantigens that arise during the formation of the membrane attack complex have been used to measure concentrations of C5b-9 (or, more correctly, SC5b-9, since the S-protein is present in the spent serum complex) in plasma and other biologic fluids. Patients with clinically active SLE have elevated plasma levels of C5b-9.[84] Levels are increased in synovial fluid from patients with rheumatoid arthritis.[85] Cerebrospinal levels of C5b-9 are increased in autoimmune neurologic diseases such as multiple sclerosis and lupus cerebritis.

CLINICAL SIGNIFICANCE

Increases in Complement Levels Due to Hypersynthesis

Elevations of complement levels occur frequently as part of the acute phase response.[86] Such elevations are accompanied by the characteristic changes in the levels of other plasma proteins, including increases in C-reactive protein, serum amyloid A protein, α_1-acid glycoprotein, and haptoglobin, and decreases in transferrin and albumin levels. Elevations of total hemolytic activity, C3, and C4 in plasma occur regularly in the active phase of virtually all rheumatic diseases, including rheumatoid arthritis, SLE, dermatomyositis and polymyositis, scleroderma, rheumatic fever, ankylosing spondylitis, and temporal arteritis. In these diseases, elevated levels are frequent, so that a level at the lower limit of normal may indicate in vivo complement activation.

Other conditions in which elevated complement levels have been observed include acute viral hepatitis, myocardial infarction, cancer, diabetes, pregnancy, sarcoidosis, amyloidosis, thyroiditis, inflammatory bowel disease, typhoid fever, and pneumococcal pneumonia. The increase in complement protein rarely exceeds twofold, compared with increases of 100- to 1000-fold commonly seen with C-reactive protein.

Decreased Concentrations Due to Hypercatabolism

Any disease associated with circulating immune complexes is likely to lead to acquired hypocomplementemia (Table 15–7), including SLE, rheumatoid arthritis, subacute bacterial endocarditis, hepatitis B surface antigenemia, pneumococcal infection, gram-negative sepsis, viremias such as measles, and recurrent parasitemias such as malaria. Essential mixed

Table 15–7. HYPOCOMPLEMENTIC STATES

Hyposynthesis
  Congenital deficiencies (see Chapter 79)
  Severe hepatic failure
  Severe malnutrition
  Glomerulonephritis*
  Systemic lupus erythematosus

Hypercatabolism
  Deficiency of control proteins
    C1 inhibitor deficiency: hereditary angioedema
    Factor I deficiency
    Factor H deficiency
  Rheumatic diseases with immune complexes
    Systemic lupus erythematosus
    Rheumatoid arthritis (with extra-articular disease)
    Systemic vasculitis
    Essential mixed cryoglobulinemia
  Infectious diseases
    Subacute bacterial endocarditis
    Infected atrioventricular shunts
    Pneumococcal sepsis
    Gram-negative sepsis
    Viremias (e.g., hepatitis B surface antigenemia,
      measles, dengue)
    Parasitemias (e.g., trypanosomiasis, malaria, babesiosis)
  Glomerulonephritis
    Poststreptococcal
    Membranoproliferative
    Idiopathic proliferative or focal sclerosing

*Usually associated with simultaneous and marked hypercatabolism.

cryoglobulinemia, a disease characterized by arthritis or arthralgias, cutaneous vasculitis, and nephritis, is invariably accompanied by profound hypocomplementemia due to classical pathway activation by the immune complexes that occur in this disease.

Systemic Lupus Erythematosus

Total hemolytic complement levels are depressed at some time in most patients with SLE, whereas levels are generally normal in patients with discoid lupus.[87] As a rule, complement depressions are associated with increased severity of disease, especially renal disease. Component analyses have demonstrated low levels of C1, C4, C2, and C3. Serial observations often reveal decreased levels preceding clinical exacerbations; reductions in C4 occur before reductions of C3, other components, and total hemolytic complement activity, but are less specific than reductions in C3.[88] As attacks subside, levels return toward normal in the reverse order, with C4 tending to remain depressed longer, even when the patient appears to be doing well clinically.

The clinical usefulness of monitoring complement levels in patients with SLE is controversial.[40, 88-91] Opinions differ greatly, with some investigators recommending complement measurements enthusiastically and others finding no value in these tests. Authors of studies with more detailed clinical characterizations of patients and longer follow-ups tend to conclude that complement determinations are both useful adjuncts in the treatment of patients with known SLE and useful tools in the diagnosis of this disease.

Rheumatoid Arthritis

Levels of total hemolytic complement activity, C3, and C4 in serum are usually normal or elevated in patients with rheumatoid arthritis. Depressed levels are associated with extra-articular manifestations of the disease, particularly vasculitis. Such patients usually also have high titers of rheumatoid factor in their sera, circulating immune complexes detectable by C1q-binding assays, and small amounts of antinuclear antibodies. Levels of complement in synovial fluid are low in patients with rheumatoid arthritis when the levels are measured by activity determination, and depression of the level of total hemolytic complement activity, C4, or C2 is most frequently found in patients who test positive for rheumatoid factor.[92] Levels of complement component protein measured in synovial fluid by radial immunodiffusion are usually normal because of the presence of antigenically intact but functionally inactive complement fragments that have not been cleared from the joint space. Cleavage fragments of C3 in synovial fluid include C3c and C3d, high proportions of C3d in relation to total C3, electrophoretically converted forms of C3,

and increased C3a, Bb, and C5b-9 by radioimmunoassay.[81, 83, 85, 93] The abundant evidence for intra-articular activation of the complement system in rheumatoid arthritis is helpful in understanding the pathogenesis of the disease process, but synovial fluid complement levels are of little value as a diagnostic test.

References

1. Williams RC: Immune Complexes in Clinical and Experimental Medicine. Cambridge, Harvard University Press, 1980.
2. Theofilopoulos AN, Dixon FJ: The biology and detection of immune complexes. Adv Immunol 28:89, 1979.
3. Schifferli JA, Ng YC, Peters DK: The role of complement and its receptor in the elimination of immune complexes. N Engl J Med 315:488, 1986.
4. MacLennan IC: Germinal centers. Annu Rev Immunol 12:117, 1994.
5. Thorbecke GJ, Amin AR, Tsiagbe VK: Biology of germinal centers in lymphoid tissue. FASEB J 8:832, 1994.
6. Knight SC, Stagg AJ: Antigen-presenting cell types. Curr Opin Immunol 5:374, 1993.
7. Szakal AK, Kapasi ZF, Masuda A, Tew JG: Follicular dendritic cells in the alternative antigen transport pathway: Microenvironment, cellular events, age and retrovirus related alterations. Semin Immunol 4:257, 1992.
8. Lin CT, Shen Z, Boros P, Unkeless JC: Fc receptor-mediated signal transduction. J Clin Immunol 14:1, 1994.
9. Fridman WH: Regulation of B-cell activation and antigen presentation by Fc receptors. Curr Opin Immunol 5:355, 1993.
10. van de Winkel JG, Capel PJ: Human IgG Fc receptor heterogeneity: Molecular aspects and clinical implications. Immunol Today 14:215, 1993.
11. Heyman B: The immune complex: Possible ways of regulating the antibody response. Immunol Today 11:310, 1990.
12. Hebert LA: The clearance of immune complexes from the circulation of man and other primates. Am J Kidney Dis 17:352, 1991.
13. Morgan BP, Walport MJ: Complement deficiency and disease. Immunol Today 12:301, 1991.
14. Davies KA, Schifferli JA, Walport MJ: Complement deficiency and immune complex disease. Springer Semin Immunopathol 15:397, 1994.
15. Von Pirquet CE: Allergy. Arch Intern Med 7:259, 1911.
16. Germuth FGJ: A comparative histologic and immunologic study in rabbits of induced hypersensitivity of the serum sickness type. J Exp Med 97:257, 1953.
17. Dixon FJ, Vazquez JJ, Weigle WO, Cochrane CG: Pathogenesis of serum sickness. AMA Arch Pathol 65:18, 1958.
18. Sylvestre DL, Ravetch JV: Fc receptors initiate the Arthus reaction: Redefining the inflammatory cascade. Science 265:1095, 1994.
19. Batsford SR: Cationic antigens as mediators of inflammation. APMIS 99:1, 1991.
20. Morrison SL, Smith RIF, Wright A: Structural determinants of human IgG function. Immunologist 2:119, 1994.
21. Cacoub P, Musset L, Lunel Fabiani F, Perrin M, Leger JM, Thi Huong Du L, Wechsler B, Bletry O, Opolon P, Huraux JM: Hepatitis C virus and essential mixed cryoglobulinaemia. Br J Rheumatol 32:689, 1993.
22. Agnello V, Chung RT, Kaplan LM: A role for hepatitis C virus infection in type II cryoglobulinemia. N Engl J Med 327:1490, 1992.
23. Schutzer SE, Coyle PK, Dunn JJ, Luft BJ, Brunner M: Early and specific antibody response to OspA in Lyme disease. J Clin Invest 94:454, 1994.
24. Schutzer SE, Coyle PK, Belman AL, Golightly MG, Drulle J: Sequestration of antibody to Borrelia burgdorferi in immune complexes in seronegative Lyme disease. Lancet 335:312, 1990.
25. McDougal JS, Hubbard M, Strobel PL, McDuffie FC: Comparison of five assays for immune complexes in the rheumatic diseases: Performance characteristics of the assays. J Lab Clin Med 100:705, 1982.
26. Nydegger UE, Svehag SE: Improved standardization in the quantitative estimation of soluble immune complexes making use of an international reference preparation: Results of a collaborative multicentre study. Clin Exp Immunol 58:502, 1984.
27. McDougal JS, Hubbard M, McDuffie FC, Strobel PL, Smith SJ, Bass N, Goldman JA, Hartman S, Myerson G, Miller S, et al: Comparison of five assays for immune complexes in the rheumatic diseases: An assessment of their validity for rheumatoid arthritis. Arthritis Rheum 25:1156, 1982.
28. Reynolds WJ, Yoon SJ, Emin M, Chapman KR, Klein MH: Circulating immune complexes in rheumatoid arthritis: A prospective study using five immunoassays. J Rheumatol 13:700, 1986.
29. Roberts-Thomson RJ, Neoh SH, Bradley J, Milazzo SC: Circulating and intra-articular immune complexes in rheumatoid arthritis: A comparative

study of the C1q binding and monoclonal rheumatoid factor assays. Ann Rheum Dis 39:438, 1980.

30. Abrass CK, Nies KM, Louie JS, Border WA, Glassock RJ: Correlation and predictive accuracy of circulating immune complexes with disease activity in patients with systemic lupus erythematosus. Arthritis Rheum 23:273, 1980.

31. Valenzuela R, Bergfeld WF, Deodhar SD: Interpretation of Immunofluorescent Patterns in Skin Diseases. Chicago, American Society of Clinical Pathologists Press, 1984, p 66.

32. Wener MH, Mannik M, Schwartz MM, Lewis EJ: Relationship between renal pathology and the size of circulating immune complexes in patients with systemic lupus erythematosus. Medicine 66:85, 1987.

33. Huston KA, Gupta RC, Donadio JVJ, McDuffie FC, Ilstrup DM: Circulating immune complexes in systemic lupus erythematosus: Association with other immunologic abnormalities but not with changes in renal function. J Rheumatol 5:423, 1978.

34. Andrews BS, Ascher MS, Barada FAJ, Davis JS: The Raji cell radioimmunoassay in patients with systemic lupus erythematosus: Clinical significance and relationships to other serologic variables assessed by discriminant analysis. J Rheumatol 12:718, 1985.

35. Mackel SE, Tappeiner G, Brumfield H, Jordon RE: Circulating immune complexes in cutaneous vasculitis: Detection with C1q and monoclonal rheumatoid factor. J Clin Invest 64:1652, 1979.

36. Seibold JR, Medsger JAJ, Winkelstein A, Kelly RH, Rodnan GP: Immune complexes in progressive systemic sclerosis (scleroderma). Arthritis Rheum 25:1167, 1982.

37. Siminovitch K, Klein M, Pruzanski W, Wilkinson S, Lee P, Yoon SJ, Keystone E: Circulating immune complexes in patients with progressive systemic sclerosis. Arthritis Rheum 25:1174, 1982.

38. Moxley G, Ruddy S: Immune complexes and complement. In Kelley WN, Harris ED, Jr., Ruddy S, Sledge CB (eds): Textbook of Rheumatology, 4th ed. Philadelphia, WB Saunders, 1993, p 188.

39. Morrow WJW, Isenberg DA, Todd-Pokropek A, Parry HF, Snaith ML: Useful laboratory measurements in the management of systemic lupus erythematosus. Q J Med 51:125, 1982.

40. Sturfelt G, Johnson U, Sjoholm AG: Sequential studies of complement activation in systemic lupus erythematosus. Scand J Rheumatol 14:184, 1985.

41. Siegert CE, Daha MR, Tseng CM, Coremans IE, Van es LA, Breedveld FC: Predictive value of IgG autoantibodies against C1q for nephritis in systemic lupus erythematosus. Ann Rheum Dis 52:851, 1993.

42. Martensson U, Sjoholm AG, Sturfelt G, Truedsson L, Laurell AB: Western blot analysis of human IgG reactive with the collagenous portion of C1q: Evidence of distinct binding specificities. Scand J Immunol 35:735, 1992.

43. Jones VE, Jacoby RK, Wallington T, Holt P: Immune complexes in early arthritis. I: Detection of immune complexes before rheumatoid arthritis is definite. Clin Exp Immunol 44:512, 1981.

44. Smeenk RJ, van den Brink HG, Brinkman K, Termaat RM, Berden JH, Swaak AJ: Anti-dsDNA: Choice of assay in relation to clinical value. Rheumatol Int 11:101, 1991.

45. Smeenk R, Brinkman K, van den Brink H, Termaat RM, Berden J, Nossent H, Swaak T: Antibodies to DNA in patients with systemic lupus erythematosus: Their role in the diagnosis, the follow-up and the pathogenesis of the disease. Clin Rheumatol 9:100, 1990.

46. Mayer MM: The complement system. Sci Am 229:54, 1973.

47. Muller-Eberhard HJ: Chemistry and function of the complement system. Hosp Pract 12:33, 1978.

48. Kinoshita T: Biology of complement: The overture. Immunol Today 12:291, 1991.

49. Zaltzman AB, Van den Berg CW, Muzykantov VR, Morgan BP: Enhanced complement susceptibility of avidin-biotin–treated human erythrocytes is a consequence of neutralization of the complement regulators CD59 and decay accelerating factor. Biochem J 307:651, 1995.

50. Muller-Eberhard HJ, Schreiber RD: Molecular biology and chemistry of the alternative pathway of complement. Adv Immunol 29:1, 1980.

51. Pangburn MK, Muller-Eberhard HJ: The alternative pathway of complement. Springer Semin Immunopathol 7:163, 1984.

52. Law SK, Levine RP: Interaction between the third complement protein and cell surface macromolecules. Proc Natl Acad Sci USA 74:2701, 1977.

53. Volanakis JE: Participation of C3 and its ligands in complement activation. Curr Top Microbiol Immunol 153:1, 1989.

54. Esser AF: Big MAC attack: Complement proteins cause leaky patches. Immunol Today 12:316, 1991.

55. Bhakdi S, Tranum-Jensen J: Complement lysis: A hole is a hole. Immunol Today 12:318, 1991.

56. Volanakis JE, Kaplan MH: Interaction of C-reactive protein complexes with the complement system. II: Consumption of guinea pig complement by CRP complexes: Requirement for human C1q. J Immunol 113:9, 1974.

57. Sim RB, Reid KBM: C1: Molecular interactions with activating systems. Immunol Today 12:307, 1991.

58. Hughes-Jones NC, Gardner B: The reaction between the complement subcomponent C1q, IgG complexes and polyionic molecules. Immunology 34:459, 1978.

59. Farries TC, Atkinson J: Evolution of the complement system. Immunol Today 12:295, 1991.

60. Whaley K, Ruddy S: Modulation of C3b hemolytic activity by a plasma protein distinct from C3b inactivator. Science 193:1011, 1976.

61. Whaley K, Ruddy S: Modulation of the alternative complement pathway by beta1H globulin. J Exp Med 144:1147, 1977.

62. Lachmann PJ, Nicol P: Reaction mechanism of the alternate pathway of complement fixation. Lancet 3:465, 1973.

63. Muller-Eberhard HJ: The membrane attack complex of complement. Annu Rev Immunol 4:503, 1986.

64. Ratnoff WD, Knez JJ, Prince GM, Okada H, Lachmann PJ, Medof ME: Structural properties of the glycoplasmanylinositol anchor phospholipid of the complement membrane attack complex inhibitor CD59. Clin Exp Immunol 87:415, 1992.

65. Lachmann PJ: The control of homologous lysis. Immunol Today 12:312, 1991.

66. Bhakdi S, Kaflein R, Halstensen TS, Hugo F, Preissner KT, Mollnes TE: Complement S-protein (vitronectin) is associated with cytolytic membrane-bound C5b-9 complexes. Clin Exp Immunol 74:459, 1988.

67. Tschopp J, Masson D, Schafer S, Peitsch M, Preissner KT: The heparin binding domain of S-protein/vitronectin binds to complement components C7, C8, and C9 and perforin from cytolytic T-cells and inhibits their lytic activities. Biochemistry 27:4103, 1988.

68. Fries LF, O'Shea JJ, Frank MM: Inherited deficiencies of complement and complement-related proteins. Clin Immunol Immunopathol 40:37, 1986.

69. Ross GD: Complement and complement receptors. Curr Opin Immunol 2:50, 1989.

70. Frank MM: Complement in the pathophysiology of human disease. N Engl J Med 316:1525, 1987.

71. Kalli KR, Ahearn JM, Fearon DT: Interaction of iC3b with recombinant isotypic and chimeric forms of CR2. J Immunol 147:590, 1991.

72. Matsumoto AK, Kopicky-Burd J, Carter RH, Tuveson DA, Tedder TF, Fearon DT: Intersection of the complement and immune systems: A signal transduction complex of the B lymphocyte–containing complement receptor type 2 and CD19. J Exp Med 173:55, 1991.

73. Tanner J, Weis J, Fearon D, Whang Y, Kieff E: Epstein-Barr virus gp350/220 binding to the B lymphocyte C3d receptor mediates adsorption, capping, and endocytosis. Cell 50:203, 1987.

74. Ingalls RR, Golenbock DT: CD11c/CD18, a transmembrane signaling receptor for lipopolysaccharide. J Exp Med 181:1473, 1995.

75. Bilsland CA, Diamond MS, Springer TA: The leukocyte integrin p150,95 (CD11c/CD18) as a receptor for iC3b: Activation by a heterologous beta subunit and localization of a ligand recognition site to the I domain. J Immunol 152:4582, 1994.

76. Lappin D, Hamilton AD, Morrison L, Aref M, Whaley K: Synthesis of complement components (C3, C2, B and C1-inhibitor) and lysozyme by human monocytes and macrophages. J Clin Lab Immunol 20:101, 1986.

77. Ruddy S, Carpenter CB, Chin KW, Knostman JN, Soter NA, Gotze O, Muller-Eberhard HJ, Austen KF: Human complement metabolism: An analysis of 144 studies. Medicine 54:165, 1975.

78. Perlmutter DH, Colten HR: Molecular basis of complement deficiencies. Immunodefic Rev 1:105, 1989.

79. Campbell RD, Carroll MC, Porter RR: The molecular genetics of components of complement. Adv Immunol 38:203, 1986.

80. Schur PH: Complement studies of sera and other biologic fluids. Hum Pathol 14:338, 1983.

81. Petersen NE, Elmgreen J, Teisner B, Svehag SE: Activation of classical pathway complement in chronic inflammation: Elevated levels of circulating C3d and C4d split products in rheumatoid arthritis and Crohn's disease. Acta Med Scand 223:557, 1988.

82. Chenoweth DE, Cooper SW, Hugli TE, Stewart RW, Blackstone EH, Kirklin JW: Complement activation during cardiopulmonary bypass: Evidence for generation of C3a and C5a anaphylatoxins. N Engl J Med 304:497, 1981.

83. Moxley GF, Ruddy S: Elevated C3 anaphylatoxin levels in synovial fluids from patients with rheumatoid arthritis. Arthritis Rheum 28:1089, 1985.

84. Buyon JP, Tamerius J, Ordorica S, Young B, Abramson SB: Activation of the alternative complement pathway accompanies disease flares in systemic lupus erythematosus during pregnancy. Arthritis Rheum 35:55, 1992.

85. Brodeur JP, Ruddy S, Schwartz LB, Moxley GF: Synovial fluid levels of complement SC5b-9 and fragment Bb are elevated in patients with rheumatoid arthritis. Arthritis Rheum 34:1531, 1991.

86. Kushner I: C-reactive protein and the acute-phase response. Hosp Pract (Off Ed) 25:13, 1990.

87. Lloyd W, Schur PH: Immune complexes, complement and anti-DNA in exacerbations of systemic lupus erythematosus (SLE). Medicine 60:208, 1981.

88. Ricker DM, Hebert LA, Rohde R, Sedmak DD, Lewis EJ, Clough JD, the Lupus Nephritis Collaborative Study Group: Serum C3 levels are diagnostically more sensitive and specific for systemic lupus erythematosus activity than are serum C4 levels. Am J Kidney Dis 18:678, 1991.

89. Kerr LD, Adelsberg BR, Schulman P, Spiera H: Factor B activation prod-

ucts in patients with systemic lupus erythematosus: A marker of severe disease activity. Arthritis Rheum 32:1406, 1989.

90. Swaak AJ, Groenwold J, Bronsveld W: Predictive value of complement profiles and anti-dsDNA in systemic lupus erythematosus. Ann Rheum Dis 45:359, 1986.

91. Valentijn RM, Van Overhagen H, Hazevoet HM, Hermans H, Cats A, Daha MR, Van es LA: The value of complement and immune complex determinations in monitoring disease activity in patients with systemic lupus erythematosus. Arthritis Rheum 28:904, 1985.

92. Ruddy S, Austen KF: Activation of the complement and properdin systems in rheumatoid arthritis. Ann N Y Acad Sci 256:96, 1975.

93. Davies ET, Nasaruddin BA, Alhaq A, Senaldi G, Vergani D: Clinical application of a new technique that measures C4d for assessment of activation of classical complement pathway. J Clin Pathol 41:143, 1988.

CHAPTER 16

Helen Tighe
Dennis A. Carson

Rheumatoid Factors

Rheumatoid factors are autoantibodies directed against antigenic determinants on the Fc fragment of immunoglobulin G (IgG) molecules (Fig. 16–1). Generally associated with rheumatoid arthritis, rheumatoid factors are also present in normal individuals and are elevated in patients with a variety of other diseases. The rheumatoid factors associated with rheumatoid arthritis are generally specific for human IgG, are of higher affinity, and include not only IgM rheumatoid factors but also IgG, IgA, and IgE rheumatoid factor variants. In contrast, rheumatoid factors associated with other diseases are frequently polyspecific, of lower affinity, and of the IgM isotype.

METHODS OF DETECTION

Most methods developed for the measurement of antibodies against exogenous antigens have also been applied to the assay of rheumatoid factor. These include agglutination, precipitation, complement fixation, immunofluorescence, radioimmunoassay, and enzyme-linked immunosorbent assay (ELISA) methods, of which the last two provide the more precise quantification of IgM, IgG, and IgA rheumatoid factors.

IgM rheumatoid factors are multivalent and hence are efficient agglutinators of antigen-coated particles. Commercially available sources of these include latex beads or bentonite particles that have been passively coated with human IgG.[1] Cross-linking of the IgG-coupled latex or bentonite by IgM rheumatoid factor in serum produces a visible flocculus. Red blood cells coated with human or rabbit IgG are likewise agglutinated by IgM rheumatoid factors.[2, 3] The quantity of IgM rheumatoid factor is then expressed as the highest dilution of serum yielding detectable agglutination.

Serum IgG competes with IgG-coated particles for reaction with IgM rheumatoid factor. Through multivalent interactions, nonspecifically aggregated IgG in improperly treated sera or specific immune complexes inhibit rheumatoid factor binding to a marked degree. Such "hidden rheumatoid factors" can be revealed by separation of the IgM and IgG fractions under dissociating conditions before performance of the rheumatoid factor assays.[4] In addition, the C1q component of complement agglutinates IgG-coated particles and must be inactivated prior to the assay.[5]

Sensitive radioimmunoassay and ELISA methods have been developed for the detection of IgM rheumatoid factors.[6] One significant advantage of these methods is that they readily detect IgM rheumatoid factors in rheumatoid sera diluted 1000- to 100,000-fold. At such high dilutions, serum IgG and immune complexes infrequently compromise the accurate determination of IgM rheumatoid factor levels.

IgG rheumatoid factors are abundant in the sera, particularly the synovial fluids, of many patients with severe rheumatoid arthritis.[7–9] Unfortunately, the routine assay of IgG rheumatoid factors presents several difficulties (Table 16–1). All assays for IgM rheumatoid factor take advantage of the markedly increased avidity of pentavalent IgM rheumatoid factors for aggregated IgG as compared with monomeric IgG. With IgG rheumatoid factor, this phenomenon is not nearly as marked. In addition, high concentrations of IgG in serum and the tendency of IgG rheumatoid factors to self-associate rather than bind aggregated IgG further increase the difficulty of the assay of this antibody. IgG rheumatoid factors in rheumatoid arthritis are most definitely detected by their characteristic sedimentation profile as intermediate complexes in the analytic ultracentrifuge.[10, 11] Although both ELISA and radioimmunoassay methods have been developed for the detection of IgG rheumatoid factor, IgM rheumatoid factor must be removed or destroyed before the IgG rheumatoid factor assay to avoid false-positive results. This can be achieved by gel filtration, ion exchange chromatography, or digestion with the proteolytic enzyme pepsin. The last

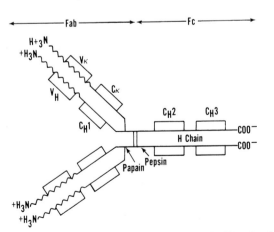

Figure 16–1. Structure of an immunoglobulin G (IgG) molecule of the G1 subclass containing kappa light chains. The antigens reacting with rheumatoid factor are in the Fc region.

241

Table 16–1. COMPARISON OF RHEUMATOID FACTORS OF THE IgM AND IgG CLASSES

Property	IgM Rheumatoid Factor	IgG Rheumatoid Factor
Valence for IgG	5	2
Intrinsic affinity for antigen (K_d, M)	10^{-4} to 5×10^{-5}	10^{-4} to 5×10^{-5}
Agglutination of IgG-coated latex particles	Strong	Weak
Enhanced binding to aggregated IgG	Marked	Moderate
Usual sedimentation constants in ultracentrifuge	19S–22S	10S–18S
Self-association	No	Yes
Binding to IgG after treatment with:		
Reducing agents	Decreased	Unchanged
Pepsin	Decreased	Unchanged or increased

Abbreviation: Ig, immunoglobulin.

technique has the additional advantage of destroying the Fc (crystallizable) portion of IgG, thereby releasing IgG rheumatoid factors trapped in self-associating complexes. The quantitative assay of IgG rheumatoid factor in serum is occasionally helpful in confirming a diagnosis of rheumatoid arthritis. In patients with rheumatoid vasculitis or the hyperviscosity syndrome, IgG rheumatoid factor levels may assist in monitoring the response to therapy.[12] However, indications for the routine clinical assay of IgG rheumatoid factor have not been well defined.

Rheumatoid factors of the IgA class have been measured in rheumatoid serum by immunoelectrophoresis, quantitative immunoabsorption, and radioimmunoassay and ELISA methods using class-specific anti-immunoglobulin reagents to distinguish them from the more abundant IgM rheumatoid factors. IgA rheumatoid factors are also found in the saliva of patients with rheumatoid arthritis and those with the sicca syndrome.[13, 14] Most salivary IgA, and presumably IgA rheumatoid factor, is produced locally. The role of IgA rheumatoid factors in chronic inflammation of the exocrine glands is not known.

INCIDENCE

Rheumatoid factor has generally been associated with rheumatoid arthritis, but the autoantibodies are also found in the sera of a variable portion of patients with other rheumatic diseases, acute and chronic inflammatory diseases, viral infections, lymphoproliferative disease, such as chronic lymphocytic leukemia, Waldenström's macroglobulinemia, and mixed cryoglobulinemia, as well as in some apparently normal individuals.[15–20] Many of these conditions are also associated with either hypergammaglobulinemia, indicative of polyclonal B lymphocyte activation, or circulating immune complexes. Table 16–2 is a partial list of diseases in which an increased incidence of rheumatoid factor has been reported. The exact incidence of rheumatoid factor in a population depends on the assay system and the titer chosen to separate positive and negative reactors. The titer of rheumatoid factor in a population, whether measured by the sensitized sheep erythrocyte agglutination test or by latex fixation, usually behaves as a continuous variable, but differs among various ethnic groups.[16, 17, 21] With increasing age, both the percentage of individuals with a particular titer and the mean titer of a population as a whole increase.[16] Some studies have shown that the prevalence of rheumatoid factors and other autoantibodies in the general population tends to decline beyond the age of 70 to 80 years.[21] This decrease may be related to an increased mortality rate among autoantibody-positive individuals.

In most nonrheumatic conditions, titers of rheumatoid factor are lower than in rheumatoid arthritis. Thus, the specificity of the rheumatoid factor reaction for rheumatoid arthritis increases with serum titer.[17] At a dilution of serum that excludes 95 percent of the normal population, results of at least 70 percent of patients with rheumatoid arthritis, as diagnosed by other criteria, are positive by latex agglutination. The

Table 16–2. SOME DISEASES COMMONLY ASSOCIATED WITH RHEUMATOID FACTOR

Rheumatic Diseases
  Rheumatoid arthritis
  Systemic lupus erythematosus
  Scleroderma
  Mixed connective tissue disease
  Sjögren's syndrome
Viral Infections
  Acquired immunodeficiency syndromes
  Mononucleosis
  Hepatitis
  Influenza
  After vaccination (may yield falsely elevated titers of antiviral antibodies)
Parasitic Infections
  Trypanosomiasis
  Kala-azar
  Malaria
  Schistosomiasis
  Filariasis
Chronic Bacterial Infections
  Tuberculosis
  Leprosy
  Yaws
  Syphilis
  Brucellosis
  Subacute bacterial endocarditis
  Salmonellosis
Neoplasms
  Tumors after radiation therapy or chemotherapy
Other Hyperglobulinemic States
  Hypergammaglobulinemic purpura
  Cryoglobulinemia
  Chronic liver disease
  Sarcoid
  Other chronic pulmonary diseases

remaining patients are considered seronegative (i.e., have rheumatoid factor titers within the normal range). Some of the latter sera, particularly from patients with juvenile rheumatoid arthritis, may contain hidden IgM rheumatoid factors.[5, 22, 23] A few have IgG rheumatoid factors in the absence of IgM. On repeated testing, some seronegative patients convert to seropositive. In general, the specificity of rheumatoid factor for rheumatoid arthritis is increased by positivity on two or more consecutive occasions, high titer, reactivity with both human and rabbit IgG, and distribution among the IgM, IgG, and IgA classes.

A variable number of adult rheumatoid patients, which in the authors' experience represent not more than 10 percent of the total, remain seronegative by the usual criteria. Analysis of these patients indicates a contributory role for rheumatoid factor in disease, since these patients generally display milder synovitis than the seropositive patients and seldom develop extra-articular rheumatoid disease.[22] Although elevated expression of rheumatoid factor may have significant effects on immune regulation through the production of immune complexes and complement activation, its absence in patients with seronegative rheumatoid arthritis argues against its being a causative factor in joint disease. This is also supported by the finding of elevated rheumatoid factor titers in other diseases, such as in congenital human immunodeficiency virus (HIV) infection, in which the infected children do not manifest clinical rheumatic disease despite the presence of circulating IgA rheumatoid factor in half the cases.[19]

IMMUNOCHEMICAL PROPERTIES

Antigenic Specificity

Polyclonal IgM rheumatoid factors from the sera of patients with rheumatoid arthritis react with a diverse array of antigenic determinants localized to the Fc portion of the IgG molecule in both the C_H2 and C_H3 domains[24-26] (see Fig. 16–1).

The rheumatoid factors derived from rheumatoid synovia may have unique subclass specificities for human IgG compared with serum-derived rheumatoid factors. The synovial antibodies bind more strongly to IgG3 than to IgG1, IgG2, and IgG4. In contrast, the serum rheumatoid factors react most strongly with IgG1, IgG2, and IgG4, and only weakly with IgG3 (Ga specificity). Monospecific human rheumatoid factors also show preferential binding to IgG3 and IgG4, whereas polyreactive rheumatoid factors tend to react equally with all subclasses.[27]

A number of years ago, it was discovered that patients with rheumatoid arthritis have significantly fewer galactose residues on their IgG Fc compared with age-matched healthy controls[28] as a result of reduced B cell galactosyltransferase activity.[29] A lack of terminal galactose residues early in disease is associated with a worse prognosis.[30] In some instances,

however, glycosylation differences in IgGs have no effect on binding of IgM rheumatoid factors, enhance binding of rheumatoid factors (particularly those of high affinity), or reduce the solubility of the immune complex.[31-33] Patients with rheumatoid arthritis differ most significantly from controls with respect to the galactosylation of IgG2 antibodies, less so for IgG1 and IgG4 antibodies, and not at all for IgG3.[34] The defect in the IgG1, IgG2, and IgG4 subclasses is intriguing, since the Ga antigenic specificity for rheumatoid factor is also present on the same subclasses.[35] Because some rheumatoid factors secreted by synovial cells react preferentially with IgG3,[27] it is possible that galactose-deficient IgG3 is produced by patients with rheumatoid arthritis but is preferentially cleared from the circulation by complexing with rheumatoid factor. In contrast to these findings, maximal binding of IgG rheumatoid factors to IgG requires intact carbohydrate residues in the $C\gamma2$–$C\gamma3$ region.[36]

Kinetics of Interaction with IgG

The affinity of rheumatoid factor for IgG depends on the source of the rheumatoid factor. Monoclonal IgM rheumatoid factors isolated from patients with mixed cryoglobulinemia or lymphoproliferative disease tend to have low affinities with a dissociation constant (K_d) in the range of 10^{-4} to 10^{-5} M.[37, 38] In contrast, patients with rheumatoid arthritis produce a high proportion of IgM rheumatoid factors that react more avidly with human IgG (K_d, 10^{-7} M).[37, 39, 40] However, even lower-affinity rheumatoid factors can produce stable complexes with IgG under appropriate conditions. For multivalent IgM rheumatoid factor, this occurs when the IgG antigen is aggregated. Although each individual antigen–antibody bond in such an IgM–IgG aggregate probably is individually of insufficient energy to yield a long-lived complex, the sum total of multiple interactions produces a stable structure.[41]

IgG rheumatoid factors have unique kinetic properties that distinguish them from all other autoantibodies and heteroantibodies, in that the antigens with which they react reside on the antibody molecule itself. Hence, IgG rheumatoid factors can self-associate and form immune complexes in the absence of exogenous antigen.[42-44] The ability of IgG rheumatoid factor to form high-molecular-weight complexes probably depends on the concentration and affinity of the autoantibody as well as the ratio of IgG rheumatoid factor to normal IgG. IgM rheumatoid factor may, in addition, enhance the formation of IgG rheumatoid factor–containing complexes by cross-linking the reversibly aggregated IgG.

ETIOLOGY

At least three types of environmental stimuli can potentially trigger active rheumatoid factor synthesis in normal adults: (1) immunization with antigen–antibody complexes during anamnestic immune responses,[45–47] (2) polyclonal B cell activation,[48, 49] and (3) cross-reactions between autologous human IgG and exogenous antigens.

Adoptive transfer experiments have elucidated the cellular requirements for the induction of rheumatoid factor synthesis during murine secondary immune responses.[46, 50] Optimal rheumatoid factor production requires the presence of T cells sensitized to the specific antigen being administered as well as antibodies against the antigen. The rheumatoid factor precursor B cells can come from nonimmunized or T cell–deficient mice. Importantly, the rheumatoid factor that is elicited during secondary immune responses is directed against the IgG isotype that is dominant in the antigen–antibody complex. These results are explainable by the ability of rheumatoid factor expressing B cells to present immune-complexed antigen to antigen-specific helper T lymphocytes. During secondary immune responses, antigen–antibody complexes are taken up and processed by rheumatoid factor precursor B lymphocytes as well as by antigen-specific B cells.[51, 52] Subsequently, peptides derived from the antigens appear on the cell surface, in association with class II histocompatibility molecules. Unlike antibodies, T cell receptors for antigens recognize small linear peptides on the cell surface. When rheumatoid factor B cells present antigenic peptides derived from immune complexes, the antigen-reactive T lymphocytes can trigger rheumatoid factor production. This phenomenon is a form of linked recognition, insofar as the helper T cell and the rheumatoid factor B cell recognize different antigens. The frequency of rheumatoid factor precursor cells in mouse spleen is remarkably high and may approach the frequency of cells producing specific antibody.[47]

Rheumatoid factors in humans develop during the course of many acute and chronic inflammatory diseases.[53, 54] Although IgM rheumatoid factors predominate in most of these conditions, IgG rheumatoid factors are occasionally produced. As in the experimental models, sustained rheumatoid factor production usually depends on the continual presence of the immunologic stimuli. A well-studied example is subacute bacterial endocarditis, in which elimination of bacteria by antibiotics leads to the subsequent decline in rheumatoid factor titers.[53, 54] With few exceptions, the nonrheumatic diseases and the animal models associated with rheumatoid factor induction are characterized by elevated levels of non–rheumatoid factor–containing immune complexes or by a diffuse elevation of serum immunoglobulins, indicating polyclonal B lymphocyte activation.

The potential importance of polyclonal B lymphocyte activation in inducing rheumatoid factor production in humans has been emphasized.[48, 49] Polyclonal B lymphocyte activators are mitogens that stimulate lymphocytes to secrete immunoglobulins in the absence of specific antigenic stimulation. They are widespread in nature and include bacterial proteins and lipopolysaccharides, *Mycoplasma* components, and certain viruses, such as the Epstein-Barr virus (EBV). Lymphocytes from many normal adults release low-affinity IgM rheumatoid factors after mitogenic stimulation by EBV.[48] These rheumatoid factors commonly express the major cross-reactive idiotypes that are found on Waldenström's macroglobulins with anti-IgG autoantibody activity and may also derive from the minor subset of B lymphocytes that express the CD5 antigen.[55]

The possibility exists that rheumatoid factors are induced by cross-reactive epitopes on foreign antigens. Herpes simplex virus and cytomegalovirus induce IgG Fc receptors on infected cells and consequently may potentially elicit anti-idiotypic antibodies with rheumatoid factor activity.[56]

GENETIC BASIS

For a number of years, investigators have been concerned with the question of the particular immunoglobulin variable (V) region genes that encode autoantibodies in disease states and in healthy individuals, and whether these are in germline configuration or are somatically mutated. Lack of mutations or limited random mutations has been assumed to indicate nonspecific polyclonal B cell activation, whereas multiple mutations usually indicate selection by antigen.

Until recently, knowledge of the structure and specificities of rheumatoid factors was largely based on monoclonal IgM rheumatoid factors isolated from patients with mixed cryoglobulinemia or lymphoproliferative diseases.[20, 57–63] Nearly 10 percent of monoclonal IgM from unrelated individuals with mixed cryoglobulinemia or Waldenström's macroglobulinemia have anti-IgG autoantibody activity.[64] These rheumatoid factors are generally encoded by a restricted set of variable region genes in germline or near to germline configuration and as such have restricted idiotypic specificities, with a relatively high percentage expressing either the 17.109 or 6B6.6 idiotypes that are markers for the human VkIIIb subgroup gene Vk325 or the VkIIIa subgroup gene Vk328.[38, 64–66] The light chain genes are preferentially associated with members of the V_H1 and V_H4 heavy chain gene families, respectively.[64, 67] Such natural antibodies have low affinity for human IgG (K_d, 10^{-4} to 10^{-5} M)[37, 38] tend to be produced by the CD5+ B lymphocyte subpopulation, and are generally polyspecific, reacting with a wide variety of both self and exogenous antigens.[37, 38, 68–70]

B cells capable of producing IgM rheumatoid factors are present in the periphery of normal individuals. These rheumatoid factors can be germline encoded and tend to cross-react with a variety of other antigens.[68, 71] Production of rheumatoid factor occurs following secondary immunization or infection[45, 53, 72] and requires the presence of both immune-complexed antigen and T cells specific for the antigen present in the immune complex.[46, 47, 50, 73] In contrast to the situation in patients with rheumatoid arthritis, rheumatoid factor production in normal people is transient and regulated. These physiologic rheumatoid factors are encoded predominantly by VkIII light chains and VhI, VhIII, or VhIV variable region genes similarly to IgM rheumatoid factors derived from mixed cryoglobulinemia patients.[74] The IgM rheumatoid factor–secreting lines derived from patients after secondary immunization have undergone extensive somatic mutation, but with no evidence of affinity maturation and with an apparent selection against amino acid replacement mutations in the antibody-combining site.[75] These data imply that, under normal circumstances, there are efficient peripheral mechanisms to prevent the expression of higher-affinity, potentially pathologic rheumatoid factors.

Many studies have analyzed rheumatoid factors derived from either the peripheral blood or synovium of patients with rheumatoid arthritis. Low-affinity, polyspecific rheumatoid factors (K_d, 10^{-4} to 5×10^{-5} M) can be derived from patients with rheumatoid arthritis.[37, 39] In contrast to normal individuals, however, these patients produce a high proportion of IgM rheumatoid factors that react avidly with human IgG (K_d, 10^{-7} M).[37, 39, 40] Monoreactive IgM rheumatoid factors can form large immune aggregates and activate complement more efficiently than the lower-affinity polyspecific rheumatoid factors.[76] Such complement activation undoubtedly contributes to joint inflammation, and there is evidence for selective enrichment of these high-affinity clones in the synovium.[77] IgM rheumatoid factor–secreting lines use many different heavy and light chain variable region genes and gene combinations. Among these are the same heavy and light chain genes found in their low-affinity counterparts but altered by somatic mutation.[39, 40, 66, 78–84] In rheumatoid arthritis, there also is a trend away from use of the VhI/IV and VkIII genes common in natural antibodies toward predominant use of VhIII genes and a wide variety of light chains including V lambda (Vλ) subgroups.[40, 79, 83–88] Together, these data indicate that the rheumatoid factors in rheumatoid arthritis have undergone antigen-induced expansion and affinity maturation, together with recruitment of new clones of B cells. Studies of IgG rheumatoid factors derived from patients with rheumatoid arthritis support this conclusion. Some IgG rheumatoid factors use the same V genes as IgM rheumatoid factors and exhibit a much greater degree of somatic mutation than IgM rheumatoid factors, indicating a further affinity maturation of the autoantibody response.[89, 90]

PHYSIOLOGIC ROLE

Most rheumatoid factor B lymphocytes in normal lymphoid tissues are in the mantle zone regions.[91] In experimental animals, antigen–antibody complexes that reach lymphoid tissues through the afferent lymphatic vessels often localize to the mantle and marginal zones.[92] Rheumatoid factor expressing B cells are able to present immune-complexed antigen to antigen-specific T cells in vitro.[52] It is likely that early in a secondary immune response, when very small amounts of antigen are available, most of the antigen arrives in the draining lymph nodes in the form of an immune complex. Low levels of immune-complexed antigen may not bind efficiently to conventional antigen-presenting macrophages. Moreover, the interaction of IgG with Fc receptors or B cells may inhibit antigen presentation.[93] Under these circumstances, IgM rheumatoid factor expressing B cells may act as highly efficient antigen-presenting cells (APCs) for immune-complexed antigen, able to enhance an antigen-specific T cell expansion early in a secondary immune response. In normal individuals, some mechanism presumably prevents long-term expression and expansion of higher-affinity rheumatoid factors induced by the antigen-specific T cells.[94]

The common appearance of IgM rheumatoid factors during acute infections also suggests that both the secreted and the surface-bound autoantibodies have an important physiologic function. The rheumatoid factors that are produced by polyclonal B lymphocyte activation can potentially amplify the early response of the humoral immune system to bacterial or parasitic exposure. IgM rheumatoid factors can cross-link low-affinity IgG antibodies aligned on a surface of a viral or bacterial particle. The net result is the formation of a relatively stable multivalent and multispecific complex.

When bound to aggregated IgG, rheumatoid factors of the IgM class activate complement remarkably efficiently.[95] If the IgG is bound to a bacterium or parasite, the end result probably is either the lysis of the invading organism or its clearance from the circulation by means of the abundant complement receptors of the reticuloendothelial system. For this reason, IgM rheumatoid factor synthesis may represent an essential component of an effective polyclonal antibody response.

Under certain conditions, complexes of IgG and antigen potently inhibit immune responses.[96] The immune complexes can bind to the FcII class of membrane receptors for the Fc fragment of IgG, which are expressed by most B lymphocytes. This interaction inhibits B lymphocyte activation by antigen and thereby impedes antibody production. Because IgM rheumatoid factors prevent immune complexes from binding to Fc receptors, they can substantially amplify IgG antibody responses.[97]

The physiologic functions of IgM rheumatoid factor are summarized in Table 16–3.

ROLE IN RHEUMATOID ARTHRITIS

In patients with rheumatoid arthritis, Sjögren's syndrome, and mixed cryoglobulinemia, rheumatoid factors persist in the circulation in the absence of any known exogenous antigenic stimulus. Understanding

Table 16–3. PHYSIOLOGIC FUNCTIONS OF IgM RHEUMATOID FACTOR

1. Cell-associated rheumatoid factor
   a. Antigen processing and presentation
2. Secreted rheumatoid factor
   a. Stabilization of low-affinity IgG antigen complexes
   b. Immune complex clearance
   c. Enhancement of opsonization

Abbreviation; Ig, immunoglobulin.

the regulation of rheumatoid factor production may therefore yield clues to the immune pathogenesis of these diseases.

As discussed previously, the rheumatoid factors produced in lymphoproliferative and autoimmune diseases are structurally dissimilar (Table 16–4). In lymphoproliferative disease, such as chronic lymphocytic leukemia, Waldenström's macroglobulinemia, and mixed cryoglobulinemia as well as in some cases of Sjögren's syndrome, the rheumatoid factors are monoclonal or oligoclonal and display cross-reactive idiotypic antigens.[61–63, 98, 99] The restricted nature of these rheumatoid factors is uncommon for antigen-driven immune responses, which typically undergo time-dependent diversification. The accumulation of somatic mutations, immunoglobulin class switching, and the recruitment of new antibody-secreting clones all contribute to antibody heterogeneity. These processes are controlled by helper T cells. In contrast, rheumatoid factor synthesis in lymphoproliferative diseases may result from unrestrained proliferation of immature B lymphocyte clones. In this regard, clinical studies have shown that a significant fraction of patients with mixed cryoglobulinemia eventually experience overt lymphoma.[98] Neoplastic transformation of B lymphocytes is an established complication of Sjögren's syndrome.[100]

In marked contrast, the rheumatoid factors in the sera of patients with rheumatoid arthritis are heterogeneous.[66, 84, 99] The autoantibodies contain light and heavy chains distributed among all the variable region subgroups and among the IgM, IgG, and IgA classes. Sequence analyses indicate that these rheumatoid factors are the products of multiple B cell clones, whose immunoglobulin genes contain many somatic

Table 16–4. COMPARISON OF RHEUMATOID FACTORS IN LYMPHOPROLIFERATIVE AND AUTOIMMUNE DISEASES

	Lymphoproliferative Disease	Autoimmune Disease
Genes	Restricted	Many
Idiotypes	Cross-reactive	Private
Somatic mutations	Limited or none	Multiple
Affinity	Low	Higher
Ig classes	Mainly IgM	All

Abbreviation: Ig, immunoglobulin.

mutations.[39, 40, 66, 77, 79, 80–82, 84, 85, 89] Altogether, the results suggest that the production of rheumatoid factors in rheumatoid arthritis is driven by helper T lymphocytes.

Rheumatoid factor expressing B cells that express low-affinity IgM rheumatoid factors are neither inactivated nor stimulated by soluble human IgG. They may, however, serve as excellent antigen-presenting cells for immune-complexed antigen, resulting in expansion of antigen-reactive T cells.[51, 52] This may account for the increase in rheumatoid factor precursor B cells that normally accompanies a secondary immune response.[73] Although there is no evidence to indicate the existence of T cells that recognize the IgG molecule itself, normal T cells reactive with exogenous antigens may be sufficient to stimulate rheumatoid factor secretion and affinity maturation of the normally low-affinity IgM rheumatoid factor response. In addition, the normal process of somatic mutation in other antibody genes may generate antibodies that cross-react with human IgG. The absence of such high-affinity rheumatoid factors in normal individuals argues strongly for the presence of a peripheral tolerance mechanism. When such a mechanism is defective, T cells capable of reacting with any antigen capable of forming an immune complex with human IgG may be able to stimulate and maintain production of high affinity rheumatoid factors. This is potentially the situation in rheumatoid arthritis.

High levels of serum rheumatoid factor are associated with a worse prognosis in rheumatoid arthritis.[101] High titers of rheumatoid factor, particularly IgG rheumatoid factor, are a risk factor for the development of vasculitis,[12, 102] whereas elevated IgA rheumatoid factors may correlate with bone erosions.[103] Although it is unlikely that prolonged production of high-affinity rheumatoid factors is responsible for the joint involvement in rheumatoid arthritis, they probably exacerbate joint inflammation and promote immune disregulation. During established disease, the synovium may convert to lymphoid granulation tissue. B lymphocytes with rheumatoid factor specificity, particularly IgG rheumatoid factor, are abundant in the rheumatoid synovium,[104] where they can lead to complement activation and contribute to the inflammatory process.[105] The synovial fluids of patients with rheumatoid arthritis, unlike their sera, frequently have markedly depressed complement levels and contain high-molecular-weight IgG aggregates as detected by analytic ultracentrifugation or cryoprecipitation.[9] Partial isolation and characterization of the immune complexes from rheumatoid synovial fluids and tissues have yielded IgG rheumatoid factors, sometimes complexed with IgM rheumatoid factors, in the absence of other known antigens.[9, 106, 107] Consequently, the synovium becomes a major source of the rheumatoid factors, which appear in copious amounts in the circulation of patients with rheumatoid arthritis, although the lymphoid tissues such as bone marrow also produce the autoantibody.[108] A number of provocative reports have indicated alternative mechanisms by which some rheumatoid factors may affect immune regulation. For example, both monoclonal and polyclonal rheumatoid factors can cross-react weakly with human β_2-microglobulin, a member of the immunoglobulin supergene family, at residues 57 to 63,[109, 110] and with some HLA molecules.[111] β_2-Microglobulin shares considerable sequence homology and three-dimensional structure with immunoglobulin domains.

As efficient antigen-presenting cells, rheumatoid factor B lymphocytes may also increase the chance of T cell autosensitization to self-components that are released from necrotic joint tissues, such as collagen, proteoglycans, and heat-shock proteins. In this way, the abnormal conglomeration of activated rheumatoid factor B cells at synovial sites would create a vicious circle that promotes T cell–dependent joint inflammation through a variety of mechanisms.

References

1. Singer JM, Plotz CM: The latex fixation test. I: Application to the serologic diagnosis of rheumatoid arthritis. Am J Med 21:888, 1956.
2. Waaler E: On the occurrence of a factor in human serum activating the specific agglutination of sheep blood corpuscles. Acta Pathol Microbiol Scand 17:172, 1940.
3. Rose HM, Ragan C, Pearce E, Lipman MO: Differential agglutination of normal and sensitized sheep erythrocytes by sera of patients with rheumatoid arthritis. Proc Soc Exp Biol Med 68:1, 1949.
4. Allen JC, Kunkel HG: Hidden rheumatoid factors with specificity for native γ globulin. Arthritis Rheum 9:758, 1966.
5. Nykanen M, Paluson T, Aho K, Sahi T, Von Essen R: Improved immunoturbimetric method for rheumatoid factor testing. J Clin Pathol 46:1065, 1993.
6. Gripenberg M, Wafis F, Isomaki H, Lindes E: A simple enzyme immunoassay for the demonstration of rheumatoid factor. J Immunol Methods 31:109, 1979.
7. Winchester RJ, Kunkel HG, Agnello V: Occurrence of γ-globulin complexes in serum and joint fluid of rheumatoid arthritis patients: Use of monoclonal rheumatoid factors as reagents for their demonstration. J Exp Med 134:2865, 1971.
8. Hannestad K: Presence of aggregated γ-globulin in certain rheumatoid synovial effusions. Clin Exp Immunol 2:511, 1967.
9. Winchester RJ, Agnello V, Kunkel HG: Gamma globulin complexes in synovial fluids of patients with rheumatoid arthritis: Partial characterization and relationship to lowered complement levels. Clin Exp Immunol 6:689, 1970.
10. Schrohenloher RE: Characterization of the γ-globulin complexes present in certain sera having high titers of anti–γ-globulin activity. J Clin Invest 45:501, 1961.
11. Chodirker WB, Tomasi TB: Low molecular weight rheumatoid factor. J Clin Invest 42:876, 1963.
12. Scott DGI, Bacon TA, Allen C, Elson CJ, Wallington T: IgG rheumatoid factor, complement and immune complexes in rheumatoid synovitis and vasculitis: Comparative and serial studies during cytotoxic therapy. Clin Exp Immunol 43:54, 1981.
13. Dunne JV, Carson DA, Spiegelberg HL, Alspaugh MA, Vaughan JH: IgA rheumatoid factor in the sera and saliva of patients with rheumatoid arthritis and Sjögren's syndrome. Ann Rheum Dis 38:161, 1979.
14. Elkon KB, Delacroix DL, Gharevi A, Vauman JP, Hughes GR: Immunoglobulin A and polymeric IgA rheumatoid factors in systemic sicca syndrome: Partial characterization. J Immunol 129:577, 1982.
15. Kunkel HG, Simon HJ, Fudenberg H: Observations concerning positive serologic reactions for rheumatoid factor in certain patients with sarcoidosis and other hyperglobulinemic states. Arthritis Rheum 1:289, 1958.
16. Mikkelson WM, Dodge HJ, Duff IV, Kato H: Estimates of the prevalence of rheumatic disease in the population of Tecumseh, Michigan, 1950–60. J Chron Dis 20:351, 1967.
17. Lawrence JS: Rheumatism in Populations. London, William Heinemann, 1977.
18. Procaccia S, Lazzarin A, Colucci A, Gasparini A, Forcellini P, Lanzanova D, Foppa CU, Novati R, Zanussi C: IgM, IgG, and IgA rheumatoid factors and circulating immune complexes in patients with AIDS and AIDS-related complex with serological abnormalities. Clin Exp Immunol 67:236, 1987.
19. Jarvis JN, Taylor H, Iobidze M, Dejonge J, Chang S, Cohen F: Rheumatoid factor expression and complement activation in children congenitally infected with human immunodeficiency virus. Clin Immunol Immunopathol 67:50, 1993.
20. Chen PP, Carson DA: New insights on the physiological and pathological rheumatoid factors in humans. In Coutinho A, Kazatchkine MD (eds): Autoimmunity: Physiology and Disease. New York, Wiley-Liss, 1994, pp 247–266.
21. Hooper B, Whittingham S, Mathews JD, Mackay IR, Curnow DH: Autoimmunity in a rural community. Clin Exp Immunol 12:79, 1972.
22. Masi AT, Maldonado-Cocco JA, Kaplan SB, Feigenbaum SL, Chandler RW: Prospective study of the early course of rheumatoid arthritis in young adults. Semin Arthritis Rheum 5:299, 1976.
23. Moore TL, Donner RW, Weiss TD, Baldassare AR, Zuckner J: Specificity of hidden 19S 19M rheumatoid factor in patients with juvenile rheumatoid arthritis. Arthritis Rheum 24:1283, 1981.
24. Natvig JB, Gaardner PI, Turner MW: IgG antigens of the Cγ2 and Cγ3 homology regions interacting with rheumatoid factors. Clin Exp Immunol 12:177, 1972.
25. Sasso EH, Barver CV, Nardella FA, Yount WJ, Mannik M: Antigenic specificities of human monoclonal and polyclonal IgM rheumatoid factors: The Cγ2-Cγ3 interface region contains the major determinants. J Immunol 140:3098, 1988.
26. Williams RC, Malone CC: Rheumatoid-factor–reactive sites on CH2 established by analysis of overlapping peptides of primary sequence. Scand J Immunol 40:443, 1994.
27. Robbins DL, Skilling J, Benisek WF, Wistar R Jr: Estimation of the relative avidity of 19S IgM rheumatoid factor secreted by rheumatoid synovial cells for human IgG subclasses. Arthritis Rheum 29:722, 1986.
28. Parekh RB, Dwek RA, Sutton BJ, Fernandes D, Leung A, Stanworth D, Rademacher TW, Mizuochi T, Taniguchi T, Matsuta K, Takeuchi F, Nagano Y, Miyamoto T, Kobata A: Association of rheumatoid arthritis and primary osteoarthritis with changes in the glycosylation pattern of total serum IgG. Nature 316:452, 1985.
29. Axford JS, Mackenzie L, Lydyard PM, Hay FC, Isenberg DA, Roitt IM: Reduced B-cell galactosyltransferase activity in rheumatoid arthritis. Lancet 2:1486, 1987.
30. Van Zeben D, Rook GAW, Hazes JMW, Zwinderman AH, Zhang Y, Ghelani S, Rademacher TW, Breedveld FC: Early agalactosylation of IgG is associated with a more progressive disease course in patients with rheumatoid arthritis: Results of a follow-up study. Br J Rheumatol 33:36, 1994.
31. Tsuchiya N, Endo T, Matsuta K, Yoshinoya S, Aikawa T, Kosuge E, Takeuchi F, Miyamoto T, Kobata A: Effects of galactose depletion from oligosaccharide chains on immunological activities of human IgG. J Rheumatol 16:285, 1989.
32. Newkirk MM, Lemmo A, Rauch J: Importance of IgG isotype, and not state of glycosylation, in determining human rheumatoid factor binding. Arthritis Rheum 33:800, 1990.
33. Soltys AJ, Hay FC, Bond A, Axford JS, Jones MG, Randen I, Thompson KM, Natvig JB: The binding of synovial tissue–derived human monoclonal immunoglobulin M rheumatoid factor to immunoglobulin G preparations of differing galactose content. Scand J Immunol 40:135, 1994.
34. Tsuchiya N, Endo T, Shiota M, Kochibe N, Ito K, Kobata A: Distribution of glycosylation abnormality among serum IgG subclasses from patients with rheumatoid arthritis. Clin Immunol Immunopathol 70:47, 1994.
35. Jefferis R, Mageed R: The epitope specificity and idiotype of monoclonal rheumatoid factors. Scand J Immunol Suppl 75:89, 1988.
36. Newkirk MM, Rauch J: Binding of human monoclonal IgG rheumatoid factors to Fc is influenced by carbohydrate. J Rheumatol 20:776, 1993.
37. Burastero SE, Casali P, Wilder AL, Notkins AL: Monoreactive high affinity and polyreactive low affinity rheumatoid factors are produced by CD5+ B cells from patients with rheumatoid arthritis. J Exp Med 168:1979, 1988.
38. Chen PP, Silverman GS, Liu MF, Carson DA: Idiotypic and molecular characterization of human rheumatoid factors. Chem Immunol 48:63, 1990.
39. Harindranath N, Goldfarb IS, Ikematsu H, Burastero SE, Wilder RL, Notkins AL, Casali P: Complete sequences of the genes encoding the VH and VL regions of low and high affinity monoclonal IgM and IgA1 rheumatoid factors produced by CD5+ B cells from a rheumatoid arthritis patient. Int Immunol 3:865, 1991.
40. Mantovani L, Wilder RL, Casali P: Human rheumatoid B-1a (CD5+ B) cells make somatically hypermutated high affinity IgM rheumatoid factors. J Immunol 151:473, 1993.
41. Eisenberg R: The specificity and polyvalency of binding of a monoclonal rheumatoid factor. Immunochemistry 13:355, 1976.
42. Pope RM, Teller DC, Mannik M: The molecular basis of self-association of antibodies to IgG (rheumatoid factors) in rheumatoid arthritis. Proc Natl Acad Sci USA 71:517, 1974.

43. Nardella FA, Teller DC, Mannik M: Studies on the antigenic determinants in the self-association of IgG rheumatoid factor. J Exp Med 154:112, 1981.

44. Lu EW, Deftos M, Tighe H, Carson DA, Chen PP: Generation and characterization of two monoclonal self-associating IgG rheumatoid factors from a rheumatoid synovium. Arthritis Rheum 35:101, 1992.

45. Welch MJ, Fong S, Vaughan J, Carson D: Increased frequency of rheumatoid factor precursor B lymphocytes after immunization of normal adults with tetanus toxoid. Clin Exp Immunol 51:299, 1983.

46. Nemazee DA, Sato VL: Induction of rheumatoid antibodies in the mouse: Regulated production of autoantibody in the secondary humoral response. J Exp Med 158:529, 1983.

47. Van Snick J, Coulie P: Rheumatoid factors and secondary immune responses in the mouse. I: Frequent occurrence of hybridomas secreting IgM anti-IgG autoantibodies after immunization with protein antigens. Eur J Immunol 13:890, 1983.

48. Slaughter L, Carson DA, Jensen FC, Holbrook TL, Vaughan JH: In vitro effects of Epstein-Barr virus on peripheral blood mononuclear cells from patients with rheumatoid arthritis and normal subjects. J Exp Med 148:1429, 1978.

49. Izui S, Eisenberg RA, Dixon FJ: IgM rheumatoid factors in mice injected with bacterial lipopolysaccharide. J Immunol 122:2096, 1979.

50. Coulie PG, Van Snick J: Rheumatoid factor (RF) production during anamnestic immune responses in the mouse: III. Activation of RF precursor cells is induced by their interaction with immune complexes and carrier-specific helper T cells. J Exp Med 161:88, 1985.

51. Roosnek E, Lanzavecchia A: Efficient and selective presentation of antigen-antibody complexes by rheumatoid factor B cells. J Exp Med 175:487, 1991.

52. Tighe H, Chen PP, Tucker R, Kipps TJ, Roudier J, Jirik FR, Carson DA: Function of B cells expressing a human IgM rheumatoid factor autoantibody in transgenic mice. J Exp Med 177:109, 1993.

53. Williams RC, Kunkel HG: Rheumatoid factor, complement and conglutinin aberrations in patients with subacute bacterial endocarditis. J Clin Invest 41:666, 1962.

54. Carson DA, Bayer AS, Eisenberg RA, Lawrance S, Theofilopoulos A: IgG rheumatoid factor in subacute bacterial endocardosis: Relationship to IgM rheumatoid factor and circulating immune complexes. Clin Exp Immunol 31:100, 1978.

55. Casali P, Notkins AL: CD5⁺ lymphocytes, polyreactive antibodies and the human B cell repertoire. Immunol Today 10:364, 1989.

56. Tsuchiya N, Williams RC Jr, Hutt-Fletcher LM: Rheumatoid factors may bear the internal image of the Fc-binding protein of herpes simplex virus type I. J Immunol 144:4742, 1990.

57. Kunkel HG, Agnello V, Joslin FG, Winchester RJ, Capra JD: Cross idiotypic specificity among monoclonal IgM proteins with anti-γ-globulin activity. J Exp Med 137:331, 1973.

58. Capra JD, Kehoe JM: Structure of antibodies with shared idiotypy: The complete sequence of the heavy chain variable regions of two immunoglobulin M anti-gamma globulins. Proc Natl Acad Sci USA 71:4032, 1974.

59. Carson DA, Fong S: A common idiotope on human rheumatoid factors identified by a hybridoma antibody. Mol Immunol 20:1081, 1983.

60. Chen PP, Goni F, Houghten RA, Fong S, Goldfien R, Vaughan JH, Frangione B, Carson DA: Characterization of human rheumatoid factors with seven antiidiotypes induced by synthetic hypervariable region peptides. J Exp Med 162:487, 1985.

61. Carson DA, Chen PP, Kipps TJ, Radoux V, Jirik FR, Goldfien RD, Fox RI, Silverman GJ, Fong S: Idiotypic and genetic studies of human rheumatoid factors. Arthritis Rheum 30:1321, 1987.

62. Liu M-F, Robbins DL, Crowley JJ, Sinha S, Kozin F, Kipps TJ, Carson DA, Chen PP: Characterization of four homologous L chain variable region genes that are related to 6B6.6 idiotype positive human rheumatoid factor L chains. J Immunol 142:688, 1989.

63. Kipps TJ, Tomhave E, Chen PP, Fox RI: Molecular characterization of a major autoantibody-associated cross-reactive idiotype in Sjogren's syndrome. J Immunol 142:4261, 1989.

64. Crowley JJ, Goldfien RD, Schrohenloher RE, Spiegelberg HL, Silverman GJ, Mageed RA, Jefferis R, Koopman WJ, Carson DA, Fong S: Incidence of three cross-reactive idiotypes on human rheumatoid factor paraproteins. J Immunol 140:3411, 1988.

65. Chen PP, Fong S, Goni F, Silverman GJ, Fox RI, Liu MF, Frangione B, Carson DA: Cross-reacting idiotypes on cryoprecipitating rheumatoid factor. Springer Semin Immunopathol 10:35, 1988.

66. Schrohenloher R, Accavitti MA, Brown AS, Koopman WJ: Monoclonal antibody 6B6.6 defines a cross-reactive kappa light chain idiotope on human monoclonal and polyclonal rheumatoid factors. Arthritis Rheum 33:187, 1990.

67. Silverman GJ, Schrohenloher RE, Accavitti MA, Koopman WJ, Carson DA: Structural characterization of the second major cross-reactive idiotype group of human rheumatoid factors. Arthritis Rheum 33:1347, 1990.

68. Nakamura M, Burastero SE, Notkins AL, Casali P: Human monoclonal

69. Hardy RR: Variable gene usage, physiology and development of Ly-1 + (CD5 +) B cells. Curr Opin Immunol 4:181, 1992.

70. Riboldi P, Kasaian MT, Mantovani L, Ikematsu H, Casali P: Natural antibodies. In Bona CA, Siminovitch K, Zanetti M, Theophilopoulos AN (eds): The Molecular Pathology of Autoimmune Diseases. Philadelphia, Gordon and Breach, 1993, pp 45.

71. Casali P, Burastero SE, Nakamura M, Inghirami G, Notkins AL: Human lymphocytes making rheumatoid factor and antibodies to ssDNA belong to the Leu-1 + B cell subset. Science 236:77, 1987.

72. Levine PR, Axelrod DA: Rheumatoid factor isotypes following immunization. Clin Exp Rheumatol 3:147, 1985.

73. Nemazee D: Immune complexes can trigger specific T cell–dependent autoanti-IgG antibody production in mice. J Exp Med 161:242, 1985.

74. Thompson KM, Randen I, Borretzen M, Forre O, Natvig JB: Variable region usage of human monoclonal rheumatoid factors derived from healthy donors following immunization. Eur J Immunol 24:1771, 1994.

75. Borretzen M, Randen I, Zdarsky E, Forre O, Natvig JB, Thompson KM: Control of autoantibody affinity by selection against amino acid replacements in the complementarity-determining regions. Proc Natl Acad Sci USA 91:12917, 1994.

76. Sato Y, Sato R, Watanabe H, Kogure A, Watanabe K, Nishimaki T, Kasukawa R, Kuraya M, Fujita T: Complement activating properties of mono-reactive and polyreactive IgM rheumatoid factors. Ann Rheum Dis 52:795, 1993.

77. Hakoda M, Ishimoto T, Hayashimoto S, Inoue K, Taniguchi A, Kamatani N, Kashiwazaki S: Selective infiltration of B cells committed to the production of monoreactive rheumatoid factor in synovial tissue of patients with rheumatoid arthritis. Clin Immunol Immunopathol 69:16, 1993.

78. Carson DA, Chen PP, Kipps TJ, Roudier J, Silverman GJ, Tighe H: Regulation of rheumatoid factor synthesis. Clin Exp Rheumatol 7(Suppl 3):69, 1989.

79. Pascual V, Victor K, Randen I, Thompson K, Steinitz M, Forre O, Fu SM, Natvig JB, Capra JD: Nucleotide sequence analysis of rheumatoid factors reactive antibodies derived from patients with rheumatoid arthritis reveals diverse use of VH and VL gene segments and extensive variability in CDR3. Scand J Immunol 36:349, 1992.

80. Lee KL, Bridges SL, Koopman WJ, Schroder HW: The immunoglobulin kappa light chain repertoire expressed in the synovium of a patient with rheumatoid arthritis. Arthritis Rheum 35:905, 1992.

81. Randen I, Brown D, Thompson KM, Hughes-Jones N, Pascual V, Victor K, Capra JD, Forre O, Natvig JB: Clonally related IgM rheumatoid factors, undergo affinity maturation in the rheumatoid synovial tissue. J Immunol 14:3296, 1992.

82. Soto-Gil RW, Olee T, Klink BK, Kenny TP, Robbins DL, Carson DA, Chen PP: A systematic approach to defining the germline gene counterparts of a mutated autoantibody from a patient with rheumatoid arthritis. Arthritis Rheum 35:356, 1992.

83. Sasso EH: Immunoglobulin V region genes in rheumatoid arthritis. Rheum Dis Clin North Am 18:809, 1992.

84. Youngblood K, Fruchter L, Ding G, Lopez J, Bonagura V, Davidson A: Rheumatoid factors from the peripheral blood of two patients with rheumatoid arthritis are genetically heterogeneous and somatically mutated. J Clin Invest 93:852, 1994.

85. Victor KD, Randen I, Thompson K, Forre O, Natvig JB, Fu SM, Capra JD: Rheumatoid factors isolated from patients with autoimmune disorders are derived from germline genes distinct from those encoding the Wa, Po, and Bla cross-reacting idiotypes. J Clin Invest 87:1603, 1990.

86. Robbins DL, Kenny TP, Coloma MJ, Gavilondo-Cowley JV, Soto-Gil RW, Chen PP, Larrick JW: Serologic and molecular characterization of a human monoclonal rheumatoid factor derived from rheumatoid synovial cells. Arthritis Rheum 33:1188, 1990.

87. Ermel RW, Kenny TP, Chen PP, Robbins DL: Molecular analysis of rheumatoid factors derived from rheumatoid synovium suggest an antigen-driven response in inflamed joints. Arthritis Rheum 36:380, 1993.

88. Ermel RW, Kenny TP, Wong A, Solomon A, Chen PP, Robbins DL: Preferential utilization of a novel Vλ3 gene in monoclonal rheumatoid factors derived from the synovial cells of rheumatoid arthritis patients. Arthritis Rheum 37:860, 1994.

89. Randen I, Pascual V, Victor K, Thompson KM, Forre O, Capra JD, Natvig JD: Synovial IgG rheumatoid factors show evidence of an antigen driven immune response and shift in the V gene repertoire compared to IgM rheumatoid factors. Eur J Immunol 23:1220, 1993.

90. Deftos M, Olee T, Carson DA, Chen PP: Defining the genetic origins of three rheumatoid synovium-derived IgG rheumatoid factors. J Clin Invest 93:2545, 1994.

91. Axelrod O, Silverman GJ, Dev V, Kyle R, Carson DA, Kipps TJ: Idiotypic cross-reactivity of immunoglobulins expressed in Waldenström's macroglobulinemia, chronic lymphocytic leukemia, and mantle zone lymphocytes of secondary B-cell follicles. Blood 77:1484, 1991.

rheumatoid factor-like antibodies from CD5 (Leu-1) + B cells are polyreactive. J Immunol 140:4180, 1988.

92. Kumararatne DS, Bazin H, MacLennan ICM: Marginal zones: The major B cell compartment of rat spleens. Eur J Immunol 11:858, 1981.

93. Phillips NE, Parker DC: Fc-dependent inhibition of mouse B cell activation by whole anti-μ antibodies. J Immunol 130:602, 1983.

94. Tighe H, Heaphy P, Baird S, Weigle WO, Carson DA: Human immunoglobulin (IgG) induced deletion of IgM rheumatoid factor B cells in transgenic mice. J Exp Med 181:599, 1995.

95. Sabharwal UK, Vaughan JH, Fong S, Bennett PH, Carson DA, Curd JG: Activation of the classical pathway of complement by rheumatoid factors. Arthritis Rheum 25:161, 1982.

96. Rigley KP, Harnett MM, Klaus GGB: Cross-linking of surface immunoglobulin Fcγ receptors on B lymphocytes uncouples the antigen receptors from the associated G protein. Eur J Immunol 19:481, 1989.

97. Panoskaltis A, St. Clair NR: Rheumatoid factor blocks regulator Fc signals. Cellular Immunol 123:177, 1989.

98. Brouet JC, Clauvel JP, Danon F, Klein M, Seligman M: Biological and clinical significance of cryoglobulins: A report of 86 cases. Am J Med 57:775, 1974.

99. Fong S, Chen PP, Gilbertson TA, Weber JR, Fox RI, Carson DA: Expression of three cross reactive idiotypes on rheumatoid factor autoantibodies from patients with autoimmune diseases and seropositive adults. J Immunol 137:122, 1986.

100. Talal N, Bunim J: The development of malignant lymphoma in Sjögren's syndrome. Am J Med 36:529, 1964.

101. Masi AT, Maldonado-Cocco JA, Kaplan SB, Geigen-Baum SL, Chandler RW: Prospective study of the early course of rheumatoid arthritis in young adults. Semin Arthritis Rheum 5:299, 1976.

102. Westedt ML, Herbrink P, Molenaar JL, de Vries E, Verlaan P, Stijnen T, Cats A, Lindeman J: Rheumatoid factors in rheumatoid arthritis and vasculitis. Rheumatol Int 5:709, 1985.

103. Arnason JA, Jonsson TH, Brekkan A, Sigurjonsson K, Valdimarsson H: Relation between bone erosions and rheumatoid factor isotypes. Ann Rheum Dis 46:380, 1987.

104. Youinou PY, Morrow JW, Lettin AWF, Lydyard PM, Roitt IN: Specificity of plasma cells in the rheumatoid synovium. I. Immunoglobulin class of antiglobulin-producing cells. Scand J Immunol 20:307, 1984.

105. Brown BP, Nardella FA, Mannik M: Human complement activation by self-associated IgG rheumatoid factors. Arthritis Rheum 25:1101, 1982.

106. Winchester RJ: Characterization of IgG complexes in patients with rheumatoid arthritis. Ann NY Acad Sci 256:73, 1975.

107. Mannik M, Nardella FA: IgG rheumatoid factors and self-association of these antibodies. Clin Rheum Dis 11:551, 1985.

108. Panush RS, Bittner AK, Sullivan M, Katz P, Longley S: IgM rheumatoid factor elaboration by blood, bone marrow and synovial mononuclear cells in patients with rheumatoid arthritis. Clin Immunol Immunopathol 57:387, 1985.

109. Williams RC Jr, Malone CC, Harley JB: Rheumatoid factors from patients with rheumatoid arthritis react with Des-Lys58-b2m, modified β2-microglobulin. Arthritis Rheum 34:916, 1993.

110. Van Eyndhoven WG, Malone CC, Williams RC Jr: Changes in rheumatoid factor and monoclonal IgG antibody specificity after site-specific mutations in antigenic region of β2-microglobulin. Clin Immunol Immunopathol 72:362, 1994.

111. Williams RC, Malone CC: Human IgM rheumatoid factors react with class I HLA molecules. Arthritis Rheum 36:S265, 1993.

CHAPTER 17

Antinuclear Antibodies

Stanford L. Peng
John A. Hardin
Joe Craft

Antinuclear antibodies (ANAs) constitute a diverse group of antibody specificities found most prominently in systemic lupus erythematosus (SLE), systemic sclerosis, mixed connective tissue disease, and Sjögren's syndrome. Related antibodies targeting cytoplasmic autoantigens characteristically appear in polymyositis and adult dermatomyositis and have generally been grouped with the ANAs because they appear to have similar structures and etiologic factors. Collectively referred to as the *ANA diseases* (Table 17–1), these illnesses are typified by cellular autoimmunity to intracellular antigens, stressing the role of ANAs as tools for diagnosis. Such autoantibodies, however, appear in a variety of infectious, inflammatory, and neoplastic diseases as well as in normal individuals. Therefore, the clinician must carefully dissect the clinical utility of the ANA test. This chapter describes the more common ANA specificities—outlining their history, methods of detection, clinical disease associations, and the molecular biology of their target autoantigens—in an effort to establish clearly the clinical efficacy of testing for these antibodies. Several recent reviews have served as references for this chapter.[1–3]

HISTORY

Autoantibodies against intracellular antigens have cultivated a collaboration between clinical immunology and molecular biology. In the first formal description of an ANA-related phenomenon in 1948, the concentrated bone marrow specimens of patients with SLE were found to contain "LE" cells,[4] which were subsequently used as an adjunct tool in the diagnosis of SLE, drug-induced lupus, Sjögren's syndrome, and rheumatoid arthritis.[5] The LE cell was soon discovered to be due to a plasma factor,[6] autoantibody against deoxyribonucleoprotein,[7] which acted as an opsonin for the phagocytosis of antibody-sensitized nuclei by polymorphonuclear neutrophils.

In 1957, the new technique of indirect immunofluorescence allowed the development of the fluorescent ANA (FANA) test, which offered a more sensitive assay for autoimmunity in SLE and other diseases, and thus brought on a new method of choice for the screening of autoimmune disease.[8] The introduction of immunodiffusion permitted a finer distinction of autoantibody specificities to soluble components of whole cells[9] and subsequently led to the identification of new ANA specificities, including Sm,[10] nuclear ribonucleoprotein (nRNP),[11–15] SS-A (Ro), and SS-B (La).[16–18]

Later studies brought further biologic significance to these findings by demonstrating that these autoantigens play prominent roles in cellular homeostasis: small nuclear ribonucleoproteins (snRNPs), for example, targets of the anti-Sm and anti-nRNP antibodies, play essential roles in the splicing of pre–messenger ribonucleic acid (pre-mRNA).[19] These discoveries subsequently led to the elucidation of many autoantigens (the most prominent are listed in Table 17–2), many of which have yet to be fully characterized. As a result of such clinical–biochemical concordances, ANAs not only have served as helpful diagnostic markers in autoimmune diseases but also have greatly aided molecular biologic studies on intracellular metabolism.

DETECTION

Immunofluorescence

The indirect immunofluorescence ANA (FANA) test provides a highly sensitive screening method for ANA detection. Test sera at varying dilutions are incubated with substrate cells, and bound antibodies are detected by fluorescein-conjugated anti–human immunoglobulin (Ig), followed by visualization through a fluorescence microscope. The test's reliability depends primarily on the choice of substrate, which can vary from rodent liver or kidney frozen sections to cultured proliferating cell lines, most commonly the human epithelial tumor line HEp-2. Although tissue sections possess the advantage of eliminating interference from blood group antibodies, heterophile antibodies, or passenger viruses, cultured cell lines are a more reliable substrate because of their higher concentration of nuclear and

Table 17–1. ANTINUCLEAR ANTIBODY (ANA) DISEASES

Disease	Patients with ANAs (%)
Systemic lupus erythematosus	99
Drug-induced lupus	100
Systemic sclerosis	97
Mixed connective tissue disease	93
Polymyositis and dermatomyositis	78
Sjögren's syndrome	96

Table 17–2. DIAGNOSTIC CHARACTERISTICS OF THE ANTINUCLEAR ANTIBODIES (ANAs)

Specificity	ANA Pattern	Other Tests	Primary Rheumatic Disease Associations
Nuclear			
Chromatin-associated antigens			
dsDNA	Rim, homogeneous	RIA, ELISA, CIF, Farr	SLE
ssDNA or dsDNA	Rim, homogeneous	RIA, ELISA, CIF	SLE
ssDNA	Undetectable	ELISA	SLE, DILE, RA
Histones		IB, RIA, ELISA	
H1, H2A, H2B, H3, H4	Homogeneous, rim		SLE, DILE, RA, PBC, Scl
H3	Large speckles		SLE, UCTD
Ku	Diffuse-speckled nuclear/ nucleolar*	ID, IPP, IB	SLE, PM/Scl overlap
PCNA/Ga/LE-4	Nuclear or nucleolar speckles*	ELISA, ID, IB, IPP	SLE
Spliceosomal components	Speckled	ID, ELISA, IB, IPP	
Sm			SLE
U1 snRNP			SLE, MCTD
U2 snRNP			SLE, MCTD, overlap
U4/U6 snRNP			SS, Scl
U5 snRNP			SLE, MCTD
U7 snRNP			SLE
U11 snRNP			Scl
Other ribonucleoproteins			
Ro(SS-A)	Speckled or negative†	ID, ELISA, IB, IPP	SS, SCLE, NLE, SLE, PBC, Scl
La(SS-B/Ha)	Speckled	ID, ELISA, IB, IPP	SS, SCLE, NLE, SLE
Mi-2	Homogeneous	ID, IPP	DM
p80-coilin	Speckled		SS
MA-I	Speckled*		SS
Nucleolar			
RNA polymerases	Punctate	IPP, IB	
RNAP I	Nucleolar		Scl
RNAP II	Nuclear or nucleolar‡		Scl, SLE, overlap
RNAP III	Nuclear or nucleolar‡		Scl
Ribosomal RNP	Nucleolar, cytoplasmic	ID, IB, IPP, ELISA	SLE
Topoisomerase I (Scl-70)	Diffuse, grainy nuclear or nucleolar spots	ID, IB, ELISA	Scl
U3 snoRNP (fibrillarin)	Clumpy	IB, IPP	Scl
Th snoRNP (RNase MRP)	Diffuse with sparse nuclear spots	IPP	Scl
NOR 90 (hUBF)	10–20 discrete nuclear spots*	IB, IPP	Scl
PM-Scl (PM-1)	Homogeneous nuclear or nucleolar	ID, IPP, IB	PM, DM, Scl, overlap
Cytoplasmic			
tRNA synthetases			
tRNA^His (Jo-1)	Diffuse	ID, IPP, IB, ELISA, AAI	PM, DM
tRNA^Thr (PL-7)	Diffuse	ID, IPP, IB, ELISA, AAI	PM, DM
tRNA^Ala (PL-12)	Diffuse	ID, IPP, IB, ELISA, AAI	PM, DM
tRNA^Gly (EJ)	Diffuse	ID, IPP, IB, ELISA, AAI	PM, DM
tRNA^Ile (OJ)	Diffuse	ID, IPP, IB, ELISA, AAI	PM, DM
Signal recognition particle (SRP)	?	IPP, IB	PM
KJ	?	ID, IB	Myositis
Elongation factor 1α (Fer)	?	IPP	Myositis
tRNA^Ser (Mas)	?	IPP	Myositis

Adapted from Fritzler MJ: Immunofluorescent antinuclear antibody test. *In* Rose NR, de Macario EC, Fahey JL, et al (eds): Manual of Clinical Laboratory Immunology. Washington, DC, American Society for Microbiology, 1992, p 724.

*Cell cycle dependent.

†In cell studies, Ro RNP associates with cytoplasmic fractions (see O'Brien CA, Wolin SL: Genes Dev 8:2891, 1994).

‡May also stain nucleoli because of an association with antibodies to RNA polymerase I.

Abbreviations: AAI, aminoacylation inhibition; CIE, counterimmunoelectrophoresis; CIF, *Crithidia luciliae* immunofluorescence; DILE, drug-induced lupus erythematosus; DM, dermatomyositis; ELISA, enzyme-linked immunosorbent assay; Farr, Farr radioimmunoassay; IB, immunoblot; ID, immunodiffusion; IPP, immunoprecipitation; MCTD, mixed connective tissue disease; NLE, neonatal lupus erythematosus; overlap, overlap syndromes; PBC, primary biliary cirrhosis; PM, polymyositis; RA, rheumatoid arthritis; RIA, radioimmunoassay; Scl, systemic sclerosis; SCLE, subacute cutaneous lupus erythematosus; SLE, systemic lupus erythematosus; SS, Sjögren's syndrome; UCTD, undifferentiated connective tissue disease.

cytoplasmic antigens.[20] Indeed, substrates tend to remain comparable in their ability to detect common ANAs but differ substantially in the quantitation of antibody titer.[21] Additional sources of variability include the subjective nature of the test, the quality of reagents used, and the microscope used for visualization. Thus, although the FANA assay remains a widely used diagnostic test, results must be interpreted in light of the particular method used by individual clinical laboratories.

Because different ANAs have different intracellular targets, some clinically useful information can be obtained by observing the fluorescence pattern in the nucleus, nucleolus, or cytoplasm (Figs. 17–1 and 17–2; see Table 17–2). Nuclear patterns include homogeneous, rim, or speckled staining; nucleolar patterns include discrete speckled, grainy speckled, and clumpy staining.[1] Unfortunately, however, FANA testing does not typically yield clear-cut diagnostic information. Fluorescent patterns vary with serum dilution: Sera containing antibodies to histones and snRNPs, for example, may produce the homogeneous pattern of anti-histone antibodies at lower dilutions but the speckled pattern of anti-snRNP antibodies at higher dilutions. In addition, normal individuals, usually older persons and women, produce positive FANA results at a frequency of 5 percent, although their titer generally remains below 1:320 and the pattern is often homogeneous. Conversely, in rare instances, patients with SLE have negative FANA

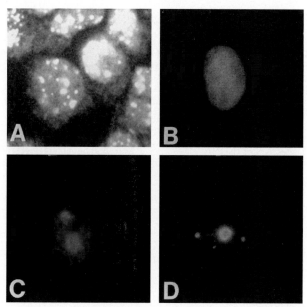

Figure 17–2. The fluorescent antinuclear antibody test: specificities of systemic sclerosis. A, Discrete speckled nuclear pattern of anti-kinetochore (centromere) antibodies. B, Grainy nuclear and nucleolar patterns of anti–topoisomerase I (Scl-70) antibodies. C, Diffuse nucleolar and sparse nucleoplasmic patterns of anti-Th (RNase MRP, 7-2) antibodies. D, Punctate nucleolar staining of anti-RNA polymerase antibodies. (A, From the Clinical Slide Collection on the Rheumatic Diseases, copyright 1991; used by permission of the American College of Rheumatology.)

results if they possess isolated anti-Ro antibodies and/or if the test uses rat or mouse tissues, which contain very low concentrations of Ro antigen. Additional false-negative results occur for sera with isolated anti–single-stranded DNA (anti-ssDNA) or cytoplasmic specificities. Such phenomena warrant further caution in the interpretation of FANA titer and pattern[1, 20] and suggest that the FANA test, although an effective screen, requires additional confirmation.

Immunodiffusion

The double-immunodiffusion Ouchterlony technique provides a crude method for the detection and confirmation of autoimmune serum specificity by the comparison of precipitin activity with prototype antisera. It consists of the placement of control and test sera in agarose wells adjacent to disrupted rabbit or calf tissue extract, which contains extractable nuclear antigens (ENAs) but which retains little DNA and DNA-associated proteins because of the insolubility of chromatin. Over the next 24 to 48 hours, the antibodies and antigens diffuse outward from the wells, forming precipitin lines as the autoantibodies bind their epitopes and form an insoluble lattice. Sera that share specificity with the prototype sera produce precipitin lines that fuse with those of the prototype; heterologous specificities spur across one another or form lines of nonfusion (Fig. 17–3).

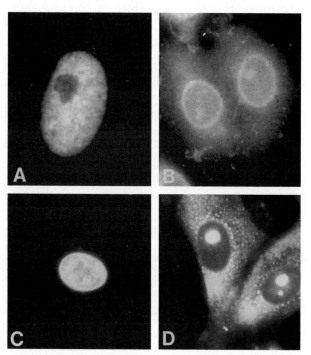

Figure 17–1. The fluorescent antinuclear antibody test: specificities of systemic lupus erythematosus. A, Speckled nuclear pattern of anti-Sm antibodies. B, Nuclear rim pattern of anti-DNA antibodies. C, Homogeneous nuclear pattern of anti-DNA antibodies. D, Discrete cytoplasmic and nucleolar pattern of anti-ribosome antibodies.

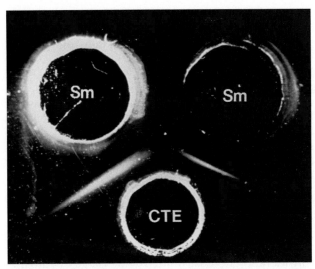

Figure 17–3. The immunodiffusion assay for the detection of anti-Sm autoantibodies. CTE, calf thymus extract. (From Craft J: Antibodies to snRNPs in systemic lupus erythematosus. Rheum Dis Clin North Am 18:311, 1992.)

Immunodiffusion remains insensitive in comparison with other assays, requiring large quantities (0.1 mg) of IgG and IgM to form visible precipitin lines. In addition, this method does not detect antibodies directed against rare or unstable antigens, such as the nucleolar Th and U3 RNPs, as well as insoluble antigens, such as DNA and histones. At the same time, immunodiffusion can detect autoantibodies to all soluble ENAs, such as snRNPs, Ro, and La; chromatin components that dissociate from DNA in saline buffer, such as topoisomerase I, proliferating cell nuclear antigen, and Ku; and soluble nucleolar components, such as PM-Scl (Table 17–3).[1] In addition, because it does not require special instrumentation or highly purified antigen, immunodiffusion has gained wide acceptance in clinical studies. Thus, although immunodiffusion provides a simple, straightforward

Table 17–3. DETECTION OF MAJOR AUTOANTIGENS BY IMMUNODIFFUSION

Detectable	Undetectable
snRNPs	Double-stranded DNA
Ro	Single-stranded DNA
La	Histones
Ku	Deoxyribonucleoprotein
PCNA	Centromere (kinetochore)
Ribosomes	RNA polymerases
Topoisomerase I	Th snoRNP (RNase MRP, 7-2 RNA)
PM/Scl	U3 snoRNP (fibrillarin)
tRNA synthetases	NOR 90 (hUBF)
Ki/SL	Signal recognition particle
Mi-2	MA-I
Ma	p80-coilin

Abbreviations: snRNP, small nuclear ribonucleoprotein; snoRNP, small nucleolar ribonucleoprotein; PCNA, proliferating cell nuclear antigen; tRNA, transfer RNA; NOR, nucleolar organizer region.

method for the detection of specific autoantibodies, its repertoire, lengthy time requirements, and low sensitivity compared with newer assays limit its widespread use.

Counterimmunoelectrophoresis

The counterimmunoelectrophoresis technique modifies the immunodiffusion technique to generate somewhat greater sensitivity. Acidic antigens, such as DNA or RNA, are electrophoresed from a cathode (negative) well, and antibodies are electrophoresed from an anode (positive) well. A precipitin line forms as specific autoantibodies encounter antigen, similar to immunodiffusion. Counterimmunoelectrophoresis requires less antibody (0.01 to 0.05 mg) but cannot measure basic proteins or antibodies that move cathodally by endosmosis, such as IgM or IgA.[22] Because this technique also provides limited sensitivity with a limited repertoire of autoantibody detection, it has largely become supplanted by other methods of ANA detection.

Enzyme-Linked Immunosorbent Assay

The enzyme-linked immunosorbent assay (ELISA) provides a highly sensitive and rapid technique for the detection of ANAs and determination of antibody specificity. Test sera are incubated in wells precoated with purified target antigen; bound antibodies are detected by means of an enzyme-conjugated anti–human immunoglobulin antibody, followed by color visualization with the appropriate enzyme substrate. Although these assays require highly purified antigen, many clinical laboratories have begun to use ELISAs for the routine determination of ANA specificity after positive FANA results. Indeed, their popularity has further resulted from the commercial availability of ELISA kits for the detection of specific autoantibodies, as well as the cloning and bacterial overexpression of recombinant autoantigens, such as Sm, U1 snRNP, Ro, La, transfer RNA (tRNA) synthetases, and topoisomerase I, making easier the development of various specificity-determining ELISAs.[1] Unfortunately, ELISAs produce some false-positive results, and confirmation sometimes requires further testing. Nevertheless, the ELISA plays a prominent role in the identification of ANAs.

Immunoprecipitation

Radioimmunoprecipitation assays provide sensitive, specific means by which to determine autoantibody specificity. In these techniques, radiolabeled cell extracts are incubated with test sera, and the resulting autoantibody–autoantigen complexes are precipitated by an insoluble carrier, such as protein A–conjugated sepharose. Subsequent resolution by electrophoresis and visualization by autoradiography allow for the detection of radiolabeled proteins or nucleic acids bound by the autoimmune serum (Fig. 17–4).[23] Through the use of radiolabeled extracts, this technique increases the sensitivity of detection of antibodies against minor cellular components, such as the Ro autoantigen,[24] as well as of more abundant antigens, such as the U1 snRNP.[25] In addition, with the use of whole cell extracts, simultaneous specificities are tested at once. Still, immunoprecipitations use radioactivity and are a more laborious procedure than ELISA or immunodiffusion. Its use has thus remained predominantly in research settings but may occasionally offer important information in determining and confirming serum specificities not defined by other assays.

Immunoblot

Western blotting techniques provide particularly efficacious information about antibody specificity. These assays use autoimmune sera as probes against membranes containing electrophoretically resolved purified or crude antigens. Bound antibodies are detected by an enzyme-linked anti–human immunoglobulin antibody and substrate-dependent color de-

velopment.[26] Such resolution of various autoantigens allows determination of all relevant polypeptides targeted by a given serum. Unfortunately, immunoblot techniques remain somewhat less sensitive than ELISA and are more laborious. In addition, some autoantigens possess conformational epitopes that are disrupted by gel electrophoresis, as in the case of the Ro autoantigen.[27] Thus, like immunoprecipitation assays, immunoblotting techniques remain predominantly confined to research settings but sometimes are used to determine or confirm the specificity of difficult sera.

Anti-DNA Antibody Tests

Anti-DNA antibodies warrant special diagnostic consideration because of their wide range of autoantigenic epitopes and their concomitant assay difficulties. Antibodies that recognize denatured ssDNA bind the free purine and pyrimidine base sequences and appear in several different diseases, including SLE, drug-induced lupus, chronic active hepatitis, infectious mononucleosis, and rheumatoid arthritis.[1] Other anti-DNA epitopes remain specific for SLE: some high-titer anti-DNA antibodies recognize native double-stranded DNA (dsDNA), binding the deoxyribose

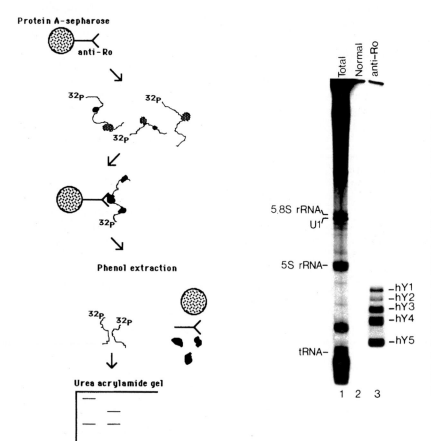

Figure 17–4. The immunoprecipitation assay for the detection of anti-Ro autoantibodies. On the left side of the figure, antibodies from a patient with systemic lupus erythematosus (SLE) are bound to sepharose beads coated with protein A; the latter binds the Fc portion of immunoglobulin of the IgG class. Antibody-coated beads are then mixed with a soluble extract, previously labeled in vivo with phosphorus 32 (^{32}P), which tags nucleic acids. Radiolabeled RNAs (as part of a ribonucleoprotein [RNP] particle) can then be immunoprecipitated via their antigenic proteins, phenol-extracted to remove proteins (Ro proteins and immunoglobulins), and fractionated by gel electrophoresis. The right side of the figure contains the radiolabeled RNAs found in a total human (HeLa) cell extract (lane 1), and those immunoprecipitated by a normal control serum (lane 2) and a serum containing anti-Ro antibodies (lane 3). As shown, the Ro RNP contains four small RNAs in human cells, the hY RNAs (hY2 is a breakdown product of hY1).

phosphate backbone; rarer conformation-dependent anti-DNA antibodies bind dsDNA in the left-handed helical Z form.[28] With these differences in epitope and disease associations, anti-DNA assays must clearly distinguish between ssDNA and dsDNA substrates. Two methods to ensure the use of native dsDNA are (1) digestion with S1 nuclease, which removes overhanging ssDNA ends, and (2) chromatography on a hydroxyapatite column, which separates large single-stranded segments from dsDNA. Unfortunately, native DNA may spontaneously denature, especially when bound to plastic ELISA plates; this may account for the results of several reports of a relative lack of specificity of anti-dsDNA antibodies for SLE.[1] Reliable assays, therefore, must ensure the integrity of the dsDNA substrate.

Two assays offer greater assurance for anti-dsDNA testing. The Farr radioimmunoassay, which resembles immunoprecipitation assays, involves the binding of autoantibodies to radiolabeled dsDNA in solution. Precipitation of the antibody–DNA complexes by ammonium sulfate allows a quantitation of the percentage of incorporated (antibody-bound) radioactive dsDNA. Normal sera typically bind a small fraction of added DNA (usually less than 20 percent), whereas SLE sera often bind nearly 100 percent of added DNA. The specificity of this assay, however, still depends on the quality of dsDNA and the removal of contaminating ssDNA, but because the assay requires autoantibodies to bind antigen in solution, the Farr assay is generally considered the gold standard for anti-dsDNA analysis.[1] One alternative to the Farr assay, the *Crithidia luciliae* test, provides an inherently reliable dsDNA substrate. In this assay, the hemoflagellate *C. luciliae* serves as a substrate for indirect immunofluorescence. Its kinetoplast, a modified giant mitochondrion, contains a concentrated focus of stable, circularized dsDNA without contaminating RNA or nuclear proteins, providing a sensitive and specific fluorescence substrate by which to establish anti-dsDNA activity. For these reasons, many laboratories have adopted the *Crithidia* immunofluorescence test for routine use.[29] Farr radioimmunoassays and *C. luciliae* immunofluorescence tests thus provide effective, complementary mechanisms to distinguish anti-ssDNA from anti-dsDNA activities.

DISEASES ASSOCIATED WITH ANTINUCLEAR ANTIBODIES

Systemic Lupus Erythematosus

Antinuclear antibodies are a hallmark of SLE. The FANA results are positive in over 99 percent of patients,[30] and although most autoantigens targeted by SLE sera reside in the nucleus, SLE can evoke specificities against a seemingly endless range of antigens in various cellular locations. Still, these autoantigens can be broadly categorized into chromatin-associated antigens versus ribonucleoproteins (Table 17–4 lists

Table 17–4. ANTINUCLEAR ANTIBODIES IN SYSTEMIC LUPUS ERYTHEMATOSUS

Antibody Specificity	Prevalence (%)
Chromatin-Associated Antigens	
dsDNA	73
Histone	50–70
Chromatin	88
Ku	20–40
PCNA	3–6
RNA polymerase II	9–14
Ribonucleoproteins	
snRNPs	
Sm core	20–30
U1 snRNP	30–40
U2 snRNP	15
U5 snRNP	?
U7 snRNP	?
Ro(SS-A)	40
La(SS-B)	10–15
Ribosomes	
P0, P1, P2 protein	10–20
28S rRNA	?
S10 protein	?
L5 protein	?
L12 protein	?

Abbreviations: dsDNA, double-stranded DNA; PCNA, proliferating cell nuclear antigen; snRNP, small nuclear ribonucleoprotein.

major specificities). Significant individual specificities are discussed below.

Chromatin-Associated Antigens

Anti-DNA antibodies remain one of the most widely recognized specificities in SLE. Recent studies have suggested, however, that more physiologic forms of DNA may provide relevant information about the pathogenesis and antibody response in lupus. In support of such views, SLE sera may target several DNA-associated molecules, such as histones; investigators have recently found higher prevalences of antibodies that recognize nucleosomes, which contain both DNA and histone proteins, rather than DNA alone.[31] In fact, anti-chromatin antibodies, reactive against native chromatin, appear at the highest described frequency for autoantibodies in SLE (88 percent), providing further support for a role of native structures in the genesis of the autoantibody response.[32] Still, most of the clinical literature about anti-chromatin autoantibodies remains linked to classic anti-DNA and anti-histone antibodies.

Anti-DNA. Anti-DNA antibodies include anti-ssDNA antibodies, which target the purine and pyrimidine bases of denatured DNA; anti-dsDNA antibodies, which target the ribose phosphate backbone of native DNA; and anti–Z-DNA antibodies, which target the left-handed helical Z form of DNA. Detection of anti-dsDNA antibodies usually involves FANA testing, in which these antibodies produce nuclear staining in a homogeneous or rim pattern, followed by confirmation by means of ELISA, *C. luciliae* immunofluorescence, or Farr radioimmunoassay. Anti-ssDNA antibodies, on the other hand, do not elicit positive FANA results and therefore require separate testing, such as ELISA, for detection.[20]

Although many diseases produce anti-ssDNA activity, only SLE sera possess high-titer anti-dsDNA or anti–Z-DNA activity. Anti-dsDNA antibodies appear in 73 percent of SLE patients, whereas low titers appear much less often in normal persons and patients with Sjögren's syndrome, rheumatoid arthritis, and other disorders.[1] In SLE, anti-DNA antibodies strongly correlate with nephritis and disease activity; they appear to contribute to disease pathology through high avidity to DNA, renal antigen cross-reactivity, complement fixation, or immune complex formation.[33] On the other hand, some reports describe lupus nephritis in the absence of anti-DNA antibodies, and others describe persistence of high-titer anti-DNA antibodies in the absence of renal injury,[1] suggesting that other antibody specificities may contribute to end-organ disease. Indeed, some studies suggest that the observed anti-DNA activities of these antibodies are experimental artifacts and that these antibodies instead recognize antigens distinct from DNA.[34] Furthermore, other investigators have found that these antibodies cross-react with other antigens, such as snRNPs or foreign proteins, suggesting that the immunologically relevant antigen for anti-DNA antibodies may not in fact be DNA.[35–37] Thus, although most investigators agree that antibodies reactive with DNA correlate strongly with lupus nephritis, they do not necessarily concur about precise pathogenic or etiologic roles.

Anti-histone (Nucleosome). Anti-histone antibodies target the protein components of nucleosomes, the DNA–protein complexes that form the substructure of transcriptionally inactive chromatin. Each nucleosome consists of approximately 140 base-pairs (bp) of chromatin DNA wrapped around a central core of the histone proteins H1, H2A, H2B, H3, and H4.[38] These antibodies may be detected by FANA, ELISA, or immunoblot; non-H3 anti-histone antibodies produce a homogeneous or rim nuclear pattern by FANA, whereas H3 anti-histone antibodies produce large speckles.[20] In the 50 to 70 percent of SLE patients with anti-histone antibodies, the antibodies target predominantly the H1 and H2B proteins, followed by H2A, H3, and H4,[39] usually in association with anti-dsDNA. These antibodies appear uniformly in drug-induced lupus,[40] in which they associate with anti-ssDNA antibodies, and they appear at lower frequency in other diseases, such as rheumatoid or juvenile arthritis, primary biliary cirrhosis,[33] scleroderma,[41–43] Epstein-Barr virus infection,[44] Chagas' disease,[45] schizophrenia,[46] sensory neuropathy,[47] monoclonal gammopathies,[48] and cancer.[49] Some researchers consider anti-histone antibodies to be sensitive markers for drug-induced lupus, and autoantibodies against native chromatin structures to be specific for SLE. Because of the wide clinical spectrum in which anti-histone antibodies appear, however, studies have not consistently upheld

any significant clinical correlations for anti-histone antibodies, unlike anti-DNA antibodies. One study, however, suggests that these antibodies may correlate with disease activity.[50]

Anti-Ku. Antibodies to the Ku antigen target a 10S chromatin-associated heterodimer that regulates the catalytic activity of a p350 DNA-dependent protein kinase implicated in DNA repair and V(D)J recombination.[51, 52] Ku controls these processes through the recognition of dsDNA termini, nicks, and gaps,[53, 54] perhaps by kinase-dependent regulation of transcription factors and RNA polymerases I and II.[55] It includes two subunits, p70 and p80, each targeted in various diseases. In FANA, anti-Ku antibodies demonstrate cell cycle–dependent diffuse nuclear and nucleolar staining, reflective of its biologic activity.[56] Originally described in scleroderma-polymyositis overlap syndrome,[57] anti-Ku has been found in the sera of 20 to 40 percent of patients with SLE (perhaps in association with anti–RNA polymerase II [RNAP II] antibodies[58]), in over 20 percent of sera from patients with primary pulmonary hypertension, and in over 50 percent of sera from patients with Graves' disease.[33, 59] The significance of these antibodies remains largely uninvestigated, although one study suggested that anti-p70 antibodies correlate with features of scleroderma-polymyositis overlap, whereas anti-p80 antibodies correlate with features of scleroderma or SLE.[60]

Anti–PCNA/Ga/LE-4. Antibodies against the proliferating cell nuclear antigen (PCNA), a 36-kD accessory factor for DNA polymerase delta, appear specifically in 3 to 6 percent of patients with SLE. These antibodies can be detected by FANA testing, which reveals variable speckled nucleoplasmic and nucleolar patterns depending on the cell cycle state of the stained cell. The clinical significance of these antibodies is unclear.

Anti-RNAP. Anti-RNA polymerase (anti-RNAP) antibodies target the eukaryotic RNA polymerases, which constitute three classes of synthetic enzymes containing two distinct high-molecular-weight polypeptides as well as at least six smaller subunits. RNA polymerase I synthesizes ribosomal RNA precursors in the nucleolus; RNA polymerase II transcribes some small nuclear RNA genes and all protein-encoding genes; and RNA polymerase III synthesizes some small nuclear RNAs as well as the 5S ribosomal RNA (rRNA) and tRNAs.[61] By FANA, these antibodies produce punctate nucleolar staining in resting cells and dots in areas of condensed chromosomes in metaphase cells.[62] Although anti–RNAP I antibodies originally were described in SLE, mixed connective tissue disease, and rheumatoid arthritis,[63] subsequent work has suggested that these antibodies are specific for scleroderma.[64] Anti–RNAP II antibodies, however, appear in 9 to 14 percent of patients with SLE and overlap syndromes, where they tend to be accompanied by anti-Ku or anti-RNP antibodies.[58, 65] Because of the paucity of information regarding these antibodies, their significance in SLE remains purely observational.

Ribonucleoproteins

Anti-snRNP. In SLE, autoantibodies against small nuclear ribonucleoproteins (snRNPs) generally target the RNAs or proteins of the spliceosome, a complex of ribonucleoprotein particles involved in the splicing of pre-mRNA. These particles include the U1, U2, U4/U6, U5, U7, U11, and U12 snRNPs, each of which consists of its respective uridine-rich (thus "U") small nuclear RNA (snRNA) and a set of polypeptides, including a common core of Sm polypeptides (B/B', D1, D2, D3, E, F, and G) and particle-specific polypeptides.[66] All anti-snRNP antibodies produce a distinct speckled nuclear pattern on FANA testing, reflective of the focal distribution of spliceosomal snRNPs in the nucleoplasm[67]; individual particle or protein epitopes can be determined by immunoprecipitation or immunoblot.[68] Anti-Sm antibodies target proteins of the Sm core, including B/B' and one of the D polypeptides; they are specific antibodies in the diagnosis of SLE, although they appear in only 20 to 30 percent of patients. Their presence has been associated with milder renal and central nervous system disease, organic brain syndrome, disease flares, or paradoxically more active disease, but additional studies have not upheld these findings, reporting no correlations with disease manifestations.[68]

Other specific anti-snRNP antibodies target polypeptides or RNAs particular to respective U snRNPs. Anti–U1 snRNP (anti-nRNP or anti–U1 RNP, historically), for example, targets the 70K, A, or C polypeptides specific to the U1 snRNP. These antibodies occur in 30 to 40 percent of SLE patients and are associated with disease activity, myositis, esophageal hypomotility, Raynaud's phenomenon, lack of nephritis, arthralgias and arthritis, sclerodactyly, and interstitial changes on chest radiographs.[69] Anti–U1 snRNP also constitutes a substantial portion of the immune response in mixed connective tissue disease, in which all patients demonstrate the antibody.

Other anti-snRNP antibodies, targeting U2,[70] U5,[71] or U7[72] snRNP–specific proteins, have been described in SLE but with low frequency. Likewise, some studies have suggested nonrheumatologic disease associations for the anti-snRNP antibodies, such as with monoclonal gammopathies[73] and psychiatric diseases,[74] but these findings are unconfirmed. Thus, although anti-Sm has generally remained a specific marker for SLE and anti–U1 snRNP maintains strong associations with SLE and mixed connective tissue disease, many studies continue to report disease associations with other anti-snRNP specificities, whose significances await determination.

Anti-Ro(SS-A) and Anti-La(SS-B). These two antibody specificities target distinct ribonucleoprotein particles. Ro is composed of 60- and 52-kD protein components as well as small RNAs known as the hY1, hY3, hY4, and hY5 RNAs. Extensive molecular biologic work in the past decade has been unable to fully define the biologic role of the Ro ribonucleoproteins, although the 60-kD protein contains a zinc-finger motif, and the 52-kD protein resembles the *rfp* protein, a homolog of the transforming protein *ret*, and *rpt-1*, a murine transcription factor.[75] Recent work suggests that 60-kD Ro may partake in a discard pathway for 5S rRNA precursors.[76]

On the other hand, the molecular biology of La, a 43- to 52-kD ribonucleoprotein, has been explored with greater success, concluding that the La ribonucleoprotein partakes in both the transcription termination of RNA polymerase III and the translation initiation of some mRNAs.[77, 78] These two particles likely exist physiologically in a complex: Ro RNAs are transcribed by RNA polymerase III, allowing a potential association with La. In addition, antibodies to Ro and La often appear in association with one another; in fact, animals immunized with La demonstrate both anti-La and anti-Ro antibodies, suggesting the operation of intermolecular epitope spreading in the antibody response.[79] Anti-Ro antibodies have posed difficulty in detection in the past, sometimes giving negative results by FANA testing because of the low concentration of Ro in substrate cells; under optimal conditions, however, both antibody specificities produce a speckled nuclear fluorescent pattern, even though biochemical studies suggest that Ro resides in the cytoplasm.[1, 76]

Although most commonly associated with Sjögren's syndrome, anti-Ro activity is seen in about 40 percent of SLE patients, and anti-La activity is seen in 10 to 15 percent. In SLE, anti-La correlates with late-onset SLE, secondary Sjögren's syndrome, the neonatal lupus syndrome, and the major histocompatibility complex (MHC) class II genes human leukocyte antigen (HLA) DR3, DQ1, and DQ2, as well as with protection from anti-Ro–associated nephritis.[80, 81] On the other hand, anti-Ro is associated with photosensitive skin rash, pulmonary disease, and lymphopenia; less discussed associations include the presence of rheumatoid factors; nephritis, thrombocytopenia; anti-La; complement (particularly C4) deficiencies; HLA-DQ1, DQ2, DR3, and DR2; and particular T cell receptor polymorphisms.[82, 83] One recent study suggested that anti–52-kD antibodies correlate with Sjögren's syndrome; anti–52-kD and anti–60-kD antibodies with SLE; and anti–60-kD antibodies with rheumatoid arthritis and other connective tissue diseases.[84] Further significant clinical associations of anti-Ro antibodies include the neonatal lupus syndrome, Sjögren's syndrome–SLE overlap, subacute cutaneous lupus erythematosus, and primary biliary cirrhosis; less described disease associations include multiple myeloma, rheumatoid arthritis, polymyositis, and scleroderma.[82]

Anti-ribosome. Anti-ribosome antibodies in SLE target protein or RNA components of the eukaryotic 80S ribosome, the ribonucleoprotein complex involved in the translation of mRNA into protein. The mammalian ribosome includes two subunits of 40S and 60S, composed of 28S, 18S, 5.8S, and 5S rRNAs in addition to at least 80 different proteins.[85] Anti–ribosomal P protein (anti-P) antibodies target the P0,

P1, and P2 alanine-rich ribosomal proteins (38, 19, and 17 kD, respectively), which are part of the large 60S subunit. Antibodies against these antigens produce FANA staining in both the cytoplasm, where protein translation occurs, and the nucleolus, where ribosome biogenesis occurs. The antibodies are found in 10 to 20 percent of SLE patients and have proved to be highly specific for SLE. Although analyses of SLE populations have failed to reveal definite clinical associations with anti-P antibodies, correlations with lupus psychosis have been found. Correlations with active disease, liver disease, renal disease, and the SLE-specific anti-Sm antibodies have also been suggested.[86, 87] Other less prevalent anti-ribosome antibodies target rRNA, such as the 28S rRNA, or other ribosomal proteins, such as the S10, L5, and L12 subunit proteins.[86] The clinical significance of these latter antibodies remains unclear, although some studies suggest that all anti-ribosome antibodies appear in association with each other, and so may represent a cluster of disease autoantibodies.[88, 89]

Anti-RNA. Autoantibodies that bind deproteinized ribonucleic acid have been described for anti–U snRNAs and anti-rRNAs.[1] Because their prevalence and disease associations have not been well characterized, their significance remains largely unknown.[90] One study, however, suggests that these antibodies associate with SLE, overlap syndromes, or both.[91]

Other Autoantibodies. A large number of other autoantibody specificities have been described in SLE, including antibodies to Ki (reactive with an undefined 32-kD autoantigen and associated with lupus plus sicca syndrome),[92] the nuclear matrix,[93] 90- or 70-kD heat-shock proteins,[94–96] neutrophil cytoplasmic antigens (p-ANCA, c-ANCA),[97, 98] carbonic anhydrase,[99] cyclophilin,[100] hn-RNP A1,[101] fimbrin,[102] microfilaments,[103] nuclear lamina,[104] and Su (which has been suggested as specific to SLE).[105] Because comprehensive studies have not been performed for many of these specificities, their clinical significance remains undetermined.

Systemic Sclerosis (Scleroderma)

Antinuclear antibodies against nucleolar antigens characterize the autoantibody response in systemic sclerosis. Positive FANA results, sometimes speckled in appearance, appear in 97 percent of sera.[106] Unlike SLE sera, however, systemic sclerosis sera usually contain monospecific autoantibody specificities, targeting such structures as the kinetochore, topoisomerase I, or RNA polymerases (Table 17–5 lists major specificities).[2]

Anti-kinetochore (Centromere). Anti-kinetochore antibodies target integral components of the mitotic spindle apparatus, which promotes chromosome separation during mitosis. Although these specificities were initially named "anti-centromere antibodies" (ACAs),[107] refined ultrastructural studies have defined the centromere as the primary constriction of mitotic

Table 17–5. ANTINUCLEAR ANTIBODIES IN SYSTEMIC SCLEROSIS

Antibody Specificity	Prevalence (%)
Kinetochore (centromere)	22–36
Topoisomerase I	22–40
RNA polymerases	4–23
U3 snoRNP (fibrillarin)	6–8
Th snoRNP (RNase MRP, 7-2 RNA)	4–11
PM-Scl	3
NOR 90 (hUBF)	?

Abbreviations: snoRNP, small nucleolar ribonucleoprotein; NOR, nucleolar organizer region; hUBF, human upstream binding factor.

chromosomes containing the genetic locus for partitioning and have defined the kinetochore, whose components are targeted by these antibodies, as the specialized trilaminar structure to which the spindle microtubules attach.[108] These autoantibodies target at least four centromere (kinetochore) antigens (CENPs)—CENP-B (the predominant kinetochore autoantigen recognized by all ACA sera), CENP-A, CENP-C, and CENP-D—which provide essential roles in the packaging of centromere DNA through various protein–protein and protein–nucleic acid interactions.[2, 64, 108] These antibodies produce weak fluorescent speckled patterns with titers below 1:32 when metabolically inactive cells, such as rodent tissues, are used as substrate; laboratories that use such FANA substrates as a screening test may therefore report such sera as negative.[2, 64] Screening for ACA therefore typically involves immunofluorescence of mitotically active cells, such as HEp-2 cells, or ELISA.[109]

ACAs are found in 22 to 36 percent of patients with systemic sclerosis. Their presence correlates with Raynaud's phenomenon; CREST (calcinosis, Raynaud's phenomenon, esophageal dysmotility, sclerodactyly, and telangiectasias, for which as many as 98 percent of patients have ACA[110]); and limited skin involvement. Several studies have reported significant prevalences of ACAs in diffuse scleroderma (22 to 36 percent) and scleroderma with proximal skin involvement (26 percent),[64] as well as Hashimoto's thyroiditis with Raynaud's syndrome,[111, 112] primary biliary cirrhosis associated with systemic sclerosis,[113, 114] and rheumatoid arthritis.[64, 115] In addition, ACA predicts the development of mat-like telangiectasias, signs of systemic sclerosis,[116] and pulmonary or vascular disease in systemic sclerosis[41, 117] and is associated with HLA-DR1, -DR4, and -DRw8.[118, 119] Despite these occasional associations with other diseases, most investigators consider ACAs specific for systemic sclerosis, CREST, and primary and secondary Raynaud's phenomenon.[64]

Anti–topoisomerase I (Scl-70). Anti–Scl-70 autoantibodies predominantly target the catalytic carboxy-terminal region of DNA topoisomerase I, a 100-kD helicase that relieves superhelical strain during the transcription or replication of DNA.[120, 121] Although studies to reveal the true molecular weight of anti–

Scl-70 have caused much dispute in the past, most workers now agree that the initial 70-kD protein recognized by these sera represents a proteolytic product of the intact helicase.[1] This specificity produces a diffusely grainy nucleoplasmic and nucleolar staining pattern on FANA testing; typical follow-up testing involves immunodiffusion, immunoblot, or ELISA.[122] Anti–topoisomerase I antibodies appear in 22 to 40 percent of patients with systemic sclerosis and generally predict diffuse cutaneous disease and proximal skin involvement,[123, 124] longer disease duration or association with cancer,[112] pulmonary fibrosis,[125] digital pitting scars, and cardiac involvement[1] as well as association with HLA-DR5, -B8, -DR3, -DR52, -DRw11, and -DR2.[118, 123, 126–128] In conjunction with ACAs, anti-topoisomerase antibodies constitute major diagnostic tools in the subclassification of diffuse versus limited systemic sclerosis.[1]

Anti-RNA Polymerases. Anti-RNAP antibodies target the eukaryotic RNA polymerases. These antibodies appear in 4 to 23 percent of scleroderma patients and are associated with diffuse cutaneous involvement.[129–131] Although anti–RNAP II antibodies appear in other diseases, such as SLE or overlap syndrome, and may be associated with other autoantibody specificities against Ku or ribonucleoproteins, anti-RNAP I and III antibodies remain specific for scleroderma.[58, 65, 130]

Anti-fibrillarin (U3 snoRNP). Anti-fibrillarin antibodies predominantly target the N^G,N^G-dimethylarginine–rich 34-kD protein of the U3 small nucleolar ribonucleoprotein (snoRNP), termed *fibrillarin* for its association with the nucleolar fibrillar component.[132, 133] FANA testing reveals clumpy nucleolar staining in resting cells and significant condensed chromosome staining in metaphase cells.[62] Anti-fibrillarin antibodies appear in 6 to 8 percent of scleroderma patients; although their clinical significance remains unclear, they appear to associate with diffuse disease, as well as lung and heart involvement.[62, 130]

Anti-Th snoRNP (RNase MRP; 7-2 RNA). Anti-Th antibodies bind the Th small nucleolar ribonucleoprotein, now known to be identical to the mitochondrial RNA processing (MRP) RNase MRP, which contains the 7-2 RNA.[134] This ribonucleoprotein resides predominantly in the nucleus and is implicated in the processing of precursor tRNAs as well as in ribosome biogenesis and mitochondrial DNA replication.[135–137] This specificity, present in 4 to 11 percent of scleroderma patients, may predict limited cutaneous disease, puffy fingers, small-bowel involvement, hypothyroidism, and reduced arthritis or arthralgias[138, 139]; comprehensive studies have not been performed, however.

Anti–NOR 90 (hUBF). Anti–NOR 90 antibodies were originally named for their immunoblotting of a 90-kD protein doublet and immunofluorescent staining of nucleolar organizer regions (NORs), which constitute the secondary constriction sites on chromosomes 13, 14, 15, 21, and 22. These sites consist of multiple rRNA gene clusters around which nucleoli reform after mitosis.[140] More recently, the molecular target of these antibodies has been demonstrated as the RNA polymerase transcription factor hUBF (human upstream binding factor), which exists as spliced variants of 97 and 94 kD.[141, 142] These sera produce 10 to 20 tiny discrete spots per nucleolus on FANA testing, changing to nucleoplasmic staining in a cell cycle–dependent fashion.[142] Although generally associated with scleroderma, anti-hUBF antibodies have been demonstrated in patients with SLE, Sjögren's syndrome, rheumatoid arthritis, and cancer[142]; their overall clinical significance and prevalence remain unknown.

Anti–PM-Scl. Anti–PM-Scl antibodies, typically identified by immunodiffusion, target a complex of at least 11 nucleolar proteins, of which the 100-, 70- to 75-, and 37-kD proteins predominate.[143–146] Three percent of scleroderma patients possess this antibody, which produces homogeneous nucleolar staining on FANA testing. Its presence associates with myositis–scleroderma overlap, without SLE features: 50 percent of anti–PM-Scl antibody–positive patients have the overlap, and 25 percent of the overlap patients have the antibody.[146] Also, anti–PM-Scl appears to be associated with arthritis, skin lesions of dermatomyositis, calcinosis, mechanic's hands, eczema, and HLA-DR3 and DR4[146, 147]; compared with other ANA-positive patients, anti–PM-Scl antibody–positive patients have a higher incidence of muscle, tendon, and renal disease.[148]

Other Autoantibodies. Other antibodies sometimes found in scleroderma include anti-histone,[41, 128] anti–nucleolar B23,[149] anti–carbonic anhydrase,[150] anti-laminin,[151] anti-hsp90,[152] anti-Ku,[2] anti-Ro,[153] anti-centriole,[154] anti–neutrophil cytoplasmic antibodies (ANCA),[155] anti-tRNA,[156] anti-microfilament,[103] anti–nuclear lamina,[104] anti-trimethylguanosine,[157] anti–U1 snRNP,[158] anti–U4/U6 snRNP,[159] and anti–U11 snRNP.[160] The significance of these findings is unclear.

Inflammatory Muscle Diseases

Inflammatory muscle diseases are a diverse group of illnesses often characterized by autoantibody responses against cytoplasmic antigens. Although between 40 and 80 percent of patients with polymyositis or dermatomyositis have positive FANA results,[161] up to 90 percent of patients with inflammatory muscle diseases as a whole have autoantibodies to cellular antigens.[162] Autoantibodies in myositis are generally categorized into myositis-specific autoantibodies (MSAs), found almost exclusively in inflammatory myositis, and those associated with overlap syndromes that include myositis. MSAs include the anti-synthetase antibodies, anti–signal recognition particle, and anti–Mi-2; overlap antibodies include anti-snRNP and anti–PM-Scl (Table 17–6 lists major specificities).[3]

Anti-synthetase. The anti-synthetase MSAs constitute a group of highly antigen-specific, disease-associated reactivities that produce cytoplasmic FANA. At

Table 17–6. ANTINUCLEAR ANTIBODIES IN INFLAMMATORY MUSCLE DISEASES

Antibody Specificity	Prevalence (%)
Myositis-Specific Antibodies	
Anti-tRNA synthetases	
Histidyl (Jo-1)	20
Threonyl (PL-7)	1–5
Alanyl (PL-12)	1–5
Glycyl (EJ)	1–5
Isoleucyl (OJ)	1–5
Mi-2	8 (15–20% of patients with dermatomyositis)
Signal recognition particle	4
KJ	<1
Other Associated Antibodies	
snRNPs	
U1 snRNP	12
U2 snRNP	3
Ro	10
PM-Scl	8
Ku	1
Elongation factor 1α (Fer)	1
tRNA^{Ser} (Mas)	1

Abbreviations: tRNA, transfer RNA; snRNP, small nuclear ribonucleoprotein.

least five different anti-synthetase activities target different aminoacyl-tRNA synthetases, cytoplasmic enzymes that catalyze the binding of amino acids to their respective tRNAs. These include anti–Jo-1, PL-7, PL-12, EJ, and OJ, which target the synthetases for histidine, threonine, alanine, glycine, and isoleucine, respectively, and which produce characteristic tRNA immunoprecipitation patterns.[163] Anti–OJ represents the only specificity targeting a class I tRNA synthetase (isoleucyl); the other anti-synthetase antibodies target class II tRNA synthetases.[164, 165] Some of these antibodies target the tRNA anticodon loop,[166] explaining their ability to specifically inhibit synthetase enzymatic activity, but other epitopes may be conformational.[167] These antibodies may therefore be identified by FANA, ELISA, immunoprecipitation, or immunoblot testing as well as by inhibition of in vitro aminoacylation reactions.[3]

Although the individual prevalences of these antibodies vary, their clinical associations remain similar. Anti–Jo-1, the most common, appears in 30 percent of patients with polymyositis or dermatomyositis,[161, 168–170] whereas the non–Jo-1 autoantibodies vary in prevalence from 1 to 5 percent, depending on geographic location.[3] Polymyositis appears more commonly with anti–Jo-1, and dermatomyositis is more common with the other synthetases, but these specificities together correlate with the "anti-synthetase syndrome," which includes interstitial lung disease, arthritis, Raynaud's phenomenon, mechanic's hands, hyperkeratotic lines, sclerodactyly, facial telangiectasia, calcinosis, and sicca.[3, 169, 171, 172] Some studies have suggested an association with HLA-DR3 and -DRw52[173] as well as HLA-DQA1*0501 and

-DQA1*0401.[174, 175] One study has associated anti–threonyl tRNA synthetase antibodies with fetal loss, severe relapsing myositis, and pregnancy.[176] Despite these common associations, different anti-synthetase antibodies have not been found within a single patient. Indeed, the anti-synthetases present a unique immunologic phenomenon: their autoantigens are each associated with the same syndrome and perform similar cellular functions, yet these specificities never cross-react or appear simultaneously in a single patient.

Anti-SRP. Anti-SRP MSAs target the signal recognition particle (SRP), the cytoplasmic ribonucleoprotein involved in the translocation of nascent proteins across the endoplasmic reticulum. They occur in 4 percent of myositis patients in the absence of other MSAs and are associated with acute onset, severe disease, resistance to therapy, cardiac involvement, and a higher mortality rate, as well as with HLA-DR5, -DRw52, and -DQA1*0301, but with a lower frequency of interstitial lung disease and arthritis.[161, 174, 177]

Anti–Mi-2. Anti–Mi-2 antibodies represent MSAs that target a nuclear antigen, eliciting homogeneous nuclear fluorescence on FANA testing. Their target remains largely uncharacterized, but recent studies demonstrate that the autoantigen includes a 240-kD non-nucleolar protein whose sequence suggests nucleic acid–binding properties and a 218-kD nuclear protein whose sequence suggests helicase activity; additional proteins of 150, 72, 65, 63, 50, and 34 kD also appear to compose the autoantigen.[178, 179] Anti–Mi-2 occurs in 15 to 20 percent of dermatomyositis patients, but more than 95 percent of patients with anti–Mi-2 have dermatomyositis rather than polymyositis. In addition, anti–Mi-2 has been associated with the "shawl" and "V" signs of dermatomyositis as well as with HLA-DR7, -DRw52, and -DQA1*0201.[161, 174, 180] Thus anti–Mi-2 appears to be generally associated with greater dermatologic involvement.

Anti-snRNP. Generally present in overlap syndromes, anti-snRNP antibodies in inflammatory muscle diseases consist predominantly of anti–U1 snRNP-specific antibodies, although a few anti-Sm and anti–U2 snRNP-specific antibodies have been described. Anti–U1 snRNP antibodies generally associate with mixed connective tissue disease (including features of polymyositis or dermatomyositis, scleroderma, and SLE); SLE–myositis overlap; myositis–scleroderma overlap; undifferentiated features (Raynaud's phenomenon, puffy fingers, arthritis) later progressing to myositis; and possibly response to corticosteroids.[181] Anti–U2 snRNP antibodies associate with myositis and sclerodactyly, sometimes with SLE, usually without interstitial lung disease.[70, 168] These antibodies may coexist with MSAs.[161, 171, 172]

Anti–PM-Scl. Anti–PM-Scl antibodies target at least three poorly defined associated proteins. Eight percent of patients with polymyositis possess this antibody. As stated earlier, their presence is associated with myositis–scleroderma overlap, without SLE features: 50 percent of anti–PM-Scl antibody–positive patients have the overlap, and 25 percent of the overlap patients have the antibody.[146] Anti–PM-Scl also appears to be associated with arthritis, dermatomyositis skin lesions, calcinosis, mechanic's hands, eczema, and HLA-DR3 and HLA-DR4.[146, 147] Unlike anti-snRNP antibodies in myositis overlap syndromes, PM-Scl and MSA autoantibodies are mutually exclusive.[146, 147]

Other Overlap Antibodies. Other antibodies associated with myositis in overlap syndromes include several specificities found in other diseases. Anti-Ku antibodies, found more commonly in patients with SLE and scleroderma, have been described in Japanese but not United States patients with myositis–scleroderma overlap.[168] Anti–U3 RNP (fibrillarin) antibodies are associated with an increased incidence of inflammatory myositis, especially the diffuse type, among scleroderma patients.[182] Anti-Ro and anti-La antibodies, typically associated with SLE and Sjögren's syndrome, may appear occasionally, but their association with myositis remains unclear.[161]

Miscellaneous Antibodies. Other autoantibodies rarely found in inflammatory muscle diseases include anti-KJ, which blocks in vitro translation[183]; anti-Mas, which precipitates a serine tRNA as well as a nonsynthetase protein[184]; anti-Fer, which targets translation elongation factor 1α[185]; antibody to a 56-kD Syrian hamster nucleoprotein, which remains uncharacterized in terms of both molecular biology and clinical significance; anti-hsp60, anti-hsp73, and anti-hsp90, the antigens of which include three heat-shock proteins involved in the cellular stress response[186–188]; and anti-laminin and anti-microfilament, which target nuclear and cytoplasmic cytoskeletal proteins.[103, 189] The significance of these antibodies remains unclear.

Sjögren's Syndrome

Antinuclear antibodies are a common finding among patients with Sjögren's syndrome. The incidence of positive FANA results approximates 96 percent,[190] and primary autoimmune targets include the Ro and La autoantigens, although other less characterized specificities have also been found (Table 17–7 lists prominent specificities).

Anti-Ro/SS-A and Anti-La/SS-B. These two antibodies target two nuclear ribonucleoproteins presumed to associate with each other and to be involved in RNA metabolism. Anti-Ro antibodies appear in approximately 40 to 95 percent of patients with Sjögren's syndrome and are associated with extraglandular manifestations such as neurologic involvement,[191] vasculitis,[192] glandular dysfunction,[193, 194] anemia, lymphopenia, thrombocytopenia, anti-La antibodies, rheumatoid factor, hypergammaglobulinemia, and HLA-B8 and -DR3, as well as heterozygosity at HLA-DQ1 and -DQ2.[82] Anti-La antibodies appear in as many as 87 percent of patients with Sjögren's syndrome and are associated with extraglandular manifestations, such as neurologic involvement and vasculitis,[192] glandular dysfunction,[194] purpura, leukopenia, lymphopenia, hypergammaglobulinemia, rheumatoid factor,[190] and with HLA-B8 and HLA-DR3.[195]

Anti–MA-I. Anti–MA-I antibodies target a 200-kD protein localized to the mitotic apparatus in dividing cells. During interphase, it produces fine speckled nucleoplasmic staining with nucleolar sparing, which changes to bright staining of centrosome rims and proximal spindles during metaphase. It appears in 8 percent of patients with Sjögren's syndrome, but its clinical significance remains unknown. This specificity may be similar or identical to anti-NuMA, which targets a 240-kD coiled-coil protein localized at the mitotic apparatus, but such conclusions await further biochemical characterization.[75, 196]

Anti–p80-coilin. Anti–p80-coilin antibodies target an 80-kD nuclear protein associated with coiled bodies, noncapsular nuclear bodies of 0.3 to 1 μm enriched in spliceosomal machinery.[197, 198] They appear in 4 percent of patients with Sjögren's syndrome, but their clinical significance remains unclear.

Miscellaneous Antibodies. Other ANAs described in patients with Sjögren's syndrome include perinuclear anti–neutrophil cytoplasmic antibodies (p-ANCA), classically associated with polyarteritis nodosa but found in 40 percent of patients with Sjögren's syndrome[199]; anti–mitochondrial antibodies and anti–pyruvate dehydrogenase antibodies, typically associated with primary biliary cirrhosis but found in 6.6 and 27 percent of patients with Sjögren's syndrome, respectively[200]; ACAs, typically associated with scleroderma but found infrequently in Sjögren's syndrome[201, 202]; anti–U4/U6 snRNP, described in a single Sjögren's syndrome patient[203]; anti-microfilament[103]; anti–carbonic anhydrase[204]; anti–nuclear lamina[104]; and anti–Golgi apparatus.[205]

Miscellaneous Diseases

ANAs have also been found among several other conditions both related and unrelated to rheumatologic illnesses. These include, to name but a few, such conditions as liver disease,[206] hepatitis infection,[207] leprosy,[208] silicone gel implants,[209] schizophrenia,[210] dementia,[211] opticomyelitis,[212] interstitial cystitis,[213] multiple sclerosis,[214] Henoch-Schönlein purpura,[215] juvenile rheumatoid arthritis,[216] polymorphous light

Table 17–7. ANTINUCLEAR ANTIBODIES IN SJÖGREN'S SYNDROME

Antibody Specificity	Prevalence (%)
Ro	40–95
La	87
MA-I	8
p80-coilin	4

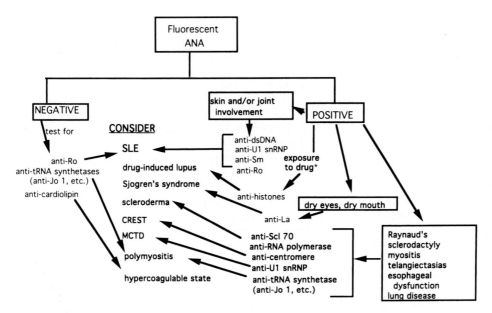

Figure 17–5. Algorithm for the use of antinuclear antibodies (ANAs) in the diagnosis of connective tissue disorders. SLE, systemic lupus erythematosus; tRNA, transfer RNA; MCTD, mixed connective tissue disease; CREST, calcinosis, Raynaud's, esophageal motility disorders, sclerodactyly, and telangiectasias (scleroderma with limited skin involvement); snRNP, small nuclear ribonucleoprotein; dsDNA, double-stranded DNA. See text.

eruption,[217] mercury intoxication,[218] atopic dermatitis,[219] myasthenia gravis,[220] eosinophilia-myalgia syndrome,[221] and pregnancy.[222] Even with the vast numbers of such diverse reports of ANAs in unexpected situations, these studies lack comprehensive analyses of the significance of the antibodies in these states. Therefore, the role of such ANAs in the clinical evaluation of such patients remains largely unexplored.

CLINICAL EVALUATION OF ANTINUCLEAR ANTIBODIES

Figure 17–5 is an algorithm for the rheumatologic evaluation of a patient for ANAs. In general, the FANA test serves as a screen, with subsequent specific autoantigen testing depending on the clinical situation. A negative FANA result usually indicates the absence of ANAs, arguing against the diagnosis of one of the ANA-associated diseases (see Table 17–1). Still, if the clinical picture strongly suggests connective tissue disease, further investigation can involve specific assays for antigens that commonly are negative on FANA testing, such as Ro, Jo-1, or cardiolipin. On the other hand, because some specific ANAs possess diagnostic significance, positive FANA results usually warrant follow-up with specialized assays. Thus, if SLE is suspected, further work may assay for anti-DNA, anti-Sm, anti–U1 snRNP, and anti-Ro antibodies. Similarly, if mixed connective tissue disease, Sjögren's syndrome, scleroderma, or polymyositis is suspected, the serum may be tested, respectively, for anti–U1 snRNP; anti-Ro or anti-La; anti-topoisomerase I, anti-centromere, or anti-nucleoli; or anti-tRNA synthetases. Positive results in these more specialized assays do not alone signify specific diseases but instead add weight to diagnoses that should rely heavily on other clinical information.

SUMMARY

Antinuclear antibodies encompass a wide range of nuclear, nucleolar, and cytoplasmic autoantigen specificities. In general, different autoantibodies associate with different rheumatologic diseases, but their correlations are not absolute. For instance, autoantibodies in SLE predominantly target intranuclear components of chromatin and ribonucleoproteins, such as DNA or small nuclear ribonucleoproteins, but several nucleolar and cytoplasmic autoantigens have also been described in SLE, such as RNA polymerases or ribosomes. Similarly, autoimmune responses in scleroderma generally target nucleolar structures, such as topoisomerase I or kinetochores, but may also less frequently include nuclear or cytoplasmic antigens such as Ku or histones. In the inflammatory muscle diseases, autoantigens consist primarily of cytoplasmic particles but secondarily include intranuclear and nucleolar targets as well. Sjögren's syndrome produces autoantibodies directed mostly against the ribonucleoproteins Ro and La, yet other nuclear, nucleolar, and cytoplasmic specificities abound. Therefore, although particular ANA specificities may help direct the clinical evaluation of patients because of their particular disease associations, their correlations are not absolute, and these antibodies retain an adjunct role in rheumatologic diagnosis. Rather, clinical acumen directs the utility of the test for ANAs.

References

1. Craft J, Hardin JA: Antinuclear antibodies. *In* Kelley WN, Harris ED, Ruddy S, Sledge CB (eds): Textbook of Rheumatology, 4th ed. Philadelphia, WB Saunders, 1993, p 164.
2. Lee B, Craft JE: Molecular structure and function of autoantigens in systemic sclerosis. Int Rev Immunol 12:123, 1995.
3. Targoff IN: Immune manifestations of inflammatory muscle disease. Rheum Dis Clin North Am 20:857, 1994.

4. Hargraves MM, Richmond H, Morton R: Presentation of two bone marrow elements: The "tart" cell and "L.E. cell." Proc Staff Meet Mayo Clin 23:25, 1948.
5. Beck J: Antinuclear antibodies: Methods of detection and significance. Mayo Clin Proc 44:600, 1960.
6. Haserick JR, Bortz DW: Normal bone marrow inclusion phenomena induced by lupus erythematosus plasma. J Invest Dermatol 13:47, 1949.
7. Holman HR, Kunkel HG: Affinity between the lupus erythematosus serum factor and cell nuclei and nucleoprotein. Science 126:162, 1957.
8. Friou GJ: Clinical application of lupus serum nucleoprotein reaction using fluorescent antibody technique. J Clin Invest 36:890, 1957.
9. Deicher HRG, Holman HR, Kunkel HG: The precipitin reaction between DNA and a serum factor in systemic lupus erythematosus. J Exp Med 109:97, 1959.
10. Tan EM, Kunkel HG: Characteristics of a soluble nuclear antigen precipitating with sera of patients with systemic lupus erythematosus. J Immunol 96:464, 1966.
11. Mattioli M, Reichlin M: Characterization of a soluble nuclear ribonucleoprotein antigen reactive with SLE sera. J Immunol 107:1281, 1971.
12. Reichlin M, Mattioli M: Correlation of a precipitating reaction to an RNA protein antigen and a low prevalence of nephritis in patients with systemic lupus erythematosus. N Engl J Med 286:908, 1972.
13. Sharp GC, Irvin WS, Tan EM, Gould RG, Holman HR: Mixed connective tissue disease—an apparently distinct rheumatic disease syndrome associated with a specific antibody to an extractable nuclear antigen (ENA). Am J Med 52:148, 1972.
14. Sharp GC, Irvin WS, Northway JD, et al: Specificity of antibodies to extractable nuclear antigens (ENA) in mixed connective tissue disease (MCTD) and systemic lupus erythematosus (SLE). Arthritis Rheum 15:125, 1972.
15. Northway JD, Tan EM: Differentiation of antinuclear antibodies giving speckled staining patterns in immunofluorescence. Clin Immunol Immunopathol 1:140, 1972.
16. Clark G, Reichlin M, Tomasi TB: Characterization of a soluble cytoplasmic antigen reactive with sera from patients with systemic lupus erythematosus. J Immunol 102:117, 1969.
17. Mattioli M, Reichlin M: Heterogeneity of RNA protein antigens reactive with sera of patients with systemic lupus erythematosus: Description of a cytoplasmic nonribosomal antigen. Arthritis Rheum 17:421, 1974.
18. Alspaugh MA, Tan EM: Antibodies to cellular antigens in Sjögren's syndrome. J Clin Invest 55:1067, 1975.
19. Lerner MR, Steitz JA: Antibodies to small nuclear RNAs complexed with proteins are produced by patients with systemic lupus erythematosus. Proc Natl Acad Sci USA 76:5495, 1979.
20. Fritzler MJ: Immunofluorescent antinuclear antibody test. In Rose NR, de Macario EC, Fahey JL, Friedman H, Penn GM (eds): Manual of Clinical Laboratory Immunology. Washington, DC, American Society for Microbiology, 1992, p 724.
21. Molden DP, Nakamura RM, Tan EM: Standardization of the immunofluorescent test for autoantibody to nuclear antigens (ANA): Use of reference sera of defined antibody specificity. Am J Clin Pathol 82:47–66, 1984.
22. Reichlin M: Antinuclear antibodies. In Kelley WN, Harris ED, Ruddy S, Sledge CB (eds): Textbook of Rheumatology, 3rd ed. Philadelphia, WB Saunders, 1989, p 208.
23. Craft J, Hardin JA: Immunoprecipitation assays for the detection of soluble nuclear and cytoplasmic nucleoproteins. In Rose NR, de Macario EC, Fahey JL, Friedman H, Penn GM (eds): Manual of Clinical Laboratory Immunology. Washington, DC, American Society for Microbiology, 1992, p 747.
24. St. Clair EW, Burch JA Jr, Saitta M: Specificity of autoantibodies for recombinant 60-kd and 52-kd Ro autoantigens. Arthritis Rheum 37:1373–1379, 1994.
25. Evans J, Arguelles E, Harley J, et al: Antibodies to ribonucleoproteins in SLE (abstr). Arthritis Rheum 31:S54, 1988.
26. Chan EKL, Pollard KM: Autoantibodies to ribonucleoprotein particles by immunoblotting. In Rose NR, de Macario EC, Fahey JL, Friedman H, Penn GM (eds): Manual of Clinical Laboratory Immunology. Washington, DC, American Society for Microbiology, 1992, p 755.
27. Boire G, Lopez-Longo F-J, Lapointe S, Menard H-A: Sera from patients with autoimmune disease recognize conformational determinants on the 60-kd Ro/SS-A protein. Arthritis Rheum 34:722, 1991.
28. Thomas TJ, Thomas T: Polyamine-induced Z-DNA conformation in plasmids containing (dA-dC)ₙ·(dG-dT)ₙ inserts and increased binding of lupus autoantibodies to the Z-DNA form of plasmids. Biochem J 298:485, 1994.
29. Ballou SP: Crithidia luciliae immunofluorescence test for antibodies to DNA. In Rose NR, de Macario EC, Fahey JL, Friedman H, Penn GM (eds): Manual of Clinical Laboratory Immunology. Washington, DC, American Society for Microbiology, 1992, p 730.
30. Tan EM, Cohen AS, Fries JF, et al: The 1982 revised criteria for the classification of systemic lupus erythematosus. Arthritis Rheum 25:1271, 1982.
31. Massa M, De Benedetti F, Pignatti P, et al: Anti–double stranded DNA, anti-histone, and anti-nucleosome IgG reactivities in children with systemic lupus erythematosus. Clin Exp Rheumatol 12:219, 1994.
32. Burlingame RW, Boey ML, Starkebaum G, et al: The central role of chromatin in autoimmune responses to histones and DNA in systemic lupus erythematosus. J Clin Invest 94:184, 1994.
33. Reeves WH, Satoh M, Jingson W, Chou C-H, Ajmani AK: Antibodies to DNA, DNA-binding proteins and histones. Rheum Dis Clin North Am 20:1, 1994.
34. Zack DJ, Yamamoto K, Wong AL, et al: DNA mimics a self-protein that may be a target for some anti-DNA antibodies in systemic lupus erythematosus. J Immunol 154:1987, 1995.
35. Reichlin M, Martin A, Taylor-Albert E, et al: Lupus autoantibodies to native DNA cross-react with the A and D snRNP polypeptides. J Clin Invest 93:443, 1994.
36. Klinman DM, Shirai A, Conover J, et al: Cross-reactivity of IgG anti–DNA-secreting B cells in patients with systemic lupus erythematosus. Eur J Immunol 24:53, 1994.
37. Zhang W, Reichlin M: IgM anti-A and D snRNP proteins and IgM anti-dsDNA are closely associated in SLE sera. Clin Immunol Immunopathol 74:70, 1995.
38. Felsenfeld G: Chromatin as an essential part of the transcriptional mechanism. Nature 355:219, 1992.
39. Hardin JA, Thomas JO: Antibodies to histones in systemic lupus erythematosus: Localization of prominent autoantigens on histones H1 and H2B. Proc Natl Acad Sci USA 80:7410, 1983.
40. Rubin RL, Bell SA, Burlingame RW: Autoantibodies associated with lupus induced by diverse drugs target a similar epitope in the (H2A-H2B)-DNA complex. J Clin Invest 90:165, 1992.
41. Martin L, Pauls JD, Ryan JP, et al: Identification of a subset of patients with scleroderma with severe pulmonary and vascular disease by the presence of autoantibodies to centromere and histone. Ann Rheum Dis 52:780–784, 1993.
42. Sato S, Fujimoto M, Ihn H, et al: Antigen specificity of antihistone antibodies in localized scleroderma. Arch Dermatol 130:1273, 1994.
43. Sato S, Ihn H, Kikuchi K, et al: Antihistone antibodies in systemic sclerosis: Association with pulmonary fibrosis. Arthritis Rheum 37:391, 1994.
44. Garzelli C, Incaprere M, Bazzichi A, et al: Epstein-Barr virus–transformed human B lymphocytes produce natural antibodies to histones. Immunol Lett 39:277, 1994.
45. Bonfa E, Viana VS, Barret AC, et al: Autoantibodies in Chagas' disease: An antibody cross-reactive with human and Trypanosoma cruzi ribosomal proteins. J Immunol 150:3917, 1993.
46. Chengappa KN, Carpenter AB, Yang ZW, et al: Elevated IgG anti-histone antibodies in a subgroup of medicated schizophrenic patients. Schizophr Res 7:49, 1992.
47. Monestier M, Fasy TM, Bohm L, et al: Anti-histone antibodies in subacute sensory neuropathy. J Neurol Oncol 11:71, 1991.
48. Shoenfeld Y, el-Roeiy A, Ben-Yehuda O, et al: Detection of anti-histone activity in sera of patients with monoclonal gammopathies. Clin Immunol Immunopathol 42:250, 1987.
49. Kamei M, Kato M, Mochizuki K, et al: Serodiagnosis of cancers by ELISA of anti-histone H2B antibody. Biotherapy 4:17, 1992.
50. Viard JP, Choquette D, Chabre H, et al: Anti-histone reactivity in systemic lupus erythematosus sera: A disease activity index linked to the presence of DNA: Anti-DNA immune complexes. Autoimmunity 12:61, 1992.
51. Gottlieb TM, Jackson SP: The DNA-dependent protein kinase: Requirement for DNA ends and association with Ku antigen. Cell 72:131, 1993.
52. Taccioli GE, Gottlieb TM, Blunt T, et al: Ku80: Product of the XRCC5 gene and its role in DNA repair and V(D)J recombination. Science 265:1442, 1994.
53. Paillard S, Strauss F: Analysis of the mechanism of interaction of simian Ku protein with DNA. Nucleic Acids Res 19:5619, 1991.
54. Suwa A, Hirakata M, Takeda Y, et al: DNA-dependent protein kinase (Ku protein–p350 complex) assembles on double-stranded DNA. Proc Natl Acad Sci USA 91:6904, 1994.
55. Kuhn A, Stefanovsky V, Grummt I: The nucleolar transcription activator UBF relieves Ku antigen–mediated repression of mouse ribosomal gene transcription. Nucleic Acids Res 21:2057, 1993.
56. Reeves WH: Antibodies to the p70/p80 (Ku) antigens in systemic lupus erythematosus. Rheum Dis Clin North Am 18:391, 1992.
57. Mimori T, Akizuki M, Yamagata H, et al: Characterization of a high molecular weight acidic nuclear protein recognized by autoantibodies in sera from patients with polymyositis–scleroderma overlap. J Clin Invest 68:611, 1981.
58. Satoh M, Ajmani AK, Ogasawara T, et al: Autoantibodies to RNA polymerase II are common in systemic lupus erythematosus and overlap syndrome. J Clin Invest 94:1981, 1994.
59. Isern RA, Yaneva M, Weiner E, et al: Autoantibodies in patients with primary pulmonary hypertension: Association with anti-Ku. Am J Med 93:307, 1992.

60. Suwa A: Studies on the antigenic epitopes reactive with autoantibody in patients with PSS–PM overlap syndrome. Keio Igaku 67:865, 1990.

61. Mosrin C, Thuriaux P: The genetics of RNA polymerases in yeasts. Curr Genet 17:367–373, 1990.

62. Reimer G, Rose KM, Scheer U, et al: Autoantibody to RNA polymerase I in scleroderma sera. J Clin Invest 79:65, 1987.

63. Stetler DA, Jacob ST: Phosphorylation of RNA polymerase I augments its interaction with autoantibodies of systemic lupus erythematosus patients. J Biol Chem 259:13629–13632, 1984.

64. Rothfield NF: Autoantibodies in scleroderma. Rheum Dis Clin North Am 18:483, 1992.

65. Satoh M, Kuwana M, Ogasawara T, et al: Association of autoantibodies to topoisomerase I and the phosphorylated (IIO) form of RNA polymerase II in Japanese scleroderma patients. J Immunol 153:5838, 1994.

66. Baserga SJ, Steitz JA: The diverse world of small ribonucleoproteins. In Gesteland RF, Atkins JF (eds): The RNA World: The Nature of Modern RNA Suggests a Prebiotica RNA World. Cold Spring Harbor, NY, Cold Spring Harbor Laboratory Press, 1993.

67. Matera AG, Ward DC: Nucleoplasmic organization of small nuclear ribonucleoprotein particles in cultured human cells. J Cell Biol 121:715, 1993.

68. Peng SL, Craft J: Antibodies to spliceosomal snRNPs. In Shoenfeld Y, Peter JB (eds): Textbook of Autoantibodies. Netherlands, Elsevier, 1996 (in press).

69. Snowden N, Hay E, Holt PJL, et al: Clinical course of patients with anti-RNP antibodies. J Rheumatol 20:1256, 1993.

70. Craft J, Mimori T, Olsen TL, et al: The U2 small nuclear ribonucleoprotein particle as an autoantigen: Analysis with sera from patients with overlap syndromes. J Clin Invest 81:1716–1724, 1988.

71. Craft J: Antibodies to snRNPs in systemic lupus erythematosus. Rheum Dis Clin North Am 18:311, 1992.

72. Pironcheva G, Russev G: Characterization of the protein moiety of U7 small nuclear RNP particles. Microbios 77:41, 1994.

73. Abu-Shakrah M, Krupp M, Argov S, et al: The detection of anti–Sm-RNP activity in sera of patients with monoclonal gammopathies. Clin Exp Immunol 75:349, 1989.

74. de Vries E, Schipperijn AJ, Breedveld FC: Antinuclear antibodies in psychiatric patients. Acta Psychiatr Scand 89:289, 1994.

75. Chan WKL, Andrade LEC: Antinuclear antibodies in Sjögren's syndrome. Rheum Dis Clin North Am 18:551, 1992.

76. O'Brien CA, Wolin SL: A possible role for the 60-kD Ro protein in a discard pathway for defective 5S rRNA precursors. Genes Dev 8:2891, 1994.

77. Tröster H, Metzger TE, Semsei I, et al: One gene, two transcripts: Isolation of an alternative transcript encoding for the autoantigen La/SS-B from a cDNA library of a patient with primary Sjögren's syndrome. J Exp Med 180:2059–2067, 1994.

78. Gottlieb E, Steitz JA: The RNA binding protein La influences both the accuracy and the efficiency of RNA polymerase III transcription in vitro. EMBO J 8:841, 1989.

79. Topfer F, Gordon T, McCluskey J: Intra- and intermolecular spreading of autoimmunity involving the nuclear self-antigens La (SS-B) and Ro (SS-A). Proc Natl Acad Sci USA 92:875, 1995.

80. St. Clair EW: Anti-La antibodies. Rheum Dis Clin North Am 18:359, 1992.

81. Wasicek CA, Reichlin M: Clinical and serological differences between systemic lupus erythematosus patients with antibodies to Ro versus patients with antibodies to Ro and La. J Clin Invest 69:835, 1982.

82. Harley JB, Scofield RH, Reichlin M: Anti-Ro in Sjögren's syndrome and systemic lupus erythematosus. Rheum Dis Clin North Am 18:337, 1992.

83. Scofield RH, Frank MB, Neas BR, et al: Cooperative association of T cell beta receptor and HLA-DQ alleles in the production of anti-Ro in systemic lupus erythematosus. Clin Immunol Immunopathol 72:335, 1994.

84. Lopez-Longo FJ, Rodriguez-Mahou M, Escalona M, et al: Heterogeneity of the anti-Ro (SSA) response in rheumatic diseases. J Rheumatol 21:1450, 1994.

85. Warner JR: The nucleolus and ribosome formation. Curr Opin Cell Biol 2:521, 1990.

86. Elkon KB, Bonfa E, Brot N: Antiribosomal antibodies in systemic lupus erythematosus. Rheum Dis Clin North Am 18:377, 1992.

87. Hulsey M, Goldstein R, Scully L, et al: Anti–ribosomal P antibodies in systemic lupus erythematosus: A case-control study correlating hepatic and renal disease. Clin Immunol Immunopathol 74:252, 1995.

88. Sato T, Uchiumi T, Arakawa M, et al: Serological association of lupus autoantibodies to a limited functional domain of 28S ribosomal RNA and to the ribosomal proteins bound to the domain. Clin Exp Immunol 98:35, 1994.

89. Elkon KB, Bonfa E, Weissbach H, et al: Antiribosomal antibodies in SLE, infection and following deliberate immunization. Adv Exp Med Biol 347:81, 1994.

90. Tsai DE, Keene JD: In vitro selection of RNA epitopes using autoimmune patient serum. J Immunol 150:1137, 1993.

91. van Venrooij WJ, Hoet R, Castrop K, et al: Anti-(U1) small nuclear RNA antibodies in anti–small nuclear ribonucleoprotein sera from patients with connective tissue diseases. J Clin Invest 86:2154, 1990.

92. Yamanaka K, Takasaki Y, Nishida Y, et al: Detection and quantification of anti-Ki antibodies by enzyme-linked immunosorbent assay using recombinant Ki antigen. Arthritis Rheum 35:667, 1992.

93. Fritzler MJ, Salazar M: Diversity and origin of rheumatologic autoantibodies. Clin Microbiol Rev 4:256, 1991.

94. Kindas-Mugge I, Steiner G, Smolen JS: Similar frequency of autoantibodies against 70-kD class heat-shock proteins in healthy subjects and systemic lupus erythematosus patients. Clin Exp Immunol 92:46, 1993.

95. Conroy SE, Gaulds GB, Williams W, et al: Detection of autoantibodies to the 90 kDa heat shock protein in systemic lupus erythematosus and other autoimmune diseases. Br J Rheumatol 33:923, 1994.

96. Minota S, Koyasu S, Yahara I, et al: Autoantibodies to the heat-shock protein hsp90 in systemic lupus erythematosus. J Clin Invest 81:106, 1988.

97. Pauzner R, Urowitz M, Gladman D, et al: Antineutrophil cytoplasmic antibodies in systemic lupus erythematosus. J Rheumatol 21:1670, 1994.

98. Schnabel A, Csernok E, Isenberg DA, et al: Antineutrophil cytoplasmic antibodies in systemic lupus erythematosus. Arthritis Rheum 38:633, 1995.

99. Itoh Y, Reichlin M: Antibodies to carbonic anhydrase in systemic lupus erythematosus and other rheumatic diseases. Arthritis Rheum 35:73, 1992.

100. Kratz A, Harding MW, Craft J, et al: Autoantibodies against cyclophilin in systemic lupus erythematosus and Lyme disease. Clin Exp Immunol 90:422, 1992.

101. Montecucco C, Caporali R, Cobianchi F, et al: Antibodies to hn-RNP A1 in systemic lupus erythematosus: Clinical association with Raynaud's phenomenon and esophageal dysmotility. Clin Exp Rheumatol 10:223, 1992.

102. De Mendonca Neto EC, Kumar A, Shadick NA, et al: Antibodies to T- and L-isoforms of the cytoskeletal protein, fimbrin, in patients with systemic lupus erythematosus. J Clin Invest 90:1037, 1992.

103. Girard D, Senécal J-L: Anti-microfilament IgG antibodies in normal adults and patients with autoimmune diseases: Immunofluorescence and immunoblotting analysis of 201 subjects reveals polyreactivity with microfilament-associated proteins. Clin Immunol Immunopathol 74:193, 1995.

104. Konstantinov K, Foisner R, Byrd D, et al: Integral membrane proteins associated with the nuclear lamina are novel autoimmune antigens of the nuclear envelope. Clin Immunol Immunopathol 74:89, 1995.

105. Treadwell EL, Alspaugh MA, Sharp GC: Characterization of a new antigen-antibody system (Su) in patients with systemic lupus erythematosus. Arthritis Rheum 27:1263, 1984.

106. Bernstein RM, Steigerwald JC, Tan EM: Association of antinuclear and antinucleolar antibodies in progressive systemic sclerosis. Clin Exp Immunol 48:43, 1982.

107. Moroi Y, Peebles C, Fritzler MJ, et al: Autoantibody to centromere (kinetochore) in scleroderma sera. Proc Natl Acad Sci USA 77:1627, 1980.

108. Earnshaw WC, Tomkiel JE: Centromere and kinetochore structure. Curr Opin Cell Biol 4:86–93, 1992.

109. Rothfield NF, Whitaker D, Bordwell B, et al: Detection of anticentromere antibodies using cloned autoantigen CENP-B. Arthritis Rheum 30:1416, 1987.

110. Fritzler MJ, Kinsella TD, Garbutt E: The CREST syndrome: A distinct serologic entity with anticentromere antibodies. Am J Med 69:520, 1980.

111. Earnshaw WC, Bordwell B, Marino C, et al: Three human chromosomal autoantigens are recognized by sera from patients with anticentromere antibodies. J Clin Invest 77:426, 1986.

112. Weiner ES, Earnshaw WC, Senecal FL, et al: Clinical associations of anticentromere antibodies and antibodies to topoisomerase I: A study of 355 patients. Arthritis Rheum 31:378, 1988.

113. Bernstein RM, Callender ME, Neuberger JM, et al: Anticentromere antibody in primary biliary cirrhosis. Ann Rheum Dis 41:612, 1982.

114. Makinen D, Fritzler M, Davis P, et al: Anticentromere antibodies in primary biliary cirrhosis. Arthritis Rheum 26:914, 1983.

115. Carcia-Del Torre I, Miranda-Mendez L: Studies of antinuclear antibodies in rheumatoid arthritis. J Rheumatol 9:603, 1982.

116. Weiner ES, Hildebrandt S, Senecal J, et al: Prognostic significance of anticentromere antibodies and anti–topoisomerase I antibodies in Raynaud's disease. Arthritis Rheum 34:68, 1991.

117. Herrick AL, Heaney M, Hollis S, et al: Anticardiolipin, anticentromere and anti-Scl-70 antibodies in patients with systemic sclerosis and severe digital ischaemia. Ann Rheum Dis 53:540, 1994.

118. Genth E, Mierau R, Genetzky P, et al: Immunogenetic associations of scleroderma-related antinuclear antibodies. Arthritis Rheum 33:657, 1990.

119. McHugh NJ, Whyte J, Artlett C, et al: Anti-centromere antibodies (ACA) in systemic sclerosis patients and their relatives: A serological and HLA study. Clin Exp Immunol 96:267, 1994.

120. Hsieh TS: DNA topoisomerases. Curr Opin Cell Biol 4:396–400, 1992.

121. Kato T, Yamamoto K, Takeuchi H, et al: Identification of a universal B cell epitope on DNA topoisomerase I, an autoantigen associated with scleroderma. Arthritis Rheum 36:1580–1587, 1993.

122. Hildebrandt S, Weiner ES, Senecal JL, et al: Autoantibodies to topoisomerase I (Scl-70): Analysis by gel diffusion, immunoblot, and enzyme-linked immunosorbent assay. Clin Immunol Immunopathol 57:399, 1990.

123. Steen VD, Powell DL, Medsger TA: Clinical correlations and prognosis based on serum autoantibodies in patients with systemic sclerosis. Arthritis Rheum 31:196, 1988.

124. van Venrooij WJ, Stapel SO, Houben H, et al: A marker antigen for diffuse scleroderma. J Clin Invest 75:1053, 1985.

125. Briggs DC, Vaughan RW, Welsh KI, et al: Immunogenetic prediction of pulmonary fibrosis in systemic sclerosis. Lancet 338:661, 1991.

126. Hietarinta M, Ilonen J, Lassila O, et al: Association of HLA antigens with anti–Scl-70 antibodies and clinical manifestations of systemic sclerosis. Br J Rheumatol 33:323, 1994.

127. Morel PA, Chang HJ, Wilson JW, et al: Severe systemic sclerosis with anti–topoisomerase I antibodies is associated with an HLA-DRw11 allele. Hum Immunol 40:101, 1994.

128. Satoh M, Akizuki M, Kuwana M, et al: Genetic and immunological differences between Japanese patients with diffuse scleroderma and limited scleroderma. J Rheumatol 21:111, 1994.

129. Hirakata M, Okano Y, Pati U, et al: Identification of autoantibodies to RNA polymerase II: Occurrence in systemic sclerosis and association with autoantibodies to RNA polymerases I and III. J Clin Invest 91:2665–2672, 1993.

130. Okano Y, Steen VD, Medsger TA Jr: Autoantibody reactive with RNA polymerase III in systemic sclerosis. Ann Intern Med 119:1005–1013, 1993.

131. Kuwana M, Kaburaki J, Mimori T, et al: Autoantibody reactive with three classes of RNA polymerases in sera from patients with systemic sclerosis. J Clin Invest 91:1399, 1993.

132. Lischwe MA, Ochs RL, Reddy R, et al: Purification and partial characterization of a nucleolar scleroderma antigen (Mr = 34,000; pI, 8.5) rich in NG, NG-dimethylarginine. J Biol Chem 260:14304–14310, 1985.

133. Ochs RL, Lischwe MA, Spohn WH, Busch H: Fibrillarin: A new protein of the nucleolus identified by autoimmune sera. Biol Cell 54:123–133, 1985.

134. Gold HA, Topper JN, Clayton DA, et al: The RNA processing enzyme RNase MRP is identical to the Th RNP and related to RNase P. Science 245:1377, 1989.

135. Altman S, Kirsenborn L, Talbot S: Recent studies of ribonuclease P. FASEB J 7:7–14, 1993.

136. Kiss T, Marshallsay C, Filipowicz W: 7-2/MRP RNAs in plant and mammalian cells: Association with higher order structures in the nucleolus. EMBO J 11:3737–3746, 1992.

137. Li K, Smagula CS, Parson WJ, et al: Subcellular partitioning of MRP RNA assessed by ultrastructural and biochemical analysis. J Cell Biol 124:871–882, 1994.

138. Okano Y, Medsger TA Jr: Autoantibody to Th ribonucleoprotein (nucleolar 7-2 RNA protein particle) in patients with systemic sclerosis. Arthritis Rheum 33:1822, 1990.

139. Kipnis RJ, Craft J, Hardin JA: The analysis of antinuclear and antinucleolar autoantibodies of scleroderma by radioimmunoprecipitation assays. Arthritis Rheum 33:1431–1437, 1990.

140. Ochs RL, Lischwe MA, Shen E, et al: Nucleologenesis: Composition and fate of prenucleolar bodies. Chromosoma 92:330–336, 1985.

141. Chan EKL, Imai H, Hamel JC, Tan EM: Human autoantibody to RNA polymerase I transcription factor hUBF: Molecular identity of nucleolus organizer region autoantigen NOR-90 and ribosomal RNA transcription upstream binding factor. J Exp Med 174:1239–1244, 1991.

142. Imai H, Fritzler MJ, Neri R, et al: Immunocytochemical characterization of human NOR-90 (upstream binding factor) and associated antigens reactive with autoimmune sera: Two MR forms of NOR-90/hUBF autoantigens. Mol Biol Rep 19:115, 1994.

143. Alderuccio F, Chan EKL, Tan EM: Molecular characterization of an autoantigen of PM-Scl in the polymyositis/scleroderma overlap syndrome: A unique and complete human cDNA encoding an apparent 75-kD acidic protein of the nucleolar complex. J Exp Med 173:941–952, 1991.

144. Ge Q, Frank MB, O'Brien CA, et al: Cloning of a complementary DNA coding for the 100-kD antigenic protein of the PM-Scl autoantigen. J Clin Invest 90:559–570, 1992.

145. Ge Q, Wu Y, Trieu EP, et al: Analysis of fine specificity of anti–PM-Scl autoantibodies (abstr). Arthritis Rheum 35:S71, 1992.

146. Oddis CV, Okano Y, Rudert WA, et al: Serum autoantibody to the nucleolar antigen PM-Scl: Clinical and immunogenetic associations. Arthritis Rheum 35:1211–1217, 1992.

147. Marguerie C, Bunn CC, Copier J, et al: The clinical and immunogenetic features of patients with autoantibodies to the nucleolar antigen PM-Scl. Medicine 71:327–336, 1992.

148. Reimer G, Steen VD, Penning CA, et al: Correlates between autoantibodies to nucleolar antigens and clinical features in patients with systemic sclerosis (scleroderma). Arthritis Rheum 31:525, 1988.

149. Li X, McNeilage LJ, Whittingham S: Autoantibodies to the major nucleolar phosphoprotein B23 define a novel subset of patients with anticardiolipin antibodies. Arthritis Rheum 32:1165, 1989.

150. Itoh Y, Reichlin M: Antibodies to carbonic anhydrase in systemic lupus erythematosus and other rheumatic diseases. Arthritis Rheum 35:73, 1992.

151. Cohen DE, Kaufman LD, Varma AA, et al: Anti-laminin autoantibodies in collagen vascular diseases: The use of adequate controls in studies of autoimmune responses to laminin. Ann Rheum Dis 53:191, 1994.

152. Conroy SE, Faulds GB, Williams W, et al: Detection of autoantibodies to the 90 kDa heat shock protein in systemic lupus erythematosus and other autoimmune diseases. Br J Rheumatol 33:923, 1994.

153. Parodi A, Puiatti P, Rebora A: Serological profiles as prognostic clues for progressive systemic sclerosis: The Italian experience. Dermatologica 183:15, 1991.

154. Sato S, Fujimoto M, Ihn H, Takehara K: Antibodies to centromere and centriole in scleroderma spectrum disorders. Dermatology 189:23, 1994.

155. Endo H, Hosono T, Kondo H: Antineutrophil cytoplasmic autoantibodies in 6 patients with renal failure and systemic sclerosis. J Rheumatol 21:864, 1994.

156. Miyachi K, Takano S, Mimori T, et al: A novel autoantibody reactive with a 48 kDa tRNA associated protein in patients with scleroderma. J Rheumatol 18:373, 1991.

157. Okano Y, Medsger TA Jr: Novel human autoantibodies reactive with 5'-terminal trimethylguanosine cap structures of U small nuclear RNA. J Immunol 149:1093, 1992.

158. Hietarinta M, Lassila O, Hietaharju A: Association of anti–U1RNP- and anti–Scl-70-antibodies with neurological manifestations in systemic sclerosis (scleroderma). Scand J Rheumatol 23:64, 1994.

159. Okano Y, Medsger TA Jr: Newly identified U4/U6 snRNP-binding proteins by serum autoantibodies from a patient with systemic sclerosis. Arthritis Rheum 33:1822, 1990.

160. Gilliam AC, Steitz JA: Rare scleroderma autoantibodies to the U11 small nuclear ribonucleoprotein and to the trimethylguanosine cap of U small nuclear RNAs. Proc Natl Acad Sci USA 90:6781, 1993.

161. Love LA, Leff RL, Fraser DD, et al: A new approach to the classification of idiopathic inflammatory myopathy: Myositis-specific autoantibodies define useful homogeneous patient groups. Medicine 70:360–374, 1991.

162. Reichlin M, Arnett FC: Multiplicity of antibodies in myositis sera. Arthritis Rheum 27:1150–1156, 1984.

163. Targoff IN: Autoantibodies to aminoacyl-transfer RNA synthetases for isoleucine and glycine: Two additional synthetases are antigenic in myositis. J Immunol 144:1737–1743, 1990.

164. Raben N: Autoimmunity to histidyl-transfer RNA synthetase: A case study. Ann Intern Med 122:718, 1995.

165. Schimmel P: Classes of aminoacyl-tRNA synthetases and the establishment of the genetic code. Trends Biochem Sci 16:1–3, 1991.

166. Bunn CC, Mathews MB: Autoreactive epitope defined as the anticodon region of alanine transfer RNA. Science 238:1116–1119, 1987.

167. Raben Nichols RC, Jain A, et al: Expression of recombinant human histidyl-tRNA synthetase, an autoantigen, in baculovirus-transfected insect cells (abstr). Arthritis Rheum 35:S170, 1992.

168. Hirakata M, Mimori T, Akizuki M, et al: Autoantibodies to small nuclear and cytoplasmic ribonucleoproteins in Japanese patients with inflammatory muscle disease. Arthritis Rheum 35:449–456, 1992.

169. Marguerie C, Bunn CC, Beynon HLC, et al: Polymyositis, pulmonary fibrosis and autoantibodies to aminoacyl-tRNA synthetase enzymes. Q J Med 77:1019–1038, 1990.

170. Oddis CV, Medsger TA Jr, Cooperstein LA: A subluxing arthropathy associated with the anti-Jo-1 antibody in polymyositis/dermatomyositis. Arthritis Rheum 33:1640–1645, 1990.

171. Targoff IN, Arnett FC: Clinical manifestations in patients with antibody to PL-12 antigen (alanyl-tRNA synthetase). Am J Med 88:241–251, 1990.

172. Targoff IN, Trieu EP, Miller FW: Reaction of anti-OJ autoantibodies with components of the multi-enzyme complex of aminoacyl-tRNA synthetases in addition to isoleucyl tRNA synthetase. J Clin Invest 91:2556–2564, 1993.

173. Goldstein R, Duvic M, Targoff IN, et al: HLA-D region genes associated with autoantibody responses to Jo-1 (histidyl-tRNA synthetase) and other translation-related factors in myositis. Arthritis Rheum 33:1240–1248, 1990.

174. Gurley RC, Love LA, Targoff IN, et al: Associations among myositis-specific autoantibodies (MSA) and HLA-DQA1 alleles (abstr). Arthritis Rheum 34:S137, 1991.

175. Reveille JD, Targoff IN, Mimori T, et al: MHC class II alleles associated with myositis (abstr). Arthritis Rheum 35:S84, 1992.

176. Satoh M, Ajmani AK, Hirakata M, et al: Onset of polymyositis with autoantibodies to threonyl-tRNA synthetase during pregnancy. J Rheumatol 21:1564–1566, 1994.

177. Targoff IN, Johnson AE, Miller FW: Antibody to signal recognition particle in polymyositis. Arthritis Rheum 33:1361–1370, 1990.

178. Seelig HP, Moosbrugger I, Ehrfeld H, et al: The major dermatomyositis-specific Mi-2 autoantigen is a presumed helicase involved in transcriptional activation. Arthritis Rheum 38:1389–1399, 1995.

179. Nilasena DS, Trieu EP, Targoff IN: Analysis of the Mi-2 autoantigen of dermatomyositis. Arthritis Rheum 38:123–128, 1995.

180. Targoff IN, Nilasena DS, Trieu EP, et al: Clinical features and immunologic testing of patients with anti-Mi-2 antibodies (abstr). Arthritis Rheum 33:S72, 1990.

181. Lundberg I, Nennesmo I, Hedfors E: A clinical, serological, and histopathological study of myositis patients with and without anti-RNP antibodies. Semin Arthritis Rheum 22:127–138, 1992.

182. Okano Y, Steen VD, Medsger TA Jr: Autoantibody to U3 nucleolar ribonucleoprotein (fibrillarin) in patients with systemic sclerosis. Arthritis Rheum 35:1211–1217, 1992.

183. Targoff IN, Arnett FC, Berman L, et al: Anti-KJ: A new antibody associated with the myositis/lung syndrome that reacts with a translation-related protein. J Clin Invest 84:162–172, 1989.

184. Gelpi C, Sontheimer EJ, Rodriguez-Sanchez JL: Autoantibodies against a serine tRNA–protein complex implicated in cotranslational selenocysteine insertion. Proc Natl Acad Sci USA 89:9739–9743, 1992.

185. Targoff IN, Hanas J: The polymyositis-associated Fer antigen is elongation factor 1a (abstr). Arthritis Rheum 32:S81, 1989.

186. Appelboom T, Kahn MF, Mairesse N: Anti-73 kDa heat shock protein (hsp 73) in mixed connective tissue disease (MCTD) (abstr). Arthritis Rheum 36:S252, 1993.

187. Jarjour WN, Jeffries BDM, Davis JS, et al: Autoantibodies to human stress proteins: A survey of various rheumatic and other inflammatory diseases. Arthritis Rheum 34:1133–1138, 1991.

188. Minota S, Koyasu S, Yhara I, et al: Autoantibodies to the heat-shock protein hsp90 in systemic lupus erythematosus. J Clin Invest 81:106–109, 1988.

189. Cohen DE, Kaufman LD, Varma AA, et al: Anti-laminin autoantibodies in collagen vascular diseases: The use of adequate controls in studies of autoimmune responses to laminin. Ann Rheum Dis 53:191–193, 1994.

190. Harley JB, Alexander EL, Bias WB, et al: Anti-Ro (SS-A) and anti-La (SS-B) in patients with Sjögren's syndrome. Arthritis Rheum 29:196, 1986.

191. Alexander EL, Razenbach MR, Kumar AJ, et al: Anti-Ro (SS-A) autoantibodies in central nervous system disease associated with Sjögren's syndrome (CNS-SS): Clinical, neuroimaging, and angiographic correlates. Neurology 44:899–908, 1994.

192. Molina R, Provost TT, Alexander EL: Two types of inflammatory vascular disease in Sjögren's syndrome: Differential association with seroreactivity to rheumatoid factor and antibodies to Ro/SSA and with hypocomplementemia. Arthritis Rheum 28:1251, 1985.

193. Tsuzaka K, Fujii T, Akizuki M, et al: Clinical significance of antibodies to native or denatured 60-kd or 52-kd Ro/SS-A proteins in Sjögren's syndrome. Arthritis Rheum 37:88–92, 1994.

194. Tsuzaka K, Ogasawara T, Tojo T, et al: Relationship between autoantibodies and clinical parameters in Sjögren's syndrome. Scand J Rheumatol 22:1–9, 1993.

195. Hietaharju A, Korpela M, Ilonen J, Frey H: Nervous system disease, immunological features, and HLA phenotype in Sjögren's syndrome. Ann Rheum Dis 51:506–509, 1992.

196. Yang CH, Lambie EJ, Snyder M: NuMA: An unusually long coiled-coil related protein in the mammalian nucleus. J Cell Biol 116:1303–1317, 1992.

197. Chan EK, Takano S, Andrade LE, et al: Structure, expression and chromosomal localization of human p80-coilin gene. Nucleic Acids Res 22:4462–4469, 1994.

198. Carmo-Fonseca M, Ferreira J, Lamond AI: Assembly of snRNP-containing coiled bodies is regulated in interphase and mitosis: Evidence that the coiled body is a kinetic nuclear structure. J Cell Biol 120:841–852, 1993.

199. Fukase S, Ohta N, Inamura K, et al: Diagnostic specificity of anti-neutrophil cytoplasmic antibodies (ANCA) in otorhinolaryngological diseases. Acta Otol Laryngol 511:204–207, 1994.

200. Skopouli FN, Barbatis C, Moutsopoulos HM: Liver involvement in primary Sjögren's syndrome. Br J Rheumatol 33:745–748, 1994.

201. Renier G, Le Normand I, Carrere F, et al: Anticentromere autoantibodies and sicca syndrome. Br J Rheumatol 33:193, 1994.

202. Chan HL, Lee YS, Hong HS, Kuuo TT: Anticentromere antibodies (ACA): Clinical distribution and disease specificity. Clin Exp Dermatol 19:298–302, 1994.

203. Fujii T, Mimori T, Hama N, et al: Characterization of autoantibodies that recognize U4/U6 small nuclear ribonucleoprotein particles in serum from a patient with primary Sjögren's syndrome. J Biol Chem 267:16412–16416, 1992.

204. Nishimori I, Bratanova T, Toshkov I, et al: Induction of experimental autoimmune sialoadenitis by immunization of PL/J mice with carbonic anhydrase II. J Immunol 154:4865–4873, 1995.

205. Kooy J, Toh BH, Pettitt JM: Human autoantibodies as reagents to conserved Golgi components: Characterization of a peripheral, 230-kDa compartment-specific Golgi protein. J Biol Chem 267:20255–20263, 1992.

206. Imai H, Nakano Y, Kiyosawa K, et al: Increasing titers and changing specificities of antinuclear antibodies in patients with chronic liver disease who develop hepatocellular carcinoma. Cancer 71:26, 1993.

207. Gutierrez A, Chinchilla V, Espasa A, et al: Transient detection of antinuclear and anti–smooth muscle antibodies in hepatitis A virus infection. Am J Gastroenterol 90:171, 1995.

208. Garcia-De La Torre I: Autoimmune phenomena in leprosy, particularly antinuclear antibodies and rheumatoid factor. J Rheumatol 20:900, 1993.

209. Bridgees AJ: Autoantibodies in patients with silicone implants. Semin Arthritis Rheum 24:54, 1994.

210. Sirota P, Firer MA, Schild K, et al: Autoantibodies to DNA in multicase families with schizophrenia. Biol Psychol 33:450, 1993.

211. Mecocci P, Ekman R, Parnetti L, et al: Antihistone and anti-dsDNA autoantibodies in Alzheimer's disease and vascular dementia. Biol Psychol 34:380, 1993.

212. Kira J, Goto I: Recurrent opticomyelitis associated with anti-DNA antibody. J Neurol Neurosurg Psychol 57:1124, 1994.

213. Ochs RL, Stein TW Jr, Peebles CL, et al: Autoantibodies in interstitial cystitis. J Urol 151:587, 1994.

214. Barned S, Goodman AD, Mattson DH: Frequency of anti-nuclear antibody in multiple sclerosis. Neurology 45:384, 1995.

215. Garber ME, Mohr BW, Calabrese LH: Henoch-Schönlein purpura associated with anti-Ro (SSA) and antiphospholipid antibody syndrome. J Rheumatol 20:1964, 1993.

216. Lawrence JM III, Moore TL, Osborn TG, et al: Autoantibody studies in juvenile rheumatoid arthritis. Semin Arthritis Rheum 22:265, 1993.

217. Kiss M, Husz S, Dobozy A: The occurrence of antinuclear, anti-SSA/Ro and anti-SSB/La antibodies in patients with polymorphous light eruption. Acta Derm Venereol 71:341, 1991.

218. Schrallhammer-Benkler K, Ring J, Przybilla B, et al: Acute mercury intoxication with lichenoid drug eruption followed by mercury contact allergy and development of antinuclear antibodies. Acta Derm Venereol 72:294, 1992.

219. Taniguchi Y, Yamakami A, Sakamoto T, et al: Positive antinuclear antibody in atopic dermatitis. Acta Derm Venereol 176:62, 1992.

220. Lindsey JW, Albers GW, Steinman L: Recurrent transverse myelitis, myasthenia gravis, and autoantibodies. Ann Neurol 32:407, 1992.

221. Varga J, Maul GG, Jimenez SA: Autoantibodies to nuclear lamin C in the eosinophilia-myalgia syndrome associated with L-tryptophan ingestion. Arthritis Rheum 35:106, 1992.

222. Kiuttu J, Hartikinen-Sorri AL, Makitalo R: Occurrence of antinuclear antibodies in an unselected pregnancy population. Gynecol Obstet Invest 33:21, 1992.

CHAPTER 18

Jean-Michel Dayer
William P. Arend

Cytokines and Growth Factors

An important advancement in basic science over the past 10 to 20 years has been a greater understanding of how cells communicate with each other. During embryogenesis as well as in normal functioning of the mature organism, soluble molecules transmit information between cells. These mediators are released by cells of origin in response to specific signals and influence the response and function of target cells largely through exerting a positive or negative influence on gene expression. In addition to playing an important role in normal physiology, unregulated or excess effects of these soluble polypeptides are thought to be involved in mediating pathophysiologic events in many autoimmune and inflammatory diseases.

These molecules of cell communication are known as interleukins (ILs), interferons (IFNs), growth factors, and colony-stimulating factors (CSFs). *Cytokine*, a generic term, refers to factors released from cells. *Lymphokines*, implying an origin from lymphocytes and *monokines*, are derived from monocytes. Cytokines are involved in the growth and differentiation of normal cells, primarily of the hematopoietic system or of mesenchymal origin. An important general principle is that each cytokine exhibits multiple effects, opposing and antagonizing or supplementing and synergizing with other cytokines. Thus, a biologic response observed in cell culture in vitro or in a tissue in vivo represents the net effects of multiple factors.

Cytokines are particularly important as local mediators of intercellular communication in normal or diseased tissues. These factors may act on the same cell that produced them in an *autocrine* fashion or on adjacent cells in a *paracrine* fashion. Autocrine stimulation can occur in two ways: (1) a released cytokine can interact with cell surface receptors, or (2) an intracellular factor can bind with internal structures without ever being secreted. Cytokines may also function in an *endocrine* fashion through exerting effects at a distance from the tissue of origin. In addition, some cytokines may remain associated with the cell surface and act in an *intracrine* fashion through direct cell contact. By all mechanisms, cytokines bind to specific receptors on target cells and induce intracellular signal transduction pathways. The resultant biologic responses to soluble or membrane-bound cytokines are determined by changes in gene transcription, messenger ribonucleic acid (mRNA) translation, and protein synthesis and secretion.

This chapter focuses on the effects of cytokines on specific stages or processes in acute and chronic inflammation occurring in autoimmune and inflammatory diseases rather than on each cytokine in isolation. Particular emphasis is placed on regulation of cytokine effects, a subject that has been recently reviewed.[1-5]

INDUCTION OF CYTOKINE PRODUCTION

Induction by Soluble Factors

Cytokines are produced by multiple cells, including all cells of the mononuclear phagocyte system, lymphocytes, epithelial cells, endothelial cells, fibroblasts, and chondrocytes. Most cells do not produce cytokines constitutively but require contact with specific factors to induce transcription and translation. One of the exceptions is tumor necrosis factor-α (TNF-α), where transcription may preexist in some cells, with stimuli being required only to induce translation.

For some cytokines, separate stimuli are required by specific cells to induce transcription or translation; that is, the complement fragment C5a stimulates IL-1 transcription in monocytes but bacterial lipopolysaccharides (LPSs) are necessary for induction of translation and protein production. In addition, the state of differentiation of a cell may influence the requirements for and response to a particular cytokine-inducing factor. For example, the production of IL-1 receptor antagonist (IL-1Ra) by monocytes requires stimulation with LPS, adherent immunoglobulin G (IgG), or other cytokines, including granulocyte-macrophage CSF (GM-CSF). In contrast, alveolar macrophages produce IL-1Ra constitutively and are not responsive to LPS or IgG but produce more IL-1Ra after culture in GM-CSF.

The effects of cytokine-inducing factors have been studied primarily in vitro, and full extrapolation to in vivo events may not be appropriate. Cells in tissues in intact organisms are exposed to a complex environment that may not be completely reproduced by in vitro culture conditions. It is important to determine the production of particular cytokines by the in vivo injection of specific stimuli in animals or humans.

A full listing of all soluble factors that may stimulate production of all cytokines by all cells is beyond the scope of this chapter. An example for one cytokine is given in Table 18–1, which lists the factors stimulating IL-1Ra production by monocytes.[4] In general, po-

Table 18–1. INDUCERS OF IL-1Ra PRODUCTION IN MONOCYTES

IL-1, IL-2, IL-4, IL-6, IL-10, and IL-13
GM-CSF, TGF-β, IFN-α, and IFN-γ
Bacterial lipopolysaccharide (LPS), phorbol myristate acetate (PMA) and β-glucan
Adherent IgG and aggregated IgG
Products of the human cytomegalovirus immediate early genes
Acute-phase proteins (C-reactive protein, α₁-antitrypsin and α₁-acid glycoprotein)

Modified from Arend WP, Malyak M, Jenkins JK, Smith MF Jr: Interleukin-1 receptor agonist. *In* Aggarwal BB, Gutterman JU (eds): Human Cytokines: Handbook for Basic and Clinical Research. Vol 2. Boston, Blackwell Science, 1996, pp 146–167.
Abbreviations: IL, interleukin; GM-CSF, granulocyte-macrophage colony-stimulating factor; TGF, transforming growth factor; IFN, interferon; Ig, immunoglobulin.

tent soluble stimuli for many cytokines include LPS and other bacterial components, viral proteins, complement fragments, and cytokines themselves.

Soluble factors may exert both stimulatory and inhibitory effects on cytokine production by a particular cell. The opposing effects of cytokines on stimulating the production of other cytokines is summarized in Table 18–2.[1] Thus, in diseased tissues, where many cytokines and other soluble factors may be present, the net production of a particular cytokine may be determined both by the nature and the stage of differentiation of the cells and by which cytokines may predominate in the extracellular environment.

In this chapter, the more important stimuli for specific cytokines are mentioned in regard to the role of that cytokine in a pathophysiologic process. The major process to be discussed is rheumatoid synovitis, although mechanisms in other rheumatic diseases are mentioned.

Induction by Direct Cell-Cell Contact

In inflammatory tissue, such as in an inflamed synovium (synovitis), both resident and infiltrated cells are in close proximity. In addition to soluble factors,

Table 18–2. OPPOSING EFFECTS OF CYTOKINES

Stimulator	Cell Responses	Inhibitor
IL-1	T-cell production of IL-2	TGF-β
TGF-β	Collagen synthesis by fibroblasts	IFN-γ, TNF-α
IL-1, TNF-α	Protease synthesis by macrophages	IL-4, IFN-γ
IFN-γ	MHC class II antigen expression	IFN-α, IFN-β, TGF-β
IL-1, TNF-α	Production of IL-1, IL-6, IL-8, TNF-α, and GM-CSF by macrophages	IL-4, IL-10
IL-4	IgE production by B cells	IFN-γ

From Arend WP: Inibiting the effects of cytokines in human diseases. Adv Intern Med 40:365, 1995.

T lymphocytes, monocyte-macrophages, and synovial fibroblast-like cells, for example, can communicate by direct cell-cell contact. In cell culture systems, direct cell contact between activated T lymphocytes and monocytes can markedly stimulate the latter to produce TNF-α, IL-1β, IL-1α,[6] matrix metalloproteinase-1 (MMP-1), 92-kD gelatinase (MMP-9), and tissue inhibitor of metalloproteinase (TIMP).[7] The degree of stimulation observed is similar to or maybe even higher than that obtained by soluble LPS or phorbol myristate acetate (PMA). Monocyte stimulation is also observed using T cell clones derived from synovial tissue of patients with rheumatoid arthritis.[8] Furthermore, direct contact between activated T cells and fibroblasts or synovial cells may also induce large amounts of MMP, which may lead to tissue destruction.[9]

Some of the membrane molecules involved in this activation process are CD11b, CD11c, CD11a, and CD69, but other molecules exist, still unidentified.[10] Membrane-bound cytokines, such as TNF-α, lymphotoxin, and GM-CSF, are also involved in these processes. It is possible that interference with this cell-cell interaction results in a considerable decrease in MMP production. The direct contact between T cells and polymorphonuclear neutrophil leukocytes (PMNs) may also be relevant to the inflammatory process.[11] In either case—soluble factors or direct cell-cell contact—both cytokines and cytokine inhibitors are produced, and the balance between them is more important than their absolute values.

CYTOKINE EFFECTS IN ACUTE INFLAMMATION

Expression of Adhesion Molecules

In acute inflammation, cellular and humoral events lead to the expression of a class of cell-surface glycoproteins with the generic name of *adhesion molecules.* Most of these molecules are on the surface of endothelial cells (ECs) and leukocytes, promoting the interaction of vascular endothelial cells with activated circulating blood cells, such as PMNs, lymphocytes, monocytes, and platelets.[12–14] Stimulated by TNF-α, IL-1α, and IL-1β, endothelial cells express new or increased levels of endothelial-leukocyte adhesion molecule-1 (ELAM-1), intercellular adhesion molecules-1 and -2 (ICAM-1 and ICAM-2), and vascular cell adhesion molecule-1 (VCAM-1).

The subsequent interaction between activated endothelial cells and white blood cells (WBCs) occurs in four stages:

1. Rolling, "tethering," or primary adhesion takes place as leukocytes are trapped by a weak interaction after expression (1 to 2 hours) of endothelial cell selectin (e.g., sialyl-Lewis x, E-, L-, and P-selectins); in the joint (synovium) and the lymphoid tissue, L-selectin and its counterligand peripheral node addressin (PNAd) seem to be the most important.

2. Stimulation, activation, or triggering of leukocytes occurs next as a result of the interaction between proteoglycans on endothelial cells and the chemokine receptors on leukocytes.

3. Strong "gluing" interaction or "activation-dependent sticking" between leukocytes and endothelial cells follows (4 to 6 hours) mediated by leukocyte function-associated antigen-1 (LFA-1, or CD18), ICAM-1, ICAM-2, and very-late-activation antigen 4 (VLA-4). In the joint, central nervous system (CNS), lymph nodes, and skin, the interaction between VCAM-1 and the integrin α4β1 appears to be essential. TNF-α and IL-1 induce endothelial cells to secrete chemotactic polypeptides (chemokines), such as IL-8 and monocyte chemotactic protein-1 (MCP-1).

4. Diapedesis then occurs as secreted chemokines bind to heparan sulfate glycosaminoglycans on the endothelial cell surface. The chemokines interact preferentially with leukocytes that are bound to endothelial cell adhesion molecules, which results in increased affinity, migration, locomotion, and extravasation of the blood cells. Members of the β1 integrin family (e.g., VLA-4 and VLA-5) enable leukocytes to bind to fibronectin, and VLA-6 mediates attachment to laminin.

At a later stage, GM-CSF has an important role in autoimmune and inflammatory diseases. Produced by T cells, monocytes, fibroblasts, and endothelial cells, this glycoprotein (14 to 35 kD) enhances monocyte migration into inflamed tissue by stimulating the expression of the adhesion molecules CD18 and CD11. IL-4 acts on endothelial cells and synergizes with IL-1β to enhance lymphocyte binding by increasing the expression of VCAM-1 on vascular cells.[15] In contrast, IL-4 inhibits endothelial cell expression of other adhesion molecules that are induced by IL-1, TNF-α, or IFN-γ and that mediate binding of neutrophils.[16] Thus, IL-4 may alter the quality of cells in an inflammatory infiltrate by promoting lymphocyte migration from blood while decreasing neutrophil egress. IL-8, the most potent chemoattractant of neutrophils, induces the expression of adhesion molecules CD11b/CD18.[17] The role of cell adhesion molecules (CAMs) has not been known until recently.[18]

Cell Recruitment and Migration

Cell recruitment and migration into the synovium depend primarily on the C-X-C, C-C, and C chemokine subfamilies (Table 18–3). The term *chemokines* includes a number of cytokines (8 to 10 kD) whose amino acid sequences exhibit between 20 to 55 percent homology.[19, 20] All chemokines have four cysteine residues that form two internal disulfide loops. Three subfamilies have been identified[21]:

1. The C-X-C subfamily. The cysteine residues are separated by one amino acid (e.g., IL-8, platelet basic protein, and neutrophil-activating peptide-2 [NAP-2]).

Table 18–3. SUBFAMILIES OF CHEMOKINES

C-X-C	C-C	C
• IL-8 (= NAP-1, NCF, MDNCF)	• MCP-1	Lymphotactin
gro α/MSGA	MCP-2	
gro β/MIP-2α	MCP-3	
gro γ/MIP-2β	MCP-4	
• PBP	• MIP-1α	
β-TG	MIP-1β	
NAP-2	• RANTES	
CTAP-III	• Eotactin	
• ENA-78		
• IP-90		
• GCP-2		
• MIG		
• MIP-2		

Abbreviations: gro, growth-regulated gene product; PBP, platelet basic protein; β-TG, β-thromboglobulin; NAP-2, neutrophil-activating peptide-2; CTAP, connective tissue–activating peptide; ENA, epithelial neutrophil-activating peptide; MIG, interferon-γ-inducible gene; MCP, monocyte chemoattractant protein; MIP, macrophage inflammatory protein; RANTES, regulated upon activation, normal T expressed and presumably secreted molecule; IL, interleukin.

2. The C-C family. The two cysteine residues are adjacent (e.g., monocyte chemoattractant protein [MCP] and macrophage inflammatory protein [MIP]).

3. The C family (e.g., lymphotactin).

Up to now, five different receptors of the chemokine family have been isolated.

The C-X-C subfamily of chemokines acts on neutrophils. Their principal biologic functions are stimulation of random leukocyte movement (*chemokinesis*) and directed migration (*chemotaxis*). C-X-C is produced by activated mononuclear phagocytes, tissue cells (endothelial cells and fibroblasts), and megakaryocytes, which give rise to platelets containing stored chemokines.

C-C members are produced primarily by activated T cells and act on specific receptors on monocytes, lymphocytes, eosinophils, and basophils, but not on neutrophils.

In rheumatoid arthritis, the expression of MCP-1 protein and mRNA is localized to synovial lining cells by immunohistochemistry and in situ hybridization (Table 18–4).[3] Although synovial fibroblasts and chondrocytes as a rule do not express MCP-1 constitutively, the addition of TNF-α and IL-1 stimulates both MCP-1 mRNA and protein. The human receptor for IL-8 shares many structural characteristics with the family of membrane receptors coupled with G-proteins, including seven transmembrane hydrophobic domains.

A cytokine detected recently in the rheumatoid joint that may facilitate the access of inflammatory cells to the synovium is vascular endothelial growth factor (VEGF),[22, 23] also known as *vascular permeability factor*[24] (see later). A new interleukin, IL-16, is a potent lymphocyte chemoattractant for CD4+ T lymphocytes.[25, 26]

Table 18–4. SOME CHEMOKINES AND RHEUMATOID ARTHRITIS (RA)

Chemokine	Cellular Origin	Stimuli	Major Functions	Location
IL-8	Tissue macrophages Fibroblasts, chrondrocytes Endothelial cells PMNs and monocytes	IL-1, TNF-α	Neutrophil chemoattractant ↑ CD11b/CD18 Chemotactic and mitogenic for endothelial cells	SF: RA > OA Gout ↑ ↑

CTAP-III	Platelets		Stimulates: DNA synthesis,
			  hyaluronic acid and
			  glycosaminoglycans
				Elevated in plasma of
				  patients with RA

MCP-1	Monocytes, T lymphocytes Synovial fibroblasts (RA) Chondrocytes Tissue macrophages	IL-1, TNF-α, IFN-γ, PDGF, TGF-β, LPS constitutively	Recruitment of macrophages	SF: RA > OA

MIP-1α	Tissue macrophages
	Synovial fibroblasts
	SF monocytes
		TNF-α	Pyrogens
			Chemoattractant for monocyte-
			  macrophages and T
			  lymphocytes
				SF: RA > OA

RANTES	Synovial fibroblasts (RA)	IL-1, TNF-α, potentiation with
		  IFN-γ, down-regulation
		  with IL-4
				Chemoattractant for
				  monocytes and
				  memory cells

Adapted from Koch AE, Kunkel SL, Strieter RM: Cytokines in rheumatoid arthritis. J Invest Med 43:28, 1995.
Abbreviations: OA, osteoarthritis; PMN, polymorphonuclear neutrophil leukocytes; PDGF, platelet-derived growth factor; IL, interleukin; TNF, tumor necrosis factor; IFN, interferon; TGF, transforming growth factor; LPS, lipopolysaccharide; DNA, deoxyribonucleic acid; SF, synovial fluid.

Cell Proliferation, Differentiation and Maturation

Immune Cells

The synovium of patients with rheumatoid arthritis is infiltrated with CD4+ T lymphocytes that express surface antigens characteristic of mature memory cells (CD45 RO+).[27] Some CD4+ cells show activation markers, such as histocompatibility locus antigen DR (HLA-DR); other indicators of T cell activation, such as cell surface receptors for IL-2 (CD25) and transferrin, are underrepresented. Most synovial membrane T cells bear the α/β T cell receptor (TCR), but some CD3+ round cells in the synovium are γ/δ cells.[28] Most studies suggest that a Th1-like profile is predominant, and that the T cell population within the rheumatoid synovial membrane can produce a high level of IL-10.[29]

The following cytokines may be involved in immune cell proliferation and differentiation during inflammation.

IFN-γ, a potent immunomodulatory molecule without structural and functional similarity with IFN-α and IFN-β,[30] is secreted by activated Th1-CD4+ helper cells, CD8+ T cytotoxic cells, and natural killer (NK) cells. The mechanism by which IFNs stimulate the transcription of early genes has only now been elucidated.[31] The original identification of what was thought to be synovial IFN-γ was consistent with the presence of large amounts of HLA-DR on lining cells, macrophages, and vascular endothelium in inflamed joints.[32] However, only trace amounts of IFN-γ have been detected in the joint effusions of patients with rheumatoid arthritis.[33] IFN-γ levels are also very low

in the supernatant of synovial cell cultures. Moreover, stimulation of synovial cells with T-cell mitogens results in the production of large amounts of IFN-γ, which indicates that cells capable of producing that cytokine are present in the synovium.[33] It is not clear why IFN-γ levels are so low in the rheumatoid synovium. Because IFN-γ antagonizes the stimulatory effects of TNF-α on rheumatoid synovial fibroblast functions, including HLA-DR expression, proliferation, collagenase production,[34] and GM-CSF production, it is possible that a deficiency in IFN-γ production in the rheumatoid joint allows TNF-α effects to remain unchallenged. A clinical trial of IFN-γ treatment in rheumatoid arthritis has not exhibited beneficial effects.

IL-2 is secreted coordinately with IFN-γ by antigen-stimulated cells and is also produced by CD4+ Th1 helper T cells after stimulation. IL-2 is a major T cell growth factor (TCGF). The IL-2 receptor complex includes three chains: (1) p55 (α-chain and Tac antigen) possessing low affinity (kD, ~10 nM), (2) p70-75 (β-chain), and (3) a newly described γ-chain.[35] Abnormalities of the IL-2 and IL-2 receptor system may occur in several autoimmune diseases. Immunoassays have revealed the presence of low concentrations of IL-2 in only a minority of rheumatoid synovial fluids. Immunohistochemical analysis did not reveal any IL-2 protein in rheumatoid synovial tissue, even though IL-2 mRNA is detectable by in situ hybridization.[36] In contrast, both IL-2 protein and transcripts for IL-2 mRNA are present in other forms of chronic inflammatory synovitis.[37] The relative absence of IFN-γ and IL-2 may imply that the CD4+ cells in rheumatoid synovium are either exhausted at the time of the sampling or are part of the Th2 subset. However, IL-

4, a marker of Th2 subset, is also found at very low levels in rheumatoid synovium.[38]

The activity of IL-15 appears to be similar to that of IL-2, with both cytokines stimulating cells through part of IL-2R.[39] In contrast to IL-2 and IL-15, which act mainly on T cells, IL-14 has been described as a high-molecular-weight B cell growth factor (HMW-BCGF).[40]

The CSF family is also important during the immune and inflammatory response.[41] Human IL-3 (or multi-CSF) is a protein (14 kD) whose gene is located on chromosome 5, close to the gene for GM-CSF, IL-4, IL-5, and M-CSF-R. The receptor for human IL-3 has two chains, α and β, and is a member of the hematopoietic receptor family. The β-chain is common to GM-CSF-R and IL-5R, which may account for the competition between IL-3, GM-CSF, and IL-5 for receptor binding. IL-3 primarily enhances early progenitor cells in the bone marrow; it also stimulates monocyte cytotoxicity, promotes eosinophil survival, and induces histamine release from basophils. In rheumatic diseases, IL-3 may be responsible for the relatively high amount of mast cells reported in the rheumatoid synovium.[42]

GM-CSF, a 22-kD glycoprotein, is produced by T lymphocytes, macrophages, endothelial cells, and fibroblasts. It induces proliferation and differentiation of bone marrow precursors (macrophages, neutrophils, and eosinophils). The cell membrane-associated form of GM-CSF is also biologically active, thus playing a role in direct cell-cell contact.[43] The role of GM-CSF is discussed within the context of the inflammatory cells.

M-CSF, a heavily glycosylated protein produced by monocytes, fibroblasts, endothelial cells, and epithelial cells can be expressed constitutively, contrary to other hematopoietic factors. A spontaneous mutation (op mutation) in the M-CSF gene leads to the phenotype op/op, which exhibits a deficiency in the phagocytic system. The op/op phenotype also is associated with osteopetrosis, which can be cured by injection of recombinant M-CSF.[44] M-CSF is a potent chemotactic and differentiating factor for monocytes.

G-CSF, a protein of 19 kD, is produced by monocytes, macrophages, endothelial cells, and fibroblasts in response to IL-1, TNF-α, or IFN-γ. It promotes the differentiation of neutrophils.

The roles of IL-5, IL-7, and IL-9 in rheumatic diseases are not well defined, but they are all important in the differentiation and maturation process. IL-5 is an "Eo-CSF," in that it induces growth and differentiation of eosinophils. In the human system, the effect of IL-5 on Ig secretion by B cells is still controversial.[45] IL-7, produced spontaneously by stromal cells of the medulla and the thymus, can be considered a "lympho-CSF" because it induces the proliferation of pre-B and pre-T cells (CD4⁻/CD8⁻) in the thymus.[46] IL-9 acts as a growth factor for T cells. Produced by CD4⁺ lymphocytes in response to mitogens and antigens, IL-9 acts in synergy with IL-3 to enhance the proliferation of mastocytes.[47]

The functions of Th1 and Th2 cells are regulated by the ratio of IL-4 to IFN-γ and of IL-10 to IL-12.[48–50] Human IL-4 (15 kD) is a growth factor of activated B cells and stimulates CD23 expression (receptor of low affinity for IgE), Fcε-RII and class II MHC antigen expression on normal and malignant B cells. IL-4 regulates the production of IgG4 and IgE and can stimulate IL-4–dependent T cell clones. Th2 cells are characterized by the preferential production of IL-4 and IL-5 but not of IFN-γ and lymphotoxin (LT). Th2 cells are involved in the generation of humoral immunity. IL-4 released by Th2 cells increases antibody production by B cells and induces the switch to IgE synthesis. In addition, recruitment and activation of eosinophils are enhanced by IL-5. Thus, acute allergic inflammation or humoral immunity is primarily associated with Th2 cells. Conversely, Th1 cells are involved in cell-mediated immunity, such as delayed type hypersensitivity (DTH). IFN-γ, TNF-α, and IL-1 mediate most of these effects of Th1 cells and are particularly important in granuloma formation in such diseases as sarcoidosis and Wegener's granulomatosis.

Th1, Th2, and Th0 cells are at the origin of the cellular and cytokine network; these cells affect other cell types and, in turn, are influenced by cytokines produced by other cells. One of the characteristics of this cytokine network is the capacity for cross-regulation. Thus, by producing IL-4, Th2 cells enhance their own differentiation and suppress differentiation and growth of IFN-γ–producing cells. Conversely, IFN-γ appears to inhibit Th2 cell differentiation (Fig. 18–1).

IL-10, also known as cytokine synthesis inhibitory factor (CSIF), has a strong inhibitory effect on IFN-γ and IL-2 production by activated Th1 cells and is part of a mechanism by which Th2 cells block the effector functions of Th1.[51] IL-10 decreases the capacity of APCs to present antigens by decreasing MHC class II expression and by decreasing the production of IL-1, IL-6 and TNF-α by monocytes. High levels of IL-10 can be produced by macrophages and T cells in the synovium.[52] Similar to IL-4, IL-10 is a strong inhibitor of MMP synthesis in chronic inflammation; unlike IL-4, however, it also stimulates tissue inhibitor of MMP-1 (TIMP-1).[53] These observations argue for a possible use of IL-4 and IL-10 as antiinflammatory agents in rheumatoid arthritis.

Produced by B cells and macrophages, IL-12 induces the secretion of IFN-γ by thymic lymphocytes and by NK cells.[50] Thus, IL-12 may play an important role in the cytotoxicity of NK and lymphokine-activated killer (LAK) cells. This is why IL-12 was formerly called "cytotoxic lymphocyte maturation factor" (CLMF), or "natural killer and stimulating factor" (NKSFR). The possible therapeutic use of IL-12 in vaccination and tumor immunology is being explored.

IL-13 shares many biologic activities with IL-4 (B cell proliferation, switch to IgE and IgG4; inhibition of the production of cytokines, such as IL-6, IL-1β,

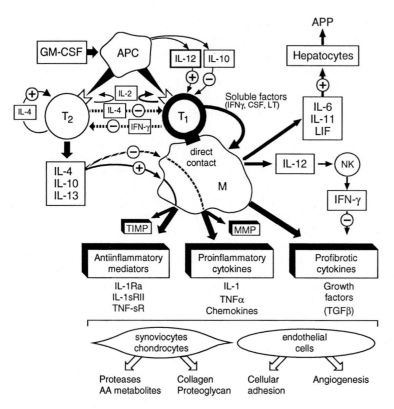

Figure 18–1. Cells and mediators in chronic inflammation: role of antigen-presenting cells (APCs) and balance between lymphocytes (T1 and T2) resulting in different cytokine profiles. Activation of monocytes (M) by direct contact or by soluble products (interferon [IFN-γ], colony-stimulating factor [CSF], lymphotoxin [LT]) leading to the production of matrix metalloproteases (MMP), tissue inhibitor of MMP (TIMP), and other mediators or cytokines by M that act on synoviocytes, chondrocytes, endothelial cells, natural killer (NK) lymphocytes, and hepatocytes, which produce acute-phase proteins (APPs). IL, interleukin; TGF, transforming growth factor; TNF, tumor necrosis factor; AA, arachidonic acid.

TNF-α, and IL-8; and increased expression of CD23.[54] IL-13 synergizes with IL-2 to increase IFN-γ production by large granular lymphocytes (LGLs). The main difference between IL-4 and IL-13 in biologic functions is expected to be at the receptor level, because, unlike IL-4R, IL-13R has not been observed on lymphocytes to date. Regulatory effects of IL-13 on macrophages and monocytes from synovial fluid of patients with inflammatory arthritis have been reported and are similar to those of IL-4.[55]

Most of the data available relate to CD4+ T cells, hence the use of the acronym Th. However, a systematic investigation of cytokine production in different pathologic conditions has been undertaken at the single-cell level. These results have revealed that CD8+ T cells are involved in inflammation and can also be divided into different subsets according to their function and pattern of cytokine production. This observation implies that the acronym Th may soon become obsolete. In conclusion, type I cytokines (IL-12, IFN-γ) drive Th0 and Th1, which, by releasing IL-2 and IFN-γ, induce predominantly the "cellular immune response." In chronic inflammation, IL-4 and IL-10 are important in decreasing the production of MMPs by fibroblasts, synovial cells, and macrophages; in addition, IL-10 stimulates TIMP production.[53]

Inflammatory Cells

The major inflammatory cells that are involved in pathophysiologic mechanisms in rheumatic diseases include PMNs, monocyte-macrophages, synovial cells, and fibroblasts.

Polymorphonuclear Leukocytes

PMNs are found in inflammatory synovial fluids and in inflamed tissues where necrosis or secondary infection may be present. Although PMNs are commonly thought to be terminally differentiated cells, they are weak producers of some cytokines, including IL-1β, IL-8, IL-1Ra, TNF-α, and GM-CSF. However, the predominance or presence of large numbers of PMNs in certain rheumatic diseases, such as in the vessel wall in necrotizing vasculitis or in rheumatoid synovial fluids, may make them an important local source of some cytokines, particularly IL-8 and IL-1Ra.[56, 57] PMNs produce increased amounts of these cytokines in response to GM-CSF or TNF-α. IL-8 is a potent chemotactic factor for other PMNs; however, other intracellular responses in PMNs are only weakly induced by exposure to exogenous cytokines.

Monocytes and Macrophages

Monocytes and macrophages exhibit diverse responses to cytokines in acute inflammation. Transforming growth factor-β (TGF-β) is chemotactic for monocytes and may contribute to the influx of these cells into the rheumatoid synovium. Monocytes and macrophages also exhibit enhanced production of IL-1β and IL-1Ra in response to stimulation by TGF-β. In addition, these cells synthesize and secrete more

IL-1β and TNF-α after exposure to either of these cytokines in the extracellular environment. As summarized in Table 18–1, many cytokines induce IL-1Ra production in monocytes. Of interest are the effects of IL-4, IL-10, and IL-13 on monocyte-macrophages to inhibit the production of inflammatory cytokines while enhancing the production of IL-1Ra. Thus, endogenous production of IL-4, IL-10, and IL-13 in the rheumatoid synovium as well as their exogenous administration may have anti-inflammatory effects and inhibit MMP production. Recent determinations of systemic and local levels of MMP and TIMP as markers of tissue destruction,[58] and of soluble adhesion molecules as markers of cell involvement in the inflammatory process, may shed new light on the relative roles of IL-1 and TNF-α in the rheumatoid disease process.[59]

Monocyte differentiation is induced by GM-CSF, and macrophage activation is stimulated by IFN-γ. Differentiated and activated macrophages are an important source of the anti-inflammatory cytokine IL-1Ra. Most studies indicate that T cell cytokines are present in only small amounts in rheumatoid synovial tissue, whereas many inflammatory cytokines and CSFs are present in abundance. Thus, GM-CSF is a more important inducer of HLA class II expression on rheumatoid synovial cells than is IFN-γ, and this effect of GM-CSF is enhanced by TNF-α.[60] Large amounts of GM-CSF are present in rheumatoid synovial fluids and cultured synovial tissue cells readily produce GM-CSF.[61] GM-CSF production is constitutive in freshly isolated rheumatoid synovial tissue macrophages, although stimulation by IL-1 and TNF-α is necessary in cultured synovial macrophages and fibroblasts.[62] CSFs also exhibit many other effects on hematopoietic cells, some of which are relevant to events in acute inflammation, such as enhancing monocyte migration and increasing expression of adhesion molecules.[63, 64] Thus, in rheumatic diseases, CSFs may be involved at two levels: induction of growth and proliferation of hematopoietic progenitor cells in the bone marrow as well as activation of mature granulocytes and monocytes locally in tissues.

Fibroblasts

Cytokines in acute inflammation also exert important effects on fibroblasts. The aggressive growth and proliferation of synovial fibroblasts in the rheumatoid joint may be due primarily to the effects of platelet-derived growth factor (PDGF) and fibroblast growth factors (FGFs).[65] These cytokines, and other local factors in the rheumatoid synovium, stimulate fibroblasts to hypertrophy and exhibit growth characteristics of invasive tumor cells. Both PDGF and FGF are found in more abundance in the joints of patients with rheumatoid arthritis compared with osteoarthritis. These cytokines may lead to a highly destructive phenotype in rheumatoid fibroblasts through binding to specific cell surface receptors and stimulating protein kinase activities.[66] Many of these effects of PDGF and FGF on rheumatoid fibroblast growth and differentiation are inhibited by TGF-β, again illustrating the self-regulatory nature of the cytokine network. In chronic inflammation, however, TGF-β contributes to tissue fibrosis through inducing collagen production by fibroblasts, as discussed later.

Induction of Acute-Phase Reactants

The acute-phase response represents the efforts of the intact organism to restore homeostasis after infection, inflammation, or other insults and consists of both local and systemic reactions.[67] The local response involves activation of PMNs, macrophages, fibroblasts, and endothelial cells with the release of various cytokines, including IL-1, TNF-α, and IL-6. These cytokines, in turn, induce the systemic response with fever, increased erythrocyte sedimentation rate (ESR), increased secretion of adrenocorticotropic hormone (ACTH) and glucocorticoids, and changes in the concentrations of various serum proteins.

Changes in the synthesis of acute-phase proteins by hepatocytes are induced primarily by IL-6.[68] IL-6 stimulates large increases in the production of C-reactive protein (CRP) and serum amyloid A (SAA) by hepatocytes, with smaller increases seen in the synthesis of ceruloplasmin, complement components C3 and C4, haptoglobin, α-1 antiprotease, ferritin, and fibrinogen. In contrast, in the acute-phase response, IL-6 decreases the hepatic synthesis of other proteins, including albumin, transthyretin, transferrin, and α-fetoprotein. Other cytokines, including IL-1, TNF-α, and TGF-β, also influence the hepatic production of acute-phase proteins, often by synergizing with IL-6; glucocorticoids also enhance the stimulatory effects of IL-6. However, the serum concentrations of these cytokines and of the acute-phase proteins are poorly correlated, indicating the complexity of this system in vivo.

IL-6, also known as "hepatocyte-stimulating factor" or B cell stimulatory factor-2, has many other important effects in acute immune and inflammatory events.[69] IL-6 is produced by numerous cells, including fibroblasts, monocytes, macrophages, endothelial cells, keratinocytes, B cells, and T cells. The major inducers of IL-6 production are bacterial or viral proteins and other cytokines, primarily IL-1 and TNF-α. IL-6 enhances Ig production by B cells; it is a potent autocrine growth factor for plasma cells in multiple myeloma and stimulates T cell growth, differentiation, and activation. IL-6 also stimulates osteoclasts and is a major contributor to the bone loss that accompanies estrogen deficiency.[70] The importance of IL-6 in local inflammatory responses is further supported by studies in mice made deficient in IL-6 production through homologous recombination.[71, 72] These mice were unable to control infections with vaccinia virus or the facultative intracellular bacterium *Listeria monocytogenes* and exhibited deficient localized inflammatory responses after tissue damage or infection. However, systemic responses to LPS were largely intact in IL-6–deficient mice.

The possible role of IL-6 in autoimmune and inflammatory diseases has been extensively examined. IL-6 concentrations are elevated in the sera of patients with systemic lupus erythematosus (SLE), and SLE monocytes spontaneously produced large amounts of IL-6 in vitro, primarily stimulated by IL-1 and TNF-α.[73] The possibility exists that autocrine IL-6 hyperactivity may contribute to the enhanced B cell function and production of autoantibodies present in patients with SLE.[74] Support for this hypothesis is derived from studies of murine lupus in which injection of anti–IL-6 antibodies prevented production of anti-DNA antibodies, reduced proteinuria, and prolonged life.[75] High IL-6 concentrations are present in the synovial fluids of patients with rheumatoid arthritis or osteoarthritis, probably derived in part from synovial macrophages and articular chondrocytes, the latter cells stimulated by IL-1 and TNF-α.[76]

Autoantibodies to IL-6 are present in the sera of patients with systemic sclerosis, but these antibodies may retain IL-6 in the circulation and lead to enhanced IL-6 biologic effects.[77] In addition, complexes of soluble IL-6 receptors and IL-6 are present in the sera of patients with juvenile rheumatoid arthritis and these complexes exhibit intact biologic effects.[78] Thus, in systemic sclerosis and juvenile rheumatoid arthritis, the presence of autoantibodies to IL-6 or of soluble IL-6 receptors paradoxically may increase and not inhibit the effects of IL-6.

Leukemia inhibitory factor (LIF) was originally defined by the ability to induce terminal differentiation of murine myeloid leukemia cells, resulting in the inhibition of their growth. LIF has a number of biologic activities, some of which overlap with those of IL-6 and IL-1. LIF induces bone resorption and the synthesis of acute-phase proteins by hepatocytes and it stimulates platelet production. Rheumatoid synovial fluid contains significantly more LIF than osteoarthritic synovial fluid, and LIF concentrations appear to correlate with leukocyte counts in synovial fluids. Synovial fibroblasts produce LIF in response to IL-1 or TNF-α. In turn, LIF induces the expression of IL-1, IL-6, and IL-8 mRNA, leading to a paracrine loop effect. LIF seems to play an important role in the regulation of bone formation and resorption.

IL-11, a 20-kD protein produced by bone marrow stromal cells, possesses lymphopoietic and hematopoietic properties.[79] IL-11 shares numerous biologic activities with IL-6 (plasmocytoma proliferation and T cell helper function for B cells). IL-11 also synergizes with IL-3 and steel factor in the differentiation of megakaryocytes. IL-11 is identical to the adipogenesis inhibitory factor (AGIF), which inhibits the differentiation of adipocytes. Viruses, histamine, TGF-β, and IL-1 stimulate IL-11 production, whereas IL-4 is inhibitory.

Induction of Angiogenesis

The development of new blood vessels is important in wound healing but may contribute to tissue dam-age in pathologic conditions, such as tumor growth, diabetic retinopathy, and rheumatoid arthritis. Increased vascularity of the rheumatoid pannus may assist the growth of this tissue with invasion into adjacent bone and cartilage. Angiogenic factors act either *directly* on endothelial cells to stimulate proliferation or *indirectly* by attracting and stimulating macrophages and other cells to release endothelial growth factors.[80] In addition to angiogenesis, endothelial cells may contribute to rheumatoid synovitis through the selective expression of adhesion molecules on high endothelial venules (HEVs), mediating the egress of PMNs, lymphocytes, and monocytes into the synovium.[81]

Angiogenesis in the rheumatoid synovium is influenced by cytokines, prostaglandins, and other small molecules. The important cytokines include acidic and basic FGFs, angiogenin, VEGF, IL-8, and TNF-α.[82]

FGF is a family of small-molecular-weight proteins that have been isolated from numerous cells and tissues. These proteins bind to heparin in the extracellular matrix.

VEGF and IL-8 also bind to heparin; this process may be important in localizing angiogenic factors to the inflamed synovium. Soluble cytokines also are important as combined antibodies to IL-8 and TNF-α inhibited by approximately 50 percent the angiogenic activity exhibited by supernatants of cultured rheumatoid synovial fibroblasts.[83]

VEGF is a 34- to 42-kD peptide originally described in the supernatants of cultured tumor cells. This potent angiogenic factor is present in rheumatoid synovial fluids in much higher concentrations than in synovial fluids from other forms of arthritis.[84] VEGF is produced by macrophages in the synovial lining layer and subsynovial tissues of patients with rheumatoid arthritis and binds to specific receptors on nearby endothelial cells.[84, 85] In addition to inducing endothelial cell proliferation, VEGF leads to increased vascular permeability and the extravasation of plasma proteins, including fibrinogen into the joint. Fibrin as well as collagens types I and III in the connective tissue matrix further enhances the growth of new blood vessels by providing a scaffold for proliferating endothelial cells.

Regulation of angiogenesis is an area of potential therapeutic intervention in rheumatoid arthritis. Cytokines present in the rheumatoid synovium, such as IL-1 and TGF-β, may act locally to inhibit growth factor–induced endothelial cell proliferation. In addition, many current therapeutic agents in rheumatoid arthritis, including glucocorticoids, methotrexate, penicillamine, and hydroxychloroquine, may inhibit angiogenesis as one of their many beneficial effects. New therapeutic approaches to inhibition of angiogenesis in rheumatoid arthritis might include the evaluation of a synthetic derivative of the antibiotic fumagillin, shown to be effective in collagen-induced arthritis in rats, both in preventing the disease and in ameliorating established arthritis.[86]

CYTOKINE EFFECTS IN CHRONIC INFLAMMATION

Induction of Tissue Destruction

One of the main features of rheumatoid arthritis is the destruction of bone and cartilage. From in vitro experiments with cultured cells and from animal models, the consensus has been reached that IL-1 and TNF-α are the main proinflammatory and destructive cytokines, acting primarily through stimulation of metalloprotease production by other cells in the inflamed synovium. The role of IL-1 and TNF-α in the mechanism of joint tissue damage in rheumatoid arthritis has recently been reviewed.[87, 88]

Interleukin-1

The term IL-1 was given to a 17-kD molecule originally described as endogenous pyrogen (EP), lymphocyte-activating factor (LAF), and mononuclear cell factor (MCF) that stimulates the production of collagenase and prostaglandin E_2 (PGE$_2$) in human synovial cells.[89] Two genes coding for two distinct proteins, IL-1α and IL-1β, were isolated.

IL-1α (17.3 kD, pI 7) is mainly cell-associated (95 percent), and IL-1β (17.3 kD, pI 7) is released into the extracellular environment after stimulation. The mature forms of human IL-1α and IL-1β share only 26 percent amino acid sequence homology. The two forms are initially synthesized as 31-kD precursor polypeptides. Only the precursor forms of IL-1 exist inside the cell, and they are present in the cytosolic fraction. The precursor form of IL-1α is biologically active, contrary to the 31-kD form of IL-1β. The active extracellular form of IL-1β results from the cleavage of the carboxy-terminal portion of the 31-kD peptide by a family of specific proteases called *IL-1β converting enzyme* (ICE). Specific inhibitors of ICE were synthesized and assessed as to their effects in an animal model of arthritis.[90] Membrane-bound IL-1α probably originates from the intracellular movement of the precursor molecule to the cell surface.

Activated monocyte-macrophages are a major source of IL-1. However, almost all cells can produce IL-1 to some extent. Activated T cells contain IL-1α, which may be membrane-associated and possibly plays a role in the initiation of the immune response. Among other cells relevant to the inflammatory response that can produce IL-1 are endothelial cells and Epstein-Barr virus-transformed B cells.

IL-1 is present mainly in macrophages of rheumatoid synovial tissue cells, either by in situ hybridization for IL-1β mRNA[91] or by immunolocalization at the pannus-cartilage junction for the protein, and in perivascular macrophages in the subsynovium.[92, 93] Cultured cells from rheumatoid synovia, where mononuclear cell infiltration predominates, produce higher levels of IL-1β than do cells from osteoarthritis synovia. The production of IL-1 by rheumatoid synovium, in contrast to the synovium in osteoarthritis, corresponds to a greater number of macrophages and degree of vascularization.[94, 95]

Although one must take caution when measuring IL-1 in extracellular compartments, peripheral monocytes from rheumatoid patients produce more IL-1 in vitro than cells from normal subjects or patients with osteoarthritis. In addition, monocytes from rheumatoid synovial fluids produce more IL-1 after in vitro stimulation than do peripheral blood cells from the same patients.[87] The presence of various substances interfering in bioassays and immunoassays, such as rheumatoid factors, IL-1Ra, and soluble IL-1 receptors, may account for the considerable variation in results between different commercial immunoassays. IL-1 is sometimes detected in very low concentrations in rheumatoid synovial fluids, and it is virtually absent in non-rheumatoid fluids.[96] In some studies, IL-1 levels in the circulation correlated with clinical and histologic parameters of disease activity in patients with rheumatoid arthritis.[96, 97]

Almost any cell perturbation is liable to induce IL-1 gene expression, particularly in monocytes. In rheumatic diseases, the stimuli for IL-1 production may include direct cell contact with activated lymphocytes, extracellular matrix elements, soluble factors, crystals, bacteria, and viruses. Among the cytokines known to stimulate IL-1 production, TNF-α appears to be particularly important,[89] but IL-1 can also induce its own production in an autocrine or paracrine fashion. In addition, leukotriene B_4 (LTB$_4$) appears to stimulate IL-1 production, whereas PGE$_2$ has the opposite effect.

Two high-affinity cell membrane receptors for IL-1 have been characterized: types I and II.[98, 99] Both IL-1α and IL-1β appear to bind to both IL-1 receptors but not with equal avidity. Type I IL-1 receptors (80 kD) are present on T cells, endothelial cells, epithelial cells, and chondrocytes. Type II IL-1 receptors (60 kD) are present on B cells, neutrophils, and macrophages. Only type I IL-1R, however, can trigger an intracellular response.

In contrast to TNF-α, the local effects of IL-1 on both immune and inflammatory cells may be more important in inflammatory joint diseases such as rheumatoid arthritis. Indeed, IL-1 effects include enhancement of T and B lymphocyte function; chemotaxis of neutrophils, lymphocytes, and monocytes; and increased expression of adhesion molecules on endothelial cells. IL-1 may further enhance chemotaxis indirectly by inducing the release of other chemoattractant cytokines. However, the most important aspect of IL-1 at the local level is its effect on tissue destruction, inducing even at low concentrations the production of collagenase, neutral proteinases, and PGE$_2$ by synovial cells, chondrocytes, and bone-derived cells.

In experimental animal models of arthritis,[87] intra-articular injection of IL-1 induces a transient infiltration of neutrophils into the joint space followed by mononuclear cells, although few cells are observed in the synovium. Collagen-induced arthritis in the mouse, an animal model of inflammatory arthritis, is accelerated by the subcutaneous infusion of IL-1. All of these observations argue strongly for the involvement of IL-1 in the processes of tissue destruction.

Tumor Necrosis Factor-α

The other principal proinflammatory cytokine is TNF-α, originally described as a monocyte product that induced tumor lysis in experimental animals and cachexia in mice (hence the name *cachectin*).[5, 100] Some properties of TNF-α overlap with those of other cytokines, such as IL-1.

The biologically active form of TNF-α is soluble and trimeric (3 × 17 kD).[101] TNF-α is produced in the cell as a 26-kD propeptide and is also present (~1 to 2 percent) within the cell membrane, where it is biologically active. The membrane form is cleaved to yield the 17-kD extracellular molecule. TNF-α gene alleles exist in New Zealand white (NZW) mice and are correlated with reduced serum TNF-α levels. It has been hypothesized that decreased TNF-α levels predispose to the SLE-like autoimmune disease seen in these mice. In fact, the administration of TNF-α reduces the severity of autoimmune diabetes in biobreeding (BB) rats.[102] Many studies have focused on the role of polymorphism of TNF-α, IL-1α and other cytokines in autoimmune diseases.[103] Patients with SLE exhibit normal circulating levels of TNF-α and a normal increase in TNF-α with infection. The complete blocking of TNF-α may lead to certain autoimmune diseases. In fact, patients with rheumatoid arthritis receiving anti–TNF-α antibodies have shown levels of autoantibodies to native DNA. An explanation for this phenomenon might be a decrease in naturally occurring apoptosis or an alteration in function of T cells that express cell-surface TNF-α.[104]

TNF-α and LT are antigenically distinct but possess 30 percent amino acid sequence homology and share the same cell surface receptor.[105, 106] TNF-α is mainly produced by monocyte-macrophages, whereas LT is mainly produced by T lymphocytes. Production of TNF-α is induced not only by LPS but also by a variety of other stimuli, including tumor promoters, viruses, and mitogens. Other cytokines that can stimulate TNF-α and LT production to a small extent are notably IFN-γ, IL-1, and the CSFs. A more powerful stimulation for TNF-α production is provided by direct cell-cell contact. IL-1 and TNF-α are usually synthesized and secreted simultaneously, although their production appears to be regulated separately and controlled by different mechanisms.

At present, there are two distinct receptors for TNF-α that belong to a superfamily of cellular and viral proteins.[107, 108] A 55-kD receptor possesses leader, extracellular, transmembrane, and intracellular domains that exhibit a high degree of sequence homology with a large number of molecules belonging to TNF-R family, such as the nerve growth factor receptor and CD40. The second TNF-α receptor (75 kD) is also a transmembranous molecule. The extracellular fragments of both TNF-α receptors can be shed and have an inhibitory effect on TNF-α biologic activities (see later).

Patients with severe rheumatoid arthritis or those with a high synovial fluid leukocyte count have elevated levels of TNF-α. Macrophages in the synovial lining layer in rheumatoid arthritis and in the subsynovium contain high levels of TNF-α, similar to IL-1. The TNF receptors are immunolocalized to both macrophages and fibroblasts in the rheumatoid synovial lining layer and to lymphocytes and endothelial cells in the subsynovium.[87]

One of the ways in which cytokines interact and influence one another's action is by transmodulation of receptor expression. TNF-α receptor mRNA and cell surface expression can be up-regulated by IFN-α, IFN-β, and IFN-γ.

The main pathologic role of TNF-α appears to be at the systemic level, where it acts on endothelial cells, as in septic shock, acute respiratory distress syndrome, and vasculitis. In rheumatic diseases, however, TNF-α stimulates collagenase and PGE$_2$ production by synovial cells or other fibroblasts and plays an important role in synovitis. The major impact of TNF-α on tissue destruction is due to the synergism between TNF-α and IL-1. In addition, TNF-α induces more IL-1 than vice versa.

An important role of TNF-α in arthritis has been established in animal studies. In mice transgenic for TNF-α, destructive arthritis developed spontaneously and the administration of monoclonal antibodies to human TNF-α prevented the development of arthritis.[109] Antibodies to IL-1 also prevented the development of arthritis in TNF-α transgenic mice. Furthermore, work in progress by the same groups has shown that transgenic mice overexpressing IL-1 also develop arthritis. The role of TNF-α has been further established in patients with collagen-induced arthritis, in whom the intra-articular administration of TNF-α has led to an aggravation of joint inflammation. In contrast, blocking TNF-α with monoclonal antibodies either before or after the onset of arthritis led to a decrease in inflammation and joint destruction.[104] The combination of monoclonal antibodies to TNF-α and to CD4 results in a greater reduction in joint inflammation and destruction in collagen-induced arthritis than observed with either agent alone. Similar results have been obtained by the infusion of recombinant human TNF receptors, administered either before the onset or during the course of the disease.[110] Biologic therapies in the treatment of autoimmune diseases and rheumatoid arthritis have been reviewed recently.[111] The initial results of studies on the administration of monoclonal antibodies to TNF-α in rheumatoid arthritis have shown short-term benefit, but longer trials are necessary.

Stimulation of Tissue Fibrosis

Enhanced tissue fibrosis is a normal reparative mechanism in response to acute inflammation. Human autoimmune and inflammatory diseases characterized by various degrees of tissue fibrosis include chronic rheumatoid synovitis and scleroderma as well as many forms of interstitial fibrosis and glomerulonephritis.

TGF-β is the major cytokine responsible for tissue fibrosis in both normal and pathologic states. The term TGF includes a family of cytokines with related activities, although the five isoforms of TGF-β are the most important in tissue repair and fibrosis.[112] These molecules consist of dimers of varying subunit peptides that are produced primarily by macrophages and platelets. TGF-β is released from cells in an inactive form, binds to matrix molecules through a noncovalently-associated protein, and probably is activated in tissues by proteases. Because the presence in the body of TGF-β is so widespread, regulation of TGF-β activity is exerted at the levels of synthesis and secretion of the latent molecule, generation of the active peptide, and expression of receptors on responding cells.

TGF-β exerts both stimulatory and inhibitory effects on target cells. The net result may depend on the presence of other cytokines that enhance or reduce the effects of TGF-β, whether TGF-β is present locally or systemically, on the concentration of the protein, and on the degree of maturation or differentiation of the target cells. In general, TGF-β is stimulatory toward resting or immature cells and in localized environments, whereas it is inhibitory toward differentiated cells and when present systemically (Fig. 18–2).[113]

TGF-β may promote inflammation locally through inducing integrin expression on monocytes and macrophages and enhancing chemotaxis of these cells as well as of PMNs and lymphocytes. Furthermore, in the rheumatoid synovium, TGF-β may stimulate numerous macrophage functions, including the production of other cytokines (IL-1, TNF-α, FGF, IL-6), phagocytic activity, and expression of Fc receptors. However, as macrophages differentiate in tissues they down-regulate their expression of TGF-β receptors and probably become less responsive to the stimulatory effects of this cytokine. The importance of the local proinflammatory effects of TGF-β early in arthritis is evidenced by the marked reduction in acute streptococcal cell wall–induced arthritis in rats after the intra-articular injection of neutralizing monoclonal antibodies for TGF-β.[114] TGF-β also may be involved in osteoarthritis as injection into the normal murine knee induced inflammation, synovial hyperplasia, osteophyte formation, and a prolonged elevation of proteoglycan synthesis and content in articular cartilage.[115]

In contrast, the anti-inflammatory effects of TGF-β include generalized immunosuppression and stimulation of tissue fibrosis. The effects of TGF-β on T cells include the generation of helper cells with the type I phenotype, thus promoting delayed type cellular

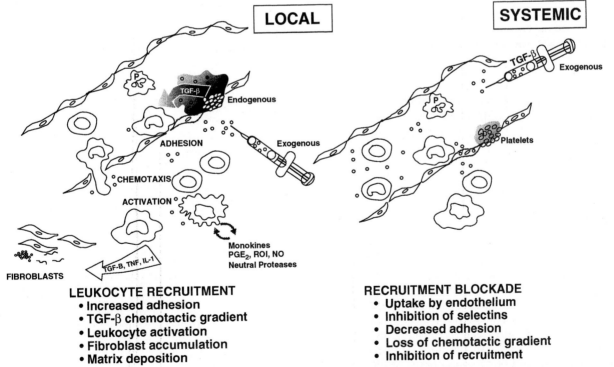

Figure 18–2. Differential regulation of inflammation by local and systemic transforming growth factor-beta (TGF-β). Summary of differential effects of TGF-β on inflammatory cell recruitment and activation after local administration and administration through the circulation. T, T lymphocyte; M, monocyte/macrophage; P, polymorphonuclear leukocyte; PGE$_2$, prostaglandin E$_2$; ROI, reactive oxygen intermediate; NO, nitric oxide; TNF, tumor necrosis factor; IL, interleukin. (From Wahl SM: Transforming growth factor beta [TGF-β] in inflammation: A cause and a cure. J Clin Immunol 12:61, 1992.)

reactions, reduction in expression of various receptors, and inhibition of proliferation of activated T cells. TGF-β enhances tissue repair through directly up-regulating fibroblast production of collagen, fibronectin, and proteoglycans. In addition, TGF-β favors fibrosis through inhibiting collagenase production by various cells while enhancing synthesis of tissue inhibitors of metalloproteinases. The possible importance of TGF-β in inducing the vascular, microvascular, and interstitial lesions in scleroderma has been reviewed.[116]

The in vivo role of TGF-β has been clarified through the recent generation of mice deficient in the production of one isoform. These TGF-β knockout mice did well for the first few weeks of life because of the residual presence of maternal TGF-β. After 2 to 3 weeks of life, however, TGF-β deficient mice developed a severe wasting syndrome characterized by the marked infiltration of various organs with immune and inflammatory cells, leading to premature death.[117–119] This cell infiltration into tissues reflects the importance of TGF-β in down-regulating endothelial cell expression of cytokine-dependent and independent adhesion molecules.[120] In addition, these TGF-β knockout mice exhibited a dysregulation of the immune system, manifested by enhanced immune responsiveness probably secondary to the absence of the antiproliferative actions of TGF-β.[121]

What are the implications for treatment of human disease of animal studies on the in vivo roles of TGF-β? Inhibition of TGF-β effects with a monoclonal antibody reduces glomerulosclerosis in animal models of nephritis.[122] This approach also is being examined in other animal models of tissue fibrosis. In addition, ongoing therapeutic trials of IFN-γ in scleroderma are based in part on the observation that this cytokine inhibits TGF-β stimulation of collagen production by fibroblasts. However, it appears that a balance normally exists in the body whereby too much or too little TGF-β may be injurious to normal cell function in various organs.[123] Interrupting this homeostasis through exogenous administration or inhibition of TGF-β may result in serious adverse consequences for protective immune and inflammatory mechanisms.

Inhibition of Repair Mechanisms

Repair mechanisms that develop simultaneously with the destructive processes in bone, cartilage, and adjacent structures of the joint may also be inhibited through the effects of cytokines and other molecules. Repair mechanisms consist of (1) impairment of immune and inflammatory cell recruitment and proliferation and (2) a decrease in synthesis of proteoglycans and collagen and of other components of the extracellular matrix.

PGE$_2$ is induced by IL-1 and TNF-α in monocyte-macrophages and synovial cells; PGE$_2$ strongly inhibits cell proliferation and collagen synthesis. However,

IL-1 can cause fibroblast proliferation if prostaglandin synthesis is inhibited, although on a molar basis it is less potent than PDGF or FGF. IL-1 alters collagen production in chondrocytes, reducing production of type II collagen and enhancing synthesis of types I and III collagen. Because type II collagen is the predominant form in articular cartilage, this effect of IL-1 may contribute to a further weakening of the joint. Cytokines and hormones that directly inhibit collagen expression by mesenchymal cells in vitro include epidermal growth factor (EGF), interferons, leukoregulin, parathyroid hormone, relaxin, and TNF-α.[2] Experimental animal models of induced arthritis have shown that IL-1 is a major inhibitor of proteoglycan synthesis,[124] consistent with in vitro experiments on human cartilage chondrocytes.[125]

REGULATION OF CYTOKINE EFFECTS

The preceding text has emphasized how cytokines may contribute to pathophysiologic events in acute and chronic inflammation. It is apparent that multiple cytokines are present in diseased tissues with often redundant, overlapping, and opposing biologic effects. Natural mechanisms exist to limit, inhibit, or regulate the effects of particular cytokines. In addition, new therapeutic approaches to autoimmune and inflammatory diseases are being evaluated that attempt to interfere with cytokine production, presence in the fluid phase, or stimulation of responding cells. These natural and contrived ways of modulating cytokine effects, including the published results of clinical trials, are summarized next. This topic is discussed in more detail in other reviews.[1, 87, 126]

Cytokine Effects at the Level of the Producing Cell

An inhibition of cytokine production may result from both the administration of specific therapeutic agents or from the effects of other cytokines (Table 18–5). Suppression of cytokine production may be one of the major anti-inflammatory effects of cortico-

Table 18–5. INHIBITION OF CYTOKINE PRODUCTION

Corticosteroids	Inhibit production of multiple cytokines
Cyclosporine	Blocks cytokine production by lymphocytes
Pentoxifylline	Inhibits TNF-α production and effects
Thalidomide	Inhibits TNF-α production
Adenosine	Blocks TNF-α production
Estrogens	Inhibit IL-6 production by osteoblasts
IL-4 and IL-10	Inhibit monocyte production of inflammatory cytokines and up-regulate production of IL-1Ra

Modified from Arend WP, Dayer J-M: Inhibition of the production and effects of interleukin-1 and tumor necrosis factor α in rheumatoid arthritis. Arthritis Rheum 38:151, 1995.
Abbreviations: TNF, tumor necrosis factor; IL, interleukin.

steroids and of the immunosuppressive drug cyclosporine. In addition, pentoxifylline, thalidomide, and analogs of adenosine may inhibit TNF-α production by macrophages. Some of these agents are currently being evaluated in clinical trials in inflammatory diseases. A specific inhibitor of a protein kinase important in LPS-induced IL-1 and TNF-α production by human monocytes in vitro has been described.[127] This unique material appears to act at the initiation of translation and represents the first observation; this suggests that regulation of cytokine production at the level of translation may be possible.

Specific inhibitors of IL-1β-converting enzyme (ICE) have been developed and are inhibitory to inflammatory events in vivo.[90] In addition, ICE is actually a family of enzymes that are also involved in Fas-mediated apoptosis and TNF-induced cytotoxicity.[128] Thus, inhibition of ICE not only may block production of active IL-1β but also may have effects on apoptosis and cytotoxicity as well. This possible approach to the treatment of human autoimmune and inflammatory diseases is under intense development.

The anti-inflammatory cytokines IL-4, IL-10, and IL-13 inhibit the production of IL-1, TNF-α, IL-6, IL-8, and GM-CSF by monocytes and macrophages, primarily by affecting transcription. The production and properties of IL-4, IL-10, and IL-13 are described earlier under proliferation and differentiation of immune cells. These cytokines are primarily products of Th2 or helper T cells and may enhance autoantibody production in addition to inhibiting monocyte responses. However, synovial macrophages may not exhibit the same changes in IL-1, TNF-α, or IL-1Ra production after stimulation by IL-4, IL-10, and IL-13 as peripheral monocytes do.[129–131]

These Th2 cytokines exhibit additional biologic properties that make them potentially interesting therapeutic agents in rheumatic diseases. IL-4 markedly suppresses production of the metalloproteinases collagenase and stromelysin by human alveolar macrophages in a manner similar to that of IFN-γ.[132] In contrast, IL-4 opposes the IFN-γ–induced production of IL-1 and TNF-α by these cells. IL-4 also inhibits the proliferation of rheumatoid synovial cells induced by IL-1β or PDGF[133] and inhibits cytokine-mediated bone resorption.[134]

The chronic tissue-destructive phase of streptococcal cell wall–induced arthritis in rats was markedly suppressed by treatment with IL-4 administered either prophylactically or during the acute arthritis.[135] The synovial tissues of the rats treated with IL-4 demonstrated increased expression of IL-1Ra mRNA. Furthermore, the deficient production of IL-1Ra, relative to that of IL-1 exhibited by rheumatoid synovial cells in vitro, is largely reversed by IL-4.[136, 137] IL-4 treatment of mice with a model of multiple sclerosis produced a marked amelioration in clinical disease accompanied by an inhibition of IL-1 and TNF-α production in the CNS.[138] However, the use of IL-4 as a therapeutic agent in human inflammatory diseases

may be limited by other in vivo effects of this cytokine.

IL-10 appears to have more potential as a therapeutic agent for human diseases. Infusion of anti–IL-10 antibodies in New Zealand black/white (NZB/NZW) F_1 mice delayed the onset of the autoimmune disease, accompanied by a decrease in the glomerulonephritis and autoantibody production.[139] Furthermore, SLE B cells produce large amounts of IL-10, and autoantibody production by SLE B cells in vitro was inhibited by antibodies to IL-10 but not IL-6.[140] These results suggest that autocrine and paracrine production of IL-10 may be an important stimulus of generalized B cell hyperactivity in patients with SLE.

IL-10 may also be an important cytokine in arthritis as synovial cells from patients with rheumatoid arthritis or osteoarthritis spontaneously produced IL-10 in vitro and neutralization of endogenous IL-10 with specific antibodies led to increased IL-1β and TNF-α production.[141] Serum and synovial fluid levels of IL-10 were increased in rheumatoid arthritis patients and correlated with serum rheumatoid factor titers.[142] This IL-10 was largely produced by non–T cells. Lastly, endogenous IL-10 may have important protective effects in immune complex–induced lung injury in rats and exogenous administration of IL-10 resulted in further anti-inflammatory effects in this model.[143, 144] A single intravenous injection of IL-10 in normal humans was well tolerated; LPS-stimulated blood cells from these individuals exhibited a marked inhibition in IL-1β and TNF-α production without any change in IL-1Ra production.[145] Further studies are necessary to evaluate the possible therapeutic efficacy of IL-10 in human diseases.

Cytokine Effects in the Fluid Phase

Natural Antibodies to Cytokines

Natural antibodies to IL-1α, IL-6, IFN, and TNF have been detected in human sera. However, few of these antibodies appear to modify the biologic activity of cytokines. Depending on their affinity, anti-cytokine antibodies can inhibit or enhance the effect of cytokines.[146] High-affinity antibodies can block binding of the cytokine to a membrane receptor and thus can inhibit the effect of that cytokine in vivo. In contrast, an antibody with low affinity might potentiate the biologic activity of a cytokine by prolonging its half-life.

Antibodies to IL-1α are commonly present in the sera of both normal subjects and patients with chronic inflammatory diseases. Only a few of the antibodies to IL-1α are specific blocking antibodies; they are mainly IgG4, which fixes complement poorly. Such autoantibodies may interfere with the determination of IL-1α by immunoassay. Anti–IL-1α antibodies have been detected in other diseases, for example, in Schnitzler's syndrome (urticaria and macroglobulinemia).[147] This study demonstrated that in the rat IgG anti–IL-1α antibodies prolonged the circulation of ^{125}I-IL-1α, probably by delaying glomerular filtration. Other studies revealed antibodies to IL-1α in the sera of 27 percent of normal subjects, 75 percent of patients with Graves' disease, and 44 percent with pernicious anemia.[148] Some studies have revealed that IgG antibodies to IL-1α can block membrane-bound IL-1α but not IL-1Ra. It is hypothesized that patients with high titers of autoantibodies to IL-1α may have less severe rheumatoid arthritis, but convincing statistical data from longitudinal studies are not yet available.

Other autoantibodies, such as specific antibodies to IL-6, were present in 10 percent of normal sera.[149] These antibodies interfere with the determination of IL-6. Again, in analogy to IL-1, anti–IL-6 antibodies belong mainly to the IgG4 subclass and can block the binding of IL-6 to its receptor.[150] It remains unclear whether in vivo these antibodies act as carriers for IL-6 or block receptor binding. However, administration of anti–IL-6 antibodies in humans has shown that IL-6 remains in the circulating pool for a longer time.

The presence of natural antibodies to IFN-γ at very low titers has been observed in normal sera[151] but at much higher titers in the sera of virus-infected patients; however, they do not appear to inhibit the antiviral activity of IFN-γ. Antibodies to IFN-α and IFN-β and neutralized antiviral activities of these interferons have also been described. The role of anti-IFN antibodies in vivo is still unclear.

Finally, antibodies to TNF-α have been detected in many pathologic conditions[152] and are of both IgM and IgG classes. Their incidence varies between 60 and 70 percent, depending on the pathologic condition, but as much as 40 percent was found in normal subjects. No convincing report exists of autoantibodies to TNF-α blocking the receptor binding of TNF-α.

Soluble Cytokine Receptors

Another potential mechanism to regulate the biology of cytokines is the presence of soluble receptors. Soluble cytokine receptors originate from (1) the proteolytic cleavage of the extramembranous part of the receptor bound to the membrane, or (2) alternative splicing of the mRNA coding for a receptor, leading to the production of a truncated receptor lacking the transmembranous and cytoplasmic regions.

The multifaceted and ambiguous biologic role of soluble receptors depends on their affinity for the ligand. Soluble receptors can have any of the following functions:

1. Biologic blocking agents, if their affinity is high and if they can be rapidly eliminated from the organism.

2. A buffer system between the inflammatory focus and the systemic pool.

3. Stabilizer or carrier of the ligand, which may potentially be released as a free molecule if the affinity is low.

4. Stimulation of target cells by binding to a homo-dimeric or heterodimeric chain capable of transducing intracellular responses.

The soluble receptors studied most are IL-1sRI, IL-1sRII, TNF-sRI (p55), TNF-sRII (p75), and IL-6Rα.

IL-1sR

Two types of single chain human IL-1 receptors belonging to the immunoglobulin gene superfamily have been cloned and possess three extracellular immunoglobulin-like domains.[98, 99] A third (accessory) chain has recently been described that markedly increases the affinity for the ligand from 2 to 0.2 nM.[153] The main structural difference between the two IL-1 receptors resides in the length of their cytoplasmic domain: type I receptor has 213 amino acids, and type II has only 29. The two receptors do not function as a heterodimeric complex, and the intracellular signal is transmitted only by the type I receptor. The type II receptor is also called a "decoy" receptor.

Consequently, IL-1 activity is counterbalanced by soluble forms of its receptors in addition to IL-1Ra. The soluble type II IL-1R (IL-1sRII) has been detected in normal human plasma,[154] synovial fluid,[155] and supernatants of several human cell lines.[156–158] Although it has not been proved conclusively that IL-1sRI occurs naturally, a circulating factor that cross-reacts with anti-sIL-RI antibodies has been found in normal human serum. The IL-1–binding characteristics of this factor differ somewhat from those of IL-1sRI, binding IL-1Ra selectively and with high affinity.[159] In contrast, IL-1β binds 10-fold more avidly to natural or recombinant human IL-1sRII compared with IL-1α or IL-1Ra.

The varying affinities of the three IL-1 ligands for cell surface and soluble IL-1 receptors make for biologic complexity. For example, the inhibitory activity of IL-1Ra is diminished by the simultaneous presence of IL-1sRI but is enhanced in the presence of IL-1sRII.[160] The simultaneous addition of IL-1Ra and IL-1sRII might be beneficial, because this combination, in contrast to IL-1Ra alone, completely abolishes the production of interstitial collagenase by human synovial cells.[160]

TNF-sR

TNF-α acts on target cells by binding to two transmembrane receptors (55 and 75 kD) with different biochemical characteristics.[107, 108] Most cell types and tissues express both TNF receptor types, which transduce different signals. TNF-R55 mediates cytotoxicity, enhances production of collagenase and other MMPs, and leads to the release of PGE$_2$ and plasminogen activator inhibitor I. TNF-R75 mediates thymocyte proliferation and cytolytic T cell proliferation. TNF-R55 possesses a "death domain," which is also found on Fas antigens, leading to enhanced apoptosis.

The two TNF receptors were identified because of the prior isolation of TNF-α–binding proteins in biologic fluids, such as urine from febrile patients and normal subjects and serum from cancer patients.[5, 161] As with TNF processing, the shedding of the extracellular domains of TNF receptors is secondary to cleavage by a metalloproteinase, as yet unidentified. Because the affinity of TNF-sR for TNF-α is similar to that of the membrane-associated receptors, its effect in vivo may be that of a modulator (buffering system) rather than an inhibitor of TNF-α. Indeed, large amounts of TNF-sR (10-fold to 100-fold that of TNF-α molar concentration) are required to overcome TNF-α activity altogether. However, biologic fluids containing very high levels of TNF-α and TNF-sR, according to immunoassays, exhibit only slight TNF activity in bioassays. Moreover, in both normal and pathologic conditions, the level of TNF-α varies between undetectable (<10 pg/ml) and several nanograms, whereas the levels of TNF-sR55 and TNF-sR75 are 10-fold higher.[162]

Elevated levels of both soluble TNF receptors are present in the circulation of patients with rheumatoid arthritis; the levels of TNF-sR55 decrease after methotrexate treatment.[163–165] The level of both TNF-sR in the circulation of arthritis patients increased transiently after surgery in a pattern suggestive of acute-phase reactants.[165] Both types of soluble TNF receptors are present in high concentrations in synovial fluid of patients with rheumatoid arthritis, particularly during the active phase of the disease.[164, 166] The levels of soluble TNF receptors are higher in synovial fluid than in the sera of rheumatoid arthritis patients, implying that they may be produced locally in the joint.

To enhance the affinity of the soluble receptor with its ligand, chimeric proteins of TNF-sR and Fc IgG domains have been generated. These fusion proteins, referred to as *immunoadhesins,* are divalent and display a higher affinity (10- to 100-fold) for TNF-α than does native TNF-sR. Immunoadhesins have been used successfully as a therapeutic agent in animal models of septic shock,[167, 168] listeriosis,[169] and collagen-induced arthritis.[170] Clinical trials with various TNF-sR preparations in patients with rheumatoid arthritis or other diseases are in progress.

Other Soluble Cytokine Receptors

Soluble receptors for many other cytokines have been described. Soluble receptors for IL-4 and IL-7 may result by synthesis from alternatively spliced mRNA, in contrast to the soluble receptors for IL-2, IL-6, TNF-α, IL-1, and IFN-γ, which result from the proteolytic cleavage of membrane-bound receptors. Markers of disease activity are the soluble IL-2 receptors, since only activated T cells release the extracellular portion of the p55 chain (α-chain) of the IL-2 receptor. This naturally occurring soluble IL-2 receptor is present only in low concentrations in the serum or urine of normal human individuals but in 10- to 100-fold higher concentrations in the serum of patients with autoimmune, inflammatory, malignant

and infectious disorders, such as human T cell lymphotropic virus type I (HTLV-1)–associated T cell leukemia, hairy cell leukemia, and non-Hodgkin's disease.[171] Because of its low affinity for IL-2, IL-2sR does not inhibit IL-2 or alter its half-life in vivo. However, this molecule is an excellent marker of T cell activation.

Receptor Antagonists

Cytokine effects also can be regulated at the level of responding cells by molecules that function as specific receptor antagonists. A naturally occurring receptor antagonist has been described only for IL-1, but structural variants of other cytokines that function as relative receptor antagonists have been derived.

By definition, a receptor antagonist binds to the specific receptor with an equal avidity as the agonist cytokine but does not stimulate target cells. At present, the only cytokine receptor antagonist that has been developed for evaluation as a therapeutic agent in human diseases is the IL-1Ra molecule, present at high levels in biologic fluids in pathologic conditions.

IL-1Ra was first described in the supernatants of monocytes cultured on adherent IgG or in the urine of patients with fever [1, 88, 126, 161, 162, 172, 173] This unique molecule is a member of the IL-1 gene family by multiple criteria. Two different isoforms of IL-1Ra have been described:

- sIL-1Ra, a 17-kD molecule that is secreted from monocytes, PMNs, and other cells
- icIL-1Ra, an 18-kD molecule that remains intracellular in keratinocytes, other epithelial cells, monocytes, and macrophages

These two forms are both transcribed from the same gene, but icIL-1Ra utilizes a different first exon with an alternate splice acceptor site in the RNA. Because the transcription of these two forms of IL-1Ra is regulated by different promoters, the characteristics of protein production are quite different. Some of the known inducers of IL-1Ra production in monocytes have been summarized in Table 18–1.

Both sIL-1Ra and icIL-1Ra bind to cell surface IL-1 receptors with equal avidity but 100- to 1000-fold excess amounts of IL-1Ra over IL-1 are necessary to effectively inhibit the stimulatory properties of IL-1 in vitro or in vivo. This requirement arises because target cells are very sensitive to IL-1 and possess excess numbers of receptors; the system must be flooded with high concentrations of IL-1Ra to prevent receptor binding of a few molecules of IL-1 per cell. Although icIL-1Ra may be released from dying cells, the biologic role of this intracellular variant remains unclear, since there appear to be no free IL-1 receptors in the cytoplasm. Administration of IL-1Ra has been evaluated extensively in in vitro systems and in animal models of disease, including models of rheumatoid arthritis, and inhibits virtually all described biologic effects of IL-1.

The presence and role of endogenous IL-1Ra in rheumatoid arthritis have recently been described.[136] This molecule is synthesized in the rheumatoid joint by macrophages in the synovial lining and subsynovial areas, although the amounts of local IL-1Ra produced appear to be deficient relative to those of IL-1.[174, 175] A possible deficiency in IL-1Ra production in rheumatoid arthritis also is supported by data from studies on IL-1β and IL-1Ra levels in serum or from production by peripheral monocytes in vitro.[176, 177] The levels of IL-1Ra in synovial fluids are higher in patients with rheumatoid arthritis than in patients with other forms of inflammatory arthritis or osteoarthritis; this IL-1Ra may be derived primarily from PMNs in these fluids.[178] Furthermore, synovial fluid IL-1Ra may be anti-inflammatory to the synovial tissue as patients with Lyme arthritis exhibited a more rapid resolution of acute knee arthritis when the synovial fluid level of IL-1Ra was much greater than that of IL-1β.[179] Therapeutic trials of systemic administration of IL-1Ra in patients with rheumatoid arthritis are still in progress. Intra-articular delivery of IL-Ra by gene transfer has been described in animals and may be a promising approach to treatment of human diseases.[180]

IL-1Ra also has been studied in other inflammatory and autoimmune diseases, including diabetes mellitus, asthma, psoriasis, graft-versus-host disease, and inflammatory bowel disease. Elevated serum IL-1Ra levels are present in patients with polymyositis/dermatomyositis, particularly in those with active myositis, with a decrease in serum IL-1Ra levels observed after treatment.[181] High serum levels of IL-1Ra are present in patients with SLE, and peripheral monocytes from SLE patients produce more sIL-1Ra in vitro after culture on adherent IgG in comparison to cells from normal individuals.[182] Alleles of the IL-1Ra gene exist as a result of a variable-length polymorphism in intron 2. An increase in allele 2 of the IL-1Ra gene has been described in association with ulcerative colitis, diabetes, psoriasis and other inflammatory dermatoses and in SLE patients with photosensitivity and discoid skin lesions.[183] This association of IL-1Ra allele 2 with extensive and severe epithelial cell diseases suggests a possible abnormality in the production of icIL-1Ra. Thus, it can be hypothesized that SLE may be characterized by excess production of sIL-1Ra but deficient production of icIL-1Ra.

Inhibition of Intracellular Responses

Another theoretical level at which cytokine effects might be blocked is after receptor binding and during activation of intracellular responses. However, potential therapeutic agents for human diseases that act at this level have not yet been clearly described. The common transcription factor NF-kB is activated in many target cells after cytokine stimulation and appears to be involved in many intracellular responses to cytokines. Inhibition of activation of NF-kB or of other signal transduction molecules is currently being explored as another possible approach to the treatment of diseases in which cytokine effects are involved in pathophysiology.

SUMMARY

We have summarized many aspects of the biology of those cytokines whose effects are exerted primarily on cells of the immune and inflammatory systems. Cytokines may play an important role in the initiation and maintenance of autoimmune and inflammatory disease as mediators of cell-cell interactions. Both agonist and antagonist effects of cytokines may be present at the same time in this disease process. The net biologic response will depend on which cytokines are present in excess. In addition, inhibitors of IL-1 and TNF-α function may be present locally, limiting the biologic effects of these potent proinflammatory cytokines.

In normal physiology, cytokines regulate the growth and differentiation of hematopoietic and mesenchymal cells in both positive and negative fashions. However, cytokines exhibit overlapping, redundant, and synergistic effects, so that multiple factors are usually involved in any particular biologic response. Cytokines exert both enhancing and inhibitory effects on immune and inflammatory cells. The cytokine network is, in large part, self-regulating through the simultaneous presence of factors with opposing properties, feedback inhibition of production, and induction of soluble cytokine receptors and specific receptor antagonists.

It is possible that in some human autoimmune or inflammatory diseases the normal cytokine balances may be disrupted. This abnormal state may occur through the unregulated production of proinflammatory factors or the inadequate exertion of anti-inflammatory cytokines or mechanisms. This chapter has emphasized the importance of natural regulatory mechanisms in the cytokine network and the development of therapeutic agents that may interrupt the effects of particular cytokines. Cytokines as therapeutic agents in human diseases are called *biologic response modifiers*. Research in this area continues to expand as new cytokines are discovered and new approaches to therapy are explored. Certainly cytokine biology has brought a new dimension to the understanding of cellular events in rheumatic diseases and holds the promise of therapeutic potential.

References

1. Arend WP: Inhibiting the effects of cytokines in human diseases. Adv Intern Med 40:365, 1995.
2. Unemori EN, Amento EP: Role of cytokines in rheumatoid arthritis. *In* Aggarwal BB, Puri RK (eds): Human Cytokines: Their Role in Disease and Therapy. Boston, Blackwell Science, 1995, pp 217–236.
3. Koch AE, Kunkel SL, Strieter RM: Cytokines in rheumatoid arthritis. J Invest Med 43:28, 1995.

4. Arend WP, Malyak M, Jenkins JK, Smith MF Jr: Interleukin-1 receptor antagonist. In Aggarwal BB, Gutterman JU (eds): Human Cytokines: Handbook for Basic and Clinical Research. Vol 2. Boston, Blackwell Science, 1996, pp 146–167.

5. Dayer J-M, Fenner H: The role of cytokines and their inhibitors in arthritis. In Emery P (ed): Baillière's Clinical Rheumatology. Vol 6. London, Baillière Tindall, 1992, pp 485–516.

6. Vey E, Zhang J-H, Dayer J-M: IFN-γ and 1,25(OH)₂D₃ induce on THP-1 cells distinct patterns of cell surface antigen expression, cytokine production, and responsiveness to contact with activated T cells. J Immunol 149:2040, 1992.

7. Lacraz S, Isler P, Vey E, Welgus HG, Dayer J-M: Direct contact between T lymphocytes and monocytes is a major pathway for induction of metalloproteinase expression. J Biol Chem 269:22027, 1994.

8. Li JM, Isler P, Dayer J-M, Burger D: Contact-dependent stimulation of monocytic cells and neutrophils by stimulated human T cell clones. Immunology 84:571, 1995.

9. Miltenburg AMM, Lacraz S, Welgus HG, Dayer J-M: Immobilized anti-CD3 antibody activates T-cell clones to induce the production of interstitial collagenase, but not tissue inhibitor of metalloproteinases, in monocytic THP-1 cells and dermal fibroblasts. J Immunol 154:2655, 1995.

10. Isler P, Vey E, Zhang J-H, Dayer J-M: Cell surface glycoproteins expressed on activated human T cells induce production of interleukin-1 beta by monocytic cells: A possible role of CD69. Eur Cytokine Netw 4:15, 1993.

11. Zhang J-H, Ferrante A, Arrigo A-P, Dayer J-M: Neutrophil stimulation and priming by direct contact with activated human T lymphocytes. J Immunol 148:177, 1992.

12. Harlan JM: Leukocyte adhesion deficiency syndrome: Insights into the molecular basis of leukocyte emigration. Clin Immunol Immunopathol 76:816, 1993.

13. Springer TA: Adhesion receptors of the immune system. Nature 346:425, 1990.

14. Bevilacqua MP: Endothelial-leukocyte adhesion molecules. Annu Rev Immunol 11:767, 1993.

15. Masinovsky B, Urdal D, Gallatin WM: IL-4 acts synergistically with IL-1β to promote lymphocyte adhesion to microvascular endothelium by induction of vascular cell adhesion molecule-1. J Immunol 145:2886, 1990.

16. Thornhill MH, Haskard DO: IL-4 regulates endothelial cell activation by IL-1, tumor necrosis factor, or IFN-γ. J Immunol 145:865, 1990.

17. Detmers PA, Powell DE, Walz A, Clark-Lewis I, Baggiolini M, Cohn ZA: Differential effects of neutrophil activating peptide-1/IL-8 and its homologues on leukocyte adhesion and phagocytosis. J Immunol 147:4211, 1991.

18. Oppenheimer-Marks N, Lipsky PE: The role of cell adhesin in the evolution of inflammatory arthritis. In Wegner CD (ed): The Handbook of Immunopharmacology: Adhesion Molecules. London, Academic Press, 1994, pp 141–161.

19. Clark-Lewis I, Sim K-S, Rajarathnam K, Gong J-H, Dewald B, Moser B, Baggiolini M, Sykes BD: Structure-activity relationships of chemokines. J Leukoc Biol 57:703, 1995.

20. Baggiolini M, Dewald B, Moser B: Interleukin-8 and related chemotactic cytokines: CXC and CC chemokines. Adv Immunol 55:97, 1994.

21. Kelner GS, Zlotnik A: Cytokine production profile of early thymocytes and the characterization of a new class of chemokine. J Leukoc Biol 57:778, 1995.

22. Klagsbrun M, d'Amore PA: Regulators of angiogenesis. Annu Rev Physiol 53:217, 1991.

23. Leung DW, Cachianes G, Kuang WJ, Goeddel DV, Ferrara N: Vascular endothelial growth factor is a secreted angiogenic mitogen. Science 246:1306, 1989.

24. Keck PJ, Hauser SD, Krivi G, et al: Vascular permeability factor, an endothelial cell mitogen related to PDGF. Science 246:1309, 1989.

25. Center DM, Cruikshank WW: Modulation of lymphocyte migration by human lymphokines: I. Identification and characterization of a lymphocyte chemoattractant factor (LCF). J Immunol 128:2562, 1982.

26. Ryan T, Cruikshank WW, Center DM: Activation of CD4 associated p56 lck by the lymphocyte chemoattractant factor: Dissociation of kinase enzymatic activity with chemotactic response. J Biol Chem 270:17081, 1995.

27. Koch AE, Robinson PG, Radosovich JA, Pope RM: Distribution of CD45RA and CD45RO T lymphocyte subsets in rheumatoid arthritis synovial tissue. J Clin Immunol 10:192, 1990.

28. Firestein GS, Zvaifler NJ: Rheumatoid arthritis: a disease of disordered immunity. In Gallin J, Goldstein I, Willis K (eds): Inflammation, 2nd ed. New York, Raven Press, 1992, pp 1–17.

29. Chomarat P, Banchereau J, Miossec P: Differential effect of interleukins 10 and 4 on the production of interleukin-6 by blood and synovium monocytes in rheumatoid arthritis. Arthritis Rheum 38:1046, 1995.

30. Young HA, Hardy KJ: Role of interferon-γ in immune cell regulation. J Leukoc Biol 58:373, 1995.

31. Darnell JE, Kerr IM, Stark GR: Jak-STAT pathways and transcriptional activation in response to IFNs and other extracellular signal proteins. Science 264:1415, 1994.

32. Hooks JJ, Moutsopoulos HM, Geis SA, et al: Immune interferon in the circulation of patients with autoimmune diseases. N Engl J Med 301:5, 1979.

33. Zvaifler NJ: Cytokine profiles in human diseases with particular attention to rheumatoid arthritis. In Lydyard PM, Brostoff J (eds): Autoimmune Disease. Oxford, Blackwell Science, 1994, pp 119–133.

34. Unemori EN, Bair M, Bauer EA, Amento EP: Stromelysin expression regulates collagenase activation in human fibroblasts. Dissociable control of two metalloproteinases by interferon-γ. J Biol Chem 266:23477, 1992.

35. Takeshita T, Asao H, Ohtani K, et al: Cloning of the gamma chain of the human IL-2 receptor. Science 257:379, 1992.

36. Firestein GS, Xu WD, Townsend K, et al: Cytokines in chronic inflammatory arthritis. I. Failure to detect T cell lymphokines (IL-2 and IL-3) and presence of macrophage colony-stimulating factor (CSF-1) and a novel mast cell growth factor in rheumatoid synovitis. J Exp Med 168:1573, 1988.

37. Howell WM, Warren CJ, Cook NJ, Cawley MI, Smith JL: Detection of IL-2 at mRNA and protein levels in synovial infiltrates from inflammatory arthropathies using biotinylated oligonucleotide probes in situ. Clin Exp Immunol 86:393, 1991.

38. Miossec P, Naviliat M, Dupuy d'Angeac A, Sany J, Banchereau J: Low levels of interleukin-4 and high levels of transforming growth factor beta in rheumatoid synovitis. Arthritis Rheum 33:1180, 1990.

39. Giri JG, Anderson DM, Kumaki S, Park LS, Grabstein KH, Cosman D: IL-15, a novel T cell growth factor that shares activities and receptor components with IL-2. J Leukoc Biol 57:763, 1995.

40. Ambrus JL, Pippin J, Joseph A, et al: Identification of cDNA for a human high-molecular-weight B cell growth factor. Proc Natl Acad Sci USA 90:6330, 1993.

41. Arai K, Lee F, Miyajima A, Miyatake S, Arai N, Yokota T: Cytokines: coordinators of immune and inflammatory responses. Annu Rev Biochem 59:783, 1990.

42. Woolley DE: Mast cells and histopathology of the rheumatoid lesion. In Balint G, et al (eds): Rheumatology: State of the Art. New York, Elsevier, 1992, pp 112–114.

43. Rasko JEJ, Gough NM: Granulocyte-macrophage colony stimulating factor. In Thomson A (ed): The Cytokine Handbook, 2nd ed. New York, Academic Press, 1994, pp 343–369.

44. Stanley ER: Colony stimulating factor-1 (macrophage colony stimulating factor). In Thomson A (ed): The Cytokine Handbook, 2nd ed. New York, Academic Press, 1994, pp 387–418.

45. Sanderson CJ: Interleukin-5. In Thomson A (ed): The Cytokine Handbook, 2nd ed. New York, Academic Press, 1994, pp 127–144.

46. Edington H, Lotze MT: Interleukin-7. In Thomson A (ed): The Cytokine Handbook, 2nd ed. New York, Academic Press, 1994, pp 169–184.

47. Renauld J-C, van Snick J: Interleukin-9. In Thomson A (ed): The Cytokine Handbook, 2nd ed. New York, Academic Press, 1994, pp 209–221.

48. Quayle AJ, Chomarat P, Miossec P, Kjeldsen-Kragh J, Førre Ø, Natvig JB: Rheumatoid inflammatory T-cell clones express mostly Th1 but also Th2 and mixed (Th0-like) cytokine patterns. Scand J Immunol 38:75, 1993.

49. Banchereau J: Converging and diverging properties of human interleukin-4 and interleukin-10. Behring Inst Mitt 96:58, 1995.

50. Trinchieri G: Interleukin-12: A cytokine produced by antigen-presenting cells with immunoregulatory functions in the generation of T-helper cells type I and cytotoxic lymphocytes. Blood 84:4008, 1994.

51. Moore KW, O'Garra A, de Waal Malefyt R, Vieira P, Mosmann TR: Interleukin 10. Annu Rev Immunol 11:165, 1993.

52. Cohen SBA, Katsikis PD, Chu C-Q, Thomssen H, Webb LMC, Maini RN, Londei M, Feldmann M: High level of interleukin-10 production by the activated T cell population within the rheumatoid synovial membrane. Arthritis Rheum 38:946, 1995.

53. Lacraz S, Nicod LP, Chicheportiche R, Welgus HG, Dayer J-M: IL-10 inhibits metalloproteinase and stimulates TIMP-1 production in human mononuclear phagocytes. J Clin Invest. 96:2304, 1995.

54. Minty A, Chalon P, Derocq JM, et al: Interleukin-13 is a new human lymphokine regulating inflammatory and immune responses. Nature 362:248, 1993.

55. Hart PH, Ahern MJ, Smith MD, Finlay-Jones JJ: Regulatory effects of IL-13 on synovial fluid macrophages and blood monocytes from patients with inflammatory arthritis. Clin Exp Immunol 99:331, 1995.

56. Beaulieu AD, McColl SR: Differential expression of two major cytokines produced by neutrophils, interleukin-8 and the interleukin-1 receptor antagonist, in neutrophils isolated from the synovial fluid and peripheral blood of patients with rheumatoid arthritis. Arthritis Rheum 37:855, 1994.

57. Malyak M, Smith MF Jr, Abel AA, Arend WP: Peripheral blood neutrophil production of interleukin-1 receptor antagonist and interleukin-1β. J Clin Immunol 14:20, 1994.

58. Yoshihara Y, Obata K, Fujimoto N, Yamashita K, Hayakawa T, Shimmei M: Increased levels of stromelysin-1 and tissue inhibitor of metalloproteinases-1 in sera from patients with rheumatoid arthritis. Arthritis Rheum 38:969, 1995.

59. Haskard DO: Cell adhesion molecules in rheumatoid arthritis. Curr Opin Rheumatol 7:229, 1995.

60. Alvaro-Garcia JM, Zvaifler NJ, Firestein GS: Cytokines in chronic inflammatory arthritis: IV. Granulocyte/macrophage colony-stimulating factor–mediated induction of class II MHC antigen on human monocytes: A possible role in rheumatoid arthritis. J Exp Med 170:865, 1989.

61. Dong Xu W, Firestein GS, Taetle R, et al: Cytokines in chronic inflammatory arthritis. II. Granulocyte-macrophage colony-stimulating factor in rheumatoid synovial effusions. J Clin Invest 83:876, 1989.

62. Alvaro-Garcia JM, Zvaifler NJ, Brown CB, et al: Cytokines in chronic inflammatory arthritis: VI. Analysis of the synovial cells involved in granulocyte-macrophage colony-stimulating factor production and gene expression in rheumatoid arthritis and its regulation by IL-1 and tumor necrosis factor-α. J Immunol 146:3365, 1991.

63. Lieschke GJ, Burgess AW: Granulocyte colony-stimulating factor and granulocyte-macrophage colony-stimulating factor. Part I. N Engl J Med 327:28, 1992.

64. Lieschke GJ, Burgess AW: Granulocyte colony-stimulating factor and granulocyte-macrophage colony-stimulating factor. Part II. N Engl J Med 327:99, 1992.

65. Lafyatis R, Remmers EF, Roberts AB, et al: Anchorage-independent growth of synoviocytes from arthritic and normal joints. Stimulation by exogenous platelet-derived growth factor and inhibition by transforming growth factor-beta and retinoids. J Clin Invest 83:1267, 1989.

66. Sano H, Engleka K, Mathern P, et al: Coexpression of phosphotyrosine-containing proteins, platelet-derived growth factor-β, and fibroblast growth factor-1 in situ in synovial tissues of patients with rheumatoid arthritis and Lewis rats with adjuvant or streptococcal cell wall arthritis. J Clin Invest 91:553, 1993.

67. Heinrich PC, Castell JV, Andus T: Interleukin-6 and the acute phase response. Biochem J 265:621, 1990.

68. Kushner I: The role of IL-6 in regulation of the acute phase response. In Revel M (ed): IL-6: Physiopathology and Clinical Potentials. New York, Raven Press, 1992, pp 163–171.

69. Akira S, Taga T, Kishimoto T: Interleukin-6 in biology and medicine. Adv Immunol 54:1, 1993.

70. Poll V, Balena R, Fattori E, et al: Interleukin-6 deficient mice are protected from bone loss caused by estrogen depletion. EMBO J 13:1189, 1994.

71. Kopf M, Baumann H, Freer G, et al: Impaired immune and acute-phase responses in interleukin-6–deficient mice. Nature 368:339, 1994.

72. Fattori E, Cappelletti M, Costa P, et al: Defective inflammatory response in interleukin 6-deficient mice. J Exp Med 180:1243, 1994.

73. Linker-Israeli M, Deans RJ, Wallace DL, et al: Elevated levels of endogenous IL-6 in systemic lupus erythematosus: A putative role in pathogenesis. J Immunol 147:117, 1991.

74. Nagafuchi H, Suzuki N, Mizushima Y, Sakane T: Constitutive expression of IL-6 receptors and their role in the excessive B cell function in patients with systemic lupus erythematosus. J Immunol 151:6525, 1993.

75. Finck BK, Chan B, Wofsy D: Interleukin 6 promotes murine lupus in NZB/NZW F1 mice. J Clin Invest 94:585, 1994.

76. Guerne P-A, Carson DA, Lotz M: IL-6 production by human articular chondrocytes: Modulation of its synthesis by cytokines, growth factors, and hormones in vitro. J Immunol 144:499, 1990.

77. Suzuki H, Takemura H, Yoshizaki K, et al: IL-6–anti-IL-6 autoantibody complexes with IL-6 activity in sera from some patients with systemic sclerosis. J Immunol 152:935, 1994.

78. de Benedetti F, Massa M, Pignatti P, et al: Serum soluble interleukin 6 (IL-6) receptor and IL-6/soluble IL-6 receptor complex in systemic juvenile rheumatoid arthritis. J Clin Invest 93:2114, 1994.

79. Paul SR, Bennett F, Calvetti JA, et al: Molecular cloning of a cDNA encoding interleukin 11, a stromal cell-derived lymphopoietic and hematopoietic cytokine. Proc Natl Acad Sci USA 87:7512, 1990.

80. Folkman J, Klagsbrun M: Angiogenic factors. Science 235:442, 1987.

81. Ziff M: Role of the endothelium in chronic inflammatory synovitis. Arthritis Rheum 34:1345, 1991.

82. Colville-Nash PR, Scott DL: Angiogenesis and rheumatoid arthritis: pathogenic and therapeutic implications. Ann Rheum Dis 51:919, 1992.

83. Koch AE, Polverini PJ, Kunkel SL, et al: Interleukin-8 as a macrophage-derived mediator of angiogenesis. Science 258:1798, 1992.

84. Koch AE, Harlow LA, Haines GK, et al: Vascular endothelial growth factor. A cytokine modulating endothelial function in rheumatoid arthritis. J Immunol 152:4149, 1994.

85. Fava RA, Olsen NJ, Spencer-Green G, et al: Vascular permeability factor/endothelial growth factor (VPF/VEGF): accumulation and expression in human synovial fluids and rheumatoid synovial tissue. J Exp Med 180:341, 1994.

86. Peacock DJ, Banquerigo ML, Brahn E: Angiogenesis inhibition suppresses collagen arthritis. J Exp Med 175:1135, 1992.

87. Arend WP, Dayer J-M: Inhibition of the production and effects of interleukin-1 and tumor necrosis factor α in rheumatoid arthritis. Arthritis Rheum 38:151, 1995.

88. Arend WP, Dayer J-M: Naturally occurring inhibitors of cytokines. In Davies ME, Dingle JT (eds): Immunopharmacology of Joints and Connective Tissue. London, Academic Press, 1994, pp 129–149.

89. Dinarello CA: The interleukin-1 family: 10 years of discovery. FASEB J 8:1314, 1994.

90. Miller BE, Krasney PA, Gauvin DM, et al: Inhibition of mature IL-1β production in murine macrophages and a murine model of inflammation by WIN 67694, an inhibitor of IL-1β converting enzyme. J Immunol 154:1331, 1995.

91. Firestein GS, Alvaro-Garcia JM, Maki R: Quantitative analysis of cytokine gene expression in rheumatoid arthritis. J Immunol 144:3347, 1990.

92. Chu CQ, Field M, Allard S, Abney E, Feldmann M, Maini RN: Detection of cytokines at the cartilage/pannus junction in patients with rheumatoid arthritis: Implications for the role of cytokines in cartilage destruction and repair. Br J Rheumatol 31:653, 1992.

93. Wood NC, Dickens E, Symons JA, Duff GW: In situ hybridization of interleukin-1 in CD14-positive cells in rheumatoid arthritis. Clin Immunol Immunopathol 62:295, 1992.

94. Yanni G, Whelan A, Feighery C, Quinlan W, Symons J, Duff G, Bresnihan B: Contrasting levels of in vitro cytokine production by rheumatoid synovial tissues demonstrating different patterns of mononuclear cell infiltration. Clin Exp Immunol 93:387, 1993.

95. Farahat MN, Yanni G, Poston R, Panayi GS: Cytokine expression in synovial membranes of patients with rheumatoid arthritis and osteoarthritis. Ann Rheum Dis 52:870, 1993.

96. Holt I, Cooper RG, Denton J, Meager A, Hopkins SJ: Cytokine interrelationships and their association with disease activity in arthritis. Br J Rheumatol 31:725, 1992.

97. Kahle P, Saal JG, Schaudt K, Zacher J, Fritz P, Pawelee G: Determination of cytokines in synovial fluids: Correlation with diagnosis and histomorphological characteristics of synovial tissue. Ann Rheum Dis 51:731, 1992.

98. Sims JE, Dower SK: Interleukin-1 receptors. Eur Cytokine Netw 5:539, 1994.

99. Sims JE, Giri JG, Dower SK: The two interleukin-1 receptors play different roles in IL-1 actions. Clin Immunol Immunopathol 72:9, 1994.

100. Brennan FM, Maini RN, Feldmann M: TNF-α—a pivotal role in rheumatoid arthritis. Br J Rheumatol 31:293, 1992.

101. Tracey KJ: Tumour necrosis factor-alpha. In Thomson A (ed): The Cytokine Handbook, 2nd ed. New York, Academic Press, 1994, pp 289–304.

102. Satoh J, Seino H, Shintani S, et al: Inhibition of type 1 diabetes in BB rats with recombinant human tumor necrosis factor-α. J Immunol 145:1395, 1990.

103. Duff GW: Molecular genetics of cytokines. In Thomson A (ed): The Cytokine Handbook, 2nd ed. London, Academic Press, 1994, pp 21–30.

104. Maini RN, Elliott MJ, Brennan FM, Feldmann M: Beneficial effects of tumour necrosis factor-alpha blockade in rheumatoid arthritis. Clin Exp Immunol 101:207, 1995.

105. Ruddle NH: Tumour necrosis factor-beta/lymphotoxin-alpha. In Thomson A (ed): The Cytokine Handbook, 2nd ed. New York, Academic Press, 1994, pp 305–318.

106. Ware CF, VanArsdale TL, Crowe PD, Browning JL: The ligands and receptors of the lymphotoxin system. In Griffiths GM, Tschopp J (eds): Pathways for Cytolysis. Berlin, Springer, 1995, pp 175–218.

107. Smith CA, Farrah T, Goodwin RG: The TNF receptor superfamily of cellular and viral proteins: activation, costimulation, and death. Cell 75:959, 1994.

108. Armitage RJ: Tumor necrosis factor receptor superfamily members and their ligands. Curr Opin Immunol 6:407, 1994.

109. Keffer J, Probert L, Cazlaris H, Georgopoulos S, Kaslaris E, Kioussis D, Kollias G: Transgenic mice expressing human tumor necrosis factor: A predictive genetic model of arthritis. EMBO J 10:4025, 1991.

110. Wooley PH, Dutcher J, Widmer MB, Gillis S: Influence of a recombinant human soluble tumor necrosis factor receptor Fc fusion protein on type II collagen-induced arthritis in mice. J Immunol 151:6602, 1993.

111. Fox DA: Biological therapies: A novel approach to the treatment of autoimmune disease. Am J Med 99:82, 1995.

112. Wahl SM: Transforming growth factor beta (TGF-β) in inflammation: A cause and a cure. J Clin Immunol 12:61, 1992.

113. Wahl SM: Transforming growth factor β: The good, the bad, and the ugly. J Exp Med 180:1587, 1994.

114. Wahl SM, Allen JB, Costa GL: Reversal of acute and chronic synovial inflammation by anti-transforming growth factor β. J Exp Med 177:225, 1993.

115. van Beuningen HM, van der Kraan PM, Arntz OJ, van den Berg WB: Transforming growth factor-β1 stimulates articular chondrocyte proteoglycan synthesis and induces osteophyte formation in the murine knee joint. Lab Invest 71:279, 1994.

116. LeRoy EC, Smith EA, Kahaleh MB, et al: A strategy for determining the pathogenesis of systemic sclerosis: Is transforming growth factor β the answer? Arthritis Rheum 32:817, 1989.

117. Shull MM, Ormsby I, Kier AB, et al: Targeted disruption of the mouse transforming growth factor-β1 gene results in multifocal inflammatory disease. Nature 359:693, 1992.
118. Kulkarni AB, Karlsson S: Transforming growth factor-β1 knockout mice: A mutation in one cytokine gene causes a dramatic inflammatory disease. Am J Pathol 143:3, 1993.
119. Boivin GP, O'Toole BA, Ormsby IE, et al: Onset and progression of pathological lesions in transforming growth factor-β1–deficient mice. Am J Pathol 146:276, 1995.
120. Cai J-P, Falanga V, Chin Y-H: Transforming growth factor-β regulates the adhesive interactions between mononuclear cells and microvascular endothelium. J Invest Dermatol 97:169, 1991.
121. Christ M, McCartney-Francis NL, Kulkarni AB, et al: Immune dysregulation in TGF-β1–deficient mice. J Immunol 153:1936, 1994.
122. Border WA, Rouslahti E: Transforming growth factor-β: The dark side of tissue repair. J Clin Invest 90:1, 1992.
123. McCartney-Francis NL, Wahl SM: Transforming growth factor β: A matter of life and death. J Leukoc Biol 55:301, 1994.
124. Van den Berg WB, Joosten LAB, Helsen M, van de Loo FAJ: Amelioration of established murine collagen-induced arthritis with anti–IL-1 treatment. Clin Exp Immunol 95:237, 1994.
125. Yaron I, Meyer FA, Dayer J-M, Bleiberg I, Yaron M: Some recombinant human cytokines stimulate glycosaminoglycan synthesis in human synovial fibroblast cultures and inhibit it in human articular cartilage cultures. Arthritis Rheum 32:173, 1989.
126. Arend WP, Dayer J-M: Cytokines and cytokine inhibitors or antagonists in rheumatoid arthritis. Arthritis Rheum 33:305, 1990.
127. Lee JC, Laydon JT, McDonnell PC, et al: A protein kinase involved in the regulation of inflammatory cytokine biosynthesis. Nature 372:739, 1994.
128. Enari M, Hug H, Nagata S: Involvement of an ICE-like protease in Fas-mediated apoptosis. Nature 375:78, 1995.
129. Hart PH, Ahern MJ, Jones CA, et al: Synovial fluid macrophages and blood monocytes differ in their responses to IL-4. J Immunol 151:3370, 1993.
130. Hart PH, Ahern MJ, Smith MD, Finlay-Jones JJ: Regulatory effects of IL-13 on synovial fluid macrophages and blood monocytes from patients with inflammatory arthritis. Clin Exp Immunol 99:331, 1995.
131. Hart PH, Ahern MJ, Smith MD, Finlay-Jones JJ: Comparison of the suppressive effects of interleukin-10 and interleukin-4 on synovial fluid macrophages and blood monocytes from patients with inflammatory arthritis. Immunology 84:536, 1995.
132. Lacraz S, Nicod L, Galve-de-Rochemonteix B, et al: Suppression of metalloproteinase biosynthesis in human alveolar macrophages by interleukin-4. J Clin Invest 90:382, 1992.
133. Dechanet J, Briolay J, Rissoan M-C, et al: IL-4 inhibits growth factor–stimulated rheumatoid synoviocyte proliferation by blocking the early phases of the cell cycle. J Immunol 151:4908, 1993.
134. Miossec P, Chomarat P, Dechanet J, et al: Interleukin-4 inhibits bone resorption through an effect on osteoclasts and proinflammatory cytokines in an ex vivo model of bone resorption in rheumatoid arthritis. Arthritis Rheum 37:1715, 1994.
135. Allen JB, Wong HL, Costa GL, et al: Suppression of monocyte function and differential regulation of IL-1 and IL-1ra by IL-4 contribute to resolution of experimental arthritis. J Immunol 151:4344, 1993.
136. Firestein GS, Boyle DL, Yu C, et al: Synovial interleukin-1 receptor antagonist and interleukin-1 balance in rheumatoid arthritis. Arthritis Rheum 37:644, 1994.
137. Chomarat P, Vannier E, Dechanet J, et al: Balance of IL-1 receptor antagonist/IL-1β in rheumatoid synovium and its regulation by IL-4 and IL-10. J Immunol 154:1432, 1995.
138. Racke MK, Bonomo A, Scott DE, et al: Cytokine-induced immune deviation as a therapy for inflammatory autoimmune disease. J Exp Med 180:1961, 1994.
139. Ishida H, Muchamuel T, Sakaguchi S, et al: Continuous administration of anti-interleukin 10 antibodies delays onset of autoimmunity in NZB/W F1 mice. J Exp Med 179:305, 1994.
140. Llorente L, Zou W, Levy Y, et al: Role of interleukin 10 in the B lymphocyte hyperactivity and autoantibody production of human systemic lupus erythematosus. J Exp Med 181:839, 1995.
141. Katsikis PD, Chu C-Q, Brennan FM, et al: Immunoregulatory role of interleukin 10 in rheumatoid arthritis. J Exp Med 179:1517, 1994.
142. Cush JJ, Splawski JB, Thomas R, et al: Elevated interleukin-10 levels in patients with rheumatoid arthritis. Arthritis Rheum 38:96, 1995.
143. Mulligan MS, Jones ML, Vaporciyan AA, et al: Protective effects of IL-4 and IL-10 against immune complex-induced lung injury. J Immunol 151:5666, 1993.
144. Shanley TP, Schmal H, Friedl HP, et al: Regulatory effects of intrinsic IL-10 in IgG immune complex-induced lung injury. J Immunol 154:3454, 1995.
145. Chernoff AE, Granowitz EV, Shapiro L, et al: A randomized, controlled trial of IL-10 in humans: Inhibition of inflammatory cytokine production and immune responses. J Immunol 154:5492, 1995.
146. Bendtzen K, Svenson M, Jønsson V, Hippe E: Autoantibodies to cytokines—friends or foes? Immunol Today 11:167, 1990.
147. Saurat J-H, Schifferli J, Steiger G, Dayer J-M, Didierjean L: Anti-interleukin-1α autoantibodies in humans: Characterization, isotype distribution, and receptor-binding inhibition—higher frequency in Schnitzler's syndrome (urticaria and macroglobulinemia). J Allergy Clin Immunol 88:244, 1991.
148. Bendtzen K, Hansen MB, Ross C, Poulsen LK, Svenson M: Cytokines and autoantibodies to cytokines. Stem Cells 13:206, 1995.
149. Hansen MB, Svenson M, Diamant M, Bendtzen K: Anti-interleukin-6 antibodies in normal human serum. Scand J Immunol 33:777, 1991.
150. Bendtzen K, Hansen MB, Diamant M, Heegard P, Svenson M: Cytokine regulation during inflammation: Modulation by autoantibodies and fever. In Bartfai T, Ottoson D (eds): Neuroimmunology of Fever. Oxford, Pergamon, 1992, pp 215–224.
151. Caruso A, Bonfanti C, Colombrita D, de Francesco M, et al: Natural antibodies to IFN-γ in man and their increase during viral infection. J Immunol 144:685, 1990.
152. Fomsgaard A, Svenson M, Bendtzen K: Autoantibodies to tumour necrosis factor α in healthy humans and patients with inflammatory diseases and gram-negative bacterial infections. Scand J Immunol 30:219, 1989.
153. Greenfeder SA, Nunes P, Kwee L, Labow M, Chizzonite RA, Ju G: Molecular cloning and characterization of a second subunit of the interleukin 1 receptor complex. J Biol Chem 270:13757, 1995.
154. Eastgate JA, Symons JA, Duff GW: Identification of an interleukin-1 beta binding protein in human plasma. FEBS Lett 260:213, 1990.
155. Symons JA, Eastgate JA, Duff GW: A soluble binding protein specific for interleukin 1β is produced by activated mononuclear cells. Cytokine 2:190, 1990.
156. Symons JA, Eastgate JA, Duff GW: Purification and characterization of a novel soluble receptor for interleukin 1. J Exp Med 174:1251, 1991.
157. Symons JA, Duff GW: A soluble form of the interleukin-1 receptor produced by a human B cell line. FEBS Lett 272:133, 1990.
158. Giri JG, Newton RC, Horuk R: Identification of soluble interleukin-1 binding protein in cell-free supernatants: Evidence for soluble interleukin-1 receptor. J Biol Chem 265:17416, 1990.
159. Svenson M, Hansen MB, Heegaard P, Abell K, Bendtzen K: Specific binding of interleukin-1 beta and IL-1 receptor antagonist (IL-1ra) to human serum: High-affinity binding of IL-1ra to soluble IL-1 receptor type I. Cytokine 5:427, 1993.
160. Burger D, Chicheportiche R, Giri JG, Dayer J-M: The inhibitory effect of human interleukin-1 receptor antagonist is enhanced by type II interleukin-1 soluble receptor and hindered by type I interleukin-1 receptor. J Clin Invest 96:38, 1995.
161. Dayer J-M, Burger D: Interleukin-1, tumor necrosis factor and their specific inhibitors. Eur Cytokine Netw 5:563, 1994.
162. Burger D, Dayer J-M: Inhibitory cytokines and cytokine inhibitors. Neurology 45(Suppl 6):S39, 1995.
163. Barrera P, Boerbooms AMT, Janssen EM, Sauerwein RW, Gallati H, Mulder J, de Boo T, Demacker PNM, van de Putte LBA, van der Meer JWM: Circulating soluble tumor necrosis factor receptors, interleukin-2 receptors, tumor necrosis factor α, and interleukin-6 levels in rheumatoid arthritis: Longitudinal evaluation during methotrexate and azathioprine therapy. Arthritis Rheum 36:1070, 1993.
164. Cope AP, Aderka D, Doherty M, Engelmann H, Gibbons D, Jones AC, Brennan FM, Maini RN, Wallach D, Feldmann M: Increased levels of soluble tumor necrosis factor receptors in the sera and synovial fluid of patients with rheumatic diseases. Arthritis Rheum 35:1160, 1992.
165. Chikanza IC, Roux-Lombard P, Dayer J-M, Panayi GS: Tumour necrosis factor soluble receptors behave as acute phase reactants following surgery in patients with rheumatoid arthritis, chronic osteomyelitis and osteoarthritis. Clin Exp Immunol 92:19, 1993.
166. Roux-Lombard P, Punzi L, Hasler F, Bas S, Todesco S, Gallati H, Guerne P-A, Dayer J-M: Soluble tumor necrosis factor receptors in human inflammatory synovial fluids. Arthritis Rheum 36:485, 1993.
167. Ashkenazi A, Marsters SA, Capon DJ, et al: Protection against endotoxic shock by a tumor necrosis factor receptor immunoadhesin. Proc Natl Acad Sci USA 88:10535, 1991.
168. Lesslauer W, Tabuchi H, Gentz R, et al: Recombinant soluble tumor necrosis factor receptor proteins protect mice from lipopolysaccharide-induced lethality. Eur J Immunol 21:2883, 1991.
169. Haak Frendscho M, Marsters SA, Mordenti J, et al: Inhibition of TNF by a TNF receptor immunoadhesin. Comparison to an anti-TNF monoclonal antibody. J Immunol 152:1347, 1994.
170. Piguet PF, Grau GE, Vesin C, Loetscher H, Gentz R, Lesslauer W: Evolution of collagen arthritis in mice is arrested by treatment with anti-tumour necrosis factor antibody or a recombinant soluble TNF receptor. Immunology 77:510, 1992.
171. Rubin LA, Nelson DL: The soluble interleukin-2 receptor: Biology, function and clinical application. Ann Intern Med 113:619, 1990.
172. Arend WP: Interleukin 1 receptor antagonist: A new member of the interleukin family. J Clin Invest 88:1445, 1991.

173. Arend WP: Interleukin-1 receptor antagonist. Adv Immunol 54:167, 1993.
174. Firestein GS, Berger AE, Tracey DE, et al: IL-1 receptor antagonist protein production and gene expression in rheumatoid arthritis and osteoarthritis synovium. J Immunol 149:1054, 1992.
175. Fujikawa Y, Shingu M, Torisu T, Masumi S: Interleukin-1 receptor antagonist production in cultured synovial cells from patients with rheumatoid arthritis and osteoarthritis. Ann Rheum Dis 54:318, 1995.
176. Chikanza IC, Roux-Lombard P, Dayer J-M, Panayi GS: Dysregulation of the in vivo production of interleukin-1 receptor antagonist in patients with rheumatoid arthritis: Pathogenetic implications. Arthritis Rheum 38:642, 1995.
177. Shingyu M, Fujikawa Y, Wada T, et al: Increased IL-1 receptor antagonist (IL-1ra) production and decreased IL-1β/IL-1ra ratio in mononuclear cells from rheumatoid arthritis patients. Br J Rheumatol 34:24, 1995.
178. Malyak M, Swaney RE, Arend WP: Levels of synovial fluid interleukin-1 receptor antagonist in rheumatoid arthritis and other arthropathies: Potential contribution from synovial fluid neutrophils. Arthritis Rheum 36:781, 1993.
179. Miller LC, Lynch EA, Isa S, et al: Balance of synovial fluid IL-1β and IL-1 receptor antagonist and recovery from Lyme arthritis. Lancet 341:146, 1993.
180. Bandara G, Mueller GM, Galea-Lauri J, et al: Intraarticular expression of biologically active interleukin-1 receptor antagonist protein by ex vivo gene transfer. Proc Natl Acad Sci USA 90:10764, 1993.
181. Gabay C, Gay-Crosier F, Roux-Lombard P, et al: Elevated serum levels of interleukin-1 receptor antagonist in polymyositis/dermatomyositis. Arthritis Rheum 37:1744, 1994.
182. Suzuki H, Takemura H, Kashiwaga H: Interleukin-1 receptor antagonist in patients with active systemic lupus erythematosus: Enhanced production by monocytes and correlation with disease activity. Arthritis Rheum 38:1055, 1995.
183. Blakemore AIF, Tarlow JK, Cork MJ, et al: Interleukin-1 receptor antagonist gene polymorphism as a disease severity factor in systemic lupus erythematosus. Arthritis Rheum 37:1380, 1994.

CHAPTER 19

John F. Penrose
K. Frank Austen

Prostaglandins, Leukotrienes, and Related Compounds

The term *eicosanoid* describes the group of bioactive lipids synthesized in cells by the oxygenation of 20-carbon polyunsaturated fatty acids, usually arachidonic acid. Every human cell studied has the potential to synthesize at least one of these compounds. Although these mediators act locally in paracrine or autocrine fashion, their synthesis and catabolism are restricted and carefully regulated. This regulation is necessary because many of the intermediates participate in normal physiologic functions at both the cellular level and tissue/organ level; an example is free arachidonic acid, which acts as a second messenger at the cellular level in potassium channel activation,[1,2] macrophage activation,[3] and cell adhesion.[4] The enzymatically derived oxygenation products provide homeostatic functions, such as regulation of sleep cycles, maintenance of gastric mucosa, vascular tone, and parturition. The major classes of bioactive lipid mediators derived from arachidonic acid include prostaglandins and thromboxanes from the enzymes of the cyclooxygenase pathways and leukotrienes and lipoxins by the actions of lipoxygenases.

BIOSYNTHESIS OF EICOSANOIDS

The generation of eicosanoids is initiated by the oxygenation of unesterified arachidonic acid (C20:4ω-6). Other polyunsaturated fatty acids may also act as substrates to provide lipid mediators, including omega-3 (ω-3) fatty acids, which are derived from fish oils. Cell membrane phospholipids typically contain arachidonic acid in the second position (sn-2) of the glycerol backbone. The initial enzymatic reaction liberating arachidonic acid from cell membrane phospholipids is catalyzed by phospholipase A_2 (PLA$_2$).[5] Specifically, PLA$_2$ hydrolyzes arachidonic acid from the preferred phospholipid substrates, 1-O-alkyl-2-acyl-sn-glycero-3-phosphoinositol and 1-O-alkyl-2-acyl-sn-glycero-3-phosphocholine. This reaction can be catalyzed with substrate fatty acids other than arachidonic acid but is less efficient. Multiple PLA$_2$ enzymes of different molecular weights have now been identified, with different physicochemical properties, such as calcium dependence and subcellular localization (Table 19–1).

Three significant mammalian classes of PLA$_2$ have been characterized.[5,6] The first two classes, referred to as *secretory PLA$_2$ enzymes*, include group I (pancreatic) PLA$_2$ and group II (nonpancreatic) PLA$_2$. Group I PLA$_2$ is a 14-kD enzyme with homology to snake venom PLA$_2$; it is found in the spleen and lung in addition to its original description in the pancreas. This enzyme is synthesized as a proenzyme and has approximately 30 percent homology to group II PLA$_2$. Group II PLA$_2$ is found in granules of mast cells and platelets as well as in inflammatory exudates (such as inflammatory synovial fluid), suggesting a role in pathophysiologic processes.[6] Inflammatory cytokines, such as interleukin (IL)-1, IL-6, and tumor necrosis factor-α (TNF-α), induce group II PLA$_2$ formation with an associated increase in prostaglandin formation; the fact that this increase can be inhibited by neutralizing antibodies and antisense oligonucleotides supports the role of group II PLA$_2$ as a pathophysiologic enzyme.[7,8] The anti-inflammatory glucocorticoid dexamethasone suppresses both induction and subsequent prostaglandin formation.[9] Group II PLA$_2$ contains many conserved amino acid sequences similar to those of group I PLA$_2$, including those in the catalytic site and calcium binding site, but group II PLA$_2$ is not found in a proenzyme form and thus must be carefully regulated to avoid cell membrane damage.

The third of the significant PLA$_2$ enzymes is the 85-kD cytosolic form. This enzyme, originally purified in monocytes and platelets, has no homology to the group I or II PLA$_2$ enzymes, is relatively specific for arachidonic acid hydrolysis from phospholipids (unlike group I and II PLA$_2$), and is activated by the concentration of calcium typically occurring in stimulus-coupled intracellular cytosolic calcium fluxes (10^{-7} to 10^{-6} M) via serine phosphorylation.[9] The full-length human complementary DNA (cDNA) for this enzyme has been isolated, and the deduced amino acid sequence reveals a motif identified as the Ca^{2+}-dependent membrane-binding domain. This motif is consistent with the observation that in stimulated cells cytosolic PLA$_2$ translocates from the cytosol to bind to the membrane compartment.[5,6,9] As with group II PLA$_2$, inflammatory cytokines also up-regulate cytosolic PLA$_2$, which is inhibited by glucocorticoids. In addition to the three well-characterized PLA$_2$ enzymes, there are also several uncharacterized PLA$_2$ enzymes with yet undefined roles.

On release of the arachidonic acid, the remain-

Table 19–1. PHYSICAL PROPERTIES OF THE MAJOR MAMMALIAN PHOSPHOLIPASE A_2 ENZYMES

Enzymes	Characteristics	Reference
Pancreatic, group I (secretory)	14 kD >1 mM Ca^{2+} required Not specific for arachidonic acid Secreted as a proenzyme Homologous to snake venom	7, 12
Nonpancreatic, group II (secretory)	14 kD >1 mM Ca^{2+} required Not specific for arachidonic acid Inducible Found in inflammatory fluids Not secreted in proenzyme form	6, 7, 9–12
Cytosolic	85.5 kD predicted from cDNA 110 kD observed by SDS-PAGE >0.1 μM Ca^{2+} required Associates with cellular membranes Specific for arachidonic acid in the sn-2 position	5, 8, 12

ing lysophospholipid, lyso–platelet-activating factor (lyso-PAF), acts as the substrate for the formation of PAF, an inflammatory mediator with bioactivity for many cell types other than platelets. Those effects that are primarily induced by PAF are transduced through the PAF receptor, which has been cloned from human leukocytes,[10] contains seven membrane-spanning domains, and transduces its signal through G proteins to activate cytosolic PLA_2. Monocytes exhibit increased chemotaxis, aggregation, superoxide generation, cytokine production, and cytotoxicity in response to PAF. After binding to the PAF receptor, PAF up-regulates the production of the inflammatory and immunoregulatory cytokines—TNF-α, IL-1, IL-2, and IL-6—in hematopoietic cells, particularly macrophages,[11–13] and up-regulates oncogenes in epidermoid carcinoma cells.[14] Granulocytes respond to PAF with minimally increased leukotriene generation. Other cells that exhibit increased bioactivity in response to PAF include B lymphocytes, natural killer (NK) cells, vascular endothelial cells, and smooth muscle cells. At the tissue level, PAF also causes airway constriction, microvascular leakage, and inflammatory cell activation; however, these effects are at least partially mediated through the release of secondary mediators, specifically cysteinyl leukotrienes.

Arachidonic acid can also be released from membrane phospholipids by the indirect action of phospholipase C to release diacylglycerol. Diacylglycerol lipase then cleaves inositol-containing phosphates,[15] thus allowing free arachidonic acid to be available for subsequent oxygenation.

After arachidonic acid is released, the cellular and tissue-specific generation of a particular eicosanoid depends on several factors:

- The presence and class of the initial cyclooxygenase or lipoxygenase

- The complement of enzymes in either the cyclooxygenase or lipoxygenase pathway
- The local cytokine environment affecting the synthesis and degradation of the metabolites
- The recruitment of circulating cells, such as mononuclear cells, neutrophils, and platelets, capable of developing a different profile of eicosanoids by means of a transcellular function in which the product of one cell is exported extracellularly for transformation by a neighboring cell
- The specific receptors and their function for a target cell

Cyclooxygenase Pathways

The products of the cyclooxygenase pathways consist of a number of biologically active lipids including prostaglandins (PG) G_2, H_2, F_2, I_2, and D_2, and thromboxane (TX) A_2 (Fig. 19–1). Prostaglandins are molecules with a 20-carbon chain in which the olefinic bonds are separated by a five-member prostane ring, whereas thromboxanes contain a six-member ring. The numeric subscript represents the number of carbon–carbon double bonds in the side chains. Because most of the prostaglandins that occur naturally have two aliphatic side chain bonds, the "2" series requires discussion. The first committed step in the biosynthesis of these compounds is catalyzed by the PGH synthase isozymes PGHS-1 and PGHS-2 and thus are a focus of therapeutic intervention. These enzymes, known also as cyclooxygenase-1 and cyclooxygenase-2, sequentially catalyze the formation of PGG_2 and PGH_2 from arachidonic acid. The prostanoids responsible for many normal homeostatic functions are formed through the action of the PGHS-1 isozyme, whereas the generation of prostanoids in inflammatory responses has been attributed to the PGHS-2 isozyme. A complex balance must be maintained between these physiologic and pathophysiologic functions, and substantial effort has been directed toward the development of drugs that specifically target the PGHS-2 isozyme, sparing PGHS-1 and its homeostatically functioning prostanoids.

PGHS-1 and PGHS-2

Although PGHS-1 and PGHS-2 both catalyze the initial reaction in the formation of the prostaglandins, they are distinct proteins, with different substrate specificities, mechanisms of regulation, tissue expression, and subcellular localizations. Moreover, they are inhibited by different anti-inflammatory agents (Table 19–2).

Each isozyme catalyzes two separate reactions. First, arachidonic acid is dioxygenated at positions C-11 and C-15 to form PGG_2, which subsequently undergoes a peroxidase reaction in which it is reduced to PGH_2. The binding constant (K_m) and maximum velocity (V_{max}) values are almost identical for the two proteins for arachidonic acid, although eico-

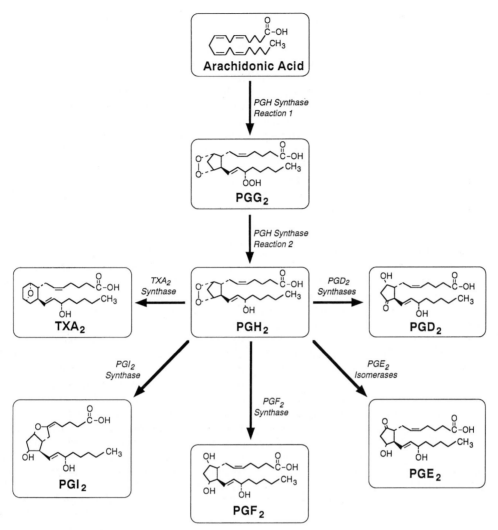

Figure 19–1. Prostaglandin biosynthesis. Arachidonic acid is the substrate for two reactions catalyzed by prostaglandin endoperoxide synthase (both the constitutive and inducible isozymes), which sequentially form prostaglandins G and H (PGG$_2$ and PGH$_2$). PGH$_2$ is the common substrate for the enzymes shown that catalyze the formation of the remainder of the prostaglandins and thromboxanes (TXA$_2$).

Table 19–2. COMPARISON OF PGHS-1 AND PGHS-2, THE ISOZYMES THAT CATALYZE THE INITIAL REACTION IN THE BIOSYNTHESIS OF THE PROSTANOIDS

Characteristic	PGHS-1	PGHS-2	Reference
Size	65.5 kD (567 amino acids)	65.5 kD	16, 17
K_m	3 μM for arachidonic acid	2.5 μM for arachidonic acid	17
Regulation	Constitutive	Inducible (phorbol ester, oncogenes, cytokines; inhibited by glucocorticoids)	19–22
Subcellular localization	Perinuclear membrane, endoplasmic reticulum	Perinuclear membrane, endoplasmic reticulum	23
Tissue localization	Platelets, endothelial cells, stomach, kidney, and most tissues	Prostate, brain, activated macrophages, fibroblasts, or synoviocytes; capable of expression in most tissues with appropriate stimulation	17
Selective inhibitors	Valeryl salicylate	6-methoxy-2-naphthyl-acetic acid (active metabolite of nabumetone), NS-398, DuP-697	17
Homology	~60 percent identical, 75 percent homologous, with conservation in heme binding sites, active site (aspirin acetylation site, serine 530), glycosylation sites, and the epidermal growth factor domain		17

sapentaenoic acid (EPA) is a better substrate for PGHS-2 than for PGHS-1. There exists 60 percent identity (and 75 percent homology) between the two isozymes, with conservation of important functional domains, including the epidermal growth factor (EGF) homology domains, heme-ligand sites, aspirin acetylation site, and glycosylation sites.[16, 17]

One important distinction between these isozymes is their genomic regulation. PGHS-1 has previously been described as constitutive in all tissues, with only a two- to fourfold range of inducibility. Recently, however, it was discovered that PGHS-1 can be transcriptionally induced several-fold in mouse mast cells primed with the cytokines c-*kit* ligand (KL) and IL-10.[18] PGHS-2, referred to as the inducible cyclooxygenase, can be induced de novo in response to multiple factors, including tumor promoters and cytokines.[19, 20]

The proposed homeostatic functions of PGHS-1 are supported by its constitutive location in many tissues, such as stomach, kidney, and smooth muscle cells. PGHS-2 is found in cells capable of inflammatory reactions (such as monocytes, synoviocytes, and fibroblasts) but can also be induced in most tissues, after stimulation by growth factors, cytokines, or hormones.

PGHS-1 is selectively inhibited by valeryl salicylate, and PGHS-2 by an experimental compound, NS-398; these reagents are useful for distinguishing the respective effects of PGHS-1 and PGHS-2. The fact that glucocorticoids completely inhibit the expression of PGHS-2, but not PGHS-1, by reducing transcription and affecting mRNA stability[21, 22] indicates that PGHS-2 belongs to a family of glucocorticoid-sensitive inflammatory response genes. Both isozymes are integral membrane proteins located at the luminal side of the endoplasmic reticulum and nuclear envelope,[23] which suggests that the prostaglandins formed may be active within the nucleus.

The formation of PGG_2 is pivotal because it acts as the common substrate for the remaining products of the pathway. The further metabolism of PGG_2 is determined by the peroxidase function of the PGHS enzyme (converting it to PGH_2) or by cell and tissue-specific isomerases that use PGH_2 as substrate to form other cyclic endoperoxides, such as TXA_2, PGI_2 (prostacyclin), PGD_2, PGE_2, PGF_2 or other prostaglandins (Table 19–3).

Prostacyclin Synthase

PGI_2 (prostacyclin) is the product formed from the action of prostacyclin synthase, a 56-kD member of the cytochrome P-450 superfamily of enzymes found predominantly in endothelial cells and vascular smooth muscle cells.[24] PGI_2 has been purified, and its cDNA has been cloned from human and bovine libraries, revealing a 1500 base-pair open reading frame encoding for a 500-amino acid polypeptide with a membrane-anchoring segment.[25] By means of its receptor-mediated activation of adenylate cyclase and subsequent increase in intracellular cyclic adenosine monophosphate (cAMP), PGI_2 causes inhibition of platelet aggregation and acts as a potent vasodilator. The generation of PGI_2 can be stimulated by thrombin, by the mechanical stretching of arterial walls, or by the 5-lipoxygenase-generated eicosanoid, LTC_4.[26] PGI_2 is an unstable molecule, and its hydroly-

Table 19–3. PHYSICAL PROPERTIES OF THE ENZYMES AND PROTEINS OF THE EICOSANOID PATHWAYS

Enzyme	K_m	pH	Protein Size (kD)	Subcellular Localization	Cofactors Required	Reference
Cyclooxygenase Enzymes						
PGD$_2$ synthase (hematopoietic)	200 μM for PGH$_2$ 300 μM for GSH	7.0	26	Cytosolic	GSH	34
PGD$_2$ synthase (brain)	8–14 μM for PGH$_2$	9.5	26	Cytosolic	GSH independent	35
PGE$_2$ Isomerase						
A	147 μM for PGH$_2$	9.6	25	Cytosolic (also membrane associated)	GSH	30, 31
B	308 μM for PGH$_2$		25			
PGF$_2$ synthase	100 μM for PGD$_2$	6.5	36	Cytosolic	NADH/NADPH	37
Prostacyclin synthase	9 μM for PGH$_2$	7.5	52	Microsomal	None	24, 25
Thromboxane synthase	12 μM for PGH$_2$	7.5	60	Microsomal	None	29
5-Lipoxygenase Enzymes and Proteins						
5-Lipoxygenase	10–20 μM for AA	7.5	80	Cytosolic	Ca^{2+} and ATP	38
LTA$_4$ hydrolase	20–30 μM for LTa$_4$	9	70	Cytosolic	None	42
LTC$_4$ synthase	5–10 μM for LTA$_4$, 3–6 mM for GSH	7.6	18	Microsomal, perinuclear membrane, endoplasmic reticulum		47, 48, 53
5-Lipoxygenase activating protein	—		18	Perinuclear membrane	None	40, 41

Abbreviations: AA, arachidonic acid; ATP, adenosine triphosphate; GSH, glutathione; LT, leukotriene; PG, prostaglandin.

sis in plasma to the inactive 6-keto-PGF$_{1\alpha}$ occurs within minutes. This characteristic, coupled with its low entry rate (0.1 ng/kg/min) into the circulatory system, makes PGI$_2$ unlikely to act as a circulating antiplatelet agent.

Thromboxane Synthase

Thromboxane synthesis involves the formation of a six-member ring, distinct from the pentane ring of prostaglandins.[27, 28] A variety of hematopoietic cells and tissues contain thromboxane synthase, a microsomal, 60-kD member of the cytochrome P-450 family, which catalyzes the formation of TXA$_2$, and a clinically insignificant additional product, 12-L-hydroxy-5,8,10-heptadecatrienoic acid (HHT). The enzyme has similar K_m values (~12 µM) for PGG$_2$ and PGH$_2$, with an optimal pH of 7.5. The cDNA and gene of this enzyme have been cloned from humans, encoding a 534-amino acid protein.[29]

TXA$_2$ is chemically unstable. Its half-life of only about 30 seconds in the plasma makes it a locally acting mediator that is then rapidly hydrolyzed (nonenzymatically) to TXB$_2$. Biologically inactive TXB$_2$ can be metabolized either by β-oxidation or by dehydrogenation, neither of which occurs in the blood or kidney. Thus, these metabolites can be measured in blood and urine and can be used as a reasonable indicator of TXA$_2$ synthesis.

PGE$_2$ Synthesis

An alternative route of metabolism of PGH$_2$ is by the opening of the cyclic endoperoxide, which forms PGE$_2$.[30] This reaction is catalyzed by microsomal enzymes and also by two glutathione (GSH)-requiring isomerases that have been identified as anionic forms of cytosolic GSH S-transferase and that have K_m values of 147 and 308 µM, respectively, and V_{max} values of 380 and 720 nmol/min/mg, respectively.[31] This reaction, as well as the formation of two other prostaglandins, PGD$_2$ and PGF$_{2\alpha}$, also occurs nonenzymatically. PGE$_2$ is the most important cyclooxygenase metabolite formed in the cells of rheumatoid synovial tissue.[32] The metabolism of PGE$_2$ occurs by means of oxidation at the C-15 position by 15-hydroxy-prostaglandin dehydrogenase and reduction of the double bond at the C-13 position by 13δ-reductase. The resultant 13,14-dihydro product has substantially less biologic activity than the parent PGE$_2$.[33]

PGD$_2$ Synthase

Prostaglandin D$_2$ is an additional isomerase product of PGH$_2$ formed by PGD$_2$ synthase. This enzymatic conversion is catalyzed by at least two isoforms of PGD$_2$ synthase—a hematopoietic form and one in the brain. The forms are clearly distinguished by amino acid composition, catalytic properties, and an-

tigenicity. A cDNA clone for the brain isozyme has been isolated from rat brain.

The GSH-dependent, cytosolic isozyme of hematopoietic origin[34] resides in spleen, mast cells, and antigen-presentation cells, such as dendritic cells, Kupffer cells, and histiocytes. This 26-kD enzyme has a K_m of 200 µM for PGH$_2$ and of 300 µM for GSH, with a pH optimum of 7.5. The brain form is a GSH-independent cytosolic member of the lipocalin family[35] with a K_m for PGH$_2$ of 6 µM at a pH optimum of 9.0. Several GSH S-transferases purified from rat tissues also catalyze the conversion of PGH$_2$ to PGD$_2$ but with lesser efficiency than the specific PGD$_2$ synthases.

PGD$_2$ is a substantial cyclooxygenase product of most tissues, including intestine, bone marrow, lung, and stomach; it is the dominant product in mast cells. The hematopoietic form of PGD$_2$ synthase is inducible in immature mouse mast cells treated with KL, as demonstrated by enzymatic function and SDS-PAGE immunoblotting of immunoreactive protein.[18]

Biologically active PGD$_2$ metabolites can be formed by dehydration to form 12δ-PGJ$_2$, or by the enzymatic action of 11-keto-reductase to produce a second prostaglandin, PGF$_{2\alpha}$.[36]

PGF$_2$ Synthase

PGF$_2$ synthesis occurs by the action of a dual function enzyme, PGF synthase, which catalyzes the reduction of PGH$_2$ to PGF$_2$ and PGD$_2$, followed by conversion to 9α, 11β-PGF$_2$ utilizing two different active sites on the same molecule. This cytosolic enzyme is a 36-kD molecule, has two isozymes that have been isolated from bovine lung and liver, is a member of the aldoreductase family, and requires NADH or NADPH as a cofactor. The 1220 bp cDNA has been cloned, which encodes for a protein of 323 amino acids, and the expressed protein has a K_m for PGD$_2$ of 100 µM at pH 6.5.[37]

Lipoxygenase Pathways

Arachidonic acid is a substrate for multiple lipoxygenases, of which at least three produce biologically active products in mammalian cells. These three lipoxygenases share 60 percent sequence similarity and catalyze the insertion of molecular oxygen into arachidonic acid at the 5-, 12-, or 15-carbon position. A histidine-rich, hydrophobic center is highly homologous in each member of the lipoxygenase family, and three of six histidines have been identified in the coordination site of iron, which is necessary for enzymatic activity. The subsequent pathways of metabolism for each of the respective lipoxygenases yield biologically active molecules (Fig. 19–2). Specifically, the leukotrienes were named as leukocyte-derived molecules containing a dihydroxylated 20-carbon backbone with three conjugated double bonds (triene). The cysteinyl leukotrienes LTC$_4$, LTD$_4$, and LTE$_4$, recognized by function before the dihydroxy leuko-

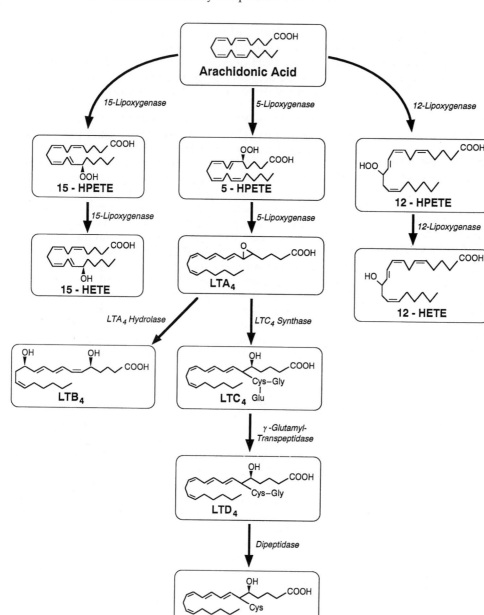

Figure 19–2. Lipoxygenase pathways of leukotriene biosynthesis. The enzymatic steps in the biosynthesis of each of the lipoxygenase pathway products are shown. Arachidonic acid is released from cell membrane phospholipids as the common precursor to 5-HPETE, 12-HPETE, and 15-HPETE. In the 5-LO pathway, LTA_4 serves as the branch point intermediate for both groups of leukotrienes.

trienes, were once called the slow-reacting substance of anaphylaxis (SRS-A). This pathway has been the focus of therapeutic targeting to inhibit both the formation of products and the receptor-mediated effects.

5-Lipoxygenase

5-Lipoxygenase (5-LO), a 78-kD soluble enzyme, catalyzes two reactions: the insertion of a single oxygen into arachidonic acid to produce 5(S)-hydroperoxy-6,8,11,14-(E,Z,Z,Z,)-eicosatetraenoic acid (5-HPETE), followed by a second function in which the dehydration of 5-HPETE forms the unstable allylic epoxide, 5S,6S-oxido-7,9,11,14(E,E,Z,Z)-eicosatetraenoic acid, known as LTA_4. The enzyme exhibits an apparent K_m of 10 to 20 μM for its substrate, arachi-

donic acid, and is facilitated by adenosine triphosphate (ATP) and Ca^{2+} in subcellular systems, although binding sequences for these factors have not been identified.[38] These reactions lead to irreversible inactivation of 5-LO. 5-HPETE may alternatively undergo an enzymatic or nonenzymatic conversion to 5-S-hydroxyeicosatetraenoic acid (5-HETE). The human cDNA and genomic sequence have been studied, revealing a 5-LO gene of fewer than 82 kb that consists of 14 exons and 13 introns. The gene contains a GC-rich promoter region but does not contain TATA or CCAAT regions. Transforming growth factor-β regulates 5-LO activity without altering its messenger RNA (mRNA) expression in granulocytes. 5-LO protein and activity have been found in human hematopoietic cells, including each of the three types of circulating granulocytes, monocytes and macrophages, and mast cells.[38] B lymphocytes (but not T lymphocytes) contain message for 5-LO as analyzed by reverse transcription polymerase chain reaction.[39]

When cells are activated, 5-LO translocates from either the nucleoplasm or the cytoplasm to the nuclear membrane,[40] where it encounters an 18-kD protein known as 5-LO activating protein (FLAP).[41] FLAP, an 18-kD perinuclear protein to which arachidonic acid is translocated for presentation to 5-LO, was purified by affinity chromatography to inhibitor analogs and bears homology only to LTC₄ synthase; together they represent a novel gene family.

The formation of LTA₄ is pivotal because it is the common precursor to the two major classes of leukotrienes: the dihydroxy leukotrienes, which include LTB₄, and the cysteinyl leukotrienes. It may also be exported for transcellular metabolism.

LTA₄ is converted to 5S,12R-(dihydroxy)-6,8,10,14-(Z,E,E,Z)-eicosatetraenoic acid (LTB₄) by LTA₄ hydrolase, a bifunctional metalloenzyme. This zinc-requiring enzyme contains two nonidentical but overlapping active sites with distinct functions—a well-characterized epoxide hydrolase activity, which converts LTA₄ into LTB₄, and a peptidase activity[42] (Fig. 19–3). LTB₄ is exported from the cell by a carrier-mediated transport system[43] to initiate extracellular biologic activity. In human polymorphonuclear leukocytes, the biologic activity of LTB₄ is attenuated before export or after reuptake by a series of oxidations of the C-20 carbon catalyzed by microsomal LTB₄ 20-hydroxylase (P-450$_{LTB}$), which sequentially converts LTB₄ to 20-hydroxy LTB₄ (20-OH LTB₄) and then to the unstable intermediate 20-aldehyde LTB₄ (20-CHO LTB₄); a 20-aldehyde dehydrogenase converts 20-aldehyde LTB₄ to 20-carboxy LTB₄ (20-COOH LTB₄).[44] LTB₄ may also be nonenzymatically hydrolyzed to inactive diastereoisomers or oxidatively degraded before excretion in the urine.[45] The biologic functions of each of the intermediates are less than the parent LTB₄, with the 20-COOH LTB₄ being totally inactive for chemotaxis and contractile responses. Cells such as monocytes, macrophages, and mesangial cells metab-

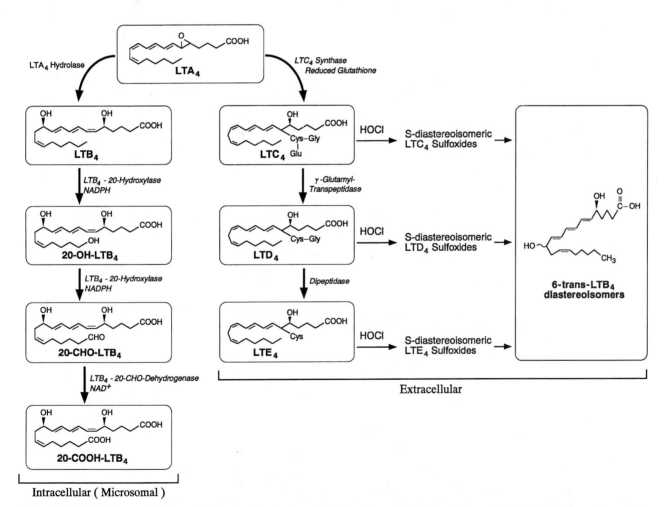

Figure 19–3. Leukotriene metabolism. The local and systemic metabolic pathways of LTB₄ and the cysteinyl leukotrienes are shown. LTB₄ metabolism occurs in the microsomal compartment of polymorphonuclear leukocytes by sequential enzymatic oxidations of the 20-carbon position, with each successive oxidation product having reduced biologic activity. The cysteinyl leukotrienes are metabolized extracellularly by both enzymatic and nonenzymatic routes.

olize LTB_4 by oxidation of the 12-carbon, and keratinocytes adduct GSH to LTB_4.[46]

Alternatively, an integral membrane enzyme, LTC_4 synthase, conjugates reduced GSH to LTA_4 to form the parent cysteinyl leukotriene, 5S-hydroxy-6R-S-glutathionyl-7,9,11,14(E,E,Z,Z)-eicosatetraenoic acid (LTC_4). LTC_4 synthase has been purified,[47] and its cDNA has been cloned,[48] revealing that its amino terminal two thirds has a sequence with 44 percent amino acid and 52 percent nucleotide homology to FLAP. LTC_4 synthase is an 18-kD protein that contains three hydrophobic regions and a domain that is highly homologous to the putative arachidonic acid–binding segment of FLAP. The K_m is 9.9 μM for LTA_4 and 1.7 mM for GSH, with a V_{max} of 4 μmol of LTC_4/mg/min[49]; however, because the calculated pI of this enzyme is 11.1, and the adduction of reduced GSH to LTA_4 occurs spontaneously at high pH, it is possible that LTC_4 synthase may act primarily to bind LTA_4 and to provide a local microenvironment for the adduction of GSH with only a mild catalytic boost. Thus, LTC_4 synthase and FLAP are members of a novel gene family, with FLAP functioning solely as an arachidonic acid–binding protein and LTC_4 synthase combining a binding function for LTA_4 with a putative enzymatic function for adducting GSH.

LTA_4 conjugation to GSH can also be catalyzed by certain cytosolic GSH S-transferases that bear no homology to LTC_4 synthase. Thus, although the function of LTC_4 synthase has been observed in endothelial cells, epithelial cells, and smooth muscle cells in vitro,[50–52] the presence of immunoreactive protein with identity to authentic hematopoietic microsomal LTC_4 synthase has been demonstrated only for certain hematopoietic cells and human lung tissue.[53]

LTC_4 metabolism to the other biologically active cysteinyl leukotrienes occurs in tissues and plasma by enzymes that cleave amino acid residues from the GSH moiety. First, γ-glutamyl transpeptidase removes glutamic acid, which forms the cysteinyl glycl derivative LTD_4.[54] LTD_4 is then converted to the final bioactive cysteinyl leukotriene, LTE_4, by dipeptidase cleavage of the glycine residue.[55] LTE_4 is excreted in the urine directly or after N-acetylation. Alternatively, cysteinyl leukotrienes are inactivated in the local extracellular environment by the interaction of released myeloperoxidase with hydrogen peroxide and chloride ion to form hypochlorous acid. The hypochlorous acid generates a chlorosulfonium ion intermediate and, subsequently, the inactive sulfoxide derivatives of each of the cysteinyl leukotrienes, which are then converted to the common biologically inactive 6-trans-LTB_4 diastereoisomers[56] (see Fig. 19–3).

12-Lipoxygenase and 15-Lipoxygenase

The 12- and 15-lipoxygenases (12- and 15-LO) continue to gain importance as the products of their reactions are recognized as biologically relevant. Multiple 12-LO species have been described, including one that overlaps structurally and functionally with 15-LO. The initial reaction product derived from arachidonic acid by the action of 12-LO is the rapidly metabolized hydroperoxyeicosatetraenoic acid, 12-HPETE. The presence of 12-LO, predominantly in platelets and other hematopoietic cells, and to a lesser degree, epithelial cells, also provides the ability to convert 5-HETE to a biologically inactive isomer of LTB_4, 5S,12S,-diHETE.[57] 12-HPETE is catalyzed to the alcohol, 12-HETE, by a peroxidase and exhibits a wide variety of functions including platelet aggregation, leukocyte chemotaxis, facilitation of macrophage adhesion, and enhancement of the metastatic potential of malignant cells.[58]

The metabolism of arachidonic acid by 15-LO occurs in a similar fashion to that by 12-LO, with 15-HPETE and, subsequently, 15-HETE being generated. 15-LO is found in a wider cellular distribution than 12-LO,[58] and 15-HETE has at least two roles that are counter to the proinflammatory processes of the leukotrienes. 15-HETE inhibits neutrophil migration, degranulation, and superoxide generation[59] through modulation of receptor-agonist cell activation.[60] 15-HETE can also serve as an alternative substrate for 5-LO, which then yields the family of lipoxins, 5S,6R,15S-trihydroxy-7,9,11,13(E,E,Z,E)-eicosatetraenoic acid (lipoxin A_4) and 5S,14R,15S-trihydroxy-6,8,10,12(E,Z,E,E)-eicosatetraenoic acid (lipoxin B_4). These unique tetraene structures, named because they are formed by the interaction of lipoxygenases, are responsible for a number of receptor-mediated biologic effects. Lipoxins act as chalones, or biologic stop signals of inflammation, in that they attenuate leukotriene-mediated functions of granulocytes, smooth muscle contraction caused by LTC_4, and LTD_4 effects in the glomerulus.[61] Lipoxin formation can also occur through the action of either 12-LO or 15-LO[62] on LTA_4 (Fig. 19–4). LTA_4, which is a pivotal common substrate for LTA_4 hydrolase or LTC_4 synthase, is exported in substantial amounts from its cell of origin.

Thus, the finding that leukotrienes and the transcellular generation of lipoxins derive from LTA_4 reveals a mechanism in which transcellular coordination of restricted enzymes may balance an inflammatory reaction by producing a specific profile of lipid mediators. The formation of lipoxins is an evolutionarily ancient process, in that the potato tuber 5-LO is capable of all of the necessary oxygenation reactions to form lipoxins from arachidonic acid in prolonged incubations with the proper conditions. In many fish species, particularly rainbow trout, lipoxins are formed in amounts four- to five-fold greater than those in mammalian cells.[63] The ability to generate lipoxins in humans has diverged evolutionarily to a two-cell system, whereas both leukotrienes and lipoxins can be generated in parallel in fish.

EICOSANOID RECEPTORS

Prostanoid Receptors

Prostanoids are not preformed. After generation, they are released by carrier-assisted diffusion to act locally on the cell of origin or on neighboring cells.

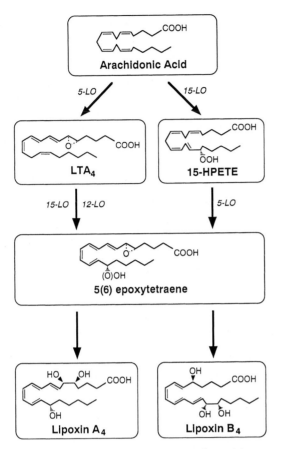

Figure 19–4. Lipoxin formation. Lipoxins are formed in mammals by the sequential action of at least two of the 5-, 12-, or 15-lipoxygenases.

mains. With the use of this information, homology screening of cDNA libraries in several species allowed the cloning of the three high-affinity EP receptors, EP1, EP2, and EP3, each defined by their rank order of affinities for PGE_2, PGE_1, and other synthetic analogs. Information from these cDNA clones defined distinctive binding specificities and distinct pathways of signal transduction.

All of the human EP receptors and most of the subtypes have been cloned. EP1 is a 42-kD, 7-transmembrane spanning protein, with a K_d of 2 nM for PGE_2.[66, 67] EP2 is a 53-kD protein with a K_d of 2.2 nM for PGE_2; PGE_2 binding was competitively inhibited by misoprostol, but not by sulprostone, consistent with the data from mouse EP2. EP2 stimulation increases intracellular cAMP but fails to transduce a rise in intracellular calcium. As determined by RNA blot analysis, EP2 is present in lungs, kidneys, pancreas, leukocytes, and immune tissues.[67, 68] EP3 has a K_d of 2.6 nM for PGE_2, a high affinity for sulprostone, and only intermediate affinity for misoprostol.[67, 69] Intracellular cAMP and Ca^{2+} both increase with binding of this receptor. The tissue distribution of EP3 is restricted to the kidney and pancreas. At least five cDNA clones from the human have been detected, with multiple variations in the EP3 receptor, which appear to be due to alternate splicing. Nomenclature is thus based on the pattern of use of secondary mediators for signal transduction, such as adenyl cyclase inhibition or enhancement, and the presence or absence of increases in intracellular calcium.[67, 70]

The FP receptor is a 40-kD 7-transmembrane domain receptor which raises intracellular calcium levels consistent with G-protein–coupled transduction. The K_d for PGF_2 is 1 nM in the expressed receptor.[67, 71]

The IP receptor is a 41-kD 7-transmembrane domain receptor that is abundantly expressed in the cardiovascular system. The K_d for iloprost is 24nM.[67]

The remaining prostanoid receptors have not been isolated in humans. They have been characterized in mice, however, and are similar to members of the rhodopsin family, each having high levels of homology in certain regions, particularly in the last of the seven transmembrane domains.[72]

Leukotriene Receptors

The leukotriene B (LTB) receptors are characterized in terms of their activation by LTB_4 and other natural and synthetic hydroxy derivatives as well as by their selective blockade by several potent and selective antagonists.[73] Although the structure of these receptors has not been fully elucidated, a 60-kD candidate protein with specific structural requirements for ligand binding has been identified. These requirements include the presence of a triene flanked by the stereospecificity of hydroxyl groups in the 5S, 12R positions. In neutrophils, LTB_4 receptors have two different affinity states, one with a K_d of 0.3 nM and the second with a K_d of 200 nM. The high-affinity receptors transduce the chemotaxis and adhesion responses, and the

Receptors for prostaglandins are termed *P receptors* based on the prostanoid to which they are most sensitive; thus, DP, EP, FP, IP, and TP receptors have been classified, with at least three subtypes of EP receptors. Receptors have been identified by pharmacologically comparing effects and potencies of various types of prostaglandins and analogs in different bioassay systems. These receptors couple (by means of G-proteins) to effectors such as adenylate cyclase and phospholipase C.

The TXA_2/PGH_2 receptor has been isolated from human platelets, and its cDNA and genomic structure have been cloned and characterized.[64, 65] This receptor is a G-protein–linked, 7-transmembrane domain rhodopsin-type receptor, encoded by a 15-kb gene containing four potential SP-1 binding promoter sites. It specifically binds the selective TXA_2 ligand 3[H]S-145 with a dissociation constant (K_d) of 0.2 nM. Other prostaglandins displaced binding, but at a level two orders of magnitude less than that of the natural ligand.

The TXA_2 receptor also shares limited homology with other receptor types, such as adrenergic and muscarinic receptors, suggesting a superfamily of receptors, all of which have signature amino acid sequences in the sixth and seventh transmembrane domains.

low-affinity receptors are responsible for secretion of granule contents and superoxide generation when stimulated with LTB$_4$.[74]

LTD$_4$ binds to high- and low-affinity receptors in microsomes of human lungs.[75] These receptors signal transduction by means of G-protein linked phospholipase C. LTE$_4$ exhibits greater potency in contracting tracheal spirals, whereas parenchymal strips contract more in response to LTD$_4$; this suggests a separate receptor for LTE$_4$ in guinea pig lungs.[76] However, LTE$_4$ and LTC$_4$ compete for binding, and LTD$_4$ antagonists attenuate the effects of LTC$_4$, which suggests that conversion of LTC$_4$ to LTD$_4$ and LTE$_4$ leads to effects through common binding sites.[77] In the case of LTC$_4$, both cytosolic and membrane-bound GSH S-transferases function as LTC$_4$ binding proteins,[78] although no specific signal transduction has been shown.

A provisional, although somewhat oversimplified classification system has been proposed in which the cysteinyl leukotriene receptors are subdivided into two categories: cys-LTR$_1$, which interact with LTD$_4$ and LTE$_4$ and which are capable of being blocked by available receptor antagonists, and cys-LTR$_2$, which interact preferentially with LTC$_4$ are narrowly distributed, and are blockade resistant. Neither cys-LTR$_1$ nor cys-LTR$_2$ represents a homogeneous population of receptors based on affinity values determined for a range of antagonists.[73]

With regard to the receptors for other lipoxygenase products, only lipoxin A$_4$ has a specific receptor. The cDNA of this inducible, high-affinity, putative serpentine receptor, related to the formyl peptide receptor, has been cloned from myeloid cells.[79]

ROLE OF LIPID MEDIATORS IN THE BIOLOGY OF INFLAMMATION

Cyclooxygenase Products

The physiologic effects of cyclooxygenase products are protean and affect every organ system. Because the control of the prostanoids is influenced by a number of physiologic conditions, two products with completely opposing effects (e.g., PGI$_2$ and TXA$_2$) may be produced by the same stimulus. Thus, the in vitro effects of lipid mediators cannot necessarily be extrapolated to in vivo situations, where various microenvironments contain a complex cytokine milieu that is likely in constant flux. For these reasons, the dominant inflammatory effects of eicosanoids and their presence in inflammatory disease states will be reviewed.

PGE$_2$ is notable for its cell biology in that as defined in vitro, it exerts both anti-inflammatory and inflammatory effects, depending on the target cell. PGE$_2$ exhibits anti-inflammatory effects on neutrophils, with reduction of superoxide generation and lysosomal enzyme release. With regard to T lymphocytes, PGE$_2$ lowers the production of IL-2 and interferon-γ, stimulates the proliferation of suppressor T lympho-

cytes, and reduces the migration of helper T lymphocytes. B cells respond to PGE$_2$ with lower immunoglobulin production and increased isotype switching.[80] Despite these immunomodulatory cellular effects, at the tissue level PGE$_2$ acts synergistically with other mediators such as bradykinin, histamine, C5a, and LTB$_4$ to increase venopermeability and sensitivity to pain, both of which contribute to the initial hyperemic phase of inflammation.[39, 81] Furthermore, PGE$_2$ is produced in rheumatoid synovium in culture,[82] where it stimulates osteoclastic activity and bone resorption[83] and inhibits monocyte-induced proliferation of human bone cells. On the basis of these in vitro culture systems, PGE$_2$ could contribute to the bony erosions and periarticular osteopenia found in inflammatory arthritides.

At the tissue level, PGI$_2$ and PGD$_2$ induce vasodilation, and this effect is counterregulated by the potent vasoconstrictor effects of PGF$_{2\alpha}$ and TXA$_2$. In addition to vasoconstriction, TXA$_2$ causes platelet activation and intravascular platelet aggregation, which enhances local inflammation by increasing the local effect of platelet-derived mediators.[28] PGD$_2$ is synthesized by antigen-presenting cells and is the major cyclooxygenase product of mast cells, inducible in committed progenitors by the cytokine KL alone or with IL-10 and IL-1.[84] PGD$_2$ exhibits a wide variety of local effects the tissue of origin, such as bronchoconstriction in the lung[85] and regulation of sleep–wake cycles in brain.[86]

Lipoxygenase Products

Neutrophils, activated by their immunoglobulin receptors or by bacterial peptides, generate LTB$_4$, which provides an amplification step for their adhesion, directed migration, and further accumulation, as well as degranulation and release of lysosomal enzymes.[87] Amplification of inflammatory processes also occurs in the presence of eosinophils, basophils, or mast cells because increased amounts of LTC$_4$ are released when these cells are subjected to immunoglobulin activation. Monocytes increase their LTB$_4$ and LTC$_4$ generation when stimulated with immunoglobulin aggregates and synthetic bacterial peptides (pretreated with cytochalasin). Monocytes are also responsive to LTB$_4$, which increases production of the inflammatory cytokine, IL-6. B lymphocytes respond to LTB$_4$ with enhanced activation, differentiation, proliferation, and immunoglobulin production.[87]

Leukotrienes stimulate cell growth in vitro. LTC$_4$ and LTD$_4$ cause epithelial and fibroblast proliferation.[88] In studies of hematopoiesis, LTB$_4$ amplifies the formation of granulocyte/macrophage colonies from human bone marrow cells, and LTC$_4$ and LTD$_4$ facilitate the activity of colony-stimulating factors.[88] Nonetheless, in mice in which the 5-LO gene was disrupted,[89] there was no recognized impairment of hematopoiesis.

With regard to the tissue effects of the leukotrienes, the cysteinyl leukotrienes were previously known as

SRS-A because of their ability to induce antihistamine-resistant contraction of nonvascular smooth muscle. The contractile effect on vascular smooth muscle has also been identified in arteries, capillaries, and venules, leading to physiologic effects such as decreased glomerular filtration secondary to renovascular constriction or glomeruloconstriction, and to negative inotropic effects on the myocardium due to coronary vasoconstriction.[88] Some of the pathophysiologic changes characteristic of bronchial asthma (smooth muscle contraction in bronchi and pulmonary parenchymal tissue, stimulation of mucus secretion, and submucosal edema) can be induced by cysteinyl leukotrienes.[88]

Because of their profound and widespread in vitro and tissue-related effects, the leukotrienes have been sought in biologic fluids in various human disease states (Table 19–4). The cysteinyl leukotrienes are present after allergen challenge in the serum, bronchial lavage fluid, and urine of patients with asthma, in the nasal secretions of those with allergic rhinitis, and in the tears of patients with conjunctivitis.[87, 88] Individuals with other pulmonary conditions, such as neonatal pulmonary hypertension and adult respiratory distress syndrome, also have LTC_4 in bronchial fluids.[87, 88] The cysteinyl leukotrienes and LTB_4 have been found in the sputum of patients with chronic obstructive pulmonary disease and cystic fibrosis.[90]

In other disease states, the rectal fluid of patients with inflammatory bowel disease contains LTB_4.[88] The skin lesions of patients with psoriasis exhibit increased LTB_4, LTC_4, and LTD_4 synthesis, and such patients have increased levels of urinary LTE_4.[88] Patients with gout, rheumatoid arthritis, and spondyloarthropathy have higher levels of arachidonic acid metabolites, particularly LTB_4, in their synovial fluid than do patients with osteoarthritis.[88] The synovial fluid in patients with rheumatoid arthritis also contains significantly higher levels of LTD_4 and LTE_4, with enhanced ability to metabolize LTC_4 to LTD_4.[82] Synovial fluid leukocytes, immune complexes, and rheumatoid factor have been correlated with LTB_4 levels in patients with rheumatoid arthritis.[91] Neutrophils in synovial fluid and peripheral blood of patients with rheumatoid arthritis generate greater amounts of LTB_4 than the same cells from unaffected individuals.[80] In patients with juvenile chronic arthritis, there is marked cysteinyl leukotriene generation, with a positive correlation between LTE_4 excretion and the number of affected joints.[92] In patients with rheumatoid arthritis, the peripheral blood mononuclear cells and the monocyte/macrophages in the synovium contribute more to the synthesis of 5-LO products and hyperalgesic 15-LO products than do the neutrophils.[93] Measurements of lipoxygenase and cyclooxygenase products generated in vitro from bone, cartilage, and synovium of patients with arthritis reveal that synovium is the predominant source of prostaglandins and leukotrienes.[82]

Lipoxins A_4 and B_4 exert significant effects on the

Table 19–4. EVIDENCE LINKING 5-LIPOXYGENASE PATHWAY PRODUCTS TO INFLAMMATORY DISEASES

Disease	5-Lipoxygenase Products Involved	Supporting Therapeutic Intervention	Reference
Asthma	LTD_4, LTE_4, and 20-OH LTB_4 in the serum or urine of patients with asthma and bronchial hyperreactivity	Zileuton, a 5-lipoxygenase inhibitor; MK-886, a FLAP inhibitor; ICI 204, 219, and MK-571, LTD_4 receptor antagonists that relieve various forms of asthma	87,* 88,* 107, 108
Adult respiratory distress syndrome	LTC_4 in bronchial fluids	—	87, 88
Neonatal pulmonary hypertension	LTC_4 in bronchial fluids	—	87, 88
Cystic fibrosis	LTB_4 and cysteinyl leukotrienes in bronchial fluids	—	90
Chronic obstructive pulmonary disease	LTB_4 and cysteinyl leukotrienes in bronchial fluids	—	90
Allergic rhinitis	LTC_4 and LTB_4 in nasal fluid	Zileuton reduces leukotriene formation and decreases symptoms	87, 88, 107
Psoriasis	LTB_4, LTC_4, and LTD_4 in skin lesion fluid	Methotrexate reduces 5-lipoxygenase products and reduces symptoms	88
Inflammatory bowel disease	LTB_4 in rectal secretions	Zileuton reduces symptoms	109
Rheumatoid arthritis	LTB_4, LTD_4, and LTE_4 in joint fluid	Methotrexate reduces LTB_4 formation and improves disease signs and symptoms; zileuton demonstrates a trend toward reduced symptoms	82, 92, 101, 102, 110
Juvenile rheumatoid arthritis	LTE_4 in urine	—	92
Gout	LTB_4 in joint fluid	—	88
Spondyloarthropathy	LTB_4 in joint fluid	Methotrexate reduces LTB_4 formation and reduces symptoms	88
Systemic lupus nephritis	LTE_4 in urine	—	88

*Reviews that record the primary sources.
Abbreviations: FLAP, 5-lipoxygenase activating protein; LT, leukotriene.

immunoregulation process of myeloid cells. They both inhibit LTB_4 binding to T lymphocytes, and lipoxin A_4 also inhibits LTB_4-induced chemotaxis of neutrophils and the subsequent inflammatory effects on venopermeability.[61] The chemotactic inhibition is accompanied by inhibition of leukocyte-endothelial adherence and transmigration.[60] Lipoxin A_4 affects the end-organ responsiveness to leukotrienes and prostaglandins by depression of LTC_4-induced smooth muscle contraction.[61]

THERAPEUTIC INTERVENTION FOR THE AMELIORATION OF EICOSANOID EFFECTS IN INFLAMMATORY DISEASES

Although the major thrust of prostaglandin research in rheumatic diseases has been toward delineating their pathophysiologic effects, a notable exception has been the pharmacologic studies with PGE_1 and some of its analogs. Given by intravenous infusion in uncontrolled studies, PGE_1 transiently improved renal function in patients with systemic lupus erythematosus and lupus nephritis, reduced circulating immune complexes in a variety of autoimmune diseases, and improved the healing of digital ulcers in patients with systemic sclerosis.

Therapeutically, intervention may be directed at different levels of the eicosanoid pathways. In the cyclooxygenase pathway, the inhibition of PGHS-1 and PGHS-2 by aspirin and other nonsteroidal anti-inflammatory drugs (NSAIDs) reduces prostaglandin synthesis.[94] Aspirin irreversibly acetylates both PGHS isozymes in their respective active sites, at serine 530 for PGHS-1 and serine 516 for PGHS-2.[94] When these amino acids are substituted, the resultant mutated proteins do not allow the formation of the normal product, PGH_2.

Because the treatment of disease with NSAIDs is often limited by adverse gastrointestinal and renal effects, selective inhibition of the inducible isozyme PGHS-2 has been sought as a way to reduce the formation of inflammatory mediators while preserving the homeostatic function of constitutively produced prostanoids. Currently available NSAIDs inhibit both PGHS isozymes, with a rank order of preference for PGHS-1 over PGHS-2.[95] The only commercially available NSAID tested that is selective for PGHS-2 is 6-methoxy-2-naphthylacetic acid, the active metabolite of nabumetone.[96] Experimental compounds such as CGP-28238,[97] DuP-697, and NS-398[98] selectively inhibit PGHS-2 in vitro. DuP-697 and NS-398 inhibit both isozymes initially, but their potencies increase with time for PGHS-2 selectively.[97, 98] NS-398 has also been demonstrated in a rat model of inflammation to be anti-inflammatory without being ulcerogenic.[99] Corticosteroids also inhibit prostaglandin synthesis (including that of rheumatoid synovium), through a variety of mechanisms, such as the decrease in cytokine-mediated PLA_2 induction and a decrease in cytokine-induced PGHS-2 generation.

An experimental model of antiphospholipid syndrome with fetal loss as the outcome is reduced by the administration of an experimental thromboxane receptor antagonist, BMS 180,291. However, prostanoids are not the sole mediators in immunologically mediated vascular disorders, as defined in a recent clinical study that showed that aspirin alone did not protect against thrombotic episodes in the antiphospholipid syndrome in general and in patients with systemic lupus erythematosus in particular.[100]

Other modalities used in the treatment of rheumatic diseases affect prostanoid generation as assessed in vitro. Oral gold therapy inhibits 5-LO by a reduction in enzymatic products and in neutrophil chemotaxis.[101] Methotrexate reduces the generation of LTB_4 by leukocytes activated in vitro without altering formation of PAF.[102]

The preferential ω-6 substrates of the cyclooxygenase and lipoxygenase pathways can be competitively inhibited by ω-3 fatty acids, and some of the eicosanoid products are attenuated in function.[103, 104] After studies in normal volunteers, a fish oil (ω-3 fatty acids)–enriched diet was given to patients with rheumatoid arthritis; the clinical benefits were statistically significant.[105] In patients with rheumatoid arthritis, eicosapentaenoic acid (EPA) resulted in a decreased ratio of arachidonic acid to EPA in neutrophil cellular lipids, a 33 percent decline in LTB_4 production by ionophore-activated neutrophils, decreased generation of PAF by monocytes, and impaired neutrophil chemotaxis to LTB_4 and bacterial peptides.[104] These anti-inflammatory effects of EPA on the 5-LO pathway are mediated through at least three processes: decrease in LTB_4 production by inactivation of LTA_4 hydrolase by LTA_5, formation of lipid products with attenuated biologic activity (TXA_3 and LTB_5), and inhibition of phosphoinositide-specific phospholipase C by incorporated EPA.[104]

Decreased production of PGE_1 and PGE_2, with increased production of PGE_3 and $PGE_{2\alpha}$, in menhaden oil–fed men is an example of PGHS inhibition. This anti-inflammatory effect on the prostanoid pathway is augmented by production of an attenuated platelet product, TXA_3.

In therapeutic intervention directed at the 5-LO pathway, pharmacologic inhibition of 5-LO, of FLAP, and of the receptor-mediated effects of LTB_4, LTD_4, and LTE_4 have been used in clinical studies (see Table 19–4). Certain 5-LO inhibitors (MK886, L-656,224, PF-5901, and tepoxalin) inhibited the production of the inflammatory cytokine IL-1 in synovial explants of patients with arthritis.[106]

The most extensive clinical data demonstrating a beneficial effect of 5-LO inhibition have been in patients with asthma and allergic diseases.[107] In aspirin-induced asthma, inhibition of the cyclooxygenase pathway is associated with activation of the 5-LO pathway and increased urinary excretion of LTE_4.[108] Zileuton, a specific 5-LO inhibitor, prevented the aspirin-induced reduction in forced expiratory volume in 1 second (FEV_1) and reduced the urinary excretion of

LTE$_4$.[107] In patients with asthma, LTD$_4$ antagonists ICI 204,219 and MK-571 and the FLAP inhibitor MK-886 partially blocked both the early and late phases of allergen- and exercise-induced airway responses.[107]

Zileuton modestly decreased the symptoms of patients with inflammatory bowel disease.[109] An oral selective LTB$_4$ receptor antagonist, SC41930, is currently in clinical trials for psoriasis and ulcerative colitis. In a 4-week, placebo-controlled trial of zileuton in patients with rheumatoid arthritis in whom NSAID therapy was withheld, the trend toward fewer painful and swollen joints and better scores on the joint swelling index did not reach statistical significance. The amount of LTB$_4$ synthesis in whole blood was reduced by 70 percent, and thus it would be prudent to consider ablation of both arms of eicosanoid synthesis in seeking to recognize the benefit of 5-LO inhibition.[110]

References

1. Kim D, Clapham DE: Potassium channels in cardiac cells activated by arachidonic acid and phospholipids. Science 244:1174, 1989.
2. Ordway RW, Walsh JV, Singer JJ: Arachidonic acid and other fatty acids directly activate potassium channels in smooth muscle cells. Science 244:1176, 1989.
3. Randriamampita C, Trautmann J: Arachidonic acid activates Ca^{2+} extrusion in macrophages. J Biol Chem 266:18059, 1990.
4. Lefkowith JB: Essential fatty acid deficiency impairs macrophage spreading and adherence: Role of arachidonate in cell adhesion. J Biol Chem 266:1071, 1991.
5. Dennis EA: Diversity of group types, regulation, and function of phospholipase A$_2$. J Biol Chem 269:13057, 1994.
6. Smith WL: Prostanoid biosynthesis and mechanisms of action. Am J Physiol 263:F181, 1992.
7. Murakami M, Austen KF: Cytokine regulation of eisosanoid synthesis. Ann NY Acad Sci 744:84, 1994.
8. Nakano T, Ohara O, Teraoka H, et al: Glucocorticoids suppress group II phospholipase A$_2$ production by blocking mRNA synthesis and post-transcriptional expression. J Biol Chem 265:12745, 1990.
9. Sharp JD, White DL, Chiou XG, et al: Molecular cloning and expression of human Ca^{2+}-sensitive cytosolic phospholipase A$_2$. J Biol Chem 266:14850, 1991.
10. Nakamura M, Honda Z, Izumi T, et al: Molecular cloning and expression of platelet-activating factor receptor from human leukocytes. J Biol Chem 266:20400, 1991.
11. Dubois C, Bissonette E, Rola-Pleszczynski M: Platelet-activating factor (PAF) stimulates tumor necrosis factor production by alveolar macrophages: Prevention by PAF receptor antagonists and lipoxygenase inhibitors. J Immunol 143:964, 1989.
12. Pignol B, Henane S, Sorlin B, et al: Effect of long-term treatment with platelet-activating factor on IL-1 and IL-2 production by rat spleen cells. J Immunol 145:980, 1990.
13. Thivierge M, Rola-Pleszczynski M: Platelet-activating factor (PAF) enhances interleukin-6 production by alveolar macrophages. J Allergy Clin Immunol 90:796, 1992.
14. Pripathi YB, Kandala JC, Guntaka R, et al: Platelet activating factor induces expression of early response genes c-fos and TIS-1 in human epidermoid carcinoma A-431 cells. Life Sci 49:176, 1991.
15. Bell RL, Kennerly DA, Dianford N, et al: Diglyceride lipase: a pathway for arachidonate release from human platelets. Proc Natl Acad Sci USA 76:3238, 1979.
16. DeWitt DL, El-Harith EA, Kraemer SA, et al: The aspirin and heme-binding site for the ovine and murine prostaglandin endoperoxide synthases. J Biol Chem 265:5192, 1990.
17. Smith WL, Meade EA, DeWitt DL: Interactions of PGH synthase isozymes-1 and -2 with NSAIDs. Ann NY Acad Sci 744:50, 1994.
18. Murakami M, Matsumoto R, Urade Y, et al: c-Kit ligand mediates increased expression of cytosolic phospholipase A$_2$, prostaglandin endoperoxide synthase-1, and hematopoietic prostaglandin D$_2$ synthase and increased IgE-dependent prostaglandin D$_2$ generation in immature mouse mast cells. J Biol Chem 270:3239, 1994.
19. Kujubu DA, Fletcher BA, Varnum BC, et al: TIS10, a phorbol ester tumor promotor inducible mRNA from Swiss 3T3 cells, encodes a novel prostaglandin synthase/cyclooxygenase homologue. J Biol Chem 266:12866, 1991.
20. Jones DA, Carlton DP, McIntyre TM, et al: Molecular cloning of human prostaglandin endoperoxide synthase type II and demonstration of expression in response to cytokines. J Biol Chem 268:9049, 1993.
21. Dewitt DL, Meade EA: Serum and glucocorticoid regulation of gene transcription and expression of the prostaglandin H synthase-1 and prostaglandin H synthase-2 isozymes. Arch Biochem Biophys 306:94, 1993.
22. Evett GE, Xie W, Chipman JG, et al: Prostaglandin G/H isoenzyme 2 expression in fibroblasts: Regulation by dexamethasone, mitogens, and oncogenes. Arch Biochem Biophys 306:169, 1993.
23. Regier MK, DeWitt DL, Schindler MS, et al: Subcellular localization of prostaglandin endoperoxide synthase-2 in murine 3T3 cells. Arch Biochem Biophys 301:439, 1993.
24. Baenziger NL, Becherer PR, Majerus PJ: Characterization of prostacyclin synthesis in cultured human smooth muscle cells, venous endothelial cells and skin fibroblasts. Cell 16:967, 1979.
25. Miyata A, Hara S, Yokoyama C, et al: Molecular cloning and expression of human prostacyclin synthase. Biochem Biophys Res Commun 200:1728, 1994.
26. Pologe LG, Cramer EB, Pawlowski NA, et al: Stimulation of human endothelial cell prostacyclin synthesis by select leukotrienes. J Exp Med 160:1043, 1984.
27. Samuelsson B, Goldyne M, Granstrom E: Prostaglandins and thromboxanes. Annu Rev Biochem 47:997, 1978.
28. Hamberg M, Svensson J, Samuelsson B: Thromboxanes: A new group of biologically active compounds derived from prostaglandin endoperoxides. Proc Natl Acad Sci USA 72:2994, 1979.
29. Ohashi K, Ruan KH, Kulmacz RJ, et al: Primary structure of human thromboxane synthase determined from the cDNA sequence. J Biol Chem 267:789, 1992.
30. Ogino N, Miyamoto T, Yamamoto S, et al: Prostaglandin endoperoxide E isomerase from bovine vesicular gland microsomes, a glutathione-requiring enzyme. J Biol Chem 252:890, 1977.
31. Ogorichi T, Ujihara M, Narumiya S: Purification and properties of prostaglandin H-E isomerase from the cytosol of human brain: Identification as anionic forms of glutathione s-transferases. J Neurochem 48:900, 1987.
32. Oates JA, Fitzgerald G, Ranch RA, et al: Clinical implications of prostaglandin and thromboxane A$_2$ formation. N Engl J Med 219:761, 1988.
33. Ferreira SH, Vane JR: Prostaglandins: Their disappearance from and release into the circulation. Nature (London) 219:868, 1967.
34. Urade Y, Fujomoto N, Ujihara M, et al: Biochemical and immunological characterization of rat spleen prostaglandin D synthetase. J Biol Chem 262:3820, 1987.
35. Shimizu T, Yamamoto S, Hayaishi O: Purification and properties of prostaglandin D synthetase from rat brain. J Biol Chem 254:522, 1979.
36. Liston TE, Roberts LJ II: Metabolic fate of radiolabeled prostaglandin D$_2$ in a normal human male volunteer. J Biol Chem 260:13172, 1985.
37. Kuchinke W, Barski O, Watanabe K: A lung type prostaglandin F synthase is expressed in bovine liver: cDNA sequence and expression in E. coli. Biochem Biophys Res Commun 183:1238, 1992.
38. Ford-Hutchinson AW, Gresser M, Young RN: 5-Lipoxygenase. Annu Rev Biochem 63:383, 1994.
39. Jakobsson PH, Steinhilber D, Odlander B, et al: On expression and regulation of 5-lipoxygenase in human lymphocytes. Proc Natl Acad Sci USA 89:23521, 1992.
40. Woods JW, Evans JF, Ethier D, et al: 5-Lipoxygenase and 5-lipoxygenase activating protein are localized in the nuclear envelope of activated human leukocytes. J Exp Med 178:1935, 1993.
41. Dixon RF, Diehl RE, Opas E, et al: Requirement of a 5-lipoxygenase activating protein for leukotriene synthesis. Nature 343:282, 1990.
42. Haeggstrom JZ, Wetterholm A, Medina J, et al: Novel structural and functional properties of leukotriene A4 hydrolase: Implications for the development of enzyme inhibitors. Adv Prostaglandin Thromboxane Leukot Res 22:3, 1994.
43. Lam BK, Gagnon L, Austen KF, et al: The mechanism of leukotriene B$_4$ export from human polymorphonuclear leukocytes. J Biol Chem 265:13438, 1990.
44. Sutyak J, Austen KF, Soberman RJ: Identification of an aldehyde dehydrogenase in the microsomes of human polymorphonuclear leukocytes that metabolizes 20-aldehyde leukotriene B$_4$. J Biol Chem 264:14818, 1989.
45. Serafin WE, Oates JA, Jubbard WC: Metabolism of leukotriene B$_4$ in the monkey: Identification of the principal nonvolatile metabolite in the urine. Prostaglandins 27:899, 1984.
46. Wheelan P, Travers JB, Morelli JG, et al: Metabolism of leukotriene B$_4$ (LTB$_4$) and 12-hydroxy-5,8,10,14-eicosatetraenoic acid (12-HETE) in human keratinocytes. Ann NY Acad Sci 744:39, 1994.
47. Penrose JF, Gagnon L, Goppelt-Struebbe M, et al: Purification of human leukotriene C$_4$ synthase. Proc Natl Acad Sci USA 89:11603, 1992.
48. Lam BK, Penrose JF, Freeman G, et al: Expression cloning of a cDNA for human leukotriene C$_4$ synthase, an integral membrane protein conjugating reduced glutathione to leukotriene A$_4$. Proc Natl Acad Sci USA 91:7663, 1994.

49. Nicholson DW, Ali A, Vaillancourt JP, et al: Purification to homogeneity and the N-terminal sequence of human leukotriene C₄ synthase: A homodimeric glutathione S-transferase composed of 18-kDa subunits. Proc Natl Acad Sci USA 90:2015, 1993.

50. Feinmark SJ: The role of the endothelial cell in leukotriene biosynthesis. Am Rev Respir Dis 146 (5, Part 2):s51, 1992.

51. Eling TE, Danilowicz RM, Kenke DC, et al: Arachidonic acid metabolism by canine tracheal epithelial cells. J Biol Chem 261:12841, 1985.

52. Feinmark SJ, Cannon J: Vascular smooth muscle cell leukotriene C₄ synthesis: Requirement for transcellular leukotriene A₄ metabolism. Biochim Biophys Acta 922:125, 1987.

53. Penrose JF, Spector J, Lam BK, et al: Purification of human lung leukotriene C₄ synthase and preparation of a polyclonal antibody. Am J Respir Crit Care Med 152:283, 1995.

54. Tate SS, Meister A: Gamma-glutamyl transpeptidase: catalytic, structural and functional aspects. Mol Cell Biochem 39:357, 1981.

55. Lee CW, Lewis RA, Corey EJ, et al: Conversion of leukotriene D₄ to leukotriene E₄ by a dipeptidase released from the specific granules of human polymorphonuclear leukocytes. Immunology 48:27, 1983.

56. Lee CW, Lewis RA, Corey EJ, et al: The myeloperoxidase-dependent metabolism of leukotrienes C₄, D₄, and E₄ to 6-trans-leukotriene B₄ diastereoisomers and the subclass-specific S-diastereoisomeric sulfoxides. J Biol Chem 258:15004, 1983.

57. Lindgren JA, Hansson G, Samuelsson B: Formation of novel hydroxylated eicosatetraenoic acids in preparations of human polymorphonuclear leukocytes. FEBS Lett 128:329, 1981.

58. Tang DG, Honn KV: 12-Lipoxygenase, 12(S)-HETE, and cancer metastasis. Ann NY Acad Sci 744:199, 1994.

59. Takata S, Matsubara M, Allen PG, et al: Remodeling of neutrophil phospholipids with 15(S)-hydroxyeicosatetraenoic acid inhibits leukotriene B₄–induced neutrophil migration across endothelium. J Clin Invest 93:499, 1994.

60. Smith RJ, Justen JM, Nidy EG, et al: Transmembrane signaling in human polymorphonuclear neutrophils: 15(S) hydroxy-(5Z,8Z,11Z,13E)-eicosatetraenoic acid modulates receptor agonist–triggered cell activation. Proc Natl Acad Sci USA 90:7270, 1993.

61. Serhan CN: Lipoxin biosynthesis and its impact in inflammatory and vascular events. Biochim Biophys Acta 1212:1, 1994.

62. Serhan CN, Sheppard KA: Lipoxin formation during human neutrophil-platelet interactions. Evidence for the transformation of leukotriene A₄ by platelet 12-lipoxygenase in vitro. J Clin Invest 85:772, 1990.

63. Pettitt TR, Rowley AF, Secombes CJ: Lipoxins are major lipoxygenase products of rainbow trout. FEBS Lett 259:168, 1989.

64. Hirata M, Hayashi Y, Ushikubi F, et al: Cloning and expression of cDNA for a human thromboxane A₂ receptor. Nature 349:617, 1991.

65. Nusing RM, Hirata M, Kakizuka A, et al: Characterization and chromosomal mapping of the human thromboxane A₂ receptor gene. J Biol Chem 268:25253, 1993.

66. Funk CD, Furci L, Fitzgerald GA, et al: Cloning and expression of a cDNA for the human prostaglandin E receptor EP1 subtype. J Biol Chem 268:26767, 1993.

67. Coleman RA, Eglen RM, Jones RL, et al: Classification of prostanoid receptors. Int Union Pharmacol Recept Compend 1, 1994.

68. An S, Yang J, Xia M, Goetzl EJ: Cloning and expression of the EP2 subtype of human receptors for prostaglandin E2. Biochem Biophys Res Commun 197:263, 1993.

69. Yang J, Xia M, Goetzl EJ: Cloning and expression of the EP3 subtype of human receptors for prostaglandin E. Biochem Biophys Res Commun 198:999, 1994.

70. Goetzl EJ, Yang J, Xia M, et al: Diverse mechanisms of specificity of human receptors for eicosanoids. Ann NY Acad Sci 744:146, 1994.

71. Abramovitz M, Boie Y, Nguyen T, et al: Cloning and expression of a cDNA for the human prostanoid FP receptor. J Biol Chem 269:2632, 1994.

72. Narumiya S: Prostanoid receptors. Ann NY Acad Sci 744:126, 1994.

73. Coleman RA, Dahlen SE, Drazen JM, et al: Classification of leukotriene receptors. Int Union Pharmacol Recept Compend 1, 1994.

74. Goldman DW, Goetzl EJ: Heterogeneity of human polymorphonuclear leukocyte receptors for leukotriene B₄: Identification of a subset of high affinity receptors that transduce the chemotactic response. J Exp Med 159:1027, 1984.

75. Rovati GE, Fiovanazzi S, Mezzetti M, et al: Heterogeneity of binding sites for ICI 198,615 in human lung parenchyma. Biochem Pharmacol 44:1411, 1992.

76. Lee TH, Austen KF, Corey EJ, et al: Leukotriene E₄–induced airway hyperresponsiveness of guinea pig tracheal smooth muscle to histamine and evidence for three separate sulfidopeptide leukotriene receptors. Proc Natl Acad Sci USA 81:4922, 1984.

77. Vegesna RV, Mong S, Crooke ST: Leukotriene D₄-induced activation of protein kinase C in rat basophilic leukemia cells. Eur J Pharmacol 147:387, 1988.

78. Metter KM, Sawyer N, Nicholson DW: Microsomal glutathione-S-transferase is the predominant leukotriene C₄ binding site in cellular membranes. J Biol Chem 269:12816, 1994.

79. Fiore S, Maddox JF, Perez D, et al: Identification of a human cDNA encoding a functional high affinity lipoxin A₄ receptor. J Exp Med 180:253, 1994.

80. Roper RL, Phipps RP: Prostaglandin E₂ regulation of the immune response. Adv Prostaglandin Thromboxane Leukot Res 22:101, 1994.

81. Ferreira SH, Nakamura M, deAbreau Castro MS: The hyperalgesic effects of prostacyclin and prostaglandin E₂. Prostaglandins 16:31, 1978.

82. Wittenberg RH, Willburger RE, Kleemeyer K, et al: In vitro release of prostaglandins and leukotrienes from synovial tissue, cartilage, and bone in degenerative joint diseases. Arthritis Rheum 36:1444, 1993.

83. Raisz LG, Pilbeam CC, Fall PM: Prostaglandins: Mechanisms of action and regulation of production in bone. Osteoporos Int 3(Suppl 1):136, 1993.

84. Murakami M, Matsumoto R, Austen KF, et al: Prostaglandin endoperoxide synthase-1 and -2 couple to different transmembrane stimuli to generate prostaglandin D₂ in mouse bone marrow–derived mast cells. J Biol Chem 269:22269, 1995.

85. Hardy CC, Robinson C, Tattersfield AE, et al: The bronchoconstrictor effect of inhaled prostaglandin D₂ in normal and asthmatic men. N Engl J Med 31:209, 1984.

86. Hayaishi O: Sleep-wake regulation by prostaglandins D₂ and E₂. J Biol Chem 263:14593, 1988.

87. Lam BK, Austen KF: Leukotrienes. Biosynthesis, release, and actions. In Gallin J, Goldstein I, Snyderman R (eds): Inflammation: Basic Principles and Clinical Correlates. New York, Raven Press, 1992, p 139.

88. Lewis RA, Austen KF, Soberman RJ: Leukotrienes and other products of the 5-lipoxygenase pathway: Biochemistry and relation to pathobiology in human diseases. N Engl J Med 323:645, 1990.

89. Xin-Sheng C, Sheller JR, Johnson EN, et al: Role of leukotrienes revealed by targeted disruption of the 5-lipoxygenase gene. Nature 372:179, 1994.

90. Zakrzewski JT, Barnes NC, Costello JF, et al: Lipid mediators in cystic fibrosis and chronic obstructive pulmonary disease. Am Rev Respir Dis 136:779, 1987.

91. Ahmadzadeh N, Shingu M, Nobunaga M, et al: Relationship between leukotriene B₄ and immunological parameters in rheumatoid synovial fluids. Inflammation 15:497, 1991.

92. Fauler J, Thon A, Tsikas D, et al: Enhanced synthesis of cysteinyl leukotrienes in juvenile rheumatoid arthritis. Arthritis Rheum 37:93, 1994.

93. Colli S, Caruso D, Stragliotto E, et al: Proinflammatory lipoxygenase products from peripheral mononuclear cells in patients with rheumatoid arthritis. J Clin Lab Med 112:357, 1988.

94. Lecomte M, Laneuville O, Ji C, et al: Acetylation of human prostaglandin endoperoxide synthase-2 (cyclooxygenase-2) by aspirin. J Biol Chem 269:13207, 1994.

95. Copeland RA, Williams JM, Giannaras J, et al: Mechanism of selective inhibition of the inducible isoform of prostaglandin G/H synthase. Proc Natl Acad Sci USA 91:11202, 1994.

96. Laneuville O, Breuer DK, Dewitt DL, et al: Differential inhibition of human prostaglandin H synthases-1 and -2 by nonsteroidal anti-inflammatory drugs. J Pharmacol Exp Ther 291:927, 1994.

97. Klein T, Nusing RM, Pfeilschifter J: Selective inhibition of cyclooxygenase-2. Biochem Pharmacol 48:1605, 1994.

98. Gierse JK, Hauser SD, Creely DP, et al: Expression and selective inhibition of the constitutive and inducible forms of human cyclooxygenase. Biochem J 305:479, 1995.

99. Masferrer JL, Zweifel BS, Manning PT, et al: Selective inhibition of inducible cyclooxygenase 2 in vivo is antiinflammatory and nonulcerogenic. Proc Natl Acad Sci USA 91:3228, 1994.

100. Khamashta MA, Cuadrado MJ, Mujic F, et al: The management of thrombosis in the antiphospholipid-antibody syndrome. N Engl J Med 332:993, 1995.

101. Elmgreen J, Ahnfelt-Ronne I, Nielson OH: Inhibition of human neutrophils by auranofin: chemotaxis and metabolism of arachidonate via the 5-lipoxygenase pathway. Ann Rheum Dis 48L:134, 1989.

102. Sperling RI, Benincaso AI, Anderson RJ, et al: Acute and chronic suppression of leukotriene B₄ synthesis ex vivo in neutrophils from patients with rheumatoid arthritis beginning treatment with methotrexate. Arthritis Rheum 35:376, 1992.

103. Lee TH, Hoover RL, Williams JD, et al: Effect of dietary enrichment with eicosapentaenoic and docosahexaenoic acids on in vitro neutrophil and monocyte leukotriene generation and neutrophil function. N Engl J Med 312:1217, 1985.

104. Sperling RI, Benincaso AI, Knoell CT, et al: Dietary ω-3 polyunsaturated fatty acids inhibit phosphoinositide formation and chemotaxis in neutrophils. J Clin Invest 91:651, 1993.

105. Sperling RI, Weinblatt M, Robin JL, et al: Effects of dietary supplementation with marine fish oil on leukocyte lipid mediator generation and function in rheumatoid arthritis. Arthritis Rheum 30:988, 1987.

106. Rainsford KD, Ying C, Smith F: Selective effects of some 5-lipoxygenase inhibitors on synovial interleukin-1 production compared with IL-1 synthesis inhibitors. Agents Actions 39:186, 1993.

107. Barnes NC, Kuitert L: Influence of leukotriene antagonists on baseline

pulmonary function and asthmatic responses. Adv Prostaglandin Thromboxane Leukot Res 22:217, 1994.

108. Israel E, Fischer AR, Rosenberg MA, et al: The pivotal role of 5-lipoxygenase products in the reaction of aspirin-sensitive asthmatics to aspirin. Am Rev Respir Dis 148:1447, 1993.

109. Rask-Madsen J, Bukhave K, Laursen LS, et al: 5-Lipoxygenase inhibitors for the treatment of inflammatory bowel disease. Agents Actions 37:46, 1992.

110. Weinblatt ME, Kremer JM, Coblyn JS, et al: Zileuton, a 5-lipoxygenase inhibitor in rheumatoid arthritis. J Rheumatol 19:1537, 1992.

CHAPTER 20

M. Amin Arnaout

Structural Diversity of Cell Adhesion Molecules and Their Role in Inflammation*

Adhesion of cells to each other and to components of the extracellular matrix plays a central role in the formation, maintenance, and remodeling of all tissues and organs throughout the life of an organism. In addition to its morphogenic and organizational functions, cell-cell and cell-matrix adhesion are essential in host defense against foreign antigens and pathogens. Like all other organ systems, the musculoskeletal system depends on highly complex and organized cell-cell and cell-matrix interactions for its formation and its structural integrity. It is also directly affected when similar interactions propel circulating inflammatory cells into muscles or joints, exacerbating the primary insult and causing more tissue injury.

Because of the vitality of the cellular processes affected by cell-cell and cell-matrix adhesion as well as their harmful potential, knowledge of the underlying cell surface molecules (cell adhesion molecules [CAMs]) is of immense biologic and medical interest. Molecular and genetic studies have identified several classes of CAMs, and the application of structural biology has recently allowed considerable refinement in our understanding of how these receptors bind to their respective ligands. This chapter reviews these advances, with an emphasis on the role of CAMs in inflammatory disorders.

CELL ADHESION MOLECULE FAMILIES

The role of cell adhesion in differential binding and sorting of cells in multicellular organisms was first reported in sponges by Wilson.[1] When mechanically dissociated cells from two different species of marine sponges were mixed together, cells from each species sought their own kind, assembled, and eventually developed into a full organism.[1] The hypothesis that specific and tightly regulated cell adhesion events occur during embryonic and neural development was later proposed by Moscona[2] and developed by Sperry[3] and Edelman.[4] It soon became evident that similar processes are used in the immune system for antigen recognition, immune surveillance,[5, 6] host defense against infections,[7] and hemostasis.[8]

A large number of molecules mediate cell adhesion in vertebrates. These can be grouped into at least six families (Fig. 20–1):

- Cadherins
- Immunoglobulin (Ig)-like proteins
- Integrins
- Selectins
- Cell surface mucins
- Cell surface proteoglycans

The classification of a certain CAM into one of these families is based on the presence of a unique structural profile or a specific adhesion-promoting domain that characterizes a particular family. In this classification, some CAMs that combine more than one function-associated domain may be included into more than one CAM family.

Cadherins

Cadherins are critical for establishing and maintaining the initial intercellular adhesive events required for formation of embryonic tissues and their stability.[9] Members of this family are detected in blastomeres of mouse embryos at the one-cell stage and are indispensable in their compaction and implantation as well as in the subsequent processes leading to morphogenesis. Antibodies to cadherins, when added to embryonic tissues, lead to severe distortion in tissue architecture as a result of disruption of cell-cell adhesion. Formation of tissues is usually accompanied by the selective induction of one or more cadherins at certain developmental stages, by their loss or redistribution when cells migrate or proliferate, and by their reinduction when cells again become stationary or stop proliferating. Cadherins also maintain tight gap junctions and intercellular spacing in adult tissues.[10]

Cadherins can be classified as *classic* and *desmosomal molecules*, on the basis of their distribution on the plasma membrane. Classic cadherins are concentrated at the *zonula adherens* cell junctions and are linked through their C-terminal cytoplasmic tails to the actin cytoskeleton through α-, β-, and γ-catenins.[11–13] Des-

*Supported by grants from the National Institutes of Health.

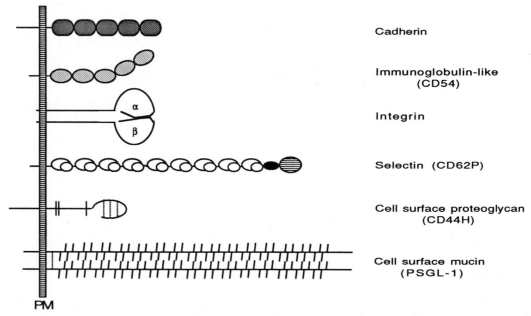

Figure 20–1. Schematic diagram of representative members of the cell adhesion molecule (CAM) families. The extracellular region of cadherins consists of five repeats (dimensions ~4.5 × 2.5 × 2.5 nm). CD54 is shown here as a representative of the immunoglobulin (Ig)-like protein family. The Ig domain, the characteristic structure of the Ig family, is depicted here as ellipsoid with dimensions of 4 × 2.5 nm. Integrins are drawn to accommodate the head and tail morphology revealed by electron microscopic studies. Dimensions of the combined head and each tail, revealed by the electron microscopic studies, are 8 × 10 nm and 15 nm, respectively. Approximately 2 nm separates the C-terminal tails of the subunits. Human P-selectin consists of a globular lectin domain (~4 × 2.5 × 2.5 nm), an epidermal growth factor (EGF) domain (see Taylor et al, 1989[253]), and nine SCRs each 4.1 nm, assembled as rod-shaped structure (based on homology with complement SCRs). Each SCR is aligned as a bead fitted into the proposed triple-loop structure (see Klickstein et al, 1987[254]). Hematopoeitic CD44 has an N-terminal PTR, stabilized by three pairs of cysteine residues (*dotted lines*), followed by a region containing multiple O-linked and chondroitin sulfate (*vertical lines*) attachment sites. The insertion of sequences encoded by exons 1–10 occurs in this region, generating the CD44 variants. P-selectin glycoprotein ligand, (PSGL-1), a dimeric transmembrane glycoprotein with a large mucin ectodomain, is depicted as a rod-like structure, with arbitrary-based carbohydrate branches, and an average extension of approximately 2.5Å/amino acid (based on the homologous structure of CD43) (see Cyster et al, 1991[157]). SCR, short consensus repeat; PTR, proteoglycan tandem repeat; PM, plasma membrane.

mosomal cadherins are found at desmosomes and link with intermediate filaments through plaque proteins, such as plakoglobin (a β-catenin homolog) and desmoplakins.[14]

Five classes of classic cadherins are known, and each exhibits a unique pattern of tissue distribution:

E- (epithelial, uvomorulin)
N- (neural)
P- (placental)
R- (retina)
B- (brain)

Desmosomal cadherins are classified into two major subgroups, *desmogleins* and *desmocollins*.[15] These differ from classic cadherins in having additional sequences in their cytoplasmic domains, resulting from alternative splicing, which probably accounts for their distinct cell junction localization and cytoskeletal associations. More than one cadherin may be expressed on a certain cell. Differential expression of cadherins during morphogenesis permits development of different spatiotemporal patterns in embryos.

Cadherin-mediated adhesion is temperature-dependent and requires Ca^{2+}, which also protects these receptors from rapid proteolysis. Cadherins interact

homophilically (i.e., identical types of cadherins on homotypic or heterotypic cells bind to each other to establish cell-cell contact). *Heterophilic* interactions (i.e., between N- and R-cadherins) of weaker avidity also occur.[16] The large extracellular region of cadherins consists of five tandem repeats of about 110 amino acids each, with the ligand-binding specificity residing in the amino-terminal domain.

The three-dimensional structure of this domain has recently been solved [17, 18] (Fig. 20–2*A*). (See Color Plate.) It is composed of a seven-stranded β-barrel structure reminiscent of the immunoglobulin fold (see later). It has three broad interfaces:

- The first appears to be involved in mediating homophilic adhesion.
- The second is involved in the Ca^{2+}-dependent association between cadherin tandem domains.
- The third, observed in one study,[18] is involved in dimer formation between two cadherins on the same cell.

Ca^{2+} is thus involved in the stable assembly of the tandem repeats rather than in directly coordinating cadherin-ligand adhesion. The assembly of cadherins into a linear zipper of receptors, as suggested by the

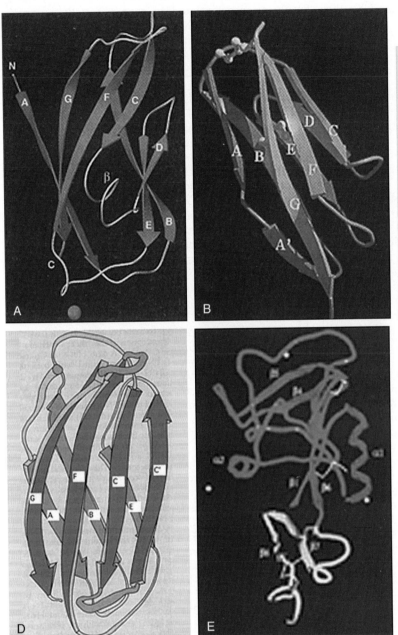
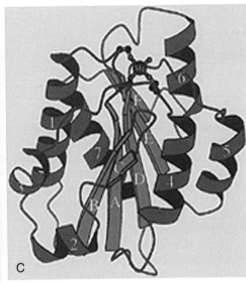

Figure 20–2. Ribbon diagrams of the structure of known adhesion domains in cellular adhesion molecule (CAM) families. (See Color Plate.)

A, The overall structure of the N-terminal cadherin domain from N-cadherin. The seven β-strands are arranged as two β-sheets connected by a quasi β-helix region. Residues from strands C, D, F, G, and β mediate homophilic cadherin-cadherin adhesion. These contact regions are far from the metal-binding site (green sphere) located near the carboxy terminus. The metal is coordinated by residues from two adjacent domains within each cadherin. Residues from β-strand A mediate dimerization of cadherins expressed on the same cell surface. The cadherin structure bears considerable similarity to the immunoglobulin (Ig) domain (see Fig. 2–2B), despite lack of any amino acid homology. (From Shapiro L, Fannon AM, Kwong PD, et al: Structural basis of cell-cell adhesion by cadherins. Nature 374:327–337, 1995. © 1995, Macmillan Magazines Limited.)

B, Structure of the immunoglobulin domain 1 of CD106. Mutational analysis has confirmed that the CD49d/CD29 (α4β1) binding site is composed of residues clustered on the CFG face, with a key asparate (Asp 40 in CD106) projecting from the distinctive CD loop. (From Jones EL, Harlos K, Bottomley MJ, et al: Crystal structure of an intern-binding fragment of vascular cell adhesion molecule-1 at 1.8 Å resolution. Nature 373:539–544, 1995. © 1995, Macmillan Magazines Limited.)

C, Structure of the A domain from integrin CD11b. The structure reveals a well-coordinated metal ion exposed on the surface of the domain. In the generated crystals, the sixth metal coordination site is provided by an acidic residue from a neighboring domain. Under physiologic conditions, the acidic residue from an integrin ligand probably completes metal coordination. (From Lee J-O, Rieu P, Arnaout MA, Liddington R: Crystal structure of the A-domain from the α-subunit of β₂ integrin complement receptor type 3 (CR3, CD11b/CD18). Cell 80:631–638, 1995. Courtesy of Cell Press.)

D, Structure of the third FN-III domain of tenascin. The structure consists of seven β-strands arranged into two β-sheets (ABE and C'CFG). The Arg-Gly-Asp sequence is located in the flexible FG loop, which projects from the protein surface. The homology of the FN-III fold to that of Ig (see Fig. 2–2B) is apparent. (From Graves BJ, Crowther RL, Chandran C: Insight into E-selectin/ligand interaction from the crystal structure and mutagenesis of the lec/EGF domains. Nature 367:532–538, 1994. © 1994, Macmillan Magazines Limited.)

E, Structure of the C-type lectin-EGF domains from E-selectin shown in red and yellow, respectively. The three Ca²⁺ positions are shown as white spheres, and the five disulfide bridges as green sticks. The left and right Ca²⁺ (neighboring α₂ and α₁ helices, respectively) are weakly coordinated. Mutagenesis studies identified a finite region in the vicinity of the upper Ca²⁺ as the most likely carbohydrate contact surface (see text). (From Leahy DJ, Hendrickson WA, Aukhil I, Erickson HP: Structure of a fibronectin type III domain from tenascin phased by MAD analysis of the selenomethionyl protein. Nature 258:987–991, 1992. © 1992, Macmillan Magazines Limited.)

structural data, may explain the strong and stable cadherin-mediated adhesion between opposing cells. Such an arrangement may also be regulated by the cytoskeletal associations described earlier, as deletion of the cytoplasmic tail in cadherins impairs cell adhesion.[19]

Immunoglobulin Supergene Family

The Ig supergene family includes a large number of proteins with diverse functions and tissue distribution.[5] Members include the antigen-specific recognition proteins, immunoglobulins, T cell receptor, and histocompatibility class I and II receptors.

The common structural feature in this family is the *Ig domain*, which is composed of 60 to 100 amino acids arranged in an antiparallel β-barrel with a hydrophobic interior and a hydrophilic exterior. A single disulfide bridge is commonly, but not invariably, found between the second and sixth β-strands. In the constant (C) region of Ig, the barrel is made up of a three-stranded β-sheet (strands C, F, G) (see Fig. 20–2B) facing a four-stranded (A, B, E, D) sheet (C1-type domain). Modifications of this basic fold include the addition of two small β-strands (C' and C'') between the two sheets (variable [V] set), deletion of the D-strand (C2-type domain), or presence of a second disulfide bridge linking the BC and FG loops (I-type domain) (see Fig. 20–2B). The face of the CFG β-sheet is the site for intercellular adhesive interactions between Ig members. The ellipsoidal (4 × 2.5 nm) Ig domain, revealed by crystallographic studies,[20] is usually encoded by one exon. In some cases, however, an intron is present, roughly separating the coding regions of the two β-sheets, which suggests that the Ig domain might have arisen by a duplication of a primordial half-domain structure. The selective advantages for preserving the Ig domain throughout evolution may relate to the known resistance of the Ig fold to proteolysis, an important consideration in promoting a stable extracellular recognition event. The Ig fold was probably first adopted in the nervous system as a cell recognition/adhesion motif prior to its use in the immune system in antigen recognition and host defense.[5, 21]

Ig members may contain one (e.g., Po and Thy1, CD1α) or more Ig domains and are expressed on the cell surface as monomers, dimers, or heterodimers. Some members, such as serum immunoglobulins and α1 Bgp, are secreted. The membrane-bound members are most often linked to the plasma membrane through a single hydrophobic region. Some are GPI-linked and some can exist in either form (e.g., CD58, neural cell adhesion molecule-1 [NCAM-1]). GPI-linked or membrane-spanning forms have equivalent functional activities (e.g., CD58, NCAM-1). Other Ig members (e.g., β2-microglobulin) are disulfide-bonded to an integral membrane protein. Although mixing of segments from different protein families is not uncommon (e.g., selectins and complement pro-

teins), this is a rare event in the extracellular portion of the Ig family. The cytoplasmic portions of the Ig family are least related to each other; they vary in length from 3 amino acids (e.g., IgM) to several hundreds and may contain domains integrated from other protein families, for example, a tyrosine kinase domain in the platelet-derived growth factor (PDGF) receptor.

Members of the Ig supergene family mediate a vast number of vital cell recognition events during morphogenesis, inflammation, hemostasis, and immunity.[5, 22–24] Ig-mediated cell adhesion involves Ca^{2+}-independent homophilic (as with NCAMs, Po protein, Thy1, L1, CD31) or heterophilic interactions. Heterophilic interactions can occur between Ig members (e.g., between CD58 and CD2, CD8, and class I HLA) or between members of the Ig family and other protein families, such as integrins and proteoglycans. Binding of Ig members to their ligands commonly involves one or more Ig domains in the protein. For example, the first two Ig domains of CD54 and CD106 mediate interaction of these proteins with integrins CD11a/CD18 (αLβ2) and CD49d/CD29 (α4β1), respectively.[25]

Immunoglobulin members can also serve as receptors for parasitic or viral proteins. For example, CD54 is a receptor for *Plasmodium falciparum*, which causes malaria,[26] and for the major group of rhinoviruses that cause the common cold.[27] CD4 is the major receptor for the human immunodeficiency virus (HIV).[28]

Integrins

Integrins are heterodimeric surface membrane receptors mediating divalent cation-dependent cell-cell and cell-matrix interactions.[25, 29–31] Each integrin consists of one α-subunit noncovalently associated with a β-subunit (Fig. 20–3). This association is required for cell-surface expression in mammalian cells. Electron microscopy of several integrin heterodimers [8, 32, 33] reveals a mushroom-like head composed of the two N-terminal halves of the α- and β-subunits (see Fig. 20–1) and two flexible tails each made up of the remaining C-terminal portion of each subunit.

Each α-subunit consists of a short cytoplasmic tail, a single membrane-spanning region, and a large N-terminal extracellular region. Alternative splicing of the cytoplasmic tails (e.g., α3 [CD49c], α6 [CD49f]) or extracellular region (e.g., PS2α and platelet IIb[CD41]) has been described.[25] The ectodomain contains seven 60-amino acid tandem repeats, three or four of which have EF-like Ca^{2+}-binding motifs (repeats 5-7 or 4-7, respectively) (see Fig. 20–3).

Some α-subunits contain additional domains between the second and third repeats (see Fig. 20–3). A second subgroup contains a conserved cleavage site near the transmembrane domain (see Fig. 20–3). The third subgroup (α4 and α9) contains neither the conserved cleavage site nor the extra domains.

Members within each subgroup are also more

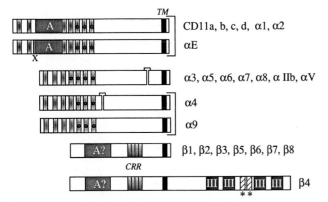

Figure 20–3. Schematic diagram showing the primary structural features of the three groups of integrin α-subunits and the two types of β-subunits in mammalian integrins. Three or four of the seven repeats in the ectodomain of the α-chains contain consensus metal-binding sites *(closed circles)*. The positions of the A-domain (A), the χ-domain (χ), the dipeptide cleavage sites (linked by disulfide bridges) in the α chains and the cysteine-rich repeats (CRR) in the β-chains are indicated. The extracellular region of the β-chains are most homologous within the A-domain–like region (see text). The cytoplasmic tail of β₄ is unique, contains four FN type III repeats and two alternative splicing segments (*).

closely related to each other when the rest of their primary sequences are compared. Members of the first and third subgroups contain three EF-like motifs, whereas members of the second subgroup have all four.

The *A-domain*, first recognized in von Willebrand factor (vWf), has been found in many structurally unrelated proteins involved in cell-cell, cell-matrix, and matrix-matrix adhesion.[34] The lack of other common features between A-domain–containing proteins suggests that the A-domain might have been the product of a primordial gene probably involved in a primitive recognition event and was later inserted into several proteins and modified to mediate specific recognition events.

Recent studies have confirmed the modular nature of the A-domain. When expressed alone as a recombinant protein, the A-domain retains specific ligand-binding functions[34] and has a specific three-dimensional structure revealed by x-ray crystallography.[35] The A-domain adopts a classic α/β fold, with six β-strands forming a central hydrophobic sheet surrounded by seven amphipathic helices (see Fig. 20–2C). The structure contains an unusual metal coordination site at its surface that is required for structural stability and metal-dependent binding to ligands.

The eight known β-subunits are homologous (40 to 48 percent) and smaller than the associated α-subunits (exception for β₄, where the domain is extended C-terminally by inclusion of fibronectin type III repeats) (see Fig. 20–3). Each β-subunit spans the membrane once and has a short C-terminal cytoplasmic tail containing binding sites for cytoskeletal proteins. The large extracellular region contains an N-terminal putative A-like domain[35] and a characteristic C-terminal cysteine-rich motif repeated four times. The β-integrin A-domain has ligand-binding functions and is

involved in the noncovalent association of the β-subunits with their α counterparts.[35] The cysteine-rich region is not essential for ligand binding and heterodimer formation. Its potential role in ligand-induced integrin signaling remains to be explored. Alternative splicing also occurs in the cytoplasmic tails of the β1-, β3-, and β4-subunits.[25]

Integrins have traditionally been divided into subfamilies based on the nature of their associated β-subunits (Fig. 20–4). The largest group is the β1-integrins, also known as very-late-activation (VLA) antigens, formed by the noncovalent association of β1 with any of ten different α-subunits, none of which belong to the A-domain α subgroup. The β1-integrins are matrix receptors mediating interactions between cells and one or more components of the extracellular matrix (see Fig. 20–4). The β1-integrins can also facilitate entry of certain viruses (e.g., foot-and-mouth virus and HIV type I) as well as certain bacteria into mammalian cells.[36–38] In addition to their role in cell-matrix adhesion, several members of the β1 subfamily also mediate cell-cell adhesion. For example, CD49d/CD29 (α4β1) mediates homotypic lymphocyte aggregation and B cell and T cell and T-endothelial cell adhesion[39, 40] and CD49c/CD29 (α3β1) is involved in homotypic aggregation of keratinocytes.[41]

Four members constitute the β2-integrins (LeuCAM or CD11/CD18).[29, 42] The β2-integrins mediate homotypic and heterotypic cell-cell interactions. Expression of this subfamily is restricted to leukocytes. CD11a/CD18 (αLβ2) is expressed on virtually all mature leukocytes. Expression of CD11b/CD18 (αMβ2) is mostly restricted to phagocytes (polymorphonuclear cells, monocytes/macrophages) and large granular lymphocytes, with some expression on CD5⁺ B cell and CD8⁺ T cell subsets. CD11c/CD18 (αXβ2) is expressed in phagocytic cells, with particularly high levels on monocyte-derived macrophages; on some B-cell lines, such as hairy cell leukemia; and on certain cloned cytotoxic T lymphocytes (CTLs). Expression of CD11d/CD18 (αDβ2) appears to be restricted to tissue macrophages and CD8⁺ T cells.

CD11a/CD18 has three known ligands—CD50 (ICAM-3), CD54 (ICAM-1), and CD102 (ICAM-2)—all members of the Ig family. CD11b/CD18, the most abundant integrin in neutrophils, can interact with several ligands, such as iC3b, the major C3 opsonin in vivo, CD54, as well as with clotting factors fibrinogen (FB) and factor X. In granulocytes and monocytes, the majority of CD11b/CD18 and CD11c/CD18 is stored in intracellular granules and is readily brought to the cell surface upon cell activation. The β2-integrins play major roles in chemotaxis, phagocytosis, adhesion to and migration across endothelium, proliferation of lymphocytes, and natural killer (NK) cell and cell-mediated killing of targets (see later).

Three integrins share the β3 (CD61) subunit (see Fig. 20–4):

- CD41/CD61 (αIIbβ3)
- CD51/CD61 (αVβ3)
- The leukocyte response integrin

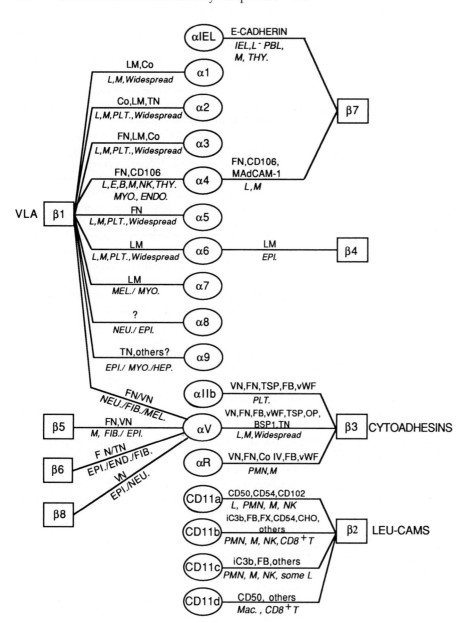

Figure 20–4. Subunit associations, distribution, and ligands of integrins. The association patterns among known subunits are shown. In each case, the ligands for a heterodimer are indicated above the line and its tissue distribution is indicated below the line in *italics.* Co, collagens; LM, laminin; FN, fibronectin; VN, vitronectin; TSP thrombospondin; TN Tenascin; FB, fibrinogen; vWf, von Willebrand factor; OP, osteopontin; FX, factor X; CHO, carbohydrates; BSP-1, bone sialoprotein-1; L, lymphocyte; M/-Mac, monocyte/macrophage; PMN, granulocytes; E, eosinophils; B, basophils; THY, thymocytes; NK, natural killer cells; PLT, platelets; IEL, intestinal intraepithelial lymphocytes; PBL, peripheral blood leukocytes; L-, L-selectin negative, respectively; EPI, epithelial cells; ENDO, endothelial cells; MYO, myocytes; NEU, neural tissue; MEL, melanoma; FIB, fibroblasts. Integrins are referred to by their subunit designation (e.g., α_1, β_3) and/or their cluster designation (CD). Some integrins are more commonly known by one designation or the other.

The β3-integrins are highly promiscuous receptors, recognizing a large number of matrix proteins (see Fig. 20–4). In platelets, CD41/CD61 accounts for 1 to 2 percent of the total platelet protein.[8] Inherited deficiency of this integrin results in a bleeding disorder (Glanzman's thrombasthenia) that is related to failure of platelets to aggregate in response to activation signals.[8]

The broadly distributed CD51/CD61 (αVβ3) interacts with multiple ligands and participates in several adhesion functions, including monocyte adhesion to endothelium,[43] bone remodeling,[44] and tumor metastasis.[45]

The leukocyte response integrin promotes phagocytosis in monocytes and perhaps in neutrophils.[46] It may be identical to a recently defined integrin on murine lymphocytes that mediates CD11a- and CD2-

independent killer-target cell adhesion.[47] The α-subunit of this receptor (αR) has not been cloned.

One or two members have been identified so far in the remaining five β subfamilies[48–53] (see Fig. 20–4). Integrins β5, β6, and β8 share the same αV-subunit and bind to vitronectin, fibronectin, or both.[54]

β5 is expressed on epithelium, fibroblasts and monocytes and is abundant on lung and pancreatic carcinomas.[55] β6 is found on epithelium, fibroblasts and human endothelial cells[56] and on epithelial-derived tumors. β8 is expressed in the kidney, brain, ovary, uterus, and placenta and is detected in certain epithelial and tumor cell lines.[57]

β4 is expressed in epithelial cells and is abundant on several colonic carcinoma cell lines,[48] which suggests that it may contribute to the metastatic potential of solid tumors.[58] It is also unique, in that its cytoplasmic tail, the longest among the β-integrin subunits, contains four fibronectin type III repeats (see Figs. 20–2D and 20–3).

Expression of the β7-subunit is restricted to leukocytes. β7-Messenger ribonucleic acid (mRNA) has been detected in T-cell, B-cell, and macrophage cell lines.[59] β7 pairs with CD49d (α4) or αE, and α4β7 is the major lymphocyte homing receptor for gut-associated lymphoid tissues, such as Peyer's patches.[60, 61] αEβ7 is expressed on most CD4⁻ CD8⁺ intraepithelial lymphocytes[62] and mediates lymphocyte adhesion to epithelial cells.[63]

In general, integrins (except for those with A-domains in their α-subunits) bind the tripeptide sequence arginine-glycine-aspartate (RGD), present in hundreds of proteins. Not every protein with an RGD sequence necessarily binds to integrins, however, because the tripeptide must be surface-exposed for accessibility as a ligand (as, for example, in fibronectin type III repeats) (see Fig. 20–2D).

Several integrins bind to a single ligand. For example, CD49c, -d, -e/CD29 (α3-5β1) and CD51/CD29 (αVβ1) bind to fibronectin; CD49a, -b, -c/CD29 (α1-3β1) binds to collagen (Co); and CD49a, -b, -f/CD29 (α1,2,6β1) binds to laminin [64–66] (see Fig. 20–3). Binding of different integrins to the same ligand is usually mediated by distinct sites in the ligand. For example, whereas CD49e/CD29 (α5βb) binds to fibronectin through its RGD-containing region, CD49d/CD29 (α4β1) binds to fibronectin in an RGD-independent manner through a leucine-aspartate-valine (LDV) sequence in the alternatively spliced CS1 site[67] of the III CS region. CD49d/CD29 (α4β1) also binds to a second site near the Hep II domain.[68] In addition, some receptors can bind, through separate regions in the receptor, to two or more distinct sites in the same ligand. Thus, three binding sites in fibrinogen (two RGD sites in the α-chain and a non-RGD site in the γ-chain) bind to three separate sites in CD61/CD41 (αIIbβ3).[8, 69, 70]

Binding of integrins to their ligands is regulated at several levels. Differentiation stimuli modulate expression of both receptors and ligands in a variety of cell types. For example, differentiation of the myeloid precursors is accompanied by expression of the β2-integrins CD11b and CD11c and several members of the β1 subfamily.[29, 30]

Activation signals acting on mature cells can also modulate expression of integrins at a transcriptional level. Thus, antigen or mitogen activation of mature lymphocytes leads to increased expression of β2-integrins and down-regulation of CD49f/CD29 (α6β1).

Increased expression of integrin can also occur without neosynthesis. Cell activation can rapidly increase expression of CD41/CD61 (αIIbβ3) in platelets and β2-integrins in neutrophils and monocytes by recruiting large amounts of presynthesized receptors, stored in intracellular organelles, to the cell surface.

In addition to these three mechanisms that regulate the quantitative expression of integrins on the cell surface, integrin function is also regulated qualita-tively. Inflammatory mediators elicit rapid conformational changes in surface-expressed integrins, switching these receptors from an inactive to an active state with an ability to bind ligands. Examples include the rapid activation of β2-integrins in leukocytes, CD41/CD61 in platelets and CD49d, -e, and -f in T cells.[71] Some integrins assume a dormant state, one that is intermediate between an inactive and an active state. Integrins expressed on memory T cells or B cells appear to be in this form and can bind ligand without cell activation, but they are further up-regulated in the presence of exogenous activation signal.[42]

Divalent cations and alternative splicing[72] also modulate integrin functions. For example, the RGD-independent binding of CD49b to collagen,[73] CD49c to fibronectin,[74] and CD49f to laminin[75] is inhibited by Ca^{2+} but increased by Mg^{2+}, which suggests that alterations in the levels of cations, perhaps in wounds, may modify usage of various integrins, even those expressed on the same cell.[76, 77]

Binding of integrins to one of several potential ligands is also regulated in a tissue-specific manner. Thus, in platelets, CD49b binds only to collagen; in other cell types, however, it also binds to laminin and fibronectin.[78]

Integrin-ligand interactions produce dramatic changes in cell morphology, migration, phagocytosis, proliferation, gene expression, and cell survival.[29, 79, 80] The diversity of these cellular events reflects the diverse signals transmitted through integrins and a highly regulated cross-talk between integrins and other receptors involved in cell growth, proliferation, motility, and gene expression. The integrin cytoplasmic tails do not have kinase or phosphatase domains or sequences that interact with G-proteins, which indicates that their dramatic effects on cell behavior must be mediated indirectly, through agonist-induced associations with signaling molecules. The nature of the intracellular signaling events set in motion upon ligation of integrins by multivalent ligands, as well as the biochemical events involved in coordinating cellular responses to stimuli generated by integrins and other receptors, is only beginning to be explored.

A number of integrin-dependent biochemical events have been described in different cell types. These include:

- Tyrosine phosphorylation[81]
- Activation of phospholipases C (PLC) and D (PLD)[82]
- Induction of Ca^{2+} transients[83]
- A rise in intracellular pH[84, 85]
- Activation of Ca^{2+}-dependent proteases[86]
- Redistribution and activation of protein tyrosine, serine-threonine, and phospholipid kinases (e.g., pp60[c-src], mitogen-activated protein [MAP] kinases, protein kinase C [PKC], PI-3, PI-4, and PIP-5 kinases)[87–90]; GTPases[91–93]; and phosphatases[94, 95]

Initiation of many of these functions requires clustering of ligand-occupied integrins by antibodies (or multivalent ligands)[96, 97] and assembly of a cytoskeleton-signaling complex. Integrin occupancy by a monomeric ligand can induce receptor redistribution to focal contacts. This function requires the cytoplasmic tail of the β-subunits, and is modified by the cytoplasmic tails of the associated α-subunits.[98-100] Integrin binding to a monomeric ligand, however, does not induce significant redistribution of cytoskeletal proteins or activation of signaling cytosolic molecules.[101] These functions require multimerization of ligand-occupied receptors. Whereas clustering of an integrin by an antibody in the absence of ligand can induce Ca²⁺ transients, activation of phospholipase D and C, the tyrosine kinase pp125[FAK], and the cytoskeletal protein tensin,[101] only clustering of the ligand-occupied integrin appears to be required for assembling the cytoskeleton into a signaling complex.[102, 103] Processing of integrin-mediated signals into diverse cell responses (e.g., migration, proliferation, gene induction) requires selective integration of such signals with those generated by other receptors known to participate in such events. The specific pathways involved in these responses and their biochemical basis represent active areas of investigation.

Selectins

Three members—L-selectin, P-selectin, and E-selectin—make up this family.[104] Each selectin consists of a short cytoplasmic tail; a single membrane-spanning region and an extracellular region consisting of a single N-terminal, C-type, Ca²⁺-dependent lectin domain; and an adjacent epidermal growth factor (EGF)-like domain, followed by a variable number of short consensus repeats (SCRs) present in several complement regulatory proteins (see Fig. 20–1). Selectins project a significant distance from the cell surface (~15 to 43 nm, depending on the number of SCRs) and are thus suited for the initial interactions between cells.

The lectin domain contains the ligand-binding site but requires the EGF motif for optimal binding. The role of the SCR domain is not clear. It may serve a spacer function, may protect the respective cell membrane from complement-induced injury, or may mediate other protein-protein interactions yet to be elucidated. The crystal structure of the C-type lectin-EGF domains of human E-selectin at 2Å resolution has been derived[105] (see Fig. 20–2E). The structure reveals that the C-type and EGF domains have very limited association. The lectin domain is ovoid, consisting of five β strands, two α helices, and an extended number of loops. It contains a Ca²⁺ ion well coordinated by the side chains of E80, N82, N105, D106, the main chain carbonyl of D106, and two water molecules, forming the typical pentagonal bipyramid coordination sphere. The side chains of the amino acids essential for ligand binding (Y48, N82, N83, E92, Y94, K11, and K113) lie on the same face as the bound Ca²⁺ and are conserved among all selectins.

Selectins bind directly to sialylated fucosylated lactose amines, such as sialyl Lewis^x (SLe^x). These decorate many cell-associated structures, such as proteins and glycosphingolipids. Biologically relevant selectin ligands are far fewer, however, because oligosaccharide clustering, presented by a more limited group of structures (e.g., certain mucins and proteoglycans), appears to be an important requirement for a biologically active selectin ligand interaction.[106] The importance of fucosylation in selectin recognition is emphasized by the fact that a genetic abnormality characterized by a general failure of fucosylation in two siblings is associated with markedly reduced selectin-mediated adhesion, so-called leukocyte adhesion deficiency type II (LAD-II).[107] Solution of the structure of a complex between the C-type lectin of mannose binding protein and mannose[108] indicates that mannose binds directly to the Ca²⁺ ion of the lectin domain. Modeling of the known structure of sialyl Lewis^x (SLe^x) shows that it can fit onto the E-selectin surface in a configuration where fucose, like mannose, can bind to Ca²⁺ directly.[105] Although direct support for this proposed docking will require solution of an E-selectin-sialyl Lewis^x complex, the available data strongly suggest that the contact region between a selectin and its ligand is rather small.

L-Selectin

L-selectin (CD62L), the first discovered member of this family, has 2 SCRs, in addition to the common C-type lectin and EGF domains. It has a transmembrane segment and a short cytoplasmic tail. A GPI-linked form of human L-selectin also exists.[109] L-selectin is constitutively expressed on a majority of bone marrow prothymocytes, immature thymocytes, naive T and B cells, a subpopulation of memory cells (CD45RO⁺), monocytes, and granulocytes. L-selectin binds to several ligands, three of which have been characterized.

Glycosylated cell adhesion molecule-1 (GlyCAM-1), mucosal addressin cell adhesion molecule-1 (MAdCAM-1), and CD34 are cell surface mucins. GlyCAM-1 is a peripheral membrane protein, whereas CD34 and MAdCAM-1 are typical membrane-spanning proteins. CD34 and MAdCAM-1 also contain Ig domains: CD34 contains one Ig domain in the membrane-proximal region, whereas MAdCAM-1 contains three Ig domains, two of which are on either side of the single mucin domain.[110]

GlyCAM-1 and CD34 are expressed on endothelium in high endothelial venules (HEVs) of peripheral lymph nodes as sialylated, fucosylated, and sulfated ligands.[111, 112] MAdCAM-1 expression is restricted to mesenteric lamina propria and the HEVs of Peyer's patches (mucosal lymphoid organs in the intestinal wall).[113] Binding of all three ligands to L-selectin takes place through the mucin domains in each structure. Interaction of L-selectin on naive T and B cells with vascular CD34 and GlyCAM-1 appears to be responsible for directing the trafficking of these leukocytes to peripheral lymph nodes (see later). Expression of these ligands on HEVs is developmentally regulated and requires mediators reaching the lymph nodes through their afferent lymph, as removal of afferent lymph changes HEV morphology from cuboidal to flat and leads to loss of expression of L-selectin ligands.[6, 114] Antigenic stimulation can restore the cuboidal phenotype of endothelia in lymph nodes as well as in nonlymphoid tissues. Although CD34 and Gly-CAM-1 are expressed in Peyer's patch HEVs and in nonlymphoid tissues, they are not properly glycosylated at these sites to serve as L-selectin ligands.[112, 113] Through interaction with MAd-CAM-1, L-selectin is also involved in targeting an L-selectin[+], integrin β7[+] subset of memory lymphocytes to the gut lamina propria. A subset of these cells (αEβ7[+]) traverses the basement membrane and settles intraepithelially, through binding to epithelial E-cadherin.[63] L-selectin may also be involved (together with CD44 and the α6 integrin[115]) in homing of bone marrow prothymocytes to the thymus.[6]

In addition to its role in the normal trafficking patterns of lymphocytes, L-selectin plays an important role in phagocyte (as well as lymphocyte) extravasation at inflammatory sites in nonlymphoid tissues (see later). The responsible L-selectin endothelial ligand has not yet been characterized. It does not appear to be a sialomucin but, rather, seems to be a heparan sulfate–containing proteoglycan.[116] L-selectin–mediated phagocyte adhesion to endothelium is enhanced by transient activation of L-selectin by inflammatory mediators and, perhaps, by the selective expression of this selectin on the tips of neutrophil pseudopodia.[117]

The subsequent rapid loss of L-selectin from the surface of activated cells may be useful in terminating adhesion through this selectin and in enhancing adhesion through integrins.[118] Loss of L-selectin in activated cells is due primarily to a proteolytic process[119] and may account for the presence of significant levels of the functional protein in serum, especially during active inflammation.[120] The mechanisms that underlie L-selectin down-regulation in thymocytes during differentiation and its re-expression on naive lymphocytes during their selective homing are unclear.

P-Selectin

Human P-selectin (CD62P) contains 9 SCRs[121] (see Fig. 20–1), whereas murine (mouse) and bovine P-selectins contain 8 and 6 SCRs, respectively.[122, 123] Two alternatively spliced forms of human P-selectin are known; one lacks the transmembrane portion (encoded by exon 14,) and the other lacks most of the seventh SCR (encoded by exon 11).[121, 124] The functional role of these variants is unknown.

A P-selectin ligand, P-selectin glycoprotein ligand (PSGL-1), is a transmembrane glycoprotein with a short cytoplasmic tail and a large mucin ectodomain.[125] PSGL-1 is expressed as a disulfide-linked dimer of 120-kD subunits. It is sialylated and fucosylated and contains potential tyrosine sulfation sites.

PSGL-1 is expressed on neutrophils, monocytes, NK cells, and lymphocyte subsets.[126] Another P-selectin ligand, recently isolated from mouse neutrophils and HL60 cells, appears to be a sialylated glycoprotein of 160 kD (80 kD reduced).[127] Its structure is unknown.

P-selectin is stored after synthesis in the Weibel-Pallade bodies of endothelial cells and in α-granules of platelets.[128] The cytoplasmic tail is important in directing newly synthesized protein to this intracellular storage compartment.[129] P-selectin is translocated to the surface within minutes after cell stimulation by inflammatory mediators such as thrombin, histamine, substance P, and membrane attack complex (MAC) of complement.[130, 131] In vitro, endothelial (but not platelet) P-selectin is rapidly internalized, disappearing after 30 minutes.[132] Oxygen free radicals induce a prolonged expression of P-selectin that does not require protein synthesis and may be due to interference with the normal internalization of this protein following its surface expression.[133] In other cases, prolonged expression can result from increased synthesis.

Tumor necrosis factor-alpha (TNF-α) has been shown to induce transcriptional activation of P-selectin with kinetics similar to those found for E-selectin.[122] This regulatory mechanism may be important in maintaining expression of P-selectin for prolonged periods, as observed in endothelium from certain vascular beds (e.g., lung, liver).[134]

P-selectin mediates adhesion between leukocytes and platelets or endothelial cells.[135] Neutrophils, monocytes, a subpopulation of memory T cells, and several carcinomas of lung, breast, and colon origin[136] express ligands that bind P-selectin. These binding events are important in leukocyte rolling and extravasation into inflamed tissues,[137] recruitment of phagocytic cells to sites of platelet thrombi, clearance of activated platelets through phagocytosis, homing of memory T cells, and tumor metastasis.[104] P-selectin also inhibits superoxide production by neutrophils, perhaps serving to protect the endothelium during its multiple encounters with the neutrophil.[138, 139] P-selectin also plays a role in a number of thrombotic and inflammatory disorders (see later), including ischemia-reperfusion injury, complement-induced lung injury,[140] monocyte adhesion to synovial microvasculature in rheumatoid arthritis,[119] and the accumulation of leukocytes at thrombotic sites.[141]

E-Selectin

E-selectin (CD62E) contains 6 SCRs. It is not found on unactivated endothelial cells, but it can be transcriptionally induced within 1 to 4 hours by bacterial products, such as lipopolysaccharides and cytokines (interleukin-1 [IL-1] and TNF-α), with the level of expression returning to baseline by 24 hours in vitro. Some of these cytokines are released by mast cells in allergic individuals after an antigenic challenge,[142] resulting in expression of E-selectin and recruitment of inflammatory cells in vivo (the late-phase response).[143] The kinetics of this response mimic closely the induction of E-selectin expression on endothelial cells in vitro. E-selectin binds in a neuraminidase-sensitive manner to neutrophils, basophils, eosinophils, monocytes, the myeloid cell lines HL60 and U937, and colonic (but not breast or lung) carcinoma cell lines.[144–146] E-selectin is also expressed on a subset of memory cells (L-selectin[+], α4β1[+], α6[+], α4β7[−]) targeted to skin.[147]

An E-selectin ligand (ESL-1) has been recently cloned.[148] ESL-1, a transmembrane protein of 150 kD, is ubiquitous, but it is sialylated and fucosylated only in myeloid cells and therefore serves as an E-selectin ligand in these cell types. In contrast to other selectin ligands, the large extracellular region of ESL-1 does not contain a mucin domain. Interestingly, it is identical to a known receptor for fibroblast growth factor (FGF). ESL-1 may normally serve as an FGF receptor, and in myeloid cells it also functions as an E-selectin receptor. The biologic relevance of ESL-1 remains to be established, because not every sialylated fucosylated glycoprotein is necessarily a selectin ligand in vivo.

Other ligands for E-selectin include a sialylated and O-glycosylated protein of about 250 kD, expressed on bovine γ/δ lymphocytes,[149] and cutaneous lymphocyte-associated antigen (CLA), which may direct lymphocyte homing to skin (see later). The structure of these ligands has not yet been elucidated.

Mucins

Mucins are a heterogeneous group of glycoproteins having in common a mucin-like segment that constitutes all or only a fraction of the protein structure. The mucin domain (~5 nm in length[150]) is a 20-amino acid sequence, rich in serines and threonines that are coupled to O-linked carbohydrate chains. Two classes of O-linked oligosaccharides are commonly found in cell surface mucins containing type 1 (Gal β3-GalNAc) or type 2 (Gal β3 [GlcNAc β6]-GalNAc) cores. The cell's lineage and its differentiation and activation states are important factors in determining the type of the core expressed. Mature granulocytes, for example, make oligosaccharides with type 2 cores.[151] T cell activation results in a switch from a type 1 to a type 2 core oligosaccharide.[152]

The cell's lineage and level of differentiation also help to determine mucin functions. For example, Gly-CAM-1 and CD34, expressed in nonlymphoid tissues and ESL-1 in nonmyeloid cells, do not serve as selectin ligands as a result of the lack of proper glycosylation in these tissues caused by differential expression of glycosyltransferases. Stage-specific alternative splicing results in three extra segments added to CD45 in B lymphocytes[153] and 1 to 3 SCRs added to platelet gpIb in platelets.[154] Several distinct repeats are also present in carcinoma—and in epithelial mucins, which contribute to their structural heterogeneity.[155, 156]

Visualization of several mucins (e.g., episialin [MUC1], submaxillary gland mucins, and CD43) by electron microscopy[157] has revealed extended conformations resulting primarily from steric interactions between oligosaccharides and adjacent amino acids. This steric restriction makes the mucin-rich region relatively resistant to proteolysis. The cell-associated forms of these rigid structures can project to significant distances from the plasma membrane (e.g., 45 nm with CD43 and 55 nm with B cell CD45[157]) and are probably the first to mediate or impede cell-cell or cell-matrix interactions. The antiadhesive role of many mucins (e.g., CD43[158]) may be the result of an extended negatively charged structure creating a repulsive field around the cell. In the presence of specific receptors (e.g., selectins), mucins can then promote adhesive rather than antiadhesive interactions.

Several mucins serve important functions in cell-cell recognition events. GlyCAM-1, MAdCAM-1, CD34, and PSGL-1 bind to various selectins through their mucin domains. Similarly, the ZP3 mucin of the zona pellucida binds in a species-specific manner to mammalian spermatozoa.[159, 160] The suitability of the mucin domain as a general ligand for selectins may have to do with its unique structure, which offers a rigid and highly concentrated cluster of sialylated fucosylated oligosaccharides. This structure provides ample opportunity for the Ca^{2+}-dependent high on-rate, high off-rate interaction that characterizes selectin binding.[161] Given the fact that the C-type lectin structure can accommodate only a single SLe^x motif at a time, carbohydrate clustering presented in the mucin domain may provide a flexible array of sugar chains that can transiently dock onto the surface of the C-type lectin per unit time. Several cell surface mucins (e.g., CD43,[162] GPIb/IX[163])are released from the cell surface after proteolytic cleavage at nonglycosylated regions in their ectodomains, and some achieve significant levels in plasma (1 to 2 μg/ml for GlyCAM-1).[164] These plasma forms may modulate cell-cell adhesion or may have additional functions yet to be discovered.

Proteoglycans

Proteoglycans are a structurally diverse family of proteins with widespread tissue distribution. Their common feature is a core protein to which one or more linear carbohydrate chains, repeating sulfated disaccharide units known as *glycosaminoglycans* (GAGs), are bound covalently.[165, 166] GAG attachment sites are often composed of multiple Ser-Gly repeats, each followed within 2 to 5 amino acids by acidic residues. In several proteins, only a single Ser-Gly is found, often sandwiched between acidic residues.[167] GAGs may be of several types, such as heparan, dermatan, chondroitin or keratan sulfate, present singly or in combination in the same proteoglycan.

Secreted, intracellular, and membrane-associated forms of proteoglycans exist. The membrane-associated forms link to the plasma membrane through typical transmembrane regions (e.g., betaglycan, thrombomodulin), a GPI-linkage (e.g., glypican[168]) or through association with other membrane proteins.[169, 170] Proteoglycans serve not only as cell adhesion molecules but also as matrix proteins,[171] cytokine receptors,[172] and growth factor receptors[173] and can act as viral receptors.[174] Binding of proteoglycans to their respective ligands is mediated by the GAG structure or the core protein.[167] A common core protein motif present in several proteoglycans, such as decorin and fibromodulin,[175] is the leucine-rich domain, a 24-amino acid motif[176] that participates in such diverse functions as cell adhesion and signaling.

Proteoglycans serve a wide variety of functions, including simple mechanical support, which is essential for maintaining tissue integrity; cell adhesion and migration; and cell differentiation and proliferation.

The role of proteoglycans in cell adhesion can be *direct* (as with CD44s, RHAMM [receptor for hyaluronate-mediated motility], and syndecans) or *indirect* (through modulating the functions of other CAMs). The extended carbohydrate chains of proteoglycans project to significant distances from the cell surface (to ~50 nm for a typical heparan sulfate chain). In addition, their net negative charge, abundance on cell surfaces (10^5 to 10^6 heparan sulfate proteoglycan molecules per cell),[166] selective membrane distribution (at focal contacts[177] or filopodia[178]), and role as storage sites for growth factors or cytokines (acidic and basic FGF, granulocyte-macrophage colony-stimulating factor [GM-CSF], IL-3, and gamma interferon [IFN-γ]) provide members of this family with a multiplicity of pathways through which they can modify, either positively or negatively, a number of cell-cell and cell-matrix interactions.[165]

Among the best characterized cell surface proteoglycans that mediate cell adhesion are the CD44 and syndecan subfamilies.

CD44

CD44 is the product of a single gene with 19 exons, 12 of which can be alternatively spliced.[179] It has a wide cell distribution and is expressed in brain, prothymocytes, immature thymocytes, mature T cells, B cells, monocytes, granulocytes, erythrocytes, fibroblasts, endothelium, keratinocytes, and carcinoma cell lines.[179] CD44s mediate cell-matrix adhesion, leukocyte homing, cell migration, and lymphocyte activation.

The basic structure of CD44, displayed in hematopoietic cells (CD44H) (see Fig. 20–1), is a type I membrane protein, 341 amino acids long. The ectodomain consists of a single N-terminal proteoglycan tandem repeat (PTR) containing five potential N-glycosylation sites, the binding site for hyaluronate.[180] PTR is also present in other proteins that bind hyaluronate, such as cartilage link protein, versecan, aggregan, RHAMM, and hyaluronectin.[181] PTR is followed by a heavily glycosylated segment containing O-linked sites and chondroitin GAG attachment sites (see Fig. 20–1). A single membrane-spanning segment is followed by a 72-amino acid cytoplasmic tail containing potential serine phosphorylation sites. Post-transcriptional RNA splicing, limited largely to CD44 variants expressed in epithelial cells, can lead to the insertion of up to ten alternative exons in tandem within the extracellular region proximal to the plasma membrane.[182] Two of these exons (v3 and v10) encode additional GAG attachment sites. Alternative splicing and variable glycosylation can potentially generate more than 1000 forms of CD44, thus accounting for the large variation in its molecular size in various tissues. Some CD44 variants do not bind to hyaluronate.[183, 184] The splicing variants also exert other effects on interaction of CD44 with substrates. For example, splice variants containing exon 3, which encodes a peptide carrying GAG of the heparan sulfate variety, binds growth factors.[185] The high level of expression of CD44 variants in epithelia indicates a primary role of these isoforms in cell-cell and cell-matrix adhesion in cells of epithelial origin, as is the case with syndecans.

In addition to its function as a major leukocyte hyaluronate receptor, hematopoeitic CD44 is involved in lymphocyte homing to lymph node, mucosal, and synovial HEVs.[186–189] Its high expression on bone marrow prothymocytes and the most immature thymocytes suggest that it also plays a role, perhaps in conjunction with L-selectin, in lymphocyte homing to primary lymphoid tissues.

CD44 also binds to a mucosal addressin through its heavily glycosylated portion[188] and enhances through its GAG motif, the adhesion of fibroblasts to collagen, sulfate, and laminin[190] as well as homotypic adhesion and migration of macrophages.[191] CD44 also facilities several heterotypic interactions, such as adhesion of T cells to sheep erythrocytes or to monocytes, CD2- or CD3-induced T cell proliferation,[192] and interaction between hematopoietic and stromal bone marrow cells during myelopoiesis and lymphopoiesis.[193] CD44 is proteolytically cleaved from granulocytes and lymphocytes activated with phorbol myristate acetate (PMA) and anti-CD44 monoclonal antibodies, respectively.[194] This may mimic the situation in vivo, since extravasating leukocytes lose CD44 during transendothelial migration.[195, 196] The cytoplasmic tail associates with several cytoskeletal proteins, thus regulating CD44 binding to hyaluronate.[179] Lymphocytes and monocytes transiently express CD44 variants that bind growth factors following mitogenic challenge or cytokine treatment.[197] Indeed, GAG-modified CD44 isolated from peripheral blood monocytes was reported to present the chemokine MIP-1β to T cells, enabling these cells to bind to CD106 in vitro. Although another heparan sulfate proteoglycan distinct from CD44 appears to serve this function in endothelial cells,[185] CD44 isoforms in particular and proteoglycans in general may also participate in the inflammatory response by presenting growth factors, cytokines, and chemokines to leukocytes.

Syndecans

Syndecans are a subfamily of heparan sulfate and chondroitin sulfate cell surface proteoglycans expressed primarily on epithelium. They are involved in tissue organization and morphogenesis.[198] At least four distinct genes have been identified. The core proteins are small (~300 amino acids), span the membrane once, and have an identical short cytoplasmic tail. The ectodomains are homologous, although less so than the transmembrane or cytoplasmic domains, contain conserved GAG attachment and N-linked glycosylation sites and a characteristic basic dipeptide proteinase site adjacent to the plasma membrane, resulting in the proteolytic release of the ectodomain from the cell. Syndecans are expressed predominantly basolaterally in mature polarized epithelia but may also localize to epithelial surfaces (in stratified epithelium). Generally lacking in circulating leukocytes, syndecans are found on pre-B cells in the bone marrow and in plasma cells. The number and type of GAG expressed on syndecans are cell-specific and responsive to growth factors.[199]

Syndecans serve dual functions as matrix receptors and as co-receptors for several growth factors.[200] Syndecans mediate metal-independent adhesion of epithelial cells through their GAG chains to collagens I, III, and V, sulfate, tenascin, and thrombospondin,[201] with thrombospondin binding preferentially to chondroitin sulfate GAG. These interactions result in the stability of epithelial cell layers. Syndecans bind several growth factors through their heparan sulfate moieties.[200]

ROLE OF CELL ADHESION MOLECULES IN LEUKOCYTE HOMING AND RECIRCULATION

The CAM families described mediate the myriad number of cell-cell and cell-matrix interactions that give organisms their form and assure their survival. The high degree of orchestration between different adhesion molecules to subserve a specific function is perhaps best exemplified in the extravasation of circulating leukocytes into tissues, a process that is essential for host survival yet can lead to significant body injury in many inflammatory and autoimmune diseases. Because of its direct relevance to the pathogenesis of commonly encountered diseases, the cell adhesion events responsible for leukocyte extravasation are reviewed here. Some reviews have described other examples of the delicate interplay among and between CAM families in morphogenesis,[202] hemostasis,[8] bone remodeling,[203] wound healing,[204] and antigen presentation.[205]

Extravasation of circulating leukocytes into tissues is an essential step in host defense against infections. The intradermal injection of a bacterial-derived product, such as lipopolysaccharide (LPS), elicits a rapid influx of neutrophils (peak, ~4 hours). A mononuclear cell infiltrate follows and predominates the site

by 48 hours. The accumulation of these phagocytic cells is instrumental in clearing the infection through phagocytosis and target cell killing and in the subsequent wound-healing process. The importance of CAMs in leukocyte influx to infected sites and phagocytosis was first recognized in patients with congenital deficiency of β2-integrins (Leu-CAM deficiency [LAD-I]).[7] These patients suffer from life-threatening infections caused by the inability of phagocytes to extravasate into infected tissues and to engulf serum-opsonized pathogens. Tissue biopsy specimens from infected areas in these patients show abundant neutrophils trapped within dilated venules, with very few exiting into the infected extravascular connective tissue. A similar profile is also observed in inherited β2-integrin deficiency in dogs[206] and cattle[207] and in CD18 knockout mice.[208] Dissection of the molecular basis for this block in extravasation was instrumental in elucidating the sequential steps required for the transendothelial migration of leukocytes and in defining the vital role of β2-integrins in this process.

Cohnheim[209] described in impressive detail the morphologic events involved in the emigration of leukocytes into tissues. In his classic ex vivo studies using frog tongue and mesentery, he observed that as the tissue became irritated under the microscope, the vessels dilated and blood flow increased transiently, then slowed down. White blood cells began to roll on the vessel wall, with some becoming adherent and then moving slowly across the endothelium into the extravascular space.[209] Refinements in the technique of intravital microscopy has allowed quantitative measurements of these leukocyte-endothelial cell interactions. As leukocytes enter postcapillary venules, they are pushed toward the endothelium by the faster-moving (at 1 to 3 mm/second) red blood cells.[210] In tissues continuously exposed to mechanical or chemical stress (e.g., skin, gut, and lung[203]), a significant proportion of leukocytes (~40 percent) establish unstable interactions with endothelium, which under flow (shear stresses of 3 to 20 dynes/cm2), force a rotational motion of the leukocyte (so-called "rolling").[211] The slower rolling speed of leukocytes (~20 to 60 μm/second) permits some to adhere firmly (i.e., to become stationary for about 30 seconds) as a prelude to emigration, a process that takes several minutes. Selectins expressed on leukocytes (L-selectin) and on vascular endothelium (P-selectin and E-selectin) mediate leukocyte rolling through interaction with cognate ligands.[104] The slower speed of rolling leukocytes enables them to bind to inflammatory mediators (presented by endothelia in free or proteoglycan-bound forms),[212] a step that leads to activation of integrin receptors. Activated integrins then mediate firm adhesion of leukocytes to endothelium.

Integrin-mediated adhesion can take place in a selectin-independent manner when flow is reduced or stopped.[107] These conditions prevail in many inflammatory states, such as ischemia-reperfusion injury, sepsis, and occlusive vascular diseases. Integrin-mediated adhesion occurs through binding of these receptors to ligands expressed on vascular endothelium (e.g., CD54 and CD102, members of the immunoglobulin family in the case of β2-integrins).

Transendothelial migration across tight junctions is also integrin-mediated. The migrating neutrophil induces endothelial cell retraction through an increase in endothelial cell intracellular Ca^{2+},[213] thus transiently loosening the tight junctions while squeezing through. CD31, a heavily glycosylated Ig member, facilitates transendothelial migration: anti-CD31 antibodies block neutrophil transmigration without affecting adhesion to endothelium. CD31 may function by facilitating homophilic adhesion between CD31 on neutrophils and on endothelial cell tight junctions.[214] This interaction may also activate integrins of the α4 and β1 subfamilies,[215] thus providing a stimulus for transmigration. Migration through the basement membrane and subendothelial tissues, which are rich in matrix proteins and hyaluronate, may involve CD44[179, 181] in addition to leukocyte integrins.

The nature and kinetics of appearance of leukocyte subpopulations at an inflammatory site (e.g., the early appearance of neutrophils in infected regions, the accumulation of eosinophils at allergic sites, or T cell subsets in rheumatoid synovium) are determined by:

- The type of inflammatory mediators present
- The nature and kinetics of the endothelial response to mediators
- The profiles of CAMs decorating leukocytes and endothelium

Monocyte chemotactic protein-1 (MCP-1) and IL-5 are selective chemokines/cytokines for monocytes and eosinophils, respectively. The lymphokines IL-4 and IFN-γ selectively up-regulate vascular CD106 and CD54, respectively. IL4-induced CD106 expression thus facilitates influx of β1-integrin expressing eosinophils and mononuclear cells but not neutrophils (that lack β1-integrins). Other mediators induce the influx of several leukocyte subtypes by increasing expression of a number of endothelial CAMs (e.g., IL-1 and TNF-α induce expression of CD54, CD106, E-selectins, and P-selectins) or by activating leukocytes (e.g., C5a, IL-8, platelet-activating factor [PAF], GM-CSF, and TNF-α activate neutrophils and monocytes).

Mediators may act additively, synergistically, or antagonistically. For example, IFN-γ together with LPS or TNF-α (but not IL-1) prolongs expression of E-selectin.[216, 217] Transforming growth factor-beta (TGF-β) and IL-4, either alone or in combination, inhibit cytokine-induced E-selectin expression.[218, 219]

Finally, differences exist in the adhesive phenotype of endothelium from different vascular beds and in its response to mediators. IL-1 and TNF-α are poor inducers of CD54 on cultured synovial-derived endothelium, in contrast to umbilical vein–derived endothelium.[220] TNF-α can up-regulate expression of CD54 and E-selectin on both arterial and venous-derived endothelium, but the inducible expression of CD106 by TNF-α is restricted to venular endothelium.[221] Other agonists, such as oxidized low-density lipopro-

tein (LDL) and lysophosphocholine, which are associated with atherogenesis, can induce CD106 (and CD54) expression on cultured arterial endothelium[222] and probably contribute to the pathogenesis of atherosclerosis.[223]

Because fewer than 1 in 100,000 lymphocytes are specific for a certain antigen, these cells must continuously circulate through the potential ports of "foreign" antigen entry (lungs, skin, and gastrointestinal tract and their draining lymph nodes) for efficient immune surveillance. Once the specific antigen is encountered on the surface of a dendritic antigen-presenting cell (APC), the naive lymphocyte is held at this site for several days, in close contact with APC. During this time, it is activated and begins to divide, and its progeny re-enter the circulation, homing back to the same site for signal amplification as well as to other sites for dissemination of the immune response. Although effector lymphocytes continue to recirculate for extended periods of time, some terminally differentiated lymphocytes (e.g., γδ intraepithelial and plasma cells) stop recirculating and take permanent residence within organs and mucosal barriers of the body. Naive lymphocytes migrate into lymphoid organs mainly across the cuboidal-shaped endothelium (HEVs), whereas only antigen-activated cells can traverse "flat" endothelium, lining other types of blood vessels.[224] Mediators, including IL-1, INF-γ, and TNF-α, present at chronic inflammatory sites, such as rheumatoid synovium, can induce an HEV-like morphology in the normally flat endothelium of nonlymphoid tissues, thus facilitating large-scale migration of lymphocytes into these sites.

As with phagocyte transendothelial emigration into an infected site, endothelial and leukocyte CAMs and mediators orchestrate the trafficking of lymphocyte subpopulations into lymphoid and nonlymphoid organs. Naive lymphocytes migrate across HEVs of peripheral and mucosal lymph nodes using a selectin-integrin cascade analogous to that of neutrophils. Naive lymphocytes, like resting neutrophils, express L-selectin on surface microvilli, and peripheral lymph node HEVs are rich in GlyCAM-1 and CD34, which explains the early observations that L-selectin is a homing receptor for peripheral lymph nodes.[225] CD54 and CD102, ligands for CD11a, and CD106, the ligand for CD49d, are expressed on peripheral lymph node HEV,[226, 227] accounting for the role of these leukocyte integrins in lymphocyte homing to these as well as other organs. Although anti-CD11a monoclonal antibodies markedly reduce lymphocyte homing to lymph node HEV, lymphocytes do localize in lymph nodes in β2-integrin deficiency, which suggests that other homing receptors—perhaps CD49d/CD29 (α4β1)—compensate for the loss of CD11a.[208]

MAdCAM-1 expression on mucosal lymphoid HEV and the lack of expression of functional GlyCAM-1 or CD34 are important determinants in directing trafficking of naive lymphocytes to mucosal lymphoid tissues. MAdCAM-1 binds L-selectin through its mucin domain and to integrin α4β7 through its N-terminal Ig domain, thus accounting for the limited dependency of lymphocyte trafficking to PP on L-selectin (see Fig. 20–4) and for the fact that mucosal lymphoid tissues in L-selectin knockout mice are populated by lymphocytes.[61, 186, 228, 229] Intravital microscopy of lymphocytes interacting with mucosal HEV reveals a rolling behavior similar to that displayed by neutrophils binding to nonlymphoid endothelium. Lymphocyte rolling is followed by firm adhesion in about 25 percent of the cells (roughly the estimated size of the pool traversing lymph nodes from the blood) and the emigration of these cells to the extravascular interstitium. Rolling, in this case, is probably mediated by the integrin α4β7 and not by a selectin.[230] Antibodies to CD11a also block by 50 to 80 percent lymphocyte migration through mucosal lymph nodes[231]; this is consistent with the function of CD11a as a nonspecific homing receptor.

Although neutrophils also adhere to HEV, they do not normally migrate across it; this suggests that HEVs generate or display mediators that trigger naive lymphocyte migration selectively. Although the nature of these lymphocyte-specific mediators is not certain, the mediators appear to function through a pertussis toxin-sensitive step.[232, 233]

Effector lymphocytes are largely L-selectin–negative, except for memory B cells,[211] but display preactivated α4- and β2-integrins. In addition, MAdCAM-1 is expressed in lesser amounts on flat endothelium than on HEV and is not properly sulfated to serve as an L-selectin ligand; this ensures a predominance of α4β7 and α4β1-integrins mediating contact, rolling, and firm adhesion in nonlymphoid tissues of the gut and in inflamed organs, respectively.[230]

High expression of CD44 on memory cells also facilitates lymphocyte adhesion and transendothelial migration.[234] Expression of intrinsically active integrins in antigen-activated cells does not appear to bypass the requirement for selectins in lymphocyte homing to skin. Memory cells that migrate to skin are L-selectin–positive[211] and selectively express CLA, which may be responsible for lymphocyte homing to skin. Expression of L-selectin may allow this activated lymphocyte subset continued access to peripheral lymph nodes that drain the skin and may also enable these cells to emigrate across flat endothelium at inflammatory sites. This probably occurs through L-selectin binding to a novel non-mucin type ligand belonging to the proteoglycan family.[235] CLA also mediates binding of lymphocytes to E-selectin induced on dermal endothelium at inflamed sites.[230] The precise leukocyte and endothelial cell adhesion profiles responsible for lymphocyte recirculation through other mucosal-associated lymphoid tissues (e.g., bronchial tree) or through lymphoid tissues induced at chronically inflamed sites (e.g., synovium) are not well characterized.

Many adhesion molecules are intrinsically expressed in synovial tissue. These include integrins β1, α5, α6, and β3; P-selectin and E-selectin; CD54; CD106; CD31; and CD44.[236, 237] Expression of CD44, CD31, CD106, and β3 is increased in rheumatoid synovium.[236, 238] Rheumatoid synovium is infiltrated with memory cells, which appear to be α4β7-positive[230]; this suggests that this receptor may also be involved in lymphocyte recirculation to HEV-like lymphoid tissues in inflamed synovium. Whether specific antigen-activated lymphocyte subsets selectively target this organ, as in the case of gut-associated lymphoid tissue, remains to be determined.

Integrins β1 and β2, CD44, and selectins that facilitate leukocyte homing into tissues continue to mediate the subsequent leukocyte interactions with other cell types in the interstitium (e.g., binding to APCs, T cell and B cell cooperation, phagocytosis, and NK cell–mediated or CTL-mediated killing). One reason for this overlap in function is that the latter interactions are, in fact, similar in many respects to leukocyte-endothelial cell interactions. All involve an initial unstable contact between two cell types, which is then stabilized in response to appropriate triggering signals, such as T cell receptor ligation by antigen class I, II complex or by local chemokines. Signals are then communicated between cells, which leads to a specific outcome (e.g., target cell killing or production of a cytokine). After this, cell-cell adhesion is actively reversed, allowing the effector cells to migrate, to seek other target cells, or to engage in other specialized functions. The commonalty in the molecular players mediating extravasation and leukocyte effector functions implies that the in vivo effects of an adhesion antagonist may not be limited to a single cellular event, such as extravasation.

CELL ADHESION MOLECULES AS TARGETS OF ANTI-INFLAMMATORY THERAPEUTICS

The excessive accumulation of activated leukocytes in tissues is a hallmark of acute and chronic inflammatory disorders. In ischemia-reperfusion injury syndromes (e.g., hemorrhagic shock, myocardial infarction, stroke, burns), neutrophilic cell infiltration into ischemic tissues after blood flow is reestablished plays a major role in injury through release of toxic chemicals from activated leukocytes. Similarly, lymphocytic infiltration characterizes many autoimmune diseases (diabetes mellitus, rheumatoid arthritis) and the rejection of allografts. Interruption of leukocyte trafficking into inflamed organs has therefore become a major focus of anti-inflammatory drug development, with its feasibility already established from the discovery and understanding of the pathophysiology of β2-integrin deficiency.[7]

Although little information is available on the role of α4β7 in inflammatory disorders, use of blocking monoclonal antibodies to selectins, β2-integrins, and CD49d/CD29 (α4β1) often results in marked attenuation of the parenchymal and microvascular dysfunctions observed in several animal models of inflammation.[140, 239] In ischemia-reperfusion syndromes, as ischemic tissues are reperfused, neutrophils aggregate, adhere to platelets and endothelium, and extravasate into tissues. Cell aggregates plug the micovasculature, reducing blood flow, which further enhances neutrophil adhesion. Endothelial cell injury caused by activated neutrophils and by ischemia is manifested by cell swelling and loss of the glycocalyx and tight junctions. This, in addition to disruption of the basement membranes, leads to leakage of plasma proteins, more edema, and further reductions in flow, thus establishing a vicious circle of inflammation and injury. In animal models of ischemia-reperfusion injury affecting the whole body,[236] myocardium,[237] skin,[238] brain,[170] intestine,[164] lungs,[240] or skeletal muscle,[180] anti-CD18 monoclonal antibodies improved perfusion of the zones of stasis surrounding wounds, preserving tissues and reducing morbidity and mortality. These effects resulted from anti-CD18–mediated inhibition of extravasation and adhesion-dependent release of toxic radicals and enzymes by neutrophils.

Similar effects have been reported using monoclonal antibodies directed against CD54,[239] a β2-integrin ligand. The latter antibodies, however, appear less effective if administered after exposure of the microvasculature to inflammatory stimuli. This is perhaps a reflection of the inability of anti-CD54 monoclonal antibodies—in contrast to anti-CD18 monoclonal antibodies—to detach already adherent leukocytes from endothelium.[181]

Anti-CD18 and anti-CD54 monoclonal antibodies also reduce inflammation and injury in animal models of allograft rejection,[221, 222, 241] antigen-induced arthritis,[242] diabetes mellitus,[243] immune complex–induced alveolitis,[67] and glomerulonephritis.[242] The inhibitory effects of anti-β2 integrin/ligand monoclonal antibodies in these models is understandably incomplete. Patients with β2-integrin deficiency display near-normal functions of mononuclear cells.[7] As already described, mononuclear leukocytes display and use multiple integrins in mediating cell adhesion, in contrast to neutrophils, which only express β2-integrins. In these and other models of immunologic injury (adjuvant arthritis,[244] ulcerative colitis,[108] experimental allergic encephalomyelitis,[245] contact hypersensitivity,[161] lung antigenic challenge),[204] use of anti-α4 monoclonal antibodies had significant anti-inflammatory effects. In fact, combination of anti-β2- and α4-integrin antibodies inhibit mononuclear leukocyte recruitment almost completely in most of the models tested.[202, 244, 246] As with anti-CD18 monoclonal antibodies, the effects observed with anti-α4 monoclonal antibodies may not be restricted to limiting leukocyte extravasation. This may explain why anti-α4 monoclonal antibodies, while effectively inhibiting T-cell–dependent contact hypersensitivity in murine models, do not appear to do so by reducing the number of infiltrating cells.[247]

Blocking monoclonal antibodies directed against L-, P- or E-selectins have also been effective in several models of ischemia-reperfusion injury,[248, 249] immune-complex diseases,[67, 222, 242] and acute inflammation.[250] In general, the protective effects observed using single anti-selectin monoclonal antibodies is partial,[164] consistent with the transient effects on leukocyte emigration into inflamed tissues observed in either P- or E-selectin knockout mice[251] and in patients with LAD-II disease.[252] The selective blockade of selectins in the experimental models described in this chapter also reveal the differential involvement of selectins in immune injury. For example, E-selectin, but not P-selectin, is important in mediating injury in IgG immune complex lung injury.[67] On the other hand, targeting P-selectin, but not E-selectin, is effective in reducing complement-induced lung injury.[222] These results suggest that the expression profile of adhesion molecules varies in different models, presumably as a function of the different mediators released. Defining these profiles in different pathologic states may facilitate more specific treatments.

SUMMARY

It is now established that cell-cell and cell-matrix interactions mediate or regulate cell differentiation, proliferation, migration, polarity, apoptosis, and many effector cell functions. Several adhesion molecule families orchestrate the multiple and complex adhesive interactions that lead to or facilitate these events. Significant progress has been made in defining the adhesion profiles of many cell types under basal conditions and in response to environmental stimuli and in understanding how these phenotypes are used in cell-cell and cell-matrix communications. Continuation of such efforts should allow the development of physical and functional cell adhesion body maps under normal and pathologic states. These maps could be used in predicting a cellular response, such as the migratory behavior of a leukocyte, platelet or tumor cell and in early interventions aimed at modifying these responses to inhibit injury, promote healing, or prevent metastasis. Much work lies ahead before this futuristic vision is accomplished. The progress made so far, however, in decoding the various cell adhesion networks has significantly advanced our understanding of the molecular basis of disease and promises to provide novel approaches to prevention and treatment.

REFERENCES

1. Wilson HV: On some phenomena of coalescence and regeneration in sponges. J Exp Zool 5:245–258, 1907.
2. Moscona AA: Cell suspensions from organ rudiments of chick embryos. Exp Cell Res 3:536–539, 1952.
3. Sperry RW: Chemoaffinity in the orderly growth of nerve fiber patterns and connections. Proc Natl Acad Sci USA 50:703–710, 1963.
4. Edelman GM: Cell adhesion and morphogenesis: The regulator hypothesis. Proc Natl Acad Sci USA 81:1460–1464, 1984.
5. Williams AF, Barclay AN: The immunoglobulin superfamily: Domains for cell surface recognition. Annu Rev Immunol 6:381–405, 1988.
6. Picker LJ, Butcher EC: Physiological and molecular mechanisms of lymphocyte homing. Annu Rev Immunol 10:561–591, 1992.
7. Arnaout MA: Leukocyte adhesion molecule deficiency: Its structural basis, pathophysiology and implications for modulating the inflammatory response. Immunol Rev 114:145–180, 1990.

8. Kieffer N, Phillips DR: Platelet membrane glycoproteins: Functions in cellular interactions. Annu Rev Cell Biol 6:329–357, 1990.

9. Takeichi M: Cadherins: A molecular family important in selective cell-cell adhesion. Annu Rev Biochem 59:237–252, 1990.

10. Gumbiner B, Simons K: A functional assay for proteins involved in establishing an epithelial occluding barrier: Identification of a uvomorulin-like peptide. J Cell Biol 102:457–468, 1986.

11. Ozawa M, Baribault H, Kemler R: The cytoplasmic domain of the cell adhesion molecule uvomorulin associates with three independent proteins structurally related in different species. EMBO J 8:1711–1717, 1989.

12. Herrenknecht K, Ozawa M, Eckerskorn C, Lottspeich F, Lenter M, Kemler R: The uvomorulin-anchorage protein α catenin is a vinculin homologue. Proc Natl Acad Sci USA 88:9156–9160, 1991.

13. Nagafuchi A, Takeichi M, Tsukita S: The 102 kD cadherin-associated protein: Similarity to vinculin and posttranslational regulation of expression. Cell 65:849–857, 1991.

14. Green KJ, Parry DAD, Steinert PM, Virata MLA, Wagner RM, Angst BD, Nilles LA: Structure of the human desmoplakins. J Biol Chem 265:2603–2612, 1990.

15. Buxton RS, Magee AI: Structure and interactions of desmosomal and other cadherins. Semin Cell Biol 3:157–167, 1992.

16. Inuzuka H, Miyatani S, Takeichi M: R-cadherin: A novel Ca($^{2+}$)-dependent cell-cell adhesion molecule expressed in the retina. Neuron 7:69–79, 1991.

17. Overduin M, Harvey TS, Bagby S, Tong KI, Yau P, Takeichi M, Ikura M: Solution structure of the epithelial cadherin domain responsible for selective cell adhesion. Science 267:386–389, 1995.

18. Shapiro L, Fannon AM, Kwong PD, Thompson A, Lehmann MS, Grubel G, Legrand J-F, Als-Nielsen J, Colman DR, Hendrickson WA: Structural basis of cell-cell adhesion by cadherins. Nature 374:327–337, 1995.

19. Gumbiner BM: Proteins associated with the cytoplasmic surface of adhesion molecules. Neuron 11:551–564, 1993.

20. Bjorkman PJ, Saper MA, Samraoui B, Bennet WS, Strominger JL, Wiley DC: Structure of the human class I histocompatibility antigen HLA-A2. Nature (Lond) 329:512–518, 1987.

21. Edelman GM: Morphoregulatory molecules. Am Chem Soc 27:3533–3545, 1988.

22. Edelman GM: Cell adhesion molecules in the regulation of animal form and tissue pattern. Cell Biol 2:81–116, 1986.

23. Dodd J, Jessell TM: Axon guidance and the patterning of neuronal projections in vertebrates. Science 242:692–699, 1988.

24. Makgoba MW, Sanders ME, Shaw S: The CD2-LFA-3 and LFA-1-ICAM pathways: Relevance to T-cell recognition. Immunol Today 10:417–422, 1989.

25. Hynes RO: Integrins: Versatility, modulation and signaling in cell adhesion. Cell 69:11–26, 1992.

26. Berendt AR, McDowall A, Craig AG, Bates PA, Sternberg MJE, Marsh K, Newbold CI, Hogg N: The binding site on ICAM-1 for *Plasmodium falciparum*–infected erythrocytes overlaps but is distinct from the LFA-1 binding site. Cell 68:71–82, 1992.

27. Greve JM, Davis G, Meyer AM, Forte CP, Yost SC, Marlor CW, Kamarck ME, McClelland A: The major human Rhinovirus receptor is ICAM-1. Cell 56:839–847, 1989.

28. Dalgleish AG, Beverley PC, Clapham PR, Crawford DH, Greaves MF, Weiss RA: The CD4 (T4) antigen is an essential component of the receptor for the AIDS retrovirus. Nature (Lond) 312:763–767, 1984.

29. Arnaout MA: Structure and function of the leukocyte adhesion molecules CD11/CD18. Blood 75:1037–1050, 1990.

30. Hemler ME: VLA proteins in the integrin family: Structures, functions, and their role on leukocytes. Annu Rev Immunol 8:365–400, 1990.

31. Ruoslahti E: Integrins. J Clin Invest 87:1–5, 1991.

32. Kelly T, Molony L, Burridge K: Purification of two smooth muscle glycoproteins related to integrin. J Biol Chem 262:17189–17199, 1987.

33. Nermut MV, Green NM, Eason P, Yamada SS, Yamada KM: Electron microscopy and structural model of human fibronectin receptor. EMBO J 7:4093–4099, 1988.

34. Michishita M, Videm V, Arnaout MA: A novel divalent cation-binding site in the A domain of the β2 integrin CR3 (CD11b/CD18) is essential for ligand binding. Cell 72:857–867, 1993.

35. Lee J-O, Rieu P, Arnaout MA, Liddington R: Crystal structure of the A-domain from the α-subunit of β2 integrin complement receptor type 3 (CR3, CD11b/CD18). Cell 80:631–638, 1995.

36. Fox G, Parry NR, Barnett PV, McGinn B, Rowlands DJ, Brown F: The cell attachment site on foot-and-mouth disease virus includes the amino acid sequence RGD (arginine-glycine-aspartic acid). J Gen Virol 70:625–637, 1989.

37. Brake DA, Debouck C, Biesecker G: Identification of an Arg-Gly-Asp (RGD) cell adhesion site in human immunodeficiency virus type I transactivating protein, tat. J Cell Biol 111:1275–1281, 1990.

38. Isberg RR, Leong JM: Multiple β1, chain integrins are receptors for invasin, a protein that promotes bacterial penetration into mammalian cells. Cell 60:861–871, 1990.

39. Takada Y, Hemler ME: The primary structure of the VLA-2/collagen receptor α2 subunit (platelet GPIa): Homology to other integrins and the presence of a possible collagen-binding domain. J Cell Biol 109:397–408, 1989.

40. Elices MJ, Osborn L, Takada Y, Crouse C, Luhowskyj S, Hemier ME, Lobb RR: VCAM-1 on activated endothelium interacts with the leukocyte integrin VLA-4 at a site distinct from the VLA-4/fibronectin binding site. Cell 60:577–584, 1990.

41. Carter WG, Wayner EA, Bouchard TS, Kaur P: The role of integrins α2β1 and α3β1 in cell-cell and cell substrate adhesion of human epidermal cells. J Cell Biol 110:1387–1404, 1990.

42. Rieu P, Arnaout MA: The structural basis and regulation of β2 integrin interactions. In Ward JC, Fantone JC, Lenfant C (eds): Lung Biology in Health and Disease. New York, Marcel Dekker, 1996, pp 1–42.

43. Murphy JF, Bordet JC, Wyler B, Rissoan MC, Chmarat P, Defrance T, Miossec P, McGregor JL: The vitronectin receptor (alpha v beta 3) is implicated in cooperation with P-selectin and platelet-activating factor, in the adhesion of monocytes to activated endothelial cells. Biochem J 304:537–542, 1994.

44. Lakkakorpi PT, Horton MA, Helfrich MH, Karhukorpi EK, Vaananen HK: Vitronectin receptor has a role in bone resorption but does not mediate tight sealing zone attachment of osteoclasts to the bone surface. J Cell Biol 115:1179–1186, 1991.

45. Brooks PC, Montgomery AM, Rosenfeld M, Reisfeld RA, Hu T, Klier G, Cheresh DA: Integrin alpha v beta 3 antagonists promote tumor regression by inducing apoptosis of angiogenic blood vessels. Cell 79:1157–1164, 1994.

46. Gresham HD, Goodwin JL, Allen PM, Anderson DC, Brown EJ: A novel member of the integrin receptor family mediates Arg-Gly-Asp-stimulated neutrophil phagocytosis. J Cell Biol 108:1935–1943, 1989.

47. Takahashi T, Nakamura T, Koyanagi M, Kato K, Hashimoto Y, Yagita H, Okumura K: A murine very late activation antigen-like extracellular matrix receptor involved in CD2- and lymphocyte function-associated antigen-1–independent killer-target cell interaction. J Immunol 145:4371–4379, 1990.

48. Suzuki S, Naitoh Y: Amino acid sequence of a novel integrin β4 subunit and primary expression of the mRNA in epithelial cells. EMBO J 9:757–763, 1990.

49. Sheppard D, Rozzo C, Starr L, Quaranta V, Erle DJ, Pytela R: Complete amino acid sequence of a novel integrin β subunit (β6) identified in epithelial cells using the polymerase chain reaction. J Biol Chem 265:11502–11507, 1990.

50. Kajiji S, Tamura RN, Quaranta V: A novel integrin (αE-β4) from human epithelial cells suggests a fourth family of integrin adhesion receptors. EMBO J 8:673–680, 1989.

51. Holzmann B, McIntyre BW, Weissman IL: Identification of a murine Peyer's patch-specific lymphocyte homing receptor as an integrin molecule with an α chain homologous to human VLA-4α. Cell 56:37–46, 1989.

52. Ramaswamy H, Hemler ME: Cloning, primary structure and properties of a novel human integrin β subunit. EMBO J 9:1561–1568, 1990.

53. Pytela R, Suzuki S, Breuss J, Erle DJ, Sheppard D: Polymerase chain reaction cloning with degenerate primers: Homology-based identification of adhesion molecules. Methods Enzymol 245:420–451, 1994.

54. Nishimura SL, Sheppard D, Pytela R: Integrin alpha v beta 8: Interaction with vitronectin and functional divergence of the beta 8 cytoplasmic domain. J Biol Chem 269:28708–28715, 1994.

55. Cheresh DA, Smith JW, Cooper HM, Quaranta V: A novel vitronectin receptor integrin (αᵥ βₓ) is responsible for distinct adhesive properties of carcinoma cells. Cell 57:59, 1989.

56. Freed E, Gailit J, van der Geer P, Ruoslahti E, Hunter T: A novel integrin β subunit is associated with the vitronectin receptor α subunit (αV) in a human osteosarcoma cell line and is a substrate for protein kinase C. EMBO J 8:2955–2965, 1989.

57. Moyle M, Napier MA, McLean JW: Cloning and expression of a divergent integrin subunit β8. J Biol Chem 266:19650–19658, 1991.

58. Falcioni R, Kennel SJ, Giacomini P, Zupi G, Sacchi A: Expression of tumor antigen correlated with metastatic potential of Lewis lung carcinoma and B16 melanoma clones in mice. Cancer Res 46:5772–5778, 1986.

59. Erle DJ, Ruegg C, Sheppard D, Pytela R: Complete amino acid sequence of an integrin beta subunit (beta 7) identified in leukocytes. J Biol Chem 266:11009–11016, 1991.

60. Hu MC-T, Crowe DT, Weissman IL, Holzmann B: Cloning and expression of mouse integrin bp(b7): A functional role in Peyer's patch-specific lymphocyte homing. Proc Natl Acad Sci USA 89:8254–8258, 1992.

61. Issekutz TB: Inhibition of in vivo lymphocyte migration to inflammation and homing to lymphoid tissues by the TA-2 monoclonal antibody: A likely role for VLA-4 in vivo. J Immunol 147:4178–4184, 1991.

62. Parker CM, Cepek K, Russell GJ, Shaw SK, Posnett D, Schwarting R, Brenner MB: A family of β7 integrins on human mucosal lymphocytes. Proc Natl Acad Sci USA 89:1924–1928, 1992.

63. Cepek KL, Shaw SK, Parker CM, Russell GJ, Morrow JS, Rimm DL,

Brenner MB: Adhesion between epithelial cells and T lymphocytes mediated by E-cadherin and the alpha E beta 7 integrin. Nature 372:190–193, 1994.

64. Hemler ME, Elices MJ, Chan BM, Zetter B, Matsuura N, Takada Y: Multiple ligand binding functions for VLA-2 (alpha 2 beta 1) and VLA-3 (alpha 3 beta 1) in the integrin family. Cell Differential Dev 32:229–238, 1990.

65. Bodary SC, Mclean JW: The integrin β1 subunit associates with the vitronectin receptor αV subunit to form a novel vitronectin receptor in human embryonic kidney cell line. J Biol Chem 265:5938–5941, 1990.

66. Vogel BE, Tarone G, Giancotti FG, Gailit J, Ruoslahti E: A novel fibronectin receptor with an unexpected subunit composition. J Biol Chem 265:5934–5937, 1990.

67. Mulligan MS, Wilson GP, Todd RF, Smith CW, Anderson DC, Varani J, Issekutz TB, Miyasaka M, Tamatani T, Rusche JR, Vaporciyan AA, Ward PA: Role of β1 and β2 integrins and ICAM-1 in lung injury after deposition of IgG and IgA immune complexes. J Immunol 150:2407–2417, 1993.

68. Wayner EA, Carter WG: Identification of multiple cell adhesion receptor for collagen and fibronectin in human fibrosarcoma cells possessing unique αβ subunits. J Cell Biol 105:1873, 1987.

69. D'Souza SE, Ginsberg MH, Burke TA, Lam SC-T, and Plow EF: Localization of an Arg-Gly-Asp recognition site within an integrin adhesion receptor. Science (Washington) 242:91–93, 1988.

70. D'Souza SE, Ginsberg MH, Burke TA, Plow EF: The ligand binding site of the platelet integrin receptor GP IIb-IIIa is proximal to the second calcium binding domain of its α subunit. J Biol Chem 265:3440–3446, 1990.

71. Arnaout MA, Spits H, Terhorst C, Pitt J, Todd RF III: Deficiency of a leukocyte surface glycoprotein (LFA-1) in two patients with Mo1 deficiency: Effects of cell activation on Mo1/LFA-1 surface expression in normal and deficient leukocytes. J Clin Invest 74:1291–1300, 1984.

72. van Kuppevelt THMSM, Languino LR, Gailit JO, Suzuki S, Ruoslahti E: An alternative cytoplasmic domain of the integrin β3 subunit. Proc Natl Acad Sci USA 86:5415–5418, 1989.

73. Staatz WD, Walsh JJ, Pexton T, Santoro SA: The α2β1 integrin cell surface collagen receptor binds to the α1(I)-CB3 peptide of collagen. J Biol Chem 265:4778–4781, 1990.

74. Elices MJ, Hemler ME: The human integrin VLA-2 is a collagen receptor on some cells and a collagen/laminin receptor on others. Proc Natl Acad Sci USA 86:9906–9910, 1989.

75. Sonnenberg A, Modderman PW, Hogervorst F: Laminin receptor on platelets is the integrin VLA-6. Nature 336:487–489, 1988.

76. D'Souza SE, Haas TA, Piotrowicz RS, Byers WV, McGrath DE, Soule HR, Cierniewski C, Plow EF, Smith JW: Ligand and cation binding are dual functions of a discrete segment of the integrin beta 3 subunit: Cation displacement is involved in ligand binding. Cell 79:659–667, 1994.

77. Grzesiak JJ, Pierschbacher MD: Shifts in the concentration of magnesium and calcium in early porcine and rat wound fluids activate the cell migratory response. J Clin Invest 95:227–233, 1995.

78. Kirchhofer D, Languino LR, Ruoslahti E, Pierschbacher MD: α2β1 integrins from different cell types show different binding specificities. J Biol Chem 265:615–618, 1990.

79. Juliano RL, Haskill S: Signal transduction from the extracellular matrix. J Cell Biol 120:577–585, 1993.

80. Boudreau N, Sympson CJ, Werb Z, Bissell MJ: Suppression of ICE and apoptosis in mammary epithelial cells by extracellular matrix. Science 267:891–893, 1995.

81. Guan J-L, Shalloway D: Regulation of focal adhesion-associated protein tyrosine kinase by both cellular adhesion and oncogenic transformation. Nature 358:690–692, 1992.

82. Fallman M, Gullberg M, Hellberg C, Andersson T: Complement receptor–mediated phagocytosis is associated with accumulation of phosphatidylcholine-derived diglyceride in human neutrophils: Involvement of phospholipase D and direct evidence for a positive feedback signal of protein kinase C. J Biol Chem 267:2656–2663, 1992.

83. Jaconi MEE, Theler JM, Schlegel W, Appel RD, Wright SD, Lew PD: Multiple elevations of cytosolic-free Ca²⁺ in human neutrophils: Initiation by adherence receptors of the integrin family. J Cell Biol 112:1249–1257, 1991.

84. Banga HS, Simmons ER, Brass LF, Rittenhouse SE: Activation of phospholipases A and C in human platelets exposed to epinephrine: Role of glycoproteins IIb/IIIa and dual role of epinephrine. Proc Natl Acad Sci USA 83:9197–9201, 1986.

85. Schwartz MA, Lechene C, Ingbar DE: Insoluble fibronectin activates the Na/H antiporter by clustering and immobilizing integrin α5β1, independent of cell shape. Proc Natl Acad Sci USA 88:7849–7853, 1991.

86. Fox JE, Taylor RG, Taffarel M, Boyles JK, Goll DE: Evidence that activation of platelet calpain is induced as a consequence of binding of adhesive ligand to the integrin, glycoprotein IIb-IIIa. J Cell Biol 120:1501–1507, 1993.

87. Juliano R: Signal transduction by integrins and its role in the regulation of tumor growth. Cancer Metastasis Rev 13:25–30, 1994.

88. Chen HC, Guan JL: Association of focal adhesion kinase with its potential substrate phosphatidylinositol 3-kinase. Proc Natl Acad Sci USA 91:10148–10152, 1994.

89. Chen Q, Kinch MS, Lin TH, Burridge K, Juliano RL: Integrin-mediated cell adhesion activates mitogen-activated protein kinases. J Biol Chem 269:26602–26605, 1994.

90. Chong LD, Traynor KA, Bokoch GM, Schwartz MA: The small GTP-binding protein Rho regulates a phosphatidylinositol 4-phosphate 5-kinase in mammalian cells. Cell 79:507–513, 1994.

91. Clark EA, Brugge JS: Redistribution of activated pp60c-src to integrin-dependent cytoskeletal complexes in thrombin-stimulated platelets. Mol Cell Biol 13:1863–1871, 1993.

92. Zhang J, Fry MJ, Waterfield MD, Jaken S, Liao L, Fox JEB, Rittenhouse SE: Activated-phosphoinositides-3-kinase associates with membrane skeleton in thrombin exposed platelets. J Biol Chem 267:4686–4692, 1992.

93. Fox JEB, Lipfert L, Clark EA, Reynolds CC, Austin CD, Brugge J: On the role of the platelet membrane skeleton in mediating signal transduction: Association of GP IIb-IIIa, pp60c-src, pp62c-yes, and the p21ras GTPase-activating protein with the membrane skeleton. J Biol Chem 268:25973–25984, 1993.

94. Arroyo AG, Campanero MR, Sánchez-Mateo P, Zapata JM, Ursa MA, del Pozo MA, Sánchez-Madrid F: Induction of tyrosine phosphorylation during ICAM-3 and LFA-1–mediated intercellular adhesion, and its regulation by the CD45 tyrosine phosphatase. J Cell Biol 126:1277–1286, 1994.

95. Frangioni JV, Oda A, Smith M, Salzman EW, Neel BG: Calpain-catalyzed cleavage and subcellular relocation of protein phosphotyrosine phosphatase 1B (PTP-1B) in human platelets. EMBO J 12:4843–4856, 1993.

96. Detmers PA, Wright SD, Olsen E, Kimball B, Cohn ZA: Aggregation of complement receptors on human neutrophils in the absence of ligand. J Cell Biol 105:1137–1145, 1987.

97. Isenberg WM, McEver RP, Philips DR, Shuman MA, Bainton DF: The platelet fibrinogen receptor: An immunogold surface replica study of agonist-induced ligand binding and receptor clustering. J Cell Biol 104:1655–1663, 1987.

98. LaFlamme SE, Akiyama SK, Yamada KM: Regulation of fibronectin receptor distribution. J Cell Biol 117:437–447, 1992.

99. LaFlamme SE, Thomas LA, Yamada SS, Yamada KM: Single subunit chimeric integrins as mimics and inhibitors of endogenous integrin functions in receptor localization, cell spreading and migration, and matrix assembly. J Cell Biol 126:1287–1298, 1994.

100. Kassner PD, Kawaguchi S, Hemler ME: Minimum α chain cytoplasmic tail sequence needed to support integrin-mediated adhesion. J Biol Chem 269:19859–19867, 1994.

101. Miyamoto S, Akiyama SK, Yamada KM: Synergistic roles for receptor occupancy and aggregation in integrin transmembrane function. Science 267:883–885, 1995.

102. Lipfert L, Haimovich B, Schaller MD, Cobb BS, Parsons JT, Brugge JS: Integrin-dependent phosphorylation and activation of the protein kinase pp125FAK in platelets. J Cell Biol 119:905–912, 1992.

103. Haimovich B, Lipfert L, Brugge JS, Shattil SJ: Tyrosine phosphorylation and cytoskeletal reorganization in platelets are triggered by interaction of integrin receptors with their immobilized ligands. J Biol Chem 268:15868–15877, 1993.

104. Lasky LA, Rosen SD: The selectins: Carbohydrate-binding adhesion molecules of the immune system. In Gallin J, Goldstein I, Snyderman R (eds): Inflammation: Basic Principles and Clinical Correlates. New York, Raven Press, 1992, pp 407–419.

105. Graves BJ, Crowther RL, Chandran C, Rumberger JM, Li S, Huang K-S, Presky DH, Familletti PC, Wolitzky BA, Burns DK: Insight into E-selectin/ligand interaction from the crystal structure and mutagenesis of the lec/EGF domains. Nature 367:532–538, 1994.

106. Varki A: Selectin ligands. Proc Natl Acad Sci USA 91:7390–7397, 1994.

107. von Adrian UH, Berger EM, Ramezani L, Chambers JD, Ochs HD, Harlan JM, Paulson JC, Etzioni A, Arfors K-E: In vivo behavior of neutrophils from two patients with distinct inherited leukocyte adhesion deficiency syndromes. J Clin Invest 91:2893–2897, 1993.

108. Weyrich AS, Ma X-L, Lefer DJ, Albertine KH, Lefer AM: In vivo neutralization of P-selectin protects feline heart and endothelium in myocardial ischemia and reperfusion injury. J Clin Invest 91:2620–2629, 1993.

109. Camerini D, James SP, Stamenkovic I, Seed B: Leu8/TQ1 is the human equivalent of the MEL-14 lymph node homing receptor. Nature 342:78–82, 1989.

110. Briskin MJ, McEvoy LM, Butcher EC: MAdCAM-1 has homology to immunoglobulin and mucin-like adhesion receptors and to IgA1. Nature 363:461–464, 1993.

111. Lasky LA, Singer MS, Dowbenko D, Imai Y, Henzel WJ, Grimley C, Fennie C, Gillett N, Watson SR, Rosen SD: An endothelial ligand for L-selectin is a novel mucin-like molecule. Cell 69:927–938, 1992.

112. Baumueter S, Singer MS, Henzel W, Hemmerich S, Renz M, Rosen SD, Lasky LA: Binding of L-selectin to the vascular sialomucin CD34. Science 262:436–438, 1993.

113. Berg EL, McEvoy LM, Berlin C, Bargatze RF, Butcher EC: L-selectin–mediated lymphocyte rolling on MAdCAM-1. Nature 366:695–698, 1993.

114. Mebius RE, Dowenko D, Williams A, Fennie C, Lasky LA, Watson SR: The expression of Gly-CAM-1, an endothelial ligand for L-selectin, is affected by afferent lymphatic flow. J Immunol 1994.

115. Imhof BA, Ruiz P, Hesse B, Palacios R, Dunon D: EA-1, a novel adhesion molecule involved in the homing of progenitor T lymphocytes to the thymus. J Cell Biol 114:1069–1078, 1991.

116. Norgard-Sumnicht KE, Varki NM, Varki A: Calcium dependent heparin-like ligands for L-selectin in nonlymphoid endothelial cells. Science 261:480–483, 1993.

117. Picker LJ, Warnock RA, Burns AR, Doerschuk CM, Berg EL, Butcher EC: The neutrophil selectin LECAM-1 presents carbohydrate ligands to the vascular selectins ELAM-1 and GMP-140. Cell 66:921–933, 1991.

118. von Andrian UH, Chambers JD, McEvoy LM, Bargatze RF, Arfors KE, Butcher EC: Two-step model of leukocyte-endothelial cell interaction in inflammation: Distinct roles for LECAM-1 and the leukocyte β2 integrins in vivo. Proc Natl Acad Sci USA 88:7538–7542, 1991.

119. Spertini O, Kansas GS, Munro JM, Griffin JD, Tedder TF: Regulation of migration by activation of the leukocyte adhesion molecule-1 (LAM-1) selectin. Nature 349:691–694, 1991.

120. Schleiffenbaum B, Spertini O, Tedder TF: Soluble L-selectin is present in human plasma at high levels and retains functional activity. J Cell Biol 119:229, 1992.

121. Johnston GI, Cook RG, McEver RP: Cloning of GMP-140, a granule membrane protein of platelets and endothelium: Sequence similarity to proteins involved in cell adhesion and inflammation. Cell 56:1033–1044, 1989.

122. Weller A, Isenmann S, Vestweber D: Cloning of the mouse endothelial selectins: Expression of both E- and P-selectin is inducible by tumor necrosis factor-alpha. J Biol Chem 267:15176–15183, 1992.

123. Strubel NA, Nguyen M, Kansa GS, Tedder TF, Bischoff J: Isolation and characterization of a bovine cDNA encoding a functional homologue of human P-selectin. BBRC 192:338, 1993.

124. Johnston GI, Bliss GA, Newman PJ, McEver RP: Structure of the human gene encoding granule membrane protein 140, a member of the selectin family of adhesion receptors for leukocytes. J Biol Chem 265:21381–21385, 1990.

125. Sako D, Chang X-J, Barone KM, Vachino G, White HM, Shaw G, Veldman GM, Bean KM, Ahern TJ, Furie B, Cumming DA, Larsen GR: Expression cloning of a functional glycoprotein ligand for P-selectin. Cell 75:1179–1186, 1993.

126. Moore KL, Patel KD, Bruehl RE, Fugang L, Johnson DA, Lichtenstein HS, Cummings RD, Bainton DF, McEver RP: P-selectin glycoprotein ligand-1 mediates rolling of human neutrophils on P-selectin. J Cell Biol 128:661–671, 1995.

127. Lenter M, Levinovitz A, Isenman S, Vestweber D: Monospecific and common glycoprotein ligands for E- and P-selectin on myeloid cells. J Cell Biol 125:471, 1994.

128. McEver RP, Beckstead JH, Moore KL, Marshall-Carlson L, Bainton DF: GMP-140, a platelet a granule membrane protein, is also synthesized by vascular endothelial cells and is localized in Weibel-Palade bodies. J Clin Invest 84:92–99, 1989.

129. Disdier M, Morrissey JH, Fugate RD, Bainton DF, McEver RP: Cytoplasmic domain of P-selectin (CD62) contains the signal for sorting into the regulated secretory pathway. Mol Biol Cell 3:309–321, 1992.

130. Hattori R, Hamilton KK, Fugate RD, McEver RP, Sims PJ: Stimulated secretion of endothelial von Willebrand factor is accompanied by rapid redistribution to the cell surface of the intercellular granule membrane protein GMP-140. J Biol Chem 264:7768–7771, 1989.

131. Hsu-Lin S-C, Berman CL, Furie BC, August D, Furie B: A platelet membrane protein expressed during platelet activation and secretion. J Biol Chem 259:9121–9126, 1984.

132. Zimmerman GA, Prescott SM, McIntyre TM: Endothelial cell interactions with granulocytes: Tethering and signaling molecules. Immunol Today 13:93–100, 1992.

133. Patel KD, Zimmerman GA, Prescott SM, McEver RP, McIntyre TM: Oxygen radicals induce human endothelial cells to express GMP-140 and bind neutrophils. J Cell Biol 112:749–759, 1991.

134. Sanders WE, Wilson RW, Ballantyne CM, Beaudet AL: Molecular cloning and analysis of in vivo expression of murine P-selectin. Blood 80:795–800, 1992.

135. Larsen E, Palabrica T, Sajer S, Gilbert GE, Wagner DD, Furie BC, Furie B: PADGEM-dependent adhesion of platelets to monocytes and neutrophils is mediated by a lineage-specific carbohydrate, LNF III (CD15). Cell 63:467–474, 1990.

136. Aruffo A, Kolanus W, Walz G, Fredman P, Seed B: CD62/P-selectin recognition of myeloid and tumor cell sulfatides. Cell 67:35–44, 1991.

137. Lawrence MB, Springer TA: Leukocytes roll on a selectin at physiologic flow rates: Distinction from and prerequisite for adhesion through integrins. Cell 65:859–873, 1991.

138. Wong CS, Gamble JR, Skinner MP, Lucas CM, Berndt MC, Vadas MA: Adhesion to GMP140 inhibits superoxide anion release human neutrophils. Proc Natl Acad Sci USA 88:2397–2401, 1991.

139. Lorant DE, Tophan MK, Whatley RE, McEver RP, McIntyre TM, Prescott SM, Zimmerman GA: Inflammatory roles of P-selectin. J Clin Invest 92:559–570, 1993.

140. Albelda SM, Smith CW, Ward PA: Adhesion molecules and inflammatory injury. FASEB J 8:504–512, 1994.

141. Palabrica T, Lobb R, Furie BC, Aronowitz M, Benjamin C, Hsu Y-M, Sajer SA, Furie B: Leukocyte accumulation promoting fibrin deposition is mediated in vivo by P-selectin on adherent platelets. Nature 359:848–851, 1992.

142. Wershil BK, Wang Z-S, Gordon JR, Galli SJ: Recruitment of neutrophils during IgE-dependent cutaneous late phase reactions in the mouse is mast cell–dependent. J Clin Invest 87:446–453, 1991.

143. Leung DYM, Pober JS, Cotran RS: Expression of endothelial-leukocyte adhesion molecule-1 in elicited late phase allergic reactions. J Clin Invest 87:1805–1809, 1991.

144. Bevilacqua MP, Pober JS, Mendrick DL, Cotran RS, Gimbrone MA Jr: Identification of an inducible endothelial-leukocyte adhesion molecule. Proc Natl Acad Sci USA 84:9238–9242, 1987.

145. Bochner BS, Lusinskas FW, Gimbrone MA, Newman W, Sterbinsky SA, Derse-Anthony CP, Klunk D, Schleimer RP: Adhesion of human basophils, eosinophils, and neutrophils to interleukin 1–activated human vascular endothelial cells: Contributions of endothelial cell adhesion molecules. J Exp Med 173:1553–1556, 1991.

146. Rice GE, Bevilacqua MP: An inducible endothelial cell surface glycoprotein mediates melanoma adhesion. Science 246:1303–1306, 1989.

147. Picker LJ, Kishimoto TK, Smith CW, Warnock RA, Butcher EC: ELAM-1 is an adhesion molecule for skin-homing T cells. Nature 349:796–799, 1991.

148. Steegmaler M, Levinovitz A, Isenmann S, Borges E, Lenter M, Kocher HP, Kleuser B, Vestweber D: The E-selectin ligand ESL-1 is a variant of a receptor for fibroblast growth factor. Nature 373:615–620, 1995.

149. Walcheck B, Watts G, Jutila MA: Bovine gamma/delta T cells bind E-selectin via a novel glycoprotein receptor: First characterization of a lymphocyte/E-selectin interaction in an animal model. J Exp Med 178:853–863, 1993.

150. Jentoft N: Why are proteins O-glycosylated? Trends Biochem Sci 15:291–294, 1990.

151. Fukuda M, Carlsson SR, Kock JC, Dell A: Structures of O-linked oligosaccharides isolated from normal granulocytes, chronic myelogenous leukemia cells, and acute myelogenous leukemia cells. J Biol Chem 261:12796–12806, 1986.

152. Piller F, Piller V, Fox RI, Fukuda M: Human T-lymphocyte activation is associated with changes in O-glycan biosynthesis. J Biol Chem 263:15146–15150, 1988.

153. Thomas ML: The leukocyte common antigen family. Annu Rev Immunol 7:339–369, 1989.

154. Lopez J, Ludwig E, McCarthy BJ: Polymorphism of human glycoprotein Iba results from a variable number of tandem repeats of a 13-amino acid sequence in the mucin-like macroglycopeptide region. J Biol Chem 267:10055–10061, 1992.

155. Gendler S, Taylor-Papadimitriou J, Duhig T, Rothbard J, Burchell J: A highly immunogenic region of a human polymorphic epithelial mucin expressed by carcinomas is made up of tandem repeats. J Biol Chem 263:12820–12823, 1988.

156. Siddiqui J, Abe M, Hayes D, Shani E, Yunis E, Kufe D: Isolation and sequencing of a cDNA coding for the human DF3 breast carcinoma associated antigen. Proc Natl Acad Sci USA 85:2320–2323, 1988.

157. Cyster JG, Shotton DM, Williams AF: The dimensions of the T lymphocyte glycoprotein leukosialin and identification of linear protein epitopes that can be modified by glycosylation. EMBO J 10:893–902, 1991.

158. Ardman B, Sikorski MA, Staunton DE: CD43 interferes with T-lymphocyte adhesion. Proc Natl Acad Sci USA 89:5001–5005, 1992.

159. Florman HM, Wassarman PM: O-Linked oligosaccharides of mouse egg ZP3 account for its sperm receptor activity. Cell 41:313–324, 1985.

160. Blobel CP, Wolfsberg TG, Turck CW, Myles DG, Primakoff P, White JM: A potential fusion peptide and an integrin ligand domain in a protein active in sperm-egg fusion. Science 356:248–252, 1992.

161. Winn RK, Liggit D, Vedder NB, Paulson JC, Harlan JM: Anti-P selectin monoclonal antibody attenuates reperfusion injury to the rabbit ear. J Clin Invest 92:2042–2047, 1993.

162. Schmid K, Hediger M, Brossmer R, Collins J, Haupt H, Marti T, Offner G, Schaller J, Takagaki K, Walsh M, Schwick H, Rosen F, Remold-O'Donnell E: Amino acid sequence of human plasma galactoglycoprotein: Identity with the extracellular region of CD43 (sialophorin). Proc Natl Acad Sci USA 89:663–667, 1992.

163. Fox JEB, Aggerbeck LA, Berndt MC: Structure of the glycoprotein Ib-IX complex from platelet membranes. J Biol Chem 263:1525–1538, 1988.

164. Barasch J, Kiss B, Prince A, Saiman L, Gruenert D, Al-Awqati Q: Defective acidification of intracellular organelles in cystic fibrosis. Nature 352:70–73, 1991.

165. Hardingham TE, Fosang AJ: Proteoglycans: Many forms and many functions. FASEB J 6:861–870, 1992.

166. Yanagishita M, Hascall VC: Cell surface heparan sulphate proteoglycans. J Biol Chem 267:9451–9454, 1992.

167. Kjellen L, Lindhal U: Proteoglycans: Structures and interactions. Annu Rev Biochem 60:443–475, 1991.

168. David G, Lories V, Decock B, Marynen P, Cassiman J-J, Van den Berghe H: Molecular cloning of a phosphatidylinositol-anchored membrane heparan sulfate proteoglycan from human lung fibroblasts. J Cell Biol 111:3165–3176, 1990.

169. Hook M, Kjellen L, Johansson S, Robinson J: Cell surface glycosaminoglycans. Annu Rev Biochem 53:847–867, 1984.

170. Gabriel SE, Clark LL, Boucher RC, Stutts MJ: CFTR and outward rectifying chloride channels are distinct proteins with a regulatory relationship. Nature 363:263–266, 1993.

171. Lee TH, Wiseniewski H-G, Vilcek J: A novel tumor necrosis factor-inducible protein (TSG-6) is a member of the family of hyaluronate binding proteins, closely related to the adhesion receptor CD44. J Cell Biol 116:545–557, 1992.

172. Andres JL, Stanley K, Cheifetz S, Massague J: Membrane-anchored and soluble forms of betaglycan, a polymorphic proteoglycan that binds transforming growth factor B. J Cell Biol 109:3137–3145, 1989.

173. Kiefer MC, Stephans JC, Crawford K, Okino K, Barr PJ: Ligand-affinity cloning and structure of a cell surface heparan sulphate proteoglycan that binds basic fibroblast growth factor. Proc Natl Acad Sci USA 87:6985–6989, 1990.

174. Shieh M-T, WuDunn D, Montgomery RI, Esko JD, Spear PG: Cell surface receptors for herpes simplex virus are heparan sulphate proteoglycans. J Cell Biol 116:1273–1281, 1992.

175. Heingard D, Oldberg A: Structure and biology of cartilage and bone matrix noncollagenous macromolecules. FASEB J 3:2042–2051, 1989.

176. Kobe B, Deisenhofer J: Crystal structure of porcine ribonuclease inhibitor, a protein with leucine-rich repeats. Nature 366:751–756, 1993.

177. Burridge K, Fath K, Kelly T, Nuckolls G, Turner C: Focal adhesions: Transmembrane junctions between the extracellular matrix and cytoskeleton. Annu Rev Cell Biol 4:487–525, 1988.

178. Garrigues HJ, Lark MW, Lara S, Hellstrom I, Hellstrom KE, Wight TN: The melanoma proteoglycan: Restricted expression on microspikes, a specific microdomain of the cell surface. J Cell Biol 103:1699–1710, 1986.

179. Lesley JR, Hyman R, Kincade PW: CD44 and its interaction with the extracellular matrix. Adv Immunol 54:271–335, 1994.

180. Green ED, Gruenebaum J, Bielinska M, Baenziger JU, Boime I: Sulfation of lutropin oligosaccharides with a cell-free system. 81:5320–5324, 1984.

181. Parkos CA, Colgan SP, Bacarra AE, Nusrat A, Delp-Archer C, Carlson S, Su DHC, Madara JL: Intestinal epithelia (T84) possess basolateral ligands for CD11b/CD18-mediated neutrophil adherence. Am J Physiol 268:C472–C479, 1995.

182. Screaton GR, Bell MV, Bell I, Jackson DG: The identification of a new alternative exon with highly restricted tissue expression in transcripts encoding the mouse Pgp-1 (CD44) homing receptor. J Biol Chem 268:12235–12238, 1993.

183. Jackson DG, Bell JI, Dickinson R, Timans J, Shields J, Whittle N: Proteoglycan forms of the lymphocyte homing receptor CD44 are alternatively spliced variants containing the v3 exon. J Cell Biol 128:673–685, 1995.

184. Stamenkovic I, Aruffo A, Amiot M, Seed B: The hematopoeitic and epithelial forms of CD44 are distinct polypeptides with different adhesion potentials for hyaluronate-bearing cells. EMBO J 10:343–348, 1991.

185. Bennett K, Jackson DG, Simon JC, Tanczos E, Peach R, Modrell B, Stamenkovic I, Plowman G, Aruffo A: CD44 isoforms containing exon v3 are responsible for the presentation of heparin-binding growth factors. J Cell Biol 128:687–698, 1995.

186. Streeter PR, Berg EL, Rouse BTN, Bargatz RF, Butcher EC: A tissue-specific endothelial cell molecule involved in lymphocyte homing. Nature (Lond) 331:41–46, 1988.

187. Stamenkovic I, Amiot M, Pesando JM, Seed B: A lymphocyte molecule implicated in lymph node homing is a member of the cartilage link protein family. Cell 56:1057–1062, 1989.

188. Goldstein LA, Zhou DFH, Picker LJ, Minty CN, Bargatze RF, Ding JF, Butcher EC: A human lymphocyte homing receptor, the hermes antigen, is related to cartilage proteoglycan core and link proteins. Cell 56:1063–1072, 1989.

189. Camp RL, Scheynius A, Johansson C, Pure E: CD44 is necessary for optimal contact allergic responses but is not required for normal leukocyte extravasation. J Exp Med 178:497–507, 1993.

190. Carter WG, Wayner EA: Characterization of the class III collagen receptor, a phosphorylated transmembrane glycoprotein expressed in nucleated human cells. J Biol Chem 263:4193–4201, 1988.

191. Green SJ, Tarone G, Underhill CB: Aggregation of macrophages and fibroblasts is inhibited by a monoclonal antibody to the hyaluronate receptor. Exp Cell Res 178:224–232, 1988.

192. Haynes BF, Telen MJ, Hale LP, Denning SM: CD44-A molecule involved in leukocyte adherence and T-cell activation. Immunol Today 10:423–428, 1989.

193. Miyake K, Medina KL, Hayashi SI, Ono S, Hamaoka T, Kincaide PW: Monoclonal antibodies to Pgp-1/CD44 block lymphohempoiesis in long term bone marrow cultures. 171:477–488, 1990.

194. Bazil V, Horejsi V: Shedding of the CD44 adhesion molecule from leukocytes induced by anti-CD44 monoclonal antibody simulating the effect of a natural receptor ligand. J Immunol 149:747–753, 1992.

195. Willerford DM, Hoffman PA, Gallatin WM: Expression of lymphocyte adhesion receptors for high endothelium in primates. Anatomic partitioning and linkage to activation. J Immunol 142:3416, 1989.

196. van Kooyk Y, Weder P, Hogervorst F, Verhoeven AJ, van Seventer G, te Velde AA, Borst J, Keizer GD, Figdor CG: Activation of LFA-1 through a Ca^{2+}-dependent epitope stimulates lymphocyte adhesion. J Cell Biol 112:345–354, 1991.

197. Mackay CR, Terpe HJ, Stauder R, Marston WL, Stark H, Gunthert U: Expression and modulation of CD44 variant isoforms in humans. J Cell Biol 124:71–82, 1994.

198. Bernfield MR, Kokenyesi R, Kato M, Hinks MT, Spring J, Gallo RL, Lose EJ: Biology of the syndecans: A family of transmembrane heparan sulphate proteoglycans. Annu Rev Cell Biol 8:365–393, 1992.

199. Rapraeger A: Transforming growth factor (type B) promotes the addition of chondroitin sulphate chains to the cell surface proteoglycan (syndecan) of mouse mammary epithelia. J Cell Biol 109:2509–2518, 1989.

200. Saksela O, Moscatelli D, Sommer A, Rifkin DB: Endothelial cell-derived heparan sulphate binds basic fibroblast growth factor and protects it from proteolytic degradation. J Cell Biol 107:743–751, 1988.

201. Saunders S, Jalkanen M, O'Farrell S, Bernfield M: Molecular cloning of syndecan, an integral membrane proteoglycan. J Cell Biol 108:1547–1556, 1989.

202. Podolsky DK, Lobb R, King N, Benjamin CD, Pepinsky B, Sehgal P, deBeaumont M: Attenuation of colitis in the cotton-top tamarin by anti-alpha 4 integrin monoclonal antibody. J Clin Invest 92:372–380, 1993.

203. Tosi MF, Zakem H, Berger M: Neutrophil elastase cleaves C3bi on opsonized Pseudomonas as well as CR1 on neutrophils to create a functionally important opsonin receptor mismatch. J Clin Invest 86:300–308, 1990.

204. Mulligan MS, Polley MJ, Bayer RJ, Nunn MF, Paulson JC, Ward PA: Neutrophil-dependent acute lung injury-requirement for P-selectin (GMP-140). J Clin Invest 90:1600–1607, 1992.

205. Collins TL, Kassner PD, Bierer BE, Burakoff SJ: Adhesion receptors in lymphocyte activation. Curr Opin Immunol 6:385–393, 1994.

206. Giger U, Boxer LA, Simpson PJ, Lucchesi BR, Todd RF3: Deficiency of leukocyte surface glycoproteins Mo1, LFA-1, and Leu-M5 in a dog with recurrent bacterial infections: An animal model. Blood 69:1622–1630, 1987.

207. Kehrli ME Jr, Ackermann MR, Shuster DE, van der Maaten MJ, Schmalsteig FC, Anderson DC, Hughes BJ: Bovine leukocyte adhesion deficiency: Beta 2 integrin deficiency in young Holstein cattle. Am J Pathol 140:1489–1492, 1992.

208. Wilson RW, Ballantyne CM, Smith CW, Montgomery C, Bradley A, O'Brien WE, Beaudet AL: Gene targeting yields a CD18-mutant for study of inflammation. J Immunol 151:1571–1578, 1993.

209. Cohnheim J: Lectures in General Pathology, 2nd ed. Vol 1. [Translated from second German edition.] London, The New Sydenham Society, 1889.

210. Schmid-schonbein GW, Usami S, Skalak R, Chien S: The interaction of leukocytes and erythrocytes in capillary and postcapillary vessels. Microvasc Res 19:45–70, 1980.

211. Breuer R, Christensen TG, Niles RM, Stone PJ, Snider GL: Human neutrophil elastase causes glycoconjugate release from the epithelial cell surfaces of hamster trachea in organ culture. Am Rev Respir Dis 139:779–782, 1989.

212. Tanaka Y, Adams DH, Hubscher S, Hirano H, Siebenlist U, Shaw S: T-cell adhesion induced proteoglycan-immobilized cytokine MIP-1 beta [see comments]. Nature 361:79–82, 1993.

213. Hunag AJ, Manning JE, Bandak TM, Ratau MC, Hanser KR, Silverstein SC: Endothelial cell cytosolic free calcium regulates neutrophil migration across monolayers of endothelial cells. J Cell Biol 120:1371–1380, 1993.

214. Muller WA, Weigl SA, Deng X, Phillips DM: PECAM-1 is required for transendothelial migration of leukocytes. J Exp Med 178:449–460, 1993.

215. Tanaka Y, Albelda SM, Horgan KJ, van Seveter GA, Shimizu Y, Newman W, Hallam J, Newman PJ, Buck CA, Shaw S: CD31 expressed on distinctive T cell subsets is a preferential amplifier of b1 integrin-mediated adhesion. J Exp Med 176:245–253, 1992.

216. Doukas J, Pober JS: IFN-γ enhances endothelial activation induced by tumor necrosis factor but not by IL-1. J Immunol 145:17127, 1990.

217. Leeuwenberg JFM, von Asmuth EJU, Jeunhomme TMAA, Buurman WA: IFN-γ regulates the expression of adhesion molecule ELAM-1 and IL-6 production by human endothelial cells in vitro. J Immunol 145:2110, 1990.

218. Thornhill MH, Haskard DO: IL-4 regulates endothelial cell activation by IL-1, tumor necrosis factor, or INF-γ. J Immunol 145:865–872, 1990.

219. Gamble JR, Khew-Goodall Y, Vadas MA: Transforming growth factor-beta inhibits E-selectin expression on human endothelial cells. J Immunol 146:4494–4503, 1993.

220. Gerritsen ME, Kelley KA, Ligon G, Perry CA, Shen C-P, Sczepanski A,

Carley WW: Regulation of the expression of intercellular adhesion molecule-1 in cultured human endothelial cells derived from rheumatoid synovium. Arthritis Rheum 36:593–602, 1993.

221. Yankaskas JR, Haizlip JE, Conrad M, Koval D, Lazarowski E, Paradiso AM, Rinehart CA, Sarkadi B, Schlegel R, Boucher RC: Papilloma virus immortalized tracheal epithelial cells retain a well-differentiated phenotype. Am J Physiol 264 (Cell Physiol. 33):C1219–C1230, 1993.

222. Mulligan MS, Warren JS, Smith CW, Anderson DC, Yeh CJ, Rudolph RA, Ward PA: Lung injury after deposition of IgA immune complexes. J Immunol 148:3086–3092, 1992.

223. Ross R: The pathogenesis of atherosclerosis: A perspective for the 1990s. Nature 362:801–809, 1993.

224. Picker LJ: Control of lymphocyte homing. Curr Opin Immunol 6:394–406, 1994.

225. Gallatin WM, Weisman IL, Butcher EC: Cell-surface molecule involved in organ-specific homing of lymphocytes. Nature (Lond) 304:30–34, 1983.

226. May MJ, Agar A: ICAM-1–independent lymphocyte transmigration across high endothelium: Differential up-regulation by interferon gamma, tumor necrosis factor-alpha and interleukin 1 beta. Eur J Immunol 22:219–226, 1992.

227. May MJ, Entwistle G, Humphries MJ, Ager A: VCAM-1 is a CS1 peptide-inhibitable adhesion molecule expressed by lymph node high endothelium. J Cell Sci 106:109–119, 1993.

228. Hamann A, Andrew DP, Jablonski-Westrich D, Holzmann B, Butcher E: Role of alpha 4-integrins in lymphocyte homing to mucosal tissues in vivo. J Immunol 152:3282–3293, 1994.

229. Hamann A, Jablonski-Westrich D, Duijevstijn A, Jonas P, Thiele HG: Homing receptors examined: Mouse LECAM-1 (MEL-14 antigen) is involved in lymphocyte migration into gut-associated lymphoid tissue. Eur J Immunol 21:2925–2929, 1991.

230. Lazarovits AI, Karsh J: Differential expression in rheumatoid synovium and synovial fluid of $\alpha\beta7$ integrin. J Immunol 151:6482–6489, 1993.

231. Hamann A, Westrich DJ, Duijevstijn A, Butcher EC, Baisch H, Harder R, Thiele HG: Evidence for an accessory role of LFA-1 in lymphocyte–high endothelium interaction during homing. J Immunol 140:693–699, 1988.

232. Sprangrude GJ, Sacchi F, Hill HR, Van Epps DE, Daynes RE: Inhibition of lymphocyte and neutrophil chemotaxis by pertussis toxin. J Immunol 135:4135–4143, 1985.

233. Bargatze RF, Butcher EC: Rapid G protein–regulated activation event involved in lymphocyte binding to high endothelial venules. J Exp Med 178:367–372, 1993.

234. Lazaar AL, Albelda SM, Pilewski JM, Brennan B, Pure E, Panettieri RJ: T lymphocytes adhere to airway smooth muscle cells via integrins and CD44 and induce smooth muscle cell DNA synthesis. J Exp Med 180:807–816, 1994.

235. Norgard-Sumnicht KE, Varki NM, Varki A: Calcium-dependent heparin-like ligands for L-selectin in non-lymphoid endothelial cells. Science 261:480, 1993.

236. Boat TF, Welsh MJ, Beaudet AL: Cystic fibrosis. In Scriver CR, Beaudet AL, Sly WS, Valle D (eds): The Metabolic Basis of Inherited Disease. New York, McGraw-Hill, 1989, pp 2649–2680.

237. Hawker PC, McKay JS, Turnberg LA: Electrolyte transport across colonic mucosa from patients with inflammatory bowel disease. Gastroenterology 79:508–511, 1980.

238. Paulson JC, Prieels JP, Glasgow LR, Hill RL: Sialyl- and fucosyltransferases in the biosynthesis of asparaginyl-linked oligosaccharides in glycoproteins: Mutually exclusive glycosylation by beta-galactoside alpha$_2$ goes to 6 sialyltransferase and N-acetylglucosaminide alpha$_1$ goes to 3 fucosyltransferase. J Biol Chem 253:5617–5624, 1978.

239. Carlos TM, Harlan JM: Leukocyte-endothelial adhesion molecules (review). Blood 84:2068–2101, 1994.

240. Lehr HA, Menger MD, Messmer K: Impact of leukocyte adhesion on myocardial ischemia/reperfusion injury mechanisms and proven facts. J Lab Clin Med 121:539–545, 1993.

241. Isobe M, Yagita H, Okumura K, Ihara A: Specific acceptance of cardiac allograft after treatment with antibodies to ICAM-1 and LFA-1. Science 255:1125–1127, 1992.

242. Mulligan MS, Johnson KJ, Todd RF III, Issekutz TB, Miyasaka M, Tamatani T, Smith CW, Anderson DC, Ward PA: Requirements for leukocyte adhesion molecules in nephrotoxic nephritis. J Clin Invest 91:577–587, 1993.

243. Hutchings P, Rosen H, O'Reilly L, Simpson E, Gordon S, Cooke A: Transfer of diabetes in mice prevented by blockade of adhesion-promoting receptor on macrophages. Nature 348:639–642, 1990.

244. Nakamura H, Yoshimura K, McElvaney NG, Crystal RG: Neutrophil elastase in respiratory epithelial lining fluid of individuals with cystic fibrosis induces interleukin-8 gene expression in a human epithelial cell line. J Clin Invest 89:1478–1484, 1992.

245. Yednock TA, Cannon C, Fritz LC, Sanchez MF, Steinman L, Karin N: Prevention of experimental autoimmune encephalomyelitis by antibodies against $\alpha4\beta1$ integrin. Nature 356:63–66, 1992.

246. Issekutz AC, Issekutz TB: Monocyte migration to arthritis in the rat utilizes both CD11/CD18 and very late activation antigen 4 integrin mechanisms. J Exp Med 181:1197–1203, 1995.

247. Nakajima H, Sano H, Nishimura T, Yoshida S, Iwamoto I: Role of vascular cell adhesion molecule 1/very late activation antigen 4 and intercellular adhesion molecule 1/lymphocyte function-associated antigen 1 interactions in antigen-induced eosinophil and T cell recruitment into the tissue. J Exp Med 179:1145–1154, 1994.

248. Gailit J, Clark RAF: Wound repair in the context of extracellular matrix. Curr Opin Cell Biol 6:717–725, 1994.

249. Paul LC, Davidoff A, Benediktsson H, Issekutz TB: The efficacy of LFA-1 and VLA-4 antibody treatment in rat vascularized cardiac allograft rejection. Transplantation 55:1196–1199, 1993.

250. Watson SR, Fennie C, Lasky LA: Neutrophil influx into an inflammatory site inhibited by a soluble homing receptor-IgG chimera. Nature 349:164–166, 1991.

251. Wolitzky B, Kwee L, Terry R, Kontgen F, Stewart C, Rumberger JM, Burns DK, Labow MA: Targeted disruption of the murine E-selectin and VCAM-1 genes. J Cell Biochem Suppl 18A:300, 1994.

252. Mayadas TN, Johnson RC, Rayburn H, Hynes RO, Wagner DD: Leukocyte rolling and extravasation are severely compromised in P-selectin-deficient mice. Cell 74:541–554, 1993.

253. Taylor HC, Lightner VA, Beyer WF Jr, McCaslin D, Briscoe G, Erickson HP: Biochemical and structural studies of tenascin/hexabrachion proteins. J Cell Biochem 41:71–90, 1989.

254. Klickstein LB, Wong WW, Smith JA, Weis JH, Wilson JG, Fearon DT: Human C3b/C4b receptor: Demonstration of long homologous repeating domains that are composed of the short consensus repeats characteristic of C3/C4 binding proteins. J Exp Med 165:1095–1112, 1987.

255. Jones EL, Harlos K, Bottomley MJ, Robinson RC, Driscoll PC, Edwards RM, Clements JM, Dudgeon TJ, Stuart DI: Crystal structure of an integrin-binding fragment of vascular cell adhesion molecule-1 at 1.8 Å resolution. Nature 373:539–544, 1995.

256. Leahy DJ, Hendrickson WA, Aukhil I, Erickson HP: Structure of a fibronectin type III domain from tenascin phased by MAD analysis of the selenomethionyl protein. Nature 258:987–991, 1992.

CHAPTER 21

Hideaki Nagase
Yasunori Okada

Proteinases and Matrix Degradation*

Proteolytic enzymes that degrade extracellular matrix (ECM) components play critical roles in many biologic processes, such as ovulation, embryo implantation, morphogenesis, and tissue involution. The breakdown of extracellular matrix affects cellular phenotype and behavior. Under normal physiologic conditions, degradation and synthesis of extracellular matrix components are precisely regulated, but when these processes are disrupted, a number of pathologic situations arise. The degradation of articular cartilage is one of the prominent features in arthritis that leads to an impairment of the joint function. This is attributed largely to an elevated production of proteinases whose activities are no longer regulated by endogenous proteinase inhibitors. This chapter describes the properties and the mechanisms of regulation of mammalian proteinases and their inhibitors that participate in the extracellular matrix.

EXTRACELLULAR MATRIX-DEGRADING PROTEINASES

Extracellular matrix macromolecules are degraded primarily by *endopeptidases (proteinases)* that cleave internal peptide bonds.[1, 2] Little evidence has been provided for the roles of *exopeptidases* in these processes. Proteinases are divided into four classes based on the functional groups involved in their catalytic mechanisms[3]:

- Aspartic proteinases
- Cysteine proteinases
- Serine proteinases
- Metalloproteinases

Inhibitors specific to each class are useful for classifying proteinases[4]:

- Aspartic proteinases: pepstatin
- Cysteine proteinases: E-64 [L-*trans*-epoxysuccinyl leucylamide(4-guanidino)butane], SH-reacting agents, such as iodoacetamide, N-ethylmaleimide
- Serine proteinases: diisopropylfluorophosphate, phenylmethylsulfonyl fluoride, 3,4-dichloroisocoumarin
- Metalloproteinases: chelating agents, such as EDTA, 1,10-phenanthroline

---

*The authors were inspired by the chapter by Z. Werb and C. M. Alexander in the fourth edition of the Textbook of Rheumatology.

The proteinases from the four classes that are likely to participate in extracellular matrix degradation are listed in Tables 21–1 and 21–2.

Aspartic Proteinases

The enzymes in the aspartic group require two aspartic acid residues as part of their catalytic site. Pepsin, renin, human immunodeficiency virus (HIV) protease, and lysosomal cathepsins D and E are examples, but *cathepsin D* is the major aspartic proteinase that is involved in matrix degradation.

Cathepsin D is found in the lysosomes of most cells. It is synthesized as a pre-proenzyme and processed to a 42-kD glycoprotein procathepsin D, which bears two N-linked oligosaccharide chains containing mannose-6-phosphate. Procathepsin D is then sorted to lysosomes through interaction with mannose-6-phosphate receptors and is stored as a 34-kD mature form.[5] Cathepsin D is released extracellularly from cells in cultured chick limb bone treated with retinol,[6] macrophages,[7] and some cancer cell lines mostly as proenzyme.[8] Cathepsin D exhibits optimal proteolytic activity against most substrates at pH 3.5. It digests cartilage aggrecan optimally at pH 5.5, but it shows little proteolytic activity at neutral pH.[2] Collagen telopeptides are susceptible to cathepsin D.[9] Although pH immediately adjacent to chondrocytes may fall as low as 5.5, several lines of evidence indicate that cathepsin D is not important in cartilage matrix resorption. A cathepsin D inhibitor, pepstatin, and an antiserum to cathepsin D do not influence cartilage degradation induced by vitamin A in cultured explants.[10] Cathepsin D is most likely to be involved in intracellular degradation of extracellular matrix.

Cysteine Proteinases

The cysteine proteinases that can degrade extracellular matrix components include cathepsins B, L, N, and S and calpains.

Cathepsins B and *L* are synthesized as proenzymes and are processed to low-molecular-weight active forms and stored in lysosomes.[11] These enzymes function optimally at acidic pH values and may digest phagocytosed materials. However, cathepsins B and

Table 21–1. PROTEINASES THAT MAY BE INVOLVED IN DEGRADATION OF EXTRACELLULAR MATRIX

Enzyme	Molecular Mass (kD)	Source	Inhibitor
Aspartic Proteinases			
Cathepsin D	34	Lysosome	Pepstatin
Cysteine Proteinases			
Cathepsin B	25	Lysosome	Cystatins
Cathepsin L	24	Lysosome	Cystatins
Cathepsin S	24	Lysosome	Cystatins
Calpain	110 (80 + 30)	Cytosol	Calpastatin
Serine Proteinases			
Neutrophil elastase	30	PMN leukocytes	α_1-PI
Cathepsin G	30	PMN leukocytes	α_1-Antichymotrypsin
Proteinase 3	29	PMN leukocytes	α_1-PI, elafin
Plasmin	94	Plasma	Aprotinin
Plasma kallikrein	115–90	Plasma	Aprotinin
Tissue kallikrein		Glandular tissues	Aprotinin, kallistatin
Tissue plasminogen activator (tPA)	67–72	Endothelial cells, chondrocytes	PAI-1, PAI-2
Urokinase (uPA)	52/33	Fibroblasts, chondrocytes	PAI-1, PAI-2, PN-1
Tryptase	160	Mast cells	Trypstatin
Chymase	26	Mast cells	α_1-PI
Metalloproteinases (MMPs)			
Interstitial collagenase (MMP-1)	52/56	Fibroblasts, chondrocytes	TIMPs
Gelatinase A (MMP-2)	72	Fibroblasts, chondrocytes	TIMPs
Stromelysin (MMP-3)	57/59	Fibroblasts, chondrocytes	TIMPs
Matrilysin (MMP-7)	28	Macrophages	TIMPs
Neutrophil collagenase (MMP-8)	75	PMN leukocyte	TIMPs
Gelatinase B (MMP-9)	92	PMN leukocytes, macrophages, fibroblasts, chondrocytes, osteoclasts	TIMPs

Modified from Nagase H, Woessner JF Jr: Role of endogenous proteinases in the degradation of cartilage matrix. *In* Woessner JF Jr, Howell DS (eds): Joint Cartilage Degradation: Basic Clinical Aspects. New York, Marcel Dekker, 1993, p 159. Reprinted by courtesy of Marcel Dekker, Inc.

Abbreviations: PMN, polymorphonuclear neutrophil leukocyte; TIMPs, tissue inhibitors of metalloproteinases; PI, proteinase inhibitor; PAI, plasminogen activator inhibitor; PN, proteinase nexin.

L are sometimes found extracellularly often as latent precursor forms, especially in activated macrophages and tumor cells.[12, 13] The secreted forms of cathepsin B are stable at neutral and alkaline pHs and have optimal activity at neutral pH.[12]

Cathepsin S is more stable than cathepsins B and L at neutral pH.[14]

Cathepsin N was described as "collagenolytic cathepsin,"[15] but it has not been clearly distinguished from cathepsins L and S.

Cathepsins B and L cleave the telopeptide regions of fibrillar collagen types I and II, resulting in depolymerization of collagen fibrils.[17, 18] Both enzymes also degrade aggrecan and collagens IX and XI at nonhelical regions at an acidic pH.[18] Cathepsin S is active against a similar spectrum of substrates but over a broad pH range. Cathepsins L and S are potent elastolytic enzymes.[11] Lysosomal cysteine proteinases secreted from osteoclasts play a key role in bone resorption by degrading collagenous bone matrix.

Calpains are cytosolic Ca^{2+}-dependent cysteine proteinases, but they also occur extracellularly and in osteoarthritic synovial fluid.[16]

Serine Proteinases

The serine group comprises the largest currently known number of proteinases. Many of the serine proteinases participate in extracellular matrix degradation either directly or by activating the precursors of matrix metalloproteinases (MMPs).

Neutrophil Elastase, Cathepsin G, and Proteinase 3

The serine proteinases are found in the azurophil granules of polymorphonuclear (PMN) leukocytes. They are synthesized as precursor forms in promyelocytes in bone marrow and are rapidly converted to active enzyme by removal of the signal peptide and then the dipeptide from the amino terminus; the mature enzymes have a molecular mass of 29 to 30 kD.[19] They digest extracellular matrix components as granule contents are discharged and promote inflammatory processes in response to chemotactic agents.

Neutrophil elastase preferentially cleaves Val-X and Ala-X bonds, whereas *cathepsin G* has chymotrypsin-like specificity. *Proteinase 3*, an autoantigen of Wegener's granulomatosis,[22] has a similar substrate specificity to elastase,[21] and both enzymes have potent elastolytic activity. Neutrophil elastase and cathepsin G cleave the telopeptide region of fibrillar collagens,[20] type IV collagen, and a number of other matrix glycoproteins.[1] Proteinase 3 degrades fibronectin, vitronectin, and collagen IV.[21] Neutrophil elastase and cathep-

Table 21–2. PROTEINASE SUSCEPTIBILITY OF EXTRACELLULAR MATRIX PROTEINS

Matrix Protein	Proteinases
Cartilage	
Aggrecan core protein	MMP-1, MMP-2, MMP-3, MMP-7, MMP-8, MMP-9, MMP-10, neutrophil elastase, cathepsin G, chymase, cathepsin B, cathepsin L, cathepsin D, calpain
Link protein	MMP-1, MMP-2, MMP-3, MMP-7, MMP-9, MMP-10, cathepsin G, cathepsin B
Collagen II	MMP-1, MMP-8
	Telopeptide only: MMP-3, neutrophil elastase, cathepsin G, cathepsin B, cathepsin L, cathepsin N
Collagen VI	Neutrophil elastase, cathepsin G, chymase, tryptase
Collagen IX	MMP-3, cathepsin B, cathepsin L
Collagen X	MMP-1, MMP-2, neutrophil elastase
Collagen XI	MMP-2
	Telopeptide only: MMP-3, cathepsin B, cathepsin L
Interstitial Connective Tissue	
Collagen I	MMP-1, MMP-8, MMP-13
	Telopeptid only: MMP-3, neutrophil elastase, cathepsin G, cathepsin B, cathepsin L, cathepsin N
Collagen III	MMP-1, MMP-8, MMP-9, MMP-3 (weak), MMP-13, neutrophil elastase
Collagen V	MMP-2, MMP-9
Collagen VI	Neutrophil elastase, cathepsin G, chymase, tryptase
Collagen VII	MMP-1, MMP-2, MMP-3, MMP-9
Fibronectin	MMP-2 (not MMP-9), MMP-3, MMP-7, MMP-10, MMP-11, neutrophil elastase, cathepsin G, plasmin, uPA, cathepsin B, cathepsin L, cathepsin S, cathepsin D
Elastin	MMP-2, MMP-3 (weak), MMP-7, MMP-9, MMP-10, MMP-12, neutrophil elastase, cathepsin L
Basement Membrane	
Collagen IV	MMP-2, MMP-3, MMP-7, MMP-9, MMP-10, neutrophil elastase, cathepsin G, chymase, plasmin, cathepsin B, cathepsin L
Heparan sulfate proteoglycan	Neutrophil elastase, chymase
Laminin	MMP-2, MMP-3, MMP-7, MMP-11 (weak), neutrophil elastase, plasmin
Entactin	MMP-1, MMP-2, MMP-7, MMP-9

sin G activate precursors of matrix metalloproteinases (proMMPs) (see later).

Mast Cell Proteinases

Mast cells contain tryptase, chymase, and cathepsin G.

Tryptase has a trypsin-like specificity but has a very limited proteolytic activity on natural substrates.[23–25] It degrades collagen VI[23] and fibronectin,[24] inactivates fibrinogen,[25] and activates prostromelysin 1 (proMMP-3).[25]

Chymase is a chymotrypsin-like monomeric enzyme of 30 kD. It has a broad spectrum of activity on extracellular matrix components and activates procollagenase (proMMP-1) and prostromelysin 1 (proMMP-3).[26, 27] It also converts angiotensin I to angiotensin II and inactivates bradykinin.[25]

Another chymotrypsin-like enzyme is found in mast cells. The enzyme has been identified as *cathepsin G*.[28]

Plasminogen Activators and Plasmin

The activation of plasminogen (90 kD) to plasmin by plasminogen activators (PAs) is one of the important regulatory steps in extracellular matrix degra-dation because plasmin not only can degrade a number of extracellular matrix macromolecules but also can activate procollagenases and prostromelysins. There are two types of plasminogen activa-tors[29, 30]: tissue-type plasminogen activator (tPA) and urokinase-type plasminogen activator (uPA).

tPA is synthesized and secreted as a proenzyme (70 kD) primarily by endothelial cells and in other cell types, such as fibroblasts, chondrocytes, and tumor cells.[29] It is the major activator of plasminogen for fibrinolysis. tPA also binds to laminin, fibronectin, thrombospondin, endothelial cell surface,[29] and lami-nin.[31]

uPA is secreted from many cell types as a 55-kD proenzyme.[29] Plasmin and plasma kallikrein convert pro-uPA into the active form. The active form of uPA consists of two chains of 30 kD and 24 kD that are linked by a disulfide bond. uPA may be further pro-cessed by plasmin to a 33-kD form, but it retains full activity. Both pro-uPA and the two-chain uPA bind to a specific uPA receptor on fibroblasts, macrophage-like cells, and neoplastic cells.[32] The receptor is a single-chain glycoprotein (50 to 60 kD) that is an-chored to the plasma membrane via a glycosyl-phos-phatidyl inositol moiety.[32] The receptor binds to the growth factor domain of uPA, which accelerates the activation of pro-uPA by plasmin; the receptor-bound uPA, in turn, accelerates the activation of the cell-associated plasminogen.[33] In addition, uPA has a limited action on fibronectin.[34]

Plasminogen, abundant in plasma, binds to fibrin and on activation by PAs, it readily digests fibrin. It also degrades a number of extracellular matrix components, including aggrecan, fibronectin, type IV collagen, and laminin.[1] An additional important function of plasmin is its ability to initiate the activation of proMMPs (see later).

Kallikreins

Two types of kallikreins are described:

1. *Plasma kallikrein* releases bradykinin from kininogens. It consists of two disulfide-linked chains (36 kD and 52 kD) and generated from a single-chain precursor, prokallikrein (88 kD) by coagulation factor XIIa or kallikrein itself.[35] The active form of kallikrein is found in rheumatoid synovial fluid at a low concentration. Plasma kallikrein activates procollagenases and prostromelysin-1.[36]

2. *Tissue kallikrein* is synthesized in glandular tissues. It generates Lys-bradykinin from kininogens and activates neutrophil procollagenase (proMMP-8).[37]

Matrix Metalloproteinases

Metalloproteinases termed *matrixins,* or *matrix metalloproteinases* (MMPs), are key ECM-degrading enzymes.[38–40] Common features of matrixins are summarized in Table 21–3.

The matrixin family comprises at least 11 different molecules. Seven of them can be classified into three subgroups based on the structural similarity and substrate specificity (Table 21–4). All matrixins except MMP-7 contain three common domains (propeptide, catalytic, and hemopexin/vitronectin-like), which are preceded by signal peptides (Fig. 21–1).

The NH$_2$-terminal *propeptide domain* (77 to 87 residues) has one unpaired cysteine in the uniquely conserved sequence PRCG[V/N]PD, which plays a critical role in maintaining the latency of proMMPs.

The *catalytic domain* (162 to 173 residues) has the zinc-binding motif HEXGHXXGXXH, in which three histidines bind to the catalytic zinc atom. Crystal structures of the catalytic domains of MMP-1[45] and

Table 21–3. PROPERTIES OF MATRIXINS

1. Contain Zn^{2+} ion essentials for catalytic activity
2. Contain the "cysteine switch" motif RRCG[V/N]PDV in the propeptide and the catalytic zinc-binding motif HEXGHXXGXXH in which three histidines bind to the Zn^{2+}
3. Require Ca^{2+} for activity and structural stability
4. Are secreted as a latent zymogen (proMMP)
5. Activated by mercurial compounds (e.g., 4-aminophenylmercuric acetate [APMA], HgCl$_2$) and by proteinases
6. Inhibited by tissue inhibitors of metalloproteinases (TIMPs)

MMP-8[46] reveal that they consist of a five-stranded β-sheet, two α-helices, and bridging loops.

The COOH-terminal *hemopexin-like domain* (202 to 213 residues) interacts with matrix and governs the substrate specificity in some cases. In addition, the two gelatinases (MMP-2 and MMP-9) contain three tandem repeats of fibronectin type II–like modules in the catalytic domain, which provide them with gelatin-binding properties.[41–43] A membrane-type MMP (MT-MMP) has a transmembrane domain in the COOH-terminal region, and the catalytic domain is exposed to the cell surface.[44]

Collagenases

The collagenases include MMP-1, MMP-8, and collagenase 3 (MMP-13).[47] Collagenases are distinguished from other MMPs by their ability to degrade triple helical regions of interstitial collagens I, II, and III at a specific site located about three-fourths the distance from the N terminal.

In addition to interstitial collagens, MMP-1 and MMP-8 digest a number of other components of extracellular matrix. MMP-1 and MMP-8 require extended amino acid sequences in substrates and favor Leu, Ile, and Met at the P$_1$' site.[48] α$_2$-Macroglobulin (α$_2$M) is an about 150-fold better as a substrate for MMP-1 than collagen I,[49] which suggests that it is a major regulator of MMP-1 activity. The catalytic domains of collagenases alone retain proteolytic activity, but they do not digest interstitial collagens.[50, 51] The C-terminal hemopexin-like domain is required for collagenolysis.

MMP-1 is synthesized by many cell types (e.g., fibroblasts, chondrocytes, osteoblasts, endothelial cells, and macrophages), but MMP-8 is found only in neutrophils. Collagenase 3 (MMP-13) occurs in breast carcinoma cells.[47] Eosinophils contain collagenolytic activity, but the enzyme has not been identified.[52]

Gelatinases

MMP-2 and MMP-9 belong to the subgroup called gelatinases. Both enzymes readily digest gelatins. They also degrade collagen IV, but their activity on collagen IV is much weaker than that on collagen V.[36] Elastin,[53] aggregan,[54] and cartilage link protein[55] are also degraded by the gelatinases. The catalytic efficiency of gelatinases depends on the length of peptide substrates.

Both MMP-2 and MMP-9 tolerate a small amino acid (e.g., Gly or Ala) at the P$_1$ site and an aliphatic or hydrophobic residue at the P$_1$' site.[56] MMP-2 is synthesized in a variety of mesenchymal cells in culture. MMP-9 is found in neutrophils, macrophages, and cancer cells. It is also produced in fibroblasts,[57] chondrocytes,[58] and T-lymphocytes[59] under stimulatory conditions.

Stromelysins

The subgroup of stromelysins comprises MMP-3 and MMP-10.[60] Both enzymes hydrolyze a number

Table 21–4. MATRIX METALLOPROTEINASES (MMPs)

Enzyme	MMP No.	M$_r$ (kD)		Matrix Substrate
		Precursor	*Active*	
Collagenases				
Interstitial collagenase (EC 3.4.24.7)	MMP-1	52 56*	41 45*	Collagens I, II, III, VII, and X; gelatins; proteoglycan; link protein; entactin
Neutrophil collagenase (EC 3.4.24.34)	MMP-8	75*	65*	Collagens I, II, and III; proteoglycan; link protein
Collagenase 3	MMP-13	65	55	Collagen I
Gelatinases				
Gelatinase A (EC 3.4.24.24)	MMP-2	72	67	Gelatins, collagens IV, V, VII, and XI; fibronectin, laminin; proteoglycan; elastin
Gelatinase B (EC 3.4.24.35)	MMP-9	92*	84*	Gelatins; collagens III, IV, and V; proteoglycan; elastin; entactin
Stromelysins				
Stromelysin 1 (EC 3.4.24.17)	MMP-3	57 59*	45 28	Proteoglycan, gelatins, fibronectin, laminin, collagens III, IV, IX, and X
Stromelysin 2 (EC 3.4.24.22)	MMP-10	57	45 28	Proteoglycan, fibronectin, laminin, collagen IV
Others				
Matrilysin (EC 3.4.24.23)	MMP-7	28	19	Proteoglycan, fibronectin, laminin, gelatins, collagen IV, elastin, entactin
Stromelysin 3	MMP-11	55	28	Weak activity on fibronectin, laminin, proteoglycan, gelatin
Metalloelastase	MMP-12	53	45 22	Elastin
Membrane-type MMP	MMP-14	63		Unknown (activates proMMP-2)

From Nagase H: Matrix metalloproteinases. *In* Hooper NM (ed): Zinc Metalloproteinases in Health and Disease. London, Taylor & Francis, 1996, p 153.
*Glycosylated.

of ECM components, including aggrecan, fibronectin, laminin, and collagen IV.[60, 61]

Collagens III, IX, and X, and telopeptides of collagens I, II, and XI, are also digested by MMP-3.[60, 62] MMP-3 shows a preference for substrates with an aliphatic or hydrophobic residue at the P$_1$' site, but the residue at the P$_1$ site has little effect.[63] MMP-3 is produced in many connective tissue cells and macrophages when they are stimulated.

MMP-10 is produced in keratinocytes in response to 12-*O*-tetradecanoyl phorbol-13-acetate (TPA), transforming growth factor-α (TGF-α), epidermal growth factor (EGF), and tumor necrosis factor-α (TNF-α).[64]

Other MMPs

Matrilysin (MMP-7), stromelysin 3 (MMP-11), macrophage metalloelastase (MMP-12), and MT-MMP do not belong to the earlier subgroups.

MMP-7 has potent proteolytic activity and digests a wide range of substrates.[61, 65]

MMP-11, although designated "stromelysin 3," is structurally distant from stromelysins 1 and 2. Recombinant mouse MMP-11 shows only weak proteolytic activity on fibronectin, laminin, proteoglycan, and gelatin,[66] but it readily inactivates α_1-PI by cleaving the Ala^{350}-Met^{351} band.[67]

MMP-12 is expressed in human lung alveolar macrophages, and it digests elastin[68]; however, information about the cell source other than macrophages and the substrate specificity is limited.

MT-MMP is expressed on the surface of the cell.[44] It activates proMMP-2, but its action on extracellular matrix is not known.

ENDOGENOUS PROTEINASE INHIBITORS

Proteinase activities are precisely controlled by endogenous inhibitors. A large number of proteinase inhibitors, whose in vivo levels usually exceed the levels of their target proteinases, are found in tissues, plasma, and body fluids. For example, about 10 percent of all plasma proteins are proteinase inhibitors.[69] Endogenous inhibitors of the ECM-degrading proteinase and their representative target enzymes are listed in Table 21–5. With the exception of α_2M, inhibitors are proteinase class-specific.

α_2-Macroglobulin

α_2-Macroglobulin is a plasma glycoprotein (725 kD) that is synthesized in the liver, by macrophages and

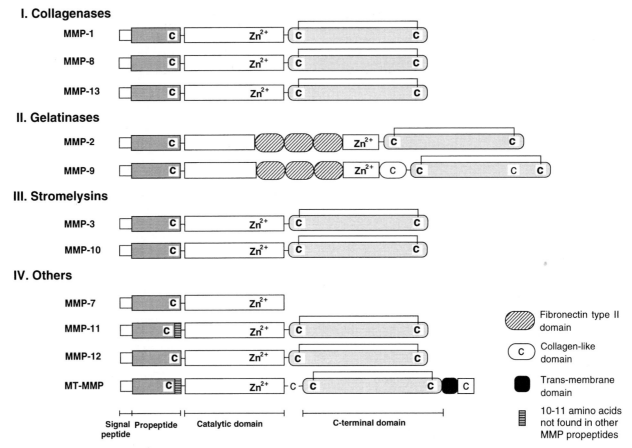

Figure 21–1. Domain structures of matrixins. MMP, matrix metalloproteinase; C (bold), conserved cysteine; Zn, zinc. (Modified from Nagase H: Matrix metalloproteinases. *In* Hooper NM: Zinc Metalloproteinases in Health and Disease. London, Taylor & Francis, 1996, p 153.)

fibroblasts. It consists of four identical subunits (185 kD) that are linked in pairs by disulfide bonds, and the pairs assemble noncovalently. This inhibitor is active against almost all endopeptidases regardless of their specificities.[70] The binding of $\alpha_2 M$ and a proteinase is initiated by proteolytic attack of the enzyme on a locus, the so-called "bait region," located near the middle of the subunit. This triggers a conformational change in the $\alpha_2 M$ molecule that in turn entraps the enzyme. Inactive proteinases do not bind to $\alpha_2 M$. The active site of the enzyme within the complex is unblocked, but it is restricted from reactions with large protein substrates. $\alpha_2 M$-proteinase complexes are rapidly cleared by macrophages, fibroblasts, and other cell types through receptor-mediated endocytosis.[71]

Another molecular feature of $\alpha_2 M$ is that each subunit contains an unusual intrachain β-cysteinyl-γ-glutamyl thiolester.[72] Thiolester bonds are also found in complement proteins C3 and C4. On proteolysis of the bait region, the thiolester bond becomes reactive with nucleophilic group of a proteinase and forms a covalent link with most of the trapped proteinases. However, the formation of an intermolecular covalent bond is not required for the inhibition of proteinases. $\alpha_2 M$ also binds to a number of growth factors and

cytokines, such as platelet-derived growth factor (PDGF), basic fibroblast growth factor (bFGF), TGF-β, insulin, interleukin-1β (IL-1β).[71]

Inhibitors of Serine Proteinases

Serpins

Human plasma contains several members of the serpin (*serine proteinase inhibitor*) super family; these proteins are homologous with human α_1-proteinase inhibitor (α_1PI).[73] Among them, α_1PI (α_1-antitrypsin), α_1-antichymotrypsin, α_2-antiplasmin, plasminogen activator inhibitors (PAIs), protein C inhibitor (PAI-3), C1-inhibitor, kallistatin, and proteinase nexin-1 (PN-1) regulate serine proteinases involved in extracellular matrix degradation (see Table 21–5).

Although many serpins are found in plasma, *PAI-1* is produced by endothelial cells, platelets, and a number of other cell types. PAI-1 inhibits both tPA and uPA, but it forms a more stable complex with tPA.[29] Secreted PAI-1 binds to the pericellular extracellular matrix, which suggests that it functions as an inhibitor of pericellular proteolysis.[74]

PAI-2 is found in plasma and is secreted from the

Table 21–5. ENDOGENOUS INHIBITORS OF THE EXTRACELLULAR MATRIX–DEGRADING PROTEINASES

Inhibitor	M_r (kD)	Source	Target Enzyme
α_2-Macroglobulin	725	Plasma, macrophages, fibroblasts	Most proteinases from all classes
Inhibitors of Serine Proteinase			
Serpins			
α_1-Proteinase inhibitor	52	Plasma, macrophages	Neutrophil elastase, cathepsin G, proteinase 3
α_1-Antichymotrypsin	58	Plasma	Cathespin G, chymotrypsin, chymase, tissue kallikrein
α_2-Antiplasmin	67	Plasma	Plasmin
Proteinase nexin-1	45	Fibroblasts	Thrombin, uPA, tPA, plasmin, trypsin, trypsin-like serine proteinase
PAI-1	45	Endothelial cell, fibroblasts, platelets, plasma	tPA, uPA
PAI-2	47	Plasma, macrophages	tPA, uPA
Protein C inhibitor	57	Plasma, urine	Active protein C, tPA, uPA, tissue kallikrein
C1-inhibitor	96	Plasma	Plasma kallikrein, C1 esterase
Kallistatin	92	Plasma; many organs, including liver, stomach, kidney, pancreas, aorta	Tissue kallikrein
Kunins			
Aprotinin	7	Mast cells	Plasmin, kallikreins
Tripstatin (rat)	6	Mast cells	Tryptase
Proteinase nexin 2 (β-amyloid protein precursor)	100	Fibroblasts	EGF binding protein, NGF-γ, trypsin, chymotrypsin, factor XIa
Others			
Secretory leukocyte proteinase inhibitor (SLPI)	15	Bronchial secretions, seminal plasma, cartilage	Neutrophil elastase, cathepsin G, chymotrypsin, trypsin
Elafin	7	Horny layers of skin	Neutrophil elastase, proteinase 3
Inhibitors of Cysteine Proteinase			
Kininogens	50–78 (light) 108–120 (heavy)	Plasma	Cysteine proteinases
Stefin A	11	Cytosol	Cysteine proteinases (not calpain)
Stefin B	11	Cytosol	Cysteine proteinases (not calpain)
Cystatin C	13	Body fluids	Cysteine proteinases (not calpain)
Cystatin S	13	Seminal plasma, tears, saliva	Cysteine proteinases (not calpain)
Calpastatin	120	Cytosol	Calpains
crmA	38	Pox virus	Interleukin-1β converting enzyme (ICE)
Metalloproteinase Inhibitors			
TIMP-1	29	Connective tissue cells, macrophages	Matrixins
TIMP-2	22	Connective tissue cells, macrophages	Matrixins
TIMP-3	21	Fibroblasts	Matrixins

Abbreviations: EGF, epidermal growth factor; TIMP, tissue inhibitor of metalloproteinase; tPA, tissue-type plasminogen activator; uPA, urokinase-type plasminogen activator; PAI, plasminogen activator inhibitor; crmA, cytokine response modifier.

cultured macrophages and macrophage-like cells. It inhibits uPA more effectively compared with tPA.

PN-1 inhibits uPA-mediated matrix degradation in fibroblast cultures. The PN-1/proteinase complex then binds to specific receptors via the PN-1 portion, which is internalized and degraded.[75]

Aprotinin

Aprotinin is a Kunitz-type pancreatic trypsin inhibitor consisting of 58 amino acids with three disulfide bonds. It is present at high levels in mast cells and inhibits plasmin and kallikreins. Homologous regions, also referred to as *kunin* domains, are found in trypstatin, plasma inter-α-inhibitor (two kunin domains), and proteinase nexin-2 (PN-2).[76] PN-2 is a

proteinase inhibitor identical to one of the forms of the Alzheimer's peptide precursor (APP).[77]

Other Inhibitors of Serine Proteinases

A 15-kD inhibitor that blocks neutrophil elastase and cathepsin G activity is found in cartilage.[84] It is identical to an inhibitor called *secretory leukocyte proteinase inhibitor* (SLPI), which is present in many secretory fluids. SLPI comprises 107 residues that are organized into two domains. The second domain contains the inhibitory capacity against elastase, cathepsin G, chymotrypsin, and trypsin.

An inhibitor termed *elafin* is isolated from horny layers of human skin. Elafin comprises 57 residues with 38 percent identity with the second domain of

SLPI.[76] It inhibits PMN elastase and proteinase 3 but not cathepsin G, chymotrypsin, or trypsin.

Inhibitors of Cysteine Proteinases

The naturally occurring cysteine proteinase inhibitors include the members of the *cystatin* superfamily, *calpastatin* and *crmA* (cytokine response modifier).

Cystatins inhibit lysosomal cysteine proteinases, but they are not effective with calpains. The superfamily consists of three subgroups.[79]

Subgroup 1 comprises *stefins A* and *B*, each with a molecular mass of 11 kD. Stefin A is found in epithelial cells and PMNs; stefin B is more widely distributed. These proteins are synthesized without a signal peptide and are confined in cells, but they are also found in extracellular fluid.

Subgroup 2 includes human *cystatins C* and *S*, each with a molecular mass of 13 kD. They occur at relatively high concentration in such secretions as seminal plasma, cerebrospinal fluid, and saliva. Cystatin C is a major secretory product of human alveolar macrophages.[80]

Subgroup 3 comprises *kininogens;* it contains three copies of group 2–like sequence. α-Cysteine proteinase inhibitors (αCPIs) isolated from human plasma are kininogens. Kininogens, therefore, participate not only in blood coagulation and inflammation but also in inhibition of cysteine proteinases.

Calpastatin is a cytosolic specific inhibitor of calpain. Human calpastatin consists of 708 amino acids.[81] The pox virus genome encodes three proteins homologous to serpins, one of which inhibits the IL-1β converting enzyme (ICE), a cysteine proteinase.[82] This serpin (crmA) modifies the infected cell's response to IL-1β.[83]

Tissue Inhibitors of Metalloproteinases

Tissue inhibitors of metalloproteinases (TIMPs) inhibit matrixins by forming a 1:1 stoichiometric complex. Three TIMPs have been identified, and they share approximately 40 percent sequence identity with each other, including 12 conserved cysteines.[39, 40, 84]

TIMP-1 is a glycoprotein (29 to 30 kD) that contains 184 amino acid residues. The N-terminal domain contains the inhibitory activity for MMPs.[85]

TIMP-2 is an unglycosylated protein (22 kD) with 194 amino acids. The solution structure of the N-terminal domain of TIMP-2 determined by nuclear magnetic resonance spectroscopy indicates that the protein has a five-stranded antiparallel β-sheet, which forms a closed β-barrel, and two short α-helices, which pack close together on the same barrel face.[86]

TIMP-3 is a 21-kD protein with 188 amino acids in humans.[87] It differs from the other two TIMPs, in that it binds tenaciously to extracellular matrix components.

Specific complexes between progelatinases and TIMPs (proMMP-2/TIMP-2 and proMMP-9/TIMP-1) are found in the medium of cultured cells.[40, 84] These complexes are formed through interaction of the C-terminal domain of progelatinase and the C terminal of TIMP. Thus, the complexes can act as MMP inhibitors.[88] Complex formation may function as a safety device because the activation of proMMP-2 and proMMP-9 is suppressed when these progelatinases are bound to the respective TIMPs. In addition to MMP inhibition activity, TIMP-1 and TIMP-2 have cell growth and erythroid-potentiating activity.[89-94]

ENZYMIC MECHANISMS OF EXTRACELLULAR MATRIX DEGENERATION

Fibrillar Interstitial Collagens

The triple-helical regions of interstitial *collagens I, II,* and *III* are extremely resistant to most proteinases, but collagenases cleave these collagens at a specific site three-fourths the distance from the N terminus to the C terminus. Collagen III is also susceptible to degradation by MMP-3,[60] MMP-9,[95] and neutrophil elastase.[96] However, the heavily cross-linked collagen fibrils are much more resistant to degradation than the soluble collagens are. The interaction of highly cross-linked fibrillar collagens with other matrix macromolecules in the tissue make them even more resistant to proteolysis. The nonhelical telopeptide regions, where both intramolecular and intermolecular cross-links occur are cleaved by a number of proteinases, including MMP-3,[60] neutrophil elastase, cathepsin G,[20] and lysosomal cysteine proteinases in vitro.[17, 18] Consequently, these enzymes can depolymerize the insoluble cross-linked collagens. Once collagen fibrils are cleaved or depolymerized, the helical structures become denatured at 37°C and become susceptible to gelatinases (MMP-2 and MMP-9).

Other Collagens

The degradation of *collagen IV,* a major structural component of basement membranes, is critical for capillary remodeling and angiogenesis as well as extravasation and intravasation of hematopoietic cells and cancer cells. MMP-2 and MMP-9 cleave collagen IV at the site about one-fourth the distance from the N terminus to C terminus of the molecule.[97] MMP-3 and MMP-7, however, are more effective at degrading collagen IV compared with gelatinases in vitro.[36, 60] Nonetheless, the pericellular concentration of MMP-2 may increase as fibroblasts and some neoplastic cells express MMP-2 receptors on cellular stimulation.[98] Neutrophil elastase, cathepsin G, chymase, plasmin, cathepsin B, and cathepsin L can degrade nonhelical regions of collagen IV.[99, 100]

Collagens II, V, VI, IX, X, and XI are found in cartilage.

Collagen IX maintains the structural integrity of cartilage; it aligns along the surface of the type II fibrils and may interact with the polyanionic glycosaminoglycan chains of aggrecan through the basic noncollagenous 4 (NC4) domain, which projects out from the surface of the fibrils. Figure 21–2 illustrates the sites at which various proteinases attack cartilage collagens.[62, 101] Collagen X is cleaved by MMP-1 and MMP-2.[102]

Collagen V, a minor component of extracellular matrix that forms hybrid collagen fibrils with other collagens, is digested by MMP-2 and MMP-9.[36]

Collagen VI is resistant to MMPs-1, 2, 3 and 9,[103] but it can be cleaved by neutrophil elastase, cathepsin G, chymase, or tryptase.[23]

Collagen VII, which forms anchoring fibrils in the skin, is susceptible to MMP-1,[104] MMP-2,[104] MMP-3, and MMP-9.

Proteoglycans

The core proteins of proteoglycans are susceptible to many proteinases. Most studies have been conducted with cartilage proteoglycan aggrecan, which forms large aggregated complexes interacting with hyaluronan and a link protein, because the loss of aggrecan is a major feature associated with various arthritides. The extended-core protein of aggrecan may be attacked by a number of proteinases in the chondroitin sulfate–rich and keratin sulfate–rich regions, but the key cleavage sites are considered to be located in the nonglobular domain that links the globular G1 and G2 domains (Fig. 21–3). A cleavage in this region releases the major glycosaminoglycan-bearing proteoglycan from the hyaluronan attachment site. While various proteinases attack this region in vitro (see Table 21–2), MMPs secreted from chondrocytes and synovial cells are thought to be the key enzymes under pathologic conditions.[54, 105, 106]

The treatment of articular cartilage explants with IL-1 releases aggrecan fragments cleaved at the Glu[373]-Ala[374] site.[107] The fragments resulting from this cleavage are found in joint fluid from patients with various inflammatory arthritides and osteoarthritis, which suggests that the enzyme called "aggrecanase" is

an important enzyme for aggrecan catabolism.[108] A high concentration of MMP-8 cleaves this bond in vitro,[109] but the cartilage-derived aggrecanase has not been identified.

Link protein stabilizes the interaction of aggrecan and hyaluronan. The proteinase-cleaved link protein increases with age. Digestion of link protein in vitro indicates that it is susceptible to a number of proteinases near the N terminus.[55, 110]

Elastin

Amorphous elastin fibers are degraded by a relatively limited number of proteinases. Neutrophil elastase and proteinase 3 released from PMN leukocytes effectively degrade elastin. Cathepsins L and S also have potent elastolytic activity.[11] The matrixins that degrade elastin include gelatinases A and B (MMP-2, MMP-9),[53] matrilysin (MMP-7)[61] and macrophage metalloproteinase (MMP-12).[68] MMP-3 has only a weak elastolytic activity.[61]

CELLULAR REGULATION OF PROTEINASE ACTIVITY

Cellular Origins of Extracellular Matrix–Degrading Proteinases

The proteinases that act on extracellular matrix components must be secreted from cells or must be bound to the cell surface. Under inflammatory conditions, not only resident cells but also infiltrated inflammatory cells produce specific proteinases. Cytokines and growth factors released by the stimulated cells also play a key role in regulating the production of ECM-degrading enzymes and their inhibitors. Table 21–6 lists the cellular origins of proteinases and their inhibitors that are involved in destruction of the joint in arthritis.

In patients with rheumatoid arthritis, synovial tissue may be the major source of proteinases. The pro-

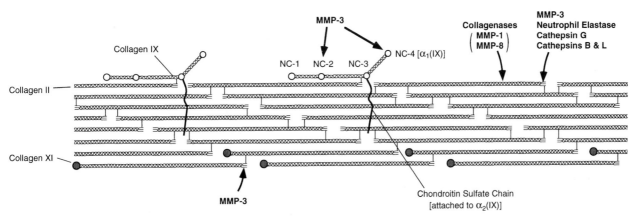

Figure 21–2. The sites of action of proteinases on fibrils of articular cartilage collagens.

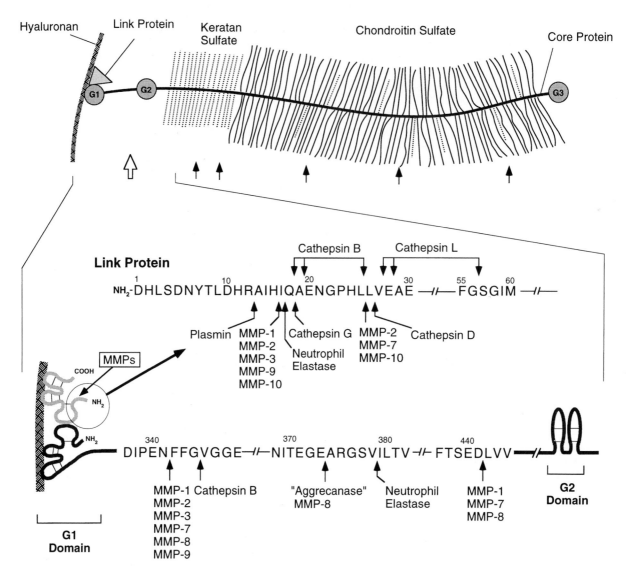

Figure 21–3. Proteolytic cleavage sites of aggrecan core protein and link protein of cartilage proteoglycan aggregates. The cleavage sites shown in the interglobular domain are derived from References 58, 114–116, and 118. The major cleavage sites are located in the region between G1 and G2 domains. Chondroitin sulfate–rich and keran sulfate–rich regions are also cleaved, generating smaller fragments. Link protein cleavage sites are derived from References 59 and 120. They are located principally on the N-terminal part of the protein. Cathepsin L cleaves the Gly[56]-Ser[57] bond located in the first disulfide-bonded loop.

Table 21–6. CELLULAR ORIGINS OF PROTEINASES AND PROTEINASE INHIBITORS IN THE JOINT

Cell Type	Proteinase	Proteinase Inhibitor
Synovial fibroblasts	MMP-1, MMP-2, MMP-3, MMP-9, MT-MMP, uPA, cathepsin B, cathepsin L, cathepsin D	TIMP-1, TIMP-2, PAI-1, PN-1
Monocytes-macrophages	MMP-1, MMP-2, MMP-7, MMP-9, MMP-12, uPA, cathepsin L, cathepsin D	TIMP-1, TIMP-2, PAI-1, α_1PI, α_2M
Endothelial cells	MMP-1, MMP-2, MMP-3, MMP-9, tPA	TIMP-1, TIMP-2, PAI-2
Mast cells	Chymase, tryptase, cathepsin G	Aprotinin
T-Lymphocytes	MMP-9	
PMN leukocytes	MMP-8, MMP-9, neutrophil elastase, cathepsin G, proteinase 3	
Chondrocytes	MMP-1, MMP-2, MMP-3, MMP-9, cathepsin B, cathepsin D, uPA, tPA	TIMP-1, TIMP-2
Osteoclasts	MMP-1, MMP-9, cathepsin B, cathepsin L	
Osteoblasts	MMP-1	

Abbreviations: MMP, matrix metalloproteinase; TIMP, tissue inhibitor of metalloproteinase; tPA, tissue-type plasminogen activator; PMN, polymorphonuclear neutrophil; PAI, plasminogen activator inhibitor; uPA, urokinase-type plasminogen activator; PN, proteinase nexin; α_2M, alpha$_2$-macroglobulin.

duction of MMP-1 and MMP-3 along with their transcripts in the lining cells is elevated.[111–116] These MMPs are secreted into the joint cavity. Inflammatory cells in the synovium include macrophages, lymphocytes, mast cells and PMN leukocytes. Macrophages produce MMP-1 and MMP-9 as well as TIMP-1 and TIMP-2. In addition, uPA and cathepsins B, L, and D can be secreted from the activated macrophages. Lymphocytes infiltrating rheumatoid synovium, mainly T lymphocytes, can synthesize and secrete MMP-9 upon appropriate stimulation. Mast cell proteinases are degranulated in response to immunoglobulin E (IgE) immune complexes. PMN leukocytes contain MMP-8 and MMP-9 in specific granules and neutrophil elastase and cathepsin G and proteinase 3 in azurophil granules. These proteinases are released extracellularly during phagocytosis of tissue debris and immune complexes. Endothelial cells produce a number of MMPs, tPA, and their inhibitors, which probably participate in tissue remodeling during angiogenesis in the synovium.

Pannus-like granulation tissue may invade the subchondral bone at the bare zone, and bone resorption occurs through the action of osteoclasts. Osteoclasts produce lysosomal cysteine proteinases, including cathepsins B and L, which can degrade highly cross-linked insoluble type I collagen in the acidic (pH 4 to 5) and hypercalcemic (40 to 50 mM Ca^{2+}) conditions of the subosteoclastic compartment. Osteoclasts produce MMP-1[117] and MMP-9.[118] The involvement of both cysteine proteinases and MMPs in osteoclastic

bone resorption is supported by studies with specific inhibitors of these proteinases.[119]

No prominent inflammatory changes occur in the synovium at early stages in osteoarthritis, but an elevated production of MMPs occurs in osteoarthritic cartilage. MMP-3 is immunolocalized in chondrocytes in the proteoglycan-depleted zone of osteoarthritic cartilage and the level of MMP-3 staining correlates directly with the histologic score.[120] Elevated production of MMP-9 and its messenger ribonucleic acid (mRNA) as well as an increase in MMP-1 and MMP-2 mRNAs is also observed in osteoarthritic cartilage.[121]

Control of MMP Gene Expression

Normal tissue extracts or cells in culture contain little or no MMP activity unless cells are stimulated with an appropriate factor. Numerous factors, including cytokines, growth factors, and chemical and physical stimuli, are stimulatory for MMP-1 production, often together with MMP-3 production (Table 21–7). The production of these MMPs is regulated at the transcriptional level.[122] However, the induction of MMP-1 and MMP-3 is not always coregulated. For example, IL-1 treatment of rheumatoid synovial fibroblasts enhances the level of MMP-3 transcripts more than of MMP-1 transcripts, whereas TNF-α and TPA are more effective for increasing MMP-1 expression than MMP-3 expression.[123] Retinoic acid, TGF-β, and glucocorticoid suppress the induced production

Table 21–7. FACTORS THAT MODULATE SYNTHESIS OF METALLOPROTEINASES (MMPs)

Enzyme	Stimulating Factor	Suppressive Factor
MMP-1	Cytokines and growth factors: IL-1; TNF-α; EGF; bFGF; PDGF; VEGF; nerve growth factor; IFN-α, IFN-β, and IFN-γ; TGF-α; leukoregulin; relaxin	Retinoic acid, glucocorticoids, estrogen, progesterone, TGF-β, transmembrane neural cell adhesion molecule, cAMP, interferon-γ
	Factors acting at cell surface: Calcium ionophore A23187; cell fusion; collagen; concanavalin A; integrin receptor antibody; crystals of urate; hydroxyapatite and calcium pyrophosphate; SPARC (osteonectin/BM40); iron; extracellular matrix metalloproteinase inducer (EMMPRIN/basigin/M6 antigen); polyhydroxyethylmethacrylate; phagocytosis	
	Chemical agents: cAMP, colchicine, cytochalasins B and D, LPS, pentoxifylline, TPA, calmodulin inhibitors, serotonin, 1,25-$(OH)_2$ vitamin D_3, platelet-activating factor serum amyloid A, β-microglobulin	
	Physical factors: heat shock, ultraviolet irradiation	
	Others: viral transformation, oncogenes, autocrine agents, aging of fibroblasts	
MMP-2	TGF-β, H-Ras transformation, extracellular matrix metalloproteinase inducer (EMMPRIN/basigin/M6 antigen)	Adenovirus E1A gene
MMP-3	*Less studied than MMP-1 induction, but stimulatory factors for MMP-1 often stimulate production of MMP-3:* IL-1, TNF-α, EGF, concanavalin A, SPARC (osteonectin/BM40), LPS, TPA, extracellular matrix metalloproteinase inducer (EMMPRIN/basigin/M6 antigen), viral transformation, oncogenes	Retinoic acid, glucocorticoids, estrogen, progesterone, TGF-β, cAMP
MMP-7	TPA, EGF, IL-1, TNF-α, LPS	
MMP-9	TGF-β, IL-1, TNF-α, TPA, LPS, SPARC (osteonectin/BM40)	

of MMP-1 and MMP-3. Interferon suppresses the IL-1–induced collagenolytic activity in human skin fibroblast. This results from the suppression of MMP-3 (collagenase activator) but not MMP-1 transcripts.[125] Other members of the matrixin family are also transcriptionally controlled (see Table 21–7).

Analysis of the 5'-flanking regions of a number of MMP genes has given insights into how these genes are regulated.[122, 125–129] The genes encoding MMP-1, MMP-3, MMP-7, MMP-9, and MMP-10 have a TATA box and a TPA-responsive element (TRE), a TGAG-TCA sequence, that binds to AP-1 proteins (Fos and Jun).[122] Small structural variations have a major effect on expressions of these genes. The enhanced expression of these MMPs by TPA, IL-1, or TNF-α is considered to be mediated by TRE in the promoter.

Many cells in culture constitutively produce MMP-2 as the 72-kD zymogen. Factors that enhance the production of MMP-1 and MMP-3 are not effective in this case. A 1.5 to 2.2-fold enhancement of MMP-2 production is observed in human gingival fibroblasts treated with TGF-β.[130] The 5'-flanking region of MMP-2 does not contain a TATA box or a TRE sequence, but it harbors an adenovirus E1A-responsive element that resembles the AP-2 binding site and two regions that function as a silencer.[131]

The expression of MMPs-1 and -3 is repressed by glucocorticoid, retinoic acid, and TGF-β. The suppression of MMP-1 transcripts by glucocorticoid results from the binding of the hormone receptor with c-Jun, which prevents the interaction between AP-1 and TRE.[132–134] The retinoic acid/retinoic acid receptor complex binds to the promoter of MMP-3, which also prevents the interaction of AP-1 and TRE.[135] TGF-β down-regulates rat MMP-3 transcription by a Fos-dependent mechanism that involves the TGF-β inhibitory element (TIE), GnnTTGGtGa sequence.[136]

Control of TIMP Gene Expression

TIMP-1 is produced in many tissues and cell types constitutively, but its production can be enhanced in response to cytokines, TGF-β, steroid hormones, oncogenic cellular transformation, and viral infection (Table 21–8). Some of these stimulatory factors also enhance the production of MMPs, but they are regulated independently.[137] For example, TGF-β, retinoic acid, progesterone, and estrogen enhance TIMP-1 production in fibroblasts, but they suppress the production of MMP-1 and MMP-3.

TIMP-2 is also constitutively expressed in various tissues and cells, but the expression of TIMP-1 and TIMP-2 is regulated differently in normal cells and transformed cells.[138–141]

TIMP-3 was originally found as a component tenaciously bound to the matrix secreted from chick embryonic fibroblasts transformed with Rouse sarcoma virus.[142] TIMP-3 transcripts in mouse fibroblasts are induced by EGF, TGF-β, TPA, and dexamethasone.[143]

Table 21–8. FACTORS THAT REGULATE EXPRESSION OF TISSUE INHIBITORS OF METALLOPROTEINASE (TIMPs)

Inhibitor	Stimulatory Factor	Suppressive Factor
TIMP-1	IL-1, IL-6, IL-11, TPA, TGF-β, lipopolysaccharide, retinoic acids, progesterone, estrogen, oncogenic cellular transformation, viral infection	Extracellular matrix interaction, cytochalasins
TIMP-2	Progesterone	TGF-β, lipopolysaccharide, gelatin, zymosan
TIMP-3	EGF, TGF-β, TPA, glucocorticoids	

Abbreviations: EGF, epidermal growth factor; TGF, transforming growth factor; TPA, 12-O-tetradecanoyl-phorbol-13-acetate.

Regulation of Expression of the Plasminogen Activator/Plasmin System

Gene expression of uPA is enhanced in a number of normal cell types and in transformed cells by agents that increase intracellular cyclic adenosine monophosphate (cAMP) levels, such as calcitonin, vasopressin, cholera toxin, and cAMP analogs; growth factors (e.g., EGF, PDGF, bFGF, vascular endothelial growth factor [VEGF]; cytokines (IL-1, TNF-α); and phorbol esters.[29, 144] Glucocorticoid or TGF-β decreases the production of uPA. Thrombin and plasmin stimulate the production of tPA by endothelial cells,[29] whereas glucocorticoids enhance it.

The expression of PAI-1 and PAI-2 is stimulated by common factors, many of which also enhance the production of uPA and tPA[29, 145] (Table 21–9). The production of PN-1 in fibroblasts is increased as treatment with phorbol esters, thrombin, and EGF.[75] The proteinase/PN-1 complex is rapidly internalized by the cells through a PN-1 receptor. Thus, PN-1 regulates the thrombin-mediated cell proliferation and uPA/plasmin-mediated degradation of extracellular matrix.

Expression of Lysosomal Proteinases

Cellular transformation is often associated with increased synthesis of cathepsin B,[12] cathepsin L,[13] and cathepsin D.[8] IL-1 stimulates chondrocytes in culture to increase intracellular cathepsin B.[146, 147] These chondrocytes resemble cells that are phenotypically modulated by serial subculture, which indicates that fibroblastic metaplasia of chondrocytes may be responsible for cathepsin B expression acting as a perpetuator of osteoarthritis.[147]

Table 21–9. FACTORS THAT REGULATE THE GENE EXPRESSION OF PLASMINOGEN ACTIVATORS AND THEIR INHIBITORS

Enzyme or Inhibitor	Stimulatory Factor	Suppressive Factor
uPA	TPA, IL-1, interferon-γ, EGF, PDGF, bFGF, VEGF, TGF-β, cholera toxin, cAMP, estrogen, calcitonin, vasopressin, disruption of E-cadherin–dependent cell-cell adhesion	Glucocorticoids, TGF-β
tPA	TPA, EGF, bFGF, VEGF, retinoic acid, glucocorticoid, cAMP, thrombin, plasmin, follicle-stimulating hormone, luteinizing hormone, gonadotropin-releasing hormone	TNF-α (endothelial cells)
PAI-1	IL-1, TNF-α, TGF-β, bFGF, VEGF, TPA, glucocorticoids	cAMP
PAI-2	TPA, LPS, TNF-α, colony-stimulating factor, cholera toxin, dengue virus	Glucocorticoids
PN-I	TPA, EGF, thrombin	

Abbreviations: PAI, plasminogen activator inhibitor; IL, interleukin; EGF, epidermal growth factor; LPS, lipopolysaccharide; bFGF, basic fibroblast growth factor; TNF, tumor necrosis factor; TGF, transforming growth factor; PDGF, platelet-derived growth factor; cAMP, cyclic adenosine monophosphate; VEGF, vascular endothelial growth factor; TPA, 12-O-tetradecanoyl-phorbol-13-acetate; tPA, tissue-type plasminogen activator; uPA, urokinase-type plasminogen activator; PN, proteinase nexin.

EXTRACELLULAR REGULATION OF MATRIX DEGRADATION

Most ECM-degrading proteinases are secreted or released from the cells as inactive zymogen except serine proteinases from granulocytes. Thus, the activation of these precursors in the extracellular space is a critical step involved in extracellular matrix degradation. Subsequently, the activated enzymes are regulated by endogenous inhibitors. Although the levels of these inhibitors are transcriptionally regulated, the inhibitor proteins may be inactivated by non-target proteinases. Another important factor that may modulate enzyme activities in the extracellular matrix involves the interaction of the secreted proteinases with specific extracellular matrix components that may serve to increase the local concentrations of specific enzymes.

Activation Mechanisms of proMMPs

The zymogens of matrixins (proMMPs) are activated in vitro by treatment with nonproteolytic agents as well as by the action of proteinases. The latency of proMMPs is maintained by interaction of the SH group of the cysteinyl residue in the conserved propeptide sequence PRCG[V/N]PD, referred to as "cysteine switch," with the zinc atom at the active site.[148, 149] This prevents the formation of a water-zinc complex that is required for the enzymatic reaction. Thus, the disruption of the Cys-Zn^{2+} interaction is essential for the zymogen activation through a stepwise processing of the propeptide (Fig. 21–4).

Activation by Nonproteolytic Agents

Agents such as thiol-modifying reagents (e.g., mercurial compounds, iodoacetamide, N-ethylmaleimide, oxidized glutathione), hypochlorous acid (HOCl), sodium dodecyl sulfate (SDS), chaotropic agents, and physical factors (heat and acid exposure) can activate many proMMPs in vitro.[40, 149] Studies on the activation of proMMP-3 by 4-aminophenylmercuric acetate (APMA) have indicated that the initial step involves the generation of a short-lived intermediate generated by removal of a part of propeptide by an intramolecular reaction[36, 40] (see Fig. 21–4).

Activation of proMMPs by Proteinases

In general, activation by proteinases also proceeds in a stepwise manner (see Fig. 21–4A). Activator proteinases initially attack the proteinase susceptible "bait" regions in the propeptides and generate intermediates. The cleavage of the propeptide destabilizes the Cys-Zn^{2+} interaction, which then renders the final activation site susceptible to a second proteolytic attack. This latter reaction is catalyzed by MMP but not by the trigger proteinase. Usually, active MMPs cannot participate in this second step unless a part of the propeptide is removed by proteolysis.[36, 40] In many cases, the bait region sequence in the propeptide dictates which proteinases can become an activator of a particular MMP.[40] Potential activators of proMMPs are listed in Table 21–10.

In vivo, the generation of plasmin by uPA and tPA may play a significant role in the activation of procollagenases, prostromelysins, and possibly other proMMPs (Fig. 21–5). The focalized activation of pro-uPA bound to the uPA receptor and the subsequent activation of plasminogen to plasmin is a mechanism that confines the site of MMP activation to the proximity of the cell surface.

When plasmin cleaves the bait region of proMMP-1, however, only about 25 percent of the potential MMP-1 activity is expressed.[150] For full activation, a specific cleavage of the Gln^{80}-Phe^{81} bond by stromelysins (MMP-3 and MMP-10) or matrilysin (MMP-7) is required.[65, 150] MMP-3 also activates progelatinase B (proMMP-9) in a stepwise manner.[36] Chymase released from mast cells directly cleaves the Phe^{81}-Val^{82} bond or Leu^{83}-Thr^{84} bond of proMMP-1,[26, 29] but MMP-1 by this process has only about 25 percent of the full activity.[27] The correct processing of the Gln^{80}-Phe^{81} bond is essential for full MMP-1 activity. Thus, the repertoire of the proteinases present in the tissue governs the degree of the collagenolytic activity.

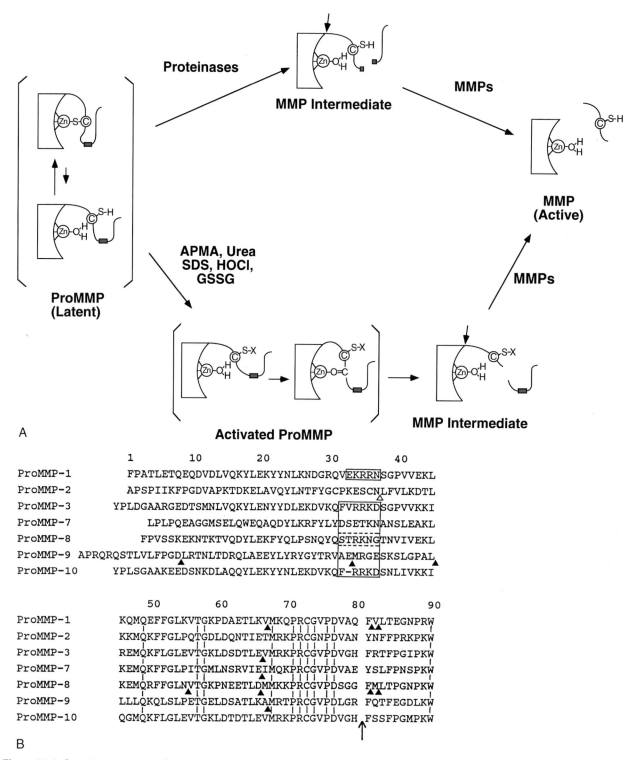

Figure 21–4. Stepwise activation of promatrixins. *A,* ProMMPs are activated in a stepwise manner by a proteinase pathway and by a conformation-induced pathway by such reagents as 4-aminophenylmercuric acetate (APMA), oxidized glutathione (GSSG), urea, sodium dodecyl sulfate (SDS), and hypochlorous acid (HOCl). In the proteinase pathway, an activator proteinase first attacks the "bait" region in the propeptide. This destabilizes the zinc-cysteine interaction. In the presence of APMA, a portion of propeptide is removed by intramolecular reaction of the proenzyme. The complete removal of the propeptide is conducted by the action of an MMP or an MMP intermediate. *B,* Cleavage sites in the propeptides of proMMPs during activation. The boxes denote the proteinase-susceptible bait region. Cleavages induced by APMA or HgCl₂ treatment is shown by ▲. The Asn³⁷-Leu³⁸ bond of proMMP-2 (△) is cleaved by the plasma membrane.[151] The final cleavage sites required for complete removal of the propeptides are indicated by ↑. Amino acid conserved in all the sequences are indicated by |. (Redrawn from Nagase H: Matrix metalloproteinases. *In* Hooper NM: Zinc Metalloproteinases in Health and Disease. London, Taylor & Francis, 1996, p 153.)

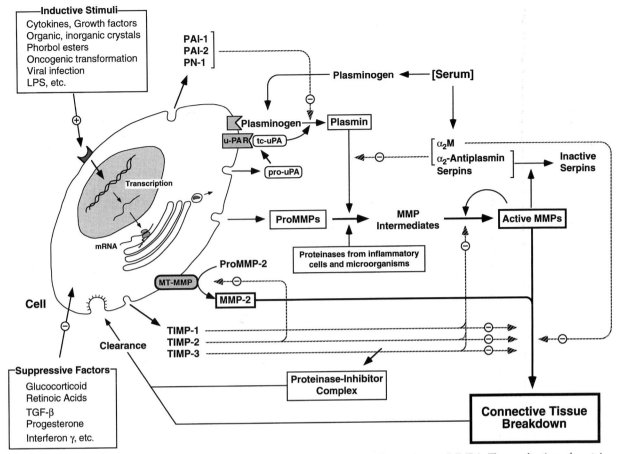

Figure 21–5. Pathways of extracellular matrix (ECM) degradation by matrix metalloproteinases (MMPs). The production of proteinases and their protein inhibitors are transcriptionally regulated by cytokines, growth factors, hormones, and other stimuli. Pro-uPA binds to the uPA receptor (U-PAR) and is activated on the cell surface to the two-chain uPA (tc-uPA), which in turn activates plasminogen on the cell surface. Plasmin then initiates activation of procollagenase and prostromelysin. Proteinases from inflammatory cells and microorganisms can also activate proMMPs. The final step of proMMP activation involves the action of MMP. MMP intermediates may bind to tissue inhibitors of metalloproteinases (TIMPs) before they are fully activated. ProMMP-2 is activated by the cell-associated membrane-type MMP (MT-MMP). This reaction is inhibited by an excess amount of TIMP-2. LPS, lipopolysaccharide; mRNA, messenger ribonucleic acid; PN, proteinase nexin; PAI, plasminogen activator inhibitor; TGF, transforming growth factor.

Activation of proMMP-2 by the Plasma Membrane

ProMMP-2 is resistant to activation by most endopeptidases.[36] An endogenous activator is found on the surface of normal or neoplastic cells treated with concanavalin A, TPA, TGF-β, the RGD-containing peptide or cells cultured on collagen.[40] The recently discovered MT-MMP has been shown to activate proMMP-2.[44] Studies by Strongin and colleagues[152] have demonstrated that MT-MMP acts as a cell surface TIMP-2 receptor. They suggest that this complex, in turn, activates proMMP-2 through the interaction of COOH-terminal domains of proMMP-2 and TIMP-2.

Balance Between Proteinases and Proteinase Inhibitors

Any imbalance between proteinases and their specific inhibitors may result in the accelerated degrada-

tion or accumulation of ECM components. Endogenous proteinase inhibitors from plasma and local tissues control proteolytic activities to provide a precise rate of tissue matrix turnover under physiologic conditions. The stepwise mechanisms of promatrixin activation also ensure that MMP activities are regulated not only after full activation of the enzyme but also during activation steps, which introduces fine tuning in the regulation of ECM proteolysis (see Fig. 21–5). The levels of proteinase inhibitors are influenced not only by changes in their synthesis in response to various stimuli but also by their inactivation or depletion. At inflammatory sites, increased proteolytic activity may destroy a number of important inhibitors. Serpins are particularly sensitive to inactivation by non-target proteinases, such as MMPs,[67, 153] cysteine proteinases, and microbial proteinases.[73] Some inactivation α_1PI and α_1-antichymotrypsin by MMP-3 may occur when the level of enzyme is elevated.[153] Elastase can potentially inactivate anti-thrombin III, α_2-antiplasmin, and C1 inactiva-

Table 21–10. ACTIVATORS OF PRO-METALLOPROTEINASES (proMMPs)

proMMP-1	Trypsin, plasmin, plasma kallikrein, chymase; MMP-3 and MMP-7 cleaves Gln^{80}-Phe^{81} bond only when a part of propeptide is removed by proteolysis
proMMP-2	MT-MMP, MMP-7 (to a lesser extent)
proMMP-3	Activated by many proteinases but not by MMPs; trypsin-like proteinases (e.g., plasmin, plasma kallikrein, tryptase, but not thrombin); chymotrypsin-like proteinases (chymase, cathepsin G, chymotrypsin); neutrophil elastase; metalloendopeptidases (thermolysin, *Pseudomonas* elastase)
proMMP-7	MMP-3 (accelerated in the presence of APMA), trypsin (partially activated by plasmin and neutrophil elastase)
proMMP-8	MMP-3, tissue kallikrein, neutrophil elastase, cathepsin G, trypsin
proMMP-9	MMP-3, trypsin (partially activated by chymotrypsin, cathepsin G, and plasmin)

Abbreviation: APMA, 4-aminophenyl mercuric acetate.

tor.[73, 154] The oxidation of Met^{358} of α_1PI by oxygen radicals generated during the respiratory burst of neutrophil and monocytes inactivates this inhibitor.[73] TIMP-1 is also inactivated by neutrophil elastase.[155]

Progelatinase-TIMP complexes can inhibit other MMPs. When this action occurs, progelatinases become available for activation.[156] This shifts the nature of the predominant matrixin activity in the tissue from one type to another. Such timing may be critical during physiologic remodeling of the matrix.

Recently, point mutations in TIMP-3 (Tyr168Cys and Ser181Cys) have shown to cause Sorsby's fundus dystrophy, a heredity macular dystrophy that causes irreversible loss of vision.[157] Thickening of the inner portion of Bruch's membrane is a hallmark of the disease, and it has been postulated that dysfunction of TIMP-3 may affect the extracellular matrix homeostasis of this membrane.

Interaction of Proteinases with Extracellular Matrix

Biochemical studies using isolated components of extracellular matrix in solution suggest that a number of them are potential substrates for specific proteinases, but the actual substrates in vivo for ECM-degrading enzymes are not well defined. Both proMMP-3 and active MMP-3 bind to collagen I through the C-terminal domain, but only active MMP-1—not proMMP-1—binds to collagen I.[50] ProMMP-2 and proMMP-9 bind to gelatin and collagen through the fibronectin-like domain.[41–43] The activation of proMMP-2 on the cell surface and the possible interaction of ECM suggest that focalized pericellular enzymic activity may be sufficient to degrade basement membrane collagen IV, although MMP-2 has only weak activity on collagen IV in solution. Plasminogen

binds to fibronectin, collagen IV, laminin, and to cell surfaces.[29, 31]

Acknowledgments

We thank Yoshifumi Itoh for drawing illustrations and Denise Byrd for secretarial assistance.

REFERENCES

1. Werb Z, Alexander CM: Proteinases and matrix degradation. In Kelley W, Harris ED Jr, Ruddy S, Sledge CB (eds): Textbook of Rheumatology, 4th ed. Philadelphia, WB Saunders, 1993, p 248.
2. Nagase H, Woessner JF Jr: Role of endogenous proteinases in the degradation of cartilage matrix. In Woessner F Jr, Howell DS (eds): Joint Cartilage Degradation: Basic Clinical Aspects. New York, Marcel Dekker, 1993, p 159.
3. Barrett AJ: An introduction to the proteinases. In Barrett AJ, Salvesen G (eds): Proteinase Inhibitors. Amsterdam, Elsevier, 1986, p 3.
4. Salvesen G, Nagase H: Inhibition of proteolytic enzymes. In Beynon RJ, Bond JS (eds): Proteolytic Enzymes: A Practical Approach. Oxford, ILS Press, 1989, p 83.
5. von Figura K, Hasklik A: Lysosomal enzymes and their receptors. Annu Rev Biochem 55:167, 1986.
6. Poole AR, Hembry RM, Dingle JT: Cathepsin D in cartilage: the immunohistochemical demonstration of extracellular enzyme in normal and pathological conditions. J Cell Sci 14:139, 1974.
7. Rossman MD, Maida BT, Douglas S: Monocyte-derived macrophage and alveolar macrophage fibronectin production and cathepsin D activity. Cell Immunol 126:268, 1990.
8. Rochefort H: Cathepsin D in breast cancer: A tissue marker associated with metastasis. Eur J Cancer 28A:1780, 1992.
9. Scott PG, Pearson CH: Cathepsin D—cleavage of soluble collagen and cross-linked peptides. FEBS Lett 88:41, 1978.
10. Hembry RM, Knight CG, Dingle JT, et al: Evidence that extracellular cathepsin D is not responsible for the resorption of cartilage matrix in culture. Biochim Biophys Acta 714:307, 1982.
11. Mason RW, Wilcox D: Chemistry of lysosomal cysteine proteinases. Adv Cell Mol Biol Membranes 1:81, 1993.
12. Mort JS, Recklies AD: Interrelationship of active and latent secreted human cathepsin B precursors. Biochem J 233:57, 1986.
13. Mason RW, Gal S, Gottesman MM: The identification of the major excreted protein (MEP) from a transformed mouse fibroblast cell line as a catalytically active precursor form of cathepsin L. Biochem J 248:449, 1987.
14. Kirschke H, Wiederanders B, Brömme D, et al: Cathepsin S from bovine spleen-purification, distribution, intracellular localization and action on proteins. Biochem J 264:467, 1989.
15. Maciewicz RA, Etherington DJ: A comparison of four cathepsins (B, L, N and S) with collagenolytic activity from rabbit spleen. Biochem J 256:433, 1988.
16. Suzuki K, Shimizu K, Hamamoto T, et al: Biochemical demonstration of calpains and calpastatin in osteoarthritic synovial fluid. Arthritis Rheum 33:728, 1990.
17. Maciewicz RA, Etherington DJ, Kos J, et al.: Collagenolytic cathepsins of rabbit spleen: A kinetic analysis of collagen degradation and inhibition by chicken cystatin. Collagen Relat Res 7:295, 1987.
18. Maciewicz RA, Wotton SF, Etherington DJ, et al.: Susceptibility of the cartilage collagens types II, IX and XI to degradation by the cysteine proteinases, cathepsins B and L. FEBS Lett 269:189, 1990.
19. Salvesen G, Enghild JJ: Zymogen activation specificity and genomic structures of human neutrophil elastase and cathepsin G reveal a new branch of the chymotrypsinogen superfamily of serine proteinases. Biomed Biochim Acta 50:665, 1991.
20. Starkey PM, Barrett AJ, Burleigh MC: The degradation of articular collagen by neutrophil proteinases. Biochim Biophys Acta 483:386, 1977.
21. Rao NV, Wehner NG, Marshall BC, et al: Characterization of proteinase-3 (PR-3), a neutrophil serine proteinase. Structural and functional properties. J Biol Chem 266:9540, 1991.
22. Campanelli D, Melchior M, Fu Y, et al.: Cloning of cDNA for proteinase 3: A serine protease, antibiotic, and autoantigen from human neutrophils. J Exp Med 172:1709, 1990.
23. Kielty CM, Lees M, Shuttleworth CA, et al: Catabolism of intact type VI collagen microfibrils: Susceptibility to degradation by serine proteinases. Biochem Biophys Res Commun 191:1230, 1993.
24. Lohi J, Harvima I, Keski OJ: Pericellular substrates of human mast

cell tryptase: 72,000 dalton gelatinase and fibronectin. J Cell Biochem 50:337, 1992.

25. Schwartz LB: The mast cell. *In* Kelley W, Harris ED Jr, Ruddy S, Sledge CB (eds): Textbook of Rheumatology, 4th ed. Philadelphia, WB Saunders, 1993, p 304.

26. Saarinen J, Kalkkinen N, Welgus HG, et al: Activation of human interstitial procollagenase through direct cleavage of the Leu[83]-Thr[84] bond by mast cell chymase. J Biol Chem 269:18134, 1994.

27. Suzuki K, Lees M, George FJ, et al: Activation of precursors for matrix metalloproteinases 1 (interstitial collagenase) and 3 (stromelysin) by rat mast-cell proteinases I and II. Biochem J 305:301, 1995.

28. Schechter NM, Wang ZM, Blacher RW, et al: Determination of the primary structures of human skin chymase and cathepsin G from cutaneous mast cells of urticaria pigmentosa lesions. J Immunol 152:4062, 1994.

29. Saksela O, Rifkin DB: Cell-associated plasminogen activation: Regulation and physiological functions. Annu Rev Cell Biol 4:93–126, 1988.

30. Pöllänen J, Stephens RW, Vaheri A: Directed plasminogen activation at the surface of normal and malignant cells. Adv Cancer Res 57:273, 1991.

31. Moser TL, Enghild JJ, Pizzo SV, et al: The extracellular matrix proteins laminin and fibronectin contain binding domains for human plasminogen and tissue plasminogen activator. J Biol Chem 268:18917, 1993.

32. Ellis V, Pyke C, Eriksen J, et al: The urokinase receptor: Involvement in cell surface proteolysis and cancer invasion. Ann NY Acad Sci 667:13, 1992.

33. Ellis V, Behrendt N, Danø K: Plasminogen activation by receptor-bound urokinase: A kinetic study with both cell-associated and isolated receptor. J Biol Chem 266:12752, 1991.

34. Quigley JP, Gold LI, Schwimmer R, et al: Limited cleavage of cellular fibronectin by plasminogen activator purified from transformed cells. Proc Natl Acad Sci USA 84:2776, 1987.

35. Heimark RL, Davie EW: Bovine and human plasma prekallikrein. Methods Enzymol 80:157, 1981.

36. Nagase H, Ogata Y, Suzuki K, et al: Substrate specificities and activation mechanisms of matrix metalloproteinases. Biochem Soc Trans 19:715, 1991.

37. Knäuper V, Krämer S, Reinke H, et al: Characterization and activation of procollagenase from human polymorphonuclear leukocytes: N-terminal sequence determination of the proenzyme and various proteolytically activated forms. Eur J Biochem 189:295, 1990.

38. Woessner JF Jr: Matrix metalloproteinases and their inhibitors in connective tissue remodeling. FASEB J 5:2145, 1991.

39. Birkedal-Hansen H, Moore WGI, Bodden MK, et al: Matrix metalloproteinases: A review. Crit Rev Oral Biol Med 4:197, 1993.

40. Nagase H: Matrix metalloproteinases. *In* Hooper NM (ed): Zinc Metalloproteases in Health and Disease. London, Taylor & Francis, 1996, p 153.

41. Collier IE, Krasnov PA, Strongin AY, et al: Alanine scanning mutagenesis and functional analysis of the fibronectin-like collagen-binding domain from human 92-kDa type IV collagenase. J Biol Chem 267:6776, 1992.

42. Murphy G, Nguyen Q, Cockett MI, et al: Assessment of the role of the fibronectin-like domain of gelatinase A by analysis of a deletion mutant. J Biol Chem 269:6632, 1994.

43. Bányai L, Tordai H, Patthy L: The gelatin-binding site of human 72 kDa type IV collagenase (gelatinase A). Biochem J 298:403, 1994.

44. Sato H, Takino T, Okada Y, et al: A novel matrix metalloproteinase expressed on invasive tumor cell surface. Nature 370:61, 1994.

45. Lovejoy B, Cleasby A, Hassell AM, et al: Structure of the catalytic domain of fibroblast collagenase complexed with an inhibitor. Science 263:375, 1994.

46. Bode W, Reinemer A, Huber R, et al: The x-ray crystal structure of the catalytic domain of human neutrophil collagenase inhibited by a substrate analogue reveals the essentials for catalysis and specificity. EMBO J 13:1263, 1994.

47. Freije JMP, Díez-Itza I, Balbin M, et al: Molecular cloning and expression of collagenase-3, a novel human matrix metalloproteinase produced by breast carcinomas. J Biol Chem 269:16766, 1994.

48. Netzel-Arnett S, Fields G, Birkedal-Hansen H, et al: Sequence specificities of human fibroblast and neutrophil collagenases. J Biol Chem 266:6747, 1991.

49. Enghild JJ, Salvesen G, Brew K, et al: Interaction of human rheumatoid synovial collagenase (matrix metalloproteinase 1) and stromelysin (matrix metalloproteinase 3) with human α₂-macroglobulin and chicken ovostatin: Binding kinetics and identification of matrix metalloproteinase cleavage sites. J Biol Chem 264:8779, 1989.

50. Murphy G, Allan JA, Willenbrock F, et al: The role of the C-terminal domain in collagenase and stromelysin specificity. J Biol Chem 267:9612, 1992.

51. Hirose T, Patterson C, Pourmotabbed T, et al: Structure-function relationship of human neutrophil collagenase: Identification of regions responsible for substrate specificity and general proteinase activity. Proc Natl Acad Sci USA 90:2569, 1993.

52. Hibbs MS, Mainardi CL, Kang AH: Type-specific collagen degradation by eosinophils. Biochem J 207:621, 1982.

53. Senior RM, Griffin GL, Flizzar CJ, et al: Human 92- and 72-kilodalton type IV collagenases are elastases. J Biol Chem 266:7870, 1991.

54. Fosang AJ, Naeme PJ, Last K, et al: The interglobular domain of cartilage aggrecan is cleaved by PUMP, gelatinases and cathepsin B. J Biol Chem 267:19470, 1992.

55. Nguyen Q, Murphy G, Hughes C, et al: Matrix metalloproteinases cleave at two distinct sites on human cartilage link protein. Biochem J 295:595, 1993.

56. Netzel-Arnett S, Sang QX, Moore WGI, et al: Comparative sequence specificities of human 72- and 92-kDa gelatinases (type IV collagenases) and PUMP (matrilysin). Biochemistry 32:6427, 1993.

57. Unemori EN, Hibbs MS, Amento EP: Constitutive expression of a 92 kDa gelatinase (type V collagenase) by rheumatoid synovial fibroblasts and its induction in normal human fibroblasts by inflammatory cytokines. J Clin Invest 88:1656, 1991.

58. Ogata Y, Pratta MA, Nagase H, et al: Matrix metalloproteinase 9 (92-kDa gelatinase/type IV collagenase) is induced in rabbit articular chondrocytes by cotreatment with interleukin 1β and a protein kinase C activator. Exp Cell Res 201:245, 1992.

59. Weeks BS, Schnaper HW, Handy M, et al: Human T lymphocytes synthesize the 92-kDa type IV collagenase (gelatinase B). J Cell Physiol 157:644, 1993.

60. Nagase H: Human stromelysins 1 and 2. Methods Enzymol 248:449, 1995.

61. Murphy G, Cockett MI, Ward RV, et al: Matrix metalloproteinase degradation of elastin, type IV collagen and proteoglycan: A quantitive comparison of the activities of 95 kDa and 72 kDa gelatinases, stromelysins-1 and -2 and punctuated metalloproteinase (PUMP). Biochem J 277:277, 1991.

62. Wu J-J, Lark MW, Chun LE, et al: Sites of stromelysin cleavage in collagen types II, IX, X and XI of cartilage. J Biol Chem 266:5625, 1991.

63. Niedzwiecki L, Teahan J, Harrison RK, et al: Substrate specificity of the human matrix metalloproteinase stromelysin and the development of continuous fluorometric assays. Biochemistry 31:12618, 1992.

64. Windsor LJ, Grenett H, Birkedal-Hansen B, et al: Cell type-specific regulation of SL-1 and SL-2 genes: Induction of the SL-2 gene but not the SL-1 gene by human keratinocytes in response to cytokines and phorbolesters. J Biol Chem 268:17341, 1993.

65. Imai K, Yokohama Y, Nakanishi I, et al: Matrix metalloproteinas 7 (matrilysin) from human rectal carcinoma cells. Activation of the precursor, interaction with other matrix metalloproteinases and enzymic properties. J Biol Chem 270:6691, 1995.

66. Murphy G, Segain J-P, O'Shea M, et al: The 28-kDa N-terminal domain of mouse stromelysin-3 has the general properties of a weak metalloproteinase. J Biol Chem 268:15435, 1993.

67. Pei D, Majmudar G, Weiss SJ: Hydrolytic inactivation of a breast carcinoma cell-derived serpin by human stromelysin-3. J Biol Chem 269:25849, 1994.

68. Shapiro SD, Kobayashi DK, Ley TJ: Cloning and characterization of a unique elastolytic metalloproteinase produced by human alveolar macrophages. J Biol Chem 268:23824, 1993.

69. Travis J, Salvesen G: Plasma proteinase inhibitors. Annu Rev Biochem 52:655, 1983.

70. Barrett AJ, Starkey PM: The interaction of α₂-macroglobulin with proteinases. Characteristics and specificity of the reaction and a hypothesis concerning its molecular mechanisms. Biochem J 133:709, 1973.

71. Borth W: α₂-Macroglobulin, a multifunctional binding protein with targeting characteristics. FASEB J 6:3345, 1992.

72. Sottrup-Jensen L: α-Macroglobulins: Structure, shape and mechanism of proteinase complex formation. J Biol Chem 264:11539, 1989.

73. Potempa J, Korzus E, Travis J: The serpin superfamily of proteinase inhibitors: Structure, function, and regulation. J Biol Chem 269:15957, 1994.

74. Laiho M, Saksela O, Keski-Oja J: Transforming growth factor-β induction of type-1 plasminogen activator inhibitor: Pericellular deposition and sensitivity to exogenous urokinase. J Biol Chem 262:17467, 1987.

75. Cunningham DD, Van Nostrand WE, Farrell DH, et al: Interactions of serine proteases with cultured fibroblasts. J Cell Biochem 32:281, 1986.

76. Salvesen G, Enghild JJ: Proteinases inhibitors: An overview of their structure and possible function in the acute phase. *In* Mackiewicz A, Kushner I, Baumann H (eds): Acute Phase Proteins: Molecular Biology, Biochemistry and Clinical Applications. Boca Raton, Fla, CRC Press, 1993, p 117.

77. Van Nostrand WE, Wagner SL, Farrow JS, et al: Immunopurification and protease inhibitory properties of protease nexin-2/amyloid beta-protein precursor. J Biol Chem 265:9591, 1990.

78. Böhm B, Deutzmann R, Burkhardt H: Purification of a serine-proteinase inhibitor from human articular cartilage: Identify with the acid-stable proteinase inhibitor of mucous secretions. Biochem J 274:269, 1991.

79. Barrett AJ, Rawlings ND, Davies ME, et al: Cysteine proteinase inhibitors of the cystatin superfamily. *In* Barrett AJ, Salvesen G (eds): Proteinase Inhibitors. Amsterdam, Elsevier, 1986, p 515.

80. Chapman HA, Reilly JJ, Yee R, et al: Identification of cystatin C, a

cysteine proteinase inhibitor, as a major secretory product of human alveolar macrophages *in vitro*. Am Rev Respir Dis 141:698, 1990.

81. Maki M, Ma H, Takano E, et al: Calpastatins: Biochemical and molecular biological studies. Biomed Biochim Acta 50:509, 1991.

82. Thornberry NA, Bull HG, Calaycay JR, et al: A novel heterodimeric cysteine protease is required for interleukin-1β processing in monocytes. Nature 356:768, 1992.

83. Ray CA, Black RA, Kronheim SR, et al: Viral inhibition of inflammation: Cowpox virus encodes an inhibitor of the interleukin-1β converting enzyme. Cell 69:597, 1992.

84. Murphy G, Willenbrock F: Tissue inhibitors of matrix metalloendopeptidases. Methods Enzymol 248:496, 1995.

85. Murphy G, Houbrechts A, Cockett MI, et al: The N-terminal domain of tissue inhibitor of metalloproteinases retains metalloproteinase inhibitory activity. Biochemistry 30:8097, 1991.

86. Williamson RA, Martorell G, Carr MD, et al: Solution structure of the active domain of tissue inhibitor of metalloproteinases-2: A new member of the OB fold protein family. Biochemistry 33:11745, 1994.

87. Silbiger SM, Jacobsen VL, Cupples RL, et al: Cloning of cDNAs encoding human TIMP-3, a novel member of the tissue inhibitor of metalloproteinase family. Gene 141:293, 1994.

88. Kolkenbrock H, Orgel D, Hecker-Kia A, et al: The complex between a tissue inhibitor of metalloproteinase (TIMP-2) and 72-kDa progelatinase is a metalloproteinase inhibitor. Eur J Biochem 198:775, 1991.

89. Gasson JC, Golde DW, Kaufman SE, et al: Molecular characterization and expression of the gene encoding human erythroid-potentiating activity. Nature 316:768, 1985.

90. Hayakawa T, Yamashita K, Kishi J, et al: Tissue inhibitor of metalloproteinases from human bone marrow stromal cell line KM 102 has erythroid-potentiating activity, suggesting its possibly bifunctional role in the hematopoietic microenvironment. FEBS Lett 268:125, 1990.

91. Stetler-Stevenson WG, Bersch N, Golde DW: Tissue inhibitor of metalloproteinase-2 (TIMP-2) has erythroid-potentiating activity. FEBS Lett 296:231, 1992.

92. Hayakawa T, Yamashita K, Tanzawa K, et al: Growth-promoting activity of tissue inhibitor of metalloproteinases-1 (TIMP-1) for a wide range of cells: A possible new growth factor in serum. FEBS Lett 298:29, 1992.

93. Hayakawa T, Yamashita K, Ohuchi E, et al: Cell growth-promoting activity of tissue inhibitor of metalloproteinases-2 (TIMP-2). J Cell Sci 107:2373, 1994.

94. Bertaux B, Hornebeck W, Eisen A Z, et al: Growth stimulation of human keratinocytes by tissue inhibitor of metalloproteinases. J Invest Dermatol 97:679, 1991.

95. Okada Y, Gonoji Y, Naka K, et al: Matrix metalloproteinase 9 (92-kDa gelatinase/type IV collagenase) from HT 1080 human fibrosarcoma cells: Purification and activation of the precursor and enzymic properties. J Biol Chem 267:21712, 1992.

96. Mainardi CL, Hasty DL, Seyer JM, et al: Specific cleavage of human type III collagen by human polymorphonuclear leukocyte elastase. J Biol Chem 255:12006, 1980.

97. Fessler LI, Duncan KG, Fessler JH, et al: Characterization of the procollagen IV cleavage products produced by a specific tumor collagenase. J Biol Chem 259:9783, 1984.

98. Emonard HP, Remacle AG, Noël AC, et al: Tumor cell surface-associated binding site for the M$_r$ 72,000 type IV collagenase. Cancer Res 52:5845, 1992.

99. Davies M, Barrett AJ, Travis J, et al: The degradation of human glomerular basement membrane with purified lysosomal proteinases: Evidence for the pathogenic role of the polymorphonuclear leucocyte in glomerulonephritis. Clin Sci Mol Med 54:233, 1978.

100. Thomas GJ, Davies M: The potential role of human kidney cortex cysteine proteinases in glomerular basement membrane degradation. Biochim Biophys Acta 990:246, 1989.

101. Gadher SJ, Eyre DR, Duance VC, et al: Susceptibility of cartilage collagens type II, IX, X and XI to human synovial collagenase and neutrophil elastase. Eur J Biochem 175:1, 1988.

102. Welgus HG, Fliszar CJ, Seltzer JL, et al: Differential susceptibility of type X collagen to cleavage by two mammalian interstitial collagenases and 72-kDa type IV collagenase. J Biol Chem 265:13521, 1990.

103. Okada Y, Naka K, Minamoto T, et al: Localization of type VI collagen in the lining cell layer of normal and rheumatoid synovium. Lab Invest 63:647, 1990.

104. Seltzer JL, Eisen AZ, Bauer, EA, et al: Cleavage of type VII collagen by interstitial collagenase and type IV collagenase (gelatinase) derived from human skin. J Biol Chem 264:3822, 1989.

105. Flannery CR, Lark MW, Sandy JD: Identification of a stromelysin cleavage site within the interglobular domain of human aggrecan: Evidence for proteolysis at this site in vivo in human articular cartilage. J Biol Chem 267:1008, 1992.

106. Fosang AJ, Last K, Knäuper V, et al: Fibroblast and neutrophil collagenases cleave at two sites in the cartilage aggrecan interglobular domain. Biochem J 295: 273, 1993.

107. Sandy JD, Neame PJ, Boynton RE, et al: Catabolism of aggrecan in

108. Sandy JD, Flannery CR, Neame PJ, et al: The structure of aggrecan fragments in human synovial fluid: Evidence for the involvement in osteoarthritis of a novel proteinase which cleaves the Glu373-Ala374 bond of the interglobular domain. J Clin Invest 89:1512, 1992.

109. Fosang AJ, Last K, Neame PJ, et al: Neutrophil collagenase (MMP-8) cleaves at the aggrecanase site E^{373}-A^{374} in the interglobular domain of cartilage aggrecan. Biochem J 304:347, 1994.

110. Nguyen Q, Liu J, Roughley PJ, et al: Link protein as a monitor *in situ* of endogenous proteolysis in adult human articular cartilage. Biochem J 278:143, 1991.

111. Okada Y, Takeuchi N, Tomita K, et al: Immunolocalization of matrix metalloproteinase 3 (stromelysin) in rheumatoid arthritis. Ann Rheum Dis 48:645, 1989.

112. Okada Y, Gonoji Y, Nakanishi I, et al: Immunohistochemical demonstration of collagenase and tissue inhibitor of metalloproteinases (TIMP) by synovial lining cells of rheumatoid synovium. Virchows Arch B Cell Pathol 59:305, 1990.

113. Firestein GS, Paine MM, Littman BH: Gene expression (collagenase, tissue inhibitor of metalloproteinases, complement, and HLA-DR) in rheumatoid arthritis and osteoarthritis synovium: Quantitative analysis and effect of intraarticular corticosteroids. Arthritis Rheum 34:1094, 1991.

114. McCachren SS: Expression of metalloproteinases and metalloproteinase inhibitor in human arthritic synovium. Arthritis Rheum 34:1085, 1991.

115. Gravallese EM, Darling JM, Ladd AL, et al: In situ hybridization studies of stromelysin and collagenase messenger RNA expression in rheumatoid synovium. Arthritis Rheum 34:1076, 1991.

116. Wolfe GC, MacNaul KL, Buechel FF, et al: Differential *in vivo* expression of collagenase messenger RNA in synovium and cartilage. Quantitative comparison with stromelysin messenger RNA levels in human rheumatoid arthritis and osteoarthritis. Arthritis Rheum 36:1540, 1993.

117. Delaissé JM, Eeckhout Y, Neff L, et al: (Pro)collagenase (matrix metalloproteinase-1) is present in rodent osteoclasts and in the underlying bone-resorbing compartment. J Cell Sci 106:1071, 1993.

118. Okada Y, Naka K, Kawamura K, et al: Localization of matrix metalloproteinase 9 (92-kilodalton gelatinase/type IV collagenase = gelatinase B) in osteoclasts: Implications for bone resorption. Lab Invest 72:311, 1995.

119. Eeckhout Y, Delaissé JM, Ledent P, et al: The proteinases of bone resorption. *In* Glauert A (ed): The Control of Tissue Damage. Belgium, Elsevier Science, 1988, p 297.

120. Okada Y, Shinmei M, Tanaka O, et al: Localization of matrix metalloproteinase 3 (stromelysin) in osteoarthritic cartilage and synovium. Lab Invest 66:680, 1993.

121. Mohtai M, Smith RL, Schurman DJ, et al: Expression of 92-kD type IV collagenase/gelatinase (gelatinase B) in osteoarthritic cartilage and its induction in normal human articular cartilage by interleukin 1. J Clin Invest 92:179, 1993.

122. Matrisian LM: Matrix metalloproteinase gene expression. Ann N Y Acad Sci 732:42, 1994.

123. MacNaul KL, Chartrain N, Lark M, et al: Discoordinate expression of stromelysin, collagenase and tissue inhibitor of metalloproteinases-1 in rheumatoid human synovial fibroblasts: Synergistic effects of interleukin-1 and tumor necrosis factor-α on stromelysin expression. J Biol Chem 265:17238, 1990.

124. Unemori EN, Bair MJ, Bauer EA, et al: Stromelysin expression regulates collagenase activation in human fibroblasts: Dissociable control of the two metalloproteinases by interon-γ. J Biol Chem 266:23477, 1991.

125. Gutman A, Wasylyk B: The collagenase gene promoter contains a TPA and oncogene-responsive unit encompassing the PEA3 and AP-1 binding sites. EMBO J 9:2241, 1990.

126. Wasylyk C, Gutman A, Nicholson R, et al: The c-Ets oncoprotein activates the stromelysin promoter through the same elements as several non-nuclear oncoproteins. EMBO J 10:1127, 1991.

127. Gaire M, Magbanua Z, McDonnell S, et al: Structure and expression of the human gene for the matrix metalloproteinase matrilysin. J Biol Chem 269:2032, 1994.

128. Sato H, Seiki M: Regulatory mechanism of 92 kDa type IV collagenase gene expression which is associated with invasiveness of tumor cells. Oncogene 8:395, 1993.

129. Sato H, Kita M, Seiki M: v-Src activates the expression of 92-kDa type IV collagenase gene through the AP-1 site and the GT box homologous to retinoblastoma control elements. J Biol Chem 268:23460, 1993.

130. Overall CM, Wrana JL, Sodek J: Transcriptional and post-transcriptional regulation of 72-kDa gelatinase/type IV collagenase by transforming growth factor-β1 in human fibroblasts. Comparisons with collagenase and tissue inhibitor of matrix metalloproteinase gene expression. J Biol Chem 266:14064, 1991.

131. Frisch SM, Morisaki JH: Positive and negative transcriptional elements of the human type IV collagenase gene. Mol Cell Biol 10:6524, 1990.

132. Jonat C, Rahmsdorf HJ, Park KK, et al: Antitumor promotion and antiinflammation: Down-modulation of AP-1 (Fos/Jun) activity by glucocorticoid hormone. Cell 62:1189, 1990.

133. Yang-Yen H-F, Chambard JC, Sun YL, et al: Transcriptional interference between c-Jun and the glucocorticoid receptor: Mutual inhibition of DNA binding due to direct protein-protein interaction. Cell 62:1205, 1990.

134. Schüle R, Rangarajan P, Kliewer S, et al: Functional antagonism between oncoprotein c-Jun and the glucocorticoid receptor. Cell 62:1217, 1990.

135. Nicholson RC, Mader S, Nagpal S, et al: Negative regulation of the rat stromelysin gene promoter by retinoic acid is mediated by an AP1 binding site. EMBO J 9:4443, 1990.

136. Kerr LD, Miller DB, Matrisian LM: TGF-β1 inhibition of transin/stromesin gene expression is mediated through a Fos binding sequence. Cell 61:267, 1990.

137. Edwards DR, Rocheleau H, Sharma RR, et al: Involvement of AP1 and PEA3 binding sites in the regulation of murine tissue inhibitor of metalloproteinase-1 (TIMP-1) transcription. Biochim Biophys Acta 1171:41, 1992.

138. DeClerck YA, Darville MI, Eeckhout Y, et al: Characterization of the promoter of the gene encoding human tissue inhibitor of metalloproteinases-2 (TIMP-2). Gene 139:185, 1994.

139. Stetler-Stevenson, WG, Brown PD, Onisto M, et al: Tissue inhibitor of metalloproteinases-2 (TIMP-2) mRNA expression in tumor cell lines and human tumor tissues. J Biol Chem 265:13933, 1990.

140. Shapiro SD, Kobayashi DK, Welgus HG: Identification of TIMP-2 in human alveolar macrophages. Regulation of biosynthesis is opposite to that of metalloproteinases and TIMP-1. J Biol Chem 267:13890, 1992.

141. Imada K, Ito A, Itoh Y, et al: Progesterone increases the production of tissue inhibitor of metalloproteinases-2 in rabbit uterine cervical fibroblasts. FEBS Lett 341:109, 1994.

142. Staskus PW, Masiarz FR, Pallanck LJ, et al: The 21-kDa protein is a transformation-sensitive metalloproteinase inhibitor of chicken fibroblasts. J Biol Chem 266:449, 1991.

143. Leco KJ, Khokha R, Pavloff N, et al: Tissue inhibitor of metalloproteinases-3 (TIMP-3) is an extracellular matrix-associated protein with a distinctive pattern of expression in mouse cells and tissues. J Biol Chem 269:9352, 1994.

144. Keski-Oja J, Koli K, Lohi J, et al: Growth factors in the regulation of plasminogen-plasmin system in tumor cells. Seminars Thromb. Hemostasis 17:231, 1991.

145. Andreasen PA, Georg B, Lund LR, et al: Plasminogen activator inhibitors: Hormonally regulated serpins. Mol Cell Endocrinol 68:1, 1990.

146. Baici A, Lang A: Effect of interleukin-1β on the production of cathepsin B by rabbit articular chondrocytes. FEBS Lett. 277:93, 1990.

147. Baici A, Lang A, Hörler D, et al.: Cathepsin B in osteoarthritis. Cytochemical and histochemical analysis of human femoral head cartilage. Ann Rheum Dis 54:289, 1995.

148. Holz RC, Salowe SP, Smith CK, et al: EXAFS evidence for a "cysteine switch" in the activation of prostromelysin. J Am Chem Soc 114:9611, 1992.

149. Springman EB, Angleton EL, Birkedal-Hansen H, et al: Multiple modes of activation of latent human fibroblast collagenase: Evidence for the role of a Cys^{73} active-site zinc complex in latency and a "cysteine switch" mechanism for activation. Proc Natl Acad Sci USA 87:364, 1990.

150. Suzuki K, Enghild JJ, Morodomi T, et al: Mechanisms of activation of tissue procollagenase by matrix metalloproteinase 3 (stromelysin). Biochemistry 29:10261, 1990

151. Strongin AY, Marmer BL, Grant GA, et al: Plasma membrane-dependent activation of the 72-kDa type IV collagenase is prevented by complex formation with TIMP-2. J Biol Chem 268:14033, 1993.

152. Strongin AY, Collier I, Bannikov G, et al: Mechanism of cell surface activation of 72-kDa type IV collagenase. Isolation of the activated form of the membrane metalloprotease. J Biol Chem 270:5331, 1995.

153. Mast AE, Enghild JJ, Nagase, H, et al: Kinetics and physiologic relevance of the inactivation of α_1-proteinase inhibitor, α_1-antichymotrypsin, and antithrombin III by matrix metalloproteinases-1 (tissue collagenase), -2 (72-kDa gelatinase/type IV collagenase), and -3 (stromelysin). J Biol Chem 266:15810, 1991.

154. Brower MS, Harpel PC: Proteolytic cleavage and inactivation of α_2-plasmin inhibitor and C1-inactivator by human polymorphonuclear leukocyte elastase. J Biol Chem 257:9849, 1982.

155. Okada Y, Watanabe S, Nakanishi I, et al: Inactivation of tissue inhibitor of metalloproteinases by neutrophil elastase and other serine proteinases. FEBS Lett 229:157, 1988.

156. Itoh Y, Binner S, Nagase H: Steps involved in activation of the complex of pro-matrix metalloproteinase 2 (progelatinase A) and tissue inhibitor of metalloproteinases (TIMP)-2 by 4-aminophenylmercuric acetate. Biochem J 308:645, 1995.

157. Weber BHF, Vogt G, Pruett R, et al: Mutations in the tissue inhibitor of metalloproteinases-3 (TIMP-3) in patients with Sorsby's fundus dystrophy. Nature Genetics 8:352, 1994.

Evaluation of the Patient

CHAPTER 22

Peter Tugwell
Maarten Boers

Clinical Epidemiology of the Rheumatic Diseases

Evaluation of the rheumatology patient requires a mastery of, and the ability to apply, the generic concepts of evidence-based medicine. *Evidence-based medicine* refers to the objective review and application of available published data to the assessment and management of patients.[1, 2] Evidence-based medicine focuses on the application of the principles of epidemiology to clinical medicine. This reflects a paradigm shift from relying predominantly on anecdotal and personal experience to the insistence on incorporating a new step, namely review of the published evidence on the accuracy of the presenting symptoms, the physical findings, the predictive value of laboratory and x-ray results, and the prognosis with, versus without, therapy with its attendant tradeoffs of benefit versus potential harm in the context of the patient's preferences.

This chapter describes a systematic approach to incorporating the available evidence into patient evaluation by categorizing the different components into "bite-sized" chunks.

HISTORY AND PHYSICAL EXAMINATION

The history and physical examination play a crucial role in labeling patients, classifying their illnesses, determining the severity of each illness, and identifying the risk of good and bad outcomes (prognosis) with and without different therapeutic interventions. Diagnosis is also needed to identify risk in the preclinical situation before the patient becomes ill.

Sackett and colleagues[1] described four diagnostic strategies:

1. *Pattern recognition:* the instantaneous realization that the patient's presentation conforms to a previously learned pattern. It is usually visual (e.g., swan neck deformity, podagra). This is an intuitive process that is difficult to explain or teach to others.

2. *Arborization using algorithms:* the progression of the diagnostic process down only one of a large number of potential preset paths by a method in which the response to each diagnostic inquiry automatically determines the next inquiry, and ultimately the correct diagnosis. In contrast to the pattern recognition approach, the algorithm strategy has to be logical, since it must be spelled out before the patient is seen.

3. *Exhaustive:* the complete history and physical. This is a two-stage process: First, all the data that may possibly be pertinent are collected. Then, only when this stage is complete, the second stage is undertaken, which involves searching through the data for the diagnosis. This extremely time-intensive approach is the method of the novice and is abandoned with experience.

4. *Hypothetico-deductive:* the formulation, from the earliest clues about the patient, of a short list of potential diagnoses, followed by the performance of those clinical maneuvers that will best rule out or rule in the potential diagnoses. This approach is used not only by expert clinicians but even by medical students on arrival at medical schools; both groups generate their first hypothesis within 20 to 50 seconds of hearing the main complaint, formulate about six hypotheses, and selectively gather historical and physical information to support working hypotheses.[3] A key element is the mastery of highly directed but unbiased selection, acquisition, and interpretation of the clinical and laboratory data that will best shorten the list of hypotheses. The skills and competencies of evidence-based medicine are essential to this.

The subroutines for history taking and physical examination are covered elsewhere in this text and in books devoted to physical examination. The following section addresses three key themes usually omitted in such texts:

1. The underappreciated power of clinical observa-

tion in determining the diagnosis, prognosis, and therapeutic responsiveness of patients.

2. The inconsistencies that undermine the power of the clinical examination as well as the magnitude and causes of these inconsistencies.

3. Ways to minimize these errors.

Power of Clinical History and Physical Examination

Clinical evaluation is far more powerful than laboratory evaluation in establishing diagnoses, prognoses, and therapeutic plans for most patients. Crombie[4] documented that 88 percent of diagnoses in a general practice were established by the end of a brief patient history and physical examination; Sandler[5] showed that in a general medical clinic 56 percent of patients had been assigned correct diagnoses by the end of the history, and this figure rose to 73 percent by the end of the physical examination. The practice of rheumatology is unlikely to be different.

Prognosis can also be determined as or even more effectively through clinical examination, as with laboratory tests. Pincus and Callahan[6] showed that in patients with rheumatoid arthritis the number of inflamed joints and the number of activities of daily living affected discriminate as effectively as any laboratory test between patients with good versus poor prognoses for long-term disability and mortality.

CLINICAL DISAGREEMENT

Clinical evaluation can be powerful only if observations are made reliably. *Reliability* of a measure can be defined as the extent to which another measurement yields the same result when the object being measured has not changed. The problem with clinical observations is that clinicians often disagree on an observation. For instance, Ritchie and colleagues considered the Ritchie index of painful joints "invalid if observations are made on the same patient by different clinicians."[7] In other words, the interobserver reliability is low. Clinicians can also disagree with themselves on further examination (intraobserver [un]reliability).

Whether such agreement matters depends on the size of the other sources of variability in the measurement. The signal of the measurement should come from the process within the patient that one is attempting to measure (e.g., rheumatoid arthritis disease activity, measured by an index of painful joints). All the other sources of variability can be termed *noise,* or error. These include the observer, the setting, patient factors apart from the disease process, interaction between the patient and the observer, and the measurement tool. For instance, a patient in a stressful environment examined by an unfriendly observer is likely to report more pain than a patient who is at ease. All the sources of noise act together to obscure the signal. They can do so randomly, so that the

scatter around the true signal increases but the mean estimate (if the examination were repeated) remains the same, or they can cause bias, so that the estimate of the true signal is distorted in one direction. In the earlier example, an observer who uses extreme pressure will elicit much more joint pain than his or her "average" colleague, causing a biased reading of the "true" joint pain in that patient.

The signal-to-noise ratio is an expression of the importance of *random* noise on a measurement. Bias can be expressed only if the truth is known (gold standard) or assumed (by a so-called construct). In the absence of bias, a large signal-to-noise ratio implies that the signal can be distinguished clearly above the noise. In such a case, observer disagreement (and other sources of variability) is irrelevant to the measurement result. An example of this is several observers' reading the results of erythrocyte sedimentation rate (ESR) tubes: they might disagree within a range of 2 to 3 mm, but this difference is irrelevant if the clinician is looking for differences of 10 mm or more. Unfortunately, in rheumatology, the signal-to-noise ratio is usually smaller. This means sources of variability must be made explicit, and strategies must be developed to reduce them.

Measurement of disagreement can be quite straightforward: ask two clinicians to score a salient clinical feature as present or absent in a representative sample of patients, and set up a two-by-two table. A popular way of judging the level of agreement in yes/no (nominal) variables is Cohen's kappa.[8] Kappa relates the actual amount of agreement beyond chance to the potential amount of agreement beyond chance. Kappa can range from -1 (absolute disagreement) through 0 (only chance agreement) to $+1$ (absolute agreement). A kappa of 0.6 is considered fair; anything above 0.8 is considered good. Kappa can be adapted for use in measures with ordinal scales (e.g., a five-point Likert scale: poor–mediocre–average–fair–good).[9] In the case of variables expressed on a continuous scale, a measure called *intraclass correlation coefficient* is used. This coefficient has the same meaning as kappa and also ranges from -1 to $+1$. This coefficient differs from the standard (Pearson) correlation coefficient, the latter being only a measure of linear association. Although standard correlation coefficients are sometimes used to measure agreement, such use is not recommended. For example, if observer "A" consistently scores one point higher than observer "B," correlation is perfect but agreement (intraclass correlation) is zero (0).

This example yields results that, strictly speaking, are valid only in that specific situation. Measurement of agreement and other sources of variability that is more generalizable involves using more than two observers and often a comparison of different assessment techniques. Variability is then usually measured in a repeated measures design; patients are repeatedly examined by different observers in a random order, and the variability components are assessed by analysis of variance. These components include variability due to differences between patients, between observers, and between time periods; and a residual term including all variability that cannot be explained.

Good examples of this process are the exercises performed by Bellamy and associates for measures in use in clinical trials of rheumatoid arthritis,[10] ankylosing spondylitis,[11] and osteoarthritis.[12] For instance, they showed that in a group of patients with rheumatoid arthritis who were selected for inclusion in a nonsteroidal anti-inflammatory drug (NSAID) trial, 70 to 80 percent of the variability in measures such as joint counts could be ascribed to differences between patients and up to 10 percent could be attributed to the experienced observers. With less experienced observers, one would expect the latter percentage, and probably the total variability, to be greater.

Sackett and colleagues[1] summarized six strategies for preventing or minimizing clinical disagreement:

1. Matching the diagnostic environment to the diagnostic task—for example, a quiet examination room with proper lighting.

2. Seeking corroboration of key findings—repeating key elements of the examination, having other "blind" colleagues examine the patient, corroborating important findings with documents and witnesses, and confirming key findings with diagnostic tests.

3. Reporting evidence as well as inference—for example, recording "pain, swelling, warmth" first and "arthritis" thereafter. This allows cross-checking by others and provides a basis for back reasoning when diagnostic inferences prove wrong.

4. Using technical aids where appropriate and applying these in a standardized manner (see later).

5. Arranging for independent interpretation of observational diagnostic test data. Expectation is a potent source for bias in assessment, and independent, preferably blind interpretation can remedy this. Such interpretation is not always feasible and in its extreme can be inappropriate: radiologists will not perform radiography on patients if relevant clinical information is missing. It is unclear, however, how much clinical data should be offered.

6. Applying the social as well as the biologic sciences of medicine. In history taking and physical examination, behavioral skills are key elements to obtaining the right information. It is likely that they are also a major source of variability between observers.

To these six strategies, we add two that are especially important in research:

7. Standardizing the measurement by agreeing beforehand on the procedure and the possible results. In the series by Bellamy and colleagues,[10–12] standardization of measurement technique was achieved by discussion of key areas, such as warmup, demonstration of the maneuver to the patient, positioning and clothing, anatomic reference points, verbal encouragement, criteria for conflict resolution, technical aspects of instruments, and methods of reading instruments and of recording results. An important and beneficial effect of this procedure was observed in most outcome variables tested.

8. Minimizing the number of observers (e.g., in a multicenter trial, have one observer per center).

DIAGNOSTIC PROCEDURES

As in other areas of medicine, rheumatologists are confronted with ever-increasing possibilities to order diagnostic tests; tests can also be used to prognosticate or to evaluate the effects of therapy. The knowledge of whether to use a test in a specific situation, and how to interpret the result, must come from a critical appraisal of the literature.

The Evidence-Based Medicine Working Group recently published a series of updated *Users' Guides to the Medical Literature.* For articles about diagnostic tests, the guides suggest criteria that help select and interpret the results[13, 14] (Table 22–1). The general questions returning in each set of guides are:

• Are the results of the study valid?
• What were the results?
• Will the results help me in caring for my patients?

We will explore this strategy with some examples. In the first example, you are having difficulty deciding whether hydroxychloroquine and diclofenac are providing adequate control of the activity of a patient with rheumatoid arthritis. Although her joint counts and the ESR have improved by 50 percent, her morning stiffness has not improved. You recall seeing an article assessing the usefulness of morning stiffness to distinguish active rheumatoid arthritis from inactive arthritis.[15] Applying the criteria listed in Table 22–1, the first question is, Are the results of the study valid?, with its two components of whether there was (1) an independent blind comparison with a reference standard, and (2) an appropriate spectrum of patients to whom the diagnostic test was applied that is comparable to the situation in which the test will be used. Both of these criteria are satisfied: the study included 48 patients with active rheumatoid arthritis and 45 patients with inactive disease.

To diagnose rheumatoid arthritis, the opinion of the patient's physician was used, similar to the process of the revised American College of Rheumatology (ACR) criteria. This was necessary because morning stiffness is in fact an ACR criterion, so that selection on the basis of ACR criteria was not possible. To distinguish active from inactive rheumatoid arthritis, two methods were used—the treating physician's subjective opinion and whether he or she intended to start (or change existing) disease-modifying antirheumatic therapy. The research nurse interviewing the patients about morning stiffness was blind to the diagnosis and the level of disease activity. Thus, the reference standard (diagnosis and activity status) was available in all patients. The researchers provided sufficient detail about their test—a structured interview on morning stiffness by a blinded observer.

Table 22–1. USERS' GUIDES FOR AN ARTICLE ABOUT PROGNOSIS AND DIAGNOSTIC TEST

Diagnostic Test	Prognosis

I. Are the results of the study valid?
 	
  A. Primary guides:
    1. Was there an independent, blind comparison with a reference standard?
    2. Did the patient sample include an appropriate spectrum of patients to whom the diagnostic test will be applied in clinical practice?
  B. Secondary guides:
    1. Did the results of the test being evaluated influence the decision to perform the gold standard?
    2. Were the methods for performing the test described in sufficient detail to permit replication?
 	
II. What are the results?
 	
  Are likelihood ratios for the test results presented or data necessary for their calculation provided?
 	
III. Will the results help me in caring for my patients?
 	
  A. Will the reproducibility of the test results and its interpretation be satisfactory in my setting?
  B. Are the results applicable to my patient?
  C. Will the result change my management?
  D. Will patients be better off as a result of the test?
	I. Are the results of the study valid?
	
	  A. Primary guides:
	    1. Was there a representative and well-defined sample of patients at a similar point in the course of the disease?
	    2. Was follow-up sufficiently long and complete?
	
	  B. Secondary guides:
	    1. Were objective and unbiased outcome criteria used?
	    2. Was there adjustment for important prognostic factors?
	
	II. What are the results?
	
	  A. How large is the likelihood of the outcome event(s) in a specified period of time?
	  B. How precise are the estimates of likelihood?
	
	III. Will the results help me in caring for my patients?
	
	  A. Were the study patients similar to my own?
	  B. Will the results lead directly to selecting or avoiding therapy?
	  C. Are the results useful for reassuring or counseling patients?

From Jaeschke R, Guyatt G, Sackett DL for the Evidence-Based Medicine Working Group: Users' guides to the medical literature. III: How to use an article about a diagnostic test. A: Are the results of the study valid? *and* B: What are the results and will they help me in caring for my patients? JAMA 271:389–391, 703–707, 1994; and Laupacis A, Wells G, Richardson S, Tugwell P for the Evidence-Based Medicine Working Group: Users' guides to the medical literature. V: How to use an article about prognosis. JAMA 272:234–237, 1994.

Results: The criteria in Table 22–1 require that the results allow likelihood ratios to be calculated. This article does permit this. Likelihood ratios can be calculated for both negative and positive results of tests. This example calls for the likelihood ratio of a positive result. This is calculated as the true-positive rate (or sensitivity; i.e., the percentage of people with the disease who test positive), divided by the false-positive rate (or 1-specificity; i.e., the percentage of people without the disease who test positive). Without the mathematics, a likelihood ratio expresses how much more likely it is for a person to have a positive test with the disease than without it. The higher the likelihood ratio, the better the test discriminates between health and disease.

In this study, the tests were not nominal—that is, not of the yes/no, normal/abnormal type. Duration and severity of morning stiffness are continuous variables. To transform such variables into nominal variables, cutoff points must be chosen, and the choice can influence the test characteristics. Usually, choosing a cutoff point so that the test is highly sensitive (i.e., able to spot all cases with disease) comes with the tradeoff that the test becomes less specific (i.e., tends to spot a lot of cases without the disease). To express the whole range of choices in cutoff points rather than choosing one arbitrary point, the researchers drew so-called receiver-operator curves (Fig. 22–1). These curves plot sensitivity (true-positive rate) against 1-specificity (false-positive rate) for every cutoff point. At each point, likelihood ratios can be calculated directly.

The curves tell us that both severity of greater than 4 cm (assessed by a 10-cm visual analog scale) and duration of morning stiffness of longer than 4 hours may be helpful in distinguishing active from inactive rheumatoid arthritis. The data on duration of stiffness, even though there was a 50 percent difference between active and inactive groups, did not achieve statistical significance; the severity scores did, however. The likelihood ratio of a severity of greater than 4 cm on the visual analog scale is calculated as follows:

$$\frac{\text{sensitivity}}{100 - \text{specificity}} = \frac{61}{30} = 2$$

This means that this severity score of more than 4 cm on the 10-cm visual analog scale is twice as likely in patients with active rheumatoid arthritis as in patients with the inactive form. This is of some use for a patient such as that described, for whom the other signs are equivocal and the prior probability of activity is over 50 percent. For example, if you judge that without this degree of morning stiffness you would estimate the need to change therapy to control progressive active disease at 60 percent, the application of this likelihood ratio of 2 to this patient would increase the probability to over 80 percent. This can be calculated through fairly time-consuming mathematics or tables.[1] An increasingly popular way of applying this uses a nomogram and is demonstrated in the next example.

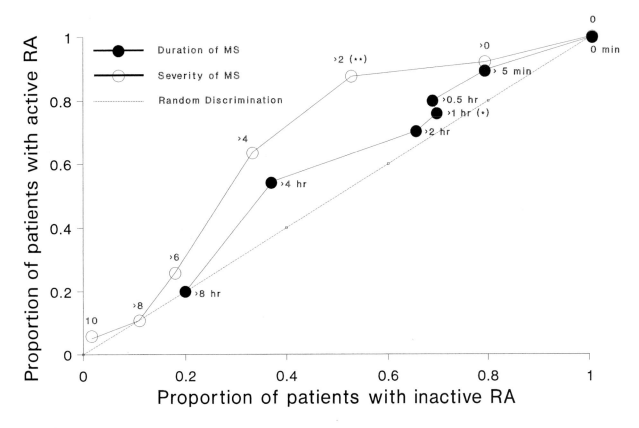

* Morning stiffness, duration > 1 hr: sensitivity = 78%, specificity = 30%
** Morning stiffness, VAS > 2: sensitivity = 85%, specificity = 44%

Figure 22–1. Receiver-operator curves of the performance of (1) Visual Analogue Scale (VAS) score of morning stiffness and (2) duration to maximum improvement of morning stiffness (MS) in discrimination between active and inactive rheumatoid arthritis (RA). (From Hazes JMW, Hayton R, Silman AJ: A reevaluation of the symptom of morning stiffness. J Rheumatol 20:1138–1142, 1993.)

Application of Likelihood Ratios to Clinical and Laboratory Data Using a Nomogram

A 33-year-old woman with a vague history of joint pains in her hands 3 months earlier presents with a 3-month history of an intermittent red malar rash that lasts a few days at a time and that is associated with exposure to the sun. The 1982 ACR criteria study[16] provided information collected in the appropriate fashion to satisfy the validity criteria data in Table 22–1 by comparing the proportions of a large number of proposed symptoms and signs and some laboratory tests found in patients with lupus versus findings from other patients presenting to a rheumatologist. The study reported a sensitivity of 57 percent (i.e., 57 percent of patients with true lupus had malar rashes) and a specificity of 96 percent (i.e., only 4 percent of rheumatology patients with other rheumatic diseases had malar rashes). The likelihood ratio can be calculated as follows:

$$\frac{\text{sensitivity}}{100 - \text{specificity}} = \frac{59}{4} = 14.75$$

By using the nomogram in Figure 22–2, one can see

how much this increases the probability that the patient has true lupus. Because the occurrence of lupus in the population is about one in 1000 persons, even though this likelihood ratio is relatively high, the likelihood that this patient has true lupus is increased only to 1.4 percent. On further questioning, the patient also has a definite history of photosensitivity, with a rash developing on exposed areas after minimal exposure to the sun during the past 12 months. This symptom has a sensitivity of 43 percent and a specificity of 96 percent, giving a likelihood ratio of 10.75. As can be seen on Figure 22–2, this raises the probability of true lupus from 1.4 percent to 13 percent. The antinuclear antibody result is weakly positive at 1:64; this has a sensitivity of 99 percent and a specificity of 49 percent, providing a likelihood ratio of 1.94. As Figure 22–2 shows, this further increases the probability of true lupus from 13 percent to 23 percent. The patient's anti–double-stranded DNA titer comes back positive at a titer of 40 percent binding; this was not reported in the 1982 ACR criteria but was evaluated in the same manner by Juby and colleagues.[17] They reported a sensitivity of 20 percent and a specificity of 99 percent, giving a likelihood ratio of 20. Applying this to the nomogram in Figure

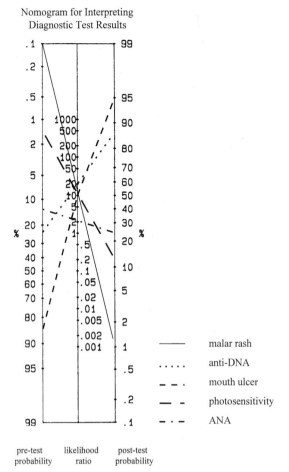

Nomogram for Interpreting
Diagnostic Test Results

| pre-test | likelihood | post-test |
| probability | ratio | probability |

——— malar rash

· · · · · anti-DNA

— — · mouth ulcer

— — photosensitivity

— · — ANA

Figure 22–2. Use of likelihood ratios in diagnosis. *Step 1:* For patient described, the pre-test probability was 0.1 percent, and the likelihood ratio for malar rash is 14.75. Anchor a straight edge at 0.1 percent on the left side (pre-test probability), direct the straight edge through the central column (likelihood ratio) at 14.75. The post-test probability can then be read off on the right side as 1.4 percent. *Step 2:* The same approach is used for each subsequent symptom, sign, and laboratory result; that is, for photosensitivity, the pre-test probability is now 1.4 percent so the straight edge is directed from 1.4 percent on the pre-test column through the likelihood ratio column at 10.75, giving a post-test probability of 13 percent. This is then repeated for antinuclear antibody (ANA), anti-DNA, and mouth ulcers.

22–2 shows that the patient now has a likelihood of true lupus of 85 percent. The following week, when the patient returns, she has a painful mouth ulcer on her soft palate with surrounding erythema; this has a sensitivity of 27 percent and specificity of 96 percent, giving a likelihood ratio of 6.75, which raises the likelihood of true lupus to 94 percent: the diagnosis is made!

This example shows how important the underlying prevalence or pretest probability is, with the most information being obtained only if the pretest probability is higher than 10 percent. The clinical symptoms and signs are critical in getting to this level of probability so that the laboratory tests result in more true-positive than false-positive results. In general, with intermediate prior probabilities, likelihood ratios be-

tween 2 and 5 carry limited weight, ratios between 5 and 10 have moderate weight, and ratios above 10 are decisive.

A more detailed discussion of likelihood ratios can be found in Jaeschke and colleagues' report.[14]

PROGNOSIS

Evaluation of the patient needs to address the features that not only will lead to the correct diagnosis but also will allow estimation and discussion with the patient of the prognosis with and without therapeutic intervention. *Prognosis* refers to the possible outcomes of a disease and the frequency with which they can be expected to occur. There are a number of different outcomes of interest in estimating prognosis and the potential impact of therapy on them; they can be conveniently summarized by a series of d's: death, disability (physical function), distress (e.g., pain, stiffness), dysfunction (psychosocial functioning), disharmony (family function), drug side effects, and dollar costs.[18, 19] Because most rheumatologic diseases are chronic, the distress and disability components are important. Prognostic factors are patient characteristics that can help predict a patient's outcome. They are usually distinguished from *risk factors* (i.e., patient characteristics that are associated with the development of disease).

We can distinguish prognosis per se—that is, prognosis without or with current standard therapy—from prognosis with a therapy that is the subject of evaluation. Randomization to different prognostic factors is usually impossible (e.g., gender) or unethical (e.g., education or no education). Therefore, the best study design to identify prognostic factors and their strength is a cohort study, in which well-defined groups of patients (having or not having the factor of interest) who have not yet experienced the outcome are observed over time to monitor the outcome of interest.

A less rigorous approach is the *case-control study*, in which patients with the outcome (*cases*) are compared with patients who resemble the cases but that have not had the outcome (*controls*). The comparison focuses on the presence or absence of the prognostic factors of interest. This design is prone to biases but can sometimes be the only source of information, especially if the disease or outcome is rare or the follow-up period is long.

To critically appraise an article on prognosis, the same questions can be asked as before: Are the results of the study valid?, What are the results?, Will the results help me in caring for my patients?[20] (see Table 22–1).

The use of the guides can be explored by considering an article by Wolfe and colleagues[21] on the mortality associated with rheumatoid arthritis. The article described the determinants and causes of death in an open cohort of 3501 patients with rheumatoid arthritis who were followed up prospectively for up to 35 years.

First, we must study the selected patient sample. The patients described came from four data banks: a university clinic being the only referral center, a private clinic, a tertiary university referral center, and a closed community-derived cohort recruited by newspaper advertisements at a single time. The baseline characteristics were extensively described. The main problem, as the researchers themselves admitted, was that the patients had not been recruited at a similar point in the course of their disease; that is, they did not constitute an inception cohort. This is a feature of many, possibly all, of the studies on rheumatoid arthritis mortality with long follow-up. However, all patients in whom rheumatoid arthritis was diagnosed within a specified time entered the study and were observed prospectively.

Next, we must look at the quality of the follow-up. The follow-up period was a mean of almost 16 years in one center (905 patients) and 5.7 to 7.2 years in the other centers. Loss to follow-up was very low in two centers (2 to 4 percent) and high in the two others (10 to 35 percent). However, mortality status of several patients could be ascertained by the United States National Death Index.

As the outcome criterion, the study used death, one of the few truly objective outcome measures. To adjust for important prognostic factors, the investigators computed standardized mortality ratios through comparison with the age- and sex-matched general United States and Canadian population. Cox's proportional hazard models studied several potential prognostic variables.

Results: In this setting, patients with rheumatoid arthritis had at least a two-fold risk of death compared with the general population. The estimates are precise because of the large number of deaths (over 25 percent) in the study period, but they vary between the centers, probably as a result of the referral pattern. Apart from age and gender, education level, smoking, and hypertension were important non–rheumatoid arthritis prognostic indicators. Rheumatoid arthritis–related factors included rheumatoid factor positivity, nodules, disease activity markers (ESR and joint count), and disability.

How to apply these results in one's practice? The patients are representative of patients in a rheumatology clinic. They cannot be used as a guide to specific therapy, but they can be used to argue that aggressive treatment should be tried in patients in this group, especially if they carry one or more of the indicators of poor prognosis.[22] Proof of the efficacy of such therapies, however, must come from randomized trials and prospective cohort studies.

Therapy: Impact on Prognosis, Risk, and Responsiveness

To incorporate these results into the evaluation of the patient, not only do the risk of the key outcomes need to be estimated as described earlier, but the likely responsiveness to therapy of the patient must be assessed. The issue here is how to assess generalizability—that is, the application of the results of published trials to the patient being evaluated to decide if the therapy should be recommended to the patient. A literature search should be conducted to find the best evidence of the benefits and side effects of the therapeutic options.

A number of meta-analyses have been published that summarize the magnitude of benefit of different therapies.[23, 24] An international data base incorporating critical appraisal and meta-analysis of all the trials in rheumatology, the Cochrane Database of Systematic Reviews, is being developed as one of the modules of the Cochrane Collaboration.[25, 26]

In the absence of a systematic overview that incorporates critical appraisal, the best articles available should be subjected to a review of their quality and applicability to the patient of interest using critical appraisal strategies, such as those described in Sackett and Guyatt and colleagues.[1, 27, 28] Another recent advance has been the development of consensus on the different assessments of the clinical, laboratory, and quality-of-life endpoints that are important to the rheumatologist and patient and that are sensitive to small but important changes. From the early 1980s, scientists have recognized flaws in the measurements performed in clinical trials on rheumatoid arthritis. The problems with existing measures have been their validity, their relation to individual patient outcomes, and their multitude. As a result, a series of consensus conferences were organized, the most recent being those of the OMERACT initiative. The OMERACT I conference in Maastricht, The Netherlands, in 1992 recommended a core set of measures to be used as a minimum in all clinical trials on rheumatoid arthritis. This was a compromise between earlier drafts from the European League of Organizations for Rheumatology and the ACR. These measures include acute-phase reactants, disability, pain, patient global assessment, physician global assessment, swollen joint count, tender joint count, and radiographic studies of joints in any trial of 1 year or longer. The core set was later endorsed by the International League of Organizations for Rheumatology and the World Health Organization.[30] The conference also stimulated thinking on ways to combine measures into an index, such as by developing improvement criteria. Consequently, the ACR formulated its preliminary criteria for improvement in rheumatoid arthritis,[31] namely an improvement by more than 20 percent in both swollen and tender joint counts, plus in three of five of the following endpoints: patient global assessment, pain, functional status, physician global assessment, and acute-phase reactant (ESR or C-reactive protein).

The OMERACT II conference in Ottawa, Canada, in 1994 focused on the importance of measuring health status, toxicity, and economics in rheumatoid arthritis and other musculoskeletal disorders.[32] Since then, the OMERACT initiative has been widening further into other musculoskeletal diseases (osteoarthritis, osteoporosis) and into new promising areas of measurement (psychosocial measures). Thus, there will be a standardized set of assessment measures that a physician treating a patient can use to assess whether the patient is similar to those in the published meta-analyses in data bases such as that of Cochrane, and that he or she can use to assess whether the patient has improved or other therapeutic options need to be explored.

In conclusion, the assessment of prognosis with therapy is often a two-step affair, involving assessing the evidence from trials or other studies and then relating these trials to cohort studies in which long-term outcomes are assessed. Often, treatment arms from randomized clinical trials are followed as a cohort after the trial and can thus contribute to the necessary long-term data. The other side of the coin, however—toxicity—also requires careful attention and incorporation into the evaluation of the patient.

ASSESSMENT OF ETIOLOGY AND ADVERSE EFFECTS OF THERAPY

Evaluation of the patient unfortunately includes passing judgment on whether a current or past therapy has been itself responsible for new symptoms or signs—that is, toxicity. It has been claimed that 4 percent of admissions to acute general hospitals are the result of adverse drug reactions. Aspirin, other nonsteroidal agents, and prednisone appear frequently on lists of drugs reported as causing severe reactions in adverse drug systems. Attribution of the signs, symptoms, and abnormal laboratory tests is often difficult. Indeed, even clinical pharmacologists disagree about whether a given patient has had an adverse reaction; when three such professionals reviewed the records of 500 patients thought by their attending physicians to have suffered adverse drug reactions, they disagreed on which drug was likely to be responsible in 36 percent of cases, on whether the drug reaction really caused the admission in 57 percent of cases, and on whether an adverse drug reaction contributed to death in 71 percent of the patients who died.[33] Rheumatologists need to equip themselves with the skills to assess the likelihood that a drug taken by the patient caused an adverse effect.

Levine and colleagues[34] published guidelines distilled from the work of a number of methodologists and based on the application by Sir Bradford Hill of Koch's postulates to epidemiologic studies of causation. The steps they recommended are as follows:

1. Decide whether there is good evidence that the drug causes the adverse effect of interest. We will use the example of whether NSAIDs truly cause clinically significant gastrointestinal events.[35]
   a. Seek the best articles in the literature that explicitly associate the drug of interest with the clinical presentation. To decide which article is likely

to provide the best information, select the articles with the strongest design: in descending order—randomized trials, cohort studies, case-control studies, case series, case reports.

Although randomized trials give the best data, it is unusual for clinical trials in rheumatology to have a sufficiently large sample size to have enough cases of rare side effects. For example, to be 95 percent confident of observing one or more adverse effects from a drug, the study needs to include three times the reciprocal of the true adverse event rate. That is, for our example, if the true rate of a severe gastrointestinal hemorrhage from a new NSAID is one in 100, 300 patients need to be studied to be 95 percent confident of seeing a single case. The recent MUCOSA (Misoprostol Ulcer Complications Outcomes Safety Assessment)[36] trial compared 4439 patients randomly assigned to receive whichever of ten specified NSAIDs the patient had been taking plus placebo versus 4404 patients who were prescribed misoprostol in addition to their NSAIDs. It showed that this size sample is occasionally attainable but is prohibitively expensive to undertake for all drugs. Before this study was done, all the randomized studies concentrated on endoscopy to detect erosions and ulcers and then made assumptions on the proportion of these that would have resulted in serious events; the estimates of this risk varied widely, so information was needed from other designs.

The cohort design is more commonly used. In this design, patients being treated with a given medication are followed up over time along with patients who are not taking the medication. The groups are then evaluated to determine whether a particular outcome occurred in the group taking the medication versus the group not taking it. The ARAMIS (Arthritis, Rheumatism and Aging Medical Information System) data base is the largest prospectively followed chart, recording some 2700 patients that have been observed for 9525 years.[37] For our example, this data base identified 116 patients with 128 gastrointestinal events that required hospitalization; all but nine were taking NSAIDs at the time. Unfortunately, there are insufficient patients without any NSAID exposure; so, although this data base allows relative risks of different NSAIDs compared with each other to be estimated, it does not allow an estimation of the relative risk of this side effect compared with no NSAID therapy. Seven other cohort studies in the literature, however, compare NSAID use with nonuse.[38] With all these cohort designs, there is the concern that confounding factors may influence the findings; for example, more recent or more expensive drugs may be given preferentially to patients who cannot tolerate their previous NSAIDs; thus, these patients would be more likely to have side effects than those doing well on the older drug.

Case-control studies are at even greater risk of significant bias. For example, patients who come in complaining of a gastrointestinal symptom or sign are more likely to be investigated. Nine case-control studies of the association between NSAIDs and serious gastrointestinal events have been published.[38]

Thus, within each of these designs, it is important to decide whether it is reasonable to accept that the estimation of exposure and determination of outcome was free of bias.

b. Assess whether the strength of association is both clinically and statistically significant. *Strength* here means the odds favoring the outcome of interest (serious gastrointestinal event in our example) with, as opposed to without, exposure to the putative cause (NSAIDs). If the treatment is harmless, the relative odds should be 1.0; relative risks of greater than 2.0 are usually judged clinically important unless the event is extremely rare (occurring less often than one in 1000 cases) when higher risks may be acceptable because the risk in absolute numbers is small.

c. Assess whether it meets the rules of evidence for causation:

(1) *Consistency*—positive: All the studies described here show a risk greater than 1.

(2) *Temporal sequence*—positive: The cohort and trial provide clear evidence that the gastrointestinal event succeeded the taking of the drug.

(3) *Dose-response gradient*—negative: The relation with dose is not clear for NSAIDs, although it is for aspirin.

(4) *Reversibility:* Does removal of the putative cause result in a reduction or disappearance of the endpoint that is thought to be caused by the putative causative agent? The results of the MUCOSA study[36] described earlier in step 1 support this conclusion; the incidence of serious ulcer complications (perforation, bleeding, and gastric outlet obstruction were 36 percent less common among the patients receiving misoprostol than among those receiving placebo (25 of 4404 misoprostol patients versus 42 of 4439 placebo patients).

(5) Credibility of the association clinically, biologically, and epidemiologically. This has four elements: first, have plausible competing explanations been ruled out? For example, new NSAIDs may be used preferentially in patients who experience side effects from the established drugs, thus putting these patients at increased risk of a higher frequency of side effects. Second, do the findings from laboratory research, including animal research, support the association? Mucosal lesions that resemble the erosions produced by NSAIDs are produced in rabbits by depleting endogenous prostaglandins, one of the postulated mechanisms for NSAID-induced ulcers.[39] Third, the epidemiologic credibility is satisfied if the association is consistent with our understanding of the distribution of causes and outcomes in humans; increases in NSAID sales are closely correlated with the increase in hospitalizations for gastric ulcer complications.[40]

2. Apply this to the patient. The decision for action depends on two components:

a. Based on the approach described here, how certain is it that the drug in question was responsible for the adverse effect?

b. What are the alternate courses of action?

CONCLUSION

Rational evaluation of the patient should include consideration of the use of the different concepts of clinical epidemiology in support of the use of evidence-based medicine. This approach to gathering, assessing, and applying the evidence also encourages ongoing review of clinical skills and their application to diagnosis and patient management; the patient will benefit.

References

1. Sackett DL, Haynes RB, Guyatt GH, Tugwell P: Clinical Epidemiology: A Basic Science for Clinical Medicine, 2nd ed. Boston, Little, Brown & Co, 1991.
2. Guyatt GH: Users' guides to the medical literature. JAMA 270:2096–2097, 1993.
3. Neufeld VR, Norman GR, Feightner JW, Barrows HS: Clinical problem-solving by medical students: A cross-sectional and longitudinal analysis. Med Educ 15:315, 1981.
4. Crombie DL: Diagnostic process. J Coll Gen Practit 6:579, 1963.
5. Sandler G: The importance of the history in the medical clinic and the cost of unnecessary tests. Am Heart J 100:928, 1980.
6. Pincus T, Callahan LF: Rheumatology function tests: Grip strength, walking time, button test and questionnaires document and predict longterm morbidity and mortality in rheumatoid arthritis. J Rheumatol 19:1051–1057, 1992.
7. Ritchie DM, Boyle JA, McInnes JM, et al: Clinical studies with an articular index for the assessment of joint tenderness in patients with rheumatoid arthritis. Q J Med 37:393–406, 1968.
8. Cohen J: A coefficient of agreement for nominal scales. Educ Psychol Meas 20:37–47, 1960.
9. Cohen J: Weighted kappa: Nominal scale agreement with provision for scaled disagreement or partial credit. Psychol Bull 70:213–220, 1968.
10. Bellamy N, Anastassiades TP, Buchanan WW, et al: Rheumatoid arthritis antirheumatic drug trials: I. Effects of standardization procedures on observer-dependent outcome measures. J Rheumatol 18:1893–1900, 1991.
11. Bellamy N, Buchanan WW, Esdaile JM, et al: Ankylosing spondylitis drug trials: I. Effects of standardization procedures on observer-dependent outcome measures. J Rheumatol 18:1701–1708, 1991.
12. Bellamy N, Carette S, Ford PM, et al: Osteoarthritis antirheumatic drug trials: I. Effects of standardization procedures on observer-dependent outcome measures. J Rheumatol 19:436–443, 1992.
13. Jaeschke R, Guyatt G, Sackett DL for the Evidence-Based Medicine Working Group: Users' guides to the medical literature: III. How to use an article about a diagnostic test. A: Are the results of the study valid? JAMA 271:389–391, 1994.
14. Jaeschke R, Guyatt G, Sackett DL for the Evidence-Based Medicine Working Group: Users' guides to the medical literature: III. How to use an article about a diagnostic test. B: What are the results and will they help me in caring for my patients? JAMA 271:703–707, 1994.

15. Hazes JMW, Hayton R, Silman AJ: A reevaluation of the symptom of morning stiffness. J Rheumatol 20:1138–1142, 1993.
16. Tan EM, Cohen AS, Fries JF, et al: The 1982 revised criteria for the classification of systemic lupus erythematosus (SLE). Arthritis Rheum 25:1271–1277, 1982.
17. Juby A, Johnston C, Davis P: Specificity, sensitivity and diagnostic predictive value of selected laboratory-generated autoantibody profiles in patients with connective tissue diseases. J Rheumatol 18:354–358, 1991.
18. Kohn R, White KL: Health Care: An International Study. Toronto, Oxford University Press, 1978.
19. Fries JF: Towards an understanding of patient outcome measurement. Arthritis Rheum 26:697–702, 1983.
20. Laupacis A, Wells G, Richardson S, Tugwell P for the Evidence-Based Medicine Working Group: Users' guides to the medical literature: V. How to use an article about prognosis. JAMA 272:234–237, 1994.
21. Wolfe F, Mitchell DM, Sibley JT, et al: The mortality of rheumatoid arthritis. Arthritis Rheum 37:481–494, 1994.
22. Pincus T: The case for early intervention in rheumatoid arthritis. J Autoimmun 5:209–226, 1992.
23. Felson DT, Anderson JJ, Meenan RF: Use of short-term efficacy/toxicity tradeoffs to select second-line drugs in rheumatoid arthritis. Arthritis Rheum 35:1117–1125, 1992.
24. Tugwell P, Bennett K, Gent M: Methotrexate in rheumatoid arthritis. Ann Intern Med 107:358–366, 1987.
25. Sackett DL: Cochrane's legacy. Lancet 340:1131–1132, 1992.
26. Robinson A: Research, practice and the Cochrane Collaboration. Can Med Assoc J 152:883–889, 1995.
27. Guyatt GH, Sackett DL, Cook DJ for the Evidence-Based Medicine Working Group: Users' guides to the medical literature: II. How to use an article about therapy or prevention. A: Are the results of the study valid? JAMA 270:2598–2601, 1993.
28. Guyatt GH, Sackett DL, Cook DJ for the Evidence-Based Medicine Working Group: Users' guides to the medical literature: II. How to use an article about therapy or prevention. B: What were the results and will they help me in caring for my patients? JAMA 271:59–63, 1994.
29. Boers M, Tugwell P for the OMERACT Committee: OMERACT conference on outcome measures in RA clinical trials. J Rheumatol 20:528–592, 1993.
30. Boers M, Tugwell P, Felson DT, et al: World Health Organization and International League of Associations for Rheumatology core endpoints for symptom modifying antirheumatic drugs in rheumatoid arthritis clinical trials. J Rheumatol 21:86–89, 1994.
31. Felson DT, Anderson JJ, Boers M, et al: American College of Rheumatology preliminary criteria for improvement in rheumatoid arthritis patients. Arthritis Rheum 38:727–735, 1995.
32. Boers M, Brooks P, Tugwell P for the OMERACT Committee: OMERACT II: Proceedings of the Second Conference on Outcome Measures in Rheumatology. J Rheumatol 22:980–1430, 1995.
33. Koch-Weser J, Sellers EM, Zacest R: The ambiguity of adverse drug reactions. Eur J Clin Pharmacol 11:75, 1977.
34. Levine M, Walter S, Lee H, et al for the Evidence-Based Medicine Working Group: Users' guides to the medical literature: IV. How to use an article about harm. JAMA 271:1615–1619, 1994.
35. Podrebarac T, Tugwell P: A reader's guide to the evaluation of causation. Postgrad Med J 72:131–137, 1996.
36. Silverstein F, Graham D, Wyn-Davies H, et al: Reduction by misoprostol of clinically detected serious gastrointestinal complications associated with non-steroidal anti-inflammatory drug use in older patients with rheumatoid arthritis. Ann Intern Med 1995 123:241–249, 1995.
37. Fries JF, McShane DJ: ARAMIS (American Rheumatism Association Medical Information System). West J Med 145:798–804, 1986.
38. Gabriel SE, Jaakkimainen L, Bombardier C: Risk for serious gastrointestinal complications related to use of non-steroidal anti-inflammatory drugs. Ann Intern Med 115:787–796, 1991.
39. Redfern JS, Feldman M: Role of endogenous prostaglandins in preventing gastrointestinal ulceration: Induction of ulcers by antibodies to prostaglandins. Gastroenterology 96:596–605, 1989.
40. Gabriel SE, Bombardier C: NSAID-induced ulcers: An emerging epidemic? J Rheumatol 17:1–4, 1990.

CHAPTER 23

Kevin G. Moder
Gene G. Hunder

Examination of the Joints

HISTORY IN THE PATIENT WITH MUSCULOSKELETAL DISEASE

Obtaining a detailed description of a patient's musculoskeletal symptoms is important because it provides much of the information needed for making a diagnosis. The goal of the interview is to understand precisely what the patient means when describing the symptoms. In obtaining a history of the patient's illness, the physician must probe for details on the sequence and severity of symptoms and patterns of progression, exacerbation, or remission. The effects of associated diseases and other life stressors must be elucidated. The functional impact of the disease on the patient also must be determined.

The effects of current or previous therapy on the course of the illness are important. Assessment of compliance is extremely important; even an ideal therapeutic regimen will fail if the patient does not comply with the outlined program. Therefore, it is vital to communicate to the patient the anticipated effect and the timing of this effect when a new medication is introduced. Often, patients decide that a medication is ineffective when in reality they have not had an adequate course of therapy. This is especially likely to happen when the physician is trying to assess the efficacy of slow-acting agents.

The patient's behavior often provides clues to the illness and the patient's response to it. It is important to determine whether the patient is reacting appropriately to an illness. Occasionally, patients are either overly concerned or inappropriately unconcerned about their symptoms. Additionally, the physician should recognize that a patient's understanding of the illness affects his or her response to it.

Pain

Pain is the symptom that most commonly brings the patient with musculoskeletal disease to the physician. Pain is a complex, subjective sensation that is difficult to define, explain, or measure. The patient's response to pain is affected by current emotional state as well as by previous experiences, including observations of pain in others.

It is critical for pain to be localized anatomically. The examiner must fully understand the patient's localization of pain. Sometimes patients use terms in a nonanatomic manner. For example, a patient complaining of "hip" pain may actually be describing pain in the buttock or thigh. To clarify the location, it is often helpful to ask the patient to point to the area of pain with one finger. If the pain is in a joint, an articular disorder is likely to be present. Pain between joints may suggest bone or muscle disease or referred pain. Pain in bursal areas, in fascial planes, or along tendons, ligaments, or nerve distributions suggests disease in these structures. Pain arising from deeper structures is often less focal than pain originating from superficial tissues. Pain in small joints of the hands or feet tends to be more accurately localized than pain in larger, more proximal joints, such as the shoulder, hip, and spine. When pain is diffuse, variable, poorly described, or unrelated to anatomic structures, fibromyalgia, malingering, or psychologic problems should be suspected.

The character of pain is also helpful in understanding the patient's illness. For example, "aching" in a joint area suggests an arthritic disorder, whereas "burning" in an extremity may indicate a neuropathy. It is also important to ask about the severity of pain. Many physicians find it helpful to ask the patient to describe severity on a numerical scale of 1 to 10. Descriptions of "intolerable" or "excruciating" pain in a patient who otherwise is able to carry out normal activities provide a clue that emotional factors may be amplifying symptoms.

Determining whether pain is present at rest is also useful. Joint pain both at rest and with movement is more suggestive of an inflammatory process, whereas pain that is present primarily during activity can indicate a mechanical disorder, such as degenerative arthritis. As discussed next, the time of day at which pain or stiffness occurs can also yield valuable information.

Stiffness

"Stiffness" has different meanings for different patients. Some equate it with pain or fatigue; others equate it with soreness, weakness, or restrictions of movement. Most rheumatologists define stiffness as discomfort perceived when the patient attempts to move the joints after a period of inactivity. When it occurs, stiffness, or "gelling," usually develops after several hours of inactivity. Mild stiffness may resolve within a few minutes. When severe, as in rheumatoid arthritis or polymyalgia rheumatica, the stiffness may persist for many hours.

Morning stiffness can be a prodromal symptom of rheumatoid arthritis, and it is one of the American College of Rheumatology criteria for the diagnosis of rheumatoid arthritis (see Chapter 56). Morning stiffness associated with noninflammatory joint diseases is almost always of short duration (usually less than ½ hour) and of less severity than the stiffness of inflammatory joint disease. In addition, in mechanical or degenerative joint disease, the degree of stiffness is related to the extent of overuse of the damaged joint, and stiffness usually subsides within a few days if use of the affected joint is adequately limited. Although lack of stiffness does not exclude the possibility of a systemic inflammatory disease, such as rheumatoid arthritis, its absence is uncommon. Stiffness from neurologic disorders, such as Parkinson's disease, also occurs, although the "limbering up" component is usually lacking.

Limitation of Motion

Patients with rheumatic disorders frequently tell of limitation of motion. This symptom must be differentiated from stiffness, because stiffness is usually transient but true limitation in motion is fixed and not variable from hour to hour. It is important to determine the extent of disability resulting from lack of motion. The length of time that restricted motion has been present can be useful in predicting whether interventions, such as medications and physical therapy, might reestablish normal joint motion. The physician should also ascertain whether both active and passive motion are limited in a joint. Frequently, patients are unable to differentiate these, but usually the physician can determine the difference at the time of the physical examination. It is helpful also to know whether limitation of motion began abruptly, which may suggest a mechanical derangement (such as a tendon rupture), or gradually, which is more common with inflammatory joint disease.

Swelling

Joint swelling is an important finding in patients with rheumatic disease. True joint swelling (true arthritis) helps to narrow the differential diagnosis in a patient who experiences arthralgias. The interviewer needs to determine where and when the swelling occurs. Often it is difficult for patients to recognize swelling, and not infrequently, patients describe a feeling of swelling when an actual effusion is not present. A description of the exact location of the swelling helps in understanding whether the swelling conforms to an anatomically discrete area, such as a particular joint, bursa, or extra-articular area. An obese person may interpret normal collections of adipose tissue over the medial aspects of the elbow or knee and lateral aspect of the ankle as swelling.

Information about onset, persistence, and factors that influence the swelling is also useful. Discomfort with use of the swollen part may indicate synovitis or bursitis because of tension on these tissues during motion of a joint. However, when inflamed tissues are not put under stress during joint movement, pain is minimal; for example, movement of the knee is generally painless in patients with prepatellar bursitis. Swelling in a confined area, such as a synovial sac or bursa, is most painful when it has developed rapidly; a similar degree of swelling that has developed slowly is often much more tolerable.

Weakness

Many patients report weakness, and it is important to ascertain exactly what they mean by this. Often, patients use the term "weakness" to describe fatigue. When weakness is present, a loss of motor power or muscle strength is nearly always objectively demonstrable on physical examination. The examiner must determine whether there is true weakness or "give way" weakness, in which the patient initially gives good effort with good strength and then suddenly gives way. In addition, the distribution and duration of weakness are important. In musculoskeletal disorders, weakness is usually persistent rather than intermittent. Initially, good strength with subsequent weakness can be a clue to neuromuscular disorders, such as myasthenia gravis. Muscle weakness from inflammatory myopathies usually occurs in a proximal distribution (i.e., shoulders and hips rather than hands and feet). Significant distal involvement suggests some other process, such as inclusion body myositis or a neurologic disorder.

Fatigue

Fatigue is a common complaint of patients with musculoskeletal disease. Fatigue can be defined as an inclination to rest even though pain and weakness are not limiting factors. It is a normal phenomenon after various degrees of activity but should resolve after rest. In rheumatic diseases, fatigue may be prominent even when the patient has not been active. Typically, if the systemic rheumatic disease abates, so does the fatigue. Malaise often occurs with fatigue but is not synonymous with it. Malaise is an indefinite feeling of lack of health, which frequently occurs at the onset of an illness. Both fatigue and malaise can occur without identifiable organic disease, and anxiety, tension, stress, and emotional factors can contribute.

Patients with inflammatory arthritis may use the terms "fatigue" and "weakness" interchangeably and often confuse stiffness with these. Fatigue can be differentiated from stiffness and weakness if the physician remembers that stiffness is a discomfort during movement and weakness is an inability to move normally, especially against resistance. Fatigue is an inclination to rest not because of muscle weakness or pain but from a sense of exhaustion.

SYSTEMATIC METHOD OF EXAMINATION

As with other parts of the general physical examination, a systematic method of examining joints is the quickest and easiest way to obtain a thorough assessment of the status of the joint. Many rheumatologists begin with the joints of the upper extremities and proceed to the joints of the trunk and lower extremities, but each examiner should establish his or her own routine. Gentle handling of tender and painful joints enhances cooperation by the patient and allows an accurate evaluation of the joints.[1-3]

Important Physical Signs of Arthritis

The general aim of the examination of the joints is to detect abnormalities in structure and function. The common signs of articular disease are swelling, tenderness, limitation of motion, crepitation, deformity, and instability.

Swelling

Swelling around a joint may be caused by intra-articular effusion, synovial thickening, periarticular soft tissue inflammation (such as bursitis or tendinitis), bony enlargement, or extra-articular fat pads. Familiarity with the anatomic configuration of the synovial membrane in various joints aids in differentiating soft tissue swelling due to synovitis (true articular effusion or synovial thickening) from swelling of the periarticular tissues.

A joint effusion is often visible on observation of a joint. It is helpful to compare joints of one side of the body with those on the other for evidence of symmetry (or asymmetry).

Palpable fluid in a joint without recent trauma usually indicates synovitis. The normal synovial membrane is too thin to palpate, whereas the thickened synovial membrane in many chronic inflammatory arthritides, such as rheumatoid arthritis, may have a "doughy" or "boggy" consistency. In some joints, such as the knee, the extent of the synovial cavity can be delineated on physical examination by compressing the fluid into one of the extreme limits of synovial reflection. The edge of the resulting bulge may thus be palpated more easily. If this palpable edge is within the anatomic confines of the synovial membrane and disappears on release of the compression, the distention usually represents synovial effusion; if the edge persists, distention indicates a thickened synovial membrane. However, reliable differentiation between synovial membrane thickening and effusion is not always possible by physical examination. Occasionally, intrasynovial loose bodies or plicae are palpated.

Tenderness

Tenderness is an unusual sensitivity to touch or pressure. Localization of tenderness by palpation may also help to determine whether the pathologic site is intra-articular or periarticular, such as in a fat pad, tendon attachment, ligament, bursa, or muscle or in the skin. It is also useful to palpate noninvolved structures to help assess the significance of tenderness. For example, finding a single tender point in a person with generalized tender points elsewhere on the body is less helpful than finding a single tender point in an otherwise asymptomatic patient.

Limitation of Motion

Because limitation of motion is a common manifestation of articular disease, it is important to know the normal type and range of motion of each joint. Comparison with an unaffected joint of the opposite extremity helps in the evaluation of individual variations. Restriction in joint motion may result from limitation in the joint itself or from disease in the periarticular structures. In patients with joint disease, passive range of motion is often greater than the active type, possibly because of pain, weakness, or the state of the articular or periarticular structures. The patient must be relaxed during the examination, because increased muscle tension may produce what appears to be significantly decreased range of motion. Stressing passive joint motion at the extremes of flexion and extension may also help in assessing joint tenderness.

Crepitation

Crepitation is a palpable or audible grating or crunching sensation produced by motion. It may or may not be accompanied by pain. Crepitation occurs when roughened articular or extra-articular surfaces are rubbed together by active motion or by manual compression. *Fine* crepitation is often palpable over joints involved by chronic inflammatory arthritis and usually indicates roughening of the opposing cartilage surfaces as a result of erosion or granulation tissue. *Coarse* crepitation, also due to irregularity of the cartilage surfaces, may be caused by either inflammatory or noninflammatory arthritis. *Bone-on-bone* crepitus produces a palpable and audible "squeak" of higher frequency.

Crepitation from within a joint should be differentiated from cracking sounds caused by the slipping of ligaments or tendons over bony surfaces during motion. The latter are usually less significant to the diagnosis of joint disease and may be heard over normal joints. In scleroderma, a distinct coarse, creaking, leathery crepitation may be palpable or audible, especially over tendon sheaths.

Deformity

Deformity is the malalignment of joints and may be manifested by a bony enlargement, articular subluxation, contracture, or ankylosis in nonanatomic positions. Deformed joints do not function normally, frequently restrict activities, and may be associated with pain, especially when put to stressful use. However, a deformed joint on occasion may be of cosmetic concern but may retain good functional use. In these cases, surgical correction should be approached with caution, because it is usually better to have a joint that functions satisfactorily than a cosmetically acceptable joint that does not.

Instability

Joint instability is present when the joint has greater than normal movement in any plane. "Subluxation" refers to partial displacement of the articular surfaces in a joint with some surface-to-surface contact. A dislocated joint has lost all cartilage surface-to-surface contact. Instability is best determined when the examiner supports the joint between two hands and stresses the adjacent bones in directions in which the normal joint does not move. Again, the patient should be relaxed during the examination, because muscle tension may serve to stabilize an otherwise unstable joint. For example, a knee with a deficient ligament might appear stable if the patient contracts the quadriceps muscles during evaluation.

Other Aspects of Examination

Muscle testing is discussed in Chapter 26. Examination of the cervical spine and the low back is discussed in Chapters 27 and 29, respectively.

Recording the Joint Examination

A permanent record of the joint examination is important not only in evaluating the extent and activity of arthritic disease but also in determining the efficacy of interventions. Many different recording methods have been described.

Abbreviations for each joint can be used, such as PIP for the proximal interphalangeal joints. A simple method, called the "S-T-L" system, records the degree of swelling (S), tenderness (T), and limitation of motion (L) of each joint on the basis of a quantitative estimate of gradation.

Grades range from 0 (normal) to 4 (highly abnormal). The scoring of the degree of swelling and tenderness is semiqualitative, but the examiner should try to be consistent from patient to patient and over time. A score of 1 indicates a small effusion or mild tenderness, whereas a 3 denotes a large effusion or significant tenderness. In limitation of motion, grade 1 indicates about 25 percent loss of motion; grade 2, about 50 percent loss; grade 3, about 75 percent loss; and grade 4, ankylosis. For example, a moderately swollen, mildly tender second right metatarsopha-

langeal joint with unlimited motion would have an abbreviated score of R_2MTP: $S_2T_1L_0$.

If many joints are abnormal, a table can be constructed with a column for each S, T, and L and the findings recorded for each joint. In a patient with limited disease, it is easier to record in narrative form only the joints that are abnormal. Examiners with more experience may add additional degrees to the scoring system, such as $+$ and $-$, after each numeral (for example, $1+$) to give a wider scale. Alternatively, one may use intermediate scores, such as 1 to 2, to further widen the scale. However, use of the basic system suffices in most instances. When more accuracy is desired, one can estimate and record the degrees of motion in a joint or measure the motion in joints with a goniometer.

A useful option for recording the results of the joint examination, especially in patients with multiple joint involvement, is a schematic skeleton with marked articulations on which the status of individual joints is recorded (Fig. 23–1).

The degree of disease activity can be assessed by calculating the total number of tender or swollen joints, or of both, and using the value obtained as a joint count or joint index. Systems that may be inefficient and cumbersome for daily office use but that have value in academic studies include measurement of the size of joints by tape measure or jeweler's rings,

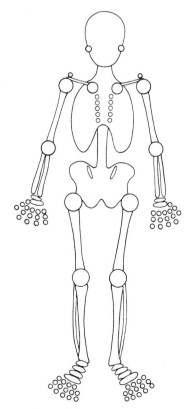

Figure 23–1. Skeleton diagram for recording joint examination findings. (From Polley HF, Hunder GG: Rheumatologic Interviewing and Physical Examination of the Joints, 2nd ed. Philadelphia, WB Saunders, 1978.)

determination of the degree of warmth by thermography, and measurement of the amount of tenderness with a dolorimeter.

Although the previously described tests and examinations can give a physical description of the joints, they do not necessarily measure function. A sense of joint function can be assessed in part by *grip strength testing*. The patient's grip strength can be measured while the patient squeezes a partially inflated (20 mm Hg) sphygmomanometer cuff or through use of a dynamometer. Tests are available that attempt to measure functional use of joints by determining the patient's speed and ability in the performance of other coordinated functions, such as the time needed to walk 50 feet. All of these functional tests, however, have an inherent tendency toward variability. For observations on qualities such as joint tenderness and grip strength, interobserver variation is often greater than intraobserver observation.[4, 5] There may also be significant intraobserver variation in observing the same patient, even over a short interval. Furthermore, biologic factors, such as circadian changes in joint size and grip strength among rheumatoid patients during a 24-hour interval, contribute to variability.[6] These tests are best suited for clinical trials, tending to be less useful in follow-up of individual patients.

EXAMINATION OF SPECIFIC JOINTS

Temporomandibular Joint

The temporomandibular joint is formed by the condyle of the mandible and the fossa of the temporal bone just anterior to the external auditory canal. Swelling in this joint is difficult to see. The joint is palpated by placing a finger just anterior to the external auditory canal and asking the patient to open and close the mouth and to move the mandible from side to side. Because of normal differences in soft tissue thickness, synovial thickness or swelling of minimal or moderate degree can be detected most easily if the synovitis is unilateral or asymmetric when the other side is used for comparison. Vertical movement of the temporomandibular joint can be measured by determining the space between the upper and the lower incisor teeth with the patient's mouth wide open. This distance is normally 3 to 6 cm. Lateral movement can be determined by using incisor teeth as landmarks. Audible or palpable crepitus or clicking may be noted in patients with and without evidence of severe arthritis.

Many forms of arthritis can affect the temporomandibular joints, including juvenile and adult rheumatoid arthritis. If these joints are affected in children, bone growth of the mandible may be arrested, with resultant micrognathia. Some patients without inflammatory arthritis describe arthralgias of the temporomandibular joint, and many of these patients have the *temporomandibular joint syndrome*. This syndrome is thought by some to result from bruxism and is likely a form of myofascial pain.

Cricoarytenoid Joint

The paired cricoarytenoid joints are formed by the articulation of the base of the small pyramidal arytenoid cartilage and the upper posterolateral border of the cricoid cartilage. The vocal ligaments (true vocal cords) are attached to the arytenoid cartilages. The cricoarytenoid joints are normally very mobile diarthrodial joints that move both medially and laterally and rotate during the opening and closing of the vocal cords. These joints are examined by direct or indirect laryngoscopy. Erythema, swelling, and lack of mobility during phonation may result from inflammation of the joints. The cricoarytenoid joints may be affected in rheumatoid arthritis, trauma, and infection. Involvement in rheumatoid arthritis is more common than clinically apparent. Symptoms may include hoarseness and a sense of fullness or discomfort in the throat that is worse on speaking or swallowing. Significant airway obstruction has been reported only rarely.

Sternoclavicular, Manubriosternal, and Sternocostal Joints

The medial ends of the clavicles articulate on each side of the sternum at its upper end to form the sternoclavicular joints. The articulations of the first ribs and the sternum (sternocostal joints) are immediately caudad. The articulation of the manubrium and body of the sternum is at the level of the attachment of the second costal cartilage to the sternum. The third through seventh sternocostal joints articulate distally along the lateral borders of the sternum. The sternoclavicular joints are the only articulations in this group that are always diarthrodial; the others are amphiarthroses or synchondroses. The sternoclavicular joints are the only true points of articulation of the shoulder girdle with the trunk. These joints lie beneath the skin; therefore, synovitis is usually visible and palpable. These joints have only slight movement, which cannot be accurately measured.

Involvement of the sternoclavicular joints is common in ankylosing spondylitis, rheumatoid arthritis, and degenerative arthritis, but it frequently remains unrecognized. The sternoclavicular joint may be the site of septic arthritis, especially in drug abusers. Tenderness of the manubriosternal or costosternal joint is much more frequent than actual swelling. Tenderness of these joints without actual swelling has been termed "costochondritis," and the term "Tietze's syndrome" may be used if swelling is observed or palpated.

Acromioclavicular Joint

The acromioclavicular joint is formed by the lateral end of the clavicle and medial margin of the acromion process of the scapula. Bony enlargement of this joint secondary to degenerative arthritis may be seen in middle-aged or older persons, but soft tissue swelling is not usually visible or palpable. Tenderness over the joint and pain with adduction of the arm across the chest suggest involvement of this joint. Arthritis of the acromioclavicular joint is usually secondary to trauma that leads to degenerative disease. The joint usually is not significantly affected by rheumatoid arthritis. Movement occurs at this joint during shoulder motion, but the extent of motion is difficult to measure accurately.

Shoulder

See Chapter 28.

Elbow

The elbow joint (see also Chapter 107) is composed of three bony articulations. The principal one is the humeroulnar joint, which is a hinge joint. The radiohumeral and proximal radioulnar articulations allow rotation of the forearm (Fig. 23–2).

To examine the elbow joint, the examiner places a thumb between the lateral epicondyle and the olecra-

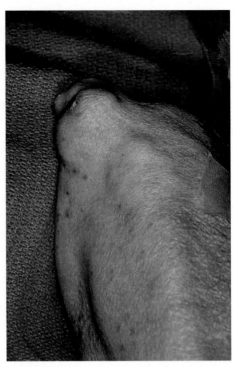

Figure 23–3. Multiple rheumatoid nodules over the extensor surface of the elbow.

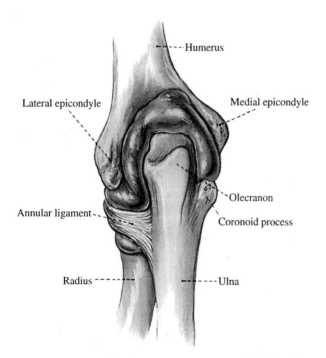

Figure 23–2. Posterior aspect of the elbow joint showing the distribution of the synovial membrane. (From Polley HF, Hunder GG: Rheumatologic Interviewing and Physical Examination of the Joints, 2nd ed. Philadelphia, WB Saunders, 1978.)

non process in the lateral paraolecranon groove and places one or two fingers in the corresponding groove medial to the olecranon. The patient's elbow should be relaxed and moved passively through flexion, extension, and rotation. One should also carefully examine the skin about the elbow joint. In patients with rheumatoid arthritis, one may be able to palpate or observe nodules (Fig. 23–3). In patients with psoriasis, plaques are often present over the extensor surface of the elbow.

Limitation of motion and crepitus may be noted. Synovial swelling is most easily palpated as it bulges under the examiner's thumb when the elbow is passively extended. Synovial membrane can sometimes be palpated over the posterior aspect of the joint between the olecranon process and the distal humerus. Synovitis is commonly associated with limitation of joint extension.

The olecranon bursa overlies the olecranon process of the ulna. Olecranon bursitis is common after chronic local trauma and in rheumatic diseases, including rheumatoid arthritis and gout. A septic olecranon bursitis may also occur. Olecranon bursitis usually appears as a swelling over the olecranon process, which often is tender and may be erythematous. Sometimes there is a large collection of fluid over the area that is palpable as a cystic mass, and often aspiration and drainage may be required.

The medial and lateral epicondyles of the humerus are tendinous attachment sites. These areas may be tender without other objective signs of inflammation in conditions thought to result from overuse, such as "tennis elbow" (*lateral epicondylitis*) and "golfer's elbow" (*medial epicondylitis*). In addition to localized tenderness on palpation, discomfort can be elicited in medial epicondylitis by resisted flexion of the supinated wrist. In lateral epicondylitis, supination of the forearm or extension of the pronated wrist against resistance elicits pain localized to the lateral epicondyle. Treatment with ice, forearm splints, anti-inflammatory medications, rest, and, occasionally, local injections is usually helpful.

Muscle function of the elbow can be assessed by testing flexion and extension. The prime movers of flexion are the biceps brachii (C-5 and C-6), brachialis (C-5 and C-6), and brachioradialis (C-5 and C-6) muscles.* The prime mover of extension is the triceps brachii muscle (C-7 and C-8).

Wrist and Carpal Joints

The wrist is a complex joint formed by several articulations among the radius, ulna, and carpal bones. The true wrist, or radiocarpal articulation (see also Chapter 106), is a biaxial ellipsoid joint formed proximally by the distal end of the radius and the triangular fibrocartilage and distally by a row of three carpal bones, the scaphoid (navicular), lunate, and the triquetrum (triangular) (Fig. 23–4). The distal radioulnar joint is a uniaxial pivot joint. The midcarpal joints are formed by the junction of the proximal and distal rows of the carpal bones. The midcarpal and carpometacarpal articular cavities often communicate. The intercarpal joints refer to the articulations between the individual carpal bones.

Movements of the wrist include palmar flexion (flexion), dorsiflexion (extension), radial deviation, ulnar deviation, and circumduction. Pronation and su-

*The level of spinal cord innervation of specific muscles is shown in parentheses after each muscle.

pination of the hand and forearm occur primarily at the proximal and distal radioulnar joints. The only carpometacarpal joint that moves to a significant degree is the carpometacarpal joint of the thumb. This joint is saddle-shaped (sellar) and possesses three degrees of freedom. Crepitus at this joint is common, as it is frequently involved in degenerative arthritis.

The wrist can normally be extended to about 70 or 80 degrees and flexed to 80 or 90 degrees. Ulnar and radial deviation should allow 50 degrees and 20 to 30 degrees of movement, respectively. Loss of dorsiflexion is the most incapacitating functional impairment of wrist motion.

The long flexor tendons of the forearm musculature cross the palmar surface of the wrist and are enclosed in the flexor tendon sheath under the flexor retinaculum (transverse carpal ligament). The flexor retinaculum and the underlying carpal bones form the carpal tunnel. The median nerve runs through the carpal tunnel superficial to the flexor tendons. The extensor tendons of the forearm pass under the extensor retinaculum and are enclosed in a synovial sheath.

The palmar aponeurosis (fascia) spreads out into the palm from the flexor retinaculum. *Dupuytren's contracture* is a fibrosing condition affecting the palmar aponeurosis, which becomes thickened and contracted and may draw one or more fingers into flexion at the metacarpophalangeal joint. The fourth finger is frequently affected first.

Swelling of the wrist may be due to inflammation involving the sheaths of the tendons crossing the wrist or the wrist joint itself, or both. When swelling is due to tenosynovitis, the outpouching tends to be more localized and is altered by flexion and extension of the fingers. Articular swelling tends to be more diffuse, protruding anteriorly and posteriorly from under the tendons.

Synovitis of the wrist joint is more reliably detected by palpation over the dorsal surface. Because of the

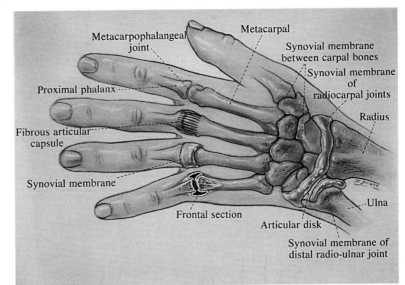

Figure 23–4. Relationship of the synovial membranes of the wrist and carpal and metacarpal joints to the surrounding bony structures. (From Polley HF, Hunder GG: Rheumatologic Interviewing and Physical Examination of the Joints, 2nd ed. Philadelphia, WB Saunders, 1978.)

structures overlying both surfaces of the wrist, accurate localization of the synovial margins is difficult. To examine the wrist, the physician should palpate the joint gently between the thumbs and fingers. Prominence or thickening of the synovium may be noted and, if significant, has the characteristics of true synovitis.

A *ganglion* is a cystic enlargement arising from a joint capsule; it characteristically occurs on the dorsum of the wrist between the extensor tendons.

Subluxation of the ulna may occur secondary to chronic inflammatory arthritis. The subluxed ulna appears as a prominence on the dorsolateral wrist and may press against the extensor tendons, especially those of the fourth and fifth digits. Potentially, these tendons may rupture.

Trigger fingers can be detected by palpating crepitus or nodules along the tendons in the palm while the patient slowly flexes and extends the fingers. Usually, the patient states that the affected finger catches or locks with movement.

Stenosing tenosynovitis occurs commonly at the radial styloid process (*de Quervain's tenosynovitis*) and characteristically involves the long abductor and short extensor tendons of the thumb. Usually, pain is localized to the radial side of the wrist, and tenderness is often elicited by palpation near the radial styloid process. The Finkelstein test for de Quervain's tenosynovitis is done by having the patient make a fist with the thumb in the palm of the hand. The examiner moves the patient's wrist into ulnar deviation. If severe pain occurs over the radial styloid, the test result is positive and the cause of the pain is stretching of thumb tendons in the stenosed tendon sheath.

Carpal tunnel syndrome, discussed in detail in Chapters 39 and 106, results from pressure on the median nerve in the carpal tunnel.

Muscle function of the wrist can be measured by testing flexion and extension as well as supination and pronation of the forearm. Prime movers in wrist flexion are the flexor carpi radialis (C-6 and C-7) and flexor carpi ulnaris (C-8 and T-l) muscles. Each of these muscles can be tested separately. To test the flexor carpi radialis, the examiner provides resistance to flexion at the base of the second metacarpal bone in the direction of extension and ulnar deviation. To test the flexor carpi ulnaris, resistance is applied at the base of the fifth metacarpal in the direction of extension and radial deviation. The prime extensions of the wrist are the extensor carpi radialis longus (C-6 and C-7), extensor carpi radialis brevis (C-6 and C-7), and extensor carpi ulnaris (C-7 and C-8) muscles.

The radial and ulnar extensor muscles can also be tested separately. Prime movers in supination of the forearm are the biceps brachii (C-5 and C-6) and supinator (C-6). Prime movers in pronation are the pronator teres (C-6 and C-7) and pronator quadratus (C-8 and T-l).

Metacarpophalangeal, Proximal, and Distal Interphalangeal Joints

The metacarpophalangeal joints are hinge joints. Lateral collateral ligaments that are loose in extension tighten in flexion, thereby preventing lateral movement of the digits. The extensor tendons that cross the dorsum of each joint strengthen the articular capsule. When the extensor tendon of the digit reaches the distal end of the metacarpal head, it is joined by fibers of the interossei and lumbricales and expands over the entire dorsum of the metacarpophalangeal joint and onto the dorsum of the adjacent phalanx. This expansion of the extensor mechanism is known as the *extensor hood.*

The proximal and distal interphalangeal joints are also hinge joints. The ligaments of the interphalangeal joints resemble those of the metacarpophalangeal joints. When the fingers are flexed, the bases of the proximal phalanges slide toward the palmar side of the heads of the metacarpal bones. The metacarpal heads form the rounded prominences of the knuckle, with the metacarpal joint spaces lying about 1 cm distal to the apices of the prominences.

The skin on the palmar surface of the hand is relatively thick and covers a fat pad between it and the metacarpophalangeal joint. The pad makes it difficult to palpate the palmar surface of the joint.

To examine the metacarpophalangeal joints, one should palpate over the dorsal aspect and sides of each joint, with the more proximal joints in 20 to 30 degrees of flexion. In examining the small joints, one may find it especially helpful to compare one joint with another to detect subtle synovitis. Gentle lateral compression, with force applied at the base of the second and fifth metacarpophalangeal joints, often elicits tenderness if synovitis is present. This maneuver has been termed the "squeeze test" by some.

The proximal and distal interphalangeal joints are best examined by gentle palpation over the lateral and medial aspects of the joint, where the flexor and extensor tendons do not interfere with assessment of the synovial membrane. Alternatively, the joint can be compressed anteroposteriorly by the thumb and index finger of one of the examiner's hands while the other thumb and index finger palpate for synovial distention medially and laterally.

Bunnell's test is useful in differentiating synovitis of the proximal interphalangeal joints from spasm of the intrinsic muscles (see Chapter 25).

Swelling of the fingers may result from articular or periarticular causes. Synovial swelling usually produces symmetric enlargement of the joint itself, whereas extra-articular swelling may be diffuse and extend beyond the joint space (Fig. 23–5). Asymmetric enlargement, involving only one side of the digit or joint, is less common and usually indicates an extra-articular process. Diffuse swelling of an entire digit may result from tenosynovitis and is more commonly seen in the spondyloarthropathies, such as Reiter's syndrome and psoriatic arthritis. The term "sausage digit" applies to this sort of dactylitis. Chronic swelling and distention of the metacarpophalangeal joints tend to produce stretching and laxity of the articular capsule and ligaments. Because of this laxity, combined with muscle imbalance and other forces, the extensor

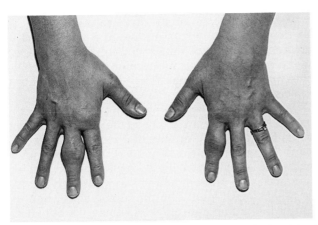

Figure 23–5. Severe fusiform swelling of the right third proximal interphalangeal joint (grade S4) and left second proximal interphalangeal joint (grade S3). Asymmetric involvement like this can occur in rheumatoid arthritis, but more typically the synovitis is symmetric. (From Polley HF, Hunder GG: Rheumatologic Interviewing and Physical Examination of the Joints, 2nd ed. Philadelphia, WB Saunders, 1978.)

tendons of the digits eventually slip off the metacarpal heads to the ulnar sides of the joints. The abnormal pull of the displaced tendons is one of the factors that cause ulnar deviation of the fingers in chronic inflammatory arthritis.

Swan neck deformity refers to the appearance of a finger affected by flexion contracture of the metacarpophalangeal joint, hyperextension of the proximal interphalangeal joint, and flexion of the distal interphalangeal joint. These changes are produced by contraction of the interossei and other muscles that flex the metacarpophalangeal joints and extend the proximal interphalangeal joints. This deformity is characteristic of rheumatoid arthritis but may be seen in other chronic arthritides (Fig. 23–6).

The term *boutonnière deformity* is used to describe

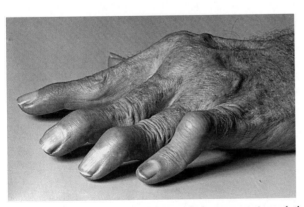

Figure 23–6. Swan neck deformity with hyperextension of the proximal interphalangeal joints and flexion of the distal interphalangeal joints of the second, third, and fourth digits of the hand. The fifth digit displays the boutonnière deformity, with flexion at the proximal interphalangeal joint and hyperextension at the distal interphalangeal joint. (From Polley HF, Hunder GG: Rheumatologic Interviewing and Physical Examination of the Joints, 2nd ed. Philadelphia, WB Saunders, 1978.)

a finger with a flexion contracture of the proximal interphalangeal joint associated with hyperextension of the distal interphalangeal joint. The deformity is relatively common in rheumatoid arthritis and results when the central slip of the extensor tendon of the proximal interphalangeal joint becomes detached from the base of the middle phalanx, allowing palmar dislocation of the lateral bands. The dislocated bands cross the fulcrum of the joint and then act as flexors instead of extensors of the joint.

Another abnormality is "telescoping," or shortening, of the digits produced by resorption of ends of the phalanges secondary to destructive arthropathy. This deformity may be seen in the arthritis mutilans form of psoriatic arthritis. Shortening of the fingers is associated with wrinkling of the skin over involved joints and also is called "opera-glass hand," or *main en lorgnette.*

A *mallet finger* results from avulsion or rupture of the extensor tendon at the level of the distal interphalangeal joint. With this deformity, the patient is unable to extend the distal phalanx, which resides in a flexed position. This deformity frequently results from traumatic injuries.

Murphy's sign is a test for lunate dislocation. The patient is asked to make a fist. Usually, the third metacarpal is more prominent than the second and fourth. If the third metacarpal is level with the second and fourth, the test result is positive for lunate dislocation.

Involvement of the distal interphalangeal joints in rheumatoid arthritis is uncommon. However, bony hypertrophy or osteophytic changes are commonly seen at both the distal and the proximal interphalangeal joints in patients with degenerative arthritis. Enlarged bony, hypertrophic distal interphalangeal joints are called "Heberden's nodes," and similar changes at the proximal interphalangeal joints are called "Bouchard's nodes" (Fig. 23–7). These are usually easily differentiated from the synovitis of inflammatory arthritis because on palpation the enlargement is hard or bony. Additionally, signs of inflammation are minimal. Furthermore, Heberden's and Bouchard's nodes should be easily differentiated from rheumatoid nodules, but occasionally patients confuse them when describing swellings over joints. One should also be aware of other causes of nodules on the hands, including tophaceous gout and, rarely, multicentric reticulohistiocytosis.

The patient's fingernails should be inspected for evidence of clubbing or other abnormalities. Often in patients with psoriatic arthritis ridging, onycholysis or nail pitting is present.

A crude but sometimes useful assessment of hand function can be made by asking the patient to make a fist. An estimate of the patient's ability to form a full fist can be recorded as a "percent" fist, with 100 percent being a complete fist. A fist of 75 percent indicates that the patient can touch the palm with the fingertips. The ability to oppose fingers, especially the thumb, is critical to hand function because of the

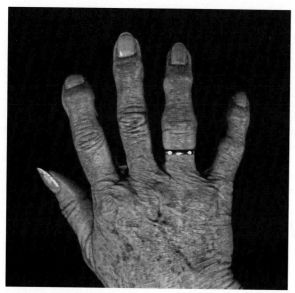

Figure 23–7. Bony hypertrophy at the second, third, fourth, and fifth distal interphalangeal joints (Heberden's nodes) and the fourth and fifth proximal interphalangeal joints (Bouchard's nodes).

necessity to grasp or at least pinch for objects. For patients who cannot form a full fist, the ability or inability to pinch or oppose fingers can also be demonstrated by having them try to pick up a small object.

Strength of the hands can be crudely assessed by asking the patient to firmly grip two or more of the examiner's fingers. Grip strength can be measured more accurately with a dynamometer or by having the patient squeeze a partially inflated sphygmomanometer (at 20 mm Hg).

It is sometimes useful to test strength of the fingers separately. The prime movers of flexion of the second through fifth metacarpophalangeal joints are the dorsal and palmar interosseus muscles (C-8 and T-1). The lumbrical muscles (C-6, C-7, and C-8) flex the metacarpophalangeal joints when the proximal phalangeal joints are extended. The flexors of the proximal interphalangeal joints are the flexor digitorum superficialis muscles (C-7, C-8, and T-1), and the flexor of the distal interphalangeal joints is the flexor digitorum profundus muscle (C-7, C-8, and T-1).

The prime extensors of the metacarpophalangeal joints and interphalangeal joints of the second through fifth fingers are the extensor digitorum communis (C-6, C-7, and C-8), the extensor indicis proprius (C-6, C-7, and C-8), and the extensor digiti minimi (C-7) muscles. The interossei and lumbrical muscles simultaneously flex the metacarpophalangeal joints and extend the interphalangeal joints. The dorsal interosseus muscles (C-8 and T-1) and abductor digiti minimi (C-8) abduct the fingers, whereas the palmar interosseus muscles adduct the fingers.

The thumb is moved by a number of muscles. The prime flexor of the first metacarpophalangeal joint is the flexor pollicis brevis muscle (C-6, C-7, C-8, and T-

1). The prime flexor of the interphalangeal joint is the flexor pollicis longus muscle (C-8 and T-1). The metacarpophalangeal joint of the thumb is extended by the extensor pollicis brevis muscle, and the prime extensor of the interphalangeal joint is the extensor pollicis longus muscle (C-6, C-7, C-8, and C-9).

The prime abductors of the thumb are the abductor pollicis longus (C-6 and C-7) and the abductor pollicis brevis (C-6 and C-7) muscles. Motion takes place primarily at the carpometacarpal joint. The prime mover in thumb adduction is the adductor pollicis muscle (C-8 and T-1). Motion takes place primarily at the carpophalangeal joint. The prime movers in opposition of the thumb and fifth fingers are the opponens pollicis (C-6 and C-7) and opponens digiti minimi (C-8 and T-1) muscles.

Sensation and nerve injuries in the upper extremity are discussed in Chapters 39 and 107.

Hip

The hip is a spheroidal or ball-and-socket joint formed by the rounded head of the femur and the cup-shaped acetabulum (see also Chapter 110). Stability of the joint is ensured by the fibrocartilaginous rim of the glenoid labrum and the dense articular capsule and surrounding ligaments, including the iliofemoral, pubofemoral, and ischiocapsular ligaments that reinforce the capsule. Support is also supplied by the powerful muscle groups that surround the hip. The primary hip flexor, the iliopsoas muscle, is assisted by the sartorius and the rectus femoris muscles. Hip adduction is accomplished by the three adductors— the longus, brevis, and magnus—and the gracilis and pectineus muscles. The gluteus medius is the major hip abductor, whereas the gluteus maximus and hamstrings extend the hip. Several clinically important bursae are located about the hip joint. Anteriorly, the iliopsoas bursa lies between the psoas muscle and the joint surface. The trochanteric bursa lies between the gluteus maximus muscle and the posterolateral greater trochanter, and the ischiogluteal bursa overlies the ischial tuberosity (Fig. 23–8).

Examination of the hip should begin with an observation of the patient's stance and gait. The patient should stand in front of the examiner so that the anterior iliac spines are visible. Pelvic tilt or obliquity may be present, related to a structural scoliosis, anatomic leg length discrepancy, or hip disease. Hip contractures may result in abduction or adduction deformities. To compensate for an adduction contracture, the pelvis is tilted upward on the side of the contracture. This allows the legs to be parallel during walking and weight bearing. With a fixed abduction deformity, the pelvis becomes elevated on the normal side during standing or walking. This causes an apparent shortening of the normal leg and forces the patient to stand or walk on the toes of the normal side or to flex the knee on the abnormal leg.

Viewed from behind, with the legs parallel, the

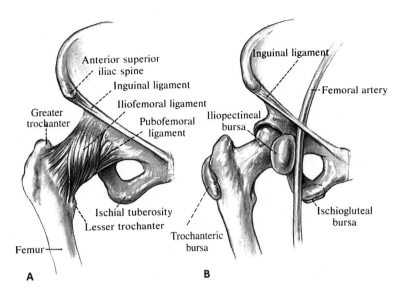

Figure 23–8. *A,* Hip and adjacent structures. *B,* Relationship of distended bursae to the hip joint. (From Polley HF, Hunder GG: Rheumatologic Interviewing and Physical Examination of the Joints, 2nd ed. Philadelphia, WB Saunders, 1978.)

patient with hip disease and an adducted hip contracture may have asymmetric gluteal folds due to pelvic tilt, with the diseased side elevated. In this situation, the patient is unable to stand with the foot of the involved leg flat on the floor. In abduction contracture, the findings are reversed; with both legs extended and parallel, the uninvolved side is elevated.

A hip flexion deformity commonly occurs in diseases of the hip. Unilateral flexion of the hip in the standing position reduces weight bearing on the involved side and relaxes the joint capsule, causing less pain. This posture is best noted by observing the patient from the side. A hyperlordotic curve of the lumbar spine compensates for lack of full hip extension.

The patient with possible hip disease should be observed walking. With a normal gait, the abductors of the weight-bearing leg contract to hold the pelvis level or elevate the non–weight-bearing side slightly. Two abnormalities of gait may be commonly observed in patients with hip disease. The most common seen with a painful hip is the *antalgic* (limping) gait. A person with this gait leans over the diseased hip during the phase of weight bearing on that hip, placing the body weight directly over the joint to avoid painful contraction of the hip abductors. In a *Trendelenburg* gait, with weight bearing on the affected side, the pelvis drops and the trunk shifts to the normal side. Although the antalgic gait usually is seen with painful hips and the Trendelenburg gait with weak hip abductors, neither gait is specific and either may accompany a painful hip. A mild Trendelenburg gait is common in normal persons.

Trendelenburg's test, which assesses the stability of the hip together with the ability of the hip abductors to stabilize the pelvis on the femur, is a measure of the strength of the gluteus medius hip abductor. The patient is asked to stand and to bear weight on only one leg. Normally, the abductors hold the pelvis level

or the nonsupported side slightly elevated. If the non–weight-bearing side drops, the test result is positive for weakness of the hip abductors, especially the gluteus medius on the weight-bearing side. This result is nonspecific and may be observed in primary neurologic or muscle disorders and in a variety of hip diseases that lead to weakness of the hip abductors.

In the supine position, a hip flexion contracture is suggested by persistence of lumbar lordosis and pelvic tilt that mask the contracture by allowing the involved leg to remain in contact with the examination table. The *Thomas test* demonstrates the flexion contracture. During this test, the opposite hip is fully flexed to flatten the lumbar lordosis and fix the pelvis. The involved leg should then be extended toward the table as far as possible. The flexion contracture of the diseased hip becomes more obvious and can be estimated in degrees from full extension. Leg length discrepancy is measured with the patient supine and the legs fully extended. Each leg is measured from the anterior superior iliac spine to the medial malleolus. A difference of 1 cm or less is unlikely to cause any abnormality of gait and may be considered normal. In addition to true leg length asymmetries, apparent leg length discrepancies may result from pelvic tilt or abduction or adduction contractures of the hip.

The range of motion of the hip includes flexion, extension, abduction, adduction, internal and external rotation, and circumduction. The degree of flexion permitted varies with the manner in which it is assessed. When the knee is held flexed at 90 degrees, the hip normally flexes to an angle of 120 degrees between the thigh and long axis of the body. If the knee is held in extension, the hamstrings limit hip flexion to about 90 degrees. Abduction is measured with the patient supine and the leg in an extended position perpendicular to the pelvis. Pelvic stabilization is achieved by placing one arm across the pelvis with the hand on the opposite anterior iliac spine. With the other hand, the examiner grasps the patient's ankle and abducts the leg until the pelvis begins to move. Abduction to about 45 degrees is normal. It is helpful to compare one side with the other, as the normal range of motion may vary somewhat. Alternatively, the examiner can stand at the foot of the table, grasp both ankles, and simultaneously abduct both legs. Abduction is commonly limited in hip joint disease. Adduction is tested by grasping the ankle and raising the leg off the examination table by flexing the hip enough to allow the tested leg to cross over the opposite leg. Normal adduction is about 20 to 30 degrees. Hip rotation may be tested with both hip and knee flexed to 90 degrees or with the leg extended. Normal hip external rotation and internal rotation are to 45 and 40 degrees, respectively. Rotation between the flexed and the extended hips is also different because of the increased stabilization of the joint by the surrounding ligaments in the extended position. Rotation decreases with extension. To test hip rotation, the examiner grasps the extended leg above the ankle and rotates it externally and internally from the neutral position. Limitation of internal rotation of the hip is a sensitive indicator of hip joint disease.

Extension is tested with the patient in the prone position. Estimating hip extension can be difficult because some of the apparent motion arises from hyperextension of the lumbar spine, pelvis rotation, motion of the buttock soft tissue, and flexion of the opposite hip. The examiner can partially immobilize the pelvis and lumbar spine by placing one arm across the posterior iliac crest and lower lumbar spine. Placing the other hand under the thigh with the knee flexed, the examiner hyperextends the thigh. Normal extension ranges from 10 to 20 degrees. Limitation of extension is often secondary to a hip flexion contracture.

Swelling about the hip can rarely be discerned on examination.

Patrick's test, or the *fabere sign*, is a commonly used test to screen for hip disease. During this test, the patient lies supine and the examiner flexes, abducts, and externally rotates the patient's test leg so that the foot of that leg is on top of the opposite knee. The examiner then slowly lowers the test leg toward the examining table. A negative result occurs when the test leg falls at least parallel to the opposite leg; a positive result occurs when the test leg remains above the opposite leg. A positive result to Patrick's test may be indicative of hip disease, iliopsoas spasm, or sacroiliac disease.

Two useful screening tests for congenital hip disease in the pediatric population are *Ortolani's sign* and the *Galeazzi sign*. In the Ortolani maneuver, the examiner flexes the hips and grasps the legs of a supine infant so that the examiner's thumbs are against the inner thighs and fingers are draped over the outer (lateral) side of the thighs. With gentle traction, the hips are abducted and laterally rotated. Usually, resistance is felt at 30 to 40 degrees of lateral rotation and abduction. For a positive test result, a

click is felt before abduction to the normal 70 degrees can be attained. Ortolani's test should not be done repeatedly, because it can lead to damage of the articular cartilage on the femoral head.

The Galeazzi sign is useful for assessing unilateral congenital hip dislocation in children younger than 18 months. The child is instructed to lie supine with the knees and hips flexed to 90 degrees. Normally, both knees should reside at the same level; the result is positive if one knee is higher than the other.

The iliotibial band is a part of the fascia lata extending from the iliac crest, sacrum, and ischium over the greater trochanter to the lateral femoral condyle, tibial condyle, and fibular head and along the lateral intermuscular system, separating the hamstrings from the vastus lateralis. The tensor fascia latae may cause an audible snap as it slips over the greater trochanter if the weight-bearing leg moves from hip flexion and adduction to a neutral position, as in climbing stairs. Most commonly observed in young women, the "snapping" hip usually does not cause any significant degree of pain. *Ober's test* evaluates the iliotibial band for contracture. The patient lies in the side position with the lower leg flexed at the hip and knee. The examiner abducts and extends the upper leg with the knee flexed at 90 degrees. The hips should also be slightly extended to allow the iliotibial band to pass over the greater trochanter. The examiner slowly lowers the limb with the muscles relaxed. A positive result, indicative of an iliotibial band contracture, occurs if the leg does not fall back to the tabletop level.

A common cause of lateral hip pain is *trochanteric bursitis*. Often, patients with this condition note pain and tenderness when they attempt to lie on the affected side at night or to walk up and down stairs. The greater trochanter should be palpated for tenderness and compared with the opposite side. In a patient with trochanteric bursitis, this area is usually exquisitely tender. The pain of trochanteric bursitis is aggravated by actively resisted abduction of the hip. Aching and tenderness over the buttock area may be secondary to an ischial bursitis. Another cause of lateral and posterior hip (buttock) discomfort is pain at muscle and tendon insertion sites.

Anterior hip and groin pain may be secondary to hip disease, most commonly degenerative arthritis. Decreased range of motion should be noted in these cases. Another cause is iliopsoas bursitis; swelling and tenderness may be noted in the middle one third of the inguinal ligament lateral to the femoral pulse. This pain is aggravated by hip extension and reduced by flexion. The bursitis may be a localized problem or represent extension of hip synovitis or even a synovial cyst to the bursa. This differentiation cannot be made on physical examination. If the patient is tender in the region of the iliopsoas bursa but no swelling is palpable, one should also consider tendinitis of the iliopsoas muscle. The inguinal region should be carefully palpated for other abnormalities, such as hernias, femoral aneurysms, adenopathy, tumor, and psoas abscess or masses.

Muscle strength testing should include the hip flexors, extensors, abductors, and adductors. The primary hip flexor is the iliopsoas muscle (L-2 and L-3). Flexion may be tested with the patient sitting at the edge of a table. The examiner exerts downward pressure against the thigh proximal to the knee while the patient attempts to flex the hip. The pelvis may be stabilized by the examiner's other hand placed on the ipsilateral iliac crest. Alternatively, with the patient supine and holding the leg in 90 degrees of flexion at the hip, the examiner may attempt to straighten the hip. Hip extension is tested with the patient lying prone. The primary hip extensor is the gluteus maximus muscle (L-5 and S-1). With the knee flexed to remove hamstring action, the patient is instructed to extend the hip and thigh off the surface of the table as the examiner places one forearm across the posterior iliac crest to stabilize the pelvis and applies downward pressure to prevent the lateral trunk muscles from raising the pelvis and leg off the table. Abduction may be tested with the patient prone or supine. The patient should abduct the thigh and leg against resistance from the examiner applied at the mid-thigh level. The primary adductor is the adductor longus (L-3 and L-4). The examiner holds the upper leg proximal to the knee in slight abduction while the patient resists and attempts to adduct the leg.

Abduction and adduction may also be tested in the two legs simultaneously. The patient lies supine with the legs fully extended and the hips moderately abducted. In the test for abduction, the patient actively pushes out against the examiner's resistance against the lateral malleoli. Adduction is tested by movement against resistance at the medial malleoli.

Knee

The knee is a compound condylar joint with three articulations: the patellofemoral and the lateral and medial tibial femoral condyles with their fibrocartilaginous menisci. The knee is stabilized by its articular capsule, the ligamentum patella, medial and lateral collateral ligaments, and anterior and posterior cruciate ligaments. The collateral ligaments provide medial and lateral stability, whereas the cruciates provide anteroposterior support and rotatory stability.

Normal knee motion is a combination of flexion or extension and rotation. The tibia internally rotates with flexion and externally rotates on the femur with extension. The surrounding synovial membrane is the largest of the body's joints; it extends up to 6 cm proximal to the joint as the suprapatellar pouch beneath the quadriceps femoris muscle. There are several clinically significant bursae about the knee, including the superficial prepatellar bursa, the superficial and deep infrapatellar bursae, the pes anserine bursa distal to the medial tibial plateau, and the posterior medial semimembranous and posterolateral gastrocnemius bursae (Fig. 23–9). Knee extension is provided for primarily by the quadriceps femoris muscle and flexion by the hamstrings. The biceps femoris externally rotates the lower leg on the femur, whereas the popliteus and semitendinous muscles are involved with internal rotation.

Examination of the knees should always include observation of the patient standing and walking. Deviation of the knees, including *genu varum* (lateral deviation of the knee joint with medial deviation of the lower leg), *genu valgum* (medial deviation of the knee with lateral deviation of the lower leg), and *genu recurvatum*, is most easily appreciated in the standing patient. The patient should also be observed walking for evidence of gait abnormalities.

The patient should be asked about symptoms of locking, catching, or "give way." *Locking* is the sudden loss of ability to extend the knee; it is usually painful and may be associated with an audible noise, such as a click or pop. It often implies significant intra-articu-

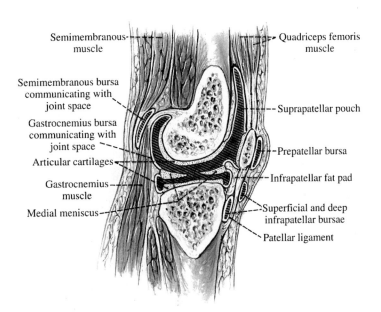

Figure 23–9. Sagittal section through the knee showing relation of the joint to adjacent structures. (From Polley HF, Hunder GG: Rheumatologic Interviewing and Physical Examination of the Joints, 2nd ed. Philadelphia, WB Saunders, 1978.)

lar disease, including loose bodies and cartilaginous tears.

Catching refers to a subjective sensation of the patient that the knee might lock; the patient may experience a momentary interruption in the smooth range of motion of the joint but is able to continue with normal motion after this brief "catch." Catching usually implies less significant disorder than true locking, and it may occur because of a variety of pathologic conditions.

True "give way" implies that the knee actually buckles and "gives out" in certain positions or with certain activities. Many patients state that their leg "gives out," but it is important to ask them exactly what they mean by this. Often, patients experience a sensation that their knee is about to give out and thus is unstable, but it actually is not. Other patients may use this term to describe severe pain that occurs and necessitates their stopping an activity. True "give way" implies a significant intra-articular abnormality, such as an unstable joint from ligamentous injury or incompetence.

Asymmetry from swelling or muscle atrophy may be noted on inspection. Patellar alignment should be noted, including high-riding or laterally displaced patellae. The examiner should inspect the knee from behind to identify popliteal swelling due to popliteal, or Baker's, cyst, which is most commonly a medial semimembranous bursal swelling. If the calves appear asymmetric, calf circumference should be measured and compared bilaterally. Popliteal cysts may rupture and dissect down into the calf muscles, producing enlargement and palpable fullness. Edema may be present if the cyst causes secondary venous or lymphatic obstruction. Acute rupture or dissection of a popliteal cyst can mimic thrombophlebitis, with local pain, heat, redness, and swelling. This cause of unilateral calf swelling is probably more common in patients with rheumatoid arthritis than in those with deep venous thrombosis. The two may not be distinguishable on physical examination alone.

In the supine position, inability to extend the knee fully may be related to a flexion contracture or a large synovial effusion. Suprapatellar swelling with fullness of the distal anterior thigh that obliterates the normally depressed contours along the side of the patella usually indicates a knee joint effusion or synovitis. Localized swelling over the surface of the patella is generally secondary to prepatellar bursitis.

Quadriceps femoris muscle atrophy often develops in chronic arthritis of the knee. Atrophy of the vastus medialis is the earliest change and may be appreciated by comparing the two thighs for medial asymmetry and circumference. The thigh circumference should be measured at 15 cm above the knee to avoid spurious results from suprapatellar effusions.

The knee should be palpated with the joint relaxed. The examination is usually best accomplished with the patient supine and the knees fully extended and not touching. Palpation should begin over the anterior thigh approximately 10 cm above the patella.

To identify the superior margin of the suprapatellar pouch, which is an extension of the knee joint cavity, the examiner should palpate the tissues by moving distally toward the knee. Swelling, warmth, thickness, nodules, loose bodies, and tenderness should be noted. A thickened synovial membrane has a boggy, doughy consistency that differs from the surrounding soft tissue and muscle. It is usually palpated earlier over the medial aspect of the suprapatellar pouch and medial tibiofemoral joint. To enhance detection of knee fluid, any fluid in the suprapatellar pouch is compressed with the palm of one hand placed just proximal to the patella. The synovial fluid forced into the inferior distal articular cavity is then palpated with the opposite thumb and index finger laterally and medially to the patella. If the examiner alternates compression and release of the suprapatellar pouch, the synovial thickening can be differentiated from a synovial effusion. An effusion intermittently distends the joint capsule under the thumb and index finger of the opposite hand, whereas synovial thickening does not. The examiner should not compress the suprapatellar pouch too firmly or push the tissues distally, because the patella or normal soft tissue, including the fat pads, will fill the palpated space and can be misinterpreted as synovitis or joint swelling. With a large effusion, the patella can be subjected to ballottement by pushing it posteriorly against the femur with the right forefinger while maintaining suprapatellar compression with the left hand.

At the other extreme, effusions as small as 4 to 8 ml can be detected by eliciting the bulge sign. This test is performed with the knee extended and relaxed. The examiner strokes or compresses the medial aspect of the knee proximally and laterally with the palm of one hand to move the fluid from the area. The lateral aspect of the knee is then tapped or stroked, and a fluid wave or bulge is noted to appear medially (Fig. 23–10). A so-called spontaneous bulge sign occurs if, on compression along the medial side of the joint space, fluid reaccumulates without any pressure or compression along the lateral side of the joint.

The medial and lateral tibiofemoral joint margins are palpated for tenderness and bony lipping or exostosis, as can be seen in degenerative joint disease. The joint margins can be palpated easily with the hip flexed to 45 degrees, the knee flexed to 90 degrees, and the foot resting on the examining table. Tenderness localized over the medial or lateral joint margin may represent articular cartilage disease, medial or lateral meniscal disease, or medial or lateral collateral ligament injury. Tenderness can also be caused by disease in the underlying bony structures.

Bursitis can be another cause of localized tenderness about the knee, and the two most common sites are the pes anserine and prepatellar bursae. Exquisite local tenderness can usually be elicited if a bursitis is present. Occasionally, mild swelling is also appreciated. The prepatellar bursa can become quite swollen. It is important not to mistakenly interpret this swelling as knee joint synovitis. Usually, the two can be

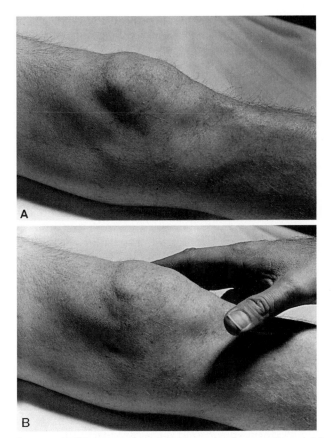

Figure 23–10. Demonstration of the bulge sign for a small synovial effusion in the knee. *A,* The synovial fluid is to be moved from the shaded, depressed area on the medial aspect of the knee. *B,* Bulge appears in previously shaded area after lateral aspect of the knee is tapped. (From Polley HF, Hunder GG: Rheumatologic Interviewing and Physical Examination of the Joints, 2nd ed. Philadelphia, WB Saunders, 1978.)

differentiated, in that the bursal margins can be outlined by palpation and other features of true joint effusion, such as the bulge sign, are absent.

Patellofemoral articulation abnormality is another common cause of knee pain.[7] It is more common in women because of the wider **Q** angle caused by the broader female pelvis. The **Q** angle is the angle formed between the quadriceps and the patellar tendon. Patients with patellofemoral disorder may experience stiffness in the knee after a period of flexion (the "moviegoer sign") or have particular difficulty when climbing stairs. Some patients have a sensation of catching as the patella moves over the distal femur.

The patella is best palpated with the knee extended and relaxed. The patella is compressed and moved so that its entire articular surface comes into contact with the underlying femur. Slight crepitation may be heard in many normally functioning knees. Pain with crepitation may suggest patellofemoral degenerative arthritis or chondromalacia patellae. Retropatellar pain occurring with active knee flexion and extension and secondary to patellofemoral disease may be differentiated from tibiofemoral articular pain. To test this, the

examiner should attempt to lift the patella away from the knee while passively moving the knee through range of motion. Painless motion during this maneuver indicates that the patellofemoral joint is the likely source.

Additionally, the *patellar grind test* is useful in patients with significant patellofemoral disease. During this test, the examiner compresses the patella distally away from the femoral condyles while instructing the patient to isometrically contract the quadriceps. Sudden patellar pain and quadriceps relaxation indicate a positive result. However, this test frequently has false-positive results.

Patellar stability should also be assessed. The *Fairbanks apprehension test* is done with the patient supine, the quadriceps relaxed, and the knee in 30 degrees of flexion. The examiner slowly pushes the patella laterally. A sudden contraction of the quadriceps and a distressed reaction from the patient indicate a positive apprehension test result. The result usually is positive in a patient who has had previous patellar dislocations. The patella can also be examined for subluxation while the knee is moved through a range of motion from full flexion to extension.

The *plica syndrome* also occasionally causes symptoms suggestive of patellofemoral disease.[8] Plicae are bands of synovial tissue, most often located on the medial side of the knee. If they are present, a tender band-like structure may be palpated parallel to the medial border of the patella. During flexion and extension, a palpable or audible snapping may be heard and the patient may experience symptoms of catching. Many plicae, however, are asymptomatic, and they are common enough to be considered a normal variant.

The normal knee range of motion should be from full extension (0 degrees) to full flexion (120 to 150 degrees). Some normal persons may be able to hyperextend to up to 15 degrees. Loss of full extension due to a flexion contracture often accompanies chronic arthritis of the knee. In advanced arthritis, such as that in some patients with rheumatoid arthritis, posterior subluxation of the tibia on the femur may be observed.

Ligamentous instability is tested by application of valgus and varus stress to the knee and by use of the *drawer test.* The knee should be extended and relaxed. The *abduction,* or *valgus, test* is performed by stabilizing the lower femur while placing a valgus stress on the knee by abducting the lower leg with the other hand placed proximal to the ankle. Separation of the medial joint line with the knee fully extended indicates a tear of the medial compartment ligaments and the posterior cruciate ligament. The test is then done with the knee in 30 degrees of flexion. If the result is negative at 0 degrees but positive at 30 degrees, the instability is caused by a tear of the medial compartment ligaments, with the posterior cruciate ligament remaining intact. The *adduction,* or *varus, test* is then performed with the knee extended and again at 30 degrees of flexion. Separation of the lateral joint line indicates a tear of the lateral compartment ligament, again either associated or not associated with a posterior cruciate ligament tear.

The degree of ligamentous laxity observed during testing can be graded on a scale of 1 to 3.[9] The joint surfaces separate 5 mm or less in mild (grade 1) instability, 5 to 10 mm in moderate (grade 2) instability, and more than 10 mm (grade 3) instability. In patients with trauma, opening of the joint space indicates ligamentous instability secondary to rupture or stretching of the ligaments. However, in chronic arthritis of the tibiofemoral compartment, apparent medial or lateral separation may be due to the "pseudolaxity" created by loss of cartilage and bone. If the ligaments are intact, the resulting degree of valgus or varus displacement with stressing is no greater than that in the normal knee.

The drawer test is performed with the hip flexed to 45 degrees and the knee to 90 degrees.[10, 11] To stabilize the knee, the examiner either sits on the foot while grasping the posterior calf with both hands or supports the lower leg between his or her lateral chest wall and forearm.

The *anterior drawer test* is performed by pulling the tibia forward. More than 6 mm of movement is abnormal and may indicate an anterior cruciate tear or laxity. However, anterior subluxation may represent more complex instability. Rotatory instability of the knee may also exist. A positive anterior drawer test result, in which the lateral tibial plateau subluxes forward while the medial stays in normal position, can indicate anterolateral rotatory instability. If both plateaus sublux, the middle third of the medial lateral capsular ligaments may be torn. If subluxation is not present with the tibia internally rotated, the posterior cruciate ligament is intact. A positive anterior drawer test result with the leg in external rotation signals a tear of the medial capsular ligament. The *Lachman test*, a modification of the anterior drawer sign, tests for one-plane anterior instability. At least six variations of this test have been described. In the original test, the patient lies supine with the tested knee between full extension and 30 degrees of flexion. The femur is stabilized by one hand of the examiner while the other hand pulls the proximal aspect of the tibia forward. A positive result is indicated by a "soft" feeling rather than a firm endpoint when the tibia moves forward on the femur. A positive Lachman result may indicate an anterior cruciate injury or disease in the posterior oblique ligament or arcuate popliteus complex.

The *posterior drawer test* may be done with the patient positioned similarly to that for the anterior drawer test, but the examiner pushes the tibia toward the patient. A positive test result suggests damage to the posterior cruciate ligament.

During the complete joint examination, tests for meniscal injury should also be done. Signs and symptoms suggestive of a meniscal tear include locking during joint extension, clicking or popping during motion, and localized tenderness along the medial or lateral joint line. For examination of the menisci, the medial and lateral joint line should be palpated with the lower leg internally rotated and the knee flexed to 90 degrees. Localized tenderness over the medial and lateral joint lines suggests involvement of the medial and lateral menisci, respectively.

McMurray's test evaluates for evidence of meniscal tear, especially in the posterior half of the menisci. The patient's knee is placed in full flexion, and the examiner places one hand over the knee with the fingers along the side of the knee over the joint line and the thumb along the other side. The other hand holds the leg at the ankle and is used to rotate the lower leg medially and apply varus stress. This test can be done repeatedly with the knee in gradually decreasing degrees of flexion. A palpable or audible snap suggests a tear of the medial meniscus. To test for a lateral meniscal injury, the examiner in a similar fashion can laterally rotate the tibia and apply valgus stress. A positive lateral test result may also indicate a tear of the popliteus tendon, which can accompany a lateral meniscal tear.

The *Apley grind test* also evaluates for a torn meniscus. With the patient lying prone and the knee flexed to 90 degrees, the examiner places downward compression on the foot while medially and then laterally rotating the tibia on the femur. Pain elicited during this maneuver suggests a meniscal tear. The examiner then performs the *distraction test* by placing his or her knee on the patient's posterior thigh to stabilize the leg while applying an upward distractive force on the foot. Pain from rotating the tibia suggests ligament damage. A simple hyperflexion test is also useful in screening for meniscal damage. If the examiner can hyperflex the knee to more than 135 degrees without eliciting pain, significant cartilaginous injury is not likely to be present. If pain occurs with hyperflexion, the patient is sometimes able to localize it medially or laterally, often at the site of the meniscal injury. Although helpful, however, none of these tests for meniscal injury is completely reliable when the result is verified by arthroscopy. Tenderness along the joint line is most sensitive but not as specific as manipulative tests, such as McMurray's test.[12]

Muscle strength testing includes testing flexion supplied by the hamstrings, that is, the biceps femoris, semitendinosus, and semimembranosus (L-5 to S-3), and extension supplied by the quadriceps femoris (L-2, L-3, and L-4). For best results, the patient is prone and attempts to flex the knee from 90 degrees to beyond. The ankle should be kept in neutral position or dorsiflexed to remove gastrocnemius action. With the leg externally rotated, the biceps femoris, which inserts on the fibula and lateral tibia, is primarily tested, whereas flexion with internal rotation tests the semitendinosus and semimembranosus muscles, which insert on the medial side of the tibia. Extension is tested with the patient sitting upright with the knee fully extended. The examiner stabilizes the thigh with downward pressure just proximal to the knee and places downward pressure at the ankle to test the knee extensors.

Ankle

The true ankle is a hinged joint, and movement is limited to plantar flexion and dorsiflexion. The joint is formed by the distal ends of the tibia and fibula and proximal aspect of the body of the talus. Inversion and eversion occur at the subtalar joint (see Chapter 31). The tibia forms the weight-bearing portion of the ankle joint, and the fibula articulates on the side of the tibia. The malleoli of the tibia and fibula extend downward beyond the weight-bearing part of the joint and articulate with the sides of the talus. The malleoli provide medial and lateral stability by enveloping the talus in a mortise-like fashion.

The articular capsule of the ankle is lax on the anterior and posterior aspects of the joint, allowing extension and flexion, but is tightly bound bilaterally by ligaments. The synovial membrane of the ankle on the inside of the capsule usually does not communicate with any other joints, bursae, or tendon sheaths.

The medial and lateral ligaments surrounding the ankle also contribute to medial and lateral stability of the joint. The deltoid ligament, the only ligament on the medial side of the ankle, is a triangle-shaped fibrous band that tends to resist eversion of the foot. It may be torn in eversion sprains of the ankles. The lateral ligaments of the foot consist of three distinct bands forming the posterior talofibular, the calcaneofibular, and the anterior talofibular ligaments. These

ligaments may be injured in inversion sprains of the ankle. All tendons crossing the ankle joint lie superficial to the articular capsule and are enclosed in synovial sheaths for part of their course across the ankle.

On the anterior aspect of the ankle, the tendons and synovial tendon sheaths of the tibialis anterior, extensor digitorum longus, peroneus tertius, and extensor hallucis longus overlie the articular capsule and synovial membrane.

On the medial side of the ankle posteriorly and inferiorly to the medial malleolus lie the flexor tendons and tendon sheaths of the tibialis posterior, digitorum longus, and flexor hallucis longus (Fig. 23–11). All three of these muscles plantar flex and supinate the foot. The tendon of the flexor hallucis longus is located more posteriorly than the other flexor tendons and lies beneath the Achilles tendon for part of its course. The calcaneus tendon (Achilles tendon), the common tendon of the gastrocnemius and soleus muscles, inserts into the posterior surface of the calcaneus, where it is subject to external trauma, various inflammatory reactions, and irritations from bony spurs beneath it.

On the lateral aspect of the ankle, posteriorly and inferiorly to the lateral malleolus, a synovial sheath encloses the tendons of the peroneus longus and peroneus brevis. These muscles extend (plantar flex) the ankle and evert (pronate) the foot. Each of the tendons adjacent to the ankle may be involved separately in traumatic or disease processes.

Three sets of fibrous bands, or retinacula, hold down the tendons that cross the ankle in their passage to the foot. The extensor retinaculum consists of a

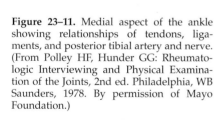

Figure 23–11. Medial aspect of the ankle showing relationships of tendons, ligaments, and posterior tibial artery and nerve. (From Polley HF, Hunder GG: Rheumatologic Interviewing and Physical Examination of the Joints, 2nd ed. Philadelphia, WB Saunders, 1978. By permission of Mayo Foundation.)

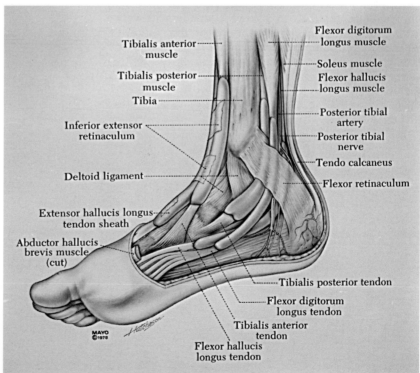

superior part (transverse crural ligament) in the anterior and inferior portions of the leg and an inferior part in the proximal portion of the dorsum of the foot. The flexor retinaculum is a thickened fibrous band on the medial side of the ankle. On the lateral side of the ankle, the peroneal retinaculum forms a superior and an inferior fibrous band. These bands bind down tendons of the peroneus longus and peroneus brevis as they cross the lateral aspect of the ankle.

Synovial swelling of the ankle joint is most likely to cause fullness over the anterior or anterolateral aspect of the joint, because the capsule is more lax in this area. Mild swelling of the joint may not be apparent on inspection because of the many structures crossing the joint superficially. Efforts should be made to differentiate between superficial linear swelling localized to the distribution of the tendon sheaths from more diffuse fullness and swelling due to involvement of the ankle joint. Similarly, synovitis of the intertarsal joints is difficult to observe. Intertarsal joint synovitis may produce an erythematous puffiness or fullness over the dorsum of the foot.

From the normal position of rest, in which there is a right angle between the leg and foot, labeled 0 degrees, the ankle normally allows about 20 degrees of dorsiflexion and about 45 degrees of plantar flexion. Inversion and eversion of the foot occur mainly at the subtalar and other intertarsal joints. From the normal position of the foot, the subtalar joint normally permits about 20 degrees of eversion and 30 degrees of inversion. To test the subtalar joint, the examiner grasps the calcaneus with one hand and attempts to invert and evert it, holding the ankle motionless.

A general assessment of muscular strength of the ankle can be obtained by asking the patient to walk on the toes and heels. If the patient can satisfactorily walk on both the toes and the heels, the muscle strength of the flexors and extensors of the ankle can be considered normal. However, many entities, including pain, can prevent the patient from satisfactorily doing this. In these instances, it is desirable to test muscles individually.

Prime movers in plantar flexion of the ankle are the gastrocnemius (S-1 and S-2) and the soleus (S-1 and S-2) muscles. The prime mover in dorsiflexion is the tibialis anterior muscle (L-4, L-5, and S-1). The tibialis posterior muscle (L-5 and S-1) is the prime mover in inversion. During testing of the tibialis posterior muscle, the patient's foot should be in plantar flexion. The examiner applies graded resistance on the medial border of the forefoot while the patient attempts to invert the foot. The prime movers in eversion of the foot are the peroneus longus (L-4, L-5, and S-1) and peroneus brevis (L-4, L-5, and S-1) muscles.

Foot

See Chapter 31.

References

1. Polley HF, Hunder GG: Rheumatologic Interviewing and Physical Examination of the Joints, 2nd ed. Philadelphia, WB Saunders, 1978.
2. Hoppenfeld S: Physical Examination of the Spine and Extremities. New York, Appleton-Century-Crofts, 1976.
3. Magee DJ: Orthopedic Physical Assessment, 2nd ed. Philadelphia, WB Saunders, 1992.
4. Ritchie DM, Boyle JA, McInnes JM, et al: Clinical studies with an articular index for the assessment of joint tenderness in patients with rheumatoid arthritis. Q J Med 37:393–406, 1968.
5. Lee P, Baxter A, Dick WC, et al: An assessment of grip strength measurement in rheumatoid arthritis. Scand J Rheumatol 3:17–23, 1974.
6. Boardman PL, Hart FD: Clinical measurement of the anti-inflammatory effects of salicylates in rheumatoid arthritis. Br Med J 4:264–268, 1967.
7. Carson WG Jr, James SL, Larson RL, et al: Patellofemoral disorders: Physical and radiographic evaluation: Part I. Physical examination. Clin Orthop 185:165–177, 1984.
8. Hardaker WT, Whipple TL, Bassett FH III: Diagnosis and treatment of the plica syndrome of the knee. J Bone Joint Surg Am 62:221–225, 1980.
9. Hughston JC, Andrews JR, Cross MJ, et al: Classification of the knee ligament instabilities. Part I. The medial compartment and cruciate ligaments. J Bone Joint Surg Am 58:159–172, 1976.
10. Katz JW, Fingeroth RJ: The diagnostic accuracy of ruptures of the anterior cruciate ligament comparing the Lachman test, the anterior drawer sign, and the pivot shift test in acute and chronic knee injuries. Am J Sports Med 14:88–91, 1986.
11. Jonsson T, Althoff B, Peterson L, et al: Clinical diagnosis of ruptures of the anterior cruciate ligament: A comparative study of the Lachman test and the anterior drawer sign. Am J Sports Med 10:100–102, 1982.
12. Anderson AF, Lipscomb AB: Clinical diagnosis of meniscal tears: Description of a new manipulative test. Am J Sports Med 14:291–293, 1986.

CHAPTER 24

W. Joseph McCune
Joseph Golbus

Monarticular Arthritis

With rare exceptions, any joint disorder is capable of presenting initially as monarthritis. Monarthritis therefore represents a diagnostic challenge to even the most experienced clinician. In fact, it often remains incompletely understood after initial evaluation. Nonetheless, it is almost always possible to identify patients who require vigorous evaluation and treatment to prevent rapid disease progression, such as those with suspected septic arthritis. One can then proceed in a measured and systematic manner with the remainder of patients, in whom the short-term clinical course and response to simple therapeutic measures may provide additional useful information. This chapter is intended to aid the clinician (1) in distinguishing true arthritis from syndromes that also present with pain in the surrounding joint structures, (2) in narrowing the list of diagnostic possibilities based on the clinical presentation, and (3) in effectively using diagnostic tests. Special attention is given to common entities that present as acute inflammatory arthritis suggesting joint sepsis.

DIFFERENTIAL DIAGNOSIS

Confronted with a patient complaining of pain or swelling in the region of a single joint, the physician must first attempt to localize the anatomic site of the abnormality. Joint pain can be the result of abnormalities in the joint itself, adjacent bone, surrounding ligaments, tendons, bursae, or soft tissues. It can also be referred, resulting from nerve root impingement or an entrapment neuropathy or even pathology in another joint. Pain from hip arthritis, for example, can be referred entirely or partially to the knee.

Arthritis involving a diarthrodial joint causes stiffness, reduced range of motion, and pain during normal use. With few exceptions (e.g., the patellofemoral joint in chondromalacia[1]) intra-articular abnormalities can be detected during both passive and active range of motion. The history and physical examination are extremely important in determining the cause of the arthritis. Inflammatory forms of arthritis are characterized by stiffness of the joint that is most noticeable in the morning (morning stiffness) or after a period of inactivity ("gelling") and that improves with motion. Inflammatory arthritis is often associated with systemic symptoms, such as fever or malaise. Joint pain due to mechanical factors usually worsens with activ-

ities, improves with rest, and is not associated with systemic symptoms.

On physical examination, it is important to compare the abnormalities (e.g., swelling, warmth, redness) with findings in the contralateral joint. Effusions almost always result from intra-articular pathology, although they may accompany osteomyelitis, fractures, or tumors.[2] The presence of excess synovial fluid does not specifically indicate joint inflammation unless the white blood cell count is elevated. The range of disorders causing monarthritis is listed in Table 24–1.

The conditions discussed in the following sections may be confused with arthritis (Table 24–2).

Internal Derangements (Particularly of the Knee or Shoulder)

Torn menisci or ligaments or loose bodies may episodically wedge into the joint, producing clicking, locking, or a "giving way." These conditions may precede or accompany degenerative arthritis and can also be a consequence of inflammatory arthritis when fronds of proliferative synovium become lodged within the joint. Symptoms are frequently intermittent. They can often be elicited on physical examination by repeatedly flexing and extending the joint in various degrees of internal and external rotation.[3]

Bone Pain

Pain in bone usually results from involvement by a disease process of either the periosteum or the marrow space, as the result of sensory nerves located in these areas. Bone pain is commonly caused by fractures, osteomyelitis, or periosteitis, such as occurs in pulmonary hypertrophic osteoarthropathy, hemoglobinopathies, hematologic malignancy,[4] primary or metastatic bone tumors, and occasionally in infiltrative processes such as Paget's disease. Characteristically, bone pain is accompanied by tenderness to pressure over involved periosteum or pain on weight bearing. When symptoms are longstanding, radiographs are typically abnormal. Paget's disease may be associated with both bone pain and arthritic symptoms as the result of expansion and deformity of subchondral bone and cartilage, particularly in the hips and knees.[5]

371

Table 24–1. DIFFERENTIAL DIAGNOSIS OF
MONARTICULAR ARTHRITIS

Usually Monarticular	Often Polyarticular
Common	
Septic arthritis	Rheumatoid arthritis
Bacterial	Osteoarthritis
Tuberculous	Psoriatic arthritis
Fungal	Reiter's syndrome (idiopathic
Lyme disease	and human immuno-
Crystal disease	deficiency virus)
Gout	Calcium pyrophosphate
Pseudogout	deposition disease
Internal derangement	Chronic articular hemorrhage
Ischemic necrosis	Most juvenile rheumatoid
Hemarthrosis	arthritis and juvenile
Coagulopathy	spondylitis
Warfarin (Coumadin)	Erythema nodosum/sarcoid
Trauma or overuse	Serum sickness
Pauciarticular juvenile	Acute hepatitis B
rheumatoid arthritis	Rubella
Neuropathic	Henoch-Schönlein purpura
Congenital hip dysplasia	Systemic lupus erythematosus
Osteochondritis dissecans	Lyme disease
Reflex sympathetic dystrophy	Parvovirus
Hydroxyapatite deposition	Dialysis arthropathy
Hemoglobinopathies	Other crystal-induced
Loose body	arthropathies
Palindromic rheumatism	
Paget's disease involving joint	
Stress fracture	
Osteomyelitis	
Osteogenic sarcoma	
Metastatic tumor	
Synovial osteochondromatosis	
Rare	
Pigmented villonodular	Undifferentiated connective
synovitis	tissue disease
Plant thorn synovitis	Relapsing polychondritis
Familial Mediterranean fever	Enteropathic disease
Synovioma	Ulcerative colitis
Synovial metastasis	Regional enteritis
Intermittent hydrarthrosis	Bypass arthritis
Pancreatic fat necrosis	Whipple's disease
Gaucher's disease	Chronic sarcoidosis
Behçet's disease	Hyperlipidemias types II
Regional migratory	and IV
osteoporosis	Still's disease
Giant cell arteritis or	Pyoderma gangrenosum
polymyalgia rheumatica	Pulmonary hypertrophic
Sea urchin spine	osteoarthropathy
Amyloidosis (myeloma)	Chondrocalcinosis-like
	syndromes due to
	ochronosis,
	hemochromatosis, Wilson's
	disease
	Rheumatic fever
	Paraneoplastic syndromes

Tendinitis or Bursitis

Findings of tendinitis or bursitis are usually localized to one area around the joint.[6] There is local tenderness and often pain that increases with active motion more than with passive motion of the joint. This is because active motion stresses the involved periarticular structures more than does passive motion. An exception to this rule is supraspinatus tendinitis of the shoulder, in which passive and active motion may produce similar pain, and there may be no localized tenderness. The clinical findings seen with tendinitis or bursitis can usually be reduced or eliminated by local instillation of lidocaine. The presence of a puncture site, a history of glucocorticoid injection, an adjacent source of infection such as an ulcerated rheumatoid nodule,[7] or severe inflammation may signify infectious bursitis.[8] Isolated tendinitis is less commonly due to hematogenous spread of infection except in disseminated gonococcal disease, which commonly presents with dorsal tenosynovitis of the wrists[9] or brucellosis.[10] Infected olecranon or prepatellar bursae commonly mimic septic arthritis.

Neuropathic Pain

Compression or irritation of peripheral nerves may produce pain referred to the region of joints, such as pain radiating from the wrist to the palmar surface of the first four digits in carpal tunnel syndrome,[11] pain in the hip region in lumbosacral radiculopathies, or shoulder pain with brachial plexopathies. Such symptoms are usually in the distribution of a peripheral nerve and tend to follow an irregular time course, with sudden exacerbations, particularly at night. Maneuvers that compress the affected nerve at the site of injury, such as straight leg raising or percussion of the median nerve at the wrist, are helpful when they exactly reproduce the patient's pain in the distribution of a peripheral nerve (see Chapter 39). Diffuse polyneuropathies may produce pain that is poorly localized and that superficially resembles joint pain in a stocking-glove distribution. Pain that localizes exactly to a joint in the setting of a polyneuropathy may be related to neuropathic joint disease or reflex sympathetic dystrophy, or may have an unrelated cause.[12]

Soft Tissue Infections

Soft tissue infections may simulate arthritis, particularly when they occur in the region of deeply buried joints that are difficult to examine. Hip pain may result from cellulitis, pyomyositis, psoas or retroperitoneal abscesses, or intrapelvic pathology, such as diverticulitis. Fever and the acute onset of hip pain and stiffness with normal radiographs and synovial fluid findings suggest soft tissue or bone infection. Pain referred to the sacroiliac joint may result from similar conditions and perirectal abscesses. Infectious processes in these locations present with unremitting severe pain, marked elevation of the erythrocyte sedimentation rate, and variably severe systemic toxicity.[13, 14] Physical examination may reveal muscular rigidity and guarding, local tenderness, increased girth of the affected limb, or draining sinuses. Im-

Table 24–2. REGIONAL PERIARTICULAR SYNDROMES

Region	Periarticular Syndrome	Monarticular Syndrome
Jaw	Temporomandibular joint dysfunction (myofascial pain syndrome)	Temporal arteritis Molar dental problems Parotid swelling Preauricular lymphadenitis
Shoulder	Subacromial bursitis Long-head bicipital tendinitis Rotator cuff tear	Pancoast tumor Brachial plexopathy Cervical nerve root injury
Elbow	Olecranon bursitis Epicondylitis	Ulnar nerve entrapment
Wrist	Extensor tendinitis (including deQuervain's tenosynovitis) Gonococcal tenosynovitis	Carpal tunnel syndrome
Hand	Palmar fasciitis (Dupuytren's contracture) Ligamentous or capsular injury	
Hip	Greater trochanteric bursitis Adductor syndrome Ischial bursitis Fascia lata syndrome	Meralgia paresthetica Deep infection Paget's disease Neoplasm
Knee	Anserine bursitis Prepatellar bursitis Meniscal injury Ligamentous tear-laxity Baker's cyst	Neoplasm Osteomyelitis
Ankle	Peroneal tendinitis Achilles tendinitis Retrocalcaneal bursitis Calcaneal fasciitis Sprain Erythema nodosum	Hypertrophic pulmonary osteoarthropathy Tarsal tunnel syndrome
Foot	Plantar fasciitis Pes planus ("fallen arches")	Morton's neuroma Vascular insufficiency Cellulitis

aging studies, such as radionuclide scanning, ultrasound, computed tomography (CT) or magnetic resonance imaging (MRI), may be essential in identifying deep infections.

Muscular Pain Syndromes (Myofascial Pain, Fibromyalgia)

Myofascial pain syndromes consist of local areas of tenderness in muscle (trigger points) that cause pain in characteristic regional zones. These can result in a variety of complaints, including headache; jaw, neck, or low back pain; and, occasionally, joint pain, particularly in the shoulder.

PATIENT HISTORY

Is the Arthritis Acute or Chronic?

Extremely rapid onset of pain (over seconds or minutes) suggests an internal derangement, fracture, trauma, or loose body. Acute onset over several hours to 2 days is typical of most forms of inflammatory arthritis, particularly bacterial infection and crystal-induced synovitis. When a careful history reveals longstanding symptoms in a joint, it is important to

distinguish exacerbations of preexisting disease (e.g., worsening of degenerative joint disease with excessive use) from a second superimposed process (e.g., infection).[15]

Is the Underlying Process Mechanical or Inflammatory?

The question of an inflammatory versus a mechanical process is most reliably answered by the synovial fluid white blood cell count (Table 24–3). Waxing and waning of disease activity unrelated to patterns of use, including fluctuations of pain and swelling, protracted morning stiffness, and gelling, suggest inflammation. Pain that occurs only after use, improves with rest, and involves weight-bearing joints, suggests mechanical disease.

Is the Arthritis Truly Monarticular?

Careful inquiry may elicit evidence of antecedent or coincident involvement of additional joints. A history of inflammatory symptoms in multiple joints for more than a month suggests a chronic, noninfectious inflammatory condition. Diffuse arthralgias of shorter duration may accompany the onset of many illnesses,

Table 24–3. SYNOVIAL FLUID AND ASSOCIATED LABORATORY FINDINGS IN MONARTICULAR ARTHRITIS

Synovial Fluid White Blood Cell Count	Predominant Cell	Appearance	Viscosity	Microorganisms	Crystals	RBC	Glucose	Protein	Complement	Cartilage Debris	Other
0–200											
Normal	M	Clear	↑	–	–	–	90%	1.5–2	–	–	Small amount not demonstrable on physical examination
0–2000											
Osteoarthritis	M	Clear	↑	–	+/– Occasional CPPD	–	–	–/↑	–	+	Radiographs positive in advanced disease; synovial fluid findings variable
Structural	M	Clear	↑	–	–	+/–	–	–/↑		+	MR scan, arthrogram, (knee) arthroscopy
Internal derangement						+/–					Marked radiographic changes
Neuropathic						+++/–					MR scan, CT scan
Osteochondritis dissecans							–				MR scan, bone scan, radiograph in advanced cases
Ischemic necrosis							–				Radiograph
Traumatic	RBC	Cloudy Bloody	↑	–	–	+++	–	↑/↑↑↑	–		
2000–10,000											
Pigmented villonodular synovitis	RBC	Brown Bloody	→	–	–	++	→	↑↑		–	Synovial biopsy
Amyloid	M	Slightly turbid		–	–						Congo red: synovial fluid Monoclonal gammopathy
Enteropathic arthritis	M/P	Slightly turbid		–	–	–					Positive stool occult blood LE cells
Systemic lupus erythematosus	M	Slightly turbid	↑	–	–	–			→		Serum autoantibodies

5000–50,000

Disease	Cells	Appearance			Crystals					Other tests
Juvenile rheumatoid arthritis	P	Slightly turbid	↓	—	—	—	—	↑/↑↑	−/↓	Synovial fluid leukocytes may be ≥100,000 Serum: + ANA (50%) + rheumatoid factor (<20%)
Sarcoidosis	P	Slightly turbid	↓	—	—	—	—			Chest radiographs, slit lamp examination
Reiter's syndrome	P	Slightly turbid	↓↓	—	—	—	↓	↑/↑↑	↑	Negative rheumatoid factor, ANA positive sign
Psoriatic arthritis	P	Slightly turbid	↓↓	—	—	—	↓			
Rheumatoid arthritis	P	Turbid	↓↓	—	—	—	↓↓	↑/↑↑↑		Serum (+) rheumatoid factor (50–80%) + ANA
Tuberculous arthritis	M	Turbid	↓↓	+/−	—	—	↓↓	↑↑/↑↑↑	→	PPD usually positive unless anergic Synovial biopsy essential

10,000–150,000

Disease	Cells	Appearance			Crystals					Other tests
CPPD pseudogout	P	Turbid	↑↓	−	CPPD (approximately 60%)	—	↓	↑	+/−	Repeated crystal examinations Radiographs: chondrocalcinosis
Gout	P	Turbid	↑	−	Monosodium urate (>90%)	—	↓	↑↑		Serum uric acid unreliable
Gonococcal infection	P	Turbid to pus	↓↓	+/−	—	—	↓↓	↑↑↑		Synovial fluid culture 20–50% positive Culture portals of entry Urogenital Gram stain
Nongonococcal bacteria	P	Turbid to pus	↓↓↓	+	—	—	↓↓	↑↑↑		Gram stain–gram-positive organisms Synovial fluid, blood cultures

Abbreviations: M, mononuclear; P, polynuclear; RBC, red blood cell; ANA, antinuclear antibodies; CPPD, calcium pyrophosphate dihydrate; LE, lupus erythematosus; MR, magnetic resonance; CT, computed tomography; PPD, purified protein derivative.

especially systemic infections. Truly migratory disease, in which there is only one inflamed joint but a clear-cut history of recent inflammatory arthritis of other joints occurring sequentially suggests gonococcal arthritis or rheumatic fever. Coexistence of symptoms in the axial skeleton may provide a clue to presence of a spondyloarthropathy.[15–17]

APPROACH TO THE PATIENT WITH ACUTE INFLAMMATORY MONARTHRITIS

The evaluation of an acute inflammatory monarthritis deserves special emphasis, because immediate benefit may result from identification and treatment of the underlying disease. In most cases, the physician must make a working diagnosis of infection, crystal-induced arthritis, or the onset of a potentially chronic inflammatory arthropathy. Each of these disorders is capable of presenting with an explosive onset of inflammation over a few hours, but the "hyperacute" presentation is most typical of infection or crystal disease. As a rule, the diagnosis of gout can be made immediately in almost all affected patients by aspirating joint fluid and examining it with use of polarizing microscopy. Calcium pyrophosphate crystals can sometimes be more difficult to identify. The diagnosis of pseudogout is often uncertain until repeated aspirations are performed and culture results are negative. The finding of chondrocalcinosis on radiography, however, can increase one's clinical suspicion. Infectious arthritis can be diagnosed by Gram stain in some patients and can be proved by culture in most within 48 hours. The presence of other conditions may be suggested by extra-articular disease features, but often laboratory testing and continued observation are needed before the diagnosis can be made with certainty. The following observations are intended to aid in the differential diagnosis of these entities.

Infectious Arthritis

In evaluating an acutely inflamed joint, one must first ask, Is the likelihood of septic arthritis sufficient to hospitalize the patient and intervene immediately? Joint sepsis produces dramatic inflammation followed quickly by irreversible destruction of cartilage and bone (see Chapter 90). It may also be the initial sign of a life-threatening systemic infection. In healthy adults, the signs are usually obvious. The patient complains of intense local pain and may resist attempts to examine the affected joint. Infected peripheral joints are swollen, warm, very tender, and sometimes red, and they have markedly restricted range of motion. As a general rule, large joints are more frequently affected than small ones in the absence of local trauma or peripheral vascular disease.[8] Unfortunately, persons at highest risk for joint sepsis are those in whom confounding factors obscure symptoms or

blunt the inflammatory response. Infection should be strongly suspected in less acutely sick-appearing patients when both systemic risk factors—such as corticosteroid therapy, immunodeficiency or immunosuppression, diabetes, intravenous drug abuse, or a remote focus of infection (e.g., pulmonary, cardiac, or genitourinary)—*and* local pathology—such as inflammatory arthritis, effusions, penetrating trauma, previous injection of corticosteroids, or a prosthetic joint—are present.

Although the clinical picture is never diagnostic of a particular infectious agent, certain presentations are characteristic: *Gonococcal infection* rarely escapes attention, since it tends to present as an inordinately painful monarthritis or polyarthritis, or as a painful, diffuse tenosynovitis in an otherwise healthy individual.[18] Skin lesions ranging from macules to pustules and vesicles are well described[14, 19] but are usually subtle and most easily identified in retrospect when they disappear during treatment. *Meningococcal arthritis* occasionally presents with clinical and Gram stain findings identical to those of gonococcal disease.

The large increase in intravenous drug abuse in the past few decades has resulted in a dramatic increase in associated *septic arthritis* through the introduction of infectious material into the intravascular space with subsequent hematogenous spread to the joints. Under unusual conditions, direct inoculation can also occur. These infections are most commonly due to *Staphylococcus aureus* and gram-negative organisms, especially *Pseudomonas*. They commonly occur in unusual locations compared with septic arthritis in other populations. There is a marked predilection for infections in the fibrocartilaginous joints of the skeleton.

Lyme arthritis presents as a true inflammatory arthritis weeks to months after initial exposure and after the development of the early syndrome of fevers, arthralgias, lymphadenopathy, and rash. This curable infection should be suspected in patients with compatible symptoms, a history of travel to endemic areas, or coexistent neurologic or cardiac abnormalities. If infection is suspected, serum antibodies to *Borrelia burgdorferi* should be obtained.

Viral illnesses, including hepatitis B, infectious mononucleosis, parvovirus, rubella, and rubella vaccination, rarely present as monarticular synovitis.

A number of arthritic syndromes that closely mimic known rheumatic diseases have now been described in association with human immunodeficiency virus (HIV) infection.[20] Most of these are polyarticular and present as arthralgias rather than true arthritis. Opportunistic infections in individuals infected with human immunodeficiency virus (HIV) can develop both within one joint and in contiguous bone. In addition to the more typical organisms, such as *S. aureus*, other less common microorganisms have been cultured from fluids of septic joints in patients with HIV infection, including *Sporothrix schenkii, Cryptococcus neoformans,* several *Salmonella* species, *Ureaplasma urealyticum,* and *Campylobacter fetus* (see Chapter 77).

Crystal-Induced Arthritis

Crystal-induced arthritis commonly presents as acute monarticular arthritis. It is particularly likely when there is a history of recurrent, self-limited attacks of inflammation of the same joint. Fortunately, the most fulminant arthropathy, gout, is also the most easily and reliably diagnosed: monosodium urate crystals can be identified in at least 95 percent of acute joint effusions by polarized microscopy, and even in some asymptomatic joints.[21] Calcium pyrophosphate crystals, on the other hand, are often not identified initially in patients who are later diagnosed as having pseudogout.[22] Hydroxyapatite crystals present a particular problem in diagnosis, since they are reliably identified only by electron microscopy or alizarin red stain.[23] Occasionally, in patients with renal failure and an acute monarthritis, calcium oxalate crystals can be identified in joint fluid aspirates. As a general rule, identification of crystals in joint fluid does not prove the absence of coexistent infection. Crystal-induced arthropathies are particularly common and difficult to manage in patients who are uremic or undergoing dialysis.

Gouty arthritis is said to be definitely present when intracellular non-birefringent, needle-shaped (sodium urate) crystals are identified in synovial fluid, and to be probably present if the crystals are extracellular. The most characteristic clinical features are extremely rapid onset of severe pain and inflammation with extension of the inflammatory process into the surrounding tissues, producing the appearance of cellulitis. Desquamation of overlying skin may occur as the attack subsides. In the ankle, the initial phases visually resemble the periarthritis of erythema nodosum, but the pain is much more severe.[24]

Podagra is characteristic but not pathognomonic of gout,[25] and first attacks of gout can occur in other large joints or in the small joints of the upper extremities (see Chapter 80).

Calcium pyrophosphate dihydrate deposition is associated with acute or chronic inflammatory arthritis and may be superimposed on osteoarthritis.[22] Pseudogout can be diagnosed by the finding of weakly positive, rhomboid-shaped birefringent crystals in the white blood cells of synovial fluid aspirates (see Chapter 81). One can also be suspicious of the diagnosis in an elderly person with an acute monarthritis of the knee or wrist and chondrocalcinosis on x-ray, in whom there are no obvious reasons to suspect infection.

Other Causes of Acute Inflammatory Arthritis

Patients Who Do Not Appear Toxic

If a patient does not have one of the foregoing disorders, there is a significant likelihood that the cause will remain elusive for a time and that the physician will be obliged to make a practical decision about how aggressively to pursue a diagnosis. The initial work-up under these circumstances should be as focused as possible so that a satisfactory result can be achieved with the greatest possible economy of patient discomfort and medical resources.

Juvenile Rheumatoid Arthritis. Although most children with juvenile rheumatoid arthritis presenting with monarticular disease eventually experience involvement of additional joints, about 25 percent have isolated monarthritis that may recur intermittently into adulthood. Antinuclear antibodies are more frequent than is rheumatoid factor; both monarticular disease and antinuclear antibodies correlate with the development of iritis.[26]

Rheumatoid Arthritis. This may present with acute or insidious onset of monarthritis. A detailed history often reveals gradual onset of fatigue or arthralgias. Physical examination may reveal unsuspected involvement of other joints, particularly the metatarsophalangeal joints.

Palindromic Rheumatism Versus Early Rheumatoid Arthritis. Episodic inflammation with total resolution of symptoms is often a prelude to rheumatoid arthritis,[27] particularly in patients who are rheumatoid factor–positive.

Seronegative Spondyloarthropathies. These were mentioned previously in the context of monarthritis accompanied by axial skeleton stiffness or pain.

Neuropathic Arthropathy (Charcot Joints). Neuropathic arthropathy should be suspected in patients with diabetes who present with a subacute or chronic monarthritis of the ankle or foot, usually with swelling and effusion, but with little pain. The arthritis develops most commonly in those with peripheral neuropathy and sensory loss. The radiographic picture is usually pathognomonic.

Hemarthroses. These may result from trauma, synovial hemangiomas, excessive anticoagulation, or inherited coagulopathies.

Patients Who Show Significant Signs of Systemic Illness

Enteropathic Arthritis. Whipple's disease, which is quite rare, can present with a monarticular arthritis when the bowel disease is not evident. Regional enteritis and ulcerative colitis are more likely to be symptomatic when arthritis develops[28] (see Chapter 62).

Systemic Autoimmune Disease. Systemic lupus erythematosus occasionally presents with monarticular arthritis, although polyarthritis is more common. Monarticular or large joint pain in a steroid-treated lupus patient suggests avascular necrosis[29] or infection. Sarcoidosis often presents as arthritis of the ankles, wrists, or knees, usually bilateral, which may be associated with erythema nodosum or hilar adenopathy.[30] Henoch-Schönlein purpura,[31] Takayasu's disease,[32] overlap syndromes,[33] polymyalgia rheumatica,[34] and giant cell arteritis[35] can all present with monarticular or polyarticular arthritis, although polyarthritis is the rule in many of these disorders.

Familial Mediterranean fever typically causes exquisitely painful monarthritis with moderately impressive physical findings.[36, 37] The combination of fever and an evanescent rash suggests Still's disease[38] or rheumatic fever.[39]

CHRONIC INFLAMMATORY MONARTICULAR ARTHRITIS

Many disorders that can present as acute monarticular inflammation progress to polyarticular involvement, remit, and relapse, or spontaneously resolve. Persistent monarticular inflammation raises special concern that a more narrow spectrum of disorders is present, particularly chronic infections or tumors. Synovial biopsy and arthroscopy may be useful in identifying the cause of chronic monarthritis (see Chapter 36).

Chronic infections result from slow-growing organisms or the presence of foreign bodies in the joint. Typically there are persistent signs of inflammation, including stiffness, pain, and warmth, and characteristically there is synovial thickening regardless of whether an effusion is present.

Tuberculosis, which is undergoing a resurgence in the United States, almost always affects a single diarthrodial joint[40] (see Chapter 91). A positive tuberculin test may be the only clue. Infection with atypical mycobacteria or *Candida,* coccidioidomycosis, or blastomycosis can produce similar syndromes.

Chronic infections may also result from penetrating wounds or the introduction of foreign bodies. Superficially located joints on the hands and the feet are most likely to be penetrated during normal activity, often without awareness on the part of the individual. Sporotrichosis should be suspected in a gardener with involvement of a hand joint, especially if there is surrounding soft tissue reaction.[41]

Tumors should always be suspected when there is chronic monarticular inflammation, particularly pigmented villonodular synovitis.[42] Metastasis to synovium from solid tumors or joint involvement by hematologic malignancies is rare. Tumors involving periarticular structures can mimic arthritis.

NONINFLAMMATORY MONARTICULAR ARTHRITIS

Structural joint disease *should be suspected* when there is little synovial inflammation in proportion to the degree of destruction of bone and cartilage, and the synovial fluid white blood cell count is less than 2000 cells/mm³. Truly noninflammatory fluid, however, contains less than 200 cells/mm³. An internal derangement of the knee is suggested by a history of trauma, episodes of joint locking or "giving way," and tenderness at the joint margin. It may be confirmed by MRI or arthroscopy, which demonstrates meniscal or ligamentous tears.

Osteoarthritis frequently presents as monarthritis, particularly in the knee, hip, acromioclavicular joint, first radiocarpal joint, or first metatarsophalangeal joint (hallux rigidus). Elderly patients with osteoarthritis may have inflammatory joint effusions that contain calcium pyrophosphate crystals.[25] In monarticular disease, a predisposing factor—such as congenital dysplasia of the hip, trauma to or prior surgical removal of ligaments or fibrocartilage from the knee, prior inflammatory arthritis or infections, occupational stress, or extreme obesity—should be sought.

Hip symptoms in a young patient suggest *congenital dysplasia of the hip* or a *slipped capital femoral epiphysis.*[43, 44] Spontaneous osteonecrosis may occur in the hip (Legg-Calvé-Perthes disease), metatarsal bones (Freiberg's disease), capitellum of the humerus, or carpal lunate. Osteochondritis dissecans should be suspected in a child or teenager who, after minor trauma, has relatively severe knee pain followed by mechanical dysfunction.[45]

Rapid development of "osteoarthritis" should lead to consideration of the possibility of a fracture related to osteopenia, an adjacent destructive process such as metastatic tumor, or avascular necrosis.

Osteonecrosis is a common cause of monarthritis of the hip, shoulders, and knees in young people with systemic diseases who require corticosteroid therapy. It also occurs in a variety of other conditions, such as alcoholism, barotrauma, hemoglobinopathies, diabetes, hyperlipidemia, hyperuricemia, and systemic lupus erythematosus.

DIAGNOSTIC STUDIES

Synovial Fluid Analysis

The primary purpose of synovial fluid analysis is to answer the following questions:

* Is the effusion inflammatory?
* Is it infected?
* Does it contain intracellular or extracellular crystals?

Even a few drops of fluid can be sufficient to obtain a white blood cell count and differential count, crystal analysis, and culture. No other tests are needed (see Chapter 41).

Cultures

If septic arthritis is a possibility, blood, synovial fluid, and urine cultures are indicated. As mentioned, gonococcal cultures are indicated in almost all patients: Cervicourethral, rectal, and pharyngeal cultures should be placed on Thayer-Martin medium. Cultures from normally sterile sites, including the synovial cavity, tenosynovial space, and intracutaneous lesions, should be placed on chocolate agar without added preservative. Occasionally, cultures of synovium yield bacteria, although other synovial fluid cultures are sterile (see Chapter 90).

Radiography

Plain radiographs of the affected and contralateral joints should almost always be obtained in patients with symptoms of more than several weeks' duration. They may also be helpful in patients with an acute arthritis in whom infection or crystal disease is suspected. In those with no prior joint complaints, frequent findings are soft tissue calcification and evidence of intra-articular pathology not known to the patient, such as osteoarthritis, chondrocalcinosis, or loose bodies. Occasionally, an unsuspected bony lesion (e.g., a fracture) or evidence of osseous or hematologic malignancy, osteomyelitis, or Paget's disease may be detected. Care should be taken to include enough surrounding bone in the radiograph to identify such lesions.

Nuclear Medicine

Radionuclide scans are useful primarily because of their sensitivity. They are used when it is important to search for a site of infection that cannot be detected or localized by other means, such as in deeply buried joints that are difficult to examine, fibrocartilaginous joints in which range of motion is poorly tested, and the spine (see Chapter 42).

Magnetic Resonance Imaging

Magnetic resonance has been shown to be superior to other imaging modalities in the diagnosis of ischemic necrosis of bone[46] and possibly Legg-Calvé-Perthes disease,[47] particularly in early cases. In the knee, MRI provides a more accurate and noninvasive alternative to arthrography for detection of meniscal and cruciate ligament injuries.[48, 49] Because of its superior definition of soft tissue pathology, it is useful in investigating deep infections about the hip, such as psoas abscesses, which may mimic arthritis.[50] Although superior in most cases to CT in detecting subchondral bone and marrow involvement by tumor or osteomyelitis, it does not provide the ability to survey the entire body that is characteristic of radionuclide scans.

Synovial and Bone Biopsy

Synovial biopsy may play a role in the diagnosis of chronic unexplained monarticular arthritis.[51] Tuberculous or fungal synovitis is more frequently identified by staining and culture of open biopsy material than by similar studies of synovial fluid. Closed needle biopsy or arthroscopic biopsy of the knee is preferable to open biopsy because of reduced morbidity. In acute inflammatory arthritis, a surgical biopsy is indicated in the diagnosis of infection of fibrocartilaginous joints, such as the sacroiliac and sternoclavicular joints, and probably the symphysis pubis if an initial attempt at aspiration is not diagnostic.[52] General anesthesia is often required for pain control. If osteomyelitis is suspected, one should consider obtaining a bone biopsy specimen before initiating antibiotic therapy.

References

1. Radin EL: Chondromalacia of the patella. Bull Rheum Dis 34:1, 1984.
2. Lagier R: Synovial reaction caused by adjacent malignant tumors: Anatomicopathological study of three cases. J Rheumatol 4:65, 1977.
3. Feagin JA Jr: The office diagnosis and documentation of common knee problems. Clin Sports Med 8:453, 1989.
4. Isenberg DA, Schoenfield Y: The rheumatologic complications of hematologic disorders. Semin Arthritis Rheum 12:348, 1983.
5. Altman RD: Paget's disease of bone (osteitis deformans). Bull Rheum Dis 34:1, 1984.
6. Larsson LG, Baum J: The syndromes of bursitis. Bull Rheum Dis 34:1, 1984.
7. Viggiano DA, Garrett JC, Clayton ML: Septic arthritis presenting as olecranon bursitis in patients with rheumatoid arthritis. J Bone Joint Surg 62A:1011, 1980.
8. Ho G Jr, Su EY: Antibiotic therapy of septic bursitis. Arthritis Rheum 24:905, 1981.
9. McCord WC, Nies KM, Louie JS: Acute venereal arthritis. Arch Intern Med 137:858, 1977.
10. Gotuzzo E, Alarcon GS, Bocangera TS, Carrillio C, Guerra JC, Rolands I, Espinoza LR: Articular involvement in human brucellosis: A retrospective analysis of 304 cases. Semin Arthritis Rheum 12:245, 1982.
11. Dorwart BB: Carpal tunnel syndrome: A review. Semin Arthritis Rheum 14:134, 1984.
12. Putten J: Neurological Differential Diagnosis. New York, Springer-Verlag, 1980.
13. Gibson RK, Rosenthal SJ, Lukert BP: Pyomyositis. Am J Med 11:421, 1982.
14. Kallen PS, Louie JS, Nies KM, Bayer AS: Infectious myositis and related syndromes. Am J Med 11:421, 1982.
15. Goldenberg DL: Infectious arthritis complicating rheumatoid arthritis and other chronic rheumatic disorders. Arthritis Rheum 32:496, 1989.
16. Resnick D, Niwayana G: Reiter's disease. In Diagnosis of Bone and Joint Disorders, 2nd ed. Philadelphia, WB Saunders, 1988.
17. Resnick D, Niwayana G: Psoriatic arthritis. In Diagnosis of Bone and Joint Disorders, 2nd ed. Philadelphia, WB Saunders, 1988, pp 1218–1251.
18. Seifert MH, Warin AP, Miller A: Articular and cutaneous manifestations of gonorrhea: Review of sixteen cases. Ann Rheum Dis 33:140, 1974.
19. Goldenberg DL, Reed JI: Bacterial arthritis. N Engl J Med 312:764, 1985.
20. Rynes RI, Goldenberg DL, DiGiacomo R, et al: Acquired-immunodeficiency syndrome–associated arthritis. Am J Med 84:810–816, 1988.
21. Bomalaski JS, Lluberas G, Schumacher HR Jr: Monosodium urate crystals in the knee joint of patients with asymptomatic nontophaceous gout. Arthritis Rheum 29:1480, 1986.
22. Masuda I, Ishikawa K: Clinical features of pseudogout attack: A review of fifty cases. Clin Orthop Rel Res 229:123, 1988.
23. Gatter RA: A Practical Handbook of Joint Fluid Analysis. Philadelphia, Lea & Febiger, 1984.
24. Yu T: Diversity of clinical features in gouty arthritis. Semin Arthritis Rheum 13:360, 1984.
25. McCarty DJ: Calcium pyrophosphate dihydrate crystal deposition disease—1975. Arthritis Rheum 19:275, 1976.
26. Chylack LT Jr: The ocular manifestations of juvenile rheumatoid arthritis. Arthritis Rheum 20(Suppl):224, 1976.
27. Schumacher HR: Palindromic onset of rheumatoid arthritis. Arthritis Rheum 25:361, 1982.
28. Weiner SR, Utsinger P: Whipple disease. Semin Arthritis Rheum 15:157, 1986.
29. Zizic TM, Hungerford DS, Stevens MB: Ischemic bone necrosis in systemic lupus erythematosus. Medicine 59:134, 1980.
30. Spilberg I, Siltzbach LE, McEwen C: The arthritis of sarcoidosis. Arthritis Rheum 12:126, 1969.
31. Cream JJ, Gumpel JM, Peachey RDG: Schönlein-Henoch purpura in the adult. QJ Med 39:461, 1970.
32. Hall S, Barr W, Lie JT, Stanson AW, Kazmier FJ, Hunder GG: Takayasu arthritis. Medicine 64:89, 1985.
33. Bennett RM, O'Connell DJ: Mixed connective tissue disease: A clinicopathologic study of 20 cases. Semin Arthritis Rheum 10:25, 1980.

34. Healey L: Long-term follow-up of polymyalgia rheumatica: Evidence for synovitis. Semin Arthritis Rheum 23:322, 1984.
35. Ginsberg WW, Cohen MD, Hall SB, Vollertsen RS, Hunder GG: Seronegative polyarthritis in giant cell arthritis. Arthritis Rheum 28:1362, 1985.
36. Meyerhoff J: Familial Mediterranean fever: Report of a large family, review of the literature, and discussion of the frequency of amyloidosis. Medicine 59:66, 1980.
37. Sohar E, Pras M, Gafni J: Familial Mediterranean fever and its articular manifestations. Clin Rheum Dis 1:195, 1975.
38. Larson EB: Adult Still's disease. Medicine 63:82, 1984.
39. Ben-Dov I, Berry E: Acute rheumatic fever in adults over the age of 45 years: An analysis of 23 patients together with a review of the literature. Semin Arthritis Rheum 10:100, 1980.
40. Nathanson L, Cohen W: A statistical and roentgen analysis of two hundred cases of bone and joint tuberculosis. Radiology 36:550, 1940.
41. Wilson DE, Mann JJ, Bennett JE, Utz P: Clinical features of extracutaneous sporotrichosis. Medicine 63:25, 1984.
42. Docken WP: Pigmented villonodular synovitis. Semin Arthritis Rheum 9:1, 1979.
43. Wilson PD, Jacobs B, Schecter L: Slipped capital femoral epiphysis. J Bone Joint Surg 14:549, 1967.
44. Ponseti IV, McClintock R: The pathology of slipping of the upper femoral epiphysis. J Bone Joint Surg 38A:71, 1956.
45. Pappas AM: The osteochondroses. Pediatr Clin North Am 14:549, 1967.
46. Thickman D, Axel L, Kresel HY, Steinberg M, Chen H, Velchick M, Fallon M, Dalinka M: Magnetic resonance imaging of avascular necrosis of the femoral head. Skeletal Radiol 15:133, 1986.
47. Scoles TV, Yoon YS, Makley JT, Kalamchi A: Nuclear magnetic resonance imaging in Legg-Calvé-Perthes disease. J Bone Joint Surg 66:1357, 1984.
48. Turner DA, Prodromos CC, Petasnick JP, Clark JW: Acute injury of the ligaments of the knee: Magnetic resonance evaluation. Radiology 154:717, 1985.
49. Reicher MA, Hartzman S, Duckwiler GR, Bassett LW, Anderson LJ, Gold RH: Meniscal injuries: Detection using MR imaging. Radiology 159:753, 1986.
50. Weintraub JC, Cohen JM, Maravilla KR: Iliopsoas muscles: MR study of normal anatomy and disease. Radiology 156:435, 1985.
51. Schumacher HR: Joint pathology in infectious arthritis. Clin Rheum Dis 4:33, 1978.
52. Gordon G, Kabins SA: Pyogenic sacroiliitis. Am J Med 69:50, 1980.

CHAPTER 25

John S. Sergent

Approach to the Patient with Pain in More Than One Joint

The approach to patients with polyarticular pain is not fundamentally different from the approach to patients with any other medical problem. With a careful history, a good physical examination, and appropriate laboratory tests and radiographs, a physician can establish the diagnosis and begin appropriate therapy in almost all cases.

Chronic pain in and around multiple joints is the most common symptom complex resulting in referral to a rheumatologist for consultation, amounting to 58 percent in a personal series. This is in accord with the experience of others.[1]

The evaluation of chronic polyarthritis is not only the most common intellectual exercise facing the rheumatologist but also one of the most rewarding. In most of the conditions to be discussed, it is the skilled, experienced physician, using the "tools" of history and physical examination, who can formulate a correct diagnosis and treatment plan. Although radiographs and certain laboratory tests are helpful, they should be used primarily as adjuncts.[2] This chapter presents a logical methodology for dealing with patients who present with chronic polyarticular pain.

HISTORY, PHYSICAL EXAMINATION, AND LABORATORY TESTS

History

As Mackenzie and others have pointed out, the clinical history is "by far the most important diagnostic tool"[3] in the evaluation of polyarticular disorders. A number of items deserve special attention.

Onset. One should direct attention early to the nature of the first symptoms. This is not always easy, especially if months or years have passed, because most patients prefer to talk about their current symptoms. It is also difficult because most patients think of arthritis as a disease, rather than a symptom or finding, and in their histories they may discuss all the joint problems of a lifetime, even obviously traumatic ones.

Course. The physician must determine what has occurred since the onset of symptoms and at what rate. Chronic arthritis may be relentlessly progressive from the onset, or it may be intermittent, with periods of partial or complete remission. In addition, as individual joints become involved, the process may be either "migratory" or "additive." The term *migratory polyarthritis* implies that previously involved joints become asymptomatic as new joints become inflamed; that is, the disease appears to migrate from joint to joint.

Specific Joint Symptoms. These features include locking, giving way without warning, palpable or audible crepitation, warmth, and swelling.

Systemic Symptoms. Patients who seek a physician's help because of joint pain often do not perceive, unless asked, relationships between joint pain and other complaints, such as fever, night sweats, weight loss, and generalized muscle stiffness. History of these symptoms should be sought specifically and, when possible, quantified.

Rheumatic Disease Systems Review. In addition to systemic symptoms, patients with arthritis must be asked specifically about conditions associated with various forms of arthritis, including rash (photosensitive, psoriatic, purpuric, or petechial), areas of alopecia, Raynaud's phenomenon, sicca syndrome, uveitis, scleritis, oral and genital ulcers, urethritis or cervicitis, symptoms of inflammatory bowel disease, and pleuropericardial symptoms.

Patient History. Previous diagnoses are not always correct. Therefore, a childhood history of rheumatic fever, for example, needs to be explored, since a number of children who have been labeled as having rheumatic fever in fact had Still's disease or another form of juvenile chronic polyarthritis; the reverse is also true. Special importance should be given to events of the immediate weeks or months preceding the onset of joint disease, including sore throats, febrile illnesses, venereal disease, sexual contacts, diarrhea, rashes, and uveitis.

Family History. In addition to asking about any type of arthritis, one should inquire about a family history of any associated condition, such as psoriasis, uveitis, or inflammatory bowel disease. In patients suspected of having ankylosing spondylitis, it is important to obtain the history of any family members with chronic back pain and then to attempt to determine the nature of that condition.

Physical Examination

A complete physical examination is essential. Special consideration must be given to searching for such

Table 25–1. LABORATORY TESTS IN POLYARTHRITIS

Test	Significance	
	Positive	*Negative*
Rheumatoid factor	Helpful in young persons, in whom background positivity is low	Prognostic significance only, not helpful in individual cases
Antinuclear antibody	High titer, suggestive of a rheumatic disease	Virtually rules out active systemic lupus
Uric acid	Elevated levels, indicating that gout is possible	If repeated levels are normal, gout unlikely
Antistreptolysin O	Recent streptococcal exposure	Rheumatic fever unlikely
HLA-B27	Possibly marginally useful in early-onset ankylosing spondylitis	No benefit
Anti-*Borrelia*	Only helpful if pretest probability is high	Chronic Lyme disease unlikely

features as small patches of psoriasis, psoriatic nails, oral and genital ulcers, funduscopic changes, murmurs, rubs, bruits, peripheral pulses. A careful neurologic examination is also warranted.

The details of a complete musculoskeletal examination are reviewed in Chapter 23. Each joint should be examined for warmth, synovial thickening, effusions, crepitation, deformity, and tenderness. Both active and passive range of motion should be tested. The spinal examination should include the range of motion of the cervical and lumbar regions, chest expansion, tenderness of the spinous processes and sacroiliac joints, abnormal curves, and muscle spasm.

Laboratory Tests

Nonspecific tests of inflammation include hematocrit, erythrocyte sedimentation rate, C-reactive protein, and white blood cell count. Tests sometimes helpful in specific diseases are shown in Table 25–1. They must be ordered wisely because the background false-positive rate can be quite high.

If obtainable, synovial fluid should be examined as described in Chapter 41. The primary benefit of synovial fluid examination is to differentiate among osteoarthritis, inflammatory arthritis, and infection. Rarely are tests indicated other than appearance, total white blood cell count and differential, crystal examination, and culture.

Radiographic Features

Important radiographic features that may help in patient evaluation include cartilage loss, erosions, periarticular osteoporosis, osteophytes, periostitis, and soft tissue changes. In many cases, properly chosen radiographs are virtually diagnostic or eliminate certain diseases from further consideration.

APPROACH TO THE PATIENT WITH POLYARTHRITIS

Once other causes of joint pain (see later) have been eliminated and the clinician is confident that polyarthritis is present, a logical, stepwise approach can lead to the correct diagnosis in nearly all cases (Table 25–2). The first problem is usually to determine whether the arthritis is inflammatory.

Historical features that support an inflammatory process include prolonged and severe morning stiffness, fever, weight loss, and spontaneous joint swelling. Physical examination often reveals local warmth and synovial thickening as well as frank effusions. Laboratory findings of inflammation include anemia, an elevated sedimentation rate or C-reactive protein level, and thrombocytosis.

Table 25–2 shows a classification of polyarthritis

Table 25–2. CLASSIFICATION OF POLYARTHRITIS

Inflammatory
Peripheral polyarticular
   Rheumatoid arthritis
   Systemic lupus erythematosus
   Viral arthritis
   Psoriatic arthritis (occasionally)
Peripheral pauciarticular
   Psoriatic arthritis
   Reiter's syndrome
   Rheumatic fever
   Polyarticular gout
   Enteropathic arthritis
   Behçet's disease
   Bacterial endocarditis
Peripheral with axial involvement
   Ankylosing spondylitis (especially juvenile onset)
   Reiter's syndrome
   Enteropathic arthritis
   Psoriatic arthritis

Noninflammatory (Osteoarthritis)
Hereditary
   Osteoarthritis of the hands
   Primary generalized osteoarthritis
Traumatic osteoarthritis
   Osteoarthritis following local injury
   Osteoarthritis of the knees in obese people
   Chondromalacia following aggressive exercise programs
   Osteoarthritis in the elderly
Metabolic diseases (may have an unusual pattern)
   Hemochromatosis
   Ochronosis
   Acromegaly
Idiopathic

that is based on two features: the presence or absence of inflammation and the number and pattern of joint involvement.

Polyarticular Peripheral Arthritis

Rheumatoid Arthritis. This condition, of course, is the prototype of this group of diseases (see Chapter 44). Rheumatoid arthritis accounts for about one fourth of all patients referred to rheumatologists.[1]

Typically beginning in multiple small joints of the hands and feet in a symmetric fashion, rheumatoid arthritis has many variations, even including months or years of recurrent monarthritis (palindromic rheumatism)[4] before a typical pattern evolves. The symmetry of rheumatoid arthritis is sometimes overemphasized, and it must be appreciated that this is a general, rough symmetry. It is rare for rheumatoid arthritis to cause extensive damage to one hand, for example, and to completely spare the other.

The arthritis of rheumatoid arthritis is typically additive, with sequential involvement of groups of joints. Most joints remain more or less symptomatic as new joints are involved. The earliest joints involved are usually small joints of the hands and feet, but the distal interphalangeal joints are spared until late in the course.

Although arthritis is usually the presenting feature of rheumatoid arthritis, occasional patients have extra-articular features of the disease at roughly the same time or even earlier. Episcleritis, subcutaneous nodules, and pleural effusions are the most frequent early extra-articular features of the disease.

Systemic Lupus Erythematosus (SLE). SLE (see Chapter 64) often presents as chronic polyarthritis, and may often be confused with rheumatoid arthritis in such patients. The arthritis is typically intermittent, may be extremely painful, and is almost never erosive. Mixed connective tissue disease may cause an identical arthritis.

Scleroderma. Scleroderma often begins as painful swollen hands, with early contractures as prominent features. Indeed, the combination of puffy hands and Raynaud's phenomenon is often termed *undifferentiated connective tissue disease* in recognition of the fact that the condition of such patients may evolve into systemic lupus, scleroderma, mixed connective tissue disease, or rheumatoid arthritis. Some individuals may remain in the undifferentiated state for many years.

Psoriatic Arthritis. Although typically pauciarticular at onset, psoriatic arthritis may evolve into a polyarticular disease that resembles rheumatoid arthritis (see Chapter 61). This presents particular diagnostic problems in children, whose disease may resemble pauciarticular juvenile chronic arthritis at onset and may then evolve into a pattern resembling polyarticular juvenile or adult rheumatoid arthritis.[5]

Gonococcal Arthritis. Unlike the monarthritis typical of most septic joint diseases, gonococcal arthritis usually presents with fever, tenosynovitis, and papular or pustular skin lesions. As it evolves over several days, it may gradually involve one or more joints in a frankly purulent arthritis (see Chapter 90).

Viral Arthritis. Viral arthritis, including that due to the human immunodeficiency virus (HIV) can cause impressive polyarticular pain, often lasting for weeks or months (see Chapter 78). Parvovirus B19 is the prototype,[6] but similar symptoms have been reported with rubella,[7] mumps,[8] hepatitis B,[9] and other viruses. Acquired immunodeficiency syndrome (AIDS), Reiter's syndrome, psoriatic arthritis, and a painful polyarthritis possibly specific for HIV have been described. In such patients, the arthritis is frequently the presenting manifestation of HIV infection.[10] Another presentation of HIV infection resembles systemic lupus erythematosus, with fever, rash, polyarthritis, proteinuria, and hematologic abnormalities.[11] Infectious polyarthritis may complicate HIV infection.

Pauciarticular Peripheral Arthritis

In general, the term *pauciarticular* is used to describe arthritis that affects four or fewer joints, although certain latitude may be taken, such as counting the midfoot or wrist as a single joint. In addition, this term is usually limited to the early phase of the disease, since many of these conditions gradually become polyarticular as the course progresses.

Psoriatic Arthritis. This condition may precede skin disease in a minority of patients and usually begins as an asymmetric pauciarticular disease, often including distal interphalangeal joints. In many cases, entire digits are involved with arthritis and periostitis, producing the "sausage digit" appearance. The arthritis is typically asymmetric (Fig. 25–1), and occasional patients show severe damage of one group of joints with no involvement of the contralateral side (see Chapter 61).

Reiter's Syndrome. Reiter's syndrome (arthritis, conjunctivitis, and skin or mucosal lesions) may present in a manner similar to that of psoriatic arthritis but with a greater predilection for the lower extremity. The arthritis is often asymmetric and is frequently associated with involvement of the heel and other entheses or the sacroiliac joints (see Chapter 60).

Adult Rheumatic Fever. Apparently increasing in frequency of occurrence, this disorder often causes a painful pauciarticular disease, which is most prominent in the larger joints of the lower extremities. The typical migratory pattern of childhood rheumatic fever is uncommon in adults,[12] and the response to aspirin is less dramatic. Finally, although some fever is usually present, carditis is uncommon, and other features, such as chorea, rash, and subcutaneous nodules, are rare. In addition, the presentation in adults may be less acute, with a more insidious arthritis developing over several days or 1 to 2 weeks.

Gout. Unfortunately, gout all too often presents to the rheumatologist as undiagnosed chronic polyarthritis (see Chapter 80). Particularly confusing can

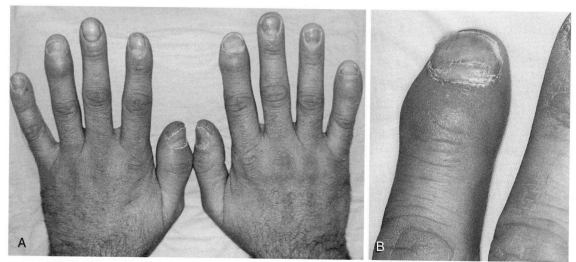

Figure 25–1. *A, B,* Psoriatic arthritis. Note the asymmetry of the distal interphalangeal joint involvement and the associated psoriatic nail disease.

be the syndrome of acute and chronic gouty arthritis superimposed on osteoarthritis of the finger joints.[13] Examination of synovial fluid or material draining from a tophus will yield the diagnosis.

Calcium Pyrophosphate Deposition Disease (CPDD). CPDD is most easily recognized when it presents as an acute monarthritis (pseudogout). It has many forms, however, including a chronic polyarthritis (see Chapter 81).

Behçet's Disease. Uncommon in the United States, Behçet's disease almost invariably causes chronic polyarthritis limited to a few joints. It is characterized by painful acute flareups associated with oral, genital, and ophthalmologic manifestations.

Enteropathic Arthritis. This is the arthritis associated with inflammatory bowel disease and characteristically involves large joints of the lower extremity or the lumbosacral spine (see Chapter 62).

Relapsing Polychondritis. This condition usually causes severe inflammation of the ears, nose, and sclera and is associated with a pauciarticular arthritis of the knees or wrists (see Chapter 85).

Sarcoidosis. Sarcoidosis causes a number of articular problems. The most frequent is an oligoarthritis of the knees or ankles in association with erythema nodosum and bilateral hilar adenopathy. Joint effusions are rare. Occasionally, in patients with long-standing sarcoidosis, a chronic, destructive polyarthritis resembling rheumatoid arthritis may develop (see Chapter 87). In many of these patients, lytic bone disease is visible on radiographs.

Lyme Disease. The arthritis of Lyme disease is usually monarticular or oligoarticular, but a chronic symmetric polyarthritis has also been described.[14]

Bacterial Endocarditis. The arthritis of bacterial endocarditis is also typically monarticular or oligoarticular, usually in the lower extremities. Polyarthralgias are common, however, and the frequent association of positive rheumatoid factor test results can add to the diagnostic difficulties.[15]

Amyloid Arthropathy. Amyloid arthropathy may include virtually all joints, but pauciarticular involvement of the upper extremities is most frequent. Bilateral shoulder disease may cause joint enlargement known as the "shoulder pad" sign. This finding, especially in association with carpal tunnel syndrome and purpura in skin folds, should always prompt one to suspect primary amyloidosis. The amyloidosis caused by β_2-microglobulin deposition in chronic dialysis patients may present with an impressive destructive arthritis of large joints, especially the knees, shoulders, and hips[16] (see Chapter 86).

Inflammatory Polyarthritis with Axial Involvement

Early involvement of the axial skeleton can be an extremely important clue to the correct diagnosis of inflammatory polyarthritis. For that reason, it may be very helpful to question the patient carefully about neck and lumbar spine pain and prolonged stiffness to rule out unusual presentations of ankylosing spondylitis, Reiter's syndrome, or other spondyloarthropathies (see Chapters 59 to 62).

Ankylosing Spondylitis. This disease is the prototype of this group of diseases. Although it typically begins in the patient's late teens or early 20s with back pain and stiffness, when it begins in juveniles or young teenagers, peripheral arthritis is common and may precede back symptoms by months or years. The arthritis involves predominantly the lower extremities and includes knees, ankles, and feet in most patients.[17]

Reiter's Syndrome. Although only one quarter to one third of patients with Reiter's syndrome have overt back symptoms on presentation, most of these patients will have either unilateral or bilateral sacroiliitis and spine disease during the course of the disease.[18]

Enteropathic Arthritis. The arthritis of inflammatory bowel disease, enteropathic arthritis may present as either axial or peripheral arthritis, or the two may coexist.[19] The axial arthritis is identical to ankylosing spondylitis and is strongly associated with HLA-B27. Once present, the spondylitis runs a progressive course regardless of the activity of the bowel disease.[20] Spondylitis typically develops at around the same time as the bowel disease but may precede it by years.

Psoriatic Arthritis. This condition may cause both an axial and a peripheral arthritis, but the axial disease is rarely an important presenting manifestation (see Chapter 61).

Whipple's Disease. Whipple's disease typically causes a polyarthritis similar to Reiter's syndrome, with sacroiliitis plus a peripheral arthritis usually involving only a few joints at a time.

Noninflammatory Polyarthritis (Osteoarthritis)

Many of the features that support the diagnosis of noninflammatory polyarthritis are simply the absence of features that suggest inflammation. A number of specific findings, however, are helpful in establishing a diagnosis of osteoarthritis (see Chapter 83).

The patient usually describes a history of pain primarily during and after use of the affected joints, with minimal pain at rest and only minimal morning stiffness. Physical examination often reveals coarse crepitation, and loose bodies and other debris may be palpable while the joint is moved through its range of motion. Bony osteophytes may be palpable, especially in the fingers.

Results of routine tests of inflammation are normal unless another disease is present. Because osteoarthritis increases in frequency with advancing age, positive test results for rheumatoid factor become less valuable in older people.

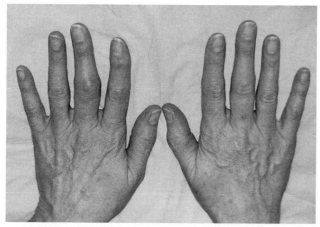

Figure 25–2. Osteoarthritis. Although the left third proximal interphalangeal joint is involved most severely, the right is also involved, and there are several early Heberden's nodes. The patient is a 60-year-old secretary who has moderate soreness in these joints at the end of the day.

The ultimate diagnostic test for osteoarthritis is the radiograph. A number of important biochemical changes in cartilage precede radiographic changes, but for all practical purposes, symptomatic osteoarthritis is nearly always accompanied by radiographic changes (see Chapter 42) and presents as specific syndromes.

Osteoarthritis of the Hands. A hereditary disease much more prevalent in women (see Chapter 83), this typically develops within a few years of menopause and is often associated with mild inflammation for the first year or two that a particular joint is involved. The joints may intermittently be warm and tender. After 1 or 2 years, the evidence of inflammation, if any, gradually subsides, and the typical osteophytes of Heberden's and Bouchard's nodes develop in the distal and proximal interphalangeal joints, respectively. The disease is strikingly symmetric, although the degree of involvement may vary somewhat (Fig. 25–2).[21]

Primary Generalized Osteoarthritis. A rare, hereditary disease with a high frequency of osteoarthritis of multiple joints, primary generalized osteoarthritis usually begins in middle age and involves "typical" joints, such as the hips, knees, and hands.[22]

Osteoarthritis Secondary to Metabolic Diseases. This is being increasingly recognized as particular patterns of osteoarthritis have been described in association with several disorders.

Hemochromatosis. Hemochromatosis, an underdiagnosed but relatively common disorder,[23] may present with osteoarthritis involving the metacarpophalangeal joints, especially the second and third. Apparent osteoarthritis of weight-bearing and large non–weight-bearing joints also is seen (see Chapter 88).

Calcium Pyrophosphate Deposition Disease. CPPD may be associated with generalized osteoarthritis, including severe involvement of unusual joints, such as the wrist and patellofemoral joint (see Chapter 81).

Hypothyroidism. Hypothyroidism is associated with symmetric, noninflammatory, highly viscous effusions, frequently in joints with preexisting osteoarthritis (see Chapter 96).

Acromegaly. Acromegaly causes polyarthritis as a result of bone and cartilage overgrowth, with the most severe involvement being in the hips and spine (see Chapter 96).

Chondromalacia. Chondromalacia of the patella has multiple causes, but as a clinical presentation, it is usually seen in physically active young and middle-aged women. Physical findings include small effusions, laxity of the patellar ligaments, and patellofemoral crepitation (see Chapter 83).

Other. *Obesity* causes a number of joint problems, the most common of which is bilateral osteoarthritis of the knees, especially in women.[24] Various *developmental defects*, such as congenitally shallow acetabulae, are often asymptomatic until osteoarthritis develops later in life.

Table 25–3. DIFFERENTIAL DIAGNOSIS OF POLYARTICULAR PAIN

Polyarthritis	Neuropathies
Tendinitis	Diseases of the spine
Muscle disorders	Primary bone diseases
Polymyalgia rheumatica	Periostitis
Vasculitis	Fibrositis
Vaso-occlusive disease	Malingering

DIFFERENTIAL DIAGNOSIS

Arthritis Versus Arthralgia. Table 25–3 lists the major nonarticular considerations in patients with chronic polyarticular pain. The first challenge to the physician is to differentiate between arthritis, arthralgia, and periarticular inflammation.

Tendinitis and Related Disorders. These include painful shoulder syndromes, tennis elbow (lateral epicondylitis), golfer's elbow (medial epicondylitis), trochanteric bursitis, prepatellar bursitis, Achilles tendinitis, and tendinitis along the radial aspect of the wrist (de Quervain's disease). In these syndromes, pain is often maximal at the beginning of an activity and then starts to subside as the activity is continued (see Chapter 28). A thorough history, including a description of job and sports activities, is essential. In many cases, physical examination reveals areas of local tenderness near, but distinct from, the joint. Pain may be exacerbated by movement of the affected structures against resistance. In tendinitis, swelling, if present, is usually minimal and limited to tendon sheaths and bursae, rather than joints.

Thickening of tendons and subcutaneous tissues in patients with diabetes can cause a variety of clinical features, including Dupuytren's contractures and, especially in patients with juvenile onset diabetes, the *diabetic stiff hand syndrome*[25] (Fig. 25–3).

Muscle Disorders. Although weakness predomi-

nates in most of these conditions, and arthritis therefore is not a serious consideration, occasional patients present with periarticular pain as a primary complaint (see Chapter 73).

Polymyalgia Rheumatica. Because many patients with polymyalgia rheumatica (see Chapter 69) have preexisting polyarticular disorders, such as osteoarthritis and tendinitis, it may require skill and experience to differentiate among these problems. Several authors[26–28] have pointed out the difficulty of distinguishing polymyalgia rheumatica from older-onset rheumatoid arthritis and have stressed that in the early stages it may be impossible to tell them apart.

Vasculitis. Frank arthritis is an uncommon manifestation of systemic vasculitis. Joint pain, however, may be deep, aching, and constant (see Chapter 68).

Vaso-occlusive Diseases. The vaso-occlusive diseases include atherosclerosis, cholesterol emboli, emboli from cardiac sources such as a myxoma, diabetes, Raynaud's disease, Buerger's disease, and the antiphospholipid syndrome, which rarely present with polyarticular pain without some other manifestations of disease. Patients with cholesterol emboli may present with polyarthralgias, myalgias, renal disease, elevated erythrocyte sedimentation rates, eosinophilia, and positive test results for rheumatoid factor and antinuclear antibody.[29]

Neurologic Diseases. The neurologic diseases include peripheral neuropathies, compression neuropathies such as the carpal tunnel syndrome, and infiltrative diseases such as amyloidosis and Waldenström's macroglobulinemia. Pain is usually associated with paresthesias and is usually worse at night. Although patients may localize pain to joints, it is more typically diffuse, and examination reveals no objective joint abnormalities (see Chapter 39).

Diseases of the Spine. A variety of diseases of the neck and spine, including spinal stenosis (congenital or acquired), spondylolisthesis, and tumors of the lower cord and cauda equina, may present in a similar fashion. The pain is usually primarily in the buttocks and is worse with certain postures or activities. In spinal stenosis, for example, pain is typically that of *neurogenic claudication,* with aching in the buttocks and thighs brought on by certain activities—often worse going down hills or steps (see Chapters 27 and 29).

Primary Bone Diseases and Malignancy. Metastatic tumors and myeloproliferative disorders may masquerade as polyarticular arthritis. In childhood, sickle cell crises and leukemia are especially likely to present as widespread joint pain, and any large series of children with the initial diagnosis of juvenile rheumatoid arthritis contains a small percentage who ultimately are found to have leukemia.[30] In adults, myeloma and a variety of widely metastatic cancers present as bone and joint pain. In childhood leukemia, joint effusions, warmth, and tenderness may be present (see Chapter 98). These objective findings are rare in adults.

Other widespread bone diseases, especially osteo-

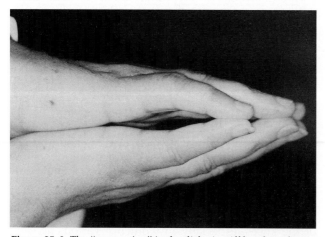

Figure 25–3. The "prayer sign" in the diabetic stiff hand syndrome. As a result of progressive thickening of tendons, joint capsules, and subcutaneous tissues, progressive stiffness and flexion contractures develop in these patients.

necrosis (see Chapter 101), may occasionally resemble polyarticular arthritis. When osteonecrosis involves peripheral joints, such as the knee and ankle, swelling and tenderness may be impressive.[31] It is not uncommon to see stress fractures in runners or other weekend athletes mimicking polyarthritis in the feet and ankles.

Periostitis. Periostitis, especially as part of the syndrome of *hypertrophic pulmonary osteoarthropathy,* may cause severe widespread joint pain, tenderness, and warmth. Careful examination reveals tenderness not only around joint structures but also along the shafts of the involved long bones (see Chapter 97).

Fibromyalgia and Psychogenic Pain Syndromes. Objective examination of these patients reveals nothing other than areas of tenderness, usually in typical trigger points (see Chapter 34).

SUMMARY

Polyarticular arthritis, the most common indication for rheumatologic consultation, represents a challenge to the skills and experience of the clinician. By careful history and physical examination along with appropriate tests, however, the physician can almost always establish the correct diagnosis and institute appropriate therapy. In an era of increasing demand that medicine demonstrate that it is cost-effective, the bedside skills required to evaluate these patients prove valuable indeed.

References

1. Hooker RS, Brown JB: Rheumatology referral patterns. HMO Practice 4:61, 1990.
2. Pauker SG, Kassirer JP: Medical progress: Decision analysis. N Engl J Med 316:250, 1987.
3. Mackenzie AH: Differential diagnosis of rheumatoid arthritis. Am J Med 85(suppl 4):2, 1985.
4. Hannonen P, Mottonen T, Oka M: Palindromic rheumatism: A clinical survey of sixty patients. Scand J Rheumatol 16:413, 1987.
5. Southwood TR, Petty RE, Malleson PN, et al: Psoriatic arthritis in children. Arthritis Rheum 32:1007, 1989.
6. Woolf AD, Campion GV, Chishick A, et al: Clinical manifestations of human parvovirus B19 in adults. Arch Intern Med 149:1153, 1989.
7. Chambers RJ, Bywaters EG: Rubella synovitis. Ann Rheum Dis 22:263, 1963.
8. Gordon SC, Lauter CB: Mumps arthritis: A review of the literature. Rev Infect Dis 6:338, 1984.
9. Sergent JS: Extrahepatic manifestations of hepatitis B infection. Bull Rheum Dis 33:1, 1983.
10. Winchester R: AIDS and the rheumatic diseases. Bull Rheum Dis 39:1, 1990.
11. Kopelman RH, Zolla-Pazner S: Association of human immunodeficiency virus infection and autoimmune phenomenon. Am J Med 84:82, 1988.
12. Wallace MR, Garst PD, Papadimos TJ, et al: The return of acute rheumatic fever in young adults. JAMA 262:2557, 1989.
13. Lally EV, Zimmerman B, Ho G Jr, et al: Urate-mediated inflammation in nodal osteoarthritis: Clinical and roentgenographic correlations. Arthritis Rheum 32:86, 1989.
14. Steere AC, Schoen RT, Taylor E: The clinical evolution of Lyme arthritis. Ann Intern Med 107:725, 1987.
15. Churchill MA, Geraci JE, Hunder GG: Musculoskeletal manifestations of bacterial endocarditis. Ann Intern Med 87:754, 1977.
16. Alfrey AC: Beta$_2$-microglobulin amyloidosis. Nephrol Lett 6:27, 1989.
17. Khan MA: Editorial comment. J Rheumatol 16:634, 1989.
18. Lionarons RJ, van Zoeren M, Verhagen JN, et al: HLA-B27–associated reactive spondyloarthropathies in a Dutch military hospital. Ann Rheum Dis 45:141, 1986.
19. Gravallese EM, Kantrowitz FG: Arthritic manifestations of inflammatory bowel disease. Am J Gastroenterol 83:703, 1987.
20. Burgos-Vargas R, Clark P: Axial involvement in the seronegative enteropathy and arthropathy syndrome and its progression to ankylosing spondylitis. J Rheumatol 16:192, 1989.
21. Cushnaghan J, Dieppe P: Study of 500 patients with limb joint osteoarthritis. I: Analysis by age, sex, and distribution of symptomatic joint sites. Ann Rheum Dis 50:8, 1991.
22. Ala-Kokko L, Baldwin CT, Moskowitz RW, Prockop DJ: Single base mutation in the type II procollagen gene (COL2A1) as a cause of primary osteoarthritis associated with a mild chondrodysplasia. Proc Natl Acad Sci USA 87:6565, 1990.
23. Edwards CQ, Griffen LM, Goldgar D, et al: Prevalence of hemochromatosis among 11,065 presumably healthy blood donors. N Engl J Med 318:1355, 1988.
24. Felson DT, Anderson JJ, Naimark A, et al: Obesity and knee osteoarthritis: The Framingham study. Ann Intern Med 109:18, 1988.
25. Kapoor A, Sibbitt WL Jr: Contractures in diabetes mellitus: The syndrome of limited joint mobility. Semin Arthritis Rheum 18:168, 1989.
26. Healey LA: Late-onset rheumatoid arthritis vs. polymyalgia rheumatica: Making the diagnosis. Geriatrics 43:65, 1988.
27. Deal CL, Meenan RF, Goldenberg DL, et al: The clinical features of elderly-onset rheumatoid arthritis. Arthritis Rheum 28:987, 1985.
28. Healy LA: Polymyalgia rheumatica and seronegative RA may be the same entity. J Rheumatol 19:270, 1991.
29. Cappiello RA, Espinoza LR, Adelman H, et al: Cholesterol embolism: A pseudovasculitic syndrome. Semin Arthritis Rheum 18:240, 1989.
30. Kunnamo I, Kallio P, Pelkonen P, et al: Clinical signs and laboratory tests in the differential diagnosis of arthritis in children. Am J Dis Child 141:34, 1987.
31. Lotke PA, Steinberg ME: Osteonecrosis of the hip and knee. Bull Rheum Dis 35:1, 1985.

CHAPTER 26

Weakness

Anthony S. Felsovanyi

Weakness implies a reduced standard of muscular performance compared with the norm. The physician in a clinical situation in which weakness constitutes the presenting symptom needs to determine whether he or she is dealing with global weakness or reduced function of certain muscle groups. The patient's complaint usually refers to reduced functional capacity, such as rising from a chair, stair climbing, or performing specific tasks; exercising the affected muscle groups may be necessary to document the presence of a deficit. Because weakness and fatigue are common complaints of patients with psychosomatic illness, a patient's perception of weakness at variance with clinical findings (Table 26–1) may suggest a functional cause, such as a depressive disorder or a conversion reaction.

This presentation reviews muscle weakness and certain of its aspects as they relate to clinical rheumatology.

CLASSIFICATION OF WEAKNESS BY ETIOLOGY (Table 26–2)

Myopathies

With clinical evaluation of muscle weakness, one must consider the patient's age; nutritional status; lifestyle, including drug abuse; state of present health; medical history, including potential exposure to infectious diseases, environmental or occupational toxins, and medications; idiosyncratic reactions; and family history.

The rate of onset of symptoms often gives good leads about etiology. A history of sudden onset may imply a toxic event on any motoneuron level, such as botulism, or a sudden change in potassium, magnesium, calcium, or phosphorus blood level. Acute events that arise from upper or lower neuron pathology, such as hemorrhage or infarction, may present as regional weakness; sensory, reflex, and other changes in neurologic examination usually localize the level of injury.

Guillain-Barré syndrome and other demyelinizing disorders may have a subacute onset, and the same may apply to the primary proximal inflammatory myopathies.

Endocrinopathies, which produce proximal muscle weakness, have a gradual onset, as do genetic disorders, such as the dystrophies and metabolic storage diseases that affect the neuromuscular junction. These afflictions may be associated with an acute or chronically recurrent course, including myasthenia gravis with cranial nerve involvement, paraneoplastic neuropathies, and acute toxic events, such as organophosphate poisoning.

Involutional Weakness

Sarcopenia is the age-related loss of skeletal muscle mass that results in decreased strength and aerobic capacity.[1] Age-related loss of muscle power appears to be the result of atrophic changes due to denervation of muscle fibers. This is coupled with an increased susceptibility to, and reduced recovery potential from, minor traumatic injuries, including muscle contraction injury.[2] There is a 30 percent reduction in muscle mass by the seventh or eighth decade of life. This also is related to reduced physical activity. Age-related decline in muscle mass involves loss of fibers with little regenerative capacity. Certain exercise, specifically resistance training, may prevent or postpone the onset of sarcopenia and its concomitant metabolic decline associated with increased fat deposits and osteopenia.[3] Disuse atrophy in younger patients, which results in decreased diameter of individual fiber, is generally reversible.[3]

Table 26–1. CLINICAL FINDINGS IN NEUROMUSCULAR SYNDROMES

	Primary Myopathy	Peripheral Neuropathy	Lower Motor Neuron Dysfunction	Upper Motor Neuron Dysfunction
Reflexes	Normal	↓ – 0	↓ – 0	↑
Atrophy	0	+	+	±
Fasciculation	0	0	+	0
Pain	±	±	+	0
Spasm	0	0	±	±

Table 26–2. CLASSIFICATION AND DISTRIBUTION OF NEUROMUSCULAR SYNDROMES ASSOCIATED WITH WEAKNESS

Generalized Primary Myopathies

Involutional
  Sarcopenia
  Disuse atrophy
  Malnutrition
Systemic diseases (acute and chronic)
Infectious inflammation
Connective tissue inflammation
Ischemic
  Cardiopulmonary
  Peripheral
Genetic (mitochondrial)
Anemia
Organ failure (liver, kidney)
Metabolic-endocrine dysfunction

Proximal Muscle Weakness

Muscular dystrophies: Duchenne's, Becker's limb girdle
Inflammation: polymyositis, dermatomyositis, inclusion body myositis, vasculitis, rheumatoid arthritis, sarcoid, human immunodeficiency virus infection
Toxic: chloroquine, cholchicine, cyclosporine, D-penicillamine, or acetaldehyde (ethanol) use
Metabolic: glycogen and lipid storage diseases
Endocrine: thyroid or parathyroid disorders, adrenal insufficiency, hyperaldosteronism, steroid myopathy (Cushing's disease), acromegaly, diabetes mellitus
Mineral: potassium, calcium, magnesium, or phosphorus imbalance
Neuromuscular dysfunction: myasthenia gravis, Eaton-Lambert syndrome, organophosphate toxicity

Distal Muscle Weakness

Myotonic dystrophies
Vasculitis, polymyositis, sarcoid (rare)

Peripheral Neuropathies As Expressed by Symmetric Mononeuritis, Multiple Mononeuritis

Genetic: Charcot-Marie-Tooth disease
Nutritional: beri-beri, anemia
Toxic: heavy metal, gold, acetaldehyde
Ischemic: vasculitis, postphlebitic
Metabolic: diabetes mellitus, myxedema
Demyelinizing: chronic (multiple sclerosis)
Demyelinizing: acute (e.g., Guillain-Barré syndrome)
Inflammatory: rheumatoid arthritis, vasculitis
Infiltrative: amyloid, carcinomatosis
Post-traumatic
Entrapment
Degenerative

Anterior Horn Involvement

Polio
Myelitis
Demyelinizing disorders
Degenerative disorders
Entrapment
Radiculitis (diabetes mellitus)
Infection
Neoplastic
Genetic

Cerebral Involvement

Genetic
Ischemic: thrombosis, embolism, bleed
Inflammation: infection, immunologic (including paraneoplastic)
Neoplastic
Traumatic
Toxic
Degenerative

Poor Nutrition

Various degrees of malnutrition have a profound effect on muscle mass and performance. Nutritional weakness may be caused by general caloric deprivation as well as by specific nutritional deficits (e.g., amino acids, minerals, and micronutrients). The cause may be lack of food; an inability to ingest, absorb, assimilate, or utilize certain foodstuffs; or an increased metabolic demand from physical activity, accelerating growth, pregnancy, or hypermetabolism. In adolescents and young adults, anorexia nervosa or bulimia may lead to fatal wasting from malnutrition.

Special Aspects of Poor Nutrition and Muscle Weakness

Respiratory muscles, stressed and at times fatigued as a result of chronic respiratory disease, appear to be especially vulnerable to nutritional deprivation; the resulting atrophy of inspiratory muscles reduces the respiratory drive, thereby promoting atelectasis and secondary infection as well as aggravating respiratory insufficiency.

Other nutritional manipulation may greatly benefit patients with certain muscle disorders, such as substi-

tuting carnitine for deficient patients and providing high-calorie diets for patients with dystrophies or acid maltase deficiencies.[4] The clinician treating patients with acute respiratory insufficiency by mechanical respiration must aim for a careful nutritional balance, since overnutrition with carbohydrates creates carbon dioxide retention, and caloric deprivation perpetuates respiratory muscle weakness and atrophy and thereby delays weaning from the respirator.[5] In addition, many patients with acute and chronic respiratory diseases are treated with corticosteroids, a major cause of muscle atrophy, including the diaphragm.

PHYSICAL FINDINGS (Fig. 26–1)

Inspection

Simple inspection of a patient who complains of weakness can convey some information as to age and nutritional and developmental status. Occasionally, speech and voice suggest some bulbar involvement. Engorged and tender temporal arteries alert the examiner to the possible presence of *granulomatous arteritis*. Facial appearance may suggest the high levels of tumor necrosis factor associated with advanced

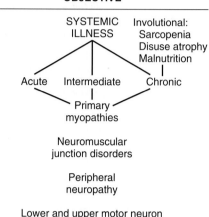

Figure 26–1. Diagnoses of muscle weakness according to subjective symptoms or objective findings of neuromuscular disease.

wasting disease, or it may indicate depressive or *parkinsonism*, or *myotonias, facioscapulohumeral dystrophy*, or *hyperthyroidism* or *hypothyroidism*. A cushingoid facies indicates *corticosteroid toxicity* or *ethanol abuse*. Pigmental stigmata of *adrenal insufficiency* may be present. Examination of the mouth and tongue may point to micronutrient deficiencies, or amyloid deposits, or certain genetic muscle disorders.

Distribution

Primary myopathy is likely to reveal preservation of reflexes and muscle bulk and proximal weakness and symmetric distribution, with occasional bulbar involvement. When the muscular end-plate is affected, it may include extraocular, bulbar, and proximal limb musculature as well as diurnal fluctuations in strength. *Distal myopathies* are uncommon and of unknown etiology and usually involve slowly progressive muscle degeneration. *Inclusion body myopathy* and, rarely, *polymyositis* initially present with distal distribution.[6]

Peripheral nerve involvement has distal distribution, frequently symmetric, may show some muscle atrophy, and may be accompanied by motor and sensory dysfunction with decreased reflexes. *Weakness of axonal origin* presents with early and profound muscle atrophy, muscle cramps, and fasciculation. Reflexes may be modified by *upper motor neuron* involvement. *Autonomic dysfunction* (e.g., orthostasis) in younger patients signifies central nervous system disease.

LABORATORY EVALUATION OF MYOPATHIES

Laboratory studies, including blood count, chemical panel, urinalysis, and other studies as indicated,

may shed further light on intercurrent acute or chronic illness. If the patient's weakness appears to be generalized, a chronic underlying disease is likely to be present, such as *diabetes mellitus* (with wide fluctuations of blood sugar), *chronic uremia, hepatic failure, chronic respiratory or congestive heart failure, metastatic cancer, tuberculosis* and *human immunodeficiency virus* (in advanced stages of illness), or other chronic, wasting afflictions. A greatly elevated erythrocyte sedimentation rate may indicate an inflammatory disorder such as *vasculitis*, an obscure *infectious process, neoplasia*, or certain connective tissue disorders; the last may be further defined through serologic studies.

Specific laboratory investigations of muscular weakness should include the study of muscle enzymes that leak from damaged muscle fibers. Creatinine kinase lends itself readily for study, and a clinically significant elevation of its MM fraction confirms acute muscular stress from severe exercise or active pathology. Such measurements may also be useful in following the clinical course and therapy. The MB isoform of creatine kinase is elevated moderately in severe skeletal muscle inflammation.

Electrophysiologic studies in the form of electromyography (EMG) and evaluation of nerve conduction can provide much functional information. Myopathies, peripheral neuropathy, and anterior horn cell pathology can be diagnosed on the basis of EMG findings. EMG in neuropathies reveals fibrillations characteristic of denervated muscle fibers and the loss of whole motor units. In contrast, myopathies show characteristic changes in action potentials due to destruction of individual muscle fibers. Axon loss may reduce the electrical amplitude, whereas destruction of myelin sheathing of nerves may slow conductivity.[6]

Myosonography (ultrasound) is an intriguing, relatively new diagnostic modality in myology that complements magnetic resonance (MR) imaging as well as MR spectroscopy and that is proving valuable in directing sites for muscle biopsy. In a study of 70 patients with various myopathic afflictions, the ultrasound sensitivity of 82.9 percent compared with an EMG sensitivity of 92.4 percent. Positive and negative predictive values were 95.1 and 89.2 percent, respectively, with an accuracy of 91.3 percent; this included patients with *polymyositis, dermatomyositis, inclusion body myositis,* and *granulomatous muscle disease.* Degenerative changes, fatty infiltrates, atrophy, and other pathologic features can be clearly delineated.[7] Echography has also been used successfully to measure individual muscle size and function, such as extraocular musculature and pelvic muscles in micturition disorders.[8–10]

Directed needle biopsy of muscle may confirm the presence of pathology and, at times, classify such pathology by detailed tissue analysis (e.g., *inclusion body myositis* in the treatment of refractory *polymyositis.*) Biopsy can also uncover cases of *neurogenic atrophy.*[11]

MR imaging can be helpful in evaluating various atrophic, dystrophic, and hypertrophic muscular conditions as well as tumors, abscesses, and other abnormalities. This mode of tissue visualization has lately proved to be most helpful in elucidating *entrapment and compression myopathies.*[12]

MR spectroscopy is primarily a research tool. As such, it clarifies physiologic functions and effect of stress on muscle metabolism, and it may monitor effects of therapeutic interventions.[13]

The medical history and physical examination of a patient with weakness and the choices of specific laboratory studies should clarify many clinical situations.

Fatigue

Another form of weakness involves the concept of "fatigue." It represents a reduction in force after a series of muscle contractions. Fatigue after stressful muscle exertion may be a physiologic event, or it may be due to physical deconditioning, nutritional deficiency, or changes in atmospheric environment as well as debilitating disease. Fatigue is also a common subjective complaint with many emotional disturbances, including depression and anxiety states. Among the diseases associated with fatigue, congestive heart failure, initially subtle in onset, may be a frequent cause as the result of inadequate tissue oxygenation. Skeletal myopathy, probably due to ischemic cell damage, has been documented in this setting. Prolonged training in chronic heart failure has been shown to improve skeletal muscle function, exercise capacity, and clinical symptoms in small controlled trials.[14]

Respiratory muscle fatigue, a concept mentioned earlier in the context of nutritional requirements, has important clinical implications, especially in patients with respiratory failure. Both inspiratory and expiratory respiratory training have proved helpful. Hypoxemia and hypophosphatemia contribute to early respiratory muscle fatigue; they are amenable to low-flow oxygen therapy and to the correction of low serum phosphate levels.[15] Patients with chronic heart failure have increased muscle fatigability and dyspnea because of underperfusion and deconditioning (skeletal muscle atrophy). Decreased perfusion reduces the force of muscular contraction and exercise tolerance. Reduced lung compliance due to chronic pulmonary congestion and fibrosis leads to increased respiratory muscle workload, fatigue, and dyspnea.[16] Another study of respiratory muscle fatigue suggests that a fatigued diaphragm can transfer much of its workload to the inspiratory rib cage muscles.[17]

Neuromuscular Junction Disorders

Neuromuscular junction disorders commonly present chronically or periodically with skeletal muscle weakness or easy fatigability. The clinical presentation of these afflictions can be easily misinterpreted as a depressive illness or other stress-related emotional reactions. The hallmark of such disorders is *myasthenia gravis,* which is caused by an autoimmune mediated block of acetylcholine receptors. More than 80 percent of afflicted patients demonstrate antibodies against acetylcholine receptors (AChRs).[18] Clinically, 90 percent of patients experience double vision and eyelid weakness, which are the presenting complaints in 50 percent of such cases. In 20 percent of patients, only extraocular muscles are affected. The Tensilon therapeutic test for myasthenia gravis is only 60 percent diagnostically accurate in cases of the pure oculomotor variety. This disease may be responsive to corticosteroids or anticholinesterase manipulations. The cause of clinical predilection for eye muscle is unknown.[19] Bulbar involvement is common. Myasthenia gravis frequently occurs in combination with hyperthyroidism or connective tissue diseases. There is a 75 percent incidence of thymus involvement, mostly in the form of hyperplasia, with a 15 percent occurrence of thymoma. Evaluation should include assessment of the degree and distribution of muscle weakness, including comparative unilateral exercise testing and electrodiagnostic studies. Because of the frequency of respiratory muscle involvement, it is also important to obtain baseline ventilatory function studies. Additional tests include an anti-AChR antibody titer and computed tomographic thymus studies to rule out the presence of a thymoma. Detailed treatment modalities for this disorder, including decisions about thymectomy, immunosuppression, and plasmapheresis, are beyond the scope of this presentation.

Paraneoplastic myasthenic (Eaton-Lambert) syndromes present with somewhat similar attacks of weakness and muscle fatigue. Unlike the situation with myasthenia gravis, physical effort may improve muscle strength and the affliction spares the cranial nerves;

dysautonomia is a frequent concurrence in this setting. In more than 60 percent of such patients, neoplasia eventually becomes apparent. The symptoms of Eaton-Lambert syndrome may precede tumor occurrence by years. The most usual neoplasm in this setting is oat cell (small cell) carcinoma of the lung.[20]

Acute toxicity from botulism affects both skeletal muscle and cranial nerves; *Clostridium botulinum*–contaminated food, and, rarely, *C. botulinum*–infected wounds are the sources of illness. The incubation period may be several days to several weeks for the wound infection variety. Fulminant gastrointestinal symptoms and signs of autonomic neuropathy are frequently prominent. Toxin from the site of infection can usually be identified. The disease can be treated with specific antitoxin.

Peripheral Neuropathies

As the cause of weakness in affected muscles, peripheral neuropathies may be of a genetic, toxic, inflammatory, infectious, metabolic, paraneoplastic, degenerative, ischemic, or post-traumatic etiology, including entrapment and compression neuropathies and local as well as axonal autoimmune phenomena. They may occur symmetrically or unilaterally; they may secondarily affect any muscle or muscle group; and they may cause pain, cramping, sensory deficits, depression of reflexes, and dystrophic changes.

Spinal Cord Disease

Diseases of the spinal cord have many causes. Space-occupying lesions—whether neoplastic, hemorrhagic, or due to edema or plaque formation—produce pronounced compressive symptoms because of the confined space of the spinal canal. Myelitis usually affects limbs symmetrically, whereas affliction of the upper neurons is, with few exceptions, unilateral.[21] Weakness, acute or gradual, or paralysis of the affected limb may accompany many spinal injuries and cause local pain or neurologic deficits, depending on the nature of the pathologic process. Affected limbs may also show dystrophic changes, suppressed reflexes, fasciculation, and muscle cramps. Radicular pathology frequently is caused by entrapment, painful weakness, and disability. Diabetic neuropathy may present as unilateral radiculitis. Guillain-Barré syndrome may mimic acute myelitis.[21, 22] A complete history and physical examination, MR visualization, a nuclear white blood cell scan (if abscess or discitis is suspected), as well as EMG with nerve conduction studies and a lumbar puncture (if indicated), can provide further clinical information.

Upper Neuron Pathology

Upper neuron pathology usually produces unilateral deficits—weakness or paralysis of affected limbs with spastic features, including exaggerated reflexes. Hoffman's and Babinski's signs are likely to be positive. Weakness may be global or focal, depending on the underlying abnormality.

Psychogenic Weakness and Fatigue

Primary or secondary psychiatric afflictions that present with weakness frequently are accompanied by sensory somatization in the form of aches and pains. Details of these phenomena are covered in other clinical texts.

WEAKNESS IN RHEUMATOLOGIC DISORDERS

Global muscle weakness, as it relates to rheumatologic disorders, implies systemic illness, such as vasculitis of all varieties, duration, and distribution, including renal involvement with uremia, severe anemia, and other manifestations. Erythrocyte sedimentation rate, appropriate serologic evaluation, tissue studies, and various imaging modalities can define the clinical situation.

Local muscle weakness about affected joints is frequently the result of disuse atrophy, although inflammatory conditions of the joint, joint capsule, and related structures may extend to adjacent muscle fibers or lead to a variety of entrapment neuropathies. The latter can be identified and localized electromyographically by ultrasonography or MR imaging.

Primary inflammatory myositis, as an expression of a rheumatic disorder, is usually of proximal distribution, with preservation of muscle bulk and deep reflexes. Myopathic pain accompanying muscle weakness may thus be myositic, neuritic, or vasculitic (or ischemic). Rheumatic disease with axial skeletal involvement commonly presents with multiple distal sensory disturbances in addition to weakness accompanied by inflammatory or more often neuropathic findings of entrapment.

It is important to differentiate muscular weakness from muscular stiffness in rheumatic disease. The latter occurs most commonly after prolonged rest (morning stiffness) and improves with ambulation. Subjective perception of swollen legs with radicular pain may suggest dorsal column involvement, and weak aching muscles may be confused with polymyositis.[23]

A number of drugs of therapeutic importance in rheumatology can cause primary or secondary muscle weakness. Differentiating their toxic or idiosyncratic myopathic effects constitutes a great challenge in clinical rheumatology.

Steroid myopathy may occur in two forms: (1) generalized muscle atrophy and rhabdomyolysis after short-term treatment with large doses of corticosteroids, and (2) proximal limb muscle weakness after extended treatment with moderate doses. Either form of toxicity may be accompanied by respiratory muscle weakness.[24–26] The therapeutic use of corticosteroids in inflammatory myopathies may give rise to serious dilemmas when the cause of disease progression has to be evaluated.

The following additional drugs used in the treatment of rheumatic diseases may produce myotoxic reactions: chloroquine and hydrochloroquine can cause proximal muscle weakness; gold salts may rarely produce secondary muscle weakness due to peripheral neurotoxicity; D-penicillamine can cause dermatomyositis[27] and myasthenia gravis[28] with long-term use.

SUMMARY

Some clinical aspects of weakness have been discussed in terms of reduced muscular performance both as a subjective perception and as a clinical finding. Consideration of a patient's genetics, age, and lifestyle, as well as the clinical approach to the diagnosis of underlying diseases and the potential toxicity of some therapeutic interventions, has been presented.

References

1. Evans WJ, Campbell WW: Sarcopenia and age-related changes in body composition and functional capacity. J Nutr 123(Suppl):465, 1993.
2. Brooks SV, Faulkner JA: Skeletal muscle weakness in old age: Underlying mechanisms. Med Sci Sports Exerc 26:432, 1994.
3. Fiatarone MA, O'Neill EF, Ryan ND, et al: Exercise training and nutritional supplementation for physical frailty in very elderly people. N Engl J Med 330:1769, 1994.
4. Aldrich TK: Nutritional factors in the pathogenesis and therapy of respiratory insufficiency in neuromuscular diseases. Monaldi Arch Chest Dis 48:327, 1993.
5. Christman JW, McCain RW: A sensible approach to nutritional support of mechanically ventilated critically ill patients. Intens Care Med 19:129, 1993.
6. Drachman DB: Weakness. In Harvey AM, Johns RJ, McKusick VA, Owens AH Jr, Ross RS (eds): Principles and Practice of Medicine, 22nd ed. Norwalk, Conn, Appleton & Lange, 1988, p 1081.
7. Reimers CD: Myosonographic findings in inflammatory muscular disease. Z Rheumatol 52:105, 1993.
8. Reimers CD, Fleckenstein JL, Witt TN, et al: Muscular ultrasound in idiopathic inflammatory myopathies of adults. J Neurol Sci 116:82, 1993.
9. Demer JL, Kerman BM: Comparison of standardized echography with magnetic resonance imaging to measure extraocular muscle size. Am J Ophthalmol 118:351, 1994.
10. Martan A, Halaska M, Drbohlav P, et al: Ultrasound of the urinary bladder neck: changes before and after pelvic floor muscle exercise (abstr). Cesk Gynekol 59:121, 1994.
11. Drachman DB: Weakness. In Harvey AM, Johns RJ, McKusick VA, Owens AH Jr, Ross RS (eds): Principles and Practice of Medicine, 22nd ed. Norwalk, Conn, Appleton & Lange, 1988, p 1081.
12. Beltran J, Rosenberg ZS: Diagnosis of compressive and entrapment neuropathies of the upper extremity: Value of MR imaging. Am J Roentgenol 163:525, 1994.
13. Kent-Braun JA, Miller RG, Weiner MW: Magnetic resonance spectroscopy of human muscle. Radiol Clin North Am 32:313, 1994.
14. Ferrari R, Bernocchi P, Boraso A, et al: Congestive heart failure from cardiac muscle to skeletal muscle. Cardiologia 38:45, 1993.
15. Yamaguchi M: Clinical study on respiratory muscle training for chronic respiratory failure (abstr). Nippon Kyobu Shikkan Gakkai Zasshi 30:1459, 1992.
16. Yan S, Sliwinski P, Gauthier AP, et al: Effect of global inspiratory muscle fatigue on ventilatory and respiratory muscle responses to CO_2. J Appl Physiol 75:1371, 1993.
17. Yan S, Lichros I, Zachynthinos S, et al: Effect of diaphragmatic fatigue on control of respiratory muscles and ventilation during CO_2 rebreathing. J Appl Physiol 75:1364, 1993.
18. Drachman DB, Adams RN, et al: Functional activities of autoantibodies to anti–acetylcholine receptors and the clinical severity of myasthenia gravis. N Engl J Med 307:769, 1982.
19. Sommer N, Nidans A, Weller M: Ocular myasthenia gravis. Doc Ophthalmol 84:309, 1993.
20. Newsome-Davis J: Diseases of the neuromuscular junction. In Asbury AK, McKhan GM, McDonald WI (eds): Diseases of the Nervous System. Philadelphia, WB Saunders, 1986, p 269.
21. Young WB: The clinical diagnosis of myelopathy. Semin Ultrasound CT MR 15:250, 1994.
22. Nobuhiro Y: Pathogenesis of axonal Guillain-Barre syndrome: Hypothesis. Muscle Nerve 17:680, 1994.
23. Ferguson IT, Hollingworth P: Neurologic complications of rheumatic diseases. In Maddison PJ, Isenberg DA, Woo P, Glass DN (eds): Oxford Textbook of Rheumatology. Oxford, UK, Oxford University Press, 1993, p 107.
24. Ellis EF: Steroid myopathy. J Allergy Clin Immunol 76:431, 1985.
25. Dekhuizen PN, Decramer M: Steroid induced myopathy and its significance to respiratory disease: A known disease rediscovered. Eur Respir J 5:997, 1992.
26. Bolton CF: Muscle weakness and difficulty in weaning from the ventilator in the critical care unit (editorial). Chest 106:1, 1994.
27. Klaassen CD: Heavy metals and heavy-metal antagonists. In Gilman AG, Rall TW, Nies AS, Taylor P (eds): The Pharmacologic Basics of Therapeutics, 8th ed. New York, Pergamon Press, 1990, p 1611.
28. Gordon RA, Burnside JW: Penicillamine-induced myasthenia gravis in rheumatoid arthritis. Ann Intern Med 87:578, 1977.

CHAPTER 27

Neck Pain

Kenneth K. Nakano

In medicine, pain is a universal clinical problem encountered by every physician who cares for patients.[1] Pain has been defined by the International Association for the Study of Pain as an "unpleasant sensory and emotional experience associated with actual or potential tissue damage."[2] Additionally, pain involves behavioral, motivational, affective, cognitive, and spiritual phenomena as well as nociceptive neuropathic phenomena. Thus, achieving relief of pain may necessitate assessments and interventions in a multidimensional fashion.

The pain pathway, consisting of the classic three-neuron chain, appears to be a dual system at each level, and the sensation of pain is thought to arrive in the central nervous system (CNS) with the discriminative component of pain ("first pain") carried separately from the affective-motivational component of pain ("second pain").[3] In addition to spinal control mechanisms of pain transmission, descending pathways that originate in three major areas—cortex, thalamus, and brainstem—can modify functions at the spinal level. A close relationship prevails between somatic pain pathways and visceral pathways at every level of the nervous system; this relationship accounts for the transmission of visceral pain as well as for autonomic responses to somatic pain and somatic responses to visceral pain.[4]

Identifying the origin of the pain is the first essential step in the diagnostic process. To do this, the physician must have a detailed knowledge of anatomy and physiology and of the nature and distribution of pain from each structure.[5, 6] An attempt must then be made to correlate the type of pain with the clinical signs.

In clinical practice, neck pain occurs slightly less frequently than does low back pain; a major difference is that neck pain is less disabling, seldom compromising work capacity.[7] Neck stiffness exists as a common disorder, occurring in up to 30 percent of the 25- to 29-year-old age group in the United States working population.[8] For the work population over 45 years of age, this figure rises to 50 percent. Episodes of "simple" stiff neck last 1 to 4 days and seldom require medical care in most people. Radicular pain to the shoulder and arm occurs later in life than does stiff neck, with a frequency of up to 10 percent in the 25- to 29-year-old age group, subsequently rising to 25 to 40 percent after age 45 years. Overall, 45 percent of working men experience at least one attack of stiff neck, 23 percent report at least

one attack of radiculopathy, and 51 percent suffer both these symptoms at some time during their working career.

Neck pain occurs in all occupational groups. Stiffness of the neck appears first, followed by headache and shoulder-arm-hand pain (brachial neuralgia).[8] Investigations have reported that up to 12 percent of women and 9 percent of men experience neck pain with or without associated arm pain at any time, and that 35 percent of the population can recall an episode of neck pain.[7] A history of neck stiffness and arm pain was elicited in 80 percent of a population of male industrial and forest workers. In a series of male workers in a broad spectrum of jobs, the number with neck pain was modified to 51 percent, but only 5.4 percent had experienced work loss as a consequence of the pain.[7]

A great deal of literature suggests that neck and upper limb pain is diagnosed with increased frequency in Japan and in Australia. In the Japanese experience, the condition appears to have prominent attention among the working population[9, 10] and has been referred to as the *occupational cervicobrachial syndrome*. The apparent high frequency of this condition in Japanese workers is the result of a large number of uncontrolled studies of the syndrome among workers in a country where a high proportion of the population is employed. The condition is identical in every way in workers and in nonworkers, so labeling it "occupational" is unjustified and misleading. The increased focus may have given the false impression of a workforce epidemic rather than an event that is an ubiquitous feature of human life.[11] In the Australian experience, a soft tissue injury termed repetition strain injury achieved a good deal of attention[12, 13]; in this concept, the "injury" was inferred by the presence of a pain, but the tissue injured was never identified. The pain was in workers, so the condition was termed "occupational," but nonworkers with this condition were left out of the equation. "Strain" was simply assumed because the patient was working, and "repetition" was never quantified.[14] Some of the original supporters of the repetition strain injury diagnosis now propose a novel neurogenic basis for that syndrome.[15]

FUNCTIONAL ANATOMY AND PATHOPHYSIOLOGY

The pain-sensitive structures of the neck include the ligaments, nerve roots, articular facets and cap-

Table 27–1. STRUCTURES THAT CAUSE NECK PAIN

Acromioclavicular joint
Heart and coronary artery disease
Apex of lung, Pancoast's tumor, bronchogenic cancer (C3, C4, C5 nerve roots in common)
Diaphragm muscle (C3, C4, C5 innervation)
Gallbladder
Spinal cord tumor
Temporomandibular joint
Fibrositis and fibromyositis syndromes (upper thoracic spine, proximal arm and shoulder)
Aorta
Pancreas
Disorders of any somatic or visceral structure (produces cervical nerve root irritation)
Peripheral nerves
Central nervous system (posterior fossa lesions)
Hiatus hernia (C3, C4, C5)
Gastric ulcer

sules, muscle, and dura. Pain in the neck region can originate from many tissue sites (Table 27–1) and can result from a number of mechanisms (Table 27–2). Normal function of the cervical spine requires physiologic movements of the joints, bones, spinal cord, nerve roots (through the intervertebral foramina), muscles, ligaments, tendons, fascia, sympathetic nervous system, and the vascular supply to all these structures. Because most structures in the neck have the potential to become pain sensitive, a knowledge of the dermatome pattern of pain distribution is necessary in clinical diagnosis and therapy.

The neck is the most complicated articular system in the body and most mobile segment of the spine. Through a cylinder that connects the head to the thorax pass structures that require the greatest protection and that possess the least: the carotid and vertebral arteries, the spinal cord, and the spinal nerve roots. The head, weighing 6 to 8 pounds, balances on the 7 cervical vertebrae in a flexible chain held together by 14 apophyseal joints, 5 intervertebral discs; 12 joints of Luschka; and a system of ligaments (anterior longitudinal [AL], posterior longitudinal [PL], ligamentum flavum, interspinous, and ligamentum nuchae and muscle (14 paired anterior, lateral, and posterior) (Figs. 27–1, 27–2). Thirty-seven separate joints carry out the myriad movements of the head and neck in relation to the trunk and serve specialized sense organs.

The shape and mode of articulation of the joints influence the axes and range of movement of the neck. The neck normally moves more than 600 times each hour, whether one is awake or asleep. The cervical spine is subject to stress and strain with daily activities such as sitting, lying down, speaking, rising, walking, turning, and gesturing. The articular surfaces of the vertebral bodies are covered by plates of avascular hyaline cartilage and united by intervertebral discs. The intervertebral discs increase in area from below the axis (C2) downward, and cervical lordosis results from their wedge shape (see Figs. 27–1, 27–2). The thickness of the discs varies; the two deepest discs lie below the sixth and fifth vertebrae,

Table 27–2. CERVICAL SPINE SYNDROMES

Localized Neck Disorders

Osteoarthritis (apophyseal joints, C1–3 levels most often)
Rheumatoid arthritis (atlantoaxial)
Juvenile rheumatoid arthritis
Sternocleidomastoid tendinitis
Acute posterior cervical strain
Pharyngeal infections
Cervical lymphadenitis
Osteomyelitis (staphylococcal, tuberculosis)
Meningitis
Ankylosing spondylitis
Paget's disease
Torticollis (congenital, spasmodic, drug-involved, hysterical)
Neoplasms (primary or metastatic)
Occipital neuralgia (greater and lesser occipital nerves)
Diffuse idiopathic skeletal hyperostosis
Rheumatic fever (infrequently)
Gout (infrequently)

Lesions Producing Neck and Shoulder Pain

Postural disorders
Rheumatoid arthritis
Fibrositis syndromes
Musculoligamentous injuries to neck and shoulder
Osteoarthritis (apophyseal and Luschka)
Cervical spondylosis
Intervertebral osteoarthritis
Thoracic outlet syndrome
Nerve injuries (serratus anterior, C3–4 nerve root, long thoracic nerve)

Lesions Producing Predominantly Shoulder Pain

Rotator cuff tears and tendinitis
Calcareous tendinitis
Subacromial bursitis
Bicipital tendinitis
Adhesive capsulitis
Reflex sympathetic dystrophy
Frozen shoulder syndromes
Acromioclavicular secondary osteoarthritis
Glenohumeral arthritis
Septic arthritis
Tumors of the shoulder

Lesions Producing Neck and Head Pain with Radiation

Cervical spondylosis
Rheumatoid arthritis
Intervertebral disc protrusion
Osteoarthritis (apophyseal and Luschka joints; intervertebral disc; osteoarthritis)
Spinal cord tumors
Cervical neurovascular syndromes
  Cervical rib
  Scalene muscle
  Hyperabduction syndrome
  Rib-clavicle compression

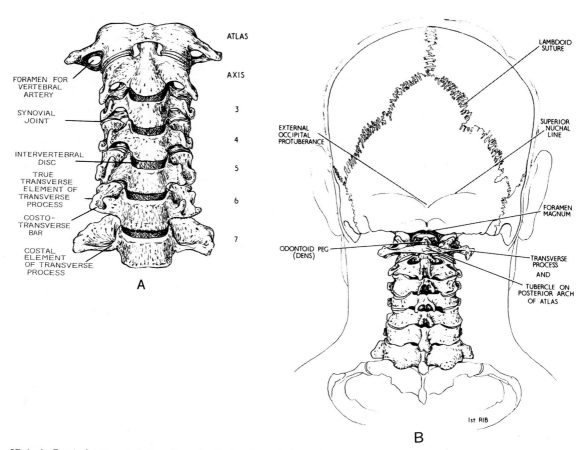

Figure 27–1. *A*, Cervical spine. Anterior view of articulated cervical vertebrae. *B*, Posterior view of the skull, seven cervical vertebrae, and first thoracic vertebra.

respectively. Each intervertebral disc consists of fibrocartilage and contains a nucleus pulposus, which changes in shape but cannot be compressed.[16]

AL and PL ligaments extend upward to the occipital bone and downward into the sacrum, joining the vertebral bodies. The AL ligament attaches to the bodies and becomes tightly fixed at the discs (see Fig. 27–2). A sudden extending force may rupture it and lead to severe hyperextension associated with damage to the spinal cord. The PL ligament attaches to the discs and adjacent bones but not to the center.

The specialized atlanto-occipital and atlantoaxial joints are controlled by intersegmental muscles. The head and atlas move together around the odontoid peg and the upper articular facets of the axis (see Fig. 27–1), the long transverse processes of the atlas providing the levers used in rotation. The anterior surface of the odontoid articulates with the posterior surface of the anterior arch of the atlas. The total excursion of the head can be measured in flexion, extension, rotation, and lateral flexion (Table 27–3). The overall range of movement in the sagittal plan (flexion and extension) approximates 90 degrees, with about three fourths due to extension. About 10 degrees of flexion and 25 degrees of extension occur at the atlanto-occipital joints. In this range of movement, the ligaments help protect the spinal cord from damage by the normal, fractured, or dislocated odontoid process. The lower parts of the cervical spine contribute to the remainder of full range in this plane. The maximal range of movement between individual vertebrae occurs between the fourth and fifth vertebrae in young children and between the fifth and sixth vertebrae in teenagers and adults. The total range of rotation of the head and neck encompasses 80 to 90 degrees. Approximately 35 to 45 degrees occurs at the atlantoaxial joint and is associated with a screwing movement of the upper vertebra on the lower vertebra, a movement that reduces the cross-sectional area of the spinal canal. Lateral flexion does not occur in isolation but accompanies some rotation. There usually is about 30 degrees of lateral mobility on both

Table 27–3. AGE AND THE NORMAL CERVICAL SPINE MOTION

Age (yr)	Flexion–Extension (degrees)	Lateral Rotation (degrees)	Lateral Flexion (degrees)
<30	90	90	45
31–50	70	90	45
>50	60	90	30

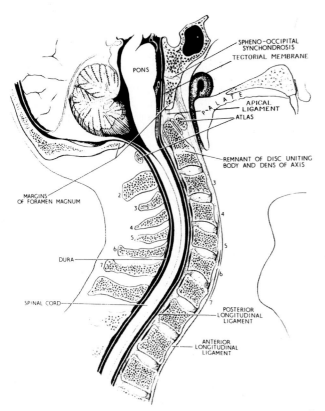

Figure 27–2. Sagittal view of the lower head and neck to show the relationship of the spinal cord and brainstem to the bones, ligaments, and joints between the bodies of the cervical vertebrae. The cervical lordosis can be seen as well as the relationship of the anterior and posterior longitudinal ligaments to intervertebral discs and the ligaments at the craniovertebral junction.

sides in the lower cervical spine. The spinal canal shortens on the side of the concavity of the spine and lengthens on the side of the convexity.

With age, the nucleus pulposus becomes vulnerable to acute and chronic trauma. With loss of disc substance, the annulus fibrosus may bulge into the spinal canal, and because of its eccentric position, the nucleus pulposus tends to prolapse backward if any tear develops in the annulus fibrosus. The most common sites for both types of herniation are the mobile regions (i.e., C5-6 and C6-7). With degenerative changes, the disc space narrows and the spinal column shortens. The intervertebral foramina become narrowed, movements become restricted, and unusual mechanical strains on the synovial joints result. These changes may be confined to a localized area or may become widespread in generalized degenerative disease. The formation of osteophytes leads to encroachment on the spinal canal and intervertebral foramina. The canal may also be further narrowed by bulging of the ligamentum flavum. Changes in the caliber of the vertebral arteries can result because of the degenerative changes in the joints of the cervical spine. Arterial branches that supply joints and nervous tissue can be distorted at rest and further obstructed with movement. With severe vertebral artery

stenosis, syncope occasionally results from rotation of the head.

The lower six cervical vertebrae articulate with each other at five points, two zygapophyseal and two uncovertebral (neurocentral) joints and one intervertebral disc. The upper two cervical vertebrae articulate at the odontoid peg, the two zygapophyseal joints and the intervertebral joint. The former are synovial joints and can be affected by various arthritic diseases and by the natural forces of the aging process. The articular cartilage may suffer from a synovitis that thins the articular cartilage and exposes the underlying bone to the disease process. If the repair process can outpace the destruction, normal bone will be laid down. If the destruction prevents this, disordered articular bone will be laid down in the form of osteophytes. The uncovertebral joints have no articular cartilage or synovial membrane and are pseudoarthroses. They are not affected by arthritis in the true sense, but their reaction to attrition ultimately leads to osteophyte formation without synovitis. All the joints are supplied with sensory nerves and nutrient vessels on the segmental basis as well as with sympathetic pain fibers. Pain from these joints is non-neurologic and felt locally; it is derived mostly from the joint capsule rather than the synovium or bone. Articular cartilage in all joints is avascular and aneural and cannot give rise to pain. The LF and interspinous ligaments are also insensitive to pain. The PL ligament is sensitive to stretch through the fibers of the recurrent meningeal nerve of Luschka and can give rise to midline non-neuralgic pain. The AL ligament is pain sensitive, but the nerve supply is still not fully defined.

The emerging nerve root is invested in dura to the outer border of the intervertebral foramina and is also supplied by the recurrent meningeal nerve. If the dura and its nerve are stretched, the accompanying nutrient vessels can be narrowed and promptly cause ischemic neuralgic pain. The production of upper limb neuralgia, with or without paresthesias, by stretching the arm at the shoulder can lead to an incorrect diagnosis of local joint or soft tissue pain. The nerve root is anchored firmly to the intervertebral foramina by the dura and does not glide in or out of the dura or the intervertebral foramina during movement of the neck. The dura accordians on extension and unfolds and tightens on flexion, placing traction on the nerve root and blood supply. Because the nerve root fills only about one fifth of the intervertebral foramina, it follows that cervicobrachial neuralgia is more commonly due to irritation, inflammation, and ischemia than to physical compression. As it leaves the intervertebral foramina, the nerve root is bounded above and below by the two vertebra pedicles, medially by the uncovertebral joint and laterally by the zygapophyseal joint. Involvement of these joints is the most common cause of cervicobrachial neuralgia.

The main load-bearing structure of the neck is the intervertebral disc, and the uncovertebral and zygapophyseal joints evolved as limiters of movement to protect the spinal cord rather than as load bearers.

The intervertebral disc consists of a tough fibroelastic envelope that has a blood supply and can therefore undergo repair. It has a nerve supply that is highly sensitive to stretching, and discogenic pain is non-neuralgic and felt locally. The nucleus pulposus has no nerve supply; this desiccation is painless. As it dries out, it loses volume; as it loses volume, it loses height. Because the nucleus pulposus is incompressible, the annulus fibrosis bulges under pressure from the head above. These changes are physiologic and not necessarily pathologic. As the disc loses height, it places increased pressure on the uncovertebral and zygapophyseal joints, which are now converted into load-bearing joints, a function for which they are not designed. Because these joints have a surface area inadequate for the imposed pressure, they become irritated. The irritation can lead to inflammatory disease, and attempts to repair the joints can cause the formation of osteophytes. The emerging roots get caught up in the inflammation, which can also cause perineural fibrosis and microvascular obliteration.

Mere bony changes do not necessarily correspond with the segmental level of neurologic damage. Two reasons exist for this:

1. The disproportionate growth of the spinal cord and column: The first thoracic segment of the spinal cord lies opposite the seventh cervical vertebra (see Fig. 27–2), and upper rootlets of the lower cervical and first thoracic nerves cross over two intervertebral discs, whereas the lower rootlets of these two nerves normally cross over only one disc.

2. Severe degeneration of the discs may shorten the vertebral canal to such an extent that the spinal cord, which remains unaltered in length, drops down relative to the bones. The spinal nerve roots may then become acutely folded as they travel toward the inter-vertebral foramina, the lowest roots becoming the most severely affected.

Familiarity with the distribution of sensory, motor, and autonomic components in segmental nerves is necessary for localization of neurologic segments in the clinical examination (Fig. 27–3, Table 27–4). For practical purposes, the lower fibers of the cervical plexus supply the top of the shoulder; C5 and C6 nerve roots supply the lateral side of the arm and forearm; C6, C7, and C8 nerve roots innervate the hand; and C8 extends into the forearm. The T1 segment innervates the medial side of the arm and forearm. Visceral pain can be referred in some instances to well-defined segmental areas (Fig. 27–4); for example, pain at the point of the shoulder (C3-4) may be associated with acute cholecystitis. The segmental supplies of individual muscles are listed in Table 27–4.

Nerve Root Compression

A radicular nerve normally occupies 20 to 25 percent of the intervertebral foramen. There may be considerable variation in the anatomy of the lower cervical nerves and their root pouches, and with increasing age, they become relatively fixed and vulnerable to damage. Two types of disc lesions cause pressure on the radicular nerves or nerve roots: a dorsolateral protrusion that does not invade the intervertebral foramina but compresses the intrameningeal nerve roots against the vertebral laminae, and an intraforaminal protrusion from the uncinate part of the disc that compresses the radicular nerve against the articular process. The extent of root compression depends on the angulation of the radicular nerve and its location in the foramen, as well as the size and position

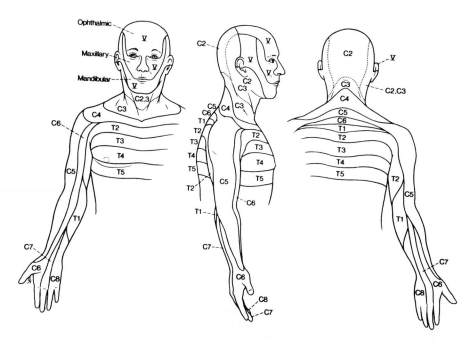

Figure 27–3. Dermatome distribution of nerve fibers from C1 through T5 carrying senses of pain, heat, cold, vibration, and touch to the head, neck, arm, hand, and thoracic area. The sclerotomes and myotomes are similar but with some overlap. Pain arising from structures deep to the deep fascia (myotome and sclerotome) do not precisely follow the dermatome distribution.

Table 27–4. NERVES AND TESTS OF PRINCIPAL MUSCLES

Nerve	Nerve Roots	Muscle	Test
Accessory	Spinal	Trapezius	Elevation of shoulders
			Abduction of scapula
	Spinal	Sternocleidomastoid	Tilting of head to same side with rotation to opposite side
Brachial plexus		Pectoralis major	
	C5, C6	Clavicular part	Adduction of arm
	C7, C8, T1	Sternocostal part	Adduction, forward depression of arm
	C5, C6, C7	Serratus anterior	Fixation of scapula during forward thrusting of the arm
	C4, C5	Rhomboid	Elevation and fixation of scapula
	C4, C5, C6	Supraspinatus	Initiate abduction arm
	(C4), C5, C6	Infraspinatus	External rotation arm
	C6, C7, C8	Latissimus dorsi	Adduction of horizontal, externally rotated arm, coughing
Axillary	C5, C6	Deltoid	Lateral and forward elevation of arm to horizontal
Musculocutaneous	C5, C6	Biceps	Flexion of supinated forearm
		Brachialis	
Radial	C6, C7, C8	Triceps	Extension of forearm
	C5, C6	Brachioradialis	Flexion of semiprone forearm
	C6, C7	Extensor carpi radialis longus	Extension of wrist to radial side
Posterior interosseous	C5, C6	Supinator	Supination of extended forearm
	C7, C8	Extensor digitorum	Extension of proximal phalanges
	C7, C8	Extensor carpi ulnaris	Extension of wrist to ulnar side
	C7, C8	Extensor indicis	Extension of proximal phalanx of index finger
	C7, C8	Abductor pollicis longus	Abduction of first metacarpal in plane at right angle to palm
	C7, C8	Extensor pollicis longus	Extension of first interphalangeal joint
	C7, C8	Extensor pollicis brevis	Extension of first metacarpophalangeal joint
Median	C6, C7	Pronator teres	Pronation of extended forearm
	C6, C7	Flexor carpi radialis	Flexion of wrist to radial side
	C7, C8, T1	Flexor digitorum superficialis	Flexion of middle phalanges
	C8, T1	Flexor digitorum profundus (lateral part)	Flexion of terminal phalanges, index and middle fingers
	C8, T1	Flexor pollicis longus (anterior interosseous nerve)	Flexion of distal phalanx, thumb
	C8, T1	Abductor pollicis brevis	Abduction of first metacarpal in plane at right angle to palm
	C8, T1	Flexor pollicis brevis	Flexion of proximal phalanx, thumb
	C8, T1	Opponens pollicis	Opposition of thumb against 5th finger
	C8, T1	1st and 2nd lumbricals	Extension of middle phalanges while proximal phalanges are fixed in extension
Ulnar	C7, C8	Flexor carpi ulnaris	Observation of tendons while testing abductor digiti minimi
	C8, T1	Flexor digitorum profundus (medial part)	Flexion of distal phalanges of ring and little fingers
	C8, T1	Hypothenar muscles	Abduction and opposition of little finger
	C8, T1	3rd and 4th lumbricals	Extension of middle phalanges while proximal phalanges are fixed in extension
	C8, T1	Adductor pollicis	Adduction of thumb against palmar surface of index finger
	C8, T1	Flexor pollicis brevis	Flexion of proximal phalanx, thumb
	C8, T1	Interossei	Abduction and adduction of fingers

of the protrusion. Marginal lipping of the vertebrae and narrowing of the discs lead to secondary osteophyte formation of the articular processes and consequent posterolateral narrowing of the foramen.

Blood Supply

Variations in the pattern of blood vessels in the cervical spinal cord exist, but the main blood supply comes through a few major articular arteries. The anterior and posterior spinal arteries act more as connecting links than as main channels of blood. The blood supply to the spinal cord may be impaired in patients with cervical spondylosis when one or more radicular arteries become compressed. The resultant ischemia may be either continuous or intermittent, and sometimes the maximal impairment occurs only when the head is in a certain position (usually extension). The vertebral arteries vary in size, and one (usually the left) may be larger than the other. The vertebral arteries lie within the vertebral canal, on

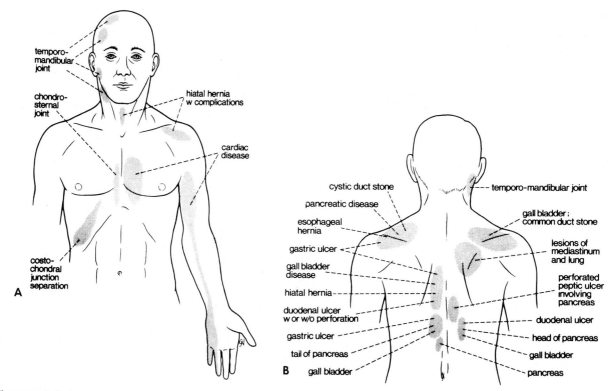

Figure 27–4. Patterns of reflexly referred pain from visceral and somatic structures. Anterior distribution *(A)*; posterior distribution *(B)*.

their medial aspect closely related to the neurocentral joint, and pass immediately anterior to the emerging cervical nerve roots. Each nerve root receives a small arterial branch. Spondylotic changes of the cervical vertebrae may displace the artery laterally and, in severe cases, posteriorly as well. The degree of displacement depends on the size and position of the body prominence that arises as a result of spondylosis.

Atheroma of the vertebral artery also may be important in the production of symptoms. Cerebellar infarction may result from a critical reduction of blood flow to the vertebral artery in the neck. When the blockage occurs in the cervical part of the vertebral artery, the cerebellar infarcts tend to be bilateral, approximately symmetric, and in the territory of the superior cerebellar artery. Most often, the obstruction is incomplete, and blood flow is reduced only when the patient turns or extends the head. Rotation and extension of the head to one side can obstruct the contralateral vertebral artery, and in patients with atherosclerosis, rotation and extension of the head can produce posterior circulation abnormalities such as nystagmus, vertigo, weakness, dysarthria, drop attacks, and the Babinski response. An anterior spinal artery–spinal cord syndrome results from either compromise of the anterior spinal artery or compression of one of the main radicular arteries by osteophytes or adhesions associated with nerve root-sleeve fibrosis. In diseases that involve the major blood vessels (e.g., arteriosclerosis, diabetes, syphilis), the blood

supply of the spinal cord may be impaired, especially if the condition is associated with spondylosis.

CLINICAL EVALUATION

The essential means in the diagnosis and management of cervical pain include patient history and the general physical and neurologic examinations. Radiologic study plus neuroimaging and neurophysiologic procedures assist in confirming the clinical formulation. It is often best to group the symptoms into functional units.

Pain

Pain is the most common symptom of cervical spine disorders (Fig. 27–5). Clinically, the approach to pain is to define it in terms of type of onset, distribution, frequency, constancy versus intermittency, duration, quality, association with neurologic symptoms and signs, localization, and various associated features. Cervical nerve root irritation causes well-localized areas of pain (see Fig. 27–3), whereas poorly defined areas of pain arise from irritation of deep connective tissue structures, muscle, joint, bone, or disc. The patient's ability to describe the pain provides the examiner with essential clues to diagnosis. Retro-orbital, temporal, and occipital pain reflects a referral pattern from the atlas, axis, C3, and their

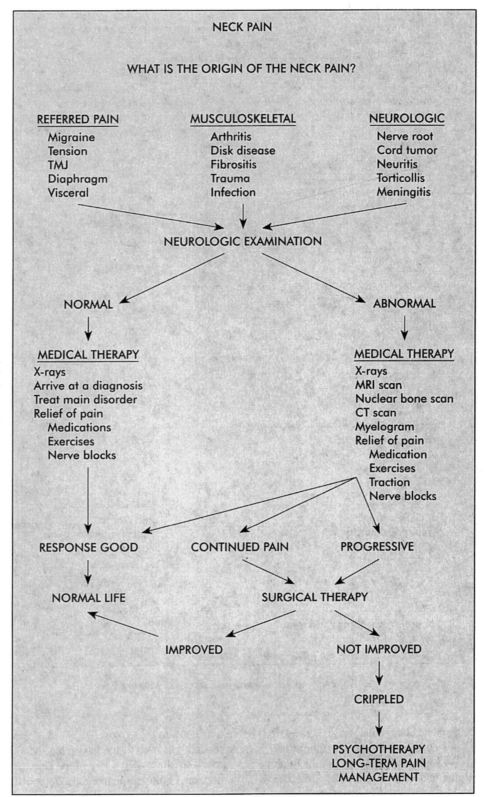

Figure 27–5. Neck pain algorithm for diagnosis and therapy. TMJ, temporomandibular joint; CT, computed tomography; MRI, magnetic resonance imaging. (From Nakano NKK: Neck and back pain. *In* Stein JH (ed): Internal Medicine, 4th ed. St. Louis: Mosby, 1994, pp 1033–1041).

surrounding structures. In cervical spine disorders, pain may radiate to the upper thoracic spine, shoulder, or scapular regions or into one or both upper limbs. Additionally, this pain may be produced, relieved, or exaggerated by various normal movements of the cervical spine. The areas of pain designation may be tender (i.e., transverse process spinous process, apophyseal joints, or anterior vertebral bodies). Sensory symptoms can be classed as somatic and autonomic, with the somatic complaints being the most common.

Somatic pain due to nerve root irritation is appreciated by the sufferer in two distinct forms, which often coexist. Neuralgic pain is caused by irritation of the dorsal sensory root. It is experienced as a "lightning" or "electric" sensation and is referred to dermatomal areas. It is felt mainly in the upper limb, scapula, and the trapezius ridge, and is often associated with numbness or paresthesias. It is common for the pain to be felt more proximally and the paresthesias to be felt more distally, but the two usually overlap. Myalgic pain is caused by irritation of the ventral motor root. It is experienced as a deep, boring, unpleasant sensation, which is frequently poorly localized because it is referred to sclerotomal areas. The sensory topography of the ventral root myalgic pain therefore conforms somewhat to the muscles supplied by that root, whereas dorsal root neuralgic pain conforms more with the territory of the peripheral nerves supplied by that root. Neuralgic and myalgic pains are not always felt in precise anatomic zones, because muscle groups and bordering areas of skin have overlapping sensory supplies; also, pain can radiate up or down a spinal segment by recruitment within the spinal column.

Paresthesias

Numbness and tingling follow the segmental distribution of the nerve roots (see Fig. 27–3) in cervical spine disorders; however, these symptoms often occur without demonstrable sensory change. Paresthesias that involve the face, head, or tongue suggest involvement of the upper three nerve roots of the cervical plexus, whereas numbness of the neck, shoulders, arm, forearms, and fingers indicates involvement of the C5 to T1 nerve roots. Sensory root involvement can also produce numbness, which is usually incomplete and often experienced as a feeling of swelling or soddenness that can inadvertently be accepted and then misinterpreted as soft tissue swelling. Complete numbness is more likely to be accompanied by signs of sensory loss and indicates a more serious nerve or root lesion.

Weakness

Muscular weakness, hypotonia, and fasciculation indicate a lower motor neuron disorder secondary to an anterior radiculopathy. More than one root innervates a given muscle, and the appearance of muscle weakness and atrophy suggests dysfunction of several roots. Pain and guarding produce functional weakness. On the other hand, a motor deficit may elicit sensory symptoms—a feeling of heaviness of the limbs. Motor symptoms are usually vague and consist of complaints of clumsiness or unexpectedly dropping things, early fatigue, or a sensation of insufficient power or gripping. A pseudomotor symptom is loss of coordination of power, and in this instance, the problem is sensory and due to disordered proprioception with often partial numbness.

Autonomic Symptoms

Autonomic symptoms are not as common but can be most distressing physically and are often dismissed as emotional or functional. The patient may complain of a feeling of flushing or coldness due to vasomotor instability or even Raynaud's phenomenon. Tachycardia or faintness, dysphagia, blurred vision, lacrimation, eye pain, drooping eyelids, and migraine can all lead to misdiagnosis.

Articular Symptoms

Articular symptoms are felt in the joints and can be grouped as articular and pseudoarticular. Articular symptoms arise from the neck owing to the underlying pathology and include local pain, stiffness made worse with disuse and in bed, grating, clicking, and a feeling of "sand" in the neck. Pseudoarticular symptoms are felt in the shoulder and elbow as the result of referred pain and of the gelling effect on muscles that accompanies myalgic sensory pain. Stiffness with consequent limitation of motion of the neck, shoulder, elbow, wrist, and even fingers may occur subsequent to injury response, articular involvement, nerve root irritation, or reflex sympathetic dystrophy. Tenosynovitis and tendinitis often accompany syndromes of the cervical spine and may involve the rotator cuff, tendons about the wrist or hand with stenosis or fibrosis of tendon sheaths, and palmar fascia. To further complicate matters, these symptoms are often accompanied by trigger zones over the affected joints, which give rise to the false impression of local pathology in the joints, ligaments, tendons, or muscles.

Vascular Symptoms

Vascular symptoms are related to the underlying cause and not specifically to the nerve root irritation. Compression of the vertebral arteries by osteophytes or a prolapsed disc in the bony vertebral canals can intensify the symptoms on neck movement and also by sleep posture.

Headache and Occipital Neuralgia

Head pain appears commonly and is characteristic of cervical spine disorders; it results from nerve root or sympathetic nerve compression, vertebral artery pressure, autonomic dysfunction, and posterior occipital muscle spasm, as well as osteoarthritic changes of the apophyseal joints of the upper three cervical vertebrae. Occipital headache occurs commonly in the age group in which spondylosis appears and becomes associated with pain in the neck and upper limbs. The pain may, in turn, spread to the eye region and become dull rather than pulsating. It is aggravated by strain, sneeze, and cough, as well as by movements of the head and neck.

Pseudoangina Pectoris

A lesion at C6 and C7 may produce neurologic or myalgic pain with tenderness in the precordium or scapular region, causing confusion with angina pectoris. Pain from C6 and C7 may become compressive, may increase with exercise, may refer down the arm, or may be aggravated by neck movement or be associated with torticollis or muscle spasm in the neck. Differentiation of heart disease from radiculopathy can be done in the presence of other neurologic signs of C6 and C7 dysfunction (e.g., muscle weakness, fasciculation, sensory changes). Difficulty will arise in clinical situations in which true angina and pseudoangina coexist, however.

Eye Symptoms

Blurring of vision relieved by changing neck position, increased tearing, pain in one or both eyes, retroorbital pain, and descriptions of the eyes being "pulled backward" or "pushed forward" may be reported by patients with cervical spine disorders. These symptoms result from irritation of the cervical sympathetic nerve supply to eye structures through the plexuses that surround the vertebral and internal carotid arteries and their branches.

Ear Symptoms

Changes in equilibrium develop with irritation of surrounding sympathetic plexuses, vertebral artery vascular insufficiency, or both. Gait disturbances with or without associated tinnitus and altered auditory acuity result from vascular insufficiency secondary to vasospasm or compression of the vertebral arteries by cervical structures.

Throat Symptoms

Dysphagia results from muscle spasm, anterior osteophyte compression of pharynx esophagus, or abnormalities of cervical cranial nerve and sympathetic communications.

Miscellaneous Symptoms

Occasionally, bizarre symptoms appear in patients with cervical spine disorders. Dyspnea (inability to take a deep breath or get enough air) results from a deficit in C3 to C5 (innervation of the respiratory muscles). Cardiac palpitations and tachycardia associated with unusual positions or hyperextension of the neck appear with irritation of the C4 nerve root, which innervates the diaphragm and pericardium, or of the cardiac sympathetic nerve supply. Nausea and emesis, ill-defined pain, and paresthesias may accompany spinal cord compression. Drop attacks with abrupt loss of proprioception and collapse without loss of consciousness may suggest posterior circulation insufficiency.

CLINICAL EXAMINATION

A general physical and neurologic examination yields objective information from the precise identification of the pain-sensitive structure and the mechanism of pain production. Systematic examination of patients with cervical spine syndromes includes the head, neck, upper thoracic spine, shoulders, arms, forearms, wrists, and hands with the patient fully undressed. The clinician observes the patient's posture, movements, facial expression, gait, and various positions (e.g., sitting, standing, supine). As the patient walks into the office, the clinician observes the patient's head position and how naturally and rhythmically the head and neck move with body movement.

The neck should be inspected for normal anatomic position of the hyoid bone, thyroid cartilage, and thyroid gland, and presence of normal cervical lordosis and scars or pigmentation. Palpation of bony structures in the neck should be done with the patient supine to relax the overlying muscles. To palpate the anterior neck, the examiner stands at the patient's side and supports the neck from behind with one hand, palpating with the other, relaxing the spine as much as possible.

The horseshoe-shaped hyoid bone lies above the thyroid cartilage and is at the level of the C3 vertebra. With the index finger and thumb (pincer-like), the examiner feels the stem of the horseshoe; as the patient swallows, the hyoid bone moves up and then down. The thyroid cartilage possesses a superior notch and a flaring upper portion (at the C4 level), whereas the lower border lies at the C5 level. Below the lower border of the thyroid cartilage, the examiner palpates the first cricoid ring (opposite the C6 vertebra); this is the upper border of the trachea and is just superior to the site of emergency tracheotomy. The cricoid ring moves with swallowing. About 2 to

3 cm lateral to the first cricoid ring, the carotid tubercle, the carotid tubercle, the anterior tubercle of the transverse process of C6, can be felt. The carotid arteries lie adjacent to the tubercle, and their pulsation can be appreciated. The transverse process of C1 lies between the angle of the jaw and the styloid process of the skull. Because it is the broadest transverse process of the cervical spine, palpation is facilitated. Normal anatomic movements of the atlanto-occipital and atlantoaxial joints and bony structures can be appreciated by a lateral sliding movement, holding the atlas between the thumb and index finger by the transverse processes.

The posterior landmarks of the cervical spine include the occiput, inion, superior nuchal line, mastoid process, spinous processes of each vertebra, and apophyseal joints. The examiner palpates the occiput, then the inion, marking the center point of the superior nuchal line (the line feels like a transverse ridge extending outward on both sides of the inion). The round mastoid process sits at the lateral edge of the superior nuchal line (see Fig. 27–1B). The spinous process of the axis (C2) can be palpated below the indented area immediately under the occiput. As each spinous process from C2 to T1 is palpated, the examiner notes the cervical lordosis. The C7 (vertebra prominens) and T1 spinous processes are larger than the others. Alignment of the spinous processes should be recorded. The apophyseal joints can be felt as small, rounded domes deep to the trapezius muscles about 2.5 cm lateral to the spinous processes. To palpate these joints, the patient must be relaxed, since spasm and tension preclude access on examination. The joint involved can be determined by lining up with the hyoid bone at C3, the thyroid cartilage at C4 and C5, and the first cricoid ring at C6. These joints often become tender with osteoarthritis, especially in the upper cervical spine, whereas the C5-6, C6-7 level is most often involved in cervical spondylosis.

Examination of the soft tissues in the neck should be divided into two anatomic areas—anterior and posterior. The anterior portion is bordered laterally by the two sternocleidomastoid muscles, superiorly by the mandible, and inferiorly by the suprasternal notch (an upside-down triangle). The posterior aspect includes the entire area posterior to the lateral border of the sternocleidomastoid muscle. The supine position appears optimal in the examination. The sternocleidomastoid muscle can be examined anteriorly by asking the patient to turn the head to the opposite side; the muscle then stands out and can be palpated from origin to insertion. The opposite muscle can be compared for any discrepancies in size, bulges, or strength. Hyperextension injuries overstretch the muscle with resultant hemorrhage into the tissue. Localized swelling may be due to hematomas. In torticollis, the sternocleidomastoid muscles will be involved. The lymph node chain resides along the medial border of the sternocleidomastoid muscle and normally cannot be palpated. Small, tender lymph nodes can be palpated if enlarged secondary to infections (throat, ear), metastases, or tumor. Enlarged

lymph nodes may, in turn, produce torticollis. The thyroid gland overlies thyroid cartilage in an H pattern, the bar being the isthmus with the two lobes situated laterally. Normally, the thyroid gland is smooth and palpable without enlargement. Diffuse enlargement of the thyroid gland, cysts, or nodules or tenderness from thyroiditis should be recorded. The carotid arteries, best felt near the carotid tubercle on C6, should be examined separately because of the carotid reflex secondary to simultaneous palpation.

Posteriorly, with the patient sitting, the clinician examines the trapezius muscle, lymph nodes, greater occipital nerves, and superior nuchal ligament. The trapezius muscle extends from the inion to the spinous process of T12 and inserts laterally in a continuous arc into the clavicle, the acromion, and the spine of the scapula. The trapezius should be felt from origin to insertion, beginning high on the neck. Flexion injuries may traumatize the trapezius, and hematomas in the muscle occur frequently. Furthermore, the trapezius is the site of focal points of pain and tenderness in fibrositis syndromes. The two trapezius muscles should be palpated bilaterally and simultaneously while assessing for tenderness, lumps, swelling, or asymmetry of the two muscles. The lymph node chain lies at the anterolateral border of the trapezius and normally cannot be palpated. The greater occipital nerves sit laterally to the inion, extending upward in the scalp, and can be easily palpated when tender and inflamed. A flexion–extension injury of the spine commonly produces traumatic inflammation and swelling of the occipital nerves with resultant painful occipital neuralgia, a frequent cause of headache. The superior nuchal ligament arises from the inion and extends to the C7 and T1 spinous processes. It is under the examining finger when the spinous processes are felt and may become tender, irregular, and lumpy if overstretched or injured.

As for the symptoms, the physical signs can be grouped as motor, sensory, autonomic, and articular. This grouping often assists in establishing an ordered approach to the diagnostic process.

Range of Motion

The cervical spine has a large range of motion (see Table 27–3), which in turn provides a wide scope of vision and remains essential to the sense of balance. The basic movements of the neck are flexion, extension, lateral flexion to the right and left, and rotation to the right and left. About half of the total flexion and extension of the neck occurs at the occiput-C1 level, the other half being equally distributed among the other six cervical vertebrae, with a slight increase at the C5-6 level. About half the rotation occurs at the atlantoaxial joint; the other half distributes equally among the other five vertebrae. All vertebrae share in lateral flexion. A decrease in specific motion may occur in the presence of blocking of a joint, pain, fibrous contractures, bony ankylosis, muscle spasm, mechanical alteration in joint and skeletal structures, or a tense and uncooperative patient. Other causes of muscle spasm include injury to muscles, involuntary splinting over painful joints or skeletal structures, and irritation or compression of cervical nerve roots of the spinal cord.

Because of the risk of neurologic trauma to an unstable spine or spinal cord, all range-of-motion testing of the cervical spine should not be performed in cases of acute head or cervical injury or in cases of suspected spinal cord compression. When range-of-motion testing is performed in a patient without these contraindications, it should be done in the following manner:

- Actively and to the extreme of motion (to assess muscle function and strength), as observed by the examiner
- Passively (to assess nonmobile structures, ligaments, capsules, and fascia), as the examiner moves the relaxed cervical spine through all its motions
- Against resistance (to study origin and insertions of tendon and ligaments and to assess motor strength), with each motion maximally attempted against force of the examiner's hand.

Flexion and Extension. The patient nods the head forward and touches the chin to sternum. If one of the examiner's fingers can be placed between the patient's chin and sternum, there is 10 degrees limitation of flexion; this limitation is 30 degrees if three fingers can be inserted within this area. Observation of the cervical spine curve should be done as the examiner instructs the patient to look from floor to ceiling. The arc of neck motion normally remains smooth and is not halting or irregular. In full hyperextension, the base of the occiput normally touches the spinous process of T1.

Lateral Flexion. The patient attempts to touch his or her ear to the shoulder without rotation or shoulder shrugging. Clinically normal people can laterally flex 45 degrees in either direction.

Rotation. The patient rotates the head maximally, usually being able to bring the chin into alignment with the shoulder. Normally, the motion remains smooth, whereas torticollis restricts motion.

Passive Range of Motion. The examiner asks for complete relaxation and takes the patient's head firmly in his or her hands, putting the spine through maximal flexion, extension, lateral flexion, and rotation. Passive motion may be more extensive than active motion if muscles remain stiff and painful or exhibit involuntary spasm.

Motion Against Resistance. All testing of the range of neck motion can be done with the examiner offering firm resistance to each movement. The anchorage of muscle, tendon insertion and origin, muscle strength, and muscular function should be assessed. This phase of the examination should be done with the patient seated. The primary (sternocleidomastoid muscles) and secondary (three scalenes and small prevertebral muscles) flexors of the neck can be assessed by the examiner's placing his or her left hand flat on the patient's upper sternum and placing the right (resisting) hand with the palm cupped on the patient's forehead; the patient then flexes his or her neck, slowly increasing the power to maximal pressure. The primary (paravertebral extensor mass, splenius and semispinalis capitis, and trapezius) and secondary (small intrinsic neck) extensor muscles should be assessed by the examiner's placing his or her left hand over the patient's shoulder (for stability) and placing the right palm (fingers extended) against the side of the patient's head; the patient then laterally flexes against the examiner's resistance. The rotators of the neck (sternocleidomastoid and intrinsic neck muscles) can be tested to right lateral rotation by placing the examiner's stabilizing left hand on the patient's left shoulder and the examiner's right hand along the right side of the patient's mandible, while the patient rotates against resistance. Left rotation is tested in the reverse fashion. Either sternocleidomastoid muscle functioning alone provides the main pull to the side being tested.

Motor Signs

If weakness, hypotonia, and fasciculation coexist, the clinician suspects a lower motor neuron disease, whereas weakness, hyperreflexia, and spasticity suggest an upper motor neuron disorder. Weakness of the muscles may be difficult to assess because innervation of the shoulder girdle, arm, forearm, and muscles occurs by two or more nerve roots (see Table 27–4). Wasting of muscles is uncommonly due to nerve root irritation and usually indicates either a nerve lesion or disuse atrophy. The distribution of the localized wasting and abnormal reflexes indicates the structure and the level in which the lesion resides. Wasting with vasomotor changes indicates an autonomic dystrophy. Muscular weakness has many possible causes; to narrow the choice down to one or a few, the physician must ascertain the anatomic localization of the patient's complaints.

Reflexes

Reflexes indicate the state of the nervous system and its afferent pathways (Table 27–5). Certain abnormal reflexes appear only with spasticity and paralysis; these indicate injury to the corticospinal tract. The primary deep tendon reflexes, abdominal reflexes, and plantar responses should be routinely examined; bulbocavernosus and anal reflexes should be tested in all suspected lower spinal cord (conus or cauda equina) lesions and in cases of sphincter disturbances. In eliciting the deep tendon reflexes, adequate relaxation of the patient and a mild degree of passive tension on the muscle become essential, especially in the radial (supinator) and ankle jerks. The examiner varies the tension on the muscle by manipulating the

Table 27–5. RELATION OF REFLEXES TO PERIPHERAL NERVES AND SPINAL CORD SEGMENTS

Reflex	Site and Mode of Elicitation	Response	Muscle(s)	Peripheral Nerve(s)	Cord Segment
Scapulohumeral reflex	Tap on lower end of medial border of scapula	Adduction and lateral rotation of dependent arm	Infraspinatus and teres minor	Suprascapular (axillary)	C4 to C6
Biceps jerk	Tap on tendon of biceps brachii	Flexion at elbow	Biceps brachii	Musculocutaneous	C5 and C6
Supinator jerk (also called radial reflex)	Tap on distal end of radius	Flexion at elbow	Brachioradialis (and biceps brachii and brachialis)	Radial (musculo-cutaneous)	C5 and C6
Triceps jerk	Tap on tendon of triceps brachii above olecranon, with elbow flexed	Extension at elbow	Triceps brachii	Radial	C7 and C8
Thumb reflex	Tap on tendon of flexor pollicis longus in distal third of forearm	Flexion of terminal phalanx of thumb	Flexor pollicis longus	Median	C6 to C8
Extensor finger and hand jerk	Tap on posterior aspect of wrist just proximal to radiocarpal joint	Extension of hand and fingers (inconstant)	Extensor of hand and fingers	Radial	C6 to C8
Flexor finger jerk	Tap on examiner's thumb placed on palm of hand; sharp tap on tips of flexed fingers (Trömner's sign)	Flexion of fingers	Flexor digitorum superficialis (and profundus)	Median	C7 and C8 (T1)
Epigastric reflex (exteroceptive)	Brisk stroking of skin downward from nipple in mamillary line	Retraction of epigastrium	Transversus abdominis	Intercostal	T5 and T6
Abdominal skin reflex (exteroceptive)	Brisk stroking of skin or abdominal wall in lateromedial direction	Shift of skin of abdomen and displacement of umbilicus	Muscles of abdominal wall	Intercostal, hypogastric, and ilioinguinal	T6 and T12
Cremasteric reflex (exteroceptive)	Stroking skin on medial aspect of thigh (pinching adductor muscles)	Elevation of testis	Cremaster	Genital branch of genitofemoral	L2 and L3 (L1)
Adductor reflex	Tap on medial condyle of femur	Adduction of leg	Adductors of thigh	Obturator	L2, L3, and L4
Knee jerk	Tap on tendon of quadriceps femoris below patella	Extension at knee	Quadriceps femoris	Femoral	(L2), L3, and L4
Gluteal reflex (exteroceptive)	Stroking skin over gluteal region	Tightening of buttock (inconstant)	Gluteus medius and gluteus maximus	Superior and inferior gluteal	L4, L5, and S1
Posterior tibial reflex	Tap on tendon of tibialis posterior behind medial malleolus	Supination of foot (inconstant)	Tibialis posterior	Tibial	L5
Semimembranosus and semitendinosus reflex	Tap on medial hamstring tendons (patient prone and knee slightly flexed)	Contraction of semimembranosus and semitendinosus muscles	Semimembranosus and semitendinosus	Sciatic	S1
Biceps femoris reflex	Tap on lateral hamstring tendon (patient prone and knee slightly flexed)	Contraction of biceps femoris	Biceps femoris	Sciatic	S1 and S2
Ankle jerk	Tap on tendon calcaneus	Plantar flexion of foot	Triceps surae and other flexors of foot	Tibial	S1 and S2
Bulbocavernosus reflex (exteroceptive)	Gentle squeezing of glans penis or pinching of skin of dorsum of penis	Contraction of bulbocavernosus muscle, palpable at root of penis	Bulbocavernosus	Pudendal	S3 and S4
Anal reflex (exteroceptive)	Scratch or prick of perianal skin (patient lying on side)	Visible contraction of anus	Sphincter ani externus	Pudendal	S5

joint, and reinforcement procedures enable the patient to relax completely, as by pulling one of his or her hands with the other (Jendrassik's maneuver). The tendon jerk normally occurs in only a part of each muscle, and in a myopathy, the reflex jerk may be lost in the quadriceps through wasting in the vastus internus, although the power of contraction of the remainder persists to a fair degree. Some clinically normal people show reduced reflexes, and before the examiner completes the assessment, he or she should ascertain whether other evidence of peripheral nerve (e.g., sensory loss, atrophy) or muscle disease exists.

Sensory Signs

Sensory signs include numbness, hyperalgesia, hyperpathia, and pain produced by compression, tapping, or stretching an involved nerve. Hyperalgesia is a heightened appreciation of pain, and hyperpathia is an appreciation of pain in response to a non-noxious stimulus. The physician should test both the entire upper limbs and the neck and be prepared to test and reexamine any nonanatomic distributions of sensory loss and to match the findings with known areas of distribution. In the presence of nerve root irritation, the entire peripheral nerve supplied by that nerve root can be hyperirritable. It is therefore not surprising that (for example) nerve root irritation at the level of C6 or C7 can rise to a positive brachial plexus stretch test result and a positive carpal tunnel compression test result, giving rise to the "double crush" syndrome.[17] From this, it follows that it is imperative to locate the upper level of the likely site of pathology.

Autonomic Signs

Autonomic signs are rare and can be grouped as vascular and dystrophic. To diagnose reflex sympathetic dystrophy in the absence of clear dystrophy signs is inappropriate and leads to erroneous and excessive treatment and an unduly glum prognosis. Vascular changes produce a local maldistribution of tissue perfusion that causes the skin first to become mottled blue or red. The skin will be either unduly warm or cold, and sudomotor changes produce excessive sweating or dryness. The changes can be paradoxical to normal physiology, with skin being either warm, red, and dry, or cold, pale, and sweaty. Dystrophic signs herald the next stage, with changes in hair over the site followed by glazing and thinning of the skin and loss of subcutaneous tissue. In time, and in extreme cases, the underlying joints become stiff and sore; very rarely, the entire area becomes atrophic leading to contractures.

Articular Signs

Articular signs are found relating to the underlying disease and to reflex sympathetic dystrophy, if present. The most common neck findings are restriction of movement, which may be painless, followed by pain on movement and local tenderness. The examiner may feel or even hear crepitus. A loud click may occur just once and indicates either a facet malalignment or an obstructing osteophyte. In degenerative diseases, lateral flexion is the earliest and most impaired movement; in rheumatoid arthritis, however, the first motion impaired is rotation as a result of early involvement of the synovium around the odontoid peg. A uniformly stiff neck should raise suspicion of diffuse idiopathic skeletal hyperostosis (DISH), ankylosing spondylosis, or recent trauma to the neck. The rest of the vertebral column and peripheral joints must be examined for evidence of further arthritis, and a search for extra-articular manifestations should complete the clinical assessment.

INVESTIGATIONS

The investigation of patients experiencing neck pain is constructed to evaluate the origin of the symptoms and signs, the extent of the lesion, and whether medical or surgical treatment is required. Investigations can be grouped as radiographic and neuroimaging, neurophysiologic, and laboratory studies.

Radiographic and Neuroimaging Examination

Radiographs are essential in the evaluation of a patient with a spine disorder. Clinicians should assess both the clinical and radiographic studies of their patients and not depend solely on the opinion of radiologists. Clinical correlation is necessary because gross radiologic signs and abnormalities may be associated with minimal or no clinical disturbance, whereas the reverse situation (minimal radiographic change in the presence of neurologic signs) may also occur. Routine radiographic views include (1) anteroposterior (AP) view of the atlas and axis through the open mouth; (2) AP view of the lower five vertebrae; (3) lateral views in flexion, neutral position, and extension; and (4) both right and left oblique views. Unless the junction of C7-T1 can be adequately visualized on the cross-table lateral view, a swimmer's view is often performed. After fractures and subluxations have been excluded in patients with trauma who have these nonstressed views, spinal stability may be evaluated with stressed-view radiographs in a flexion–extension series.[18] The bones should be examined, particularly for osteoporosis. The joints might reveal osteophytes with or without encroachment of the foramina or even the erosions of systemic arthritis. One must not neglect to look for congenital abnormalities, such as vertebral fusion. Ligamentous calcification might indicate degeneration, trauma, ankylosing spondylitis, or DISH. Instability in the action views might be due to trauma (such as an athletic injury) but is far more often due to constitutional ligament laxity in an unfit individual. Signs of previous surgery might give a clue to the nature of the problem.

Neuroimaging studies include computed tomography (CT), magnetic resonance imaging (MRI), and radionuclide bone scans. MRI combines the best features of these conventional techniques; it can display vertebrae, intervertebral discs, the thecal space, neural elements, blood vessels, and paraspinal structures without the use of radiographic or intravenous or intrathecal contrast agents.[19–21] Patients who undergo spinal MRI should be evaluated with at least two pulse sequences, a combination of a T1- and a T2-weighted technique.[20] Sagittal images are supplemented with axial slices through the level of clinical interest. MRI is the preferred method for the evaluation of suspected cervical radiculopathy, spinal stenosis, congenital anomalies (particularly Chiari malformations), syringomyelia, cord neoplasm, multiple sclerosis, and early disc degeneration. CT and MRI are about equivalent in the evaluation of extramedullary spinal tumors and trauma.[22, 23] Certain acutely traumatized patients must be excluded from MRI because of accompanying life support apparatus. In an unstable patient, CT remains the imaging test of choice, given MRI's limitations in terms of examination length and lack of adequate patient access. CT also assesses the specific details of osseous injuries better than does MRI. The initial imaging evaluation of a patient with cervical spine trauma is conducted with plain radiographs to detect gross fractures or dislocations. MRI has revolutionized the role of imaging in the management of patients with cervical spine injuries and spinal cord deficits. Furthermore, MRI is unique in its ability to directly delineate spinal cord injuries with the display of contusion, hematomas, lacerations, and traumatic syrinx. Additionally, MRI can portray precise locations and causes of epidural impingement on the spinal cord, including osteophytes, calcified ligaments, acutely or chronically herniated intervertebral discs, and epidural hematoma. While injury to supporting ligaments of the cervical spine can often be inferred by mechanism of injury, MRI can directly demonstrate avulsion, stripping, or disruption of ligamentous structures.[22] MRI and CT are not mutually exclusive; ideally, both studies should be performed, particularly if surgical intervention is being considered.

Radioisotope bone scans are best used for the evaluation of a possible inflammatory joint disease or metabolic disorder of the bone. It is sometimes helpful to do a full-body study in these cases and to perform radiography (and, at times, tomography) on the areas of increased uptake that might help in the overall evaluation of the patient. Three-phase studies can be helpful in the diagnosis and follow-up of reflex sympathetic vasomotor disorder and reflex sympathetic dystrophy.

Neurophysiology (Electrodiagnostic Studies)

Neurophysiology can be used to distinguish sensory and motor dysfunction of the peripheral nerves.[24] It can also be used to distinguish a lesion in the periphery from a nerve root lesion, by combining electromyography (EMG), nerve conduction studies, and somatosensory evoked responses.[25] Additionally, EMG and nerve conduction studies can be used to differentiate normal conditions from a diffuse polyneuropathy, focal entrapment neuropathy, radiculopathy, myopathy, disorder of the neuromuscular junction (e.g., myasthenia gravis), and anterior horn cell disease (e.g., amyotrophic lateral sclerosis). No single feature of the EMG provides a diagnosis (except true myotonia); rather, it requires the combined information of needle EMG coupled with nerve conduction studies and somatosensory evoked responses, as well as the clinical examination as performed by an experienced physician.

Continuous intraoperative somatosensory evoked response monitoring appears to be a practical tool for monitoring scoliosis and cervical surgery.[26] Such monitoring of cervical surgery for disc disease, spinal stenosis, spondylosis, and ossification of the posterior longitudinal ligament can be used to evaluate the integrity of the spinal cord. The complexity of interpreting somatosensory evoked response changes during surgical monitoring can be encountered by defined physiologic effects of anesthetics.

Dynamic posturography is a new neurophysiologic tool to assess the presence of vertigo of cervical origin.[27] Dynamic posturography on the sway-referenced forceplate demonstrated lower equilibrium scores in patients with vertigo or unsteadiness than in controls when recorded in neutral position of the head, in rotation, and in lateral flexion.[27] In addition, the patients with vertigo also show lower equilibrium scores in the position most prone to elicit vertigo or unsteadiness as compared with patients with only neck pain.

Cervical discography as a diagnostic method using reproduced pain appears to be unreliable for diagnosing symptomatic disk levels.[28, 29] Moreover, the investigation of neck pain by discography alone or by zygapophyseal blocks alone constitutes an inadequate approach to neck pain that fails to identify most patients whose symptoms stem from multiple elements in the three-joint complexes of the neck.[29]

Laboratory Studies

The clinical laboratory offers some help in the diagnosis and management of neck pain in specific diseases (e.g., rheumatoid arthritis hyperparathyroidism, human immunodeficiency virus–related conditions, multiple myeloma, ankylosing spondylitis, or certain metastatic malignant cancers). Cerebrospinal fluid evaluation should be done in patients with neck pain who are suspected of having infection (meningitis, meningismus) or subarachnoid hemorrhage; in the latter conditions, the cerebrospinal fluid is diagnostic.

DIFFERENTIAL DIAGNOSIS

Many clinical conditions that arise outside the cervical spine but that are perceived in or about the neck area mimic cervical nerve root irritation, muscle spasm, ligament strain, bone disease, or joint disorder. Although Table 27–1 lists multiple structures potentially causing neck pain, clinical evaluation usually differentiates between the entities. Table 27–2 summarizes various cervical spine syndromes and the associated pathogenic process.

Disorders of somatic or visceral structures that have cervical nerve root innervation (same embryologic origin) cause pain that is felt in the neck. Because these areas constitute reflexively referred pain along the segmental distribution of the nerve roots, such areas of referral are not tender on deep palpation. Areas of superficial peripheral tenderness develop because of reflex or direct sympathetic irritation secondary to vasomotor changes. Referred painful areas do not have muscle spasm and often are described as experiencing a burning or cramping sensation. Nausea, emesis, and pallor may accompany this type of pain. The visceral causes of neck and arm pain can be excluded by the history. For example, esophageal pain is usually related to food and can be promptly relieved by a liquid antacid. Cardiac pain is usually exertional and should respond to sublingual nitroglycerin. Neither of these pains is associated with paresthesias or numbness or is influenced by neck or arm posture. Shoulder pain radiates to the deltoid area; in severe cases, however, the brachial plexus can be irritated as it passes in proximity to the joint and may cause pain in the arm with paresthesias. This pain does not radiate into the neck, and examination of the shoulder usually reveals the lesion. Neck pain can cause secondary shoulder muscle tension, which can give a false impression of a local arthritis or capsulitis.

Peripheral neuropathy may produce pain both proximal as well as distal to the irritative site. With peripheral neuropathy, there is no muscle spasm. Spinal cord tumor produces a poorly localized and ill-defined neck pain, hyperreflexia, and spasticity; immobilization does not relieve the pain, and deep tenderness and local muscle spasms are absent. Furthermore, in spinal cord lesions, paralysis or weakness exists below the cord level (not dermatome) associated with sensory changes and Babinski's signs. Cerebral or subarachnoid hemorrhage, meningitis, head and neck trauma, or a central tumor produces cervical spine pain that mimics cervical spine syndromes that result in nerve root irritation. In these instances, the clinical examination, MRI scan, and cerebrospinal fluid studies differentiate among the various conditions.

Neck pain may occur in malingerers, depressed persons, patients seeking compensation, psychoneurotic individuals, and victims of motor vehicle accidents.[30–33] If these patients possess no concomitant nerve root irritation, they derive no relief from local anesthesia injected into the painful areas. Absence of muscle spasm, an antalgic position, and feigning limitation of motion should arouse the examiner's suspicion.

Skilled clinical elicitation of historical data and physical and neurologic examination constitute the principal and most reproducible means of differential diagnosis (see Fig. 27–5). In evaluating a patient with neck pain, the examiner soon realizes that there may be a syndrome of neck pain alone, head and neck pain, neck and shoulder pain, shoulder pain alone, shoulder and arm pain, or just arm, forearm, hand, or finger pain. Symptoms of altered sensation and vascular insufficiency often accompany the complaint of neck pain. Symptoms or signs in the head and upper cervical spine arise only from structures at the C1 to C4 level. An unusual example of this fact is the "crowned dens" syndrome[34] in which the patient experiences acute neck pain followed by headache that is associated with calcification surrounding the odontoid process. Rarely, canal stenosis at the level of the atlas can present with muscular weakness and wasting of the upper limbs and spastic paresis of the lower limbs.[35] Symptoms in the lower neck, shoulder, and arm arise from structures at the C4-T1 levels. When the examiner observes muscle weakness in a patient with neck pain, he or she must differentiate between nerve root compromise, myelopathy, peripheral neuropathy,[36] and a primary muscle disease.[37] Infrequently, a synovial cyst of the cervical spine presents as an extradural lesion with radicular pain or pain localized in the involved level of the spine.[38]

Headaches may be associated with a Chiari type I malformation.[39] The various types of headaches include "cough headache" attacks that last less than 5 minutes, relatively long-lasting attacks that last 3 hours to several days, and continuous headache. Unlike the short-lasting cough headache attacks, long-lasting attacks are usually not precipitated by a Valsalva-like maneuver. With discriminant analysis, this headache can be rather well differentiated from migraine and cervicogenic headache. In many respects, however, this headache resembled cervicogenic headache, often with accompanying occipital and neck pain, pain in the arm, restriction of neck movement, and dizziness. Dizziness was the most distinguishing feature in the patients with Chiari type I malformations. It has been postulated that the Chiari type I malformation may cause long-lasting headache attacks or continuous head pain by compression of the brainstem, by central spinal cord degeneration, or by intracranial hypertension. In some cases, neurosurgical treatment provided a beneficial effect on the symptoms.[39] The neck appears to play an important, but largely ignored role in the manifestations of adult benign headaches. Both patients with muscle contraction ("tension") headaches and those with common migraines have high occurrences of occipital and neck pain during headache, tender points in the upper cervical region, greatly reduced or absent cervical curve, and radiographic evidence of joint dysfunction in the upper and lower cervical spine.[40, 41]

TREATMENT

Opinions differ about the best medical treatment of neck pain and the various cervical spine syndromes. Cautious clinical, neurophysiologic, radiographic, and neuroimaging studies must precede the planning of treatment. In any therapeutic regimen, the clinician must consider the severity of the symptoms, the presence or absence of neurologic findings, and the severity of the condition as seen by neurophysiologic assessment and radiographic and neuroimaging procedures.

Medical therapy aims at the relief of pain and stiffness in the neck and upper limbs. Early mobilization exercises in patients with acute sprains often improve outcome.[42] Bed rest should be reserved for severe acute cases, chronic cases with acute exacerbation of symptoms, or patients in whom ambulatory treatment fails. For relief of pain, adequate analgesics should be prescribed. Salicylates and nonsteroidal anti-inflammatory drugs (NSAIDs) usually suffice. If severe pain develops, however, codeine, meperidine, or morphine may become necessary. Muscle relaxants or hypnotics may be used concomitantly. With complete bed rest and sufficient analgesic, NSAID, and muscle relaxant therapy, acute neck pain usually subsides in 7 to 10 days. When the acute pain subsides, the patient can commence active exercises. In cervical spondylosis and other musculoskeletal syndromes, limitation of neck movement benefits the patient, and cervical collars can be used to achieve this end. Patients with nerve root pain often find relief of their symptoms after collar use. Before prescribing a cervical collar, it is essential to assess the degree of disability, and the type of collar selected should depend on the degree of immobilization desired. Felt, foam, and rubber collars restrict gross movement, whereas plastic and plaster collars give more secure immobilization. Any collar must fit well and maintain the neck in the most comfortable position. In general, the patient should leave the collar off after about 2 months to prevent weakness and wasting of the neck muscles.

Traction, either continuous or intermittent, should be considered when bed rest fails. Continuous traction should be reserved for more severe cases with symptoms of nerve root compression. Many patients cannot tolerate traction, and some become worse with it. Analgesics and muscle relaxants can be used in doses sufficient to prevent restlessness. Intermittent traction can be applied manually or mechanically by pulley and weight with the head halter. The direction of pull should be in the most comfortable position. Treatment should be repeated daily if necessary. Occasionally, side effects of traction occur; rarely, hemianopic visual field defects develop. Traction appears unsuitable for patients with gross changes of the cervical spine visible on radiographs because of the danger of spinal cord compression or pressure on the vertebral arteries.

Exercises should be used in most regimens of treatment[43]; active exercises can be categorized as anterior neck-mobilizing exercises, shoulder-raising exercises, and muscle-strengthening exercises. Shoulder exercises, aimed at elevating the shoulder girdle and relieving drag on the nerve roots, can be combined with the use of a cervical collar. Head positioning can be used to relieve symptoms, because placing the head in certain positions relieves pain.

The role of physical therapy has recently been reviewed.[44, 45] From the outset of treatment, the patient should be encouraged to return to work or other productive activities and should be taught how to be responsible for his or her own recovery. If passive modalities are used, they must be an adjunct to the active modalities. As soon as the patient is able to continue with an active program without unbearable pain, the passive treatment should be discontinued gradually; if neck pain becomes chronic, the accompanying psychosocial dysfunction must be addressed through behavioral modification techniques, preferably in a multidisciplinary setting. Modification of the workplace, work habits, and lifestyle must be emphasized at both the acute and chronic stages. The modalities postulated earlier, as well as many physical therapy measures, unfortunately have not been clinically proved.

Catastrophes, with severe neurologic complications and even death, have sometimes occurred with neck manipulation as a treatment of neck pain.[46, 47] These complications usually result from vascular disturbances of the vertebral arteries, which appear to be particularly vulnerable at the C1 level, where they enter the skull. Rotation and hyperextension can become dangerous movements. After cervical spine fracture or dislocation, vertebral artery injury is more prevalent than commonly believed, and the possibility of vertebral artery injury should be considered during the establishment of clinical management schemes for blunt trauma of the cervical spine.[48]

Surgery appears to be appropriate for two groups of patients.[49, 50] In the first group, symptoms relate principally to the nerve roots emerging from the cervical spine, and the condition presents itself with either neck or arm pain. In the second group, a slowly progressive spinal cord syndrome involves the legs first and then the arms. One of the primary factors in the pathogenesis of radiculopathy and myelopathy is compression. Treatment is aimed at the elimination of this pressure. The most clear-cut indication for surgery is the presence of a neurologic deficit related to compression that is unrelieved by medical treatment. Recent data indicate that cervical spine surgery for neck pain is an increasingly common procedure with wide geographic variability.[51] Rational treatment of neck pain requires further definition of indications for cervical spine surgery, preferably based on firm data about the outcomes of surgical and nonsurgical care.

Radicular symptoms respond readily to surgical

treatment. In the past, the initial surgical approach was from the posterior midline, but many surgeons have recently advocated an anterior approach. In patients with defined neurologic deficits, results have been excellent in 80 to 90 percent of cases, regardless of surgical approach. This appears especially the case for patients with a centrally herniated disc.[52-54] In cases of myelopathy, the surgical approach may be either anterior or posterior.[55, 56] However, surgical repair of cervical myelopathies is less effective than in cases of acute radiculopathy, with approximately 60 to 70 percent of treated patients remaining stable or improving. In patients with a cervical bony canal diameter of 11 mm or less at several levels, a long posterior decompression may be necessary. In patients with a diffuse bulging disc or an osteophytic ridge, and in whom the bony elements are normal (or slightly small), the site of compression and approach may be anterior (several levels may be operated on at the same time). In patients with a large, centrally herniated cervical disc, the surgeon may have difficulty deciding on the appropriate approach; opinions differ as to the optimal surgical technique in these cases.[57, 58]

PATIENT EDUCATION

An important aspect in the treatment of patients with neck pain entails patient education, occupation, and some lifestyle factors.[59, 60] The clinician should define the problem, instruct the patient in the rationale of treatment, and teach the patient how to care for his or her neck in standing, sitting, driving, occupational tasks, and other activities of daily living.

SUMMARY

In the clinical evaluation and treatment of a patient who complains of neck pain, the physician should ask and answer the following questions:

1. Am I treating the right condition?
2. Am I using therapy that is correct for the mechanism of causation of pain in this patient at this time?
3. Is the patient's account of nonimprovement in keeping with the observed changes in his or her mobility, daily activities, and analgesic consumption?
4. Are there mechanical perpetuating factors?
5. Is there neurologic injury?
6. Is there an underlying systemic or metabolic disease?
7. Is there a space-occupying lesion?
8. Are there secondary gain motivational factors at work?

Many medical conditions produce neck pain both locally and in its referred aspect. Confirming the source of dysfunction in the neck, understanding the mechanism by which the symptoms occur, and recognizing the tissues capable of eliciting clinical signs assume importance. A careful, thorough history and complete physical and neurologic examination usually reveal the problem clearly. When clinicians recognize which symptoms can be reproduced and which movements and positions reproduce them, they will arrive at a working diagnosis and direct effective therapy. Following the principles established on that basis reaffirms the fact that a diagnosis need not be a diagnosis of exclusion.

References

1. Rummans TA: Symposium on pain management: Introduction. Mayo Clin Proc 69:373, 1994.
2. American Pain Society: Principles of Analgesic Use in Treatment of Acute Pain and Cancer Pain, 3rd ed. Skokie, Ill, American Pain Society, 1992.
3. Cross SA: Pathophysiology of pain: Symposium on pain management. Part I. Mayo Clin Proc 69:375, 1994.
4. Abram SE: Advances in chronic pain management since gate control. Reg Anesth 18:66, 1993.
5. Nakano KK: Neurology of Musculoskeletal and Rheumatic Disorders. Boston, Houghton Mifflin, 1979.
6. Nakano KK: Neck and back pain. In Stein JH (ed): Internal Medicine, 4th ed. St Louis, CV Mosby, 1994, pp 1033–1041.
7. Hult L: The Munkfors investigation. Acta Orthop Scand 16(Suppl):1, 1954.
8. Holt L: Frequency of symptoms for different age groups and professions. In Hirsch C, Sotterman Y (eds): Cervical Pain. New York, Pergamon Press, 1971, pp 17–20.
9. Maeda K, Horiguchi S, Hosokawa S: History of the studies on occupational cervicobrachial disorder in Japan and remaining problems. J Hum Ergol (Tokyo) 11:17, 1982.
10. Hidalgo JA, Genaida Huston R, Arantes J: Occupational biomechanics of the neck: a review and recommendations. J Human Ergol (Tokyo) 21:165, 1992.
11. Hadler NM: Industrial rheumatology: The Australian and New Zealand experience with arm pain and backache in the workplace. Med J Aust 144:191, 1986.
12. Champion GD, Cornell J, Browne CD, et al: Clinical observations of patients with the clinical syndrome "repetition strain injury." J Occup Health Safety 2:107, 1986.
13. Browne CD, Nolan BM, Faithful DK: Occupational repetition strain injuries: Guidelines for diagnosis and management. Med J Aust 140:329, 1984.
14. Lucire Y: Neurosis in the workplace. Med J Aust 145:32, 1986.
15. Cohen ML, Arroyo JF, Champion GD, et al: Hypothesis. In search of the pathogenesis of refractory cervicobrachial pain syndrome: A deconstruction of the RSI phenomenon. Med J Aust 156:432, 1992.
16. Cassady JJ, Hiltner A, Baer E: Hierarchical structure of the intervertebral disc. Clin Rheumatol 8:282, 1989.
17. Upton ARM, McComas AJ: The double crush in nerve entrapment syndromes. Lancet 2:359, 1973.
18. Davidorf J, Hoyt D, Rosen P: Distal cervical spine evaluation using swimmer's flexion–extension radiographs. J Emerg Med 11:55, 1993.
19. Bradley WG, Waluch V, Yadley RA, et al: Comparison of CT and NMR in 400 patients with suspected disease of the brain and spinal cord. Radiology 152:695, 1984.
20. Murayama S, Numaguchi Y, Robinson AE: The diagnosis of herniated intervertebral discs with MR imaging: A comparison of gradient-refocused-echo pulse sequences. AJNR 11:17, 1990.
21. Davis SJ, Teresi LM, Bradley WG Jr, et al: Cervical spine hyperextension injuries: MR findings. Radiology 180:245, 1991.
22. Mirvis SE, Wolf AL: MRI of acute cervical spine trauma. Appl Radiol 21:15, 1992.
23. Yasuyuki Y, Matsumasa T, Matsuno Y, et al: Acute spinal cord injury: Magnetic resonance imaging correlated with myelography. Br J Radiol 64:201, 1991.
24. Kimura J: Electrodiagnosis in Diseases of Nerve and Muscle: Principles and Practices, 2nd ed. Philadelphia, FA Davis, 1989.
25. Chiappa KH: Evoked Potentials in Clinical Medicine, 2nd ed. New York, Raven Press, 1990.
26. Epstein NE, Danto J, Nardi D: Evaluation of intraoperative somatosensory-evoked potential monitoring during 100 cervical operations. Spine 18:737, 1993.
27. Alund M, Ledin T, Odkvist L, et al: Dynamic posturography among patients with common neck disorder: A study of 15 cases with suspected cervical vertigo. J Vestib Res 3:383, 1993.

28. Shinomiya K, Nakao K, Shidoh S, et al: Evaluation of cervical diskography in pain origin and provocation. J Spinal Disord 6:422, 1993.
29. Bogduk N, Aprill C: On the nature of neck pain, discography and cervical zygapophyseal joint blocks. Pain 54:213, 1993.
30. Sturzenegger M, DiStefano G, Radanov BP, et al: Presenting symptoms and signs after whiplash injury: The influence of accident mechanisms. Neurology 44:688, 1994.
31. Barnsley L, Lord SM, Wallis BJ, et al: Lack of effect of intraarticular corticosteroids for chronic pain in the cervical zygapophyseal joints. N Engl J Med 330:1047, 1994.
32. Carette S: Whiplash injury and chronic neck pain. N Engl J Med 330:1083, 1994.
33. Leino P, Magni G: Depressive and distress symptoms as predictors of low back pain, neck-shoulder pain, and other musculoskeletal morbidity: A 10-year follow-up of metal industry employees. Pain 53:89, 1993.
34. Nakano KK, Newbill DC: An unusual source of acute neck pain: Calcifications surrounding the odontoid process. Straub Proc 52:13, 1987.
35. Sawada H, Akiguchi I, Fukuyama H, et al: Marked spinal stenosis at the level of the atlas. Neuroradiology 31:346, 1989.
36. Schaumburg HH, Berger AR, Thomas PK: Disorders of Peripheral Nerves, 2nd ed. Philadelphia, FA Davis, 1992.
37. Emery AEH: Population frequencies of inherited neuromuscular diseases: A world survey. Neuromuscul Disord 1:19, 1991.
38. Patel SC, Sanders WP: Synovial cyst of the cervical spine: Case report and review of the literature. AJNR 9:602, 1988.
39. Stovner LJ: Headache associated with the Chiari type I malformation. Headache 33:175, 1993.
40. Vernon H, Steiman I, Hagino C: Cervicogenic dysfunction in muscle contraction headache and migraine: A descriptive study. J Manipulative Physiol Ther 15:418, 1992.
41. Blau JN, MacGregor EA: Migraine and the neck. Headache 34:88, 1994.
42. McKinney LA. Early mobilization and outcome in acute sprains of the neck. BMJ 299:1006, 1989.
43. Rodriquez AA, Bilkey WJ, Agre JC: Therapeutic exercise in chronic neck and back pain. Arch Phys Med Rehabil 73:870, 1992.
44. Tan JC, Nordin M: Role of physical therapy in the treatment of cervical disk disease. Orthop Clin North Am 23:435, 1992.
45. Linton SJ, Hellsing AL, Andersson D: A controlled study of the effects of an early intervention on acute musculoskeletal pain problems. Pain 54:353, 1993.
46. Miller RG, Burton R: Stroke following chiropractic manipulation of the spine. JAMA 229:189, 1974.
47. Powell FC, Hanigan WC, Olivero WC: A risk/benefit analysis of spinal manipulation therapy for relief of lumbar or cervical pain. Neurosurgery 33:73, 1993.
48. Willis BK, Greiner F, Orrison WW, et al: The incidence of vertebral artery injury after midcervical spine fracture or subluxation. Neurosurgery 34:435, 1994.
49. Dunsker SB: Cervical spondylosis. In Seminars in Neurological Surgery. New York, Raven Press, 1981.
50. Jacchia GE, Innocenti M, Pavolini B, et al: Indications and results of surgical treatment of cervical disc disease by anterior and posterior approach. Chir Organi Mov 77:111, 1992.
51. Einstadter D, Kent DL, Fihn SD, et al: Variation in the rate of cervical spine surgery in Washington State. Med Care 31:711, 1993.
52. Lunsford LN, Bassonette DJ, Jannetta PJ, et al: Anterior surgery for cervical disc disease. J Neurosurg 53:1, 1980.
53. Laus M, Pignatti G, Alfonso C, et al: Anterior surgery for the treatment of soft cervical disc herniation. Chir Organi Mov 77:101, 1992.
54. Figueiredo SR, Vital JP, Dominguez ML, et al: Cervical discectomies by anterior approach. Acta Med Port 6:249, 1993.
55. Cooper PR: Posterior stabilization of the cervical spine. Clin Neurosurg 40:286, 1993.
56. Epstein N: The surgical management of ossification of the posterior longitudinal ligament in 51 patients. J Spinal Disord 6:432, 1993.
57. Murphy KP, Opitz JL, Cabanela ME, et al: Cervical fractures and spinal cord injury: Outcome of surgical and nonsurgical management. Mayo Clin Proc 65:949, 1990.
58. Snyder GM, Berhardt M: Anterior cervical fractional interspace decompression for treatment of cervical radiculopathy: A review of the first 66 cases. Clin Orthop Rel Res 246:92, 1989.
59. Jacobsson L, Lindgarde F, Manthorpe R, et al: Effect of education, occupation and some lifestyle factors on common rheumatic complaints in a Swedish group aged 50–70 years. Ann Rheum Dis 51:835, 1992.
60. Hellsing AL, Linton SJ, Kalvemark M: A prospective study of patients with acute back and neck pain in Sweden. Phys Ther 74:116, 1994.

CHAPTER 28

Thomas S. Thornhill

Shoulder Pain

Shoulder pain is one of the most common musculo-skeletal problems seen in an outpatient setting. The clinician must differentiate between pain from a local shoulder problem and that referred from another source. Owing to its role as the link between the thorax and the upper extremity and the close proximity of major neurovascular structures, the shoulder is frequently painful as an early manifestation of systemic disease. Left shoulder pain may be the initial presentation of coronary artery disease. Hepatic or splenic disease may initially present as shoulder pain. The purpose of this chapter is to provide practical guidelines for the diagnosis and treatment of painful shoulder disorders seen in a rheumatology practice. Improvements in diagnostic tests such as magnetic resonance imaging (MRI), arthrography–computed tomography (arthro-CT), sonography, and electromyography (EMG) have facilitated early diagnosis of shoulder pain. Moreover, these improved techniques have led to a better understanding of rotator cuff diseases, impingement, instability patterns, and a variety of other disorders related to shoulder pain.

A detailed analysis of shoulder problems and the treatment of major trauma are beyond the scope of this chapter and have been covered by other authors.[1-5] The conditions to be discussed here are divided, albeit artificially, into disorders of the periarticular structures, disorders of the glenohumeral joint, and regional disorders (Table 28–1).

DIAGNOSTIC AIDS

Anatomy

An understanding of the structural and functional anatomy is requisite for the clinician treating shoulder pain. One must visualize the three-dimensional relationships, the muscular function, the ligamentous and tendinous attachments, and the routing of neurovascular structures. Figure 28–1 shows the musculoskeletal and topographic localization of pain in association with common shoulder disorders. Figure 28–2 shows the relationship of the posterior musculature coursing anteriorly underneath the acromion to insert on the greater tuberosity. These muscles, combined with the subscapularis inserting on the lesser tuberosity, form the functionally important rotator cuff. By understanding the relationship between the rotator cuff and the subacromial region bounded inferiorly by the hu-

meral head and superiorly by the undersurface of the acromion, the clinician not only can visualize the problems of an impingement syndrome but also can accurately aspirate and inject this space. Knowledge of the route of the tendon of the long head of the biceps through the bicipital groove and onto the superior aspect of the glenoid helps in understanding bicipital tendinitis. Before attempting to diagnose and treat shoulder pain, the reader should review in some detail one of the many sources describing the structural and functional relationships of the shoulder girdle.[2, 3]

The introduction of arthroscopy for both the diagnosis and the treatment of shoulder problems has led to an increased understanding of the arthroscopic anatomy of the capsular region. Figure 28–3 shows the glenohumeral ligaments, which are important in maintaining the stability of the shoulder joint. Anterior stability is predominantly conferred by the infe-

Table 28–1. COMMON CAUSES OF SHOULDER PAIN

Periarticular Disorders

   Rotator cuff tendinitis/impingement syndrome
   Calcific tendinitis
   Rotator cuff tear
   Bicipital tendinitis
   Acromioclavicular arthritis

Glenohumeral Disorders

   Inflammatory arthritis
   Osteoarthritis
   Osteonecrosis
   Cuff arthropathy
   Septic arthritis
   Glenoid labrum tears
   Adhesive capsulitis
   Glenohumeral instability

Regional Disorders

   Cervical radiculopathy
   Brachial neuritis
   Nerve entrapment syndromes
   Sternoclavicular arthritis
   Reflex sympathetic dystrophy
   Fibrositis
   Neoplasms
   Miscellaneous
      Gallbladder disease
      Splenic trauma
      Subphrenic abscess
      Myocardial infarction
      Thyroid disease
      Diabetes mellitus
      Renal osteodystrophy

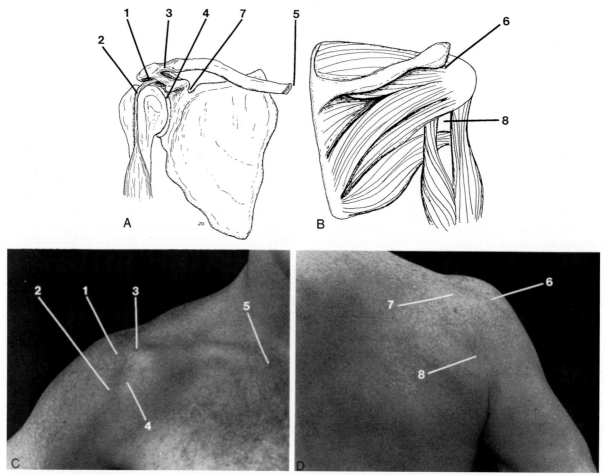

Figure 28–1. Musculoskeletal (*A* and *B*) and topographic (*C* and *D*) areas localizing pain and tenderness associated with specific shoulder problems. 1, Subacromial space (rotator cuff tendinitis/impingement syndrome, calcific tendinitis, rotator cuff tear). 2, Bicipital groove (bicipital tendinitis, biceps tendon subluxation and tear). 3, Acromioclavicular joint. 4, Anterior glenohumeral joint (glenohumeral arthritis, osteonecrosis, glenoid labrum tears, adhesive capsulitis). 5, Sternoclavicular joint. 6, Posterior edge of acromion (rotator cuff tendinitis, calcific tendinitis, rotator cuff tear). 7, Suprascapular notch (suprascapular nerve entrapment). 8, Quadrilateral space (axillary nerve entrapment). These areas of pain and tenderness frequently overlap.

rior glenohumeral ligament. The labrum serves to enlarge the contact area of the articular surface as well as to confer stability to the joint. Lesions of the labrum indicate certain instability patterns and may be a source of pain from internal derangement of the shoulder.

History

Most shoulder problems can be diagnosed by taking a detailed history. The association with trauma, the rapidity of onset, and the character and localization of the pain frequently lead the clinician to the proper diagnosis. For instance, anterior dislocations of the glenohumeral joint are usually associated with a force directed to the arm with the shoulder in an abducted and externally rotated position, whereas dislocations of the acromioclavicular (AC) joint are usually due to direct trauma to the shoulder region. The gradual onset of pain in the subacromial region

that is increased with forward elevation of the shoulder is characteristic of rotator cuff tendinitis with impingement. The presence of a snap or click on forward elevation combined with weakness frequently indicates rotator cuff tear associated with impingement. The burning quality and characteristic radiation of pain are indicative of a neuropathic process.

Physical Examination

A detailed physical and neurologic examination with particular attention to the involved extremity is essential. Careful recording of range of motion should include both active and passive forward flexion, abduction, internal and external rotation both in a neutral position and at 90 degrees of abduction, and forward elevation. Forward elevation is defined as the functional arc between forward flexion and abduction and represents the most important arc in terms of placing the hand in a functional position. Abduction

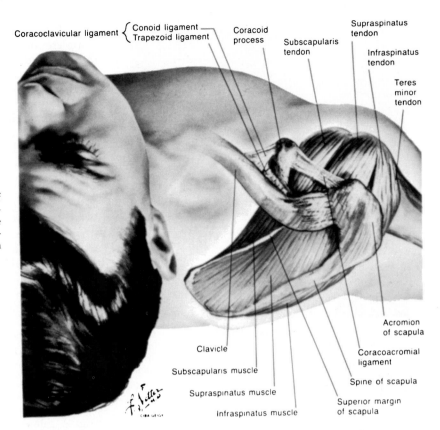

Figure 28–2. Superior view of the rotator cuff musculature as it courses anteriorly underneath the coracoacromial arch to insert on the greater tuberosity. (Reproduced by permission of Ciba-Geigy. From The Ciba Collection of Medical Illustrations, Volume 8, Part I.)

should be divided into that occurring at the glenohumeral joint and that occurring at the scapulothoracic joint. Careful recording of these values on serial examinations will aid in measuring response to therapy. The localization of tenderness can help differentiate common entities such as glenoid labral tears, rotator cuff tendinitis, and bicipital tendinitis. Although all three are associated with tenderness in the anterior aspect of the shoulder, the tenderness of rotator cuff tendinitis is generally subacromial, whereas that of bicipital tendinitis migrates laterally and superiorly as the shoulder is abducted and externally rotated.

Tenderness in the quadrilateral space or suprascapular notch is frequently associated with nerve entrapment syndromes. Neurologic examination should include sensory testing of the upper extremity with particular reference to the area innervated by the axillary nerve. Results of evaluation of all muscle systems should be graded and recorded, and the presence of atrophy or fasciculations noted.

Examination of the ipsilateral elbow, wrist, and hand is important not only in planning therapy but also in determining functional expectations.

Imaging Studies

Diagnostic confirmation, delineation of pathology, and operative planning are greatly aided by imaging studies. Because various studies define abnormalities with differing sensitivity and specificity, the clinician must order the appropriate test to confirm or refute his or her suspected diagnosis. In this era of cost accountability, clinicians must perform minimal testing and be aware of the cost of each procedure. Although charges vary among providers and don't specifically reflect true costs, relative charges are important to consider. Moreover, as the efficacy of each test varies with the diagnosis, the clinician must perform a careful history and physical examination before considering a specific imaging study.[5a, 5b]

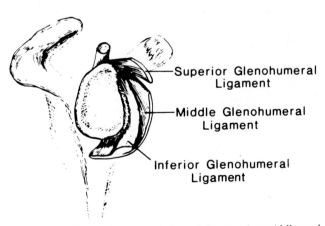

Superior Glenohumeral Ligament

Middle Glenohumeral Ligament

Inferior Glenohumeral Ligament

Figure 28–3. Schematic representation of the superior, middle, and inferior glenohumeral ligaments as visualized arthroscopically.

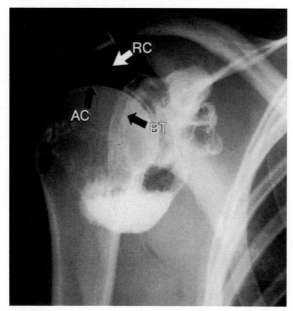

Figure 28–4. Normal double-contrast arthrogram showing the inferior edge of the rotator cuff (RC) as it courses through the subacromial space to the greater tuberosity; the tendon of the long head of the biceps (BT); and the articular cartilage of the humeral head (AC).

Plain Radiographs

For most nontraumatic painful shoulder syndromes, the use of an anteroposterior (AP) or glenohumeral view of the involved shoulder in internal and external rotation suffices. In cases of injury to the shoulder girdle, a "trauma series," involving an anteroposterior view, scapular Y view, and axillary view, has become the standard protocol. The axillary view is particularly helpful in assessing posterior or anterior subluxation of the humeral head. It has been recognized that impingement-induced rotator cuff tendinitis can be caused by or, if already present, increased by anterior subluxation.[6, 7] In such cases of suspected AC joint injury, an AP view of the shoulder with a weight held in the ipsilateral hand frequently demonstrates subluxation at the AC joint. A variety of special shoulder radiographs are available for the evaluation of specific lesions such as Bankart's lesion of the anterior inferior glenoid rim (West Point view) or a Hill-Sachs lesion (Didiee view, Hermodsson view).

Scintigraphy

Technetium Tc 99m methylene diphosphonate technetium (Tc 99m MDP) or gallium may be of diagnostic help in evaluating the painful shoulder. This benefit usually occurs in the evaluation of skeletal lesions about the shoulder joint. Bone scans are generally not helpful in the diagnosis of non-neoplastic or noninfectious shoulder disease, with the possible exception of differentiating those patients with complete rotator cuff tears that will proceed to cuff tear arthropathy.

This distinction is important, because patients with complete rotator cuff tears may do well, whereas those who develop changes of cuff tear arthropathy have progressive arthritis, pain, and significant functional impairment. The presence of synovitis and/or calcium pyrophosphate deposition disease (CPPD) may be an important factor in the pathogenesis of cuff tear arthropathy. In such cases, scintigraphy may demonstrate the increased blood flow and pooling associated with the chronic synovitis.

Arthrography

Single-contrast arthrography, double-contrast arthrography, and double-contrast arthrotomography (DCAT) are valuable tools in evaluating problems of the rotator cuff, the glenoid labrum, the biceps tendon, and the shoulder capsule.[8-11] Figure 28–4 shows a normal double-contrast arthrogram of the shoulder. Rotator cuff tears can be demonstrated by single- or double-contrast studies. The proponents of double-contrast arthrography believe that the extent of the tear, the preferred surgical approach, and the quality of the rotator cuff tissue are best determined with double-contrast studies.[9-11] Figure 28–5 demonstrates extravasation of contrast into the subacromial space from a rotator cuff tear. Arthrography can be misleading by underestimating the extent of a rotator cuff tear.

Tears of the glenoid labrum without shoulder dislocation are now being recognized as sources of anterior

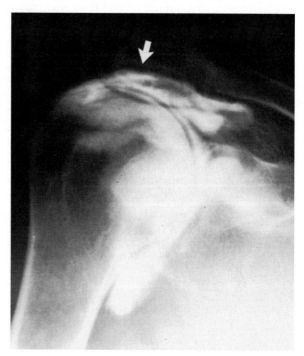

Figure 28–5. Single-contrast arthrogram demonstrating a massive rotator cuff tear with extravasation of contrast into the subacromial space (*arrow*).

shoulder pain in athletes. Glenoid labral tears (Fig. 28–6) with or without associated glenohumeral subluxation can frequently be identified by DCAT.[11, 12] Kneisl and colleagues reported on 55 patients who underwent DCAT followed by a diagnostic shoulder arthroscopy.[13] DCAT confirmed the arthroscopic findings in 76 percent of anterior labra and 96 percent of posterior labra. This test was 100 percent sensitive and 94 percent specific in diagnosing complete rotator cuff tears. Partial rotator cuff tears identified at arthroscopy were missed in 83 percent of patients undergoing DCAT. The authors felt that DCAT was better in diagnosing articular and cuff pathology in the presence of instability than with pain alone as a presenting diagnosis.[13] Shoulder arthrography can confirm a diagnosis of adhesive capsulitis by showing a contracted capsule with an obliterated axillary recess (Fig. 28–7).

The use of subacromial bursography has been reported to be beneficial in visualizing the outer surface of the rotator cuff and the subacromial space in cases of impingement.[14, 15] Fukuda and associates reported a small series of younger patients (average age 41.8 years) who underwent subacromial bursography following a negative glenohumeral arthrogram.[16] These patients demonstrated pooling of contrast medium on a bursal side tear, which was confirmed at the time of surgery. At the time of surgical exploration, these patients underwent wedge resection and primary repair of these partial tears.

It is unclear whether patients undergoing open or arthroscopic decompression for impingement require resection or repair of partial lesions. Subacromial bursography is not routinely used diagnostically and seems to be of little value in planning surgical procedures.

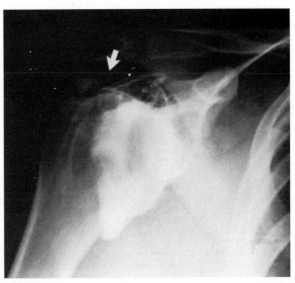

Figure 28–7. Double-contrast arthrogram in patient with calcific tendinitis (*arrow*) and adhesive capsulitis. Note the contracted capsule with diminution of the synovial space and obliteration of the axillary recess.

Computed Tomography

Computed tomography (CT) has been shown to be helpful in evaluating the musculoskeletal system. In recent years, CT combined with contrast arthrography has become a major diagnostic tool for the evaluation of glenoid labral tears, loose bodies, and chondral lesions (Fig. 28–8). Rafii and colleagues reported on the use of arthro-CT in the evaluation of shoulder derangement.[17] They found a 95 percent accuracy of arthro-CT in investigating lesions of the labrum and articular surface.[17] Blum and coworkers found that obtaining a coronal oblique section was an effective way of improving the accuracy of the arthro-CT diagnosis of labial lesions as well as demonstrating the size and presence of cuff tears.[17a] Moreover, arthro-CT may still be the best test for determining full-thickness rotator cuff tears in making a decision about surgical repair.

Ultrasound

The technologic improvement of sonographic equipment has allowed ultrasonographic study of the rotator cuff. The technique is noninvasive, is rapid, and involves no radiation exposure.[12–15] The cuff is examined in both horizontal and transverse planes, with the arm in different positions to allow visualization of different areas of the cuff in the two planes. These techniques generally provide visualization of the distal cuff, which is where most rotator cuff tears are located.[12–15] Figure 28–9 shows normal and abnormal ultrasound (US) images of the rotator cuff in both longitudinal and transverse planes. Several studies report a high sensitivity and specificity for the ultrasonographic diagnosis of a rotator cuff tear.[12, 15–17] The

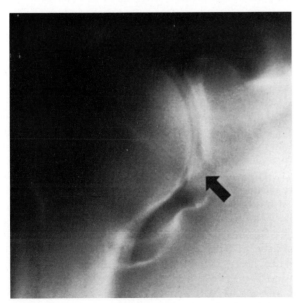

Figure 28–6. A double-contrast arthrotomogram demonstrating a tear of the anteroinferior portion of the glenoid labrum (*arrow*).

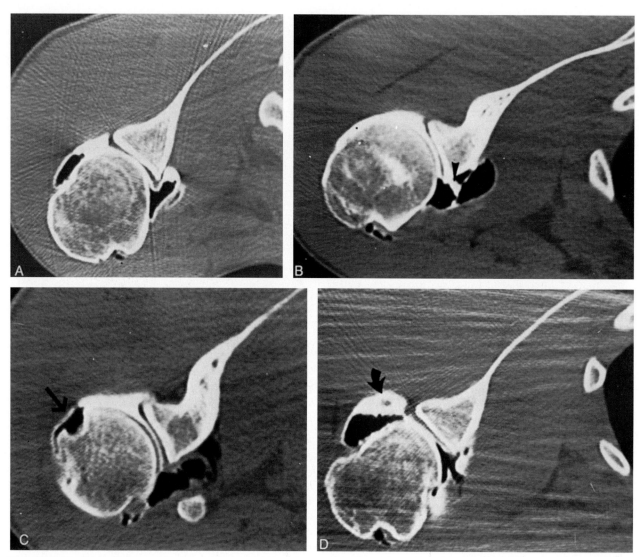

Figure 28–8. Arthrographic computed tomography (CT) scan of shoulder showing *(A)* normal findings; *(B)* tear of the anterior glenoid labrum *(arrowhead); (C)* a large defect of the articular surface of the posterior portion of the humeral head (Hill-Sachs lesion) *(arrow);* and *(D)* loose body in the posterior recess *(arrow).*

specificity and sensitivity of the procedure are reported to be greater than 90 percent as determined by both arthrographic and surgical correlation.[15, 17] This technique has also been used for the postoperative evaluation of a rotator cuff repair and for evaluation of abnormalities of the biceps tendon.[18, 19]

US of the rotator cuff requires an ultrasonographer experienced not only in performing the technique but also in interpreting the images. Abnormalities in the rotator cuff can be seen as hyperechoic areas, hypoechoic areas, or discontinuities in the cuff. US scan of associated lesions, such as calcific tendinitis or subluxation of the humeral head, and even the normal biceps tendon can be misinterpreted as a rotator cuff lesion.[20] Small echogenic areas within an injured rotator cuff may be confused with partial rotator cuff lesions. Further experience with this procedure and correlation with arthrography, arthroscopy, and open surgery should further delineate the role of this procedure in the evaluation of the painful shoulder.[21–26]

Gardelin and Perin reported US to be 96 percent sensitive in determining rotator cuff and biceps tendon pathology.[27] Mack and coworkers found US to be valuable even in evaluating the postoperative patient with recurrent shoulder symptoms.[28] In a prospective study, Hodler and associates compared US with MRI and arthrography in evaluating rotator cuff lesions in 24 shoulders.[29] Sonography identified 14 of 15 torn cuffs, MRI 10 of 15, and arthrography 15 of 15. Sonography identified 7 of 9 intact rotator cuffs, and MRI was accurate in 8 of 9 intact cuffs. Vestring and colleagues found US to be as accurate as MRI in the diagnosis of humeral head defects and joint effusions, but inferior to MRI in the diagnosis of labral lesions, rotator cuff lesions, subacromial spurs, and synovial inflammatory disease.[30] Sonography has also been re-

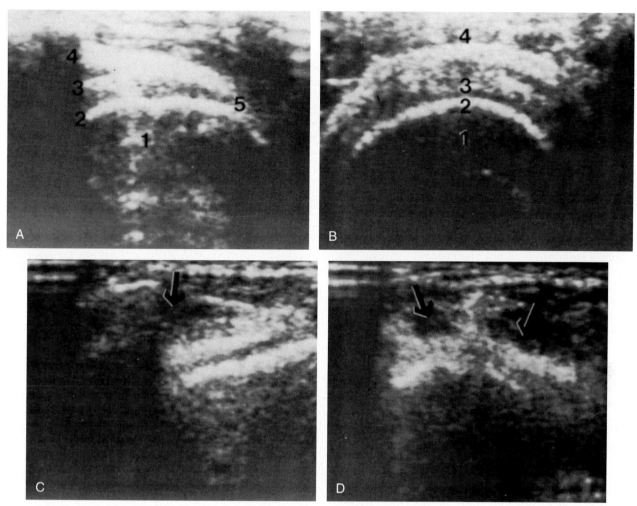

Figure 28–9. *A,* Normal longitudinal view of rotator cuff by ultrasound showing (1) humeral head, (2) the superior articular surface, (3) the rotator cuff, (4) the deltoid tendon, and (5) the tapering of the cuff to its insertion on the greater tuberosity. *B,* Transverse view of a normal intact rotator cuff covering the humeral head. *C,* Rotator cuff tear showing hypoechoic area *(arrow)* on a longitudinal view. *D,* Rotator cuff tear demonstrating hypoechoic area *(arrows)* on a transverse view.

ported to be valuable in identifying dislocation of the biceps tendon, particularly when it is associated with a full-thickness rotator cuff tear. Van Moppers and coworkers reported an 86 percent sensitivity and 91 percent specificity of US in detecting partial and total rotator cuff tears.[30a]

Ryu and colleagues used dynamic sonography to diagnose adhesive capsulitis with a sensitivity of 91 percent and a specificity of 100 percent. In this study adhesive capsulitis was confirmed by limitation of the sliding movement of the supraspinatus tendon.[30b]

In rheumatoid arthritis, US has been reported to confirm early changes of synovitis, subdeltoid bursitis, and biceps tendinitis before plain radiographic findings were observed.

US is helpful in the evaluation of an acutely injured shoulder if a rotator cuff tear is suspected. In the hands of a well-trained sonographer, US may be the most cost-effective test for initial evaluation of rotator cuff injury; however, most surgeons would require arthro-CT or MRI confirmation prior to surgical exploration.[27-31]

Arthroscopy

Diagnostic arthroscopy and arthroscopic surgery have greatly aided the diagnosis and treatment of knee injuries (see Chapter 43). In recent years these arthroscopic techniques have been applied to the diagnosis and treatment of glenohumeral and subacromial disorders. They have been recommended for evaluating glenohumeral synovitis, articular cartilage damage, and loose bodies, and particularly for diagnosing labral tears. In combination with physical examination, history, and examination under anesthesia, arthroscopy has been helpful in the diagnosis of chronic instability patterns of the glenohumeral joint. Compared with DCAT, arthroscopy has been reported to be more accurate in the diagnosis of intra-articular lesions associated with a painful shoulder.[13] An additional benefit is that arthroscopy can be used for both diagnosis and treatment of shoulder problems of the glenohumeral joint and the subacromial region. Debridement of rotator cuff tears in elderly patients, resection of the subacromial bursa, debridement of labral tears, and removal of loose bodies have become standard arthroscopic procedures in the shoulder. The use of the arthroscope for repairing torn rotator cuffs and for stabilization of the dislocating shoulder is still in the investigative phase.[32]

In the subacromial region, arthroscopy is used for both diagnosis and treatment of chronic impingement, rotator cuff tendinitis, and calcific tendinitis.

Magnetic Resonance Imaging

In recent years MRI has been used to diagnose partial- and full-thickness rotator cuff tears, impingement of the rotator cuff, synovitis, articular cartilage damage, and labral pathology associated with glenohumeral instability.[33–35] For rheumatoid arthritis, MRI is reported to be more sensitive than plain radiographs in determining soft tissue abnormalities and osseous abnormalities of the glenoid and humeral head.[36]

The best use of MRI is in the diagnosis of rotator cuff pathology. Morrison and Offstein studied 100 patients with chronic subacromial impingement syndrome using arthrography and MRI.[37] MRI was 100 percent sensitive but only 88 percent specific in confirming arthrogram-proven rotator cuff tears. Nelson and coworkers studied 21 patients with shoulder pain and found MRI to be more accurate than arthro-CT or US in identifying partial-thickness cuff tears.[38] These authors also reported MRI to be as accurate as arthro-CT in diagnosing abnormalities of the glenoid labrum.[38] Robertson stressed inter- and intraobserver variation in MRI interpretation. In this study diagnosis of full-thickness tears was reproducible, but there was greater variation in the interpretation of tendinitis and partial tears.

The characteristic MRI findings in rotator cuff tears include a hypointense gap within the supraspinatus muscle tendon complex on T1-weighted films. The presence of fluid in the subacromial bursa in symptomatic patients is indicative of pathology in the shoulder joint.[38a] Fluid in the glenohumeral joint usually is associated with cuff tears or arthritic changes.[38b] Another common finding is the absence of a demonstrable supraspinatus tendon with narrowing of the subacromial space and an increased signal in the supraspinatus tendon on T2-weighted images.[39] Seeger and colleagues, reporting on 170 MRI scans, found that T1-weighted images were highly sensitive in identifying abnormalities in the supraspinatus tendon, but that T2-weighted images were required in differentiating tendinitis from a small supraspinatus tendon tear.[40] Large, full-thickness tears, however, could be identified on both T1- and T2-weighted images.[40] Figures 28–10 and 28–11 depict common shoulder pathology as seen by MRI. Owen and associates used MRI to evaluate shoulders after surgery to identify metal, bone, and soft tissue artifacts.[40a] In this study the MRI criteria for full-thickness tears were fluid on T2-weighted images extending through the

cuff and nonvisualization of a portion of the cuff. Using these criteria, the authors reported 90 percent accuracy in diagnosing full-thickness tears. Partial tears could not be distinguished from repaired tendons.

Emig and coworkers reported MRI findings in adhesive capsulitis as including capsular and synovial thickness greater than 4 mm.[40b] Using these criteria, the authors reported a sensitivity of 70 percent and a specificity of 95 percent.

MRI is nearly as sensitive as and certainly more specific than scintigraphy in the diagnosis of osteonecrosis and neoplastic lesions about the shoulder. The combination of MRI and arthrography offers improved resolution over MRI alone, especially in diagnosing intra-articular lesions.[40c–40f] Chandnani and coworkers reported MRI arthrography to be superior to arthrography and arthro-CT in diagnosing labial pathology.[40d] Figure 28–10 depicts a normal rotator cuff and a full-thickness cuff tear as diagnosed by MRI arthrography.

Electromyography and Nerve Conduction Velocity Studies

Electromyography (EMG) and nerve conduction velocity (NCV) studies can be helpful in differentiating shoulder pain from pain of neurogenic origin (see Chapter 44). They may also be beneficial in determining the localization of neurogenic pain to a particular cervical root, the brachial plexus, or a peripheral nerve.[41, 42]

Injection

Injection of local anesthetics and glucocorticoids is a useful technique for both diagnosis and treatment of shoulder pain (see Chapter 40). The physician must have a thorough knowledge of the anatomy of the shoulder girdle and a presumptive diagnosis to direct the injection properly. Referred pain areas may be misleading. For example, in the patient with lateral arm pain due to deltoid bursal involvement from calcific tendinitis of the supraspinatus tendon, injection should be in the subacromial space and not the area of referred pain in the deltoid muscle.

It is often better to use a posterior subacromial approach in injection for rotator cuff tendinitis in a patient with anterior impingement symptoms; it is easier to enter the subacromial region posteriorly, and this approach involves less trauma to the contracted anterior structures.

The instillation of rapidly acting local anesthetics can be beneficial in determining the source of shoulder pain. Obliteration of pain, for instance, by injection of a local anesthetic along the bicipital groove can confirm a diagnosis of bicipital tendinitis. Injection of local anesthetics is somewhat less helpful in the subacromial space, owing to its extensive com-

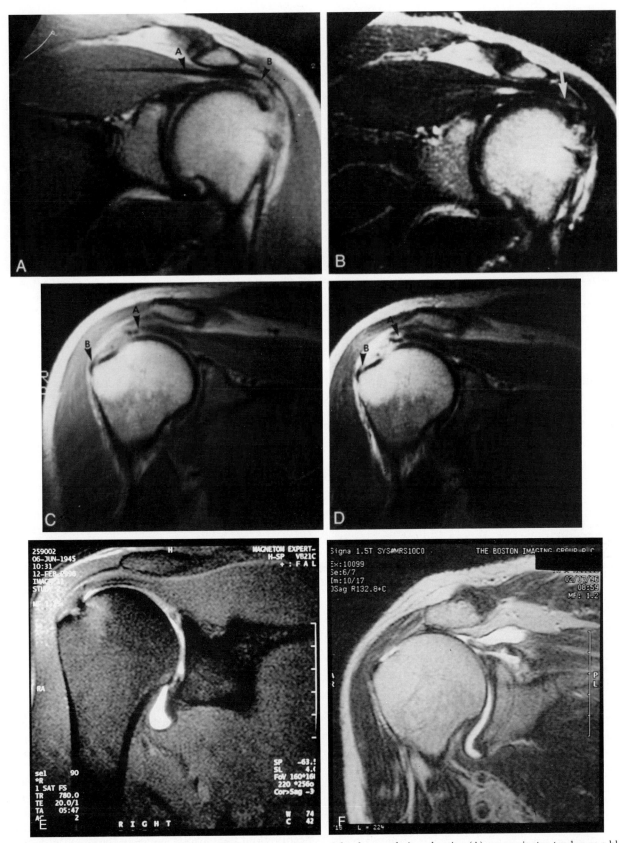

Figure 28–10. *A,* Magnetic resonance imaging (MRI) proton density–weighted coronal view showing (A) supraspinatus tendon as a black band that has an increased signal (B) as it nears insertion on the greater tuberosity. *B,* Similar view in T2-weighted image showing increased signal as gray *(arrow),* indicating partial thickness tear or tendinitis. *C,* MRI proton density–weighted coronal view showing (A) abrupt end of supraspinatus tendon as it courses right to left. From (A) to (B) is area of increased signal followed by short portion of tendon (B) inserting at greater tuberosity. *D,* Similar view in T2-weighted image showing increased signal as white (fluid density), indicating fluid in the gap of a complete rotator cuff tear. *E,* MRI arthrography showing normal rotator cuff. *F,* MRI arthrography showing chronic cuff tear with retraction.

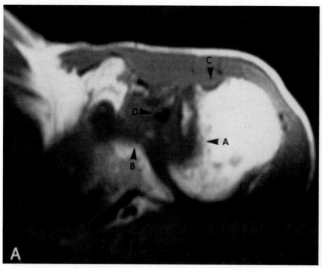 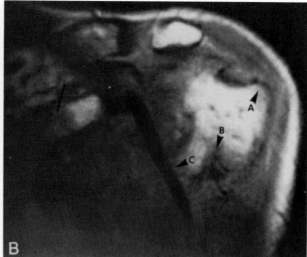

Figure 28–11. *A,* MRI T2-weighted transverse view of patient with recurrent anterior and posterior dislocation and chronic dislocation of the long head of the biceps tendon, showing (A) large reverse Hill-Sachs lesion (anterior humeral defect from posterior dislocation), (B) Bankart lesion of anterior glenoid rim indicating anterior instability, (C) the bicipital groove, and (D) the biceps tendon, which is chronically dislocated from the groove. *B,* Coronal view of same patient showing (A) greater tuberosity, (B) bicipital groove, and (C) long head of biceps tendon (broad black band) that is dislocated from the groove.

munication with the rest of the shoulder girdle, but relief of symptoms with such an injection can rule out pain from conditions such as cervical radiculopathy or an entrapment neuropathy.

Preferred Diagnostic Tests

Table 28–2 lists the relative costs of various shoulder diagnostic tests based on 1995 estimates at a single institution. The choice of a specific test depends on its sensitivity, specificity, and cost-benefit analysis. In considering arthroscopy, it must be remembered that concomitant therapy can be delivered. For instance, in patients with symptoms of internal derangement and presumed labral tears, arthroscopy can be used both to confirm and to treat (debride) the pathologic abnormality.

The history and physical examination are the most important factors in establishing diagnosis of the painful shoulder. Plain radiographs (three views) should be the first imaging study performed. Although not as sensitive as the more sophisticated tests, plain radiographs can identify arthritic change,

Table 28–2. RELATIVE COSTS OF SHOULDER DIAGNOSTIC PROCEDURES (1995)

Office visit (30 min): diagnostic examination	$ 75
Plain radiography	82
Arthrography	477
Ultrasonography	140
Magnetic resonance imaging	1000
Computed tomography	590
Tomography	328
Bone scan	500

calcifying tendinitis, established osteonecrosis, and most neoplasms. If intra-articular pathology is suspected (labral tear, capsular tear, loose body, chondral defect), arthro-CT is preferable to MRI. In diagnosing acute rotator cuff tears in the younger patient, sonography is the most cost-effective test for confirming a clinical suspicion. In cases of impingement syndrome, MRI is sensitive but involves difficulty in differentiating tendinitis, partial tears, or small complete tears. In the use of arthroscopic versus open decompression for chronic impingement, the author prefers arthrography to MRI; open decompression is favored if there is a repairable full-thickness tear.

PERIARTICULAR DISORDERS

Rotator Cuff Tendinitis/Impingement Syndrome

The majority of painful nontraumatic conditions about the shoulder joint are caused by tendinitis of the rotator cuff. Codman, in his classic text reviewing the nature of these lesions, pointed out their importance in work-related disabilities.[1] Degenerative tendinitis has been labeled pericapsulitis, subacromial bursitis, subdeltoid bursitis, supraspinatus tendinitis, rotator cuff tear, and impingement syndrome. The variation in clinical description, method of treatment, and response to treatment perhaps is due to different descriptions of the same condition at various points in the disease. Neer has clarified this condition by pointing out the various stages of the disorder.[43] Stratified into three stages, the process represents a continuum of inflammation, degeneration, and attrition of the rotator cuff by impingement on the anterior edge and undersurface of the anterior third of the acromion, the coracoacromial ligament, and occasionally the acromioclavicular joint.[44]

Investigators have come to understand the dynamic aspects of impingement, finding that normal physiologic translation and axterior laxity increase the risk of impingement. Wuelker and colleagues showed that during elevation of the glenohumeral joint from 20 to 90 degrees, there is an average 90-mm superior and 4.4-mm anterior translation.[44a] Using a similar dynamic shoulder model, investigators demonstrated peak forces of 37.8 N under the acromion during shoulder elevation and postulated this as the etiology of impingement.[44b] Kvitne and Jobe described the syndrome of anterior laxity and impingement in the throwing athlete.[44c] With forward elevation anterior laxity occurs, allowing the humeral head to sublux anteriorly and impinge on the coracoacromial arch. Posterosuperior impingement may also occur as the tendinous portions of the supraspinatus and infraspinatus muscles impinge along the posterosuperior border of the glenoid run. Ferrari and colleagues,[44d] Tirman and colleagues,[44e] and Liu and Boynton[44f] have also described posterior impingement and posterior ossification (Bennett's lesion) in the throwing athlete. The wear and attritional tears of the cuff usually occur in the supraspinatus tendon and may extend into the infraspinatus tendon and the long head of the biceps.[45] The mechanical impingement of the rotator cuff may be influenced by variations in the shape and slope of the acromion.[45, 46]

According to Neer,[43] the three stages of impingement are as follows: *Stage I, edema and hemorrhage,* usually occurs in active individuals younger than age 25 years who engage in activities requiring excessive overhead arm usage. Treatment is conservative, and the patient generally responds to rest, nonsteroidal anti-inflammatory drugs (NSAIDs), and occasional glucocorticoid injection. *Stage II, fibrosis and tendinitis,* represents the biologic response of fibrosis and thickening due to repeated episodes of mechanical impingement. This stage usually occurs in active individuals between 25 and 40 years of age. They may respond to conservative treatment as in stage I but generally experience recurrent attacks. *Stage III, rotator cuff tears, biceps rupture, and bone changes,* rarely appears before the age of 40 years. Stage III represents the attritional wear of the supraspinatus tendon, and occasionally the infraspinatus and long head of the biceps, from repeated impingement. Patients with stage III disease present with varying weakness, crepitus, and supraspinatus atrophy, depending on the extent of the tear and its chronicity.

The dominant feature of degenerative tendinitis is pain. The pain can be sudden and incapacitating or may be a dull ache. It can be focal and pinpointed as an area of tenderness along the anterior edge of the acromion (see Fig. 28–1). It also may present as a diffuse pain around the anterolateral or even posterior edge of the acromion, possibly radiating to the subdeltoid bursa. This pain can be differentiated from other nontraumatic painful conditions about the shoulder by its position and response to treatment. For instance, the tenderness from bicipital tendinitis follows the bicipital groove as the arm is externally rotated. Tenderness from a glenoid labral tear generally occurs beneath the coracoid and over the anterior edge of the glenoid. The impingement sign as illustrated in Figure 28–12 is useful in the diagnosis of rotator cuff tendinitis. Patients with stage I and even stage II disease frequently describe a catch as the arm is brought to an overhead position. The patient commonly raises the arm by abduction and rotation to bypass the painful "spot." This observation underscores the Codman paradox, which states that the arm can be brought fully overhead from an anatomic position by either external rotation and abduction in the coronal plane, or internal rotation and forward flexion in the sagittal plane.[1] In patients with focal tenderness of the supraspinatus, the pain may disappear under the edge of the acromion as the arm is abducted (Dawbarn's sign).[3] Instillation of short-acting local anesthetics into the subacromial space may obliterate the symptoms and confirm the diagnosis of degenerative tendinitis with impingement. It is important to remember that trigger point injection alone can be misleading, and that injection of the subacromial space is necessary to ensure the validity of this diagnostic test.

Radiographs in the early stages of degenerative tendinitis with impingement are normal. As the disease progresses, there may be some sclerosis, cyst formation, and eburnation of the anterior third of the acromion and the greater tuberosity. An anterior acromial traction spur may appear on the undersurface of the acromion lateral to the AC joint, representing contracture of the coracoacromial ligament. Late radiographic findings include narrowing of the

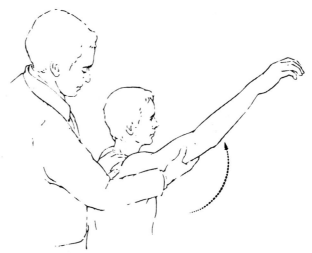

Figure 28–12. The impingement sign is elicited by forced forward elevation of the arm. Pain results as the greater tuberosity impinges on the acromion. The examiner's hand prevents scapular rotation. This maneuver may be positive in other periarticular disorders. (Reproduced with permission from Neer CS II: Impingement lesions. Clin Orthop 173:70, 1983.)

acromiohumeral gap, superior subluxation of the humeral head in relation to the glenoid, and erosive changes of the anterior acromion.[47] Arthrography and ultrasound, as discussed earlier, may be helpful in diagnosing a full-thickness tear of the rotator cuff in association with stage III disease. In some cases of untreated stage III impingement, proximal migration of the humeral head leads to a pattern of degenerative arthritis known as cuff tear arthropathy.

The choice of treatment, and frequently its result, is a function of the stage of the impingement. In stage I disease, in which there is little mechanical impingement, most patients respond to rest. It is important not to immobilize the shoulder for any period of time, as contraction of the shoulder capsule and periarticular structures can produce an adhesive capsulitis. After a period of rest, a progressive program of stretching and strengthening exercises generally restores the shoulder to normal function. Use of aspirin and other NSAIDs may shorten the symptomatic period. Modalities such as ultrasound, neuroprobe, and transcutaneous electrical nerve stimulation (TENS) are generally not helpful. Patients with stage I and stage II disease may have a dramatic response to local injection of glucocorticoids. In stage II disease, in which there is fibrosis and thickening anteriorly, it is frequently better to inject using a posterior approach. The author prefers a combination of 3 ml of 1 percent lidocaine, 3 ml of 0.5 percent bupivacaine, and 20 mg of triamcinolone. This combines a short-acting anesthetic for diagnostic purposes, a longer-acting anesthetic for analgesic purposes, and a steroid preparation in a depot form.

An integrated program of occupational and physical therapy will often preclude the need for surgery in patients with stage II disease. Job modification for individuals with impingement syndrome secondary to overuse may alleviate symptoms. A recent report of a 53-year-old woman who in 2 years stacked over 20 tons of cheese from a conveyor belt to shoulder height underscores this point. Because of poor assembly line ergonomics, this patient developed intractable impingement and was forced to take a disability pension. Management is becoming more aware of the cost savings associated with proper job ergonomics.[48, 49]

The initial rehabilitation in stage II impingement is the cessation of the repetitive overhand activity. Ice, nonsteroidal agents, and local injections may also be beneficial. The initial physical therapy includes passive, active assisted, and active range of motion combined with stretching and mobilization exercises to prevent contracture. As pain and inflammation subside, isometric or isotonic exercises are used to strengthen the rotator cuff musculature. Isokinetic training at variable speeds and in variable positions is instituted prior to returning the patient to full activity. For patients with a job-related injury, it is critical to review and modify job mechanics to prevent recurrent episodes that cause further disability and may precipitate a need for surgery.[49]

Neer has suggested that the patient with refractory stage II disease may respond to division of the coracoacromial ligament and bursectomy of the subacromial bursa.[43] Division of the coracoacromial ligament alone has been performed under a local anesthetic.

Treatment of stage III disease depends on the chronicity of the symptoms and the presence or absence of a rotator cuff tear. Neer recommends arthrography in patients over 40 years of age who fail to respond to conservative treatment or experience sudden weakness of abduction and external rotation, suggesting extension of a tear.[43] The surgical treatment of choice is an anterior acromioplasty.[44] Bosley reported a 20-year experience using total acromionectomy for treatment of impingement.[50] In this study of 34 shoulders, at 5-year follow-up 25 were excellent, 4 were good, 3 were fair, and 1 was poor. The author stressed the importance of repair of the deltoid muscle in order to achieve a good functional result. Most investigators prefer acromioplasty and feel that lateral acromionectomy or complete acromionectomy unnecessarily weakens the deltoid muscle and predisposes the patient to proximal migration of the humeral head.[47]

The indication for anterior acromioplasty is based on symptoms that fail to respond to at least 1 year of conservative therapy. There is controversy as to the role of open versus arthroscopic acromioplasty for stage II or III disease. Gartsman reviewed 154 arthroscopic acromioplasties in patients with stage II or stage III impingement.[51] Eighty-two of 89 stage II shoulders with an intact rotator cuff improved. In stage II disease involving a partial rotator cuff tear, 33 of 40 shoulders improved. In stage III disease with a complete rotator cuff tear, only 14 of 25 patients improved. It was the author's conclusion that arthroscopic acromioplasty is effective in treatment of stage II disease, but that open acromioplasty is preferable in patients with full-thickness tears.[51] Another prognostic indicator of the effectiveness of arthroscopic decompression is the presence of an osseous component of impingement. In a study of 80 arthroscopic subacromial decompressions, patients who underwent soft tissue rather than bony decompression had a better final outcome.[52]

Roye and associates recently reported their 2.7-year follow-up of arthroscopic subacromial decompression in stage II and early stage III impingement.[52a] Satisfactory results were reported in 80 to 90 percent of patients, with no difference between those with and without cuff tears. Throwing athletes (68 percent satisfactory) did not do as well as nonthrowing athletes (90 percent satisfactory). Van Hoilsbeech and colleagues reported comparable results using open decompression (OD) versus arthroscopic decompression (AD).[52b] Good to excellent results were seen in 83.1 percent of patients with AD and 81.1 percent of patients with OD; patient satisfaction was 88.3 and 94.3 percent, respectively. These results were not influenced by associated pathologies such as adhesive capsulitis, calcific tendinitis, or rotator cuff lesions. Schneider and coworkers, however, reported a higher incidence of failure with AD in patients with joint laxity.[52c] Moreover, Zvijac and associates stated that patients undergoing arthroscopic decompression for full-thickness cuff tears tended to fare worse at longer follow-up, with 84 percent showing satisfactory results at 24 months compared with only 68 percent at 45.8 months.[52d] Patients wth large tears did worse than those with small and moderate-size tears.

Arthroscopy may be of value in elderly patients with stage III disease, even with full-thickness rotator cuff tears. In elderly patients with stage III disease and no functional weakness, arthroscopic debridement without repair of full-thickness tears may be associated with a good functional result.[53, 54]

The results of open acromioplasty for impingement with an intact rotator cuff are gratifying.[55, 56] Hawkins and coworkers reported an 87 percent success rate following anterior acromioplasty in 108 patients with intact rotator cuffs.[55] In this study, the procedure was less successful in women, in patients with limited motion, in patients whose injury was due to direct trauma, and in worker's compensation claims.[55] Stuart and associates reported an overall 77 percent pain relief in 66 shoulders undergoing open acromioplasty. This study reported no significant difference in results for patients with or without an associated rotator cuff tear.[56] Bigliani and colleagues reported an 81 percent good to excellent result rate in 26 patients younger than 40 years of age who underwent open acromioplasty for subacromial impingement.[57] Bjorkenheim and colleagues reviewed 78 decompression and rotator cuff reconstructions for patients with long-standing impingement and a cuff tear.[58] In this study, 71 percent of patients were reported as excellent or satisfactory, and 29 percent were unsatisfactory. A recent review of 67 failed anterior acromioplasties found diagnostic and operative errors to be a common cause of failure.[59] The authors point out the importance of identifying associated abnormalities such as intra-articular pathology that may be overlooked during a subacromial approach. Subsequent surgery was 75 percent successful in patients not receiving worker's compensation but only 46 percent successful in the compensation group.

It is important to understand that not all torn rotator cuffs require surgical repair.[60] Wuelker and associates demonstrated in a dynamic shoulder model that the supraspinatus portion of the cuff (the area most likely to be torn in impingement) produces less torque and more joint compression than the deltoid and has no effect on humeral head depression during shoulder elevation.[60a] Not all cuff tears cause progression to superior migration and eventual cuff tear arthropathy. The indication for surgery is intractable pain and functional impairment. In elderly individuals, symptomatic treatment and physical therapy is generally sufficient, and most cuff tears are treated conservatively.[61]

Calcific Tendinitis

Although most cases of rotator cuff tendinitis represent one of the stages of mechanical impingement, there appears to be a group of patients predisposed to inflammation in this area. These patients frequently have bilateral disease and a history of other periarticular conditions such as trochanteric bursitis of the hip or symptoms of fibrositis. One particular subset of this group is made up of individuals with calcific tendinitis. Calcific tendinitis is a painful condition about the rotator cuff in association with the deposition of calcium salts, primarily hydroxyapatite.[62–64] It is most common in patients over 30 years of age and shows a predilection for females.[62, 65] Although it is more common in the right shoulder, there is at least a 6 percent incidence of bilaterality.[62] Patients with bilateral shoulder involvement often have the syndrome of calcific periarthritis, where calcium hydroxyapatite crystals are found at multiple sites.[69]

Codman pointed out the localization of the calcification within the tendon of the supraspinatus.[1] He provided a detailed description of the symptoms and natural history of this condition. In describing the phases of pain, spasm, limitation of motion, and atrophy, he noted the lack of correlation between symptoms and the size of the calcific deposit. According to Codman, the natural history includes degeneration of the supraspinatus tendon, calcification, and eventual rupture into the subacromial bursa. During the last phase, pain and decreased motion can lead to adhesive capsulitis (see Fig. 28–7).

The pathogenesis of calcific tendinitis of the supraspinatus is recognized as a degenerative process with secondary calcification within the tendon fibers.[62–64] The localization of calcium within the supraspinatus may be due to several factors. Many of these patients have an early stage of impingement, with compression of the supraspinatus tendon on the anterior portion of the acromion.[43, 44] This long-standing impingement may lead to local degeneration of the tendon fibers. In patients without impingement, the localization of the calcium within the supraspinatus may be related to the blood supply of the rotator cuff, which normally is derived from an anastomotic network of vessels from either the greater tuberosity or the bellies of the short rotator muscles.[63] The watershed of these sources is just medial to the tendinous attachment of the supraspinatus.[66] Rathburn and Macnab referred to this watershed as the "critical zone" and pointed out that during abduction this area was rendered ischemic.[67]

Gartner and Heyer classified calcific tendinitis as a *chronic initial phase* (type I), where the calcific deposit is dense and well circumscribed; a *resolving phase* (type III), where the deposit is translucent and cloudy; and an *indeterminate phase* (type II).[67a] The phase of the disease is an important prognostic indicator. In type III lesions, spontaneous resolution usually occurs in approximately 2 to 3 weeks, whereas type I and type II deposits are characterized by a more refractory course. Jim and coworkers reported that small calcific lesions are more likely to be associated with rotator cuff tears, and that cuff tears are rarely seen with larger calcific deposits.[67b]

The stimulation for calcification in calcific tendinitis has been the focus of considerable study.[63, 64, 66] Steinbrocker postulated that the process begins with necrosis and fraying of the tendon fibers, with secondary formation of a fibrinoid mass surrounded by leukocytes; this mass then serves as a template for calcification.[68] Others have suggested that the process of degeneration of the tendon causes formation of small particles consisting primarily of calcium salts.[4] The hyperemia associated with the acute episode would cause coalescence of the calcium, with formation of a liquefied calcium mass. As the increased vascularity subsides, this calcified mass would return to its "dry state."

It is also possible that the hypervascularity may, in fact, "wash out" an inhibitor substance and allow calcification to occur on the denuded fibers of the frayed tendon. It would be attractive to consider proteoglycans in this inhibitory role, because they are ubiquitous in tendons and articular cartilage, neither of which calcify in the normal state.

Uhthoff and associates have proposed that the pathogenesis of this process is not associated with inflammation or scarring, but that the primary stimulus is hypoxia, which results in transformation of portions of the tendon into fibrocartilage.[63] The chondrocytes then would mediate calcification in a way similar to that occurring in the calcifying zone of the epiphyseal plate. A subsequent study pointed out that the ultrastructure of calcifying tendinitis failed to demonstrate the arrangement or cell types seen in the epiphyseal plate.[64] The calcification occurred in extracellular matrix vesicles located in areas that had undergone fibrocartilaginous transformation. The authors pointed out the similarity to extracellular vesicles noted in other normal and pathologic conditions.[64] After calcification, the foci became surrounded by mononuclear and multinucleate cells, with phagocytized material within the cytoplasm.[63] Vascular invasion occurred as part of the repair process. With restoration of normal perfusion and oxygen tension to the tissue, the calcium could be resorbed and the tendon returned to its normal state.[63]

Calcific tendinitis has also been identified at the insertion of the long head of the biceps on the superior glenoid ring and in the long head of the biceps at the junction of the tendon and the muscle. Of 119 cases of calcific tendinitis reviewed between 1980 and 1988, 20 had calcific tendinitis in the region of the biceps tendon (9 at the glenoid insertion and 11 adjacent to the humeral shaft). In the 11 cases with distal calcification, all had small homogeneous deposits, and the major differential diagnosis was with loose bodies trapped in the biceps tendon sheath.[67]

Treatment of calcific tendinitis depends on the clinical presentation and the presence of associated impingement. These patients can have an acute inflammatory reaction that may resemble gout. The acute inflammation can be treated with local glucocorticoid injection or the use of nonsteroidal agents, or both. On occasion the use of ultrasound may be

of some benefit. If there is associated impingement, treatment depends on the stage of presentation. The radiographic appearance of the calcification can direct and perhaps predict the response to therapy. In the resorptive phase, the deposits appear floccular, suggesting that the process is in the phase of repair and that a conservative program is indicated. Those patients with discrete calcification, and perhaps associated adhesive capsulitis (see Fig. 28–7), may be at a stable phase at which the calcium produces a mechanical block and is unlikely to be resorbed. In these patients mechanical removal of the calcific deposits and correction of associated pathologic lesions may be necessary. Percutaneous disruption of the calcified areas may be performed using a needle directed by fluoroscopy. This technique allows lavage and injection but will not treat associated impingement. Subacromial arthroscopy allows the mechanical needle disruption of calcific deposits under direct visualization. Moreover, this technique can be combined with arthroscopic removal of the inflamed bursa and decompression of associated impingement. In many cases of refractory calcific tendinitis associated with impingement, open acromioplasty, subacromial bursectomy, and decompression are indicated.

Ark and colleagues reviewed the results of arthroscopic removal of calcific deposits.[68a] In this study of 23 patients, 13 had partial calcium removal; in time the removal was complete. Results were good in 11 patients (50 percent), satisfactory in 9 (41 percent), and unsatisfactory in 2 (9 percent).

Rotator Cuff Tear

Spontaneous tear of the rotator cuff in an otherwise normal individual is rare.[43] It can occur in patients with rheumatoid arthritis or lupus as part of the pathologic process with invasion from underlying pannus. Metabolic conditions such as renal osteodystrophy or agents such as glucocorticoids are occasionally associated with spontaneous cuff tears. Most patients report a traumatic episode, such as falling on an outstretched arm or lifting a heavy object. The usual presenting symptoms are pain and weakness of abduction and external rotation. There may be associated crepitus and even a palpable defect. Longstanding tears are generally associated with atrophy of the supraspinatus and infraspinatus muscles. It may be difficult to differentiate a partial-thickness cuff tear from a painful tendinitis. Plain radiographs are helpful only during a later stage of the process, when there may be narrowing of the acromiohumeral gap, proximal subluxation of the humeral head, and even erosion on the undersurface of the acromion.[71] Sonography or MRI is helpful in evaluating acutely torn rotator cuffs. Arthrography, however, is more selective in differentiating full-thickness tears from partial tears. The overlap in the diagnosis of complete tears and incomplete lesions makes development of a rational form of treatment difficult. DePalma reported that 90 percent of patients with rotator cuff tears respond to conservative measures such as rest, analgesics, anti-inflammatory agents, and physiotherapy.[72]

During the acute phase of pain the arm may be supported in a sling, but early restoration of motion is important to prevent adhesive capsulitis. Instillation of glucocorticoids into the subacromial bursa may provide dramatic relief of symptoms.

Surgical treatment depends on the patient's symptoms, the functional demand, and the etiology of the tear. Most acute tears represent the extension of a tear associated with chronic impingement.[43] Patients in this group who fail to respond to conservative means should be treated by an anterior acromioplasty with rotator cuff repair.

In elderly patients whose pain and weakness do not create a functional problem, a conservative program is preferable. Wolfgang pointed out that surgical results are less satisfactory with increased patient age.[73] Earnshaw and associates reviewed 37 patients who had undergone rotator cuff repair and found that overall 65 percent showed good results.[74] Patients in the fourth and fifth decades of life generally did well, but only 60 percent of patients in the sixth and seventh decades had good results. In their study, the mechanism of injury, the extent of the tear, and the timing of repair had no influence on the outcome. The authors pointed out that most shoulders showed radiographic progression of proximal subluxation despite surgical repair. In this small series, good functional results were reported in 2 patients with irreparable tears and in some patients with postoperative arthrograms showing leakage of contrast. The authors concluded that relief of impingement and debridement of the edge of the tear were important determinants in the relief of symptoms.[74]

Acute traumatic tears of the rotator cuff in active patients may occur without long-standing impingement. These tears can occur with an acute episode and even can be associated with other pathologic changes, such as dislocation or fracture. The presence of weakness to initiation of abduction and external rotation in a neutral position following injury suggests the possibility of an acute rotator cuff tear. Acute full-thickness rotator cuff tears associated with functional weakness should be considered for immediate surgical repair.

The surgical approach, technique of repair, and postoperative management are beyond the scope of this discussion and are well covered in other sources.[2, 3, 72, 74, 75]

Bicipital Tendinitis and Rupture

Bicipital tendinitis, subluxation of the biceps tendon within the bicipital groove, and rupture of the long head of the biceps are generally associated with anterior shoulder pain.

The long head of the biceps is an intracapsular and extrasynovial structure. It passes through the bicipital groove and over the head of the humerus and inserts on the superior rim of the glenoid (see Fig. 28–1A).[76] The biceps tendon aids in flexion of the forearm, supination of the pronated forearm if the elbow is flexed, and forward elevation of the shoulder.[3] As it crosses the humeral head, the biceps tendon is fixed within the bicipital groove. Meyer described a bony ridge on the lesser tuberosity and suggested that this was a source of tendon wear and eventual rupture.[77] Shallowness of this groove has been reported as a cause of subluxation and dislocation of the bicipital tendon.[78] Peterson reported a dissection study to determine the incidence of medial displacement of the biceps tendon.[79] In 77 cadaver dissections, the biceps tendon was found to be medially displaced in 5 cases (6.5 percent). Displacement was always found in association with a full-thickness tear of the supraspinatus tendon.[79] Moreover, in most cases, the tendon was displaced deep to a partially disrupted subscapularis tendon rather than over the subscapularis tendon, as commonly believed.[79]

Crenshaw and Kilgore reported that the early phases of bicipital tendinitis are associated with hypervascularity, edema of the tendon, and tenosynovitis.[80] Persistence of this process leads to adhesions between the tendon and its sheath, with impairment of the normal gliding mechanism in the groove. Stretching of these adhesions may be associated with chronic bicipital tendinitis.[78] The diagnosis of bicipital tendinitis is based on the localization of tenderness (see Fig. 28–1). It is often confused with impingement symptoms and, in fact, is frequently seen in association with an impingement syndrome.[43] Isolated bicipital tendinitis can be differentiated by the fact that the tender area will migrate with the bicipital groove as the arm is abducted and externally rotated.

There are many eponyms associated with tests to identify bicipital tendinitis.[3] Yergason's supination sign refers to pain in the bicipital groove when the examiner resists supination of the pronated forearm with the elbow at 90 degrees. Ludington's sign refers to pain in the bicipital groove when the patient interlocks the fingers on top of the head and actively abducts the arms.

Treatment is generally conservative and consists of rest, analgesics, nonsteroidal agents, and local injection of glucocorticoids. The use of US and neuroprobe is more beneficial in this condition than in isolated rotator cuff tendinitis. Treatment for patients with refractory bicipital tendinitis and recurrent symptoms of subluxation consists of opening the bicipital groove and resecting the proximal portion of the tendon with either tenodesis of the distal portion into the groove or transfer to the coracoid process. The proponents of tenodesis believe that it prevents proximal migration of the humeral head, whereas those who advocate transfer to the coracoid think that it maintains biceps power. Becker and Cofield reviewed the results of tenodesis of the long head of the biceps for chronic bicipital tendinitis in 54 shoulders. The authors reported initial short-term relief but found that recurrent symptoms occurred in a disproportionate number of the patients.[81]

Rupture of the long head of the biceps is easily diagnosed by the appearance of the contracted belly of the biceps muscle ("Popeye sign"). Patients frequently report a snap and acute pain in association with lifting an object. In older patients, in whom rupture is due to attrition, presentation is frequently spontaneous and is associated with few or no symptoms. Acute ruptures in young active individuals are best treated surgically with either tenodesis of the distal stump into the bicipital groove or transfer to the coracoid. Patients with long-standing symptoms of impingement and acute biceps tendon rupture are treated with anterior acromioplasty and tenodesis of the distal stump into the bicipital groove. In older patients without symptoms of impingement, a conservative program is preferable, because these patients are generally asymptomatic and have sufficient strength. Mariani and coworkers compared surgical and nonsurgical repair of a ruptured long head of the biceps tendon and found that pain relief was equivalent in both groups.[82] Residual subjective weakness at the elbow was reported in 4 of 27 patients in the surgical group and in 20 of 30 patients treated nonsurgically. The surgically treated patients returned to work later than the nonsurgical group, but 11 patients in the nonsurgical group were unable to return to full work capacity. On biomechanical testing, the nonsurgical group were found to have lost an average of 21 percent supination strength and 8 percent of elbow flexion strength. The surgical group lost no strength based on biomechanical testing.[82]

Acromioclavicular Arthritis

The majority of painful conditions about the acromioclavicular joint are caused by trauma with resultant acromioclavicular joint instability, meniscal tears, and secondary degenerative change.[83] Most of these patients have a history of direct trauma to the shoulder girdle. The pain may be generalized, but tenderness and, at times, crepitus can be palpated directly over the AC joint. The pain is increased by abduction of the arm and particularly by adducting the arm across the chest and compressing the joint.[2]

Plain radiographs may be normal unless there is a true dislocation or degenerative change. It is important to differentiate the traction spur at the insertion of the coracoacromial ligament from an osteophyte associated with degenerative change of the joint. An anteroposterior radiograph with the patient holding a weight in the ipsilateral hand may demonstrate joint instability in acute cases. Acute injuries are treated by rest, strapping, or surgical repair, depending on the degree of instability and the functional demand of the patient. Acute injuries without subluxation (grade I) or partial subluxation (grade II) are best treated by conservative means. Complete dislocations (grade III) are treated by early mobiliza-

tion, strapping to reduce the dislocation, or surgical repair according to the patient's functional demand and the surgeon's preference.[83–87]

Patients with degenerative change in the AC joint and symptoms that cannot be controlled by conservative means are best treated by debridement of the joint and resection of the distal clavicle.[84, 86] At no time should this joint be surgically fused.

GLENOHUMERAL DISORDERS

The various arthritides that affect the shoulder joint are discussed in detail in other chapters. They are reviewed here to discuss aspects unique to the glenohumeral joint. The usual symptom of intra-articular disorders is pain with motion. The pain is generalized throughout the shoulder girdle and at times referred to the neck, back, and upper arm. The usual response to pain is to decrease glenohumeral motion and to substitute increased scapulothoracic mobility. Patients with adequate elbow and scapulothoracic motion require little glenohumeral motion for activities of daily living; in fact, patients with glenohumeral arthrodesis can achieve adequate function.[87, 88] The response to pain, therefore, is diminution of motion and secondary soft tissue contractures with muscle atrophy. With increasing weakness and involvement of adjacent joints, the pain, limitation of motion, and weakness cause a substantial functional deficit.

Inflammatory Arthritis

The most common inflammatory arthritis involving the shoulder joint is rheumatoid arthritis, but other systemic disorders such as systemic lupus erythematosus (SLE), psoriatic arthritis, ankylosing spondylitis, Reiter's syndrome, and scleroderma may cause glenohumeral arthritis. The pathogenesis of the joint involvement in these conditions is discussed in detail in other chapters. All patients with significant involvement have pain. The limitation of motion is either due to splinting of the joint with secondary soft tissue contractures or attributable to primary soft tissue involvement with scarring or rupture. Plain radiographs will confirm glenohumeral involvement (Fig. 28–13A). There is narrowing of the glenohumeral joint space, with erosion and cyst formation without significant sclerosis or osteophytes. As the disease progresses, superior and posterior erosion of the glenoid with proximal subluxation of the humeral head may occur. Eventually, there may be secondary degenerative changes and even osteonecrosis of the humeral head.

Treatment is initially conservative and directed toward controlling pain, inducing a systemic remission (see Chapter 59), and maintaining joint motion by physical therapy. The use of intra-articular glucocorticoids may be beneficial in controlling local synovitis. In rheumatoid arthritis the involvement of periarticu-

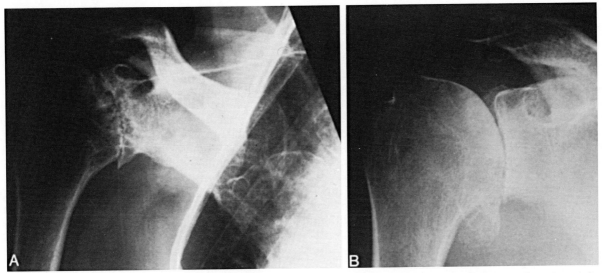

Figure 28–13. Plain radiographs. *A,* Rheumatoid arthritis with loss of joint space, cyst formation, glenohumeral erosion, and early proximal subluxation of the humerus indicating a rotator cuff tear. *B,* Osteoarthritis with narrowing of the glenohumeral joint space, sclerosis, and osteophyte formation. Note the preservation of the subacromial space, suggesting an intact rotator cuff.

lar structures with subacromial bursitis and rupture of the rotator cuff magnifies the functional deficit.

When the synovial cartilage interactions produce significant symptoms and radiographic changes that cannot be controlled by conventional therapy, glenohumeral resurfacing should be considered. The treatment of choice is an unconstrained shoulder arthroplasty of the type reported in detail in Chapter 108.[89, 90] Total shoulder arthroplasty is best performed in patients with rheumatoid arthritis before end-stage bony erosion and soft tissue contractions occur.[91, 92]

Acute inflammatory arthritis of the glenohumeral joint may also occur in association with gout, pseudogout, hydroxyapatite deposition of renal osteodystrophy, and recurrent hemophilic hemarthrosis.

Osteoarthritis

Osteoarthritis is less common in the glenohumeral joint than in the hip, its counterpart in the lower extremity. This is a result of both the non–weight-bearing characteristics of the shoulder joint and the distribution of forces throughout the shoulder girdle. Osteoarthritis is divided into those conditions associated with high unit loading of articular cartilage and those in which there is an intrinsic abnormality within the cartilage that causes abnormal wear at normal loads. Because the shoulder is normally a non–weight-bearing joint and is less susceptible to repeated high loading, the presence of osteoarthritis of the glenohumeral joint should alert the physician to consider other associated factors. Has the patient engaged in unusual activities such as boxing, heavy construction, or chronic use of a pneumatic hammer? Is there some disorder such as epiphyseal dysplasia that has created joint incongruity with high unit load-

ing of the articular cartilage? Is this a neuropathic process caused by diabetes, syringomyelia, or leprosy? Is there associated hemochromatosis, hemophilia, or gout that may have altered the ability of articular cartilage to withstand normal loading? Is unrecognized chronic dislocation responsible? Pain is the usual presentation, but it is generally not acute or associated with the spasm seen in inflammatory conditions. Plain radiographs show narrowing of the glenohumeral joint, osteophyte formation, sclerosis, and some cyst formation (Fig. 28–13B). Because the rotator cuff is generally intact, there is less bony erosion of the glenoid and proximal subluxation of the humerus. Patients with osteoarthritis of the glenohumeral joint frequently do well with functional adjustment and conservative therapy. Analgesics and nonsteroidal agents may provide symptomatic relief. The use of glucocorticoid injections is less beneficial unless there is evidence of synovitis. Patients with severe involvement who fail to respond are best treated by shoulder arthroplasty (see Chapter 108).[89–91]

Osteonecrosis

Osteonecrosis of the shoulder refers to necrosis of the humeral head in association with a variety of conditions. Symptoms are due to synovitis and joint incongruity resulting from resorption, repair, and remodeling. The pathogenesis and various causes are discussed in Chapter 101.

The most common cause of osteonecrosis of the shoulder is avascularity due to fractures through the anatomic neck of the humerus.[93] Fracture through this area disrupts the intramedullary and capsular blood supplies to the humeral head. Another common cause of osteonecrosis of the shoulder is steroid therapy in conjunction with organ transplantation, SLE, or asthma. The mechanism by which steroids are associated with osteonecrosis is unknown. There appears to be a host susceptibility, which may be genetically predetermined. Patients generally develop osteonecrosis shortly following steroid use, although symptoms may not manifest for a considerable period. At least in renal transplant patients, the association of osteonecrosis is independent of steroid dosage. The proposed pathogenesis of steroid-induced osteonecrosis includes increased free fatty acids with obliteration of intramedullary blood supply and steroid-induced vasculitis. This may elevate the intramedullary pressures within the humeral head and cause bone ischemia and death.[94] Other conditions associated with osteonecrosis of the humeral head include SLE, hemoglobinopathies, pancreatitis, and hyperbarism.

Avascular necrosis of the shoulder is common in sickle cell disease. David and associates reviewed 138 patients with sickle cell disease and reported shoulder avascular necrosis in 28 percent of patients, with only 53 percent having normal shoulder function.[95]

Early diagnosis of osteonecrosis is difficult because symptoms are often considerably delayed. Bone scans may be helpful early, before radiographic changes are present. Plain radiographs demonstrate progressive phases of necrosis and repair, as discussed in detail in Chapter 101. In the early stages, the films may be normal or show either osteopenia or bone sclerosis. A crescent sign, representing subchondral fracture or demarcation of the necrotic segment, appears during the reparative process. Patients who fail to remodel show collapse of the humeral head with secondary degenerative changes. There is often a considerable discrepancy between symptoms and radiographic involvement. Patients with extensive bony changes may be asymptomatic. Treatment should be directed by the patient's symptoms rather than the radiographs and is similar to that for osteoarthritis. Patients with severe symptoms that cannot be controlled by conservative means are best treated with an unconstrained shoulder arthroplasty or hemiarthroplasty.[89]

Cuff Arthropathy

In 1873 Adams described the pathologic changes in rheumatoid arthritis of the shoulder as well as a condition that has been referred to as Milwaukee shoulder or cuff tear arthropathy. The original lithographs of this report were recently reproduced in another article.[96] Halverson and coworkers reported that factors predisposing to this syndrome include deposition of calcium pyrophosphate dyhydrate crystals, direct trauma, chronic joint overuse, chronic renal failure, and denervation.[97] Patients with Milwaukee shoulder have been reported to have elevated levels of synovial fluid 5'-nucleotidase activity as well as elevated levels of synovial fluid inorganic pyro-

phosphate and nucleotide pyrophosphohydrolase activity.[98, 99]

Neer and colleagues have reported an unusual condition in which untreated massive tears of the rotator cuff with proximal migration of the humeral head are associated with erosion of the humeral surface.[46] The erosion of the humeral head is different from that seen in other arthritides and is presumed to be due to a combination of mechanical and nutritional factors. As the humeral head migrates superiorly, it is no longer contained and its cartilage cannot be nourished by the synovial fluid.

Patients with cuff tear arthropathies present a difficult therapeutic problem, as the bony erosion and disruption of the cuff jeopardizes the functional result from an unconstrained prosthesis.[91] In such patients a constrained total shoulder arthroplasty may be indicated.[100, 101]

It is crucial to determine which patients with massive rotator cuff tears are likely to proceed to the syndrome of cuff tear arthropathy. Patients with such tears who develop localized calcium pyrophosphate disease may be predisposed to further proximal migration and further joint destruction. This situation poses a dilemma for the treating physician. Many patients with massive rotator cuff tears remain stable and require little or no treatment. Occasionally, symptomatic patients can be treated by arthroscopic debridement of the cuff tear. If crystal deposition disease predisposes patients to proximal migration and joint destruction, joint aspiration with crystal analysis or scintigraphy to determine synovial reaction may be helpful.

Hamada and coworkers followed 22 patients with massive rotator cuff tears treated conservatively.[102] The radiographic findings included narrowing of the acromiohumeral interval and degenerative changes of the humeral head, tuberosities, acromion, acromioclavicular joint, and glenohumeral joint. Five of seven patients followed for more than 8 years progressed to cuff tear arthropathy. The authors concluded that progressive radiographic changes were associated with repetitive use of the arm in elevation, rupture of the long head of the biceps, impingement of the humeral head against the acromion, and weakness of external rotation.[102]

Septic Arthritis

Septic arthritis can masquerade as any of the conditions classified as periarticular or glenohumeral disorders. Sepsis must be included in any differential diagnosis of shoulder pain, as early recognition and prompt treatment are necessary to achieve a good functional result. The diagnosis is confirmed by joint aspiration with synovial fluid analysis and culture. Cultures should include aerobic, anaerobic, mycobacterial, and fungal studies. Septic arthritis is extensively covered in Chapters 90 to 93.

Glenoid Labral Tears

The increasing popularity of throwing sports and racket sports with individuals 25 to 60 years old has led to the recognition of tears of the glenoid labrum as a cause of anterior shoulder pain (see Fig. 28–1).

This diagnosis is easily confused with rotator cuff tendinitis or bicipital tendinitis and can best be confirmed by arthro-CT, DCAT,[11] or arthroscopy (see Fig. 28–6). Glenoid labral tears may be seen in association with anterior or even posterior instability. Labral tears can be divided into those associated with symptoms of internal derangement and those associated with instability. The SLAP (superior labrum anterior and posterior) lesion is associated with internal derangement but not instability. These tears involve the biceps tendon and labrum complex. The most common mechanism of injury is a compressive force to the shoulder as a result of a fall on an outstretched arm with the shoulder positioned in abduction and forward flexion. Depending on the size of the tear, it may be treated arthroscopically by debridement or arthroscopic stapling.[103, 104] If a glenoid labral tear is associated with instability, care must be taken in debriding the lesion, which may increase the symptoms of instability. Swimmer's shoulder, long thought to be an impingement syndrome, is often due to anterior labral changes that respond well to conservative arthroscopic debridement.[105]

Adhesive Capsulitis

Adhesive capsulitis, or "frozen shoulder," is a condition characterized by limitation of motion of the shoulder joint with pain at the extremes of motion. It was first described by Putnam in 1882[106] and later by Codman.[1] The initial presentation is pain, which is generalized and referred to the upper arm, the back, and the neck. As the pain increases, loss of joint motion ensues. The process is generally self-limiting and usually resolves spontaneously within 10 months unless there is an underlying problem.

Adhesive capsulitis is slightly more common in females than in males.[107] There is usually an underlying condition producing pain and restricted motion of the glenohumeral joint. Adhesive capsulitis may be seen as the end result of rotator cuff tendinitis, calcific tendinitis (see Fig. 28–7), bicipital tendinitis, and glenohumeral arthritis.[108, 109] It is also seen in a variety of other conditions, including apical lung tumors, pulmonary tuberculosis, cervical radiculopathy, and postmyocardial infarction.[108, 110, 111] In recent reviews of frozen shoulder, 3 of 140 patients with this syndrome had local primary invasive neoplasms.[112] Another study reviewed 3 patients presenting with the syndrome of adhesive capsulitis who subsequently were found to have neoplastic lesions of the midshaft of the humerus.[113]

DePalma reported that any condition hindering scapulohumeral motion causes muscular inactivity and predisposes the patient to adhesive capsulitis.[109] Neviaser found capsular adhesions to the underlying humeral head on surgical exploration for adhesive capsulitis.[114] Wiley described the arthroscopic findings associated with the diagnosis of primary adhesive capsulitis. These included a patchy vascular reaction around the biceps tendon and the opening into the subscapularis bursa. The capacity of the joint was reduced. In no case was the infraglenoid recess obliterated, and no adhesions were observed.[115] Morris and associates described erosions of the humeral head in association with the clinical syndrome of adhesive capsulitis.[116]

It is unclear whether the contracture of the shoulder capsule is a passive process related to lack of motion or an active process associated with capsular inflammation. Bulgen and colleagues reported an association between adhesive capsulitis and HLA-B27 antigen positivity.[117] They also reported decreased IgA levels in patients with the condition.[118] Lundberg[119] and Neviaser[114] failed to demonstrate synovitis or capsular inflammation during surgical exploration of patients with adhesive capsulitis.

Treatment of adhesive capsulitis is directed toward pain relief, restoration of function, and correction of the underlying cause. Many patients have depression or emotional lability either as an underlying problem or as a result of their pain and functional limitation. The physician must direct a long-term therapy program and reassure the patient that this condition is usually self-limiting. Because symptoms may last for a year, visits to the physical therapist become impractical, and a home program should be outlined.

Treatment of adhesive capsulitis is controversial. It is generally agreed that the disease is self-limiting and that its symptoms will improve in 1 to 2 years. Fareed and Gallivan reported good results with hydraulic distention of the glenohumeral joint using local anesthetic agents.[120] Similarly, Ekelund and Rydell found distention, manipulation, and intra-articular steroid administration to alleviate pain (91 percent of patients) and to restore motion (83 percent of patients) in patients with adhesive capsulitis.[120a] Corbeil and associates, however, in a double-blind prospective study, failed to show improved efficacy of distention arthrography with steroid injection versus steroid injection alone.[120b] In this study, more than 80 percent of patients improved with either therapy. Rizk and coworkers recently performed a prospective randomized study to assess the effect of steroid and/or local anesthetic injection in 48 patients with frozen shoulder.[121] In this study there was no significant difference in outcome between those individuals who received intrabursal injections and those receiving intra-articular injections. Moreover, steroid administration with lidocaine had no advantage over lidocaine alone in restoring shoulder motion. Transient pain relief, however, occurred in two thirds of the steroid-treated patients.[121]

Pollock and coworkers felt that shoulder arthroscopy to manipulation was helpful in that it allowed identification and correction of associated pathology such as impingement lesions and secondary subacromial space inflammation.[121a]

In patients with restriction of motion that prevents activities of daily living, a closed manipulation is indicated. This is best achieved at the time of arthrography (to confirm the diagnosis) and entails passive manipulation after the joint is inflated with a local anesthetic. The combination of inflating the joint and passive manipulation may free some adhesions and improve joint motion. On occasion, a general anesthetic is indicated for closed manipulation. Hill and Bogumill reported the results of manipulation on 17 frozen shoulders in 15 patients who did not respond to physical therapy.[122] Seventy-eight percent of the individuals working prior to their shoulder problems returned to work an average of 2.6 months following manipulation. The authors concluded that manipulation allowed patients to return to a normal lifestyle and to work sooner relative to the reported natural history of the condition.[122] Surgical intervention for adhesive capsulitis should be limited to treatment of the underlying problem such as calcific tendinitis or an impingement syndrome.

In a Swiss study Waldburger and colleagues stratified 50 cases of adhesive capsulitis in three etiologic groups; post-traumatic (40 percent), neurologic (14 percent), and idiopathic (46 percent).[122a] Bone scans were hot in 96 percent of cases. A combination of physical therapy and salmon calcitonin (100 units/day for 21 days) was significantly better in relieving pain than physical therapy alone.

Glenohumeral Instability

Dislocation of the glenohumeral joint in association with trauma has characteristic clinical and radiographic findings that are beyond the scope of this chapter and have been reviewed in detail elsewhere.[123] Anterior dislocation generally occurs with the arm in an abducted and externally rotated position, and the diagnosis is usually obvious. Posterior dislocation may be difficult to diagnose and is frequently seen in association with convulsive disorders or unusual trauma with the arm in a forward flexed and internally rotated position. There is often a significant delay in the recognition of a posterior dislocation, and this diagnosis should be suspected in patients who are unable to externally rotate from a neutral position. Recurrent subluxation without dislocation may be difficult to diagnose and be mistakenly identified as impingement with chronic rotator cuff tendinitis. Jobe and coworkers described the syndrome of shoulder pain in overhand or throwing athletes that presents as impingement but is due to anterior subluxation of the joint with the humeral head impinging on the anterior aspect of the coracoacromial arch.[124] Fu and associates divided the etiology of rotator cuff tendinitis into primary impingement of the supraspinatus tendon on the coracoacromial

arch and anterior subluxation with secondary impingement in young athletes performing overhead movements.[125]

The diagnosis of glenohumeral instability with subluxation in one or more directions is made on the basis of a detailed history, careful physical examination, and use of adjuncts such as arthrography, CT, and arthroscopy. The syndrome of multidirectional instability has been recognized in patients who are unstable in more than one direction.[126] This syndrome frequently occurs in young athletic patients, particularly in the dominant arm of pitchers, racket sport players, and swimmers. The most common presentation in these individuals is pain, often mistakenly attributed to rotator cuff tendinitis. The patient may relate a history of a minor trauma causing acute pain followed by a "dead arm" syndrome lasting for minutes or hours. Associated symptoms include a sense of instability, weakness, and even radicular symptoms suggestive of a neuropathy. There may be few, if any, positive physical findings in association with chronic subluxation or multidirectional instability. The patient may have signs of generalized ligamentous laxity, and pain may be reproduced by placing the arm in an evocative position. At times the arm may be excessively subluxed in one direction by physical examination. One particularly helpful sign is the "sulcus" sign, which refers to a subacromial indentation occurring with subluxation of the arm inferiorly with longitudinal traction or weights. Because this syndrome frequently occurs in athletes with highly developed musculature about the shoulder girdle, these physical findings of subluxation may be difficult to reproduce.[124]

Plain radiographs are generally normal, although some inferior subluxation may be reproduced by obtaining a plain radiograph with the patient carrying a weight and relaxing the shoulder musculature. Special radiographs may demonstrate Bankart's lesion (avulsion of the anterior inferior glenoid rim) or a Hill-Sachs lesion (osteochondral defect of the posterior humeral head) occurring with subluxation of the humeral head in front of the anterior glenoid rim. An arthro-CT scan may demonstrate a glenoid labral tear, laxity of the anterior glenohumeral ligaments, or a Hill-Sachs lesion (see Fig. 28–8). Arthroscopy may be of further help in delineating these pathologic abnormalities seen in association with the syndrome of multidirectional instability.

Treatment of chronic subluxation or multidirectional instability is first directed at rehabilitation. Strengthening exercises of the shoulder girdle under the supervision of an experienced therapist may control symptoms, stabilize the glenohumeral joint, and obviate the need for surgical intervention. If a conservative treatment program fails, surgery is directed at tightening the capsular structures to stabilize the glenohumeral joint.

REGIONAL DISORDERS

Because the shoulder girdle connects the thorax with the upper extremity, and the major neurovascular structures pass in close proximity to the joint, shoulder pain is a hallmark of many nonarticular conditions.

Cervical Radiculopathy

Cervical neck pain, with or without radiculopathy, may be associated with shoulder pain.[127] When cervical radiculopathy presents as shoulder pain, it is frequently due to involvement of the upper cervical roots. It can be differentiated from shoulder pain on the basis of history, physical examination, electromyographs, cervical radiographs, and myelography when indicated. Since conditions causing cervical neck pain and those causing shoulder pain, such as calcific tendinitis and cervical radiculopathy, may coexist, it is often difficult to distinguish which lesion is responsible for the symptoms. These conditions can often be differentiated by injection of local anesthetics to block certain components of the pain. Cervical neck pain is reviewed extensively in Chapter 27, so its diagnosis and treatment will not be discussed here. Hawkins and colleagues reported a study of 13 patients who underwent both subacromial shoulder decompressions or rotator cuff repairs and anterior cervical spine fusions.[128] Eight of the patients presented with nearly equal neck and shoulder pain, whereas the other 5 had predominantly neck symptoms. Following anterior cervical fusion, these 5 patients developed shoulder pain requiring subsequent surgical intervention.[128]

Brachial Neuritis

In the 1940s, Spillane[129] and Parsonage and Turner[130, 131] described a painful condition of the shoulder associated with limitation of motion. As the pain subsided and motion improved, muscle weakness and atrophy became apparent. The deltoid, supraspinatus, infraspinatus, biceps, and triceps are the most frequently involved muscles,[132] although diaphragmatic paralysis has also been reported.[131, 133] The etiology remains unclear, but the clustering of cases suggests a viral or postviral syndrome.[130, 131] Occasionally an associated influenza-like syndrome or previous vaccination has been reported.[132] Herschman and colleagues reported on acute brachial neuropathy in athletes.[134] The findings that suggest an acute brachial neuropathy include an acute onset of pain without trauma.

The prognosis for recovery is excellent, although full recovery may take 2 to 3 years. Tsiaris and co-workers reported 80 percent recovery within 2 years and more than 90 percent by the end of 3 years.[135] Malamut and colleagues pointed out the importance of differentiating this syndrome from brachial plexus stretch or direct injury to prevent unnecessary surgery.[135a]

Nerve Entrapment Syndromes

Entrapment of peripheral nerves as either a primary or a secondary process may cause pain about the shoulder girdle. The clinical picture and neurophysiology of nerve entrapment syndromes are covered in Chapter 42 and in other detailed sources.[136–138] Two entrapment neuropathies, axillary nerve entrapment and suprascapular nerve entrapment, are frequently overlooked and merit further discussion here.

The axillary nerve arises from the posterior cord of the brachial plexus and exits posteriorly through the quadrilateral space. This space is bordered superiorly by the teres major, inferiorly by the teres minor, medially by the long head of the triceps, and laterally by the humeral shaft and lateral triceps heads. After sending a sensory branch to the upper lateral cutaneous surface and a motor branch to the teres minor, the nerve courses anteriorly to innervate the deltoid.[76]

Entrapment of the axillary nerve as it exits through the quadrilateral space is an infrequent cause of pain, weakness, and atrophy about the shoulder girdle. It is most commonly seen in the dominant shoulder of young athletic individuals, such as pitchers, tennis players, and swimmers, who function with excessive overhead activity (Fig. 28–14). The pain may occur throughout the shoulder girdle and radiate down the

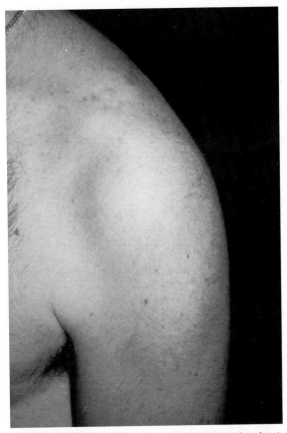

Figure 28–14. Marked anterior deltoid atrophy in the dominant arm of a professional tennis player with chronic axillary nerve entrapment.

arm in a nondermatomal pattern. It may be elicited by abduction and external rotation or by palpation of the quadrilateral space (see Fig. 28–1).

This condition represents entrapment of the axillary nerve as it leaves the posterior cord, penetrates the quadrilateral space, and moves anteriorly to innervate the deltoid. On surgical exploration, the nerve has been found to be tethered on the aponeurosis of the hypertrophied muscle or by fibrous bands encroaching on the quadrilateral space.[140]

Francel reported five patients with quadrilateral space syndrome or axillary nerve entrapment. In each case there was a history of trauma. The diagnosis was made on the basis of tenderness over the quadrilateral space, paresthesia over the lateral shoulder and upper arm, and deltoid weakness. The suprascapular nerve is a branch of the upper trunk of the brachial plexus formed by the fifth and sixth cervical nerves. It passes obliquely beneath the trapezius and crosses the scapula through the suprascapular notch.[76] The suprascapular nerve has no cutaneous sensory branches but supplies motor branches to the supraspinatus and infraspinatus muscles.

The suprascapular nerve entrapment syndrome is the result of compression and tethering of the nerve as it passes through the suprascapular notch. Rengachary and colleagues described variations in the size and shape of the fossa and the suprascapular ligament, which forms its superior border. The authors demonstrated variations in the fossa from a complete bony foramen to a smooth depression on the upper border of the scapula.[141] Patients with a true bony foramen or a deep notch should be more susceptible to the development of entrapment in this area.

The primary symptom is pain, which generally is described as a deep ache felt over the upper border and body of the scapula. The pain is well localized and does not radiate down the arm. Any activity that brings the scapula forward, such as reaching across the chest, may aggravate the pain.[142] Palpation of the suprascapular notch may elicit local tenderness (see Fig. 28–1).

Fritz and associates reported MRI to be helpful in the diagnosis of suprascapular nerve syndrome. The authors reported 21 ganglion cysts, two synovial sarcomas, one Ewing's sarcoma, one chondrosarcoma, one metastatic renal cell carcinoma, and one hematoma associated with this condition.[142a] In 40 percent of cases atrophy of both the supraspinatus and infraspinatus muscles was seen with anteriorly located masses and proximal entrapment of the nerve. In 33 percent of cases isolated atrophy of the infraspinatus muscle was found with posteriorly located masses and distal entrapment of the nerve.

Because the suprascapular nerve has no cutaneous innervation, there is no associated numbness, tingling, or paresthesias. With time, the patients develop atrophy and weakness of the supraspinatus and infraspinatus muscles.[142] This syndrome must be differentiated from rotator cuff tendinitis, which could be associated with a similar pattern of pain and muscle atrophy.[143] It also must be differentiated from brachial neuritis and a cervical radiculopathy involving the fifth and sixth roots.[144] Selective EMG determinations of the supraspinatus and infraspinatus muscles may reveal motor atrophy. Instillation of local anesthetics into the supraspinous notch may relieve the symptoms. As with axillary nerve entrapment, this syndrome is often associated with young athletic individuals with excessive overhead activity. It has also been reported in relation to trauma.[145, 146] After the diagnosis is confirmed, the treatment of choice is surgical decompression of the suprascapular notch. If the entrapment is associated with trauma, a substantial period of time should be allowed to rule out a neuropraxia, which is likely to resolve.

Sternoclavicular Pain

Occasionally, traumatic and nontraumatic conditions can cause pain about the sternoclavicular joint (see Fig. 28–1). The most common problem is ligamentous injury and painful subluxation or dislocation. This can be diagnosed by palpable instability and crepitus over the sternoclavicular joint. Sternoclavicular views may radiographically demonstrate dislocation.[84]

Inflammatory arthritis of the sternoclavicular joint has been seen in association with rheumatoid arthritis, ankylosing spondylitis, and septic arthritis. Two other conditions involving the sternoclavicular joint are *Tietze's syndrome,* a painful nonsuppurative swelling of the joint and adjacent sternochondral junctions, and *Friedreich's disease,* a painful osteonecrosis of the sternal end of the clavicle.[3]

Reflex Sympathetic Dystrophy

Since its original description by Mitchell in 1871,[147] reflex sympathetic dystrophy (RSD) has remained a poorly understood and frequently overlooked condition. Its etiology is unknown but may be related to sympathetic overflow or short-circuiting of impulses through the sympathetic system. Any clinician dealing with painful disorders must be familiar with the diagnosis and treatment of this condition. Bonica has provided an excellent review, which covers the clinical presentation, the various stages of the disease, and the importance of early intervention to ensure a successful outcome.[148]

RSD has been called causalgia, shoulder-hand syndrome, and Sudeck's atrophy. It is generally associated with minor trauma and is to be differentiated from causalgia involving trauma to major nerve trunks.[148] RSD is divided into three phases, which are important in the determination of the stage of involvement and the mode of treatment.[149] Phase 1 is characterized by sympathetic overflow with diffuse swelling, pain, increased vascularity, and radiographic evidence of demineralization. If left untreated for 3 to 6 months, this may progress to phase 2, which is characterized by atrophy. The extremity may now be cold and shiny, with atrophy of the skin and muscles. Phase 3 refers to progression of the trophic changes, with irreversible flexion contractures and a pale, cold, painful extremity. It has been speculated that phase 1 is related to a peripheral short-circuiting of nerve impulses, phase 2 represents short-circuiting through the internuncial pool in the spinal cord, and phase 3 is controlled by higher thalamic centers.[148, 149]

Steinbrocker reported that, as long as there is evidence of vasomotor activity with swelling and hyperemia, there remains a chance for recovery.[150] Once phase 2 or 3 is established, the prognosis for recovery is poor. Prompt recognition of the syndrome is important, because early intervention to control pain is mandatory. Careful supervision and reassurance are critical, because many of these patients are emotionally labile as a result of either their pain or an underlying problem. The syndrome may be remarkably reversed by a sympathetic block. Patients who receive transient relief from sympathetic blockade may be helped by surgical sympathectomy.

Veldman and Goris reported a 21 percent incidence of shoulder involvement in patients with RSD of the upper extremity.[150a] In this study, females with RSD of the upper extremity were more likely to have shoulder involvement. Falasca and colleagues reported an association of RSD and use of antiepileptic medication.[150b]

Fibrositis

Fibrositis and other diffuse musculoskeletal syndromes are characterized by multiple trigger points about the shoulder girdle. This subject is discussed in Chapter 34.

Neoplasms

Primary and metastatic neoplasms may cause shoulder pain by direct invasion of the musculoskeletal system or by compression with referred pain.[2, 138] Primary tumors are more likely to occur in younger individuals. The more common lesions have a typical distribution, such as the predilection of a chondroblastoma for the proximal humeral epiphysis or of an osteogenic sarcoma for the metaphysis.[151] The differential diagnosis of spontaneous onset of shoulder pain in older individuals should include metastatic lesions and myeloma. Neoplasms are best identified by plain radiographs, technetium Tc 99m MDP scintigraphy, and CT.

Pancoast's syndrome or apical lung tumor may present as shoulder pain owing to invasion of the brachial plexus.[109, 152, 153] With invasion of the cervical sympathetic chain, the patient may also develop Horner's syndrome.

Miscellaneous Conditions

A variety of other conditions may present as shoulder pain and should be mentioned in this discussion. Acute abdominal disorders such as gallbladder disease, splenic injuries, and subphrenic abscess can refer pain to the shoulder. The pain of acute angina and myocardial infarction may be referred to the left shoulder and down the inner aspect of the left arm. Metabolic disorders such as hypo- and hyperthyroidism,[153] diabetes mellitus,[154–156] and secondary hyperparathyroidism in association with renal osteodystrophy are infrequently associated with pain about the shoulder girdle. With the increasing number of patients undergoing long-term maintenance hemodialysis, a shoulder pain syndrome known as dialysis shoulder arthropathy has been described. This consists of shoulder pain, weakness, loss of motion, and functional limitation. The etiology and pathogenesis of this syndrome are unclear, although rotator cuff disease, pathologic fracture, bursitis, and local amyloid deposition have been implicated as causative factors.[157] To date, there are insufficient surgical or necropsy data to confirm any specific diagnosis. These patients generally respond poorly to local measures such as injection, heat, and NSAIDs but may improve with correction of underlying metabolic disorders such as osteomalacia and secondary hyperthyroidism.

References

1. Codman EA: The Shoulder: Rupture of the Supraspinatus Tendon and Other Lesions in or About the Subacromial Bursa. Boston, Thomas Todd, 1934.
2. Bateman E: The Shoulder and Neck, 2nd ed. Philadelphia, WB Saunders, 1978.
3. Post M: The Shoulder—Surgical and Non-surgical Management. Philadelphia, Lea & Febiger, 1988.
4. Cailliet R: Shoulder Pain, 2nd ed. Philadelphia, FA Davis, 1981.
5. Greep JM, Lemmens HAJ, Roos DB, Urschel HC: Pain in Shoulder and Arm: An Integrated View. The Hague, Martinus Nijhoff, 1979.
5a. Tyson LL: Imaging of the painful shoulder (review). Curr Probl Diagn Radiol 24:110–140, 1995.
5b. Green A, Norris TR: Imaging techniques for glenohumeral arthritis and glenohumeral arthroplasty. Clin Orthop 307:7–17, 1994.
6. Jobe FW, Kvitne RS, Giangarra CE: Shoulder pain in the overhand or throwing athlete: The relationship of anterior instability and rotator cuff impingement. Orthop Rev 18(9):963, 1989.
7. Dalton SE, Snyder SJ: Glenohumeral instability. Baillieres Clin Rheumatol 3:511, 1989.
8. Goldman AB: Shoulder Arthrography. Boston, Little, Brown & Co, 1982.
9. Goldman AB, Ghelman B: The double contrast shoulder arthrogram: A review of 158 studies. Radiology 127:655, 1978.
10. Mink J, Harris E: Double contrast shoulder arthrography: Its use in evaluation of rotator cuff tears. Orthop Trans 7:71, 1983.
11. Braunstein EM, O'Connor G: Double-contrast arthrotomography of the shoulder. J Bone Joint Surg 64:192, 1982.
12. el-Khoury GY, Kathol MH, Chandler JB, Albright JP: Shoulder instability: Impact of glenohumeral arthrotomography on treatment. Radiology 160:669, 1986.
13. Kneisl JS, Sweeney HJ, Paige ML: Correlation of pathology observed in double contrast arthrotomography. Arthroscopy 4:21, 1988.
14. Strizak AM, Danzig L, Jackson DW, Greenway D, Resnick D, and Staple T: Subacromial bursography. J Bone Joint Surg Am 64:196, 1982.
15. Lie S: Subacromial bursography. Radiology 144:626, 1982.
16. Fukuda H, Mikasa M, Yamanaka K: Incomplete thickness rotator cuff tears diagnosed by subacromial bursography. Clin Orthop 223:51, 1987.
17. Rafii M, Minkoff J, Bonano J, Firooznia H, Jaffe L, Golimbu C: Computed tomography (CT) arthrography of shoulder instabilities in athletes. Am J Sports Med 16:352, 1988.

17a. Blum A, Boyer B, Regent D, Simon JM, Claudon M, Mole D: Direct coronal view of the shoulder with arthrographic CT. Radiology 188:677–681, 1993.
18. Mack LA, Matsen FA, Kilcoyne RF, Davies PK, Sickler ME: US evaluation of the rotator cuff. Radiology 157:206, 1985.
19. Crass JR, Craig EV, Bretzke C, Feinberg SB: Ultrasonography of the rotator cuff. Radiographics 5:941, 1985.
20. Middleton WD, Edelstein G, Reinus WR, Melson GL, Murphy WA: Ultrasonography of the rotator cuff: Technique and normal anatomy. J Ultrasound Med 3:549, 1984.
21. Bretze CA, Crass JR, Craig EV, Feinberg SB: Ultrasonography of the rotator cuff: Normal and pathologic anatomy. Invest Radiol 20:311, 1985.
22. Crass JR, Craig EV, Thompson RC, Feinberg SB: Ultrasonography of the rotator cuff: Surgical correlation. J Clin Ultrasound 12:487, 1984.
23. Middleton WD, Edelstein G, Reinus WR, Melson GL, Totty WG, Murphy WA: Sonographic detection of rotator cuff tears. AJR Am J Roentgenol 144:349, 1985.
24. Crass JR, Craig EV, Feinberg SB: Sonography of the postoperative rotator cuff. AJR Am J Roentgenol 146:561, 1986.
25. Middleton WD, Reinus WR, Totty WG, Melson GL, Murphy WA: US of the biceps tendon apparatus. Radiology 157:211, 1985.
26. Middleton WD, Reinus WR, Melson GL, Totty WG, Murphy WA: Pitfalls of rotator cuff sonography. AJR Am J Roentgenol 146:555, 1986.
27. Gardelin G, Perin B: Ultrasonics of the shoulder: Diagnostic possibilities in lesions of the rotator cuff. Radiol Med (Torino) 74:404, 1987.
28. Mack LA, Nyberg DA, Matsen FR, Kilcoyne RF, Harvey D: Sonography of the postoperative shoulder. AJR Am J Roentgenol 150:1089, 1988.
29. Hodler J, Terrier B, von-Schulthess GK, Fuchs WA: MRI and sonography of the shoulder. Clin Radiol 43:323, 1991.
30. Vestring T, Bongartz G, Konermann W, Erlemann R, Reuther G, Krings W, Saathoff J, Drescher H, Peters PE: The place of magnetic resonance tomography in the diagnosis of diseases of the shoulder joint. Rofo Fortschr Geb Rontgenstr Neuen Bildgeb Verfahr 154:143, 1991.
30a. van Moppers MF, Veldkamp O, Roorda J: Role of shoulder ultrasonography in the evaluation of the painful shoulder. Eur J Radiol 19:142–146, 1995.
30b. Ryu KN, Lee SW, Rhee YG, Lim JH: Adhesive capsulitis of the shoulder joint: usefulness of dynamic sonography. J Ultrasound Med 12:445–449, 1993.
31. Ahovuo J, Paavolainen P, Slatis P: Diagnostic value of sonography in lesions of the biceps tendon. Clin Orthop 202:184, 1986.
32. Ogilvie-Harris DJ, D'Angelo G: Arthroscopic surgery of the shoulder. Sports Med 9:120, 1990.
33. Zlatkin, MB, Reicher MA, Kellerhouse LE, McDade W, Vetter L, Resnick D: The painful shoulder: MR imaging of the glenohumeral joint. J Comput Assist Tomogr 12:995, 1988.
34. Meyer SJ, Dalinka MK: Magnetic resonance imaging of the shoulder. Orthop Clin North Am 21:497, 1990.
35. Seeger LL, Gold RH, Bassett LW: Shoulder instability: Evaluation with MR imaging. Radiology 168:696, 1988.
36. Kieft GJ, Dijkmans BA, Bioem JL, Kroon HM: Magnetic resonance imaging of the shoulder in patients with rheumatoid arthritis. Ann Rheum Dis 49:7, 1990.
37. Morrison DS, Offstein R: The use of magnetic resonance imaging in the diagnosis of rotator cuff tears. Orthopedics 13:633, 1990.
38. Nelson MC, Leather GP, Nirschl RP, Petrone FA, Freedman MT: Evaluation of the painful shoulder: A prospective comparison of magnetic resonance imaging, computerized tomographic arthrography. J Bone Joint Surg Am 73:707, 1991.
38a. Monu JU, Pruett S, Vanarthos WJ, Pope TJ: Isolated subacromial bursal fluid on MRI of the shoulder in symptomatic patients: Correlation with arthroscopic findings. Skeletal Radiol 23:529–533, 1994.
38b. Schweitzer ME, Magbalon MJ, Frieman BG, Ehrlich S, Epstein RE: Acromioclavicular joint fluid: Determination of clinical significance with MR imaging. Radiology 192:205–207, 1994.
39. Reeder JD, Andelman S: The rotator cuff tear: MR evaluation. Magn Reson Imaging 5:331, 1987.
40. Seeger LL, Gold RH, Bassett LW, Ellman H: Shoulder impingement syndrome: MR findings in 53 shoulders. AJR Am J Roentgenol 150:343, 1988.
40a. Owen RS, Iannotti JP, Kneeland JB, Dalinka MK, Deren JA, Oleaga L: Shoulder after surgery. Radiology 186:443–447, 1993.
40b. Emig EW, Schweitzer ME, Karasick D, Lubowitz J: Adhesive capsulitis of the shoulder: MR diagnosis. AJR Am J Roentgenol 164:1457–1459, 1995.
40c. Massengill AD, Seeger LL, Yao L, Gentili A, Shnier RC, Shapiro MS, Gold RH: Labrocapsular ligamentous complex of the shoulder: Normal anatomy, anatomic variation, and pitfalls of MR imaging and MR arthrography. Radiographics 14:1211–1223, 1994.
40d. Chandnani VP, Yeager TD, DeBerardino T, Christensen K, Gagliardi JA, Heitz DR, Baird DE, Hansen MF: Glenoid labral tears: Prospective evaluation with MRI imaging, MR arthrography, and CT arthrography. AJR Am J Roentgenol 161:1229–1235, 1993.
40e. Kopka L, Funke M, Fischer U, Keating D, Oestmann J, Grabbe E: MR arthrography of the shoulder with gadopentetate dimeglumine: Influence of concentration, iodinated contrast material, and time on signal intensity. AJR Am J Roentgenol 163:621–623, 1994.
40f. Uri DS, Kneeland JB, Dalinka MK: Update in shoulder magnetic resonance imaging (review). Magn Reson Q 11:21–44, 1995.
41. Nakano KK: Neurology of Musculoskeletal and Rheumatic Disorders. Boston, Houghton Mifflin, 1979.
42. Leffert RD: Brachial plexus injuries. N Engl J Med 291:1059, 1974.
43. Neer CS II: Impingement lesions. Clin Orthop 173:70, 1983.
44. Neer CS II: Anterior acromioplasty for the chronic impingement syndrome in the shoulder: a preliminary report. J Bone Joint Surg Am 54:41, 1972.
44a. Wuelker N, Schmotzer H, Thren K, Korell M: Translation of the glenohumeral joint with simulated active elevation. Clin Orthop 309:193–200, 1994.
44b. Wuelker N, Plitz W, Roetman B: Biomechanical data concerning the shoulder impingement syndrome. Clin Orthop 303:242–249, 1994.
44c. Kvitne RS, Jobe FW: The diagnosis and treatment of anterior instability in the throwing athlete (review). Clin Orthop 2917:107–123, 1993.
44d. Ferrari JD, Ferrari DA, Coumas J, Pappas AM: Posterior ossification of the shoulder: The Bennett lesion. Etiology, diagnosis, and treatment. Am J Sports Med 22:171–175, 1994.
44e. Tirman PF, Bost FW, Garvin GJ, Peterfy CG, Mall JC, Steinbach LS, Feller JF, Crues JV III: Posterosuperior glenoid impingement of the shoulder: Findings at MR imaging and MR arthrography with arthroscopic correlation. Radiology 193:431–436, 1994.
44f. Liu SH, Boynton E: Posterior superior impingement of the rotator cuff on the glenoid rim as a cause of shoulder pain in the overhead athlete. Arthroscopy 9:697–699, 1993.
45. Neer CS II, Bigliani LU, Hawkins RJ: Rupture of the long head of the biceps related to subacromial impingement. Orthop Trans 1:111, 1977.
46. Neer CS II, Craig EV, Fukada H, Mendoza FX: Cuff tear arthropathy. Exhibit at the Annual Meeting of the American Academy of Orthopedic Surgeons, New Orleans, 1982.
47. Neer CS II, Marberry TA: On the disadvantages of radical acromionectomy. J Bone Joint Surg Am 63:416, 1981.
48. Ellman H: Occupational supraspinatus tendinitis: The rotator cuff syndrome. Ugeskr Laeger 151:2355, 1989.
49. Scheib JS: Diagnosis and rehabilitation of the shoulder impingement syndrome in the overhand and throwing athlete. Rheum Dis Clin North Am 16:971, 1990.
50. Bosley RC: Total acromionectomy: A twenty year review. J Bone Joint Surg Am 73:961, 1991.
51. Gartsman GM: Arthroscopic acromioplasty for lesions of the rotator cuff. J Bone Joint Surg Am 72:169, 1990.
52. Paulos LE, Franklin JL: Arthroscopic shoulder decompression development and application: A five year experience. Am J Sports Med 18:235, 1990.
52a. Roye RP, Grana WA, Yates CK: Arthroscopic subacromial decompression: Two- to seven-year follow-up. Arthroscopy 11:301–306, 1995.
52b. Van Hoilsbeech HE, DeRycke J, Declercq G, Martens M, Verstreken J, Fabry G: Subacromial impingement: Open versus arthroscopic decompression. Arthroscopy 8:173–178, 1992.
52c. Schneider T, Strauss JM, Hoffstetter I, Jerosch J: Shoulder joint stability after arthroscopic subacromial decompression. Arch Orthop Trauma Surg 113:129–133, 1994.
52d. Zvijac JE, Levy HJ, Lemak LJ: Arthroscopic subacromial decompression in the treatment of full thickness rotator cuff tears: A 3–6 year follow-up. Arthroscopy 10:518–523, 1994.
53. Levy HJ, Gardner RD, Lemak LJ: Arthroscopic subacromial decompression in the treatment of full-thickness rotator cuff tears. Arthroscopy 7:8, 1991.
54. Ellman H: Arthroscopic subacromial decompression: Analysis of one to three year results. Arthroscopy 3:173, 1987.
55. Hawkins RJ, Brock RM, Abrams JS, Hobekia P: Acromioplasty for impingement with an intact rotator cuff. J Bone Joint Surg 70:795, 1988.
56. Stuart MJ, Azevedo AJ, Cofield RH: Anterior acromioplasty for treatment of the shoulder impingement syndrome. Clin Orthop 260:195, 1990.
57. Bigliani LU, D'Alesandro DF, Dduralde XA, Mclveen SJ: Anterior acromioplasty for subacromial impingement in patients younger than 40 years of age. Clin Orthop 246:111, 1989.
58. Bjorkenheim JM, Paavolainen P, Ahovuo J, Slatis P: Surgical repair of the rotator cuff and surrounding tissues: Factors influencing the results. Clin Orthop 236:148, 1988.
59. Ogilvie-Harris DJ, Wiley AM, Sattarian J: Failed acromioplasty for impingement syndrome. J Bone Joint Surg Br 72:1070, 1990.
60. Rockwood CA, Jr: The shoulder: Facts, confusions and myths. Int Orthop 15:401, 1991.
60a. Wuelker N, Plitz W, Roetman B, Wirth CJ: Function of the supraspinatus muscle: Abduction of the humerus studied in cadavers. Acta Orthop Scand 65:442–446, 1994.

61. Steffens K, Konermann H: Rupture of the rotator cuff in the elderly. Z Gerontol 20:95, 1987.
62. McKendry RJR, Uhthoff HK, Sarkar K, Hyslop P: Calcifying tendinitis of the shoulder: Prognostic value of clinical, histologic, and radiographic features in 57 surgically treated cases. J Rheumatol 9:75, 1982.
63. Uhthoff HK, Sarkar K, Maynard JA: Calcifying tendinitis: A new concept of its pathogenesis. Clin Orthop 118:164, 1976.
64. Sarkar K, Uhthoff HK: Ultrastructural localization of calcium in calcifying tendinitis. Arch Pathol Lab Med 102:266, 1978.
65. Vebostad A: Calcific tendinitis in the shoulder region: A review of 43 operated shoulders. Acta Orthop Scand 46:205, 1975.
66. Moseley HF, Goldie I: The arterial pattern of the rotator cuff of the shoulder. J Bone Joint Surg Br 45:780, 1963.
67. Rathbun JB, Macnab I: The microvascular pattern of the rotator cuff. J Bone Joint Surg Br 52:540, 1970.
67a. Gartner J, Heyer A: Calcific tendinitis of the shoulder (review) [German]. Orthopade 24:284–302, 1995.
67b. Jim YF, Hsu HC, Chang CY, Wu JJ, Chang T: Coexistence of calcific tendinitis and rotator cuff tear: An arthrographic study. Skeletal Radiol 22:183–185, 1993.
68. Steinbrocker O: The painful shoulder. In Hollander JE (ed): Arthritis and Allied Conditions, 8th ed. Philadelphia, Lea & Febiger, 1972.
68a. Ark JW, Flock TJ, Flatow EL, Bigliani LU: Arthroscopic treatment of calcific tendinitis of the shoulder. Arthroscopy 8:183–188, 1992.
69. Hayes CW, Conway WF: Calcium hydroxyapatite deposition disease. Radiographics 10:1031, 1990.
70. Goldman AB: Calcific tendinitis of the long head of the biceps brachii distal to the glenohumeral joint: Plain film radiographic findings. AJR Am J Roentgenol 153:1011, 1989.
71. Kotzen LM: Roentgen diagnosis of rotator cuff tear. AJR Am J Roentgenol 112:507, 1971.
72. DePalma AF: Surgery of the Shoulder, 2nd ed. Philadelphia, JB Lippincott, 1973.
73. Wolfgang GL: Surgical repair of tears of the rotator cuff of the shoulder. Factors influencing the result. J Bone Joint Surg Am 56:14, 1974.
74. Earnshaw P, Desjardins D, Sarkar K, Uhthoff HK: Rotator cuff tears: The role of surgery. Can J Surg 25:60, 1982.
75. Post M, Silver R, Singh M: Rotator cuff tear, diagnosis and treatment. Clin Orthop 173:78, 1983.
76. Goss CM: Gray's Anatomy of the Human Body, 28th ed. Philadelphia, Lea & Febiger, 1966.
77. Meyer AW: Spontaneous dislocation and destruction of the tendon of the long head of the biceps brachii: Fifty-nine instances. Arch Surg 17:493, 1928.
78. Hitchcock HH, Bechtol CO: Painful shoulder: Observtions on the role of the tendon of the long head of the biceps brachii in its causation. J Bone Joint Surg Am 30:263, 1948.
79. Peterson CJ: Spontaneous medial dislocation of the tendon of the long biceps brachii: An anatomic study of prevalence and pathomechanics. Clin Orthop 211:224, 1986.
80. Crenshaw AH, Kilgore WE: Surgical treatment of bicipital tenosynovitis. J Bone Joint Surg Am 48:1496, 1966.
81. Becker DA, Cofield RH: Tenodesis of the long head of the biceps brachii for chronic bicipital tendinitis: Long-term results. J Bone Joint Surg Am 71:376, 1989.
82. Mariani EM, Cofield RH, Askew LJ, Li GP, Chao EY: Rupture of the tendon of the long head of the biceps brachii: Surgical versus nonsurgical treatment. Clin Orthop 228:233, 1988.
83. Wright PE: Dislocations. In Edmonson AS, Crenshaw AH (eds): Campbell's Operative Orthopedics. St Louis, CV Mosby, 1980.
84. Rockwood CA Jr: Fractures and dislocations of the shoulder: Part II. In Rockwood, CA Jr, Green DP (eds): Fractures. Philadelphia, JB Lippincott, 1975.
85. Glick J: Acromioclavicular dislocations in athletes. Orthop Rev 1:31, 1972.
86. Taylor GM, Tooke M: Degeneration of the acromioclavicular joint as a cause of shoulder pain. J Bone Joint Surg Br 59:507, 1977.
87. Cofield RH, Briggs BT: Glenohumeral arthrodesis. J Bone Joint Surg Am 61:668, 1979.
88. Rowe CR: Arthrodesis of the shoulder used in treating painful conditions. Clin Orthop 173:92, 1983.
89. Neer CS II, Watson KC, Stanton FJ: Recent experience in total shoulder replacement. J Bone Joint Surg Am 64:319, 1982.
90. Cofield RH: Unconstrained total shoulder prosthesis. Clin Orthop 173:97, 1983.
91. Thornhill TS, Karr MJ, Averill RM, Batte NJ, Thomas WH, Sledge CB: Total shoulder arthroplasty: The Brigham experience. 50th Annual Meeting of the American Academy of Orthopedic Surgeons, Anaheim, 1983.
92. Thornhill TS, Barrett WP: Total shoulder arthroplasty. In Rowe CR (ed): The Shoulder. New York, Churchill Livingstone, 1988.
93. Neer CS II: Fractures and dislocations of the shoulder: Part 1. In Rockwood CA, Green DP (eds): Fractures. Philadelphia, JB Lippincott, 1975.
94. Ficat RP, Arlet J: Ischemia and Necrosis of the Bone. Baltimore, Williams & Wilkins, 1980.
95. David HG, Bridgman SA, Davies SC, Hine AL, Emery RJ: The shoulder in sickle-cell disease. J Bone Joint Surg Br 75:538–545, 1993.
96. McCarty DJ: Robert Adams' rheumatic arthritis of the shoulder: "Milwaukee shoulder" revisited. J Rheumatol 16:668, 1989.
97. Halverson PB, Carrera GF, McCarty DJ: Milwaukee shoulder syndrome: Fifteen additional cases and a description of contributing factors. Arch Intern Med 150:677, 1990.
98. Wortmann RL, Veum JA, Rachow JW: Synovial fluid 5′-nucleotidase activity: Relationship to other purine catabolic enzymes and to arthropathies associated with calcium crystal deposition. Arthritis Rheum 34:1014, 1991.
99. Rachow JW, Ryan LM, McCarty DJ, Halverson PC: Synovial inorganic pyrophosphate concentration and nucleotide pyrophosphohydrolase activity in basic calcium phosphate deposition arthroplasty and Milwaukee shoulder syndrome. Arthritis Rheum 31:408, 1988.
100. Post M, Haskell SS, Jablon M: Total shoulder replacement with a constrained prosthesis. J Bone Joint Surg Am 62:327, 1980.
101. Post M, Jablon M: Constrained total shoulder arthroplasty: Long-term follow-up observations. Clin Orthop 173:109, 1983.
102. Hamada K, Fukuda H, Mikasa M, Kobayashi Y: Roentgenographic findings in massive rotator cuff tears: A long-term observation. Clin Orthop 254:92, 1990.
103. Snyder SJ, Karzel RP, Del-Pizzo W, Ferkek RD, Friedman MJ: SLAP lesions of the shoulder. Arthroscopy 6:274, 1990.
104. Yomeda M, Kiroka AS, Saito S, Yamamoto T, Ochi T, Shino K: Arthroscopic stapling for detached superior glenoid labrum. J Bone Joint Surg Br 73:746, 1991.
105. McMaster WC: Anterior glenoid labrum damage: A painful lesion in swimmers. Am J Sports Med 14:388, 1986.
106. Putnam JJ: The treatment of a form of painful periarthritis of the shoulder. Boston Med Surg J 107:536, 1882.
107. Lippman RK: Frozen shoulder; periarthritis; bicipital tenosynovitis. Arch Surg 47:283, 1943.
108. McLaughlin HL: The "frozen shoulder." Clin Orthop 20:126, 1961.
109. DePalma AF: Loss of scapulohumeral motion (frozen shoulder). Ann Surg 135:193, 1952.
110. Johnson JTH: Frozen shoulder syndrome in patients with pulmonary tuberculosis. J Bone Joint Surg Am 41:877, 1959.
111. Dee PE, Smith RG, Gullickson MJ, Ballinger CS: The orthopedist and apical lung carcinoma. J Bone Joint Surg Am 42:605, 1960.
112. Demaziere A, Wiley AM: Primary chest wall tumor appearing as frozen shoulder: Review and case presentations. J Rheumatol 18:911, 1991.
113. Smith CR, Binder AI, Paice EW: Lesions of the mid-shaft of the humerus presenting as shoulder capsulitis. Br J Rheumatol 29:386, 1990.
114. Neviaser JS: Adhesive capsulitis of the shoulder: A study of the pathological findings in periarthritis of the shoulder. J Bone Joint Surg 27:211, 1945.
115. Wiley AM: Arthroscopic appearance of frozen shoulder. Arthroscopy 7:138, 1991.
116. Morris IM, Mattingly PA, Thompson AJ: Radiological erosions in frozen shoulder. Br J Rheumatol 29:293, 1990.
117. Bulgen DY, Hazelman BL, Voak D: HLA-B27 and frozen shoulder. Lancet 1:1042, 1976.
118. Bulgen DY, Hazelman BL, Ward M, McCallum M: Immunological studies in frozen shoulder. Ann Rheum Dis 37:135, 1978.
119. Lundberg BJ: The frozen shoulder. Acta Orthop Scand Suppl 119:1, 1969.
120. Fareed DO, Gallivan WR Jr: Office management of frozen shoulder syndrome: Treatment with hydraulic distension under local anesthesia. Clin Orthop 242:177, 1989.
120a. Ekelund AL, Rydell N: Combination treatment for adhesive capsulitis of the shoulder. Clin Orthop 282:105–109, 1992.
120b. Corbeil V, Dussault RG, Leduc BE, Fleury J: Adhesive capsulitis of the shoulder: A comparative study of arthrography with intra-articular corticotherapy and with or without capsular distension [French]. Can Assoc Radiol J 43:127–30, 1992 282:105–109, 1992.
121. Rizk TE, Pinalls RA, Talaiver AS: Corticosteroid injections in adhesive capsulitis: Investigation of their value and site. Arch Phys Med Rehab 72:20, 1991.
121a. Pollock RG, Duralde XA, Flatow EL, Bigliani LU: The use of arthroscopy in the treatment of resistant frozen shoulder. Clin Orthop 304:30–36, 1994.
122. Hill JJ Jr, Bogumill H: Manipulation in the treatment of frozen shoulder. Orthopedics 11:1255, 1988.
122a. Waldburger M, Meier JL, Gobelet C: The frozen shoulder: Diagnosis and treatment. Prospective study of 50 cases of adhesive capsulitis. Clin Rheumatol 11:364–368, 1992.
123. Rowe CR: Dislocations of the shoulder. In Rowe CR (ed): The Shoulder. New York, Churchill Livingstone, 1988.
124. Jobe FW, Kvitne RS, Giangarra CE: Shoulder pain in the overhand or throwing athlete: The relationship of anterior instability and rotator cuff impingement. Orthop Rev 18:963, 1989.

125. Fu FH, Harner CD, Klein AH: Shoulder impingement syndrome: A critical review. Clin Orthop 269:162, 1991.
126. Neer CS, Foster CR: Inferior capsular shift for involuntary inferior and multidirectional instability of the shoulder: A preliminary report. J Bone Joint Surg 62:897, 1980.
127. Hawkins, RJ: Cervical spine and the shoulder. Instr Course Lect 34:191, 1985.
128. Hawkins RJ, Bilco T, Bonutti P: Cervical spine and shoulder pain. Clin Orthop 258:142, 1990.
129. Spillane JD: Localized neuritis of the shoulder girdle: A report of 46 cases in the MEF. Lancet 2:532, 1943.
130. Parsonage MJ, Turner JWA: Neurologic amyotrophy: The shoulder girdle syndrome. Lancet 1:973, 1948.
131. Turner JWA, Parsonage MJ: Neurologic amyotrophy (paralytic brachial neuritis): With special reference to prognosis. Lancet 2:209, 1957.
132. Bacevich BB: Paralytic brachial neuritis. J Bone Joint Surg 58:262, 1976.
133. Walsh NE, Dumitru D, Kalantri A, Roman AM Jr: Brachial neuritis involving the bilateral phrenic nerves. Arch Phys Med Rehab 68:46, 1987.
134. Hershman EB, Wilbourn AJ, Bergfield JA: Acute brachial neuropathy in athletes. Am J Sports Med 17:655, 1989.
135. Tsiaris P, Dyck PJ, Mulder DW: Natural history of brachial plexus neuropathy. Arch Neurol 27:109, 1972.
135a. Malamut RI, Marques W, England JD, Sumner AJ: Postsurgical idiopathic brachial neuritis. Muscle Nerve 17:320–324, 1994.
136. Omer GE Jr, Spinner M: Management of Peripheral Nerve Problems. Philadelphia, WB Saunders, 1980.
137. Kelly TR: Thoracic outlet syndrome: Current concepts and treatment. Ann Surg 190:657, 1979.
138. Brown C: Compressive invasive referred pain to the shoulder. Clin Orthop 173:55, 1983.
139. Bateman JE: Neurologic painful conditions affecting the shoulder. Clin Orthop 173:44, 1983.
140. Cahill BR: Quadrilateral space syndrome. In Omer GE Jr, Spinner MD (eds): Management of Peripheral Nerve Problems. Philadelphia, WB Saunders, 1980.
141. Rengachary SS, Neft JP, Singer PA, Brackett CE: Suprascapular entrapment neuropathy: A clinical, anatomical and comparative study. Neurosurgery 5:441, 1979.
142. Habermeyer P, Rappaport D, Wiedermann E, Wilhelm K: Incisura scapulae syndrome. Handchir Mikrochir Plast Chir 22:120, 1990.
142a. Fritz RC, Helms CA, Steinbach LS, Genant HK: Suprascapular nerve entrapment: Evaluation with MR imaging. Radiology 182:437–444, 1992.
143. Drez D: Suprascapular neuropathy in the differential diagnosis of rotator cuff injuries. Am J Sports Med 4:43, 1976.
144. Khalili AA: Neuromuscular electrodiagnostic studies in entrapment neuropathy of the suprascapular nerve. Orthop Rev 3:27, 1974.
145. Rask MR: Suprascapular nerve entrapment: A report of two cases treated with suprascapular notch resection. Clin Orthop 123:73, 1977.
146. Solheim LF, Roaas A: Compression of the suprascapular nerve after fracture of the scapular notch. Acta Orthop Scand 49:338, 1978.
147. Mitchell SW: Phantom limbs. Lippincott's Mag 8:563, 1871.
148. Bonica JJ: Causalgia and other reflex dystrophies. In Bonica JJ (ed): Management of Pain. Philadelphia, Lea & Febiger, 1979.
149. Evans JA: Reflex sympathetic dystrophy. Surg Gynecol Obstet 82:36, 1946.
150. Steinbrocker O: The shoulder-hand syndrome: Present perspective. Arch Phys Med 49:388, 1968.
150a. Veldman PH, Goris RJ: Shoulder complaints in patients with reflex sympathetic dystrophy of the upper extremity. Arch Phys Med Rehabil 76:239–242, 1995.
150b. Falasca GF, Toly TM, Reginato AJ, Schraeder PL, O'Connor CR: Reflex sympathetic dystrophy associated with antiepileptic drugs. Epilepsia 35:394–349, 1994.
151. Dahlin DC: Bone Tumors. Springfield, Il, Charles C Thomas, 1978.
152. Pancoast HK: Importance of careful roentgen ray investigation of apical chest tumors. JAMA 83:1407, 1924.
153. Vargo MM, Flood KM: Pancoast tumor presenting as cervical radiculopathy. Arch Phys Med Rehab 71:606, 1990.
154. Bridgman JF: Periarthritis of the shoulder and diabetes mellitus. Ann Rheum Dis 31:69, 1972.
155. Moren-Hybbinette I, Moritz U, Schersten B: The painful diabetic shoulder. Acta Med Scand 219:507, 1986.
156. Leedman PJ, Davis S, Harrison LC: Diabetic amyotrophy: Reassessment of the clinical spectrum. Aust NZJ Med 18:768, 1988.
157. Brown EA, Arnold LR, Gower PE: Dialysis arthropathy: complication of long term treatment with haemodialysis. Br Med J 292:163, 1986.

CHAPTER 29

Stephen J. Lipson

Low Back Pain

INCIDENCE AND DISABILITY

Low back pain is extremely common, is estimated to affect about 65 to 80 percent of populations sampled,[1-3] and accounts for one third of rheumatic complaints.[4] As many as 25 percent of those 30 to 50 years of age report back trouble, and it is the most common cause of disability in patients younger than 45. Particular groups, notably those doing heavy industrial labor, have a higher incidence.[5] Back pain has accounted for a 63 percent rate of sick leave among manual laborers,[6] about 500 work days lost per 1000 workers per year,[7] prolonged disability with pain of up to 3 months' duration in 87 percent of those afflicted,[8] and a 60 percent incidence of recurrent bouts of pain in the first year of an attack. Back pain accounts for 4.2 percent of all consultations in general practice in Great Britain,[4, 9] where 1.1 million persons with back pain see general practitioners for a total of 3.1 million consultations per year[10] and where it creates an annual cost of over $500 million in medical care, disability benefits, and lost work. In the United States, a family practice study over a 3-year period showed that 11 percent of men and 9.5 percent of women reported low back pain.[11] Associated risk factors are considered to be occupation, anxiety, depression, pregnancy, and cigarette smoking.[11] Over $5 billion are spent annually for diagnosis and treatment, while lost productivity, compensation payments, and litigation costs added up to more than $14 billion per year[12] in the United States in 1976. The cumulative costs of spinal disorders have escalated, with current estimates ranging from $25 billion to $100 billion annually.[12a]

OVERALL ADVANCES

The understanding of back disorders has historically been overshadowed by the syndrome of the herniated nucleus pulposus as delineated by Mixter and Barr.[13] Disc herniations, however, account for only 5 percent of back disorders[14] and do not increase in incidence with a heavy-lifting population,[15] as does low back pain. Progress in back pain research has been directed away from this limited condition. Improvement in the understanding and management of low back pain has come in several areas: recognition of the multiple factors involved in disability secondary to low back pain; better methods of elucidating

the source of the pain and therefore of attempting more specific therapy; definitions of the various syndromes and their pathologic processes; advances in radiologic imaging techniques, leading to refinements of operative indications; and, finally, improved operative techniques. It is the goal of this chapter to review these advances, except for operative techniques, in terms of patient evaluation and disease states. An intended emphasis is placed on disc degeneration. Tumors, traumatic fractures, and metabolic bone disease are not discussed.

BACK PAIN AND CLINICAL EVALUATION

Relevant Anatomy and Pain Sources

Adjacent vertebrae are connected by an articular triad composed of the intervertebral disc anteriorly and two zygoapophyseal facet joints lined with synovium posteriorly. The unit is further stabilized by the anterior longitudinal ligament on the ventral side of the intervertebral disc and the posterior longitudinal ligament on the dorsal side. The latter is thinner and consists of bands fanning out over the posterior surface of the disc and loosely attached to it. In the vertebral arches the ligamentum flavum acts as a ligament and blends into the medial superior aspect of the facet joint capsule; it may prevent the synovium from being pinched in the joint during motion and protect the spinal nerves from protrusion of the capsule into the spinal nerve foramen. The interspinous ligament runs between the posterior spinous processes and is a true ligament. The supraspinous ligament connects the spinous processes.

The muscles of the lumbar region are the sacrospinalis and multifidus muscles. The sacrospinalis attaches to the posterior surface of the sacrum and iliac crest, inserts at the lateral angulus of the ribs, and acts as the posterior longitudinal support. The multifidus covers the intervertebral facet joints, running from the mamillary and transverse processes to insert on the spinous process one or two vertebrae above. These act as rotator muscles of the spine. The abdominal muscles provide anterior support to the spine.

The innervation of the lumbar spine has been well reviewed.[16] It consists of the sinuvertebral nerve and the posterior primary ramus (Fig. 29–1). The sinuvertebral nerve, first described by Luschka,[17] arises from the anterior aspect of the spinal nerve just distal to

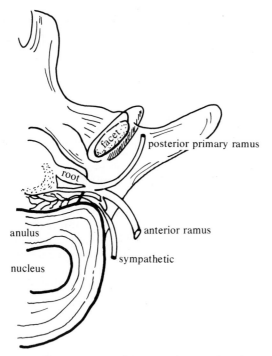

Figure 29–1. The innervation of the spine showing the relationships of the posterior primary ramus and the sinuvertebral nerve.

the spinal ganglion. After turning medially it is joined by a sympathetic branch from the ramus communicans, and the composite nerve passes through the intervertebral foramen into the spinal canal, where it branches. Adjacent to the posterior longitudinal ligament it divides into ascending, descending, and transverse branches anastomosing with branches from the contralateral side and adjacent levels above and below. The branches are believed to innervate the vertebral body, laminae, intervertebral discs at the same level and one above and below, the posterior longitudinal ligament, the internal vertebral plexus, the epidural tissues, and the dura. The normal intervertebral disc is believed to be innervated only to the extent of the outer layers of the annulus fibrosus.

The posterior primary ramus arises from the spinal nerve just lateral to the intervertebral foramen in association with the major branch, the anterior ramus. It then divides into medial and lateral branches. The medial branch descends in a notch posterior to the transverse process and is covered by the medial part of the intertransverse ligament. It immediately gives off a small branch to the inferior part of the capsule of the facet joint. The medial branch then continues caudally, innervating the dorsal musculature, anastomosing with nerves from adjacent levels, and then innervating the superior part of the capsule of the facet joint below. The lateral branches of the upper three lumbar levels have cutaneous nerves reaching as far as the greater trochanter, and the two lower lumbar posterior primary rami have no skin supply.

There have been a number of clinical experimental studies to demonstrate pain sources in the low back.

Smyth and Wright used nylon thread loops to stimulate various structures: the dura, ligamentum flavum, and interspinous ligaments were insensitive; the annulus produced back pain; and the nerve root caused sciatic pain when stimulated.[18] Kellgren injected hypertonic saline into spinal muscles and interspinous ligaments and produced back pain with sclerotomal referral.[19] Hirsch and colleagues also injected hypertonic saline into the facet joint, which produced back pain with sclerotomal referral.[20] Injection of the disc resulted in severe back pain resembling patients' attacks, whereas injection of the ligamentum flavum caused mild discomfort. Mooney and Robertson demonstrated that facet irritation produced not only back pain but also marked patterns of referred pain into the thigh and leg, depending on the level.[21] Hamstring muscle activity was enhanced, as evidenced by electromyographic findings and diminished straight leg raising. There was return of depressed reflexes when the facet was anesthetized.

Pain sources in the back, then, appear to originate from the disc and the facet joint. The root may contribute to the pain of sciatica, but it is clear that the pain pattern seen clinically can also be produced by facet joint irritation. It is because of the overlap of contributing pain sources that evaluation must be done carefully to sort out the pathologically significant anatomy; otherwise, surgical measures in particular may be aimed at noncontributing structures and fail.

Presenting Complaints

The role of history taking and physical examination in the elucidation of low back disorders cannot be overemphasized. Disc degeneration is so commonplace that more complex examinations must be selectively invoked and interpreted on the basis of clinical complaints and findings. Low back pain is age related. Back pain begins in the second decade, and the incidence increases through the fifth decade of life[1] and then decreases.[3, 22] Sciatica is rarely seen before the second decade, and it peaks in the third.[23] Back pain is increased in heavy-lifting laborers,[5] and therefore a work history is necessary both for documentation and for purposes of certifying disability. Pain presents with a number of patterns, and the history facilitates an accurate assessment of what is or is not its cause. Traditional analysis of low back pain demonstrates that the pain is usefully categorized as local, radicular, referred, or spasmodic.[24]

Local pain, presumably from a pathologic process stimulating sensory nerve endings, is usually steady, is occasionally intermittent, changes with position, is sharp or dull, and is felt in the affected part. It most often gives reflex paravertebral spasm.

Referred pain from pelvic and abdominal viscera is referred to dermatomal areas and takes on a deep and aching characteristic. Referred pain from spinal sources is noted in the sacroiliac area, buttocks, and

Table 29–1. SUMMARY OF THE CHARACTERISTICS OF LOW BACK PAIN OF VARIOUS ORIGINS

Source of Pain	Distribution	Nature	Aggravating Factors	Neurologic Changes
Spinal pain	Sclerotomal Local	Sharp Dull	Motion	None
Discogenic pain	Sclerotomal	Deep, aching	Increased intradiscal pressure, e.g., bending, sitting, Valsalva maneuver	None
Nerve root pain	Radicular	Paresthesias Numbness	Root stretching	Present
Multiple lumbar spinal stenosis pain	Radicular Sclerotomal	Paresthesias Spinal claudication pattern	Lumbar extension Walking	Present
Referred visceral pain	Dermatomal	Deep, aching	Related to affected organ	None

posterior thigh and is noted as sclerotomal pain, as the referral area has the same embryonic origin as the mesodermal tissue involved.

Radicular pain relates to a spinal nerve root distribution, worsens with root stretching maneuvers such as bending, and usually improves with rest. (If pain is worsened or not relieved by rest, particularly at night, a spinal cord tumor may be suspected.) The pain has neurologic characteristics of paresthesias and numbness, and there may be associated motor weakness. The characteristic of walking giving rise to the spinal claudication symptom of spinal stenosis should be noted, as well as the effect of sitting, which will improve spinal stenosis symptoms but worsen those of disc herniation. Bladder, bowel, and sexual function should be determined, as they are involved in central midline herniations of the disc, conus tumors, and occasionally spinal stenosis. Pain from muscular spasm will have cramping, achy characteristics, usually in the sacrospinalis and gluteus maximus. A summary of the characteristics of back pain of various origins is given in Table 29–1.

A useful analysis of back pain arises out of an evaluation of further mechanical relationships of the pain. These mechanical relationships reflect the pathophysiologic origins of the pain. Low back pain and the pain of disc herniation tend to worsen with postural positions of prolonged duration. Positions that increase intradiscal pressure exacerbate pain; those that decrease pressure improve the pain, as outlined by the intradiscal pressure measurements done by Nachemson.[70] However, it is not established that intradiscal pressure causes pain, only that this relationship exists. Another pattern of pain, commonly seen in degenerative spinal stenosis, is that of neurogenic claudication, pain produced in the back or leg by walking or by assuming an erect position. This pain tends to be more diffuse than the pain caused during root entrapment by a herniated lumbar disc. In neurogenic claudication, when the spine is in flexion, room in the lumbar canal enlarges and the pain lessens. A summary of mechanical relationships is given in Table 29–2.

A history of medications, other medical conditions, and a family history, especially of arthritic diseases, is necessary. It is useful at the initial encounter to ascertain work status, compensation, litigation, disability at work and home, and the patients' own assessments of how well they are coping with their afflictions, as these factors can markedly alter the assessment, management, and outcome of treatment.[25–28] A recent study of aircraft workers suggests that psychosocial factors are the most important determinants of work disability from low back pain.[28a]

Physical Examination

Examination is preferably done with the patient undressed. The spine and stance are inspected while the patient is standing, to note lumbar lordosis, thoracic kyphos, scoliosis, tilt from "sciatic scoliosis," flexed lower extremities to relieve root tension, muscle spasm, and skin nevi over the spine. Gait and motion are noted, including toe and heel gait, to determine muscular weakness and to observe any inconsistent or exaggerated posturing.

Forward bending is measured and can be crudely quantitated by an estimate of flexion or the distance of the fingers from the floor. Lateral bending may be asymmetric with unilateral root entrapment. Hyperextension will elicit pain from inflamed facet joints. The spine is palpated to determine local tenderness, the stepoff of spondylolisthesis, or the defect of spina bifida, and percussed to produce local pain or sciatica and, in the costovertebral angle, to elicit pain of renal

Table 29–2. MECHANICAL RELATIONSHIPS NOTED IN DISCOGENIC LOW BACK PAIN AND HERNIATED NUCLEUS PULPOSUS AS COMPARED WITH SPINAL STENOSIS

	Herniated Nucleus Pulposus/Discogenic Low Back Pain	Spinal Stenosis
Standing/walking	▼	▲
Sitting	▲	▼
Valsalva maneuver	▲	—
Bending	▲	—
Lifting	▲	—
Bed rest	▼	▼

origin. The iliac crests are palpated and may be tender, particularly over the posterior iliac spine, where local injection may give symptomatic relief. The sciatic nerve is palpated in its notch and along its course to determine hyperesthesia and tenderness. Calf tenderness may be found, reflecting sciatic hyperesthesia.

A thorough neurologic examination is done for objective signs of lumbar root involvement. In disc herniations, L5–S1 and L4–L5 are most commonly affected, followed by L3–L4. Disc herniations at L5–S1 usually involve the S1 root; L4–L5, the L5 root; and L3–L4, the L4 root. L4–L5 herniation may involve both the L5 and S1 roots, and there is a 10 percent incidence of two-level herniations.[29] The neurologic findings are summarized in Table 29–3. The findings according to level should be regarded as guidelines because, although these patterns are generally accurate as to level of entrapment, they can be misleading. The distribution of paresis in the lower extremity in herniated discs at the L4–L5 and L5–S1 levels was studied by Weber,[30] who noted that, although there is localization of paresis according to nerve root, 30 to 40 percent of other muscle groups in the lower extremity are also affected. Impairment of the knee jerk has been shown to be caused more often by L4–L5 herniations than by those at L3–L4.[31] Neurologic assessment must be done carefully, as often only subtle motor weakness is present and must be elicited by repetitive testing. This is particularly true for the gastrosoleus, which is so powerful that manual testing may not demonstrate weakness. Repetitive toe lifts with the patient standing on one foot are useful in this respect, as is examining a toe-toe and heel-heel gait. Reflexes can be enhanced by an isometric maneuver with the hands or, in the case of the ankle jerk, having the patient kneel on a chair. Sensory findings are often confusing and must be mapped carefully. It is of value to perform both pin and vibration tests to ascertain that all columns of the cord are intact.

The patient can then be placed supine, and thigh and leg girths measured for atrophy. Leg lengths are measured, as leg length inequality may be associated with back pain that can be helped symptomatically with a shoe lift. Maneuvers are then done to stretch the sciatic nerve and elicit pain. Straight leg raising is done by lifting the leg by the heel with the knee extended until the patient expresses pain and the hamstrings tighten. The site of the pain is identified, as only radicular pain, not back pain, is indicative of a herniated disc. The test is of value only with distal roots and is therefore most accurate with lesions involving the L5 and S1 roots. Young patients have a marked tendency toward a positive straight leg raising test result with disc herniations. A negative result fairly accurately rules out a disc herniation up to the age of 30, when it no longer excludes the diagnosis.[32] Variations of the test include dorsiflexion of the foot at the endpoint of straight leg raising to further stretch the sciatic nerve. Lasègue's test is done by having the hip and knee flexed and then slowly extending the knee. It can also be done with the patient seated over the side of the examining table. The crossed straight leg raising test is done by elevating the leg contralateral to the symptomatic side. Reproduction of radicular pain by this maneuver is considered the most indicative sign of disc herniation.[31]

To stretch the more proximal roots to the femoral nerve, the patient is turned prone and the Ely test for rectus femoris contracture done. The knee is flexed, and the hip is hyperextended. This motion is limited by irritation of the L3 and L4 roots. The Patrick or fabere test, to implicate the sacroiliac rather than the hip joint, is done by *f*lexing, *ab*ducting, *e*xternally *r*otating, and *e*xtending the hip (giving rise to the mnemonic *fabere*).[33] A painful response points to the sacroiliac joint as the source of the complaint.

If it is thought that the patient has too much emotional overlay, is too coached in examination by multiple previous consultations, or is guilty of outright malingering, some tests are available to help reveal this. In straight leg raising, the foot is both dorsiflexed and plantar flexed to ascertain the correct anatomic result. When the patient is sitting on the table, the knees are casually extended to note the presence of

Table 29–3. NERVE ROOT FINDINGS

Nerve Root	Pain and Dysesthesia	Weakness and Atrophy	Decreased Reflexes
L4	Posterolateral thigh across knee Anteromedial leg	Quadriceps	Knee jerk
L5	Posterior thigh Anterolateral leg Medial foot and hallus	Tibialis anterior Extensor hallucis longus Atrophied anterior compartment of the leg	None or decreased tibialis posterior
S1	Posterior thigh Posterior leg Posterolateral foot Lateral toes	Gastrosoleus	Ankle jerk
Sacral roots S2–S4	Buttocks and perineum Posterior thigh Posterior leg Plantar foot	Gluteus maximus Hamstrings Gastrosoleus Foot intrinsics and long flexors Anal and bladder sphincters	Ankle jerk Absent plantar toe responses

Lasègue's sign and to see if the patient sits back to relax sciatic tension. With the patient supine, he or she is asked to do an active straight leg raising maneuver while the examiner's hand is under the contralateral heel. A true effort will give a downward push on the opposite heel, whereas a feigned attempt will not. A true list will persist while the patient is bending forward in a chair. These and other useful tests are reviewed elsewhere.[34, 35]

An assessment of peripheral circulation should be performed, as well as an abdominal, rectal, and pelvic examination, as the source of some back pain is found in these areas. Chest expansion is measured with a tape measure as a screen for ankylosing spondylitis; it is highly significant when chest excursion is reduced to 1 inch.

Laboratory Examination

Laboratory examination provides little useful information on low back pain unless specifically utilized for the evaluation of metabolic and selective abnormalities causing back pain. There is no laboratory screening test for back pain.

Psychologic Evaluation

Back pain involves a significant number of emotional factors, and it is necessary to recognize them early in assessing pain. When personality factors are unfavorable, management will be unsuccessful no matter how skillfully performed.[27] Fortunately, identification of emotional factors can be made more objective by psychologic testing. The Minnesota Multiphasic Personality Inventory (MMPI) has been the most accurate guideline for detecting personality traits that will predict poor results.[28, 36] The hysteria (Hy) and hypochondriasis (Hs) scales of the MMPI have been shown to be the best predictors of the symptomatic result of surgery and chemonucleolysis for disc disease. A simple pain diagram has been correlated with the MMPI.[37] This makes it possible to have a quick, simple office assessment of personality traits that may confuse pain assessment. Specific examination techniques can be incorporated in the evaluation of acute and chronic low back pain. Nonorganic physical signs include superficial tenderness, simulated axial loading, distracted straight leg raising, regional motor and sensory deficits suggesting functional disturbance, and over-reaction patterns.[55] These tests cannot be used in an absolute sense to distinguish functional from organic pain[38] but help in deciding whether to pursue invasive therapy, to seek psychologic or psychiatric consultation, or, in the case of chronic pain, to initiate behavior modification by operant conditioning.[39, 40] The presence of psychologic traits of chronic pain syndromes and nonorganic physical findings indicate that traditional strategies will not succeed.

Anatomically based aid is given by the thiopental (Pentothal) interview,[41] utilizing the straight leg raising test. The patient's straight leg raising endpoint is established, and she or he is then given intravenous thiopental anesthesia until a noxious stimulus such as toe squeeze or heel cord pinching no longer produces a response. The anesthetic is allowed to wear off, and at intervals the noxious stimulus, given in the limb examined, is tested. On return of a response such as a grimace, deep sigh, or withdrawal, the straight leg raising is repeated. If there is organic disease and lumbar root irritation, an appropriate response to this noxious stimulus will be registered. In this manner, further information as to the severity and organic nature of the pain described is gained.

Radiologic Evaluation

Plain Radiographs and Common Anomalies of the Low Back

A lateral lumbosacral radiograph delivers a 2-rem skin dose, which is 15 times the exposure delivered by a chest radiograph.[42] It should therefore be obtained with some discretion. One study has shown that the risks and costs of obtaining a lumbar radiograph at the initial visit do not justify the small associated benefit.[43] Nonetheless, the lumbosacral spine film is a necessary part of early evaluation to exclude serious conditions such as tumor and infection. The anteroposterior, lateral, and coned-down lateral views are standard. Oblique views can offer additional information.[56] Early signs of disc degeneration are decreased height of the anterior disc space and anteroposterior intervertebral shift on flexion-extension lateral views.[44] The so-called vacuum sign of intranuclear gas also reflects disc degeneration.[45] Later radiographic signs of disc degeneration are further collapse of the disc space, sclerosis, and osteophyte formation. Osteophytes also occur in Reiter's syndrome, ankylosing spondylitis, and psoriatic arthritis. The presence of disc degeneration radiographically does not imply that a disc is the cause of pain. Lawrence surveyed lumbosacral spine films in persons 35 years of age and older.[46] Sixty-five percent of the males and 52 percent of the females showed disc degeneration, but in only 13 percent were there symptoms of pain. Nerve root involvement occurred in only 10 percent of those with signs of moderate to severe degeneration. In a large series of disc herniations proved at operation, the plain radiograph predicted a correct diagnosis in only 34 percent of cases.[47] Epstein found 46 percent narrowing at L5–S1 and only 25 percent narrowing at L4–L5 in 300 proved herniations.[48] Therefore, a disc can appear radiographically normal when it is symptomatic, and when a disc is symptomatic, radiography is not an accurate predictor of the symptomatic level. Plain radiographs offer little in the assessment of low back pain, and positive findings do not provide specific information as to the cause of the pain.[57, 58]

Various structural anomalies, definable on plain radiographs and associated with back pain and disc degeneration, have been reviewed.[49] A defect in the pars interarticularis (spondylolysis) increases the likelihood of symptomatic back pain by about 25 percent. Disc herniation, however, is unusual. The incidence of disc degeneration defined by discogram is increased by bilateral pars defects, and the degeneration is thought to be more rapidly progressive. Wiltse believes that unilateral pars defects increase the rate of disc degeneration.[49] Tropism, or a rotational asymmetry of the lumbosacral facets from a sagittal to a coronal direction, produces accelerated disc degeneration. Farfan and Sullivan found a 23 percent incidence of asymmetry in asymptomatic backs.[50] In symptomatic backs they found a high incidence of asymmetry and disc herniations on the side of the more coronal facet.

Scoliosis in the thoracolumbar region does not increase the incidence of low back pain in individuals up to the age of 56 years.[4, 5, 51] There is progressive disc degeneration at the apex of the curve in progressive scoliotic curves. Lumbar lordosis does increase the incidence of back pain.[1, 5] Lumbosacral tilt from a unilateral anomalous lumbosacral facet or unilateral hypoplasia of the sacrum and pelvis is not known to produce rapid disc degeneration, although it might be expected to.[49] Leg length discrepancy producing tilt is known not to cause symptoms with up to 1 to 2 cm of discrepancy.[1, 5] With greater than 4.5 cm of discrepancy, the incidence of back pain increases.[49]

Spina bifida occulta does not produce back pain.[1, 5] Transitional vertebrae are either a sacralized lumbar vertebra or a lumbarized sacral vertebra, and neither produces increased back pain.[1, 5] Five percent of people have six lumbar vertebrae, 2.5 percent have four, and the rest have the usual five.[52] Wiltse advances a guideline that the more sacralized a vertebra, the more vestigial its disc and the less likely it is to herniate.[49] If there is disc herniation, it is usually at the level above the transitional vertebra.

Bone Scan

Bone scanning with technetium-99m diphosphonate can be of use in defining the origin of back pain in some situations. It can demonstrate bony infections or tumors and is useful in detecting early evidence of ankylosing spondylitis with increased activity in the sacroiliac, facet, and costovertebral joints. A developing pars interarticularis defect, not visible on plain radiography, can be demonstrated by bone scan. Advanced degenerative disc and facet disease produces increased uptake, and bone scan yields little useful information.[53] Gallium citrate scanning offers the possibility of early diagnosis of infections.[54] Indium-labeled leukocyte imaging provides a newer technique for the early detection of infection.[59]

Myelography

Myelography is used as a preoperative investigation, not as a diagnostic technique.[29, 41] It is recommended preoperatively for two reasons: (1) it will reveal a tumor presenting as a disc herniation, which might be missed if it is not at the level examined at surgery; and (2) it more precisely localizes the site of disc herniation and root entrapment. Lateral bony root entrapments may be present with a normal myelogram. Diffuse anular bulges will give a waisted, hourglass appearance. Multiple disc herniations occur with a 5 to 10 percent incidence.[42] Myelographic information thus allows the surgeon to modify the approach so that excessive exposure will be avoided, minimizing postoperative perineural scarring. As has been previously noted, neurologic examination is not completely accurate in localizing the level of involvement. In disc herniations, neurologic symptoms associated with the two lowest spaces point to the correct level only about 60 percent of the time.[31] Neurologic signs are more accurate, reaching 75 to 80 percent.[31] Myelography is accurate 80 to 90 percent of the time,[47, 65, 66] but it is not foolproof in that lateral disc herniations are detected in only 70 to 80 percent of myelograms,[42] and 11 percent of cases of sciatica have a normal myelogram as well as a normal neurologic examination.[67] Over two thirds of disc herniations with false-negative myelography are in the L5–S1 space,[31] because the dural sac may be short or may lie away from the disc by 3 to 4 mm.

Traditional myelography was done with iodophenylundelic acid (Pantopaque), which is an oil-soluble contrast medium. The complications are numerous and include fever, headache, nausea, meningismus, backache, urinary changes, paresthesias, ileus, and acute and chronic arachnoiditis. Complications related to technique include extradural injections, epidural hematomas, contrast retention, venous intravasation, pulmonary embolism, epidermoid cyst formation, chronic dural leaks, chemical arachnoiditis secondary to the mixing of blood with Pantopaque, and others that are well reviewed.[68, 69] Complications are infrequent, but the most common are the acute, transient systemic reactions secondary to inflammation caused by the Pantopaque, the extradural or mixed injection, and retention of contrast caused by faulty technique.[68]

Water-soluble myelography has replaced oil-soluble myelography and has been used extensively in Europe. Oil-soluble contrasts are now banned in Scandinavia.[70] Meglumine[69] and, more recently, metrizamide[60] are the agents used. These water-soluble contrast media are found to fill the root sleeves more completely because of their solubility in cerebrospinal fluid and their low viscosity. Therefore, lateral disc herniations are more readily detected. These agents are less inflammatory and they are resorbed, leaving no retained contrast. The major complications are meningeal irritation, increased radicular symptoms, transient hypotension, and seizures.[69] Metrizamide is the most improved of the contrast agents but is still regarded as epileptogenic. It is reported to have 95 percent accuracy in identifying disc herniations.[70] Iohexol is the newest of the water-soluble contrast agents and has a lower frequency of adverse reactions than metrizamide.[60]

The abnormalities noted on myelography vary with the size and location of the lesion. Lateral disc herniations usually cause incomplete filling of the root sleeve, lateral dural sac indentation, and a double density of the sac (Fig. 29–2). Central midline herniations often give a complete block with ventral indentation. Sequestered free fragments may migrate and will be seen as circumscribed masses. Chronic degeneration with a diffuse annular bulge will give a waisted, hourglass appearance at the level of the disc space and osteophytes (Fig. 29–3). Artifacts encountered are from the needle, hematomas, and scarring from previous surgery.

Computed Tomography

Computed tomography (CT) has replaced many of the alternative methods of radiologic imaging. With fourth-generation scanners, the need for myelography and therefore the morbidity of investigation have decreased. CT scanning has the disadvantage of not being useful as a screening procedure, as myelography is, and it may not visualize intradural lesions unless contrast is present intrathecally. The reliability of CT scanning in detecting herniated disc appears to be well over 95 percent. A herniated disc can be easily visualized on a thin-cut CT scan, as shown in Figure 29–4. Spinal stenosis can be visualized as in Figure 29–5, with bulging of the disc, thickening of the ligamentum flavum, osteophytic entrapment from the facets, and the obliteration of epidural fat.

These techniques should be reserved for cases in which there is clinical suspicion of an anatomic lesion.[71a] Imaging techniques should not be used to search for the lesion and thereby provide a presumptive diagnosis of the cause of pain. If one uses the latter approach, false-positive results from asymptomatic degeneration will confuse the evaluation. Such degeneration in the cervical and lumbar region was found following myelography in 28 percent of patients who had no spinal symptoms but were being studied for other reasons.[72]

A study of CT scans in asymptomatic patients demonstrated abnormal findings in 35.4 percent. In pa-

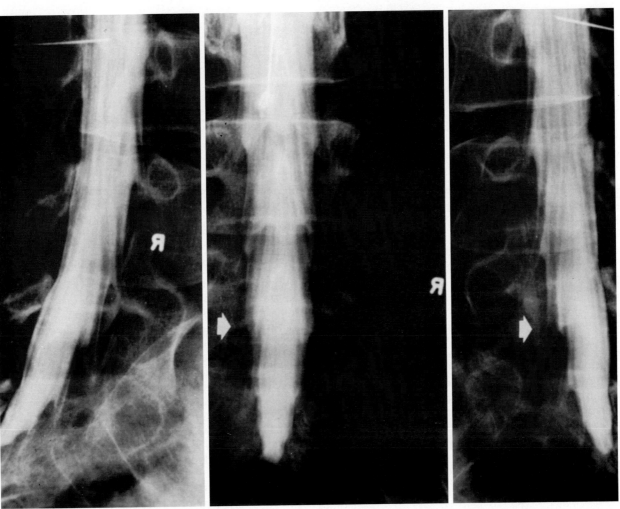

Figure 29–2. A metrizamide myelogram with L5–S1 herniated nucleus pulposus and root sleeve cutoff (arrows).

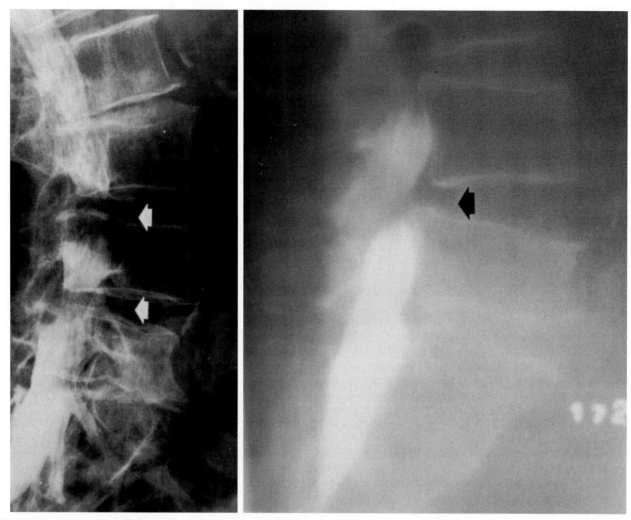

Figure 29–3. A metrizamide myelogram of a patient with degenerative spinal stenosis demonstrating central exclusion of the contrast with the hourglass configuration at the level of the discs *(arrows).* Tomography was used to enhance visualization.

tients younger than 40, 19.5 percent had a CT diagnosis of herniated disc. In patients older than 40 years, 50 percent had abnormal findings, primarily of herniated disc, spinal stenosis, and facet degeneration.[61] The studies emphasize the importance of clinical correlation.

Magnetic Resonance Imaging

Magnetic resonance imaging (MRI) offers excellent soft tissue contrast and the ability to provide multiplanar images. The vertebrae, discs, and spinal canal over an entire anatomic region can be displayed without contrast. The normal disc has increased signal intensity on T2-weighted images because of its water content. With degeneration, height and signal intensity are lost. Sagittal images are valuable in assessing disc herniation.[62] MRI may be sensitive and specific in the assessment of vertebral osteomyelitis[63] and has become the imaging modality of choice in the assessment of patients with persistent or recurrent symptoms following spinal surgery.[63a] Further studies

are needed to compare MRI and CT evaluations of low back disorders.

Other Techniques

Lumbar epidural venography has been replaced in the era of CT scanning but was previously of significant value.[71] Epidurography is a technique of injecting epidural water-soluble contrast medium to outline the dural sac and root sleeves. It is placed via the sacral hiatus, but in one series 7.5 percent of patients could not be injected successfully.[66] Subarachnoid injections carry a risk of seizure and death.

Nerve root infiltration is of value in localizing the level of root involvement.[41] It is done under image intensification with oil-soluble contrast medium injected into the sleeve for definition and lidocaine (Xylocaine) injected to determine if clinical relief of pain occurs.

Facet blocks offer both a diagnostic and a therapeutic measure for relief of back pain.[21, 53] Under image intensification a needle is placed into the facet joint.

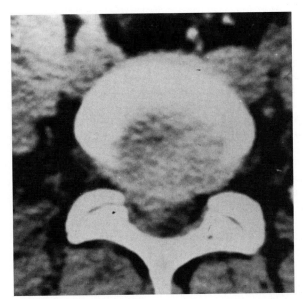

Figure 29–4. Computed tomography (CT) scan of a herniated intervertebral disc with unilateral obliteration of the root by disc material.

Water-soluble contrast can be used to outline the facet, and a local anesthetic and/or a depot steroid injected for prolonged relief of symptoms. The relief of pain is the only endpoint of significance.

DISEASE STATES

Spinal Stenosis and Lumbar Root Entrapment

Intervertebral disc degeneration is the central factor in many of the conditions of age-related degenerative

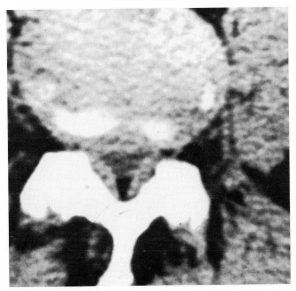

Figure 29–5. CT scan of spinal stenosis with bulging of the annulus, osteophytic overgrowth of the facet joints, and annulus thickening of the ligamentum flavum.

disease of the lumbar spine. As already noted, disc degeneration progresses with age and with progression down the lumbar spine. Mixter and Barr first emphasized the role of herniation of the nucleus pulposus in producing lumbar root entrapment.[13] Much work has focused on disc degeneration itself and lumbar root entrapment as a result of anatomic changes secondary to disc degeneration. Clinically, lumbar root entrapment is now encompassed in the broad classification of spinal stenosis,[74] which includes narrowing of the spinal canal, nerve root canals, and intervertebral foramina. The process may be local, segmental, or generalized. It may be secondary to soft tissue or bone encroachment and may involve the canal, dural sac, or both. This definition includes classic disc herniation and a variety of entrapment syndromes described by Macnab.[75] The classification of spinal stenosis is outlined in Table 29–4.[74]

Spinal stenosis was originally used to describe root entrapment caused by a congenital narrowing of the spinal canal produced by thickening of the neural arches, interpedicular narrowing, and a trefoil configuration of the canal.[76, 77] The term was subsequently extended[78, 79] to include degenerative and other changes causing root entrapment (illustrated in Fig. 29–6). Prior to their inclusion in the definition of spinal stenosis, it was already known that degenerative changes caused root entrapment,[80] and it had been shown that in an already compromised canal, small changes causing further root entrapment can have marked neurologic consequences.[81] Iatrogenic spinal stenosis has been shown to produce symptomatic narrowing of the canal by thickening of the laminae after decortication—particularly after posterior fusion. Scar tissue from laminectomy may cause compression. Epidural fat involved in lipomatosis can cause spinal stenosis.[82] Degenerative stenosis is the most common kind of spinal stenosis encountered.[83]

Clinical States

Clinical complaints involving the lumbar spine can present with backache and no nerve root entrapment,

Table 29–4. CLASSIFICATION OF SPINAL STENOSIS

Congenital
 Idiopathic
 Achondroplastic
Acquired
 Degenerative
  Central portion of the spinal canal
  Lateral portion of the spinal canal
  Degenerative spondylolisthesis
 Combined: any combination of congenital, degenerative, and disc herniations
Spondylolytic, spondylolisthetic
Iatrogenic
 Postlaminectomy
 Postfusion
 Postchemonucleolysis
Post-traumatic
Miscellaneous
 Paget's disease
 Fluorosis

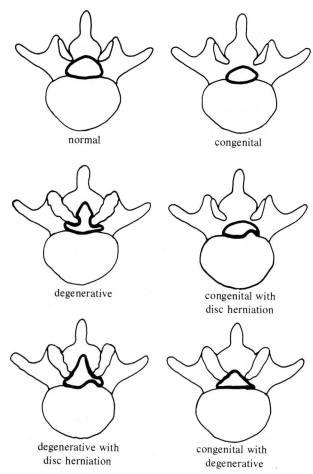

normal

congenital

degenerative

congenital with
disc herniation

degenerative with
disc herniation

congenital with
degenerative

Figure 29–6. Outlines of the cross-section of the spinal canal in different types of spinal stenosis.

percent incidence of recurrent bouts within the first year of an attack. It is managed with bed rest, analgesics, muscle relaxants, corsets, weight loss, and exercises that emphasize back stretching and abdominal strengthening. Bed rest can decrease discomfort and hasten recovery, but analgesics do not speed recovery and nonsteroidal anti-inflammatory drugs (NSAIDs) are ineffective.[85] Bed rest is recommended for 2 to 7 days. Beyond this time, and certainly beyond 2 weeks, bed rest is deleterious in the management of acute low back pain. Outlines of treatment programs vary with the treating physician but usually follow these measures.[34, 86] Spinal fusion may be warranted in cases of chronic backache, but thorough investigation of the patient, including a psychologic assessment,[86, 87] is required to give some preoperative estimate of the likelihood of success.

Lumbar Disc Herniation

Lumbar nerve root entrapment in disc degeneration was classically ascribed to disc herniation.[13] With annular radial fissures, the nucleus, as long as it is mobile, can herniate. The nomenclature describing disc herniations has been confusing, but certain patterns are established (Fig. 29–7). If the nucleus is confined by a few outer annular fibers so that it does not enter the epidural space, it may present as a concealed disc with a localized or diffuse annular bulge. If the annular fibers are disrupted so that the nucleus leaves the confines of the annulus and enters

or with nerve root involvement with or without backache. As the disc degenerates, segmental instability is produced and abnormal degrees of motion are permitted. This produces excessive motion and subluxation in the facet joints, which undergo small degrees of trauma. As the disc loses height, further subluxation of the facets occurs, and degenerative arthritis in these joints is the sequela. Disc degeneration may remain asymptomatic, may be symptomatic because of changes in the disc itself, or may be symptomatic because of trauma in the facet joints and ligaments. Root entrapment occurs when roots are involved in disc herniations or entrapment by settling structures or osteophytic processes, yielding pain with discogenic or neurogenic claudication mechanics. The differences are presumably based on different pathophysiologic mechanisms involving nociception to a radicular irritation or inflammatory phenomenon versus radicular ischemia.

Treatment

Backache without nerve involvement is managed conservatively. Pain can be prolonged, lasting up to 3 months in 87 percent of those affected,[8] and has a 60

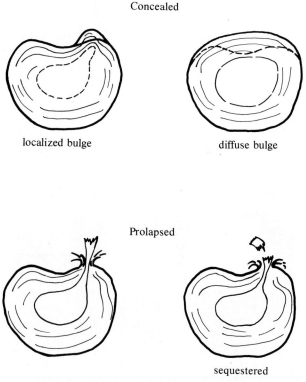

Concealed

localized bulge

diffuse bulge

Prolapsed

sequestered

Figure 29–7. A classification of disc herniations.

the epidural space, it is prolapsed. If a piece of herniated material breaks off and is free in the epidural space, it is a sequestered disc or free fragment. The mechanism of root pain is not clear. Originally it was thought to be compression, but root compression is not necessarily found at surgery. All observers agree that involved roots exhibit stages of inflammation and that these inflamed roots will reproduce sciatic symptoms when stimulated. There is biopsy substantiation of intraneural inflammation.[84] Possible mechanisms of neural damage have been reviewed by Murphy.[88]

Symptoms of disc herniation may include backache, backache and sciatica, sciatica, or those of cauda equina compression. The onset can be sudden and severe. Sciatic symptoms are radicular in nature and are exacerbated by activities such as Valsalva maneuvers and bending, which increase intradiscal pressure. Signs present are those reflecting root tension (see above). The phenomenon of sciatic scoliosis may suggest the relation of the herniation to the root. If the herniation is lateral to the root, the patient leans away from the symptomatic side. The patient leans toward the symptomatic side if the herniation is medial to the root. The clinical examination is directed toward establishing the diagnosis as accurately as possible. Neurologic symptoms give the correct level only 46 percent of the time,[47] whereas signs raise the accuracy to about 75 percent. Complete loss of a reflex is much more reliable as a diagnostic sign than simple depression.[31] A positive straight leg raising test is 75 to 80 percent diagnostically accurate, with pain on crossed straight leg raising almost pathognomonic for disc herniation. Electromyography raises diagnostic accuracy to 80 percent.[89] Plain radiographs are essentially nondiagnostic. Water-soluble myelography raises accuracy to 90 to 95 percent, as does CT imaging.

Conservative therapy for disc herniation centers on bed rest, analgesics, muscle relaxants, and anti-inflammatory medications. Pelvic traction may be of benefit in some patients. The degree of bed rest is dependent on the severity of symptoms. Once they abate, a program of exercises and back protection is started. For severe symptoms, more enforced bed rest over a 2-week period is used. Most disc herniations respond to conservative therapy, but in those that are unresponsive further measures may be needed.[89a]

Chemonucleolysis is the injection of chymopapain into the disc space. Previously it had about a 75 percent rate of good results, about the same as for laminectomy and discectomy.[90] More recent studies indicate good results in 89 percent of cases.[91] It is indicated in patients with a proven disc herniation who would otherwise be surgical candidates. The primary risk of chymopapain is allergic reaction, with anaphylaxis the most threatening form. The small risk of transverse myelitis, with irreversible paraplegia, has led to the decline in the use of chemonucleolysis in the United States. Other techniques available for symptomatic relief are facet blocks[21] and radiofrequency facet denervation.[53] Intrathecal and epidural

steroids have had some success in the symptomatic relief of discogenic pain,[92] although some authors find them no better than placebo.[93] Nerve root sleeve infiltrations with steroid may give relief.[86] Intradiscal steroids have been used.[94]

The one indisputable indication for surgery for removal of a disc is the cauda equina syndrome, in which a central midline herniation causes paralysis of the sacral roots, with bladder and bowel dysfunction and inability to walk (see Table 29–2). It occurs in about 2.4 percent of operative disc herniations.[95] The loss of bladder and bowel function is disastrous and return is limited, so this entity is a true surgical emergency. There is seldom recovery from perineal anesthesia, and bladder paralysis may have a worse rate of recovery than somatic sensory deficits.[96]

Other indications for laminectomy are marked muscular weakness and progressive neurologic deficit in spite of bed rest.[86, 87] There have been studies to dispute these indications as absolute. Andersson and Carlsson found that the time since onset, duration of symptoms, and operative findings have no relationship to the return of minor activity in foot drop secondary to disc herniation.[97] Estimates of motor return after loss from disc herniation range from 50 percent[23] to 80 percent[98] and are not different in operative compared with nonoperative patients. After 1 year of follow-up the prognosis of motor return is no better after delayed surgery than with conservative therapy. Immediate surgical treatment is regarded as adequate therapy for the pain of disc herniation, but there is some doubt as to the use of paresis as an indication.[30]

Relative indications for laminectomy are intolerable pain unrelieved by bed rest, and recurrent episodes of incapacitating pain. Laminectomy for definite disc herniation remains a highly successful procedure.[2, 67, 95] Hirsch and Nachemson reported that if disc herniation is a prolapse, 96 percent of operative patients have improvement.[67] If concealed disc herniation is found with scarring and inflammation the predominant findings, 70 percent of patients have relief regardless of whether or not the disc is removed. Improvement in these patients is a matter of degree, and only 15 percent have complete and permanent relief. The remainder are improved but have recurrent symptoms. About one third will have persistent backache after discectomy.[95] The relationship between complete prolapse and a high degree of relief after surgery has been substantiated in other series.[95] Negative explorations prolong disability.[23] The overall long-term relief of sciatica has been shown to be the same in operative versus nonoperative patients, although the operative patients achieve their degree of relief more rapidly.[23] A 10-year prospectively randomized study of operative versus nonoperative treatment of disc herniation has shown no difference in the relief of symptoms after 4 years.[64] These studies imply that a relative indication for surgery offering optimal results is the emotionally stable patient with unequivocal disc herniation who, for personal and socioeconomic reasons, cannot sustain prolonged or repeated bouts of incapacitating pain. The most common cause of surgical failure is poor initial patient selection.[99]

Adhesive radiculitis is a condition in which the nerve root is found to be extensively involved in fibrous tissue in proximity to a disc space. It is presumably the result of chronic inflammation and clinically presents with persistent sciatic pain. Neurolysis is the only treatment, but the results are variable.

Spinal Stenosis

The remainder of the lumbar root entrapment syndromes fall into the broad definition of degenerative spinal stenosis.[99a] They are predominantly bony entrapments. As these are changes resulting from more advanced disc degeneration, they usually occur in patients over age 50.[99b] Before age 50, disc herniation is the common cause of radicular pain, but over age 50 bony entrapment predominates. The entrapment may be more lateral, giving only root symptoms, or more central, giving cauda equina symptoms. Unlike those with disc herniations, patients with spinal stenosis syndromes have a long history of back pain and more recent history of sciatica. There is often a claudicating character to the pain, with pain experienced in the back or in the legs while walking. The pain is not relieved by standing still but rather by flexing the back, as in sitting. Therefore, these patients can walk up hills more easily than down and can bicycle, but cannot tolerate lumbar extension. These changes are usually progressive. There may be bowel and bladder symptoms, with the latter mimicking prostatic bladder outlet obstruction. These patients do not give marked root tension signs, such as with straight leg raising, and may have multiple levels of root involvement. Radiographs reveal changes of degenerative disc disease, with disc height narrowing, facet subluxation and degeneration, retrolisthesis, and pseudospondylolisthesis. Visualization of the cross-section of the spinal canal is difficult but can be done with transverse axial tomography,[100] and CT[101] has dramatically lessened the difficulty. Myelography[83] reveals the canal diameter. In the anteroposterior dimension it is normally a minimum of 14 to 15 mm.[102, 103] Degenerative stenotic changes are noted centrally at the discs, producing hourglass waisting of the contrast column by a thickened ligamentum flavum and bulging degenerative discs (see Fig. 29–3). Peripherally the facets produce "cutoff" root sleeves by subluxation and osteophyte formation, leading to canal and foraminal encroachment. Water-soluble contrast media give better definition of lateral entrapment by filling the root sleeve more fully. CT scan (see Fig. 29–5) easily demonstrates the entrapment via disc, bone, and ligamentum flavum.

Macnab has described a variety of root entrapment syndromes resulting from degenerative changes.[41, 75, 86] Central stenosis can occur with the bulging degenerative disc and posteriorly with a "shingling" overlap of the laminae, thickening of the ligamentum flavum, and subluxation and osteophyte formation in the facet joints. Subarticular entrapment occurs when the superior articular facet enlarges and compresses the root against a bulging disc or against the dorsum of a vertebral body. Foraminal encroachment occurs in the foramen where the superior facet lies in close relationship to the root. With subluxation and osteophytic outgrowths from the facet and the vertebral body, the root may be entrapped. Pedicular kinking occurs when there is loss of disc height, particularly asymmetrically, where the root is kinked by the descending pedicle and commonly is entrapped between a bulging disc and a pedicle about it. Extraforaminal entrapment occurs after the root has left the foramen, where it may be involved in diffuse or discrete annular bulge and, in the case of L5, trapped by the corporotransverse ligament against the sacral ala.

For patients with mild symptoms and disability or those who are not operative candidates for medical reasons, epidural steroid injections may be useful. One study, however, found that approximately 50 percent of patients with radicular symptoms received temporary relief with steroid injection and that long-term relief occurred in fewer than 25 percent of patients.[103a] The treatment of all these spinal stenosis syndromes with severe symptoms is surgical, with emphasis placed on adequate decompression of the entrapped roots.[75, 104] When the symptoms are severe, they tend not to improve. If symptoms are not severe, regimens of back protection, isometric exercises, back supports, and anti-inflammatory medications are used. Operation is withheld until symptoms are no longer tolerable. Neurologic changes are not usually severe enough to warrant surgery. The symptomatic relief offered by adequate surgical decompression is considered particularly good,[104] with positive results expected in about 85 percent of patients.[104a]

Systemic Inflammatory Disease of the Low Back

Rheumatoid arthritis is known to involve the lumbar spine. An increased incidence of subluxation and disc narrowing, apophyseal destruction, and osteoporosis has been found in rheumatoid patients.[105] Rheumatoid erosions in facet joints have been demonstrated by stereoscopic radiographic examination.[106]

The inflammatory spondyloarthropathies, of which ankylosing spondylitis is the prototype, produce back pain of a diffuse and often severe nature.[107–111] They are discussed in detail in Section VIII.

Hyperostotic spondylosis, described by Forestier and Rotes-Querol,[112] is a disease of new bone formation in the thoracic and thoracolumbar spine. The spine stiffens and spurs form at multiple levels, often causing a bony ankylosis more marked on the right side of the spine. The disc spaces remain intact.[113] There may be subperiosteal new bone formation in the pelvis.[114] The cause is unknown, but there is associated glucose intolerance, diabetes, and obesity.[115]

Infections

Pyogenic Vertebral Osteomyelitis

Hematogenous osteomyelitis has a predilection for the vertebral column,[116, 117] and pyogenic vertebral osteomyelitis has a predilection for older adults.[118] This is believed to be attributable to the marked vascularity of adult vertebra[116] with seeding of the capillary beds at the end-plate, whereas the disc has no vascular channels in the adult.[119] An associated causative factor is that the incidence of urinary tract infections rises in adults, and these organisms may be seeded to the vertebrae by Batson's plexus—the vertebral, ascending lumbar, and sacral veins—freely communicating with the external vertebral, internal vertebral, and intraosseous vertebral veins.[120, 121] Pyogenic infection then starts in the vertebral body and frequently involves the next body by spread to the epidural space and formation of an abscess, with compression, fracture, and collapse of the involved vertebra and spinal cord vascular compromise. These complications, plus bacteremia, accounted for most of the deaths in the older literature. Mortality now is expected to be less than 10 percent.[122, 122a]

Staphylococcus aureus traditionally has been the responsible organism, but gram-negative bacilli, especially related to genitourinary manipulations, are increasingly common.[118, 123–125]

Patients present with backache of slow onset with or without radicular symptoms, low-grade fever, night sweats, and weight loss.[126] Paravertebral and hamstring spasms are present. Diabetes is frequently associated and should be sought.[117, 127] The erythrocyte sedimentation rate (ESR) is elevated, but the white blood cell count may be normal. Early radiographic signs are an eroded subchondral end-plate, followed by involvement of the adjacent vertebra and loss of disc height. There is progressive loss of disc height over 6 to 8 weeks, progressive bony destruction, and reactive bone formation. Serial radiographs help to confirm the diagnosis.[128] Bone scan is useful in early detection. Multiple blood cultures and urine cultures should be obtained to determine the responsible organism. A biopsy for culture, either closed Craig needle biopsy or open biopsy, is strongly advised, especially if blood cultures are negative. Antibiotics are recommended for 6 weeks,[118] with monitoring of blood levels of the appropriate antibiotic to achieve bactericidal levels. The ESR can be used to follow the disease course.[127, 129] Bed rest is used during the treatment period, and a plaster jacket is used for 3 months. Fusion occurs in half the patients within 1 year, and in most patients the disc space is obliterated over 2 years.

Disc Space Infections

Disc space infections can result from any procedure inoculating the disc space. The most common is disc excision, the incidence of which is estimated to be 1 to 2.8 percent.[130, 131] The hallmark of the disease is severe, excruciating pain, which may have an onset as late as 3 months postoperatively; in some cases, however, postoperative pain may not disappear but increase. There is marked muscle spasm. Laboratory evidence is not present or is obscured by the recent operation, although an elevated ESR after operation normally falls over a period of 3 months. Aspiration biopsy of the disc space is needed to determine the specific organism and its antibiotic sensitivity. Radiographic signs include dissolution of the subchondral bone, but these signs lag clinical signs by 2 to 3 weeks. There is a progression of loss of disc space height and sclerotic bony reaction.[132] Bone scan is of no diagnostic value because of operative changes. The disc space often becomes fused when infected.[133] Treatment is with antibiotics and cast immobilization.

Disc space infections in children are different from pyogenic vertebral osteomyelitis and offer a different prognosis.[134] They also differ from adult postoperative disc space infections. The child is irritable and has progressive backache or a limp, or refuses to walk. Night pain is common. There is paravertebral spasm. Early radiographic findings are absent. Later, progressive loss of disc space height with irregularity of the vertebral end-plates is seen. The ESR is elevated. *Staphylococcus aureus* is the most common organism. Gallium bone scan may be useful for early detection.[54] Treatment is aimed toward 6 to 12 weeks of immobilization in a body jacket or spica cast. Antibiotics are not necessarily indicated and may not affect prognosis. They should be used when pain is not relieved by immobilization, when paravertebral spasm does not subside, or if the ESR remains elevated and the child is systematically ill. Aspiration biopsy is recommended if there are progressive symptoms despite prolonged immobilization.

Other Infections of the Spine

Nontubercular granulomatous infections of the spine are widely reported and have been reviewed by Pritchard.[135] Blastomycosis in the vertebrae infects the disc space, adjacent bodies, and frequently the adjacent ribs. Cryptococcosis of the spine is uncommon and is thought to be hematogenous in origin. It produces little periosteal reaction and has lucent lesions. Actinomycosis may involve the anterior and posterior elements and has a tendency toward paravertebral abscesses. The vertebral body produces a "soap bubble" radiographic appearance, and the disc is spared. Coccidioidomycosis usually causes multiple vertebral lesions with relative sparing of the disc space. Brucellosis has a spondylitic form with involvement of the disc and adjacent vertebra.

Tuberculosis of the spine is now found primarily in Third World countries. The spine accounts for about half the cases of bone and joint tuberculosis. There is a predilection for L1 to be the involved vertebra, and this is thought to be due to invasion by bacteria transported from the urinary tract via Batson's plexus.[136] The vertebral body is invaded, and the disc is spared. The primary symptom is insidious backache, increasing over many months. Constitutional symptoms can usually be elicited and paravertebral spasm with an acute kyphosis is found on examination. The ESR is elevated. Radiographs initially reveal osteopenia, followed by erosion on each side of the disc. Vertebral collapse follows, producing a variety of radiographic signs described by Hodgson[136] as concertina collapse, aneurysmal syndrome, lateral deviation, bony bridging, reversal of height to width ratio of the body, and wedging of the intervertebral disc. Paraplegia is a relatively frequent complication. Management is with multiple-drug therapy; there is debate about the role of surgery and immobilization.[135] Long-term results were equally good in patients treated with chemotherapy and those undergoing anterior spinal fusion in a 10-year study. Surgery does have the advantage of better maintaining vertebral height and reducing kyphosis. Anterior surgery is indicated for neurologic deficit, instability, and failed medical therapy.

Syphilitic spondylitis is rare and occurs secondary to gummatous destruction with vertebral collapse and a great deal of reactive bone. The more common manifestation is that of destructive change with excessive bony reaction from Charcot's neuropathic arthropathy, usually at the thoracolumbar junction.

Hydatid disease of bone is rare. The midthoracic spine is usually involved, and the vertebral body is permeated by cysts, which often progress into the spinal canal. Vertebral collapse is common because of pathologic fractures. The incidence of paraplegia is high, as is the mortality.[139]

Spondylolysis and Spondylolisthesis

Spondylolysis indicates a separation at the pars interarticularis, permitting slippage or "olisthesis." Spondylolisthesis designates a slipping of one vertebra forward on the one below. A classification of spondylolysis and spondylolisthesis has been proposed[140] (Table 29–5). Spondylolysis and, more frequently, spondylolisthesis can be involved with back pain. As previously noted, a pars interarticularis defect increases the incidence of back pain.[49] A vertebra

Table 29–5. CLASSIFICATION OF SPONDYLOLYSIS AND SPONDYLOLISTHESIS

Dysplastic: congenital abnormalities of the upper sacrum or the arch of L5 allow the olisthesis
Isthmic: a pars interarticularis lesion of one of three types:
  Lytic: fatigue fracture of the pars
  Elongated, but intact pars
  Acute fracture
Degenerative: secondary to long-standing intervertebral instability
Traumatic: secondary to bony fractures in areas other than the pars
Pathologic: secondary to generalized or local bone disease

---

may slip forward on the one below as a whole, or it may separate at the isthmus and slip. The entire unit may slip with subluxated posterior facets in degenerative spondylolisthesis or pseudospondylolisthesis. The slippage is graded either as a percentage of subluxation or as I to IV by quarterly increments of slipping.

In the dysplastic type there is congenital dysplasia of the upper sacrum or the neural arch of L5, and the lowest free lumbar vertebra slips forward, usually in adolescence. The pars may remain unchanged, and the slippage will not exceed 25 percent, preventing cauda equina paralysis. Usually the pars elongates or separates. Dysplastic changes of the upper sacrum with inadequate development of the L5–S1 facets most commonly produce the instability.[141] The pars is often dysplastic, and the sacrum and L5 may have a wide spinal bifida, giving rise to a high-grade slippage. It appears to be twice as common in girls as in boys.[140]

Isthmic spondylolisthesis involves a lesion in the pars interarticularis. The lytic lesion is a separation of the pars and is a fatigue fracture.[142] It is the most common type in patients younger than 50 years and is rarely seen in those younger than 5 years. The incidence in white children is 5 percent at 7 years and increases to 5.8 percent by 18 years of age, mostly during the 11- to 15-year age period.[140] There is a hereditary component,[143] with the incidence increasing to 35 percent in families in which one member has spondylolysis or spondylolisthesis. Female gymnasts have been noted to have a fourfold increase in pars defects and spondylolisthesis,[144] and football interior linemen have an even higher incidence over the normal population.[145] Of the mechanical forces involved—flexion overload, unbalanced shear forces, and forced rotation—it is not yet known[146, 147] which is primarily responsible for the slippage.

Elongation of the pars without separation represents the same disease as the lytic lesion, but with repeated microfractures healing in an elongated position. The pars may taper out and then separate, in which case the defect is reclassified as lytic. Acute pars fractures are secondary to trauma and usually involve only spondylolysis without slippage.

Degenerative spondylolisthesis is secondary to degenerative disc disease; with intersegmental instability[80] producing a local spinal stenosis. It is seldom seen before the age of 50, is ten times more frequent at L4 than at L5 or L3, is six times more frequent in women, and is three times more frequent in blacks. Sacralization is four times more frequent in individuals with degenerative spondylolisthesis than in the general population. It does not occur with spina bifida or isthmic spondylolisthesis, and the slippage is never more than 30 percent. A predisposing factor is a straight, stable lumbosacral joint putting more stress on the L4–L5 facets. The disc and ligaments degenerate and allow hypermobility and facet degeneration, permitting forward slipping.[148]

Traumatic spondylolisthesis is caused by a fracture

in the posterior elements other than the pars, such as a facet or pedicle.[140]

Pathologic spondylolisthesis is due to a local or generalized bone disease in the pedicle, pars, or facets, where the forward forces are inadequately opposed and forward slippage results. It is found in osteopetrosis with pars fractures giving spondylolysis, arthrogryposis in Eskimos,[149] Paget's disease with pars elongation, syphilis secondary to gummas,[150] neurogenic arthropathies, tuberculous spondylitis, giant cell tumors of the posterior elements, and metastatic tumors.[141] Spondylolysis and spondylolisthesis aquisita are known to occur at the upper end of lumbar spine fusions[151–156] and have been reported below a thoracolumbar scoliosis fusion.[157] These are complications not seen with lateral fusions.[140]

Management of spondylolisthesis is age and lesion dependent. Wiltse and Jackson have provided guidelines for the management of children with spondylolisthesis.[158] A child, especially one younger than 10 years, who is found to have an isthmic spondylolisthesis is examined, and radiographs are obtained every 4 months for a year, then every 6 months up to the age of 15 years, and then annually until growth is completed. This is especially important in girls, who have twice the incidence of high-grade olisthesis (slippage). In cases with up to 25 percent slippage and without symptoms, the child is followed and advised to avoid a career of heavy labor. In those with up to 50 percent slippage without symptoms, avoidance of traumatic sports is recommended. Those children with symptoms, but recovery by conservative measures, are followed. In a child with greater than 50 percent slippage, fusion is recommended regardless of symptoms. A child with persistent symptoms regardless of degree of slippage is advised to undergo fusion. A child younger than 10 years with a 50 percent slippage is often given fusion. Slippage usually occurs before 18 years of age if it is going to occur and rarely past 25 years of age. The most rapid slippage is between 9 and 15 years of age.[159] The onset of pain may be sudden and produce a "listhetic crisis" with the sudden onset of backache. On examination, a rigid lumbar spine, spastic scoliosis, flattened sacrum, and often hamstring spasm are found. There is usually no nerve root involvement; but if such involvement is present, laminectomy and possibly decompression will be required in addition to lumbosacral fusion.[86] A prospective study of spondylolisthesis demonstrated that the incidence was 44 percent at age 6, decreasing to 6 percent by adulthood. Progression of the slippage was unusual, and pain was not a factor in the population studied. No restriction of activities was recommended.

The presence of a pars defect does not mean that it is the cause of back pain. Macnab examined a large series of patients with backache and found a 7.6 percent incidence of pars defects, similar to the overall incidence in asymptomatic individuals.[86] Dividing these patients by age, he showed that for those older than 40 years of age the incidence is the same as in the general population. However, about 19 percent of symptomatic individuals younger than 26 years of age had a defect. Therefore, if the patient is younger than 26, the defect is probably the cause of the back pain. Between ages 26 and 40 it is possibly the cause. In persons older than 40 years it is rarely the cause.

Root irritation can occur with lytic spondylolisthesis through a variety of mechanisms. The neural arch of L5 may rotate forward on the sacrum and encroach on the foramen. Small ossicles and traction spurs make foraminal encroachment worse. Bony entrapment, described by Macnab,[86] occurs with forward and downward descent. The pedicles may kink the roots. Disc degeneration with bulging may cause entrapment lateral to the foramen. The corporotransverse ligament of L5 may compress the L5 root against the sacral ala with descent of L5. Disc herniation of L4–L5 may involve the L5 root. Disc degeneration itself may be painful, and in patients older than 35 years of age lumbodorsal disc degeneration may be symptomatic.[86] Therefore, clinical evaluation with myelography and root sleeve injection is necessary in the older patient with back pain and spondylolisthesis. Foraminotomy may be necessary with fusion if there is a long history of backache. In this case discography is used to determine the upper extent of the fusion. If there is L4–L5 degeneration or the slip is greater than 50 percent, an L4–S1 fusion is indicated.

In adults older than 40 years with painful spondylolisthesis, Gill's procedure of removal of the loose posterior elements has been successful.[161] In adults without evidence of root entrapment and minimal slip, Newman recommends direct repair of the defect.[162]

Degenerative spondylolisthesis is a form of local spinal stenosis and a result of disc degeneration. It produces root entrapment and cauda equina symptoms with back pain, sciatic symptoms, and occasionally spinal claudication symptoms. Ten percent of Rosenberg's series came to decompression.[148] The question of fusion is unresolved. Guidelines of management are essentially those for degenerative disc disease and spinal stenosis.

Nonspinal Sources of Back Pain

Back pain can occur from disorders of the abdominal, retroperitoneal, and pelvic viscera, but it is rarely the only symptom. Pain is referred in a dermatomal distribution from viscera and is not aggravated by activity or relieved by rest, as is most pain of spinal origin. Peptic ulcer disease; gastric, duodenal, and pancreatic tumors; retroperitoneal lymphoma; sarcoma; and colonic tumors all can give rise to back pain. Retroperitoneal bleeding in anticoagulated patients can cause back pain. In the pelvis, endometriosis and uterine, cervical, and bladder invasive carcinoma may produce back pain, and tumors invading the lumbosacral plexus give rise to radicular pain. Sacral menstrual pain occurs, and uterine malposition and prolapse can give rise to sacral pain on standing. Fibroids may cause back pain. Chronic prostatitis can result in sacral pain. Renal pain is located in the costovertebral angle and frequently radiates to the groin and testis.

Abdominal aortic aneurysm may give rise to back pain, which is particularly acute during dissection. Intermittent claudication of peripheral vascular disease may mimic sciatic pain and can be confused with spinal stenosis, but can be differentiated by the relief of vascular claudication pain on standing still.

References

1. Horal J: The clinical appearance of low back disorders in the city of Gothenburg, Sweden. Acta Orthop Scand Suppl 118:1, 1969.
2. Hirsch C: Efficiency of surgery in low-back disorders. J Bone Joint Surg 47:991, 1965.
3. Kelsey JL, White AA: Epidemiology and impact of low back pain. Spine 5:133, 1980.
4. Wood PHN, MacLeish CL: Digest of data on the rheumatic diseases: 5. Morbidity in industry and rheumatism in general practice. Ann Rheum Dis 33:93, 1974.
5. Hult L: The Munk Fors investigation. Acta Orthop Scand Suppl 16, 1954.
6. Anderson JAD: Back pain in industry. In Jayson M (ed): The Lumbar Spine and Back Pain. London, Sector, 1976.
7. Glover JR: Prevention of back pain. In Jayson M (ed): The Lumbar Spine and Back Pain. London, Sector, 1976.
8. Berquist-Ullman M, Larsson U: Acute low back pain in industry. Acta Orthop Scand Suppl 170, 1977.
9. Wood PHN: Epidemiology of back pain. In Jayson M (ed): The Lumbar Spine and Back Pain. London, Sector, 1976.
10. Benn RT, Wood PHN: Pain in the back: An attempt to estimate the size of the problem. Rheum Rehab 14:121, 1975.
11. Frymoyer JW, Pope MH, Cogtanza MC, Rosa JC, Goggin JE, Wilder DG: Epidemiologic studies of low back pain. Spine 5:419, 1980.
12. Akeson WH, Murphy RW: Low back pain. Clin Orthop 129:2, 1977.
12a. Cats-Baril WL, Frymoyer JW: The economics of spinal disorders. In Frymoyer JW (ed): The Adult Spine. New York, Raven Press, 1991, p 103.
13. Mixter WJ, Barr JS: Rupture of the intervertebral disc with involvement of the spinal canal. N Engl J Med 211:210, 1934.
14. Hirsch C: Etiology and pathogenesis of low back pain. Isr J Med Sci 2:362, 1966.
15. Kelsey JL: An epidemiological study of acutely herniated lumbar intervertebral discs. Rheum Rehab 14:144, 1975.
16. Edgar MA, Ghadially JA: Innervation of the lumbar spine. Clin Orthop 115:35, 1976.
17. Luschka H: Die Nerven des menschlichen Wibelkanales. Verlag der H Lappschen Buchhandelung PV 4850:8:1, 1850.
18. Smyth MJ, Wright VJ: Sciatica and the intervertebral disk: An experimental study. J Bone Joint Surg Am 40:1401, 1958.
19. Kellgren JH: Observations on referred pain arising from muscle. Clin Sci 3:175, 1938.
20. Hirsch C, Ingelmark B, Miller M: The anatomical basis for low back pain. Acta Orthop Scand 33:1, 1963.
21. Mooney V, Robertson J: The facet syndrome. Clin Orthop 115:149, 1976.
22. Nachemson AL: The natural course of low back pain. In White AA, Gordon SL (eds): AAOS Symposium on Idiopathic Low Back Pain. St Louis, CV Mosby, 1982, p 46.
23. Hakelius A: Long term follow-up in sciatica. Acta Orthop Scand Suppl 129, 1972.
24. Mankin HJ, Adams RD: Pain in the back and neck. In Thorn GW, Adams RD, Braunwald E, Isselbacher KJ, Petersdorf RG (eds): Harrison's Principles of Internal Medicine, 8th ed. New York, McGraw-Hill, 1977.
25. Macnab I: The "whiplash syndrome." Orthop Clin North Am 2:389, 1971.
26. Wilfling FJ, Klonoff H, Kokan P: Psychological, demographic and orthopaedic factors associated with prediction of outcome of spinal fusion. Clin Orthop 90:153, 1973.
27. White AWM: The compensation back. Appl Ther 8:871, 1966.
28. Wiltse LL, Rocchio PD: Preoperative psychologic tests as predictors of success of chemonucleolysis in the treatment of low-back syndrome. J Bone Joint Surg Am 57:478, 1975.
28a. Bigos SJ, Battie MC, Spengler DM, Fisher LD, Fordyce WE, Hansson

TH, Nachemson AL, Wortley MD: A prospective study of work perceptions and psychosocial factors affecting the report of back injury. Spine 16:1, 1991.
29. Rothman RH, Simeone FA: Lumbar disc disease. In Rothman RH, Simeone FA (eds): The Spine. Philadelphia, WB Saunders, 1975.
30. Weber H: The effect of delayed disc surgery on muscular paresis. Acta Orthop Scand 46:631, 1975.
31. Hakelius A, Hindmarsh J: The significance of neurologic signs and myelographic findings in the diagnosis of lumbar root compression. Acta Orthop Scand 43:239, 1972.
32. Sprangfort E: Lasègue's sign in patients with lumbar disc herniation. Acta Orthop Scand 42:459, 1971.
33. Hoppenfeld S: Physical Examination of the Spine and Extremities. New York, Appleton-Century-Crofts, 1976.
34. Finneson BE: Low Back Pain. Philadelphia, JB Lippincott, 1973.
35. Wiltse LL: Lumbosacral strain and instability. In American Academy of Orthopedic Surgeons: Symposium on the Spine. St Louis, CV Mosby, 1969.
36. Caldwell AB, Chase C: Diagnosis and treatment of personality factors in low back pain. Clin Orthop 129:141, 1977.
37. Ransford AO, Cairns D, Mooney V: The pain drawing as an aid to the psychologic evaluation of patients with low back pain. Spine 1:127, 1976.
38. Sternbach RA: Psychologic aspects of chronic pain. Clin Orthop 129:150, 1977.
39. Fordyce WE, Fowler RS, Lehman JF, DeLateur BJ, Sand PL, Trieschmann RB: Operant conditioning in the treatment of chronic pain. Arch Phys Med Rehab 54:399, 1973.
40. Anderson TP, Cole TM, Gullickson G, Hudgens A, Roberts AH: Behavior modification of chronic pain: A treatment program by a multidisciplinary team. Clin Orthop 129:97, 1977.
41. Macnab I: Surgical treatment of degenerative disc disease of the lumbar spine. In McKibbin B (ed): Recent Advances in Orthopaedics. Edinburgh, Churchill Livingstone, 1975.
42. Park W: Radiological investigation of the intervertebral disc. In Jayson M (ed): The Lumbar Spine and Back Pain. London, Sector, 1976.
43. Liang M, Komaroff AL: Roentgenograms in primary care patients with acute low back pain: A cost-effective analysis. Arch Intern Med 142:1108, 1982.
44. Harris RI, Macnab I: Structural changes in the lumbar intervertebral discs: Their relationship to low back pain and sciatica. J Bone Joint Surg Br 36:304, 1954.
45. Edeiken J, Pitt MJ: The radiologic diagnosis of disc disease. Orthop Clin North Am 2:405, 1971.
46. Lawrence JS: Disc degeneration: its frequency and relationship to symptoms. Ann Rheum Dis 28:121, 1969.
47. Hakelius A, Hindmarsh J: The comparative reliability of preoperative diagnostic methods in lumbar disc surgery. Acta Orthop Scand 43:234, 1972.
48. Epstein B: The Spine: A Radiological Text and Atlas, 3rd ed. Philadelphia, Lea & Febiger, 1969.
49. Wiltse LL: The effect of common anomalies of the lumbar spine upon disc degeneration and low back pain. Orthop Clin North Am 2:569, 1971.
50. Farfan HF, Sullivan JD: The relation of facet orientation to intervertebral disc failure. Can J Surg 10:179, 1967.
51. Collis DK, Ponseti IV: Long term followup of patients with idiopathic scoliosis not treated surgically. J Bone Joint Surg Am 51:425, 1969.
52. Roche MB, Rowe GG: The incidence of separate neural arch and coincident bone variations. Anat Rec 109:233, 1951.
53. Shealy CN: Facet denervation in the management of back and sciatic pain. Clin Orthop 115:157, 1976.
54. Norris SH, Ehrlich MG, McKusick K, Provine H: The radioisotope study of an experimental model of disc space infection. J Bone Joint Surg Br 60:281, 1978.
55. Waddell G, McCulloch JA, Kummel E, Venner RM: Nonorganic physical signs in low-back pain. Spine 5:117, 1980.
56. Gehweiler JA Jr, Daffner RH: Low back pain: The controversy of radiologic evaluation. Am J Radiol 140:109, 1983.
57. Frymoyer JW, Newberg A, Pope MH, Wilder DG, Clements J, MacPherson B: Spine radiographs in patients with low-back pain: An epidemiological study in men. J Bone Joint Surg Am 66:1048, 1984.
58. Witt I, Vestergaard A, Rosenklint A: A comparative analysis of x-ray findings of the lumbar spine in patients with and without lumbar pain. Spine 9:298, 1984.
59. Merkel KB, Brown ML, Dewanjee MK, Fitzgerald RH Jr: Comparison of indium-labeled-leukocyte imaging with sequential technetium-gallium scanning in the diagnosis of low-grade musculoskeletal sepsis: A prospective study. J Bone Joint Surg Am 67:465, 1985.
60. Hindmarsh T, Ekholm SE, Kido DK, Sahler L, Sands M: Lumbar myelography with iohexol and metrizamide: A double-blind clinical trial. Acta Radiol 25:365, 1984.
61. Wiesel SW, Tsourmas N, Feffer HL, Citrin CM, Patronas N: A study of

computer assisted tomography, I. The incidence of positive CAT scans in an asymptomatic group of patients. Spine 9:549, 1984.

62. Modic MT, Pavilcek W, Weinstein MA, Boumphrey F, Ngo F, Hardy R, Duchesneau PM: Magnetic resonance imaging of intervertebral disk disease: Clinical and pulse sequence considerations. Radiology 152:103, 1984.

63. Modic MT, Feiglin DH, Piraino DW, Boumphrey F, Weinstein MA, Duchesneau PM, Rehm S: Vertebral osteomyelitis: Assessment using MR. Radiology 157:157, 1985.

63a. Djukic S, Lang P, Morris J, Hoaglund F, Genant HK: The postoperative spine: Magnetic resonance imaging. Orthop Clin North Am 21:603, 1990.

64. Weber H: Lumbar disc herniation: A controlled, prospective study with ten years of observation. Spine 8:131, 1983.

65. Friberg S, Hult L: Comparative study of Abrodil myelogram and operative findings in low back pain and sciatica. Acta Orthop Scand 20:303, 1951.

66. Luyendijk W, Van Voorthuisen AE: Contrast examination of the spinal epidural space. Acta Radiol Scand 5:1051, 1966.

67. Hirsch C, Nachemson A: The reliability of lumbar disc surgery. Clin Orthop 29:189, 1963.

68. Post MJD, Brown MD, Gargano FP: The technique and interpretation of lumbar myelograms. Spine 2:214, 1977.

69. McNeill TW, Huncke B, Kornblatt I, Stiehl J, Kahn HA: A new advance in water-soluble myelography. Spine 1:72, 1976.

70. Nachemson A: The lumbar spine: An orthopaedic challenge. Spine 1:59, 1976.

71. Macnab I, St Louis EL, Grabias SL, Jacob R: Selective ascending lumbo-sacral venography in the assessment of lumbar-disc herniation. J Bone Joint Surg Am 58:1093, 1976.

71a. Deyo R, Bigos SJ, Maravilla KR: Diagnostic imaging procedures for the lumbar spine. Ann Intern Med 111:865, 1989.

72. Hitselberger WA, Witten RM: Abnormal myelograms in asymptomatic patients. J Neurosurg 32:132, 1970.

73. Mathews JA: Epidurography—A technique for diagnosis and research. In Jayson M (ed): The Lumbar Spine and Back Pain. London, Sector, 1976.

74. Arnoldi CC, Brodsky AE, Cauchoix J, Crock HV, Dommisse GF, Edgar MA, Gargano FP, Jacobson RE, Kirkaldy-Willis WH, Kurihara A, Langerskjold A, Macnab I, McIvor GWD, Newman PH, Paine KWE, Russin LA, Sheldon J, Tile M, Urist MR, Wilson WE, Wiltse LL: Lumbar spinal stenosis and nerve root entrapment syndrome: Definition and classification. Clin Orthop 115:4, 1976.

75. Macnab I: Negative disc exploration: An analysis of causes of nerve-root involvement in sixty-eight patients. J Bone Joint Surg Am 53:891, 1971.

76. Verbeist H: A radicular syndrome from developmental narrowing of the lumbar vertebral canal. J Bone Joint Surg Br 36:230, 1954.

77. Verbeist H: Further experiences on the pathological influence on the developmental narrowness of the lumbar vertebral canal. J Bone Joint Surg 37:576, 1955.

78. Kirkaldy-Willis WH, Paine KWE, Cauchoix J, McIvor GWD: Lumbar spinal stenosis. Clin Orthop 99:30, 1974.

79. Schatzker J, Pennal GF: Spinal stenosis. A cause of cauda equina compression. J Bone Joint Surg Br 50:606, 1968.

80. Macnab I: Spondylolisthesis with an intact neural arch: The so-called pseudospondylolisthesis. J Bone Joint Surg Br 32:325, 1950.

81. Schlesinger EB, Taveres JM: Factors in the production of "cauda equina" syndromes in lumbar discs. Trans Am Neurol Assoc 78:263, 1953.

82. Lipson SJ, Naheedy MH, Kaplan MM, Bienfang DC: Spinal stenosis caused by epidural lipomatosis in Cushing's syndrome. N Engl J Med 302:36, 1980.

83. McIvor GWD, Kirkaldy-Willis WH: Pathologic and myelographic changes in the major types of lumbar spinal stenosis. Clin Orthop 115:72, 1976.

84. Lindahl O, Rexed G: Histologic changes in spinal nerve roots of operated cases of sciatica. Acta Orthop Scand 20:215, 1951.

85. Wiesel JW, Cuckler JM, DeLuca F, James F, Zeide MS, Rothman RH: Acute low back pain: An objective analysis of conservative therapy. Spine 5:324, 1980.

86. Macnab I: Backache. Baltimore, Williams & Wilkins, 1977.

87. Wiltse LL: Surgery for intervertebral disk disease of the lumbar spine. Clin Orthop 129:22, 1977.

88. Murphy RW: Nerve roots and spinal nerves in degenerative disk disease. Clin Orthop 129:47, 1977.

89. Knuttson B: Comparative value of electromyographic, myelographic and clinical neurological examination in diagnosis of lumbar root compression syndrome. Acta Orthop Scand Suppl 49, 1961.

89a. Curd JG, Thorne RP: Diagnosis and management of lumbar disk disease. Hosp Pract (Off Ed) 24:135, 1989.

90. Nordby EJ, Brown MD: Present status of chymopapain and chemonucleolysis. Clin Orthop 129:79, 1977.

91. McCulloch JA: Chemonucleolysis: Experience with 2000 cases. Clin Orthop 146:128, 1980.

92. Brown FW: Management of diskogenic pain using epidural and intrathecal steroids. Clin Orthop 129:72, 1977.

93. Snoek W, Weber H, Jorgensen B: Double blind evaluation of extradural methylprednisolone for herniated lumbar discs. Acta Orthop Scand 48:635, 1977.

94. Feffer HL: Therapeutic intradiscal hydrocortisone. A long term study. Clin Orthop 67:100, 1969.

95. Spangfort EV: The lumbar disc herniation: A computer aided analysis of 2,504 operations. Acta Orthop Scand Suppl 142:1, 1972.

96. Scott RJ: Bladder paralysis in cauda equina lesions from disc prolapse. J Bone Joint Surg 47:224:1, 1965.

97. Andersson H, Carlsson CA: Prognosis of operatively treated lumbar disc herniation causing foot extensor paralysis. Acta Chir Scand 132:501, 1966.

98. Weber H: An evaluation of conservative and surgical treatment of lumbar disc protrusion. J Oslo City Hosp 20:81, 1970.

99. Spengler DM, Freeman C, Westbrook R, Miller JW: Low back pain following multiple spine procedures: Failure of initial selection? Spine 5:356, 1980.

99a. Haglund MM, Schumacher JM, Loeser JD: Spinal stenosis: An annotated bibliography. Pain 35:1, 1988.

99b. Lipson S: Spinal stenosis. Rheum Dis Clin North Am 14:613, 1988.

100. Sheldon JJ, Russin LA, Gargano FP: Lumbar spinal stenosis: Radiographic diagnosis with special reference to transverse axial tomography. Clin Orthop 115:53, 1976.

101. Hammerschlag SB, Wolpert SM, Carter BL: Computed tomography of the spinal canal. Radiology 121:361, 1976.

102. Eisenstein S: Measurements of the lumbar spinal canal in 2 racial groups. Clin Orthop 115:53, 1976.

103. Paine KWE, Huang PWH: Lumbar disc syndrome. J Neurosurg 37:75, 1972.

103a. Rosen CD, Kahanovitz N, Bernstein R, Viola K: A retrospective analysis of the efficacy of epidural steroid injections. Clin Orthop 228:270, 1988.

104. Wiltse LL, Kirkaldy-Willis WH, McIvor GWD: The treatment of spinal stenosis. Clin Orthop 115:83, 1976.

104a. Nakai O, Ookawa A, Yamaura I: Long-term roentgenographic and functional changes in patients who were treated with wide fenestration for central lumbar stenosis. J Bone Joint Surg Am 73:1184, 1991.

105. Lawrence JS, Sharp J, Ball J, Bier F: Rheumatoid arthritis of the lumbar spine. Ann Rheum Dis 23:205, 1964.

106. Sims-Williams H, Jayson MIV, Baddeley H: Rheumatoid involvement of the lumbar spine. Ann Rheum Dis 36:524, 1977.

107. West HF: The aetiology of ankylosing spondylitis. Ann Rheum Dis 8:143, 1949.

108. Lawrence JS: The prevalence of arthritis. Br J Clin Pract 17:699, 1963.

109. deBlecourt JJ, deBlecourt-Meindersma T: Hereditary factors in rheumatoid arthritis and ankylosing spondylitis. Ann Rheum Dis 20:215, 1961.

110. Schlosstein L, Terasaki PI, Bluestone R, Pearson CM: High association of HL-A antigen W27 with ankylosing spondylitis. N Engl J Med 288:704, 1973.

111. Brewerton DA, Caffrey M, Hart FD, James DCO, Nicholls A, Sturrock RD: Ankylosing spondylitis and HL-A-27. Lancet 1:904, 1973.

112. Forestier J, Rotes-Querol J: Senile ankylosing hyperostosis of the spine. Ann Rheum Dis 9:321, 1950.

113. Vernon-Roberts B, Pirie CJ, Trenwith V: Pathology of the dorsal spine in ankylosing hyperostosis. Ann Rheum Dis 33:281, 1974.

114. Harris J, Carter AR, Glick RN, Storey GO: Ankylosing hyperostosis: Clinical and radiological features. Ann Rheum Dis 33:210, 1974.

115. Julkunen H, Heinonen OP, Pyorala K: Hyperostosis of the spine in an adult population: Its relation to hyperglycemia and obesity. Ann Rheum Dis 30:605, 1971.

116. Wiley AM, Trueta J: The vascular anatomy of the spine and its relation to pyogenic vertebral osteomyelitis. J Bone Joint Surg Br 41:796, 1959.

117. Stone DB, Bonfiglio M: Pyogenic vertebral osteomyelitis: A diagnostic pitfall for the internist. Arch Intern Med 112:491, 1963.

118. Waldvogel FA, Medoff G, Swartz MN: Osteomyelitis: A review of clinical features, therapeutic considerations and unusual aspects (third of three parts). N Engl J Med 282:316, 1970.

119. Crock HV, Yoshzava H, Kame SK: Observations on the venous drainage of the human vertebral body. J Bone Joint Surg Br 55:528, 1973.

120. Batson OV: The function of the vertebral veins and their role in the spread of metastasis. Ann Surg 112:138, 1940.

121. Batson OV: The vertebral vein system. AJR Am J Roentgenol 78:195, 1957.

122. Musher DM, Thorsteinsson SB, Minuth JN, Luchi RJ: Vertebral osteomyelitis: Still a diagnostic pitfall. Arch Intern Med 136:105, 1976.

122a. Wisneski RJ: Infectious disease of the spine: Diagnostic treatment considerations. Orthop Clin North Am 22:491, 1991.

123. Stauffer RN: Pyogenic vertebral osteomyelitis. Orthop Clin North Am 6:1015, 1975.

124. Wedge JH, Onyschak AF, Robertson DE, Kirkaldy-Willis WH: Atypical manifestations of spinal infections. Clin Orthop 123:155, 1977.

125. Ross PM, Fleming JL: Vertebral body osteomyelitis: Spectrum and natural history. Clin Orthop 118:190, 1976.
126. Bonfiglio M, Lange TA, Kim YM: Pyogenic vertebral osteomyelitis. Clin Orthop 96:234, 1973.
127. Garcia A, Grantham SA: Hematogenous pyogenic vertebral osteomyelitis. J Bone Joint Surg Am 42:429, 1960.
128. Guri JP: Pyogenic osteomyelitis of the spine: Differential diagnosis through clinical and roentgenographic observations. J Bone Joint Surg Am 28:29, 1946.
128a. Appel B, Moens E, Lowenthal A: MRI of the spine and spinal cord: Infectious and inflammatory pathology. J Neuroradiol 15:325, 1988.
129. Griffiths HED, Jones DM: Pyogenic infection of the spine. J Bone Joint Surg Br 53:383, 1971.
130. Ford LT, Key JA: Postoperative infection of the intervertebral disc space. South Med J 48:1295, 1955.
131. Pilgaard S: Discitis (closed space infection) following removal of lumbar intervertebral disc. J Bone Joint Surg Am 51:713, 1969.
132. Thibodeau AA: Closed space infection following removal of lumbar intervertebral disc. J Bone Joint Surg Am 50:400, 1968.
133. Sullivan CR, Bickel WH, Svien HJ: Infections of vertebral interspaces after operations on the intervertebral disks. JAMA 166:1973, 1958.
134. Boston HC, Bianco AJ, Rhodes KH: Disk space infections in children. Orthop Clin North Am 6:953, 1975.
135. Pritchard DJ: Granulomatous infections of bones and joints. Orthop Clin North Am 6:1029, 1975.
136. Hodgson AR: Infectious disease of the spine. In Rothman RH, Simeone FA (eds): The Spine. Philadelphia, WB Saunders, 1975.
137. Medical Research Council Working Party in Tuberculosis of the Spine: A 10-year assessment of a controlled trial comparing debridement and anterior spinal fusion in the management of tuberculosis of the spine in patients on standard chemotherapy in Hong Kong. J Bone Joint Surg Br 64:393, 1982.
138. Lifeso RM, Weaver P, Harder EH: Tuberculous spondylitis in adults. J Bone Joint Surg Am 67:1405, 1985.
139. Alldred AJ, Nisket NW: Hydatid disease of bone in Australasia. J Bone Joint Surg Br 46:260, 1964.
140. Wiltse LL, Newman PH, Macnab I: Classification of spondylolysis and spondylolisthesis. Clin Orthop 117:30, 1976.
141. Taillard WF: Etiology of spondylolisthesis. Clin Orthop 117:30, 1976.
142. Wiltse LL, Widell EH, Jackson DW: Fatigue fracture: The basic lesion in isthmic spondylolisthesis. J Bone Joint Surg Am 57:17, 1975.
143. Wiltse LL: Etiology of spondylolisthesis. Clin Orthop 10:45, 1957.
144. Jackson DW, Wiltse LL, Cirincione RJ: Spondylolysis in the female gymnast. Clin Orthop 117:68, 1976.
145. Ferguson RJ: Low-back pain in college football linemen. J Bone Joint Surg Am 56:1300, 1974.
146. Farfan HF, Osteria V, Lamy C: The mechanical etiology of spondylolysis and spondylolisthesis. Clin Orthop 117:40, 1976.
147. Troup JDG: Mechanical factors in spondylolisthesis and spondylolysis. Clin Orthop 117:59, 1976.
148. Rosenberg NJ: Degenerative spondylolisthesis. J Bone Joint Surg Am 57:4, 1975.
149. Petajan J, Momberger G, Aase J, Wright DG: Arthrogryposis syndrome (Kusokwim disease) in the Eskimo. JAMA 209:1481, 1969.
150. Karaharjii E, Hummuksela M: Possible syphilitic spondylitis. Acta Orthop Scand 44:289, 1973.
151. Anderson CE: Spondyloschisis following spine fusion. J Bone Joint Surg Am 38:1142, 1956.
152. Harris RI, Wiley JJ: Acquired spondylolisthesis as a sequel to spine fusion. J Bone Joint Surg Am 45:1159, 1963.
153. Unander-Scharin L: A case of spondylolisthesis lumbalis aquisita. Acta Orthop Scand 19:536, 1950.
154. DePalma AF, Marme PJ: Spondylolysis following spine fusion. Clin Orthop 15:208, 1959.
155. Harrington PR, Tullos HS: Spondylolisthesis in children. Clin Orthop 79:75, 1971.
156. Strayer LM, Risser JC, Waugh TR: Results of spine fusion for scoliosis twenty-five years or more after surgery. J Bone Joint Surg Am 51:205, 1969.
157. Tietjen R, Morgenstern JM: Spondylolisthesis following surgical fusion for scoliosis. Clin Orthop 117:176, 1976.
158. Wiltse LL, Jackson DW: Treatment of spondylolisthesis and spondylolysis in children. Clin Orthop 117:92, 1976.
159. Laurent LE, Einola S: Spondylolisthesis in children and adolescents. Acta Orthop Scand 82:45, 1961.
160. Frederickson BE, Baker D, McHolick WJ, Yuan HA, Lubicky JP: The natural history of spondylolysis and spondylolisthesis. J Bone Joint Surg Am 66:699, 1984.
161. Osterman K, Lindholm TS, Laurent LE: Late results of removal of the loose posterior element (Gill's operation) in the treatment of lytic lumbar spondylolisthesis. Clin Orthop 117:121, 1976.
162. Newman PH: Surgical treatment for spondylolisthesis in the adult. Clin Orthop 117:106, 1976.

CHAPTER 30

Michael F. Dillingham
N. Nichole Barry
John V. Lannin

Hip and Knee Pain

Recent pressures on the cost of health care have mandated an emphasis on nonsurgical care for orthopedic and musculoskeletal conditions, limiting resources for patients' medical visits, diagnostics, and treatment. The physician is beset not only with decreasing resources but also with patients' expectations of a speedy return to high activity levels. For the efficient evaluation of hip and knee pain in this setting, the internist's precise algorithmic approach to diagnosis must be coupled with the orthopedist's and physiatrist's specific knowledge. The differential diagnosis of such pain entails a subset analysis of the disorders affecting the lower limb and of systemic disease manifestations.

KNEE PAIN

Relevant Anatomic Features

Knowledge of topographic anatomy remains the key to diagnosis of pain in the knee. Pain in a knee joint or the surrounding soft tissue is only infrequently referred. Rather, the area tender to palpation usually correlates with local pathology. Information on intra-articular anatomy is relevant and can easily be obtained by arthroscopy. For example, Figure 30–1 shows the relation of a normal medial meniscus to the femur and tibia as seen by arthroscopy; Figure 30–2 shows the patella in relation to the femoral trochlea; and Figure 30–3 shows an osteoarthritic medial compartment with a meniscal tear. Arthroscopy has tremendously enhanced our understanding of the intra-articular environmental patterns of injury secondary to overload and trauma. Moreover, this procedure has expanded our knowledge of the natural history of knee pathology, improved the correlation between topographic findings and intra-articular anatomy, and provided the opportunity for the diagnosis of knee pain through direct observation.

At least some knowledge of the mechanics of joint load is necessary for the diagnosis of knee pain. The knee can be conceptually separated into the medial and lateral tibiofemoral compartments and the patellofemoral compartment. An abnormal articular surface, whether the result of a destructive process owing to inflammatory disease, age, overuse, repetitive microtrauma, macrotrauma, or a combination of these factors, does not distribute load normally, and the abnormal focus of load in the joint is perceived by the patient as pain.[1] The physician must be aware of the factors that influence joint load and thus the development of symptoms—among these diverse factors are ligament competence, muscular strength, and type and volume of activity and exercise. Exercise and rehabilitation programs are more aggressive, precise, and effective when based on a knowledge of these factors.[2]

History and Physical Examination

The physical examination of the knee should be conducted with the patient's comfort and relaxation in mind. Otherwise, reflex guarding or postural muscle activation may alter or impede the examination.

With the patient supine, the knee and surrounding muscles should be relaxed. Acute trauma, tense effusion, mechanical derangement, or localized acute areas of articular inflammation may all inhibit complete relaxation. A pillow placed under the knee for support often contributes to relaxation. In some cases, aspiration of a tense effusion or hematoma is required for comfort.

Once the patient is comfortable, the knee and surrounding structures should be examined for any abnormality, effusion, or deformity as well as for patellar and tibiofemoral alignment. Palpation should be performed with a secure knowledge of topographic anatomy and the relevant underlying structures. Withdrawal of the fat pad in knee flexion facilitates palpation of the condyles. The lateral joint line is best palpated in varus flexion, or the "figure-four position" (Fig. 30–4). Methodical palpation of the patellar tendon and parapatellar areas is vital. Small variations in the sites exhibiting tenderness may have significant diagnostic implications.

The range of motion must be checked actively and, if necessary, passively (gently). During the range-of-motion examination, palpation for crepitus of the articular surfaces, the snapping or catching of a scar or plica (a redundant fold of the synovium) and tenderness of the hamstring tendons and iliotibial band may also be performed. The location of any finding should be noted.

Special attention should be paid to the patella. An abnormal tilt, lateralization, and an alta (high-riding) or baja (low-riding) position should be noted, and the patella should be tracked through the range of motion. In addition, the relative tension of the medial

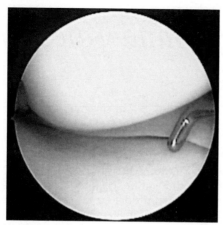

Figure 30–1. Normal meniscus as seen by arthroscopy, with the surface of the femoral condyle above and the tibial plateau below.

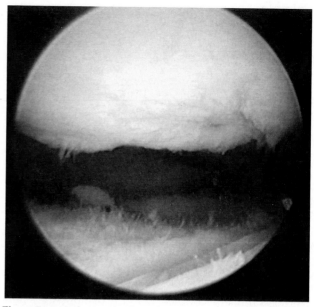

Figure 30–3. Arthroscopic view of osteoarthritis of the medial compartment of the knee, with the surface of the femoral condyle above and the tibial plateau below.

and lateral structures of the patella should be assessed by mobilization. Vigorous patellar compression is painful to even a normal patient and is therefore relatively worthless in establishing a diagnosis of patellofemoral overload or degenerative arthritis or in implicating the patella as a pain generator.

An assessment of the stability of the knee is a crucial part of the basic examination. Application of valgus and varus stress to the knee in a 30-degree flexed position and in full extension stretches the medial and lateral collateral ligaments, respectively. Some laxity will be evident in the 30-degree position but should diminish as the knee is brought to full extension. A comparison with the opposite knee should always be made. The competence of the anterior cruciate ligament can be assessed by anterior displacement of the tibia on the femur with the knee in 20 to 30 degrees of flexion (the Lachman maneuver). The lack of solid resistance to anterior displacement beyond 2 to 3 mm, especially when compared with the resistance of the opposite knee, strongly suggests compromise of the anterior cruciate ligament. A posterior stress in the same position will test

the posterior cruciate ligament. More sophisticated maneuvers exist for the assessment of instabilities, some of which involve rotary manipulation.[3] Learning the advanced aspects of knee ligament examination requires repetition and coaching and thus may be hampered by the limited number of appropriate patients.

Hamstring flexibility should be noted via a straight leg raise, which also stretches the sciatic nerve and its branches. Neurologic examination should include palpation of the tibial nerve in the popliteal space with the knee extended, the peroneal nerve, and any other area of neurogenic discomfort.

Imaging

Some type of imaging should be included in the evaluation of most patients with significant knee complaints.

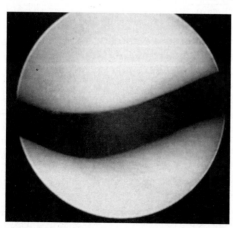

Figure 30–2. Articular surface of the patella (above) in relation to the trochlea (below), as seen by arthroscopy.

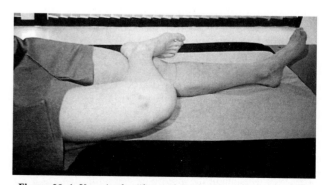

Figure 30–4. Knee in the "figure-four position" (varus flexion).

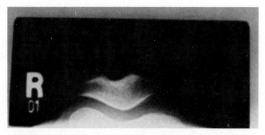

Figure 30–5. Merchant's view (modified axial view of the patella).

Plain Radiography

A series of simple non–weight-bearing anteroposterior (AP) and lateral radiographs can evaluate gross fracture changes, excessively superior or inferior patellar position, severe arthritic changes, spurring, some "loose bodies," gross bone-density changes, and calcifications. The inclusion of weight-bearing on the AP view adds valuable information regarding articular surface abnormalities, which are seen as the joint collapses. These views are best obtained in 30 degrees of flexion, a position that allows maximal contact between the femoral condyles and the tibia.[4] A notch view may be added for evaluation of osteochondral defects.

A modified axial patellar, or Merchant's, view (Fig. 30–5), allows an approximation of patellar alignment and a reasonable estimate of arthritic changes.[5] The alignment shown on these views is approximate because the patient is relaxed and static and the position of the patella is not being influenced by muscle activity. A complete knee series typically includes a standing AP, a lateral, a notch, and a Merchant's view but can be modified on an individual basis to include other useful views. For example, an oblique projection of the tibial plateaus may reveal plateau fractures not appreciated on an AP view.

Finally, a long cassette view including the hip, knee, and ankle allows simple calculation of the mechanical axis and the weight-bearing line. This information is valuable in diagnosis and treatment and especially in the evaluation of a patient as a candidate for osteotomy,[6] an underutilized procedure for osteoarthritis and traumatic arthritis associated with angular deformity (Fig. 30–6).

Scintigraphy

Technetium-99 scans have traditionally been used for load analysis. A positive scan reflects an increase in blood flow in reaction to acute or chronic overload in a given area[7] (Fig. 30–7). Although relatively inexpensive and sensitive, this method is not very specific. The specificity of the bone scan can be greatly surpassed by the use of short tau inversion recovery (STIR) or fat-suppression sequences on magnetic resonance imaging (MRI), which dramatically reveal fluid in bone.[8, 9] An MRI study limited to STIR sequences—with sagittal, coronal, or axial views, or a combination

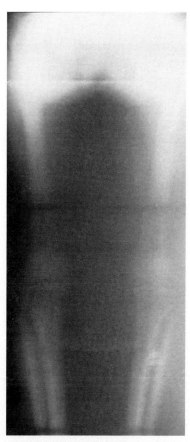

Figure 30–6. Fifty-one–inch cassette view illustrating axial alignment and calculation of the mechanical varus/valgus angle of the knees and the weight-bearing line.

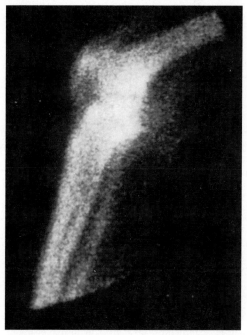

Figure 30–7. Technetium-99 bone scan (medial view) illustrating increased uptake in the knee of a patient with osteoarthritis.

of these, as indicated by clinical impression—can be ordered for comparable cost. In addition, significant information about surrounding soft tissue is gained by the latter method. The MRI will not show a pattern of synovitis that would be revealed by a bone scan, however.[10] The use of the bone scan for the evaluation of reflex sympathetic dystrophy is presently being challenged by the noninvasive limited MRI scan.[8]

Arthrography

The longtime mainstay of advanced knee imaging, arthrography evolved from modest beginnings in 1905 (pneumarthrography first used in Germany)[11] to a sophisticated double-contrast technique by 1948.[12] Operator dependent and at times uncomfortable, arthrography has been supplanted by MRI for non-surgical, noninvasive evaluation except when MRI is contraindicated. Arthrography can detect meniscal changes, articular defects, loose bodies, large synovial abnormalities, plicae, and cruciate ligament abnormalities[13] (Fig. 30–8).

Computed Tomography

Computed tomography (CT) is rarely used in the evaluation of knee pain except for the specific examination of bone, as in a fracture or a tumor (Fig. 30–9).

Ultrasonography

Ultrasonography of the lower limb is used primarily to evaluate fluid-filled spaces. It is also employed

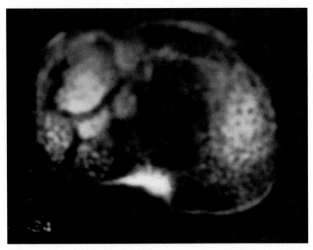

Figure 30–9. Computed tomography (CT) scan of the knee revealing a complex fracture of the tibial plateau (axial view).

to detect thrombi in phlebitis. Post-traumatic hematomas and seromas and popliteal cysts can be identified and, if necessary, aspirated under direct ultrasonographic control[14] (Fig. 30–10).

Arthroscopy

Arthroscopy is the ultimate tool for the evaluation of joint intra-articular topography. Performed with

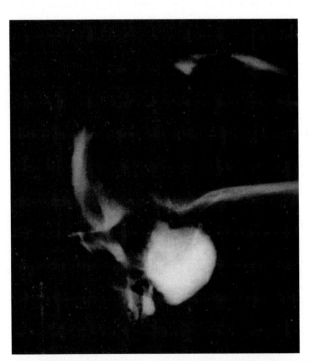

Figure 30–8. Arthrograph of a knee in flexed position (medial view). Contrast is in the joint space; the large posterior collection of contrast suggests Baker's cyst.

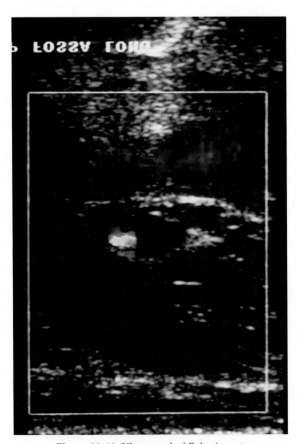

Figure 30–10. Ultrasound of Baker's cyst.

the patient under local or light epidural anesthesia, it allows direct visualization of articular congruence throughout the active range of motion with different muscle loads. Arthroscopy also permits direct evaluation of the effects of surgical manipulations such as patellar realignment. Both because it has dramatically advanced the diagnosis and treatment of knee pathology and because its associated cost and morbidity have decreased, the indications for arthroscopy have expanded greatly.[15] However, because this procedure reveals neither subchondral changes nor alterations within soft tissue, nonlacerated menisci, or certain portions of the joint, enthusiasm for simple diagnostic arthroscopy as a substitute for MRI needs to be tempered.[15] Arthroscopy is certainly indicated as a diagnostic aid when chronic knee pain is resistant to diagnosis.

Magnetic Resonance Imaging

A noninvasive modality of unprecedented precision and scope, MRI, which postdates the revolution in arthroscopic technique, has changed the algorithm for the diagnosis of pain in peripheral joints. Its development continues, with increasing technical capacity, broader application, and better understanding of which particular images are useful in a given case. The pictures are simply software-derived re-formations, and the type and number of cuts are operator dependent. Use of the "standard series" in every case is not required and can be quite costly. The application of new technology and the use of the most appropriate or the use of modified studies, or both, can help contain cost while retaining precision.

MRI has proved useful in imaging articular surface and subchondral bone changes and edema in arthritis and in post-traumatic and postoverload bone stress reactions, effusions, synovial abnormalities, menisci,

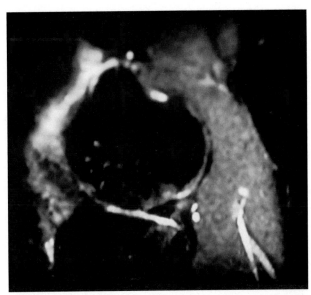

Figure 30–12. Short tau inversion recovery (STIR) image of the knee (sagittal view). High signal intensity from bone edema in the femoral condyle indicates an area of force overload.

plicae, intra-articular and extra-articular ligaments, medial and lateral retinacular changes, patellar position, meniscal and popliteal cysts, intra-articular ganglions, ganglions of tendons, and intraosseous cysts.[16] It reveals edema in tendons as a result of inflammation or trauma as well as tears of menisci, muscles, tendons, and ligaments[17] (Fig. 30–11). MRI elucidates neurogenic postexercise and post-traumatic changes or fluid collections[18] and is also used to assess nerves and tumors.[19] This technique so precisely depicts the intra-articular, subchondral, and periarticular structures that it is often a major factor in decisions regarding medical and surgical treatments. Finally, MRI is an invaluable teaching aid to the patient and the physician, providing a picture of the pathology.

In general, T1 images offer the best anatomic detail, and T2 images permit a better evaluation of fluid.[19] Fat suppression images show marrow fluid/edema very well, with good anatomic detail.[19] STIR images show muscle, tendon, joint, and marrow fluid best of all and thus are quite useful for the detection of bone trauma or overload (Fig. 30–12). Some loss of detail in the bone is encountered with STIR.[20]

Contrast Magnetic Resonance Imaging

Contrast MRI is extremely valuable in several settings. The injection of intra-articular solution may facilitate the visualization of certain intra-articular structures such as a plica or medial shelf. The plical tissue sits on subchondral bone in the axial view and is not easily differentiated from the sclerotic subchondral bone of the femoral condyle unless it is "floated" up by contrast in the axial view (Fig. 30–13). Articular surface defects and osteochrondral lesions are also best defined by contrast MRI.[21]

Simple saline solution is a satisfactory and inexpen-

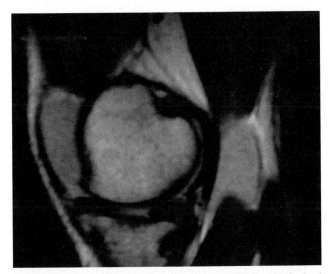

Figure 30–11. Magnetic resonance imaging (MRI) (sagittal view) revealing a tear of the posterior medial meniscus as a line of increased uptake through the meniscus.

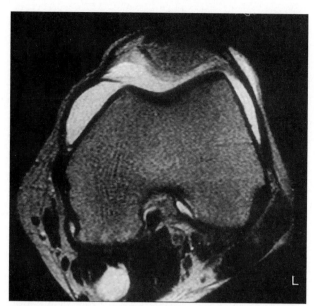

Figure 30–13. Contrast MRI of the knee (axial view) illustrating a plica or medial shelf. The redundant fold of synovium is seen to the left of the patella as a line of low uptake outlined by contrast within the joint space.

sive contrast agent, especially when used with T2 imaging.[21, 22] The use of gadolinium is controversial and is certainly not necessary in all cases.

Electromyography/Nerve Conduction Velocity Studies

In the setting of knee pain, electromyography (EMG) and nerve conduction velocity (NCV) studies assess not only local nerve entrapment but also radiculopathy and other proximal or distal causes of neurogenic pain. For correct diagnosis, the electromyographer must be able and willing to conduct a comprehensive study and to interpret the resulting data and provide a true consultation.

Differential Blocks

Diagnostic injection is most frequently performed to delineate local nerve irritation, to determine whether pain is extra-articular in origin (e.g., referable to the tibiofibular joint), or to identify specific periarticular soft tissue sites or bursae as the source of pain. Occasionally, fluoroscopy is used to enhance precision.

Disorders Generating Knee Pain

Anterior Knee Pain

Bursitis

The prepatellar bursa normally covers the patella and portions of the patellar tendon. With macrotrauma (e.g., a blow) or repetitive microtrauma (e.g.,

repeated kneeling), the bursa can become inflamed, fill with fluid, and enlarge in volume and area. Eventually, if this condition is not treated, bands and "loose bodies" of scar tissue may develop. The patient with prepatellar bursitis presents with pain on flexion or direct pressure and reports pain with walking or running. On physical examination, a soft tissue enlargement—sometimes warm, tender, and erythematous—is found anterior to the patella. Signs of acute inflammation require aspiration and synovial fluid analysis to rule out septic bursitis. Cultures of bursal fluid may need review before corticosteroids are administered. Treatment usually is nonsurgical, consisting of measures to prevent repetitive trauma, compression, use of oral nonsteroidal anti-inflammatory drugs (NSAIDs), and rest. If this conservative treatment fails, aspiration and corticosteroid injection may be considered. Occasionally surgical excision is necessary.[23]

Disorders of the Patellar Tendon and Related Structures

Like all tendons, the patellar tendon is subject to inflammation (tendinitis), degeneration (microtears, tendinosis), and macrotears (partial or complete). The patellar tendon serves as a site of attachment for the patella and is subject to large tension loads, especially with high-impact activities such as jumping or running. Overload of the patellar tendon may also result from simple activities of daily living if the quadriceps muscle is weak or inhibited.[24] The patient presents with anterior knee pain that is exacerbated by jumping, cutting, running, squatting, and sometimes even walking. Inflammation or tearing is most common at the tendon's point of origin at the distal pole of the patella; damage and pain at this site are commonly referred to as *jumper's knee.*[25] Bone tension overload (stress fracture or reaction) commonly occurs distally at the point of the tendon's insertion on the tibia in adolescents (Osgood-Schlatter's disease)[26] and proximally at its origin on the patella in highly active individuals. Occasionally, a frank tendon rupture or fracture at the distal pole of the patella occurs.[25]

Information on the inciting activity is useful in diagnosis and treatment. Careful palpation serves to determine the site of maximal pain, which is usually along the tendon or at its origin on the patella. MRI reveals tendon changes consistent with inflammation or tears and bone stress reactions.[27]

Initial treatment targets symptoms and includes rest, compressive bracing, use of NSAIDs, and muscle strengthening, with an emphasis on eccentric quadriceps work to shield the involved structures from stress.[24] Because corticosteroid injection may weaken the tendon and predispose it to rupture, this mode of treatment should be used only rarely, with injection of the peritendinous sheath alone, after the patient is advised of the risks.[28] For several weeks after a steroid injection, the patient should avoid strenuous activity that may stress the patellar tendon and increase the risk of rupture.

Surgical repair and debridement are sometimes necessary for chronic tendinitis/tendinosis. Incomplete tears that do not heal or that remain symptomatic may also require surgical repair. MRI performed early in cases that start with a specific event and in refractory cases identifies partial tears that will not improve with the passage of time and physical therapy.[28]

Plicae

During development of the fetus, the knee is divided into compartments by tissue septa that eventually disappear in humans (but not in many other animals). In some people, remnants of these septa, or plicae, remain in one of three areas: the medial parapatellar area, the infrapatellar area of the fat pad, and the suprapatellar area underneath the quadriceps tendon (Fig. 30–14). The medial parapatellar remnant plica (medial shelf) is by far the most common and problematic. Since the plica runs along the knee capsule, the patient generally presents with medial or inferior medial parapatellar pain. Other symptoms may include snapping, catching, or giving way as the plica moves across the medial condyle during flexion and extension. Anterior knee pain is sometimes more diffuse, and an effusion sometimes develops.[29] Plicae often begin to cause symptoms in the second decade of life.[30] Plicae also may become symptomatic in patients who are physically active and in those who have experienced a trauma.[29] Unfortunately, plicae are often dismissed as growing pains or misdiagnosed as chondromalacia of the patella.

In many cases, physical examination reveals tenderness to palpation in the medial parapatellar and medial fat pad areas. Occasionally, a snap can be felt

medially during flexion.[29] In the differential diagnosis, medial patellofemoral degenerative arthritis is most commonly considered; also considered are medial capsular fibrosis, anteromedial meniscal tears and ganglionic cysts of the anterior knee, and tibiofemoral arthritis.[30] MRI with contrast or with saline solution injected intra-articularly will differentiate the plica from other conditions on the axial view.[29] Treatment consists of resection.[30, 31] Nonsurgical therapy generally gives only temporary relief.

Medial Fibrosis

Medial fibrosis presents as chronic medial parapatellar pain and tenderness. Despite longstanding symptoms, the MRI is usually normal. The affected patients have often limited their activity for years owing to persistent pain and generally have undergone unsuccessful nonsurgical intervention. Arthroscopy may appear normal and reveals a "minor plica" or medial capsular fibrosis. In more than 200 patients treated with arthroscopic release of the inferomedial parapatellar tissues in the area of the medial patellotibial ligament, pain has been relieved; this relief has been maintained with increased activity in approximately 80 percent of cases.[32] The differential diagnosis via imaging work-up is the same as for a plica.

Patellofemoral Arthritis/Overload

A common source of anterior knee pain is patellofemoral arthritis. This condition is often described as *chondromalacia*—a broad, nonspecific term that conveys neither the importance of mechanics in its development nor its significance to the patient.[33]

Patellar biomechanics are highly specific. The patella absorbs load across approximately one fourth of its surface area at any time, the exact site varying with the degree of flexion of the knee.[34] The same is true of the femoral groove (trochlea). With the knee in full extension, the patella sits above the femoral joint surface on the suprapatellar fat. The load on the patella increases with increasing flexion. Accordingly, symptoms tend to arise from activities of daily life that involve flexion, such as squatting, rising from a seated position, climbing stairs or hills, and running. Exercises involving knee extension impose the maximum load near full extension and therefore tend to cause pain at that point. Thus, rehabilitation for patellofemoral arthritis now emphasizes the use of knee flexion or press (closed chain) exercises, or both, rather than knee extension (open chain) exercises.[35]

Factors predisposing to patellofemoral arthritis include repetitive flexion in work or sports, congenital or traumatic malalignment, malpositioning (baja or alta), and malformation (flattening of the trochlea or patellar maldevelopment). All of these conditions reduce the contact surface area, thereby resulting in increased stress and osteoarthritis.[36] Any factor that significantly weakens the quadriceps muscle (especially the vastus medialis oblique) may result in malalignment of the patella and predispose to patello-

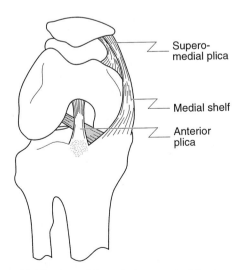

Supero-
medial plica

Medial shelf

Anterior
plica

Figure 30–14. Diagram of the anterior aspect of the knee showing the position of a synovial plica. (From Johnson DP, Eastwood DM, Witherow PJ: Symptomatic synovial plicae of the knee. J Bone Joint Surg 75A:1486, 1993; with permission.)

femoral arthritis.[35] The destructive aspects of inflammatory arthritis can also affect the patellofemoral joint.

Physical examination may reveal lateral tilt of the patella, tightness of lateral or medial retinacular tissues, lateral tracking, patella alta or baja, parapatellar tenderness, or subpatellar crepitus on extension or flexion.[35] Vigorous compression of the patella against resistance may cause pain; however, this pain may not reflect patellar pathology. It is important to realize that patellar pain will be local and does not radiate to other areas of the knee.

Options for treatment are similar to those for any osteoarthritic joint. The focus is on the modification of abnormal patterns or degrees of load and stress. One option is relative rest, which implies the modification of lifestyle in a way that minimizes the inciting or overload activity. Another is shock absorption, with specific training (very specific physical therapy and strengthening exercises) to shield the joint from stress during flexion activity.[35] The patient should be counseled on how to maintain an exercise program on his or her own once physical therapy has been completed. Third, surgical realignment or local manipulation of the articular surface, with drilling or burring, results in relocation or wider distribution of the patellar load. Multiple surgical techniques, some of which involve drilling or burring, are available for patellar realignment.[37, 38] Fourth, biologic resurfacing—a relatively new approach—utilizes chondrocyte reimplantation after growth and tissue culture. Other techniques employing biologic resurfacing are being developed.[39] Finally, total joint replacement is an option, but limited replacement of the patellofemoral joint has a very narrow range of indication.

All of these techniques directly address the issue of force per area/overload. Arthroscopic debridement as well as treatment with oral or injectable medications focus on pain relief or reduction of synovitis, therefore enhancing comfort, increasing function, and in some cases providing an opportunity for rehabilitation. They do not, however, address the fundamentals of abnormal load distribution.

Tibiofemoral Arthritis/Overload

Arthritic changes in the anterior condyles or anterior tibial plateau may cause anterior knee pain. Although this etiology is at times difficult to differentiate from a patellar or trochlear etiology, the diagnosis can generally be based on localized tenderness on palpation or imaging.[4, 7, 10, 14]

Arthrofibrosis

Knees that lack a full range of motion after surgery, trauma, or inflammation or as the result of osteoarthritis have two specific and unique pain generators. First, the fibrous tissue itself can be painful during an inflammatory phase that, depending on an individual's genetics, may last for many months. Treatment consists of anti-inflammatory medication and physi-

cal therapy. If this approach fails to relieve pain and increase range of motion to a satisfactory degree, then surgical release may be necessary. Although it is preferable to perform surgery after the inflammatory phase, it is not always possible to wait.

Second, the techniques of physical therapy, especially aggressive use of passive range of motion, may lead to compressive joint overload, bone stress, and pain. It is critical that therapists be aware of this possibility. Distraction of the joint, with extension and careful compression at end-range of flexion, is an important component of therapy. MRI may show the stress reaction on fat suppression or STIR.

Causes of Anterior Thigh Pain

Anteriorly distal thigh pain can be referred from the hip or can be neurogenic. A good history and a physical examination that includes the structures and joints above and below usually eliminate this source of confusion.

Mediolateral Knee Pain

Specificity in categorizing mediolateral knee pain according to the topographic anatomy of the knee is critical. For example, joint line pain should refer to pain on palpation on what is confidently felt to be the joint line. It is important to be aware that a 1-cm difference in any direction can change the differential. A thorough physical examination is crucial.

Meniscal Abnormalities

Both menisci are subject to abnormalities that can create joint line pain on palpation and with manipulation. The patient may describe catching or locking of the knee that at times can be elicited on examination. An effusion may also be noted. Although the patient may describe more diffuse knee pain, the hallmark of a meniscal tear—and often the only finding on examination—is tenderness along the joint line.

In the younger population, meniscal tears are related to activity and are therefore traumatic in origin. With increasing age, degenerative tears predominate as the internal architecture of the meniscus fails. Not all degenerative tears are symptomatic. The treatment for a symptomatic tear, regardless of its etiology, is generally surgical. Certain degenerative tears present as pain and a palpable mass at the joint line, most frequently involving the lateral meniscus. The mass may be a ganglionic cyst but usually connects directly to the meniscus.[40] Treatment consists of arthroscopic debridement of the meniscus and cyst.[41]

Chondrocalcinosis can increase the likelihood of meniscal tears as the calcific deposits make the menisci brittle. In addition, the liberation of calcium salts in the knee at the time of arthroscopy often generates troublesome significant postoperative synovitis.[42, 43]

One of the most important functions of the menisci is load distribution. The removal of menisci may reduce the area of forced distribution at the posterior tibia by more than half.[44] Multiple studies dating from 1948 onward[45] have demonstrated that meniscectomy, especially in a young population, correlates with an earlier-than-anticipated appearance of degenerative arthritis, which is aggravated in knees with significant valgus or varus alignment.[46–50] Therefore, if at all possible, menisci should be repaired in persons who have not yet reached middle age; if the meniscus is not degenerative, it can often be repaired even in early middle age.[51] A delay in diagnosis can eliminate the possibility of successful repair. Preservation of the meniscus with synovectomy[52] offers a unique opportunity to prevent degenerative arthritis. Imaging should be aggressively pursued in candidates for repair.

When repair is not feasible, the smallest possible portion of the meniscus should be removed to alleviate symptoms and prevent further tears. The utility of meniscal allograft is not yet clear.[53] Long-term studies of irradiated grafts have shown high rates of failure. As of this writing, no long-term study on nonirradiated grafts has been reported.

Tibiofemoral Arthritis

Degenerative or traumatic arthritis of either the medial or the lateral compartment may present as joint line pain, effusion, stiffness, or an insidious impairment of flexion or extension. Often, more than one compartment is involved, and the result is diffuse pain.

Moderate to severe changes can be diagnosed not only by examination but also by standing AP radiography, which often is best done at 30 degrees of flexion to load the area of greatest loss of articular cartilage, revealing narrowing.[4] MRI will show articular cartilage defects (particularly if an effusion is present) and bone edema on fat suppression or STIR in areas of bone overload.[19]

Options for treatment include those described for patellofemoral arthritis. Rehabilitation and arthroscopic debridement can delay—or in some cases eliminate—the need for other interventions.[54] Tibial or femoral osteotomy is significantly underused and may delay for years or eliminate the need for joint replacement. Osteotomy can be done on patients as old as their early 70s, if they are fit enough to undergo rehabilitation, and allows a much wider range of function than joint replacement. Certain conditions that may cause presenting symptoms similar to those of osteoarthritis or post-traumatic arthritis include osteochondritis dissecans, osteonecrosis, and chondrolysis.

Osteochondritis dissecans is a developmental abnormality in which a fragment of subchondral bone and the overlying articular material spontaneously detach. This abnormality can involve any joint surface of the knee and generally affects relatively young patients. It may be painless and be manifested only by locking as the fragment of subchondral bone catches.

More commonly, it causes pain, often along the joint line or in the patellofemoral area, depending on the location of the lesion[55] (Fig. 30–15) (see Color Plate). The diagnosis is frequently made by routine radiography but may require MRI. Treatment in the early phases is variable, but an attempt should be made to repair lesions that are loose or have nearly come loose.[55]

Osteonecrosis, a frank aseptic necrosis of a portion of the condyle, presents as joint line pain that is often more severe and intense than the pain typically associated with osteoarthritis. A recalcitrant effusion may be documented. Treatment is the same as for osteoarthritis. However, the diagnosis must be made as early as possible, since attempts at rehabilitation and nonsurgical care commonly fail and osteotomy or joint replacement is almost always required.[56, 57]

Chondrolysis, an acute loss of the articular cartilage surface somewhere within the knee, typically follows immediately on trauma and often affects younger patients. It presents as sudden onset of severe pain (often associated with a traumatic event) or as an effusion recalcitrant even to repetitive steroid injections. Arthroscopy may reveal severe synovitis that is considered to be secondary to the great volume of articular cartilage debris within the knee. Reduction of synovitis often requires arthroscopic lavage to eliminate this debris. After arthroscopic lavage, treatment is the same as for osteoarthritis of the particular area involved.[58]

Bursitis

Any of the multiple bursae about the knee can become inflamed. Around the joint line are three bursae that are occasional sources of pain. On the medial side of the knee, a bursa is present over the semimembranous tendon (one of the medial hamstrings that is inserted below the level of the posteromedial joint line). The site of insertion of the hamstrings along the proximal medial tibia is the pes anserinus. The pes anserine bursa lies between the aponeurosis of these tendons and the medial collateral ligament, approxi-

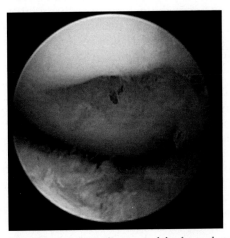

Figure 30–15. Osteochondritis dissecans of the femoral condyle, as seen by arthroscopy. (See Color Plate.)

mately 5 cm below the anteromedial joint line.[59] The most common site of bursitis, however, is the iliotibial band area. Examination reveals tenderness above the lateral joint line and perhaps extending to the joint line itself. The iliotibial band is often tight and may click as it passes over the lateral femoral condyle. Iliotibial bursitis is associated with overuse and with running, bicycling, or other vigorous endurance sports.[59] Treatment for all bursitis is conservative, including stretching, anti-inflammatory medication, or injection of corticosteroids. On very rare occasions, bursectomy or partial release of the overlying tendons (e.g., a tight iliotibial band) is necessary.

Tendinitis

Tendinitis commonly involves the medial hamstrings. It may be associated with degeneration of the tendon and some snapping. Tenderness of the affected tendon leads to the diagnosis. Treatment modalities include rest from inciting activities, oral anti-inflammatory medication, and physical therapy for stretching and strengthening. The patient should be advised that a degenerative medial hamstring tendon may rupture.[59]

Tibiofibular Arthritis

The tibiofibular joint, although rarely a pain generator, should be considered a source of lateral knee pain, especially if degenerative change is evident on radiography. If the injection of lidocaine into the joint eliminates the pain, this joint is the source of the pain. Generally, tibiofibular arthritis is treated with steroid injection. If pain persists, surgical treatment involving enucleation of the fibular head is an option.[60]

Stress Reaction

The same type of bone stress reaction/stress fracture condition that occurs in the distal tibia (often described as *shin splints*) can also develop around the knee, typically on the tibial side. The diagnosis is made partly by exclusion of other causes and partly by history, since the patient often has high levels of use and load (e.g., a long distance runner) or a recent history of trauma. The diagnosis can be made by an MRI via STIR or fat suppressor images.[61]

Posterior Knee Pain

Any affliction of the joint in its posterior recesses, including arthritis, synovitis, meniscal abnormalities, and inflammation of any of the posterior tendons, can cause posterior knee pain. Posterior cruciate trauma and posterior capsular trauma are also possible sources of such pain. Tibial neuritis can cause posterior pain.

Two sources of posterior knee pain deserve specific mention. Of cysts that present in the popliteal space, the most common is the popliteal or Baker's cyst (see Figs. 30–8 and 30–10). Rising off the posteromedial capsule, this type of cyst is frequently associated with synovitis of any etiology and the subsequent effusion. Symptoms result from compression of the fluid-filled cyst as the knee is flexed or from inflammation in the cyst itself. MRI has permitted the recognition of other cysts in the area (often of gastrocnemius origin) that produce symptoms locally by inflammation or compression.[19] Thus, posterior knee pain of unknown etiology requires MRI if symptoms persist. The cysts identified may be treated with aspiration or, more definitively, with surgical excision.

NEUROGENIC PAIN

Pain from tibia, peroneal, or saphenous nerve entrapment or pathology is often misinterpreted as knee pain or radiculopathy. Local nerve tenderness, with reproduction of symptoms with nerve stretch, is common. The history often includes local deep aching or paresthesias with radiation of discomfort.

HIP PAIN

The diagnosis of hip pain is a problem commonly encountered not only by musculoskeletal experts (such as rheumatologists and orthopedists) but also frequently by family practitioners and internists on the front lines of primary care. Identification of the cause of this discomfort is complicated by the fact that different patients mean different things by "hip pain." A 50-year-old laborer may say that his hip hurts, although the source of his problem turns out to be sciatica from a disc herniation in his lower back. A 50-year-old jogger may complain of a pulled muscle in his groin—not even mentioning hip pain—and yet have early osteoarthritis of the hip. Referred pain patterns are, in fact, common with hip pathology. The anatomic source of an ache in the distal thigh or knee may be the hip joint. The hip joint and its periarticular structures are relatively deep and therefore relatively inaccessible to evaluation by manual elicitation of tenderness.

Relevant Anatomic Features

The practitioner evaluating a patient with hip pain should attempt to find the anatomic source of the pain by eliciting a history and conducting a physical examination. Having tentatively identified the source, the physician should then define the pathophysiologic condition responsible for the pain.

Pathology in four general anatomic areas is considered. The first category is intra-articular hip joint pathology, which includes processes that affect the articular cartilage (such as osteoarthritis), the synovium (such as rheumatoid arthritis or pigmented villonodular synovitis), the intra-articular soft tissue structures (such as tearing or infolding of the labrum), and the bones forming the joints (such as avascular necrosis affecting the femoral head and trauma). The second category is pathology of the extra-articular bony structures around the hip joint, which includes any process of the femoral shaft (such as fracture or tumor) and any process affecting the pelvic bones (including pelvic fracture, stress fracture, and osteitis pubis). The third category is pathology of the extra-articular soft tissues, which includes muscular pathology, soft tissue overuse syndromes (such as tendinitis/bursitis), and local nerve processes (such as meralgia paresthetica). The fourth category is pathology outside the hip area that can refer to the hip, which includes lumbosacral radiculopathy, femoral and inguinal hernias, and intrapelvic pathology (e.g., endometriosis or lymphoma).

The broad categories of entities to be considered once the anatomic source of pain has been identified include:

- Infections, such as septic arthritis and osteomyelitis
- Degenerative conditions, such as osteoarthritis
- Metabolic conditions, such as Paget's disease of the femur or pelvis
- Inflammatory conditions, such as rheumatoid arthritis, synovial chondromatosis, and pigmented villonodular synovitis
- Neurogenic conditions, such as radiculopathy and local nerve entrapment
- Traumas, such as femoral neck fractures and stress or insufficiency fractures
- Overuse syndromes, such as tendinitis and osteitis pubis
- Tumors, such as metastatic disease to the femoral neck or pelvis
- Vascular conditions, such as avascular necrosis of the femoral head and claudications with pain referred to the hip and leg

History

The history of the patient with hip pain is the key to the source of the pain. Some patients respond well to an open-ended question like "What kind of trouble are you having?" The patient who answers, "Well, Doc, I was lifting 100-pound bags of cement, putting in a sidewalk over the weekend, and started getting pain in my back. It went down to my hip and seemed to go all the way down into my foot, along with some numbness and tingling in my foot," has, in a few sentences, revealed the cause of his hip pain to be referred radiculopathy. Specifically, certain questions can be very helpful.

How did the pain begin and how long ago? If a patient has experienced a gradual increase in pain and a gradual diminution of function over 5 years, she or he is more likely to have an arthritic hip than acute tendinitis or a fracture. A patient training for a marathon who has rapidly increased his or her running program and now has acute groin pain is most likely to have an overuse syndrome, such as a stress fracture or tendinitis.

Where is the pain located? A patient whose "hip pain" begins in the low back and radiates down the buttock and the back of the leg to the side of the calf and lateral side of the foot is more likely to have referred radiculopathy than an arthritic hip joint. In contrast, the patient with pain deep in the groin or the front of the hip that radiates down the thigh to the knee and is accompanied by hip initiation stiffness and pain with weight bearing is more likely to have an arthritic hip than high lumbar radiculopathy.

What is your hip's range of motion? A patient who has lost the ability to cut toenails or tie shoes or who notes that his or her leg turns outward when it is raised or when he or she rides a bicycle is likely to have hip joint pathology such as osteoarthritis or avascular necrosis and is developing contractures.

Are you less able to participate in the activities of daily living as a result of your pain? A patient who now has to climb stairs with the single-step gait of a 2-year-old or who has to lift her or his leg with hands to get in and out of a car is likely to have severe osteoarthritis of the hip.

Have you had any related symptoms in the past? Since lumbosacral radiculopathy frequently causes pain referred to the hip, the patient should be asked about prior low back pain and about previous numbness, tingling, or weakness of the foot or leg.

In addition to these specific points, a general medical history is important. A patient with a history of prolonged oral steroid treatment for ulcerative colitis who now has groin pain or limitation of motion of the hip may well have avascular necrosis of the femoral head. A patient who has a history of breast cancer and now has insidious pain in the hip and thigh may have metastasis of the tumor. A thin runner who states that she has had menstrual irregularities or amenorrhea and now has hip or pelvic pain may have insufficiency stress fractures.

Physical Examination

The physical examination of the hip contributes important diagnostic information. The patient's gait should be assessed for signs of antalgic limp, Trendelenburg's weakness, steppage gait, footdrop, and other abnormalities. Range-of-motion examination of the hip in the supine position is revealing. Flexion of the uninvolved hip with the knee to the chest and extension of the involved hip (the Thomas test) may reveal a flexion contracture. Lack of internal rotation or pain with internal rotation is frequently a sign of hip joint pathology (e.g., osteoarthritis, avascular necrosis, or inflammatory synovitis). A patient who has neither pain nor limitation of internal rotation but who has tenderness to palpation posterior to the trochanter is much more likely to have trochanteric bursitis than hip osteoarthritis. "Hip-irritability signs" are informative. A patient who cannot raise a straight leg off the table against gravity or who cannot hold the leg straight against resistance, experiencing pain in the groin or thigh during the maneuver, is likely to have primary hip joint pathology.

The results of local palpation are somewhat difficult to interpret. Palpation of the inguinal region is frequently uncomfortable even when the hip is normal. However, gentle palpation should be attempted and may be helpful in distinguishing among osteitis pubis; pubic ramus fractures; ischial tendinitis, bursitis, or fractures; posterior trochanteric bursitis or abductor tendinitis; and iliac crest tensor fascia lata tendinitis. Palpation of the groin or inguinal region may reveal a femoral or inguinal hernia. Significant lymphadenopathy may be indicative of infection or lymphoma.

A thorough neurologic examination is helpful. An absent knee-jerk reflex accompanied by quadriceps weakness and thigh pain may reflect L4 radiculopathy causing referred pain. As in most musculoskeletal conditions, examination of the opposite (uninvolved) side may be valuable for comparison.

Diagnostic Testing

Once the history has been elicited and the physical examination performed, additional testing may be considered. Nowadays, physicians are frequently subject to a number of forces influencing their management decisions: patients, who want fast diagnoses, relief of pain, and restoration of function; insurance companies, government agencies, and patients, who want low-cost medical care; a litigious society, which demands accuracy and quality of treatment with minimal risk; and physicians themselves, who want to make a good living. In the best-case scenario, common sense and an effort to do what is right for the patient will ultimately determine which tests are conducted.

Plain Radiography

Plain radiographs of the hip and pelvis are frequently helpful. An AP pelvic radiograph and a "frog-leg" lateral-hip film may reveal fractures, joint space narrowing indicative of articular cartilage loss, spurs or osteophytes indicative of arthritic change, segmental radiolucency or sclerotic changes of the femoral head indicative of avascular necrosis, calcifications indicative of synovial chondromatosis, or soft tissue calcification indicative of calcific tendinitis. When to order a plain film is a judgment call. For example, plain films are not necessary at the first visit of a 25-year-old flight attendant who has recently increased her aerobic workouts at the gym, who has a 2-week history of soreness over her abductor muscles, and whose physical examination shows no limitation of the hip's range of motion, no hip-irritability signs, and local tenderness over her tensor fascia lata origin.

Scintigraphy

Technetium-99m methylene diphosphonate (99mTc-MDP) bone scanning has been valuable in the past for detecting areas of stress reaction and bone turnover and has been quite sensitive in picking up some conditions that are not necessarily revealed by plain radiographs such as stress fractures,[62] early avascular necrosis of the femoral head,[63] osteoid osteoma,[64] and occult fractures of the hip in the elderly.[65] With increasing frequency, however, MRI is being used in place of bone scan. The bone scan is still helpful in searching for metastatic lesions because a generalized skeletal survey can be done. Moreover, it remains useful in settings where MRI is contraindicated (e.g., for a patient who has a cardiac pacemaker).

Arthrography

Arthrography is now rarely conducted in the management of adults with hip pain, having generally been supplanted by advanced imaging techniques such as MRI. Nevertheless, arthrography may still be valuable in the demonstration of labral pathology.[66] It is certainly useful in confirming the interarticular localization of an injection when differential injections are being administered, and it continues to have a role in the diagnosis of infection and in loosening of the prosthesis in the patient with a painful total joint replacement.[67]

Computed Tomography

CT of the hip and pelvis is probably most useful in the assessment of fractures, particularly complex acetabular and pelvic fractures. It can also serve as an adjunct in planning reconstructive procedures; it is helpful in the fabrication of custom implants and in the construction of models for reconstructions such as osteotomy.[68]

Magnetic Resonance Imaging

MRI has dramatically facilitated the diagnosis of hip pain, and the indications for its use continue to expand.[69] Although its value depends on both the quality of the image and the skill of the interpreter, MRI has become the standard technique for the diagnosis of several hip conditions.

The diagnosis of aseptic necrosis of the femoral head is made earlier by MRI than by any other technique, including bone scan, CT scan, and plain films[70] (Fig. 30–16). As information gained by MRI accumulates, new staging classifications of avascular necrosis are being developed.[71, 72] MRI is the method of choice for the diagnosis of occult hip fracture in the elderly and, despite its expense, can be cost-effective for this purpose. For instance, the diagnosis of an occult femoral neck fracture within the first 24 hours by MRI makes it unnecessary to wait for positive bone scan results and thus may obviate several days of hospitalization or a delay in treatment.[73] MRI is currently the best test for the diagnosis of transient osteonecrosis of the hip.[74] It is also the most valuable test for the staging of both bony and soft tissue tumors around the hip.[75] MRI is frequently helpful in documenting synovitis of the hip joint by revealing effusion and sometimes (e.g., in pigmented villonodular synovitis) accurately shows synovial change.[76] At present, MRI is the most accurate method for diagnosis of stress

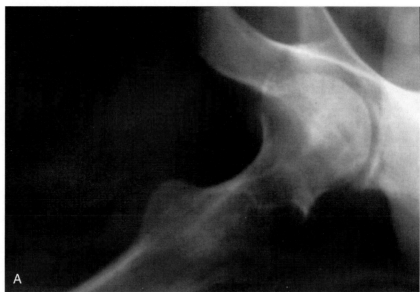

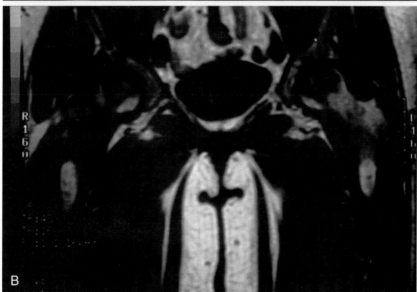

Figure 30–16. Aseptic necrosis of the femoral head—plain film (*A*) and MRI scan (*B*).

fractures around the hip and pelvis. MRI is sometimes useful in distinguishing pathologic conditions owing to soft tissue overuse such as tendinitis, bursitis, and degenerative tendinosis, but its value in this setting still depends on its resolution and its interpretation by the clinician.[77]

Arthroscopy

Hip arthroscopy can be a valuable tool for the diagnosis and treatment of a painful hip.[78] Even when the arthroscopist is experienced, the procedure is demanding because the hip joint is large and deep and thus is less accessible than more superficial joints such as the knee and shoulder.[79] Hip arthroscopy is useful, however, in several circumstances. There is a role for hip arthroscopy in the removal of loose bodies—whether from osteochondritis dissecans or an iatro-genic source. Hip arthroscopy techniques have reportedly been used to remove fragmented methylmethacrylate cement in total joint replacement.[80] Several reports have described the use of arthroscopic lavage in the treatment of septic arthritis of the hip.[81, 82] The diagnosis of torn or painful inverted labrum may be confirmed and some labral pathologic conditions debrided by hip arthroscopy.[66] As techniques improve and experience accumulates, the indications for this procedure will probably broaden.

Electromyography and Nerve Conduction Velocity Studies

EMG and NCV studies are used in the differential diagnosis of hip pain to evaluate referred lumbosacral plexopathies and to assess local nerve entrapment or nerve damage from trauma, surgery or other disease states.

Injections

Differential block of the hip joint can be a valuable adjunct in differentiating intra-articular hip joint pain generated from other sources. This procedure is best undertaken in the fluoroscopy suite, with arthrography used to confirm the location of the injection. The technique may be particularly useful in distinguishing intra-articular hip pathology from referred lumbosacral radiculopathy.[83] Like most injection techniques, differential hip block is limited by a placebo effect. Differential injection can also be helpful in distinguishing among painful soft tissue conditions. Iliopsoas tenography can help demonstrate snapping hip pathology.[84] Dye injection along the iliopsoas tendon sheath under fluoroscopy sometimes reveals the snapping of the iliopsoas tendon over the pelvic brim and, accompanied by lidocaine or corticosteroid injection, may help prove that the tendon condition is the pain generator.

Disorders Causing Hip Pain

Intra-articular Disorders

Intra-articular disorders of the femoral head acetabular joint account for a significant portion of cases of hip pain. The presentation of these disorders is variable but frequently includes pain deep in the groin or thigh and involves the anterior hip more than the posterior. The patient often reports that the pain is worse with weight-bearing; commonly has true passive loss of motion, with internal rotation and extension particularly affected; and frequently has hip-irritability signs, such as pain on forced internal rotation and pain on straight-leg raising against resistance. Plain radiography is generally helpful in this situation, sometimes revealing narrowing and osteophytes associated with osteoarthritis, fractures of the femoral neck, and mottling or even collapse with the crescent sign of avascular necrosis.

Osteoarthritis of the hip joint, inflammatory arthritis, avascular necrosis of the femoral head, and septic hip joint are covered extensively in other portions of this book and are not discussed here. The other prominent causes of intra-articular hip disease are discussed briefly.

Labral Pathology

Hip pain accompanied by a painful mechanical snap can have a number of causes (see "Snapping Hip," later in this chapter). One intra-articular cause of hip pain with snapping is a tear of the acetabular labrum.[66] The patient with acetabular labral tear is frequently a young, active adult with a history of trauma ranging from relatively minor twists, slips, and falls to more violent injuries, such as those incurred in an automobile accident. Most patients present with pain or discomfort deep in the anterior groin, and these symptoms are frequently exacerbated by pivoting or twisting. In addition, most patients describe a click or mechanical catch associated with their discomfort.

On physical examination, patients most commonly have a normal range of motion or only mild limitation. Fitzgerald described his experience with 55 patients whose acetabular labral tears were treated at the Mayo Clinic and Wayne State University from 1974 to 1993.[66] He found that the predominant physical finding on examination was reproduction of hip pain, with or without a painful click. A special maneuver of the hip during the examination—acute flexion with external rotation and full abduction followed by extension with internal rotation and adduction—precipitated pain, sometimes with a click, in patients with anterior labral tears. Full flexion, adduction, internal rotation, and then extension of the hip with abduction and external rotation reproduced pain, with or without a click, in patients with posterior labral tears.

Routine radiography generally yields normal results. Ikeda and associates described the management of torn acetabular labra in young patients with developmental acetabular dysplasia.[85] These patients may have an unusually high incidence of torn acetabular labra secondary to hypertrophy of the labrum associated with dysplasia as well as the abnormal increased load from the femoral head on the uncovered acetabulum in the area of the superior labrum. Hence, plain radiographs may show acetabular dysplasia.

Fitzgerald reported that arthrography was useful in two ways.[66] With the injection of local anesthetic, relief of the sharp catching hip pain confirmed an intra-articular source. With the injection of dye, the labral tear was visualized in 44 of 50 hips.

Initial treatment of the patient with a labral tear may be nonsurgical, with activities restricted and NSAIDs administered in an effort to reduce or eliminate the inflammation of the hip. However, given the mechanical nature of the problem, this effort may fail and surgery may be required. An acetabular labral tear may be seen by hip arthroscopy, and portions of the internal labrum may be resectable. However, visualization is limited and resection of the labrum technically difficult; hence, open resection of the torn labrum through a formal arthrotomy may be needed. Fitzgerald reported that dislocation of the hip was necessary for adequate resection of the labrum. Of the 45 patients undergoing open arthrotomy, however, only 1 developed osteonecrosis, and this patient had received prednisone for an unrelated illness. Hence, with cautious application of a transtrochanteric or anterior approach, dislocation and resection of the labrum appear to be safe and generally effective.

Fractures

Hip fractures are a common source of hip pain. Such fractures, which are most commonly intracapsular breaks involving the peritrochanteric region of the femur, are most frequently sustained by the elderly population. The result is substantial morbidity or even death. Patients' quality of life can be significantly diminished, and their management generally costs millions of dollars a year. As the population of the United States ages over the next few decades, the incidence of hip fracture probably will increase markedly, and the management of this problem will become even more important.[86] Surgical and medical management of hip fractures are beyond the scope of this chapter. We simply reiterate that aggressive management, with an emphasis on stabilization and early mobilization (aimed at reducing the problems associated with prolonged recumbency), is recommended.

A hip fracture in an elderly patient who presents to the emergency room after falling, is unable to walk, and exhibits shortening and rotation of the leg can usually be diagnosed easily by history, physical examination, and confirmatory radiograph. More difficult is the diagnosis of an occult fracture. Typically, an elderly patient presents to the physician's office or the emergency room after a fall; physical examination does not reveal the typical shortening or malrotation deformity of a displaced fracture but does document hip-irritability signs with pain on passive motion (particularly internal rotation). The patient clinically resembles patients with the more easily diagnosed displaced hip fractures. Plain radiographs may show osteoporosis but do not show fracture lines or trabecular disruption and, thus, are often read as normal. Many patients with occult fractures are unable to walk and are admitted to the hospital, treated with bed rest, and reevaluated over the next few days. Technetium bone scanning has been used to detect occult hip fractures (Fig. 30–17).[62] However, a frequent recommendation has been to delay bone scanning for as long as 72 hours to optimize the chances of detecting the fracture. Although bone scanning is highly sensitive, uptake may be increased[87] for reasons other

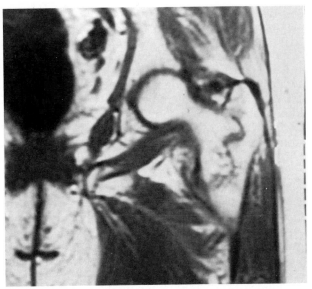

Figure 30–18. STIR image of an occult fracture of the hip; note areas of increased intensity.

than fracture (e.g., degenerative joint disease, tumor, and infection[88]).

Several studies have described the use of MRI in the diagnosis of occult fractures of the hip.[65, 73, 89, 90] A fracture may appear as low signal bands on both T1-weighted and T2-weighted sequences and as areas of increased intensity on STIR imaging (Fig. 30–18). The cited advantages of MRI over bone scanning include its noninvasive nature, its ability to detect occult fractures within 24 hours, and its high degree of sensitivity and specificity. Aggressive treatment of patients in whom occult fractures are documented may diminish the morbidity associated with bed rest, and those patients with negative MRI results may be more rapidly mobilized and discharged from the hospital. Hence, although more costly than bone scanning, MRI is preferable in several respects.[89]

In a study of 37 patients admitted to the hospital with hip pain and normal radiographs, Evans and colleagues showed by MRI that 8 patients had undisplaced femoral neck fractures; 6 of the 8 fractures were picked up by isotope scan, whereas the other 2 were not.[91] The remaining 29 patients had no evidence of a fracture and remained asymptomatic months after the injury.

Quinn and McCarthy described the diagnostic efficacy of coronal T1-weighted hip MRI in the diagnosis of occult fractures in 20 consecutive patients whose plain radiographs gave indeterminate results despite the clinical suspicion of a fracture.[73] The prospective accuracy of MRI was 100 percent. Of 13 patients with fractures, 8 had peritrochanteric fractures and 5 had femoral neck fractures. The cost of the single T1-weighted MRI scan was $48—much lower than that of a radionuclide bone scan ($455) or a CT scan ($797). The authors concluded that the savings from a shorter

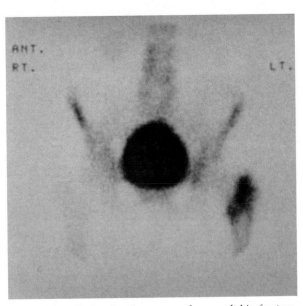

Figure 30–17. Technetium bone scan of an occult hip fracture.

duration of hospitalization alone offset the cost of imaging.

The failure to diagnose occult hip fracture creates the potential for worse outcomes, as patients who go on to displace an undiagnosed fracture may require more extensive procedures, may endure greater morbidity, and may entail more costs. For example, an elderly patient with a nondisplaced femoral neck fracture picked up by MRI may carefully be managed without surgery or perhaps with limited internal fixation accomplished percutaneously with cannulated screws, whereas that same patient who has a completely displaced femoral neck fracture may require prosthetic replacement, suffering greater morbidity and sustaining greater costs.

Not all patients with a presentation suggesting occult hip fracture actually have "surgical fractures" of the femoral neck or peritrochanteric area; some instead have isolated greater trochanter fractures or pelvic fractures such as of the pubic rami, which can be managed without surgery. Thus, the recommendation for a person whose history and examination findings are typical of hip fracture but whose radiographs are normal is to undergo MRI within the first 24 hours. T1-weighted coronal sections alone are likely to be diagnostic and may be preferable to a full MRI series.

Stress Fractures

Another cause of hip pain may be a stress fracture of the bone. There are two types of stress fracture. *Insufficiency fractures* occur in diseased bone that is involved in routine activity, and these typically affect older persons with osteopenic bone.[84, 92] *Fatigue fractures* occur in normal healthy bones repeatedly subjected to high-level stress that is not great enough on any individual occasion to cause acute traumatic fracture but that cumulatively causes fatigue failure of the bone. The latter fractures are most likely in young healthy persons involved in new activities (e.g., military recruits participating in training or athletes intensifying their training regimens). The popularity of athletics and workouts in the United States has resulted in an increase in rates of fatigue stress fractures among young patients.[93] Around the hip, such fractures can occur in the femoral neck and pelvic rami. Like occult fractures in the elderly, stress fractures in young athletes can be hard to diagnose and are commonly missed, occasionally with disastrous consequences.[94] Since a displaced femoral neck fracture in a young person often results in nonunion or avascular necrosis, it is important to maintain a high index of suspicion and to detect these fractures before they become displaced. The diagnosis can generally be made by either MRI or technetium bone scan (Fig. 30–19).

Devas described two categories of femoral neck stress fractures. In *transverse fractures*, the fracture line is perpendicular to the neck and extends to the superior surface. Because these are considered tension

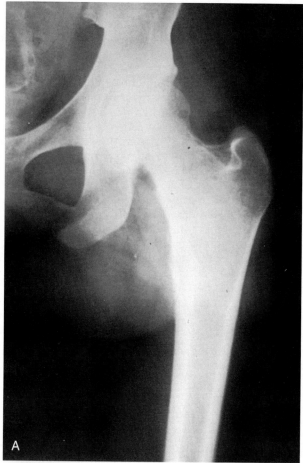

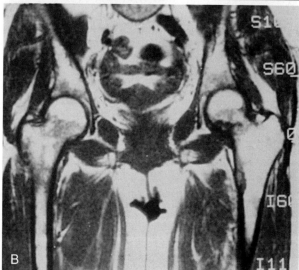

Figure 30–19. Displaced femoral neck fracture—plain film (*A*) and MRI technetium bone scan (*B*).

fractures at risk for displacement, their immediate internal fixation is recommended. In *compression fractures*, the showing fracture line or callus appears at the inferior part of the femoral neck. The risk of displacement is thus thought to be lower and the fracture to be more amenable to nonsurgical management consisting of limitations on activity and protective weight-bearing.[95]

Blikenstaff and Morris[96] divided femoral neck stress fractures into three categories: (1) a periosteal callus with no definitive fracture line; (2) a nondisplaced fracture line; and (3) a displaced fracture. They recommended that type 1 be treated with protective weight-bearing, type 3 with reduction and internal fixation, and type 2 possibly with either method. Some authors have recommended internal fixation of all femoral neck fractures because of a low associated morbidity and a high reliability in preventing displacement.

Transient Osteoporosis

Transient osteoporosis of the hip has been described in numerous reports and under various names, including *regional migratory osteoporosis* and *transient regional osteoporosis*.[74, 97–104] The causes of this syndrome are unknown, and it is unclear whether it represents a single clinical entity or a group of entities with similar clinical presentations. Most cases have affected young and middle-aged men or pregnant women in the third trimester. The presentation frequently consists of the sudden or gradual onset of dull, aching pain in the region of the hip joint, typically including the groin and thigh and sometimes accompanied by minor trauma. Patients are not likely to have risk factors for avascular necrosis. Physical examination generally shows some hip irritability with pain on passive range of motion, particularly rotational maneuvers. The condition is typically exacerbated by weight-bearing. Radiographs characteristically show demineralization of the femoral head and neck, although no radiologic abnormalities may be seen early on. Findings on routine laboratory examination are frequently normal. Technetium isotope studies characteristically demonstrate increased uptake within the femoral head. MRI typically shows decreased signal intensity on T1-weighted images and increased signal intensity on T2-weighted images, with a so-called bone marrow edema pattern (Fig. 30–20).[103] There may be effusion in the joint, but there is usually no erosion or cartilage involvement. In most cases, the problem is self-limiting; generally, pain resolves and function returns within 2 to 6 months. Plain radiographs show gradual remineralization of bone with resolution.

To a certain extent, the diagnosis is one of exclusion, as more serious problems need to be ruled out. In its early stages, osteonecrosis can produce similar MRI findings; ultimately, however, in osteonecrosis, MRI shows the T2-weighted double-line sign. The possibility of hip infection needs to be considered. An aspirate of synovial fluid is occasionally evaluated, although in transient osteoporosis of the hip the aspirate may be sterile. Inflammatory arthritis, infiltrative tumors, and trauma are also considered. Some patients experience a recurrence or the involvement of other joints, including the opposite hip, the knee, the foot or ankle, and (rarely) the upper extremities (e.g., shoulder and wrist) and are categorized as having transient regional osteoporosis.

Treatment is basically supportive, entailing activity modification; occasional protective weight-bearing during the active phase of the disease; maintenance of range of motion, with gradual ambulation as comfort allows and as the process progresses; and use of NSAIDs or other mild analgesics for pain relief. It has not been demonstrated that the use of corticosteroids speeds resolution.[99]

Periarticular Disorders

Hip pain whose origins lie not in the hip joint itself but in structures around the hip joint is difficult to diagnose and manage. The presenting patient is frequently young and athletic and has a "chronic groin pull." The symptoms may be diffuse and nonspecific. Plain films and more sophisticated imaging techniques, such as bone scanning and MRI, may yield results that are virtually normal. Thus, an unsatisfactory diagnosis of "soft tissue strain" is often made. Treatment is complicated by the absence of a good understanding of the etiology and pathophysiology of the problem.

Snapping Hip

Not uncommonly, patients present with hip pain accompanied by a biomechanical snapping sensation. These patients are usually relatively young, are frequently athletes or dancers, and may give a history of trauma or repetitive overuse activity, such as running. The numerous causes of this problem[105] fall into three categories: external, internal, and intra-articular.

External Snapping Hip. External causes are thought to be most common and involve thickening of the posterior part of the iliotibial band or of the anterior border or the gluteus maximus, with snapping over the greater trochanter. The thickened band lies posterior to the greater trochanter when the hip is in extension and snaps forward over the greater trochanter with flexion. Repetitive overuse can cause inflammation and subsequent irritation and thickening of the greater trochanteric bursa underneath

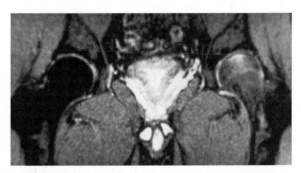
Figure 30–20. "Bone marrow edema pattern" in STIR MRI in transient osteoporosis of the hip.

the iliotibial tract, with consequent worsening of pain and snapping.

Occasionally, snapping hip follows total hip replacement or surgery involving the iliotibial band at the knee. Patients report that the hip pops out of place or dislocates; they generally perceive the problem to be in the area of the greater trochanter—a description that helps to distinguish this type of snapping from the internal and intra-articular types. The snapping is frequently detectable when the examiner places a hand over the greater trochanter and walks along with the patient. The iliotibial band can often be felt to pop over the greater trochanter if the patient lies on the unaffected side with the affected hip adducted, keeps the knee in extension (thus keeping the fascia lata tight), and then actively flexes and extends the hip.

Diagnostic testing usually is not helpful or necessary. Treatment is initially nonsurgical, consisting of stretching of the iliotibial band, reduction of inflammation (e.g., with ice and NSAIDs), occasional injection of corticosteroid, and short-term activity modification. If the pain remains significant, surgical treatment can be undertaken. A number of papers have described the procedures that can be used. These authors' preference is bursectomy and Z-plasty, as described by Brignall and Stainsby.[106] All eight patients so treated by these latter authors experienced complete resolution of snapping and substantial pain relief.

Internal Snapping Hip. In 1951, Nunziata and Blumenfeld reported three cases of deep painful anterior hip snapping believed to be secondary to the slipping of the psoas tendon over the iliopectineal eminence.[107] Two of the patients involved obtained good relief from iliopsoas lengthening. Anatomic dissection performed more recently at the University of Missouri[108] showed that the iliac and psoas muscles converge as they pass through a groove between the iliopectineal eminence and the anterior inferior iliac spine. When the hip moves from full flexion, abduction, and external rotation to extension, adduction, and internal rotation, the larger part of the iliopsoas tendon remains in this groove but moves from the lateral to the medial side of the femoral head over the anterior capsule. This motion can result in painful snapping of the iliopsoas over the femoral head and hip capsule; this event may irritate and inflame the iliopsoas tendon and iliopsoas bursa between the anterior capsule and the tendon, causing inflammation, thickening, and exacerbation of the snapping.

Patients presenting with this problem frequently report a painful snapping sensation that they perceive to be in the anterior hip and groin. This snapping may occur several times a day and may limit the individual's participation in sports. Most patients can demonstrate the phenomenon at will. An examiner can sometimes reproduce the snap by having the patient lie supine, flex and abduct the hip, and then bring it back into a position of extension and abduction. Sometimes the snap can be felt or blocked by the application of pressure over the iliopsoas tendon with the hand at the level of the femoral head.

Diagnostic testing may be helpful in the evaluation of internal snapping. Iliopsoas bursography or iliopsoas tenography is most useful.[108] Under fluoroscopic control, a spinal needle is inserted over the superomedial quadrant of the femoral head, advanced until bone is contacted, and then retracted 5 mm. Contrast material is injected. If the iliopsoas bursa is defined, the tendon is sometimes seen as a filling defect and, with motion of the hip, can be seen to pop. With luck, an iliopsoas tenogram can be done by drawing the needle back just a few millimeters, injecting contrast, and filling the tendon sheath. Again, the hip can be examined under fluoroscopy while being voluntarily moved by the patient. If a painful pop occurs as the tendon moves from lateral to medial, a painful snapping tendon can be diagnosed.

Initial treatment is nonsurgical, with stretching of the iliopsoas in extension, use of NSAIDs, and modification of activities until symptoms diminish. If symptoms persist, surgical treatment can be undertaken. Jacobson and Allen reported the results of fractional lengthening of the iliopsoas tendon in 18 symptomatic cases.[108] Nearly all patients were able to return to their preoperative level of participation in sports and other activities. Five of 6 patients reported a recurrence of symptoms but said that the frequency in snapping and intensity of pain were dramatically reduced. Only 1 of 13 patients interviewed stated that she would not repeat the procedure; this woman had no postoperative decrease in snapping and actually had a slight increase in pain.

Intra-articular Snapping Hip. Intra-articular snapping may be caused by tearing of the acetabular labrum, as described earlier in this chapter (see "Labral Pathology"). Other causes include traumatic loose body, synovial chondromatosis, and post-traumatic femoral head defects.[105] Patients with an intra-articular lesion frequently have pain as their primary complaint, with clicking as a secondary complaint. The physical examination for acetabular labrum is described in the section just cited. Plain radiographs may reveal a loose body or possible hip dysplasia associated with a torn labrum. Intra-articular injection may be informative if pain is relieved in the anesthetic phase, and contrast may demonstrate torn labrum pathology.[66]

Bursitis

Frequently, patients present to the clinician's office with pain on the side of the hip over or posterior to the greater trochanteric area. Although this symptom could have numerous causes, three major entities are commonly seen in this setting in clinical practice: (1) referred pain from the low back with sciatica; (2) referred pain from intra-articular hip pathology, most often osteoarthritis; and (3) local soft-tissue inflammation, frequently called *trochanteric bursitis*. Since no findings are pathognomonic for trochanteric bursitis, the diagnosis is generally based on clinical impression.

There are three trochanteric area bursae. The most clinically relevant is the gluteus maximus bursa, which separates the gluteus maximus from the greater trochanter. The other two bursae are smaller and separate the greater trochanter from the gluteus medius and the gluteus minimus, respectively. The patient is most often middle-aged, female, and heavy. Pain is typically located along the lateral side of the upper thigh, frequently radiates from the buttock down toward the knee, is characteristically aggravated by activity such as walking or stair climbing, is typically worse at night, and prevents patients from lying on the affected side.

Physical examination reveals localized tenderness over the greater trochanter that is best elicited by palpation with the patient lying on the unaffected side. Trochanteric bursitis is commonly associated with other pathologic conditions. In 1986, Schapira and coworkers described a study of 72 patients with a clinical diagnosis of trochanteric bursitis; 91.6 percent of these patients had associated problems, including osteoarthritis of the same hip (44.5 percent), lumbar spondyloarthrosis (38.8 percent), and rheumatoid arthritis (8.3 percent). Findings related to these other conditions can make it hard to determine by physical examination whether trochanteric pain is localized or referred. Furthermore, as has already been mentioned, no finding is pathognomonic for trochanteric bursitis.[109] Plain radiographs may show peritrochanteric calcification. Localized increase in uptake on technetium bone scanning has been reported, but the results of this test generally do not influence treatment recommendations.[110] MRI occasionally shows trochanteric bursitis, but again, these results may not alter clinical recommendations and thus may not be warranted except to rule out other pathologic conditions.[77]

Some younger patients may develop traumatic bursitis owing to overuse (e.g., in running) or to local direct trauma. Treatment is generally nonsurgical. NSAIDs and local anti-inflammatory measures such as icing may be palliative. The benefits of physiotherapy, including ultrasound, are anecdotal and sporadic.[109] Local corticosteroid injection is frequently effective:[109] In Schapira and coworkers' paper, 71 percent of patients recovered after a single injection and 93 percent benefited from one or two injections. Raman and Haslock found trochanteric bursitis by clinical evaluation in 15 of 100 patients with rheumatoid arthritis.[111] In this study, two thirds of the patients with bursitis obtained pain relief from a single corticosteroid injection, and the rest responded to a second injection. Surgical exploration and excision of the bursa may be considered for the rare recalcitrant cases.

Another source of bursitic hip pain is iliopsoas bursitis.[112–115] The iliopsoas bursa is the largest synovial bursa in the body and is localized anterior to the hip joint between the iliopsoas muscle and the ante-

rior capsule of the hip. Fourteen percent of adult cadavers dissected by Chandler had a communication from the hip joint into the iliopsoas bursa. This type of communication is markedly more prevalent among patients with associated underlying hip disease, including rheumatoid arthritis, osteoarthritis, avascular necrosis, and synovial chondromatosis. Enlargement of the iliopsoas bursa may present as pain in the anterior groin, as an anterior hip or inguinal mass, or occasionally as a compression syndrome with neurogenic involvement or venous obstruction with swelling of the leg.[115]

The differential diagnosis of hip bursitis includes lymphadenopathy, tumors, hernias, and vascular malformations. Tuberculous infections have been reported in the iliopsoas bursa. Plain radiographs may reveal underlying hip disorders. Ultrasound may be an economical way to demonstrate a fluid-filled mass. CT/arthrography can demonstrate communication between the hip joint and the bursa, and the lesion can be well defined on MRI. Treatment depends on the nature of the symptoms and of the underlying or associated conditions. Aspiration of the bursa with corticosteroid injection is sometimes effective. Occasionally, resection of the bursa is indicated.

Osteitis Pubis

Osteitis pubis is an inflammatory condition of unknown etiology affecting the pubic symphysis and surrounding muscular attachments. Osteitis pubis has been reported in association with complications of suprapubic surgery and in association with peripartum urinary tract infections.[116] However, most recent reports have described its occurrence in athletes.[117] An athlete's variety of symptoms at presentation may lead to a delay in the diagnosis of osteitis pubis. These symptoms include pain in the groin, medial thigh, testicles, hips, or lower abdomen. It may well be that a number of underlying conditions initiate the process and that compensatory mechanisms (e.g., an adductor strain) then increase the shear stress across the symphysis pubis, leading to mechanical irritation, inflammation, and (ultimately) bony resorption.

Patients may have tenderness at the symphysis or pubic rami, but associated tenderness of other adjacent muscle groups may confuse the issue. Plain radiographs may show changes typical of osteitis pubis, with osteolysis at the joint; however, these radiologic changes may not be evident early on. Technetium bone scanning is likely to give positive results.[118] MRI—particularly fat-suppression sequences—may document stress around the symphysis but may also detect adjacent areas of pathology or help identify other conditions (e.g., pubic stress fracture). Limited STIR sequences may be economical for the monitoring of changes in the stress reaction with treatment.[18]

The initial focus of treatment is the reduction of inflammation. Rest from the inciting activity is required, with cross-training used to maintain aerobic fitness. NSAIDs or even oral corticosteroids may be used. Intra-articular cortisone injection may be of value when other methods are not working. Once the stress has been reduced across the symphysis and the inflammation diminished, a stretching and strengthening program emphasizing abdominal, hip, and short-arc closed chain exercises is instituted.[117] Unfortunately, recurrence is not uncommon. Surgical intervention can be considered for the rare recalcitrant cases.

A differential diagnosis must be undertaken in evaluating groin pain in an athlete and should include osteitis pubis, stress fracture to the pubic or ischial rami or femoral neck, hernias, isolated muscle tears or strains in the adductor abdominal muscles, apophysitis or bony avulsion injuries, genitourinary infection, or urolithiasis. In rare cases, seronegative spondyloarthropathy, such as ankylosing spondylitis or Reiter's syndrome, is sought.[117]

Regional Disorders

The source of hip pain quite commonly is the hip joint or the immediate periarticular structures. Hence, only a high index of suspicion may prompt a thorough examination of other areas of anatomy. Nevertheless, such an examination can be crucial in an evaluation of hip pain.

Lumbosacral Radiculopathy

The need for a "regional" approach is illustrated by hip pain arising from lumbosacral pathology. (Chapter 30 provides a more comprehensive discussion.) A typical diagnostic dilemma is exemplified by a 50-year-old who presents with posterior buttock and side-of-hip pain. Although it can have a number of causes, such pain is most likely attributable to lumbosacral radiculopathy, owing to local soft tissue inflammation (e.g., trochanteric bursitis), or referred from intra-articular hip pathology (e.g., osteoarthritis). Certain features of the patient's history may help to distinguish among the choices. Referred radicular pain is frequently worsened by prolonged sitting and sometimes by lying flat, whereas intra-articular hip pathology is usually relieved by rest and lack of weight-bearing. The neurologic nature of the referred pain may be apparent in the patient's description of its character: burning and tingling symptoms are uncharacteristic of intra-articular discomfort. Pain that radiates from the hip all the way down into the foot and is accompanied by tingling or weakness is more frequently neurogenic than of hip joint origin. Comprehensive physical and neurologic evaluations are frequently helpful; if a patient has a true flexion or external rotation contracture of the hip joint, with limitation of internal rotation and hip irritability on these maneuvers, the pain is more likely to be attributable to intra-articular hip pathology than to be lumbar-referred. True motor loss and reflex changes are more likely signs of lumbar radiculopathy. Local tenderness over the trochanter and the lumbar area and

relief of pain by anesthetic and cortisone injection are hallmarks of trochanteric bursitis; and their absence warrants consideration of other referred sources of pain. The situation is complicated by the fact that patients may have pathology in both areas. A 75-year-old patient with an osteoarthritic hip may well have concomitant lumbosacral spinal stenosis, with mixed symptoms and signs.

An EMG can be included in the work-up to look for signs of radiculopathy or nerve entrapment. MRI frequently reveals disc herniation, nerve impingement, and bony spinal stenosis impingement. Differential injections can be extremely helpful in distinguishing referred lumbar radicular pain from hip joint or periarticular pain. Particularly valuable are selective nerve root blocks, epidural corticosteroid injection, local soft tissue bursal injection, and intra-articular hip injection.

Traycoff described 18 patients with a clinical diagnosis of trochanteric bursitis who did not respond to local injection.[83] Their work-up included contrast-enhanced CT or MRI, EMG, and root blocks. Referred lumbar radicular pain was thought to be the source of discomfort in 61 percent of patients.

Miscellaneous Disorders

A variety of miscellaneous disorders can cause pain referred to the hip. Local nerve entrapments may cause referred pain (see Chapter 39). For example, entrapment of lateral cutaneous branches of the iliohypogastric nerve and the subcostal nerves can produce pain in the upper lateral thigh. Meralgia paresthetica is anterolateral thigh pain secondary to entrapment of the lateral femoral cutaneous nerve.[119] Femoral and inguinal hernias can produce pain in the inguinal and hip areas and can generally be diagnosed by history and physical examination. Tumors, particularly lymphomas, can be manifested in the hip and inguinal regions. The proximal femur and the pelvis are common sites of metastatic bone disease. Low intrapelvic pathology (e.g., ovarian pathology or intrapelvic or extrapelvic endometriosis) sometimes presents as hip pain.[120]

References

1. Radin EL, Rose RM: Role of subchondral bone in the initiation and progression of cartilage damage. Clin Orthop 213:34, 1986.
2. Saal J, Dillingham MF: Nonoperative treatment and rehabilitation of disc, facet, and soft-tissue injuries in athletes. In Hershman E (ed): The Lower Extremity and Spine in Sports Medicine, 2nd ed. St. Louis, Mosby–Year Book, 1994.
3. Feagin JA: The office diagnosis and documentation of common knee problems. Clin Sports Med 8:453, 1989.
4. Messieh SS, Fowler PJ, Munro T: Anteroposterior radiographs of the osteoarthritic knee. J Bone Joint Surg 72B:639, 1990.
5. Merchant AC: Classification of patellofemoral disorders. Arthroscopy 4:235, 1988.
6. Moreland JR, Bassett LW, Hanker GJ: Radiographic analysis of the axial alignment of the lower extremity. J Bone Joint Surg 69A:745, 1987.
7. McCrae F, Shouls J, Dieppe P, et al: Scintographic assessment of osteoarthritis of the knee joint. Ann Rheum Dis 51:938, 1992.
8. Schietzer ME, Mandel S, Schwartzman RJ, et al: Reflex sympathetic

dystrophy revisited: MR imaging findings before and after infusion of contrast material. Radiology 195:211, 1995.

9. Rankine JJ, Smith FW, Scotland TR: Case report: Short tau inversion recovery (STIR) sequence MRI appearances of reflex sympathetic dystrophy. Clin Radiol 50:188, 1995.

10. Rosenthall L: Nuclear medicine techniques in arthritis. Rheum Dis Clin North Am 17:585, 1991.

11. Werndorff R, Robinson I, cited by Werndorff R: Employment of oxygen in bone and joint disease. J Iowa Med Soc 17:240, 1929.

12. Lindblom K: Arthrography of the knee: Roentgenographic and anatomic study. Acta Radiol (Suppl) 47:1, 1948.

13. Wolfe R: Knee Arthrography: A Practical Approach. Philadelphia, WB Saunders, 1984.

14. Ostergaard M, Court-Payen M, Weislander S, et al: Ultrasonography in arthritis of the knee: A comparison with MR imaging. Acta Radiol 36:19, 1995.

15. Dillingham MF, Mishra A: Arthroscopy. In Kelley WN (ed): Textbook of Internal Medicine, 3rd ed. Philadelphia, JB Lippincott, 1997.

16. Burk DL, Mitchell DG, Rifkin MD, et al: Recent advances in magnetic resonance imaging of the knee. Radiol Clin North Am 28:379, 1990.

17. Tehranzadeh J, Kerr R, Amster J: Magnetic resonance imaging of tendon and ligament abnormalities. Skeletal Radiol 21:79, 1992.

18. Tuite MJ, DeSmet AA: MRI of selected sports injuries: Muscle tears, groin pain, and osteochondritis dissecans. Semin Ultrasound CT MR 15:318, 1994.

19. Stoller D: Magnetic Resonance Imaging in Orthopedics and Rheumatology. Philadelphia, JB Lippincott, 1989.

20. Newberg AH, Wetzner SM: Bone bruises: Their patterns and significance. Semin Ultrasound CT MR 15:396, 1994.

21. Chandnani VP, Ho CH, Chu P, et al: Knee hyaline cartilage evaluated with MR imaging: A cadaveric study involving multiple imaging sequences and intra-articular injection of gadolinium and saline solution. Radiology 178:557, 1991.

22. Ho C, M.D.: Personal communication.

23. Kerr DR: Prepatellar and olecranon arthroscopic bursectomy. Clin Sports Med 12:137, 1993.

24. Mangine-Eifert M, Brewster C, Wong M, et al: Patellar tendonitis in the recreational athlete. Orthopedics 15:1359, 1992.

25. Nichols CE: Patellar tendon injuries. Clin Sports Med 11:807, 1992.

26. Tachdjian OM: Pediatric Orthopedics, 2nd ed. Philadelphia, WB Saunders, 1990, p 1010.

27. Davies SG, Baudouin CJ, King JB, et al: Ultrasound, computed tomography, and magnetic resonance imaging in patellar tendonitis. Clin Radiol 43:52, 1991.

28. Leadbetter WB, Pekka PA, Lane GJ, et al: The surgical treatment of tendinitis. Clin Sports Med 11:679, 1992.

29. Tindel NL, Nisonson B: The plica syndrome. Orthop Clin North Am 23:613, 1992.

30. Johnson DP, Eastwood DM, Witherow PJ: Symptomatic synovial plica of the knee. J Bone Joint Surg 75A:1485, 1993.

31. Dorchak JD, Barrack RL, Kneisl JS, et al: Arthroscopic treatment of symptomatic synovial plica of the knee. Am J Sports Med 19:503, 1991.

32. Dillingham, unpublished data.

33. Kelly MA, Insall JN: Historical perspectives of chondromalacia patellae. Orthop Clin North Am 4:517, 1992.

34. Reilly D, Martens M: Experimental analysis of the quadriceps muscle force and patellofemoral joint reaction force for various activities. Acta Orthop Scand 43:126, 1972.

35. Zappala FG, Taffel CB, Scuderi GR: Rehabilitation of patellofemoral disorders. Orthop Clin North Am 23:555, 1992.

36. Tria AJ, Palumbo RC, Alicea JA: Conservative care for patellofemoral pain. Orthop Clin North Am 23:545, 1992.

37. Fu FH, Maday MG: Arthroscopic lateral release and the lateral compression syndrome. Orthop Clin North Am 23:601, 1992.

38. Fulkerson JP, Schutzer SF: After failure of conservative treatment for painful patellofemoral malalignment: Lateral release or realignment? Orthop Clin North Am 17:283, 1986.

39. Kolettis GT, Stern SH: Patellar resurfacing for patellofemoral arthritis. Orthop Clin North Am 23:665, 1992.

40. Glasgow MM, Allen PW, Blakeway C: Arthroscopic treatment of cysts of the lateral meniscus. J Bone Joint Surg 75B:299, 1993.

41. Mills CA, Henderson IJ: Cysts of the medial meniscus: Arthroscopic diagnosis and management. J Bone Joint Surg 75B:293, 1993.

42. Fisseler-Eckhoff A, Muller KM: Arthroscopy and chondrocalcinosis. Arthroscopy 8:98, 1992.

43. Zarins B, McInerney VK: Calcium pyrophosphate and pseudogout. Arthroscopy 1:8, 1985.

44. Baratz ME, Fu FH, Mengato R: Meniscal tears: The effect of meniscectomy and of repair on intra-articular contact areas and stress on the human knee. Am J Sports Med 14:270, 1986.

45. Fairbank TJ: Knee joint changes after meniscectomy. J Bone Joint Surg 30B:664, 1948.

46. Allen PR, Denham RA, Swan AV: Late degenerative changes after meniscectomy. J Bone Joint Surg 66B:666, 1984.

47. Lynch MA, Henning CE, Glick KR: Knee joint surface changes, longterm follow-up meniscus tear treatment in stable anterior cruciate ligament reconstruction. Clin Orthop 172:148, 1983.

48. McGinty JB, Guess LF, Marvin RA: Partial or total meniscectomy, a comparative analysis. J Bone Joint Surg 59A:763, 1977.

49. Tapper EM, Hoover NW: Late results after meniscectomy. J Bone Joint Surg 51A:517, 1969.

50. Yocum LA, Kerlan RK, Jobe FW, et al: Isolated lateral meniscectomy. J Bone Joint Surg 61A:338, 1979.

51. Scott GA, Jolly BL, Henning CE: Combined posterior incision and arthroscopic intra-articular repair of the meniscus. J Bone Joint Surg 68A:847, 1986.

52. O'Meara PM: The basic science of meniscus repair. Orthop Rev 22:681, 1993.

53. Veltri DM, Warren RF, Wickiewicz TL, et al: Current status of allograft transplantation. Clin Orthop 303:44, 1994.

54. Rand JA: Role of arthroscopy in osteoarthritis of the knee. Arthroscopy 7:358, 1991.

55. Garrett JC: Osteochondritis dissecans. Clin Sports Med 10:569, 1991.

56. Motohashi M, Morii T, Koshino T: Clinical course and roentgenographic changes of osteonecrosis in the femoral condyle and conservative treatment. Clin Orthop 266:156, 1991.

57. al-Rowaih A, Lindstrand A, Bjorkengren A, et al: Osteonecrosis of the knee. Acta Orthop Scand 62:19, 1991.

58. Bradley J, Dandy DJ: Osteochondritis dissecans and other lesions of the femoral condyles. J Bone Joint Surg 71B:518, 1989.

59. Safran MR, Fu FH: Uncommon causes of knee pain in the athlete. Orthop Clin North Am 26:547, 1995.

60. Sutro CJ, Sutro WH: The clinical importance of articulations of the fibula. Bull Hosp J Dis Orthop Inst 42:68, 1982.

61. Fredericson M, Bergman AG, Hoffman KL, et al: Tibial stress reaction in runners: Correlation of clinical symptoms and scintigraphy with a new magnetic resonance imaging grading system. Am J Sports Med 23:472, 1995.

62. Geslien GE, Thrall JH, Espinosa JL, et al: Early detection of stress fractures using 99m-Tc-polyphosphate. Radiology 121:683, 1976.

63. Mont MA, Hungerford DS: Non-traumatic avascular necrosis of the femoral head. J Bone Joint Surg 77A:259, 1995.

64. Cohen I, Rzetelny V: Osteoid osteoma of the acetabulum. Clin Orthop 304:204, 1994.

65. Rizzo PF, Gould ES, Lyden JP, et al: Diagnosis of occult fractures about the hip: Magnetic resonance imaging compared with bone scanning. J Bone Joint Surg 75A:395, 1993.

66. Fitzgerald RH: Acetabular labrum tears. Clin Orthop 311:60, 1995.

67. Kraemer WJ, Saplys R, Waddel JP, et al: Bone scan, gallium scan, and hip aspiration in the diagnosis of infected total hip arthroplasty. J Arthroplasty 8:611, 1993.

68. Gill K, Bucholz RW: The role of computerized tomographic scanning in the evaluation of major pelvic fractures. J Bone Joint Surg 66A:34, 1984.

69. Pitt MJ, Lund PJ, Speer DP: Imaging of the pelvis and hip. Orthop Clin North Am 21:545, 1990.

70. Fordyce MJ, Solomon L: Early detection of avascular necrosis of the femoral head by MRI. J Bone Joint Surg 75B:365, 1993.

71. Sugano N, Ohzono K, Masuhara K, et al: Prognostication of osteonecrosis of the femoral head in patients with systemic lupus erythematosus by magnetic resonance imaging. Clin Orthop 305:190, 1994.

72. Lafforgue P, Dahan E, Chanaud C, et al: Early-stage avascular necrosis of the femoral head: MR imaging for prognosis in 31 cases with at least 2 years of follow-up. Radiology 187:199, 1993.

73. Quinn SF, McCarthy JL: Prospective evaluation of patients with suspected hip fracture and indeterminate radiographs: Use of T1-weighted MR images. Radiology 187:469, 1993.

74. Rhodes I, Matzinger MA: Residents' corner: Answer to case of the month. Transient osteonecrosis of the hip. Can Assoc Radiol J 44:399, 1993.

75. Aboulfia AJ, Malawer M: Surgical management of pelvic and extremity osteosarcoma. Cancer 71(Suppl):3358, 1993.

76. Boyd AD, Sledge CB: Evaluation of the hip with pigmented villonodular synovitis. A case report. Clin Orthop 275:180, 1992.

77. Caruso FA, Toney MA: Trochanteric bursitis. A case report of plain film, scintigraphic, and MRI correlation. Clin Nucl Med 19:393, 1994.

78. Byrd JW: Hip arthroscopy utilizing the supine position. Arthroscopy 10:275, 1994.

79. Glick JM, Sampson TG, Gordon RB, et al: Hip arthroscopy by the lateral approach. Arthroscopy 3:4, 1987.

80. Mah ET, Bradley CM: Arthroscopic removal of acrylic cement from unreduced hip prosthesis. Aust N Z J Surg 62:508, 1992.

81. Bould M, Edwards D, Villar RN: Arthroscopic diagnosis and treatment of septic arthritis of the hip joint. Arthroscopy 9:707, 1993.

82. Chung WK, Slater GL, Bates EH: Treatment of septic arthritis of the hip by arthroscopic lavage. J Pediatr Orthop 13:444, 1993.

83. Traycoff RB: "Pseudotrochanteric bursitis": The differential diagnosis of lateral hip pain. J Rheumatol 18:1810, 1991.

84. Schaberg JE, Harper MC, Allen WC: The snapping hip syndrome. Am J Sports Med 12:361, 1984.
85. Ikeda T, Awasya C, Suzuki A, et al: Torn acetabular labrum in young patients. Arthroscopic diagnosis and management. J Bone Joint Surg 70B:13, 1988.
86. Falch JA, Ilebekk A, Slungaard U: Epidemiology of hip fractures in Norway. Acta Orthop Scand 56:12, 1985.
87. Matin P: The appearance of bone scans following fractures, including immediate and long-term studies. J Nucl Med 20:1227, 1979.
88. Lewis SL, Rees JS, Thomas GV, et al: Pitfalls of bone scintigraphy in suspected hip fractures. Br J Radiol 64:403, 1991.
89. Haramati N, Staron RB, Barax C, et al: Magnetic resonance imaging of occult fractures of the proximal femur. Skeletal Radiol 23:19, 1994.
90. Guanche CA, Kozin SH, Levy AS, et al: The use of MRI in the diagnosis of occult hip fractures in the elderly: A preliminary review. Orthopedics 17:327, 1994.
91. Evans PD, Wilson C, Lyons K: Comparison of MRI with bone scanning for suspected hip fracture in elderly patients. J Bone Joint Surg 76B:158, 1994.
92. Tountas AA: Insufficiency stress fractures of the femoral neck in elderly women. Clin Orthop 292:202, 1993.
93. Matheson GO, Clement DC, McKenzie JE, et al: Stress fractures in athletes: A case study of 320 cases. Am J Sports Med 15:46, 1987.
94. Johansson C, Ekenman I, Tornkvist H, et al: Stress fractures in the femoral neck in athletes. Am J Sports Med 18:524, 1990.
95. Devas MB: Stress fractures of the femoral neck. J Bone Joint Surg 47B:728, 1965.
96. Blikenstaff LP, Morris JM: Fatigue fractures of the femoral neck. J Bone Joint Surg 48A:1031, 1966.
97. Potter H, Moran M, Schneider R, et al: Magnetic resonance imaging in diagnosis of transient osteoporosis of the hip. Clin Orthop 280:223, 1992.
98. Urbanski SR, deLange EE, Eschenroeder HC: Magnetic resonance imaging of transient osteoporosis of the hip. J Bone Joint Surg 73A:451, 1991.
99. Lakhanpal S, Ginsburg WW, Luthra HS, et al: Transient regional osteoporosis: A study of 56 cases and review of the literature. Ann Intern Med 106:444, 1987.
100. Grimm J, Higer HP, Benning R, et al: MRI of transient osteoporosis of the hip. Arch Orthop Trauma Surg 110:98, 1991.
101. Ben-David Y, Bornstein J, Sorokin Y, et al: Transient osteoporosis of the hip during pregnancy. A case report. J Reprod Med 36:672, 1991.
102. Daniel WW, Sanders PC, Alarcon GS: The early diagnosis of transient osteoporosis by magnetic imaging. A case report. J Bone Joint Surg 74A:1262, 1992.
103. Hayes CW, Conway WF, Daniel WW: MR imaging of bone marrow edema pattern: Transient osteoporosis, transient bone marrow edema syndrome, or osteonecrosis. Radiographics 13:1001, 1993.
104. Schapira D: Transient osteoporosis of the hip. Semin Arthritis Rheum 22:98, 1992.
105. Allen WC, Cope R: Coxa saltans: The snapping hip revisited. J Am Acad Orthop Surg 3:303, 1995.
106. Brignall CG, Stainsby GD: The snapping hip. Treatment by Z-plasty. J Bone Joint Surg 73B:253, 1991.
107. Nunziata A, Blumenfeld I: Cadera a resorte: A proposito de una variedad. Prensa Med Argent 38:1997, 1951.
108. Jacobson T, Allen WC: Surgical correction of the snapping iliopsoas tendon. Am J Sports Med 18:470, 1990.
109. Schapira D, Nahir M, Scharf Y: Trochanteric bursitis: A common clinical problem. Arch Phys Med Rehabil 67:815, 1986.
110. Allwright SJ, Cooper RA, Nash P: Trochanteric bursitis: Bone scan appearance. Clin Nucl Med 13:561, 1988.
111. Raman D, Haslock I: Trochanteric bursitis—A frequent cause of "hip" pain in rheumatoid arthritis. Ann Rheum Dis 41:602, 1982.
112. Toohey AK, LaSalle TL, Martinez S, et al: Iliopsoas bursitis: Clinical features, radiographic findings, and disease associations. Semin Arthritis Rheum 20:41, 1990.
113. Generini S, Matucci-Cerinic M: Iliopsoas bursitis in rheumatoid arthritis. Clin Exp Rheumatol 11:549, 1993.
114. Meaney JF, Cassar-Pullicino VN, Etherington R, et al: Ilio-psoas bursa enlargement. Clin Radiol 45:161, 1992.
115. Lertourneau L, Dessureault M, Carette S: Rheumatoid iliopsoas bursitis presenting as unilateral femoral nerve palsy. J Rheumatol 18:462, 1991.
116. Lentz SS: Osteitis pubis: A review. Obstet Gynecol Surv 50:310, 1995.
117. Batt ME, McShane JM, Dillingham MF: Osteitis pubis in collegiate football players. Med Sci Sports Exerc 27:629, 1995.
118. Burke G, Joe C, Levine M, et al: Tc-99m bone scan in unilateral osteitis pubis. Clin Nucl Med 19:535, 1994.
119. Macnicol MF, Thompson WJ: Idiopathic meralgia paresthetica. Clin Orthop 254:270, 1990.
120. Moeser P, Donofrio P, Karstaedt N, et al: MRI findings of sciatic endometriosis. Clin Imaging 14:64, 1990.

CHAPTER 31

Robert J. Scardina
Bruce T. Wood

Ankle and Foot Pain

Various acute and chronic arthritic conditions affect the foot and ankle, representing local or systemic processes that are monoarticular, polyarticular, or migratory in nature. Virtually all rheumatic disorders can be the cause of foot symptoms and pain, including inflammatory, degenerative, metabolic, neuropathic, enthesopathic, infectious, and traumatic disorders.[1]

Accurate patient history and physical examination with appropriate, selective laboratory and imaging studies are initial requisites. A thorough working knowledge of foot and ankle anatomy and of the mechanics of the primary functions of the foot and ankle are essential for diagnosis and successful treatment, both conservative and surgical.

This chapter addresses the uniqueness of the foot-ankle mechanical complex, pertinent elements of the physical examination, and radiographic and newer imaging methods of particular usefulness in the diagnosis of foot and ankle rheumatologic pathology. Major rheumatic diseases are covered emphasizing regional clinical manifestations, radiographic findings, and conservative treatment. Less common arthritides that display frequent and significant foot and ankle involvement are also mentioned, but in less detail. The interested reader is referred to Chapter 112 for additional detailed information beyond the scope and intent of this chapter.

ANATOMY AND BIOMECHANICS

Demands are made on the foot to respond in specific active and passive fashions throughout the gait cycle. The overall position, intrinsic configuration, and focal areas of weight bearing of the foot change in a precise and predictable sequence through a progression from heel strike to foot flat to midstance to heel lift to toe off. Deviations from these normal requirements commonly lead to pain as a result of dynamic or structural deformity, excessive intra-articular compressive or load forces, or excessive tension forces on supporting and controlling soft tissue structures.[2]

Structurally, the foot can be separated into three regions: forefoot (metatarsals and phalanges), midfoot (cuneiforms, navicular, and cuboid) and hindfoot (talus and calcaneus) (Fig. 31–1). Major joints include the ankle and subtalar, midtarsal, and metatarsophalangeal (MTP) joints. Individual osseous components are united or supported by more than 100 ligaments that maintain structural integrity and joint congruency, and that are intended to allow motion in only normal planes and within normal ranges. During standing and locomotion, extrinsic and intrinsic musculotendinous units stabilize, accelerate, or decelerate the foot, ankle, or lower leg. To meet the requirements of each gait event or phase, they act either predominantly or subordinately with other associated soft tissue structures. In the presence of neurovascular integrity and adequate cutaneous and subcutaneous coverage and protection (especially the fat pads of the heel and forefoot), this intricate repetitive cascade of events and integration of structures allows for pain-free, efficient locomotion, dampening impact forces at heel strike (through ankle plantar flexion and subtalar pronation), adapting to unevenness in terrain (through subtalar and midtarsal pronation), while ultimately converting the foot into a rigid lever (through subtalar supination) for active propulsion.

Joints

The ankle (talocrural) joint is a synovium-lined hinge composed of the superior (trochlear) surface of the talus secured into a mortise formed by the distal articular aspect of the tibia and fibula and connected by dense collateral and syndesmotic ligaments.[3] Although some obliquity exists in its true axis of motion, for practical purposes, this joint can be considered to function in the sagittal plane. Normal non–weight-bearing range of motion from the perpendicular is 10 to 20 degrees of dorsiflexion and 40 to 65 degrees of plantar flexion; normal ambulation requires a minimum of 10 degrees of dorsiflexion and 30 degrees of plantar flexion.

Unlike the ankle, the subtalar (talocalcaneal) joint has an axis that runs oblique to the three cardinal body planes (i.e., frontal, sagittal, transverse). Hence, subtalar motion is overtly triplanar. Non–weight-bearing motions include pronation (dorsiflexion, abduction, eversion) and supination (plantar flexion, adduction, inversion), and when combined with the lower leg in weight bearing, a universal joint effect becomes apparent.[4]

During locomotion and stance, pronation is evidenced by eversion of the calcaneus, abduction of the foot, and collapse of the medial longitudinal arch. Inversion of the calcaneus, adduction of the foot, and a rise in the medial longitudinal arch indicate supina-

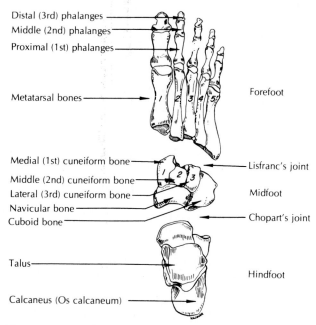

Distal (3rd) phalanges
Middle (2nd) phalanges
Proximal (1st) phalanges

Metatarsal bones

Forefoot

Medial (1st) cuneiform bone
Middle (2nd) cuneiform bone
Lateral (3rd) cuneiform bone
Navicular bone
Cuboid bone

Lisfranc's joint

Midfoot

Chopart's joint

Talus

Hindfoot

Calcaneus (Os calcaneum)

Figure 31–1. Dorsal view showing individual osseous components of the forefoot, midfoot, and hindfoot. (From Rockwood CA, et al [eds]: Fractures: Vols 1 and 2. Fractures in Adults, 3rd ed. Philadelphia, JB Lippincott, 1991, pp 2042–2043.)

tion. Clinical evaluation of the subtalar joint—performed by assessing frontal plane motion of the posterior aspect of the calcaneus—is difficult to reproduce consistently, and methods vary between investigators.[5] Normal non–weight-bearing range of motion is 25 to 30 degrees of inversion and 10 to 15 degrees of eversion, with requisites for normal ambulation (4 to 6 degrees of both inversion and eversion) falling within this range, allowing the foot to assume a plantigrade position on the ground during its total contact phase.

The midtarsal joints (talonavicular, calcaneocuboid) are under the direct influence of the subtalar position, leading to more overall foot mobility (subtalar pronation) or rigidity (subtalar supination). For clinical examination purposes, this joint is evaluated in the frontal plane (up to 20 degrees maximum), with slight oblique or transverse plane motion also depending on subtalar position. This locking and unlocking mechanism of the midtarsal joint dependent on the subtalar joint is critical for shock absorption and accommodation to changes in terrain. The MTP joints have essentially two functions during gait. At heel lift, they passively dorsiflex, and during toe off and propulsion, they provide stability against the ground with the assistance of the plantar intrinsic and lower leg extrinsic long toe flexor musculature. Normal walking requires 65 to 75 degrees of dorsiflexion of the first MTP joint and 60 to 65 degrees of dorsiflexion of the lesser MTP joints.

Musculature

Musculotendinous structures influence the foot and ankle by providing stability, acceleration, and deceler-

ation, depending on the requirements of each specific gait event or phase. In general, extrinsic muscles are divided into four compartments: anterior, lateral, posterior/deep, and posterior/superficial. The anterior group dorsiflexes the foot and toes during the swing phase of gait and decelerates the foot at heel strike. The lateral group provides stability from foot flat to just before toe off. The superficial posterior group decelerates, stabilizes, and accelerates during the stance phase, also influencing coincidental knee motions. The posterior tibial muscle of the deep posterior group is of vital importance in decelerating necessary subtalar pronation from heel strike to foot flat.[6]

The intrinsic muscles of the foot consist of four layers of plantar muscles and two superficial dorsal muscles. The plantar intrinsic muscles stabilize the MTP joints or assist deep extrinsic muscle function. Superficial to the intrinsic muscles, the plantar aponeurosis (fascia) spans the inferior calcaneus to the inferior MTP joints in three separate bands (medial, middle, lateral), providing support to the longitudinal arch of the foot, especially at heel lift as a windlass mechanism.

PHYSICAL EXAMINATION

A standardized, sequential approach to physical examination of the foot and ankle is essential to establishing a diagnosis. The examination follows a complete history that elicits the region, provocative and palliative influences, quality, severity, and duration of the pain. The goal is to identify the structure or structures involved—bone, articular surface, synovium, ligament, tendon, adventitious subcutaneous structures, skin, or a combination. A thorough physical examination includes evaluation of the vascular, neurologic, dermatologic, and musculoskeletal systems of the foot and ankle.

Inspection

The foot and ankle should be observed bilaterally in three different modes: non–weight bearing, standing, and walking. The examiner should check for evidence of asymmetry, deformity (including relation of forefoot to hindfoot), edema, articular swelling, subcutaneous nodules, bursae, erythema, and cutaneous changes (e.g., plantar or digital hyperkeratoses, nail changes, ulcers), all of which may suggest rheumatologic disease but must be differentiated from other local or systemic processes. Observations about standing include identification of alterations in shape (including medial longitudinal arch height, anterior foot splay, and accentuation of non–weight-bearing deformity), malalignment (especially of the hindfoot), and width (base) of stance.[7] Visual gait analysis (with the foot shod and unshod) involves identifying abnormalities at each gait cycle event, including a final propulsive phase with active push-off, angle of gait (i.e., toe-in or toe-out), and base of gait. Any evidence of antalgia may negate the significance of these observations.

Whenever possible, the patient's shoe gear should be examined. Areas and patterns of sole and heel wear and heel counter deformation may be of diagnostic value, especially when correlated with gait observations.

Palpation

Off-weight-bearing, specific areas of the foot and ankle should be palpated for tenderness or pain, temperature increase, and induration or thickening of soft tissues. These areas include the ankle joint, Achilles tendon, heel (both inferior and posterior), osseous prominences or deformities of the midfoot and forefoot, plantar fat pads of the heel and forefoot, and the MTP and interphalangeal joints proper.

Joint effusion of the ankle is best appreciated along the anterior joint line, medially and laterally. MTP joints may be examined by dorsoplantar pressure individually or simultaneously with collateral compression of all five metatarsals (Bayles' test) (Fig. 31–2).[8]

Range of Motion

Major joints of the foot-ankle complex should be taken through full excursion, with total range of motion, aberrations of direction, excess or limitation, quality (lax or firm), endpoint (soft or hard), crepitus, and coincidental elicitation of pain noted. The examiner should be cognizant of potential causes of both limited range of motion (e.g., muscle splinting due to articular pain or active synovitis, tarsal coalition, muscle or tendon contracture, fibrous or bony ankylo-

sis) and excessive range of motion (e.g., ligamentous laxity, tendon dysfunction, or rupture) associated with rheumatologic and other systemic diseases.

RADIOGRAPHY AND ADVANCED IMAGING STUDIES

Plain radiographic evaluation is a common and useful tool in the evaluation of foot and ankle pain, especially when undertaken in a systematic fashion. Foot views should be taken in a weight-bearing position (normal angle and base of stance and gait), including bilateral (for comparison) dorsoplantar, oblique, lateral, and forefoot axial views. The ankle is evaluated separately with anteroposterior, lateral, and mortise views. Magnification enhancement may be helpful before considering more sophisticated and expensive studies.[9]

When faced with the need for more sophisticated types of imaging studies, four methods lend well anatomically to the foot and ankle: magnetic resonance imaging (MRI), bone scans, computed tomography (CT), and contrast studies. MRI aids in the diagnosis of soft tissue, joint, and bone changes in arthritis by providing extremely detailed and differentiated images. In rheumatoid arthritis, MRI is useful in early disease detection as well as for follow-up.[10] Radionuclide imaging is highly sensitive, differentiating bone from soft tissue pathology, determining distribution, and following disease course (serial scans).[11] In feet with rheumatoid arthritis, radionuclide imaging can assist in differentiation of stress fractures, vasculitis, enthesopathy, and osteomyelitis. CT scanning is used primarily to identify the location and extent of positional deformity and post-traumatic or degenerative arthritis of the ankle, subtalar, and midtarsal joints.[12] Contrast studies (arthrography and tenography) are useful in visualizing ankle joint pathology (osteochondral lesions, fractures, synovial irregularities), and hindfoot–ankle tendon pathology, especially peroneal and posterior tibial tenosynovitis as a manifestation of inflammatory joint disease.

RHEUMATOID ARTHRITIS

More than 90 percent of patients with rheumatoid arthritis ultimately have foot-ankle manifestations, with ankle involvement rivaling the forefoot in some studies.[13] Patterns of involvement include 3:1 female to male ratio and a predominance in the 40- to 60-year-old age category.

Foot symptoms develop from two distinct processes: (1) synovial proliferation creating capsular and ligamentous distention that leads to subluxation and dislocation, and (2) cartilage erosion resulting in joint destruction and structural deformity.[14] Both processes occur in the forefoot or hindfoot (usually sparing the lesser tarsus) and lead to alterations in gait patterns and locomotion, including reduced velocity, shuffling

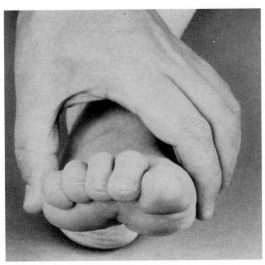

Figure 31–2. Bayles' (forefoot squeeze) test is performed by applying collateral compression along the metatarsal shafts, proximal to the metatarsophalangeal joints.

gait, shortened stride length, and absence of normal heel-toe pattern.[15] Articular symptoms are usually symmetric, and, as such, require differentiation from lymphoproliferative (and other systemic) disorders.[16]

Clinical Presentation

Onset of rhematoid arthritis in the foot is usually insidious, beginning with localized joint swelling and stiffness after rest, initially alleviated somewhat by movement. The MTP and proximal interphalangeal joints may also be tender to palpation and passive motion, with associated warmth and erythema. The subtalar and ankle joints have painful effusions and are accompanied by findings in the joints of the forefoot. Over time, joint erosions lead to fixed structural deformities, including dorsal subluxations or dislocations of the MTP joints. Lateral drift of the lesser toes and hammertoe deformities develop, with associated anterior displacement of the plantar fat pads, commonly leading to metatarsalgia, painful calluses, or ulcerations.[17] Subcutaneous nodules may be detected beneath prominent metatarsal heads and the heel. Other deformities, such as hallux valgus and bunions, may be mechanically induced sequelae of hindfoot hyperpronation and calcaneovalgus.[18]

Radiographic Findings

Radiographic and imaging findings are in keeping with the rate of disease progression, generally demonstrating increased involvement within 3 years of onset.[19] Progressively, joint and subchondral erosions become evident, as do non–joint-destructive deformities on clinical examination (e.g., MTP dislocations, hammertoes, hallux valgus) (Fig. 31–3). Erosive processes tend to progress from lateral to medial (frequently sparing the first MTP joint), and dorsal deformities progress from medial to lateral in the lesser MTP joints.

Treatment

During the acute, painful inflammatory initial stages, before deformity develops, any preexisting structural or dynamic deformities should be addressed, especially hyperpronation with calcaneovalgus; with time, the disease process will only accentuate these deformities. Physical therapy, including assist devices (canes and walkers), active and passive exercise, and application of moist heat, commonly provides a measure of pain relief and maintains mobility. As tolerated, passive and active (particularly isometric) exercises, especially of the ankle, subtalar, and MTP joints, are important for the maintenance of muscle tone, strength, and joint mobility. Various types of foot and foot-ankle night splints stabilize or

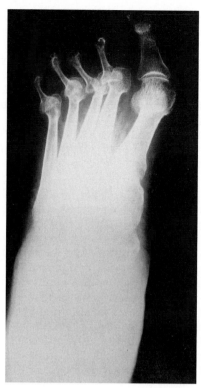

Figure 31–3. Anteroposterior view of a rheumatoid foot with lesser metatarsophalangeal (MTP) joint dislocations, interphalangeal joint erosions, but general sparing of first MTP joint involvement.

prevent potential contractures and secondary deformity.

Biomechanical therapy consists of various foot or foot-ankle orthoses, including in-shoe padding and inserts, custom shoe gear, and shoe modifications.[20, 21] Reducing or eliminating functional limitations and pain while allowing limited ambulation is the primary goal. As a general rule, shoes should be lightweight, flexible, and modifiable to conform to deformity in each dimension. Insole material should provide cushioning, particularly in the heel and forefoot regions. To facilitate putting on and removing footwear (especially in patients with hand involvement), a Velcro closure (as opposed to laces) may be helpful. Jogging shoes provide a practical, economical, and readily available answer in certain situations. Appropriately fitted specialty shoe gear, either commercially available (in-depth) or custom molded, is generally indicated for patients with more severe stable deformities in the chronic disease state.[22, 23] Finally, modifications of the traditional shoe gear (if generally appropriate for the overall foot structure) can often provide a quick, inexpensive, and convenient method of treatment.

In instances of refractory monarticular joint pain or isolated inflamed bursae or tendon sheaths, injection therapy with soluble corticosteroid preparations can prove particularly helpful. For small (i.e., interphalangeal and MTP) joints, tuberculin syringes are most helpful. The MTP joints are entered either dorsomedially or dorsolaterally, with avoidance of the extensor tendon and distraction used to facilitate entry. A standard 3-mL syringe with a 25-gauge needle is used for the subtalar joint, entering the sinus tarsi in an anterolateral to posteromedial oblique fashion. Ankle joint access is usually achieved through an anteromedial approach with the joint in slight gravity plantar flexion; the needle is inserted medial to the anterior tibial tendon and directed posterolaterally. The other tarsal joints, with the exception of the talonavicular joint, are difficult to inject. Aspiration (for the purposes of collecting synovial fluid for analysis) is performed routinely when possible before instillation of corticosteroid preparations.

Another nonsurgical alternative, particularly for refractory acute ankle pain in the absence of joint destruction, is radiation synovectomy.[24]

Juvenile Rheumatoid Arthritis

Patients with juvenile rheumatoid arthritis can present significant challenges in preventing, correcting, or accommodating foot deformities. Early detection of structural changes and initiation of appropriate biomechanical measures (e.g., shoe gear, orthoses, splints) and physical therapy are essential. More physically active patients should be observed for development of deformity in the hindfoot and midfoot, where, in contrast to the adult calcaneovalgus deformity, equinovarus occurs more commonly. To achieve and maintain reasonable functional alignment, corrective measures must be initiated early, before development of fixed deformity. Accordingly, both active and passive range of motion and strengthening exercises should be started promptly, as pain tolerance permits. After fibrous or bony ankylosis is present, conservative therapy is ineffective and surgical intervention is generally necessary.[25, 26]

OSTEOARTHRITIS

Osteoarthritis (degenerative joint disease) is the most common arthropathy seen in clinical practice, including a significant incidence in the foot and ankle. Weight-bearing joints are usually involved, particularly the first MTP, first metatarsocuneiform, tarsometatarsal (Lisfranc's), talonavicular, subtalar, and ankle joints. Associated deformities include hallux valgus and bunion, hallux limitus or rigidus, dorsal midfoot exostoses, fixed hindfoot malalignments (calcaneovalgus and varus), and ankle arthritis. Each may lead to progressive severe, functional disability with weight bearing and ambulation.

Clinical Presentation

Symptoms and deformity of osteoarthritis develop slowly over years either secondary to repetitive exces-sive abnormal forces (microtrauma) on otherwise normal joints or as sequelae to overt intra-articular macrotrauma, especially of the hindfoot and ankle. Passive and active joint pain, stiffness relieved by rest (in early stages), and bony enlargement (proliferative osteophytosis) precede eventual bony ankylosing and fixed deformity.

Radiographic Findings

As with other rheumatic disorders, radiographic findings in osteoarthritis parallel the stage and extent of the disease process. Initially, uneven joint space narrowing is observed with subchondral sclerosis, followed by osteophyte formation with loose bodies, and finally periarticular cysts and ankylosis.

Types of Conditions

Bunion or Hallux Valgus

Usually attributable to an inward deviation of the first metatarsal, a painful bump develops on the medial first metatarsal head, accompanied by lateral (and valgus) malposition of the hallux (Fig. 31–4).[27] Hindfoot (subtalar) hyperpronation is the most common mechanical cause. Secondary lesser digital crowding leads to hammertoe formation and retro-

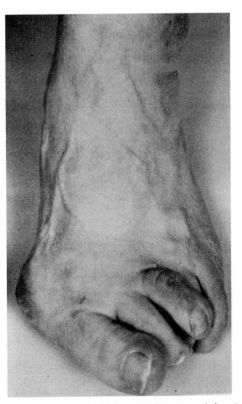

Figure 31–4. Hallux abductovalgus and bunion deformity with secondary lesser digital crowding, hammertoes, and metatarsophalangeal joint dislocation (Fig. 31–3).

grade metatarsal prolapse producing plantar forefoot pain (metatarsalgia and capsulitis). Foot–shoe incompatibility over bony prominences eventually creates painful bursae.

Hallux Limitus and Rigidus

Hallux limitus and rigidus present as a painful bump on the dorsal first MTP joint as a result of restriction of the first MTP range of motion. Causes include direct trauma and a variety of predisposing structural abnormalities, such as a relatively long first toe or metatarsal, hypermobility or fixed elevation of the first metatarsal, and excessive midstance pronation.[28] Four clinical and radiographic stages range from soft tissue limitation in the absence of radiographic findings to marked circumferential enlargement of the joint, painful synovitis, and sclerosis with loss of joint space and absolute rigidity (Fig. 31–5).[29]

Lisfranc's (Tarsometatarsal) Arthritis

Most often the result of traumatic hyperflexion or extension, subtle radiographic changes in the presence of diffuse swelling are commonly overlooked and underappreciated in tarsometatarsal arthritis. Injury involves soft tissue, dislocation, cartilage, and fracture, most often in combination. CT scanning is helpful in detecting subtle joint changes, both positional and destructive. Despite closed or open reduc-

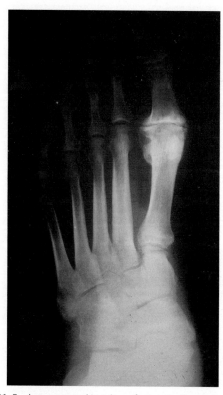

Figure 31–5. Anteroposterior view demonstrating severe hallux limitus (rigidus) with joint space narrowing and flattening, osteophytic ridging, and pronounced subchondral sclerosis.

tion, gross injury and deformity often progress to arthritis that requires arthrodesis.[30, 31]

Subtalar and Ankle Arthritis

Intra-articular fracture and osteochondral injury of these primary weight-bearing joints lead to degenerative joint disease, often even after early surgical intervention. Pain, synovitis, and restricted motion are typical sequelae.[32, 33]

Treatment

The treatment goal is to minimize or eliminate pain and disability, and limited weight bearing and temporary immobilization may be needed initially. Custom orthoses and shoe modifications realign, limit motion, or accommodate deformity, and various impact-attenuating materials help reduce ankle and subtalar pain.[34] Injection (corticosteroid) therapy and physical therapy have a place in acute and chronic phases.

GOUT

Gout often manifests first in the foot with severe pain. Most often, these acute attacks are monarticular and involve the first MTP joint of the foot, although the hallux interphalangeal, midtarsal, and ankle joints are sometimes involved. Onset is acute (frequently nocturnal), with exquisite pain accompanied by erythema, warmth, and swelling, resembling septic arthritis or cellulitis.

If untreated, attacks usually last for days, with symptoms resolving slowly and temporarily preventing the use of conventional shoe gear. Typically, patients are symptom free between attacks. Chronic recurrent attacks result in joint destruction, accompanying deformity, and ankylosis with painful ambulation. Positional joint changes or subluxations are uncommon except for transverse lateral deviation of the hallux due to loss of ligamentous integrity in the hyperpronated foot.

Radiographic Findings

Radiographs taken during acute bouts of gout reveal joint effusions with juxta-articular increased soft tissue density, generally in the absence of joint space narrowing. After repetitive attacks, tophaceous deposits erode both articular cartilage and subchondral bone in the region of capsular attachments. Eventually, cartilage erosions lead to painful irregular joint space narrowing, which ultimately results in restricted motion. Subchondral erosions (usually medial) present in association with a classic "overhanging edge" of periosteal new bone at the joint line level (Martel's sign), which is atypical of other arthritides.

Treatment

Treatment consists of two phases: resolution of pain and management of hyperuricemia in an attempt to prevent future attacks and potential irreversible joint damage. As an alternative to acute phase medical management, a posterior tibial nerve block (with a long-acting local anesthetic such as bupivacaine) can provide immediate pain relief and create a hyperemic flush of the synovial joint fluid. Painful tophi, joint disease, and deformity usually require surgical treatment.

NEUROPATHIC OSTEOARTHROPATHY

Whereas most inflammatory, degenerative, and other rheumatic disorders that affect the foot or ankle produce pain as well as deformity and disability, etiologic and coexistent insensitivity is the hallmark of neuropathic osteoarthropathy. Motor, sensory, and especially autonomic neuropathy all contribute to the process. Absence (or significant diminution) of pain and proprioception allow foot and ankle articulations to exceed normal ranges of motion, resulting in instability, subluxation, and deformity. The most common cause of neuropathic osteoarthropathy in the adult foot and ankle by far is diabetes mellitus, with other causes including leprosy, chronic alcoholism, spinal cord injury, peripheral nerve injury, and congenital insensitivity to pain.[35]

Clinical Presentation

Although often unrecognized by the patient, incidental minor trauma is the usual precipitating factor.[36, 37] The process follows in three distinct phases (development, coalescence, and reconstruction), all with characteristic clinical and radiographic features. In the initial acute phase, erythema, diffuse edema, warmth, hypermobility, and joint effusions are evident and must be differentiated from symptoms of osteoarthritis or infection. This is followed by alteration in foot shape, with the development of a midfoot rocker-bottom deformity or prolapse of the medial ankle. Early changes, if not addressed immediately, lead to abnormal focal bony prominences susceptible to inordinate weight-bearing pressures and possible ulceration.

Radiographic Findings

Radiographically, each phase can demonstrate a combination of both atrophic and hypertrophic changes (due to autonomic and sensory pathology) of bone and cartilage, resulting in destruction, periosteal reaction, consolidation, and gross deformity.[35]

Treatment

In the absence of significant malalignment and deformity, the treatment of choice in the early stages consists of non–weight bearing and immobilization, followed by judicious protective weight bearing. The goal is to maintain reasonable foot architecture and a plantigrade attitude while the process runs its course (usually 3 to 4 months). For chronic, stable deformity (especially in the plantar foot), custom-molded shoes with soft insoles and a rocker-type outside sole are used. Severe deformity of the foot or ankle unresponsive to this type of treatment often requires surgical intervention (arthrodesis or resection).

NONARTICULAR RHEUMATISM

Three major nonarticular rheumatic conditions give rise to pain and disability about the foot and ankle: fasciitis, bursitis, and tendinitis. They are generally well localized on palpation to the involved structure, are easily differentiated from joint disease per se, and most often are due to functional or structural abnormalities or overuse.

Plantar Fasciitis

One of the most common foot complaints encountered in clinical practice, plantar fasciitis occurs most frequently in individuals 35 years of age and older and is characterized by deep aching inferior heel pain, usually poorly localized by the patient. The consistent, if not pathognomonic, pattern is pain most pronounced with the first step in the morning (or after sitting), known as poststatic dyskinesia. Palpation is a key to diagnosis through localization of the point of maximal tenderness, either over the medial tubercle of the calcaneus or beneath the heel centrally, consistent with the origins of the plantar fascia bands. This enthesopathy occurs both in planus (flat) feet and cavus (high-arched) feet, since both forms produce undue tension and subsequent tears (microscopic) at the fascia-bone junction. Radiographs may reveal an inferior traction exostosis and are helpful in ruling out spur fracture, stress fracture of the calcaneal body, and stigmata of inflammatory joint disease.

Treatment methods include orthoses (for hindfoot alignment or heel cushioning) (Fig. 31–6), nonsteroidal anti-inflammatory drugs (NSAIDs) (indomethacin and piroxicam are most effective), ankle-foot orthoses–type night splints, and Achilles tendon stretching and physical therapy treatments (phonophoresis, iontophoresis). Injection of local anesthetic or corticosteroid preparations, under sterile technique with a fine-gauge needle from a medial approach, is often curative when followed by orthotic management.[38]

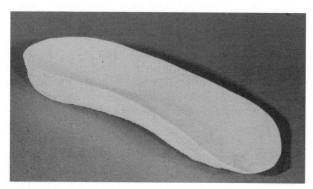

Figure 31–6. Soft orthosis commonly used in the management of plantar fasciitis.

Bursitis

There are only three anatomic bursae in the foot: infracalcaneal, retrocalcaneal (between calcaneus and Achilles tendon), and postcalcaneal (between Achilles tendon and overlying skin).[39] Adventitious bursae develop most commonly in the region of bunion and bunionette (fifth MTP) deformities as well as over posterior interphalangeal joints (hammertoes), primarily as the result of foot-shoe incompatibility. Both anatomic and adventitious bursae become inflamed in response to excessive pressure or friction.

Treatment involves removal of the inciting external factor, rest, ice, protective padding, or surgical correction of underlying deformity if it is otherwise unresponsive. Injection therapy should be performed with precision and in limited fashion to avoid atrophy of fat pads or rupture of neighboring tendons.

Tendinitis

The posterior tibial, Achilles, and peroneal tendons are most commonly involved in tendinitis. Hyperpronation, creating excessive and prolonged tensile forces, leads to posterior tibial dysfunction. The Achilles tendon is susceptible to similar forces and pathology in pes cavus and overuse (athletic) activities, as are the peroneals to a lesser degree. Treatment is directed at symptoms (rest, temporary immobilization, NSAIDs, ice, and addressing biomechanical abnormalities with custom orthoses). The use of injection treatment (corticosteroids) is discouraged, because tendon rupture may rapidly ensue.

OTHER RHEUMATIC DISORDERS

Seronegative Spondyloarthropathies

Ankylosing spondylitis, psoriatic arthritis, and Reiter's syndrome constitute the seronegative spondyloarthropathies, a group of acute and chronic arthritides. All three involve not only synovial but also extrasynovial tissues, including joint capsule, entheses, and periosteum.

Ankylosing spondylitis, although primarily a disease of the axial skeleton, can affect the foot. Most common sites of involvement include the inferior and posterior calcaneus, presenting as plantar fasciitis and Achilles tendinitis, followed by periosteal reaction and fibrotic tissue ossification, which result in classic spurs. Alternatively, inflammatory erosions of the posterior calcaneus (from retrocalcaneal bursitis) may occur. MTP joint destruction accompanied with periosteal new bone formation is far less common.[40]

Psoriatic arthritis involves the feet in a small percentage of patients with psoriasis. In a symmetric more than asymmetric fashion, the distal interphalangeal and, to a lesser extent, MTP joints are involved. The latter pattern may resemble rheumatoid arthritis. Nail pitting usually occurs in the toes with distal interphalangeal joint involvement. A whittled joint destructive process ("pencil-in-cup" appearance), especially in the hallux, is a late-stage radiographic finding. Similar to ankylosing spondylitis, inferior and posterior calcaneal erosions may also be seen.[41]

In patients with Reiter's syndrome, joints of the foot and ankle are usually involved asymmetrically. The plantar skin may show lesions (keratoderma blennorrhagicum) that are virtually indistinguishable from those of pustular psoriasis. The arthritic changes closely resemble those of psoriatic arthritis, with large, fluffy, painful calcaneal exostoses ("lover's heel").[42, 43] Treatment is largely directed at symptoms, involving the use of NSAIDs along with moderate exercise, physical therapy, supportive or accommodative orthoses, and injection therapy (corticosteroids), particularly for enthesopathies of Reiter's syndrome and psoriatic arthritis.

Systemic Lupus Erythematosus

A chronic inflammatory rheumatic disease, systemic lupus erythematosus may affect the foot in a fashion closely resembling rheumatoid arthritis. Nonerosive joint involvement with pain and swelling can precede pathology in other organ systems by years, making accurate diagnosis all the more difficult. As in rheumatoid arthritis, symmetric involvement of the proximal interphalangeal joints of the foot is a common presentation. Unlike in rheumatoid arthritis, however, the hammertoe deformities are reducible, with bony or fixed ankylosis occurring rarely.[44]

Scleroderma

Foot involvement in scleroderma leads to pain, ischemic skin changes, and fixed deformity. Early involvement resembles that of rheumatoid arthritis, with pain and swelling, especially in the digits. Progressive, severe stiffness due to contracture, fibrosis, and atrophy of the skin and subcutaneous structures develops, leading to rigid digital deformity. Characteristically, as adherence to underlying tissues develops, the skin becomes firm, immobile, and shiny. Severe ischemia from arteritis and Raynaud's phenomenon commonly results in painful distal digital necrosis or ulceration. Osteopenia, articular cartilage destruction, cortical thinning, and bone resorption in the distal phalangeal tufts are typical radiographic findings. Punctate digital calcific deposits may be observed in areas of focal pressure.

SUMMARY

An integrated team approach that involves rheumatologist, orthopedist, podiatrist, physical therapist, and orthotist is essential to the overall evaluation, treatment, and management of foot and ankle pathology in rheumatic disease. As a combined effort, early diagnosis and conservative treatment can prevent, delay, or minimize the onset of pain, deformity, or functional disability. Lifestyle modifications and realistic goals must be appreciated by the clinician and patient alike. However, when faced with failure of conservative measures and resultant joint destruction with pain or deformity and severe locomotor limitations, the possibilities of surgical treatment of the foot and ankle must be considered.[45]

References

1. Yale I: The Arthritic Foot and Related Connective Tissue Disorders. Baltimore, Williams & Wilkins, 1984.
2. Sgarlato TE (ed): A Compendium of Podiatric Biomechanics. San Francisco, California College of Podiatric Medicine, 1971, pp 115–116.
3. Clemente CD (ed): Gray's Anatomy of the Human Body. Philadelphia, Lea & Febiger, 1985, pp 409–413.
4. Inman VT: The subtalar joint. In Inman VT (ed): The Joints of the Ankle. Baltimore, Williams & Wilkins, 1976, pp 35–44.
5. Milgrom C, Giladi M, Simkin A, et al: The normal range of subtalar inversion and eversion in young males as measured by three different techniques. Foot Ankle 6:143–145, 1985.
6. Root M, Orien W, Weed J: Muscle function of the foot during locomotion. In Normal and Abnormal Function of the Foot. Los Angeles, Clinical Biomechanics Corp, 1977, pp 181–220.
7. Mann RA: Principles of examination of the foot and ankle. In Surgery of the Foot, 5th ed. St Louis: CV Mosby, 1986, pp 31–49.
8. Rigby AS, Wood PH: The lateral metacarpophalangeal/metatarsophalangeal squeeze: An alternative assignment criterion for rheumatoid arthritis. Scand J Rheumatol 20:115–120, 1991.
9. Weissman SD: Joint diseases. In Radiology of the Foot, 2nd ed. Baltimore, Williams & Wilkins, 1989, pp 289–315.
10. Forrester DM: Arthritis. In Kricun ME (ed): Imaging of the Foot and Ankle. Rockville, Md, Aspen Publishers, 1988, pp 129–157.
11. Brower AC: Imaging of rheumatic disorders. In Brandt KD (ed): Diagnostic Studies in Rheumatology. Summit, NJ, Ciby-Geigy Corp, 1992, pp 44–53.
12. Seltzer SE, Weissman BN, Braunstein EM, et al: Computed tomography of the hindfoot with rheumatoid arthritis. Arthritis Rheum 28:1234–1241, 1985.
13. Michelson J, Easley M, Wigley FM, et al: Foot and ankle problems in rheumatoid arthritis. Foot Ankle Int 15:608–613, 1994.
14. Calabro J: Juvenile rheumatoid arthritis. Clin Podiatr Med Surg 5:57–76, 1988.
15. Platto MJ, O'Connell PG, Hicks JE, et al: The relationship of pain and deformity of the rheumatoid foot to gait and an index of functional ambulation. J Rheumatol 18:38–43, 1991.
16. Menon N, Madhok R: Symmetrical polyarthritis is not always rheumatoid. Ann Rheum Dis 53:631–632, 1994.
17. Geppert MJ, Sobel M, Bohne WH: The rheumatoid foot: Part 1. Forefoot. Foot Ankle 13:550–558, 1992.
18. Stockley I, Betts RP, Rowley DI, et al: The importance of the valgus hindfoot in forefoot surgery in rheumatoid arthritis. J Bone Joint Surg 72B:705–708, 1990.
19. van der Heijde DM, van Leeuwen MA, van Riel PC, et al: Biannual radiographic assessments of hands and feet in a three-year prospective followup of patients with early rheumatoid arthritis. Arthritis Rheum. 35:26–34, 1992.
20. Wu KK: Foot ulcers in rheumatoid arthritis. In Foot Orthoses: Principles and Clinical Applications. Baltimore, Williams & Wilkins, 1990, pp 292–301.
21. Berenter RW, Kosai DK: Various types of orthoses used in podiatry. Clin Podiatr Med Surg 11:219–229, 1994.
22. Kaye RA: The extra-depth toe box: A rational approach. Foot Ankle Int 13:146–150, 1994.
23. White J: Custom shoe therapy: Current concepts, designs, and special considerations. Clin Podiatr Med Surg 11:259–270, 1994.
24. Barnes CL, Shortkroff S, Wilson M, et al: Intra-articular radiation treatment of rheumatoid synovitis of the ankle with dysprosium-165 ferric hydroxide macroaggregates. Foot Ankle Int 15:306–310, 1994.
25. Schaller J: Chronic arthritis in children. Clin Orthop 182:79, 1983.
26. Swann M: Juvenile chronic arthritis. Clin Orthop 219:38–49, 1987.
27. O'Connor PL, Baxter DE: Bunions. In Gould JS (ed): The Foot Book. Baltimore, Williams & Wilkins, 1988, pp 206–218.
28. Smith TF, Malay DS, Ruch JA: Hallux limitus and rigidus. In McGlamry ED (ed): Comprehensive Textbook of Foot Surgery. Baltimore, Williams & Wilkins, 1987, pp 238–251.
29. Durrant MN, Siepert KK: Role of soft tissue structures as an etiology of hallux limitus. J Am Podiatr Med Assoc 83:173–180, 1993.
30. Stenström A: The treatment of tarsometatarsal injuries. Foot Ankle 11:117–123, 1990.
31. Faciszewski T, Burks RT, Manaster BJ: Subtle injuries of the Lisfranc joint. J Bone Joint Surg 72A:1519–1522, 1990.
32. Walter JH, Spector A: Traumatic osteoarthritis of the ankle joint secondary to ankle fractures. J Am Podiatr Med Assoc 81:399–404, 1991.
33. Good RP: Arthrodesis and arthroplasty. In Hamilton WC (ed): Traumatic Disorders of the Ankle. New York, Springer-Verlag, 1984, pp 255–268.
34. Garcia AC, Dura JV, Ramiro J, et al: Dynamic study of insole materials simulating real loads. Foot Ankle Int 15:311–323, 1994.
35. Sanders LJ, Frykberg RG: Diabetic neuropathic osteoarthropathy: The Charcot foot. In Frykberg RG (ed): The High Risk Foot in Diabetes Mellitus. New York, Churchill Livingstone, 1991, pp 297–338.
36. Young MJ, Marshall A, Adams JE, et al: Osteopenia, neurological dysfunction, and the development of Charcot neuroarthropathy. Diabetes Care 18:34–38, 1995.
37. Slowman-Kovacs SD, Braunstein EM, Brandt KD: Rapidly progressive Charcot arthropathy following minor joint trauma in patients with diabetic neuropathy. Arthritis Rheum 33:412–417, 1990.
38. Davis PF, Severud E, Baxter DE: Painful heel syndrome: Results of nonoperative treatment. Foot Ankle Int 15:531–535, 1994.
39. Cailliet R: Painful conditions of the heel. In: Foot and Ankle Pain, 2nd ed. Philadelphia, FA Davis, 1983, pp 139–147.
40. Bartolomei FJ: Pedal radiographic manifestations of the seronegative spondyloarthritides: Part III. Ankylosing spondylitis. J Am Podiatr Med Assoc 76:380–385, 1986.
41. Bartolomei FJ: Pedal radiographic manifestations of the seronegative spondyloarthritides: Part II. Psoriatic arthritis. J Am Podiatr Med Assoc 76:266–274, 1986.
42. Bartolomei FJ: Pedal radiographic manifestations of the seronegative spondyloarthritides: Part I. Reiter's syndrome. J Am Podiatr Med Assoc 76:189–198, 1986.
43. Sebes JI: The significance of calcaneal spurs in rheumatic diseases. Arthritis Rheum 32:338–340, 1989.
44. Reilly PA, Evison G, McHugh NJ, et al: Arthropathy of the hands and feet in systemic lupus erythematosus. J Rheumatol 17:777–784, 1990.
45. Kirkup J: Rheumatoid arthritis and ankle surgery. Ann Rheum Dis 49:837–844, 1990.

CHAPTER 32

The Eye and Rheumatic Diseases

Robert S. Weinberg

Ocular involvement in rheumatic disease is common; it may be either the initial presentation of the systemic disease or a later problem for a patient with an already diagnosed rheumatic disease. Ocular findings may be similar in a variety of diseases, and a thorough history can be important in linking the ocular finding with the systemic disease. In some cases, therapy for the systemic illness is likely to improve the ocular problem; in other patients, management of the ophthalmic condition may require additional medication. Although ocular involvement may vary in extent and severity, three problems appear to occur with high frequency in patients with rheumatic disease: tear dysfunction, uveitis, and scleritis. Table 32–1 indicates the disease entities most commonly associated with specific ocular findings.

TEAR DYSFUNCTION

Keratoconjunctivitis sicca, or "dry eye syndrome," is common and may be seen in otherwise healthy individuals. Because a normal tear film is essential for both good vision and ocular comfort, symptoms of tear deficiency may vary greatly, from complaints of blurred vision to those of ocular burning or itching to foreign body sensation and redness. Some patients may complain of constant ocular discomfort; more commonly, however, ocular discomfort increases as the day progresses. Awareness by the rheumatologist of the spectrum of problems caused by inadequacies in the tear film can help facilitate better patient management.

The tear film consists of three layers: the *mucin* layer, produced by conjunctival goblet cells; the *aqueous* layer, produced by the lacrimal gland and accessory lacrimal glands; and the *lipid* layer, produced mainly by the meibomian glands in the lids. Symptoms may occur because of abnormalities in any of the layers. The term tear dysfunction applies to problems with the tear film in general. In patients with connective tissue disease, aqueous tear deficiency is the most common tear problem. These patients frequently have increased ocular symptomatology late in the day. Exposure to smoke, chemicals, or cold may increase symptoms. Occasionally, these patients have epiphora, or excessive tearing, a reflex in response to drying of the ocular surface. Many patients with aqueous tear deficiency have no associated systemic disease.

Aqueous tear production decreases with age and may decrease during pregnancy, with oral contraceptive use, and after menopause. Decreased aqueous tear production, therefore, may be seen in conditions in which estrogen levels may be elevated or depressed, suggesting the possibility that hormones other than estrogen may affect tear production.[1]

Dryness of the mouth and oropharynx consequent to salivary gland atrophy is a frequent associated finding. The combination of xerostomia and keratoconjunctivitis sicca is commonly referred to as the *sicca syndrome.*[2] When associated with rheumatoid arthritis or another connective tissue disorder, the triad is known as *Sjögren's syndrome* (see Chapter 58).

In Sjögren's syndrome, lymphocytic infiltration of the lacrimal gland increases, with helper T cells and IgG-secreting B lymphocytes. Secretory epithelial tissue atrophies and is replaced by fibrous connective tissue.[3] These changes in the lacrimal glands cause a decreased elaboration of the aqueous component of the tears. The tear film may become more viscous.

The eyes often appear slightly to moderately red and irritated (Fig. 32–1) (see Color Plate). On slit-lamp biomicroscopic examination, tiny, punctate gray opacities are seen that stain with fluorescein solution. This epithelial keratopathy is most prominent in the portion of the cornea located in the interpalpebral fissure. Because this area is not covered by the lids during most of the waking hours, it is particularly subject to drying.

Additional ophthalmic findings in keratoconjunctivitis sicca include mucus strands, filamentary keratitis, and rarely corneal ulceration. The conjunctival goblet cells are stimulated to secrete an overabundance of mucus. A common finding is the presence of rope-like strands of mucus on the cornea or on the surface of the conjunctiva, with the complaint of foreign body sensation. Foreign body sensation may also be caused by epithelial filaments, plaques of desquamated corneal epithelium that remain attached to the cornea in a condition known as filamentary keratitis. Infectious corneal ulcers resulting in corneal opacification and decreased visual acuity may occur in areas of corneal drying.

The diagnosis of keratoconjunctivitis can be made on the basis of a compatible history and slit-lamp

Table 32–1. OCULAR FINDINGS IN RHEUMATIC DISEASES

Disease	Tear Dysfunction	Uveitis	Scleritis	Other
Sjögren's syndrome	x			
Rheumatoid arthritis	x		x	
Juvenile rheumatoid arthritis		x		
Systemic lupus erythematosus	x		x	
Systemic sclerosis	x			
Mixed connective tissue disease	x		x	
Relapsing polychondritis	x		x	
Wegener's granulomatosis	x	x	x	Retinal vasculitis Keratitis
Polyarteritis nodosa	x		x	
Seronegative spondyloarthropathies		x	x	
Sarcoidosis	x	x		
Behçet's disease		x	x	
Lyme disease		x		Conjunctivitis

biomicroscopic findings. Testing to confirm the diagnosis can be extensive but is frequently not necessary. Tear film stability and integrity may be tested with a slit-lamp biomicroscope. The *Schirmer test* of tear secretion may be helpful in confirming a diagnosis of aqueous tear dysfunction or keratoconjunctivitis sicca. Although there are many variables, including the patient's age, wetting of 5 mm or less in 5 minutes is considered abnormal. Laboratory tests available to analyze the tear film include measurement of tear film osmolality, tear lysozyme, and tear lactoferrin. Tear lysozyme production and tear lactiferrin levels decrease with lacrimal gland destruction. Conjunctival impression cytology and lacrimal biopsy may provide tissue confirmation of the diagnosis.[4]

Treatment

Unfortunately, management of the underlying rheumatic disease usually does not affect the symptoms caused by tear deficiency. Therapeutic options for treating aqueous tear deficiency include tear replacement, lubrication, and tear preservation.

A large number of tear substitutes are available without prescription. These preparations vary in pH, viscosity, and the presence or absence of preservatives. Many patients who use artificial tears frequently experience ocular irritation as a result of preservatives present in the preparations. A commonly used regimen to determine whether tear substitutes will relieve a patient's symptoms is to begin tear supplementation every 2 hours while awake and then decrease the frequency to that which the patient finds is as comfortable as the every-2-hour regimen. Sustained-release hydroxyproplycellulose rods (Lacriserts) placed in the inferior conjunctival cul-de-sac can provide relief of symptoms for some patients, particularly if tear substitutes are also used. Bedtime application of an ocular ointment to the conjunctiva can be helpful for patients who have discomfort on awakening. Tear production decreases during sleep, and some patients are more comfortable using an ointment lubricant at bedtime. Tears leave the eye through the puncta, located in the nasal aspects of the upper and lower lids, and pass through the canaliculi into the nasolacrimal sac. Tear preservation with punctal occlusion, of one or both puncta in each eye, either temporarily or permanently, can decrease ocular symptoms in some patients who find no relief with the frequent use of tear substitutes or who cannot use tear substitutes frequently enough.

Because none of the regimens for treating the dry eye syndrome works in all patients, research into finding new therapies is ongoing. These investigations include the development of new artificial tear preparations, the use of epidermal growth factor to strengthen the ocular surface epithelium, and immunotherapy with topical cyclosporine and interferon-α.[5]

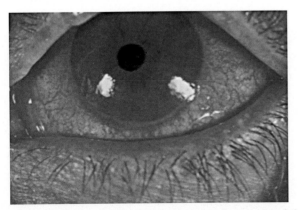

Figure 32–1. Keratoconjunctivitis sicca. Intense hyperemia of the conjunctival vessels accounts for the prominent redness. Dryness of the corneal epithelium causes the reflection from the photographic flash to be dull and irregular rather than normally sharp and highly polished. (See Color Plate.)

UVEITIS

The term uveitis means intraocular inflammation. Uveitis may be classified in various ways to more accurately describe the part of the eye that is involved or the severity of the intraocular inflammation. Four commonly used classifications are employed to describe uveitis, but a combination of all classifications is useful clinically:

1. The *temporal* classification relates to the time of onset, with *acute* uveitis being of less than 3 weeks' duration and *chronic* uveitis being of greater than 3 weeks duration.

2. An *etiologic* classification relates to causation, with the terms infectious, malignant, and autoimmune frequently used.

3. A *symptomatic* classification indicates a degree of severity, ranging from mild to severe uveitis.

4. An *anatomic* classification, utilizing clinical ophthalmologic examination to determine the part of the eye primarily or most severely involved, is perhaps the most useful. The uveitis then may be termed *anterior* or *posterior*, depending on whether the anterior segment of the eye or the posterior segment is involved. *Iritis* refers to a uveitis that is primarily anterior, with little or no inflammation in the vitreous cavity. *Iridocyclitis* indicates anterior chamber and anterior vitreous inflammation. *Retinitis* means uveitis that primarily affects the retina. *Choroiditis* signifies a uveitis that mainly affects the choroid. *Panuveitis* is involvement of all parts of the eye.

The uveitis associated with rheumatic diseases is most often anterior in the eye, and hence the term iritis or iridocyclitis usually applies. Patients with anterior uveitis usually complain of pain, redness, and photophobia. Patients with posterior uveitis, on the other hand, complain of blurred vision and floating spots. The primary exceptions in the uveitis associated with rheumatic disease are juvenile rheumatoid arthritis, sarcoidosis, and Behçet's disease. Patients with juvenile rheumatoid arthritis may be asymptomatic, yet have marked intraocular inflammation but no ocular redness. Because sarcoidosis and Behçet's disease can cause panuveitis, any portion of the eye may be involved; therefore, symptoms may vary widely.

Management of the uveitis associated with rheumatic diseases requires close cooperation between the rheumatologist and the ophthalmologist. Although therapy with topical corticosteroids is usually the mainstay of most uveitis therapy, intraocular inflammation may subside or may be more easily controllable in response to therapy directed toward the underlying systemic disease. Untreated uveitis may lead to permanent loss of vision. It must be emphasized to patients that cataract formation may be a result of untreated intraocular inflammation, or may be a side effect of appropriate therapy with corticosteroids. Fortunately, cataract extraction is extremely successful, even in patients with uveitis. However, the sequelae of untreated uveitis, namely secondary glaucoma and optic nerve damage, may not be as readily managed.

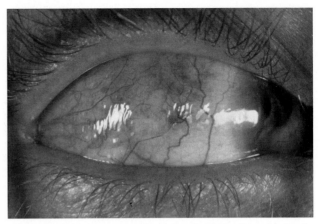

Figure 32–2. Episcleritis. Localized episcleral injection with overlying conjunctival injection adjacent to areas with no vascular congestion. (See Color Plate.)

SCLERITIS AND EPISCLERITIS

Anatomy

The sclera is composed of three layers—the episcleral tissue, the sclera proper, and the lamina fusca. The episclera is a loose structure of fibrous and elastic tissue continuous superficially with overlying Tenon's capsulae. The episclera merges with the sclera, but it has many small blood vessels, unlike the sclera, which is almost avascular. Episcleral vessels are not seen readily in the uninflamed eye but are easily seen when the eye is inflamed. The sclera itself consists of fibrous tissues, arranged in bundles of collagenous fibers and elastic fibers.

Episcleritis means inflammation of the episclera. Pain is usually not present, or it may be minimal. The presenting complaint is usually ocular redness (Fig. 32–2) (see Color Plate). Scleritis, inflammation of the sclera, is usually very painful, and the presenting complaint is most often ocular redness with severe pain in the eye or periorbita (Fig. 32–3) (see Color Plate). Although episcleritis may be seen in patients with rheumatic disease, most patients with episcleritis

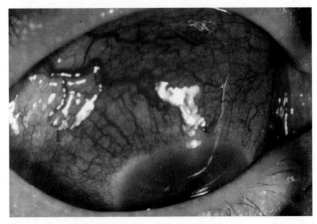

Figure 32–3. Diffuse scleritis. Diffuse scleritis in a patient with rheumatoid arthritis. There is intense vascular engorgement, overlying conjunctival injection, but no discharge. (See Color Plate.)

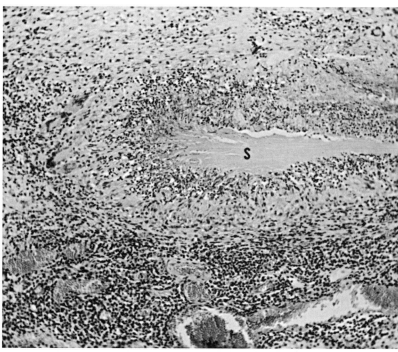

Figure 32–4. Granulomatous scleritis. In this field only a small island of necrotic sclera (S) remains. It is being attacked and surmounted by polymorphonuclear neutrophils and a mantle of epithelioid cells. Several well-developed giant cells are present at the left side of the field, directly opposite the scleral fragment. The granulomatous inflammatory reaction is surrounded, in turn, by an outpouring of inflammatory cells consisting chiefly of plasma cells and lymphocytes. These are seen best in the lower portion of the field. (Hematoxylin & eosin stain, ×115.) Armed Forces Institute of Pathology Negative No. 57–1163. (Courtesy of Lorenz E. Zimmerman, M.D.)

have no underlying connective tissue disease. Approximately 50 percent of patients with scleritis have a systemic connective tissue disease.[6]

Pathology

The characteristic histologic picture in rheumatoid scleritis is a zonal type of granulomatous inflammatory reaction (Fig. 32–4). A central area of necrotic scleral collagen is surrounded by a palisade of epithelioid cells and giant cells. These epithelioid and giant cells, in turn, are surrounded by a mantle of chronic inflammatory cells, chiefly plasma cells and lymphocytes, which often involve the overlying episclera and the underlying uvea. In eyes with scleromalacia perforans (Figs. 32–5 and 32–6) (see Color Plates), the nongranulomatous component of the inflammatory reaction is often inconspicuous. In simple episcleritis and in most cases of nodular episcleritis, the usual histologic changes consist of hyperemia, edema, and infiltration by lymphocytes and plasma cells. On pathologic examination, however, some rheumatoid episcleral nodules have exhibited all the features of subcutaneous rheumatoid nodules.

Treatment

Episcleritis is usually self-limited but does respond to topical corticosteroid therapy. Scleritis therapy re-

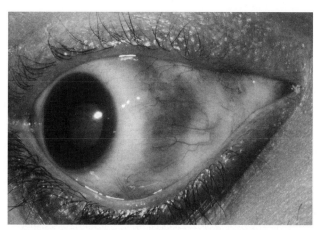

Figure 32–5. Scleromalacia. Therapy for scleritis can decrease scleral inflammation. Once active inflammation has decreased, the sclera may be thin and translucent, appearing bluish-gray. (See Color Plate.)

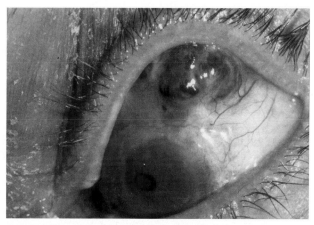

Figure 32–6. Scleromalacia perforans. Severe scleral thinning and translucency with bulging of underlying uveal tissue in a patient with severe rheumatoid arthritis. (See Color Plate.)

quires the use of systemic agents for relief of pain, preservation of vision, and prevention of ocular tissue destruction. A team approach between the ophthalmologist and the rheumatologist is frequently required to provide the ideal therapeutic milieu. Therapy for scleritis usually begins with the use of systemic nonsteroidal anti-inflammatory agents. If these do not relieve pain, targeting the first symptom to respond to appropriate therapy, systemic corticosteroids, often in high doses, is the next line of approach. In steroid-unresponsive patients or in such patients as those with insulin-dependent diabetes, for whom high doses of systemic corticosteroid may be dangerous, antimetabolites and alkylating compounds may provide good results. The most effective of these drugs, cyclophosphamide, may be required for prolonged periods to quiet severe scleral inflammation.

RHEUMATOID ARTHRITIS

In patients with rheumatoid arthritis, estimates of the incidence of scleritis vary from 0.15 to 6.3 percent.[7] In a retrospective study of patients with scleritis and episcleritis, the mean age of patients with rheumatoid scleritis and rheumatoid episcleritis was in the sixth decade. In patients with rheumatoid scleritis, both eyes were involved in 25 of 37 cases (68 percent).[8] In rheumatoid arthritis, scleritis and episcleritis generally occur in patients whose arthritis is of longer duration than that of rheumatoid control patients. These patients usually have more widespread systemic disease, particularly of the cardiovascular and respiratory systems, and have radiologic evidence of more advanced joint disease than do rheumatoid control patients. Subcutaneous granulomatous nodules and atrophy of the skin are more common in patients with rheumatoid scleritis and episcleritis compared with rheumatoid control patients.[8]

JUVENILE RHEUMATOID ARTHRITIS

Juvenile rheumatoid arthritis differs from the adult form in terms of its ocular involvement. In juvenile rheumatoid arthritis, the triad of ocular lesions consists of anterior uveitis, band keratopathy, and secondary cataract. In adults with rheumatoid arthritis, uveitis occurs no more often than it does in the general population. Scleritis is rarely, if ever, seen in patients with juvenile rheumatoid arthritis. Tear dysfunction, too, is unusual in juvenile rheumatoid arthritis.

Risk factors for the development of uveitis are young age, female sex, antinuclear antibody positivity, rheumatoid factor seronegativity, and pauciarticular onset. The uveitis usually involves the anterior segment of the eye and is therefore an iritis or iridocy-

clitis. Iridocyclitis occurred in 36 of 210 patients (17 percent) with juvenile rheumatoid arthritis in one retrospective study.[9] Children with Still's disease do not generally develop uveitis.[6]

Band keratopathy is not pathognomonic of juvenile rheumatoid arthritis. It occurs in a variety of other disorders and results from deposition of calcium in Bowman's layer of the cornea, beginning at the nasal and temporal limbus and extending centrally (Fig. 32–7). Cataract is frequently present, with incidences ranging from 22 to 46 percent in various retrospective studies.[10, 11] Management of these two problems may necessitate surgical intervention. Calcific band keratopathy may require chelation of the calcium with edetate disodium. Cataract extraction may be done successfully, especially if surgery is delayed until ocular inflammation is minimized.

SYSTEMIC LUPUS ERYTHEMATOSUS

Ocular involvement in systemic lupus erythematosus most commonly occurs as cotton-wool patches in the retina. Tear dysfunction frequently develops, and patients may also have scleral disease, similar to that seen in other forms of connective tissue disease. The cotton-wool spots seen in lupus (Fig. 32–8) are grayish-white, soft, fluffy exudates, usually near retinal arterioles, and occurring in the inner layers of the retina. Cotton-wool spots are small, usually about one third of a disc in diameter, and are most frequently located in the posterior part of the retina; they can also occur in other conditions, such as anemia, connective tissue diseases, hypertension, dysproteinemia, and leukemia.[12]

Pathologic examination of cotton-wool spots shows disciform thickening of the retinal nerve fiber layer. In this region, some of the nerve fibers have been interrupted, leading to formation of cytoid bodies. These are globular structures, 10 to 20 μm, and resemble a cell. Cotton-wool spots are an ophthalmologic

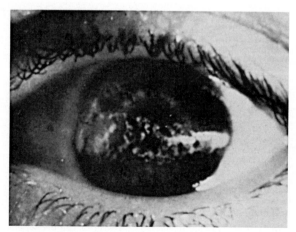

Figure 32–7. Band keratopathy in a 12-year-old girl with severe juvenile rheumatoid arthritis.

feature, whereas a cytoid body is a histologic feature of a cotton-wool spot.[12]

Inner retinal layer hemorrhages are also seen in the retinopathy associated with systemic lupus erythematosus. They do not necessarily signify the presence of systemic hypertension, but like the cotton-wool spots, they are a manifestation of vasculitis.

RELAPSING POLYCHONDRITIS

Ocular involvement in relapsing polychondritis can include keratitis and retinal vasculitis, but scleritis is the most frequent ocular presentation. A retrospective study of 11 patients showed that immunosuppressants, such as azathioprine and cyclophosphamide, were more effective than systemic corticosteroids alone or in combination with dapsone in controlling inflammation.[13]

WEGENER'S GRANULOMATOSIS

Ocular involvement may be the initial presenting complaint in a patient with Wegener's granulomatosis, occurring in up to 50 percent of patients.[6] Proptosis, secondary to retrobulbar granulomatous inflammation, can present acutely and bilaterally[14] and was present in 18 percent of reported cases. Other reported ocular findings include conjunctivitis, episcleritis, scleritis, keratitis, retinal vasculitis, and uveitis. In some patients, ring ulcers of the cornea are the initial sign of Wegener's granulomatosis (Fig. 32–9) (see Color Plate). Serum antineutrophil cytoplasmic antibodies (ANCAs) have been shown to be sensitive and specific for the scleritis seen in Wegener's granulomatosis.[15, 16]

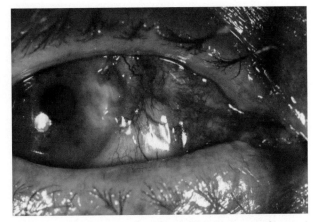

Figure 32–9. Scleritis and keratitis in Wegener's granulomatosis. Localized keratitis at the limbus, adjacent to an area of localized scleritis in Wegener's granulomatosis. The corneal thinning is approximately 90 percent with a high risk of corneal perforation. (See Color Plate.)

POLYARTERITIS NODOSA

Ocular involvement is uncommon in polyarteritis nodosa. However, tear dysfunction, scleritis, and choroidal angiitis have been reported, with retinal and choroidal vasculitis the most common problems.[6, 16]

SARCOIDOSIS

Sarcoidosis may affect any part of the eye or ocular adnexa. Ocular involvement may be the presenting problem in 7 percent of patients with sarcoidosis, but is usually seen in approximately 50 percent of patients with the disease. Uveitis is the most common form of intraocular involvement in sarcoidosis. The uveitis may be difficult to classify because sarcoid uveitis may be acute or chronic; anterior, posterior, or diffuse; and bilateral or unilateral. Retinal perivasculitis, with inflammation especially in the midperipheral fundus, accounts for the ophthalmoscopic picture known as "candle wax drippings." Conjunctival nodules, scleritis, and lacrimal gland involvement all have been present in a patient with sarcoid ocular disease (Fig. 32–10). The lacrimal gland and conjunctiva are readily available for biopsy. At the Medical College of Virginia, lacrimal gland biopsies were performed on 60 patients who had uveitis, compatible with a diagnosis of sarcoidosis. Thirty-three percent of the biopsy specimens contained noncaseating, epithelioid tubercles, affording a tissue diagnosis of sarcoidosis. In the same study, 11 of 50 other patients (22 percent) who did not have uveitis but who had been referred for lacrimal gland biopsy because of systemic or roentgenographic findings suggestive of sarcoidosis had abnormal biopsy findings.

Biopsy of the conjunctiva or lacrimal gland may be safer and less expensive than other invasive procedures, such as biopsy of a scalene lymph node, medi-

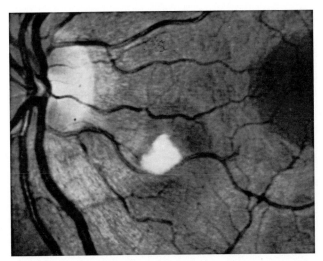

Figure 32–8. A typical cotton wool spot in a young woman with systemic lupus erythematosus. The lesion is situated along the upper border of a retinal arteriole, about midway between the optic nerve head and the macula.

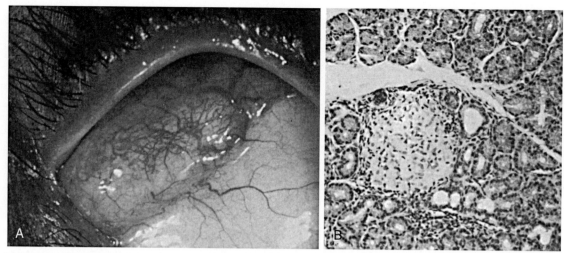

Figure 32–10. Sarcoidosis of the lacrimal gland. *A,* The right upper lid is partially everted for photographic purposes, and the patient is directing her gaze inferonasally. The palpebral lobe of the lacrimal gland is moderately to markedly enlarged. *B,* Biopsy of the lacrimal gland revealed many discrete, noncaseating epithelioid cell tubercles of the type seen near the center of the field. (Hematoxylin & eosin stain, ×150.)

astinoscopy, or transbronchial biopsy of the lung. Biopsy of the conjunctiva or lacrimal gland may be done using only topical anesthesia at the slit-lamp biomicroscope, and no sutures are required. A second biopsy procedure may easily be done. If tissue confirmation is required to confirm a clinical diagnosis of sarcoidosis, conjunctival or lacrimal gland biopsy may be performed prior to other more invasive procedures and may obviate the need for additional diagnostic procedures.

SERONEGATIVE SPONDYLOARTHROPATHIES

Ankylosing spondylitis, psoriatic arthritis, Reiter's disease, and inflammatory bowel disease have common ocular presentations. Acute anterior uveitis is the most frequent ocular manifestation in these seronegative spondyloarthropathies. Patients characteristically present with the sudden onset of pain, redness, and photophobia, usually in one eye. Scleritis and episcleritis may also be seen but are less common. Because the uveitis may be severe, systemic or periocular corticosteroids may be required in addition to topical corticosteroids. As in other entities in which scleral inflammation is seen, systemic therapy is necessary for management.

LYME DISEASE

Although conjunctivitis may be the most frequent ocular finding in patients with Lyme disease, episcleritis, keratitis, iritis, choroiditis, retinal edema, papilledema, and pseudotumor cerebri have all been reported. Ocular findings, fortunately, are rare.[17, 18] The conjunctivitis may be transient, occurring in stage I. Uveitis occurs in stage II. Topical corticosteroid ther-

apy is effective in treating the conjunctivitis and anterior uveitis, but systemic therapy with appropriate antibiotics is also required.[19]

BEHÇET'S DISEASE

Ocular Behçet's disease most commonly manifests as recurrent, acute, severe iridocyclitis. Panuveitis with vitreous cellular reaction and retinal vasculitis with retinal ischemia may result in profound visual loss in patients with Behçet's disease (Fig. 32–11) (see Color Plate). Therapy for the intraocular inflammation may require systemic corticosteroids, cytotoxic agents, colchicine, or cyclosporine.[20]

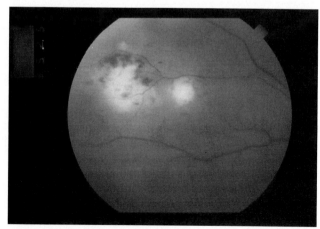

Figure 32–11. Retinal ischemia in Behçet's disease. Areas of white retinal ischemia in the mid-periphery of the retina in a patient with Behçet's disease. Ischemic areas are partially surrounded by retinal hemorrhages. (See Color Plate.)

References

1. Warren DW: Hormonal influences on the lacrimal gland. Int Ophthalmol Clin 34:19–25, 1994.
2. Farris RL: Sjögren's syndrome. *In* Gold DH, Weingeist TA (eds): The Eye in Systemic Disease. Philadelphia, JB Lippincott, 1990, pp 70–71.
3. Micheff AK, Glerow JP, Wood RL: Autoimmunity of the lacrimal gland. Int Ophthalmol Clin 34:1–18, 1994.
4. Nelson JD: Diagnosis of keratoconjunctivitis sicca. Int Ophthalmol Clin 34:37–56, 1994.
5. Tsubota K: New approaches to dry-eye therapy. Int Ophthalmol Clin 34:115–129, 1994.
6. Hakin KN, Watson PG: Systemic associations of scleritis. Int Ophthalmol Clin 31:111–130, 1991.
7. Watson PG, Hazleman BL: The Sclera and Systemic Disorders. London, WB Saunders Company, Ltd, 1976, p 220.
8. McGavin DD, Williamson J, Forrester JV, Foulds WS, Buchanan WW, Dick WC, Lee P, Macsween RN, Whaley K: Episcleritis and scleritis: A study of their clinical manifestations and association with rheumatoid arthritis. Br J Ophthalmol 60:192, 1976.
9. Chylack LT, Bienfang DC, Bellows AR, Stillman JS: Ocular manifestations of juvenile rheumatoid arthritis. Am J Ophthalmol 79:1026, 1975.
10. Kanski JJ: Anterior uveitis in juvenile rheumatoid arthritis. Arch Ophthalmol 95:1794, 1977.
11. Wolf MD, Lichter HR, Ragsdale CG: Prognostic factors in the uveitis of juvenile rheumatoid arthritis. Ophthalmology 94:1242, 1987.
12. Ferry AP: Retinal cotton wool spots and cytoid bodies. Mt Sinai J Med 39:604, 1972.
13. Hoang-Xuan T, Foster CS, Rice BA: Scleritis in relapsing polychondritis. Ophthalmology 97:892–898, 1990.
14. Haynes BF, Fishman ML, Fauci AS, Wolff SM: The ocular manifestations of Wegener's granulomatosis: Fifteen years experience and review of the literature. Am J Med 63:131, 1977.
15. Soukiasian SH, Foster CS, Niles JL, Raizman MB: Diagnostic value of antineutrophil cytoplasmic antibodies in scleritis associated with Wegener's granulomatosis. Ophthalmology 99:125–132, 1992.
16. Pulido JS, Goeken JA, Nerad JA, Sobol WM, Folberg R: Ocular manifestations of patients with circulating antineutrophil cytoplasmic antibodies. Arch Ophthalmol 108:845–850, 1990.
17. Flach AJ, Lavoie PE: Episcleritis, conjunctivitis, and keratitis as ocular manifestations of Lyme disease. Ophthalmology 97:973, 1990.
18. Karma A, Seppala I, Mikkila H, Kaakkola S, Viljanen M, Tarkkanen H: Diagnosis and clinical characteristics of ocular Lyme borreliosis. Am J Ophthalmol 119:127–135, 1995.
19. Winterkorn JMS: Lyme disease: Neurologic and ophthalmic manifestations. Surv Ophthalmol 35:191–204, 1990.
20. Weinberg RS: Selected inflammatory diseases of the skin and eye. Ophthalmol Clin North Am 5:215–226, 1992.

CHAPTER 33

Nicholas A. Soter
Andrew G. Franks, Jr.

Cutaneous Manifestations of Rheumatic Diseases

The presence of skin lesions is especially noteworthy in patients with rheumatic diseases. Thus, the integument should be assessed with the same precision that is devoted to an examination of the joints and musculoskeletal system.

RHEUMATOID ARTHRITIS

The most frequently recognized cutaneous lesion in patients with rheumatoid arthritis is the *rheumatoid nodule*. This lesion occurs over areas subjected to trauma or pressure, especially the ulnar aspect of the forearm and the lumbosacral area. Rheumatoid nodules vary in size, are firm in consistency, may be movable or fixed to underlying structures, and may ulcerate after trauma. They occur in approximately 20 percent of patients with rheumatoid arthritis, especially in individuals with severe forms of the disease and rheumatoid factor.

The skin is often pale, translucent, and atrophic, especially over the fingers and toes. The swelling of the proximal interphalangeal joints with atrophic skin may mimic the appearance of sclerodactyly. Palmar erythema is a frequent feature. Some patients manifest telangiectases of the nail folds. Raynaud's phenomenon may occur as a blue coloration over the distal portions of the fingers and toes. Occasionally, erythematous papules and plaques are present on the extremities that histologically contain neutrophilic infiltrates without vasculitis.[1] Pyoderma gangrenosum may occur in individuals with severe rheumatoid arthritis.

Vasculitis in patients with rheumatoid arthritis appears as a variety of syndromes.[2] Frequently involved are the small arteries, such as the vasa nervorum and the digital arteries, and the cutaneous features include digital gangrene and nail fold infarcts. Patients with nodular and erosive disease and high titers of rheumatoid factor are particularly susceptible to arteritis. Occasional patients experience involvement of the medium rather than the small arteries. The nodular lesions in these instances resemble those of polyarteritis nodosa.

A common form of necrotizing vasculitis in the skin of patients with rheumatoid arthritis involves the venules and is recognized as purpuric papules. The venular lesions are associated with severe articular disease, which is generally but not invariably seropositive. Arteritic, arteriolar, and venular lesions may coexist in the same patient.

SJÖGREN'S SYNDROME

The dermatologic manifestations in patients with Sjögren's syndrome either reflect glandular dysfunction with desiccation of the skin and mucous membranes or represent involvement of blood vessels. Dry skin *(xerosis)* is present in approximately 50 percent of these individuals. The mucous membranes of the eyes, oral cavity, and vagina usually are involved in the sicca complex. A burning sensation of the eyes may occur with erythema, pruritus, decreased ability to form tears, and the accumulation of inspissated, rope-like material at the inner canthus. The oral cavity and tongue may be red and dry with oral erosions and decreased amounts of saliva. Scale of the lips and fissures at the angles of the mouth may be noted; the teeth readily decay. Vaginal involvement results in burning, pruritus, and dyspareunia. Enlargement of parotid and accessory salivary glands is frequently noted. Raynaud's phenomenon may be present.

Necrotizing vasculitis of venules occurs in patients with Sjögren's syndrome and appears as episodes of either palpable purpura or urticaria. The venular lesions are present over the lower extremities, appear after exercise, and are associated with hyperpigmentation and cutaneous ulcers. Anti-Ro (SS-A) antibodies are noted in the majority of individuals with primary Sjögren's syndrome, especially when it is associated with systemic or cutaneous necrotizing vasculitis.[3] Because Sjogren's syndrome occurs in association with other conditions, such as hypergammaglobulinemic purpura, systemic lupus erythematosus, scleroderma, biliary cirrhosis, and lymphoproliferative disorders, the dermatologic features may reflect the presence of the coexistent disorder.

REITER'S SYNDROME

Reiter's syndrome, which occurs primarily in men, consists of a tetrad of features that include conjunctivitis, urethritis, arthritis, and skin lesions. Postdysenteric forms of Reiter's syndrome often are not diagnosed, owing to the lack of the classic tetrad of features. An association between infection with human immunodeficiency virus (HIV) and Reiter's syndrome has been noted.[4]

The conjunctivitis and urethritis tend to be transient in contrast to the more persistent arthritis and skin manifestations. Approximately 50 to 80 percent of patients experience mucocutaneous alterations with involvement of the acral regions, especially the soles, toes, and fingers. The most characteristic skin lesions, which are rare, begin as vesicles on erythematous bases, become sterile pustules, and evolve to manifest keratotic scale; these are known as *keratoderma blennorrhagica* (Fig. 33–1) (see Color Plate). In addition, keratotic papules and plaques, which are reminiscent of psoriasis, occur on the scalp and elsewhere on the skin. Indeed, there have been patients reported with both Reiter's syndrome and psoriasis, yet the skin lesions in these two disorders are often difficult or impossible to distinguish clinically and histologically. Sterile pustules may develop beneath the nail plate; onychodystrophy frequently is noted.

Conjunctivitis, which occurs in 50 percent of patients, is usually bilateral. Balanitis occurs in 25 percent of individuals and appears as papules and plaques with scale over the glans penis. Mouth erosions have been noted.

PSORIATIC ARTHRITIS

Psoriasis appears as erythematous papules and plaques with layers of silver-white scale that are sharply demarcated from adjacent uninvolved skin. Individual lesions may heal with transient hyperpigmentation or hypopigmentation.

Psoriasis occurs in two distinct forms; one form is

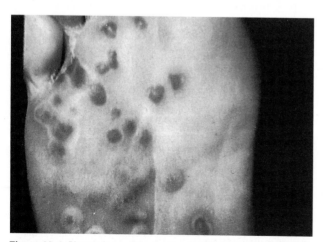

Figure 33–1. Keratoderma blennorrhagica. Vesicles and pustules of the sole in a patient with Reiter's syndrome. (From Soter NA, Franks AG Jr: Cutaneous manifestations of rheumatic diseases: An update. *In* Kelley WN, et al: Textbook of Rheumatology, 4th ed. Philadelphia, WB Saunders. Update No. 15, pp 1–24, 1995.) (See Color Plate.)

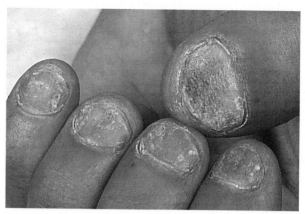

Figure 33–2. Psoriasis. Onychodystrophy of the nail plate with pits. (From Soter NA, Franks AG Jr: Cutaneous manifestations of rheumatic diseases: An update. *In* Kelley WN, et al: Textbook of Rheumatology, 4th ed. Philadelphia, WB Saunders. Update No. 15, pp 1–24, 1995.)

hereditary, with an onset in the second and third decades, and the other is sporadic, with an onset in the sixth decade.[5] Psoriasis may occur over any portion of the integument, especially the scalp, elbows, knees, lumbosacral area, gluteal cleft, and glans penis. The oral mucosa and tongue are infrequently involved. Considerable numbers of small, drop-like plaques, designated as *guttate psoriasis*, may occur after infections.[6] At times, fissures and scale of the distal portions of the fingers may be a prominent manifestation. The skin lesions often appear at sites of trauma (*Koebner reaction* or *isomorphic phenomenon*). Although the stimulus is usually mechanical, excess exposure to sunlight and allergic reactions to the administration of drugs have been implicated.

The nails are frequently affected; the extent of involvement varies in severity and may include one or several nails. The nail plate manifests a translucent quality with a yellow or brown coloration. There may be subungual accumulations of keratotic material, which frequently contains *Candida* or *Pseudomonas* species; however, dermatophyte infections are rare. The most widely recognized alteration of the nail plate is the presence of discrete pits (Fig. 33–2).

Generalized erythroderma or exfoliative dermatitis may develop spontaneously or occur after systemic illness, the administration of medications, or prolonged exposure to the sun.

Pustular types of psoriasis are uncommon; they may occur in a generalized form or in a form localized to the palms and soles.

In patients with *generalized* pustular psoriasis (Fig. 33–3), the onset is sudden with pyrexia, myalgia, and arthralgia. The skin lesions consist of superficial pustules that may evolve into larger purulent areas; existing psoriatic plaques may also contain sterile pustules. The episodes of pustules may continue to appear over intervals of days to weeks. It has been suggested that patients with psoriatic arthritis are

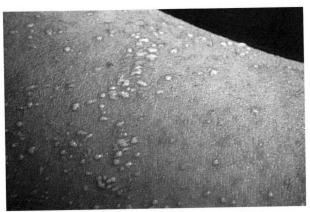

Figure 33–3. Psoriasis. Generalized pustules. (From Soter NA, Franks AG Jr: Cutaneous manifestations of rheumatic diseases: An update. *In* Kelley WN, et al: Textbook of Rheumatology, 4th ed. Philadelphia, WB Saunders. Update No. 15, pp 1–24, 1995.)

more susceptible to generalized pustular psoriasis than are patients without arthritis.

Localized pustular psoriasis of the palms and soles is bilateral and recalcitrant without systemic manifestations. Onychodystrophy is common, and the plaques of ordinary psoriasis may be found elsewhere on the body.

There are increased numbers of *Staphylococcus aureus* organisms on the lesional skin of patients with psoriasis. Scale has been suggested as a source of hospital infection. Surgical intervention through psoriatic plaques, such as in prosthetic joint replacement, also has been associated with increased risk of local infection.[7]

Psoriasis may occur in association with various forms of inflammatory arthritis,[8] including asymmetric oligoarthritis, symmetric arthritis, spondyloarthritis, and arthritis mutilans. The presence of psoriasis in patients with rheumatoid arthritis is considered to be the coincidental association of two common disorders. Onychodystrophy in patients with symmetric psoriatic arthritis may help to differentiate them from patients with rheumatoid arthritis.

Psoriasis has been reported in individuals with acquired immunodeficiency syndrome (AIDS).[9]

RELAPSING POLYCHONDRITIS

The manifestations of relapsing polychondritis include auricular chondritis, nasal chondritis, and arthritis. The chondritis is characterized by the sudden onset of redness, swelling, and tenderness, which are limited to the cartilaginous portions of the affected sites, and by resolution in 1 to 2 weeks. There may be reoccurrences over weeks to months. This inflammatory process results in floppy ears and nasal deformities. Less frequent skin manifestations include urticaria, angioedema, palpable purpura, livedo reticularis, and panniculitis.

An association of spondyloarthritis with polychondritis has been reported in three patients. Other features of the disease include uveitis, optic neuritis, and aortic insufficiency.[10]

LUPUS ERYTHEMATOSUS

Lupus erythematosus may occur as a systemic disease or as a disorder in which the lesions are restricted to the skin. The term *discoid lupus erythematosus* has been used to refer to disease restricted to the skin as well as to the gross appearance of the atrophic skin lesions, irrespective of whether systemic disease is present. The term *subacute cutaneous lupus erythematosus* defines a systemic form with symmetric, nonscarring skin lesions.[11] When lupus erythematosus initially is restricted to the skin, particularly involving only the head and neck, available data suggest that these individuals are at low risk for the development of systemic disease. However, widespread cutaneous involvement is more likely to be associated with extracutaneous manifestations.

At some time during the course of disease, the skin is involved in approximately 80 percent of patients with lupus erythematosus. The most widely recognized manifestation is an erythematous eruption (butterfly rash) over the malar areas of the face, which occurs in patients with systemic lupus erythematosus (SLE) (Fig. 33–4). Rarely, bullous skin lesions (Fig. 33–5) (see Color Plate) that contain infiltrates of neutrophils occur in the superficial dermis.[12]

The discoid skin lesions in patients with lupus erythematosus are identified by their characteristic PASTE features (follicular *p*lugs, *a*trophy, *s*cale, *t*elangiectases, and *e*rythema). The pigmentary alterations are especially prominent in black patients, in whom the cosmetic alterations may be disfiguring. The cutaneous lesions are usually multiple and occur over any portion of the body; however, the nasolabial folds usually are spared. In some individuals, there is a predilection for sun-exposed areas. The skin lesions are usually asymptomatic, but pruritus may occur.

The skin lesions in subacute cutaneous lupus erythematosus are symmetric and predominantly affect the neck, the extensor surfaces of the arms, and the upper portions of the trunk. The cutaneous lesions may resemble psoriasis or may appear as annular and polycyclic configurations.[11] Although subacute SLE originally was thought to be associated with mild systemic features, one study suggests that the prevalence of severe systemic disease in subacute cutaneous lupus erythematosus may be similar to that in SLE.[13] There is an association with HLA-B8 and DR3 as well as anti-Ro and anti-La antibodies.

A variant of cutaneous lupus erythematosus, called *tumid* lupus erythematosus (Fig. 33–6) (see Color Plate), is present as erythematosus, indurated papules, plaques, and nodules without surface changes.[14] Systemic features are absent. *Hypertrophic* lupus erythematosus is a rare variant.

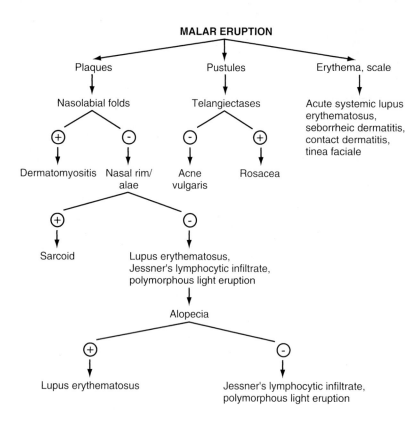

MALAR ERUPTION

Plaques → Nasolabial folds
- (+) → Dermatomyositis
- (−) → Nasal rim/alae
  - (+) → Sarcoid
  - (−) → Lupus erythematosus, Jessner's lymphocytic infiltrate, polymorphous light eruption → Alopecia
    - (+) → Lupus erythematosus
    - (−) → Jessner's lymphocytic infiltrate, polymorphous light eruption

Pustules → Telangiectases
- (−) → Acne vulgaris
- (+) → Rosacea

Erythema, scale → Acute systemic lupus erythematosus, seborrheic dermatitis, contact dermatitis, tinea faciale

Figure 33–4. Clinical algorithm for distinguishing diagnosis of a malar eruption must be confirmed by appropriate cultures, serology, and/or biopsy.

Alopecia is common in patients with lupus erythematosus; it occurs in both scarring and non-scarring forms. Recession of the frontal hairline, progressing to diffuse hair loss without scars, may occur, especially in people with subacute cutaneous lupus erythematosus or with SLE.

Although telangiectases tend to develop over the nail folds in many patients with subacute or systemic forms of lupus erythematosus, this sign also occurs in patients with rheumatoid arthritis, dermatomyositis, and scleroderma. Whereas these telangiectases usually are linear in patients with SLE and rheuma-

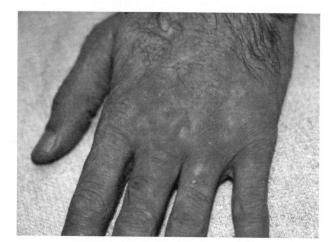

Figure 33–5. Systemic lupus erythematosus. Note bulla over the dorsum of the hand. (From Soter NA, Franks AG Jr: Cutaneous manifestations of rheumatic diseases: An update. *In* Kelley WN, et al: Textbook of Rheumatology, 4th ed. Philadelphia, WB Saunders. Update No. 15, pp 1–24, 1995.) (See Color Plate.)

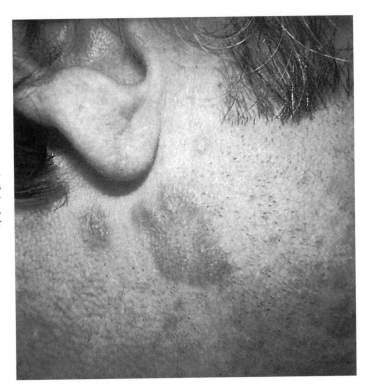

Figure 33–6. Tumid lupus erythematosus. Erythematous, indurated plaques. (From Soter NA, Franks AG Jr: Cutaneous manifestations of rheumatic diseases: An update. *In* Kelley WN, et al: Textbook of Rheumatology, 4th ed. Philadelphia, WB Saunders. Update No. 15, pp 1–24, 1995.) (See Color Plate.)

toid arthritis, polygonal mats with areas of vascular dropout develop in patients with dermatomyositis and scleroderma.

Necrotizing vasculitis of venules may occur during exacerbations of systemic disease and may appear as either palpable purpura or urticaria.[15] Involvement of larger arterial blood vessels may be present as peripheral gangrene. In addition, flat purpura and petechiae may occur as manifestations of thrombocytopenia or of the administration of corticosteroid preparations. Raynaud's phenomenon is reported to occur in 10 to 30 percent. Livedo reticularis may be present as a reticulate, erythematous mottling of the skin.

Photosensitivity occurs in at least one third of patients with SLE and may be associated with flares of both the cutaneous and the systemic manifestations of the disease.

The oral and lingual lesions are more common in patients with SLE and consist of erythematous patches, dilated blood vessels, and erosions, which are frequently painful. Ulcers of the nasal septum and palate may occur.

A rare skin manifestation is panniculitis (lupus profundus),[16] which appears as firm, deep nodules that have a predilection for the face, upper arms, and buttocks. The overlying skin may be normal, erythematous, atrophic, or ulcerated. Healing results in a depressed scar.

Alterations in the integument are prominent features that aid in the classification of patients with SLE. Noteworthy features include the presence of an erythematous macular eruption, atrophic plaques with follicular plugs, photosensitivity, and oral or nasopharyngeal ulcers. Alopecia and Raynaud's phenomenon are excluded, owing to their lack of specificity and sensitivity as discriminating factors.

Direct immunofluorescence techniques have been applied to the study of the skin of patients with lupus erythematosus as an aid in diagnosis and prognosis.[17] This procedure is known as the *lupus band test* (Fig. 33–7). In the skin lesions of both systemic and cutaneous lupus erythematosus, immunoglobulins and complement proteins are deposited in a granular pattern along the dermoepidermal junction in 90 to 95 percent of patients, whereas these immunoreactants are detected in uninvolved non–sun-exposed skin of approximately 50 percent of patients with systemic but not cutaneous lupus erythematosus—an important distinguishing feature. When uninvolved sun-exposed skin is examined, the lupus band test is usually negative in those with the cutaneous form but is positive in about 80 percent of those with the systemic form.

The types of immunoglobulin (Ig) detected in the deposited materials include mainly IgG and IgM. Complement proteins from both the classical activation and the amplification pathways are deposited at the same site, notably Clq, C4, C3, properdin, and B as well as those of the terminal membrane attack complex (MAC), C5b-C9.

It has been suggested that the deposition of immunoreactants in uninvolved non–sun-exposed skin of patients with SLE can be correlated with renal dis-

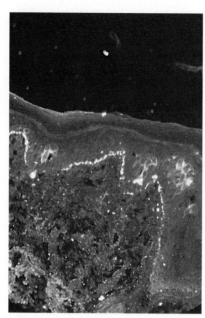

Figure 33–7. Positive lupus band test. Note granular deposits of immunoglobulin G (IgG) along the basement membrane zone. Vascular staining is also present. (×25.) (Courtesy of Dr. Jean-Claude Bystryn.)

ease.[18] In a longitudinal analysis of 10 years' duration that attempted to assess the relation between the deposition of cutaneous immunoreactants and renal disease in SLE, an initial positive lupus band test identified patients with renal disease and a decreased survival.[19] Also, it appears that the specificity and predictive value of the lupus band test depend, at least in part, on the nature and number of the immunoreactants detected at the dermal-epidermal junction.

MIXED CONNECTIVE TISSUE DISEASE

Mixed connective tissue disease is a disorder with clinical features of SLE, scleroderma, and/or polymyositis in association with circulating antibody to a soluble ribonuclear protein (nRNP). The inflammation and swelling of the fingers and hands, which leads to sausage-shaped digits and progresses to sclerodactyly, is characteristic, as is the associated Raynaud's phenomenon with periungual suffusion. There may be dilated and tortuous corkscrew periungual telangiectases with alternating avascular areas or dropout. The cutaneous features suggest discoid and subacute cutaneous disease in half of the reported cases. Hair loss may be gradual but leads to non-scarring alopecia. Pigmentary disturbances with hyperpigmentation and hypopigmentation, similar to those observed in scleroderma, often are noted. Truncal scleroderma is rare and should provoke a search for systemic sclerosis. Cutaneous vasculitis presents as livedoid vasculitis, palpable purpura, tender nodules along blood

vessels, and ulcers. Mucous membrane erosions of the lips, tongue, and buccal area may be observed. Prominent polygonal telangiectases may be found on the face along with swelling of the eyelids; these changes sometimes suggest the heliotrope alteration of dermatomyositis. Calcinosis cutis and subcutaneous nodules are less severe than are those associated with dermatomyositis.[20] Patients with mixed connective tissue disease are considered to have a good prognosis with a low incidence of renal disease.

NECROTIZING VASCULITIDES

Necrotizing angiitis or *vasculitis* refers to disorders in which there is segmental inflammation with fibrinoid necrosis of the blood vessels. Clinical syndromes are based on criteria[21] that include the gross and histologic appearance of the vascular lesions, the caliber of the affected blood vessels, the frequency of involvement of specific organs, and the presence of hematologic, serologic, and immunologic abnormalities. Although all sizes of blood vessels may be affected, necrotizing vasculitis of the skin in most instances involves venules and has been called *cutaneous necrotizing venulitis* and *leukocytoclastic vasculitis*. The cutaneous vascular lesions may occur in association with coexistent chronic diseases, may be precipitated by infections or drugs, or may develop for unknown reasons[22] (Table 33–1). Although the cutaneous manifestations are polymorphous, the most characteristic lesion is an erythematous papule, in which the erythema does not blanch when the skin is pressed (*palpable purpura*) (Fig. 33–8) (see Color Plate). Urticaria or angioedema,[23] nodules, pustules, vesicles, ulcers, necrosis, and livedo reticularis may occur. Occasionally, subcutaneous edema may be present in the area of the vascular lesions.

The vascular eruption most often appears on the

Table 33–1. CUTANEOUS NECROTIZING VENULITIS

Associated chronic disorders
  Rheumatoid arthritis
  Sjögren's syndrome
  Systemic lupus erythematosus
  Hypergammaglobulinemic purpura
  Paraneoplastic vasculitis
  Cryoglobulinemia
  Ulcerative colitis
  Cystic fibrosis
Precipitating events
  Infections
  Drug-induced reactions
Idiopathic disorders
  Henoch-Schönlein syndrome
  Chronic urticaria-angioedema and variants
  Erythema elevatum diutinum
  Nodular vasculitis
  Livedoid vasculitis
  Genetic C2 deficiency
  Acute hemorrhagic edema

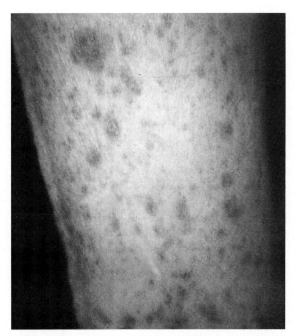

Figure 33–8. Necrotizing venulitis. Palpable purpura distributed over the lower extremities. (See Color Plate.)

lower extremities and frequently over the dependent portions of the body or areas under local pressure. The lesions may occur anywhere on the skin but are uncommon on the face, palms, soles, and mucous membranes. The skin lesions occur in episodes that may recur for various periods of time ranging from weeks to years. Palpable purpuric lesions persist from 1 to 4 weeks and then resolve, leaving hyperpigmentation or atrophic scars. An episode of cutaneous vascular lesions may be attended by pyrexia, malaise, arthralgias, or myalgias. When present, associated systemic involvement of the small blood vessels most commonly occurs in joints, muscles, peripheral nerves, gastrointestinal tract, and kidneys.

Involvement of large blood vessels occurs in *polyarteritis nodosa,* which is recognized in the skin as nodular lesions and ulcers over an artery,[24] and *giant cell (temporal) arteritis,* which is present as erythema overlying the affected vessel. Both *Wegener's granulomatosis*[25] and allergic angiitis and granulomatosis *(Churg-Strauss syndrome)* affect large and small vessels; the skin lesions in both disorders are present as erythematous nodules with or without necrosis and a variety of less specific erythematous, edematous, purpuric, papular, pustular, and necrotic lesions. Systemic necrotizing vasculitis accompanied by skin lesions but not corresponding to any diagnostic category is referred to as *systemic polyangiitis.*[26]

The term *paraneoplastic vasculitis*[27] has been used to describe patients with cutaneous necrotizing venulitis associated with malignant conditions, which include Hodgkin's disease, lymphosarcoma, adult T cell leukemia, myelofibrosis, mycosis fungoides, acute and chronic myelogenous forms of leukemia, IgA my-

eloma, diffuse large-cell leukemia, hairy-cell leukemia, squamous cell bronchiogenic carcinoma, prostate carcinoma, and colon carcinoma.

Cryoglobulins[28] may occur in patients with cutaneous necrotizing venulitis with and without concomitant connective tissue and lymphoproliferative disorders, in patients with hepatitis A, B, and C virus infections,[29–31] and idiopathically. Antineutrophil cytoplasmic antibodies have been noted in patients with polyarteritis nodosa, Churg-Strauss syndrome, systemic polyangiitis, and Wegener's granulomatosis. The most common cutaneous feature in patients with antineutrophil cytoplasmic antibodies is palpable purpura.

The most commonly recognized infectious agents are hepatitis B virus,[29] group A streptococci, *Staphylococcus aureus,* and *Mycobacterium leprae.*[32] In hepatitis B virus disease, transient urticaria may be present early in the course and represents vasculitis.[29] HIV infection has been associated in a limited number of patients with cutaneous vasculitis.[33]

The most commonly incriminated medications are sulfonamides, thiazides, penicillin, and serum. Cutaneous vasculitis has developed after the administration of granulocyte colony-stimulating factor (G-CSF)[34] and radiocontrast media. The literature consists of case reports rather than prospective or retrospective studies.

In perhaps 50 percent of instances the cause of cutaneous necrotizing venulitis remains unknown. The *Henoch-Schönlein syndrome* is the most widely recognized subgroup. A history of upper respiratory tract symptoms and signs is occasionally obtained. The syndrome, which occurs predominantly in children and less frequently in adults, includes involvement of the skin, joints, gastrointestinal tract, and kidneys. IgA is deposited around blood vessels in the skin, synovium, kidneys, and gastrointestinal tract.

Urticarial vasculitis affects mainly women and is associated with episodic arthralgias. General features include fever, malaise, myalgia, and enlargement of the lymph nodes, liver, and spleen. Specific organ involvement may include the kidneys, in the form of glomerulitis or glomerulonephritis; the gastrointestinal tract, in the form of nausea, vomiting, diarrhea, and pain; the respiratory tract, as laryngeal edema and chronic obstructive pulmonary disease; the eyes, as conjunctivitis, episcleritis, and uveitis; and the central nervous system, as headaches and benign intracranial hypertension (pseudotumor cerebri).

Patients also have been described under the appellations unusual systemic lupus erythematosus–like syndrome, hypocomplementemic urticarial vasculitis, and atypical erythema multiforme.

Erythema elevatum diutinum[35] consists of erythematous papules, plaques, and nodules predominantly disposed over the buttocks and extensor surfaces and is often accompanied by arthralgias. Associated conditions include IgA monoclonal gammopathy, multiple myeloma, and myelodysplasia.

Nodular vasculitis occurs as painful red nodules over

the lower extremities, especially the calves. Recurrent episodes are common, and ulcers at times may occur. *Erythema induratum*, which has been associated with tuberculosis, represents a form of nodular vasculitis. A female patient with antiphospholipid antibodies and cutaneous nodules that showed vasculitis and thrombosis has been reported.[36]

Livedoid vasculitis[37] occurs in women as recurrent, painful ulcers of the lower legs associated with a persistent livedo reticularis that often is deep purple in color. Healing results in sclerotic pale areas surrounded by telangiectases that have been called *atrophie blanche*. Livedoid vasculitis may be idiopathic, or it may occur in patients with SLE who develop central nervous system involvement[38]; antiphospholipid antibodies have been detected in both groups of patients.[39] Moreover, a clinical syndrome of livedo reticularis and transient cerebral ischemia with circulating antiphospholipid antibodies has been reported.[40]

Acute hemorrhagic edema[41] occurs in children and appears as painful, edematous areas with petechiae and ecchymoses on the head and distal extremities. Systemic features usually are absent. This form of vasculitis must be differentiated from Henoch-Schönlein syndrome, with which it has been confused in the past.

DERMATOMYOSITIS–POLYMYOSITIS

Patients with dermatomyositis usually have skin involvement several months before the onset of proximal muscular weakness. The early skin lesions are often nonspecific. The cutaneous lesions appear either as transient macular erythema, which is the more common presentation, or as persistent violaceous plaques. The violaceous erythema of dermatomyositis is often accompanied by scale and/or atrophy.

The sun-exposed areas and extensor surfaces are frequently involved. Photosensitivity[42] (Fig. 33–9) (see Color Plate) is prominent over the malar region of the face and the "V" area of the neck and chest. The lesions are initially flat, but they may become raised and edematous with a purple-red hue. In contradistinction to lupus erythematosus, the malar eruption usually involves the nasolabial folds. As the disease progresses, the intensity of the eruption diminishes and may be replaced by a reticulated, hyperpigmented and hypopigmented atrophy and a network of fine telangiectases known as *poikiloderma*. Poikiloderma is rarely found in other connective tissue diseases. Raynaud's phenomenon may be associated with sclerodactyly in about one third of patients. Mucous membrane changes with erythema, scars, and ulcers may mimic SLE; however, nasal or palatal perforation is rare.[43]

The heliotrope eruption is a lilac or erythematous coloration of and around the eyelids with or without periorbital edema. The edema can occur independently. *Gottron's sign* is a flat or raised purple-red area over the interphalangeal joints of the hands, olecra-

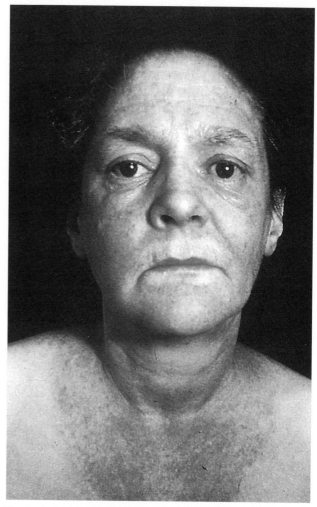

Figure 33–9. Dermatomyositis. Photosensitivity. (From Soter NA, Franks AG Jr: Cutaneous manifestations of rheumatic diseases: An update. *In* Kelley WN, et al: Textbook of Rheumatology, 4th ed. Philadelphia, WB Saunders. Update No. 15, pp 1–24, 1995.) (See Color Plate.)

nons, patellae, and malleoli that evolves into atrophic plaques with telangiectases and pigmentary alterations (Fig. 33–10). Linear extensor erythema characteristically follows the course of the extensor tendons or body surfaces alone. A distinctive shawl pattern of erythema on the upper back and shoulders also is characteristic (Fig. 33–11) (see Color Plate). *Mechanic's hand* with scale and fissures of the lateral aspects of the fingers may be found in up to one third of patients and resembles contact dermatitis. Periungual suffusion with dilated corkscrew vessels alternating with areas of avascularity may be prominent and are often associated with a cuticular overgrowth pattern.

Calcinosis cutis (Fig. 33–12) is rarely observed in connective tissue diseases other than dermatomyositis and scleroderma. The calcinosis in dermatomyositis is usually more extensive than it is in scleroderma and extends into both muscle and subcutaneous tissues. These changes are observed more frequently when the disease begins in childhood. Calcification

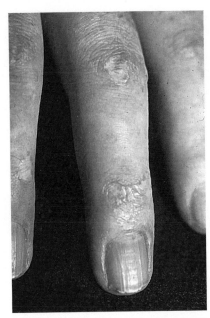

Figure 33–10. Dermatomyositis. Atrophic plaques with telangiectases and pigmentary alterations over the intephalangeal joints of the fingers. (From Soter NA, Franks AG Jr: Cutaneous manifestations of rheumatic diseases: An update. *In* Kelley WN, et al: Textbook of Rheumatology, 4th ed. Philadelphia, WB Saunders. Update No. 15, pp 1–24, 1995.)

occurs especially over the shoulders, elbows, and buttocks and, in contrast to scleroderma, is rare over the fingers. Cutaneous ulcers and sinuses may develop after the extrusion of deposited calcium. Raynaud's phenomenon is rare in children, although a child may often manifest facial erythema and necrotizing vasculitis involving the gastrointestinal tract that leads to intestinal perforation.

Certain patterns of dermatositis-polymyositis may be associated with myositis-specific autoantibodies. Anti-Jo-1 is associated with a predominance of Raynaud's phenomenon, severe onset of myositis, arthritis, interstitial lung disease, and mechanic's hand. Anti–Mi-2 antibodies are associated with classic der-

matomyositis with the "V sign," shawl sign, and cuticular overgrowth.

SCLERODERMA

Scleroderma may occur as a systemic disorder or as various localized forms that primarily affect the skin. The most common type is *morphea*, in which the skin lesions are present as circumscribed areas of atrophy with an ivory color in the center and a violet hue at the periphery. The lesions of morphea commonly persist for years; however, they may disappear spontaneously and heal with or without residual pigmentary alterations.

Linear scleroderma appears in a band-like distribution. The lower extremities are most frequently affected. In addition to the skin, underlying muscles and bones may be involved. Linear scleroderma begins most frequently during the first two decades of life. It has been associated with abnormalities of the axial skeleton, especially occult spina bifida. Other variants of scleroderma include frontal or frontoparietal involvement of the head known as *en coup de sabre*, which is characterized by an atrophic furrow that extends below the plane of the skin and progressive facial hemiatrophy *(Parry-Romberg syndrome)*.

Although proximal cutaneous involvement is characteristic in systemic scleroderma, cutaneous alterations of the face and hands may be especially prominent. Features include a mask-like, expressionless face with a fixed stare, inability to wrinkle the forehead, tightening of the skin over the nose with a beak-like appearance, and restriction of the mouth with radial folds and loss of tissue such that the teeth are prominent. An early sign is indolent nonpitting edema over the dorsa of the fingers, hands, and forearms. Sclerodactyly is noted with tapered fingers over which the skin is atrophic; flexion contractures may be present, especially about the fingers, elbows, and knees. When calcification occurs in association with *Raynaud's* phenomenon (Fig. 33–13), *e*sophageal abnormalities, *s*clerodactyly, and *t*elangiectases, the clinical symptom

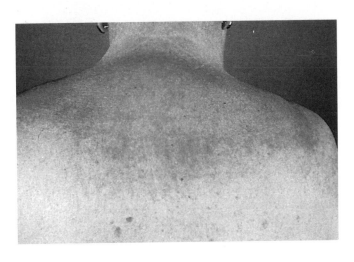

Figure 33–11. Dermatomyositis. Shawl pattern of erythema on the upper back. (From Soter NA, Franks AG Jr: Cutaneous manifestations of rheumatic diseases: An update. *In* Kelley WN, et al: Textbook of Rheumatology, 4th ed. Philadelphia, WB Saunders. Update No. 15, pp 1–24, 1995.) (See Color Plate.)

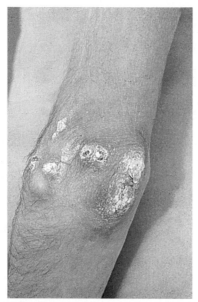

Figure 33–12. Dermatomyositis. Calcinosis cutis. (From Soter NA, Franks AG Jr: Cutaneous manifestations of rheumatic diseases: An update. *In* Kelley WN, et al: Textbook of Rheumatology, 4th ed. Philadelphia, WB Saunders. Update No. 15, pp 1–24, 1995.)

complex is known as the *CREST* syndrome. Although this form of scleroderma has been alleged to pursue a more benign course, pulmonary hypertension and biliary cirrhosis have been reported.

Telangiectases occur commonly on the nail folds; square telangiectatic macules may involve the face, lips, tongue, and hands. Other features may include generalized hyperpigmentation and alopecia.

Disorders with cutaneous sclerosis that should be considered in the differential diagnosis of scleroderma include eosinophilic fasciitis,[44] porphyria cutanea tarda, papular mucinosis (scleromyxedema), lichen sclerosus et atrophicus, melorheostosis, the

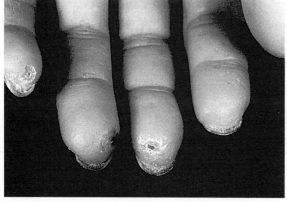

Figure 33–13. Scleroderma. Ulcers and scars of the tips of the digits in an individual with Raynaud's phenomenon. (From Soter NA, Franks AG Jr: Cutaneous manifestations of rheumatic diseases: An update. *In* Kelley WN, et al: Textbook of Rheumatology, 4th ed. Philadelphia, WB Saunders. Update No. 15, pp 1–24, 1995.)

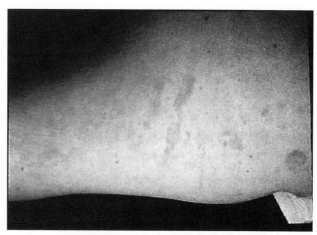

Figure 33–14. Juvenile rheumatoid arthritis. Salmon-colored lesions on the arm. (From Soter NA, Franks AG Jr: Cutaneous manifestations of rheumatic diseases: An update. *In* Kelley WN, et al: Textbook of Rheumatology, 4th ed. Philadelphia, WB Saunders. Update No. 15, pp 1–24, 1995.) (See Color Plate.)

chronic form of graft-versus-host disease,[45] and eosinophilia–myalgia syndrome related to L-tryptophan ingestion.[46]

JUVENILE RHEUMATOID ARTHRITIS

Cutaneous eruptions occur in association with juvenile rheumatoid arthritis *(Still's disease).* The most frequently recognized form is an evanescent, erythematous eruption that accompanies the late afternoon temperature rise in 25 to 40 percent of patients, especially boys. The skin lesions (Fig. 33–14) (see Color Plate) appear as small erythematous or salmon-colored macules and papules that are distributed over the face, trunk, and extremities. They are usually not pruritic, and once formed, they do not move or enlarge. The lesions occur when the disease is active, subside with remission, heal without residua, and are not related to prognosis. Subcutaneous nodules may occur and must be differentiated from the subcutaneous form of granuloma annulare.

RHEUMATIC FEVER

During the 1980s, an increased prevalence of rheumatic fever occurred in the United States.[47, 48] A variety of erythematous eruptions have been noted in patients with rheumatic fever. The most specific eruption is *erythema marginatum,* which occurs in 5 to 13 percent of patients. It appears as transient erythematous rings, usually with raised margins, that rapidly spread peripherally to form polycyclic or geographic outlines and that leave a pale or pigmented center. The essential feature is the rapid spread, which may be 2 to 10 mm in 12 hours. The lesions occur on the trunk and proximal portions of the extremities; they are rarely pruritic. The flat or macular form is known as *erythema circinatum.* Both erythema marginatum and circinatum are usually associated with carditis and are unaffected by treatment of the underlying disease. Small, multiple subcutaneous nodules may be noted, especially in patients with carditis. A rare manifestation is *erythema papulatum,* which appears as indolent, asymptomatic papules, especially over the elbows and knees.

LYME BORRELIOSIS

Lyme borreliosis is a multisystem disorder caused by the spirochete *Borrelia burgdorferi* and transmitted by the tick *Ixodes dammini.* The clinical manifestations occur in three stages. Early infection consists of regional lymphadenopathy and mild constitutional features. The cutaneous hallmark, which occurs in 60 to 80 percent of patients, is the expanding erythematous skin lesion *erythema migrans,* which is recognized as an expanding ring with partial central clearing (Fig. 33–15) (see Color Plate). The lesion may enlarge up to 20 to 60 cm over days to weeks and fades within 3 to 4 weeks.[49] The average diameter is 15 cm. Approximately 50 percent of patients have one or more annular lesions, urticaria, and morbilliform eruptions. The skin manifestations clear without treatment.

The second stage develops within days to weeks. The cutaneous features include erythema migrans, lymphocytoma cutis, urticaria, and macular erythema associated with other systemic manifestations.

Late cutaneous features have included atrophic or scleroderma-like lesions.

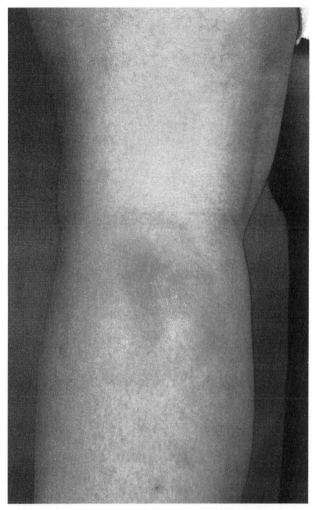

Figure 33–15. Lyme borreliosis. Erythema migrans. (From Soter NA, Franks AG Jr: Cutaneous manifestations of rheumatic diseases: An update. *In* Kelley WN, et al: Textbook of Rheumatology, 4th ed. Philadelphia, WB Saunders. Update No. 15, pp 1–24, 1995.) (See Color Plate.)

AMYLOID

Amyloid may be present as a primary cutaneous disease, may occur with multiple myeloma or genetic disorders, may be associated in a secondary fashion with chronic inflammatory conditions, or may be restricted to a single tissue site, which includes forms localized to the skin. Skin lesions occur in primary amyloid; secondary amyloid is rarely accompanied by skin lesions. It is noteworthy, however, that clinically uninvolved skin may contain amyloid deposits in both primary and secondary types, which suggests that a skin biopsy of such uninvolved skin can have a high diagnostic yield.

The skin lesions appear as firm, translucent papules that occur on the face (especially about the eyes), neck, intertriginous areas, and extremities. They vary in color from rose to yellow to brown; pruritus is absent. A conspicuous feature is hemorrhage; in fact,

the tendency for purpura development is the basis for a diagnostic maneuver, in which purpura occurs after a blunt instrument is used to traumatize the lesions. Ecchymoses may occur in the absence of papules. Macroglossia is present in 25 to 40 percent of patients; the surface of the tongue may be smooth, or it may contain papules or nodules or manifest ulcers and purpura (Fig. 33–16).

Localized cutaneous amyloidosis may be present as macules, papules, or nodules. *Macular amyloidosis* consists of pruritic brown macules distributed over the upper back and extremities. *Lichen amyloidosis* appears as pruritic, discrete, multiple papules and plaques distributed over the anterior aspects of the lower legs. Localized nodular amyloidosis presents as single or multiple nodules on the face, trunk, or genitalia. These lesions are indistinguishable from those lesions associated with systemic amyloidosis. These patients should be followed up carefully, be-

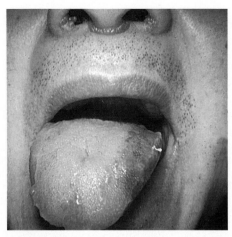

Figure 33–16. Amyloid. Macroglossia with purpura. (From Soter NA, Franks AG Jr: Cutaneous manifestations of rheumatic diseases: An update. *In* Kelley WN, et al: Textbook of Rheumatology, 4th ed. Philadelphia, WB Saunders. Update No. 15, pp 1–24, 1995.)

cause systemic amyloidosis and paraproteinemia occasionally develop.

SARCOID

Skin lesions of sarcoid[50] occur in 25 percent of patients with sarcoid, and erythema nodosum occurs in 30 percent. The most characteristic lesions observed in the United States are yellow-brown to violaceous papules and plaques with a predilection for the face, especially the alae nasi and the periocular areas. Similar lesions may be widely distributed over the trunk and extremities. The papules may arise in a scar, a valuable diagnostic sign. Livid purple plaques have been described on the nose (nasal rim lesions), cheeks, and lobes of the ears; these lesions are known as *lupus pernio*, which is associated with involvement of the respiratory tract[51] and kidneys. Other skin manifestations include an ichthyosiform dermatosis over the lower legs, subcutaneous calcification, and areas of hypopigmentation. In rare instances, ulcers occur over the lower legs, especially in black women.

PANNICULITIS

Panniculitis is the term used to describe disorders in which inflammation occurs in the subcutaneous tissue. Panniculitis of all types is recognized as erythematous or violaceous nodules that may or may not ulcerate. When the inflammation is localized in septa, it is designated *septal* panniculitis; inflammation localized in the fat lobules is classified as *lobular* panniculitis.

Erythema nodosum is the most widely recognized form of panniculitis.[52] The age and sex distribution for erythema nodosum vary throughout the world,

depending on the eliciting etiologic agents, which include a variety of infections, medications, and systemic diseases (Table 33–2).

The clinical eruption appears as tender, erythematous nodules over the extensor aspects of the lower extremities, which may be accompanied by fever, chills, malaise, and leukocytosis. The erythema evolves into a violet-blue color and contused appearance during the second week. Individual nodules usually resolve spontaneously in 3 to 6 weeks without ulcers or scars. Patients with erythema nodosum often experience arthralgias, which may persist after the cutaneous lesions have resolved. Episcleral lesions also may occur.

Weber-Christian disease is the term applied to a relapsing form of idiopathic panniculitis associated with systemic manifestations. The cutaneous lesions occur as recurrent episodes of erythematous, sometimes tender, subcutaneous nodules that appear at intervals of weeks to months. The lesions are symmetric in distribution, and the thighs and lower legs usually are affected. Occasionally, necrosis of the overlying skin occurs, and an oily yellow-brown liquid is discharged. Individual nodules involute over the course of a few weeks, resulting in hyperpigmented and atrophic scars. The episodes of cutaneous lesions usually are accompanied by malaise, fever, and arthralgias. Nausea, vomiting, abdominal pain, weight loss, and hepatomegaly also may occur.

Physical trauma of a thermal, mechanical, or chemical nature can result in panniculitis. The most common physical factors are exposure to cold or direct physical or chemical trauma; sometimes these traumatic factors are factitious and are consequent to self-induced lesions.

Table 33–2. CAUSES OF ERYTHEMA NODOSUM

Infections
  β-hemolytic streptococci
  Tuberculosis
  Yersinia infections
  Leptospirosis
  Tularemia
  Mycoplasma pneumoniae
  Leprosy
  Blastomycosis
  Coccidioidomycosis
  Histoplasmosis
  Infectious mononucleosis
  Lymphogranuloma venereum
  Cat-scratch disease
  Paravaccinia
  Psittacosis
Drugs
  Oral contraceptives
  Sulfonamides
Systemic Disorders
  Ulcerative colitis
  Regional enteritis
  Sarcoidosis
  Behçet's syndrome
  Malignant conditions

Lobular panniculitis may be associated with pancreatic carcinoma or pancreatitis. Painful erythematous nodules may appear in any location, but there is a predilection for the legs. The nodules occasionally drain an oily substance. Arthritis occurs in about 60 percent of the cases, and a polyserositis can be manifested as pleuritis, pericarditis, or synovitis.

Panniculitis may be a sign of underlying systemic diseases, such as lupus erythematosus, lymphomas and leukemia, sarcoidosis, and fungal and bacterial infections. Panniculitis occurring after jejunoileal bypass surgery has been reported.

PARVOVIRUS ARTHROPATHY

Parvovirus B19 infection in children is a viral disorder with cutaneous features known as *erythema infectiosum* (Fifth disease) and arthritis. The eruption begins with confluent, erythematous, and edematous plaques over the malar eminences (slapped cheeks). The facial eruption fades over 1 to 4 days; then erythematous macules or papules with a lace-like or reticulated appearance develop on the trunk and extensor surfaces of the extremities.

Rheumatologic manifestations of human parvovirus B19 infection in adults have been described as polyarthralgia and polyarthritis, with a chronic disease pattern sometimes suggesting seronegative rheumatoid arthritis.[53] Although the typical dermatologic features of parvovirus B19 in children are generally not found in adults, a malar rash mimicking lupus erythematosus has been described.[54] Other cutaneous manifestations in adults include palpable purpura, pustules, and desquamation of the palms and soles. Acral pruritus, pain, petechiae, edema, and erosions may develop; these features are known as the glove and sock syndrome.[55]

References

1. Sanchez JL, Cruz A: Rheumatoid neutrophilic dermatitis. J Am Acad Dermatol 22:922, 1990.
2. Glass DN, Soter NA, Schur PH: Rheumatoid vasculitis. Arthritis Rheum 19:950, 1976.
3. Alexander EL, Arnett FC, Provost TT, Stevens MB: Sjögren's syndrome: Association of anti-Ro (SS-A) antibodies with vasculitis, hematologic abnormalities, and serologic hyperreactivity. Ann Intern Med 98:155, 1983.
4. Winchester R, Brancato L, Itescu S, Skovron ML, Solomon G: Implications from the occurrence of Reiter's syndrome and related disorders in association with advanced HIV infection. Scand J Rheumatol 74:89, 1988.
5. Henseler T, Christophers E: Psoriasis of early and late onset: Characterization of two types of psoriasis vulgaris. J Am Acad Dermatol 13:450, 1985.
6. Honig PJ: Guttate psoriasis associated with perianal streptococcal disease. J Pediatr 113:1037, 1988.
7. Stern SH, Insall JN, Windsor RE, Inglis AE, Dines DM: Total knee arthroplasty in patients with psoriasis. Clin Orthop 248:108, 1989.
8. Kammer GM, Soter NA, Gibson DJ, Schur PH: Psoriatic arthritis: A clinical, immunologic and HLA study of 100 patients. Semin Arthritis Rheum 9:75, 1979.
9. Johnson TM, Duvic M, Rapini RP, Rios A: AIDS exacerbates psoriasis. N Engl J Med 313:1415, 1985.
10. Pazirandeh M, Ziran BH, Khandelwal BK, Reynolds TL, Kahn MA: Relapsing polychondritis and spondyloarthropathies. J Rheumatol 15:630, 1988.
11. Sontheimer RD, Thomas JR, Gilliam JN: Subacute cutaneous lupus erythematosus—a cutaneous marker for a distinct LE subset. Arch Dermatol 115:1409, 1979.
12. Hall RP, Lawley TJ, Smith HR, Katz SI: Bullous eruption of systemic lupus erythematosus: Dramatic response to dapsone therapy. Ann Intern Med 97:165, 1982.
13. Cohen MR, Crosby D: Systemic disease in subacute cutaneous lupus erythematosus: A controlled comparison with systemic lupus erythematosus. J Rheumatol 21:1665, 1994.
14. Franks AG Jr: Identifying dermatologic manifestations of lupus erythematosus. J Musculoskel Med 5:59, 1988.
15. O'Loughlin S, Schroeter AL, Jordon RE: Chronic urticaria-like lesions in systemic lupus erythematosus: A review of 12 cases. Arch Dermatol 114:879, 1978.
16. Peters SM, Su DWP: Lupus erythematosus panniculitis. Med Clin North Am 73:1113, 1989.
17. Harrist TJ, Mihm MC Jr: The specificity and clinical usefulness of the lupus band test. Arthritis Rheum 23:479, 1980.
18. Gilliam JN, Cheatum DE, Hurd ER, Stastny P, Ziff M: Immunoglobulin in clinically involved skin in systemic lupus erythematosus: Association with renal disease. J Clin Invest 53:1434, 1974.
19. Davis BM, Gilliam JN: Prognostic significance of subepidermal immune deposits in uninvolved skin of patients with systemic lupus erythematosus: A 10-year longitudinal study. J Invest Dermatol 83:242, 1984.
20. Gilliam JN, Prystowsky SD: Mixed connective issue disease syndrome: Cutaneous manifestations of patients with epidermal nuclear staining and high titer serum antibody to ribonuclease-sensitive extractable nuclear antigen. Arch Dermatol 113:583, 1977.
21. Sanchez NP, Van Hale HM, Su WP: Clinical and histopathologic spectrum of necrotizing vasculitis: Report of findings in 101 cases. Arch Dermatol 121:220, 1985.
22. Soter NA: Cutaneous necrotizing venulitis. In Frank MM, et al (eds): Samter's Immunological Diseases, 5th ed. Boston, Little, Brown & Company, 1995, pp 865–876.
23. Soter NA: Chronic urticaria as a manifestation of necrotizing venulitis. N Engl J Med 296:1440, 1977.
24. Diaz-Perez JL, Winkelmann RK: Cutaneous periarteritis nodosa. Arch Dermatol 110:407, 1974.
25. Francès C, Du LTH, Piette J-C, Saada V, Boisnic S, Wechsler B, Blétry O, Godeau P: Wegener's granulomatosis: Dermatological manifestations in 75 cases with clinicopathologic correlation. Arch Dermatol 130:861, 1994.
26. Leavitt RY, Fauci AS: Polyangiitis overlap syndrome: Classification and prospective experience. Am J Med 81:79, 1986.
27. Sánchez-Guerrero J, Gutiérrez-Ureña S, Vidaller A, Reyes E, Iglesias A, Alarcón-Segovia D: Vasculitis as a paraneoplastic syndrome: Report of 11 cases and review of the literature. J Rheumatol 17:1458, 1990.
28. Cohen SJ, Pittelkow MR, Su WPD: Cutaneous manifestations of cryoglobulinemia: Clinical and histopathologic study of seventy-two patients. J Am Acad Dermatol 25:21, 1991.
29. Dienstag JL, Rhodes AR, Bhan AK, Dvorak AM, Mihm MC Jr, Wands JR: Urticaria associated with acute viral hepatitis type B. Ann Intern Med 89:34, 1978.
30. Inman RD, Hodge M, Johnston MEA, Wright J, Heathcote J: Arthritis, vasculitis and cryoglobulinemia associated with relapsing hepatitis A virus infection. Ann Intern Med 105:700, 1986.
31. Hearth-Holmes M, Zahradka SL, Baethge BA, Wolfe RE: Leukocytoclastic vasculitis associated with hepatitis C. Am J Med 90:765, 1991.
32. Murphy GF, Sanchez NP, Flynn TC, Sanchez JL, Mihm MC Jr, Soter NA: Erythema nodosum leprosum: Nature and extent of the cutaneous microvascular alterations. J Am Acad Dermatol 14:59, 1986.
33. Weimer CE Jr, Sahn EE: Follicular accentuation of leukocytoclastic vasculitis in an HIV-positive man: Report of a case and review of the literature. J Am Acad Dermatol 24:898, 1991.
34. Jain KK: Cutaneous vasculitis associated with granulocyte colony-stimulating factor. J Am Acad Dermatol 31:213, 1994.
35. Katz SI, Gallin JI, Hertz KC, Fauci AS, Lawley TJ: Erythema elevatum diutinum: Skin and systemic manifestations, immunologic studies, and successful treatment with dapsone. Medicine 56:443, 1977.
36. Renfro L, Franks AG Jr, Grodberg M, Kamino H: Painful nodules in a young female. Arch Dermatol 128:847, 1992.
37. Stiefler RE, Bergfeld WF: Atrophie blanche. Int J Dermatol 21:1, 1982.
38. Yasue T: Livedoid vasculitis and central nervous system involvement in systemic lupus erythematosus. Arch Dermatol 122:66, 1986.
39. Stephansson EA, Scheynius A: Immunological studies of cutaneous vasculitis and primary antiphospholipid syndrome. Eur J Dermatol 3:289, 1993.
40. Grattan CEH, Burton JL, Boon AP: Sneddon's syndrome (livedo reticularis and cerebral thrombosis) with livedo vasculitis and anticardiolipin antibodies. Br J Dermatol 120:441, 1989.
41. Legrain V, Lejean S, Taïeb A, Guillard J-M, Battin J, Maleville J: Infantile acute hemorrhagic edema of the skin: Study of ten cases. J Am Acad Dermatol 24:17, 1991.
42. Cheong WK, Hughes GR, Norris PG, Hawk JL: Cutaneous photosensitivity in dermatomyositis. Br J Dermatol 131:205, 1994.

43. Franks AG Jr: Important cutaneous markers of dermatomyositis. J Musculoskel Med 5:39, 1988.

44. Schulman LE: Diffuse fasciitis with eosinophilia: A new syndrome? Trans Assoc Am Phys 88:70, 1975.

45. Hood AF, Soter NA, Rappeport J, Gigli I: Graft-versus-host reaction: Cutaneous manifestations following bone marrow transplantation. Arch Dermatol 113:1087, 1977.

46. Silver RM, Heyes MP, Maize JC, Quearry BS, Vionnet-Fuasset M, Sternberg EM: Scleroderma, fasciitis, and eosinophilia associated with the ingestion of tryptophan. N Engl J Med 322:874, 1990.

47. Veasy LG, Wiedmeier SE, Orsmond GS, Ruttenberg HD, Boucek MM, Roth SJ, Tait VF, Thompson JA, Duly JA, Kaplan EL, Hill HR: Resurgence of acute rheumatic fever in the intermountain areas of the United States. N Engl J Med 316:421, 1987.

48. Griffiths SP, Gersony WM: Acute rheumatic fever in New York City (1969–1988): A comparative study of two decades. J Pediatr 116:882, 1990.

49. Asbrink E, Hovmark A: Lyme borreliosis: Aspects of tick-borne *Borrelia burgdorferi* infection from a dermatologic viewpoint. Semin Dermatol 9:277, 1990.

50. Olive KE, Kataria YP: Cutaneous manifestations of sarcoidosis: Relationship to other organ system involvement, abnormal laboratory measurements, and disease course. Arch Intern Med 145:1811, 1985.

51. Jorizzo JL, Koufman JA, Thompson JN, White WL, Shar GG, Schreiner DJ: Sarcoidosis of the upper respiratory tract in patients with nasal rim lesions: A pilot study. J Am Acad Dermatol 22:439, 1990.

52. Hannuksela M.: Erythema nodosum. Clin Dermatol 4:88, 1986.

53. Naides SJ, Scharosch LL, Foto F, Howard EJ: Rheumatologic manifestations of human parvovirus B19 infection in adults. Arthritis Rheum 33:1297, 1990.

54. Kalish RA, Knopf AN, Gary GW, Canoso JJ: Lupus-like presentation of human parvovirus B19 infection. J Rheumatol 19:169, 1992.

55. Halasz CL, Cormier D, Den M: Petechial glove and sock syndrome caused by parvovirus B19. J Am Acad Dermatol 27:835, 1992.

Special Issues of the Rheumatic Diseases

CHAPTER **34**

Robert M. Bennett

The Fibromyalgia Syndrome

Fibromyalgia is a readily recognized syndrome of widespread musculoskeletal pain and fatigue, often associated with a multiplicity of other symptoms. As a primary disorder, it is one of the commonest reasons for rheumatology referrals. Whereas there is a widening acceptance of the fibromyalgia syndrome as a clinical reality, there is confusion regarding its designation as a distinctive entity. For instance, fibromyalgia does not fit the concepts of the "classical medical model," in that it does not fulfill the equivalent of Koch's postulates. On the other hand, the classical medical model has not proved productive in facilitating the understanding of disorders that bridge the gray area of psyche and soma. The account of the fibromyalgia syndrome given here strives to be pragmatic and to provide some brief insights into contemporary research.

CLINICAL FEATURES

The core *symptom* of the fibromyalgia syndrome is chronic widespread pain (Fig. 34–1).[1] The pain is thought to arise from muscle; however, most patients with the disorder also have tender skin. Fibromyalgia pain typically waxes and wanes in intensity; flares are associated with unaccustomed exertion, soft tissue injuries, lack of sleep, cold exposure, and psychologic stressors. Many patients describe increased pain with cold, damp weather, in particular low-pressure fronts; however, these claims have not been objectively verified.[2] Fibromyalgia pain is predominantly axial in distribution, but pain in the hands and feet is not uncommon and may lead to a misdiagnosis of "early" rheumatoid arthritis.[3]

Although most patients have widespread body pain, typically one or two locations are the major foci. These pain centers often shift to other locations, often in response to new biomechanical stresses or trauma.

Many patients describe a feeling of swelling in the soft tissues; this is often localized to the area of joints, leading to self-diagnosis of arthritis. Stiffness is a prominent feature in most fibromyalgia patients and can further reinforce the impression of early arthritis. Most patients with this array of pain symptomatology have multiple tender points[4]—the core *physical finding* of the fibromyalgia syndrome (see Diagnosis and Differential Diagnosis later).

Fibromyalgia is more than a muscle pain syndrome, in that most patients have an array of other somatic complaints.[5] Nearly all patients with fibromyalgia experience severe fatigue, poor sleep, and postexertional

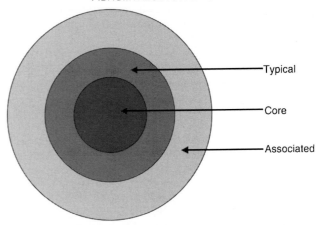

FIBROMYALGIA SYNDROME

Typical

Core

Associated

Figure 34–1. All fibromyalgia patients, by definition, have a history of widespread musculoskeletal pain and the physical finding of multiple tender points—the *core* features. Most patients also report fatigue, stiffness, skin tenderness, postexertional pain, and fragmented sleep—the *typical* features. Many patients have a confusing spectrum of other symptoms, such as spastic colon, poor memory, headaches, Raynaud's phenomenon, dizziness, fluid retention, restless legs, bruising, bladder irritation, and paresthesias—the *associated* features.

pain.[1] Other symptoms include tension-type headaches, cold intolerance, sicca symptoms, unexplained bruising, fluid retention, chest pain, jaw pain, dyspnea, dizziness, abdominal pain, paresthesias, and low-grade depression and anxiety.[6–12] Some symptoms relate to specific syndromes whose prevalence appears to be increased; these include irritable bowel syndrome, migraine, premenstrual syndrome, Raynaud's phenomenon, female urethral syndrome, and restless leg syndrome.[13–16]

EPIDEMIOLOGY

Two epidemiologic studies, one from Europe and the other from the United States, have provided important information on the community prevalence of widespread musculoskeletal pain and fibromyalgia. Croft and colleagues, using a postal survey in the north of England, found widespread pain in 13 percent of all responders, regional pain in 43 percent, and no pain history in 44 percent.[17] When subjects with widespread pain were examined, 81.5 percent had 11 or more tender points and 14.7 percent had no tender points. Women had more tender points than men, with 90 percent of subjects having more than 11 tender points being female; however, 60 percent of all patients with a history of widespread pain had fewer than 11 tender points. The authors concluded that a combination of widespread pain and a high number of tender points was one end of a continuous spectrum of pain status and myalgic foci. Furthermore, in the general population, the tender point count did not necessarily correlate with widespread pain but did correlate with depression, fatigue, and poor sleep—independently of pain status. Thus, an arbitrary cutoff of 11 tender points may be inappropriate in the analysis of pain complaints and tender points of population surveys.

In a similar study by Wolfe and coworkers in Wichita, Kansas,[18] the prevalence of widespread musculoskeletal pain was more common in women and increased progressively from ages 18 to 70, with a 23 percent prevalence in the seventh decade. When patients with widespread pain were examined for tender points, 25.2 percent of women and 6.8 percent of men had 11 or more tender points. There was an almost linear increase in the prevalence of fibromyalgia up to the eighth decade (Fig. 34–2). These findings are contrary to the widespread notion that fibromyalgia is predominantly a disorder of young and middle-aged women. The overall (M + F) prevalence of fibromyalgia in the total Wichita population was 2 percent, with a prevalence of 3.4 percent in women and 0.5 percent in men. Psychologic distress was just as high in the community as in the rheumatology clinic. This observation suggests that psychologic issues are not necessarily the reason that *subjects* with widespread pain become *patients* with fibromyalgia.

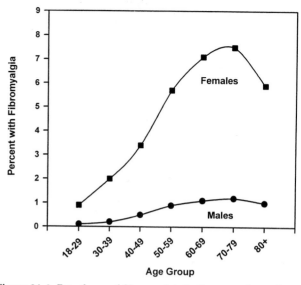

Figure 34–2. Prevalence of fibromyalgia in the general population. An epidemiologic study from Wichita, Kansas, indicated a progressive increase in the prevalence of fibromyalgia up to the eighth decade. The overall population prevalence was 2 percent, with a prevalence of 3.4 percent in all women and of 0.5 percent in all men. (Adapted from Wolfe F, Ross K, Anderson J, et al: The prevalence and characteristics of fibromyalgia in the general population. Arthritis Rheum 38:19–28, 1995. Used with permission of the American College of Rheumatology.)

DIAGNOSIS AND DIFFERENTIAL DIAGNOSIS

The 1990 American College of Rheumatology guidelines for diagnosing fibromyalgia specify a history of widespread pain of 3 months or more.[1] "Widespread" is defined as pain in an axial distribution with pain of both left and right sides of the body and pain above and below the waist. Thus, axial pain and pain in three body segments would qualify as fibromyalgia. In addition, to meet the diagnostic criteria, pain must be present in 11 or more out of 18 specified tender point sites on digital palpation with an approximate force of 4 kg (the amount of pressure required to blanch a thumbnail). The locations of the 18 tender points are shown in Figure 34–3. Symptoms and signs such as sleep disturbance, fatigue, stiffness, skin fold tenderness, and cold intolerance are common in fibromyalgia patients, but their inclusion did not improve diagnostic accuracy. The recommended number of tender points (i.e., 11 or greater) was originally derived from a receiver operating curve and relates to the number giving the best sensitivity and specificity.

In clinical practice, the diagnosis of fibromyalgia can be entertained when fewer than 11 tender points are present. In such cases, it is useful to palpate other areas that are commonly tender, including the infraspinatus, the upper portion of the latissimus dorsi, the scapular insertion of the levator scapulae, the humeral insertion of the deltoid, the interossei muscles in the first web space of the hand, the junction of the tensor fascia latae and iliotibial tract, the junction of the soleus and Achilles' tendon, and the origin of

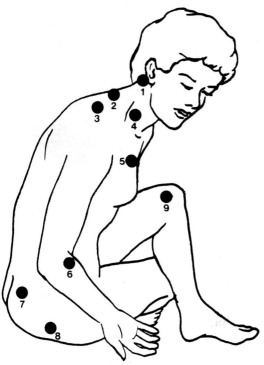

Figure 34–3. Tender point location. The nine paired tender points recommended by the 1990 American College of Rheumatology Criteria Committee for establishing a diagnosis of fibromyalgia are (1) insertion of nuchal muscles into occiput; (2) upper border of trapezius—midportion; (3) muscle attachments to upper medial border of scapula; (4) anterior aspects of the C5, C7 intertransverse spaces; (5) second rib space about 3 cm lateral to the sternal border; (6) muscle attachments to lateral epicondyle—about 2 cm below bony prominence; (7) upper outer quadrant of gluteal muscles; (8) muscle attachments just posterior to greater trochanter; and (9) medial fat pad of knee proximal to joint line. A total of eleven or more tender points in conjunction with a history of widespread pain is characteristic of the fibromyalgia syndrome.

the foot flexor muscles from the medial aspect of the calcaneum.

In general, designated tender points are more tender than control areas (i.e., the distal dorsal third of forearm, the thumbnail, and the midfoot of the midpoint of the dorsal third metatarsal). It is now appreciated, however, that such a differentiation cannot be used to *exclude* fibromyalgia or indicate malingering. The 1990 criteria suggested abolishing the distinction between primary and secondary fibromyalgia. This notion is important, because some fibromyalgia patients receive extensive workups to *exclude* another diagnosis. The multiple symptomatology of fibromyalgia patients is often confusing to physicians not familiar with the fibromyalgia construct.[5] Some common misdiagnoses are shown in Table 34–1.

CONSEQUENCES AND PROGNOSIS

The essential feature of fibromyalgia, namely chronic musculoskeletal pain, often affects a patient's

quality of life severely.[19] The consequences of muscular pain and fatigability influence motor performance. Henriksson and associates have noted that everyday activities take longer in patients with fibromyalgia, because they need more time to get started in the morning and often require extra rest periods during the day.[20] Patients have difficulty with repetitive sustained motor tasks unless frequent time-outs are taken. Tasks may be well tolerated for short periods of time, but they become aggravating factors when carried out for prolonged periods.[21] Prolonged muscular activity, especially under stress or in uncomfortable climatic conditions, was reported to exacerbate the symptoms of fibromyalgia. The adaptations that fibromyalgia patients have to make in order to minimize their pain experience has a negative impact on both vocational and avocational activities. Several long-term follow-up studies have indicated that fibromyalgia symptomatology is persistent over many years.[22–24]

ASSOCIATED ISSUES

The pervasive symptomatology of fibromyalgia patients, the lack of a well-defined pathophysiologic basis, and the issue of causality have generated several side issues.

Causation

Patients frequently attribute an "event" to the onset of their symptoms. Attribution and rationalization are common human traits, and *correlation* does not equal *causation*. Events that have been linked to the onset of fibromyalgia include flu-like illness, human immunodeficiency virus (HIV) infection, parvovirus infection, Lyme disease, toxic oil syndrome, persistent stress, chronic sleep disturbance, and physical trauma.[25–32]

Chronic Fatigue Syndrome and Related Syndromes

Patients with the *chronic fatigue syndrome* are very similar to fibromyalgia patients.[33] Characteristically,

Table 34–1. MISDIAGNOSES THAT MAY BE GIVEN TO PATIENTS WHO EVENTUALLY ARE FOUND TO HAVE THE FIBROMYALGIA SYNDROME

Systemic lupus erythematosus/ rheumatoid arthritis	Inflammatory bowel disease
Early spondyloarthropathy	Sciatica
Multiple sclerosis	Neuropathy
Depression	Interstitial cystitis
Hypochondriasis	Metabolic myopathy
Somatoform pain disorder	Inflammatory myopathy
Malingering	Alzheimer's disease
Hypothyroidism	Meniérè's disease
	Polymyalgia rheumatica

patients with chronic fatigue syndrome have an acute onset of symptoms after an infectious illness, with subsequent persistence of debilitating fatigue and postexertional malaise.[34] Other prominent symptoms include myalgias, sleep disturbances, cognitive impairment, and features suggestive of infections, such as low-grade fevers, pharyngitis, and adenopathy. Despite the attribution of a viral etiology, an infectious cause has never been convincingly demonstrated. About 75 percent of patients meeting the diagnostic criteria of chronic fatigue syndrome also meet the diagnostic criteria for fibromyalgia.

Similar to both fibromyalgia and chronic fatigue syndrome is the *syndrome of multiple chemical sensitivities*. There is no agreed on definition for this syndrome, but it is generally perceived as a multisystem disorder that follows exposure to diverse chemicals at doses below those usually known to cause adverse effects in humans. In one comparative study of multiple chemical sensitivities, chronic fatigue syndrome, and fibromyalgia, all three syndromes were remarkably similar in their demographic profiles and clinical characteristics.[35]

Myofascial Pain and Repetitive Strain

Muscle pain following unaccustomed exertion or soft tissue injury is a universal occurrence. Musculoskeletal pain goes with the "territory" for ballet dancers, musicians, and manual laborers.[36] When does such *expected* muscle pain become a medical disorder? Littlejohn and colleagues have described the epidemic of *repetitive strain syndrome* in Australia that appeared to be driven by generous compensation laws but subsided when these laws were changed.[37]

With increasing age, the musculoskeletal system becomes less tolerant of unaccustomed stresses and repetitive injuries.[38] Hence, with the evolution of time, the continued performance of a job involving repetitive activity may cause unacceptable levels of pain. What is considered *unacceptable* depends on many factors, such as individual coping styles, concomitant illnesses, job satisfaction, and opportunities for compensation. For some patients who have regional pain that is related to the work environment or following an acute trauma, a fibromyalgia syndrome may develop later. The treating physician is then asked to render an opinion as to causality. Currently, such questions cannot be answered with *scientific* precision and need to be answered in terms of *reasonable medical probability*.[39] Contemporary studies on the neurophysiology of pain, in particular the concept of *neuroplasticity* (described later), offer an explanation for the evolution of a regional pain syndrome into a total body pain syndrome.[40]

Secondary Fibromyalgia

Fibromyalgia often occurs in association with other rheumatic disorders and other chronic pain states. For

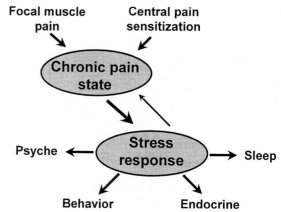

Figure 34–4. Model for symptom generation in fibromyalgia patients. The diverse symptoms of the fibromyalgia syndrome cannot be explained in terms of the classical *medical model*. It is envisaged that persistent focal muscle pain, arising from muscle microlesions, eventually leads to a state of enhanced central pain perception. Depending on a person's response to the burden of chronic pain, secondary physiologic changes and symptoms are generated as part of a generalized stress response. In some patients, the secondary responses, such as catastrophizing, behavioral or deconditioning, and endocrine or growth hormone deficiency, provide a positive feedback loop that amplifies the chronic pain state.

instance, fibromyalgia has been described in about 25 percent of patients with rheumatoid arthritis,[41] 30 percent of patients with systemic lupus erythematosus (SLE),[42] and 50 percent of patients with Sjögren's syndrome.[43] In general, the second rheumatic condition is usually well established and the diagnosis is obvious. In other words, fibromyalgia does not usually antedate rheumatoid arthritis or SLE. One possible exception to this rule is Sjögren's syndrome in some patients.[44]

PATHOPHYSIOLOGY

Considering the total spectrum of the fibromyalgia syndrome (see Fig. 34–1), it is evident that there can be no single unifying pathology. According to the rheumatologic paradigm, widespread pain and multiple tender points are the core features.[1]

The major peripheral pain component of fibromyalgia appears to arise from nociceptors in muscle.[45] Many patients also have a centrally mediated *allodynia* (a pain sensation evoked by light touch) with or without hyperalgesia.[46] Prolonged, unremitting pain is often a major stressor. Thus, one paradigm for trying to understand the fibromyalgia syndrome is to causally link chronic pain and associated stress, which in turn leads to changes affecting the psyche, neuroendocrine system, sleep, and behavior (Fig. 34–4).[47–49] Possible pathophysiologic mechanisms are reviewed in light of this hypothesis.

Muscle Studies

The notion that muscles are a peripheral source of pain in fibromyalgia is based on the following features:

- The patient's attribution to the site of pain[50]
- Increased pain following exertion (typically delayed 24 hours)[49]
- Reduced pain following epidural blockade[51]
- Characteristic myalgic foci (tender points)[1]
- Focal reduction in levels of high-energy phosphates[52]
- Reduced regional pain following trigger point injections[53]
- Focal disruption of muscle oxygenation at tender point areas[54]
- Focal areas of increased electromyographic (EMG) activity on needling of tender point areas[55]

The last four observations suggest that the origin of pain from fibromyalgia muscles is of *focal* rather than *global* origin. Biopsy specimens of trigger point areas in patients with chronic trapezius myalgia and patients with fibromyalgia have shown some *quantitative* changes from normal subjects but no distinct *qualitative* changes. For instance, Henriksson's group described lower levels of high-energy phosphates in both fibromyalgia tender points and myalgic trigger points.[52] It has been hypothesized that focal *muscle microlesions* arise as a result of disordered capillary blood flow and that the subsequent release of algesic molecules (e.g., substance P, bradykinin, K^+ ions, and prostaglandins), sensitizes peripheral *nociceptors* (free nerve endings) to stimuli that were previously perceived as innocuous.[56] Based on the observation that fibromyalgia patients typically describe a delayed onset of pain after unaccustomed exertion, Bennett has hypothesized that the focal microlesions may be a result of postexertional muscle microtrauma.[49] Increased sarcolemmal levels of calcium are the postulated mechanism of postexertional muscle microtrauma.[57] Nuclear magnetic resonance (NMR) spectroscopy has shown an increased prevalence of phosphodiester peaks in fibromyalgia patients compared with those in controls.[58] Phosphodiesters are formed as a result of lipid peroxidation of cell membranes and arise as a consequence of calcium-activated muscle damage.

Multiple muscle studies, including biopsies, electromyography, muscle enzyme analyses, exercise laboratory testing, and NMR spectroscopy, have been unable to show any *global* defect of muscles in fibromyalgia patients.[50, 58–61] However, Elert and associates reported that the muscles of fibromyalgia patients engaging in repetitive muscular activity showed increased EMG activity during a relaxation phase—a time during which the muscles should be electrically silent.[62] The relaxation phase between active muscle contractions is important for permitting normal blood flow, and one study has reported reduced blood flow in exercising fibromyalgia muscle.[60]

Neurophysiology of Muscle Pain

Muscle pain differs from cutaneous pain in several ways:

1. It is usually described as aching or cramping rather than sharp or stabbing.
2. It is poorly localized, whereas cutaneous pain is localized with great accuracy.
3. It is generally referred to other deep somatic structures (muscles, fascia, tendons, ligaments, and joints), whereas cutaneous pain is not referred.

Myogenic pain arises from free nerve endings, or nociceptors, that are responsive to mechanical stretching and squeezing, chemical stimuli (e.g., substance P, bradykinin, K^+ ions), and ischemic muscle contractions.[45] Nociceptor discharge travels to the dorsal root ganglion by thin myelinated (group 3) or unmyelinated (group 4) nerve fibers. The dorsal root ganglia, receiving nociceptive information from muscles, also receive additional input from cutaneous receptors. This phenomenon, called "input convergence," probably accounts for the experience of skin pain and tenderness in patients with fibromyalgia.

It is apparent that patients with severe fibromyalgia have a reduction in pain threshold (allodynia), an increased response to painful stimuli *(hyperalgesia)*, and an increase in the duration of pain after nociceptor stimulation (persistent pain). It has been hypothesized that reduced serotonin levels in the central nervous system (CNS) play a role in these phenomena.[63] Fibromyalgia patients commonly describe an antecedent regional pain syndrome, with the subsequent spread of pain and hyperalgesia to previously uninvolved tissues. This history is counterintuitive to most physicians' notions of neurophysiology. Indeed, the apparent implausibility of pain spread to uninjured areas has often led to the patient being labeled as a malingerer. There is now persuasive evidence that chronic noxious stimuli *sensitize* the central neural structures involved in pain perception.[45, 64–66] This central sensitization, called "neuroplasticity", is probably relevant to the pain experience of fibromyalgia patients.[40]

Arroyo and Cohen, using the technique of electrocutaneous stimulation, reported that the upper limbs of fibromyalgia patients could be characterized as regions of secondary hyperalgesia.[46] Animal experiments have shown that *pathologic* pain results from cellular and molecular changes that bring about an increased transcription of genes encoding algesic neurotransmitters.[40, 45] Increased levels of substance P in the cerebrospinal fluid of fibromyalgia patients may be an example of such increased neurotransmitter production.[67]

Sleep Disturbances

Patients with fibromyalgia sleep poorly. They describe themselves as being light sleepers and as awakening frequently. Moldofsky and others originally reported that such disturbed sleep had an electroencephalographic correlate in the form of an alpha intrusion during stage 4 sleep (delta sleep).[68] Recent

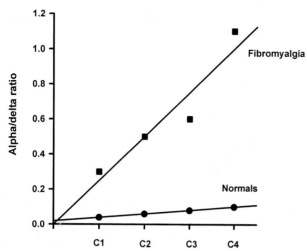

Figure 34–5. Progression of alpha intrusion with sleep cycles. Alpha rhythm (7.6 to 11.4 Hz) on polysomnography often fragments the usual delta rhythm (0.4 to 4.2 Hz) of slow-wave sleep in patients with fibromyalgia—"alpha-delta sleep." This electroencephalographic finding correlates with nonrestorative sleep. In the graph, the ratio of alpha to delta rhythms in successive sleep cycles (C1 to C4) increases progressively in fibromyalgia patients compared with healthy controls (Adapted from Branco J, Atalaia A, Paiva T: Sleep cycles and alpha-delta sleep in fibromyalgia syndrome. J Rheumatol 21:1113–1117, 1994.)

research supports these findings (Fig. 34–5), but it is now appreciated that alpha-delta sleep is not universally present or specific for fibromyalgia.[69]

There are several reasons for the sleep disturbances (Table 34–2). Sleep apnea is particularly common in male fibromyalgia patients[70] but may be more common than is generally recognized in female fibromyalgia patients. The clinical correlates of sleep apnea in women are an "underslung" jaw, a vaulted palette, underweight, and a small oropharyngeal space.[71] Rapid eye movement (REM) sleep is also reduced by about 50 percent in fibromyalgia patients.[69] Interestingly, such REM deficits have been shown to compromise short-term memory in healthy volunteers; memory loss is a common complaint of fibromyalgia patients. Fibromyalgia patients have an altered chro-

Table 34–2. CAUSES OF SLEEP DISTURBANCE IN PATIENTS WITH FIBROMYALGIA

Psychophysiologic insomnia
Poor sleeping habits
Sleep disruption by newborn baby
Pain
Restless leg syndrome
Sleep apnea
Rhinitis
Esophageal reflux
Nocturia
Narcolepsy
Sleeping partner's snoring
Circadian rhythm disorder
Rapid eye movement sleep behavioral disorder

nobiology that is probably related to sleep dysfunction.[72] They typically have a short period of reduced pain and increased energy for accomplishing daily tasks. This window of opportunity occurs at about midday and lasts 2 to 4 hours. By comparison, healthy individuals have good energy levels throughout most of the day, with a mild downswing in the late afternoon.

Neuroendocrine Abnormalities

McCain and colleagues initially described neuroendocrine changes in fibromyalgia patients.[73] Compared with rheumatoid patients, patients with fibromyalgia exhibited a reduced excretion of urinary free cortisol but a paradoxical blunting of the normal evening cortisol trough. Crofford and others have found somewhat similar changes in the hypothalamic-pituitary-adrenal (HPA) axis.[74] Levels of insulin growth factor, or IGF-1 (somatomedin-C), a growth hormone–related peptide, are low in about one third of fibromyalgia patients.[75] This finding may be the result of disturbed stage 4 sleep—the sleep stage that usually coincides with maximum growth hormone production. It seems likely that these neuroendocrine changes, occurring in a subset of fibromyalgia patients, are a secondary rather than a primary problem. The extent to which they affect the symptomatology of patients is not clear.

Psychologic Issues

Studies of clinic patients have shown that fibromyalgia is usually associated with considerable psychologic distress.[76] This is most frequently manifested as varying degrees of depression, anxiety, panic attacks, poor coping mechanisms, and exacerbation of symptoms by stressful situations. About 20 percent of patients with fibromyalgia have major depression, and almost 50 percent have a lifetime history of depression.[12, 77] They also report more problems in dealing with stress and in being satisfied with the quality of their life.[19, 78] Some fibromyalgia patients have been sexually abused as children[79]; such experiences can adversely affect a person's interpretation of pain experiences in adult life.[80] A subset of patients develop maladaptive pain behavior (sometimes called *operant conditioning*) in which they unconsciously perpetuate their sick role by entrenched ideas about the therapeutic values of inactivity. In general, it is thought that the psychologic problems encountered by fibromyalgia patients are secondary to having fibromyalgia rather than vice versa (see Fig. 34–4).[81, 81a] Although fibromyalgia is clearly associated with varying degrees of psychopathology, the weight of contemporary opinion suggests that it cannot be regarded *solely* as a psychiatric diagnosis.[76]

TREATMENT

While readily recognizable, fibromyalgia cannot be considered a distinctive disease entity in terms of a specific pathophysiology. Rather, it is a complex spectrum of problems with considerable variation from patient to patient. This implies that there is no one treatment strategy that is effective in all patients. This singular fact makes the management of fibromyalgia patients both challenging and time-consuming.

Education and Support

In general, treating physicians should reassure the patient that fibromyalgia does not cause crippling or reduced life expectancy and that they are prepared to provide empathic and continuing support. As in any chronic incurable condition, education is an important resource.[82] Patients need to understand that their symptoms cannot be eradicated in toto and that the aim of treatment is to make them more functional but not to eliminate all pain.[83] The role of the physician needs to be recast to that of a supportive "coach," and the role of the patient needs to be proactive.

Psyche

Patients with poor coping strategies often tend to catastrophize adverse life events, which they perceive as being helpless to influence. Psychologic intervention, in terms of improving the internal locus of control and imparting more effective problem solving, is important for such patients. Techniques of cognitive-behavioral therapy seem particularly well suited to bring about these changes and may be enhanced when taught as a part of group therapy.[84, 85] Specific psychologic problems, such as depression, anxiety, alcoholism, and childhood abuse, need to be recognized early and treated appropriately.

Sleep

A careful analysis of sleep should be undertaken to identify any treatable causes of sleep disturbance (see Table 34–2). Patients with sleep apnea usually require treatment with continuous positive airway pressure (CPAP) or surgery. Patients with restless leg syndrome or nocturnal myoclonus are greatly helped by levodopa/carbidopa (Sinemet, 10/100 mg at suppertime) or clonazepam (Klonopin, 0.5 or 1.0 mg at bedtime).[86] Most patients with fibromyalgia seem to derive some benefit from low dosages of tricyclic compound drugs to help with sleep.[87–89] It is worthwhile experimenting with several different compounds with respect to their anticholinergic and antihistamine profiles, because individuals vary greatly in their ability to tolerate and benefit from such medications. Patients who cannot tolerate these drugs may benefit from the cautious use of benzodiazepine-like medications, such as aprazolam,[90] zolpidem,[90a] and zopiclone.[91]

Pain

Attempts to break the pain cycle in order to enable patients to be more functional are especially important. In general, most fibromyalgia patients do not derive a great deal of benefit from nonsteroidal anti-inflammatory drugs, although such agents may take the edge off the pain enough to be therapeutically worthwhile.[92] Prednisone is ineffective.[93] Narcotic analgesics may provide some initial benefit but should be used sparingly and for a defined period only under special circumstances. Tramadol (Ultram), a pain medication with a low potential for addiction that prevents the reuptake of noradrenaline at the level of the spinal cord inhibitory pain neurons, has recently been approved by the Food and Drug Administration. Its use in fibromyalgia needs to be evaluated.

Physical modalities, such as heat, massage, acupuncture, and passive stretching, often provide short-term palliative relief. When the patient has a major focus of regional pain, it may be worthwhile trying a course of trigger point injections using 1 percent procaine or lidocaine.[94] The technique of Fluori-Methane spray and stretch, which can be taught to family members, is a strategy that can minimize repetitive office visits for pain management.[94]

Exercise

Patients with fibromyalgia cannot afford *not* to exercise.[60, 95] However, musculoskeletal pain and severe fatigue are powerful conditioners for inactivity. All patients need to have a home program with muscle stretching, gentle strengthening, and aerobic conditioning. Several points should be stressed about exercise:[96]

1. Exercise is health training, not sports training.
2. Exercise should be non–impact loading.
3. Aerobic exercise should be done three to four times a week at about 70 percent of maximum pulse rate for 20 to 30 minutes. This should be the aim; it may take 6 to 12 months to achieve this level.

Regular exercise needs to become part of the patient's usual lifestyle; it is not merely a 3- to 6-month program to restore a patient to health.

Regular stretching exercises are essential and are best taught by a physical therapist or exercise physiologist. Suitable aerobic exercises include regular walking, a stationary bicycle, or a Nordic track (initially with the patient not using the arm component). Patients who are deconditioned or incapacitated should be started with water therapy using a buoyancy belt (e.g., the Aqua-jogger). The patient should be seen regularly and encouraged to continue with the exercise program. In this respect, the use of an exercise log that is inspected every 2 to 4 months can provide a positive reinforcement to become active.

Multidisciplinary Team Therapy

Because patients with fibromyalgia are often polysymptomatic, they can be very demanding of the physician's time. In the current era of cost-effective medicine, it is often difficult to accommodate the needs of these patients. One solution to this dilemma is to bring together a team of interested health professionals (nurse practitioners, clinical psychologists, exercise physiologists, mental health care workers, and social workers) who are prepared to offer a team approach.[97-99] In this way, groups of 10 to 30 patients can be seen in designated sessions several times a month. Patients usually appreciate meeting others who share similar problems, and the dynamics of group therapy are often a powerful aid to cognitive-behavioral modifications. Such groups can be encouraged to develop a sense of camaraderie in solving mutual problems.

The comprehensive team approach to management of patients with fibromyalgia is now being developed in many academic and nonacademic environments. The effectiveness of this approach has recently been demonstrated in the program at Oregon Health Sciences University.[100]

References

1. Wolfe F, Smythe HA, Yunus MB, Bennett RM, Bombardier C, Goldenberg DL, Tugwell P, Campbell SM, Abeles M, Clark P, Fam AG, Farber SJ, Fiechtner JJ, Franklin CM, Gatter RA, Hamaty D, Lessard J, Lichtbroun AS, Masi AT, McCain GA, Reynolds WJ, Romano TJ, Russell IJ, Sheon RP: The American College of Rheumatology 1990 criteria for the classification of fibromyalgia: Report of the Multicenter Criteria Committee. Arthritis Rheum 33:160–172, 1990.
2. de Blecourt AC, Knipping AA, de Voogd N, van Rijswijk MH: Weather conditions and complaints in fibromyalgia. J Rheumatol 20:1932–1934, 1993.
3. Reilly PA, Littlejohn GO: Peripheral arthralgic presentation of fibrositis/fibromyalgia syndrome. J Rheumatol 19:281–283, 1992.
4. Campbell SM, Clark S, Tindall EA, Forehand ME, Bennett RM: Clinical characteristics of fibrositis: I. A "blinded," controlled study of symptoms and tender points. Arthritis Rheum 26:817–824, 1983.
5. Bennett RM: Confounding features of the fibromyalgia syndrome: A current perspective of differential diagnosis. J Rheumatol Suppl 19:58–61, 1989.
6. Deodhar AA, Fisher RA, Blacker CVR, Woolf AD: Fluid retention syndrome and fibromyalgia. Br J Rheumatol 33:576–582, 1994.
7. Pellegrino MJ: Atypical chest pain as an initial presentation of primary fibromyalgia. Arch Phys Med Rehabil 71:526–528, 1990.
8. Caidahl K, Lurie M, Bake B, Johansson G, Wetterqvist H: Dyspnoea in chronic primary fibromyalgia. J Intern Med 226:265–270, 1989.
9. Blasberg B, Chalmers A: Temporomandibular pain and dysfunction syndrome associated with generalized musculoskeletal pain: A retrospective study. J Rheumatol Suppl 19:87–90, 1989.
10. Dinerman H, Goldenberg DL, Felson DT: A prospective evaluation of 118 patients with the fibromyalgia syndrome: Prevalence of Raynaud's phenomenon, sicca symptoms, ANA, low complement, and Ig deposition at the dermal-epidermal junction. J Rheumatol 13:368–373, 1986.
11. Gerster JC, Hadj Djilani A: Hearing and vestibular abnormalities in primary fibrositis syndrome. J Rheumatol 11:678–680, 1984.
12. Burckhardt CS, O'Reilly CA, Wiens AN, Clark SR, Campbell SM, Bennett RM: Assessing depression in fibromyalgia patients. Arthritis Care Res 7:35–39, 1994.
13. Yunus M, Masi AT, Calabro JJ, Miller KA, Feigenbaum SL: Primary fibromyalgia: Clinical study of 50 patients with matched normal controls. Semin Arthritis Rheum 11:151–171, 1981.
14. Wallace DJ: Genitourinary manifestations of fibrositis: An increased association with the female urethral syndrome. J Rheumatol 17:238–239, 1990.
15. Bennett RM, Clark SR, Campbell SM, Ingram SB, Burckhardt CS, Nelson DL, Porter JM: Symptoms of Raynaud's syndrome in patients with fibromyalgia: A study utilizing the Nielsen test, digital photoplethysmography, and measurements of platelet alpha 2-adrenergic receptors. Arthritis Rheum 34:264–269, 1991.
16. Veale D, Kavanagh G, Fielding JF, Fitzgerald O: Primary fibromyalgia and the irritable bowel syndrome: Different expressions of a common pathogenetic process. Br J Rheumatol 30:220–222, 1991.
17. Croft P, Schollum J, Silman A: Population study of tender point counts and pain as evidence of fibromyalgia. Br Med J 309:696–699, 1994.
18. Wolfe F, Ross K, Anderson J, Russell IJ, Hebert L: The prevalence and characteristics of fibromyalgia in the general population. Arthritis Rheum 38:19–28, 1995.
19. Burckhardt CS, Clark SR, Bennett RM: Fibromyalgia and quality of life: A comparative analysis. J Rheumatol 20:475–479, 1993.
20. Henriksson CM: Long-term effects of fibromyalgia on everyday life: A study of 56 patients. Scand J Rheumatol 23:36–41, 1994.
21. Waylonis GW, Ronan PG, Gordon C: A profile of fibromyalgia in occupational environments. Am J Phys Med Rehabil 73:112–115, 1994.
22. Felson DT, Goldenberg DL: The natural history of fibromyalgia. Arthritis Rheum 29:1522–1526, 1986.
23. Ledingham J, Doherty S, Doherty M: Primary fibromyalgia syndrome—an outcome study. Br J Rheumatol 32:139–142, 1993.
24. Bengtsson A, Backman E, Lindblom B, Skogh T: Long term follow-up of fibromyalgia patients: Clinical symptoms, muscular function, laboratory tests—an eight year comparison study. J Musculoskel Pain 2:67–80, 1994.
25. Asch ES, Bujak DI, Weiss M, Peterson MGE, Weinstein A: Lyme disease: An infectious and postinfectious syndrome. J Rheumatol 21:454–461, 1994.
26. Magnusson T: Extracervical symptoms after whiplash trauma. Cephalalgia 14:223–227; discussion, 181–182, 1994.
27. Lapossy E, Maleitzke R, Hrycaj P, Mennet W, Muller W: The frequency of transition of chronic low back pain to fibromyalgia. Scand J Rheumatol 24:29–33, 1995.
28. Culclasure TF, Enzenauer RJ, West SG: Post-traumatic stress disorder presenting as fibromyalgia. Am J Med 94:548–549, 1993.
29. Greenfield S, Fitzcharles MA, Esdaile JM: Reactive fibromyalgia syndrome. Arthritis Rheum 35:678–681, 1992.
30. Simms RW, Zerbini CA, Ferrante N, Anthony J, Felson DT, Craven DE: Fibromyalgia syndrome in patients infected with human immunodeficiency virus. Am J Med 92:368–374, 1992.
31. Leventhal LJ, Naides SJ, Freundlich B: Fibromyalgia and parvovirus infection. Arthritis Rheum 34:1319–1324, 1991.
32. Alonso-Ruiz A, Hoz-Martinez A, Zea-Mendoza AC: Fibromyalgia syndrome as a late complication of toxic oil syndrome. J Rheumatol 12:1207–1208, 1985.
33. Goldenberg DL, Simms RW, Geiger A, Komaroff AL: High frequency of fibromyalgia in patients with chronic fatigue seen in a primary care practice. Arthritis Rheum 33:381–387, 1990.
34. Komaroff AL, Buchwald D: Symptoms and signs of chronic fatigue syndrome. Rev Infect Dis 13:S8–S11, 1991.
35. Buchwald D, Garrity D: Comparison of patients with chronic fatigue syndrome, fibromyalgia, and multiple chemical sensitivities. Arch Intern Med 154:2049–2053, 1994.
36. Hoppmann RA, Patrone NA: A review of musculoskeletal problems in instrumental musicians. Semin Arthritis Rheum 19:117–126, 1995.
37. Littlejohn GO: Fibrositis/fibromyalgia syndrome in the workplace. Rheum Dis Clin North Am 15:45–60, 1989.
38. Editorial: Ageing at work: Consequences for industry and individual. Lancet 340:87–88, 1993.
39. Bennett RM: Disabling fibromyalgia: Appearance versus reality. J Rheumatol 20:1821–1824, 1993.
40. Coderre TJ, Katz J, Vaccarino AL, Melzack R: Contribution of central neuroplasticity to pathological pain: Review of clinical and experimental evidence. Pain 52:259–285, 1993.
41. Wolfe F, Cathey MA, Kleinheksel SM: Fibrositis (fibromyalgia) in rheumatoid arthritis. J Rheumatol 11:814–818, 1984.
42. Middleton GD, McFarlin JE, Lipsky PE: The prevalence and clinical impact of fibromyalgia in systemic lupus erythematosus. Arthritis Rheum 37:1181–1188, 1994.
43. Vitali C, Tavoni A, Neri R, Castrogiovanni P, Pasero G, Bombardieri S: Fibromyalgia features in patients with primary Sjögren's syndrome: Evidence of a relationship with psychological depression. Scand J Rheumatol 18:21–27, 1989.
44. Bonafede RP, Downey DC, Bennett RM: An association of fibromyalgia with primary Sjögren's syndrome: A prospective study of 72 patients. J Rheumatol 22:133–136, 1995.

45. Mense S: Nociception from skeletal muscle in relation to clinical muscle pain. Pain 54:241–289, 1993.
46. Arroyo JF, Cohen ML: Abnormal responses to electrocutaneous stimulation in fibromyalgia. J Rheumatol 20:1925–1931, 1993.
47. Yunus MB: Towards a model of pathophysiology of fibromyalgia: Aberrant central pain mechanisms with peripheral modulation [editorial]. J Rheumatol 19:846–850, 1992.
48. Bennett RM: Beyond fibromyalgia: Ideas on etiology and treatment. J Rheumatol Suppl 19:185–191, 1989.
49. Bennett RM: The origin of myopain: An integrated hypothesis of focal muscle changes and sleep disturbance in patients with the fibromyalgia syndrome. J Musculoskel Pain 1:95–112, 1993.
50. Bengtsson A, Henriksson KG, Jorfeldt L, Kagedal B, Lennmarken C, Lindstrom F: Primary fibromyalgia: A clinical and laboratory study of 55 patients. Scand J Rheumatol 15:340–347, 1986.
51. Bengtsson M, Bengtsson A, Jorfeldt L: Diagnostic epidural opioid blockade in primary fibromyalgia at rest and during exercise. Pain 39:171–180, 1989.
52. Bengtsson A, Henriksson KG, Larsson J: Reduced high-energy phosphate levels in the painful muscles of patients with primary fibromyalgia. Arthritis Rheum 29:817–821, 1986.
53. Jaeger B, Skootsky SA: Double blind, controlled study of different myofascial trigger point injection techniques. Pain 31:S292, 1987.
54. Lund N, Bengtsson A, Thorborg P: Muscle tissue oxygen pressure in primary fibromyalgia. Scand J Rheumatol 15:165–173, 1986.
55. Durette MR, Rodriquez AA, Agre JC, Silverman JL: Needle electromyographic evaluation of patients with myofascial or fibromyalgic pain. Am J Phys Med Rehabil 70:154–156, 1991.
56. Henriksson KG: Chronic muscular pain: Aetiology and pathogenesis. Baillieres Clin Rheumatol 8:703–719, 1994.
57. Armstrong RB, Warren GL, Warren JA: Mechanisms of exercise-induced muscle fibre injury. Sports Med 12:184–207, 1991.
58. Jubrias SA, Bennett RM, Klug GA: Increased incidence of a resonance in the phosphodiester region of 31P nuclear magnetic resonance spectra in the skeletal muscle of fibromyalgia patients. Arthritis Rheum 37:801–807, 1994.
59. Simms RW, Roy SH, Hrovat M, Anderson JJ, Skrinar G, LePoole SR, Zerbini CA, de Luca C, Jolesz F: Lack of association between fibromyalgia syndrome and abnormalities in muscle energy metabolism. Arthritis Rheum 37:794–800, 1994.
60. Bennett RM, Clark SR, Goldberg L, Nelson D, Bonafede RP, Porter J, Specht D: Aerobic fitness in patients with fibrositis: A controlled study of respiratory gas exchange and 133xenon clearance from exercising muscle. Arthritis Rheum 32:454–460, 1989.
61. Yunus MD, Kalyan-Raman UP, Masi AT, Aldag JC: Electromicroscopic studies of muscle biopsy in primary fibromyalgia syndrome: A controlled and blinded study. J Rheumatol 16:97–101, 1989.
62. Elert JE, Rantapää Dahlqvist SB, Henriksson-Larsen K, Gerdle B: Increased EMG activity during short pauses in patients with primary fibromyalgia. Scand J Rheumatol 18:321–323, 1989.
63. Russell IJ: Neurohormonal aspects of fibromyalgia syndrome. Rheum Dis Clin North Am 15:149–168, 1989.
64. Hoheisel U, Mense S: Response behavior of CAT dorsal horn neurones receiving input from skeletal muscle and other deep somatic tissues. J Physiol 426:265–280, 1990.
65. Dubner R: Hyperalgesia and expanded receptive fields. Pain 48:3–4, 1992.
66. Dickenson AH, Sullivan AF: NMDA receptors and central hyperalgesic states. Pain 46:344–345, 1991.
67. Russell IJ, Orr MD, Littman B, Vipraio GA, Alboukrek D, Michalek JE, Lopez Y, MacKillip F: Elevated cerebrospinal fluid levels of substance P in patients with the fibromyalgia syndrome. Arthritis Rheum 37:1593–1601, 1994.
68. Moldofsky H, Scarisbrick P, England R, Smythe H: Musculoskeletal symptoms and non-REM sleep disturbance in patients with "fibrositis syndrome" and healthy subjects. Psychosom Med 37:341–351, 1975.
69. Branco J, Atalaia A, Paiva T: Sleep cycles and alpha-delta sleep in fibromyalgia syndrome. J Rheumatol 21:1113–1117, 1994.
70. May KP, West SG, Baker MR, Everett DW: Sleep apnea in male patients with the fibromyalgia syndrome. Am J Med 94:505–508, 1993.
71. Guilleminault C, Stoohs R, Kim YD, Chervin R, Black J, Clerk A: Upper airway sleep-disordered breathing in women. Ann Intern Med 122:493–501, 1995.
72. Moldofsky H: Chronobiological influences on fibromyalgia syndrome: Theoretical and therapeutic implications. Baillieres Clin Rheumatol 8:801–810, 1994.
73. McCain GA, Tilbe KS: Diurnal hormone variation in fibromyalgia syndrome: A comparison with rheumatoid arthritis. J Rheumatol Suppl 19:154–157, 1989.
74. Crofford LJ, Pillemer SR, Kalogeras KT, Cash JM, Michelson D, Kling MA, Sternberg EM, Gold PW, Chrousos GP, Wilder RL: Hypothalamic-pituitary-adrenal axis perturbations in patients with fibromyalgia. Arthritis Rheum 37:1583–1592, 1994.
75. Bennett RM, Clark SR, Campbell SM, Burckhardt CS: Low levels of somatomedin C in patients with the fibromyalgia syndrome: A possible link between sleep and muscle pain. Arthritis Rheum 35:1113–1116, 1992.
76. Yunus MB: Psychological aspects of fibromyalgia syndrome: A component of the dysfunctional spectrum syndrome. Baillieres Clin Rheumatol 8:811–837, 1994.
77. Hudson JI, Goldenberg DL, Pope HG Jr, Keck PE Jr, Schlesinger L: Comorbidity of fibromyalgia with medical and psychiatric disorders. Am J Med 92:363–367, 1992.
78. Uveges JM, Parker JC, Smarr KL, McGowan JF, Lyon MG, Irvin WS, Meyer AA, Buckelew SP, Morgan RK, Delmonico RL, Hewett JE, Kay DR: Psychological symptoms in primary fibromyalgia syndrome: Relationship to pain, life stress, and sleep disturbance. Arthritis Rheum 33:1279–1283, 1990.
79. Taylor ML, Trotter DR, Csuka ME: The prevalence of sexual abuse in women with fibromyalgia. Arthritis Rheum 38:229–234, 1995.
80. Scarinci IC, McDonald-Haile J, Bradley LA, Richter JE: Altered pain perception and psychosocial features among women with gastrointestinal disorders and history of abuse: A preliminary model. Am J Med 97:108–118, 1994.
81. Gamsa A: The role of psychological factors in chronic pain: II. A critical appraisal. Pain 57:17–29, 1994.
81a. Aaron CA, Bradley LA, Alaron GS, Alexander RW, Triana-Alexander M, Martin MY, Alberts KR: Psychiatric diagnoses in patients with fibromyalgia are related to health care seeking behavior rather than illness. Arthritis Rheum 39:436–445, 1996.
82. Burckhardt CS, Mannerkorpi K, Hedenberg L, Bjelle A: A randomized, controlled clinical trial of education and physical training for women with fibromyalgia. J Rheumatol 21:714–720, 1994.
83. Rosen NB: Physical medicine and rehabilitation approaches to the management of myofascial pain and fibromyalgia syndromes. Baillieres Clin Rheumatol 8:881–916, 1994.
84. Goldenberg DL, Kaplan KH, Nadeau MG, Brodeur C, Smith S, Schmid CH: A controlled study of a stress-reduction, cognitive-behavioral treatment program in fibromyalgia. J Musculoskel Pain 2:53–66, 1994.
85. Nielson WR, Walker C, McCain GA: Cognitive behavioral treatment of fibromyalgia syndrome: Preliminary findings. J Rheumatol 19:98–103, 1992.
86. Montplaisir J, Lapierre O, Warnes H, Pelletier G: The treatment of the restless leg syndrome with or without periodic leg movements in sleep. Sleep 15:391–395, 1992.
87. Goldenberg DL: A review of the role of tricyclic medications in the treatment of fibromyalgia syndrome. J Rheumatol Suppl 19:137–139, 1989.
88. Bennett RM, Gatter RA, Campbell SM, Andrews RP, Clark SR, Scarola JA: A comparison of cyclobenzaprine and placebo in the management of fibrositis: A double-blind controlled study. Arthritis Rheum 31:1535–1542, 1988.
89. Carette S, Bell MJ, Reynolds WJ, Haraoui B, McCain GA, Bykerk VP, Edworthy SM, Baron M, Koehler BE, Fam AG, Bellamy N, Guimont C: Comparison of amitriptyline, cyclobenzaprine, and placebo in the treatment of fibromyalgia. Arthritis Rheum 37:32–40, 1994.
90. Russell IJ, Fletcher EM, Michalek JE, McBroom PC, Hester GG: Treatment of primary fibrositis/fibromyalgia syndrome with ibuprofen and alprazolam: A double-blind, placebo-controlled study. Arthritis Rheum 34:552–560, 1991.
90a. Moldofsky H, Lue FA, Moudy C, Roth-Schechtner B, Reynolds WJ: The effect of zolpidem in patients with fibromyalgia: Double-blind, placebo-controlled, modified crossover study. J Rheumatol 23:529–533, 1996.
91. Drewes AM, Andreasen A, Jennum P, Nielsen KD: Zopiclone in the treatment of sleep abnormalities in fibromyalgia. Scand J Rheumatol 20:288–293, 1991.
92. Simms RW: Controlled trials of therapy in fibromyalgia syndrome. Baillieres Clin Rheumatol 8:917–934, 1994.
93. Clark S, Tindall E, Bennett RM: A double blind crossover trial of prednisone versus placebo in the treatment of fibrositis. J Rheumatol 12:980–983, 1985.
94. Travell JG, Simons DG: Myofascial Pain and Dysfunction: The Trigger Point Manual. Baltimore, Williams & Wilkins, 1983.
95. McCain GA, Bell DA, Mai FM, Halliday PD: A controlled study of the effects of a supervised cardiovascular fitness training program on the manifestations of primary fibromyalgia. Arthritis Rheum 31:1135–1141, 1988.
96. Clark SR: Prescribing exercise for fibromyalgia patients. Arthritis Care Res 7:221–225, 1994.
97. Bennett RM: A multidisciplinary approach to treating fibromyalgia. In Vaeroy H, Merskey H (eds): Progress in Fibromyalgia and Myofascial Pain. New York, Elsevier, 1993, p 393.
98. Masi AT: Management of fibromyalgia syndrome: A person-centered approach. J Musculoskel Med 11:27–37, 1994.
99. Bennett RM: Multidisciplinary group program to treat fibromyalgia patients. In Goldenberg DL (ed): Rheum Dis Clin North Am 22(2):351–367, 1996.
100. Bennett RM, Burckhardt CS, Clark SR, O'Reilly CA, Wiens AN, Campbell SM: Group treatment of fibromyalgia: A 6-month outpatient program. J Rheumatol 23:521–528, 1996.

CHAPTER 35

Joel M. Kremer

Nutrition and Rheumatic Diseases

Although it has been appreciated for some time that disease processes can interfere with adequate nutrition, we are only now beginning to understand how altered nutritional status contributes to the pathogenesis of disease. As a corollary, it is now known that certain dietary manipulations can result in improvements in the inflammatory disease process. These principles represent an evolution of thinking from the relatively recent past when contributors to the field believed it extremely unlikely that dietary manipulation could affect patients with inflammatory disease. Appreciation of the possible role of nutritional manipulation in inflammatory disease has increased, however, along with the understanding of immunity, eicosanoid metabolism, and cellular biology. Epidemiologic studies have confirmed the role of diet in other disease processes, such as vascular and gastrointestinal disease.[1, 2] Surprisingly, improvements in mortality from cardiovascular disease in some large population studies are not linked solely to favorable changes in cholesterol, hypertension, or smoking profiles, but also to alteration of other biologic processes through the intake of dietary fatty acids.[3] Paralleling the emergence of data on the role of diet in disease states is the realization that our current dietary habits are altered from those that our species have adapted to during almost the entire span of human history (Table 35–1).[4, 5] Circumstantial evidence has linked an increased incidence of cancer and cardiovascular and gastrointestinal disease to high-fat, low-fiber diets.

ROLE OF PROTEIN ENERGY MALNUTRITION AND METABOLIC RESPONSE TO INFLAMMATION

The catabolic effect of inflammatory disease is multifactorial and may lead to weight loss through a variety of mechanisms. Fever is associated with increased energy expenditure and thus increased caloric requirements to maintain body weight. Catecholamine-mediated increases in lipolysis and hepatic and muscular glycogenolysis occur along with hyperglycemia and hypoinsulinemia to increase energy substrates in the acute phase response to injury.[6] After a few days, hyperinsulinemia and increased protein catabolism occur in what Blackburn and Bistrian

called the adaptive phase of metabolic response to stress or injury.[6] The increased amino acids may then serve as precursors for hepatic production of acute phase reactants and gluconeogenesis. Increased production of eicosanoids and cytokines associated with the inflammatory state lead to an enhanced catabolic effect and increased protein breakdown.

Weight loss of 5 to 10 percent is associated with little functional impairment,[7] although it should be considered to be of potential clinical significance if it occurs over a period of 1 to 6 months, respectively. Protein-calorie malnutrition is subdivided into marasmus and kwashiorkor. *Marasmus* is defined as a weight below 80 percent of ideal weight calculated from standardized tables of height and weight with preservation of serum protein levels and immune function. *Kwashiorkor* may be associated with a similar degree of weight loss, but has the additional factor of lowered serum protein levels and compromised immune function. Patients with the hypoalbuminemic malnutrition of kwashiorkor have a significantly higher mortality rate as a result of infections and other metabolic stress.

Table 35–1. COMPARISON OF THE LATE PALEOLITHIC DIET, CURRENT AMERICAN DIET, AND U.S. DIETARY RECOMMENDATIONS

	Late Paleolithic Diet	Current American Diet	U.S. Senate Select Committee Recommendations*
Total dietary energy (%)			
Protein	34	12	12
Carbohydrate	45	46	58
Fat	21	42	30
P:S ratio	1.41	0.44	1
Cholesterol (mg)	591	600	300
Fiber (g)	45.7	19.7	30–60
Sodium (mg)	690	2300–6900	1100–3300
Calcium (mg)	1580	740	800–1200
Ascorbic acid (mg)	392.3	87.7	45

From Eaton SB, Konner M.: Paleolithic nutrition: A consideration of its nature and current implications. N Engl J Med 312:283, 1985. Reprinted with permission from *The New England Journal of Medicine.*
*Select committee on Nutrition and Human Needs, United States Senate: Dietary Goals for the United States. Washington, DC, Government Printing Office, 1977.
Abbreviation: P:S, polyunsaturated:saturated fats.

521

ROLE OF NUTRITION

Rheumatoid Arthritis

Interest in the possible role of nutrition in the pathogenesis of the rheumatic diseases is not new. An early study analyzed dietary intake in the period preceding the onset of rheumatoid arthritis in an attempt to determine whether altered nutrition could be linked to the development of disease.[8] Information obtained from patient recall indicated that there were no significant dietary differences between patients with arthritis and the population at large. A later investigation compared the nutritional status of patients with rheumatoid arthritis to those with osteoarthritis.[9] Patients with osteoarthritis were found to be 15 pounds overweight on average, whereas patients with rheumatoid arthritis were an average of 10.3 pounds underweight. The groups did not differ in intake of protein, fat, carbohydrate, vitamins, or minerals, although both groups had a high prevalence of deficient vitamin intake.

More recent investigations have assessed nutrition in patients with rheumatoid arthritis using a 3-day food record, a reliable method of diet assessment. Deficient dietary intake of folic acid, zinc, magnesium, and pyridoxine have been reported by two independent groups of investigators.[10, 11] Intake of other nutrients, including fat, protein, and carbohydrate, was reported to be similar to age-matched subjects in one investigation.[10]

A nutritional assessment of 50 patients with rheumatoid arthritis involved anthropometric measurements, including triceps skin fold thickness and body mass index calculated from height, weight, and upper arm muscle circumference, as well as biochemical measurements of nutrition.[12] Patients were judged to be malnourished if they had a reduction in one anthropometric measurement in conjunction with a reduction in two or more biochemical indices. By these criteria, 13 patients (26 percent) were malnourished. When the dietary history was assessed, no differences in dietary intake could be found between these individuals and those with normal nutritional status. Malnourished patients were more likely to have severe rheumatoid arthritis than those without malnutrition. In addition, significantly lower values were obtained for all anthropometric measurements in the patients with rheumatoid arthritis compared with a control population. Decreased weight and triceps skin fold thickness occurred twice as frequently as a significant reduction in upper arm muscle circumference. Because dietary intake was judged to be adequate in these patients, it was suggested that the increased demand of the inflammatory state placed a greater burden on the metabolism of certain essential nutrients. Rheumatoid cachexia has been reported in patients with elevated serum levels of tumor necrosis factor-α (TNF-α).[13]

Juvenile Rheumatoid Arthritis

Dietary assessments of children with juvenile rheumatoid arthritis were reported in two Swedish studies.[14, 15] Biochemical measures and anthropometric measurements were examined in 26 11- to 16-year-old girls with juvenile chronic arthritis and matched healthy control subjects. Arm muscle circumference and serum creatinine levels were lower in the children with arthritis. Significant inverse correlations were observed between disease activity and concentrations of albumin, prealbumin, and retinol-binding protein. Using the same definition of malnutrition as in the study of adult patients with rheumatoid arthritis previously discussed,[12] the researchers found that five girls with chronic arthritis (19 percent) fit the definition of malnutrition. The intake of calories and protein did not differ from the control population. An analysis of nutrient intake by means of a 4-day dietary history in the same population failed to reveal any significant differences from controls. Children with arthritis were, however, observed to derive a greater percentage of their energy requirements from fat and a lower percentage from carbohydrates than did controls. Another study observed increased spinal bone mass in children with arthritis given supplemental calcium and vitamin D.[16]

Independent investigations have thus reached similar conclusions about the nutritional status of patients with rheumatoid and juvenile chronic arthritis: Patients with active disease require increased dietary energy and protein and frequently exhibit deficiencies in micronutrients, including selenium, zinc, magnesium, vitamin C, and vitamin A. They have a high intake of fat, particularly saturated fatty acids, which could have significant effects on immune function. These nutritional alterations are at times associated with frank malnutrition. The appreciation of the less than optimal dietary and nutritional status of patients with rheumatic disease is poor among most practitioners who treat these conditions. It is therefore apparent that considerable potentials exist for improving general well-being, with a greater attention to the overall nutritional status of patients with rheumatic problems.

FREE RADICALS AND NUTRITION

A compound with unpaired free electrons is termed a *free radical*, and some of the most reactive of these compounds contain oxygen. Free radicals extract electrons from stable compounds in an attempt to stabilize themselves, and in the process they create new free radicals.[17] The rapidly proliferating cells of the immune system are uniquely prone to oxidative damage from free radicals, which can also affect the activity of thromboxane, prostaglandin, and leukotriene species.[18]

The phospholipid bilayer of cell membranes contains polyunsaturated fatty acids, which can be common sites for free radical reactions (Fig. 35–1). Membrane damage from lipid peroxidation results in the formation of unstable lipid peroxyl radicals, which can further damage the membrane in a snowball-like effect.[17] Potentially toxic products of lipid membrane peroxidation include malondialdehyde, volatile substances such as ethane and pentane, cross-linked membrane lipids, conjugated dienes, and protein-lipid adducts.[19]

Free radicals are also essential to normal immune competence.[20, 21] Intracellular free radical production is part of the host response necessary for the killing of invading microorganisms. Free radical reactions are associated with the release of arachidonic acid and the conversion of arachidonate to eicosanoids and subsequent eicosanoid metabolism.[22] These substances are in turn essential in the functioning of a normal immune system.[23] When considering the production and modulation of free radicals, therefore,

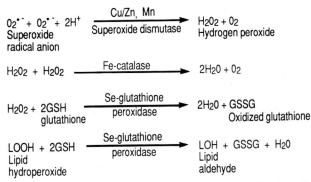

Figure 35–2. Antioxidant metalloenzyme reactions. Nutritionally essential elements are not antioxidants until they are incorporated into their metalloenzyme ligand. Cu, copper; Zn, zinc; Mn, manganese; Fe, iron; Se, selenium. (From Bendich A: Antioxidant micronutrients and immune functions. Ann NY Acad Sci 587:168–180, 1990.)

the critical issue is the balance between potentially destructive reactions and naturally occurring free radical generation, which is essential for normal immune competence.

Several naturally occurring enzymes inactivate reactive oxygen molecules. Antioxidant metalloenzymes interfere with the production of free radicals by inactivating precursor molecules. Superoxide dismutase exists in two forms, either of which can inactivate the superoxide anion. There is a manganese-containing superoxide dismutase in mitochondria and a copper-zinc–containing superoxide dismutase in the cytoplasm (Fig. 35–2). Both of these reactions produce hydrogen peroxide (H_2O_2). An iron-containing catalase found in cytoplasmic peroxisomes catalyzes the decomposition of H_2O_2 to oxygen and water. Selenium is an essential component of two glutathione peroxidases that inactivate H_2O_2, lipid peroxides, and phospholipid peroxides.

The nutritionally essential mineral elements copper, zinc, iron, manganese, and selenium are not antioxidants until they are incorporated into the antioxidant enzymes.[17] Further addition of these elements to the system by dietary intake does not enhance the activity of the antioxidative enzymes once the system is saturated. Circulating levels of these enzymes are lower than intracellular concentrations. The balance between extracellular free radical formation and release and antioxidant enzyme protection may be important in the inflammation and tissue destruction of several immune-mediated inflammatory diseases.

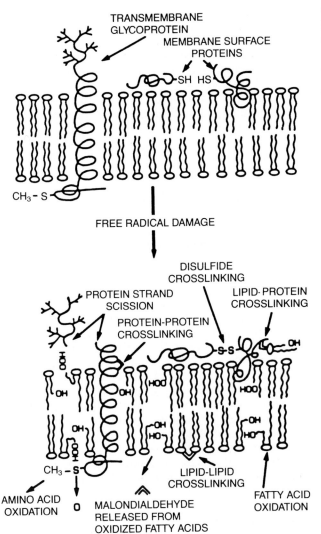

Figure 35–1. Free radical damage to lipid membranes and proteins associated with cell membranes. (From Bendich A: Antioxidant micronutrients and immune functions. Ann NY Acad Sci 587:168–180, 1990.)

ANTIOXIDANT VITAMINS

Beta-Carotene

The carotenoids are red-yellow pigments found in all photosynthesizing plants. There are more than 500 carotenoids, but only a small number of these compounds can be synthesized to vitamin A. Cleavage of beta-carotene, however, results in two molecules of vitamin A, which makes it unique among the carotenoids. In contrast to vitamin A, beta-carotene is a potent antioxidant and can also function as an immunostimulant. Enhancement of activation markers of human peripheral blood mononuclear cells was observed in vitro after exposure to carotenoids.[24] In models of animal tumorigenesis, both cytotoxic T lymphocyte functions and macrophage secretion of TNF were increased following carotenoid administration.[25] These findings are part of a body of evidence that suggests that carotenoid ingestion is associated with important chemoprotective effects that are separate from their provitamin A activity.

Vitamin E

Vitamin E (α-tocopherol) is the major lipid soluble antioxidant found in cells. Vitamin E protects the unsaturated double bonds of the fatty acids in the phospholipid bilayer from oxidation. It accomplishes this by donating electrons to lipid peroxide and other radicals, and in this way can interrupt the chain reaction of free radical damage to the cell membrane. The antioxidant activity of vitamin E is regenerated by electron donation from vitamin C, glutathione, and other antioxidants.

Vitamin E is critical to maintaining the normal function of the immune system. T cells are more susceptible to membrane peroxidative damage than B cells, and peroxidative damage has been associated with the loss of certain T cell receptor activities.[26] T cells are therefore more sensitive to vitamin E status, even though the vitamin E content of both T and B lymphocytes is more than ten times that found in red blood cells.[27] The macrophage membrane expresses decreased Ia antigen in the vitamin E–deficient state. Phagocytic function is diminished in the presence of vitamin E deficiency in both animal and human studies.[28]

Vitamin C

Vitamin C (ascorbic acid) is water soluble and is important in decreasing free radical reactions in both intracellular and extracellular fluids. It is also required for the hydroxylation of proline and lysine in the production of collagen and is involved in several enzymatic reactions in the formation of neuropeptides. Neutrophils and mononuclear cells maintain concentrations of vitamin C that are approximately 150 times that found in serum.[29] Vitamin C has been shown to increase neutrophil and monocyte chemotaxis in vitro in experimental models.[30]

Plasma and platelet ascorbic acid levels have been demonstrated to be low in patients with rheumatoid arthritis who take high doses of aspirin.[31] The decrease was thought to be from either impaired tissue uptake or increased urinary excretion. Lowered ascor-

bate levels may be caused by superoxide-associated oxidation at inflammatory sites. Scorbutic guinea pigs develop lesions resembling rheumatoid arthropathy, prompting a suggestion that synovial vitamin C deficiency could contribute to rheumatoid synovitis.[31] An early study of vitamin C supplementation in patients with rheumatoid arthritis failed to show any effect.[32]

Free radicals derived from phagocytes are autotoxic to cells in their immediate environment, causing inhibition of chemotaxis, phagocytosis, and antimicrobial activity.[33] Reactive oxygen species also inhibit proliferation of T and B lymphocytes as well as the cytotoxic activity of natural killer cells.[34] Neutrophil-derived production of hydrogen peroxide and hypochlorous acid (HOCl) are the most potent mediators of immunosuppression.[35] At physiologically relevant concentrations, ascorbate protects neutrophil metabolic activity and function from HOCl-, but not H_2O_2-, mediated inhibition.[36] Ascorbate is the first-line plasma antioxidant in the defense against phagocyte-derived reactive oxidants; only when it is depleted does lipid peroxidation occur.[37] By neutralizing granulocyte-derived HOCl, ascorbate maintains host defenses by sustaining the function of phagocytes and bystander lymphocytes by protecting them from oxidative damage.[36] Vitamin C may also enhance immune responses indirectly by maintaining optimal levels of vitamin E. It does this by donating an electron to the α-tocopherol molecule to reestablish the latter's antioxidant activity.

Vitamin D

Dietary deficiency of vitamin D may contribute to osteopenia in patients with rheumatoid arthritis and has been linked to cortical thinning and spontaneous fractures of long bones in this condition.[38] Vitamin D supplementation may have some beneficial effect in the treatment of psoriasis.[39] 1,25-dihydroxyvitamin D_3 has inhibitory effects in vitro on psoriatic fibroblast proliferation[40] and has been shown to inhibit the effects of interleukin (IL)-1B on prostaglandin production from human fibroblasts. It has significant effects on the T lymphocyte proliferative response to mitogen stimulation[41] and has demonstrated effects on cytokine production.[42] 1,24-dihydroxyvitamin D_3 can potentiate the inhibitory effects of cyclosporine on helper T cells from patients with rheumatoid arthritis.[43] An open, uncontrolled study using increasing dosages of 1,25(OH)$_2$D$_3$ over 6 months showed significant improvement in several clinical parameters of psoriatic arthritis disease activity in a small number of patients who completed the study.[44]

TRACE ELEMENTS

Before considering the effects of certain trace elements on the immune response and inflammatory disease, it is appropriate to first examine certain related areas of their metabolism and processing. Copper, zinc, and iron are bound to metalloproteinases, which are metal-binding proteins found within the intestinal mucosa.[45] Because these different metals compete for binding with the same proteins, there may be a reciprocal relation between high dietary levels of certain elements and a deficiency in others.[46]

Increased circulating levels of the cytokines IL-1, IL-6, and TNF may affect the availability of trace elements by inducing the production of increased metalloproteinases within the liver and intestine. This increased metalloproteinase production results in sequestration of these elements so that they are less readily available to peripheral tissues.[46] Thus, the diets of patients with inflammatory disease may have adequate iron and zinc but inadequate levels at metabolically important sites, with iron bound to increased cytokine-induced ferritin within the macrophages and liver and zinc bound to the excess metalloproteinases in liver and gut.[47] Teleologically, the cytokine-induced decreased concentrations of iron and zinc may have enhanced host defenses against infection or parasitism, since iron is required for bacterial replication and zinc has a natural anti-inflammatory role.[48]

Zinc

Zinc has been known to be an essential element for growth for more than 100 years. It is essential for a large and diverse collection of enzymes involved in multiple areas of normal metabolic functioning. Only iron exceeds zinc in total body tissue concentrations. It is considerably less reactive and less toxic than copper. Dietary sources include protein derived from meat, fish, or dairy products, and total body storage reserves are thought to be somewhat limited. Absorption of zinc is diminished by ingestion of copper or iron. As is the case with iron and copper, increased cytokine production in inflammatory disease can result in increased binding of zinc to metallothioneins and decreased serum and leukocyte zinc concentrations.[48] This situation may be compounded in patients who regularly consume iron supplements, since this interferes with zinc absorption.

The unexpected incidence of autoimmune disease after treatment with D-penicillamine has been linked to the ability of D-penicillamine to chelate zinc, as well as magnesium and pyridoxine.[49] Zinc can function as a lymphocyte mitogen when added in vitro to experimental systems.[50] The process of activation is thought to be initiated through monocyte processing of a zinc–transferrin complex. Zinc has been demonstrated to enhance natural killer cell activity in vitro in the presence of interferon-α or -γ.

The rationale for trials using zinc in inflammatory diseases has been summarized by Whitehouse.[51] It is derived from a collection of evidence showing the following:

- A tendency for decreased zinc concentrations at critical tissue stores in inflammatory disease
- Decreased absorption associated with iron therapy
- The importance of zinc to normal immune functioning
- The tendency of certain drugs such as D-penicillamine and corticosteroids to suppress zinc concentrations
- Depressed oral intake of zinc in dietary surveys[10, 11] and serum measurements of patients with rheumatoid arthritis
- The anti-inflammatory effect of zinc complexes in chronic models of inflammation[52]

The clinical studies of zinc supplementation, however, have yielded unconvincing mixed results.[53] Because zinc plays an important role as a cofactor in collagen synthesis, it has been proposed that zinc deficiency contributes to altered collagen metabolism in the osteoporosis seen in patients with rheumatoid arthritis. Researchers in the field retain a good deal of interest in the potential role of zinc therapy in the rheumatic diseases.

Selenium

Selenium was recognized to be an essential nutrient in 1957. It exerts a myriad of effects on the immune system and functions through several different pathways that have been extensively reviewed.[54] Spallholz and colleagues[55] summarized its three major functions: (1) reduction of organic and inorganic peroxides; (2) metabolism of hydroperoxides, which are intermediate steps in the metabolism of prostaglandins and leukotrienes derived from arachidonic acid; and (3) modulation of the respiratory burst through the control of superoxide (O_2^-) and hydrogen peroxide generation.

The effect of selenium on immune function is derived from the selenium-dependent enzymes glutathione peroxidase and phospholipidhydroperoxide. The former is responsible for antioxidant activities in reactions described earlier in this chapter in the section on free radicals and nutrition (see Fig. 35–2). Both enzymes participate in the reduction of prostaglandin (PG) G_2 in the arachidonic acid cascade leading to the production of thromboxane A_2, prostacyclin, and prostaglandins.[55] They also participate in the production of leukotrienes and lipoxins through the reduction of the hydroperoxy intermediates.[56] Eicosanoid synthesis is significantly diminished in the absence of selenium.[57] It is likely that both the anti-inflammatory and immune-modulating effects of selenium are mediated by means of the effect of its ligand enzymes on the production of eicosanoids and the reduction of hydroperoxides. Dietary supplementation of selenium is associated with increased production of superoxide in an animal model.[58] It may therefore exert cytotoxic, protective, or modulatory effects in different biologic systems.

Because selenium's ligand enzyme glutathione peroxidase catalyzes the reduction of peroxides and increased levels of these reactive elements are found in serum and synovial fluid of some patients with rheumatoid arthritis, there has been some interest in the selenium status of these patients as well as those with other arthritic conditions. There are conflicting reports of selenium–glutathione peroxidase status in patients with rheumatoid arthritis.[59, 60] Selenium has been administered to patients with rheumatoid arthritis[61] and osteoarthritis[62] without apparent effect. A reduction in serum selenium has been found in patients with systemic sclerosis.[63] Patients with rheumatoid arthritis but not osteoarthritis showed an improved pain score in one study of selenium supplementation.[64]

Copper

Copper is an essential nutrient for biologic systems, including the immune system. Copper is the third largest trace element found in human tissues after iron and zinc. Free copper ion is rapidly complexed to specific ligands, through which it expresses its biologic activity. Most serum copper is bound to ceruloplasmin, which increases as part of the acute phase response.

The mechanisms of the effects of copper on the immune system are unknown, although several hypotheses are plausible. As mentioned, along with zinc and manganese, copper is a cofactor in the enzyme superoxide dismutase, which has an essential role in inhibiting free radical damage in tissues and the immune system (see Fig. 35–2). Altered glutathione levels have also been reported in copper-deficient rats.[65] The circulating cuproenzyme ceruloplasmin also has antioxidant properties. Increased levels of ceruloplasmin produced as a result of the acute phase response to inflammation may directly scavenge superoxide, although this is thought to be inefficient.[51] Of more importance, ceruloplasmin can oxidize Fe(II) to Fe(III), thus inhibiting the Fe(II)–catalyzed reactions of lipid peroxidation and the scavenging of reactive hydroxyl radicals. It also transports copper for synthesis of intracellular copper-zinc superoxide dismutase, which is critical in the reduction of highly reactive oxygen free radical species.

Two copper-dependent enzymes present within lymphocytes are important in immune function: cytochrome C oxidase and sulfhydryl oxidase. The former acts in intracellular energy metabolism, and the latter is located in lymphocyte plasma membranes and is a cofactor in pentamer immunoglobulin M (IgM) formation and B cell differentiation.[66]

Iron

Asymptomatic tissue iron deficiency is the most common nutritional deficiency in the world. It occurs along with the more severe iron deficiency anemia and is particularly common in infants, children, and pregnant and menstruating females. Iron-deficient populations have a high rate of infectious diseases, which may paradoxically be worsened with iron supplementation. This is thought to be due to the improved replication of many microorganisms that also require iron for optimal growth.[67]

Iron has many well-documented effects on immune function. The iron-containing enzyme catalase is found in cytoplasmic peroxisomes and catalyzes the decomposition of hydrogen peroxide to water and O_2, protecting the cellular environment from free radical–induced damage (see Fig. 35–2). Like zinc, serum levels of iron decrease in inflammation and infection, probably by a mechanism of cytokine-stimulated withdrawal from the circulation and enhanced synthesis of ferritin.[67] The immune effects of iron may be at least partially mediated through alterations in prostaglandin synthesis. Prostaglandin endoperoxide synthase is an iron-dependent enzyme critical in the synthesis of prostaglandin species.[67] Because PGE_2 can in turn regulate the production of IL-1, impaired prostaglandin production secondary to iron deficiency could effect the production of this important cytokine. The precise mechanism responsible for the effects of iron on the immune response has not been established and may have to do with a general role in cellular growth and protein synthesis as well as more specific effects on the immune system.

FATTY ACIDS

Background

Certain long-chain fatty acids are deemed essential in our diet because their deficiency can result in severe growth retardation and death. Early experiments showed that rats fed a fat-free diet failed to grow or reproduce and eventually died. Linoleic acid was found to be the primary essential fatty acid, together with its derivative ω-6 fatty acid compounds. The ω-3 fatty acids have also been found to be essential. They represent the largest species of fatty acids in the cerebral cortex and retina and can be derived only from the diet. Animals lack two important desaturase enzymes that are present in plants and phytoplankton and that convert the monounsaturate oleic acid to linoleic acid and linoleic acid to α-linolenic acid. Once animals and humans consume linoleic acid or α-linolenic acid, the basic ω-6 and ω-3 fatty acids, they can then be metabolized to the longer-chain fatty acids, including arachidonic, eicosapentaenoic acid (EPA), and docosahexaenoic acid (DHA).

Because of the mammalian inability to interconvert ω-3 and ω-6 fatty acids, the composition of phospholipids in cellular membranes is determined by nutritional intake.[68] The fatty acids found in the membrane bilayer are substrates for the production of prostaglandin and leukotriene species essential for many biologic activities, including modulation of the inflammatory and immune response. It is becoming widely recognized that reproducible metabolic alterations in these pathways can be engineered by consistent modifications in dietary fatty acid content. These fatty acid–induced changes have been documented in trials in animals[69] and normal humans,[70] as well as in large epidemiologic studies of populations that consume relatively homogeneous diets.[71]

Fatty acids are designated with a number followed by a colon, another lesser number, a lowercase *n* and yet another number; for example, 18:2 n-6. The first number designates the number of carbon atoms in the molecule. The number appearing after the colon represents the number of double bonds. The number after the *n* indicates the position of the first double bond starting from the methyl or *omega* (n = ω) end of the fatty acid chain. Linoleic acid, 18:2 n-6, thus has 18 carbons and two double bonds, and the first double bond is found six carbon atoms from the terminal methyl group. It is therefore an ω-6 fatty acid. In discussing fatty acid dietary studies in inflammatory disease, we will consider ω-6 and ω-3 intervention separately.

Omega-6 Fatty Acids

By far the most common fatty acid constituents in the Western diet are the ω-6 fatty acids. They are derived predominantly from terrestrial sources and are ubiquitous in plant seeds. Linoleic acid (18:6 n-6) is essential to life as it is the precursor of arachidonic acid (20:4 n-6) (Fig. 35–3). Arachidonate is present in cellular membranes, where it is esterified to phospholipids in the 2 position. It is released by phospholipase A_2 to form the eicosanoid derivatives of the prostaglandin and leukotriene families through the enzymes cyclooxygenase and 5-lipoxygenase, respectively, which catalyze the insertion of molecular oxygen into arachidonic acid. Gamma-linolenic acid (GLA; 18:3 n-6) is found in seeds from the evening primrose and borage plants. It may be converted by an elongase enzyme to dihomogammalinolenic acid (DGLA; 20:3 n-6). DGLA is oxidized by cyclooxygenase to PGE_1 (Fig. 35–4), a monoenoic prostaglandin that has altered biologic activities from the dienoic PGE_2. For example, PGE_1 can inhibit platelet aggregation in humans and rats in vivo and in vitro, whereas PGE_2 cannot.[72] PGE_1 dietary supplementation can suppress inflammation and joint tissue injury in several animal models of inflammation[73] and can inhibit neutrophil function. GLA dietary supplementation can suppress acute and chronic inflammation in several experimental animal models.

Animal Studies

The subcutaneous air pouch model of inflammation was used to assess response to monosodium urate crystals or Freund's adjuvant in Sprague-Dawley rats

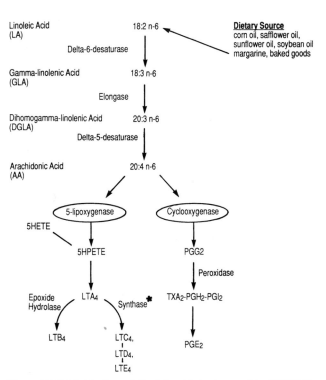

Classical Pathway of Dietary Fatty Acid Derived Eicosanoid Metabolism

Figure 35–3. Metabolism of linoleic acid to eicosanoids. 5-HPETE, 5S-hydroperoxyeicosatetraenoic acid; 5-HETE 5S-hydroperoxyeicosatetraenoic acid; LT, leukotriene; PG, prostaglandin; TXA_2, thromboxane A_2; PGI_2, prostacylin I_2. Synthase is also known as glutathione S transferase.

that consumed diets enriched with either safflower oil as a source of linoleic acid or borage seed oil as a source of GLA.[74] Animals that consumed GLA had a marked reduction of neutrophil exudate and lysosomal enzyme activity compared with those fed sunflower oil. PGE_2 and leukotriene B_4 ($LTBO_4$) concentrations were significantly diminished in pouch exudates in the GLA-fed rats. The fatty acid profiles in the serum and inflammatory cells from animals that consumed primrose oil exhibited significant increases in GLA and DGLA.

When DGLA is added to human synovial cells grown in tissue culture, IL-1B–stimulated growth is suppressed five-fold compared with cells grown in medium supplemented with arachidonic acid.[75] Cells incubated with DGLA exhibited a 14-fold increase in PGE_1 and a 70 percent decrease in PGE_2 compared with cells in control medium. The increase in PGE_1 concentrations was associated with significantly enhanced levels of cyclic adenosine monophosphate (cAMP), which the researchers suggested was responsible for the antiproliferative effects. The inhibiting effect could be blocked by indomethacin, lending further support to PGE_1 mediation of growth suppression.

Gamma-Linolenic Acid Derived Alterations in Eicosanoid Metabolism

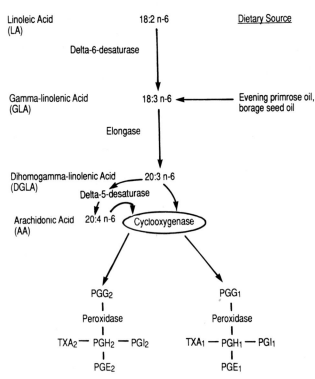

Figure 35–4. Metabolism of gamma-linolenic acid (GLA) to prostaglandin species with one double bond. Dihomogamma-linolenic acid (DGLA) cannot be converted to a leukotriene compound. Instead, it is converted by 15-lipoxygenase to 15-hydroxy DGLA (reaction not shown), which can inhibit 5-lipoxygenase activities. (See Ziboh and Chapkin, Arch Dermatol 123:1686, 1987.)

Human Studies

Studies of dietary supplementation with GLA in humans have shown somewhat mixed results. An open study of only 20 patients with rheumatoid arthritis treated with GLA in combination with various vitamins showed no significant changes of any clinical or laboratory parameters over 12 weeks.[76] An investigation that compared evening primrose oil to olive oil as a source of GLA in 20 patients with rheumatoid arthritis over 13 weeks failed to show any significant difference between groups.[77]

In a well-designed study, investigators treated patients with rheumatoid arthritis with 1.4 g of GLA daily over 24 weeks.[78] They observed a clinically important reduction in both the tender and swollen joint counts of 36 and 28 percent, respectively; the placebo group showed no improvement in these parameters. It had previously been demonstrated that GLA can inhibit IL-2 production by peripheral blood mononuclear cells in vitro[79] and may reduce the expansion of activation markers on T lymphocytes.[80] The precise mechanism of the improvements observed was not studied.[78]

Omega-3 Fatty Acids

Omega-3 fatty acids have their first double bond at the third carbon atom from the methyl end of the molecule. The primary dietary source of this class of fatty acids in human diets is fish and other marine sources, which derive the ω-3 fatty acids from phytoplankton and zooplankton at the base of the food chain. EPA (20:5 n-3) (Fig. 35–5) and DHA (22:6 n-3) are the ω-3 fatty acids derived from marine sources. Omega-3 fatty acids may also occur naturally in terrestrial sources in the form of α-linolenic acid (18:3 n-3) commonly found in chloroplasts of green leaves and in some plant oils, including flax, canola, and soybean oils. The ability to synthesize the longer chain ω-3 fatty acids EPA and DHA from α-linolenic acid is slow in humans and may diminish even further with aging or certain disease states[81] as a result of a loss of the δ-6 and δ-5 desaturase enzyme activity. The shorter chain ω-3 fatty acids must also compete for these enzymes with the much larger amounts of

n-3 Fatty Acid Derived Alterations in Eicosanoid Metabolism

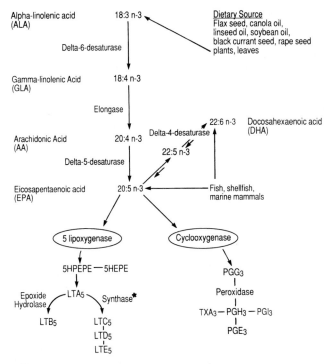

* Also known as glutathione S-Transferase

Figure 35–5. Metabolism of omega-3 fatty acids to eicosanoids. α-Linolenic acid (ALA) is derived from terrestrial sources and eicosapentaenoic acid (EPA) and docosahexaenoic acids (DHA) are derived from marine sources. Omega-3 fatty acids are converted to prostaglandin species with three double bonds and leukotriene species with five double bonds. They also compete with arachidonic acid as the substrate for cyclooxygenase and may selectively inhibit the epoxide hydrolase enzyme converting LTA_4 to LTB_4. 5-HPEPE, 5S-hydroperoxyeicosapentaenoic acid; 5-HEPE, 5S-hydroxyeicosapentaenoic acid; LT, leukotriene; PG, prostaglandin; TXA_3, thromboxane A_3; PGI_3, prostacyclin I_3.

ω-6 fatty acids found in the typical Western diet. The ω-6 fatty acids can competitively inhibit the formation of EPA and DHA from α-linolenic acid.[3] The primary source of ω-3 fatty acids in the Western diet is therefore nonterrestrial, a reversal of the pattern of most of human prehistory, in which large sources of ω-3 fatty acids were obtained in hunter-gatherer societies through consumption of wild game.[4] Fat of wild animals contains about 9 percent EPA and five times more polyunsaturated fat per gram than is found in domestic livestock,[82] which contains almost undetectable amounts of EPA. Throughout most of human history, hunter-gatherer societies consumed a higher percentage of polyunsaturated fat, more ω-3 fatty acids, more fiber, and less total fat than are found in the present Western diet (see Table 35–1). Our current dietary fatty acid intake must be properly viewed as a relatively recent alteration of longstanding dietary patterns that humans had adapted to over tens of thousand of years. Speculation has thus arisen about the possible influence of our changing dietary patterns on the development of some major chronic diseases of industrialized society.[4]

EPA can be metabolized through both the cyclooxygenase and 5-lipoxygenase metabolic pathways to form end-products with altered biologic activity. EPA is acted upon by cyclooxygenase to form thromboxane A3 (TXA3) and prostacyclin I3 (PGI3) (see Fig. 35–5).[83] PGI3 retains its antiaggregatory platelet activity, but thromboxane (TX) A3 is not nearly as potent as TXA2 in inducing platelet aggregation. This may partially account for the diminished risk of cardiovascular morbidity and mortality that is associated with fish consumption.[2, 3] EPA is also metabolized to PGE3, a compound with less inflammatory activity than PGE2.[84] PGE2 stimulates osteoclast activity, resulting in bone resorption, a process of significance in rheumatoid arthritis. The dienoic prostaglandins also increase vascular permeability in a synergistic effect with serotonin and bradykinin.[84] PGE series prostaglandins have important functions in blood pressure regulation, fertility, and modulation of the immune response. Omega-3 fatty acid ingestion has been documented to have significant effects in all of these areas[3, 84] as well as cardiovascular health and well being. Moreover, the E series prostaglandins are not localized to specific tissues, as is the case with thromboxane and prostacyclin, which are limited to platelets and vascular endothelium, respectively. Therefore, the effect of altering PGE content in any specific site varies depending on the tissue where the synthesis takes place.[85]

Of possibly greater importance than the altered end-products of ω-3 fatty acid ingestion is their ability to inhibit arachidonate metabolism. They can inhibit the synthesis of arachidonic acid from its linoleic acid substrate,[86] possibly through competition for the 2 position occupied by arachidonate in membrane phospholipids. EPA also directly competes with arachidonic acid as the substrate for cyclooxygenase and inhibits its metabolism into eicosanoids.[87] Omega-3 fatty acid ingestion thus results in the production of compounds with altered biologic activity as well as a decrease in the usual amounts of biologically active arachidonate derivatives.

Ingestion of EPA is associated with the production of leukotrienes with five double bonds such as LTB5 (see Fig. 35–5), which has greatly attenuated proinflammatory activities.[88] LTB5 is usually undetectable in humans who consume a Western diet. Simultaneous with the production of small amounts of LTB5 from stimulated neutrophils of normal persons who consume fish oil, large decreases occur in the production of neutrophil LTB4.[89] Neutrophil chemotaxis was significantly suppressed in these subjects after 6 weeks of fish oil ingestion and returned to normal after the supplements were discontinued.

Other investigators have found evidence of a selective inhibition of the epoxide hydrolase enzyme (see Fig. 35–5) in neutrophils from normal persons[88] and patients with rheumatoid arthritis[90] who consume fish oil because of unaltered quantities of 5-hydroxyeicosatetraenoic acid and 5-hydroxyeicosapentaenoic acid relative to the corresponding arachidonic acid product generated before dietary supplementation.

Chemotactic activity of neutrophils from patients with rheumatoid arthritis who had ingested fish oil was found to be enhanced compared with the pretreatment state.[90] This seems paradoxical in view of the suppression of neutrophil chemotaxis after fish oil ingestion in normal persons.[89] The improved chemotaxis in patients with rheumatoid arthritis represents a partial correction of a reduced chemotactic activity of peripheral blood neutrophils of persons with this disease. Platelet activating factor (PAF)–acether generation of stimulated monocytes is significantly diminished[89] after fish oil ingestion, suggesting an ω-3 fatty acid–induced inhibitory effect of phospholipase A2 activity on substrate alkyl phospholipids, which affects PAF generation. This is of considerable interest in the context of inflammation in that PAF can stimulate TNF as well as other cytokines in endothelial tissue[91] and is 1000 times more potent than histamine in inducing changes in vascular permeability.[92] Evidence suggests that PAF can also modulate T cell and monocyte function.[93]

Omega-3 fatty acid ingestion is associated with significant changes in the fatty acid profiles of cellular lipids. Neutrophil arachidonic acid content is reduced by 33 percent and EPA content is enhanced 20-fold compared with presupplement values obtained in patients with rheumatoid arthritis who ingested fish oil.[90] Omega-3 fatty acid ingestion is thus associated with reproducible changes in the biochemical composition of cell membranes of neutrophils and monocytes as well as striking alterations in the production of the metabolic end products of a myriad of inflammatory and immunologically active compounds that may influence the course of rheumatic disease.

The lipid bilayer of cellular membranes is composed primarily of phospholipids and cholesterol (Fig. 35–6). Because cellular receptors, enzymes, and

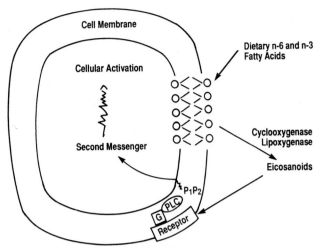

Figure 35–6. Potential role of dietary fatty acids in the function of the membrane phospholipid bilayer of cells. Dietary fatty acids will be incorporated into the phospholipid bilayer of cells, where they can be metabolized to eicosanoids. Biologically modified eicosanoids derived from feeding omega-3 or omega-6 fatty acids may have a role in modulating receptor-ligand activity and cellular activation to various stimuli. Fatty acid changes in the lipid bilayer may also result in changes in membrane fluidity that could have potential effects on the function of other receptor-related membrane activities. The stimulated receptor transmits a signal via a G-protein to phospholipase C (PLC), which splits phosphatidylinositol-4,5-biphosphate (PIP_2) to products that eventually lead to second-messenger generation and cellular activation (biochemical steps not shown). (Modified from Weber PC: Membrane phospholipid modification by dietary ω-3 fatty acids: Effects on eicosanoid formation and cell function. *In* Karnovsky, ML [ed]: Biological Membranes: Aberrations in Membrane Structure and Function. New York, Alan R Liss, 1988, pp 263–274. Copyright © 1988 Wiley-Liss. Reprinted by permission of Wiley-Liss, A Division of John Wiley & Sons, Inc.)

transport proteins are embedded in the phospholipid bilayer, a change in its structure could have significant implications for cellular function that extend beyond the alterations in eicosanoid and PAF-acether biosynthesis described herein. One investigation demonstrated a significant reduction of IL-1 from monocytes of normal volunteers ingesting fish oil for 6 weeks.[93] The precise mechanism of this effect is speculative, but it may be associated with membrane changes in phospholipid fatty acid content, leading to diminished amounts of eicosanoid products, such as LTB_4.

Animal Studies

Dietary modifications containing ω-3 fatty acids reduce the severity of diffuse proliferative glomerulonephritis in several autoimmune strains of mice, including NZBxNZWF1, BxSB/Mpj, and MRL/lpr.[69, 94] Dietary ω-3 fatty acids reduce the severity of glomerulonephritis even when they are withheld until after the renal disease has begun to evolve.[94] Not all observed effects of fish oil have been beneficial in the laboratory; an increased incidence of arthritis was observed in rats immunized with type II collagen who consumed a fish oil–enriched diet compared

with animals ingesting beef tallow, although the severity of the arthritis was the same in each group.[95] An increased incidence of necrotizing vasculitis was noted in renal arteries of MRL/lpr mice with systemic lupus erythematosus–like disease, even while their glomerulonephritis was alleviated on a fish oil diet.[94] Studies indicate that a mixture of ω-3 fatty acids containing both EPA and DHA may be more effective than either of these ω-3 fatty acids by themselves.[96]

Human Studies

A pilot study published in 1985 suggested a possible beneficial effect of dietary supplementation with ω-3 fatty acids in patients with rheumatoid arthritis.[97] In a subsequent investigation, patients received 2.8 g of EPA and 1.8 g of DHA in a blinded crossover format in which subjects received fish oil derived ω-3 fatty acids or olive oil for a period of 14 weeks before crossing over to receive the opposite dietary supplement.[98] Patients were observed to have a highly statistically significant decrease in the number of tender joints after they took fish oil in contrast to when they consumed olive oil. Fatigue, which was quantitated as the time interval from awakening to the first feeling of tiredness, also lessened significantly in patients who consumed fish oil. All of 12 clinical parameters measured favored fish oil, although only two achieved statistical significance. LTB_4 from stimulated neutrophils decreased by 57.8 percent in patients who consumed the fish oil ω-3 supplement compared with olive oil. A significant correlation was observed between the decrease in the number of tender joints and the decrease in neutrophil LTB_4 production in individual patients.

LTB_4 production from stimulated neutrophils was significantly reduced at week 4 in patients taking fish oil, even though significant clinical improvement did not occur until week 12.[99] There is thus an asynchrony between ω-3–induced decreases in neutrophil LTB_4 production that occur after only 4 to 6 weeks[89, 90, 99] and the clinical benefits, which are delayed until at least week 12.[97–99] This might be due, in part, to the delayed suppressive effects of fish oil ingestion on the production of IL-1.[93]

The effects of different doses of fish oil versus olive oil were studied in a 6-month randomized, double-blind, parallel investigation of 49 patients with active rheumatoid arthritis.[100] Fish oil supplements were supplied according to body weight, not as a uniform dose as in previous studies. A "low-dose" group consumed 27 mg/kg/day of EPA and 18 mg/kg/day of DHA. A "high-dose" group ingested exactly twice that amount. Patients maintained their background medications and diets without change, as in the previously described studies in patients with rheumatoid arthritis. Multiple clinical parameters improved from baseline in the groups consuming fish oil, with statistically significant improvements in joint swelling and tenderness scores, morning stiffness and physician evaluation of global disease activity occurring with significantly greater frequency in the high-dose group. Significant decreases were also observed in stimulated neutrophil production of LTB_4 and monocyte IL-1, and the greatest decreases in IL-1 were observed in the patients consuming the higher dose of fish oil.

It thus appears that the beneficial effects of ω-3 fatty acid ingestion in humans with inflammatory disease may be dose-dependent, as in the autoimmune animal model,[96] and studies of the antihypertensive effects of fish oil ingestion in humans.[101] Significant clinical benefits were observed more commonly after 18 and 24 weeks of fish oil ingestion. Fish oil dietary supplementation has not been effective in patients with stable lupus nephritis[102] or osteoarthritis,[103] but it does appear to offer a protective effect in the prevention of renal transplant rejection[104] and treatment of IgA nephropathy.[105]

Vascular Diseases

The role of ω-3 fatty acids in cardiovascular disease is well established and has been recently reviewed.[3] Effects of ω-3 fatty acids that may improve the status of individuals with impaired circulation include the following:

- improved rheologic status secondary to increased erythrocyte deformability
- decreased plasma viscosity
- a more favorable vascular response to ischemia
- a reduced vasospastic response to catecholamines and angiotensin
- increased levels of tissue plasminogen activator
- increased endothelial-dependent relaxation of arteries in response to bradykinin, serotonin, adenine diphosphate, and thrombin

Fish oil dietary intervention thus differs from present interventions for vascular disease because of the potential for beneficial benefits at multiple physiologic loci.

In an investigation of the effect of fish oil ingestion in patients with Raynaud's phenomenon, 32 patients with primary or secondary disease consumed daily dietary supplements of 3.96 g of EPA and 2.64 g of DHA or olive oil for 12 weeks.[106] Digital systolic blood pressure and blood flow were evaluated by a strain gauge plethysmograph in room air and in water baths of different temperatures. Results showed significant improvements in the time to onset of symptoms and in digital systolic pressure in the cold water baths in patients with primary, but not secondary, Raynaud's phenomenon. The mechanism of these benefits was not studied.

ALLERGIC ARTHRITIS

The idea that rheumatologic disease might be etiologically linked to ingestion of food is not a new one.[107, 108] The idea has gained some support from sporadic but convincing case reports of the reproducible onset of joint symptoms shortly after the ingestion of certain foodstuffs. Patients with Behçet's syndrome had striking exacerbations of disease within 48 hours of ingestion of English walnuts.[109] Lymphocytes from these patients also had significantly decreased reactivity to a walnut extract ex vivo within 2 days of ingestion of English walnuts, and leukocyte incorporation of tritiated thymidine after mitogen stimulation was increased.[109] A hypersensitivity to certain foods has been speculated to be the cause of at least some cases of palindromic rheumatism[108] and was documented to occur in a report of an individual with a hypersensitivity to sodium nitrate in food preservatives.[110] L-Canavanine, a nonprotein amino acid found in alfalfa, has been linked to exacerbations of systemic lupus erythematosus in both monkeys[111] and humans.[112]

For a response to food to be plausibly linked to a hypersensitivity reaction resulting in articular symptoms, it is necessary to implicate an altered intestinal permeability that would allow passage of intact food antigens into the circulation. Circumstantial evidence exists to link arthritis to damaged intestinal function in ulcerative colitis,[113] Crohn's disease,[114] and the polyarthritis that follows jejunal bypass surgery for obesity.[115] Moreover, immune complexes that contain intact food antigens complexed to IgE or IgG have been documented in normal and atopic subjects[116] and have been observed to cause bronchospasm and pruritus in allergic individuals. A study of intestinal permeability that used oral ^{51}Cr-EDTA (edetic acid) showed that patients with rheumatoid arthritis who took nonsteroidal anti-inflammatory drugs (NSAIDs) exhibited abnormalities, whereas patients not taking NSAIDs did not have abnormal permeability.[117] Indium-III–labeled leukocyte scans showed ileocecal inflammation in six of nine patients taking NSAIDs.

A food antigen can be convincingly linked to arthritis if a flare of clinical symptoms occurs within 48 hours of a blinded challenge with the putative offending antigen. An elimination diet in which a patient totally discontinues ingestion of the food in question with total clearing of articular symptoms would also provide implicative evidence, albeit weaker than a flare after a blinded challenge. Two cases have been reported involving significant flares in articular symptoms after ingestion of milk or dairy products.[118, 119] The challenges were open[118] and blinded,[119] and symptoms peaked within 24 to 48 hours. IgE antibodies to milk were demonstrated using the radioallergosorbent test in one patient,[118] and large amounts of IgG$_4$ antimilk antibodies directed to α-lactalbumin were detected in the other.[119] A flare in articular disease manifestations has also been documented after blinded challenges with shrimp and nitrates.[120]

Interest in the possible role of food intolerance in the etiology of arthritic symptoms has been renewed[121, 122] as a result of these case reports. It is difficult to assess the incidence of this syndrome in that patients may not necessarily be aware of possible sensitivities to commonly ingested foods in their diet. Because of the small number of documented cases of food intolerance in the literature, however, the syndrome is probably rare.

References

1. Hirai A, Terano T, Saito H, et al: Eicosapentaenoic acid and platelet function in Japanese. *In* Lovenburg W, Yamori Y (eds): Nutritional Prevention of Cardiovascular Disease. New York, Academic Press, 1984, pp 231–239.
2. Kromhout D, Bosschieter EB, de Lezenne Coulander C: The inverse relation between fish consumption and 20-year mortality from coronary heart disease. N Engl J Med 312:1205–1209, 1985.
3. Leaf A, Weber PC: Cardiovascular effects of n-3 fatty acids. N Engl J Med 318:549, 1988.
4. Eaton SB, Konner M: Paleolithic nutrition: A consideration of its nature and current implications. N Engl J Med 312:283, 1985.
5. Hecht A: Hocus-pocus as applied to arthritis. FDA Consumer 14:24, 1980.
6. Blackburn GL, Bistrian BR: Nutritional care of the injured and/or septic patient. Surg Clin North Am 56:1195, 1976.
7. Silberman H, Eisenberg D: Consequences of malnutrition. *In* Parenteral and Enteral Nutrition for the Hospitalized Patient. East Norwalk, Conn, Appleton-Century-Crofts, 1982, pp 1–18.
8. Bayles TB, Richardson H, Hall FC: The nutritional background of patients with rheumatoid arthritis. N Engl J Med 229:319, 1943.
9. Eising L: Dietary intake in patients with arthritis and other chronic diseases. J Bone Joint Surg 45A:69, 1963.
10. Kowsari B, Finnie SK, Carter RL, et al: Assessment of the diet of patients with rheumatoid arthritis and osteoarthritis. J Am Diet Assoc 82:657, 1983.
11. Bigaouette J, Timchalk MA, Kremer J: Nutritional adequacy of diet and supplements in patients with rheumatoid arthritis who take medications. J Am Diet Assoc 87:1687, 1987.
12. Helliwell M, Coombes EJ, Moody BJ, et al: Nutritional status in patients with rheumatoid arthritis. Ann Rheum Dis 43:386, 1984.
13. Roubenoff R, Roubenoff R, Ward L, Holland S, Hellmann D: Rheumatoid cachexis: Depletion of lean body mass in rheumatoid arthritis. Possible association with tumor necrosis factor. J Rheumatol 19:10:1505–1510, 1992.
14. Johansson U, Portinsson S, Akesson A, et al: Nutritional status in girls with juvenile chronic arthritis. Hum Nutr Clin Nutr 40C:57, 1986.
15. Portinsson S, Akesson A, Svantesson H, et al: Dietary assessment in children with juvenile chronic arthritis. J Hum Nutr Diet 1:133, 1988.
16. Warady B, Lindsley R, Robinson R, Lukert B: Effects of nutritional supplementation on bone mineral status of children with rheumatic diseases receiving corticosteroid therapy. J Rheumatol 21:3:530–535, 1994.
17. Bendich A: Antioxidant nutrients and immune functions. Adv Exp Med Biol 262:1–12, 1990.
18. Tengerdy RP, Mathias MM, Nockels CF: Effect of vitamin E on immunity and disease resistance. *In* Prasad KN (ed): Vitamins, Nutrition and Cancer. Basel, Karger, 1984, pp 118–122.
19. Halliwell B, Gutteridge JMC: Lipid peroxidation: A radical chain reaction. *In* Free Radicals in Biology and Medicine. Oxford, Clarendon Press, 1985, pp 139–189.
20. Fidelius RK: The generation of oxygen radicals: A positive signal for lymphocyte activation. Cell Immunol 113:175, 1988.
21. Dornand J, Gerber M: Inhibition of murine T-cell responses by antioxidants: The targets of lipoxygenase pathway inhibitors. Immunology 68:384, 1989.
22. Austen KF, Soberman RJ: Perspectives on additional areas for research in leukotrienes. N. Y. Ann Acad Sci 524:xi, 1988.
23. Goodwin JS, Behrens T: Role of lipoxygenase metabolites of arachidonic acid in T cell activation. Ann N Y Acad Sci 524:201, 1988.
24. Bendich A: A role for carotenoids in immune function. Clin Nutr 7:113, 1988.
25. Boxer LA: Functional effects of leukocyte antioxidants on polymorphonuclear leukocyte behavior. Adv Exp Med 262:19–34, 1990.
26. Grever MR, Thompson VN, Balcerzak SP, et al: The effect of oxidant stress on human lymphocyte cytotoxicity. Blood 56:284, 1980.
27. Hatam CJ, Cayden HJ: A high performance lipid chromatographic method for the determination of tocopherol in plasma and cellular elements of the blood. J Lipid Res 20:639, 1979.
28. Boxer LS, Oliver JM, Spielberg SP, et al: Protection of granulocytes by vitamin E in glutathione synthetase deficiency. N Engl J Med 301:901, 1979.
29. Moser J, Weber F: Uptake of ascorbic acid by human granulocytes. Int J Vitam Nutr Res 54:47, 1983.
30. Goetzl EJ, Wasserman SI, Gigli I, Austen KF: Enhancement of random

31. migration and chemotactic response of human leukocytes by ascorbic acid. J Clin Invest 53:813, 1974.
31. Sahud MA, Cohen R: Effect of aspirin ingestion on ascorbic acid levels in rheumatoid arthritis. Lancet 1:937, 1971.
32. Hall MG, Darling RC, Taylor FH: The vitamin C requirement in rheumatoid arthritis. Ann Intern Med 13:415, 1939.
33. Baehner RL, Boxer A, Allen JM, et al: Autooxidation as a basis for altered function by polymorphonuclear leukocytes. Blood 50:327, 1977.
34. El-Hag A, Lipsky PE, Bennett M, et al: Immunomodulation by neutrophil myeloperoxidase and hydrogen peroxide: Differential susceptibility of human lymphocyte functions. J Immunol 136:3420, 1986.
35. El-Hag A, Clark RA: Immunosuppression by activated human neutrophils: Dependence on the myeloperoxidase system. J Immunol 139:2406, 1987.
36. Anderson R, Smit M, Joone GK, VanStaden AM: Vitamin C and cellular immune functions. Ann N Y Acad Sci 587:34–48, 1990.
37. Frei BR, Stocker R, Ames BN: Proc Natl Acad Sci 85:9748, 1988.
38. Maddison PJ, Bacon PA: Vitamin D deficiency, spontaneous fractures and osteopenia in rheumatoid arthritis. Br Med J 4:433, 1974.
39. Smith EL, Pincus SH, Donovan L, et al: A novel approach for the evaluation and treatment of psoriasis. J Am Acad Dermatol 19:516, 1988.
40. MacLaughlin JA, Gange W, Taylor D, et al: Cultured psoriatic fibroblasts from involved and uninvolved sites have a partial but not absolute resistance to the proliferation-inhibition activity of 1,25-dihydroxyvitamin D3. Proc Natl Acad Sci USA 82:5409, 1985.
41. Rigby WFC, Stacy T, Ganger MW: Inhibition of T lymphocyte mitogenesis by 1,25-dihydroxyvitamin D3 (calcitriol). J Clin Invest 74:1451, 1984.
42. Ghalla AK, Amento EP, Krane SM: Differential effects of 1,25-dihydroxyvitamin D3 on human lymphocytes and monocyte/macrophages: Inhibition of interleukin-2 and augmentation of interleukin-1 production. Cell Immunol 98:311, 1986.
43. Gepner P, Amor B, Fournier C: 1,25-dihydroxyvitamin D3 potentiates the in vitro inhibitory effects of cyclosporin A on T cells from rheumatoid arthritis patients. Arthritis Rheum 32:31, 1989.
44. Huckins D, Felson DT, Holick M: Treatment of psoriatic arthritis with oral 1,25-dihydroxyvitamin D3: A pilot study. Arthritis Rheum 33:1732, 1990.
45. Fukushima T, Iijima Y, Kosaka F: Endotoxin-induced zinc accumulation by liver cells is mediated by metallothionein synthesis. Biochem Biophys Res Commun 152:874–878, 1988.
46. Cousins RJ: Absorption, transport and hepatic metabolism of copper and zinc: Special reference to metallothionein and ceruloplasmin. Physiol Rev 65:238–309, 1985.
47. Kluger MJ, Rothenburg BA: Fever and reduced iron: Their interaction as a host defense response to bacterial infection. Science 203:374, 1979.
48. Svenson KLG, Hallgren R, Johansson E: Reduced zinc in peripheral blood cells from patients with inflammatory connective tissue diseases. Inflammation 9:189, 1985.
49. Seelig MS: Auto-immune complications of D-penicillamine: A possible result of zinc and magnesium depletion and of pyridoxine inactivation. J Am Coll Nutr 1:207, 1982.
50. Ruhl J, Kirshner H: Monocyte-dependent stimulation of human T cells by zinc. Clin Exp Immunol 32:484, 1978.
51. Whitehouse MW: Trace element supplements for inflammatory disease. *In* Dixon J, Furst D (eds): Second Line Agents in the Rheumatic Diseases. New York, Marcel Dekker, 1991.
52. Whitehouse MW, Rainsford KD, Taylor RM, Vernon-Roberts B: Zinc monoglycerolate: A slow-release source of zinc with anti-arthritic activity in rats. Agents Actions 31:47, 1990.
53. Cimmino MA, Mazzucotelli A, Rovetta G, Cutolo M: The controversy over zinc sulfate efficacy in rheumatoid and psoriatic arthritis. Scand J Rheumatol 13:191, 1984.
54. Spallholz JE: Anti-inflammatory immunologic and carcinostatic attributes of selenium in experimental animals. Adv Exp Med Biol 135:43, 1981.
55. Spallholz JE, Boyland LM, Larsen HS: Advances in understanding selenium's role in the immune system. Ann N Y Acad Sci 587:123–139, 1990.
56. Ursini F, Maiorino M, Gregolin C: The selenoenzyme phospholipid hydroperoxide glutathione peroxidase. Biochem Biophys Acta 839:62, 1985.
57. Bryant RW, Bailey JM, King JC, Levander OA: Altered platelet glutathione peroxidase activity and arachidonic acid metabolism during selenium repletion in a controlled human study. *In* Spallholz JE, Martin JL, Ganther HE (eds): Selenium in Biology and Medicine. Westport, Conn, AVI, 1981, pp 395–399.
58. Spallholz JE, Boylan LM: Effect of dietary selenium on peritoneal macrophage chemiluminescence. Fed J 3:A778, 1989.
59. Sonne M, Helleberg L, Jenson PT: Selenium status in patients with rheumatoid arthritis. Scand J Rheumatol 14:318, 1985.
60. Borgland M, Akesson A, Adesson B: Distribution of selenium and glutathione peroxidase in plasma compared in healthy subjects and rheumatoid arthritis patients. Scand J Clin Lab Invest 48:27, 1988.
61. Tarp U, Overvad K, Thorling EB, Grandal H, Hansen JC: Selenium treatment in rheumatoid arthritis. Acta Pharmacol Toxicol 59 (Suppl 7):382, 1986.

62. Hill J, Bird HA: Failure of selenium-ACE to improve osteoarthritis. Br J Rheumatol 29:211, 1990.

63. Herrick A, Rieley F, Schofield D, Hollis S, Braganza J, Jayson M: Micronutrient antioxidant status in patients with primary Raynaud's phenomenon and systemic sclerosis. J Rheumatol 21:8:1477–1483, 1994.

64. Wagner E, Gruber FO: The trace element selenium in rheumatic diseases (abstract P-682). Rio de Janeiro, XVII ILAR Congress of Rheumatology, 1989.

65. Allen KGD, Arthur JR, Morrice PC, et al: Copper deficiency and tissue glutathione concentration in the rat. Proc Soc Exp Biol Med 187:38, 1988.

66. Roth RA, Koshland ME: Identification of a lymphocyte enzyme that catalyzes pentamer immunoglobulin M assembly. J Biol Chem 256:4633, 1981.

67. Sherman AR: Influence of iron on immunity and disease resistance. In N Y Acad Sci 587:140–146, 1990.

68. Weber PC: Membrane phospholipid modification by dietary n-3 fatty acids: Effects on eicosanoid formation and cell function. In Karnovsky ML (ed): Biological Membranes: Aberrations in Membrane Structure and Function. New York, Alan R Liss, 1988, pp 263–274.

69. Prickett JD, Robinson DR, Steinberg AD: Dietary enrichment with the polyunsaturated fatty acid eicosapentaenoic acid prevents proteinuria and prolongs survival in (NZB × NZW) F1 mice. J Clin Invest 68:556, 1981.

70. Lee TH, Hoover RL, Williams JD, et al: Effect of dietary enrichment with eicosapentaenoic and docosahexaenoic acids on in vitro neutrophil and monocyte leukotriene generation and neutrophil function. N Engl J Med 312:1217, 1985.

71. Shekelle RB, Missell LV, Paul O, et al: Fish consumption and mortality from coronary heart disease. N Engl J Med 313:820, 1985.

72. Willis AL, Comai K, Kuhn DC, et al: Dihomogammalinolenate suppresses platelet aggregation when administered in vitro or in vivo. Prostaglandins 7:509, 1974.

73. Zurier RB: Prostaglandins, immune responses, and murine lupus. Arthritis Rheum 25:804–809, 1982.

74. Tate GA, Mandell BF, Karmali RA, et al: Suppression of monosodium urate crystal-induced acute inflammation by diets enriched with gammalinolenic acid and eicosapentaenoic acid. Arthritis Rheum 31:1543, 1988.

75. Baker DG, Krakauer KA, Tate G, et al: Suppression of human synovial cell proliferation by dihomogammalinolenic acid. Arthritis Rheum 32:1273, 1989.

76. Hansen TM, Lerche A, Kassis V, et al: Treatment of rheumatoid arthritis with prostaglandin E1 precursors cis-linoleic acid and gamma-linolenic acid. Scand J Rheumatol 12:85, 1983.

77. Jantti J, Nikkari T, Solakivi T, et al: Evening primrose oil in rheumatoid arthritis: Changes in serum lipids and fatty acids. Ann Rheum Dis 48:124, 1989.

78. Leventhal LJ, Boyce EG, Zurier RB: Treatment of rheumatoid arthritis with gammalinolenic acid. Ann Intern Med 119:9:867–873, 1993.

79. Santoli D, Zurier RB: Prostaglandin E precursor fatty acids inhibit human IL-2 production by a prostaglandin E–independent mechanisms. J Immunol 143:1303–1309, 1989.

80. Santoli D, Philips PD, Zurier RB: Suppression of interleukin 2–dependent human T cell growth by prostaglandin E (PGE) and their precursor fatty acids: Evidence for a PGE-independent mechanism of inhibition by the fatty acids. J Clin Invest 85:424–432, 1990.

81. Lands WEM: Fish and Human Health. Orlando, Fla, Academic Press, 1986, p 103.

82. Crawford MA: Fatty-acid ratios in free-living and domestic animals. Lancet 1:1329, 1968.

83. Fischer S, Weber PC: Prostaglandin I3 is formed in vivo in man after dietary eicosapentaenoic acid. Nature 307:165, 1984.

84. Robinson DR, Tateno S, Balkrishna P, Hirai A: Lipid mediators of inflammatory and immune reactions. In Karnovsky ML (ed): Biological Membranes: Aberrations in Membrane Structure and Function. New York, Alan R Liss, 1988, pp 295–303.

85. Ferretti A, Flanagan VP: Modification of prostaglandin metabolism in vivo by longchain omega-3 polyunsaturates. Biochem Biophys Acta 1045:299, 1990.

86. Holman RT: Nutritional and metabolic interrelationships between fatty acids. Fed Proc 23:1062, 1964.

87. Simopoulos AP, Kifer RR, Martin RE (eds): Health Effects of Polyunsaturated Fatty Acids in Seafoods. New York, Academic Press, 1986.

88. Lee TH, Mencia-Huerta JM, Shih C, et al: Characterization and biologic properties of 5,12-dihydroxy derivatives of eicosapentaenoic acid, including leukotriene B5 and the double lipoxygenase product. J Biol Chem 259:2383, 1984.

89. Lee TH, Hoover RL, Williams JD, et al: Effect of dietary enrichment with eicosapentaenoic and docosahexaenoic acids on in vitro neutrophil function. N Engl J Med 312:1217, 1985.

90. Sperling RI, Weinblatt M, Robin JL, et al: Effects of dietary supplementation with marine fish oil on leukocyte lipid mediator generation and function in rheumatoid arthritis. Arthritis Rheum 30:988, 1987.

91. Dulioust A, Salem P, Vivier E, et al: Immunoregulatory functions of PAF-acether (Platelet-Activating Factor) in Biological Membranes: Aberrations in Membrane Structure and Function. New York, Alan R Liss, 1988, pp 87–96.

92. Humphrey DM, McManase L, Satouchi K, et al: Vasoactive properties of acetyl glyceryl ether phosphorylcholine and analogs. Lab Invest 46:422, 1982.

93. Endres S, Chorbani R, Kelley VE, et al: The effects of dietary supplementation with n-3 polyunsaturated fatty acids on the synthesis of interleukin-1 and tumor necrosis factor by mononuclear cells. N Engl J Med 320:265, 1989.

94. Robinson DR, Prickett JD, Makoul GT, Steinberg AD, Colvin RB: Dietary fish oil reduces progression of established renal disease in (NZB × NZW) F1 mice and delays renal disease in BXSB and MRL/1 strains. Arthritis Rheum 29:539–546, 1986.

95. Prickett JD, Trentham DE, Robinson DR: Dietary fish oil augments the induction of arthritis in rats immunized with type II collagen. J Immunol 132:725–729, 1984.

96. Robinson DR, Tateno S, Knoell C, et al: Dietary marine lipids suppress murine autoimmune disease. J Intern Med 225 (Suppl 1):211, 1989.

97. Kremer JM, Bigauoette J, Michalek AU, et al: Effects of manipulating dietary fatty acids on clinical manifestations of rheumatoid arthritis. Lancet 1:184, 1985.

98. Kremer JM, Jubiz W, Michalek A, et al: Fish-oil fatty acid supplementation in active rheumatoid arthritis: A double blinded, controlled cross-over study. Ann Intern Med 106:498, 1987.

99. Cleland LG, French JK, Betts WH, et al: Clinical and biochemical effects of dietary fish-oil supplements in rheumatoid arthritis. J Rheumatol 15:1471–1475, 1988.

100. Kremer JM, Lawrence DA, Jubiz W, et al: Dietary fish oil and olive oil supplementation in patients with rheumatoid arthritis: Clinical and immunologic effects. Arthritis Rheum 33:810, 1990.

101. Knapp HR, FitzGerald GA: The antihypertensive effects of fish oil: A controlled study of polyunsaturated fatty acid supplements in essential hypertension. N Engl J Med 320:1037, 1989.

102. Clark WF, Parbtani A, Naylor CD, Levinton CM, Muirhead N, Spanner E, Huff MW, Philbrick DJ, Holub BJ: Fish oil in lupus nephritis: Clinical findings and methodological implications. Kidney Int 44:75–85, 1993.

103. Stammers T, Sibbald B, Freeling P: Efficacy of cod liver oil as an adjunct to non-steroidal anti-inflammatory drug treatment in the management of osteoarthritis in general practice. Ann Rheum Dis 51:128–129, 1992.

104. Homan van der Heide JJ, Bilo HJG, Donker JM, Wilmink JM, Tegzess AM: Effect of dietary fish oil on renal function and rejection in cyclosporine-treated recipients of renal transplants. N Engl J Med 329:11:769–773, 1993.

105. Donadio JV Jr, Bergstralh EJ, Offord KP, Spenser DC, Holley KE, et al: A controlled trial of fish oil in IgA nephropathy. N Engl J Med 331:18:1194–1199, 1994.

106. DiGiacomo RA, Kremer JM, Shah DM: Fish oil supplementation in patients with Raynaud's phenomenon: A double-blind controlled prospective study. Am J Med 86:158, 1989.

107. Lewis P, Taub SJ: Allergic synovitis due to ingestion of English walnuts. JAMA 106:214–244, 1936.

108. Zeller M: Rheumatoid arthritis food allergy as a factor. Ann Allergy 7:200, 1947.

109. Marquardt JC, Snyderman R, Oppenheim JJ: Depression of lymphocyte transformation and exacerbation of Behçet's syndrome by ingestion of English walnuts. Cell Immunol 9:263, 1973.

110. Epstein S: Hypersensitivity to sodium nitrate: A major causative factor in case of palindromic rheumatism. Ann Allergy 27:343, 1969.

111. Malinow MR, Bardana EJ, Pirofsky B, et al: Systemic lupus erythematosus–like syndrome in monkeys fed alfalfa sprouts: Role of a non protein amino acid. Science 216:415, 1982.

112. Roberts JL, Hayashi JA: Exacerbation of SLE associated with alfalfa ingestion (letter). N Engl J Med 308:1361, 1983.

113. Wright V, Watkinson G: The arthritis of ulcerative colitis. Br Med J 2:670, 1965.

114. von Potter WN: Regional enteritis. Gastroenterology 26:347, 1954.

115. Wands JR, LaMont JT, Mann E, Isselbacher K: Arthritis associated with intestinal by-pass procedure for morbid obesity. Complement activation and character of circulating cryoproteins. N Engl J Med 294:121, 1976.

116. Paganelli R, Levinsky RJ, Brostoff J, et al: Immune complexes containing food proteins in normal and atopic subjects after oral challenge and effect of sodium cromoglycate on antigen absorption. Lancet 1:1270, 1979.

117. Bjarnason I, So A, Levi AJ, et al: Intestinal permeability and inflammation in rheumatoid arthritis: Effects of non-steroidal anti-inflammatory drugs. Lancet 2:1171, 1984.

118. Parke EL, Hughes GRV: Rheumatoid arthritis and food: A case study. BMJ 282:2027, 1981.

119. Panush RS, Stroud RM, Webster EM: Food-induced (allergic) arthritis. Arthritis Rheum 29:220, 1986.

120. Panush RS: Food induced ("allergic") arthritis: Clinical and serologic studies. J Rheumatol 17:291, 1990.

121. Darlington LG: Does food intolerance have any role in the aetiology and management of rheumatoid disease? Ann Rheum Dis 44:801, 1985.

122. Panush RS: Possible role of food sensitivity in arthritis. Ann Allergy 19 (Suppl):31, 1988.

CHAPTER 36

Psychosocial Management of Rheumatic Diseases

Liv Marit Smedstad
Matthew H. Liang

The humane and effective care of patients with chronic rheumatic illnesses requires that the physician attend to the psychologic needs of the patient.[1,2] Psychologic impairment is an intrinsic component of all diseases, and managing it will enhance the medical, surgical, and rehabilitation program. Making psychosocial problems a legitimate concern without being able to "fix" them is a source of comfort for patients and their families. For most rheumatic disorders, patients and their physicians are involved in a lifelong relationship in which the vagaries of the disease and normal life interact in a complex manner.

THE EXPERIENCE OF RHEUMATIC ILLNESS

For those with chronic rheumatic diseases, the most mundane activities of daily life cannot be taken for granted.[3-5] It is difficult to capture the suffering and frustration of an existence characterized by pain and loss of physical capacity with numbers alone. Patients' expressions about how a rheumatic disorder affects their lives and what helps them evoke common themes.

Arthritis is boring—in the clinical sense. I am tired of talking about this ache and that pain, or the newest wonder drug. What remains the most striking and frustrating aspect of this illness for me is that I, more fortunate than many people with arthritis, look well. People compliment my healthy appearance, applaud my swimming regimen and active lifestyle. And yet some days I feel so bad that I become angry. I am angry that no one can see my pain, that people cannot tell that with every other walking step comes a pulse of pain that won't quit. That by late afternoon in my office, my elbows are so stiff and throbbing that I just want to go home and rest. But I rarely do. I never miss a day of work because of this.

The anger, which is really an anger towards the effects of disease on my body, spills out, sometimes into my interactions with strangers, often with people I care about. Arthritis makes me feel self-indulgent. Arthritis, with me, appears to be nothing at all. So I am awkward having it as an excuse for behavior I believe I would not otherwise have developed.

Beyond the physical waxing and waning of flares and remissions, arthritis has contributed to my becoming who I am. It has made me a cautious person, difficult, unpredictable, and unrevealing. I am curious, desire to be logical and reasonable, but am intensely critical of myself and too demanding of others. All these qualities, found a place in the little girl diagnosed with JRA [juvenile rheumatoid arthritis] at the age of six, so afraid of the

judgments of others, and grew into the woman who underwent TJR [total joint replacement] surgery at the age of 27, intent on trying to push herself out there with everyone else. My nature, set against my strengths and fears, and sometimes foolishness represent another chronic struggle, to choose what's good for my body without compromising what's good for my soul, knowing that some choices have cost me, feeling satisfied with other choices that have been made based on the acceptance of my abilities.

I used to believe that "my arthritis" was separate from myself. I have come to understand, after 30 years of living with JRA, that this is no less a part of me than my fingers, my voice. My appreciation for pain, especially that which goes unseen, for recognizing the reality of potential (not everyone can be whatever they want), and for the ability to work at accepting one's limitations, has, and still does, guide my perspective. Everything about who I am is wrapped in and around this illness.

Catherine Morlino, age 35,
with JRA since 6, and
Editorial Assistant, *Arthritis and Rheumatism*

Beyond the obvious day-to-day discomfort, the most significant effect on my life from the spondylitis is that which it has on my self-image. This image is directly related to how I feel at any given moment. When I feel good, and am essentially unaware of symptoms, I am who I always have been—young, energetic, capable. But when my symptoms are present, my self-image changes—I am aging, tentative, dependent, tinged with self-pity and regret. I am more willing to accept, rather than strive. In short, my confidence in my life and myself is reduced by how I feel physically.

Despite this, a part of me rebels against this lowered self-esteem. It effectively refuses to accept the disease, to admit to not being able to do things I once did with ease or even skill. These two conflicting personae—the hesitant, reflective sick person, and the unaccepting person who does what he wants despite how he feels—arise from each other in a constant, uninterrupted shifting pattern. The self-pity, which is the last stage of my "sick person," awakens my "healthy person." When he is eventually confronted with a task, however mundane, which symptoms prevent him from doing, the "sick person" reemerges and the cycle begins anew. Maintaining equilibrium about my condition—emotional balance—is essential, and the best way to maintain it is to understand the disease, as it affects you, in a realistic manner, including realistic expectations of the future. It is thus most important that the treating physician be open and honest with the patient regarding treatment, diagnosis, prognosis, and symptoms.

Michael J. Brooks,
a lawyer with spondylitis since age 20

As health professionals, we usually deal with the negative impacts of diseases. However, we must realize that patients persevere and stay active and experience satisfaction with their lives[6–8] and that some even inspire the healthy with their accomplishments.

PSYCHOLOGIC FRAMEWORK

With rheumatic disease, as with other chronic illnesses, the vagaries of the disease interact with the patients' stage in life; their life experience, personality, and home and work environment; and their social and cultural systems. The interaction of these factors defines the meaning of the disease to the patient (the "illness experience"). People with chronic rheumatic diseases experience a series of adaptations. The responses seen in acute life-threatening illnesses (shock, anger, denial, resignation, and acceptance) are mirrored in the course of having a chronic disease. Reaction to the initial diagnosis is influenced by the degree of incapacity and the immediate threat to the patient's lifestyle. Patients with insidious-onset rheumatoid arthritis or systemic lupus erythematosus (SLE) may be relieved to have a diagnosis after frustrating efforts to have their condition diagnosed or after a lack of sympathy for their symptoms. Patients commonly ask themselves, "Why did this happen to me?" and attempt their own explanation as a way of rationalizing their illness or relieving uncertainty. The disease may be attributed to emotional or physical trauma, or punishment for some misdeed in search for causal explanations, and represents a common adaptive reaction.

Denial is another common reaction that may help the patient to adapt to the disease. At this stage, the most helpful approach is to provide support, reassurance, a plan, and a discussion of what to expect.

During periods of stable or quiescent disease activity, resignation and acceptance are more prominent adaptive mechanisms. During exacerbations, anger, denial, and anxiety and depression may recur. Anger, frequently toward the bearer of bad news, may manifest itself in demanding behavior or noncompliance.

IMPACT OF RHEUMATIC DISEASE AT DIFFERENT STAGES IN LIFE

A patient's adjustment to having chronic arthritis occurs against a background of one's stage in life. For the physician, sensitivity to the psychologic meaning of the illness starts with an awareness of the usual concerns and growth and development issues in that stage.

Arthritis commonly occurs during infancy between 2 and 4 years of age. The critical developmental milestone during this period is that the child must bond to the mother; the resultant physical satisfaction and warmth lay the foundation for developing trust in others. Other critical developmental tasks are to gain new motor and mental skills and a basic control of self and environment, which promote a sense of confidence and mastery. Between ages 3 and 6 years, a child begins to explore a wider environment and to

develop a conscience. Between ages 6 and 12 years, a child begins to explore the world beyond the home at school, to master intellectual and social skills, and to show an increase in physical strength.

One fourth of children with rheumatic disorders experience psychosocial problems in addition to the impaired function and delayed physical growth that may occur with inflammatory arthritis. Systemic illness and polyarthritis in the child may limit parents in providing physical warmth and comfort. Rheumatic disorders also limit the child's involvement in the school—the most important social experience in youth—which may lead to social isolation and psychosocial growth retardation. A study by Stoff and coworkers suggests that school achievement in children with rheumatic diseases was related more to inattention and distractibility than to impaired mobility or fatigue.[9] Young children may react to pain by passivity, protest, or vocal or facial expressions, and, unless asked specifically, they might not express their pain verbally.[10, 11]

Normal family dynamics are challenged.[12] A healthy sibling may feel abandoned because of the interest shown in the child with illness, which increases sibling rivalry and conflict. The father may be frequently uninvolved with the day-to-day health care of his child and may feel estranged and bewildered by the experience. Parents and teachers may overprotect and deprive the child of the chance to be strong and to feel independent. Children with less obvious physical impairment, such as monarticular or pauciarticular disease, may have more psychosocial problems than children with more extensive disease.[13] The latter group may have a legitimized disability, with allowances made for them by adults; children with minimal disease may not be perceived as sick or disabled, and this discrepancy may cause conflict in roles and interpersonal relationships. Less functional incapacity, higher family income, and higher educational level of the mother are factors that lessen the impact of a child's illness on the family.[12]

Public law 94–142 (The Education for All Handicapped Children Act) emphasizes mainstreaming and mandates that support services be available in schools for all children. Because arthritis disorders are rare in childhood, the school system, the teachers, or the school nurse is not likely to have experience in helping such patients. Ensuring smooth integration into the school usually requires follow-up by the health care team to educate school personnel in the nuances of the disease.

Polyarthritis affects the critical issues of adolescence; these include separation from parents and home, career training, career choice, achieving economic independence, peer relationships, and finding a mate.[14] Adolescence is normally a tumultuous time for young people and their families, and with the additional stress of a chronic illness, many problems become manifest. Adolescents with arthritis may refuse to take their pills or to do prescribed exercises.[15, 16] This "push–pull" conflict, characteristic of adolescents, can create many problems for parents and health care providers and requires a coordinated, consistent approach to management. The adolescent must be treated as an adult whenever possible. The physical examination should be done without the parent in the room. Giving some young patients choices from a menu of equivalent therapy or control over when treatment is administered is another way to treat and make them feel like adults. Adolescents do not want to appear different from their peers, and the use of devices, aids, or splints might be encouraged at home or at night as a tradeoff between what is necessary and what is responsive to their feelings.

Spondylitis disability seen in patients with ankylosing spondylitis, spondylitis associated with Reiter's disease, psoriasis, and inflammatory bowel disease are dominated by stiffness and restrictive movement of the spine with occasional involvement of the shoulder, hip, or knee; difficulties in sitting or standing for extended periods; stiffness and fatigue on awakening; a male predominance; and onset in young and middle-aged adults. Spondylitis disability is usually compatible with good function except when it involves peripheral joints. Iritis, or associated systemic diseases such as inflammatory bowel disease, may be even more limiting in some patients. Spondylitis in young adult males may affect self-esteem, body image, leisure and athletic activities in general, and peer and sexual relationships in particular.

Patients with spondylitis are frequently lost to follow-up, perhaps because the disease is insidious and generally compatible with good function. Compliance with physical therapy programs to maintain or improve spinal mobility is poor unless the routine is perceived as being useful and, most importantly, unless it is incorporated into normal activities. In Reiter's disease, the connection with venereal infection and urethritis may raise anxiety or guilt about intercourse in patients or their partners.

For adults, childbearing is a crucial issue. Adult women with systemic rheumatic disorders must confront the uncertainty of the effect of pregnancy on their usual activity or other organ involvement and how the challenge of motherhood will affect the physical demands of child rearing. A wish for children can be present even in disabled rheumatic patients, whereas the number of children regarded as feasible depends largely on the availability of help with child care and the patient's own coping strategies.[17] Counseling women who wish to become pregnant includes providing medical information and problem solving after delivery.

In late midlife, rheumatic disorders may intensify the perception of aging and accelerate physical dependence. After midlife, the dominant issue is maintaining one's independence. Old age is the time when people look forward to activities previously deferred because of work or family commitments, and a chronic illness may accelerate dependency.

Osteoarthritis is the most common rheumatic condition of late middle-aged patients, the elderly, and the oldest old. The disability associated with osteoarthritis unfolds slowly, paralleling the aging process. Indeed, many patients (and physicians) assume that musculoskeletal symptoms from osteoarthritis are an inevitable part of aging. In old-old age, osteoarthritis is the major cause of dependence and being homebound.[18] The impact of osteoarthritis can be particularly devastating because old age is often a time of many losses, especially general health, friends, family, and financial independence. Nevertheless, substantial depressive symptomatology appears to be no greater in elderly persons with osteoarthritis than in the general population of similar age.[19]

COMMON PSYCHOLOGIC PROBLEMS

Most systemic rheumatic diseases, such as rheumatoid arthritis and seronegative polyarthritis, are characterized by chronicity, unpredictability, potential disability, pain, and constitutional symptoms. Consequently, common psychologic problems include the fear of becoming disabled and dependent, uncertainty about the disease process, altered body image, devaluation of self, frustration, and depression. Early in the course of the disease, most patients experience the fear of becoming disabled or helpless. Seeing other patients or knowing someone with handicapping arthritis can be frightening to a person with a newly diagnosed condition. The most useful approach for the physician is to be frank, give information to demystify the illness, and discuss the range of treatments available. The way in which patients resolve the dilemma of independence versus dependence depends on disease activity, the degree of social support, the presence of financial resources, and their capacity to receive and ask for help. Having the ability to modify a work schedule, to hire additional help, or to work part-time aids adjustment. In time, most patients discover that they can gain more independence by both acknowledging and accepting help from others.

A patient's reaction may center on a specific loss, such as physical limitations, and abstract losses, such as expectations for the future, self-image, and self-esteem. Grief over such losses may lead to depressive symptoms. Prolonged grief or clinical depression may require antidepressant medication or referral for psychotherapy. Indications for a referral include impaired function, vegetative symptoms, sleep disturbance, loss of appetite, and ruminating, intractable hopelessness, or suicidal ideation.

Chronic pain is a major stress in rheumatic patients and plays a key role in psychologic well-being and disability.[20] Over time, pain is distracting and demoralizing and leads to lowered tolerance, irritability, and loss of concentration. A vicious circle may be set up in which the pain leads to inactivity and withdrawal, which in turn reinforces the pain. Nevertheless, considering the chronic pain experienced by people with various forms of chronic arthritis, few become chronic pain patients or patients who use narcotic analgesics and have lifestyles dominated by pain behavior.

Sexuality may be altered by pain, discomfort, and constitutional symptoms (e.g., fatigue), and poor self-image from deformities or medications, such as steroids. The unaffected partner may fear causing discomfort to the partner with arthritis, who may view unwillingness to engage in sexual activity as a loss of attraction. Systemic symptoms impair libido. A physician can legitimize the subject by raising the issue or by appropriate referral if sexuality is a concern.

Patients with rheumatoid vasculitis or with rheumatoid arthritis and extra-articular manifestations, SLE, or other systemic vasculitides face uncertainty and the potential life-threatening nature of the disease. The symptoms and functional capacity of those with rheumatoid arthritis may change from day to day and even from morning to afternoon.

Fatigue is a common and incapacitating symptom in many systemic rheumatic conditions but particularly in SLE and rheumatoid arthritis. Its importance is frequently underestimated by physicians, and its management can be haphazard. Depression, disease activity, anemia, deconditioning, and disturbed sleep are potential contributing factors, and the physician should attempt to find treatable causes. In patients with lupus or other rheumatic disorders with a paucity of physical signs, morning stiffness and fatigue need to be explained to the family and other contacts because the patient may not have anything visible to validate the symptoms to others. The patient may be able to work but may have less energy for other activities. This difficulty can be mitigated to a degree if the patient can explain the problem without feeling guilty about being unable to fulfill commitments.

In patients with SLE, neuropsychiatric manifestations (e.g., psychoaffective disorders, psychosis, cognitive disorders, and organic brain syndrome) are described. Cognitive dysfunction manifested by impaired short-term memory, concentration, and word finding seems to be a common feature of SLE.[21, 22] Psychologic profiles, as measured by the Minnesota Multiphasic Personality Inventory (MMPI), do not show differences between patients with SLE, rheumatoid arthritis, or other chronic disorders.[4] In the individual patient, whether the manifestation is due to SLE itself, a side effect of treatment, a reaction to having a serious illness, or a concomitant psychiatric disorder, it is always a challenge to sort out. When a specific cause can be found, it is treated; for serious psychiatric symptoms, psychotherapy or pharmacotherapy is necessary. Some patients with chronic rheumatic disorders attempt to conceal their disability for fear that their arthritis will make them less attractive to others or will cost them a job. In many situations, denial and acting no differently from others are the most healthy behaviors. Patients who maintain their own identity, as distinct from that of an "arthritis patient," seem to adapt better, function better, and to be in a better psychologic state. On the other hand,

concealment of symptoms may not allow others to help or to understand what the patient is going through. The physician should try to make the patient not feel pitied and to help friends and relatives to understand that talking about the disorder will not upset the patient.

PSYCHOLOGIC RESEARCH

Earlier work focused on a unique rheumatoid personality and on the psychologic factors that were thought to induce rheumatoid arthritis, but a critical review of the evidence casts doubt on this hypothesis.[5] Fibrositis has been considered a psychosomatic illness or as having a psychologic cause, but the evidence is similarly wanting.[23] However, it is possible that stress modifies the expression of the disease or lowers the patient's pain threshold. Tantalizing studies link psychologic phenomena with immune functions.[24, 25] During the past decades, a number of studies have addressed the global impact of disease on the patient and his or her psychologic and social well-being. These areas are briefly reviewed next.

Psychosocial Impact

Few diseases cause patients to suffer as much pain and discomfort over a prolonged period as arthritis.[23, 24] Although patients with chronic rheumatic disorders have a greater burden imposed on them than healthy individuals, several longitudinal studies suggest that psychologic and physical adaptation among patients with arthritis and other chronic illnesses is remarkably effective. Patients with rheumatoid arthritis appear to have no more depression as measured by psychologic testing than do individuals with other chronic diseases.[6, 26] Although there are setbacks and stress, given guidance, support and time, many, perhaps more than is generally appreciated, do well despite physical impairment. For health care providers, this is a reminder that medicalizing problems, overmanaging, and making patients more dependent may undermine their coping skills and the innate resourcefulness of patients and their families.

COMPLIANCE

Estimates of self-reported nonadherence to medications range from 22 to 67 percent and to physical therapy range from 33 to 66 percent.[27, 28] In contrast to the vast descriptive literature, little attention has been paid to evaluating strategies to enhance compliance.[29] Because prescribed arthritis regimens are rarely curative and their side effects are neither predictable nor trivial, noncompliance may be the best solution for the patient. Not surprisingly, noncompliance is increased when patients doubt a regimen's effectiveness, when they have erroneous beliefs about the medication,[30] or when they need to take the medication in multiple doses. Furthermore, the patient and the physician may differ in regard to what is an acceptable risk in treatment; a physician may be more willing than a patient to risk serious side effects on behalf of the patient for a particular expected benefit.[31]

The literature on compliance in other illness shows that adherence is improved under these circumstances:

• When the patient and physician agree on the problem, the disease model, and the treatment goals
• When the patient perceives a threat and an effective treatment exists
• When there is a simple technique for self-monitoring
• When there is social reinforcement
• When the regimen is not disruptive to normal patterns of activities
• When the disease is of more recent onset

The patient can identify potential barriers to carrying out the recommendations that can be overcome. Writing down the prescribed regimen is a simple and effective way to enhance compliance. The most significant predictor of compliance is a strong physician-patient relationship.[32]

PSYCHOEDUCATIONAL TECHNIQUES

A number of psychoeducational approaches for treating pain, disability, and psychologic distress have been evaluated in controlled studies.[33–35] These include:

• Educational approaches
• Group psychotherapy
• Structured group support
• Electromyography or alpha biofeedback training
• Relaxation training

These techniques teach patients to recognize and alter the association between environmental stimuli and pain and to place therapy under control of the patient.

Cognitive-behavioral interventions are considered self-control programs and emphasize the patient's role in reducing pain and disability and in appraising efficacy. Biofeedback training has been used in patients with chronic arthritis pain and with Raynaud's phenomenon and disease. A substantial body of evidence shows that a variety of psychoeducational interventions reduce pain and improve function and psychologic well-being.[33, 34, 36–40] A behavioral component added to an educational program increases its effectiveness, and even "experienced" patients, observed by specialists and who have had the disease for years, appear to gain knowledge about their disease and its treatment with organized patient education programs. The cost-effectiveness and durability of the results are suggested by a study by Lorig and associates that demonstrated reduced use of medical

services and reduced pain 4 years after participation in a self-management program.[41]

Controlled studies of health education have shown that although experimental groups adopt more of the desired behaviors and exhibit improvement in health outcome, the relationship between the performance of behaviors and health outcomes is not clear.[42] Participants in such programs are taught various skills and may only use those that are applicable or effective for them. Training in coping skills also gives patients a sense of control and mastery that can improve their coping with the disease or their perceptions of the disease.

A study using lay instructors and health professionals for a program modeled after the self-management program of Lorig and associates[43] showed that patient educational programs improved participants' knowledge of arthritis and compliance with therapeutic exercise compared to a nonintervention control group. The groups led by professional instructors had the same outcome as those led by lay instructors. However, neither intervention was any more effective than nonintervention in lessening pain, improving function, enhancing social support, or lessening depression.[44]

A randomized clinical trial evaluated three interventions in patients with rheumatoid arthritis:

1. A biofeedback-assisted cognitive-behavioral psychologic intervention.
2. A structured group social support therapy group.
3. A control group.

The psychologic intervention produced statistically significant reductions in pain behavior and in the Rheumatoid Activity Index at 3 months. Relaxation training was believed to be the most important component of the intervention. Anxiety was reduced at the 6-month follow-up.[45] In another study, education alone was compared with a cognitive-behavioral approach in patients with osteoarthritis. The results demonstrated that these two modes produced similar effects with respect to health outcomes and psychologic variables.[46]

In a randomized clinical trial in a Veterans Administration Hospital population with rheumatoid arthritis, a 12-month cognitive-behavioral pain management group, an attention-placebo group, and a control group were evaluated.[47] The group receiving psychologic intervention showed significantly greater use of coping strategies and more confidence in their ability to manage pain. However, the impact of the program on disease activity, functional status, or psychologic status was minimal and only in the most compliant group.

Structured group support for patients with rheumatic disease and their families provides a milieu to verbalize and share concerns, to learn about the disease, to realize that others have similar experiences and emotional reactions, and to strengthen coping strategies through problem solving. Though diverse, all programs have educational goals and emphasize communication skills, coping, and mutual support; however, some focus more on one aspect than another. Groups emphasizing psychologic support are usually led by psychologists, social workers, or health professionals with special training.

The supportiveness of one's social relations correlates with other psychosocial, behavioral, and physiologic indicators of health. However, clinical trials show that increasing social support alone produces mixed results.[48, 49] These negative studies may be a result of weak interventions, insensitive outcome measures, or small sample sizes. On the other hand, two successful interventions show their potential benefits.

Patients with osteoarthritis were contacted monthly in person, by phone, or both, for a year by a trained research assistant and engaged in dialogue about medications, joint pain, next clinic appointment, and barriers to keeping the appointment.[50] Pain and physical disability improved in patients contacted by telephone, and those who received either the telephone call or both interventions were significantly better than those who did not receive a call. An analysis of a subset of patients who had radiographic evidence of knee osteoarthritis and whose antirheumatic therapy did not change was done.[63] Patients contacted by telephone experienced significantly less pain and improved physical function. Notably, the improvement in joint pain was as marked as that achieved with a nonsteroidal anti-inflammatory drug.

An 8-week, randomized, controlled study was conducted of 102 patients with osteoarthritis of one or both knees. The control group received standard medical care; the intervention group received, in addition, supervised fitness walking and educational sessions three times per week designed to enhance physical activity, functional status, and optimal medication use to minimize pain.[52] The program significantly improved functional status without worsening pain, triggering flares, or increasing the use of medication. Self-efficacy beliefs of the patient's ability to manage symptoms other than pain due to osteoarthritis also improved.

SUMMARY

Psychologic and social problems constitute an integral feature of chronic rheumatic diseases and are a key to understanding how these diseases affect the individual patient. Patients and their advocates must find ways of dealing with the psychosocial consequences. These include a commitment to dealing with these consequences, a caring attitude, and an understanding of how the life cycle interacts with a chronic illness, how social factors modify the resultant handicap, and how specific interventions might be employed to ameliorate these effects. Psychologic and educational interventions can provide substantial benefits to people with chronic arthritis.

References

1. Rogers MP, Liang MH, Partridge AJ: Psychological care of adults with RA. Ann Intern Med 96:344–348, 1982.
2. Daltroy LH: Doctor-patient communication in rheumatological disorders. Baillieres Clin Rheumatol 7:221–239, 1993.
3. Bradley LA: Psychological aspects of arthritis. Bull Rheum Dis 35:1–12, 1985.
4. Liang MH, Rogers M, Larson M, Eaton HM, Murawski BJ, Taylor JE, Swafford J, Schur PH: The psychosocial impact of systemic lupus erythematosus and rheumatoid arthritis. Arthritis Rheum 27:13–19, 1984.
5. Baum J: A review of the psychological aspects of rheumatic diseases. Semin Arthritis Rheum 11:352–361, 1982.
6. Cassileth BR, Lusk EJ, Strouse TB, Miller DS, Brown LL, Gross PA, Tenaglia AN: Psychosocial status in chronic illness: A comparative analysis of six diagnostic groups. N Engl J Med 311: 506–511, 1984.
7. Burckhardt CS, Archenholtz B, Bjelle A: Quality of life of women with systemic lupus erythematosus: A comparison with women with rheumatoid arthritis. J Rheumatol 20:977–981, 1993.
8. Daltroy LH, Larson MG, Eaton HM, Partridge AJ, Pless IB, Rogers MP, Liang MH: Psychosocial adjustment in juvenile arthritis. J Pediatr Psychol 17:277–289, 1992.
9. Stoff E, Bacon ML, White PH: The effects of fatigue, distractibility, and absenteeism on school achievement in children with rheumatoid diseases. Arthritis Care Res 2:49–53, 1990.
10. Beales JC, Keen JH, Holt PJ: The child's perception of the disease and the experience of pain in juvenile chronic arthritis. J Rheumatol 10:16–18, 1983.
11. Vandvik IH, Eckblad G: Relationship between pain, disease severity and psychosocial function in patients with juvenile chronic arthritis (JCA). Scand J Rheumatol 19:295–302, 1990.
12. McCormick MC, Stemmoer MM, Athreya BH: The impact of childhood rheumatic diseases on the family. Arthritis Rheum 29:872–879, 1986.
13. McAnarney ER, Pless IB, Satterwhite B, Friedman SB: Psychological problems in children with chronic juvenile arthritis. Pediatrics 53:523, 1974.
14. Miller JJ, Spitz PW, Simpson U, Williams GF: The social function of young adults who had arthritis in childhood. J Pediatr 100:378–382, 1982.
15. Rapoff MA: Compliance with treatment regimens for pediatric rheumatoid diseases. Arthritis Care Res 2:S40–S47, 1989.
16. Hayford JR, Ross CK: Medical compliance in juvenile rheumatoid arthritis: Problems and perspectives. Arthritis Care Res 1:190–197, 1989.
17. Østensen M: Counselling women with rheumatic disease—how many children are desirable? Scand J Rheumatol 20:121–126,1991.
18. Badley EM, Tennant A: Disablement associated with rheumatic disorders in a British population: Problems with activities of daily living and level of support. Br J Rheumatol 32:601–608, 1993.
19. Dexter P, Brandt K: Distribution of depressive symptoms in osteoarthritis. J Rheumatol 21:279–286, 1994.
20. Affleck G, Tennen H, Urrows S, Higgins P: Individual differences in the day-to-day experience of chronic pain: A prospective daily study of rheumatoid arthritis patients. Health Psychol 10:419–429, 1991.
21. Ginsburg KS, Wright EA, Larson MG, Fossel AH, Albert M, Schur PH, Liang MH: A controlled study of the prevalence of cognitive dysfunction in randomly selected patients with systemic lupus erythematosus. Arthritis Rheum 35:776–782, 1992.
22. Fisk JD, Eastwood B, Sherwood G, Hanly JG: Patterns of cognitive impairment with systemic lupus erythematosus. Br J Rheumatol 32:458–462, 1993.
23. Bradley LA, Anderson HO, Young LD, McDaniel LK: Is psychological disturbance highly associated with primary fibrositis? Evidence that primary fibrositis is not a form of "psychogenic rheumatism." Behav Med Abstr 6:145–147, 1985.
24. Parker JC, Smarr KL, Angelone EO, et al: Psychological factors, immunologic activation, and disease activity in rheumatoid arthritis. Arthritis Care Res 5:196–201, 1992.
25. Reichlin S: Neuroendocrine-immune interactions. N Engl J Med 329:1246–1253, 1993.
26. Hawley DJ, Wolfe F: Depression is not more common in rheumatoid arthritis: A 10-year longitudinal study of 6,153 patients with rheumatic disease. J Rheumatol 20:2025–2031, 1993.
27. Ferguson K, Bole GG: Family support, health belief, and therapeutic compliance in patients with rheumatoid arthritis. Patient Counsel Health Educ 1:101–105, 1979.
28. Bradley LA: Adherence with treatment regimens among rheumatoid arthritis patients: Current status and future directions. Arthritis Care Res 2:S33–S39, 1989.
29. Waggoner CD, LeLieuvre RB: A method to increase compliance to exercise regimens in rheumatoid arthritis patients. J Behav Med 4:191–201, 1981.
30. Lorish CD, Richards B, Brown S Jr: Perspective of the patient with rheumatoid arthritis on issues related to missed medication. Arthritis Care Res 3:78–84, 1990.
31. Pullar T, Wright V, Feely M: What do patients and rheumatologists

regard as an 'acceptable' risk in the treatment of rheumatic disease? Br J Rheumatol 29:215–218, 1990.

32. Feinberg J: The effect of patient-practitioner interaction on compliance: A review of the literature and application in rheumatoid arthritis. Patient Educ Counseling 11:171–187, 1988.

33. Winfield JB and the ACR/AHPA/AF/NAAB Task Force on Arthritis Patient Education: Arthritis patient education: Efficacy, implementation, and financing. Arthritis Rheum 32:1330–1333, 1989.

34. Mullen PD, Laville EA, Biddle AK, Lorig K: Efficacy of psycho-educational interventions on pain, depression, and disability with arthritic adults: A meta-analysis. J Rheumatol 15:33–39, 1987.

35. DeVellis RF, Blalock SJ: Psychological and educational interventions to reduce arthritis disability. Bailleres Clin Rheumatol 7:397–416, 1993.

36. Shearn MA, Fireman BH: Stress management and mutual support group in rheumatoid arthritis. Am J Med 78:771–775, 1985.

37. Schwartz JH, Marcus R, Gordon R: Multidisciplinary group therapy for rheumatoid arthritis. Psychosomatics 19:289–293, 1978.

38. Strauss GD, Spiegel JS, Daniels M, Spiegel T, Landsverk J, Roy-Byrne P, Edelstein C, Ehlhardt J, Falke R, Hinden L, Zackler L: Group therapies for rheumatoid arthritis: A controlled study of two approaches. Arthritis Rheum 29:1203–1209, 1986.

39. Kaplan S, Kozin F: A controlled study of group counselling in rheumatoid arthritis. J Rheumatol 8:91–99, 1981.

40. Gross M, Brandt KD: Educational support groups for patients with ankylosing spondylitis: A preliminary report. Patient Counsel Health Educ 3:6–12, 1981.

41. Lorig KR, Mazonson PD, Holman HR: Evidence suggesting that health education for self-management in patients with chronic arthritis has sustained health benefits while reducing health care costs. Arthritis Rheum 36:439–446, 1993.

42. Lorig K, Seleznick M, Lubeck D, Ung E, Chastain RL, Holman HR: The beneficial outcomes of the arthritis self-management course are not adequately explained by behavior change. Arthritis Rheum 32:91–95, 1989.

43. Lorig K, Lubeck D, Kraines RG, Seleznick M, Holman HR: Outcomes of self-help education for patients with arthritis. Arthritis Rheum 28:680–685, 1985.

44. Cohen JL, Sauter S, DeVellis RF, DeVellis BM: Evaluation of arthritis self-management courses led by lay persons and by professionals. Arthritis Rheum 29:388–393, 1986.

45. Bradley LA, Young LD, Anderson KO, McDaniel LK, Pisko EJ, Samble EL, Morgan TM: Effects of psychological therapy on pain behavior of rheumatoid arthritis patients: Treatment outcomes and six-month follow-up. Arthritis Rheum 30:1105–1114, 1987.

46. Calfas KJ, Kaplan RM, Ingram RE: One-year evaluation of cognitive-behavioral intervention in osteoarthritis. Arthritis Care Res 5:202–209, 1992.

47. Parker JC, Frank RG, Beck NC, Smarr KL, Buescher KL, Phillips LR, Smith EI, Anderson SK, Walker SE: Pain management in rheumatoid arthritis patients: A cognitive-behavioral approach. Arthritis Rheum 31:593–601, 1988.

48. Potts M, Brandt KD: Analysis of education-support groups for patients with rheumatoid arthritis. Patient Counsel Health Educ 4:161–166, 1983.

49. Parker JC, Singsen BH, Hewett JE, Walker SE, Hazelwood SE, Hall PJ, Holstein DJ, Rodon CM: Educating patients with rheumatoid arthritis: A prospective analysis. Arch Phys Med Rehabil 65:771–774, 1984.

50. Weinberger M, Tierney WM, Booher P, Katz BP: Can the provision of information to patients with osteoarthritis improve functional status? A randomized, controlled trial. Arthritis Rheum 32:1577–1583, 1989.

51. Rene J, Weinberger M, Mazzuca SA, Brandt KD, Katz BP: Reduction of joint pain in patients with knee osteoarthritis who have received monthly telephone calls from lay personnel and whose medical treatment regimens have remained stable. Arthritis Rheum 35:511–515, 1992.

52. Kovar PA, Allegrante JP, MacKenzie CR, Peterson MGE, Gutin B, Charlson ME: Supervised fitness walking in patients with osteoarthritis of the knee: A randomized, controlled trial. Ann Intern Med 116:529–534, 1992.

CHAPTER 37

Evan Calkins

Some Aspects of Rheumatic Disease in the Older Patient

The fields of rheumatology and geriatrics are becoming increasingly intertwined, largely because of three factors. First, arthritis, or, more broadly, musculoskeletal disease, is the most frequently encountered and, for many, most bothersome complaint of older people.[1] Second, rapid growth in both the numbers and the percentage of older people in society means that an increasing component of the practice of all physicians, especially rheumatologists, will focus on geriatric patients. Third, it seems almost inevitable that changes in the pattern of medical practice in the United States will place increasing responsibility for coordinating care on a single physician, with other physicians and care providers serving in adjunctive capacities. The rheumatologist who wishes to directly influence ongoing patient management will also need to assume the role of primary care provider.[2] For the large segment of his or her practice with older people, this will require a thorough understanding of the concepts and knowledge base of geriatrics.

BIOLOGY OF AGING

Aging is a continuous process that involves sequential changes in the composition, function, and structure of cells, organs, and the entire organism.[3, 4] Figure 37–1 schematically depicts the lifetime curve of the physiologic function and structure of many, possibly most, components of the body. At genesis or birth, certain components are at negligible levels (e.g., the diameter of the myofibrils of the human heart[5]); others start at high levels (e.g., the number of cells per given weight or volume of certain organs, such as the brain,[6] skin,[7] or cartilage.[8] Rapid changes occur during early developmental life and extend through youth and adolescence. Most structures and functions achieve their peak by the time the person reaches his or her mid-20s. From that point on, with few exceptions, the curve pursues a pattern of progressive decline, gradually approaching the minimal level required for maintenance of life (indicated schematically by the horizontal dotted line in Fig. 37–1).

The general shape of the curve is the same for everyone, but individual variations are large. In addition, genetic factors may cause shifts in the curve, sometimes resulting in premature organ failure or death. Certain diseases, toxic exposures, and habits that affect health—occurring either throughout life

(e.g., lifetime habit of smoking) or during a short interval (e.g., exposure to industrial toxins, or a viral encephalitis occurring in someone with a predisposition to Parkinson's disease[9])—also result in more rapid declines. There is debate about the extent to which these changes represent what might be called "normal aging," or the accumulating effect of disease.[10, 11] Accordingly, an emphasis on primary, secondary, and tertiary prevention in both older and younger persons has emerged as an important goal of geriatric medicine.[12, 13] A major factor that underlies the vulnerability, loss of physical reserve, and declining health status of older people is physical inactivity.[14, 15] It has been suggested that many of the risk factors that have been attributed to aging may be more precisely attributed to the decreased physical activity that frequently accompanies the aging process. Although muscle-building exercise cannot totally ablate age-related declines in muscle function,[16] it can enhance the efficiency of muscle metabolism at any age[17–19] and, in this way, can contribute substantially to improving the functional and emotional status of older persons, including those with arthritis.

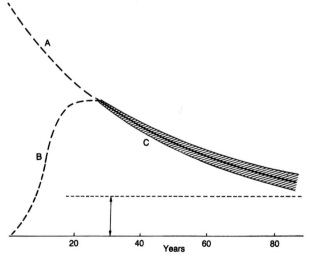

Figure 37–1. Schematic representation of normal development and aging (A–C). A and B represent changes during early life, as referred to in the text. C represents the gradual but inevitable declines accompanying aging. The *shaded area* reflects the different rates occurring in different individuals. The horizontal *dotted line* represents the functional level required for continued life. (From Katz P, Dube D, Calkins E: Aging and disease. *In* Calkins E, Davis PJ, Ford AB [eds]: The Practice of Geriatrics. Philadelphia, WB Saunders, 1986, p 2.)

Because the presence of musculoskeletal disease is one of the factors that inhibits the overall physical activity of older persons, the prevention and effective treatment of musculoskeletal problems, combined with an effort to reverse or retard age-related declines in muscle function, appears to have major significance not only for patient comfort, mobility, and capacity for independent life but also for overall health and survivorship.

PRACTICAL APPLICATIONS OF THE BIOLOGY OF AGING

Practice Concepts Relevant to All Older Persons

While seemingly in good health, most older people have little functional reserve and, with this, reduced capacity for homeostasis. A relatively minor intercurrent event, such as a fall, may lead to a cascade of organ system failure. Preventive care is important. Apparently minor intercurrent illnesses should be taken seriously. Steps should be taken to avoid overstressing uninvolved organ systems.

These principles apply equally to psychologic and social aspects of function. Behavior-oriented preventive care includes maintenance of important interpersonal relationships and attention to possible overburdening of care providers. Relocations are difficult for older people to accept. These alone may trigger a cascade of psychosocial and physiologic decline. It is important to avoid hospitalization whenever possible.

Most older persons are already experiencing fears and limitations that they themselves recognize but do not wish to reveal to others, including their physicians.[20] These include fear of underlying disease and fear of possible hospitalization or institutionalization in a nursing home. In general, older people do not complain excessively.

Objective assessment tools are available to measure the functional capacity of older patients. Slightly different from the instruments that have been developed for the assessment of function and status of patients with arthritis, these instruments are extremely helpful in prioritizing needs of older persons and in designing comprehensive ongoing care. Examples include the mini-mental status examination[21] for cognitive function and, for overall physical function, instruments to assess the activities of daily living,[22] the instrumental activities of daily living,[23] physical performance,[24, 25] and overall function and well-being (the MOS Short Form Health Survey—SF-36).[26]

The major goal of geriatric medicine is maintenance of function—physical, cognitive, and social. In addition to multifaceted assessment, clinical diagnosis, and medical treatment, geriatric medicine relies on interdisciplinary teams and coordination of multiple levels of care (i.e., acute in-hospital care, emergency care, geriatric assessment units,[27] nursing home care, and home care).

The age-related changes in organ function mentioned earlier often are not clinically apparent or reflected in the usual clinical studies. An important example is the decline in renal function that occurs throughout life in almost everyone.[10] Although renal function may appear to be normal (i.e., normal urinalysis, blood urea nitrogen level, and serum creatinine concentration), serial estimations of creatinine clearance show a significant decline in about 65 percent of older people.

Applications Especially Relevant to the Practice of Rheumatology

Altered Presentation and Incidence of Rheumatic Diseases

One of the classic concepts of geriatric medicine is that the clinical expression of many disease states in older people is strikingly different from that in persons at midlife.[28] Because most textbooks focus on patients in early and middle adulthood, consideration of disease in the elderly in "textbook presentations" is often conspicuous by its absence (e.g., patients with ischemic heart disease who experience no pain, lobar pneumonia in the absence of fever, fecal impaction as a cause of fever). In rheumatology, many diseases tend to occur in people who are in the later stages of life (e.g., osteoarthritis, Sjögren's syndrome, polymyalgia rheumatica, giant cell arteritis, calcium pyrophosphate deposition disease, Paget's disease), and the textbook descriptions relate primarily to older patients. Other rheumatic diseases, such as rheumatoid arthritis and gout, occur in persons in widely different age groups, and the clinical manifestations in older patients may differ from those in younger persons.[28–36]

Because of the wide variability of most of these diseases among persons of any age, however, these differences have relatively little value in practice with individual patients (except for disseminated lupus erythematosus, in which they are particularly clear-cut.)[31–33] What *is* important in rheumatologic practice with older patients is the frequency with which musculoskeletal symptoms leading to referral or self-referral of older patients to the rheumatologist reflect a wide variety of conditions, many of them with serious implications, that *are not usually regarded as falling within the constellation of rheumatic disease*. Examples include multiple myeloma, carcinomatosis, hypothyroidism, hyperparathyroidism, Parkinson's disease, neuropathy due to diabetes mellitus, alcoholism, and pernicious anemia. Differential diagnosis requires a broad understanding of many aspects of clinical medicine, including ones that fall outside of the frame of reference of traditional rheumatology. Also, in older persons without any evidence of rheumatic or inflammatory disease, certain diagnostic tests (e.g., erythrocyte sedimentation rate, assays for rheumatoid factor and antinuclear antibody) frequently exhibit levels that would be of clinical significance in younger individuals.[37, 38]

Multiple Diseases

Equally challenging for the consultant rheumatologist is the fact that chronic diseases rarely occur alone in older patients. Although an occasional elderly person has only one disease, or even none, most older people suffer simultaneously from multiple chronic diseases—often multiple rheumatic diseases. This tendency is a reflection of the concurrent age-related declines in physiologic function in all organ systems, as well as the fact that, in the past half century, medical science has yielded effective treatment for many acute, formerly lethal, conditions, while little progress has been made in the prevention and treatment of many chronic diseases, such as osteoarthritis, that linger, often in multiples, as a person ages.[39]

The symptoms of the rheumatic diseases are themselves relatively nonspecific—pain (often diffuse), stiffness, weakness, numbness, and paresthesias in the extremities and, for systemic diseases, constitutional symptoms, such as weight loss. When a person is affected by a single disease, the product of these nonspecific symptoms provides specificity and the correct diagnosis can be reached relatively easily. When the patient has several diseases, each of which may be characterized by any or none of these nonspecific manifestations, the pattern becomes much more difficult to analyze and interpret and presents a special challenge to the careful clinician.

Use of Drugs

A patient with multiple diseases presents potential challenges not only in diagnosis but also in treatment, especially regarding use of drugs. The omnipresent threat of adverse reaction to drugs, often serious and sometimes fatal, is an important component of geriatric rheumatologic practice. According to Fries and colleagues, gastropathy associated with one of the most commonly used groups of medications, the nonsteroidal anti-inflammatory drugs (NSAIDs), may be the most frequent drug side effect in the United States.[40] Whether the high frequency of adverse reaction to drugs among older people is due to age itself or to other factors, such as the presence of multiple diseases (leading to prescriptions for numerous drugs) or disease-related declines in renal or hepatic function, is not clearly understood.[41] A recent report suggested that physical disability may be an important predisposing factor to NSAID-related gastropathy and that regular physical activity decreases the risk of this outcome.[42] Nevertheless, some of the reasons for the high frequency of adverse reaction to drugs in older persons are clear[43–48] and are summarized in Table 37–1.

Unfortunately, the number of drugs that constitute modern pharmacologic management, the frequency of introduction of new agents, and the potential for any drug to cause substantial harm through any of several mechanisms outlined earlier combine to make it almost impossible to recall all of the potential toxic

Table 37–1. SOME REASONS FOR INCREASED DRUG TOXICITY AMONG OLDER PATIENTS

1. Inherent toxicity of the drug itself (chemical or immunologic)
2. Altered pharmacodynamics: varied end-organ responsiveness as a result of the aging process[44]
3. Altered pharmacokinetics: alterations in distribution, excretion, or detoxification of drugs secondary to age-related or disease-related changes of kidney and liver; changes in binding of drugs to α-1 acid glycoprotein and albumin[43]
4. Nutritional insufficiency, including protein-calorie malnutrition
5. Polypharmacy: simultaneous prescriptions for numerous medications in response to the simultaneous occurrence of several acute and chronic diseases
6. Drug interaction: administration of one drug may enhance the potential of toxicity of a second agent because of alterations in renal clearance, catabolism, or protein binding of the second agent or to increase sensitivity or responsiveness of tissue receptors. Pharmacokinetics of methotrexate can be altered by simultaneous administration of chloroquine, salicylate, and many NSAIDs. Coadministration of sulfasalazine with methotrexate or trimethoprim-sulfamethoxazole leads to additive toxicity.[45]
7. Presence of conditions that would exaggerate potential adverse effects of drug therapy (i.e., warfarin in patients who fall or NSAIDs in patients with a history of peptic ulcer or previous upper gastrointestinal bleeding)
8. Compliance error: confusion regarding older patients' instructions in taking different medications, each at a different daily schedule; confusion enhanced by receipt of prescriptions from several physicians simultaneously

Abbreviation: NSAIDs, nonsteroidal anti-inflammatory drugs.

effects of the agents one is using. Table 37–2 lists some general principles that can prove helpful in decreasing the frequency of adverse drug reactions in clinical practice with older patients.[43]

Nonpharmacologic Therapy

Many physicians working under tight time constraints, especially primary care physicians as well as many patients themselves, think of medical care in terms of diagnosis and prescribing "the right drug" or, all too frequently, "one more drug." One of the major contributions a consulting rheumatologist or geriatrician can bring to patient care is an apprecia-

Table 37–2. GUIDELINES FOR PRESCRIBING DRUGS TO ELDERLY PATIENTS

1. Take a careful drug history, including any use of over-the-counter medications.
2. Become familiar with the effects of age on the pharmacology of the drugs prescribed.
3. Strive to make a diagnosis before treatment.
4. In general, use smaller initial doses in the elderly.
5. Adjust the dose according to the patient's response.
6. Review the drugs and the treatment plan regularly, and simplify the therapeutic regimen whenever possible.
7. Be alert to the possibility of drug-induced illness and that of interactions between disease states and drugs.

Modified with permission from Montamat SC, Cusack BJ, Vestal RE: Management of drug therapy in the elderly. New England Journal of Medicine 321:307, 1989.

tion of the significant benefits of well-designed comprehensive care, extending far beyond the prescription of systemic medication. Examples include appropriate attention to psychologic aspects, which often contribute substantially to musculoskeletal pain and disability[49, 50]; appropriate exercise[51–53] and other methods of physical therapy[54]; careful injection of joints, bursae, and tendon sheaths; rest; postural therapy[55]; good shoes; and appropriate use of assistive devices, including a cane. Details about most of these approaches are described in other chapters of this book and elsewhere.[56, 57] Gaining some expertise in the field of orthopedic medicine can be an advantage for both rheumatologists and primary care physicians who treat geriatric patients with rheumatologic disease.

Time Factor

Both geriatrics and rheumatology relate to patients with chronic illness. However, a special point of emphasis in geriatrics—important but less emphasized in rheumatology—is the perspective of the entire life course. This is exemplified by the problem of osteoporosis. For many physicians, concerned primarily with chronic disease, the chief points of emphasis are efforts to combat postmenopausal osteoporosis through appropriate use of estrogens and other agents, including diphosphonate,[58] and to minimize osteoporosis in patients receiving longstanding, low-dose prednisone therapy.[59] For the geriatrician, however, the initial point of concern focuses on adolescent children. The period coincidental with and immediately after sexual maturation is the only time in life when increased doses of calcium result in an increased mineral density of the skeleton.[60] The most effective means of combating postmenopausal osteopenia is not confined to the administration of estrogens to high-risk patients early in menopause, but reflects equally, or even more, the extent of the reservoir of calcium in the skeleton before the process begins. This in turn is directly related to the lifestyle and dietary habits of the patient during his or her adolescent years. As stated by Dixon, "Good bones should last a lifetime."[61]

Thus, the field of geriatrics brings to general medicine and also to rheumatology an enhanced awareness of the importance of a healthy life (intrauterine, neonatal, early childhood, adolescent, and young adult life as well as old age) as a major determinant of the ability of the individual to thrive during the challenge of later years.

In a practical way, these considerations influence decision making in the various phases of life. For a rheumatologist caring for a patient with active rheumatoid arthritis in his or her early thirties, the achievement of a true remission represents an important goal, worth a considerable investment in time and care and, if necessary, relatively short-term use of selected potentially toxic drugs. For a person in his or her 80s, with early active rheumatoid arthritis, the achievement of a true remission is of less importance. What *is* important is to restore the person, in the shortest possible time, to a level of physical functioning that permits him or her to retain relatively independent life in the community and to maintain the social context essential to this objective. Thus, one should avoid a long course of treatment with an agent, such as hydroxychloroquine (Plaquenil), whose effectiveness requires an interval of months. Instead, emphasis is placed on measures such as early initiation of low-dose prednisone therapy, which, even though it may pose considerable risk, is likely to restore overall function and to achieve it in the shortest possible interval.

Empowering the Patient

Philip Wood has stated: "We cannot expect major reductions in the scale of problems for which some help from the health and social services will be needed. The strategic goals should be towards policies of enablement, seeking ways of maximizing the ability of old people to handle their health and other problems."[62]

Thus, the physician caring for older patients should never overlook the benefits that can be achieved through patient education[63] and support programs. The PACE program, developed by the Arthritis Foundation and available in most communities, provides an excellent avenue to greater empowerment and social support as well as an introduction to the potential benefits of well-designed exercises. *The Moisture Seekers Newsletter*, published monthly by the Sjögren's Syndrome Foundation,* provides an outstanding array of background information for patients with sicca syndrome, and other informational materials are available through the Arthritis Foundation.

SUMMARY

Although geriatrics and rheumatology share many concepts and tools, there are important differences. Geriatrics brings a greater sensitivity to the developmental concepts of life and, with this, greater emphasis on prevention, multifaceted assessment, and comprehensive care of the illnesses that afflict older people. High priority is also assigned to therapeutic approaches directed toward maintenance of function and preservation of independence. In view of the increasing size of the older population and the new roles that professionals in the field of rheumatology are being called on to play, an appreciation of the attitudes, knowledge, and skills required for the treatment of geriatric patients becomes important in the future of rheumatology.

---

*Sjögren's Syndrome Inc., 333 North Broadway, Jericho, NY 11753.

References

1. National Center for Health Statistics: Current estimates from the National Health Survey: United States 1966. Vital Health Statistics Series 10:164, 1987.
2. American College of Rheumatology Executive Group: Bulletin on Healthcare Reform: Managed Care and the Rheumatologist. Atlanta, American College of Rheumatology, 1993.
3. Abrass IB: The biology and physiology of aging. West J Med 153:641, 1990.
4. Williams ME: Clinical implications of aging physiology. Am J Med 76:1049, 1984.
5. Dogliotti Z: Physiological and pathological aging. Z Anat Entwicklungsgesch 76:716, 1931. [Mentioned in Finch CE, Hoflick L: Handbook of Biology of Aging. New York, Van Nostrand Reinhold, 1977, p 686.]
6. Brody H: Organization of the cerebral cortex. III: A study of aging in the human cerebral cortex. J Comp Neurol 102:511, 1955.
7. Andrew W, Behnke RH, Sato T: Changes with advancing age in the cell population of the human dermis. Gerontologica 10:1, 1965.
8. Mankin HJ, Brandt KD: Biochemistry and metabolism of articular cartilage in osteoarthritis. In Moskowitz RW, Howell DS, Goldberg VM, et al (eds): Osteoarthritis: Diagnosis and Medical/Surgical Management, 2nd ed. Philadelphia, WB Saunders, 1984, pp 109–154.
9. Ben-Shlomo Y, Finnan F, Allwright S: The epidemiology of Parkinson's disease in the Republic of Ireland: Observations from routine data sources. Ir Med J 86:190, 1993.
10. Lindeman RD, Tobin J, Shock NW: Longitudinál studies on the rate of decline of renal function with age. J Am Geriatr Soc 33:278, 1985.
11. Evans JG, Williams TF: Introduction. In Oxford Textbook of Geriatric Medicine. Oxford, UK, Oxford University Press, 1992, p xv.
12. German PS, Fried LP: Prevention and the elderly: Public health issues and strategies. Annu Rev Public Health 10:319, 1989.
13. Buchner DM, Wagner EH: Preventing frail health (rev). Clin Geriatr Med 8:1, 1992.
14. Wagner EH, LaCroix AZ, Buchner DM, et al: Effects of physical activity on health status in older adults. I: Observational studies (rev). Annu Rev Public Health 13:451, 1992.
15. Pendergast DR, Fisher NM, Calkins E: Cardiovascular, neuromuscular, and metabolic alterations with age leading to frailty (rev). J Gerontol 48:61, 1993.
16. Heath GW, Hagberg JM, Ehsani AA, et al: A physiological comparison of young and old endurance athletes. J Appl Physiol 51:634, 1981.
17. Fisher NM, Pendergast DR, Calkins E: Muscle rehabilitation in impaired elderly nursing home residents. Arch Phys Med Rehab 72:181, 1991.
18. Fiatarone MA, Evans WJ: The etiology and reversibility of muscle dysfunction in the aged (rev). J Geriontol 48:77, 1993. Special issue.
19. Buchner DM, Bersford SA, Larson EB, et al: Effects of physical activity on health status of older adults II. Annu Rev Public Health 13:469, 1992.
20. Levkoff SE, Cleary PD, Wetle T: Illness behavior in the aged: Implications for clinicians. J Am Geriatr Soc 36:622, 1988.
21. Folstein MF, Folsein S, McHugh PR: "Minimental state": A practical method for grading the cognitive state of patients for the clinician. J Psychiatric Res 12:189, 1975.
22. Katz S, Downs TD, Cash HR, et al: Progress in development of the index of ADL. Gerontologist 10:20, 1970.
23. Lawton MP, Brody EM: Assessment of older people: Self-maintaining and instrumental activities of daily living. Gerontologist 9:179, 1969.
24. Reuben DB, Siu AL: An objective measure of physical function of elderly outpatients: The physical performance test. J Am Geriatr Soc 38:1105, 1990.
25. Nelson E, Wasson J, Kirk J, et al: Assessment of function in routine clinical practice: Description of the COOP chart method and preliminary findings. J Chron Dis 40(Suppl 1):55S, 1987.
26. Ware JE Jr, Sherbourne CD: The MOS 36-Item Short-Form Health Survey (SF-36). 1: Conceptual framework and item selection. Med Care 30:473, 1992.
27. Rubenstein LZ, Josephson KR, Wieland GD, et al: Effectiveness of a geriatric evaluation unit: A randomized clinical trial. N Engl J Med 311:1664, 1994.
28. Deal CL, Meenan RF, Goldenberg DL, et al: The clinical features of elderly onset rheumatoid arthritis: A comparison with younger-onset disease of similar duration. Arthritis Rheum 28:987, 1985.
29. Healey LA: Rheumatoid arthritis in the elderly. Clin Rheum Dis 12:173, 1986.
30. Wilkins E: Osteoarthritis and articular chondrocalcinosis in the elderly. Ann Rheum Dis 42:280, 1983.
31. Maddison PJ: Systemic lupus erythematosus in the elderly. J Rheum 14 (Suppl 13):182, 1987.
32. Reveille JD, Bartolucci A, Alarcon GS: Prognosis in systemic lupus erythematosus: Negative impact of increasing age at onset, black race, and thrombocytopenia as well as causes of death. Arthritis Rheum 33:37, 1990.
33. Cervera R, Khamashta MA, Font J, et al: Systemic lupus erythematosus: Clinical and immunologic pattern of disease expression in a cohort of 1,000 patients. The European Working Party on Systemic Lupus Erythematosus. Medicine 72:113, 1993.
34. Holti G, Schuster S: Scleroderma in the elderly (letter). Br Med J 282:1400, 1981.
35. Campbell SM: Gout: How presentation, diagnosis, and treatment differ in the elderly (rev). Geriatrics 43:71, 1988.
36. Strickland RW, Tesar JT, Berne HH, et al: The frequency of the sicca syndrome in the elderly population. J Rheumatol 14:766, 1987.
37. Hayes GS, Stinson IN: Erythrocyte sedimentation rate and age. Arch Ophthalmol 94:939, 1976.
38. Hallgren HM, Buckley CE II, Gilbertson VA, Yunis EJ: Lymphocyte phytohemagglutinin responsiveness, immunoglobulins, and autoantibodies in aging humans. J Immunol 111:1101, 1973.
39. Gruenberg EM: The failures of success. Milbank Mem Q Health Soc 55:3, 1977.
40. Fries JF, Miller SR, Spitz PW, et al: Toward an epidemiology of gastropathy associated with nonsteroidal anti-inflammatory drug use. Gastroenterology 96:647, 1989.
41. Gurwitz JH, Avorn J: The ambiguous relation between aging and adverse drug reactions (rev). Ann Intern Med 114:956, 1991.
42. Pahor M, Guralnik JM, Salive ME, et al: Physical activity and risk of severe gastrointestinal hemorrhage in older persons. JAMA 272:595, 1994.
43. Montamat SC, Cusack BJ, Vestal RE: Management of drug therapy in the elderly. N Engl J Med 321:303, 1989.
44. Feely J, Coakley D: Altered pharmacodynamics in the elderly. Clin Geriatr Med 6:269, 1990.
45. Wolfe F, Cathey MA: The effect of age on methotrexate efficacy and toxicity. J Rheumatol 18:973, 1991.
46. Llewellyn JG, Pritchard MH: Influence of age and disease state on nonsteroidal anti-inflammatory drug–associated gastric bleeding. J Rheumatol 15:691, 1988.
47. Griffin MR, Piper JM, Daugherty JR, et al: Nonsteroidal anti-inflammatory drug use and increased risk for peptic ulcer disease in elderly persons. Ann Intern Med 114:257, 1991.
48. Beers MH, Ouslander JG: Risk factors in geriatric drug prescribing: A practical guide to avoiding problems. Drugs 37:105, 1989.
49. Lichtenberg PA, Swensen CH, Skehan MW: Further investigation of the role of personality, life style and arthritic severity in predicting pain. J Psychosomatic Res 30:327, 1986.
50. Keefe FJ, Caldwell DS, Queen KT, et al: Pain coping strategies in osteoarthritis patients. J Consult Clin Psychol 55:208, 1987.
51. Fisher NM, Pendergast DR, Gresham GE, Calkins E: Muscle rehabilitation: Its effect on the muscular and functional performance of patients with knee osteoarthritis. Arch Med Rehab 72:367, 1991.
52. Galloway MT, Jokl P: The role of exercise in the treatment of inflammatory arthritis (rev). Bull Rheum Dis 42:1, 1993.
53. Kovar PA, Allegrante JP, MacKenzie CR, et al: Supervised fitness walking in patients with osteoarthritis of the knee: A randomized, controlled trial. Ann Intern Med 116:529, 1992.
54. De Lisa JA, Currie DM, Gans BM, et al: Rehabilitation Medicine: Principles and Practice. Philadelphia, JB Lippincott, 1988.
55. Stankovic R, Johnell O: Conservative treatment of low back pain: A prospective randomized trial: McKenzie method of treatment versus patient education in "mini-back school." Spine 15:120, 1990.
56. Moskowitz RW, Howell DS, Goldberg VM, et al: Osteoarthritis: Diagnosis and Medical/Surgical Management, 2nd ed. Philadelphia, WB Saunders, 1992.
57. Dorman TA, Ravin TH: Diagnosis and Injection Techniques in Orthopedic Medicine. Baltimore, Williams & Wilkins, 1991.
58. Liberman VA, Weiss S, Broll J, et al: Effect of oral alendronate on bone mineral density and the incidence of fractures in post-menopausal osteoporosis. N Engl J Med 333:1437, 1995.
59. Mulder H, Struys A: Intermittent cyclical etidronate in the prevention of corticosteroid-induced bone loss. Br J Rheumatol 33:348, 1994.
60. Lloyd T, Andon MB, Rollings N, et al: Calcium supplementation and bone mineral density in adolescent girls. JAMA 270:841, 1993.
61. Dixon ASJ: Health of the nation and osteoporosis. Ann Rheum Dis 51:914, 1992.
62. Wood PHN: Epidemiology of joint and connective tissue disorders. In Evans JG, Williams TF (eds): Oxford Textbook of Geriatric Medicine. Oxford, UK, Oxford University Press, 1992, p 355.
63. Winfield JB: Arthritis patient education: Efficacy, implementation and financing. The ACR/AHPA/AF/NAAB Task Force on Arthritis Patient Education. Arthritis Rheum 32:1330, 1989.

CHAPTER 38

Sports Medicine

Scott A. Lintner
John A. Feagin, Jr.
Arthur L. Boland

Sports medicine involves the study of the physiologic, psychologic, and pathologic aspects of athletics and exercise. As sport and exercise have taken a greater role in everyday life, the injuries that often accompany them have become more common.

Hippocrates, the father of medicine, is credited with the first description of a surgical treatment of shoulder instability suffered during gymnastic exercises.[11] Galen served as the physician to the gladiators of Pergamum from 158 to 161 A.D., thus becoming the first known team physician. He was active in anatomic and physiologic research through animal dissections and published many works about exercise and physiology.[2] After the fall of the Roman empire, Muslim physicians translated and then adopted many of the writings of Galen. Avicenna, considered the father of Muslim medicine, compiled his *Canon of Medicine,* which was considered the medical standard from the 12th to the 17th centuries. It contains information on sports medicine and rehabilitation.[3] Geronimo Mercuriali published "Artis Gymnasticae Apud Antiguas Celeberrimas, Nostris Temporibus Ignoratae" in 1569. This is the first illustrated book of sports medicine.[4] In America, sports medicine began with pioneers such as Hitchcock, Darling, Nichols, Stevens, and Quigley.[5, 6]

Injuries resulting from recreational and competitive athletics are common. Acute musculoskeletal injuries can occur in any age group and may lead to a functional disability if not promptly diagnosed and treated appropriately. Repetitive athletic activities may insidiously injure periarticular soft tissues, tendons, and bursae, producing pain and gradual limitation of motion and function. To recognize and manage these traumatic and overuse injuries, one must be familiar with the specific anatomic features of the involved area, the common mechanisms of injury, the relevance of the clinical signs and symptoms, the acceptable treatment options, and the physical demands of a specific athletic activity or sport.

This chapter provides a general overview of the anatomic areas commonly involved in athletic injuries and considers the common pathologic conditions that afflict these regions, with corresponding diagnostic and treatment strategies. It is not meant to cover all the anatomic areas and their associated injuries.

GENERAL PRINCIPLES

More so than with most conditions, successful diagnosis and treatment of athletic injuries require a thorough history and physical examination. Obtaining the history of the patient's chief complaint usually provides a clue to the eventual diagnosis. How the symptoms relate to the patient's daily, recreational, and occupational activities should be determined. A history of trauma, time course of symptom onset, and previous medical or surgical treatment should be documented. General medical health and involvement of litigation or worker's compensation may also be important.

After a careful history is obtained, a complete and thorough physical examination should be performed. The physical examination methods for many anatomic areas are specific to that region and to certain injuries within that region.[7]

THE SHOULDER

Chief Complaint

The two most common complaints involving the shoulder are pain and instability. For pain, the onset, location, character, and exacerbating or relieving factors should be determined. The patient may point to the acromioclavicular (AC) joint as a source of pain. Pain over the deltoid is often found in patients with rotator cuff tendinitis. Pain over the top of the shoulder may be referred from the cervical spine. Many patients complain of night pain, which is in rotator cuff disease. Other conditions that cause night pain are degenerative joint disease, infection, and tumors.

Complaints of instability can cover a wide range of clinically evident conditions. Patients may relate a known dislocation that required manipulative reduction or complain of a feeling of slipping or sliding or of the arm going "dead." Pain may also be the only complaint in some athletes with subtle instability.

Instability has been separated into two groups: (1) *t*raumatic and *u*nidirectional with a *B*ankart lesion, which usually requires *s*urgical intervention for maintenance of stability (TUBS), and (2) *a*traumatic and *m*ultidirectional, commonly with *b*ilateral involvement, which usually responds to *r*ehabilitation, but if surgery is indicated, an *i*nferior capsular shift is the procedure of choice (AMBRI).[8]

The direction of the instability is ascertained by questioning or by examining previous radiographs of dislocations (Fig. 38–1). Anterior instability is usually symptomatic when the arm is abducted and exter-

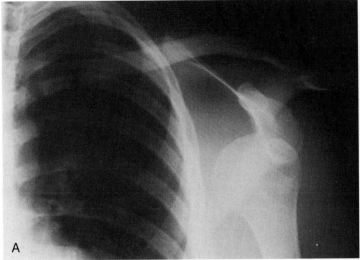

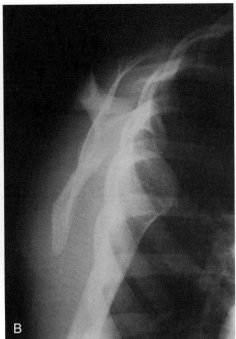

Figure 38–1. Radiographs of an acute anterior shoulder dislocation. *A,* Anteroposterior view. *B,* Scapular lateral projection.

nally rotated. Posterior instability is often symptomatic with forward flexion and internal rotation, with or without adduction. Inferior instability becomes symptomatic with an inferior force, such as carrying a suitcase. The circumstances that surround episodes of instability may also provide a clue to the direction of instability.

A decrease in the usual range of motion is another common complaint in shoulder injuries. It often represents a reaction to pain with resultant stiffness. Poor active motion may represent rotator cuff disease. An absolute decrease in passive motion is a sign of adhesive capsulitis. A posterior shoulder dislocation must be ruled out; it can cause a limitation of external rotation and is often overlooked, sometimes with disastrous consequences.

The common complaint of weakness raises a number of diagnostic possibilities. The examining physician should be sure that there truly is muscle weakness and not strength inhibition secondary to pain. Rotator cuff disease is a common condition that results in weakness. Neurologic diseases, either central or peripheral, often present as weakness.

A sensation of grinding or catching is another complaint in the shoulder. This may represent subacromial inflammation and scarring, a rotator cuff tear, labral tears, intra-articular loose bodies, or an impingement.

Physical Examination

Examination of the shoulder is complex and requires practice and experience. It should be performed carefully and systematically and should include inspection, palpation, range of motion testing, muscle strength testing, neurologic evaluation, and laxity testing.

Laxity Test

Laxity testing of the glenohumeral joint is one of the most difficult and demanding portions of the physical examination. There are numerous methods of testing for laxity as well as a number of special tests for assessing it. Increased laxity does not necessarily indicate instability. The shoulders may or may not be symmetric on laxity examination and still not be unstable (Lintner SA, Speer KP, Levy A, et al. Duke University, unpublished data, 1995). It is only with the addition of symptoms of instability that differences in laxity become potentially pathologic.

Laxity testing can be performed with the patient in the sitting or supine position. When the patient is sitting, the humeral head is grasped between the thumb and index and long fingers. A compressive force is applied toward the glenoid at the same time that an anterior and then a posterior force is applied.

The amount of translation is graded on a scale of 0 to 3. Zero indicates a trace of translation; 1 shows that the humeral head rides up on but not over the glenoid rim; 2 signifies that the humeral head rides up and over the glenoid rim but reduces when the force is removed; and 3 indicates that the humeral head rides up and over the glenoid rim and remains dislocated even after removal of the translatory force (Fig. 38–2). An inferior force is applied to the glenohumeral joint by pulling on the adducted arm. The amount of translation of the head is estimated by

GRADE   GLENOHUMERAL   CLINICAL
                TRANSLATION

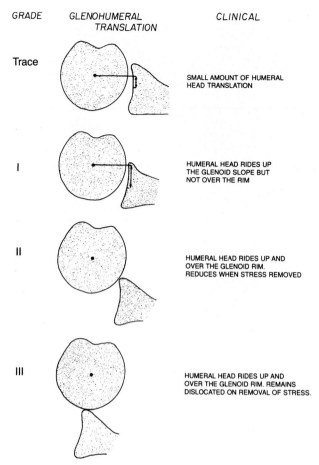

Trace

SMALL AMOUNT OF HUMERAL
HEAD TRANSLATION

I

HUMERAL HEAD RIDES UP
THE GLENOID SLOPE BUT
NOT OVER THE RIM

II

HUMERAL HEAD RIDES UP AND
OVER THE GLENOID RIM.
REDUCES WHEN STRESS REMOVED

III

HUMERAL HEAD RIDES UP AND
OVER THE GLENOID RIM. REMAINS
DISLOCATED ON REMOVAL OF STRESS.

Figure 38–2. Clinical evaluation of translation of the humeral head within the glenoid fossa utilizing the load and shift test. (From Rockwood CA Jr, Matsen FA III [eds]: The Shoulder. Philadelphia, WB Saunders, 1990, p 168.)

palpating the movement of the humeral head inferiorly in relation to the anterior acromion.

Inferior laxity is also graded from 0 to 3, 0 indicating minimal inferior translation, 1 signifying up to 1 cm of translation, 2 indicating 1 to 2 cm of translation, and 3 indicating more than 2 cm of inferior translation.

The laxity examination can also be performed with the patient supine. The degree of translation is graded using the same scale. The anterior-posterior translation is performed by abducting the arm 30 degrees and flexing it forward 30 degrees, and the arm is maintained in neutral rotation. The anterior and posterior force is applied to either the humeral head or the proximal humeral diaphysis.

Apprehension Test

Another physical examination performed to assess clinical stability is the apprehension test. For this maneuver, the patient is placed supine and the arm is abducted to 90 degrees, with maximal external rotation applied passively. This position may cause feelings of impending instability. The patient may grimace or make an attempt to limit further rotation. The production of pain without instability is not a positive result even though pain is often present.

Relocation Test

The relocation test is used in cases of suspected instability. For this test the apprehension test is performed, with the addition of an anteriorly directed force applied to the humeral head. This usually results in an increase in symptoms if instability is present. After the anterior force is removed, a posteriorly directed force is applied. The patient is questioned about the change in symptoms with this posterior force. The test result is positive when the instability symptoms are alleviated with posterior pressure.

Pathology of the Shoulder Commonly Found in the Athlete

Acromioclavicular Joint

The acromioclavicular joint is often injured in contact sports. The mechanism is usually a blow to or fall on the top of the shoulder. The patient usually complains of pain at the acromioclavicular joint as well as pain with active or passive shoulder elevation. On examination, tenderness and swelling over the acromioclavicular joint are observed. A deformity may exist in the more severe injuries.

The acromioclavicular joint injuries were originally classified into three types.[9] Rockwood[10] added three further descriptions for injuries not found in the original classification. The complete injury classification is as follows:

- *Type I:* The acromioclavicular ligaments are sprained, but the coracoclavicular ligaments are intact.
- *Type II:* The acromioclavicular ligaments are disrupted with a proximal migration of the distal clavicle; the coracoclavicular ligaments are sprained but intact.
- *Type III:* The acromioclavicular and coracoclavicular ligaments are disrupted, with obvious elevation (25–100 percent) of the distal clavicle; the trapezius and deltoid attachments on the distal end of the clavicle may also be disrupted.
- *Type IV:* This category includes the same pathology as a type III injury, but the clavicle is displaced posteriorly through the fascia of the trapezius.
- *Type V:* This category is the same as a type III injury but with even greater elevation of the clavicle (100–300 percent).
- *Type VI:* This classification includes a disruption of the acromioclavicular and coracoclavicular ligaments with inferior displacement of the distal clavicle.

Radiographs should be obtained to rule out a fracture of the clavicle. Comparison views of the uninjured shoulder and weighted stress views often are helpful in determining the extent of the injury.[11]

Treatment of acromioclavicular joint injuries is somewhat controversial, especially for the more severe injuries. Treatment of type I injuries is nonoperative and includes ice and rest with use of a sling as needed. The patient can return to activities when full painless range of motion is present. Type II injuries are also usually treated nonoperatively, with similar treatment as in type I injuries. Bergfeld[12] and colleagues have suggested that type I and II injuries may be more troublesome than originally thought. A sling usually is sufficient, but plaster cast and more elaborate immobilization devices have also been used.[13] Criteria for returning to activities in type II injuries are the same as for type I injuries.

The treatment of type III injuries is more controversial. Nonoperative treatment involves the use of a sling or harness as in type I and II injuries. Operative treatment involves acromioclavicular joint fixation or coracoclavicular ligament reconstruction or fixation. Good functional results have been reported after operative and nonoperative treatment.[14] If nonoperative methods of treatment fail and the acromioclavicular joint remains symptomatic, a late reconstruction or resection arthroplasty of the distal clavicle can be performed.[15]

The treatment of type IV, V, and VI injuries is less controversial, with most experts[16, 17] recommending open reduction and internal fixation.

The acromioclavicular joints of athletes are also prone to degeneration and distal clavicle osteolysis. Osteolysis is especially common in sports that require repetitive overhead activity and weight lifting (Fig. 38–3).[18] This condition may lead to arthritic changes in the acromioclavicular joint with accompanying pain and disability. The symptoms may respond to anti-inflammatory medication or injection but frequently require surgical resection of the distal clavicle for relief.[19]

Glenohumeral Instability

In the form of either subluxations or dislocations, glenohumeral instability is common in athletes.[20] The patient may complain of recurrent episodes of instability or of a single event. A careful history and physical examination are crucial to determining the cause and direction of the instability. The type of sport involved may provide a clue to the mechanism as well.

The physical examination of instability, previously addressed, is often diagnostic in patients with suspected glenohumeral instability. Great care should be taken during this portion of the examination if underlying instability is suspected.

The proper radiographic work-up for patients suspected of having instability is crucial. Anteroposterior and axillary lateral views should be obtained and may be sufficient to determine whether the shoulder is dislocated. Additional approaches to investigate instability include the West Point lateral view, which identifies glenoid rim changes that may occur with instability,[21] and the Stryker notch view, which helps to identify the characteristic Hill-Sachs lesion often seen in the humeral head following anterior dislocations.[22] Magnetic resonance imaging (MRI) is useful in detecting soft tissue injuries (Fig. 38–4) that occur with instability that may not be evident of plain radiographs (Lintner SA, Speer KP, Duke University, unpublished data, 1995).

In treating shoulder instability, one should make every effort to determine the underlying cause. In athletes with acute traumatic dislocations, a reduction should be performed as quickly as possible. The affected shoulder should be immobilized after reduction, but the duration and efficacy of immobilization are controversial.[23] Some investigators[24] recommend surgical treatment for athletes at the first dislocation.

If the patient and physician choose a nonoperative course of treatment, a period of immobilization of 3 to 8 weeks is usually undertaken. After this period, a gradual program of regaining motion and strength is initiated. Emphasis is placed on the rotator cuff muscles, especially the internal and external rotators.[25]

A common form of instability seen in the athletic population is the AMBRI type. It is especially common in overhead throwing athletes,[25] who often pre-

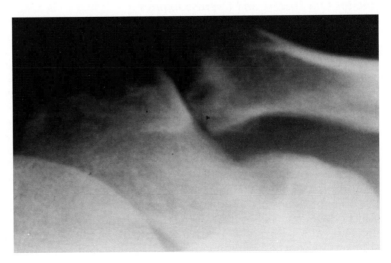

Figure 38–3. Radiograph demonstrating acromioclavicular joint narrowing and subchondral cystic changes in the distal clavicle.

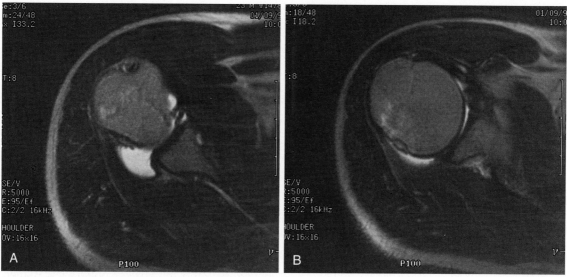

Figure 38–4. An MRI study of the shoulder 3 days following an acute anterior dislocation and manipulative reduction. *A,* A large effusion as well as an injury to the anterior inferior glenoid labrum (Bankart's lesion) is present. *B,* A large bone bruise is present in the posterior superior humeral head in the area of a Hill-Sachs lesion.

sent with pain as the chief complaint. It is the examining physician's role to distinguish the instability as the source of the pain. The pain is often secondary to impingement that occurs as the delicate kinematics of the shoulder become dysfunctional because of the underlying instability.[25] Patient may also have suffered an injury to the glenoid labrum, which can contribute to symptoms. This form of instability usually responds favorably to vigorous physical therapy and rehabilitation.[25] Activity modification, rest, anti-inflammatory medications, stretching, and strengthening of the rotator cuff and scapular stabilizers are important points to be addressed in a comprehensive rehabilitation program. A thorough trial of therapy, lasting 6 to 12 months, should be initiated.[25] Nonoperative therapy occasionally fails, and the patient continues to have pain and disability, at which point surgical intervention may be indicated.

Rotator Cuff Disease and Overuse Injuries

Overuse injuries of the rotator cuff are caused by sporting activities that require repetitive overhead or throwing movements. The injuries that involve the rotator cuff in athletes often have a different etiology than do those in nonathletes. Primary bony impingement is thought to be the etiology of the impingement syndrome.[26, 27] In athletes, demands are made of the rotator cuff and the static glenohumeral stabilizing structures that may overwhelm their capabilities. Eccentric overload secondary to overuse and fatigue may result in dysfunction of the rotator cuff and result in fiber failure.[28] This dysfunction may lead to the phenomenon of secondary impingement,[25] in which the bony architecture is not pathologic, but the cuff failure causes a relative narrowing of the subacromial space. Static shoulder instability con-

tributes to secondary impingement by further requiring the cuff to function as a dynamic glenohumeral stabilizer.

In athletes with suspected impingement, the common complaint is pain that is difficult for the patients to pinpoint but that is commonly located in the area of the lateral deltoid or deltoid tuberosity.[8] Pain with overhead activities and night pain are also common complaints. Weakness, stiffness, or a feeling of "catching" may also be present. The patient should be questioned as to which activities cause the symptoms.

In performing the physical examination, one should take care to inspect for atrophy that may indicate a complete cuff tear. Palpation often elicits tenderness along the anterior edge of the acromion and the supraspinatus tendon. Range-of-motion testing often reveals a painful arc of motion, typically between 60 and 120 degrees of forward motion.[29] Strength testing is important, since weakness beyond that caused by pain, especially weakness to resisted external rotation, is a sign of rotator cuff disease. Stability testing should be performed carefully to determine whether instability may be playing a role in the impingement process.

Signs of impingement can be sought in two ways. In the first method, pain is referable to the anterior acromion region with passive forward flexion, usually at between 60 and 120 degrees.[30] The second method, described by Hawkins and Hobeika,[31] involves passively flexing the arm forward to 90 degrees and then forcibly internally rotating the shoulder. In a positive result, the patient experiences pain in the area of the anterior acromion. The supraspinatus test can be performed to assess the integrity of the supraspinatus musculotendinous unit. This test is performed by having the patient forward flex the maximally internally rotated extended arm in the plane of the scapula against resistance. Pain or weakness is considered a positive sign.

Diagnostic testing should begin with routine radiography. This is frequently normal but may reveal evidence of impingement, such as sclerosis on the undersurface of the acromion or sclerosis or subchondral cyst formation in the area of the supraspinatus insertion on the greater tuberosity.[32] If a tear of the rotator cuff is suspected, a double-contrast arthrogram is helpful (Fig. 38–5).[33] MRI with or without contrast also helps in the diagnosis of cuff pathology and provides additional information about the other soft tissues surrounding the glenohumeral joint.[34]

Diagnostic testing can also include injecting the subacromial space with 10 mL of 1 percent lidocaine, after which the patient is reexamined. A positive result is one in which the symptoms are relieved with the injection.[27]

Treatment of rotator cuff injuries should be based on the underlying cause. The main form of treatment is nonoperative.[36] An acute traumatic injury usually responds to rest followed by an accelerated rehabilitation program. An early return to activities should be anticipated in these injuries. Primary impingement usually presents at a later age and may respond to a rehabilitation program, but surgical decompression of the subacromial space is usually necessary.

Secondary impingement from either overuse or underlying instability often responds to nonoperative treatment. The treatment program should consist of rest and activity modification. The athlete may continue to train but should avoid aggravating activities. Nonsteroidal anti-inflammatory medications are usually prescribed, especially during the initial 2 to 4 weeks of treatment.[36] A steroid injection can be given during the acute phase if the physician is certain that it enters the subacromial space and not the cuff tendon tissue. Ice or another form of cryotherapy can be used and appears to be most beneficial after workouts and therapy. Therapeutic modalities, such as ultrasound and diathermy, may also have a role in the treatment program.

Strengthening and stretching are the mainstays of treatment of athletic patients with rotator cuff disease.[25] An emphasis should be placed on maintaining full range of motion. Strengthening of the rotator cuff and scapular stabilizing muscles is vital. As symptoms decrease, sports-specific training can begin within the limits of comfort. Return to high-level or competitive participation should be gradual and based on symptoms. Full return is allowed when range of motion is full and painless and when high-level sports-specific activities can be performed with no symptoms.

THE ELBOW

Chief Complaint

Athletes with injuries to the elbow usually complain of pain. Because the elbow is a skeletally congruent joint with inherent stability, complaints of instability are much less common than in the shoulder. Instability in the elbow usually presents as pain. Difficulty with range of motion is another common complaint.

When the history is being obtained, care should be taken to ask about the history of trauma, the location of the symptoms, and sport- or occupation-specific activities.

Physical Examination

Inspection of the elbow should begin with the examination of the region—instability, limitation in range of motion, erythema, ecchymosis, or deformity. Palpation is usually accomplished easily because little tissue surrounds the joint. Palpation should proceed in a systematic fashion. The lateral supracondylar ridge and epicondyle are easily palpable. The radial head and olecranon can be felt. An effusion of the elbow joint is detectable in the center of the triangle formed by the lateral epicondyle, the radial head, and the tip of the olecranon (Fig. 38–6).[37] The olecranon and proximal ulna are subcutaneous and are easily palpated. On the medial aspect of the elbow, the medial epicondyle and ulnar notch are assessed. The ulnar nerve can be felt immediately behind the medial epicondyle. The nerve can be palpated with passive elbow flexion and extension to assess its stability. The medial collateral ligament complex is the primary stabilizer to valgus stress and can be palpated with the elbow in 30 degrees of flexion just distal and anterior to the medial epicondyle.

The range of motion of the elbow is easily measurable and should be obtained bilaterally. The normal flexion and extension is from 0 to about 145 degrees.

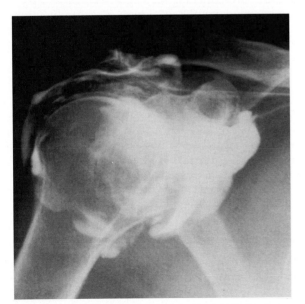

Figure 38–5. Arthrogram of a patient with chronic impingement and rotator cuff tear demonstrating extension of contrast material into the subacromial space.

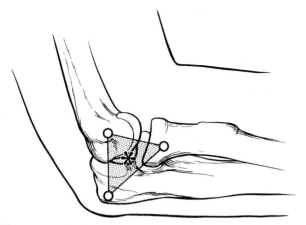

Figure 38–6. The landmarks for aspiration of the elbow joint are the radial head, lateral epicondyle, and tip of the olecranon. A needle inserted into the center of the triangle *(asterisk)* penetrates only the anconeus muscle and capsule before entering the joint. (From Rockwood CA Jr, Green DP: Fractures in Adults, 3rd ed. Philadelphia, JB Lippincott, 1991, p 634.)

Some amount of hyperextension is often evident and should not be considered pathologic.[38, 39] Pronation and supination are measured. Normal pronation is approximately 75 degrees, and supination is about 85 degrees. Range of motion required for most daily activities is 30 to 130 of flexion–extension and 50 degrees of pronation–supination.[40]

Muscle strength in flexion, extension, pronation, and supination is tested and graded. The examiner can assess stability of the elbow by applying varus and valgus stress while the elbow is in about 30 degrees of flexion. A side-to-side comparison is made.

Pathology of the Elbow Commonly Found in the Athlete

Epicondylitis

Commonly called "tennis elbow," epicondylitis is a condition of pain and tenderness in the region of the epicondyle. Although common in tennis players,[41–43] about 95 percent of cases occur in patients other than tennis players.[44, 45] Racquet sports such as tennis and squash seem to cause more symptoms laterally, whereas golf, rowing, and baseball affect the medial side more often.[46] This condition represents an overuse injury to the soft tissue attaching to and surrounding the humeral epicondyles. The lateral epicondyle is affected seven to 20 times more often than the medial.[47] The patient frequently gives a history of repetitive use with flexion–extension or pronation–supination. The backhand stroke in tennis has been implicated, but an exact mechanism is unclear.[48] The most accepted theory is that mechanical overload is placed on the common tendinous insertions at the respective epicondyles. Repeated contractions eventually cause small tears, which induce a healing response. This cycle is repeated when the person contin-

ues the offending activities. There does not appear to be an inflammatory component.[49, 50]

On physical examination, there is tenderness over the lateral epicondyle and at the insertion of the extensor carpi radialis brevis in lateral epicondylitis. Resisted wrist extension often elicits pain, as does resisted long finger extension. Results of the chair test, as described by Gardner,[51] are usually positive.

Medial epicondylitis is characterized by tenderness over the medial epicondyle, pain with resisted wrist flexion and pronation. Pain with making a fist and a decrease in grip strength are also common findings.[46] Radiographs are usually normal, but evidence of valgus extension overload may be identifiable in the throwing athlete with medial elbow symptoms.[52]

When one is making the diagnosis of epicondylitis, the differential diagnosis should include local or proximal neurologic pathology and intra-articular derangement. If the diagnosis of epicondylitis is in doubt, further work-up, such as cervical spine radiography or electrodiagnostic studies, may be indicated.

The treatment of epicondylitis is conservative, with rest and activity modification the most important components.[53] A short course of immobilization may be helpful during the acute phase. Prolonged immobilization should be avoided. Anti-inflammatory medications are useful, as are ultrasound, iontophoresis, and cryotherapy. Injection of corticosteroids and local anesthetics should be considered if there is no response to this initial therapy. Injections have met with mixed results and are not without the inherent risks.[54] Counterforce bracing was introduced in 1965[55] and appears to act by reducing the muscle activity and force acting at the insertion point.[56, 57]

Rehabilitation continues with a muscle-strengthening and a flexibility program. Passive stretching and isometric strengthening are begun as soon as they can be performed painlessly. There is a gradual return to resistance exercises performed concentrically and eccentrically as symptoms allow. Through training, the patient returns to a normal functional level of strength and flexibility; at this point, sport-specific activities are initiated. Return to sports should be gradual and guided by comfort.

Ensuring that the proper equipment and technique are used is an important consideration in the treatment and prevention of epicondylitis. Patients with chronic cases of epicondylitis may require 6 to 12 months to become free of symptoms before returning to sports. In refractory cases that do not respond to conservative care, surgical treatment is indicated.[58]

Olecranon Bursitis

Acute or chronic irritation may result in swelling and pain in the olecranon bursae. Aspiration often relieves the pain and swelling, but care should be taken to use proper sterile technique. When the aspirate is not bloody, cell counts and cultures should be obtained. Gout, rheumatoid arthritis, and infection must be excluded. After aspiration, a compressive wrap is applied and is usually sufficient to prevent reaccumulation of the fluid. Elbow pads may be needed to prevent further injury and recurrences. Chronic cases of recurrent olecranon bursitis with fibrosis of the bursae may require surgical excision.

KNEE

Chief Complaint

Knee injuries are common in sports. The musculotendinous units, ligamentous structures, articular cartilage, and meniscal cartilage are all susceptible to injury. Patients may complain of instability, generalized or sport-specific pain, a catching or locking sensation, a loss of previous range of motion, or chronic swelling.

When obtaining the history from an athlete with a knee injury, the examiner should recall that the mechanism of injury plays an important role. The athlete should be questioned about whether the injury involved contact, what position the leg was in, whether the foot was stationary or free, whether he or she heard a pop, whether he or she was able to continue playing, how much time had passed until swelling developed, and whether there is a history of injury or disability. The answers to these questions often make the diagnosis.

Physical Examination

Physical examination of the knee, like that of the shoulder, often requires repetition and practice by the examining physician, who must gain confidence and accuracy. As in the shoulder, the opposite (well) leg should be used as the control. The patient should be dressed in shorts and positioned comfortably to facilitate the examination.

Inspection of the knee, first the uninvolved knee and then the injured knee, is the first step in the examination. The skin should be examined for abrasion, lacerations, and contusions that might give information about the direction, force, and mechanism of the injury. The shape of the joint, upper and lower limb segments, their general alignment, and muscle size and tone should be observed. Size, condition, and location of scars should also be recorded.

Palpation can begin in various areas, and the examiner should develop a system with which he or she is comfortable. The areas that need to be palpated include the entire medial and lateral joint lines, the tibial tubercle, the patellar tendon, the inferior pole of the patella, the peripatellar soft tissues, and the insertion of the pes anserinus. It should be assessed whether effusion is present. Palpation can be performed in full extension, at 90 degrees of flexion, or in the figure 4 position (Fig. 38–7).

Range-of-motion examination in the knee is not as simple. The knee is not a hinge joint in that it has six degrees of freedom. Motion of the injured knee should be checked in flexion–extension as well as in tibial internal and external rotation; the motion should be compared with that of the opposite knee. The mobility of the patella and symptoms associated with translation should also be checked.

Stability of the knee can be examined through a variety of techniques. Varus-valgus stability is examined by placing a varus or valgus load on the knee with variable degrees of flexion. Stability at full extension–hyperextension, at 0 degrees and at 30 degrees, should be recorded. Anterior-posterior stability can be examined by the use of the anterior and posterior drawer maneuvers. The most specific test for determining the integrity of the anterior cruciate ligament is *Lachman's test*.[59] This test is performed at 20 to 30 degrees of knee flexion with the patient supine or prone. The *pivot shift test* or one of the many variants (Losee test, MacIntosh test, Slocum test, flexion rotation drawer test, and jerk test) can be performed to determine the functional stability of the knee. For an accurate result in tests assessing stability, it is vital that the patient be relaxed and comfortable.

Pathology of the Knee Commonly Found in the Athlete

Lesions of the Meniscus

Meniscal tears are common sport and non-sport injuries. The number of acutely torn menisci is estimated at 61 per 100,000 people.[59] The medial meniscus is torn more frequently than the lateral meniscus in most sports except wrestling.[60] A disruption of the anterior cruciate ligament (ACL) is usually associated with acute tears of the lateral meniscus and chronic tears of the medial meniscus.

The mechanism of injury for most meniscal tears is a compressive, rotational, and shearing force.[58, 61] Shearing forces tend to result in longitudinal tears, which account for up to 90 percent of the tears in young patients; horizontal degenerative tears occur more commonly in older patients.[62, 63] Multiple tears and complex tears are not uncommon.

The history of a meniscal tear is not consistent or definitive from one athlete to another. Patients often notice a sudden onset of pain or change in knee symptoms, frequently after a twisting-type injury. They usually have some degree of swelling in the knee. An effusion that occurs quickly, within 6 to 8 hours, indicates an acute hemarthrosis. The etiology may include an osteochondral fracture, disruption of the anterior cruciate ligament, a patellar dislocation, a collateral ligament injury, or a peripheral meniscal tear in the vascular zone. Delayed swelling may be caused by a more central meniscal tear or a chondral cartilage injury. Other patients may describe a sharp, stabbing pain in the knee, commonly on flexion. They may relate a history of a catching or locking sensation

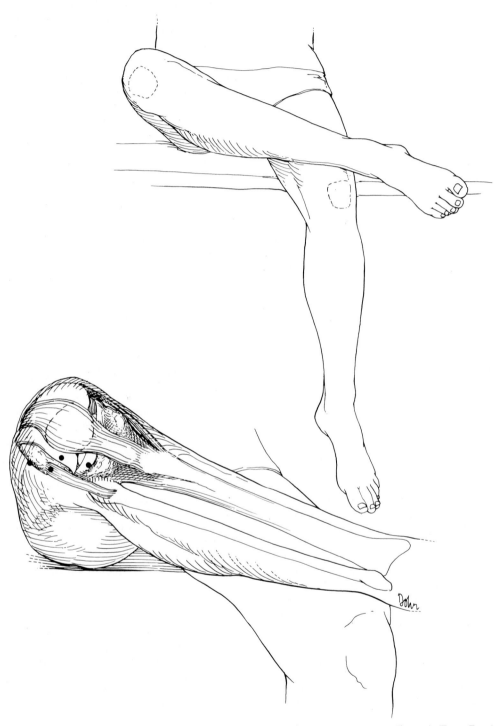

Figure 38–7. The figure 4 position *(top)*. Schematic drawing of the relations of anatomic structures *(bottom)*. (From Feagin JA Jr [ed]: The Crucial Ligaments, 2nd ed. New York, Churchill Livingstone, 1994, p 21.)

or actual episodes in which full extension is not possible.[64] Giving way of the knee is another common complaint and may indicate a meniscal tear, patellofemoral instability, or ligamentous instability.

The physical examination of a patient with a meniscal tear usually reveals characteristic findings. An effusion is common but nonspecific and may represent other pathology.[65] Joint line tenderness is one of the most reliable signs of a meniscal tear and is best assessed in the figure-4 position or at 90 degrees of flexion.[64, 65] Assessment of range of motion is important, since inability to regain full extension may indicate a locked displaced bucket-handle meniscus tear. Pain with squatting or with forced passive flexion is also a common and reliable physical finding. Other provocative tests that can be performed are the McMurray test, the Helfet test, and the Apley Grind test in the hopes of reproducing the symptoms.[66–69]

Radiographic studies should include routine anteroposterior, lateral, tunnel, and Merchant's patellofemoral views. Plain radiographs do not show a tear of the meniscus but may help to rule out the other causes of knee pain and to provide an estimation of knee alignment. Double-contrast arthrography had been the standard previously, with an accuracy of 60 to 97 percent. Accuracy is higher on the medial than on the lateral side.[70–74] MRI has become the gold standard for noninvasive detection of meniscal tears. Accuracy of detection is approximately 95 percent,[74, 75] but different magnet sizes may alter the results.[76] The MRI scan is useful not only for assessing meniscal tissues but also for evaluating the other soft tissues and bony structures about the knee joint (Fig. 38–8). Diagnostic arthroscopy[77, 78] may be indicated when other evaluations prove negative and the symptoms

remain. Drawbacks include the risk of an invasive procedure and the added expense, but there is the benefit of potentially having the opportunity to address the pathology at the time of diagnosis.

After the diagnosis of a torn meniscus has been made, a decision must be reached about treatment options. Tears that are minimally symptomatic can be left alone if the patient desires. Arthroscopy is usually needed to determine whether tears are amenable to nontreatment, resection, or repair. Injuries likely to heal without treatment are small peripheral tears in the vascular zone of the meniscus. When surgery is indicated, it is usually performed arthroscopically. A judgment can be made at this time as to whether to resect the torn portion or to perform a meniscal repair. The ideal injury to repair is a simple tear in the vascular portion of the meniscus. A variety of techniques can be used with similar success, with a healing rate of 75 to 100 percent based on various criteria. Nonreparable meniscal tears are complex tears or tears in the nonvascular zone. During resection of the meniscal tear, the unstable portion is removed, but as little tissue as possible should be excised. Total meniscectomies are not usually performed or indicated.

Ligamentous Injuries

Ligamentous injuries may involve one of the four major ligaments or ligament complexes that support and provide for normal kinematics of the human knee joint:[79] (1) the anterior cruciate ligament (ACL), (2) the posterior cruciate ligament (PCL), (3) the medial collateral ligament (MCL), and (4) the lateral collateral ligament (LCL). Anatomic descriptions and functions of these are described elsewhere.

Injuries to the ligament of the knee are common in sports. Ligament injuries are generally graded on a scale of three degrees. A *first-degree* sprain involves microscopic damage to the ligament structure, but the ligament functions appropriately and there is no instability evident. Usually, the symptoms are pain and tenderness. A *second-degree* sprain involves structural damage to the ligament with clinically evident instability. There is usually more pain, tenderness, and swelling than a first-degree injury. In a *third-degree* injury, the ligament is completely disrupted. Total loss of function and instability is usually obvious. Swelling may be greater, but pain often is less in complete injuries because of discontinuity of the ligament fibers.[59] When more than one ligament is injured, the findings on both the history and the physical examination may be confusing.

Anterior Cruciate Ligament

Injuries to the ACL interrupt the main restraint to anterior translation of the tibia on the femur. The ACL provides rotatory stability by tightening with tibial internal rotation and aids in the normal kinematics and complexities of knee motion.[80] The ACL

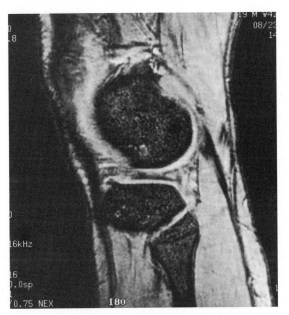

Figure 38–8. An MRI study of the knee showing an increased signal in the body of the meniscus that communicates with the articular surface indicating a tear.

can be injured by various mechanisms—hyperextension, relative tibial internal rotation with external rotation of the body on a fixed foot, deceleration, and in conjunction with other ligament injuries due to severe varus or valgus stresses. The examining physician should listen carefully to patients as they describe the incident of injury or previous injuries. In the history of a suspected ACL injury, the patient has often heard or felt a pop. After the injury occurs, the athlete usually cannot continue the activity. With this history, there is a 70 percent chance that an ACL disruption has occurred.[81] An acute knee effusion often occurs within 6 to 12 hours. With such a history, there is an 85 percent chance that an ACL tear is the cause.[82]

The physical examination of an athlete with an ACL tear varies slightly, depending on the interval between the time of injury and the examination. First, the uninvolved knee should be examined. Presence of an effusion and range of motion should be documented. Failure to obtain full extension equal to the opposite limb may be caused by a displaced bucket-handle meniscal tear. Tenderness may be present over the joint lines; this suggests a meniscal tear or a bone bruise. Bone bruises usually occur in the posterior lateral tibial plateau and the mid-portion of the lateral femoral condyle secondary to the force of injury.[83] The maneuver that confirms the diagnosis of an ACL tear is a difference in anterior translation of the injured compared with the opposite knee. If the difference is greater than 3 mm of anterior translation, a diagnosis of an ACL disruption is accurate 90 percent of the time.[81, 84, 85] Two tests that measure anterior tibial displacement are Lachman's test and the anterior drawer test. Lachman's test is a good indicator of anterior tibial translation.[86, 87] The technique for performing the test is well described and easily mastered after some practice. Other examination techniques used to diagnose ACL tears include the pivot shift test and its variations. These techniques measure the instability in a more complex fashion than Lachman's test does and are more difficult to master.

Radiographic views should include routine anteroposterior and lateral radiographs. A patellofemoral view is also indicated because patellar dislocation can cause an acute hemarthrosis. A small fragment of bone may be attached to the ligament as it is avulsed from its insertion site.[88] *Segond's fracture* is an avulsion fracture of the lateral capsule off the lateral tibial plateau and is consistent with an ACL injury.[89, 90] MRI is the preferred radiographic method of diagnosis and is about 95 percent accurate in diagnosing ACL pathology.[91] There is no need to perform MRI if the clinical diagnosis is clear and uncomplicated. The clinical presence of a meniscal tear may warrant MRI, especially if a displaced bucket-handle tear is suspected. MRI is also able to detect other intra-articular pathology commonly present with ACL disruptions (Fig. 38–9).[83]

Repairs with augmentation or reconstruction of the ACL have produced consistently good results.

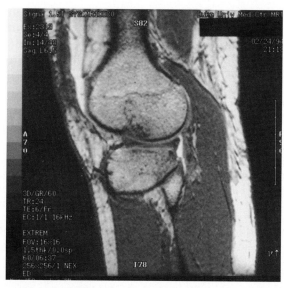

Figure 38–9. An MRI study of a knee that has sustained an acute disruption of the anterior cruciate ligament. This illustrates a bone bruise of the lateral femoral condyle—a bruise in the characteristic area for an athlete with this injury.

Stronger grafts, improved techniques and instrumentation, and a better understanding of anatomic and surgical principles have helped to improve results. Despite these results, not every ACL disruption should be treated surgically. Recreational athletes willing to modify their activities may never require surgery. Bracing can be helpful but may not eliminate sports-related instability. The decision of treatment is left to the patients after been informed of their options. Athletes who want to return to their previous level of sports participation, especially pivoting and jumping activities, should give serious consideration to surgical treatment.

Nonoperative treatment involves an organized and supervised rehabilitation program that focuses on range of motion, especially extension, and early control of pain and swelling. This is followed by muscle strengthening and flexibility training. The athlete should be informed of the risks of meniscal and chondral injuries that may occur late if the ACL is treated conservatively. There is always the option of treating the injury nonoperatively with the knowledge that surgery can be performed later if conservative therapy does not provide satisfactory stability at the desired level of activity.

Posterior Cruciate Ligament

Injuries to the PCL (the main restraint to posterior translation of the tibia on the femur) are much less common in athletes than injuries to the ACL.[92] The reported incidence of PCL injuries varies from about 3.5 percent[93] to 20 percent[94, 95] of knee ligament injuries treated surgically. An injury to the PCL usually occurs by one of four mechanisms:

- The anterior tibia is forced posteriorly in the flexed knee, such as striking the knee against the dashboard in a motor vehicle accident.
- A fall in which the person lands on the tibial tubercle, forcing the tibia posteriorly.
- Hyperflexion by itself.[96, 97]
- A posterior force is applied against a hyperextended knee with the foot fixed.

In the last instance, multiple ligaments usually are injured.[98]

In a patient with a PCL tear, a trivial injury that was virtually ignored by the athlete may be the cause, especially in an isolated PCL injury.[99] There may be a history of an acute effusion, but it is less frequent and less severe than in acute ACL disruptions. Patient complaints are often those of pain and stiffness.[100] The patient may also complain of patellofemoral pain, instability, or pain after prolonged activity.[101, 102]

On physical examination, acute injuries to the PCL are often overlooked. Inspection of the skin may provide evidence of a blow to the tibial tubercle. There may be full range of motion and minimal joint effusion.[92, 100, 102] With the knee flexed to 90 degrees, the tibia subluxes posteriorly. This produces the posterior *sag sign* that is characteristic for a PCL injury. The *posterior drawer test* may be used, but it has had mixed results in accuracy of diagnosis of PCL tears.[103, 104] Daniel and associates[105] introduced the *quadriceps active drawer test* to help in the clinical diagnosis of PCL injuries. During this test, the contraction of the quadriceps causes anterior translation and reduction of the posteriorly displaced tibia when the patient is placed supine with the knee flexed 70 to 90 degrees. This test is reported to be more sensitive for diagnosing PCL tears than the posterior drawer maneuver.[105]

Radiographic tests for a PCL injury are the same as for a suspected ACL injury. Bony avulsion fractures may be evident on the plain radiographs. An MRI scan usually confirms the diagnosis if the history and physical examination are not conclusive (Fig. 38–10).

Treatment of PCL injuries is somewhat controversial. Few studies are available to document long-term results in a controlled fashion using similar patients and similar methods. Isolated PCL injuries can be treated nonoperatively with reported good results.[106, 107] The nonoperative treatment of the PCL injuries is similar to that of the ACL, with an organized therapy and rehabilitation program being implemented. Bony avulsion injuries are probably best treated with primary surgical repair. The treatment of combined knee ligament injuries that involve the PCL is beyond the scope of this chapter, but most are best treated surgically.

Medial Collateral Ligament

Injuries of the MCL are common in athletic endeavors, especially in contact sports. The MCL is one of several structures of the knee that provide medial support and resistance to valgus stress and external

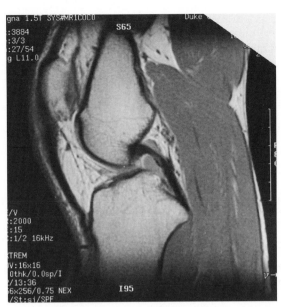

Figure 38–10. An MRI slice illustrating the intra-articular course of the normal uninjured posterior cruciate ligament.

rotation. The history of a patient with an MCL injury may include a noncontact twisting event; in more severe injuries, a lateral valgus force has usually been applied. If the athlete can continue playing, the injury is less severe. The presence and location of pain in the knee should be questioned and recorded.

Injuries to the MCL can be classified by the graded system: 0 is no opening, I is 1 to 4 mm, II is 5 to 9 mm, and grade III is greater than 10 mm.[108] An actual displacement or medial instability with valgus stress is also used to classify these injuries. *Stress testing* can be performed in various positions of knee flexion. At 0 degrees, there should be no valgus instability unless the MCL, PCL, and posterolateral capsule are disrupted. At 30 degrees of knee flexion, there is valgus instability if the MCL has been injured despite the status of the other ligament complexes in the knee. A valgus injury not only can injure the MCL but also may disrupt the cruciate ligaments; therefore, a thorough examination for cruciate integrity should always be performed.

Radiographs should include at least anteroposterior, lateral, and patellofemoral views. Fractures, avulsions of the MCL (Pellegrini-Stieda lesion), dislocations, loose bodies, or osteochondral injuries may be evident. MRI can be useful in detecting MCL injuries and identifying any other associated knee pathology.

In treating MCL injuries, it is important to ensure that the proper and complete diagnosis has been made. In isolated grade I and II injuries, nonoperative treatment is standard. Nonoperative treatment usually involves some form of bracing in conjunction with a rehabilitation program that emphasizes return of full motion, strengthening, and sports-specific exercises.[109] Treatment of grade III injuries is somewhat controversial. Some experts[110, 111] recommend and report good results with surgical management; others[112–114] recommend and report good results with nonoperative therapy. The nonoperative management of grade III injuries is similar to that of grades I and II, with the realization that the time to return to sport is longer.

Lateral Collateral Ligament

Injuries to the LCL involve not only the LCL but also other ligaments, resulting in complex patterns of instability.[115] The LCL is just one of many structures that form the complex stabilizing mechanism on the lateral aspect of the knee. An injury to the lateral side of the knee is not as common as the medial side and is less likely to be an isolated ligamentous injury.[116–118]

The history of a lateral-side injury often involves severe trauma and force. An attempt to determine the mechanism of injury should always be made. Care should be taken to investigate whether a dislocation has occurred, because this may warrant further diagnostic studies.[119]

The physical examination should be performed as previously described for other knee injuries when ligamentous lesions are suspected. The LCL is easily palpable with the knee in the figure-4 position. Varus stress testing is performed at 0 and 30 degrees of flexion. The grading system is the same as for MCL injuries. There are many special tests to perform for combined instabilities involving the lateral side. The status of the remaining ligaments of the knee should be assessed and documented. A full neurologic examination should be performed on the involved limb; lateral-side injuries have a high incidence of nerve injury.[120, 121]

Routine plain radiographs should be obtained as part of the original set of tests. Stress radiographs can be obtained, but care should be taken to prevent further injury. MRI can also be used to evaluated these injuries. The MRI scan may reveal that more than one structure is involved and which structures are complicating the injury.

An examination with the patient anesthetized is one of the most helpful methods to diagnose these complex injuries accurately. A surgical referral is indicated in these instances. If there has been a disruption of a primary ligamentous knee restraint, a surgical evaluation is recommended.

Treatment of lateral-side injuries is surgical except in the most mild of injuries. Unlike medial-side injuries, lateral ligament tears do not respond well to nonoperative treatment.[122]

Patellar Tendinitis

Patellar tendinitis (jumper's knee) is a common affliction of younger athletes. It tends to be a chronic and persistent problem related to activities that involve repetitive jumping or running, and sports with high demand on the quadriceps. Although it is an "-itis," histologic studies[123, 124] have not revealed evidence of cellular inflammation. This process appears to be a tendinopathy histologically, with areas of necrosis, degeneration, and fibroblastic regeneration.

The patient's history usually involves complaints of pain at the inferior pole of the patella and reveals participation in a jumping sport, such as basketball. The onset of pain is gradual, with no single precipitating event. Going up stairs or a deep squat may reproduce the symptoms. There is often a history of overuse, an increase in training, or a change in training habits.

On physical examination, the tenderness at the inferior pole of the patella is demonstrated by the examiner's pushing down on the superior pole of the patella in the extended knee; the inferior pole tilts upward. As with other examinations, the opposite extremity should be palpated for comparison.

Routine radiographs usually show no abnormalities. In Sinding-Larsen-Johansson syndrome, irregular calcifications may be present at the inferior pole. In a skeletally mature patient, irregular calcifications usually are not present. MRI reveals thickening of the tendon near the attachment at the inferior pole of the patella (Fig. 38–11). There may also be intratendinous degenerative changes.

Treatment of jumper's knee is usually conservative. Blazina and colleagues[125] divided the process into three stages based on symptoms:

- Stage 1 is pain after activity only without functional impairment.
- Stage 2 is pain during and after activity, but the athlete is able to perform at an acceptable level.
- Stage 3 is prolonged pain during and after activity with a corresponding decrease in performance level.

Treatment is based on the severity of the symptoms. The basic treatment consists of rest, cryotherapy, anti-inflammatory medications, strengthening and flexibility exercises, and an elastic support sleeve. Duration of treatment depends on the symptomatic response. Steroid injections are usually not indicated and may be detrimental. For refractory symptoms, surgical intervention with debridement of the degenerative tendon may be indicated. Return to sporting activities is possible when symptoms are eliminated and flexibility and strength have returned to normal.

LOWER LEG

Medial Tibial Stress Syndrome

Overuse injuries to the lower leg are common, especially in activities that involve running and jumping. The two most common injuries to the leg are stress fractures and medial tibial stress syndrome (*shin splints*).

The more accurate term medial tibial stress syndrome (MTSS) is used to describe pain over the posteromedial border of the tibia in the mid-distal third of the leg.[126] The patient usually complains of pain on

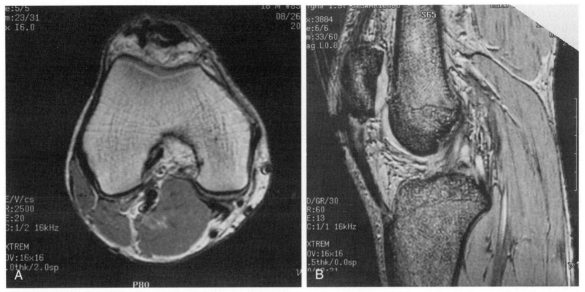

Figure 38–11. An MRI scan of an athlete's knee with patellar tendinitis (jumper's knee). *A,* An axial image at the level of the distal pole of the patella showing an intratendinous increased signal indicating degeneration. *B,* A sagittal image showing that the patellar insertion of the tendon is thickened with areas of high signal (i.e. degeneration).

initial exertion that may be relieved with continued activity. The pain often returns after completion of the workout and is more severe than the pain at startup. As the condition progresses, symptoms may continue throughout the duration of the activity. MTSS is an overuse injury; it usually occurs after there has been a change in the amount or type of activity.[127]

The physical examination is consistent in the findings of tenderness along the posteromedial border of the mid-distal tibia. Swelling or induration of the soft tissues is often present. In examination of a patient with suspected MTSS, alignment of the feet should be checked, particularly the amount of pronation, because there is an association between excessive pronation and development of MTSS.[128]

Radiographic studies should include anteroposterior and lateral views. These are usually normal, but hypertrophy of the posterior cortex may be present. A bone scan is the most useful test in evaluating MTSS. There is usually a characteristic diffuse and elongated area of uptake along the posteromedial border of the tibia, especially on the delayed images. This is in contrast to *stress fractures* (see later), in which there is usually a discrete and more intense area of increased activity.[129] This area of increased uptake in MTSS appears to correlate with the medial tibial attachment of the soleus muscle.[130]

The primary treatment of MTSS, as in other overuse syndromes, is rest. Changes in training techniques and routines need to be addressed. Non-impact activities can be implemented to help maintain aerobic fitness levels. Water activities, such as water running and swimming, are excellent; a limited amount of bicycling is also acceptable. Anti-inflammatory medications and cryotherapy are most beneficial in the acute stages. If excessive foot pronation appears to be an underlying problem, custom shoe orthotics should be prescribed. The most important phase of treatment is prevention of recurrence of symptoms when training resumes. To ensure a complete cure, a gradual and structured return to activities is vital.

Stress Fractures

Stress, or fatigue, fractures are common overuse injuries that occur in running and jumping sports. The tibia is the most commonly involved bone in athletes.[131] The overall incidence of stress fractures is about 0.12 percent in the athlete and 4 to 15.6 percent in the population as a whole.[131, 132] The etiology of stress fractures is multifactorial. Activity level and intensity, gender, bone density, and hormonal and dietary factors all influence the susceptibility to stress fractures. Hyperpronation, as in MTSS, is associated with an increased risk of tibial stress fractures.[131]

On physical examination, stress fractures are easily confused with MTSS. The tenderness may be more localized to a focal area. Foot alignment is important and should be examined as in MTSS. Distinction between the diagnoses can be made radiographically, particularly on bone scans.

Plain radiographs are often normal, but a lucent line may occasionally be evident and located at the point of tenderness. Periosteal reaction, cortical thickening, or scalloping may be present.[133] Bone scan remains the most sensitive method of detecting stress fractures.[129, 133] The bone scan pattern reveals a more distinct, intense, and linear area of uptake than that seen in MTSS.

Treatment is the same as that for MTSS. Orthotic

use to correct foot alignment is indicated if excessive pronation is considered a contributing factor. Prevention of recurrences is important. Prevention is emphasized in a number of articles, with researchers[131, 134, 135] reporting that recurrence rates approach 10 percent. Activity modification remains the mainstay of therapy. Surgical intervention is rarely indicated, even for fractures resistant to nonoperative measures or multiple recurrences.

Other Causes of Lower Leg Pain

Other less common causes of lower leg pain include chronic exertional compartment syndrome, popliteal artery entrapment, muscular strains, and neurologic and vascular abnormalities.

FOOT AND ANKLE

Ankle Sprains

Ankle sprains are the most common injury in sports activities. Inversion injuries are more common than eversion injuries.[136-138] Proper diagnosis and treatment are important in providing a quick, safe return to activities and in preventing long-term disability. Ankle sprains are graded by using the 0 to III system described for MCL injuries.

The lateral ligaments of the ankle are injured much more often than the medial deltoid ligament complex. There are three major ligaments on the lateral side of the ankle. The *anterior talofibular ligament* prevents inversion and anterior translation of the talus, especially in plantar flexion. The *calcaneofibular ligament* prevents inversion and anterior translation, especially in dorsiflexion. The *posterior talofibular ligament* is rarely injured and functions primarily in preventing inversion. The tibia and fibula are connected and stabilized by the interosseous membrane and syndesmotic ligaments (anterior and posterior tibiofibular ligaments) distally. The medial side of the ankle is stabilized by the deltoid ligament complex, which comprises four closely associated ligaments and which prevents eversion of the ankle.

A patient with an ankle sprain usually has a history of a twisting injury to the ankle. The patient often recalls stepping on another player's foot, landing wrong, or stepping in a hole. There is usually an immediate onset of pain and some degree of swelling. Weight bearing is painful and difficult. The patient often relates hearing a pop at the time of injury.

On examination of the injured ankle, the physician usually sees swelling over the injured side, but it is not uncommon to observe diffuse swelling that involves the entire ankle. The presence of ecchymosis is variable and usually appears later. The ankle should be palpated over the specific sites of the ligaments to determine areas of maximal tenderness. The entire fibula and medial malleolus should be pal-

pated. Crepitus indicates a fracture and may alter the treatment plan. Subluxation of the peroneal tendons can be confused with an ankle sprain, but usually there is tenderness and swelling over the tendon sheath posterior to the fibula. An avulsion fracture at the base of the fifth metatarsal should also be excluded. Range of motion should be assessed. Evertor and invertor muscle function should be checked. Stability testing, such as the anterior drawer and talar tilt tests, are usually painful in acute injuries and can be performed later. The syndesmosis may be injured and can be tested with the *squeeze test* and *Cotton's test*.[139, 140] Differentiating a syndesmotic or high sprain from a low ankle sprain is important. A high sprain usually has a longer rehabilitation and return to activity time.

Treatment of ankle sprains is conservative, with the goal of preventing loss of motion and strength in the ankle. Cryotherapy, compression, elevation, and weight bearing as tolerated are the mainstays of early treatment. For more severe injuries, a short period of immobilization may be necessary during the acute phase of swelling and inflammation. Crutches can be used, as necessary, for ambulation. Range of motion and weight bearing should be encouraged as rapidly as the patient can tolerate the movement and ambulation. As comfort improves, strengthening of the peroneal muscles should be initiated. Proprioceptive training on a tilt board helps to improve balance and dynamic ankle control.

Aggressive treatment usually brings about a functional return within 1 to 2 weeks. Syndesmotic injuries can be expected to result in a longer period of disability. The decision to return to sports is guided by the ability to perform sport-specific demands on an ankle that has full motion and good strength. If the risk of re-injury is high, the patient should have the ankle taped or may find an orthosis beneficial.[141, 142] Chronic symptomatic ankle instability should be approached nonoperatively with an aggressive rehabilitation program. If this fails, surgical stabilization may be indicated.

Ankle Fractures

Radiographic evaluation of ankle fractures should include anteroposterior, lateral, and mortise views. Fractures of the distal fibula and medial malleolus must be ruled out. Talar dome or tibial plafond fractures may be present. If there is pain and tenderness at the proximal fibula, full-length anteroposterior and lateral radiographs of the lower leg should be obtained to rule out *Maisonneuve's fracture* (a fracture of the proximal fibula resulting from a total disruption of the syndesmosis.) Stress radiographs are not indicated in acute injuries but may be useful in evaluating chronic ankle instability. If stress radiography is performed, stress views of both ankles should be obtained for comparison (Fig. 38–12).

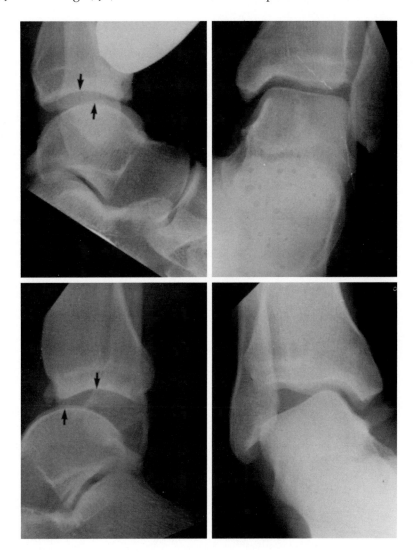

Figure 38–12. Stress radiograph of the ankle, revealing excessive anterior subluxation of the talus in the lower left film and instability on inversion in the lower right film. The normal contralateral ankle is depicted under stress in the upper two films.

SUMMARY

The practice of sports medicine requires a thorough understanding of anatomy and physiology. Proper treatment results from a proper diagnosis and an appreciation for the demands placed on the body by the athlete. A sound patient-doctor relationship and proper rehabilitation techniques help achieve the goal of a safe and effective return to sports. Restoration of adequate strength, endurance, and flexibility through rehabilitation also helps achieve this goal. The practicing physician must give this goal as much dedication and interest as is given to formulating an accurate diagnosis and treatment plan.

References

1. Hippocrates: The Genuine Works of Hippocrates. [Translation by F. Adams.] Baltimore, Williams & Wilkins, 1939, pp 212–214.
2. Snook GA: The father of sports medicine. Am J Sports Med 6:128–131, 1978.
3. Adams JW: Development of sports medicine. N C Med J 55:488–492, 1994.
4. Peltier LF: Geronimo Mercuriali and the first illustrated book on sports medicine. Clin Orthop 198:21–25, 1985.
5. Snook GA: The history of sports medicine: Part I. Am J Sports Med 12:252–254, 1984.
6. Darling EA: The effects of training. Boston Med Surg J 141:205–233, 1899.
7. Hoppenfeld S: Physical Examination of the Spine and Extremities. New York, Appleton & Lange, 1976.
8. Hawkins RJ, Bokor DJ: Clinical evaluation of shoulder problems. In Rockwood CA, Matsen FA (eds): The Shoulder. Philadelphia, WB Saunders, 1990, pp 150–177.
9. Tossy JD, Mead NC, Sigmond HM: Acromioclavicular separations: Useful and practical classification for treatment. Clin Orthop 28:111–119, 1963.
10. Rockwood CA Jr: Injuries to the acromioclavicular joint. In: Fractures in Adults, Vol 1, 2nd ed. Philadelphia, JB Lippincott, 1984, pp 860–910.
11. Bearden JM, Hughston JC, Whatley GS: Acromioclavicular dislocation: A method of treatment. Am J Sports Med 1:5–17, 1973.
12. Bergfeld JA, Andrish JT, Clancy WG: Evaluation of the acromioclavicular joint following first- and second-degree sprains. Am J Sports Med 6:153–159, 1978.
13. Urist MR: Complete dislocation of the acromioclavicular joint: The nature of the traumatic lesion and effective methods of treatment with an analysis of 41 cases. J Bone Joint Surg 28A:813–837, 1946.
14. Taft TN, Wilson FC, Oglesby JW: Dislocation of the acromioclavicular joint: An end result study. J Bone Joint Surg 69A:1045–1051, 1987.
15. Mumford EB: Acromioclavicular dislocation. J Bone Joint Surg 23A:799–802, 1941.
16. Patterson WR: Inferior dislocation of the distal end of the clavicle. J Bone Joint Surg 49A:1184–1186, 1967.
17. Nieminen S, Aho AJ: Anterior dislocation of the acromioclavicular joint. Ann Chir Gynaecol 73:21–24, 1984.

18. Cahill BR: Osteolysis of the distal part of the clavicle in male athletes. J Bone Joint Surg 64A:1053–1058, 1982.

19. Morrison IS: Post traumatic osteolysis of the acromial end of the clavicle. Australas Radiol 22:183–186, 1978.

20. Henry JH, Genung JA: Natural history of glenohumeral dislocation revisited. Am J Sports Med 10:135–137, 1982.

21. Rokous JR, Feagin JA, Abbott HG: Modified axillary roentgenogram: A useful adjunct in the diagnosis of recurrent instability of the shoulder. Clin Orthop 82:84–86, 1972.

22. Hall RH, Isaac F, Booth CR: Dislocations of the shoulder with special reference to accompanying small fractures. J Bone Joint Surg 41A:489–494, 1959.

23. Kiviluoto O, Pasila M, Jaroma H, et al: Immobilization after primary dislocation of the shoulder. Acta Orthop Scand 51:915–919, 1980.

24. Arciero RA, Wheeler JH, Ryan JB, et al: Arthroscopic Bankart repair versus nonoperative treatment for acute, initial anterior shoulder dislocations. Am J Sports Med 22:589–594, 1994.

25. Jobe FW, Tibone JE, Jobe CM, et al: The shoulder in sports. In Rockwood CA, Matsen FA (eds): The Shoulder. Philadelphia, WB Saunders, 1990, pp 961–990.

26. Neer CS II: Anterior acromioplasty for the chronic impingement syndrome in the shoulder: A preliminary report. J Bone Joint Surg 54A:41–50, 1972.

27. Neer CS II: Impingement lesions. Clin Orthop 173:70–77, 1983.

28. Fowler PJ: Shoulder injuries in the mature athlete. Adv Sports Med Fitness 1:225–238, 1988.

29. Hawkins RJ, Kennedy JC: Impingement syndromes in athletes. Am J Sports Med 8:151–158, 1980.

30. Kessel L, Watson M: The painful arc syndrome. J Bone Joint Surg 59B:166–172, 1977.

31. Hawkins RJ, Hobeika PE: Physical examination of the shoulder. Orthopedics 6:1270–1278, 1983.

32. Weiner DS, MacNab I: Superior migration of the humeral head: A radiological aid in the diagnosis of tears of the rotator cuff. J Bone Joint Surg 52B:524–527, 1970.

33. Brems J: Rotator cuff tear: Evaluation and treatment. Orthopedics 11:69–81, 1988.

34. Evancho AM, Stiles RG, Fajman WA, et al: MR imaging diagnosis of rotator cuff tears. Am J Radiol 151:751–754, 1988.

35. Rockwood CA Jr, Burkhead WZ, Brna J: Subluxation of the glenohumeral joint: Response to rehabilitative exercise—traumatic versus atraumatic instability. Orthop Trans 10:220, 1986.

36. Hawkins RJ, Hobeika PE: Impingement syndrome in the athletic shoulder. Clin Sports Med 2:391–405, 1983.

37. Regan WD, Morrey BF: The physical examination of the elbow. In Morrey BF (ed): The Elbow and Its Disorders, 2nd ed. Philadelphia, WB Saunders, 1993, pp 73–85.

38. Boone DC, Azen SP: Normal range of motion of joints in male subjects. J Bone Joint Surg 61A:756–759, 1979.

39. Wagner C: Determination of the rotary flexibility of the elbow joint. Eur J Appl Physiol 37:47–59, 1977.

40. Morrey BF, Askew LJ, An KN, Chao EY: A biomechanical study of normal functional elbow motion. J Bone Joint Surg 63A:872–877, 1981.

41. Nirschl RP: Prevention and treatment of elbow and shoulder injuries in the tennis player. Clin Sports Med 7:289–308, 1988.

42. Nirschl RP, Pettrone FA: Tennis elbow: The surgical treatment of lateral epicondylitis. J Bone Joint Surg 61A:832–839, 1979.

43. Priest JD, Braden V, Gerberich JG: The elbow and tennis. Part I. Physician Sports Med 8:80–83, 1980.

44. Coonrad RW: Tennis elbow. Instr Course Lect Am Acad Orthop Surgeons 35:94–101, 1986.

45. Werner CO: Lateral elbow pain and posterior interosseous nerve entrapment. Acta Orthop Scand 174(Suppl):1–62, 1979.

46. Jobe FW, Ciccotti MG: Lateral and medial epicondylitis of the elbow. J Am Acad Orthop Surgeons 2:1–8, 1994.

47. Leach RE, Miller JK: Lateral and medial epicondylitis of the elbow. Clin Sports Med 6:259–272, 1987.

48. Roles NC, Maudsley RH: Radial tunnel syndrome: Resistant tennis elbow as a nerve entrapment. J Bone Joint Surg 54B:499–508, 1972.

49. Regan W, Wold LE, Coonrad R, et al: Microscopic histopathology of chronic refractory lateral epicondylitis. Am J Sport Med 20:746–749, 1992.

50. Sarkar K, Uhthoff HK: Ultrastructure of the common extensor tendon in tennis elbow. Virchows Arch A Pathol Anat Histopathol 386:317–330, 1980.

51. Gardner RC: Tennis elbow: Diagnosis, pathology and treatment. Clin Orthop 72:248–253, 1970.

52. Wilson FD, Andrews JR, Blackburn TA: Valgus extension overload in the pitching elbow. Am J Sports Med 11:83–88, 1983.

53. Binder AI, Hazleman BL: Lateral humeral epicondylitis: A study of natural history and the effect of conservative therapy. Br J Rheumatol 22:73–76, 1983.

54. Price R, Sinclair H, Heinrich I: Local injection treatment of tennis elbow: Hydrocortisone, triamcinolone and lignocaine compared. Br J Rheumatol 30:39–44, 1991.

55. Froimson AI: Treatment of tennis elbow with forearm support band. J Bone Joint Surg 53A:183–184, 1971.

56. Groppel JL, Nirschl RP: A mechanical and electromyographical analysis of the effects of various joint counterforce braces of the tennis player. Am J Sports Med 14:195–200, 1986.

57. Snyder-Mackler L, Epler M: Effect of standard and Aircast® tennis elbow bands on integrated electromyography of forearm extensor musculature proximal to the bands. Am J Sports Med 17:278–281, 1989.

58. O'Donoghue DH: Treatment of Athletic Injuries, 3rd ed. Philadelphia, WB Saunders, 1976, pp 630–640.

59. Feagin JA Jr: Principles of diagnosis and treatment. In The Crucial Ligaments, 2nd ed. New York, Churchill Livingstone, 1994, pp 9–25.

60. Baker BE, Peckham AC, Pupparo F, et al: Review of meniscal injury and associated sports. Am J Sports Med 13:1–4, 1985.

61. Smillie IS: Injuries of the Knee Joint, 4th ed. Baltimore, Williams & Wilkins, 1970, p 33.

62. Northmore-Ball MD, Dandy DJ: Long-term results of arthroscopic partial meniscectomy. Clin Orthop 167:34–42, 1982.

63. Scott GA, Jolly BL, Henning CE: Combined posterior incision and arthroscopic intra-articular repair of the meniscus: An examination of factors affecting healing. J Bone Joint Surg 68A:847–861, 1986.

64. Shakespeare DT, Rigby HS: The bucket-handle tear of the meniscus: A clinical and arthrographic study. J Bone Joint Surg 65B:383–387, 1986.

65. Anderson AF, Lipscomb AB: Clinical diagnosis of meniscal tears: Description of a new manipulative test. Am J Sports Med 14:291–293, 1986.

66. Apley G: The diagnosis of meniscus injuries. J Bone Joint Surg 29:78–84, 1947.

67. Helfet AJ: Disorders of the Knee. Philadelphia, JB Lippincott, 1982, pp 117–129.

68. Henning CE, Lynch MA, Glick KR: Physical examination of the knee. In Nicholas JA, Hershman EB (eds): The Lower Extremity and Spine in Sports Medicine. St Louis, CV Mosby, 1985, pp 685–689.

69. McMurray TP: The semilunar cartilages. Br J Surg 29:407–414, 1942.

70. Daniel D, Daniels E, Aronson D: The diagnosis of meniscus pathology. Clin Orthop 163:218–224, 1982.

71. Gilles H, Seligson D: Precision in the diagnosis of meniscal lesions: A comparison of clinical evaluation, arthrography, and arthroscopy. J Bone Joint Surg 61A:343–346, 1979.

72. Ireland J, Trickey EL, Stoker DJ: Arthroscopy and arthrography of the knee: A critical review. J Bone Joint Surg 62B:3–6, 1980.

73. Nicholas JA, Freiberger RH, Killoran PJ: Double-contrast arthrography of the knee: Its value in the management of two hundred and twenty-five knee derangements. J Bone Joint Surg 52A:203–220, 1970.

74. Polly DW, Callaghan DD, Sikes RA, et al: The accuracy of selective magnetic resonance imaging compared with the findings of arthroscopy of the knee. J Bone Joint Surg 70A:192–198, 1988.

75. Jackson DW, Jennings LD, Maywood RM, et al: Magnetic resonance imaging of the knee. Am J Sports Med 16:29–47, 1988.

76. Silva NG, Silver D: Tears of the meniscus as revealed by magnetic resonance imaging. J Bone Joint Surg 70A:199–202, 1988.

77. Dandy DJ: Arthroscopic Surgery of the Knee. London, Churchill Livingstone, 1981.

78. Johnson LL: The Comprehensive Examination of the Knee. St Louis, CV Mosby, 1977.

79. Brantigan OC, Voshell AF: Ligaments of the knee joint. J Bone Joint Surg 23A:44–66, 1941.

80. Markolf KL, Mensch JS, Amstutz HC: Stiffness and laxity of the knee—the contributions of the supporting structures: A quantitative in vitro study. J Bone Joint Surg 58A:583–594, 1976.

81. Hirshman HP, Daniel DM, Miyasaka K: The fate of unoperated knee ligament injuries. In Daniel DM, Akeson WH, O'Connor JJ (eds): Knee Ligaments: Structure, Function, Injury, and Repair. New York, Raven Press, 1990, pp 481–503.

82. Daniel DM, Stone ML, Sachs R, et al: Instrumented measurement of anterior knee laxity in patients with acute anterior cruciate ligament disruption. Am J Sports Med 13:401–407, 1985.

83. Speer KP, Spritzer CE, Bassett FH III: Osseous injury associated with acute tears of the anterior cruciate ligament. Am J Sports Med 20:382–389, 1992.

84. Daniel DM, Stone ML: KT-1000 anterior–posterior displacement measurements. In Daniel DM, Akeson WH, O'Connor JJ (eds): Knee Ligaments: Structure, Function, Injury, and Repair. New York, Raven Press, 1990, pp 427–447.

85. Shoemaker SC, Daniel DM: The limits on knee motion: In vitro studies. In Daniel DM, Akeson WH, O'Connor JJ (eds): Knee Ligaments: Structure, Function, Injury, and Repair. New York, Raven Press, 1990, pp 153–161.

86. Torg JS, Conrad W, Kalen V: Clinical diagnosis of anterior cruciate ligament instability in the athlete. Am J Sports Med 4:84–93, 1976.

87. Johnson T, Althoff B, Peterson L, et al: Clinical diagnosis of ruptures of the anterior cruciate ligament: A comparative study of the Lachman test and the anterior drawer sign. Am J Sports Med 10:100–102, 1982.

88. Kennedy JC: The Injured Adolescent Knee. Baltimore, Williams & Wilkins, 1979, pp 103–120.
89. Lynch MA, Henning CE, Glick KR: Knee joint surface changes: Long-term follow-up meniscus tear treatment in stable anterior cruciate ligament reconstructions. Clin Orthop 172:148–153, 1983.
90. Cockshott WP, Racoveanu NT, Burrows DA, et al: Use of radiographic projections of the knee. Skeletal Radiol 13:131–133, 1985.
91. Mink JH, Levy T, Crues JH: Tears of the anterior cruciate ligament and menisci of the knee: MR evaluation. Radiology 167:769–774, 1988.
92. Clancy WG, Shelbourne KD, Zoellner GB: Treatment of knee joint instability secondary to rupture of the posterior cruciate ligament. J Bone Joint Surg 65A:310–322, 1983.
93. O'Donoghue DH: Surgical treatment of injuries to ligaments of the knee. JAMA 169:1423–1431, 1959.
94. Bianchi M: Acute tears of the posterior cruciate ligament: Clinical study and results of operative treatment in 27 cases. Am J Sports Med 11:308–314, 1983.
95. Clendenin MB, DeLee JC, Heckman JD: Interstitial tears of the posterior cruciate ligament. Orthopaedics 3:764–772, 1980.
96. Fowler PJ, Messieh SS: Isolated posterior cruciate ligament injuries in athletes. Am J Sports Med 15:553–557, 1987.
97. Fowler PJ: The classification and early diagnosis of knee joint instability. Clin Orthop 147:15–21, 1980.
98. Kennedy JC, Hawkins RJ, Willis RB, et al: Tension studies of human knee ligaments: Yield point, ultimate failure, and disruption of the cruciate and tibial collateral ligaments. J Bone Joint Surg 58A: 350–355, 1976.
99. Bergfeld JA: Diagnosis and nonoperative treatment of acute posterior cruciate ligament injury. Instr Course Lect 208, 1990.
100. DeLee JC, Bergfeld JA, Drez D Jr, et al: The posterior cruciate ligament. In DeLee JC, Drez D Jr (eds): Orthopaedic Sports Medicine. Philadelphia, WB Saunders, 1994, p 1380.
101. Cross MJ, Powell JF: Long-term follow-up of posterior cruciate ligament rupture: A study of 116 cases. Am J Sports Med 12:292–297, 1984.
102. Dandy DJ, Pusey RJ: The long-term results of unrepaired tears of the posterior cruciate ligament. J Bone Joint Surg 64B:92–94, 1982.
103. Moore HA, Larson RL: Posterior cruciate ligament injuries: Results of early surgical repair. Am J Sports Med 8:68–78, 1980.
104. Savatsky GJ, Marshall JL, Warren RF, et al: Posterior cruciate ligament injury. Orthop Trans 4:293, 1980.
105. Daniel DM, Stone ML, Barnett P, et al: Use of the quadriceps active test to diagnose posterior cruciate ligament disruption and measure posterior laxity of the knee. J Bone Joint Surg 70A:386–391, 1988.
106. Tietjens BB: Posterior cruciate ligament injuries (abstr). J Bone Joint Surg 67B:674, 1985.
107. Parolie JM, Bergfeld JA: Long-term results of nonoperative treatment of isolated posterior cruciate ligament injuries in the athlete. Am J Sports Med 14:35–38, 1986.
108. Hughston JC, Andrews JR, Cross MJ, et al: Classification of knee ligament instabilities. Part I: The medial compartment and cruciate ligaments. J Bone Joint Surg 58A:159–172, 1976.
109. Dersherd GL, Garrick JC: Medial collateral ligament injuries in football: Nonoperative management of grade I and grade II sprains. Am J Sports Med 9:365–368, 1981.
110. Collins HR: Reconstruction of the athlete's injured knee: Anatomy, diagnosis, treatment. Orthop Clin North Am 2:207–230, 1971.
111. Müller W: The Knee: Form, Function and Ligament Reconstruction. New York, Springer-Verlag, 1983, pp 168–189.
112. Indelicato PA, Hermansdorfer J, Huegel M: The non-operative management of complete tears of the medial collateral ligament of the knee in intercollegiate football players. Clin Orthop 256:174–177, 1990.
113. Indelicato PA: Non-operative treatment of complete tears on the medial collateral ligament of the knee. J Bone Joint Surg 65A:323–329, 1983.
114. Kannus P: Long-term results of conservatively treated medial collateral ligament injuries of the knee joint. Clin Orthop 226:103–112, 1988.
115. Hughston JC, Andrews JR, Cross MJ, et al: Classification of knee ligament instabilities. Part II: The lateral compartment. J Bone Joint Surg 58A:173–179, 1976.
116. Abbot LC, Saunders BM, Bost FC, et al: Injuries to the knee joint. J Bone Joint Surg 26A:503–521, 1941.
117. Smillie IS: Injuries to the Knee Joint, 2nd ed. Edinburgh, Livingstone, 1950.
118. Hughston JC: Acute knee injuries in athletes. Clin Orthop 23:114–133, 1962.
119. DeLee JC, Riley MB, Rockwood CA: Acute straight lateral instability of the knee. Am J Sports Med 11:404–411, 1983.
120. Platt H: On the peripheral nerve complications of certain fractures. J Bone Joint Surg 10:403–414, 1924.
121. Towne LC, Blazina ME, Marmor L, et al: Lateral compartment syndrome of the knee. Clin Orthop 76:160–168, 1971.
122. Kannus P: Non-operative treatment of grade II and III sprains of the lateral ligament compartment of the knee. Am J Sports Med 17:83–88, 1989.
123. Ferretti A, Ippolito E, Mariani P, et al: Jumper's knee. Am J Sports Med 11:58–62, 1983.
124. Roels J, Martens M, Mulier JC, et al: Patellar tendinitis (jumper's knee). Am J Sports Med 6:362–368, 1978.
125. Blazina ME, Kerlan RK, Jobe FW, et al: Jumper's knee. Orthop Clin North Am 4:665–678, 1973.
126. Mubarak SJ, Gould RN, Lee YF, et al: The medial tibial stress syndrome: A cause of shin splints. Am J Sports Med 10:201–205, 1982.
127. Andrish JT, Bergfeld JA, Walheim JA: A prospective study on the management of shin splints. J Bone Joint Surg 56A:1697–1700, 1974.
128. Messier SP, Pittala KA: Etiologic factors associated with selected running injuries. Med Sci Sports Exerc 20:501–505, 1988.
129. Rupani H, Holder L, Espinola D, Engin S: Three–phase radionuclide bone imaging in sports medicine. Radiology 156:187–196, 1985.
130. Michael RH, Holder LE: The soleus syndrome: A cause of medial tibial stress (shin splints). Am J Sports Med 13:87–94, 1985.
131. Matheson GO, Clement DB, McKenzie DC, et al: Stress fractures in athletes: A study of 320 cases. Am J Sports Med 15:46–58, 1987.
132. Orava S, Hulkko A: Stress fractures in athletes. Int J Sports Med 8:221–226, 1987.
133. Rosen PR, Micheli LJ, Treves S: Early scintigraphic diagnosis of bone stress and fractures in athletic adolescents. Pediatrics 70:11–15, 1982.
134. Giladi M, Ziv Y, Aharonson Z, et al: Comparison between radiography, bone scan, and ultrasound in the diagnosis of stress fractures. Milit Med 149:459–461, 1984.
135. Milgrom C, Giladi M, Chisin R, et al: The long-term follow up of soldiers with stress fractures. Am J Sports Med 13:398–400, 1985.
136. Balduini FF, Tetzlaff J: Historical perspectives on injuries of the ligaments of the ankle. Clin Sports Med 1:3–12, 1982.
137. Garrick JM: The frequency of injury, mechanism of injury, and epidemiology of ankle sprains. Am J Sports Med 5:241–242, 1977.
138. McConkey JP: Ankle sprains, consequences and mimics. Med Sport Sci Exerc 23:39–55, 1987.
139. Hopkinson WJ, St Pierre P, Ryan JB, et al: Syndesmosis sprains of the ankle. Foot Ankle 10:325–330, 1990.
140. Stiehl JB: Complex ankle fracture dislocations with syndesmosis diastasis. Orthop Rev 14:499–507, 1990.
141. Bunch RP, Bednarski K, Holland D, et al: Ankle joint support: A comparison of reusable lace-on braces with taping and wrapping. Physician Sports Med 13:59–62, 1985.
142. Rovere GD, Clarke TJ, Yates CS, et al: Retrospective comparison of taping and ankle stabilizers in preventing ankle injuries. Am J Sports Med 16:228–233, 1988.

CHAPTER 39

Entrapment Neuropathies and Related Disorders

Kenneth K. Nakano

The term *peripheral entrapment* describes the mechanical irritation by which a specific peripheral nerve becomes locally injured in a vulnerable anatomic site.[1, 2] Peripheral nerve entrapment may result from a number of mechanisms, including pressure (compression), stretch, friction, and angulation. The pathophysiology of the nerve entrapment syndromes differs owing to this variety. Additional clinical circumstances influence these disorders, including the patient's age and the presence of underlying systemic diseases (e.g., diabetes mellitus, rheumatologic diseases).[3] Compression on the nerve within a closed space can occur wherever a peripheral nerve passes through an opening in fibrous tissue or through an osseofibrous canal (e.g., cubital tunnel), soft tissue swelling (e.g., rheumatoid arthritis), an anomalous or hypertrophied muscle[4] (e.g., the pronator teres syndrome), a constricting scar or ligament, a bony deformity, or a mass (e.g., benign or malignant tumor, ganglion, synovial cyst) (Table 39–1). Damage to a peripheral nerve may result from high pressure exerted for a short time (e.g., acute radial nerve palsy) or from moderate or low pressure exerted for long periods of time or intermittently (e.g., tardy ulnar palsy).

The basic anatomy of peripheral nerves includes a composition of axons of sensory, motor, and autonomic neurons combined with supporting elements. Schwann cells ensheath the neuronal processes and can be classified as either *myelinated* or *unmyelinated*. The Schwann cell wraps multiple layers of its cell membrane around the axon, producing a myelin sheath (Fig. 39–1). For unmyelinated nerve cells, several axons share the same Schwann cell and lie in a simple invagination of the Schwann cell membrane. An individual Schwann cell makes only a single segment of myelin for a single axon, and this segment of myelin is termed an internode. The nodes of Ranvier are between the internodal segments of myelin where the axon is not covered by Schwann cells. In the normal situation, the internodal segments of a single axon are all approximately the same length and the nodes themselves are quite short.

Generally, the small axons are unmyelinated and the large axons are myelinated; the larger the axon, the thicker its myelin sheath. A *fascicle* is composed of several nerve axons running together to form a subunit of the entire nerve, and between the fibers of

Table 39–1. ENTRAPMENT NEUROPATHIES

Nerve	Entrapment Syndrome
Upper Limbs	
Median	Carpal tunnel
	"Pseudo-carpal-tunnel" (sublimis)
	Digital nerve
	Anterior interosseous nerve
	Pronator teres
	Ligament of Struthers
	Double-crush
Ulnar	Guyon's canal
	Digital nerve
	Cubital canal
	"Tardy ulnar palsy"
	Double-crush
Radial	Saturday night palsy
	Posterior interosseous nerve
	"Tennis elbow"
Musculocutaneous	Coracobrachialis
Suprascapular	Suprascapular foramen
	Infraspinatus branch
Dorsal scapular	Scalenus medius
Long thoracic	Serratus anterior palsy
Brachial plexus	Thoracic outlet syndrome
	Scalenus anticus
	Cervical rib
	Costoclavicular
	Hyperabduction
Lower Limbs	
Sciatic	Pyriformis
	Popliteal (Baker's) cyst
Common peroneal	Hereditary compression neuropathy
	Ganglion
	Leprosy
	Popliteal (Baker's) cyst
Posterior tibial	Popliteal (Baker's) cyst
	Tarsal tunnel
	Medial and lateral plantar nerve
	Interdigital nerve
Femoral	Pressure by space-limiting process
Saphenous	Subsartorial (Hunter's) canal
Lateral femoral cutaneous	Meralgia paresthetica
Obturator	Obturator canal
	Osteitis pubis
Ilioinguinal	Anterior superior iliac spine
Genitofemoral	Adhesions after surgery

From Nakano KK: Entrapment neuropathies. Muscle Nerve 1:264, 1978.

an individual fascicle resides endoneural connective tissue. Surrounding each fascicle is connective tissue circularly arranged (termed the *perineurium*), whereas the connective tissue that binds the individual fasci-

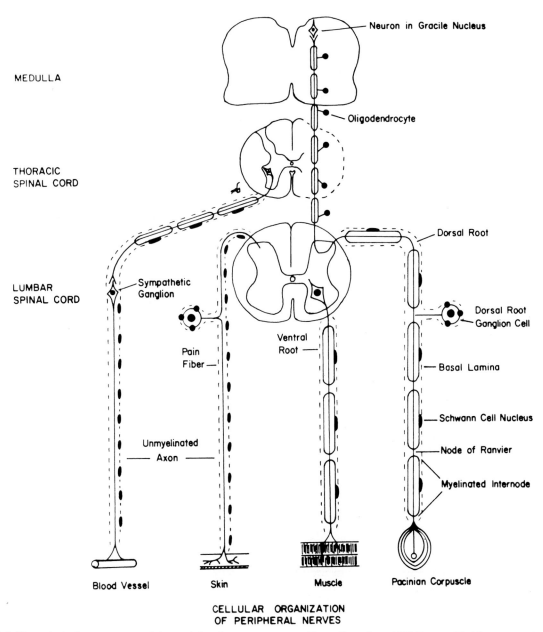

MEDULLA

THORACIC
SPINAL CORD

LUMBAR
SPINAL CORD

— Neuron in Gracile Nucleus

— Oligodendrocyte

Sympathetic
Ganglion

Pain
Fiber —

Ventral
Root —

Unmyelinated
— Axon

Dorsal Root

Dorsal Root
Ganglion Cell

— Basal Lamina

— Schwann Cell Nucleus

— Node of Ranvier

— Myelinated Internode

Blood Vessel   Skin   Muscle   Pacinian Corpuscle

CELLULAR ORGANIZATION
OF PERIPHERAL NERVES

Figure 39–1. The principal components of the peripheral nervous system. (From Shaumburg HH, Berger AR, Thomas PK: Disorders of Peripheral Nerves, 2nd ed. Philadelphia, FA Davis, 1992.)

cles into the nerve trunk is called the epineurium (Fig. 39–2).

The connective tissue plays an important protective role; the epineurial areolar connective tissue protects the nerve from compression.[5] The initial events with longitudinal tension on the nerve trunk are stretching out of the undulations in the epineurium and perineurium, leaving the nerve axons tension free. Action potentials transmit information along axons from one area of the body to another and travel continuously along the surface of unmyelinated fibers. Among myelinated fibers, the action potential jumps from node to node by saltatory conduction rather than by traveling all along the intervening axon cell membrane underneath the internode. The larger the axonal di-

ameter and the thicker the myelin sheath, the faster the action potential can be propagated.

Three important terms are used to describe types of nerve injury[6]:

1. *Neurapraxia* is a segmental block of axonal conduction whereupon a nerve can conduct action potential above and below a certain area but not across the same region. Although the nerve is in continuity, it does not function, and this phenomenon results from a focal region of demyelination. If severe myelin injury exists in a local area, action potential cannot propagate through the area.

2. *Axonotmesis* refers to loss of continuity of the nerve axons, but with continuity of the connective

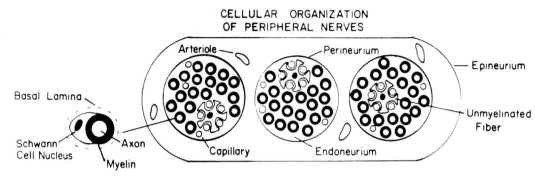

CELLULAR ORGANIZATION
OF PERIPHERAL NERVES

PERIPHERAL NERVE
COMPONENTS

Figure 39–2. A diagram of a peripheral nerve in cross section. The nerve contains three fascicles. The figure on the left represents a high magnification of a myelinated axon in cross-section. (From Shaumburg HH, Berger AR, Thomas PK: Disorders of Peripheral Nerves, 2nd ed. Philadelphia, FA Davis, 1992.)

tissue sheath; this process leads to wallerian degeneration of the distal part of the nerve and is characterized by breakdown of the axon into ovoids with secondary degeneration of the myelin sheath of the axon.

3. *Neurotmesis* occurs not only when the axons are destroyed but also when the connective tissue is damaged, a process that is more severe than axonotmesis. There is less chance for regrowth in the appropriate direction as a result of the loss of the continuity of the supporting elements of the nerve; in this circumstance, the nerve may not grow much beyond the site of injury and may ball up into a neuroma.[5]

Entrapment neuropathies are most often characterized physiologically by focal slowing and histologically by a segmental demyelination and remyelination. Peripheral nerve entrapment syndromes appear to result from direct mechanical injury (Fig. 39–3), such as chronic low pressure or friction (e.g., carpal tunnel syndrome). Additional minor roles in the production of nerve damage may be played by ischemia, damage to the blood-brain barrier, and fibrosis.

In addition to the clinical examination (Table 39–2), the evaluation of patients with peripheral nerve entrapments should include various electrophysiologic studies, such as electromyography (EMG), nerve conduction velocity (NCV) studies, and somatosensory evoked responses (SERs) (Table 39–3). These electrodiagnostic procedures are valuable under four circumstances:

1. When the clinical diagnosis is uncertain.

2. In following the course of patients with entrapment neuropathies being treated conservatively.

3. In detecting or excluding a coexisting condition such as a radiculopathy or subclinical polyneuropathy.

4. Preoperatively.

It should be cautioned that in the initial evaluation of patients with entrapment syndromes, detailed electrophysiologic studies should be performed in a well-established clinical neurophysiology laboratory.[7–10]

Neuroimaging computerized technology in the form of computed tomography (CT), magnetic resonance imaging (MRI), and ultrasound has assisted in the diagnosis and planning of surgical approaches to certain peripheral entrapment syndromes (Figs. 39–4 and 39–5).[11, 12]

Many physicians, including neurologists, neurosurgeons, orthopedic surgeons, physiatrists, hand surgeons, rheumatologists, sports medicine specialists, and internists with specific interest in neurologic diseases, deal with the peripheral nerve entrapment syndromes daily. Entrapment neuropathies occur commonly, and the clinician must have a method of evaluating, assessing, and treating patients with these syndromes (Fig. 39–6) (see p. 570).[1, 2, 13] Peripheral nerve entrapments produce focal disturbances of nerve function. The differential diagnosis of peripheral nerve entrapments therefore revolves around other conditions that may damage nerves in a focal manner[14]; these disorders include degenerative, he-

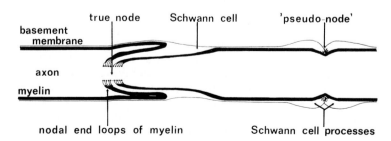

Figure 39–3. Diagram of affected nerve fiber in the paranodal region showing invagination of one paranode by the adjacent one. This is followed by paranodal demyelination. The direction of invagination is toward uncompressed tissue. (From Ochoa J, Fowler TJ, Gilliat RW: Changes produced by a pneumatic tourniquet. *In* Desmedt JE (ed): New Developments in Electromyography and Clinical Neurophysiology. Vol 2. Basel, Karger, 1973, pp 174–180.)

Table 39–2. CHARACTERISTIC FEATURES ASSOCIATED WITH VARIOUS NERVE ENTRAPMENTS

Nerve	Primary Clinical Involvement
Median	Thumb and thenar eminence
Anterior interosseous	Flexor pollicis longus, pronator quadratus, flexor digitorum profundus to index and middle fingers; normal sensation
Ulnar	Small finger and hypothenar eminence
Musculocutaneous	Biceps
Radial	Wrist drop; sensory loss in the dorsum of the thumb
Posterior interosseous	Wrist drop; normal sensation
Suprascapular	Abduction and rotation of glenohumeral joint
Dorsal scapular	Winging of scapula on wide abduction of arm
Long thoracic	Winging of lower scapula
Femoral	Absent knee jerk; weak knee extension and hip flexion
Saphenous	Sensory loss in the medial knee and leg
Lateral femoral cutaneous	Sensory loss in the lateral thigh
Obturator	Weak hip adduction; sensory loss in the upper medial thigh
Ilioinguinal	Direct hernia; sensory loss in the iliac crest, crural area
Genitofemoral	Altered cremasteric reflex; sensory loss in the femoral triangle
Peroneal	Foot drop; sensory loss in the dorsum of the foot
Posterior tibial	Sensory loss in the medial heel; weakness of intrinsic muscles of foot
Sural	Sensory loss over lateral foot
Sciatic	Pain down lateral thigh; ankle jerk often absent; foot drop

From Nakano KK: Entrapment neuropathies. Muscle Nerve 1:265, 1978.

reditary (i.e., hereditary neuropathy with liability to pressure palsies [HNLPP]),[15, 16] vascular, inflammatory, and metabolic diseases.[10] The physician must be alert to the possibilities of diagnostic confusion, as the following conditions may resemble entrapment neuropathies: polyneuropathies (symmetric, asym-

metric, demyelinating), brachial plexopathy, radiculopathy, amyotrophic lateral sclerosis (ALS), and connective tissue and vasospastic conditions (Raynaud's phenomenon, peripheral neuropathies with vasomotor changes, reflex sympathetic dystrophy [RSD]).[17, 18]

The different entrapment neuropathies are discussed herein according to the peripheral nerves that they involve.

UPPER LIMBS

Median Nerve

The median nerve derives from spinal roots at C6, C7, C8, and T1. It arises in outer and inner heads from the upper and lower secondary trunks of the brachial plexus. The median nerve controls the following movements: pronation of the forearm by the pronator quadratus (PQ) and pronator teres (PT); flexion of the hand by the flexor carpi radialis (FCR) and palmaris longus (PL); flexion of the thumb and index and middle fingers by the superficial and deep flexors; and opposition and abduction of the thumb. The sensory supply of the median nerve serves the radial side of the palm of the hand, and the palmar surfaces of the thumb, index and middle fingers, and the neighboring half of the ring finger. Except for articular branches to the elbow joint, the nerve has no branches above the elbow. Because associated lesions involve blood vessels, vasomotor disturbances occur with median nerve lesions. Causalgia syndromes often result after median nerve injuries.

Carpal Tunnel Syndrome

The commonest entrapment neuropathy occurs in the carpal tunnel of the hand, at the point where the median nerve passes in company with the flexor tendons of the fingers (see Figs. 39–4 and 39–5). In most cases of carpal tunnel syndrome (CTS), the clinical symptoms and the physical findings are specific

Table 39–3. SUMMARY OF THE EMG-NCV FINDINGS BY LOCATION OF DISEASE IN THE MOTOR UNIT

	Location						
		Nerve Root					
Study	Spinal Cord: Anterior Horn Cell	Anterior Motor Root	Dorsal Pre-	Ganglion Post-	Peripheral Nerve	Neuromuscular Junction	Muscle
MNCV	N	N	N	N	+	N	N
SNAP	N	N	N	±	+	N	N
EMG	+	+	N	N	+	±	+
Repetitive stimulation	±	N	N	N	±	+	N
F wave	+	+	N	N	+	N	N
H reflex	+	+	+	+	+	N	N
SER	N	N	+	+	+	N	N

From Nakano KK: Neurology of Musculoskeletal and Rheumatic Disorders. Boston, Houghton Mifflin Professional Publishers, 1979. Copyright © 1979, John Wiley & Sons, Inc.

Abbreviations: N, normal; MNCV, motor nerve conduction velocity; SNAP, sensory nerve action potential; EMG, electromyography; SER, somatosensory evoked response.

Key: +, abnormal; ±, occasional abnormality.

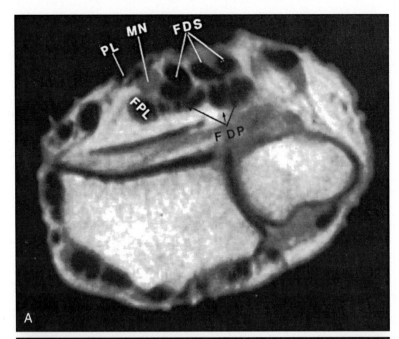

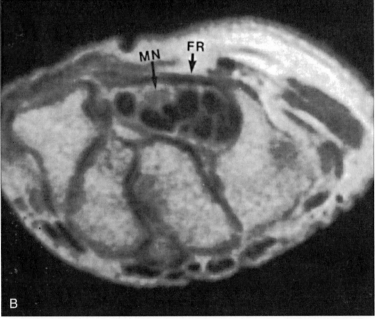

Figure 39–4. Normal wrist anatomy. Axial, T1-weighted images of wrist at the level of the distal radius *(A)* and the hook of the hamate *(B)* from a normal subject. *A,* the median nerve (MN) is easily located beneath the palmaris longus (PL). The flexor pollicis longus (FPL), flexor digitorum profundus (FDP), and flexor digitorum superficialis (FDS) surround the median nerve. *B,* The palmaris longus terminates in the flexor retinaculum (FR). The flexor retinaculum spans the carpal tunnel in relatively straight configuration from the hook of the hamate to the tubercle of the trapezium. The median nerve is rounded, shows no significant increase in cross-sectional area relative to *A,* and maintains some relationship with tendons. (From Magnetic Resonance Update. Wrist pain: Carpal tunnel syndrome. Miller Freeman, Inc., 1992.)

(Table 39–4). Patients report numbness, tingling, and pain in the hand, which often worsens at night or after use of the hand. Some individuals complain of pain radiating proximally into the forearm and arm. In the early stages, examination frequently reveals no abnormality; with greater severity of median nerve compression, the patient may experience sensory loss over some or all of the digits innervated by the median nerve and weakness of thumb abduction.

Clinical assessment includes *Tinel's sign* (paresthesia in the median territory elicited by gentle tapping over the carpal tunnel) and *Phalen's maneuver* (appearance or worsening of paresthesia with maximal passive wrist flexion for 1 minute). Reverse *Phalen testing* (passive wrist and finger extension for 1 minute) yielded higher intracarpal canal hydrostatic pressure and prolonged sensory latencies and altered amplitudes when compared with traditional Phalen's or modified Phalen's maneuvers[19]; when conducted in the proper clinical setting, these tests can provide useful information.[20, 21]

Electrodiagnostic testing is important for accurate diagnosis; the sensitivity of sensory nerve conduction testing improves with sequential measurements at short distances over the course of the nerve in the palm.[22, 23] One should use caution in performing electrodiagnostic studies, since approximately half of patients with CTS possess abnormalities of the contralat-

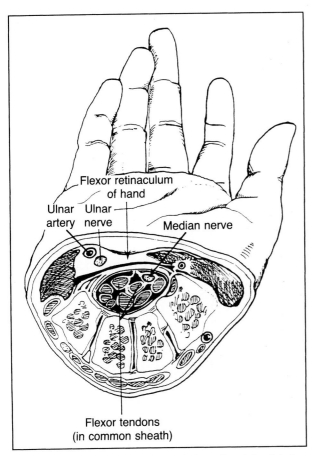

Figure 39–5. Transverse section through the palm of the right hand at the level of the distal carpal tunnel, showing the median nerve and flexor tendons within the tunnel. The flexor retinaculum is incised during the release of the carpal tunnel. The ulnar nerve and artery are superficial to it. (Reproduced with permission from Dawson DM: Entrapment neuropathies of the upper extremities. New England Journal of Medicine 329:2014, 1993. Copyright 1993, Massachusetts Medical Society. All rights reserved.)

eral median nerve; therefore, NCV values in patients should be compared with reference data obtained among "normals" along with the involved patient's own ulnar and radial latency values. In addition, the electromyographer must consider the normal control data, limb temperature, age,[24, 25] body mass index (BMI),[26] and forearm mixed median NCV.[27] EMG of the limb muscles as well as the paraspinal cervical muscles should usually be done in order to consider in the differential diagnosis the presence of coexisting disease (namely, radiculopathy due to cervical spine disease, diffuse peripheral neuropathy, proximal nerve lesions). In patients with CTS, no other tests than EMG-NCV studies provide higher diagnostic accuracy. However, false-positive and false-negative results do occur; many of the apparent false-positive results occur in patients who have measurable abnormalities of NCV but no symptoms (e.g., the high rate of abnormalities in the contralateral hands of patients with CTS). On the other hand, only rarely do patients who have typical symptoms of CTS have normal

EMG-NCV results, yet respond to carpal tunnel surgical release.[28]

Neuroimaging computerized studies (CT, MRI),[11, 12, 29] other clinical tests (e.g., tethered median nerve stress test,[30] and provocative work simulation machines[31]) and pressure measurements within the carpal tunnel[32] have been advocated and used in the diagnosis and management of CTS. At this time, thermography has limited clinical value in the differential diagnosis of CTS[33]; although thermography can show clear abnormalities in CTS, there is difficulty in the diagnosis of bilateral cases with this procedure.

Various conditions that may be associated with CTS include diabetes,[10] rheumatoid arthritis,[34] hypothyroidism, amyloid,[35] gout,[36] acromegaly, pregnancy and lactation,[37] renal failure with chronic hemodialysis,[38] lipoma of the flexor digitorum superficialis (FDS),[39] fascia of the FDS,[40] ganglion cysts,[41] the daily activities[42, 43] and athletics[44] of paraplegics, gonococcal tenosynovitis,[45] pigmented villonodular synovitis,[46] Lyme borreliosis,[47] arterial anomalies (including aneurysms of the median nerve),[48, 49] trauma, including motor vehicle accidents,[50] sports,[51, 52] and other previously known inflammatory reactions involving tendons and connective tissues of the wrist.[18]

Epidemiologic studies indicate that the prevalence of CTS is common; a review of the medical records of people having symptoms compatible with CTS and excluded from other illnesses in Rochester, Minnesota, revealed a prevalence of 125 per 100,000 population during a 5-year period (1976–1980).[53] In one survey of physicians in 1988, it was estimated that 515 of every 100,000 patients sought medical care for CTS

Table 39–4. SYMPTOMS AND SIGNS OF CARPAL TUNNEL SYNDROME IN 1016 PATIENTS

Symptom or Sign	%
Median paresthesias	100
Nocturnal paresthesias	71
Proximal extension of pain	38
Tinel's sign	
Positive	55
Negative	29
Unknown	17
Phalen's test	
Positive	53
Negative	23
Unknown	24
Sensation on sensory examination	
Decreased	28
Normal	36
Unknown	36
Thenar muscle strength	
Decreased	18
Normal	42
Unknown	41
Thenar muscle bulk	
Wasted	18
Normal	31
Unknown	50

Modified from Spinner RJ, Bachman JW, Amadio PC: The many faces of carpal tunnel syndrome. Mayo Clin Proc 64:829, 1989.

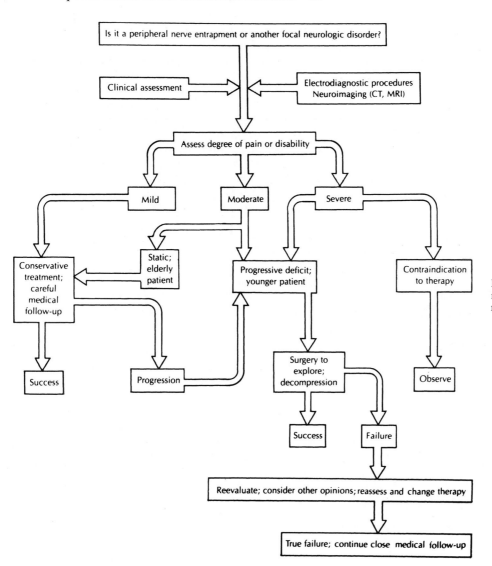

Figure 39-6. Clinical decision making in cases of entrapment neuropathies.

and in half of these, it was thought that the CTS was occupational in origin.[54] It appears that repetitive use of the hands in certain occupations can precipitate CTS in some individuals,[55, 56] but there may be an ethnic difference, as noted in a study comparing American and Japanese industrial workers.[57] Some studies indicate a difference in prevalence when cases are industrial or covered by a workman's compensation health plan[58]; in the state of Washington, the frequency of CTS in work compensation cases was 15 times greater compared with that in the general population. Furthermore, a larger percentage of men were affected with CTS (60 versus 25 percent), and the peak age of onset was younger (37.4 versus 51 years).

It appears that the frequency of CTS is increased among frozen food processors, including shellfish packers,[53] dental hygienists, electronic-parts assemblers, musicians and those in the performing arts,[59] and meatpackers.[60] Among certain meatpackers in Illinois, 15 percent underwent CTS release owing to their apparent "industrial" occupational exposure. The use

of vibrating tools or machines, awkward wrist positions, use of highly repetitive wrist movements, and great force may be correlated or confused with CTS.[61] In people with hand-arm vibration syndrome (HAVS), Raynaud's phenomenon to some extent, numbness or tingling in the fingers exposed to cold or vibration (even the steering wheel of a car), and reduced grip strength and aches or pains in the upper limbs are typical. CTS can be distinguished from HAVS if all factors (e.g., anatomic, associated physiologic and medical conditions, work exposure history, and ulnar nerve involvement) are evaluated. A review of relevant studies of all musculoskeletal disorders of the upper limb in the workplace found only 3 of 49 studies to be sufficiently well designed[62]; therefore, further controlled and larger studies are needed to answer the question of the workplace as a cause of CTS.

Carpal tunnel syndrome can be diagnosed reliably by the experienced clinician after a patient history, physical examination, and neurologic examination.[1, 2, 13] In the differential diagnosis of CTS, the clinician must exclude a cervical radiculopathy, which often can be identified by the occurrence of proximal radiation of pain above the shoulder, paresthesias with coughing or sneezing, or a pattern of motor or sensory disturbances beyond the territory of the median nerve. Occasionally, the thoracic outlet syndrome (TOS) may be of concern. Transient ischemic attacks (TIAs) or pure sensory strokes (e.g., a lesion of the medial lemniscus of the mid to lower pons) may present with confusing symptoms, but usually there is absence of pain during an episode of numbness.[63] Because no more than half of patients with CTS can reliably report the location of their paresthesias[64] and owing to anomalous anatomy of peripheral nerves,[4, 5] ulnar neuropathies must be considered in certain clinical presentations. In an occupational setting the *overuse syndrome* may become a common diagnostic problem. In this "cumulative trauma syndrome," one experiences muscle pain and ache, tendinitis, fibrositis, epicondylitis, and psychologic problems that may contribute to the symptoms; apparently, more than half of all occupational illnesses in the United States have been accounted for by the overuse syndrome since 1989.[65] It is believed that automation and specialization in the workplace, with concentration of the workload on a few smaller groups of muscles, explains the higher prevalence of overuse syndrome in certain occupational environments. Overall, CTS probably accounts for a minority of cases of the overuse syndrome; however, the frequency of both CTS and overuse syndrome appears to increase in parallel in workers who are at risk.[66]

Early diagnosis and treatment become important because delay can result in irreversible median nerve damage with persistent symptoms and permanent disability. Nonsurgical treatment would be advised for patients with mild symptoms, intermittent symptoms, or an acute flare-up of CTS from a specific injury. Some types of nonsurgical therapy include:

1. Avoiding the activities that precipitate the condition.
2. Splinting the wrist firmly in the neutral position for night and day use.[67]
3. Local steroid injection by an experienced clinician.
4. A brief course of either oral steroids or nonsteroidal anti-inflammatory drugs (NSAIDs).
5. A trial of diuretics, particularly when the CTS symptoms appear premenstrually.

For mild night CTS symptoms, a removable volar wrist splint with the wrist in a neutral position often alleviates all symptoms. If symptoms persist or recur, additional treatment is indicated; local steroid injections or a trial of oral medications may be recommended for mild, persistent symptoms; for the elderly; or for poor surgical risk patients who complain of pain from the CTS. Local steroid injections often relieve pain but may not change the other symptoms of CTS; patients with thenar atrophy or muscle weakness or those with advanced sensory loss should not receive local steroid injections.

Surgical treatment demands care and skill and is one of the most successful operations that can be performed on the hand; furthermore, it is reliably good and may now be obtained with resulting low morbidity by means of several minimally invasive techniques performed through limited incisions that involve less extensive exposure than the "classic" open procedure.[68–70] These include flexor tenosynovectomy without transverse carpal ligament (TCL) division, endoscopic release of the TCL, and subcutaneous TCL division with a two-incision technique. Complications of CTS surgery and poor results are usually related to poor surgical technique.[71]

Indications for surgical therapy of CTS include:

1. Failure of nonoperative treatment or clinical evidence of thenar atrophy.
2. Persistent sensory loss.
3. Re-exploration when the patient does not respond to CTS release or has recurrent CTS.

Surgery with a carbon dioxide laser may offer an alternative technique in treatment of some patients with CTS,[72] but some reports indicate that lasers may affect nerve conduction.[73]

Anterior Interosseous Nerve Syndromes

The anterior interosseous nerve (AIN) is a purely motor branch of the nerve that arises from the median nerve 5 to 8 cm distal to the lateral epicondyle and supplies the flexor pollicis longus (FPL), the pronator quadratus (PQ), and the flexor digitorum profundus (FDP) of the index and middle fingers (Fig. 39–7).[74] It contains no fibers of superficial sensation but does supply deep pain and proprioception to some deep tissues, including the wrist joint. Trauma, inflammation,[74] or anatomic variations may cause AIN paralysis; acute localized neuritis may be more common than trauma or compression.[75]

Patients often complain of a nonspecific pain in the forearm or elbow, frequently demonstrating weakness of the FPL, PQ, and FDP1 or FDP2 on examination. Sometimes only the FPL or the FDP1 is involved; in the latter situation, one must rule out tendon ruptures of the FPL or the FDP1, which occasionally develop in rheumatoid arthritis.[34] In a person with AINS, routine motor and sensory NCV of the radial, median, and ulnar nerves is normal[74]; however, the latency and duration of the evoked action potential from elbow to PQ are prolonged and EMG demonstrates denervation in the PQ, FPL, and the FDP1, FDP2 muscles.

Treatment depends on the cause; penetrating wounds require immediate exploration and surgical repair, impending Volkmann's contracture demands immediate surgical decompression. In spontaneous cases of AIN syndrome (AINS), the initial step in management includes avoiding activity that exacerbates the symptoms, resting the affected upper limb, and taking NSAIDs. If no improvement occurs within

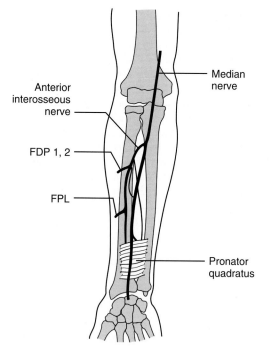

Figure 39–7. Diagram of the anterior interosseous nerve, a purely motor branch of the median nerve in the forearm. The anterior interosseous nerve supplies the flexor digitorum profundus of the index and middle fingers (FDP 1,2), the flexor pollicis longus (FPL), and the pronator quadratus muscles. (From Nakano KK: Neurology of Musculoskeletal and Rheumatic Disorders. Boston, Houghton Mifflin Professional Publishers, 1979, p 191. Copyright © 1979, John Wiley & Sons, Inc.)

8 to 12 weeks, surgical exploration by an experienced hand surgeon should be considered. In cases of partial lesions of AINS, a longer trial of nonsurgical therapy may be warranted.

Pronator Teres Syndrome

The pronator teres syndrome (PTS) in which entrapment of the median nerve occurs at the level of the pronator teres muscle, producing pain and tenderness of the proximal forearm as well as paresthesias of the hand, is relatively rare.[76] Patients with the PTS demonstrate weakness of the FPL and of the abductor pollicis brevis (APB), whereas pronation of the forearm remains normal. NCV studies reveal slowing in the proximal forearm but normal distal motor latencies and sensory action potential at the wrist.

Causes of the PTS include trauma, fracture, muscle hypertrophy in vascular structures.[1] Nonsurgical treatment is indicated in cases of PTS with mild, intermittent symptoms associated with strenuous use of the involved limb, especially repeated elbow flexion and pronation. Use of NSAIDs and splints on the elbow and wrist often proves beneficial in conjunction with avoidance of exacerbating activities. Surgical therapy is indicated in cases of persistent or progressive symptoms and signs of nerve dysfunc-

tion. Adequate exploration and decompression both distally and proximally are required.

Rarely, median neuralgia can be caused by a brachial pseudoaneurysm as a neurovascular complication of an antebrachial arteriovenous fistula or complication of blood donation.[77] Other instances in which the median nerve can be involved include entrapment beneath the bicipital aponeurosis[78] or beneath an anomalous muscle in the distal half of the arm,[79] following physeal fractures of the distal radius,[114] after operative treatment of intra-articular distal humerus fracture with intact supracondylar process, and compression in the proximal forearm.[79]

Ligament of Struthers Entrapment

On rare occasions, the median nerve may become entrapped by a ligament of Struthers (LS) (i.e., a fibrous band from a supratrochlear spur or supracondylar process at the distal anteromedial humerus).[80, 81] This structure encloses a foramen, the other boundaries of which are the median intermuscular septum and the distal and anterior surface of the medial humeral condyle. The median nerve and brachial artery pass through this foramen. Entrapment of the median nerve by the LS occurs in the upper-arm area, simulating a PTS.[1, 3] In a true PTS, the innervation to the pronator teres muscle is often spared whereas entrapment above the elbow weakens the PT muscle. In the LS entrapment, palpation and routine radiographs demonstrate a spur about 5 cm above the median epicondyle. Careful EMG of the pronator teres and of more distal median-innervated muscles, as well as NCV studies from above and below the elbow and from elbow to wrist, can localize the deficit as proximal to the pronator teres muscle. Because the brachial artery has been entrapped along with the median nerve, the radial pulse often decreases or disappears when the forearm is fully extended or supinated. Surgery appears to benefit cases in which focal entrapment by a fibrous band produces a proximal median neuropathy.

Digital Nerves in the Hand

Prolongations of the median nerve end as interdigital nerves, and these provide sensation to the index fingers and to part of the middle fingers. An anastomosis between the median and ulnar nerves forms the interdigital nerve to the middle and ring fingers. An entrapment of the interdigital nerve may occur in the intermetacarpal tunnel of the hand region if trauma or a mass (tumors, osteophytes, cysts) obstructs the passageway. When the finger is hyperextended and spread laterally, the interdigital nerve draws tightly against the edge of the deep transverse metacarpal ligament. Direct trauma, phalangeal fracture, and tenosynovitis may also produce this entrapment.[1, 3] Alteration in the flexor tendon sheath complex or in the lumbrical muscle can result from arthritis, from an inflammatory response of the metacarpophalangeal joint, or, infrequently, from a tumor. Patients with an interdigital neuropathy complain of pain in one or two fingers.

Clinical examination reveals hyperpathia or anesthesia, secondary vasomotor changes, and acute tenderness of the interdigital nerve upon palpation at the palmar surface of the interdigital web between the metacarpal heads. Spreading the affected finger away from the affected web space in hyperextension is usually painful for the patient. Local infiltration of steroids may assist in diagnosis, and repeated injections may relieve the entrapment. Neurolysis should be considered in patients with a cyst or tumor and in those with severe neuropathy who do not respond to other measures. Additionally, chronic trauma to the hands, as seen in woodchoppers, musicians, laborers, and staplers, should be avoided if possible.

Palmar Cutaneous Nerve

Isolated entrapment of the palmar cutaneous branch of the median nerve can be caused by a ganglion compressing the nerve within its tunnel,[82] and decompression and excision of the ganglion reportedly can relieve symptoms. Furthermore, neuroma of the palmar cutaneous nerve (PCN) can cause pain after CTS surgery with secondary diminished wrist range of motion and reduced grip[83]; resection and implantation of the PCN have been shown to reduce pain and allow patients to return to their prior jobs.

Ulnar Nerve

The ulnar nerve is the major branch of the lower secondary trunk of the brachial plexus. Its fibers arise from the C8 and T1 segments; and it has both motor and sensory functions. Motor functions provided by the ulnar nerve include flexion and abduction of the wrist and flexion of the ring and little fingers, abduction and apposition of the little finger, adduction of the thumb, and adduction and abduction of the fin-

gers. The sensory portion of the ulnar nerve supplies the skin on the palmar and dorsal surfaces of the little finger, the inner half of the ring finger, and the ulnar side of the hand. Dissociated paresis of the muscles supplied by the ulnar nerve results from partial lesions of the nerve in the arm or forearm. Irritative lesions may be accompanied by pain, but injuries to the ulnar nerve only infrequently result in causalgia. The diagnosis of ulnar nerve lesions requires clinical findings in areas corresponding to the distribution of the ulnar nerve, while EMG-NCV studies localize the precise area of entrapment and the degree of abnormality.

Ulnar Nerve Entrapment in the Region of the Elbow

Entrapment of the ulnar nerve in the region of the elbow is the second most frequent upper limb compression neuropathy. As the ulnar nerve passes through the ulnar groove in the vicinity of the medial epicondyle of the elbow, it is subject to several types of compressive injuries. Causes, in approximate order of prevalence, include the following:

- Cubital tunnel syndrome (CUBTS)
- External compression
- Previous fracture and scarring
- Recurrent subluxation of the ulnar nerve
- Entrapment

A CUBTS can occur where the ulnar nerve passes the aponeurosis of origin of the flexor carpi ulnaris muscle (FCU)[84, 85] (Fig. 39–8).[86] In certain individuals, the aponeurosis is drawn taut over the ulnar nerve, particularly with elbow flexion; the point of constriction lies 1.5 to 3.5 cm distal to the medial epicondyle.

External compression results from repeatedly resting the elbow on a flat surface, especially if the ulnar groove is shallow. Persons subjected to immobility (e.g., anesthesia, coma, restrained positions) appear at risk for prolonged pressure on the ulnar nerve.[87] Previous fracture may damage the elbow, and scarring can compromise the ulnar nerve.

Figure 39–8. Elbow anatomy illustrating the relationship of the ulnar collateral ligament and flexor carpi ulnaris to the nerve. (Redrawn from Kincaid JC: AAEM Minimonograph No. 31: The electrodiagnosis of ulnar neuropathy at the elbow. Rochester, Minn, American Association of Electromyography and Electrodiagnosis [AAEE], October 1988. Muscle Nerve 11:1005, 1988.)

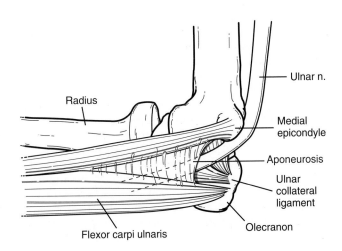

Recurrent subluxation of the ulnar nerve, which can roll anteriorly over the medial epicondyle, may contribute to ulnar neuropathies, especially in the throwing athlete.[88] Compression of the ulnar nerve can occur at the elbow in association with synovial cysts.[89] Rarely, a CUBTS is caused by an abnormal insertion of the medial head of the triceps brachii muscle onto the medial epicondyle of the elbow.[90] Also, a high ulnar nerve palsy may be caused by the arcade of Struthers or entrapment may occur distal to the CUBT (more than 4 cm beyond the medial epicondyle) in the flexor-pronator aponeurosis.

Clinically, patients with a CUBTS experience onset of or increase in one or more of the symptoms of pain, numbness, or tingling with the elbow flexion test (full elbow flexion with full extension of the wrists for 3 minutes).[91] If weakness occurs, it will affect functions of the hand, including finger abduction, thumb abduction, pinching of the thumb and forefinger, and, eventually, power grip. Athletes[88] and performing artists[59] who require very fine control of the fingers may note a decline in performance with minimal ulnar compression.

Electrodiagnostic testing includes both motor and sensory NCV studies; the site of the abnormality is located by sequentially assessing ulnar nerve conduction across the elbow segment. EMG should test the intrinsic muscles of the hand as well as forearm, arm, and paraspinal muscles to verify that no other condition exists, since other conditions can present with numbness of the little finger and motor weakness. Cervical radiculopathy of the C8 nerve root can cause radiating paresthesias in the hand. Rarely, a brachial plexus lesion (e.g., metastatic tumor) or a thoracic outlet syndrome can mimic symptoms of an ulnar neuropathy. The ulnar nerve can be constricted at the wrist rather than the elbow by repeated trauma to the palm or by a mass (tumor or ganglion).

Treatment depends on the cause and severity of the ulnar nerve compression and on the length of time the symptoms have been present. Nonsurgical therapy appears to be indicated for the patient with intermittent symptoms, acute or chronic mild neuropathy, or mild neuropathy associated with an occupational cause. Treatment entails avoidance of repetitive flexion and extension of the elbow, resting the elbow, or splinting the elbow in extension. For intermittent symptoms associated with repetitive flexion-extension, a change of activity may alleviate the condition. For a mild neuropathy produced by a blow or chronic pressure, splinting the elbow in an extended position may prove helpful. A bivalved long-arm cast can be fabricated for a more prolonged period. Splinting may be continued for 2 or 3 months, especially if the symptoms remain intermittent or improve. As long as symptoms or signs do not progress, and particularly as long as there exists no motor involvement or objective sensory loss, surgical intervention will not be necessary. Careful clinical follow-up is important, and the patient should be checked for development of motor deficit, atrophy, or weakness, since develop-

ment of any of these findings calls for a change in the therapeutic program.

Surgical techniques in the treatment of ulnar neuropathies at the elbow remain controversial,[92, 93] however; the best results of surgery occur in patients with mild signs and symptoms, but poor results develop in patients with severe atrophy. Medial epicondylectomy for ulnar neuropathy at the elbow provided symptomatic improvement in 98 per cent of 46 patients undergoing this operation, but only 54 percent showed improved motor strength.[92] In patients with an ulnar neuropathy at the elbow and an associated anconeus epitrochlearis muscle, surgical treatment with excision of the anconeus epitrochlearis and cubital tunnel release without anterior transposition of the ulnar nerve has been successful.

Ulnar Nerve Entrapments at the Wrist

Ulnar nerve entrapment occurs less frequently at the wrist in Guyon's canal than at the elbow.[93, 94] Since no tendons pass through Guyon's canal, there should be no tenosynovium to entrap the nerve. In rare instances, however, the tenosynovium within the carpal tunnel bulges and compresses the ulnar nerve proximal to the canal, thereby producing symptoms that clinically simulate an ulnar neuropathy at the elbow. On examination, however, one finds normal motor function of the FCU and of the FDP to the ring and little fingers. Additionally, the sensory loss is confined to the palmar branch while the dorsum of the hand has normal sensation (the dorsal cutaneous branch lies proximal to the wrist).

The diagnosis is confirmed if prolonged motor and sensory terminal latencies are demonstrable in the ulnar nerve of the affected hand. A ganglion is the most likely cause of entrapment in Guyon's canal; however, trauma, rheumatoid arthritis, long-distance bicycling ("handlebar palsy"),[95] masses (including ganglions and rarely tuberculoma),[96] anomalies,[97] or inflammation can produce similar clinical symptoms.

Treatment of ulnar nerve compression at the wrist depends on the origin and duration of the condition responsible. For mild compressions associated either with a single traumatic event or with chronic trauma, conservative treatment should be initially prescribed. Avoidance of the trauma, with or without splinting, often results in complete return of function. For patients not responding to nonsurgical care, surgical exploration, decompression, and neurolysis are indicated. If the hook of the hamate bone is fractured, it should be excised along with decompression and neurolysis of the nerve. Ganglia and other soft tissue masses should be removed.[93]

Dorsal Sensory Branch Compression

Isolated neuropathy of the dorsal sensory branch (DSB) of the ulnar nerve is associated with blunt trauma, laceration, or tight restraints; tightly applied handcuffs may produce a neuropathy of the dorsal ulnar cutaneous nerve.[98] Treatment in most cases of blunt trauma includes protecting the area of injury, and symptoms usually subside within a few weeks. In conditions of painful neuromas following a laceration, surgical exploration may be considered. If the involved nerve is entrapped in scar tissue, neurolysis may prove beneficial.

Digital Ulnar Nerves

The interdigital nerves to the ring and little fingers arise as prolongations of the ulnar nerve. The nerve to the middle and ring fingers is formed by an anastomosis between the median and ulnar nerve. Mechanisms and etiologic factors similar to those discussed for median digital neuropathies apply to ulnar digital entrapment syndromes. Clinical examination demonstrates a characteristic pattern of sensory loss and pain. Treatment is similar to that for other interdigital entrapments.

Radial Nerve

The radial nerve arises from the posterior secondary trunk of the brachial plexus (C5-C8); it is predominantly motor and innervates the extensors of the forearm, wrist, and fingers as well as the supinator of the forearm. The sensory supply of the radial nerve includes a small area on the posterior radial surface of the hand and the first and second metacarpals of the thumb, index, and middle fingers. Entrapments of the radial nerve or its branches in the forearm or wrist result in clinical findings related to the site of the lesion.

High Radial Nerve Compression

High radial nerve compressions occur proximal to the elbow prior to the division of the posterior interosseous branch and the sensory branch. Most of these radial nerve lesions are traumatic (shoulder dislocations, humeral neck fractures)[99] or secondary to pressure (e.g., crutches).[100] A lesion localized to the region of the spiral groove may produce an acute retrohumeral radial neuropathy,[101] and a high radial nerve palsy may follow strenuous muscular activity (i.e., the radial nerve becomes constricted by the lateral head of the triceps muscle).[102] Furthermore, a compressive radial nerve palsy has been reported after military training (e.g., shooting a rifle for 3 hours).[103]

Therapy for traumatic radial nerve compression is generally conservative, as most patients with radial nerve paresis secondary to compression recover spontaneously. Treatment of a compression lesion of a high radial nerve should include a cock-up splint made of plaster or plastic for the wrist joint. This splint should be applied if the paresis lasts longer than a week. In long-lasting weakness, a spring-loaded extensor brace for the fingers may be used. In humeral fractures requiring surgical exploration, the radial nerve should also be explored at the time of surgery, and in displaced fractures of the distal part of the humerus early exploration is necessary because of the high frequency of radial nerve entrapment between the fracture fragments.

Posterior Interosseous Nerve Syndrome

The posterior interosseous nerve syndrome (PINS) is an entrapment of the deep branch of the radial nerve just distal to the elbow joint (Fig. 39–9).[104] Motor weakness of the extensors of the wrist and fingers (sparing the extensor carpi radialis longus and brevis) is seen. Infrequently, the PINS occurs after excision of the radial head, as an isolated paralysis of the descending branch, in association with congenital hemihypertrophy, and rarely secondary to vasculitis[105] or a myxoma.[106]

The proper diagnosis of the PINS can be established by careful clinical examination and electrodiagnosis. The rheumatoid patient with PINS shows evidence of elbow synovitis with pain, limitation of movement, and elbow spasm. A positive tenodesis effect is noted with PIN paralysis. When the wrist is passively flexed, the metacarpophalangeal joints extend, showing that the extensor tendons are intact. In patients with ruptured extensor tendons, the ends of the tendons are distal to the wrist and therefore a negative tenodesis is seen. The most important physical finding is radial deviation of the wrist on dorsiflexion from noninvolvement of the extensor carpi radialis longus (ECRL) and extensor carpi radialis brevis (ECRB), with paralysis of the extensor carpi ulnaris (ECU). One also finds that, even with partial paralysis, the digits that extend show marked weakness; EMG confirms the diagnosis, as there will be denervation changes in the muscles supplied by the PIN, including the extensor digitorum communis (EDC), ECU, extensor digitorum minimi (EDM), extensor indicis proprius (EIP), abductor pollicis longus (APL), extensor pollicis brevis (EPB), and extensor pollicis longus (EPL).

Treatment in most cases is surgical. Ganglia, tumors, and lipomas should be removed surgically, and the PIN should be freed from any compressive bands or other constricting structures.

Resistant Tennis Elbow

The PIN may be entrapped and may mimic lateral epicondylitis in resistant tennis elbow.[1, 3] Treatment includes surgical exploration with release of the extensor carpi radialis tendon origin and removal of any constricting vascular or fibrous band. According to one report, 30 percent of 111 cases of resistant tennis elbow experienced relief of PIN symptoms following surgery.[107]

Superficial Radial Nerve Lesions

The superficial radial nerve can be damaged by lacerations or compression around the wrist because

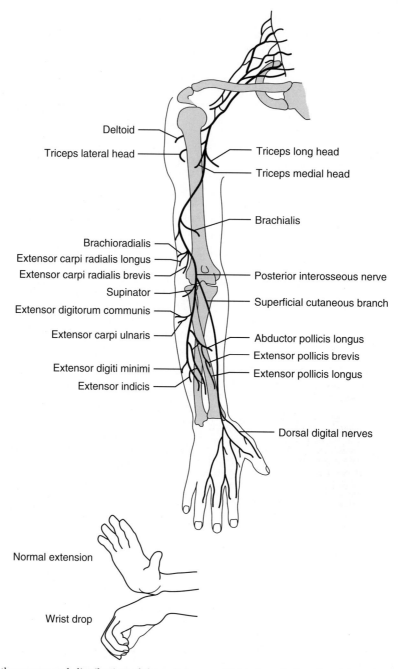

Deltoid

Triceps lateral head

Triceps long head

Triceps medial head

Brachialis

Brachioradialis

Extensor carpi radialis longus

Extensor carpi radialis brevis

Posterior interosseous nerve

Supinator

Superficial cutaneous branch

Extensor digitorum communis

Extensor carpi ulnaris

Abductor pollicis longus

Extensor pollicis brevis

Extensor digiti minimi

Extensor pollicis longus

Extensor indicis

Dorsal digital nerves

Normal extension

Wrist drop

Figure 39–9. Diagram of the course and distribution of the radial nerve. Wrist drop *(bottom figure)* is a sign of a proximal radial nerve lesion. (From Nakano KK: Entrapment neuropathies of rheumatoid arthritis. Orthop Clin North Am 6:837–860, 1975.)

of its superficial position. Infrequently, the nerve can be compressed by handcuffs, a tightly fitting wristwatch, or other straps and bandages around the wrist. *Wartenberg's disease* is an entrapment of the superficial branch of the radial nerve in the forearm, and *de Quervain's disease* can be associated in 50 percent of these cases.[108]

Conservative treatment yields excellent to good results in 71 percent of cases with Wartenberg's disease, although operations are successful in 74 percent.[108] It is important to differentiate Wartenberg's disease

prior to surgery for tenosynovitis in order to avoid postoperative complications.

Radial Digital Nerve

Infrequently a palmar ganglion produces diminished sensation in the distribution of the radial digital nerve of the thumb.[109] Surgical excision using an extensile incision has been successful in treating this condition.

Thoracic Outlet Syndromes

Brachial plexus lesions result more often from birth injuries, trauma, anesthesia, and surgical and medical procedures. MRI may be useful in certain disorders of the brachial plexus.[110, 111] Bony, fascial, and muscular structures can interfere with functions of the neurovascular bundle located in the thoracic outlet. Although the clinician may commonly encounter patients who report tingling of the hands with shoulder abduction or elevation, neurogenic thoracic outlet syndrome (TOS) with measurable neurologic deficit is rare. Neurogenic TOS is caused by abnormal bands crossing the brachial plexus, often inserting on the rudimentary cervical rib; paresthesias commonly precede the development of persistent pain, atrophy, or muscle weakness. The anatomic territories affected include those of the ulnar nerve and the medial cutaneous nerve of the forearm.

The pathophysiology of reversible, positionally dependent paresthesias remains unknown. A change in pulse with arm abductions is not a reliable indicator of the TOS, because a change will be found in 15 percent of normal persons. Moreover, a "pseudoneurogenic" TOS has been reported in a patient with multifocal right cerebral infarctions who presented with focal atrophy and weakness secondary to the central lesion, thus simulating a TOS.[112] Electrodiagnostic testing shows no abnormalities in patients with the more common reversible paresthesias; however, in true neurogenic TOS the following findings are present:

1. Low amplitude of the median nerve motor response.
2. Low or relatively low amplitude of the ulnar sensory action potential.
3. Normal low or normal amplitude of the ulnar motor nerve response.
4. Normal amplitude of the median sensory action potential (Fig. 39–10).[113]

Two types of nonsurgical therapy include (1) a corset and restraints to prevent elevation of the arms or the hands placed behind the head and (2) a set of exercises designed to correct slumping shoulder posture, to increase range of motion of the neck and shoulders, to strengthen the rhomboid and trapezius muscles, and to provide behavior modification.[114]

Surgical treatment carries some risk[115] and should be reserved for rare cases in which there is documented worsening of neurologic functions. The clinician must consider the following criteria: (1) signs of muscle wasting in the involved hand, (2) intermittent paresthesias replaced by sensory loss, and (3) incapacitating pain. First-rib resection through the transaxillary approach has been commonly used.[116] Alternatively, exploration from above, usually with removal of the anterior scalene muscle, and exploration of the thoracic outlet have been used.[117] This latter supraclavicular procedure possesses the advantage that a cervical rib, if present, will be directly within the field of operation. Additionally, constricting bands may be found passing from a rudimentary rib, or from the transverse process of C7, to attach to the first rib.

There are some disadvantages to the supraclavicular approach:

1. The surgical scar is cosmetically less acceptable than a transaxillary approach.
2. Temporary damage to the phrenic nerve or to the long thoracic nerve from retraction during the extensive dissection may result.
3. More surgical dissection may be required with this procedure.

Suprascapular Nerve

The suprascapular nerve is purely motor and arises from the upper trunk of the brachial plexus, which is formed from the roots of C5 and C6; it passes down behind the plane of the brachial plexus to the upper border of the scapula. At the superior border of the scapula, the nerve passes through the suprascapular notch; this notch is roofed over by the transverse scapular ligament which converts the notch into a foramen. After passing through the notch, the suprascapular nerve reaches the posterior aspect of the scapula in the supraspinous fossa. In this region, it supplies the supraspinatus muscle and gives off articular branches to the glenohumeral and acromioclavicular joints. From this point, it winds around the lateral edge of the scapular spine, the spinoglenoid

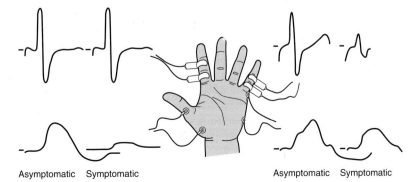

Figure 39–10. Median and ulnar amplitude changes with true neurogenic thoracic outlet syndrome. (Redrawn from Wilbourn AJ: Case Report No. 7: True neurogenic thoracic outlet syndrome. Rochester, Minn, American Association of Electromyography and Electrodiagnosis (AAEE), October 1982.)

Asymptomatic   Symptomatic   Asymptomatic   Symptomatic notch, to reach its destination in the infraspinatus muscle.

Suprascapular nerve entrapment occurs when the nerve's passage through the suprascapular foramen is compromised and results in pain and weakness or atrophy of the supraspinatus and infraspinatus muscles.[118, 119] Suprascapular nerve syndromes may occur with exertion at sports activities (e.g., volleyball,[120, 121] baseball[122]), Latin dancing,[123] work exertion (especially with heavy objects lifted overhead),[124, 125] masses[126] (e.g., ganglions,[126, 127] sarcomas, metastatic cancer, hematoma), as a complication during some surgeries in predisposed positions,[128] with certain exercises, in an athrodesed shoulder, and with primary shoulder dislocations and humeral neck fractures.[129]

Electrodiagnostic studies are helpful in the diagnosis of the lesion or entrapment. MRI scans have been useful in the evaluation of patients with suprascapular nerve entrapments.[127]

Treatment depends on the cause and duration of the symptoms. Observation and conservative care are indicated in cases of acute blunt trauma with or without scapular fracture. In the case of a severe comminuted fracture of the scapula with obvious involvement of the scapular notch, earlier surgical exploration may be considered. For patients who are experiencing repetitive minor trauma, avoiding the trauma generally corrects the problem. Whenever persistent signs and symptoms exist or in cases of spontaneous onset without known cause, surgical exploration may be indicated.

Dorsal Scapular Nerve

The dorsal scapular nerve arises primarily from spinal segment C5 and innervates the levator scapulae and the rhomboids. Following trauma and in rare entrapments, there will be weakness of the rhomboideus major and minor and the levator scapulae as well as a tendency of the vertebral border of the scapula (particularly the lower portion) to be displaced dorsally, forming a prominence under the skin, and the scapula will shift laterally.[3]

Treatment should be directed toward the cervical spine. Sedation, muscle relaxants, analgesics, and physical therapy are indicated, since this syndrome is secondary to scalene hyperactivity caused by inadequacy of the spinal stabilization system. In severe cases, surgical neurolysis may be considered.

Long Thoracic Nerve

The long thoracic nerve originates from the undivided anterior primary rami of C5, C6, and C7 after they emerge from the intervertebral foramina; it traverses the neck behind the cords of the brachial plexus, enters the medial aspect of the axilla, and continues downward to the lateral wall of the thorax

to reach the serratus muscle. The long thoracic nerve follows a straight course and becomes fixed by the scaleni and muscle slips of the serratus anterior. Because of the long thoracic nerve's straight anatomic course and fixation, it can be stretched; this occurs most often in heavy laborers or after direct trauma.[1] In this condition, the shoulder girdle displaces slightly backward while the lower scapula demonstrates undue winging. In most patients, recovery from this syndrome occurs within 6 months of the original stretch injury.

Musculocutaneous Nerve

Rarely an injury affects the musculocutaneous nerve (MCN) in the vicinity of the lateral cord of the upper trunk of the brachial plexus. In a person with MCN injuries, flexion of the forearm at the elbow is weakened because of biceps and brachialis involvement, but the disability is not severe because the brachioradialis and pronator teres muscles take part in producing this movement. With the forearm in pronation, flexion at the elbow becomes impossible; sensation is reduced along the lateral border of the forearm.[1, 3] Very occasionally, the MCN may become entrapped by the coracobrachial muscle or may even be ruptured by violent extension of the forearm. Surgical exploration may be necessary to differentiate a nerve entrapment from a nerve rupture. If coracoid mobilization becomes necessary during surgery, the MCN and its branches should be identified and protected, keeping in mind the variations in anatomy and the level of penetration.

Axillary Nerve

Most lesions of the axillary nerve are traumatic (namely, a blow on the tip of the shoulder after motor vehicle accidents, football injuries, or anterior dislocations of the shoulder). The *quadrilateral space syndrome* occurs secondary to compression of the axillary nerve by fibrous bands in the quadrilateral space and is a cause of shoulder pain[130]; MRI scanning can confirm atrophy of the teres minor muscle.

The treatment of an axillary nerve injury depends on the cause.[131] A poor prognosis for full recovery may result from stretch injuries of the distal portions of the brachial plexus and the shoulder will sag with deltoid atrophy.

LOWER LIMBS

Sciatic Nerve

The sciatic nerve originates from undivided primary rami at L4, L5, S1, S2, and S3 and can be divided into component parts: tibial, common peroneal, and the nerve to the hamstring muscles. As a single trunk, the sciatic nerve leaves the pelvis by way of the greater sciatic foramen. After emerging in the gluteal region, it courses laterally and then downward to lie in the hollow midway between the ischial tuberosity and the greater trochanter, where it is covered by the gluteus maximus muscle. In the thigh region, the sciatic nerve is at the inferior aspect of the buttock, where it occupies a superficial position and descends in the plane between the adductor magnus and hamstring muscles. Above the popliteal fossa, the sciatic nerve terminates by forming the tibial and common peroneal nerve. In the medial side of the sciatic trunk is the nerve to the hamstrings, which innervates the adductor magnus, semimembranosus, semitendinosus, and the long head of the biceps femoris muscles. The short head of the biceps is supplied by the common peroneal nerve.

Sciatic nerve entrapments are uncommon, and most patients complaining of symptoms traceable to the sciatic nerve suffer from trauma and after hip fracture and arthroplasty[132] or have disease of the lumbosacral spine (e.g., spinal stenosis,[133] degenerative disease, rheumatoid arthritis, osteoarthritis, ankylosing spondylitis, intravertebral tumor, and metastatic disease). Rarely, sciatic neuropathies appear during correction of knee flexion deformities, as a complication of a prolonged position during surgical procedures, and secondary to a pelvic mass (namely, "cyclic sciatic"[134]). At times a high sciatic lesion can mimic a peroneal neuropathy at the fibular head.[135] A variation in the course of the sciatic nerve involves its passage between parts of the piriformis muscle (the division of the nerve that becomes the peroneal trunk is usually the one that deviates). True compression of the sciatic nerve may occur from the piriformis muscle, a myofascial band in the distal portion of the thigh between the biceps femoris and the adductor magnus, a Baker's cyst,[1, 3] secondary to atraumatic gluteal compartment syndrome,[136] muscle fibrosis after intramuscular injections and anticoagulation complications, and after trauma (e.g., hip operation or needle biopsy or sitting on hard surfaces).

Treatment of the piriformis syndrome consists of operating on the piriformis muscle, removing one of the heads of origin, and releasing any constriction. Other causes of slowly progressive sciatic palsy should be treated according to the condition that caused the symptoms.

Peroneal Nerve

Palsy of the common, deep, or superficial peroneal nerves secondary to trauma or undue pressure can be seen in either medical (leprosy, HNLPP) or surgical patients (fractures and perioperative complications) and infrequently as an obstetric complication during childbirth; an entrapment infrequently causes a peroneal palsy. The most vulnerable spot for compression occurs where the nerve winds around the neck of the fibula near its division into the deep and superficial peroneal nerves.

The mechanism of damage to the peroneal nerves at the head of the fibula is a compression causing a neuropraxic lesion. Compressive causes of peroneal nerve damage include improperly applied plaster casts, tight stockings, bandages, other constrictive garments, and, rarely, cysts.[137] Unconsciousness from drug overdosage, anesthesia, or acute illness with stupor or coma renders patients susceptible to a peroneal compressive neuropathy.

Treatment in most cases of peroneal neuropathies is nonsurgical. With motor disturbance, bracing with a plastic orthosis molded to the posterior calf and projecting in the shoe on to the plantar surface of the foot provides stability. With this type of brace, a compressive lesion of the peroneal nerve can be monitored for several months before a surgical approach needs to be considered. Surgical therapy should be considered in those patients with a slowly progressive disturbance of peroneal nerve function in whom there is pain and progressive motor and sensory loss, entrapment neuropathy, ganglion, cyst, or other tumor. In such conditions, relatively early exploration is indicated, since little would be gained by further delay and a simple entrapment is unlikely.

Anterior Tarsal Tunnel Syndrome

The anterior tarsal tunnel syndrome (ATTS) is a rarely reported entrapment neuropathy of the deep peroneal nerve under the extensor retinaculum at the ankle.[138] The roof of the tunnel is the inferior extensor retinaculum; the floor is the fascia overlying the talus and navicular. Within the tunnel are four tendons, an artery, a vein, and the deep peroneal nerve. Patients with an ATTS present with foot pain and dysesthesias while NCV studies show prolonged peroneal distal latencies with reduced amplitude from the extensor digitorum brevis (EDB). EMG abnormalities are confined to the EDB; however, the electrodiagnostician must beware of an accessory peroneal nerve that does not go through the tunnel, thus masking the EMG findings in the EDB, and when fibrillation potentials appear in the EDB secondary to shoe wear or other localized trauma as well as to prolonged peroneal latencies in cool limbs.

Nonsurgical therapy includes a comfortable foot position, by splint, rest, or a combination of both. Surgical release of the entrapment may be needed, and it is necessary to trace the nerve far enough proximally to exclude a lesion in the ankle under the extensor retinaculum.

Posterior Tibial Nerve

Posterior Tarsal Tunnel Syndrome

In a person with the posterior tarsal tunnel syndrome (PTTS), the posterior tibial nerve becomes entrapped at the level of the medial malleolus, the point from which the nerve supplies sensory innervation to the sole of the foot and motor innervation to the intrinsic muscle of the foot (Fig. 39–11).[139, 140] Pain in the sole of the foot is the primary symptom of PTTS.

Nonsurgical therapy begins with removal of any irritating process and bracing the foot with a medial arch support. Anti-inflammatory medications work against local phlebitis or tenosynovitis. Surgery may be needed in as many as 60 percent of cases of PTTS; the surgical approach involves a curved incision below the medial malleolus, extending beyond the distal limit of the retinaculum. The lacinate ligament and the retinaculum are opened, and the nerve is freed. The release and dissection of the nerve must be carried as far distally as possible, typically to the level of its bifurcation into the plantar nerves.[139]

Medial and Lateral Plantar Nerve Syndrome

A partial PTTS (either a medial or a lateral plantar nerve deficit in the foot) alerts the clinician to the possibility of a process distal to the flexor retinaculum. Symptoms include weakness and burning of the feet. Conservative measures, including rest and local steroid injection into the appropriate area, should be taken initially. Surgery should be considered if the symptoms or signs progress or if the exact level of compression is not certain.

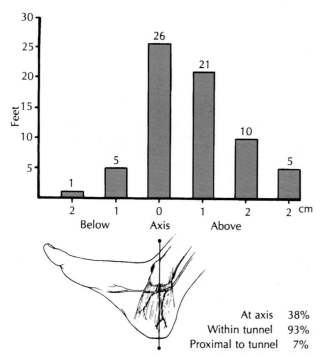

Figure 39–11. Distribution of posterior tibial nerve branching. (From Havel PE, Elbraheim NA, Clark SE, et al: Tibial nerve branching in the tarsal tunnel. Foot Ankle 9:117, 1988. © 1988, Orthopaedic Foot Society.)

Interdigital Nerves

The medial and lateral plantar nerves terminate in the interdigital nerves. *Morton's neuroma* may occur at the region of the interdigital nerve in the third and fourth interspaces of the foot and become a source of lower limb pain. Initial conservative management consists of padding the metatarsal head or changing to shoes that cause less lateral pinching. Occasionally, a surgical excision of the nerve is required; this is done by an incision over the web space between the toes; the branch of the nerve is identified and tracked proximally until the branch point at which the two digital nerves are formed from the proper interdigital nerve.

Sural Nerve

The sural nerve originates from an anastomotic branch of the tibial nerve; this branch joins the peroneal anastomotic nerve and extends down the back of the leg to the outer side of the foot. The sural nerve is subject to laceration or compressive lesions primarily at the level of its exit through fascia, with subsequent paresthesias radiating into the lateral part of the foot.[141] Since the sural nerve can be a site for nerve biopsy, clinical symptoms similar to lacerations and compressive lesions may ensue after such a biopsy. If initial avoidance of continued irritation and rest of the affected area do not produce resolution of the symptoms, surgical exploration may be considered.

Lateral Femoral Cutaneous Nerve

The lateral femoral cutaneous nerve (LFCN) is derived from the L2 and L3 nerve roots and emerges from the lateral border of the psoas major muscle to cross the iliacus muscle; it goes forward to the lateral end of the inguinal ligament and at first lies under the iliacus fascia. It then enters into and runs between the fascial layers just before going through a tunnel in the lateral attachment of the inguinal ligament to the anterior superior iliac spine. Beyond its opening in the inguinal ligament, the nerve is beneath the deep fascia of the upper thigh for a short portion of its course, piercing it to reach its final subcutaneous and intracutaneous position. About 12.5 cm below the anterior superior iliac spine, the nerve divides into anterior and posterior branches. The anterior branch innervates the skin of the anterior and lateral aspects of the thigh as far as the knee. The posterior branch innervates the skin over the lateral and posterior portions of the thigh from the trochanteric region to the middle of the thigh.

Meralgia paresthetica is where entrapment of the LFCN occurs as it passes underneath or through the inguinal ligament at its origin on the anterior iliac spine.[142, 143] Other causes of the LFCN dysfunction include leprosy,[144] tumor of the psoas,[145] and complications of laparoscopic procedures and surgery.[146–149]

Nonsurgical therapy consists of avoiding any new or recently started exercises and removing constricting binders, corsets, or tight belts. If pregnancy or weight gain appears to be a provocative factor, the passage of time and weight reduction improve symptoms. In certain conditions, local nerve blocks may be beneficial. Surgical procedures should be considered if the symptoms are relatively long-lasting or very painful. Surgery consists of release of the entrapment at the level of the nerve's exit under the inguinal ligament. If the LFCN is severed, unpleasant paresthesias will increase.

Femoral Nerve

The femoral nerve arises from the L2, L3, and L4 nerve roots and traverses the psoas muscle in a lateral direction; in the pelvis it then pursues its way in the fossa between the psoas and iliacus muscles. Immediately under Poupart's ligament, the femoral nerve reaches the extensor side of the thigh, where, a few centimeters below, it divides into motor and sensory terminal branches. The motor branches of the femoral nerve innervate the quadriceps (rectus femoris, vastus medialis, vastus lateralis, vastus intermedius), sartorius, and pectineus muscles. Sensory branches divide as the anterior femoral cutaneous nerve (supplies the anterior aspect of the thigh), the medial femoral cutaneous nerve (innervates part of the medial aspect of the thigh), and the long saphenous nerve (along with the infrapatellar branch supplies the medial tibial surface of the leg, reaching to the medial malleolus and medial edge of the foot).

Femoral nerve lesions produce weakness and atrophy of the quadriceps muscle, reduction in the knee reflex on the affected side, and a sensory loss over the anterior thigh and medial calf. Entrapments of the femoral nerve occur rarely, and more common causes of femoral neuropathy include trauma (penetrating, blunt, and stretch injuries), diabetes mellitus, vascular disease; infrequently, entrapment may occur during surgical procedures,[150, 151] after renal transplantation,[152] and as a complication of cardiac catheterization[153] or malignancies, infections, or hemorrhage in either the psoas or iliacus compartments.[154]

Treatment usually does not require surgery in entrapments; most pelvic lesions in the femoral triangle at the region of the inguinal ligament are treated by waiting if a vascular process is suspected or by medical management if a tumor or other mass lesion is the cause. Treatment of a femoral neuropathy may necessitate a long leg brace, including a spring-loaded knee assist to produce knee extension so that the patient may walk safely. Alternatively, if the lesion is expected to be of short duration, assistance with a crutch will suffice.

Saphenous Nerve

The saphenous nerve is one of three sensory branches of the femoral nerve; it has a long course through the adductor canal, penetrating fascia above the level of the knee and supplying the medial calf, the medial malleolus, and a small portion of the medial part of the arch of the foot. Entrapments, trauma, or surgical procedures may produce a saphenous neuropathy. Treatment is usually symptomatic (i.e., rest, NSAIDs, and physical therapy).

Ilioinguinal Nerve

The point of entrapment of the ilioinguinal nerve is located slightly medial to the anterior iliac spine near its exit from the superficial inguinal ring, where it lies almost directly superior to the pelvic tubercle. Clinically, the patient complains of burning pain over the lower abdomen, radiating down into the inner portion of the upper thigh and into the scrotum or labia majora. Causes of an ilioinguinal nerve syndrome include trauma (blow to the abdominal wall), a surgical incision or procedure,[155–157] or a scar; rarely this entrapment can occur with scleroderma.[158]

Conservative measures include rest and anti-inflammatory medications. Neurolysis is indicated in severely affected patients who experience persistent pain.

Genitofemoral Nerve

The genitofemoral nerve supplies the skin over the upper thigh below the femoral triangle and the lower lateral scrotum or labia and descends through the pelvis over the iliac muscle near the obturator nerve. In retroperitoneal processes, such as tumor, infection, and, rarely, during laparoscopic varicocelectomy,[159] the genitofemoral nerve may be involved. If adhesions entrap the nerve, relief of symptoms can be provided by surgery.

Obturator Nerve

The clinical symptoms of obturator neuropathy are sensory, including paresthesias, sensory loss, and radiating pain in the medial thigh. Most obturator nerve lesions are traumatic, resulting from pelvic and acetabular fractures,[160] gunshot wounds, and pelvic laparoscopic procedures,[161] and can be stimulated during extracorporeal shock wave lithotripsy.[162] Also, a benign schwannoma of the retroperitoneal space[163] as well as pelvic cancers[164] can produce an oburator neuropathy. Initial therapy includes rest, appropriate analgesic, and NSAIDs. Rarely, surgical exploration and epineural repair may become necessary.[165]

Pudendal Nerve

In patients with the Alcock syndrome, temporary penile insensitivity is due to compression of the pudendal nerve within the Alcock canal.[166] Other causes of pudendal palsy have included a complication of intramedullary nailing of the femur[167] induced by a fracture table.[168]

MISCELLANEOUS ENTRAPMENT SYNDROMES

Double Crush Syndromes

The double crush hypothesis attempts to explain the clinical observation that patients with distal compression neuropathies also frequently have had signs of more proximal nerve injury.[169] Furthermore, the double crush hypothesis suggests that serial constraints to axoplasmic flow, each of which is insufficient to cause changes in function by itself, can be additive in causing ultimate dysfunction of the nerve.

Degenerative cervical spine disease, with variable degrees of spondylosis, is a common clinical condition. When a patient becomes symptomatic from the cervical spine disorder and develops a concomitant entrapment neuropathy (especially CTS and ulnar neuropathies), confusion may arise not only in diagnosis but also with therapy. A comparison of neurologic examination and testing at rest and then subsequent to provocation of the patient's symptoms may allow the clinician to quantify an abnormality that corresponds to the patient's symptoms.[170] An expansion of the double crush concept includes increased vulnerability of the nerve to compression when predisposed by a metabolic injury to nerve fibers (the metabolic insult, such as diabetes mellitus, being one of the "crushes"). Moreover, a "reverse double crush" describes the circumstance in which a preexisting distal lesion predisposes to the development of symptoms following proximal injury. With the use of electrodiagnostic studies and MRI techniques these syndromes can often be discerned. Usually, the patient with the double crush syndrome responds when treatment is directed toward both processes (i.e., a cervical spine syndrome as well as the more distal entrapment neuropathy). When the etiologic factor appears work-related, it appears prudent to modify the patient's work habits and consider job modifications.

Rectus Abdominis Syndrome

Any of the branches of intercostal nerves T7 to T12 may be entrapped rarely within the substance of the rectus muscle, leading to localized pain in the abdominal wall that becomes exaggerated by pressure over the rectus muscle or by elevating one leg while the patient is in a supine position. Conservative measures, including local steroid injections, often provide relief of symptoms.

Pseudoradicular Syndromes

In undiagnosed persistent leg pain, the pseudoradicular syndrome may be considered.[171] Of 4000 patients with lower limb pain referred to a medical center for evaluation of suspected lumbar radiculopathy, 36 patients were found to have peripheral nerve entrapments as the sole cause of their leg pain; nine patients had femoral nerve entrapments proximal to the inguinal ligaments, seven had saphenous nerve entrapments about the knee, 20 had peroneal nerve entrapments at or above the popliteal fossa, and nine had tibial nerve entrapments in the popliteal space.[171] The diagnosis was made on the basis of selective spinal and nerve blocks as well as electrodiagnostic tests. Thirty-two patients underwent surgical exploration and external neurolysis (12 with peroneal, nine with tibial, seven with saphenous, and four with femoral nerve lesions). Prior to lumbar spine surgery, peripheral nerve lesions should be ruled out.

Compartment Syndromes

Compartment syndromes occur in specific clinical situations as a serious potential complication of trauma to the extremities.[172–175] Increases in intracompartmental tissue pressure follow from increases in fluid pressure, plus the contribution of cells, fibers, gel, and matrices, and result in increased venous pressure that decreases the arteriovenous pressure gradient leading to reduced local blood flow and neuromuscular function. The increased frequency of compartment syndromes correlates with prevalence of limb trauma, drug[176] and alcohol abuse, limb surgery,[177] limb ischemia, the lithotomy position, and physical exertion of the muscles after sports[178] or in forced situations (e.g., military training).[179] Rarely, compartment syndromes can appear as a complication of human immunodeficiency virus (HIV) infection,[180] leukemia,[181] hypothyroidism,[182] gemfibrozil medication in chronic renal failure,[183] polyarteritis nodosa,[184] hemophilia,[185] theophylline toxicity with rhabdomyolysis,[186] secondary to pressure monitoring devices,[187] Ehlers-Danlos syndrome,[188] infusion pumps, diabetes insipidus,[189] and secondary to a popliteal artery entrapment. Factors that reduce the tolerance of limbs for increased tissue pressure include hypotension, hemorrhage, arterial occlusion, and limb elevation.

The clinical features of compartment syndromes include (1) tense compartment envelope, (2) severe pain in excess of that clinically expected for the specific condition, (3) pain on passive stretch of the muscles in the compartment, (4) muscle weakness within the compartment, and (5) altered sensation in the distribution of the nerves coursing through the compartment. Anatomic locations within the body in

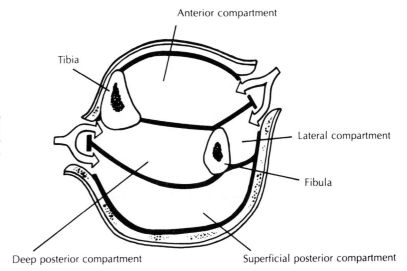

Figure 39–12. Cross-section through the upper third of the left calf. (From Lagerstrom CF, Reed RL II, Rowlands BJ, Fischer RP: Early fasciotomy for acute clinically evident post-traumatic compartment syndrome. Am J Surg 158:36–39, 1989.)

which the compartment syndromes may occur include:

- Leg (Fig. 39–12), anterior, lateral, and posterior (superficial and deep)
- Thigh (Fig. 39–13), quadriceps muscle
- Buttock, gluteal muscles[190]
- Hand, interosseous muscles
- Forearm, dorsal and volar
- Arm, deltoid, biceps, and triceps[191]
- Foot[192]
- Scapula[193]

Treatment aims at minimizing neurologic deficits by promptly restoring local blood flow and avoiding compression. Nonsurgical measures include eliminating external envelopes, maintaining local arterial pressures, and preserving peripheral nerve function. The objective of surgery is to decompress limiting envelopes and debride nonviable tissue (Fig. 39–14).[172, 173, 194] Other medical conditions that may be confused with compartment syndromes include infection or inflammation, arterial occlusion, and primary nerve injury, entrapment, or both. Careful clinical examination, tissue pressure measurements,[172, 194] direct

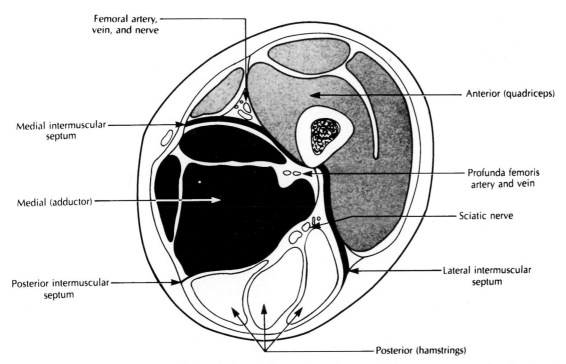

Figure 39–13. Cross-sectional anatomy of the thigh, demonstrating the anterior (quadriceps), posterior (hamstrings), and medial (adductor) compartments. (From Schwartz JT, Brumback RJ, Lakatos R, Poka A, Bathon GH, Burgess AR: Acute compartment syndrome of the thigh: A spectrum of injury. J Bone Joint Surg 71A:392, 1989.)

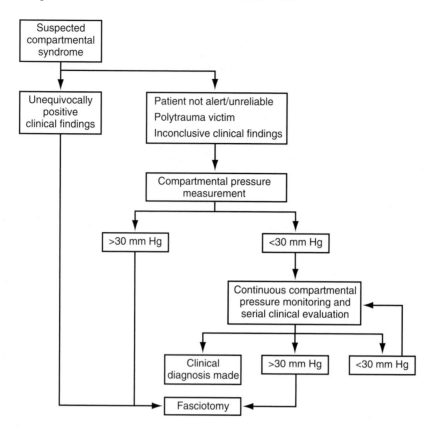

Figure 39–14. Algorithm used in the diagnosis and treatment of an acute compartment syndrome of the lower leg, secondary to a tibial fracture. (Redrawn and modified from Bourne RB, Rorabeck CH: Compartment syndromes of the lower leg. Clin Orthop 240:97, 1989.)

nerve stimulation, electrodiagnostic studies, Doppler sonography, arteriography, venography, and MRI assist in differentiating between these conditions and the various true compartment syndromes.

Repetitive Strain Disorder, Occupation-Related Syndromes, and Neuromuscular Disorders Affecting the Performing Arts

Clinically, it becomes useful to place patients in whom this type of diagnosis can be considered into three categories.[195] The first category includes patients in whom the diagnosis of repetitive strain disorder is beyond doubt, such as peritendinitis crepitans (de Quervain's disease), a tender swelling in which the radial wrist extensors cross under the abductor pollicis longus and extensor pollicis brevis, described in washerwomen and autoworkers in England. Also included in this group, but having less defined pathophysiology are musicians,[59] dancers,[196] keyboard operators, and avid athletes (joggers, cross-country skiers, sailboard enthusiasts, rock climbers, and those participating in other sports activities). When the pain arises in the arm and shoulder in this last group of individuals, it is best conceptualized as a form of fatigue.

Within the second category are patients who have "genuine" problems that are mistakenly believed to be caused by their employment but that are in fact just part of many of the natural processes that affect the human body. Indeed, some forms of usage can exacerbate the symptoms of some regional musculo-skeletal illness (e.g., CTS). Apparently, sociopolitical phenomena allow some of these patients to attribute symptoms to their work.

The third, and apparently the smallest category, includes those who realize that their symptoms, if indeed they exist, are not caused by their work but hope to establish such a relation in order to get financial or other reward.

An optimal approach to treatment of repetitive strain disorders combines physical and psychologic techniques.

Overuse Syndromes

The overuse syndromes are symptom complexes defined as injuries caused by the cumulative effects on tissues of repetitive physical stresses that exceed physiologic limits.[197] Among musicians and dancers, the overuse syndromes originate in the constant repetition of intense practice of a musical instrument or dancing, respectively.[59, 196] This situation most commonly affects the muscle-tendon units, and the usual symptom is pain while one is playing the instrument or dancing and, not long thereafter, disability. In the initial stages, the pain subsides when the activity stops. During later advanced stages (after severe or prolonged injury to the muscle-tendon unit) pain persists, and if injury continues, accurate performance may become impossible.

Musicians playing keyboard instruments must repeat movements of extension, flexion, and rotation of their fingers. Overuse or misuse problems with the extensors of the fingers and wrist, the lumbrical muscles, and the interosseous muscles of the dominant hand can easily develop (Table 39–5). Viola and violin players can develop problems in the fingers, hands, and wrists compounded by the awkward position in which the instrument must be held. Rotation of the neck to the left and abduction and external rotation of the left shoulder predispose the cervical spine and left shoulder to pain in these points. Viola and cello players may have the same digital and manual difficulties, and they have the added risk of development of paresthesias in the legs. Wind instrument players may suffer overuse that affects the embouchure (position of the lips), the soft palate, and the muscles of the pharynx, leading to inadequate volume, imperfect control, and, at times, inaccuracy of intonation.[197]

It appears that overuse leads to muscle-fiber injury. Muscle biopsy studies from players with overuse syndrome show glycogen depletion and acute degenerative changes in muscle fibers, edema of the perimysium and areolar tissues, interstitial hemorrhage, thrombosis of venules, and margination of leukocytes around arterioles.[197] Additional changes include hypertrophy of type 2 muscle fibers, an increased number of central nuclei, and mitochondrial abnormalities.

The overuse syndromes and peripheral nerve entrapments may overlap because hypertrophy of small muscle groups can cause compression of nerves at various anatomic sites (Table 39–6). An important clinical difference between entrapment neuropathies and the overuse syndromes is that the former produce weakness, sensory changes, or both in addition to discomfort, pain, and loss of ability to play or dance accurately. Among the entrapment syndromes, CTS is the one most often seen in musicians, even though subjective symptoms of a thoracic outlet syndrome may be a more common complaint. Other rare entrapment syndromes include entrapment of the median nerve in the pronator teres or in the forearm (AINS). The ulnar nerve can be entrapped at the elbow or wrist, especially in flute players. Rarely does the radial nerve become involved among musicians. Most authorities recommend rest for the overuse syndromes.[59, 197]

Table 39–6. INSTRUMENTALISTS: 1979–1992: PERIPHERAL NERVE DISORDERS

Disorder	n
Thoracic outlet syndromes	45
Carpal tunnel syndrome	36
Median, other	7
Ulnar, elbow	29
Ulnar, other	5
Cervical radiculopathy	17
Digital neuropathy	7
Radial neuropathy	2
Cranial neuropathy	9
Other	11
Total	168

From Lederman RJ: Neuromuscular problems in the performing arts. AAEM Minimonograph No. 43. Rochester, Minn, American Association of Electrodiagnostic Medicine, 1994, p 6.

Dystonia

Dystonia has been defined as a movement disorder characterized by sustained muscle contractions, frequently causing repetitive movements, twisting, or abnormal postures.[198] A classic example of a focal dystonia is "writer's cramp." Electrodiagnostic studies have demonstrated abnormalities of muscle control, with concurrent contraction of both agonist and antagonist muscle groups, and abnormalities in the normal reflex inhibition of antagonist muscles.[198] As many as 15 percent of instrumental performers experience focal dystonias in one form or another.[59, 197] These individuals initially report loss of coordination while playing an instrument, often accompanied by curling or extension of fingers during passages that require rapid and forceful finger movements.

Once the disorder develops, the loss of motor control progresses slowly over years and is not accompanied by sensory symptoms. There is no firm evidence that relates focal dystonias to an overuse injury preceding the dystonia. When a physician is confronted by a painless hand problem suggesting some features of an entrapment syndrome, focal dystonia should be considered when loss of motor function is characterized by some loss of voluntary motor control. A diagnosis of hysteria must be excluded in these patients.

Perioperative Nerve Lesions

Perioperative nerve lesions (PONLs) refer to focal neuropathies that result from acute trauma during surgical procedures.[199] In the differential diagnosis, events that are only indirectly related to a medical procedure as well as others that are only coincidental are included. There appears to be no specific pattern of pathophysiologic mechanisms. The following syndromes are discussed according to the clinical setting in which they occur.

Table 39–5. INSTRUMENTALISTS: 1979–1992

Diagnoses	Strings, No. (%)	Keyboard, No. (%)	Wind, No. (%)	Percussion, No. (%)
Musculoskeletal	257 (69)	157 (67)	56 (45)	10 (53)
Peripheral nerve	73 (20)	56 (24)	35 (28)	4 (20)
Focal dystonia	18 (5)	10 (4)	19 (15)	3 (16)
Other	21 (8)	12 (5)	14 (11)	2 (11)

From Lederman RJ: Neuromuscular problems in the performing arts. AAEM Minimonograph No. 43. Rochester, Minn, American Association of Electrodiagnostic Medicine, 1994, p 5.

Brachial Plexus Palsy in Surgery

The brachial plexus appears to be the most susceptible of all nerve groups to damage from poor positioning during anesthesia. Stretching appears to be the usual cause of injury; the plexus has a relatively long course, traveling from the vertebral foramina to the axilla, and it lies in close proximity to a number of mobile bony structures. Most patients with brachial plexus stretch injuries recover within 3 months; recovery, however, may be prolonged for more than a year. Although surgery is not indicated in most cases, some studies suggest improvement in motor function after certain types of brachial plexus injury. MRI evaluation may provide clinical information on distal as well as proximal lesions of the brachial plexus and may assist in defining both the nature and the extent of injury.[110, 111] Open heart surgery by a median sternotomy approach can give rise to a brachial plexus palsy. In this clinical situation, it is not clear that improper positioning always produces the palsy. Serious neurologic complications can develop from a surgical procedure for TOS; causalgia may develop with relatively few neurologic deficits on clinical examination.

Ulnar Nerve Palsy

Among the most common focal peripheral neuropathies are those involving the ulnar nerve; intraoperative positional damage to the ulnar nerve in anatomic variants has been reported. In case of increased mobility of the ulnar nerve at the elbow, it has been recommended that the arm be placed in supination with the elbow extended and carefully padded at the time of surgical procedures. Other cases occur during the postoperative period, or symptoms that previously had been mild or transient may abruptly become obvious and disabling. Since ulnar nerve disorders are often heterogeneous, some reflecting longstanding trauma and some reflecting entrapment in the cubital tunnel, it appears that various factors play a role in postoperative ulnar neuropathies.

Ulnar nerve lesions during surgical procedures may reflect the additive effects of positioning as well as a subclinical compression of preexisting neuropathy at the cubital tunnel. Furthermore, diabetic patients may be more susceptible to compressive neuropathies.

Peroneal Nerve

Peroneal nerve palsies can occur with knee arthroplasties, and this complication appears most commonly in those with prior severe knee deformities. Positioning or use of certain appliances may also produce a peroneal neuropathy.

Sciatic Nerve, Obturator Nerve, and Femoral Nerve

Sciatic, obturator, or femoral nerve injury may occur after cardiac surgery, cardiac catheterization,[153] or total hip arthroplasty; rarely, patients have had one or more nerves embedded in methylmethacrylate. In diabetic patients, sciatic nerve palsy may occur more often with surgical procedures. Hematoma formation may be a potential source of femoral neuropathy during renal transplantation.

Lateral Femoral Cutaneous Nerve

Meralgia paresthetica may occur after iliac bone grafting, complication of a groin flap, and after laparoscopic procedures and surgery.[146-149] In these instances, there appears to be injury to the LFCN where it passes close by the iliac crest.

Iliohypogastric Nerve, Ilioinguinal Nerve, and Genitofemoral Nerve

Hernia repair, lower abdominal surgery, or gynecologic surgery may injure these three nerves as they traverse the lower abdominal wall.[155-157] In patients suffering longstanding pain or paresthesias as a result of injury to one of these nerves of the lower abdomen, a surgical exploration may be warranted.

Obstetric Injuries

During vaginal delivery, infrequently a painless unilateral lower limb weakness may develop; often this is a footdrop, suggesting a partial sciatic nerve injury. Other clinical presentations include weakness of knee extension and reduction of knee reflex, indicating a femoral neuropathy. Although these disorders may be due to pressure on the lumbosacral plexus by the fetal head, the cause may be multivariate.[200]

CONCLUSIONS

In addition to a careful clinical history as well as a thorough general physical and neurologic examination, the evaluation of any patient with suspected peripheral nerve entrapment syndrome, PONL, compartment syndrome, or overuse syndrome should include electrodiagnostic studies (in particular EMG and NCV), appropriate radiographs, use of current neuroimaging techniques (i.e., CT, MRI), and laboratory studies in patients believed to have systemic illnesses (e.g., connective tissue diseases, diabetes mellitus, uremia). Diagnosis and therapy can be effected early if a thorough clinical evaluation commences when the patient initially complains of symptoms. It is vitally important to distinguish the correct diagnosis of repetitive strain disorders so that appropriate diagnosis and therapy can be rendered. As more knowledge accumulates, additional information concerning mechanisms of pathophysiology and therapy for the entrapment neuropathies, focal nerve lesions and PONLs, and overuse syndromes will become available.

References

1. Nakano KK: Entrapment neuropathies. Muscle Nerve 1:264, 1978.
2. Dawson DM, Hallet M, Millender LH: Entrapment Neuropathies, 2nd ed. Boston, Little, Brown & Co, 1990.
3. Nakano KK: Neurology of Musculoskeletal and Rheumatic Disorders. Boston, Houghton Mifflin. 1979.
4. Gutmann L: AAEM Minimonograph No. 2: Important anomalous innervations of the extremities. Muscle Nerve 16:339–347, 1993.
5. Sunderland S: Nerves and Nerve Injuries, 2nd ed. Edinburgh, Churchill Livingstone, 1978.
6. Seddon HJ: Three types of nerve injury. Brain 66:237, 1943.
7. Iyer VG: Understanding nerve conduction and electromyographic studies. Hand Clin 9:2373, 1993.
8. Levin KH: Common focal mononeuropathies and their electrodiagnosis. J Clin Neurophysiol 10:181, 1993.
9. Hennessey WJ, Falco FJE, Braddon RL: Median and ulnar nerve conduction velocities: Normative data for young adults. Arch Phys Med Rehabil 75:259, 1994.
10. Johnson EW: Sixteenth Annual AAEM Edward H. Lambert Lecture: Electrodiagnostic aspects of diabetic neuropathies: Entrapments. Muscle Nerve 16:127, 1993.
11. Mesgarzadeh M, Schneck CD, Bonakdarpour A: Carpal tunnel: MR imaging. Part I. Normal anatomy. Radiology 171:743, 1989.
12. Mesgarzadeh M, Schneck CD, Bonakdarpour A, et al: Carpal tunnel: MR imaging: Part II. Carpal tunnel syndrome. Radiology 171:749, 1989.
13. Dawson DM: Entrapment neuropathies of the upper extremities. N Engl J Med 329:2013, 1993.
14. Shaumburg HH, Berger AR, Thomas PK: Disorders of Peripheral Nerves, 2nd ed. Philadelphia, FA Davis, 1992.
15. Verhalle D, Lofgren A, Nelis E, et al: Deletion of CMT1A locus on chromosome 17p11.2 in hereditary neuropathy with liability to pressure palsies. Ann Neurol 35:704, 1994.
16. Felice KJ, Poole RM, Blaivas M, et al: Hereditary neuropathy with liability to pressure palsies masquerading as slowly progressive polyneuropathy. Eur Neurol 34:173, 1994.
17. Seale KS: Reflex sympathetic dystrophy of the lower extremity. Clin Orthop 243:80, 1989.
18. Olney RK: AAEM Minimonograph No. 38. Neuropathies in connective tissue disease. Muscle Nerve 15:531, 1992.
19. Werner RA, Bir C, Armstrong TJ: Reverse Phalen's maneuver as an aid in diagnosing carpal tunnel syndrome. Arch Phys Med Rehabil 75:783, 1994.
20. Spinner RJ, Bachman JW, Amadio PC: The many faces of carpal tunnel syndrome. Mayo Clin Proc 64:829, 1989.
21. Katz JN, Larson MG, Sabra A, et al: The carpal tunnel syndrome: Diagnostic utility of the history and physical examination findings. Ann Intern Med 112:321, 1990.
22. Nathan PA, Srinivasan H, Doyle LS, et al: Location of impaired sensory conduction of the median nerve in carpal tunnel syndrome. J Hand Surg 15B:89, 1990.
23. Kimura J: The carpal tunnel syndrome: Location of the conduction abnormalities within the distal segment of the median nerve. Brain 102:619, 1979.
24. Hennessey WJ, Falco FJE, Braddon RL, et al: The influence of age on distal latency comparisons in carpal tunnel syndrome. Muscle Nerve 17:1215, 1994.
25. Deymeer F, Jones HR Jr: Pediatric median mononeuropathies: A clinical and electromyographic study. Muscle Nerve 17:755, 1994.
26. Werner RA, Albers JW, Franzblau A, et al: The relationship between body mass index and the diagnosis of carpal tunnel syndrome. Muscle Nerve 17:632, 1994.
27. Hanson S: Does forearm mixed nerve conduction velocity reflect retrograde changes in carpal tunnel syndrome? Muscle Nerve 17:725, 1994.
28. Grundberg AB: Carpal tunnel decompression in spite of normal electromyography. J Hand Surg 8A:348, 1983.
29. Sugimoto H, Miyaji N, Ohsawa T: Carpal tunnel syndrome: Evaluation of median nerve circulation with dynamic contrast enhanced MR images. Radiology 190:459, 1994.
30. LaBan MM, MacKenzie JR, Semerick GA: Anatomic observations in carpal tunnel syndrome as they relate to the tethered median nerve stress test. Arch Phys Med Rehabil 70:44, 1989.
31. Braun RM, Davidson K, Doehr S: Provocative testing in the diagnosis of carpal tunnel syndrome. J Hand Surg 14A:195, 1989.
32. Szabo RM, Chidgey LK: Stress carpal tunnel pressures in patients with carpal tunnel syndrome and normal patients. J Hand Surg 14A:624, 1989.
33. So YT, Olney RK, Aminoff MJ: Evaluation of thermography in the diagnosis of selected entrapment neuropathies. Neurology 39:1, 1989.
34. Nakano KK: The entrapment neuropathies of rheumatoid arthritis. Orthop Clin North Am 6:837, 1975.
35. Kyle RA, Eilers SG, Linscheid RL, et al: Amyloid localized to tenosyno-

36. Chuang HL, Wong CW: Carpal tunnel syndrome induced by tophaceous deposits on the median nerve: Case report. Neurosurgery 34:919, 1994.
37. Wand JS: The natural history of carpal tunnel in lactation. J R Soc Med 82:349, 1989.
38. Chanard J, Bindi P, Lavaud S, et al: Carpal tunnel syndrome and type of dialysis membrane. Br Med J 298:867, 1989.
39. Brand MG, Belberman RH: Lipoma of the flexor digitorum superficialis causing triggering at the carpal canal and median nerve compression. J Hand Surg 13A:342, 1988.
40. Shimizu K, Iwasaki R, Hoshikawa H, et al: Entrapment neuropathy of the palmar cutaneous branch of the median nerve by the fascia of flexor digitorum superficialis. J Hand Surg 13A:581, 1988.
41. Kerrigan JJ, Bertoni JM, Jaeger SH: Ganglion cysts and carpal tunnel syndrome. J Hand Surg 13A:763, 1988.
42. Gellman H, Chandler DR, Petrasek J, et al: Carpal tunnel syndrome in paraplegic patients. J Bone Joint Surg 70:517, 1988.
43. Burnham R, Chan M, Hazlett C, et al: Acute median nerve dysfunction from wheelchair propulsion: The development of a model and study of the effect of hand protection. Arch Phys Med Rehabil 75:513, 1994.
44. Burnham RS, Steadward RD: Upper extremity peripheral nerve entrapments among wheelchair athletes: Prevalence, location and risk factors. Arch Phys Med Rehabil 75:519, 1994.
45. DeHertogh D, Ritland D, Green R: Carpal tunnel syndrome due to gonococcal tenosynovitis. Orthopedics 11:199, 1988.
46. Chidgey LK, Szabo RM, Wiese DA: Acute carpal tunnel syndrome caused by pigmented villonodular synovitis of the wrist. Clin Orthop 228:254, 1988.
47. Steere AC: Lyme disease. N Engl J Med 321:586, 1989.
48. Widder S, Shons AR: Carpal tunnel syndrome associated with extra tunnel vascular compression of the median nerve motor branch. J Hand Surg 13A:926, 1988.
49. Wright C, MacFarlane I: Aneurysms of the median artery causing carpal tunnel syndrome. Aust N Z J Surg 64:66, 1994.
50. Coert JH, Dellon AL: Peripheral nerve entrapment caused by motor vehicle crashes. J Trauma 37:191, 1994.
51. Lorei MP, Hershman EB: Peripheral nerve injuries in athletes: Treatment and prevention. Sports Med 16:130, 1993.
52. Howse C: Wrist injuries in sport. Sports Med 17:163, 1994.
53. Stevens JC, Sun S, Beard CM, et al: Carpal tunnel syndrome in Rochester, Minnesota, 1961–1980. Neurology 38:134, 1988.
54. Occupation disease surveillance: Carpal tunnel syndrome. MMWR Morb Mortal Wkly Rep 38:485, 1989.
55. Osorio AM, Ames RG, Jones J, et al: Carpal tunnel syndrome among grocery store workers. Am J Ind Med 25:229, 1994.
56. Margolis W, Kraus JF: The prevalence of carpal tunnel syndrome symptoms in female supermarket checkers. J Occup Med 29:953, 1987.
57. Nathan PA, Takegawa K, Keniston RC, et al: Slowing of sensory conduction of the median nerve and carpal tunnel syndrome in Japanese and American industrial workers. J Hand Surg 19B:30, 1994.
58. Franklin GM, Haug J, Heyer N, et al: Occupational carpal tunnel syndrome in Washington State, 1984–1988. Am J Public Health 81:741, 1991.
59. Lederman RJ: AAEM Minimonograph No. 43: Neuromuscular problems in the performing arts. Muscle Nerve 17:569, 1994.
60. Masear VR, Hayes JM, Hyde AG: An industrial cause of carpal tunnel syndrome. J Hand Surg 11A:222, 1986.
61. Pelmear PL, Taylor W: Carpal tunnel syndrome and hand-arm vibration syndrome. Arch Neurol 51:416, 1994.
62. Stoch SR: Workplace ergonomic factors and the development of musculoskeletal disorders of the neck and upper limb: A meta-analysis. Am J Ind Med 19:87, 1991.
63. Shintani S, Tsuruoka S, Shiigai T: Pure sensory stroke caused by a pontine infarct: Clinical, radiological, and physiological features in four patients. Stroke 25:1512, 1994.
64. Loong SC: The carpal tunnel syndrome: A clinical and electrophysiological study of 250 patients. Proc Aust Assoc Neurol 14:51, 1977.
65. Rempel DM, Harrison RJ, Barnhart S: Work-related cumulative trauma disorders of the upper extremity. JAMA 267:838, 1992.
66. Liss GM, Armstrong C, Kusiak RA, et al: Use of provincial health insurance plan billing data to estimate carpal tunnel syndrome morbidity and surgery rates. Am J Ind Med 22:395, 1992.
67. Rempel D, Manojlovic R, Levinsohn DG, et al: The effect of wearing a flexible wrist splint on carpal tunnel pressure during repetitive hand activity. J Hand Surg 19A:106, 1994.
68. Singh I, Khoo KM, Krishnamoorthy S: The carpal tunnel syndrome: Clinical evaluation and results of surgical decompression. Ann Acad Med Singapore 23:947, 1994.
69. Bromley GS: Minimal-incision open carpal tunnel decompression. J Hand Surg 19A:119, 1994.
70. Erdmann MW: Endoscopic carpal tunnel decompression. J Hand Surg 19B:5, 1994.

vium at carpal tunnel release: Natural history of 124 cases. Am J Clin Pathol 91:393, 1989.

71. Murphy RX Jr, Jennings JF, Wukich DK: Major neurovascular complications of endoscopic carpal tunnel release. J Hand Surg 19A:114, 1994.

72. Bergman RS, Murphy BJ, Foglietti MA: Clinical experience with the CO_2 laser during carpal tunnel decompression. Plast Reconstr Surg 81:933, 1988.

73. Baxter GD, Walsh DM, Allen JM, et al: Effects of low intensity infrared laser irradiation upon conduction in the human median nerve in vivo. Exp Physiol 79:227, 1994.

74. Nakano KK, Lundergan C, Okihiro MM: Anterior interosseous (AIN) syndromes: Diagnostic methods and alternative therapies. Arch Neurol 34:477, 1977.

75. Wertsch JJ: AAEM case report No. 25: Anterior interosseous syndromes. Muscle Nerve 15:977, 1992.

76. Morris HH, Peters BH: Pronator syndrome: Clinical and electrophysiological features in seven cases. J Neurol Neurosurg Psychiatry 35:461, 1976.

77. Popovsky MA, McCarthy S, Hawkins RE: Pseudoaneurysm of the brachial artery: A rare complication of blood donation. Transfusion 34:253, 1994.

78. Nelson KR, Goodheart R, Salotto A, et al: Median nerve entrapment beneath the bicipital aponeurosis: Investigation with intraoperative short segment simulation. Muscle Nerve 17:1221, 1994.

79. Olehnik WK, Manske PR, Szerzinski J: Median nerve compression in the proximal forearm. J Hand Surg 19A:121, 1994.

80. Marquis JW, Bruwer AJ, Keith HM: Supracondyloid process of the humerus. Proc Staff Meet Mayo Clin 32:691, 1957.

81. Witt CM: The supracondyloid process of the elbow. J Missouri Med Assoc 47:445, 1950.

82. al-Oattan MM, Robertson GA: Entrapment neuropathy of the palmar cutaneous nerve within its tunnel. J Hand Surg 18B:465, 1993.

83. Evans GR, Dellon AL: Implantation of the palmar cutaneous branch of the median nerve into the pronator quadratus for treatment of painful neuroma. J Hand Surg 19A:203, 1994.

84. Foberg CR, Weiss AP, Akelman E: Cubital tunnel syndrome: Part I. Presentation and diagnosis. Orthop Rev 23:136, 1994.

85. Foberg CR, Weiss AP, Akelman E: Cubital tunnel syndrome: Part II. Treatment. Orthop Rev 23:233, 1994.

86. Kinkaid JC: AAEM Minimonograph No. 31: The electrodiagnosis of ulnar neuropathy at the elbow. Muscle Nerve 11:1005, 1988.

87. Miller RG: AAEM case report No. 1: Ulnar neuropathy at the elbow. Muscle Nerve. 14:97, 1991.

88. Norkus SA, Meyers MC: Ulnar neuropathy of the elbow. Sports Med 17:189, 1994.

89. Laurencin CT, Schwartz JT Jr, Koris MJ: Compression of the ulnar nerve at the elbow in association with synovial cysts. Orthop Rev 23:62, 1994.

90. Matsuura S, Kojima T, Kinoshita Y: Cubital tunnel syndrome caused by abnormal insertion of triceps brachii muscle. J Hand Surg 19B:38, 1994.

91. Buehler MJ, Thayer DT: The elbow flexion test: A clinical test for the cubital tunnel syndrome. Clin Orthop Rel Res 233:213, 1988.

92. Goldberg BJ, Light TR, Blair SJ: Ulnar neuropathy at the elbow: Results of medial epicondylectomy. J Hand Surg 14A:182, 1989.

93. Shea JD, McClain EJ: Ulnar nerve compression syndrome at and below the wrist. J Bone Joint Surg 51A:1095, 1969.

94. Foucher G, Berard V, Snider G, et al: Distal ulnar nerve entrapment due to tumors of Guyon's canal: A series of ten cases. Handchir Mikrochir Plast Chir 25:61, 1993.

95. Richmond DR: Handlebar problems in bicycling. Clin Sports Med 13:165, 1994.

96. Nucci F, Mastronardi L, Artico M, et al: Tuberculoma of the ulnar nerve: Case report. Neurosurgery 22:906, 1988.

97. Dodds GA III, Hale D, Jackson WT: Incidence of anatomic variants in Guyon's canal. J Hand Surg 15A:352, 1990.

98. Robinson LR, Henderson M: Handcuff neuropathy involving the dorsal ulnar cutaneous nerve. Muscle Nerve 17:113, 1994.

99. de-Latt EA, Visser CP, Coene LN, et al: Nerve lesions in primary shoulder dislocations and humeral neck fractures: A prospective clinical and electromyography study. J Bone Joint Surg 76B:381, 1994.

100. Poddar SB, Gitelis S, Heydemann PT, et al: Bilateral predominant radial nerve crutch palsy: A case report. Clin Orthop 297:245, 1993.

101. Brown WF, Watson BV: AAEM case report No. 27: Acute retrohumeral radial neuropathies. Muscle Nerve 16:706, 1993.

102. Mitsunaga MM, Nakano KK: High radial nerve palsy following strenuous muscular activity: A case report. Clin Orthop 234:139, 1988.

103. Shyu WC, Lin LC, Chang MP, et al: Compressive radial nerve palsy induced by military shooting training: Clinical and electrophysiological study. J Neurol Neurosurg Psychiatry 56:890, 1993.

104. Papadopoulos N, Parachos A, Pelekis P: Anatomical observations on the arcade of Froshse and other structures related to the deep radial nerve: Anatomical interpretation of deep radial nerve entrapment neuropathy. Folia Morphol 37:319, 1989.

105. Hashizume H, Inoue H, Nagashima K, et al: Posterior interosseous nerve paralysis related to focal radial nerve constriction secondary to vasculitis. J Hand Surg 18B:757, 1993.

106. Valer A, Carrera L, Ramirez G: Myxoma causing paralysis of the posterior interosseous nerve. Acta Orthop Belg 59:423, 1993.

107. Jalovaara P, Lindholm RV: Decompression of the posterior interosseous nerve for tennis elbow. Arch Orthop Trauma Surg 108:243, 1989.

108. Lanzetta M, Foucher G: Entrapment of the superficial branch of the radial nerve (Wartenberg's syndrome): A report of 52 cases. Int Orthop 17:342, 1993.

109. Margles SW: Palmar ganglion producing diminished sensation in the distribution of the radial digital nerve of the thumb: A case not previously reported. Plast Reconstr Surg 93:1512, 1994.

110. Bilbey JH, Lamond RG, Mattrey RF: MR imaging of disorders of the brachial plexus. J Magn Reson Imaging 4:13, 1994.

111. Ochi M, Ikuta Y, Watanabe M, et al: The diagnostic value of MRI in traumatic brachial plexus injury. J Hand Surg 19B:55, 1994.

112. Simpson DM: Pseudoneurogenic thoracic outlet syndrome. Muscle Nerve 17:242, 1994.

113. Wilbourn AJ: Case report No. 7: True neurogenic thoracic outlet syndrome. Rochester, Minn, American Association of Electromyography and Electrodiagnosis (AAEE), October 1982.

114. Walsh MT: Therapist management of thoracic outlet syndrome. J Hand Ther 7:131, 1994.

115. Wilbourn AJ: Thoracic outlet syndrome: Surgery causing severe brachial plexopathy. Muscle Nerve 11:66, 1988.

116. Wood VE, Ellison DW: Results of upper plexus thoracic outlet syndrome operation. Ann Thorac Surg 58:458, 1994.

117. Cheng SW, Stoney RJ: Supraclavicular reoperation for neurogenic thoracic outlet syndrome. J Vasc Surg 19:565, 1994.

118. Kaspi A, Yanai J, Pick CG, et al: Entrapment of the distal suprascapular nerve: An anatomical study. Int Orthop 12:273, 1988.

119. Kiss G, Komar J: Suprascapular nerve compression at the spinoglenoid notch. Muscle Nerve 13:556, 1990.

120. Biundo JJ Jr, Harris MA: Peripheral nerve entrapment, occupation-related syndromes and sports injuries, and bursitis. Curr Opin Rheumatol 5:224, 1993.

121. Tengan CH, Oliveira AS, Kiimoto BH, et al: Isolated and painless infraspinatus atrophy in top-level volleyball players: Report of 2 cases and review of the literature. Arq Neuropsiquatr 51:125, 1993.

122. Glennon TP: Isolated injury of the infraspinatus branch of the suprascapular nerve. Arch Phys Med Rehabil 73:201, 1992.

123. Kukowski B: Suprascapular nerve lesion as an occupational neuropathy in a semiprofessional dancer. Arch Phys Med Rehabil 74:768, 1993.

124. Vastamaki M, Boransson H: Suprascapular nerve entrapment. Clin Orthop 297:135, 1993.

125. Arboleya L, Garcia A: Suprascapular nerve entrapment of occupational etiology: Clinical and electrophysiological characteristics. Clin Exp Rheumatol 11:665, 1993.

126. Fritz RC, Helms CA, Steinbach LS, et al: Suprascapular nerve entrapment: Evaluation with MR imaging. Radiology 182:437, 1992.

127. Skirving AP, Kozak TK, Davis ST: Infraspinatus paralysis due to spinoglenoid ganglion. J Bone Joint Surg 76B:588, 1994.

128. Shaffer JW: Suprascapular nerve injury during spine surgery: A case report. Spine 19:70, 1994.

129. de Laat EA, Visser CP, Coene LN, et al: Nerve lesions in primary shoulder dislocations and humeral neck fractures: A prospective clinical and electromyography study. J Bone Joint Surg 76B:381, 1994.

130. Linker CS, Helms CA, Fritz RC: Quadrilateral space syndrome: Findings at MR imaging. Radiology 188:675, 1993.

131. Coene LN, Narakas AO: Operative management of lesions of the axillary nerve, isolated or combined with other nerve lesions. Clin Neurol Neurosurg 94(Suppl):564, 1992.

132. Yuen EC, Olney RK, So YT: Sciatic neuropathy: Clinical and prognostic features in 73 patients. Neurology 44:1669, 1994.

133. Pritchard JW: Lumbar decompression to treat foot drop after hip arthroplasty. Clin Orthop 303:173, 1994.

134. Takata K, Takahashi K: Cyclic sciatica: A case report. Spine 19:89, 1994.

135. Katirji B, Wilbourn AJ: High sciatic lesion mimicking peroneal neuropathy at the fibular head. J Neurol Sci 121:172, 1994.

136. Hynes JE, Jackson A: Atraumatic gluteal compartment syndrome. Postgrad Med J 70:210, 1994.

137. Evans JD, Mewmann L, Frostick SP: Compression neuropathy of the common peroneal nerve caused by a ganglion. Microsurgery 15:193, 1994.

138. Andresen BL, Wertsch JJ, Stewart WA: Anterior tarsal tunnel syndrome. Arch Phys Med Rehabil 73:1112, 1992.

139. Havel PE, Elbraheim NA, Clark SE, et al: Tibial nerve branching in the tarsal tunnel. Foot Ankle 9:117, 1988.

140. Park TA, DelToro DR: The medial calcaneal nerve: Anatomy and nerve conduction technique. Muscle Nerve 18:32, 1995.

141. Bruyn RP: Occupational neuropathy of the sural nerve. Ital J Neurol Sci 15:119, 1994.

142. Benini A: Meralgia paresthetica: Pathogenesis, clinical aspects and therapy of compression of the lateral cutaneous nerve of the thigh. Schwiz Rundsch Med Prax 81:215, 1992.

143. Edelson R, Stevens P: Meralgia paresthetica in children. J Bone Joint Surg 76A:993, 1994.
144. Theubenet WJ, Finlay K, Roche P, et al: Neuritis of the lateral femoral cutaneous nerve in leprosy. Int J Lepr Other Mycobact Dis 61:592, 1993.
145. Amoiridis G, Wohrle J, Grunwald I, et al: Malignant tumour of the psoas: Another cause of meralgia paresthetica. Electromyogr Clin Neurophysiol 33:109, 1993.
146. Ferzli GS, Massaad A, Dysarz F III, et al: A study of 101 patients treated with extraperitoneal endoscopic laparoscopic herniorrhaphy. Ann Surg 59:707, 1993.
147. Eubanks S, Newman L III, Goehring L, et al: Meralgia paresthetica: A complication of laparoscopic herniorrhaphy. Surg Laparosc Endosc 3:381, 1993.
148. Rosser J: The anatomical basis for laparoscopic hernia repair revisited. Surg Laparosc Endosc 4:36, 1994.
149. Kraus MA: Nerve injury during laparoscopic inguinal hernia repair. Surg Laparosc Endosc 3:342, 1993.
150. Rosario DJ, Skinner PP, Raftery AT: Transient femoral nerve palsy complicating preoperative ilioinguinal nerve blockade for inguinal herniorrhaphy. Br J Surg 81:897, 1994.
151. Infantino A, Farden P, Pirone E, et al: Femoral nerve damage after abdominal rectopexy. Int J Colorectal Dis 9:32, 1994.
152. Jog MS, Turley JE, Berry H: Femoral neuropathy in renal transplantation. Can J Neurol Sci 21:38, 1994.
153. Kent KC, Moscucci M, Gallagher SC, et al: Neuropathy after cardiac catheterization: Incidence, clinical pattern, and long-term outcome. J Vasc Surg 19:1008, 1994.
154. Eustace S, McCarthy C, O'Byrne J, et al: Computed tomography of the retroperitoneum in patients with femoral neuropathy. Can Assoc Radiol J 45:277, 1994.
155. Miyazaki F, Shook G: Ilioinguinal nerve entrapment during needle suspension for stress incontinence. J Obstet Gynecol 80:246, 1992.
156. Woods S, Polglase A: Ilioinguinal nerve entrapment from laparoscopic hernia repair. Aust N Z J Surg 63:823, 1993.
157. Liszka TG, Dellon AL, Manson PN: Iliohypogastric nerve entrapment following abdominoplasty. Plast Reconstr Surg 93:181, 1994.
158. Langevitz P, Buskila D, Lee P: Ilioinguinal nerve entrapment in a patient with systemic sclerosis (scleroderma). Clin Rheumatol 12:540, 1993.
159. Jarow JP, Assimos DG, Pittaway DE: Effectiveness of laparoscopic varicocelectomy. Urology 42:544, 1993.
160. Mayo KA: Open reduction and internal fixation of fractures of the acetabulum: Results in 163 fractures. Clin Orthop 305:31, 1994.
161. Kavoussi LR, Sosa E, Chandhoke P, et al: Complications of laparascopic pelvic lymph node dissection. J Urol 149:325, 1993.
162. Cass AS, Doce CD, Ugarte RR: Extracorporeal shock wave lithotripsy induced stimulation of the obturator nerve. J Urol 151:144, 1994.
163. Brady KA, McCarron JP Jr, Vaughan ED Jr, et al: Benign schwannoma of the retroperitoneal space: Case report. J Urol 150:179, 1993.
164. Rogers LR, Borkowski GP, Albers JW, et al: Obturator mononeuropathy caused by pelvic cancer in 6 cases. Neurology 3:1489, 1993.
165. Vasilev SA: Obturator nerve injury: A review of management options. Gynecol Oncol 53:152, 1994.
166. Oberpenning F, Roth S, Leusmann DB, et al: The Alcock syndrome: Temporary penile insensitivity due to compression of the pudendal nerve within the Alcock canal. J Urol 151:423, 1994.
167. Brumback RJ, Ellison TS, Molligan H, et al: Pudendal nerve palsy complicating intramedullary nailing of the femur. J Bone Joint Surg 74A:1450, 1992.
168. Lyon T, Koval KJ, Kummer F, et al: Pudendal nerve palsy induced by fracture table. Orthop Rev 22:521, 1993.
169. Upton AR, McComas AJ: The double crush in nerve entrapment syndromes. Lancet 2:359, 1973.
170. MacKinnon SE: Double and multiple "crush" syndromes: Double and multiple entrapment neuropathies. Hand Clin 8:369, 1992.
171. Saal JA, Dillingham MF, Gamburd RS, et al: The pseudoradicular syndrome: Lower extremity peripheral nerve entrapment masquerading as lumbar radiculopathy. Spine 13:926, 1988.
172. Bourne RB, Rorabeck CH: Compartment syndromes of the lower leg. Clin Orthop 240:97, 1989.
173. Schwartz JT, Brumback RJ, Lakatos R, et al: Acute compartment syndrome of the thigh: A spectrum of injury. J Bone Joint Surg 71A:392, 1989.
174. Lagerstrom CF, Reed RL II, Rowlands BJ, et al: Early fasciotomy for acute clinically evident posttraumatic compartment syndrome. Am J Surg 158:36, 1989.
175. Mabee JR, Bostwick TL: Pathophysiology and mechanisms of compartment syndromes. Orthop Rev 22:175, 1993.
176. Torrens C, Marin M, Mestre C, et al: Compartment syndromes and drug abuse. Acta Orthop Belg 59:143, 1993.
177. Hak DJ, Johnson EE: The use of the unreamed nail in tibial fracture with concomitant preoperative or retrooperative elevated compartment pressure or compartment syndrome. J Orthop Trauma 8:203, 1994.
178. Hutchinson MR, Irland ML: Common compartment syndromes in athletes: Treatment and rehabilitation. Sports Med 17:200, 1994.
179. Blasier D, Barry RJ, Weaver T: Forced march–induced peroneal compartment syndrome: A case report of two cases. Clin Orthop 284:189, 1992.
180. Desai SS, McCarthy CK, Kestin A, et al: Acute forearm compartment syndrome associated with HIV induced thrombocytopenia. J Hand Surg 18A:865, 1993.
181. Veeragandham RS, Paz IB, Nadeemanee A: Compartment syndrome of the leg secondary to leukemic infiltration: A case report and review of the literature. J Surg Oncol 55:198, 1994.
182. Thacker AK, Agrawal D, Sarkari NB: Bilateral anterior tibial compartment syndrome associated with hypothyroidism. Postgrad Med J 69:881, 1993.
183. Chow CS, Chow WH: Acute compartment syndrome: An unusual presentation of gemfibrozil induced myositis. Med J Aust 158:48, 1993.
184. Hasaniya N, Katzen JT: Acute compartment syndrome of both lower legs caused by ruptured tibial artery aneurysm in a patient with polyarteritis nodosa: A case report and review of the literature. J Vasc Surg 18:295, 1993.
185. Tountas CP, Ferris FO, Cobb SW: Exertional compartment syndrome in covert mild hemophilia: A case report. Minn Med 75:27, 1992.
186. Titley OG, Williams N: Theophylline toxicity causing rhabdomyolysis and acute compartment syndrome. Intensive Care Med 18:129, 1992.
187. Vidal P, Sykes PJ, O'Shaughnessy M, et al: Compartment syndrome after use of an automatic arterial pressure monitoring device. Br J Anaesth 71:902, 1993.
188. Schmalzrieed TP, Eckardt JJ: Spontaneous gluteal artery rupture resulting in compartment syndrome and sciatic neuropathy: Report of a case in Ehlers-Danlos syndrome. Clin Orthop 275:253, 1992.
189. Geutzens G: Spontaneous compartment syndrome in a patient with diabetes insipidus. Int Orthop 18:53, 1994.
190. Yoshioka H: Gluteal compartment syndrome: A report of four cases. Acta Orthop Scand 63:347, 1992.
191. Cameron SE: Acute compartment syndrome of the triceps: A case report. Acta Orthop Scand 64:107, 1993.
192. Fakhouri AJ, Manoki A II: Acute foot compartment syndromes. J Orthop Trauma 6:223, 1992.
193. Landi A, Schoenhuber R, Funicello R, et al: Compartment syndrome of the scapula: Definition on clinical, neurophysiological and magnetic resonance data. Ann Chir Main Memb Super 11:383, 1992.
194. Schepsis AA, Martini D, Corbett M: Surgical management of exertional compartment of the lower leg: Long-term follow-up. Am J Sports Med 21:811, 1993.
195. Barton N: Repetitive strain disorder. Br Med J 299:405, 1989.
196. Bejjani FJ, Halpen N, Pio A, et al: Musculoskeletal demands on flamenco dancers: A clinical and biomechanical study. Foot Ankle 8:254, 1988.
197. Lockwood AH: Medical problems of musicians. N Engl J Med 320:221, 1989.
198. Fry H, Hallet M: Focal dystonia (occupational cramp) masquerading as nerve entrapment or hysteria. Plast Reconstr Surg 82:989, 1988.
199. Dawson DM, Krarup C: Perioperative nerve lesions. Arch Neurol 46:1355, 1989.
200. Feasby TE, Furton SR, Hahn AF: Obstetrical lumbosacral plexus injury. Muscle Nerve 15:937, 1992.

Diagnostic Tests and Procedures in Rheumatic Diseases

CHAPTER 40

Duncan S. Owen, Jr.

Aspiration and Injection of Joints and Soft Tissues

Synovial fluid analysis is an important diagnostic procedure and is thoroughly covered in Chapter (41). This chapter describes the techniques, benefits, and contraindications of soft tissue and intra-articular injection of glucocorticoids. An interesting survey was conducted by the Mayo Clinic in 1990 and directed toward former medical residents in the internal medicine program. The study revealed that 65 percent of general internists trained there after 1970 performed arthrocenteses; of these, however, 64 percent responded that they needed more training in these procedures.[1] Therefore, it is hoped this chapter will be helpful not only to rheumatologists and orthopedists but also to all physicians who perform or are interested in learning diagnostic and therapeutic injections of the musculoskeletal system.

Shortly after systemic cortisone and hydrocortisone were first used in the management of rheumatoid arthritis, Thorn in the late 1940s injected 10 mg hydrocortisone into the knee joint of a patient with rheumatoid arthritis.[2] The knee improved locally, but the patient also improved generally; it was concluded that the improvement resulted from systemic absorption of the intra-articularly injected material. No further studies of intra-articular glucocorticoid injections were done until the early 1950s.[3, 4] Ten years later, a series of more than 100,000 injections of joints, bursae, or tendon sheaths in 4000 patients was reported by Hollander and associates.[5] The researchers called attention to the usefulness of intra-articular glucocorticoids as temporary, palliative, repeatable, local adjunctive treatments for a variety of rheumatic conditions[6] and to the more prolonged benefits afforded by preparations less rapidly hydrolyzed than hydrocortisone.

MECHANISM OF ACTION OF INTRA-ARTICULAR GLUCOCORTICOIDS

The anti-inflammatory mechanisms of systemically administered glucocorticoids are still not fully under-

stood. Even less is known about the mechanisms of intra-articular glucocorticoids. Also, the mechanisms of action of systemic glucocorticoids, discussed in Chapter 50, may not be analogous to those of glucocorticoids administered intra-articularly. Early studies after intra-articular administration demonstrated a decrease in erythema, swelling, heat, and tenderness of the inflamed joints.[4] An increase in viscosity and hyaluronate concentration of the synovial fluid was also observed.[7]

One study of intra-articular glucocorticoids demonstrated a transient decrease in synovial fluid complement.[8] In another study, 12 patients received intra-articular methylprednisolone. Six patients showed no alteration of synovial fluid total hemolytic complement, C4 protein level, or rheumatoid factor titer. The other six showed a 50 percent or greater change in only one of the synovial fluid values. Most had reductions in total leukocyte counts, polymorphonuclear leukocyte counts, and acid phosphatase levels.[9]

In 1970, Dick and colleagues[10] reported the results of studies using intra-articular radioactive xenon (^{133}Xe). They observed a fall in the rate of disappearance of ^{133}Xe after an intra-articular injection of hydrocortisone hemisuccinate. They believed that glucocorticoids diminish synovial permeability. In 1979, the same laboratory reported on patients with rheumatoid arthritis[11] who were treated with intra-articular ^{113}Xe and triamcinolone hexacetonide in one group and ^{113}Xe and lidocaine in a second group. No difference in the rate of clearance of ^{113}Xe after 40 minutes was observed in the triamcinolone-treated group. Therefore, these investigators believed that triamcinolone had no immediate effect on synovial blood vessels. The lidocaine-treated group, however, showed a decrease in the rate of ^{113}Xe clearance.

Eymontt and coworkers[12] in 1982 reported the effects of intra-articular triamcinolone hexacetonide, prednisolone tebutate, and a saline administration on both synovial permeability and synovial fluid leukocyte counts in patients with symptomatic osteoarthritis. The study used a radioactive blood pool tracer, ^{99m}Tc human serum albumin. The results indicated that glucocorticoids decrease synovial permeability but produce an increase in synovial fluid leukocytes.

POTENTIAL SEQUELAE

The potential sequelae of intra-articular and soft tissue glucocorticoid injections are summarized in Table 40–1. In the late 1950s, there first appeared a few reports of a Charcot-like arthropathy attributed to intra-articular glucocorticoid therapy.[13, 14] A study by Mankin and Conger[15] in 1966 reported that intra-articularly administered hydrocortisone acetate reduced the incorporation of glycine-^{3}H into rabbit articular cartilage to approximately one third of control values within 6 hours. They related the decrease in utilization to a decrease in matrix protein synthesis caused by hydrocortisone.

In 1969, Bentley and Goodfellow[16] advised strongly against recurrent intra-articular injections of glucocorticoids because of potential severe arthropathy. In 1970, Moskowitz and associates[17] showed that intra-articular triamcinolone acetonide produced nuclear degeneration of chondrocytes and prominent cyst formation. In 1972, Mankin and coworkers[18] reported that intramuscular cortisone reduced the incorporation of glycine-^{3}H and radioactive-labeled sulfur dioxide (^{35}SO$_4$) and was associated with a progressive decline in the concentration of hexosamine. In 1975, Behrens and associates[19] found an increased number of fissures in rabbit cartilage after intra-articular injections of hydrocortisone. Hexosamine incorporation decreased, as did synthesis of proteoglycans; collagen production was reduced to one fifth. The researchers hypothesized that the antianabolic effects of the glucocorticoids cause a massive decrease in the synthesis of all major matrix components. The loss of proteoglycan content led to a decrease in cartilage stiffness such that the impact of cyclic loading with weight bearing caused death of cells, cystic degeneration of matrix, and fissuring in the midzonal areas of weight-bearing surfaces.

Completely different data were reported in 1976 by Gibson and associates.[20] They repeatedly injected the knee joints of ten *Macaca irus* monkeys with either methylprednisolone or a control solution. Minor degenerative changes of femoral condyles were shown by India ink staining and by a system of histochemical grading, but changes in the joints injected with glucocorticoids were *not* significantly different from those seen in control joints. Additionally, in 1985, Williams and Brandt[21] reported that triamcinolone hexacetonide protects against fibrillation and osteophyte formation following chemically induced articular cartilage damage. Protective effects were reported in 1989 on cartilage lesions and osteophyte formation in the Pond-Nuki dog model of osteoarthritis by Pelletier and Martel-Pelletier.[22]

In 1981, Tenenbaum and associates[23] reported on a continuing study of the long-term effects of intra-articular dexamethasone tebutate (TBA) on rabbit knee cartilage. There was an acceleration of the calcific degenerative arthropathy that occurs in mature New Zealand rabbits. Under these experimental conditions, the cartilage injury seemed limited and did not progress with repeated injections. In 1994, a group in Montreal examined the effect of intra-articular injections of methylprednisolone acetate on osteoarthritic lesions and chondrocyte stromelysin synthesis in experimental osteoarthritis. The size and incidence of osteophytes was significantly reduced. The beneficial effects may be mediated through the suppression and stromelysin synthesis.[24]

The concept of glucocorticoid arthropathy is based largely on subprimate animal studies and anecdotal case reports. Studies of primate models have shown no long-term adverse effect on cartilage.[25] Gray and associates[26] reported a case of a 51-year-old woman who received 100 glucocorticoid injections into each knee during a span of 10 years with no deleterious effects seen on knee radiographs taken before and after these treatments. A recent study by Emkey and associates[25a] suggests that intra-articular administration of corticosteroid has no net effects on bone resorption and only a transient systemic effect on bone formation. Intra-articular corticosteroid administration may be better for bone metabolism than continuous use of orally administered corticosteroid.

In 1969, Sweetnam[27] cautioned against steroid injection of inflamed tendons in athletes because of the possibility of tendon rupture. In 1954, Wrenn and coworkers[28] demonstrated a 40 percent reduction in tensile strength of a tendon after the use of glucocorticoids. (I have rarely observed a rupture of the long head of the biceps tendon or Achilles tendon following the injection of the tendon sheath for tendinitis.) Other complications include soft tissue atrophy, especially when the small joints, such as the proximal interphalangeal joints of the finger, are injected. Periarticular calcifications and ecchymoses around the atrophied areas have been reported.[27, 29] The locations

Table 40–1. POTENTIAL SEQUELAE FROM INTRA-ARTICULAR AND SOFT TISSUE GLUCOCORTICOID INJECTIONS

Radiologic deterioration of joints: "steroid arthropathy,"
   Charcot-like arthropathy, osteonecrosis—low incidence for all
Iatrogenic infection—very low incidence
Tendon rupture
Tissue atrophy, fat necrosis, calcification
Nerve damage (e.g., inadvertent injection of median nerve in
   carpal tunnel syndrome)
Postinjection flare
Uterine bleeding
Pancreatitis—rare
Erythema, warmth, diaphoresis of face and torso
Posterior subcapsular cataracts

of the calcification seemed to be related to the site of needle perforation.[30]

The intra-articular injection of corticosteroids occasionally produces what has been called a postinjection flare.[31] This increase in local inflammation may develop a few hours after injection and can last up to 48 hours. The difficulty of distinguishing this reaction from an iatrogenic infection can be worrisome. The flare is more common with the needle-shaped glucocorticoid crystals and may be a form of crystal-induced arthritis produced by synovial fluid leukocytes phagocytosing the crystals and subsequently releasing lysosomal enzymes and other mediators of inflammation. These flares, however, may be caused by preservatives in the suspension.

Systemic absorption of intra-articular glucocorticoids, or absorption from other soft tissue injections, occurs in almost all patients. Usually, this is clinically manifested (e.g., in a patient with rheumatoid arthritis) by subjective and objective improvement of inflamed joints other than the ones injected. There may also be other effects, such as eosinopenia, lymphopenia, and, depending on the glucocorticoid injected, changes in serum and urine cortisol levels. The hypothalamic-pituitary-adrenal axis may be suppressed.[32, 33] Patients with diabetes mellitus may notice a short-lived, several-fold rise in their blood glucose levels.

Prominent erythema, warmth, and diaphoresis of the face and torso may occur within minutes to hours after an intra-articular glucocorticoid injection,[34] especially with triamcinolone acetonide. Some authorities think it is an uncommon reaction, but I note it in more than 10 percent of patients injected with this medication. Some of these patients report headache. In this regard, it resembles the nitritoid reaction occasionally observed with the injection of gold salts, especially gold sodium thiomalate. These glucocorticoid reactions may last a few minutes to a few days. However, some patients are so frightened by these reactions that they refuse further injections. Local skin eruptions have also been reported.[35]

Abnormal uterine bleeding may occur after injection of glucocorticoids, especially triamcinolone acetonide. The exact mechanisms are unknown, but ovulation may be inhibited.[36, 37] Also, glucocorticoids can produce uterine bleeding in postmenopausal patients. This alarms both patient and physician.

Pancreatitis, apparently induced by injectable glucocorticoids, is rarely seen.

Cushing's syndrome is rare, but Gray and colleagues[26] observed posterior subcapsular cataracts in a number of middle-aged patients who were receiving frequent intra-articular glucocorticoid injections.

An interesting side effect of intra-articular glucocorticoids is the transient fall in serum salicylate levels in patients with rheumatoid arthritis. This probably is related to an increase in the glomerular filtration rate.[38]

PRECAUTIONS

Strict adherence to aseptic procedures is required while one is performing arthrocenteses or soft tissue injections. The physician should use the same precautions as for a lumbar spinal puncture. Iatrogenic infections may be disastrous but are rare if these precautions are taken. At the Medical College of Virginia, only one or two infections have been observed in more than 100,000 injections.

In theory, arthrocentesis may provide a focus for septic arthritis in a patient with bacteremia, such as staphylococcal endocarditis.[39] It is well known that a patient with damaged joints from, for example, rheumatoid arthritis is more susceptible to the development of spontaneous septic arthritis resulting from blood-borne bacteria. In such instances, arthrocentesis has enabled rapid diagnosis and prevented the joint from being destroyed. Routine therapeutic arthrocentesis should be avoided, however, if the patient is being treated for a condition associated with bacteremia.

Because of tissue atrophy with glucocorticoids, one should use extreme caution when injecting near peripheral nerves. For example, carpal tunnel syndrome, either idiopathic or rheumatoid arthritis-induced, may improve after glucocorticoid injection in the carpal tunnel. An injection directly into the median nerve may result in nerve necrosis or atrophy.

Gottlieb[40] reported two cases of hypodermic needle separations during arthrocentesis. He recommended that the needles be inspected after arthrocentesis to ensure that they are intact, and he advised keeping a hemostat within easy access to enable the operator to remove a separated needle from the soft tissues.

EFFICACY OF INJECTIONS

Intra-articular Injections

Despite the fact that thousands of intra-articular glucocorticoid preparations have been injected into thousands of patients, good studies of their efficacy are few.[41] The length of symptomatic improvement appears to be related to the particular preparation used. Most patients with rheumatoid arthritis benefit from an injection, but the effect may last for only days. Hydrocortisone acetate may give improvement for a few days to a week or more and prednisolone tebutate for 2 weeks or more. Triamcinolone hexacetonide, which is poorly water-soluble and one of the longest-acting agents, can provide reversal of inflammation in some patients for longer periods.[29] As with oral nonsteroidal anti-inflammatory drugs (NSAIDs), responses among patients are extremely varied. If one or two injections prove ineffective or give only short-lived benefit, there is no logic in persistently injecting the same joint.

Results of injections in osteoarthritic joints conflict, with reports ranging from outstanding benefit to no benefit.[2, 42–48] The differences may relate in part to the joint injected. For example, degenerative arthritis of the first carpometacarpal joint is a fairly common and painful condition in which there is little synovial thickening or increase in synovial fluid. The injection of glucocorticoid is often painful, probably because of the moderate or marked decrease in joint space, but dramatic improvement in symptoms usually occurs within 12 hours and may last many months. This contrasts with injection for osteoarthritis of the hip, in which it is difficult to know whether the hip joint space has been entered, even with use of the fluoroscope as a guide. Improvement of hip symptoms within 12 to 24 hours after injection probably indicates that the glucocorticoid was injected intra-articularly, but benefit often lasts only 2 days to a week. The mechanical problem of bone rubbing against bone in a weight-bearing joint may be the reason for the short-lived benefit, and repeated injections can be expected to have little efficacy.

Osteoarthritis of the knee can be quite painful and associated with large volumes of synovial fluid. Although it is the usual practice to remove as much synovial fluid as possible, the efficacy of this procedure in osteoarthritis is questionable. The glucocorticoid injection usually is associated with dramatic relief of symptoms that lasts days to weeks or more. If the injections give short-lived benefit, repeated injections are probably contraindicated because the primary problem is in the cartilage and repeated injections could hasten cartilage deterioration for reasons previously outlined.

A weight-bearing joint probably should be rested as much as possible for 48 to 72 hours after injection. Neustadt[49] recommends the use of crutches or a cane for another 3 weeks. Others advise resting all glucocorticoid-injected joints for a longer period.[50, 51] There is no consensus, however.

Nonarticular Injections

In contrast to the situation with intra-articular injections, which are used adjunctively, certain soft tissue inflammatory conditions can be more or less permanently eradicated by judicious injections of glucocorticoids with or without local anesthetics.[52–55] The conditions that receive the longest benefit from injections are those precipitated by trauma, especially when the activity causing the inflammation is avoided. For example, a patient troubled by recurrent lateral epicondylitis who derives short-lived benefit from a glucocorticoid injection into the inflamed area may experience more permanent improvement by discontinuing the precipitating physical activity, (e.g., tennis or racquetball).

Many cases of apparent tendinitis and bursitis are secondary manifestations of rheumatoid arthritis, in which injections may give outstanding, although temporary, initial benefit. In such patients, appropriate treatment of the underlying disease should be instituted and the injections must be considered as adjunctive management.

The poorly understood but apparently common "fibromyalgia" syndrome[56, 57] is associated with various "tender points" and is discussed in detail in Chapter (34). These exaggerated tender areas may respond dramatically to the injection of a local anesthetic directly into the most tender area, but the addition of a glucocorticoid in the same syringe may give more lasting relief.

TYPES OF PREPARATIONS

The original intra-articular glucocorticoid, hydrocortisone acetate, is still available, widely used, and inexpensive. Other preparations of various potency and solubility are also available (Table 40–2). Few comparative studies of the efficacy or duration of action of the various agents have been reported. As mentioned, McCarty[29] reported long-term benefits with triamcinolone hexacetonide and thinks this is the least soluble agent and produces the most prolonged effect of the agents commercially available. Such longer-acting and more potent suspensions are much more expensive than hydrocortisone. Some investigators believe that the more potent preparations are also more efficacious,[41] but the evidence for this is only moderate.

Many clinicians, over months or years of practice, have settled on a preparation that seems to have, in their opinion, good benefit and few side effects. Some prefer, for example, a preparation of a short-acting solution and a long-acting suspension of betamethasone (Celestone Soluspan). They believe that the solution works rapidly and prevents the possibility of a postinjection flare. For the same reason, others prefer to inject a short-acting solution, such as dexamethasone sodium phosphate, together with a more long-acting suspension.

Mixing the glucocorticoid suspension with a local anesthetic, particularly procaine or lidocaine, may be helpful for injecting small joints and tendon sheaths; this avoids the injection of a highly concentrated sus-

Table 40–2. GLUCOCORTICOIDS AND PREDNISONE EQUIVALENTS*

Intra-articular Preparations	Prednisone Equivalents
Betamethasone sodium phosphate and acetate suspension, 6 mg/ml (Celestone Soluspan)	10
Dexamethasone sodium phosphate, 4 mg/ml (Decadron and Hexadrol)	8
Dexamethasone acetate, 8 mg/ml (Decadron—LA)	16
Hydrocortisone acetate 25 mg/ml, (Hydrocortone)	1
Methylprednisolone acetate, 20, 40, and 80 mg/ml (Depo-Medrol)	5, 10, and 20
Prednisolone tebutate, 20 mg/ml (Hydeltra-T.B.A.)	4
Triamcinolone acetonide, 10 and 40 mg/ml (Kenalog-10 and Kenalog-40)	2.5 and 10
Triamcinolone hexacetonide, 20 mg/ml (Aristospan)	5

*One equivalent = 5 mg prednisone.

Table 40–3. AMOUNT OF INTRA-ARTICULAR GLUCOCORTICOID

Size of Joint	Examples	Range of Dosage
Large	Knees Ankles Shoulders	1–2 ml
Medium	Elbows Wrists	0.5–1.0 ml
Small	Interphalangeal Metacarpophalangeal	0.1–0.5 ml

pension into a single area, which might produce soft tissue atrophy. (Some clinicians prefer to inject the corticosteroid first; then, with the needle in the joint, the syringe is removed and the local anesthetic is injected. This technique may prevent pericapsular calcifications in small joints.) However, one must be concerned over the compatibility of the two preparations. In the Fujisawa section of the 1996 *Physicians' Desk Reference*, the following caution appears: "Aristospan suspension may be mixed with 1 percent or 2 percent lidocaine hydrochloride, using the formulations which do not contain parabens. Similar local anesthetics may also be used. Diluents containing methylparaben, propylparaben, phenol, etc., should be avoided since these compounds may cause flocculation of the steroid."[58] A review of package inserts of intra-articular glucocorticoids from the larger pharmaceutical companies revealed that most do not recommend the use of a mixture of glucocorticoids and local anesthetics that contain preservatives. Some manufacturers are less specific. In addition, flocculation has been seen with certain generic brands, but not with the brand name product.

Local anesthetic agents usually contain preservatives. Preparations without preservatives are usually more expensive and are frequently not available on the average arthrocentesis tray. Lidocaine for intravenous use does not contain preservatives. A brief survey of several rheumatologists and orthopedic surgeons throughout the United States revealed that about half used a glucocorticoid–local anesthetic mixture, and only one was aware of the potential problem of flocculation. A few orthopedists, however, reported finding "steroid chalk" in joints, especially wrists, that had been injected with the "older steroids." There is no way of knowing whether these joints had been injected with glucocorticoid–local anesthetic combinations. Also, one wonders whether the "chalk" might represent formations of hydroxyapatite, apparently from injections of only glucocorticoids.

There is no consensus concerning the amount of material that should be injected into the various sizes of joints. Some clinicians inject a smaller amount in volume of the more potent glucocorticoids, but many, probably most, inject 1 ml in the large joints and a lesser amount in the medium and small joints. Table 40–3 is a rough guide to the amount to be injected.

INDICATIONS

Intra-articular and soft tissue glucocorticoid injections are considered adjunctive therapy; rarely are they considered primary therapy. Exceptions, as mentioned, include bursitis, tendinitis, and documented gout. Table 40–4 lists the indications for intra-articular glucocorticoid injections. This therapeutic list is not in any particular order of preference or likelihood of response. Intra-articular injection of experimental drugs, including radioisotopes, is not discussed in this chapter.

Articular

Rheumatoid Arthritis, Adult and Juvenile. Rheumatoid arthritis (with the possible exception of tendinitis and bursitis) is probably the illness for which the most injections are given by rheumatologists. The efficacy of such injections is controversial, for reasons previously discussed. If systemic regimens were uniformly efficacious in patients with rheumatoid arthritis, there would be no need to inject glucocorticoids in the joints. Because this is not the case, the judicious use of intra-articular glucocorticoids may enable the patients to lead a more productive life and one of better quality. Most rheumatologists are enthusiastic about the injections.[59, 60] Injections are especially indicated when the patient has failed to respond or when there are contraindications to NSAIDs, hydroxychloroquine, gold salts, methotrexate, or other systemic agents. The injections usually enable the patient to participate more fully in physical therapy procedures. The number of injections on a single day should be limited to two, but other joints can be injected on other days. There are no data as to how often the same joint can be safely re-injected, but no more than three times a year seems prudent.

In children with rheumatoid arthritis, the number of systemic drugs that can be administered is limited. The judicious use of intra-articular glucocorticoids may prove helpful, particularly when only a few

Table 40–4. INDICATIONS FOR INTRA-ARTICULAR GLUCOCORTICOID INJECTIONS

Rheumatoid arthritis (adult and juvenile)
Crystal deposition disease (gout and pseudogout)
Systemic lupus erythematosus and mixed connective tissue disease
Acute traumatic arthritis
Osteoarthritis
Synovitis of ipsilateral knee following total hip arthroplasty
Miscellaneous conditions with joint manifestations: inflammatory bowel disease, ankylosing spondylitis, psoriatic arthritis, Reiter's disease (injections probably should be avoided in cases of Reiter's disease associated with human immunodeficiency virus infections)
Shoulder periarthritis (adhesive capsulitis, frozen shoulder)
Tietze's syndrome

joints are involved, such as in the pauci(oligo)articular type.[61]

Crystal Deposition Diseases (Gout and Pseudogout). Acute gouty arthritis (monosodium urate monohydrate crystal deposition disease) is sometimes refractory to so-called conventional regimens (i.e., colchicine and NSAIDs). If this is the case, and if phagocytosed sodium urate crystals continue to be present in the synovial fluid, complete aspiration of the inflamed joint followed by glucocorticoid injection may be helpful. One must be sure, however, that an infectious process is not the reason for the persistent inflammation.

The diagnosis of pseudogout (calcium pyrophosphate dihydrate crystal deposition disease) requires the identification of calcium pyrophosphate crystals in synovial fluid. Aspirating as much fluid as possible may alleviate not only pain but also inflammation; that is, aspiration may remove a sufficient number of crystals to reduce the inflammatory process. On occasion, however, the inflammation does not respond to this or the usual NSAIDs and intra-articular glucocorticoids prove efficacious. In older patients, especially those with even mild renal insufficiency, serious sequelae from colchicine and nonsteroidal anti-inflammatory drugs may occur. For example, NSAIDs may produce worsening renal failure, hypertension, and congestive heart failure.[62] Colchicine is an especially dangerous drug in these circumstances and may produce bone marrow abnormalities, septicemia, and death.[63] The use of intra-articular glucocorticoids seems to be a much safer regimen.

Systemic Lupus Erythematosus and Mixed Connective Tissue Disease. These diseases may be associated with polyarticular or pauciarticular synovitis that persists despite good control of the systemic disorder. Intra-articular glucocorticoids may be helpful.

Acute Traumatic "Arthritis." Acute trauma to joints is usually treated with a conservative regimen of cold packs, rest, and, after an appropriate time, an increase in activity. Many authorities believe that injuries to the soft tissue of the shoulder and ankle will cause serious sequelae if range-of-motion exercise is not instituted after a short period of rest. Intra-articular glucocorticoids may help in these situations by allowing early movement.

Osteoarthritis. Osteoarthritic joints, as previously discussed, can be extremely painful. The efficacy of intra-articular glucocorticoids is debated; on occasion, however, injections give outstanding and prolonged benefit. This is especially true if inflammation is present and if there is little cartilage loss. If one or two injections do not give benefit, there is no good reason to continue injections into the joint.

Synovitis of Knee After Hip Arthroplasty. Synovitis of the ipsilateral knee after total hip arthroplasty occurs on occasion and may resolve spontaneously after a few days. It may persist, however, and injection of the knee with a glucocorticoid usually is beneficial.

Miscellaneous. Inflammatory gastrointestinal diseases may be associated with peripheral or axial arthritis. Sometimes, depending on the type of intestinal disorder, an exacerbation of the intestinal problem is associated with an exacerbation of the joint symptoms. In certain situations, control of the intestinal disease also controls the joint disease. If the arthropathy is not helped, however, injections of intra-articular glucocorticoids may give rapid and prolonged relief. Even the sacroiliac joints are injected with good subjective benefit.[64]

Peripheral joint manifestations of other inflammatory arthritides, such as ankylosing spondylitis, psoriatic arthritis, and Reiter's disease, may also improve with intra-articular glucocorticoids. If a patient with Reiter's disease has human immunodeficiency virus (HIV) infection, intra-articular glucocorticoid injections are probably contraindicated.

Shoulder Periarthritis (Adhesive Capsulitis, Frozen Shoulder). This condition may improve, sometimes dramatically, with intra-articular and tendinous sheath glucocorticoid injections.[64-68] Many clinicians, however, combine the treatment with NSAIDs and physical therapy.

Tietze's Syndrome. Tietze's syndrome, an "illness" associated with pain and tenderness of the parasternal joints, may be helped by injections of a combination of glucocorticoid and local anesthetic.[69]

Nonarticular

Nonarticular inflammatory conditions may be greatly benefited by the injection of a glucocorticoid with or without a local anesthetic. Table 40-5 lists various soft tissue conditions that may benefit from injections.

Shoulder. The main shoulder problems are bicipital tendinitis, subacromial bursitis, and supraspinatus tendinitis. As mentioned, these problems can be primary or part of a systemic problem (e.g., rheumatoid arthritis). Injection into the specifically inflamed tendon sheath or bursa usually gives relief within a few hours. When a local anesthetic is added, however, relief is usually immediate if the correct area is injected.

The possible sequelae of intratendinous injections have already been mentioned. If the inflammatory problems involve the bicipital tendon or subacromial bursa, some physicians prefer to inject the shoulder joint directly. This seems especially true in patients with rheumatoid arthritis because arthrographic studies in these patients have frequently shown a communication between the subacromial bursa, the bicipital tendon sheath, and the shoulder joint. Thus, the drug can have a local effect in all these areas. Shoulder periarthritis was discussed earlier.

Elbow. Inflammation of the elbow epicondylar areas is common in patients who are active in sports, especially tennis and golf. Painful lateral epicondylitis is a frequent sequela of these activities. Injections into the inflamed region can give good to excellent results.

Table 40–5. INDICATIONS FOR NONARTICULAR GLUCOCORTICOID INJECTIONS

Shoulder
Bicipital tendinitis
Subacromial bursitis
Supraspinatus tendinitis
Periarthritis (adhesive capsulitis, frozen shoulder)
Elbow
Lateral epicondylitis—"tennis elbow"
Medial epicondylitis—"golfer's elbow"
Olecranon bursitis
Cubital tunnel syndrome
Wrist and Hand
Ganglion
DeQuervain's disease—stenosing tenosynovitis of extensor pollicis brevis and abductor pollicis longus
Trigger (snapping) fingers
Carpal tunnel syndrome
Hip
Trochanteric bursitis
Knee
Anserine bursitis
Prepatellar bursitis and neuritis
Pelvis
Ischial bursitis
Iliopectineal bursitis
Back
Fibromyalgia trigger points
Herniated presacral fat pads (Stockman's nodules)
Foot
Achilles tendinitis
Achilles bursitis
Calcaneal bursitis
Morton's neuroma
Tarsal tunnel syndrome

Some physicians prefer a more conservative approach.[70] Mixing the glucocorticoid with local anesthetic can give immediate benefit; when the effect of the anesthetic subsides, however, there is frequently a marked exacerbation of pain that lasts 6 to 24 hours, which apparently is a crystal-induced postinjection flare. Medial epicondylitis also can be painful and usually responds well to an injection. However, one should be careful not to inject the nearby ulnar nerve.

Olecranon bursitis may be a primary condition, probably as a result of trauma, but may be secondary to conditions such as gout, infection, and rheumatoid arthritis. Because septic olecranon bursitis is common, aspiration of the fluid and synovial fluid analysis are essential before injection of glucocorticoids. *Cubital tunnel syndrome*, an entrapment of the ulnar nerve at the elbow, may be caused by tenosynovitis. The symptoms are usually more motor-related than sensory. Injections can be administered by experienced operators, but surgical decompression is usually necessary.[71]

Wrist and Hand. A *ganglion* on the dorsal aspect of the wrist can be treated by aspiration and injection. Again, there may be considerable discomfort several hours after injection. In two thirds to three fourths of patients, the ganglia can be "cured" by this conservative approach.[31, 72]

Stenosing tenosynovitis of the extensor pollicis bre-

vis and abductor pollicis longus (de Quervain's disease) can cause considerable discomfort over the distal aspect of the radius. Conservative management with glucocorticoid and local anesthetic injection may help.[55, 73, 74] If benefit is immediate, the injection probably was in the proper area. Recurrence is common, according to some operators, but Harvey and colleagues[75] reported complete and lasting relief in 40 percent of cases.

Trigger and *snapping fingers* may be caused by a primary nonspecific hand flexor tenosynovitis or tenosynovitis with rheumatoid arthritis. Injection of glucocorticoid and local anesthetic into the tendinous sheath is efficacious in more than 90 percent of cases, and the median length of relief is 2 years.[53, 76–78] *Carpal tunnel syndrome* has multiple causes; but the rheumatoid and idiopathic types may be helped by glucocorticoid injections. Extreme care is necessary to prevent median nerve damage.[73, 79–81] Personal instruction in the technique is recommended.

Hip. *Trochanteric bursitis* can give considerable discomfort and may be relieved by injections. There are one or more bursae about the femoral trochanter at the gluteal insertion. The tender region is easily palpated unless the patient is obese.

Knee. The anserine bursa is present on the medial aspect of the knee, where the tendons of the sartorius, semitendinosus, and gracilis muscles insert on the tibia.[82] When the bursa is inflamed, there is pain, tenderness, and usually swelling over the medial anterior aspect of the tibia just below the knee. There may be associated degenerative arthritis of the knee, obesity, or a history of physical activity, such as jogging, frequent knee bending, or frequent going up and down stairs. Some authors do not consider the condition a true bursitis and classify it as *Dercum's disease* (painful adiposity) or place it in the "fibrositis syndrome" category.[56] I disagree with this opinion and consider it a commonly misdiagnosed condition. In addition, other bursae that are close by may become inflamed. Most patients benefit from injection of glucocorticoid and local anesthetic. If the material is injected in the proper place, relief is usually immediate.

Prepatellar bursitis can be secondary to trauma (e.g., "housemaid's knee") or to systemic illness, such as rheumatoid arthritis or gout. The bursitis may be asymptomatic or quite painful. Some patients request treatment for cosmetic reasons. If clinically indicated, the bursal fluid can be examined in a similar manner to synovial fluid. Injections are usually effective.[79] The prepatellar bursa is supplied by branches of the saphenous nerve. Irritation of these branches can induce a neuritis that produces pain. Injections are beneficial.[83]

Pelvis. *Ischial* or *ischiogluteal bursitis* is more common than is generally thought and may be misdiagnosed as herniated nucleus pulposus, lumbosacral strain, or thrombophlebitis.[84] The ischiogluteal bursa overlies the sciatic nerve and the posterior femoral cutaneous nerve. Therefore, the pain may radiate and the wrong diagnosis be made. Palpation over the ischial tuberosity should cause significant pain. Injections are helpful but are not recommended for the inexperienced operator.

Iliopectineal (iliopsoas) bursitis is an inflammation of the bursa that is located between the iliopsoas muscle and the iliopectineal eminence. It may communicate with the hip joint. There is tenderness over the anterior aspect of the hip in the region of the middle portion of the inguinal ligament. Hyperextension, adduction, or internal rotation of the hip elicits pain. Differential diagnoses include femoral hernia, psoas abscess, and septic arthritis of the hip. When these other diagnoses have been excluded, and if more conservative regimens have failed or are not practical, an injection of glucocorticoid with or without local anesthetic can be tried.[85]

Back. Painful subjective and objective areas of the back that may be difficult to explain anatomically. Areas tender to moderately deep palpation (the so-called tender points) may be noted, especially around the upper medial border of the trapezius, various periscapular areas, the inferior posterior cervical area, and presacral regions. The last may represent herniated presacral fat pads (Stockman's nodules). Some of these painful areas may be part of the fibrositis syndrome.[56] An injection of glucocorticoid, local anesthetic agent, or a combination of the two into the tender points frequently gives relief. The same can be said for obturator internus bursitis, which some believe is quite common.[86] Only an experienced operator should attempt this injection.

Foot. *Achilles tendinitis* may be secondary to trauma or to systemic illness, such as rheumatoid arthritis or gout. The former may be associated with rheumatoid nodules in the tendon and the latter with tophi. Rest, analgesics, and anti-inflammatory medications are preferable to injections. If little benefit is obtained from these conservative measures, a small amount of a mixture of glucocorticoid and local anesthetic may be injected into the tendon sheath.

Achilles bursitis may represent inflammation of the retrocalcaneal bursa between the calcaneus and Achilles tendon or a subcutaneous bursitis between the skin and tendon. One should not forget gout as a possible cause, and if the bursae are punctured, aspiration should be attempted and the aspirate examined with polarizing microscopy. *Reiter's syndrome* should be suspected when inflammatory fluid is aspirated from the retrocalcaneal bursa, no crystals are present, and there is no other obvious diagnosis.[87] Conservative management of nonspecific bursitis is similar to that of Achilles tendinitis. If this is ineffective, however, an injection may prove beneficial.

Calcaneal bursitis is an inflammation of the bursa at the attachment of the plantar fascia to the os calcis. Pain occurs in the center of the plantar aspect of the heel. Conservative management, such as a rubber doughnut, may help. If not, an intrabursal injection of glucocorticoid mixed with a local anesthetic usually gives good relief, although the injection frequently causes considerable pain.

Tarsal tunnel syndrome is an entrapment neuropathy of all or part of the posterior tibial nerve as it passes under the flexor retinaculum of the ankle. Burning pain and paresthesias in the affected foot are the symptoms. It may be associated with the hypermobile joint syndrome.[88] Injections by an experienced operator may help, but relief is usually temporary.[89]

An excellent review on the syndromes of bursitis by Larsson and Baum[90] suggests that glucocorticoids with local anesthetic injection is the most successful treatment.

The metatarsalgia of *Morton's neuroma* may be greatly relieved by the direct injection of a glucocorticoid–local anesthetic mixture.[91]

CONTRAINDICATIONS

The main contraindications to intra-articular glucocorticoid injections are listed in Table 40–6. As mentioned, although they are rare, iatrogenic infections do occur. Therefore, it is essential to adhere to strict aseptic procedures, and the physician must avoid inserting a needle through any areas of cellulitis and active psoriasis.

The previously mentioned bacteremia—as is seen in certain cases of pneumonia, endocarditis, and pyelonephritis—is considered a contraindication by some authorities. Therefore, if a patient hospitalized for a condition that may be associated with bacteremia concomitantly has active rheumatoid arthritis, it is probably wise not to institute therapeutic arthrocentesis and glucocorticoid injections because of the possibility of an iatrogenic infection. (If one is concerned that bacteremia may have produced septic arthritis, arthrocentesis and special studies on the synovial fluid are mandatory.)

Instability of joints possibly may be part of a Charcot-like arthropathy from multiple intra-articular glucocorticoid injections. Theoretically, further injections may make the instability worse. In general, joints such as those in the spine are considered inaccessible, and injections are contraindicated because of potential sequelae. Facet joint arthropathy, however, is believed to be a common cause of low back and cervical spine

Table 40–6. CONTRAINDICATIONS TO INTRA-ARTICULAR GLUCOCORTICOID INJECTIONS

Periarticular sepsis
Bacteremia
Unstable joints
Most spinal joints
Intra-articular fracture
Septic joint: Do *not* forget the possibility of tuberculosis.
Difficult access to nondiarthrodial joints (e.g., symphysis pubis); sternomanubrial injections may prove helpful
Marked juxta-articular osteoporosis
Failure to respond to prior injections
Blood-clotting disorders

pain. The injection of these joints by an experienced operator may give long-lasting benefit.[92, 93] In 1993, less favorable results were reported in a randomized, double-blind, placebo-controlled trial with 6 months of follow-up.[94]

Articular pain following trauma could represent an intra-articular fracture. Glucocorticoid injection is contraindicated because it has the potential to retard fracture healing.

Injection of a septic joint with a glucocorticoid can greatly increase the morbidity of the infection. Purulent appearance of synovial fluid should alert the physician to this possibility, but tuberculous synovitis, for example, can produce synovial fluid with minimal inflammatory findings, which is misleading. The possibility of infection is always present, and further studies of synovial fluid and even percutaneous synovial biopsy or arthroscopy with biopsy should be considered.

Nondiarthrodial joints, such as the symphysis pubis, are involved with certain arthritides but are difficult to inject. If the joints are accessible, injections are sometimes helpful but several punctures may be necessary.

Juxta-articular osteoporosis of a marked degree may be worsened by intra-articular glucocorticoid administration. This type of osteoporosis is seen more commonly in patients with rheumatoid arthritis, and the arthritis itself plus lack of motion in the joint may be the main cause of the osteoporosis. Theoretically, one or two glucocorticoid injections may improve the problem. If one or two glucocorticoid injections in the same joint provide no benefit, there is no sound reason to continue, since one could be producing more harm than good.

Blood clotting disorders, such as factor VIII deficiency, may produce a destructive type of arthritis. Arthrocentesis could produce both intra-articular and external hemorrhage. This problem should definitely be considered when undiagnosed synovitis is observed in a child. Arthrocentesis can be performed with caution in patients receiving anticoagulants if the joint is immobilized for 24 to 48 hours after the injection. Applying ice and wrapping the joint with an elastic bandage may be helpful.

Patients with rheumatoid arthritis who have had total joint arthroplasties, especially of the knees, may subsequently experience exacerbation of synovitis in these joints. Because of the increased incidence of infections in such joints, physicians have been reluctant to inject them with glucocorticoids. At the Medical College of Virginia, however, more than 400 joints with replacements in which recurrent rheumatoid synovitis developed have been injected with glucocorticoids with benefit and without sequelae since 1975. In these cases, synovial fluid analysis, including culture, should be performed before glucocorticoids are injected.

ANESTHESIA

As previously discussed, some physicians prefer mixing the glucocorticoid with a local anesthetic, usu-

ally procaine or lidocaine, for two reasons. First, during injection of a bursa, tendon sheath, or periarticular region, this combination usually gives immediate relief if the materials are injected in the proper space. The immediate benefit, of course, would be from the local anesthetic, not the glucocorticoid; patients should be told that they may experience further pain in an hour or two but should improve a few hours later, when the anti-inflammatory actions of the glucocorticoids begin. Second, a mixture may be preferable because the glucocorticoid is diluted and there should be less soft tissue atrophy at the sites of injection.

A physician experienced in arthrocentesis may elect not to use any anesthesia when injecting large joints. If the patient is cooperative and relaxed, and if disposable needles are used, little pain should be associated with arthrocentesis. If the physician is inexperienced or the patient is anxious and tense, a short burst of ethyl chloride spray on the skin over the joint to be injected is helpful.

Injection of a local anesthetic is the other option. First, a skin wheal should be made followed by infiltration of the subcutaneous tissue and joint capsule. After a few minutes, arthrocentesis can be done and should be painless.

TECHNIQUES FOR ARTHROCENTESES

To perform an arthrocentesis, the specific area of the joint to be aspirated is palpated and then marked with firm pressure by a ballpoint pen that has the ink cartridge and point retracted. This will leave an impression that will last 5 to 15 minutes. (The ballpoint pen technique can also be used with soft tissue injection.) Strict asepsis is important and deserves reemphasis. The area to be aspirated or injected should be carefully cleaned with a good antiseptic, such as one of the iodinated compounds. Then, the needle can be inserted through the ballpoint pen impression. I strongly recommend the operator be immunized against hepatitis B. The Council on Rheumatologic Care of the American College of Rheumatology recommends that gloves be worn and remain on the hands until the completion of the procedure, that any aspirated fluid be secured in appropriate containers, and that all materials contaminated by blood or synovial fluid be disposed of in appropriate biohazard containers.

A tray for arthrocentesis can be prepared and kept available for use. It should include the following items:

• Alcohol sponges
• Iodinated solution and surgical soap
• Gauze dressings (2 × 2)
• Sterile disposable 3-, 10-, and 20-ml syringes
• 18- and 20-gauge, 1½-inch needles
• 20-gauge spinal needles
• 25-gauge, ½-inch needles

- Plain test tubes
- Heparinized tubes
- Clean microscope slides and coverslips
- Heparin to add to heparinized tubes if a large amount of inflammatory fluid is to be placed in the tube
- Fingernail polish to seal wet preparation and slide coverslip
- Chocolate agar plates or Thayer-Martin medium
- Tryptic soy broth for most bacteria
- Anaerobic transport medium (replace periodically to keep culture media from becoming outdated)
- Tubes with fluoride for glucose
- Plastic adhesive bandages
- Ethyl chloride
- Hemostat
- Tourniquet for drawing of simultaneous blood samples
- 1 percent lidocaine

Articular

Knee. The knee is the easiest joint to inject. If fluid is to be aspirated, the patient should be in a supine position with the knee fully extended. The puncture mark is made just posterior to the medial portion of the patella, and an 18- to 20-gauge 1½-inch needle is directed slightly posteriorly and slightly inferiorly. The joint space should be readily entered and synovial fluid easily aspirated. On occasion, thickened synovium or villous projections occlude the opening of the needle, and it may be necessary to rotate the needle to facilitate aspiration of the knee when using the medial approach. An infrapatellar plica, a vestigial structure also called the ligamentum mucosum, may prevent adequate aspiration of the knee when the medial approach is used.[95] However, the plica should not adversely affect aspiration from the lateral aspect. If glucocorticoid is administered, there should be no feeling of obstruction as it is being injected. Parenthetically, a medial synovial shelf plica may become thickened and inflamed. Rovere[96] believes that this diagnosis can be made by physical examination and the plica itself injected with relief of symptoms, but others disagree. A review of the subject is presented by Schonholtz and Magee.[97]

The supine technique is illustrated in Figure 40–1. The patient should be relaxed if this technique is used. An anxious patient may tighten the patella to the point of making arthrocentesis difficult. If this is the case or if fusion or osteophytes make the medial or lateral approach to the knee joint difficult, an easy technique that usually avoids these problems is to inject the knee while the patient sits with the knee flexed. The mark is made at the medial aspect of the distal border of the patella, and the needle is directed slightly superiorly toward the joint cavity. It is usually difficult to obtain fluid with this technique.

The suprapatellar bursa, which is really an extension of the knee joint, may be distended if a large amount of synovial fluid is present. In this instance,

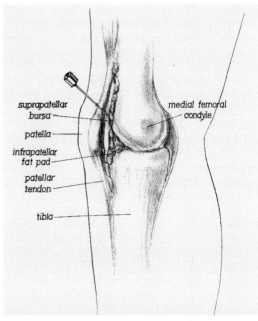

Figure 40–1. Knee arthrocentesis. The needle is inserted just posterior to the medial portion of the patella and is directed slightly posteriorly and slightly inferiorly.

the bursa may be aspirated in an easy and essentially asymptomatic fashion.

Shoulder. The shoulder arthrocentesis is most easily accomplished with the patient sitting and the shoulder externally rotated. A mark is made just medial to the head of the humerus and slightly inferiorly and laterally to the coracoid process. A 20- to 22-gauge, 1½-inch needle is directed posteriorly and slightly superiorly and laterally. One should be able to feel the needle enter the joint space. If bone is hit, the needle should be pulled back and redirected at a slightly different angle. This technique is illustrated in Figure 40–2.

The acromioclavicular joint may be palpated as a groove at the lateral end of the clavicle just medial to the shoulder. A mark is made, and a 22- to 25-gauge, ⅝- to 1-inch needle is carefully directed inferiorly. Rarely is synovial fluid obtained.

The sternoclavicular joint is most easily entered from a point directly anterior to the joint. Caution is necessary to avoid a pneumothorax. The space is fibrocartilaginous, and rarely can fluid be aspirated.

Ankle Joint. The patient should be supine and the leg-foot angle at 90 degrees. A mark is made just medial to the tibialis anterior tendon and lateral to the medial malleolus. A 20- to 22-gauge, 1½-inch needle is directed posteriorly and should enter the joint space easily without striking bone. Figure 40–3 illustrates injection of the ankle joint.

For the subtalar ankle joint, again the patient is supine and the leg-foot angle at 90 degrees. A mark is made just inferior to the tip of the lateral malleolus. A 20- to 22-gauge, 1½-inch needle is directed perpendicular to the mark. With the subtalar joint, the needle

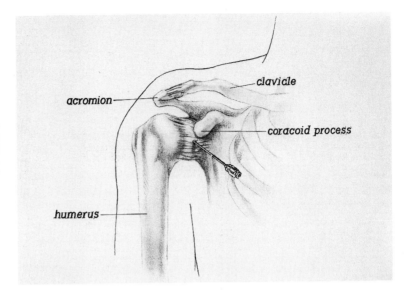

Figure 40–2. Shoulder arthrocentesis. With the shoulder externally rotated, the needle is inserted at a point just medial to the head of the humerus and slightly inferior and lateral to the coracoid process. The needle is then directed posteriorly and slightly superiorly and laterally.

may not enter the first time, and another attempt or two may be necessary. Because of this and the associated pain, local anesthesia may be helpful. Figure 40–4 illustrates injection of this joint.

Wrist. The wrist is a complex joint, but most of the intercarpal spaces communicate. A mark is made just distal to the radius and just ulnar to the so-called anatomic snuff box. Usually, a 24- to 26-gauge, ⅝- to 1-inch needle is adequate, and the injection is made perpendicular to the mark. If bone is hit, the needle should be pulled back and slightly redirected toward the thumb. This type of injection is illustrated in Figure 40–5.

First Carpometacarpal Joint. Degenerative arthritis often involves the first carpometacarpal joint. Frequently the joint space is quite narrowed, and arthrocentesis may be difficult and painful. A few simple maneuvers can make the injection fairly easy, however. The thumb is flexed across the palm toward the tip of the fifth finger. A mark is made at the base of the first metacarpal bone away from the border of the snuff box. A 22- to 26-gauge, ⅝- to 1-inch needle is inserted at the mark and directed toward the proximal end of the fourth metacarpal. This approach avoids hitting the radial artery. Figure 40–6 illustrates injection of this joint.

Metacarpophalangeal Joints and Finger Interphalangeal Joints. Synovitis in these joints usually causes the synovium to bulge dorsally, and a 24- to 26-gauge, ½- to ⅝-inch needle can be inserted on either side just under the extensor tendon mechanism. It is not necessary for the needle to be interposed between the

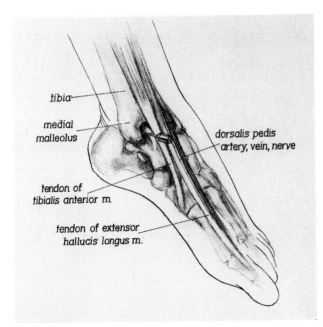

Figure 40–3. Ankle arthrocentesis. With the leg-foot angle at 90 degrees, the needle is inserted at a point just medial to the tibialis anterior tendon and just lateral to the medial malleolus. The needle is then directed posteriorly.

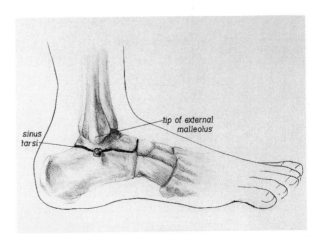

Figure 40–4. Ankle subtalar arthrocentesis. With the leg-foot angle at 90 degrees, the needle is inserted at a point just inferior to the tip of the lateral (external) malleolus, and is directed perpendicularly.

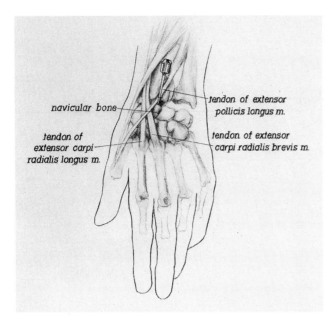

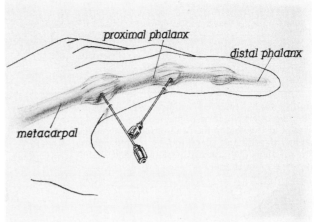

Figure 40–7. Metacarpophalangeal and finger interphalangeal arthrocenteses. With the digit straight or slightly flexed, a small and short needle is inserted on either side just under the extensor tendon mechanism. It is not necessary for the needle to be interposed between the articular surfaces.

Figure 40–5. Wrist arthrocentesis. The needle is inserted at a point just distal to the radius and just ulnar to the anatomic snuff box. It is then directed perpendicularly. If bone is hit, the needle should be pulled back and slightly redirected toward the thumb.

articular surfaces. Some physicians prefer the patient's fingers to be slightly flexed when one is injecting the metacarpophalangeal joints. It is unusual to obtain synovial fluid. When injecting glucocorticoids, consider mixing them with a small amount of local anesthetic using the precautions previously discussed. This combination distends the joint on all sides and possibly help prevent soft tissue atrophy. These injections are illustrated in Figure 40–7.

Metatarsophalangeal Joints and Toe Interphalangeal Joints. The techniques for these joints are similar to those for the metacarpophalangeal and finger interphalangeal joints, but many physicians prefer to inject more dorsally and laterally to the extensor tendons. Marking the area to be injected is helpful, as is gentle traction on the toe of each joint that is injected.

Elbow. The technique preferred by many physicians for injections into the elbow is to have it flexed at 90 degrees. The joint capsule bulges if there is inflammation. A mark is made just below the lateral epicondyle of the humerus. A 22-gauge, 1- to 1 ½-inch needle is inserted at the mark and directed parallel to the shaft of the radius or directed perpendicular to the skin. Figure 40–8 illustrates these two approaches.

Hip. The hip is a difficult joint to inject even when a fluoroscope is used as a guide. Rarely is the physician sure that the joint has been entered; synovial

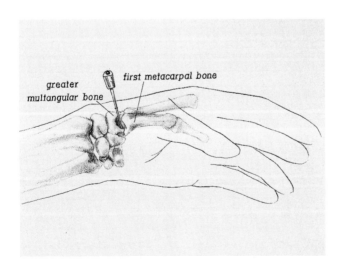

Figure 40–6. First carpometacarpal arthrocentesis. The thumb is flexed across the palm toward the tip of the fifth finger. The needle is inserted at the base of the metacarpal bone away from the border of the snuff box. It is then directed toward the proximal end of the fourth metacarpal.

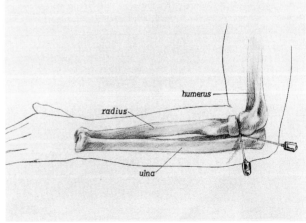

Figure 40–8. Elbow arthrocenteses illustrating parallel and perpendicular techniques. With the elbow flexed at 90 degrees, the needle is inserted just below the lateral epicondyle of the humerus and is directed parallel to the shaft of the radius; it may also be directed perpendicular to the skin.

fluid is rarely obtained. Two approaches can be used, anterior or lateral. A 20-gauge, 3½-inch spinal needle should be used for both approaches.

For the anterior approach, the patient is supine and the extremity is fully extended and externally rotated. A mark should be made about 2 to 3 cm below the anterosuperior iliac spine and 2 to 3 cm lateral to the femoral pulse. The needle is inserted at a 60-degree angle to the skin and directed posteriorly and medially until bone is hit. The needle is withdrawn slightly, and a drop or two of synovial fluid may be obtained, indicating entry into the joint space.

Many physicians prefer the lateral approach because the needle can "follow" the femoral neck into the joint. The patient is supine, and the hips should be internally rotated—the knees apart and toes touching. A mark is made just anterior to the greater trochanter, and the needle is inserted and directed medially and sightly cephalad toward a point slightly below the middle of the inguinal ligament. One may feel the tip of the needle slide into the joint. Figure 40–9 illustrates the lateral approach to the hip joint.

Temporomandibular Joint. The temporomandibular joint is palpated as a depression just below the

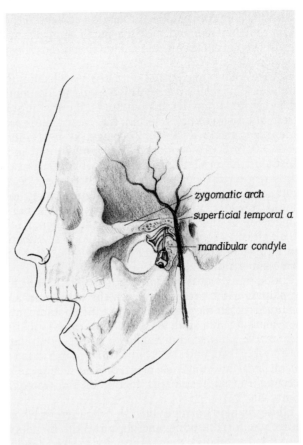

Figure 40–10. Temporomandibular arthrocentesis. With the patient's mouth open, the joint space is palpated as a depression just below the zygomatic arch and 1 to 2 cm anterior to the tragus. The needle is inserted just perpendicular to the skin and directed slightly posteriorly and superiorly.

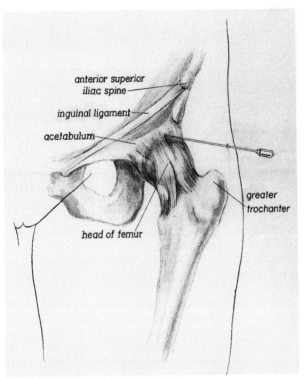

Figure 40–9. Hip arthrocentesis illustrating lateral technique. In this technique, the patient is supine with the hips internally rotated—knees apart and toes touching. The needle is inserted just anterior to the greater trochanter and is directed medially and slightly cephalad toward a point slightly below the middle of the inguinal ligament. One may feel the needle slip into the joint. For the *anterior approach,* the patient is supine and the extremity fully extended and externally rotated. A mark is made 2 to 3 cm below the anterior superior iliac spine and 2 to 3 cm lateral to the femoral pulse. The needle is inserted at a 60 degree angle to the mark and directed posteriorly and medially until bone it hit.

zygomatic arch and 1 to 2 cm anterior to the tragus. The depression is more easily palpated by having the patient open and close the mouth. A mark is made and, with the patient's mouth open, a 22-gauge, ½- to 1-inch needle is inserted perpendicular to the skin and directed slightly posteriorly and superiorly. Figure 40–10 illustrates injection of the temporomandibular joint.

Nonarticular

Shoulder. Bicipital tendinitis can be treated by injecting the shoulder joint or by injecting the tendon sheath. The tendon is tender, is easily palpated in the bicipital groove of the humerus, and can be rolled from side to side. If it is elected to inject the sheath, the point of maximal tenderness is marked. A 22-gauge, 1½-inch needle is inserted in the sheath at the mark, and a portion of 0.5 ml glucocorticoid, with or without local anesthetic, is injected at this site. The needle is then directed superiorly along the tendon, in the sheath, for about 2 to 3 cm, and more drug is injected. The needle is then partially withdrawn and redirected inferiorly along the tendon for about 2 to 3 cm, and the remainder of the material is injected. Figure 40–11 illustrates the bicipital tendon sheath injection.

Subacromial bursitis can be treated by injecting the shoulder joint or the bursa. The bursitis is frequently secondary to supraspinatus tendinitis. If only the subacromial bursa is to be injected, the most tender area is marked; using a 20- to 22-gauge, 1- to 1½-inch needle, 0.5 ml glucocorticoid, with or without local anesthetic, is injected. Calcification of the supraspinatus tendon may be present, and there may be an acute and severe pain. In this circumstance, one should consider aspirating and irrigating the bursa using a 16- to 18-gauge, 1½-inch needle. Then, 0.5 to 1.0 ml glucocorticoid, with or without local anesthetic, can be injected. Figure 40–12 illustrates the injection of the subacromial bursa.

The supraspinatus tendon can be directly injected by palpating the groove between the acromium and the humerus on the lateral aspect of the shoulder, and then marking this spot. A 20- to 22-gauge, 1- to 1½-inch needle is directed medially on a horizontal plane for about 2.5 cm, and 0.5 ml glucocorticoid and 2.5 to 4.0 ml local anesthetic is injected. The technique of injecting the supraspinatus tendon is illustrated in Figure 40–12.

Elbow. Lateral epicondylitis, so-called tennis elbow, can be painful, disabling, and chronic. With the elbow flexed and pronated, there is usually marked tenderness to palpation of a small area on the anterolateral surface of the external condyle of the humerus. This spot should be marked. A 20- to 22-gauge, 1- to 1½-inch needle is inserted about 2 cm distal to the mark; 0.5 ml glucocorticoid mixed with 4 to 4.5 ml local anesthetic is administered in several small doses by injecting the mixture, withdrawing and redirecting the needle, and reinjecting the mixture. The injection of tennis elbow is illustrated in Figure 40–13.

"Nodule." A nodule—for example, in the olecranon region or on the proximal aspect of the extensor surface of the ulna—can be a diagnostic dilemma: is it a tophus or a rheumatoid nodule? A simple punch needle biopsy should answer the question. Figure 40–14 illustrates the technique. The nodule is prepared with an antiseptic solution. Then, an 18- to 20-gauge, 1- to 1½-inch needle is inserted at a 90-degree angle and rotated. The needle is then retracted almost completely and is inserted at a 45-degree angle and again rotated (see Fig. 14A). This procedure is repeated in the three other quadrants of the nodule. The needle is removed from the nodule and slightly loosened. The syringe plunger is pulled back to the 2- to 3-ml level, the needle is tightened, and the contents are expelled onto a microscopic slide. In addition, a 25-gauge needle is used to pick out collected material from the biopsy needle (see Fig. 14B). The specimen is examined under the microscope for sodium urate crystals, preferably with the use of polarizing filters. With a little experience, the possibility of a tophus can be virtually excluded if no crystals are seen.

Wrists and Hands. Aspiration of a ganglion on the dorsal aspect of the wrist is done with an 18-gauge, 1½-inch needle. After as much material as possible is aspirated, 0.5 to 1.0 ml of an intra-articular glucocorticoid is injected.

De Quervain's disease (stenosing tenosynovitis of the extensor pollicis brevis and abductor pollicis longus) may be helped by injection. The most tender area in the region of the radial styloid is located by performing a modified Finkelstein's test—clasping the fingers over the thumb and gradually flexing the wrist in ulnar deviation. The most tender point is marked. Then, a 22-gauge, 1½-inch needle is inserted about 1 cm proximal to the most tender spot and directed almost parallel to the skin toward the styloid process. As the needle is being advanced in the tendon sheath, 0.5 ml glucocorticoid and 2.5 ml local anesthetic can be injected.

Trigger fingers are usually associated with chronic stenosing tenosynovitis of the finger flexor tendons. The main pathology usually lies over the head of the metacarpal bones in the palm, and a localized swelling may be palpated in this area. After a mark has been made over the palmar aspect of the metacarpal head, a 22-gauge, 1½-inch needle is inserted at a 45-degree angle and then directed proximally, almost parallel to the skin, and a mixture of 0.5 ml of both glucocorticoid and local anesthetic is injected. Lack of resistance during injection indicates proper needle placement.

Injections for carpal tunnel syndrome should not be done by an inexperienced operator. Theoretically, injection of a long-acting glucocorticoid directly into the median nerve will damage it. If one elects to perform the procedure, a mark is made over the carpal tunnel just on the ulnar side of the long palmar

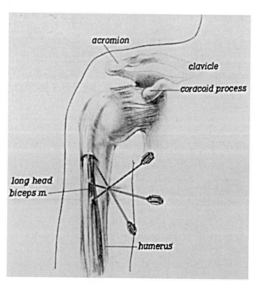

Figure 40–11. Bicipital tendon sheath injections. At the point of maximal tenderness, the needle is inserted just under the sheath and corticosteroid, with or without local anesthetic, is injected. The needle is directed superiorly and then inferiorly, with further injections at each site.

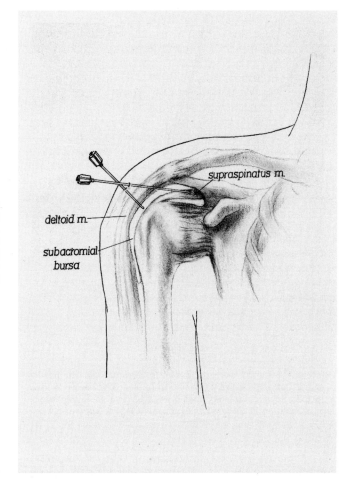

Figure 40–12. Subacromial bursa and supraspinatus tendon injections. For the subacromial bursa, the most tender area is palpated, and the needle is inserted directly into this area. To inject the supraspinatus tendon, the groove between the acromium and the humerus on the lateral aspect of the shoulder is palpated. The needle is inserted at this point and directed medially on a horizontal plane for 2.5 cm; the materials are injected at this point.

tendon. A 25-gauge, 5/8-inch needle is directed perpendicular to the mark and inserted its full length. Some operators prefer performing the injection at a 45-degree angle, directing the needle either proximally or

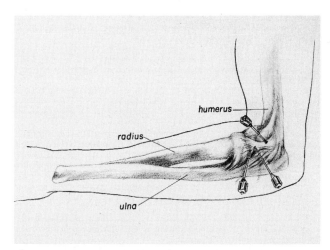

Figure 40–13. "Tennis elbow" injections. With the elbow flexed and pronated, the needle is inserted at the most tender area on the anterolateral aspect of the external condyle of the humerus. A combination of corticosteroid and local anesthetic is injected in several areas.

distally. If the needle meets obstruction, or if the patient experiences paresthesias, the needle should be withdrawn and redirected in a more ulnar fashion. An injection of 0.5 ml glucocorticoid may give benefit. The carpal tunnel can be injected again, but if relief is short-lived, surgery should be considered.

Hip. With trochanteric bursitis, there is an area that is tender to palpation in the region of the greater trochanter of the femur. After marking this area, a 20- to 22-gauge, 1½- to 3½-inch needle is inserted perpendicular to the skin directly into the tender area. Because several bursae may be inflamed, it is usually more effective to inject several areas superior and inferior to the mark with a mixture of 0.5 to 1.0 ml glucocorticoid and 4.0 to 4.5 ml local anesthetic.

Knee. Anserine bursitis produces pain on the medial aspect of the tibia. Pain from a fat pad, from another bursa, or from medial collateral ligament strain may occur in the same region. All may benefit from injection. The point of maximal tenderness is marked. A 20- to 22-gauge, 1½-inch needle is inserted perpendicular to the skin and continued until bone is hit. It is then withdrawn slightly, and 0.25 to 0.5 ml glucocorticoid and 2.5 to 4.5 ml local anesthetic is injected.

The prepatellar bursa is easily aspirated. An 18-gauge, 1½-inch needle is recommended because

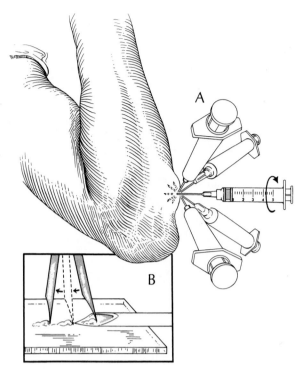

Figure 40–14. Punch-needle biopsy of forearm nodule. The needle is inserted at a 90-degree angle and is rotated. The needle is then retracted almost completely, and is inserted at a 45-degree angle. This is repeated in three other quadrants (*A*). The contents of the needle are placed on a microscopic slide (*B*) and examined.

sometimes the fluid is gelatinous and difficult to obtain through a small-bore needle. After as much fluid as possible is aspirated, 0.5 to 1.0 ml glucocorticoid is injected. On occasion, very little fluid is obtained during the initial aspiration, but a second try 24 hours after glucocorticoid injection may yield a large amount of fluid.

Pelvis. When inflamed, the ischial (ischiogluteal) bursa is usually easily palpated as a tender area when the patient is lying on his or her side with the knees flexed. This position theoretically better exposes the ischium as gluteal muscles and sciatic nerve are pulled away. The point of maximal tenderness is marked, and 0.5 to 1.0 ml glucocorticoid and 2.5 to 4.0 ml local anesthetic are mixed in a syringe with a 20-gauge, 3½-inch needle attached. It is helpful to "fix" the skin over the mark. The needle is inserted into the mark until bone is hit. The needle is withdrawn slightly and all the mixture injected; alternatively, the needle is redirected in one or two other directions and portions of the mixture injected.

Iliopectineal (iliopsoas) bursitis, as mentioned, must be differentiated from psoas abscess, femoral hernia, and septic arthritis of the hip. If one elects to inject the bursa, a 20- to 22-gauge, 3½-inch spinal needle is used. Many use the technique of hip arthrocentesis. A dose of 0.5 to 1.0 ml glucocorticoid is injected, with or without 4 to 4.5 ml local anesthetic.

Back. The fibrositis syndrome and the tender points of the back have been discussed briefly. These tender points can be marked and each injected with 0.25 ml glucocorticoid or 1 ml or more of local anesthetic or, as many physicians prefer, a combination of the two. The shorter-acting corticosteroids, in contrast to the repository forms, have been recommended.[55] The physician must be careful to avoid injury to the underlying structures.

Foot. Achilles tendinitis may respond to injection. A 22-gauge, 1½-inch needle is inserted just under the tendon sheath and a mixture of 0.25 ml glucocorticoid and 2.5 ml local anesthetic is injected. Direct injection of the tendon should be avoided.

An inflammation of the subcutaneous Achilles bursa between the skin and tendon is usually readily palpable, can be marked, and should be easily aspirated with a 20-gauge, 1-inch needle. The retrocalcaneal bursa is located between the Achilles tendon and the posterior facet of the calcaneus. A lateral or medial approach is probably best. Careful injection of either location with 0.25 to 0.5 ml glucocorticoid, with or without local anesthetic, is usually beneficial.

Calcaneal bursitis can be treated by inserting a 20-gauge, 1½-inch needle perpendicular to the plantar surface of the mid-calcaneal region, pushing the needle in until bone is hit, withdrawing it slightly, and injecting 0.5 ml glucocorticoid and 3.5 ml local anesthetic. Some operators prefer a lateral approach because it is less painful. A mark is made at the lateral and inferior borders of the calcaneus. The needle is inserted there and directed medially to the site that is most painful. The mixture is then injected.

REFERENCES

1. Nelson RL, McCaffrey LA, Nobrega FT, et al: Altering residency curriculum in response to a changing practice environment: Use of the Mayo internal medicine residency alumni survey. Mayo Clin Proc 65:809, 1990.
2. Hollander JL: Arthrocentesis and intrasynovial therapy. In McCarty DJ (ed): Arthritis and Allied Conditions, 9th ed. Philadelphia, Lea & Febiger, 1979.
3. Hollander JL: The local effects of compound F (hydrocortisone) injected into joints. Bull Rheum Dis 2:3, 1951.
4. Young HH, Ward LE, Henderson ED: The use of hydrocortisone acetate (compound F acetate) in the treatment of some common orthopedic conditions. J Bone Joint Surg 36A:602, 1954.
5. Hollander JL, Jessar RA, Brown EM Jr: Intrasynovial corticosteroid therapy: A decade of use. Bull Rheum Dis 11:239, 1961.
6. Hollander JL: Intrasynovial corticosteroid therapy in arthritis. Md State Med J 19:62, 1970.
7. Jessar RA, Ganzell MA, Ragan C: The action of hydrocortisone in synovial inflammation. J Clin Invest 32:480, 1954.
8. Hunder GG, McDuffie FC: Effect of intra-articular hydrocortisone on complement in synovial fluid. J Lab Clin Med 79:62, 1972.
9. Goetzl EJ, Bianco NE, Alpert JS, et al: Effects of intra-articular corticosteroids in vivo on synovial fluid variables in rheumatoid synovitis. Ann Rheum Dis 33:62, 1974.
10. Dick WC, Whaley K, St. Onge RA, et al: Clinical studies on inflammation in human knee joints: Xenon (Xe[133]) clearances correlated with clinical assessment in various arthritides and studies on the effect of intra-articular administered hydrocortisone in rheumatoid arthritis. Clin Sci 38:123, 1970.
11. DeCeulaer K, Balint G, El-Ghobarey A, et al: Effects of corticosteroids and local anaesthetics applied directly to the synovial vascular bed. Ann Rheum Dis 38:440, 1979.
12. Eymontt MJ, Gordon GV, Schumacher HR, et al: The effects on synovial permeability and synovial fluid leukocyte counts in symptomatic osteoarthritis after intra-articular corticosteroid administration. J Rheumatol 9:198, 1982.
13. Chandler GN, Wright V: Deleterious effect of intra-articular hydrocortisone. Lancet 2:661, 1958.

14. Chandler GN, Wright V, Hartfall SJ: Intra-articular therapy in rheumatoid arthritis: Comparison of hydrocortisone tertiary butylacetate and hydrocortisone acetate. Lancet 2:659, 1958.
15. Mankin HJ, Conger KA: The acute effects of intra-articular hydrocortisone on articular cartilage in rabbits. J Bone Joint Surg 48A:1383, 1966.
16. Bentley G, Goodfellow JW: Disorganization of the knees following intra-articular hydrocortisone injections. J Bone Joint Surg 51B:498, 1969.
17. Moskowitz RW, Davis W, Sammarco J, et al: Experimentally induced corticosteroid arthropathy. Arthritis Rheum 13:236, 1970.
18. Mankin HJ, Zarins A, Jaffe WL: The effect of systemic corticosteroids on rabbit articular cartilage. Arthritis Rheum 15:593, 1972.
19. Behrens F, Shepard N, Mitchell N: Alteration of rabbit articular cartilage by intra-articular injections of glucocorticosteroids. J Bone Joint Surg 57A:70, 1975.
20. Gibson T, Barry HC, Poswillo D, et al: Effect of intra-articular corticosteroid injections on primate cartilage. Ann Rheum Dis 36:74, 1976.
21. Williams JM, Brandt KD: Triamcinolone hexacetonide protects against fibrillation and osteophyte formation following chemically induced articular cartilage damage. Arthritis Rheum 28:1267, 1985.
22. Pelletier J-P, Martel-Pelletier J: Protective effects of corticosteroids on cartilage lesions and osteophyte formation in the Pond-Nuki dog model of osteoarthritis. Arthritis Rheum 32:181, 1989.
23. Tenenbaum J, Pritzker KPH, Gross AE, et al: The effects of intra-articular corticosteroids on articular cartilage. Semin Arthritis Rheum 11(Suppl 1):140, 1981.
24. Pelletier J-P, Mineau, F, Raynauld J-P, et al: Intra-articular injections with methylprednisolone acetate reduce osteoarthritic lesions in parallel with chondrocyte stromelysin synthesis in experimental osteoarthritis. Arthritis Rheum 37:414, 1994.
25. Gray RG, Gottlieb NL: Intra-articular corticosteroids: An updated assessment. Clin Orthop Rel Res 177:235, 1983.
25a. Emkey RD, Lindsay R, Lyssy J, et al: The systemic effect of intraarticular administration of corticosteroid on markers on bone formation and bone resorption in patients with rheumatoid arthritis. Arthritis Rheum 39:277, 1996.
26. Gray RG, Tenenbaum J, Gottlieb NL: Local corticosteroid injection treatment in rheumatic disorders. Semin Arthritis Rheum 10:231, 1981.
27. Sweetnam R: Corticosteroid arthropathy and tendon rupture (Editorial). J Bone Joint Surg 51B:397, 1969.
28. Wrenn RN, Goldner JL, Markee JL: An experimental study of the effect of cortisone on the healing process and tensile strength of tendons. J Bone Joint Surg 36A:588, 1954.
29. McCarty DJ: Treatment of rheumatoid joint inflammation with triamcinolone hexacetonide. Arthritis Rheum 15:157, 1972.
30. Gilsanz V, Bernstein BH: Joint calcification following intra-articular corticosteroid therapy. Radiology 151:647, 1984.
31. McCarty DJ Jr, Hogan JM: Inflammatory reaction after intrasynovial injection of microcrystalline adrenocorticosteroid esters. Arthritis Rheum 7:359, 1964.
32. Koehler BF, Urowitz MB, Killinger DW: The systemic effects of intra-articular corticosteroid. J Rheumatol 1:117, 1974.
33. Armstrong RD, English J, Gibson T, et al: Serum methylprednisolone levels following intra-articular injection of methylprednisolone acetate. Ann Rheum Dis 40:571, 1981.
34. Gottlieb NL, Riskin WG: Complications of local corticosteroid injections. JAMA 243:1547, 1980.
35. Konttinen YT, Friman C, Tolvanen E, et al: Local skin rash after intra-articular methylprednisolone acetate injection in a patient with rheumatoid arthritis. Arthritis Rheum 26:231, 1983.
36. Carson TE, Daane TA, Lee PA, et al: Effect of intramuscular triamcinolone acetonide on the human ovulatory cycle. Cutis 19:633, 1977.
37. Cunningham GR, Goldzieher JW, de la Pena A, et al: The mechanism of ovulation inhibition by triamcinolone acetonide. J Clin Endocrinol Metab 46:8, 1978.
38. Baer PA, Shore A, Ikeman R: Transient fall in serum salicylate levels following intra-articular injection of steroid in patients with rheumatoid arthritis. Arthritis Rheum 30:345, 1987.
39. McCarty DJ Jr: A basic guide to arthrocentesis. Hosp Med 4:77, 1968.
40. Gottlieb NL: Hypodermic needle separation during arthrocentesis. Arthritis Rheum 24:1593, 1981.
41. Fitzgerald RF Jr: Intrasynovial injection of steroids. Mayo Clin Proc 51:655, 1976.
42. Miller JH, White J, Norton TH: The value of intra-articular injections in osteoarthritis of the knee. J Bone Joint Surg 40B:636, 1958.
43. Friedman DM, Moore MF: The efficacy of intra-articular corticosteroid for osteoarthritis of the knee. Arthritis Rheum 21:556, 1978.
44. Utsinger PD, Resnick D, Shapiro RF, et al: Roentgenologic, immunologic, and therapeutic study of erosive (inflammatory) osteoarthritis. Arch Intern Med 138:693, 1978.
45. Huskinsson EC: The drug treatment of osteoarthritis. Scand J Rheumatol 43(Suppl):57, 1982.
46. Friedman DM, Moore ME: The efficacy of intra-articular steroids in osteoarthritis: A double-blind study. J Rheumatol 7:850, 1980.
47. Neustadt DH: Intra-articular steroid therapy: In Moskowitz RW, Howell DS, Goldberg VM, Mankin HJ (eds): Osteoarthritis: Diagnosis and Management. Philadelphia, WB Saunders, 1984.
48. Dieppe PA, Sathapatayavongs B, Jones HE, et al: Intra-articular steroids in osteoarthritis. Rheumatol Rehabil 19:212, 1980.
49. Neustadt DH: Intra-articular therapy for rheumatoid synovitis of the knee: Effects of the postinjection rest regimen. Clin Rheumatol Pract 3:65, 1985.
50. McCarty DJ: Intrasynovial therapy with adrenocorticosteroid esters. Wis Med J 77:S75, 1978.
51. Charkravarty K, Pharoah PDP, Scott DGI: Intra-articular steroid therapy for knee synovitis role of post injection rest. Arthritis Rheum 35:5200, 1992.
52. Henderson ED, Henderon CC: The use of hydrocortisone acetate (compound F acetate) in the treatment of post-traumatic bursitis of the knee and elbow. Minn Med 36:142, 1953.
53. Gray RG, Kiem IM, Gottlieb NL: Intratendon sheath corticosteroid treatment of rheumatoid arthritis-associated and idiopathic hand flexor tenosynovitis. Arthritis Rheum 21:92, 1978.
54. Steinbrocker O: Management of some non-articular rheumatic disorders. Mod Treat 1:1254, 1964.
55. Steinbrocker O, Neustadt DH: Aspiration and injection therapy in arthritis and musculoskeletal disorders. Hagerstown, Md, Harper & Row, 1972.
56. Smythe HA, Moldofsky H: Two contributions to understanding of the "fibrositis" syndrome. Bull Rheum Dis 28:928, 1977.
57. Brown BB Jr: Diagnosis and therapy of common myofascial syndromes. JAMA 239:646, 1978.
58. Physician's Desk Reference (Fujisawa Laboratories). Montvale, NJ, Medical Economics Company, 1996.
59. Geborek P, Mansson B, Wollheim FA, et al: Intra-articular corticosteroid injection into rheumatoid arthritis knees improves extensor muscle strength. Rheumatol Int 9:265, 1990.
60. Owen DS Jr, Weiss JJ, Wilke WS: When to aspirate and inject joints. Patient Care 24:128, 1990.
61. Hertzberger-ten CR, de Vries van der Vlugt BCM, Van Suijlekom-Smit LWA: Intra-articular steroids in pauciarticular juvenile chronic arthritis, type European J Pediatr 150:170, 1991.
62. Gurwitz JH, Avorn J, Ross-Degnan D, et al: nonsteroidal anti-inflammatory drug–associated azotemia in the very old. JAMA 264:471, 1990.
63. Roberts WN, Liang MH, Stern SH: Colchicine in acute gout: Reassessment of risks and benefits. JAMA 257:1920, 1987.
64. Steinbrocker O, Agyros TG: Frozen shoulder treatment by local injection of depot corticosteroids. Arch Phys Med 55:209, 1974.
65. Roy S, Oldham R: Management of painful shoulder. Lancet 1:1322, 1976.
66. Weiss JJ, Ting YM: Arthrography-assisted intra-articular injection of steroids in treatment of adhesive capsulitis. Arch Phys Med 59:285, 1978.
67. Kozin F: Painful shoulder and the reflex sympathetic dystrophy syndrome. In McCarty DJ (ed): Arthritis and Allied Conditions, 10th ed. Philadelphia, Lea & Febiger, 1985.
68. Lee PN, Lee M, Hag AM, et al: Periarthritis of the shoulder: Trial of treatments investigated by multivariate analysis. Ann Rheum Dis 33:116, 1974.
69. Jelenko C: Tietze's syndrome at the xiphisternal joint. South Med J 67:818, 1974.
70. Kamien M: A rational management of tennis elbow. Sports Med 9:173, 1990.
71. Clark CB: Cubital tunnel syndrome. JAMA 241:801, 1979.
72. Lapidus PW, Guidotti FP: Report on the treatment of one hundred and two ganglions. Bull Hosp Joint Dis 28:50, 1967.
73. Phalen GS: Soft tissue affection of the hand and wrist. Hosp Med 7:47, 1971.
74. Anderson BC, Manthey R, Brouns MC: Treatment of de Quervain's tenosynovitis with corticosteroid. Arthritis Rheum 34:793, 1991.
75. Harvey FJ, Harvey PM, Horsley MW: De Quervain's disease: surgical or nonsurgical treatment. J Hand Surg 15A:83, 1990.
76. Marks MR, Gunther SF: Efficacy of cortisone injection in treatment of trigger fingers and thumbs. J Hand Surg 14A:722, 1989.
77. Canoso JJ: Bursitis, tenosynovitis, ganglions, and painful lesions of the wrist, elbow, and hand. Curr Opin Rheumatol 2:276, 1990.
78. Fauno P, Anderson HJ, Simonsen O: A long-term follow-up of the effect of repeated corticosteroid injections for stenosing tenosynovitis. J Hand Surg 14B:242, 1989.
79. Blau SP: All those joint pains may not be arthritis. Drug Ther November 1976, p 144.
80. Schuchmann JA, Melvin JL, Duran RJ, et al: Evaluation of local steroid injection for carpal tunnel syndrome. Arch Phys Med Rehabil 51:253, 1971.
81. Dehaan MR, Wilson RL: Diagnosis and management of carpal tunnel syndrome, J Musculoskeletal Med, 6:47, 1989.
82. Larsson L-G, Baum J: The syndrome of anserina bursitis: An overlooked diagnosis. Arthritis Rheum 28:1062, 1985.

83. Lozen L. and DeFond, W.: Prepatellar bursal neuritis: A neglected entity. Contemp Orthop 28:237, 1994.
84. Swartout R, Compere EL: Ischiogluteal bursitis. JAMA 227:551, 1974.
85. Hucherson DC, Freeman GE Jr: Iliopectineal bursitis: a cause of hip pain frequently unrecognized. Am J Orthop 4:220, 1962.
86. Swezey RL: Obturator internus bursitis: a common factor in low back pain. Orthropaedics 16:783, 1993.
87. Canoso JJ, Wohlgethan JR, Newberg AH, et al: Aspiration of the retrocalcaneal bursa. Ann Rheum Dis 43:308, 1984.
88. Francis H, March L, Terenty T, et al: Benign joint hypermobility with neuropathy: Documentation and mechanism of tarsal tunnel syndrome. J Rheumatol 14:577, 1987.
89. Kaplan PE, Kernahan WT: Tarsal tunnel syndrome. J Bone Joint Surg 63A:96, 1981.
90. Larsson L-G, Baum J: The syndromes of bursitis. Bull Rheum Dis 36:1, 1986.
91. Strong G, Thomas PS: Conservative treatment of Morton's neuroma. Orthop Rev 16:97, 1987.
92. Roy DR, Fleury J, Fontaine SB, et al: Clinical evaluation of cervical facet joint infiltration. Can Assoc Radiol J 39:118, 1988.
93. Warfield CA: Facet syndrome and the relief of low back pain. Hosp Pract 23:41, 1988.
94. Carette S, Marcoux S, Truchon R, et al: A controlled trial of corticosteroid injection into facet joints for chronic low back pain. N Engl J Med 325:1002, 1991.
95. Hardaker WT, Whipple TL, Bassett FH: Diagnosis and treatment of the plica syndrome of the knee. J Bone Joint Surg 62A:221, 1980.
96. Rovere GD: Medial synovial shelf plica syndrome. Am J Sports Med 13:382, 1984.
97. Schonholtz GJ, Magee CM: The synovial plicae of the knee joint. Contemp Orthop 12:31, 1986.

CHAPTER 41

H. Ralph Schumacher, Jr.

Synovial Fluid Analysis and Synovial Biopsy

The actual disease process in a given joint can be defined only by direct study of that joint. Abnormal results of blood tests, such as those for rheumatoid factor, antinuclear antibodies, and elevated uric acid, can be misleading and do not establish the nature of disease in the joint. Because crystal-induced arthritis can closely mimic rheumatoid disease, at least one joint fluid specimen should be examined for crystals in most cases. Nearly 100 other diseases can also involve joints; in many, the study of fluid or tissue is the only way to establish the diagnosis. In addition, not all joints in each patient need to have the same findings. Some joints in patients with rheumatoid arthritis may be totally spared or affected only by coincidental osteoarthritis, whereas others may have a superimposed infectious arthritis.

Full information from aspiration or biopsy or both may suggest major changes in management. Unexpected findings can suggest a variety of less common but often specifically treatable causes of arthritis. Expertise in joint fluid analysis and interpretation of synovial tissue study is not widely available, and these skills should be developed by anyone specializing in the care of joint disease.

SYNOVIAL FLUID ANALYSIS

Joint fluid examination[1, 2] is even more important in the evaluation of joint disease than urinalysis is in renal disease. Analysis of joint fluid should be performed as part of the diagnostic evaluation in any patient with joint disease. Examination of joint fluid is especially important in monarticular arthritis, in which septic arthritis must be distinguished from a wide variety of possible causes (see Table 24–3). Even small amounts of joint fluid can be aspirated and systematically examined. A few drops or more of synovial fluid can often be obtained from normal joints and virtually any joint that is even equivocally swollen.[3]

Some common diseases, such as gout, pseudogout, septic arthritis, and systemic lupus erythematosus (SLE), as well as other less common diseases, can be quickly and almost definitively diagnosed by examination of joint fluid. In one study, joint fluid examination changed clinically suspected diagnoses (and of-

ten planned treatments) in about 20 percent of patients seen for initial evaluation.[4] Even if joint fluid examination is not diagnostic, it can be one of the most useful of a battery of clinical and laboratory tests used in differential diagnosis. Gross examination and leukocyte count allow narrowing of diagnostic possibilities to the diseases causing "noninflammatory" effusions; inflammatory fluids, including septic effusions; and hemarthroses (Tables 41–1 to 41–4).

Even in patients in whom the diagnosis has been established, synovial fluid analysis can show clues to a new development, such as low-grade infection in a joint of a patient with SLE or rheumatoid disease, superimposition of calcium pyrophosphate or apatite crystal deposition in osteoarthritis, or crystals of intra-articularly injected glucocorticoids that cause a transient crystal-induced synovitis.

Discrepancies between different laboratories examining the same fluids are common.[5] It is best to examine fluids personally and to be certain of quality control mechanisms established in your own laboratory.[6]

Normal joint fluid is described in detail in Chapter 1. Briefly, normal synovial fluid is an ultrafiltrate of plasma—with only small amounts of higher-molecular-weight proteins such as fibrinogen, complement, globulin, and other immunoglobulins—to which has been added hyaluronate protein produced in the synovial membrane. Normal fluid is compared with that seen in various diseases in Table 41–1.

Techniques for Arthrocentesis

The techniques used, appropriate precautions, and routes for arthrocentesis are described in Chapter 40. If no fluid is identified in the syringe after attempted aspiration, a drop of blood or tissue fluid may be found in the needle. One can use a single drop for crystal examination, Gram's stain, or culture. If no fluid is obtained and infection is suspected, the joint can be irrigated with a small amount of normal saline and this irrigating fluid can be obtained for culture.

The studies most likely to be helpful in each case should be considered before arthrocentesis and a list of priorities prepared for the fluid obtained. By no means must all tests be performed on each specimen. Because leukocyte counts can fall and artefactual crys-

Table 41–1. CLASSIFICATION OF SYNOVIAL EFFUSIONS*

Gross Examination	Normal	Noninflammatory	Inflammatory	Septic
Volume (knee)	< 1 ml	Often > 1 ml	Often > 1 ml	Often > 1 ml
Viscosity	High	High	Low	Variable
Color	Colorless to straw	Straw to yellow	Yellow	Variable
Clarity	Transparent	Transparent	Translucent	Opaque
WBCs/μL†	< 200	50–1000	1000–75,000	Often > 100,000 +
PMN†	< 25%	< 25%	Often > 50%	> 85%
Culture	Negative	Negative	Negative	Often positive
Mucin clot	Firm	Firm	Friable	Friable
Glucose (A.M. fasting)	Nearly equal to blood	Nearly equal to blood	< 50 mg/dl lower than blood	> 50 mg/dl lower than blood

*See Tables 41–2 and 41–3 for diseases in the noninflammatory and inflammatory groups.
†The white blood cell (WBC) count and polymorphonuclear neutrophil (PMN) percentage are less if organism is less virulent or partially treated.

tals may develop over several hours, the fluid should be examined promptly.[7]

Gross Examination

Gross examination can be done immediately to help plan which of the other studies are most pertinent.

Volume. The amount of effusion can help serve as one measure of the severity of arthritis and can be used for comparison with previous arthrocentesis results. Low volume does not mean absence of an important intra-articular process. Effusions may be difficult to aspirate because of thick fibrin, rice bodies, and other debris. Fluid may be loculated and not accessible by the route chosen.

Viscosity. Although estimation of viscosity is now known to be less reliable than previously thought in classification of effusions,[8] viscosity can be estimated by watching the synovial fluid as it is slowly expressed from the syringe or by manipulating several

Table 41–2. RELATIVELY NONINFLAMMATORY JOINT EFFUSIONS (LEUKOCYTE COUNT BELOW 1000/mm³)

Osteoarthritis
Traumatic arthritis
Acromegaly
Gaucher's disease
Hemochromatosis
Hyperparathyroidism
Ochronosis
Paget's disease
Mechanical derangement
Erythema nodosum
Villonodular synovitis, tumors
Aseptic necrosis
Ehlers-Danlos syndrome
Sickle cell disease
Amyloidosis
Hypertrophic pulmonary osteoarthropathy
Pancreatitis
Osteochondritis dissecans
Charcot's joints
Wilson's disease
Epiphyseal dysplasias
Glucocorticoid withdrawal

drops of fluid between the gloved thumb and finger. Fluid of normal viscosity holds together and stretches to a string of 1 to 2 inches before separating. Low-viscosity fluid drips from a syringe like water. Very viscous fluid is seen in hypothyroid effusions and in ganglia or osteoarthritic mucous cysts. Viscosity is generally decreased in inflammation (see Table 41–1) but also is low in edema fluid. Viscosity tends to parallel the concentration of hyaluronate. In purulent effusions, the massive numbers of leukocytes can make the fluid seem more viscous. Hyaluronidase or dilution with saline can be used to decrease synovial fluid viscosity before performing other tests, provided the normal values using this enzyme have been standardized in the laboratory[9] and that the dilution factor is considered.

Color and Clarity (Fig. 41–1). If print cannot be read easily through the fluid, the effusion is cloudy, and this finding should suggest an inflammatory process. The plastic of some syringes makes fluids appear falsely cloudy, so fluids should be examined in glass. Generally, the more cloudy fluids have more cells, but not all cloudy or opaque fluids are inflammatory. Microscopic examination is needed to be certain that the opacity is not due to massive numbers of crystals, lipids, fibrin, or amyloid. Chronically inflamed joints sometimes have effusions that contain rice bodies, which might also be confused grossly with pus. Rice bodies are end results of synovial proliferation and degeneration; they contain collagen, cell debris, and fibrin (Fig. 41–2; see Color Plate at the front of this volume).

Ochronotic fluid may be speckled with dark particles (ground pepper sign).[10] Black or gray debris from metal or plastic fragments after prosthetic arthroplasty can also discolor the fluid.[11]

Fluid in pigmented villonodular synovitis can be grossly bloody or may have an orange-brown color. Urate- or apatite-laden fluids can be white or yellow and pasty. Cholesterol-containing fluids may be golden. Streaks of blood are the result of injury to a small vessel during the procedure. Causes of diffusely bloody fluids are listed in Table 41–4. Lipid floating on the top of the erythrocytes is often a result of fracture to the joint. Partially treated or low-grade

Table 41–3. INFLAMMATORY JOINT EFFUSIONS (LEUKOCYTE COUNT ABOVE 1000/mm³)

Rheumatoid arthritis
Psoriatic arthritis
Reiter's syndrome
Ulcerative colitis
Regional enteritis
Post–ileal bypass arthritis
Ankylosing spondylitis
Juvenile rheumatoid arthritis
Rheumatic fever
Collagen–vascular disease
   Systemic lupus erythematosus
   Scleroderma
   Polymyositis
   Polychondritis
   Polyarteritis
Polymyalgia rheumatica
Giant cell arteritis
Sjögren's syndrome
Wegener's granulomatosis
Goodpasture's syndrome
Henoch-Schönlein purpura
Familial Mediterranean fever
Whipple's disease
Behçet's syndrome
Erythema nodosum
Sarcoidosis
Multicentric reticulohistiocytosis
Erythema multiforme (Stevens-Johnson)
Reactive arthritis
Infectious arthritis
   Parasitic
   Viral (e.g., hepatitis, mumps, rubella, human
      immunodeficiency virus)
   Fungal
   Mycoplasmal
   Bacterial (staphylococcal or gonococcal
      infection, tuberculosis, others)
   Spirochetal (Lyme disease, syphilis)
Carcinoid
Subacute bacterial endocarditis
Crystal-induced arthritis
   Gout
   Pseudogout
   Post–intra-articular steroid injection
   Apatite arthritis
   Oxalosis
Hyperlipoproteinemias
Serum sickness
Hypogammaglobulinemia
Leukemia
Hypersensitivity angiitis
Palindromic rheumatism

flammatory, or non-inflammatory (see Table 41–1). Synovial fluid leukocyte counts, along with volumes, can be used as a rough measure of the intensity of inflammation in sequential samples.

The standard leukocyte-counting chamber and techniques are used, except that ordinary counting fluid should be replaced with normal or 0.3 percent saline, which lyses erythrocytes. The acid of ordinary leukocyte-counting fluid clots synovial fluid and gives inaccurate counts. A small amount of fluid should be placed in a heparinized tube and shaken to mix it thoroughly. The count must be done promptly, since there may be some spontaneous clotting and clumping of leukocytes. Methylene blue can be added for easier identification of leukocytes. Rheumatoid arthritis fluid usually has a leukocyte count of 2000 to 75,000/mm³. Counts over 60,000 should raise a suspicion of infection. Partially treated infections or low-grade infections with gonococci, mycobacteria, and fungi often have lower leukocyte counts, however. Patients with rheumatoid disease, psoriatic arthritis, Reiter's syndrome, and crystal-induced arthritis may have leukocyte counts over 100,000 cells/mm³. Small joints, such as finger joints, may have unusually high counts, because less volume dilutes the cells in such joints.

Leukocyte counts of 200 to 2000/mm³ generally are termed *noninflammatory*. Actually, a gradation needs to be considered based on the clinical picture. More than 1000 cells/mm³ should suggest consideration of one of the inflammatory diseases shown in Table 41–3. Truly normal joint fluid usually has only 50 to 100 leukocytes so counts over 200/mm³ clearly represent at least a low-grade inflammatory response such as is seen, for example, in some patients with osteoarthritis. Patients who have predominantly degenerative arthritis, as in hemochromatosis, can have inflammatory effusions with high leukocyte counts if associated chondrocalcinosis leads to crystal-induced arthritis.

Microscopic Studies

Wet Preparation. Probably the single most important step in synovial fluid analysis is prompt mi-

infection can make the synovial fluid like any other moderately inflammatory but nonpurulent fluid. Slightly inflammatory or clear fluids are common in SLE, rheumatic fever, polymositis, and scleroderma, and can be seen in the interim between attacks of gout and pseudogout.

Leukocyte Count

The leukocyte count is an important part of synovial fluid analysis, especially because it is the major basis for classification of an effusion as septic, in-

Table 41–4. HEMARTHROSES

Trauma with or without fractures
Pigmented villonodular synovitis
Tumors
Hemangioma
Charcot's joint or other severe joint destruction
Hemophilia or other bleeding disorders
Von Willebrand's disease
Anticoagulant therapy
Myeloproliferative disease with thrombocytosis
Thrombocytopenia
Scurvy
Ruptured aneurysm
Arteriovenous fistula
Idiopathic
Intense inflammatory disease

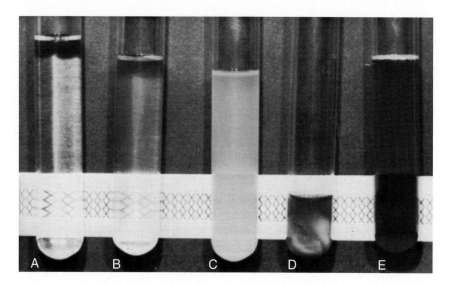

Figure 41–1. Synovial effusions. *A,* Normal or edema fluid is clear, pale yellow, or colorless. Print is easily read through the tube. *B,* Fluid from noninflammatory joint disease is yellow and clear. *C,* An inflammatory effusion is cloudy and yellow. Print may be blurred or completely obliterated, depending on the number of leukocytes. The effusion is translucent. *D,* A purulent effusion from septic arthritis contains a dense clump that does not even allow light through the many leukocytes. *E,* Hemorrhagic fluid is red. The supernatant may be darker yellow-brown (xanthochromic). A traumatic tap is less uniform and often has blood streaks.

croscopic examination of a fresh drop of synovial fluid as a wet preparation. Even if only a single drop of fluid is obtained with aspiration, it can be examined for crystals and other constituents as a wet preparation; the same fluid can then be allowed to dry for staining with Gram's stain if required. One drop of unadulterated synovial fluid is expressed from the syringe, or the fluid is transferred with a pipette or loop onto an ultraclean glass slide. The author usually examines uncentrifuged fluids, but examination of a pellet after centrifugation can help concentrate rare crystals or cells in clear-appearing fluid. Dirty slides can be washed in acetone and air dried. Lens paper used to clean slides can introduce birefringent paper fibrils.

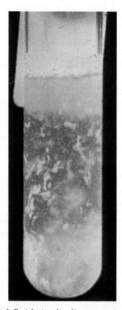

Figure 41–2. Synovial fluid rice bodies containing fibrin and debris from degenerated villi are especially common in rheumatoid arthritis but can also be seen in other conditions such as tuberculous arthritis. (See Color Plate.)

A glass coverslip is placed on the drop of synovial fluid. If any delay is expected before examination, the coverslip margins can be sealed with nail polish. This allows several hours of delay, but slides may still dry out and produce birefringent-drying artifacts if left overnight. The nail polish at the margins is birefringent with polarized light.

Regular Light Microscopy. Each joint fluid sample is first examined with regular light microscopy. Erythrocytes and leukocytes can be seen and their numbers estimated. Fragments of cartilage or synovium may contain crystals and, if numerous enough, can be concentrated by centrifugation and fixed for staining as a biopsy. Some leukocytes contain shiny, round cytoplasmic inclusions that are thought to represent distended phagosomes or lipid droplets. Such cytoplasmic inclusion-containing cells,[12] or ragocytes, were first detected in rheumatoid arthritis but are also seen in other inflammatory arthropathies. Erythrocytes may be sickled in patients with sickle cell disease or trait, but this does not establish that the current effusion is due to the sickle cell disease, although sickle cells may be phagocytized and cause inflammation.[13]

A variety of fibrillar materials can be seen in joint fluids. Some of these fibrils are fibrin, whereas others can be shown to be collagen from synovium or cartilage fragments.[14, 15] Such fibrils (and crystals) often can be seen better by lowering the condenser or closing the diaphragm to produce a partial phase effect. Both collagen and fibrin are faintly birefringent. Dark, irregularly shaped metal fragments can be seen in effusions of patients with implant arthroplasties.[11] Polymer fragments might also be seen. The rare shards of ochronotic cartilage are yellow or ochre fragments on regular light microscopy[16] (Fig. 41–3; see Color Plate at the front of this volume).

Large numbers of extracellular lipid droplets may be seen in traumatic arthritis[17]; in inflammatory effusions of various types, including some otherwise unexplained effusions; and in pancreatic fat necrosis[18]; a

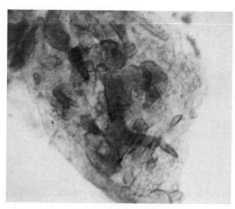

Figure 41–3. Any fragments floating in fluid should be examined. They may be cartilage or synovium and contain crystals or other diagnostic clues. Shards of golden or ochre cartilage fragments here are embedded in detached synovium found in synovial fluid in a patient with ochronotic arthropathy. (See Color Plate.)

few droplets also can simply result from the arthrocentesis. In trauma, some lipid presumably comes from marrow and synovium. Bone spicules may be found if fracture into the joint has occurred. Such spicules tend to adhere to glass and must be sought carefully.[19]

Amorphous globular and irregular material, usually without birefringence, can be seen and can be due to amyloid masses[20] in patients with primary amyloid, multiple myeloma, and Waldenström's macroglobulinemia or in patients with chronic renal failure who are treated with dialysis regimens. Congo red stains this material pink or red on the wet preparation. Apple-green birefringence is seen with polarized light. Other shiny globular or coinlike clumps can be seen from apatite aggregates in joint and bursa fluids.[21] Clumps of apatites and other calcium-containing crystals can be stained red with alizarin red S as an additional screening aid.[22]

Crystals can be seen with regular light microscopy. Urate crystals are usually 2- to 20-μm long rods or needles. Calcium pyrophosphate crystals can be thin or thick rods or rhomboids, are rarely as long as urates, and occasionally are best seen with regular light since they are often faintly birefringent. Oxalate crystals as a complication of renal failure can be pleomorphic but usually include some bipyramidal forms.[23] These and other crystals can be further differentiated with compensated polarized light.

Compensated Polarized Light Microscopy (Table 41–5).[24, 25] In a polarized light microscope, ordinary incandescent light is oriented in a single plane by a polarizer over the light source. When a second polarizer is added and rotated 90 degrees to the first, all light is blocked and the microscope field viewed through the ocular appears totally dark. If crystalline (birefringent) material is placed in the light path between the polarizers, light is deflected and split into fast and slow rays that vibrate at different angles from the incident light. The vibration planes of these two new rays are mutually perpendicular, but neither is parallel to the original ray of plane polarized light. Some of these rays now pass through the second polarizer (also termed the *analyzer*) and are brightly visible on the dark field. This brightness is common to all birefringent material.

In clinical use, different birefringent materials such as crystals can be distinguished in part by the altered behavior of light that passes through another birefringent structure (the *compensator*) placed between the first polarizer and the specimen. The compensator generally used is a first-order red plate, which eliminates green from the background and produces a background field that is rose-colored rather than black. The first-order red compensator quality and thickness can be expressed numerically as 540 nm. If the slow ray of a birefringent crystal is parallel to the slow ray from the compensator, the additive effect of a urate or pyrophosphate crystal creates a value of

Table 41–5. MORPHOLOGIC FEATURES OF SOME SYNOVIAL FLUID CRYSTALS ASSOCIATED WITH JOINT DISEASE

Crystals	Size (μm)	Morphology	Birefringence	Diseases
MSU	2–10	Needles, rods	Intensely negative	Acute and chronic gout
CPPD	2–10	Rhomboids, rods	Weakly positive	CPPD crystal deposition disease, osteoarthritis
Apatite-like clumps	5–20	Round, irregular clumps	None	Periarthritis, acute or chronic arthritis, osteoarthritis
Calcium oxalate	2–10	Polymorphic, dipyramidal shapes	Itensely or weakly positive	Renal failure
Cholesterol	10–80	Rectangles, often with missing corners; needles	Negative or positive	Chronic rheumatoid or osteoarthritic effusions
Depot glucocorticoids	4–15	Irregular rods, rhomboids	Intensely positive or negative	Iatrogenic postinjection flare
Lipid liquid crystals	2–8	Maltese crosses	Intensely positive	Acute arthritis, bursitis
Charcot-Leyden	17–25	Spindles	Positive and negative	Eosinophilic synovitis
Immunoglobulins	3–60	Polymorphic, rods	Positive and negative	Multiple myeloma, cryoglobulinemia

Abbreviations: MSU, monosodium urate; CPPD, calcium pyrophosphate dihydrate.

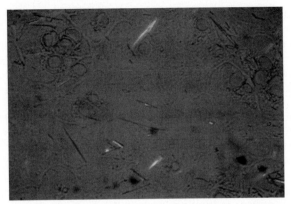

Figure 41–4. Monosodium urate crystals from a gouty synovial fluid as viewed with compensated polarized light. The crystals are yellow parallel to the axis of slow vibration marked on the compensator (negative birefringence). Do not expect to see so many crystals, as even a few can cause acute gout. (See Color Plate.)

about 700 nm and a blue color. If the same crystal is now rotated 90 degrees so that its fast ray is parallel to the compensator's slow ray, a color subtraction of the same number of nanometers gives a yellow color.

Monosodium urate crystals can be differentiated from calcium pyrophosphate dihydrate (CPPD) crystals because with urate crystals the fast ray is in the long axis of the crystal, giving a yellow color when the crystal axis is parallel to the slow ray of the compensator. This is termed a *negative optical sign* or *negative elongation.* CPPD crystals have their slow ray in the long axis of the crystal; thus, when parallel to the axis of slow vibration of the compensator, they appear blue (positive elongation).

Monosodium urate crystals of gout tend to be brightly negatively birefringent (Fig. 41–4; see Color Plate at the front of this volume). Crystals are generally identifiable within cells during active gouty arthritis. Crystals obtained from puncturing a tophus in a joint or elsewhere are often longer needles that are predominantly extracellular. Microtophi may occasionally be seen in tissue fragments found floating in

the fluid. CPPD crystals have a weaker birefringence and positive elongation (Fig. 41–5; see Color Plate at the front of this volume).

A variety of other birefringent materials are seen on polarized light examinations of joint fluids. Depot corticosteroid preparations are crystalline[26] and can contaminate fluids during injections or occasionally remain in joints or adjacent connective tissue for variable periods after local injections. These crystals can be phagocytized and occasionally induce a transient inflammation several hours after intra-articular injections (Fig. 41–6; see Color Plate at the front of this volume). Corticosteroid crystals can appear as positively or negatively birefringent rods similar in size to urates or CPPD crystals, as granules, or as irregular debris.

Cholesterol crystals can be seen in chronic joint effusions, especially in rheumatoid arthritis.[27] Crystals are usually platelike with a notch in one corner (Fig. 41–7; see Color Plate at the front of this volume) and larger than a cell, but crystals in cholesterol-laden effusions may also be needles with negative elongation. Some lipid droplets appear as positively birefringent Maltese crosses,[28] and these may be phlogistic in some cases.

Calcium hydrogen phosphate dihydrate crystals are brightly positively birefringent and have been identified in joint fluids and tissues.[29] These crystals might be confused with CPPD and can best be definitely differentiated by x-ray diffraction. Apatite crystal clumps occasionally have some birefringence. Spindle-shaped Charcot-Leyden crystals can be seen in fluids with eosinophils. Rarely, cryoglobulin (or other immunoglobulins), hemoglobin, and hematoidin derived from red blood cells are a cause of joint fluid crystals.

Most other irregular birefringent material is artifact, such as dust from the slide or glass fragments from the coverslip. Powder from rubber gloves is birefringent and generally has a Maltese cross appearance. Artifactual needle-shaped or irregular crystals can develop in time, so prompt examination of fluid is

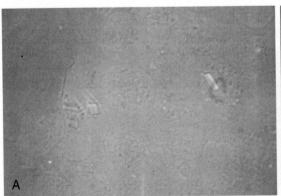
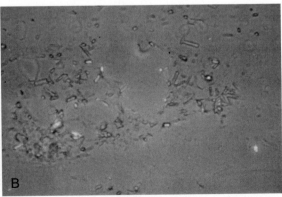

Figure 41–5. Calcium pyrophosphate dihydrate (CPPD) crystals can be needle, rod, or rhomboid shaped but usually have blunt ends *(A).* They often have fainter birefringence than is seen with urates *(B).* CPPD are blue when aligned longitudinally with the axis of slow vibration of the compensator (positive birefringence). (See Color Plate.)

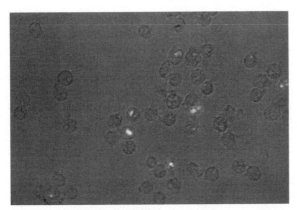

Figure 41–6. Triamcinolone acetonide (Aristospan) crystals phagocytized by synovial fluid cells after intra-articular injection. (See Color Plate.)

important. Erroneous use of an ethylene-diaminetetraacetic acid, oxalate,[30] or lithium heparin[31] anticoagulant can introduce anticoagulant-derived crystals. Such crystals can be phagocytized by white blood cells in vitro and can thus be seen intracellularly.

Commercial polarizing microscopes are readily available and should generally be used.[21] One can also obtain polarizing filters to be inserted into a regular light microscope. One filter is placed between the light source and condenser; another is placed above the objective or in the eyepiece. Filters are rotated until a black field is obtained. This produces the white birefringence that shows crystals more easily than ordinary light but cannot separate positive and negative birefringence. An effect similar to that obtained with a commercial compensated polarizing microscope can be achieved by applying two layers of cellophane tape to the top of a clean glass slide and placing this over the polarizing filter above the light source.[32] The long axis of the slide then is substituted for the axis of slow vibration of the first-order red compensator. Tapes that appear semi-opaque before use do not work. Before using such a setup, findings should be clinically compared on several crystals with findings obtained with a commercial compensator.

Absolutely definitive diagnosis of crystals can be made by x-ray diffraction, but sufficient numbers of crystals are needed for this. Uricase digestion may be helpful in that urates but not other crystals are digested with uricase.[33] Fortunately, this is rarely required. Occasionally crystals of urate or CPPD are so few or so small that they are detected only by electron microscopy.[34] Urate crystals are dissolved out in usual electron microscopic preparations, leaving only typical clefts, but CPPD crystals are not. Individual apatite crystals can be seen only by electron microscopy. Electron diffraction or electron probe elemental analysis can be performed on apatites and other basic calcium phosphates.[1] Atomic force microscopy is being tested as a means of identifying crystals by their surface molecular structure. Infrared spectroscopy using Fourier transformation or electron microscopy can

identify small amounts of crystals mixed with other predominant crystals.

Dried Smears for Staining. Synovial smears are made using one or two drops of heparinized fluid on slides in the same manner as with peripheral blood smears. If the leukocyte count is greater than approximately 2500/mm³ a good smear can generally be made from the whole fluid. Fluids with lower counts often produce better smears if the fluid is cytocentrifuged or centrifuged and the button is resuspended in a few drops of the supernatant before smearing. Smears should be made within several hours after aspiration of fluid and allowed to air dry. They can be stained the same day or the next. Some fluids with few cells can be best examined for cellular features in a wet preparation with a supravital stain.[35]

Wright's stain is the single most useful stain.[36, 37] Smears should be examined briefly under low magnifications to look for such findings as lupus erythematosus cells. Lupus erythematosus cells have so far been reported frequently in SLE and only rarely in rheumatoid arthritis, but they need not be present in typical SLE. Cartilage and synovial fragments may be seen and should be examined for any characteristic changes such as tophi. Iron-laden chondrocytes have been seen in cartilage fragments in hemochromatosis. Brown-pigmented debris or cytoplasmic granules can be seen in ochronosis. Bone marrow spicules with fat cells or other marrow elements may also be seen.

The smear is next examined carefully under oil immersion. Cells can be fairly easily separated into polymorphonuclear leukocytes (PMNs), monocytes, small lymphocytes, and large mononuclear cells. The last probably include some transformed lymphocytes, macrophages, natural killer cells, and synovial lining cells. Although classification of individual large mononuclear cells may be difficult, it is worth attempting, since transformed lymphocytes tend to be seen in rheumatoid arthritis and not in acute gout or pseudogout.[36] Most other diseases have received insufficient study. Atypical lymphocytes with nuclear indentations have been seen in human lymphotrophic virus type 1 (HTLV-1)–associated arthritis.[38] Synthetic-

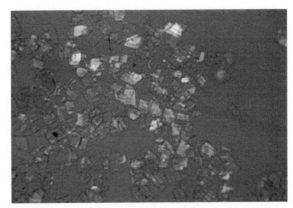

Figure 41–7. Cholesterol crystals from a chronic rheumatoid olecranon bursal effusion. These are most often flat plates with notched corners. (See Color Plate.)

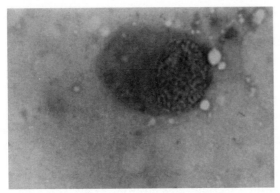

Figure 41–8. Synovial lining cell. The prominent homogeneous blue cytoplasm is typical of type B or synthetic cells. Other large cells with a nucleus:cytoplasm ratio of less than 50 percent have vacuolated cytoplasm and are either phagocytic lining cells or large monocytes (macrophages). (See Color Plate.)

type synovial lining cells (Fig. 41–8; see Color Plate at the front of this volume) typically are 20 to 40 μm in diameter, with an eccentric nucleus that occupies less than half of the cytoplasm. Some large monocyte-derived cells are similar in size, although they often have larger nuclei. Other large cells (15 to 25 μm in diameter) that have nuclei filling most of the cytoplasm are the transformed lymphocytes or lymphoblasts (Fig. 41–9; see Color Plate at the front of this volume). Both the lining cells and lymphoblasts often have prominent nucleoli. Mononuclear cells in joint fluid can now also be classified by monoclonal antibodies, and there are preliminary suggestions that this may be helpful in diagnosis.[39] The percentage of PMNs is helpful in distinguishing some diseases (see Table 41–1). Even among noninflammatory fluids, higher percentages of PMNs should raise consideration that one is seeing crystal-associated disease between acute attacks or another low-grade inflammatory disease.[35] Among the inflammatory effusions, lower PMN counts have been seen in early rheumatoid arthritis, SLE, rheumatic fever, scleroderma, and fungal and other chronic infections. Pyknotic (apop-

totic) PMNs are common; their significance has not been studied. Recent studies suggest that drugs may account for some variation in joint fluid differentials, with use of nonsteroidal anti-inflammatory drugs alone being associated with the presence of more lymphocytes in the fluid.[40] Lining cells or large monocytes can be seen to have phagocytized PMNs in a variety of diseases in which there is both exudation of neutrophils and lining cell proliferation. Such cells are common in Reiter's syndrome but are by no means diagnostic (Fig. 41–10). Typical plasma cells with or without Russell's body cytoplasmic inclusions are uncommon but have been suggested to be more common in reactive or psoriatic arthritis,[41] as have cells in mitosis. Mast cells can be seen in rheumatoid arthritis and probably other diseases but require toluidine blue or other special staining. Multinucleated cells can be seen in pigmented villonodular synovitis and multicentric reticulohistiocytosis[42] but also occasionally in rheumatoid arthritis, osteoarthritis, and other states. Dark purple inclusions in phagocytic cells can be from cell debris but also can be clumps of apatite crystals or organisms. Bacteria can occasionally be seen in cells, even with Wright's stain. Urate or CPPD crystals can often be seen in Wright-stained specimens, although the urates are dissolved out of some smears.

Eosinophils are uncommon in differential counts but have been reported after arthrography with just air or contrast medium, in angioedema, in parasitic diseases, in tumors, after radiation, in rheumatoid arthritis, and in hypereosinophilic syndrome, but also occasionally in a variety of other effusions, including infections such as Lyme disease[43] as well as in rheumatic fever. Malignant cells can occasionally be

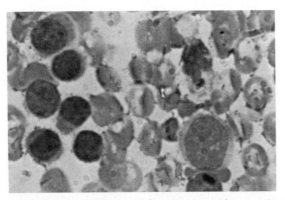

Figure 41–9. Synovial fluid small lymphocytes with one activated lymphocyte, the larger cell with nucleus filling most of the cytoplasm. (See Color Plate.)

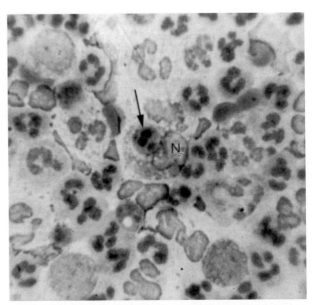

Figure 41–10. "Reiter's cell." This is a phagocytic mononuclear cell with its nucleus marked (N) that has phagocytized a polymorphonuclear leukocyte (arrow) with a pyknotic nucleus.

identified in synovial fluid with Wright's or Papanicolaou's stain or immunocytochemistry.[37, 44]

Smears for Gram's stain are made as for Wright's stain. Bacteria can be quickly classified into broad groups, but mucin and cell debris artifacts can be confusing. The absence of bacteria on Gram's stain is much too common in infection and does not exclude the possibility of a septic joint. Kinyoun carbolfuchsin stain may be helpful in evaluation of possible tuberculosis, but culture and synovial biopsy are often needed. Periodic acid–Schiff (PAS) staining may show deposits in synovial macrophages in Whipple's disease. Prussian blue staining can identify iron in synovial lining cells in pigmented villonodular synovitis or in hemochromatosis.

Special Tests

Mucin Clot Test. The mucin clot test[45] is largely of historical interest. Several drops of synovial fluid are added to about 20 ml of 5 percent acetic acid in a small beaker. Normal or osteoarthritis fluid forms a firm mass that does not fragment on shaking. A poor clot, such as can result from many inflammatory effusions, fragments easily. A poor clot generally indicates both dilution and destruction of hyaluronate protein (see Table 41–1).

Proteoglycans. Actual measurements of hyaluronate or of sulfated glycosaminoglycans presumably derived from cartilage can be made but do not yet convincingly correlate with any clinical findings.[46]

Glucose. If measured, glucose should be analyzed simultaneously on fasting serum and synovial fluid for comparison.[45] Synovial fluid glucose concentration is normally slightly less than that of blood. Equilibration between blood and synovial fluid after a meal is slow and unpredictable, so fasting levels are most reliable. Effusions for glucose should be placed in a fluoride tube to stop glucose metabolism in vitro by the synovial fluid leukocytes. A very low level of glucose in the synovial fluid suggests joint infection. Most effusions in rheumatoid arthritis have a synovial fluid glucose level of less than half that of the blood, and some are as low as in infections.

Complement. Synovial fluid complement is predominantly of value when compared with serum levels and with serum and synovial fluid protein determinations.[47] Fluid must be centrifuged promptly and the supernatant stored at −70°C if total hemolytic complement is to be measured. In rheumatoid arthritis, the serum complement level is usually normal, but the synovial fluid level is often less than 30 percent of this. In SLE and hepatitis, both serum and synovial fluid levels may be low. Synovial fluid complement levels in infectious arthritis, gout, and Reiter's syndrome may be high, but this is largely the result of elevated serum levels. Complement components C3 or C4 can also be measured by immunodiffusion in addition to or instead of hemolytic complement. Measurement of activation fragments such as C5a may be of more interest.[48] Synovial fluid complement level may be low in normal or noninflammatory fluids in which there is little escape of complement or other proteins into the joint space from the circulation.

Cultures. Prompt and careful culture of synovial fluid is important if there is any suspicion of infection. Most laboratories prefer that fluid is delivered immediately in the syringe rather than handled outside the microbiology laboratory. Try to obtain laboratory help in planning cultures needed for fastidious organisms.

Other Tests. Antinuclear antibodies, rheumatoid factor immunoglobulins, and other substances involved in immune reactions can be measured in synovial fluid, but these assays have so far added little to the studies described here. Tests for antinuclear antibodies and latex fixation tests for rheumatoid factor are occasionally positive in effusions when negative in the serum. However, the significance of such positive synovial fluid results is not established. Several causes of false-positive results for rheumatoid factor in synovial fluid have been described.[49] Immune complexes can be measured with a variety of techniques, but the implications are not clear.

Cytokines, their inhibitors, and other mediators can be measured in joint fluid, with patterns of cytokines offering potential for being clinically helpful. Soluble interkeukin-2 receptor levels may parallel disease activity in rheumatoid arthritis.[50]

The pH of normal fluid is 7.4, and this is slightly lower in inflammation.[51] Joint fluid PO_2 also falls in many inflammatory conditions. This tends to correlate with severity of leukocytosis and also with synovial fluid volume, which may lower PO_2 by affecting blood flow to the joint.[52] Relative ischemia may also be a factor in rheumatoid arthritis. Total protein normally averages only 1.7 g/dl, but this level rises with inflammation. Protein levels, however, have not been shown to be of any diagnostic value. Uric acid, electrolytes, and urea nitrogen tend to reflect the serum values. Fibrinogen and its products are normally absent, so normal fluid does not clot on standing. Bence Jones kappa light chains have been demonstrated in amyloid arthropathy secondary to multiple myeloma.

Gas chromatography on synovial fluid has been suggested as an aid in identifying bacterial products in culture-negative infections.[53] Elevated synovial fluid lactic acid measurements have been found in untreated nongonococcal septic arthritis. Succinic acid levels are also elevated in septic arthritis and tend to persist even after treatment. Neither lactic nor succinic acid is specific for infection but may complement other tests for early diagnosis of infectious arthritis. Bacterial antigens can also be sought in synovial fluid by counterimmunoelectrophoresis, and recently developed molecular probes can detect DNA or RNA sequences of a growing list of organisms.[54, 55]

SYNOVIAL BIOPSY AND PATHOLOGY

Biopsy of the synovial membrane should be considered in patients in whom the diagnosis is not clear after clinical evaluation. Synovial fluid analysis should generally be performed before consideration of a biopsy if a synovial effusion can be aspirated. Examination of synovial tissue may be the only way to make a definite diagnosis in some infectious, infiltrative, and deposition diseases of joints, such as granulomatous infections, other difficult-to-culture organisms, such as *Chlamydia* and *Neisseria,* sarcoidosis, osteochondromatosis, the rare synovial leukemia or other malignancy, multicentric reticulohistiocytosis, pigmented villonodular synovitis, hemochromatosis, Whipple's disease, ochronosis, and amyloidosis. Although the diagnosis of gout or pseudogout is best made by joint fluid analysis, occasionally these or other crystals are first found in synovial membrane when joint fluid is absent or not seen to contain crystals.[56]

Synovial membrane findings of villous proliferation, superficial fibrin, marked lining cell increase, focal necrosis, plasma cells, and lymphoid follicles may strongly suggest rheumatoid arthritis but are not specific. In rheumatoid arthritis, as with several other systemic rheumatic diseases, diagnosis is often made by accumulation of criteria. A synovial biopsy showing a definite inflammatory process may help, as, for example, in the previous American Rheumatism Association (ARA) diagnostic criteria.[57] Even if not giving a definite diagnosis, by illustrating the presence or absence of inflammation, synovial biopsy can help guide symptomatic treatment. Synovial fluid findings can help in the same way, but both inflammatory and infiltrative synovial membrane lesions are not infrequently found with noninflammatory effusions.[58] About 35 percent of needle biopsies performed in diagnostic problems are of clinical assistance.[58]

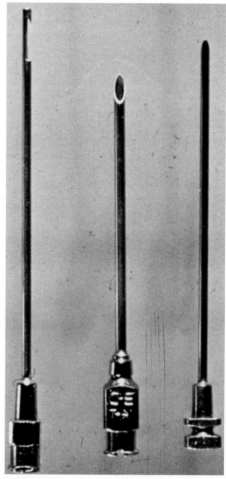

Figure 41–11. Parker-Pearson synovial biopsy needle. The hooked biopsy needle on the left is inserted through the center 14-gauge needle, and tissue is drawn into the notch proximal to the hook by suction.

Methods for Obtaining Synovium

Needle Biopsy. Probably the most popular technique for diagnostic synovial biopsy is use of the 14-gauge Parker-Pearson needle[58] (Fig. 41–11) for closed synovial biopsy. Needle synovial biopsy can be performed in the hospital or in the clinic or office. The knee is by far the most frequent joint to undergo biopsy, but synovial tissue can also be obtained successfully from shoulders, elbows, wrists, ankles, olecranon bursae, and occasionally even smaller joints if they are sufficiently swollen. The route of entry is generally that described for arthrocentesis. The procedure can be performed by a single operator with one assistant. Meperidine is occasionally used for anxious patients; young children may even need general anesthesia.

The biopsy area is widely prepared with soap and then iodine and is washed with alcohol. The operator then dons gloves and places a transparent plastic drape with a 2-inch hole over the biopsy site. The skin and subcutaneous tissue are infiltrated to the capsule with 1 percent lidocaine, using a 25-gauge needle. Caution is exercised to avoid instilling anesthetic into the joint space, which would distort the

findings of the synovial fluid analysis. Next, a 20-gauge needle is passed through the anesthetized area into the joint space. Fluid is aspirated for analysis. Four to 8 ml of 1 percent lidocaine can be instilled into the joint space, but biopsy can also be done without this if it is believed important to avoid any possible artifact that might be introduced by the local anesthetic. As the needle is withdrawn, lidocaine can be infiltrated into the needle track. The trocar is inserted, and the biopsy needle is inserted through it. The side with the hooked notch is approximated against the synovium, and suction is applied with a 20-ml Luer-Lok syringe. The needle is always directed away from the site of initial lidocaine infiltration, to avoid possible artifacts in this area. Five or more specimens (to minimize sampling error) are taken from the various parts of the joint by angling the needle without reinserting the outer needle. Suction is maintained with one hand on the syringe while the other retracts the inner needle through the outer with a slight twist. One must become familiar with the appearance of the specimens, so as not to mistake fibrin or necrotic material (yellow-white) for synovial tissue (pink). Specimens may be transferred carefully from the needle to the fixative on a small piece of sterile paper by a 25-gauge needle.

Patients are instructed to rest the joints until the following day, when they are permitted to resume usual activity, provided there has been no increased pain or swelling. Hemarthrosis and infection are rare complications. To avoid breaking off of needle tips in the joint,[59] care must be taken before biopsy to check that the needle fits easily through the trocar and that the tip is not bent or weakened. Other needles that have been used for synovial biopsy are those of Cope, Williamson and Holt,[63] and Franklin and Silverman.[61]

Other Methods of Synovial Biopsy

Arthroscopy. Arthroscopy has the advantage of identifying discrete localized lesions, which can then undergo biopsy with a needle technique under direct visualization.[62] The procedure is generally limited to larger joints, although thinner arthroscopes can be used in digits (see Chapter 43).

Open Surgical Biopsy. If one is concerned about the possibility of focal granulomas or tumors, deeper lesions such as a vasculitis in larger capsular vessels, or other lesions that might have been missed on needle biopsy, open surgical biopsy can be considered. Surgical biopsy is also useful at small joints not suitable for needle biopsy. A small incision over a metacarpophalangeal joint is effective and offers virtually no morbidity. Open biopsy even of a knee can be done with a small incision. If one wants the advantage of the full joint exploration, however, a large surgical incision and some postoperative immobilization are obviously needed.

Found Fragments of Synovial Membrane. Synovial membrane fragments can occasionally be found floating in joint fluid after arthrocentesis. These can be examined in a wet smear for crystals and can also be collected by centrifugation and fixed for processing as with any biopsy specimen.

Specimens from Previous Procedures. Tissue from a previous carpal tunnel release, meniscectomy, or other exploration may be reviewed and found to contain helpful information. Even clinically uninvolved joints may have significant inflammatory changes in rheumatoid arthritis.[63]

Methods of Handling Tissue

The multiple small pieces of synovium from needle biopsy or the large specimens obtained at operation should be distributed among several methods of handling, depending on the questions being asked. Specimens for routine light microscopy are placed into neutral buffered formalin and embedded in paraffin. Some slides should be stained with hematoxylin and eosin and other tissue saved for consideration of special stains. If gout is a possibility, a portion of the biopsy should be placed in absolute alcohol, since urates are soluble in other fixatives. Specimens then should be stained with DeGolanthal's stain for urate; unstained sections can be examined with compensated polarized light. Frozen sections of unfixed specimens can also be used for polarized light examination for urates.

Immunofluorescent or other immunocytochemical study of synovium on frozen sections has not been of any general clinical value but is of research interest. Studies have suggested that demonstration of prominent extravasated immunoglobulin may favor the diagnosis of rheumatoid arthritis.[64] Detailed characterization of mononuclear cell subsets is under study with suggestions that increased numbers of monocytes may indicate a poorer prognosis in rheumatoid arthritis, for example. Specimens for such study should be placed in OCT compound on a cryostat chuck, which is then quick-frozen by immersion in liquid nitrogen. Such specimens can also be used for molecular and in situ hybridization. This and polymerase chain reaction on frozen unembedded specimens are of increasing value in identification of *Chlamydia, Ureaplasma, Borrelia,* and other difficult-to-identify infections.[65]

Electron microscopy of synovium is also largely of research interest. For example, it can show still unexplained electron-dense deposits in vessel walls in early rheumatoid arthritis[66] and in palindromic rheumatism[64] in the syndrome of hypertrophic pulmonary osteoarthropathy[68] (Fig. 41–12). Of more immediate value, electron microscopy may be a major diagnostic aid in identifying apatite crystals (Fig. 41–13), viruses (including human immunodeficiency virus),[69] small amounts of amyloid, bacilliform bodies of Whipple's disease, chlamydial elementary bodies in Reiter's syndrome,[70] Lyme spirochetes,[71] and Gaucher's cell tubules. Any specimen for electron microscopy should be placed immediately in a fixative such as 3 percent glutaraldehyde or half-strength

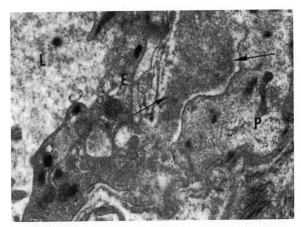

Figure 41–12. Electron-dense deposit *(arrows)* in vessel wall of synovium of patient with rheumatoid arthritis of recent onset. E, vascular endothelium; L, lumen; P, pericyte. Electron micrograph (×16,000).

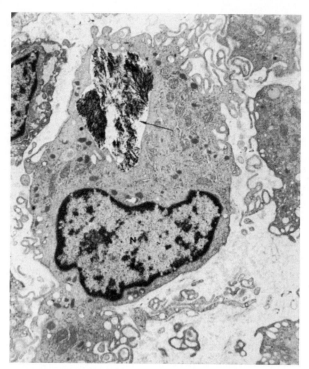

Figure 41–13. Apatite crystals *(arrow)* in vacuole of a synovial lining cell in a patient with osteonecrosis of the knee. N, nucleus of cell. Electron micrograph (×17,000).

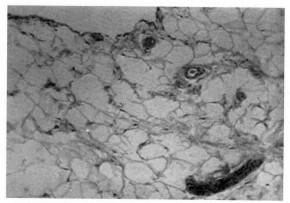

Figure 41–14. Normal synovial membrane of the knee. There is a single layer of flattened synovial cells overlying areolar connective tissue. Note the small synovial vessels immediately under the lining layer and the larger vessel in the lower right corner. (×100, hematoxylin & eosin stain.) (See Color Plate.)

Karnovsky's paraformaldehyde glutaraldehyde. Specimens should be minced into 0.5 × 0.5 mm pieces, ideally fixed for up to 4 hours, and then switched into a buffer before processing. Specimens for research involving immunocytochemical electron or light microscopic studies are best handled by gentle fixation in 2 percent glutaraldehyde for only 1 hour or by quick-freezing, respectively.

Culture of synovial membrane can sometimes be more useful than that of synovial fluid, especially with mycobacteria, fungi, and gonococci. Synovial membrane can also be grown in tissue culture for investigative purposes. Biopsy specimens so designated are placed promptly in tissue culture medium and taken to the laboratory.

Findings on Light Microscopic Examination of Synovial Biopsy Specimens

Normal. Normal synovial membrane (Fig. 41–14; see Color Plate at the front of this volume) consists of one or two layers of synovial lining cells that overlie a richly vascular areolar or fibrous connective tissue. A biopsy specimen that contains several pieces of normal synovium does not absolutely exclude intra-articular disease but should direct the search toward focal disease or extrasynovial processes. Failure to identify a characteristic lesion does not exclude diagnosable diseases. For example, gouty, tuberculous, or ochronotic synovium can show only mild proliferation or changes indistinguishable from those of rheu-

matoid arthritis in tissue adjacent to a tophus, granuloma, or typical pigmented shard.

Rheumatoid Arthritis and Spondyloarthropathies. In rheumatoid arthritis, the combination of villous hypertrophy, lining cell proliferation, infiltration by lymphocytes, and plasma cells (Fig. 41–15; see Color Plate at the front of this volume) with a tendency to form lymphoid nodules, fibrin deposition, and focal necrosis is typical. This is not diagnostic, similar changes being sometimes seen in SLE and other diseases. Especially in rheumatoid arthritis of recent onset, all the aforementioned findings may not be present, and vascular occlusion or mild vasculitis may be especially prominent.[66] Rheumatoid nodules are seen only rarely in synovium. There may be multinucleated giant cells beneath the lining cells. Effects of drugs on findings are just beginning to be studied but must be taken into consideration.[72]

Psoriatic arthritis and ankylosing spondylitis can show synovial changes indistinguishable from those in rheumatoid arthritis; large numbers of plasma cells

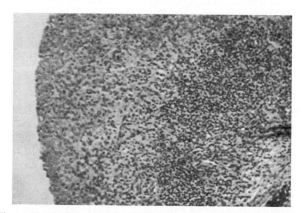

Figure 41–15. Rheumatoid arthritis synovium showing many layers of synovial lining cells on the left and infiltration of lymphocytes and plasma cells on the right. (×100, Hematoxylin & eosin stain.) (See Color Plate.)

are actually more common in spondylitis than in rheumatoid arthritis.[73] Early Reiter's syndrome has a typical superficial vascular congestion and PMN infiltration, which can, however, also be seen in some patients with early rheumatoid arthritis, familial Mediterranean fever, Behçet's disease, enteritis, and other conditions. Synovium from patients with chronic Reiter's syndrome is indistinguishable from that of patients with rheumatoid arthritis.

Collagen-Vascular Diseases. The synovial membrane in SLE typically shows less intense lining cell hyperplasia and less leukocyte infiltration than in rheumatoid arthritis,[74] although inflammation occasionally mimics rheumatoid arthritis. In polyarteritis, synovial inflammation is usually mild, and inflammatory cell infiltration of medium-sized vessel walls is only a rare finding.[75] Early scleroderma[76] shows sparse lining cells, superficial fibrin, and chronic inflammatory cell infiltration (Fig. 41–16; see Color Plate at the front of this volume). Similar findings with paucity of lining cells can be seen also in some patients with SLE, polymyositis, rheumatic fever, and certain infections. In later scleroderma, synovial fibrin and fibrosis predominate.

Infectious Arthritis and Sarcoidosis. Infection is one of the types of joint disease that can be definitively diagnosed by synovial biopsy.[77] In acute bacterial arthritis, clusters or sheets of neutrophils can be seen (Fig. 41–17). Bacteria can sometimes be demonstrated in synovium with a tissue Gram's stain. Culture results may be positive for synovial biopsy specimens when they have been negative for blood and synovial fluid.[78] In chronic or resolving infections, there are often large numbers of lymphocytes and plasma cells.

Chronic infections such as tuberculosis and fungus disease can produce focal lesions that may be missed on limited biopsies. Mycobacterial granulomas in the superficial synovium do not always show caseation (Fig. 41–18; see Color Plate at the front of this volume). Kinyoun stains can show acid-fast organisms. Staining for fungi should be attempted with Grocott-

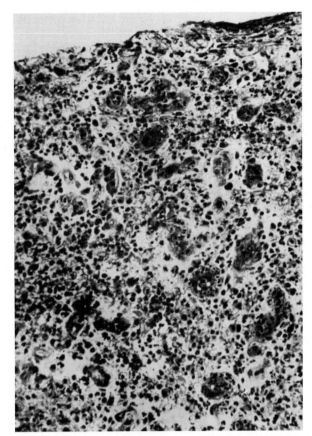

Figure 41–17. Massive infiltration of synovium with neutrophils and some lymphocytes in untreated septic arthritis of 10 days' duration. (×100, Hematoxylin & eosin stain.)

Gomori and Gridley's stains. Spirochetes can be sought in Lyme disease and secondary syphilis with fluorescent and silver stains or with electron microscopy. Monoclonal antibodies and molecular probes can also identify *Chlamydia* and many other organisms.[65, 79] Sarcoidosis can involve the synovium with typical granulomas[80]; other patients, however, especially those with erythema nodosum, more often have

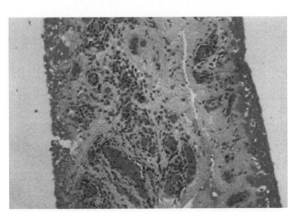

Figure 41–16. Synovial membrane in early scleroderma shows massive superficial fibrin, loss of lining cells, and infiltration with lymphocytes and plasma cells. (×100, Hematoxylin & eosin stain.) (See Color Plate.)

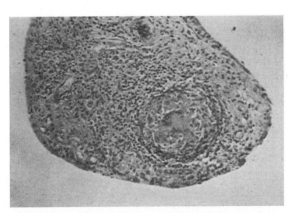

Figure 41–18. Granuloma in superficial synovium in tuberculous arthritis. Some superficial granulomas, such as this one, do not show caseation. There is also scattered chronic inflammatory cell infiltration. (×100, Hematoxylin & eosin stain.) (See Color Plate.)

predominantly periarthritis or only scattered lymphocytes in the synovium.

Infiltrative and Deposition Diseases. Infiltrative and deposition diseases have specific findings that are amenable to diagnosis by synovial biopsy.

Crystal-Induced Arthritis. Both gout and pseudogout often have tophus-like deposits in synovial membrane[81] (Fig. 41–19; see Color Plate at the front of this volume). Precautions for tissue handling to demonstrated urate tophi were described earlier. CPPD crystals are not as soluble but can be dissolved by decalcification in specimens submitted along with bone. Thus, pseudogout synovium occasionally has lucent areas where crystals were lost, as in gout. Usually only a fibrous capsule, a few histiocytes, and giant cells surround the tophi. In acute crystal-induced arthritis, there are areas of neutrophil infiltration; in chronic disease, however, large numbers of lymphocytes and plasma cells can be seen. Clumps of apatite crystals in synovium can appear as hematoxyphilic areas.[82] The tiny crystals that form these clumps are identifiable by electron microscopy. Oxalate crystals have also been found as pleomorphic birefringent bodies in synovial samples from patients undergoing hemodialysis for chronic renal failure.[83]

Amyloidosis. In patients with primary amyloidosis, multiple myeloma, and Waldenström's disease, amyloid may be deposited in the synovium. It appears pink on hematoxylin and eosin stain, and red with Congo red. The Congo red–stained material has an apple-green birefringence when viewed with plain polarized light.[84] Most amyloid has been on the synovial surface (Fig. 41–20; see Color Plate at the front of this volume) and in the interstitium, but rarely in vessel walls. Synovial amyloid deposits can also complicate hemodialysis.[85]

Ochronosis. The synovial membrane in ochronosis is embedded with brownish shards from the friable cartilage[86] (Fig 41–21; see Color Plate at the front of this volume). Macrophages adjacent to the cartilage fragments often contain pigment granules. Clusters of lymphocytes can be seen and can also be found in

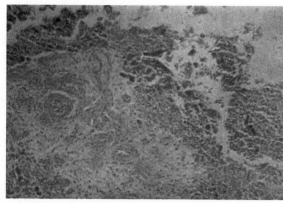

Figure 41–20. Amyloid arthritis as seen here in a patient with multiple myeloma is characterized by Congo red staining on the surface and sparing of the synovial vessels (V). (×100, Congo red stain.) (See Color Plate.)

areas of synovium in other patients with cartilage degeneration, such as in primary or secondary osteoarthritis. Cartilage and bone fragments without the ochronotic pigment can also be seen embedded in synovium in osteoarthritis, rheumatoid arthritis, and other destructive arthropathies.[87]

Hemochromatosis. Golden brown hemosiderin pigment deposition in synovial lining cells and, to a lesser degree, in deeper phagocytes is characteristic of hemochromatosis[88] and other diseases with systemic iron overload. Iron in synovium from bleeding into the joint space or extravasation or erythrocytes into tissue produces hemosiderin, mainly in deep macrophages. Iron stains blue with Prussian blue for confirmation (Fig. 41–22; see Color Plate at the front of this volume). CPPD crystals can be seen in these synovial samples as well as in several other metabolic joint diseases.

Tumors. A variety of benign and malignant tumors

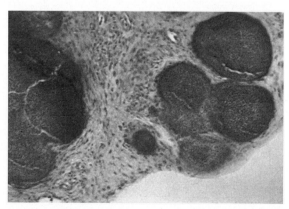

Figure 41–19. Tophus-like deposits in synovium containing positively birefringent crystals in pseudogout. (×100, Hematoxylin & eosin stain.) (See Color Plate.)

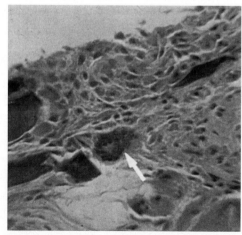

Figure 41–21. Dark, angular cartilage shards pigmented brown with homogentisic acid polymer are embedded in ochronotic synovium. Note also a giant cell (*arrow*) and mild proliferation of synovial lining cells. (×400, Hematoxylin & eosin stain.) (See Color Plate.)

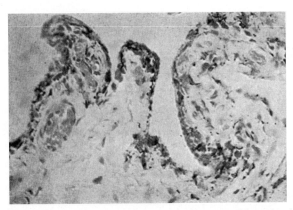

Figure 41–22. Iron stain of synovial membrane in idiopathic hemochromatosis shows blue (dark) staining predominantly in the lining cells. (×100, Prussian blue stain.) (See Color Plate.)

or tumor-like conditions can involve the synovial membrane. Metastatic malignancies are occasionally identified in synovium.[89] Blast forms or overt lymphomatous cells have been found infiltrating synovium in a few, but by no means all, patients with leukemia or lymphoma and arthritis.[90] Monoclonal populations can be established by T cell receptor gene rearrangement analysis.[91] Malignant synovioma is an extra-articular tumor that is rarely seen in joint synovium. Osteochondromas that develop in synovium can be seen as foci of metaplasia to bone and chondrometaplasia in the synovial connective tissue. Pigmented villonodular synovitis, generally involving a single joint or tendon sheath, is characterized by giant cells, foamy cells, and hemosiderin deposits predominantly in the deep synovium (Fig. 41–23; see Color Plate at the front of this volume). There is villous or nodular proliferation with areas also showing some lymphocytes and plasma cells.

Other Diseases. *Multicentric reticulohistiocytosis*[92] shows extensive infiltration of synovium with large

foamy cells or multinucleated cells with eosinophilic ground-glass cytoplasm. *Whipple's disease* synovial membrane often shows just mild lining cell hyperplasia and scattered lymphocytes and neutrophils, but PAS-positive macrophages can be seen in some cases to suggest the diagnosis.[93] Electron microscopy can show suggestions of bacilliform bodies and PCR can confirm the presence of *Trophyrema whipelli*.[94] Despite large painful effusions, early *hypertrophic osteoarthropathy* tends to have virtually no inflammatory cell infiltration in synovium but marked vascular congestion.[68] In chronic hypertrophic osteoarthropathy, infiltration is reported. *Scurvy* of the synovium shows edema, estravasation of erythrocytes, and large fibrocytes that have been unable to release their collagen precursors because of the lack of vitamin C.[95] A *familial arthropathy* with synovial coating with fibrin-like material and giant cells has been described in children.[96] Synovium in *sickle cell disease* can show obliterated vessels and occasionally some lymphocyte and plasma cell infiltration.[97]

Exogenous particles such as thorns or animal spines can occasionally penetrate into joints and be visible in biopsy specimens; they can also produce a chronic synovitis.[98] Lead particles from bullets have been identified in joints. Metallic or silicone prosthetic particles or polymethacrylate cement is also commonly found embedded in synovium of patients with joint arthroplasties or prosthetic ligaments.[99, 100]

Synovial fat necrosis and lipid-laden macrophages can be associated with *pancreatic disease*.[101] Rare, unexpected new findings occasionally are encountered if biopsy is done in undiagnosed cases. For example, an eosinophilic infiltration with fibrin deposition was found in a patient later determined to have the *hypereosinophilic syndrome*.[102]

Summary

Synovial biopsy specimens obtainable by a variety of mechanisms can give specific diagnoses in some diseases or can provide additional criteria to support diagnoses in other situations. Current studies of synovium are providing important ideas about pathogenesis and therapy. Careful consideration of the questions to be asked before performing a diagnostic biopsy allows optimal handling of the tissue.[103]

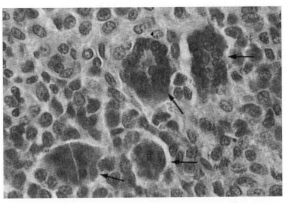

Figure 41–23. Pigmented villonodular synovitis is characterized by golden brown hemosiderin in deep macrophages, giant cells *(arrows)*, monotonous proliferation of deep cells with pale nuclei, and, not illustrated here, foam cells, lining cell hyperplasia (dark), and villous proliferation. (×400, Hematoxylin & eosin stain.) (See Color Plate.) (Courtesy of Schumacher HR: Semin Arthritis Rheum 12:32, 1982.)

References

Synovial Fluid Analysis

1. Schumacher HR, Reginato AJ: Atlas of Synovial Fluid Analysis and Crystal Identification. Philadelphia, Lea & Febiger, 1991.
2. Gatter RA, Schumacher HR: A Practical Handbook of Joint Fluid Analysis, 2nd ed. Philadelphia, Lea & Febiger, 1991.
3. Bomalaski JS, Lluberas G, Schumacher HR: Monosodium urate crystals in the knee joints of patients with asymptomatic nontophaceous gout. Arthritis Rheum 29:1480, 1986.
4. Eisenberg JM, Schumacher HR, Davidson PK, Kaufmann L: Usefulness of synovial fluid analysis in the evaluation of joint effusions. Arch Intern Med 144: 715, 1984.

5. Schumacher HR, Sieck MS, Rothfuss S, Clayburne GM, Baumgarten DF, Mochan BS, Kant JA: Reproducibility of synovial fluid analysis: A study among 4 laboratories. Arthritis Rheum 29:770, 1986.
6. Schumacher HR, Sieck MS, Clayburne G: Development and evaluation of a method for presentation of synovial fluid wet preparations for quality control testing of crystal identification. J Rheumatol 17:1369, 1990.
7. Kerolus G, Clayburne G, Schumacher HR: Is it mandatory to examine synovial fluids promptly after arthrocentesis? Arthritis Rheum 32:271, 1989.
8. Hasselbacher P: Measuring synovial fluid viscosity with a white blood cell diluting pipette. Arthritis Rheum 19:1358, 1978.
9. Palmer DG: Total leukocyte enumeration in pathologic synovial fluids. Am J Clin Pathol 49:812, 1968.
10. Hunter T, Gordon DA, Ogryzlo MA: The ground pepper sign of synovial fluid: A new diagnostic feature of ochronosis. J Rheumatol 1:45, 1974.
11. Kitridou R, Schumacher HR, Sbarbaro JL, Hollander JL: Recurrent hemarthrosis after prosthetic knee arthroplasty: Identification of metal particles in the synovial fluid. Arthritis Rheum 12:520, 1969.
12. Hollander JL, McCarthy DJ, Rawson AJ: The "RA cell," "ragocyte," or "inclusion body cell." Bull Rheum Dis 16:382, 1965.
13. Mann D, Schumacher HR: Pseudoseptic inflammatory knee effusion caused by phagocytosis of sickled erythrocytes after fracture into the knee joint. Arthritis Rheum 38:284, 1995.
14. Waggett AD, Kielty CM, Shuttleworth AC: Microfibrillar elements in the synovial joint: Presence of type VI collagen and fibrillin-containing microfibrils. Ann Rheum Dis 52:449, 1993.
15. Cheung HS, Ryan LM, Kozin F, McCarthy DJ: Identification of collagen subtypes in synovial fluid sediments from arthritic patients. Am J Med 68:73, 1980.
16. Schumacher HR, Holdsworth DE: Ochronotic arthropathy. I: Clinico-pathologic studies. Semin Arthritis Rheum 6:207, 1977.
17. Weinberg A, Schumacher HR: Experimental joint trauma: Synovial response to blunt trauma and inflammatory response to intraarticular injection of fat. J Rheumatol 8:380, 1981.
18. Gibson T, Schumacher HR, Pascual E, Brighton C: Arthropathy, skin and bone lesions in pancreatic disease. J Rheumatol 2:7, 1975.
19. Lawrence C, Seife B: Bone marrow in joint fluid: A clue to fracture. Ann Intern Med 74:740, 1971.
20. Gordon OA, Pruzanski W, Orgyzlo MA: Synovial fluid examination from the diagnosis of amyloidosis. Ann Rheum Dis 32:428, 1973.
21. Schumacher HR, Somlyo AP, Tse RL, Maurer K: Apatite crystal–associated arthritis. Ann Intern Med 87:411, 1977.
22. Paul H, Reginato AJ, Schumacher HR: Alizarin red S staining as a screening test to detect calcium compounds in synovial fluid. Arthritis Rheum 26:191, 1983.
23. Reginato AJ, Kurnik BRC: Calcium oxalate and other crystals associated with kidney disease and arthritis. Semin Arthritis Rheum 18:198, 1989.
24. Phelps P, Steele AD, McCarthy DJ: Compensated polarized light microscopy. JAMA 203:508, 1968.
25. Gatter RA: Use of the compensated polarized microscope. Clin Rheum Dis 3:91, 1977.
26. Kahn CB, Hollander JL, Schumacher HR: Corticosteroid crystals in synovial fluid. JAMA 211:807, 1970.
27. Zuckner J, Uddin J, Gantner G, Dorner RW: Cholesterol crystals in synovial fluid. Ann Intern Med 60:436, 1964.
28. Trostle DC, Schumacher HR, Medsger TA, Kappor WN: Lipid microspherule-associated acute monarticular arthritis. Arthritis Rheum 29:1166, 1986.
29. Gaucher A, Faure G, Netter P, Pourel J, Ducheille J: Identification des cristaux observes dans les arthropathies destructices de la chondrocalcinose. Rev Rheumatol 44:407, 1977.
30. Schumacher HR: Intracellular crystals in synovial fluid anticoagulated with oxalate. N Engl J Med 274:1372, 1966.
31. Tanphaichitr K, Spielberg I, Hahn B: Lithium heparin crystals simulating calcium pyrophosphate dihydrate crystals in synovial fluid (letter). Arthritis Rheum 19:966, 1976.
32. Fagan TJ, Lidsky MD: Compensated polarized light microscopy using cellophane adhesive tape. Arthritis Rheum 17:256, 1974.
33. McCarthy DJ, Hollander JL: Identification of urate crystals in gouty synovial fluid. Ann Rheumatol 54:452, 1961.
34. Honig S, Gorevic P, Hoffstein S, Weissman G: Crystal deposition disease: Diagnosis by electron microscopy. Am J Med 63:161, 1977.
35. Louthrenoo W, Sieck M, Clayburne G, et al: Supravital staining of cells in non-inflammatory synovial fluids. J Rheumatol 18:409, 1991.
36. Traycoff RB, Pascual E, Schumacher HR: Mononuclear cells in human synovial fluid: Identification of lymphoblasts in rheumatoid arthritis. Arthritis Rheum 19:743, 1976.
37. Villanueva TG, Schumacher HR: Cytologic examination of synovial fluid. Diagn Cytopathol 3:141, 1987.
38. Ijich S, Matsuda T, Maruyama I, et al: Arthritis in a human T lymphotrophic virus type I (HTLV-I) carrier. Ann Rheum Dis 49:718, 1990.
39. Poulter LW, Ai-Shakarchi HAA, Campbell FDR, Goldstein AJ, Richardson AT: Immunocytology of synovial fluid cells may be of diagnostic and prognostic value in arthritis. Ann Rheum Dis 45:584, 1986.
40. Bahremand M, Schumacher HR: Effect of medication on synovial fluid leukocyte differentials in patients with rheumatoid arthritis. Arthritis Rheum 34:1173, 1991.
41. Freemont AJ, Denton J, Chuck A, et al: Diagnostic value of synovial microscopy: A reassessment and rationalization. Ann Rheum Dis 50:101, 1991.
42. Samaan SS, Schumacher HR, Villanueva T, Levin R, Atkinson BF: Unusual immunocytochemical and ultrastructural features of synovial fluid cells in multicentric reticulohistiocytosis. Acta Cytol 38:582, 1994.
43. Kay J, Eichenfield A, Arthreya B, et al: Synovial fluid eosinophilia in Lyme disease. Arthritis Rheum 31:1384, 1988.
44. Fam AG, Voornevelt C, Robinson JB, et al: Synovial fluid immunocytology in the diagnosis of leukemic synovitis. J Rheumatol 18:293, 1991.
45. Ropes MM, Bauer W: Synovial Fluid Changes in Joint Disease. Cambridge, Mass, Harvard University Press, 1953.
46. Silverman B, Cawston TE, Page Thomas DP, et al: The sulfated glycosaminoglycan levels in synovial fluid aspirates in patients with acute and chronic joint disease. Br J Rheumatol 29:340, 1990.
47. Bunch TW, Hunder GG, McDiffie FC, O'Brien PC, Markowtiz H: Synovial fluid complement determination as a diagnostic aid in inflammatory joint disease. Mayo Clin Proc 49:715, 1974.
48. Jose PJ, Moss IK, Maini RN, Williams TJ: Measurement of the chemotactic complement fragment C5a in rheumatoid synovial fluids by radioimmunoassay: Role of C5a in the acute inflammatory phase. Ann Rheum Dis 49:747, 1990.
49. Seward CW, Osterland CK: The pattern of anti-immunoglobulin activities in serum, pleural and synovial fluids. J Lab Clin Med 81:230, 1973.
50. Moisse CP, Elhamiani M, Edmonds-Alt X: Functional studies of soluble low-affinity interleukin-2 receptors in rheumatoid synovial fluid. Arthritis Rheum 33:1688, 1990.
51. Ward TT: Acidosis of synovial fluid correlates with synovial fluid leukocytosis. Am J Med 64:933, 1978.
52. Richman AL, Su EY, Ho G: Reciprocal relationship of synovial fluid volume and oxygen tension. Arthritis Rheum 24:701, 1981.
53. Borenstein DG, Gibbs CA, Jacobs RB: Gas–liquid chromatographic analysis of synovial fluid. Arthritis Rheum 25:947, 1982.
54. Rahman MU, Cheema MA, Schumacher HR, Hudson AP: Molecular evidence for the presence of Chlamydia in the synovium of patients with Reiter's syndrome. Arthritis Rheum 35:521, 1992.
55. Vitanen AM, Arstila TP, Lahesmaa R, et al: Application of the polymerase chain reaction and immunofluorescence techniques to the detection of bacteria in Yersinia-triggered reactive arthritis. Arthritis Rheum 34:89, 1991.

Synovial Biopsy and Pathology

56. Agudelo C, Schumacher HR: The synovitis of acute gouty arthritis. Hum Pathol 4:265, 1973.
57. Ropes MW, Bennett GA, Cobbs S, et al: 1958 revision of diagnostic criteria for rheumatoid arthritis. Arthritis Rheum 2:16, 1959.
58. Schumacher HR, Kulka JP: Needle biopsy of the synovial membrane: Experience with the Parker-Pearson technique. N Engl J Med 286:416, 1972.
59. Bocanerga TS, McClelland JJ, Germain BF, et al: Intraarticular fragmentation of a new Parker-Pearson synovial biopsy needle. J Rheumatol 7:248, 1980.
60. Williamson N, Holt LPT: A synovial biopsy needle. Lancet 1:799, 1966.
61. Moon MS, Kim JM: Synovial biopsy by Franklin-Silverman needle. Clin Orthop 150:224, 1980.
62. Moreland LW, Calvo-Alen J, Koopman WJ: Synovial biopsy of the knee joint under direct visualization by needle arthroscopy. J Clin Rheumatol 1:103, 1995.
63. Soden M, Rooney M, Cullen A, et al: Immunohistologic features in the synovium obtained from clinically uninvolved knee joints of patients with rheumatoid arthritis. Br J Rheumatol 28:287, 1989.
64. Fritz P, Laschner W, Saal JG, et al: Histological classification of synovitis. Zentralblatt Algemeine Pathol Anat 135:729, 1989.
65. Beutler AM, Schumacher HR, Whittum-Hudson JA, et al: In situ hybridization for detection of inapparent infection with Chlamydia trachomatis in synovial tissue of a patient with Reiter's syndrome. Am J Med Sci 310:206, 1995.
66. Schumacher HR, Bautista BB, Krauser RE, Mathur AK, Gall EP: Histological appearance of the synovium in early rheumatoid arthritis. Semin Arthritis Rheum 23:3, 1994.
67. Schumacher HR: Palindromic onset of rheumatoid arthritis: Clinical synovial fluid and biopsy studies. Arthritis Rheum 25:361, 1982.
68. Schumacher HR: The articular manifestations of hypertrophic pulmonary osteoarthropathy in bronchogenic carcinoma. Arthritis Rheum 19:629, 1876.
69. Bentin J, Feremans W, Pasteels JL, et al: Chronic acquired immunodefi-

ciency syndrome–associated arthritis: A synovial ultrastructural study. Arthritis Rheum 33: 268, 1990.

70. Schumacher HR, Magge S, Cherian PV, et al: Light and electron microscopic studies on the synovial membrane in Reiter's syndrome. Arthritis Rheum 31:937, 1988.

71. Valesova M, Tranvsky K, Hulinska D, et al: Detection of *Borrelia* in the synovial tissue from a patient with Lyme borreliosis by electron microscopy. J Rheumatol 16:1502, 1989.

72. Haraoui B, Pelletier JP, Clouther JM, et al: Synovial membrane histology and immunopathology in rheumatoid arthritis and osteoarthritis: In vivo effects of antirheumatic drugs. Arthritis Rheum 34:153, 1991.

73. Chang CP, Schumacher HR: Light and electron microscopic observations in the synovitis of ankylosing spondylitis. Semin Arthritis Rheum 22:54, 1992.

74. Labowitz R, Schumacher HR: Articular manifestations of SLE. Ann Intern Med 74:911, 1974.

75. Smuckler NM, Schumacher HR: Chronic non-destructive arthritis associated with cutaneous polyarteritis. Arthritis Rheum 20:1114, 1977.

76. Schumacher HR: Joint involvement in progressive systemic sclerosis (scleroderma). Am J Clin Pathol 60:593, 1973.

77. Schumacher HR: Joint pathology in infectious arthritis. Clin Rheum Dis 4:33, 1978.

78. Wofsy D: Culture-negative septic arthritis and bacterial endocarditis: Diagnosis by synovial biopsy. Arthritis Rheum 23:605, 1980.

79. Espinoza LR, Aguilar JL, Espinoza CG, et al: HIV-associated arthropathy—HIV demonstration in the synovial membrane. J Rheumatol 17:1195, 1990.

80. Sokoloff L, Bunim JJ: Clinical and pathological studies of joint involvement in sacroidosis. N Engl J Med 260:841, 1959.

81. Beutler A, Rothfuss, Clayburne G, Sieck M, Schumacher HR: Calcium pyrophosphate dihydrate crystal deposition in synovium: Relationship to collagen fibers and chondrometaplasia. Arthritis Rheum 36:704, 1993.

82. Reginato AJ, Schumacher HR: Synovial calcification in a patient with collagen–vascular disease: Light and electron microscopic studies. J Rheumatol 4:261, 1977.

83. Hoffman GS, Schumacher HR, Paul H, et al: Calcium oxalate microcrystalline–associated arthritis in end-stage renal disease. Ann Intern Med 97:36, 1982.

84. Canoso JJ, Cohen AS: Rheumatological aspects of amyloid disease. Clin Rheum Dis 1:149, 1975.

85. Bardin T, Kuntz D, Zingraff J, et al: Synovial amyloidosis in patients undergoing long-term hemodialysis. Arthritis Rheum 28:1052, 1985.

86. Schumacher HR, Holdsworth DE: Ochronotic arthropathy. Semin Arthritis Rheum 6:207, 1977.

87. Resnick D, Weisman M, Goergan TG, Feldman PS: Osteolysis with detritic synovitis. Arch Intern Med 138:1003, 1978.

88. Schumacher HR: Ultrastructural characteristics of the synovial membrane in idiopathic hemochromatosis. Ann Rheum Dis 31:465, 1972.

89. Goldenberg DL, Kelley W, Gibbons RB: Metastatic adenocarcinoma of synovium presenting as an acute arthritis. Arthritis Rheum 18:107, 1975.

90. Spilberg I, Myer GJ: The arthritis of leukemia. Arthritis Rheum 15:630, 1972.

91. Yancey WB, Dolson LH, Oblon D, et al: HTLV-1 associated T-cell leukemia/lymphoma presenting with nodular synovial masses. Am J Med 89:676, 1990.

92. Krey PR, Comerford FR, Cohen AS: Multicentric reticulo-histiocytosis. Arthritis Rheum 17:615, 1974.

93. Delcambre B, Luez J, Leonardelli J, et al: Les manifestations articulaires de la maladie de Whipple. Semin Hop Paris 50:847, 1974.

94. Rubinow A, Canoso JJ, Goldenberg DL, Cohen AS: Synovial fluid and synovial membrane pathology in Whipple's disease. Arthritis Rheum 19:820, 1976.

95. Bevilaqua FA, Hasselbacher P, Schumacher HR: Scurvy and hemarthrosis. JAMA 235:1874, 1976.

96. Athreya B, Schumacher HR: Pathologic features of a recently recognized form of familial arthropathy. Arthritis Rheum 21:429, 1978.

97. Schumacher HR: Rheumatological manifestations of sickle cell disease and other hereditary hemoglobinopathies. Clin Rheum Dis 1:37, 1975.

98. Reginato AJ, Ferreiro JL, O'Connor OR, et al: Clinical and pathologic studies of 26 patients with penetrating foreign body injury to the joints, bursae and tendon sheaths. Arthritis Rheum 33:1753, 1990.

99. Kitridou RC, Schumacher HR, Sbarbaro JL, Hollander JL: Recurrent hemarthrosis after knee arthroplasty. Arthritis Rheum 12:520, 1969.

100. Christie AJ, Pierre G, and Levitan J: Silicon synovitis. Semin Arthritis Rheum 19:166, 1989.

101. Smuckler NM, Schumacher HR, Pascual E, et al: Synovial fat necrosis associated with ischemic pancreatic disease. Arthritis Rheum 22:547, 1979.

102. Brogadir SP, Goldwein MI, Schumacher HR: A hypereosinophilic syndrome mimicking rheumatoid arthritis. Am J Med 69:799, 1980.

103. Schumacher HR: Exploring the synovium in 1990. Br J Rheumatol 29:3, 1990.

CHAPTER 42

Imaging

Donald Resnick
Joseph S. Yu
David Sartoris

The routine radiographic examination is a keystone in the diagnosis and management of the patient with articular disease. In some patients, the diagnosis may initially be suggested by standard radiographic films, whereas in other patients with a known clinical diagnosis, the extent and the severity of the disease process may be documented by such techniques. Furthermore, serial radiographic examinations provide evidence of the therapeutic response of the disease process. In this chapter, we discuss routine radiographic techniques and additional imaging methods, cardinal roentgen signs of articular disease, and the radiographic findings at specific "target" areas of the major articular disorders. Because the major advances in imaging of musculoskeletal disorders since the late 1980s have involved computed tomography (CT) and magnetic resonance (MR) techniques, these two methods are emphasized in this chapter.

IMAGING TECHNIQUES AND METHODS

Plain Film Examination

Appropriately selected plain films form the initial step in the radiographic evaluation of the articular disease. The choice of radiographic projections for each anatomic area is a decision that deserves careful consideration. The need for a comprehensive examination to document the extent and configuration of the disease process must be balanced with the consideration of expense, comfort, and radiation exposure to the patient, who may be expected to have numerous radiation examinations over many years.

In most instances, multiple radiographic projections of a number of joints are indicated. Table 42–1 lists the suggested radiographic projections for the optimal evaluation of specific anatomic areas. In the patient with monoarticular or pauciarticular disease, such a protocol may be followed closely. In the patient with polyarticular disease, however, obtaining the numerous radiographic views listed in Table 42–1 would be considered excessive in almost all instances. In these patients, the initial radiographic examination should be individually tailored to as great an extent as possible.

A "tailored" arthritis series is useful in those patients with polyarthritis who have either a known or a highly likely clinical diagnosis. In this setting, plain films are selected that optimally show the major target

areas of the disease as well as additional areas of clinical significance. For example, the patient with rheumatoid arthritis requires careful radiographic evaluation of the hands, wrists, feet, knees, shoulders, and cervical spine, whereas the patient with calcium pyrophosphate dihydrate (CPPD) crystal deposition disease usually requires analysis of only the hands, wrists, knees, and symphysis pubis.

The situation often arises in which a patient has polyarthritis without a specific clinical diagnosis. In this instance, a so-called standard arthritis series is useful; projections are selected to provide adequate visualization of a large number of major target areas with a minimum of radiation exposure. A suggested standard arthritis series, consisting of 15 radiographs, is listed in Table 42–2.

The follow-up radiographic examination obtained during the course of treatment need not be as extensive as the initial survey. In many instances, it can be limited to a few symptomatic areas or areas where unsuspected progression of disease may lead to catastrophic consequences, such as the cervical spine in patients with rheumatoid arthritis.

Use of intensifying screen in a radiographic film cassette combined with double-emulsion radiographic film allows formation of a radiographic image with considerably less radiation exposure to the patient. A small decrease in radiographic resolution is the price paid for this considerable diminution in radiation exposure. Occasionally, however, in evaluating diseases such as rheumatoid arthritis, osteomyelitis, septic arthritis, or hyperparathyroidism, greater resolution may be important in establishing a diagnosis at an early stage.[1-3] In these instances, increased radiation exposure to a relatively radioresistant area of the body, such as the hand, the wrist, or the foot, may be acceptable for the important diagnostic information that is obtained. With virtually any radiographic unit, use of single-emulsion film and a nonscreen vacuum-packed cassette, referred to as the *mammographic technique*, allows high-resolution images to be obtained. Furthermore, optical or radiographic magnification can be extremely helpful. With the magnification technique, images may be obtained using microfocal spot radiographic tubes, such as those present on many angiographic units, or specially designed magnification units. It should be emphasized that these are specialized techniques and should be used only in selected clinical situations.

Radiographs of an articulation obtained during

Table 42–1. RADIOGRAPHIC PROJECTIONS

Hand	Posteroanterior, obliques
Wrist	Posteroanterior, obliques, lateral
Elbow	Anteroposterior, lateral
Shoulder	Anteroposterior with internal rotation of the humerus, anteroposterior with external rotation of the humerus
Foot	Anteroposterior, obliques, lateral (including calcaneus)
Ankle	Anteroposterior, lateral
Knee	Anteroposterior, lateral, anteroposterior in semiflexion ("tunnel"), axial patellar ("sunrise")
Hip	Anteroposterior of pelvis, anteroposterior of hip with internal rotation of leg, anteroposterior of hip with external rotation of leg ("frog leg")
Sacroiliac joint	Anteroposterior, anteroposterior with 30 degrees cephalic angulation of central ray
Lumbar spine	Anteroposterior, obliques, lateral, lateral coned down to L5–S1
Thoracic spine	Anteroposterior, lateral
Cervical spine	Anteroposterior, obliques, lateral with neck in flexion, lateral with neck in extension, "open-mouth" odontoid view

weight bearing or the application of stress or traction may provide valuable supplemental information to the plain-film radiographic examination. Weight-bearing views of the knees are especially valuable in the evaluation of patients with osteoarthritis[4] and may allow a more exact delineation of cartilaginous loss as well as abnormal varus or valgus angulation of the joint. Stress radiographs may be used to assess soft tissue and bony stability following injury to the knee, ankle, acromioclavicular joint, or first metacarpophalangeal joint.[5] Upright lateral radiographs of the lumbar spine obtained after prolonged standing may accentuate bony neural arch defects (spondylolysis) or intervertebral slippage (spondylolisthesis). Radiographs of the pelvis obtained with the patient standing on one leg at a time may demonstrate instability of the sacroiliac joint or symphysis pubis.[6]

Radiographs obtained during application of traction across a joint also may prove useful in selected circumstances. Demonstration of subtle transchondral fractures in osteonecrosis of the femoral head may be improved with this technique.[7] Such traction may also stimulate the release of gas, primarily nitrogen, into the joint cavity, an occurrence that usually will rule out the presence of a joint effusion, and allows visual-

Table 42–2. ARTHRITIS SURVEY

Area	Projection
Hand and wrist	Posteroanterior, obliques
Foot	Anteroposterior, obliques, lateral
Knee	Anteroposterior, lateral
Pelvis and hips	Anteroposterior
Thorax and shoulders	Anteroposterior
Cervical spine	Lateral with neck in flexion

ization of a portion of the cartilaginous surface. This method is mostly used in children to rule out a septic arthritis.

Conventional Tomography

Conventional tomography can aid both in the identification of subtle abnormalities and in the more precise delineation of previously identified lesions. In some anatomic areas, such as the temporomandibular joint (TMJ) and sternoclavicular and costovertebral articulations, plain radiographs are rarely adequate and conventional tomography is often indicated.

Arthrography and Bursography

Injection of radiopaque contrast material or air, or both into a joint or bursa may be essential in evaluating a number of articular disorders.[8] Contrast arthrography is most often used in the knee and shoulder to identify surgically repairable soft tissue injuries such as meniscal or rotator cuff tears. Aspiration arthrography allows confirmation of suspected joint sepsis; fluoroscopically guided intra-articular needle placement is particularly useful in recovering fluid from deep articulations such as the glenohumeral joint or the hip. Subsequent instillation of a small amount of radiographic contrast agent allows verification that the joint space was entered and may also yield important information concerning the extent of periarticular soft tissue destruction. An important indication for aspiration arthrography is evaluation of the patient with a painful total hip or knee prosthesis to differentiate conclusively between chronic infection and aseptic loosening of the prosthesis.[9] Air arthrography, usually combined with conventional tomography, often is of great value in the identification of transchondral fractures and intra-articular osteocartilaginous bodies. Arthrography also may provide a firm diagnosis in cases of pigmented villonodular synovitis[10] or idiopathic synovial osteochondromatosis.[11] Finally, arthrography can serve as a method of treatment with the "brisement" procedure, or distention arthrography in cases of adhesive capsulitis, in which the articular capsule is progressively distended with a mixture of lidocaine or bupivacaine hydrochloride and steroids until the capsule ruptures or relief of symptoms is obtained.

Bursography has its greatest value in evaluating lesions of the subacromial bursa in the shoulder.[12, 13] In this location, bursitis, intrabursal osteocartilaginous bodies, partial rotator cuff tears, and causes of shoulder impingement may be identified. At the same time, instillation of local anesthetic agents or anti-inflammatory medications directly into the bursa can serve both diagnostic and therapeutic purposes.

Computed Tomography

Introduction and Technical Considerations

In an age in which MR imaging is increasingly being employed, CT remains an excellent investigative tool for musculoskeletal disorders used either alone or in combination with MR. CT permits cross-sectional images to be displayed with excellent structural definition of both soft tissues and bones. In most circumstances, CT scans provide more than sufficient information and obviate any other imaging examination. Nevertheless, significant drawbacks limit its performance. For instance, artifacts caused by the presence of metallic objects greatly diminish image quality. Also, direct images obtainable during CT are generally in the transaxial plane. Although most CT units have software capable of reconstructing original image data in any plane or in three dimensions,[14] sometimes this requires increased patient radiation exposure or an increased examination time, and often results in a significant loss of definition in the reconstructed images.

CT frequently serves as a supplement to conventional imaging techniques. Because different factors often reduce its availability, it is of the utmost importance that clinical and imaging records be reviewed to select the most appropriate examination protocol for any given condition.

Each examination begins with a scout film covering the area of interest. It is important to note that, although CT generally is limited with regard to the initial imaging plane, the patient's body or specific regions of the body can, to some extent, be positioned in such a way that different planes other than transaxial can be produced. As a rule, the more distal the body part to be studied, the greater the number of possible planes that can be obtained. For example, transaxial views are required for the lumbar spine, whereas virtually all planes are obtainable for a hand, elbow, or foot. Positioning of the subject also may be limited by the patient's comfort, physical state, and cooperation.

The next important step relates to the choice of slice thickness and interval. Although slice thickness and interval are included as part of many standard protocols, it is important to tailor these specific aspects of the procedure whenever necessary. The choice depends primarily on the type, size, and location of the lesion, the need for further reformation of the images, the duration of the examination, and the resulting radiation exposure.

CT images are digitalized and depict various structures in terms of different densities on a standard gray scale. The distribution within the range of the gray scale can be modified to enhance soft tissue relationships or bony structures, but not both of these at the same time on one image. Generally, two sets of images are obtained at different "window" levels to optimally show bone and soft tissue structures. The relative densities of all structures are expressed in Hounsfield units (HU). Arbitrarily, gas has the lowest density, at −1000 HU, and bone or metal the highest, at +1000 HU. Water is considered neutral, with a value of 0 HU. CT depicts the shape, structure, content, and above all, the extent of a lesion with a precision far beyond that of any conventional imaging technique. It is possible to rely on the Hounsfield values to predict the nature of a given lesion, including cysts (Fig. 42–1), fat, and calcification; however, density alone should not be regarded as a precise histologic indicator. One must rely on the results of a combination of clinical, laboratory, conventional, and other imaging techniques.

In some specific clinical settings, the simultaneous use of positive or negative contrast material enhances the value of CT. In the musculoskeletal system, this has been most true for spine studies in which intrathecal positive contrast material is used. Because of the invasiveness of and the risks related to the injection of intrathecal iodinated material and the more extensive use of MR, this type of procedure has been used less frequently in the past few years. Nevertheless, injection of positive contrast material into the intrathecal space in combination with CT remains extremely useful in acute or emergency settings when patients cannot undergo an MR examination because of clinical status or because of medical equipment attached to them. Intravenous contrast material is mainly used to characterize soft tissue masses or the vascular status of a given lesion, and positive or negative contrast material (air), or both, is used frequently in articular studies in which it is particularly useful to evaluate the articular surface; to detect intra-articular bodies, such as in primary synovial osteochondromatosis; and to study other articular components. Three-dimensional reconstruction of image data is especially useful in the study of areas of complex anatomy, such as the facial bones, pelvis, spine, and hindfoot. Moreover, it has important applications in trauma, reconstructive surgery, and prosthetic design.[15, 16]

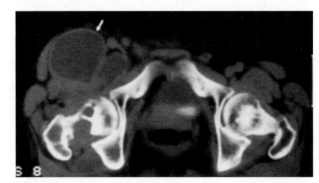

Figure 42–1. Synovial cyst of the hip in a patient with rheumatoid arthritis. Observe the erosion of the femoral head and femoral neck and a large cystic mass (*arrow*) located anterior to the hip.

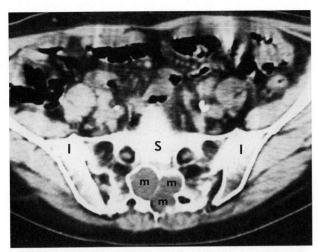

Figure 42–2. Sacral meningoceles. Computed tomography (CT) image of the sacrum demonstrates scalloped erosions from cyst-like structures exiting through the body of the sacrum. S, sacrum; I, ilium; m, meningocele.

Clinical Indications

CT is efficient and practical in studying axial structures such as the spine, pelvis, sacrum (Fig. 42–2), and sacroiliac joints, sternum and sternoclavicular joints, hip, shoulder, hindfoot (Fig. 42–3), and midfoot. The wrist and TMJ are now better studied by MR imaging. Some specific indications and applications of CT scanning are discussed briefly here.

Trauma

CT has its greatest advantage in the evaluation of the acutely traumatized patient, especially when the injury involves axial structures. It allows the identification of fractures and dislocations. It is extremely useful in the investigation of acute spinal trauma[17, 18] and, in that regard, is superior to plain films. Standard CT slices at the suspected level of injury with multiplanar reformatted images will accurately determine the extent of vertebral fractures and provide information on their stability, simultaneous dislocation, cord compression by bone fragments in the spinal canal, and the integrity of posterior elements below and above the injured level.[19–22] In most instances, this information can be obtained rapidly, without significant risk to the patient.

The value of CT also is evident in the analysis of injuries to the pelvis and hip.[23] Pelvic and sacral fractures often are difficult to assess on plain films, whereas CT depicts them and their extent with great precision. Particularly in the evaluation of the acetabulum for femoral head dislocation, loose bodies, and acetabular fragment displacement, CT again is a superior technique.

Helical (spiral) CT is a recent innovation in CT technology that allows the rapid acquisition of volumes of CT data in a time frame of 24 to 32 seconds. It has a wide range of applications and is becoming an invaluable imaging tool for the assessment of skeletal trauma, particularly in difficult structures such as the tibia, acetabulum, sacrum, and spine.[24, 25] Results of a comparison between helical and serial CT data with regard to three-dimensional image reconstruction indicate that data acquired with helical CT are far superior.[26]

Other traumatized articulations also benefit from CT evaluation. The sternum and sternoclavicular joints often are poorly demonstrated by conventional imaging techniques, but CT reveals their anatomy

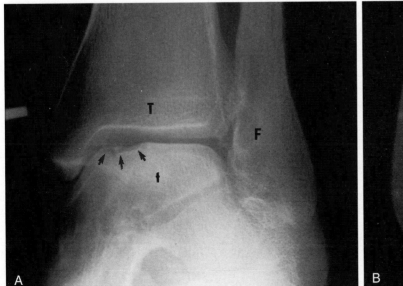
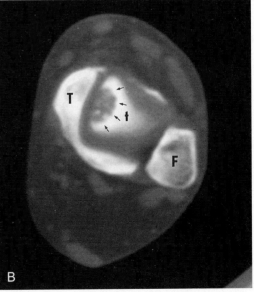

Figure 42–3. Osteochondral defect of the talar dome. *A,* Medial oblique radiograph of the left ankle shows a saucer-shaped defect in the articular surface of the talar dome medially *(arrows). B,* The extent of involvement, outlined by a rim of sclerosis, can be easily demonstrated with CT *(arrows).* T, tibia; F, fibula; t, talus.

with great precision. Furthermore, it has the advantage of providing information about the mediastinum at the same time.[27, 28] The injured glenohumeral joint is much better studied with CT than with plain films. Humeral head dislocation[29] is a frequent diagnosis. Although the diagnosis can be made on plain films, the associated bone injury and cartilaginous injuries are better assessed with CT. The Bankart deformity, a cartilaginous or bone lesion of the inferior glenoid rim cavity, and the Hill-Sachs deformity, an impaction fracture of the posterior aspect of the humeral head at the level of the coracoid process, usually indicate previous anterior glenohumeral dislocation and frequently are not detected when plain films alone are used.[30] An injury involving an occipital condyle may be radiographically occult. Three-dimensional CT images enhance the conspicuousness of the complex anatomic relationships of the craniovertebral junction.[31]

CT is of more limited use in the evaluation of trauma to the foot, hand, or elbow, although this imaging method is widely used for the assessment of calcaneal,[32] talar (Fig. 42–4), and wrist fractures and the presence of loose bodies in the elbow. MR studies have replaced CT for evaluation of traumatic damage to ligaments, articular cartilage, and menisci of the knee.

Infections

CT plays a significant role in the diagnosis of osteomyelitis. Although such a diagnosis still relies on the combination of clinical, scintigraphic, and plain-film findings, CT features characteristic of infection include single or multiple sequestra, delineation of sinus tracts, and rarely, intraosseous (pneumatocysts)[33] or soft tissue gas. Although the presence of gas always is suggestive of infection, gas density in the intervertebral disc and vertebral bodies in disc degeneration and vertebral body osteonecrosis (Kümmell's disease), respectively, are well known. CT also allows the physician to choose the most appropriate site for an eventual biopsy or aspiration.

Bone and Soft Tissue Neoplasms

MR imaging is the preferred technique in the evaluation of tumors; CT, however, remains useful in this setting.[34] CT is able to determine (1) whether the neoplasm is fatty, produces bone or cartilage, or has a nidus surrounded by bone sclerosis (osteoid osteoma) or a fluid level (e.g., cyst, giant cell tumor); or (2) the thickness of the cartilaginous cap of an osteochondroma (the thicker the cap, the more likely the presence of a chondrosarcoma).[35–37] Soft tissue neoplasms are much better studied by MR. MR is quite sensitive but not specific for these neoplasms, whereas CT is neither sensitive nor specific. On the other hand, if the presence of calcified matrix in a soft tissue neoplasm must be evaluated, the use of CT is

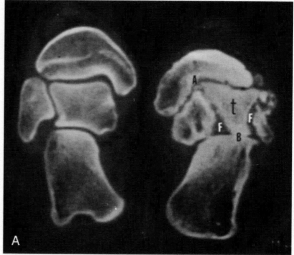

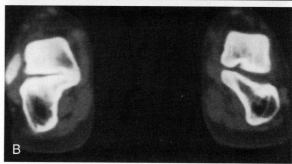

Figure 42–4. Ankle and hindfoot disease. *A,* Degenerative alterations following talar fracture. Articular irregularity and narrowing of the tibiotalar (A) and posterior subtalar (B) joints are evident in the right foot. Multiple persistent fracture lines (F) can be identified within the talus (t), indicative of nonunion. *B,* Talocalcaneal tarsal coalition. A bony bridge extending between the sustentaculum tali of the calcaneus and the middle facet of the talus is indicative of a bony coalition. Compare the appearance with that of the opposite normal side.

still recommended. Finally, CT allows accurate diagnostic biopsy if necessary.

Articular Diseases

Generally, CT is not required for the diagnosis of articular disorders, but in some instances, it may be employed to define the extent of bone involvement in these disorders. This is particularly true in joints that are difficult to assess by conventional imaging techniques, such as apophyseal, costovertebral, sternoclavicular, and temporomandibular joints.

Temporomandibular Joint. Exquisite TMJ anatomic detail can be obtained with CT using high-resolution techniques and multiplanar reconstructed images.[38] Previous studies have shown that CT findings correlate well with arthrographic and surgical abnormalities. CT can demonstrate indirect signs of internal derangement of the TMJ, such as post-traumatic alterations and meniscus dislocation.[39] MR imaging, however, is actually the preferred imaging technique for this articulation. Nevertheless, if MR is not available,

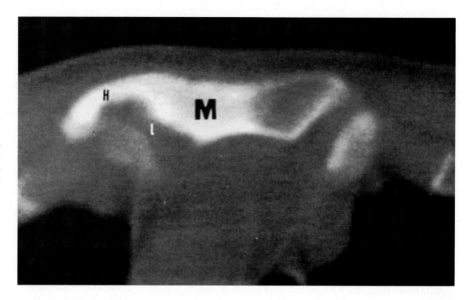

Figure 42–5. In a patient with sterno-costoclavicular hyperostosis, osteosclerosis and irregular articular margins are noted in the manubrium (M), associated with bone proliferation (H) in the soft tissues anterior to the left sternocostoclavicular joint (J).

CT is definitely the best alternative. The examination protocol should include open- and closed-mouth 1.5-mm transaxial contiguous slices, the use of bone and soft tissue window images, and coronal and sagittal reformatted images, although direct sagittal images[40–42] can be obtained with some specialized software. Direct sagittal CT has 92 percent sensitivity and 87 percent accuracy, for a predictive value of 93 percent in the diagnosis of meniscal displacement. Direct sagittal CT allows assessment of the range of motion, osseous abnormalities of the temporal eminentia and the mandibular condyle, joint space narrowing, meniscal configuration, and positional abnormalities without the technical problems and limitations of reconstructing sagittal images from transaxial slices.

Sternoclavicular Joint. The sternoclavicular joint can be affected by a wide variety of pathologic processes, ranging from trauma to inflammatory or neoplastic diseases (Fig. 42–5). CT, compared with conventional imaging techniques, is much less time consuming, is less uncomfortable for the patient, and provides detailed information about the articulation and the surrounding soft tissues. CT remains the preferred examination technique for sternoclavicular joint disorders.[27]

Lumbar Facet Joint. Facet, or zygapophyseal, joints are diarthrodial synovial articulations that can be affected by a wide variety of diseases, including inflammatory and degenerative disorders,[43, 44] trauma, and neoplasms. CT constitutes one of the best imaging modalities to investigate apophyseal joint disorders. Because these joints have varying anatomic orientations at different levels, CT is particularly well suited for their study. Furthermore, if necessary, reformatted sagittal, coronal, or oblique views can be obtained. Standard protocols include nontilted transaxial contiguous 3- to 5-mm slices. Intraspinal synovial cysts,[45, 46] which result from a herniation of the capsule of the apophyseal joint within the spinal canal, are clearly demonstrated by CT. They are seen as homogeneous, low-density posterolateral masses in the spinal canal with or without cord compression. These synovial cysts can contain a certain amount of gas. Synovial cysts have been seen in association with degenerative spondylolisthesis and osteoarthritis involving apophyseal joints with or without radiculopathy. It is important to note that the clinical manifestations of synovial cysts can mimic those of a disc herniation. CT evaluation is important because it enables the correct diagnosis and thus prevents unnecessary exploratory laminectomy. Furthermore, CT-guided intra-articular injection of glucocorticoids may lead to relief of symptoms and cause the cyst to decrease in size. In patients with ankylosing spondylitis[47] and the cauda equina syndrome, careful CT examination of the lumbar posterior elements may reveal multiple scalloped erosions involving the laminae. These result from thecal diverticula (Fig. 42–6).

Sacroiliac Joint. The contribution of CT in the investigation of sacroiliac joint disorders,[48, 49] especially sacroiliitis,[50] has been evaluated in numerous studies. Certain normal CT variants have been established by studying asymptomatic subjects prospectively. These studies showed asymmetry in the sacroiliac joints in 77 percent of asymptomatic subjects over the age of 30 years and in 87 percent of those over 40 years of age. Poor indicators of sacroiliitis consist of nonuniform iliac sclerosis, focal joint space loss, ill-defined areas of subchondral sclerosis (mostly on the iliac side), and vacuum phenomena (indicative of lack of joint effusion). Good indicators of sacroiliitis include increased subchondral sclerosis in patients under 40 years of age, unilateral or bilateral diffuse joint space loss (<2 mm), and erosions and intra-articular ankylosis. The superiority of CT over plain films and tomograms in the study of sacroiliitis is controversial. In most patients with clinical signs of sacroiliitis, high-quality radiographs of the sacroiliac joints are diagnostic. When CT is used, however, it may reveal that the disease is more advanced than had been

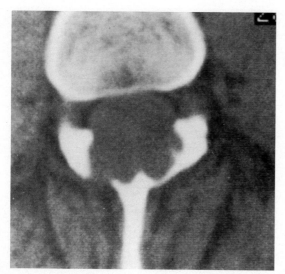

Figure 42–6. Ankylosing spondylitis and thecal diverticula. A CT image of a lumbar vertebra demonstrates scalloped erosions of the posterior elements, diagnostic of thecal diverticula.

suspected. CT also allows aspiration and arthrography of the sacroiliac joint in instances of suspected infection.[51]

Hip. CT plays little diagnostic role in the evaluation of disorders of the hip.[52] Nevertheless, CT still is useful in demonstrating the extent of synovial osteochondromatosis prior to therapy. Although CT had

been widely used to investigate the possibility of osteonecrosis of the femoral head, the emergence of MR imaging, which is a far more sensitive and specific diagnostic method for ischemic necrosis, has led to a decline in the use of CT for this indication.

Glenohumeral Joint. CT, alone or combined with arthrography, is an excellent diagnostic tool for shoulder trauma and specifically for instability of the glenohumeral joint[53, 54] (Fig. 42–7). For the investigation of soft tissue structures such as the rotator cuff, MR is the preferred imaging method.

Knee. MR imaging is better suited than CT[55] to the evaluation of soft tissue structures, and because the most common pathologic processes affecting the knee involve the menisci and ligaments, MR imaging is now the best imaging method for evaluation of a great variety of internal derangements of the knee. CT, however, represents an efficient technique for examination of the femoropatellar articulation, especially when malalignment is suspected. Different CT protocols have been described for the investigation of this problem. Dynamic investigation of this compartment can be accomplished by imaging the knee sequentially at different degrees of knee flexion (e.g., from 0 to 30 degrees of flexion). By reformatting these images, it is then possible to obtain a "cinematic" view of patellofemoral motion and thereby assess the possibility of malalignment during this motion. Some investigators have tried to evaluate the degree of lateral or medial displacement of the patella in relation to the anterior tibial tuberosity. This is done by ob-

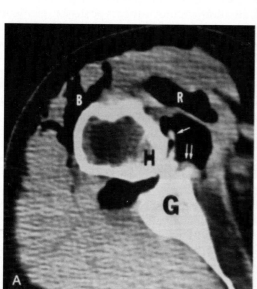
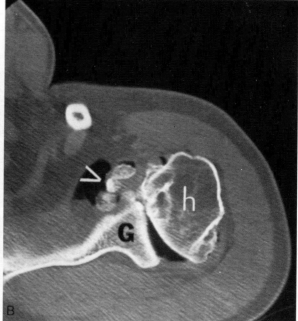

Figure 42–7. Computed air arthrotomography of the shoulder joint. *A,* Following introduction of air into the glenohumeral articulation, communication with the subacromion-subdeltoid bursa (B) is indicative of a full-thickness rotator cuff tear. The anterior portion of the cartilaginous labrum is blunted *(double arrow),* and the anterior capsular recesses (R) appear prominent owing to prior anterior dislocation. An intra-articular osteochondral body *(single arrow)* is also evident. H, humerus. *B,* In another patient, multiple intra-articular osteochondral bodies *(arrowhead)* are demonstrated, along with post-traumatic and degenerative deformity of the humeral head (h). G, glenoid.

taining contiguous 5-mm slices of the knee with the patient lying supine in a neutral position, with a lead marker placed on the anterior tibial tuberosity. Two images are then selected for each knee, one that shows the marker and one that includes both the patella and the femoral condyles. These selected images are then superimposed by a computer to ensure a common relation to the reference frame. It is then possible to measure the actual projection of the femoral groove and the patella in relation to the anterior tibial tuberosity. These measurements are corrected for any imaging magnification. Angles between the patella and the femoral groove also are measured. A more detailed description of this procedure and the normal reference values are available elsewhere.[56, 57]

Miscellaneous Regions and Disorders

Spine. Retrospective review of cervical myelograms and CT scans of patients with cervical radiculopathy secondary to disc herniation or spondylosis has indicated that CT, with or without the use of intrathecal metrizamide, is more accurate in the identification of causative lesions. In certain patients, CT can obviate cervical myelography.[58] Metrizamide CT myelography provides significant information, including improved characterization of the abnormality and lateralization, when the conventional myelogram is indeterminate. In patients with cervical myelopathy, a cross-sectional diameter of the cord equaling less than 50 percent of the subarachnoid space is predictive of poor patient response to surgical intervention.[59]

Unilateral flattening of the cord by a spondylitic mass or bulging disc in a normally wide spinal canal on CT myelography is considered nonspecific, because nerve root signs are contralateral nearly as often as they are ipsilateral to the radiologic findings. Concentric compression of the cord in a narrow canal produces long tract signs only after the cross-sectional area of the cord has been reduced by about 30 percent (to a value of 60 mm^2 or less). Strong correlation exists between the side of disc herniation with occlusion of the corresponding neural foramen and the side of nerve root symptoms. If stenosis of the spinal canal and disc herniation are considered reliable CT myelographic signs of nerve root symptoms, a specific diagnosis can be made in about 40 percent of cases.[60] Posterior displacement of the epidural veins and epidural enhancement following high-dose intravenous contrast administration provide excellent delineation of disc extrusion and may allow demarcation of free fragments. Although noninfusion scans are usually adequate, the improved anatomic information available from infusion CT may increase diagnostic certainty and, in selected cases, makes myelography unnecessary in patients with focal cervical radiculopathy.[61]

Criteria have been established for distinguishing between a herniated nucleus pulposus and a bulging annulus fibrosus by CT. In anatomically or surgically verified cases of bulging annulus, CT reveals generalized extension of the disc border beyond the vertebral body margin. A herniated nucleus pulposus, conversely, exhibits a focal, usually posterolateral, protrusion of the disc margin, which may be calcified.[62] The demonstration of intradiscal gas by CT is virtually diagnostic of degenerative disease (Fig. 42–8), because rarely is gas observed in the setting of infection.[63]

Retrospectively, poor correlation has been found between CT and myelography in the diagnosis of a slightly bulging lumbar disc. A major discrepancy rate of less than 1 percent among patients without prior surgery has been reported, and the two methods agree on definite abnormalities in 70 percent of cases.[64] CT has been shown to demonstrate normal and herniated intervertebral discs as effectively as myelography in a prospective comparative study.[65] Transaxial CT scans are most sensitive and specific, whereas sagittal reformations are helpful in evaluating the size of a disc bulge into the spinal canal (especially at the L5–S1 level) and spondylolisthesis. Coronal reformations are least informative. Myelography and sagittal reformations are equally useful in the detection of a herniated disc, but transaxial CT scans are superior to either.[66]

CT of the lumbar spine has exhibited 93 percent agreement with surgical findings in revealing the presence or absence of a herniated nucleus pulposus, including posterior disc protrusion and extruded disc fragments. Discrepancy is most likely in the setting of previous surgery, spondylolisthesis, or spinal stenosis.[67] In patients with low back pain or sciatica, CT findings also correlate well with clinical response to intra-articular facet block. CT can thus effectively differentiate between lumbar facet arthropathy and a herniated disc.[68]

CT has been shown to be useful in diagnosing posterolateral as well as central lumbar disc herniations. Because it can image the disc margin and free disc fragments irrespective of dural sac or root sheath deformity, CT is more effective than myelography for demonstrating the presence and extent of lateral disc herniation. The CT features of a lateral herniated disc include (1) focal protrusion of the disc margin; (2) displacement of epidural fat within the intervertebral foramen; (3) absence of dural sac deformity; and (4) soft tissue mass within or lateral to the intervertebral foramen.[69]

An extruded or free disc fragment commonly appears on CT scans as an epidural mass, and a normal posterior disc margin does not exclude herniation when the nuclear fragment is extruded. Free disc fragments can be differentiated from root sheath anomalies and tumors in most instances by measuring tissue densities and analyzing adjacent bone.[70] The CT appearance of conjoined nerve roots has been described, including the resemblance between this condition and herniated nucleus pulposus, as well as differentiation between the two using the "blink mode."[71] CT features of conjoined lumbar nerve roots include asymmetry of the bony spinal canal, mani-

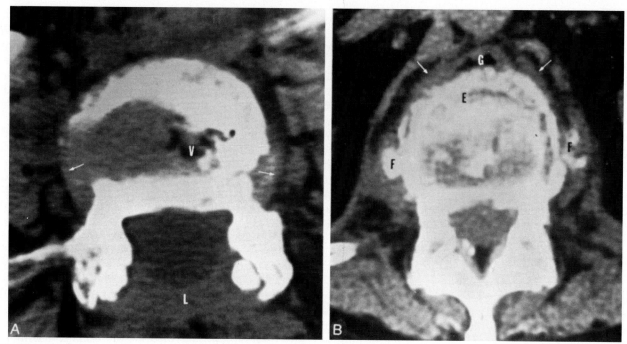

Figure 42–8. CT identification of gas as a diagnostic aid in the spine. *A*, Intradiscal gas or vacuum phenomenon (V) in association with diffuse annular bulge *(arrows)* is a classic finding of degenerative intervertebral disc disease. The site of a previous laminectomy (L) can also be appreciated. Demonstration of gas within a collapsed vertebral body by CT should suggest ischemic necrosis as the underlying etiology. *B*, Pyogenic infection of the lumbar spine. Low-density areas (G) in the soft tissues anterior to the spine are typical of gas-forming organisms. Vertebral end-plate destruction (E) with osseous fragmentation (F) is characteristic. Prevertebral soft tissue swelling *(arrows)* is also evident.

fested as slight dilation of the ipsilateral lateral recess. This alteration is not typically associated with extruded free intervertebral disc fragments and thus serves as a distinguishing feature between these two entities.[72]

Patients with unequivocal regression or disappearance of a herniated lumbar disc on follow-up CT study have been reported. More frequent use of sequential CT scans has thus been advocated to determine whether regression of herniated disc is a frequent occurrence among patients who recover with conservative therapy.[73]

CT has also been shown to be an effective noninvasive means of imaging the lumbar spine in patients with suspected recurrent disc disease. Intravenous contrast material significantly increases the diagnostic accuracy and level of confidence in differentiating between recurrent herniated disc and hypertrophic extradural scar by CT.[74] Enhancement occurs with scar but not with recurrent disc herniation. The method is advocated by some investigators for more accurate evaluation of failed back surgery and can assist in the recognition of discitis.[75]

Patient selection for chymopapain chemonucleolysis is based partially on the CT demonstration of morphologic criteria for a herniated nucleus pulposus, which favors a successful therapeutic outcome. CT studies have been found to correlate closely with objective clinical parameters used to assess therapeutic response.[76] In a prospective evaluation, changes in the size, location, shape, homogeneity, and density of the disc herniation after chemonucleolysis were uncommon on 6-week follow-up CT studies.[77] The most common findings at this time were vacuum phenomena, increased disc attenuation, and a slight decrease (1 to 3 mm) in the size of the disc herniations.[77] At 3 months, the compression produced by the herniated disc was eliminated or reduced, with development of diffuse annular bulging in most patients. No evidence for osseous alterations or epidural fibrosis has been detected by CT.[78] A successful response on 6-month follow-up CT scans has been characterized by decreased disc height, vacuum phenomena, and a more impressive decrease in the size of the disc herniations.[77]

Articular Sepsis. The diagnostic role of CT in septic arthritis is based primarily on its ability to guide proper access to joints that are difficult to image otherwise (e.g., intervertebral discs, sacroiliac joints). CT also allows evaluation of soft tissues around these anatomically complex areas and thereby excludes the presence of a periarticular abscess. CT makes diagnostic aspiration possible in difficult cases. Extension of an infectious process through an intervertebral disc to adjacent vertebral bodies with or without surrounding soft tissue abscess formation is well depicted by CT, although MR imaging often can give equal or superior information.

Congenital Diseases. CT plays an important role in the diagnosis and evaluation of many congenital diseases involving the musculoskeletal system. Examples include leg length discrepancy, femoral neck anteversion, tibial torsion, scoliosis with rotation, coalitions, and congenital hip dysplasia.[79, 80] In congenital hip dysplasia, CT can outline the interposition of the iliopsoas tendon between the femoral head and the acetabulum, which could prevent reduction of the dislocation or cause instability. CT with three-dimensional reconstructed images also is of great importance in surgical decision making and postoperative follow-up evaluation. Spinal dysraphism likewise can be evaluated by CT. Although spondylolysis and spondylolisthesis can be detected on plain radiographs, CT allows an accurate evaluation of the posterior elements of the involved vertebra and the adjacent apophyseal joints.

Magnetic Resonance Imaging

The indications for MR have increased dramatically in the last several years. Multiplanar MR imaging is extremely rewarding in the study of many musculoskeletal disorders. Newly designed surface coils are more specifically adapted to each part of the body, thereby enhancing image quality. MR imaging's advantages are its ability to depict physical differences among tissues and fluids, expressing these differences in terms of image contrast; the apparent lack of significant biologic hazard; the capacity to select any direct imaging plane closely adapted to the anatomic or pathologic structure under study; the close correlation of the images with actual normal anatomy; and outstanding sensitivity. Its main drawback is that it often lacks specificity. For many reasons, MR is employed as the sole imaging method only infrequently; in most instances, it is used as an adjunct to conventional imaging techniques or even CT. It is beyond the scope of this chapter to discuss in great detail the physics and examination protocols of MR. However, it should be mentioned that primary pulse sequences include T1- and T2-weighted spin-echo and gradient-echo methods, whereas more sophisticated sequences (such as short-flip-angle three-dimensional gradient-echo and short-time-to-echo, high-flip-angle gradient-echo techniques) may be utilized in a tailored approach.[81-83]

Spine

Anatomic areas of interest in the spine that are frequently studied with MR imaging include intervertebral discs, spinal canal, neural foramina, and apophyseal joints. In addition, a variety of axial conditions or disorders can be studied with MR, including degenerative disc disease, disc herniation, spinal stenosis, the postoperative spine, discitis, vertebral osteomyelitis, and spinal dysraphism.

Degenerative Disc Disease

The basic chemical constitution of vertebral discs is a combination of proteoglycans and collagen. The nucleus pulposus has a greater proportion of proteoglycans, whereas the surrounding annulus fibrosus has more collagen. This is reflected by different signal intensities of these structures on MR images. The disc is attached superiorly and inferiorly to the fused physeal ring of the adjacent vertebral body surfaces by strong annular fibers, and anteriorly and posteriorly it is loosely attached to the corresponding longitudinal ligaments. The normal intervertebral disc has a concave contour on a sagittal view and a symmetric appearance on a transaxial view. The annulus fibrosus shows low signal intensity (dark) with all pulse sequences, whereas the nucleus pulposus shows a moderate signal intensity (gray) on T1-weighted images and a high signal intensity (bright) on both T2-weighted and gradient-echo images. With aging, the intervertebral disc is subject to biochemical and structural changes, resulting in an imbalance in which the proteoglycans lose their close association with collagen fibers and the disc loses 15 to 20 percent of its water content. At the same time, the adjacent end-plates of the vertebral bodies become thinner.[84] When this process is more advanced, the distinction between the nucleus pulposus and the annulus fibrosus disappears as dense, disorganized, fibrous tissue replaces the normal fibrocartilaginous structure of the nucleus pulposus. Fissures then develop within the cartilaginous end-plates and granulation tissue appears in this area. A correlative study of cadavers and MR images by Yu and colleagues[85] demonstrated three types of tears in the annulus fibrosus: radial, concentric, and transverse.

These biochemical and structural changes in the intervertebral disc are reflected on MR images by a change in signal intensity, mainly a decreased signal in gradient-echo and T2-weighted images. A *bulging* disc refers to a symmetric circumferential enlargement of the disc without major disruption of the annulus fibrosus. *Protrusion* refers to an eccentric bulging of the disc, indicating a focal weakening of the annulus fibers with consequent thinning of the involved area (Fig. 42–9). This may potentially predispose to disc herniation. Disc *herniation* refers to a rupture of the annulus fibrosus with consequent extrusion of the disc through the annular defect while the extruded part remains in contact with the parent disc (Fig. 42–10). A disc *prolapse* describes a herniated disc still covered with a few remaining annular fibers.[86] Finally, *sequestration* refers to a disc fragment that is no longer in contact with the parent disc; such a fragment can be located either above or below the involved disc level. To study discal abnormality, transaxial and sagittal MR images are usually obtained. In neither plane does a normal disc project beyond the posterior margin of the vertebral bodies. Sagittal views are better suited to the analysis of disc herniation. The herniated disc has an hourglass appearance along the posterior disc margin. On transaxial views, the posterior disc margin will show some asymmetry and often a soft tissue mass displacing the adjacent nerve root or thecal sac to a varying extent.[87] Anatomic contact with the parent disc is still apparent. Sequestrated discs do not have such contact, although other findings are similar to those of a simple disc herniation. Disc fragments are more often located on the anterolateral aspect of the spinal canal because the lateral portion of the posterior longitudinal ligament is somewhat weaker than its central part.

Spinal Stenosis

Spinal stenosis is either congenital or acquired. The congenital form is related to developmental aberrations such as short pedicles, whereas the acquired form results from a reduction in diameter of the spinal canal caused by any combination of disc bulging, ligamentum flavum hypertrophy, postoperative modifications, and facet hypertrophy. The most common form of spinal stenosis that is studied by MR imaging is the acquired form.[88, 89] It is best displayed by MR using sagittal gradient-echo–pulsed images. In this sequence, the thecal sac, which displays a high-intensity signal, appears compressed or even obliterated

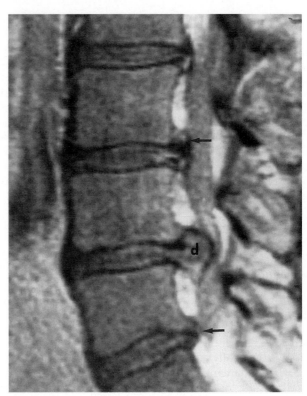

Figure 42–10. Herniation of an intervertebral disc. On this sagittal T2-weighted magnetic resonance (MR) image of the lumbar spine, observe a soft tissue mass (d) protruding into the spinal canal at the L4–5 interspace. Smaller disc bulges are present at the interspaces above and below the disc herniation *(arrows)*.

by bulging discs, osteophytes, and a hypertrophied ligamentum flavum. The resulting appearance of the thecal sac is an hourglass deformity. Multilevel disc degeneration illustrated by an abnormally low signal intensity for these discs and disc space narrowing also may be present. On transaxial images, the stenotic spinal canal has a triangular shape owing to an encroachment by hypertrophied facets.

Postoperative Spine

One of the most common and often difficult tasks in diagnostic radiology is the evaluation of patients with a failed back surgery syndrome. These are patients who have residual or recurrent back pain after back surgery.[90, 91] MR now is recognized as the imaging method of choice for analysis of the postoperative spine.[92–94] Furthermore, experience with gadolinium–diethylenetetraminepenta-acetic acid (Gd-DTPA)–enhanced MR imaging in combination with noncontrast MR imaging has revealed unprecedented sensitivity and accuracy in the investigation of such patients.[95, 96] The main causes of failed back surgery syndrome are lateral spinal stenosis, recurrent or residual disc herniation, fibrosis, scar formation, arachnoiditis, infection, surgical nerve injury, pseudomeningocele formation, and incorrect choice of level of surgery. MR studies obtained in the early postoper-

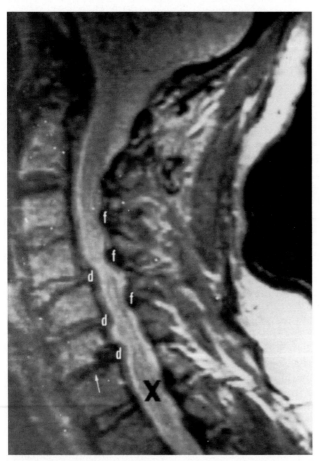

Figure 42–9. Degenerative disc disease in the cervical spine. On a T2-weighted sagittal image, irregular impingement on the thecal sac (X) by posteriorly protruding disc material (d) and ligamentum flavum thickening (f) is evident. Diminished signal intensity in the nucleus pulposus of the C6-7 disc *(arrow)* indicates desiccation related to degenerative disease. Narrowing can be appreciated at the lowest three intercervical disc levels.

ative period are exceedingly difficult to interpret. The presence of various types of materials at the site of surgery, such as gas, Gelfoam, blood, and fat graft, leads to complex imaging alterations. The topographic features and signal intensity of recurrent disc herniation and epidural scar are very similar. After a 1-month delay, however, it is easier to distinguish a scar from recurrent or residual disc herniation. Recurrent or residual disc herniation is associated with a mass that is still in contact with the parent disc. The signal intensity is the same for both herniated disc material and the parent disc on both T1- and T2-weighted images unless the herniated material has been separated, surgically or not, from the parent disc, thus becoming sequestered. Also, a discontinuity in the fibers of the annulus fibrosus can reflect the presence of disc disease, or it can be secondary to the surgical incision. Finally, herniated discs are usually well delineated and are sometimes circumscribed by a rim of low signal intensity. The margins of an epidural scar are usually poorly defined. The MR signal of a scar is either isointense or hypointense to the disc signal in T1-weighted images and hyperintense on T2-weighted images.[92] The latter tends to be attenuated months or years after surgery. Scar also causes retraction of soft tissues with displacement of the thecal sac on the same side as the surgery. With Gd-DTPA–enhanced MR imaging, epidural scar shows greater enhancement than adjacent disc or nerve root structures. Gd-DTPA is incorporated into inflammatory material, allowing clearer depiction of the scar and enabling it to be distinguished from adjacent disc and nerve roots, even if the latter are incorporated within the scar.

In some situations contrast agent is not helpful, however. In a prospective study of 15 patients who had complete resolution of symptoms after successful lumbar disc surgery, a residual mass effect on the neural elements that simulated recurrent or residual disc fragments was present in 38 percent at 3 weeks and in 12 percent at 3 months, thus limiting the interpretation of the MR examination during the first 6 months after lumbar surgery.[97]

Postsurgical Infection

Infections after back surgery are uncommon but may have severe consequences. They usually consist of vertebral osteomyelitis with or without adjacent discitis or epidural abscess. MR imaging is an excellent diagnostic method in this clinical setting. Changes that are encountered in cases of infection include confluent areas of low signal intensity in vertebral bone marrow and adjacent disc on T1-weighted images, increased signal intensity of the bone marrow and adjacent disc on T2-weighted images, the loss of the normal demarcation between vertebral body and intervertebral disc, and abnormal disc shape. Epidural abscesses (Fig. 42–11) form a mass of variable size that is usually easy to separate from the thecal sac; abscesses appear isointense to the thecal sac

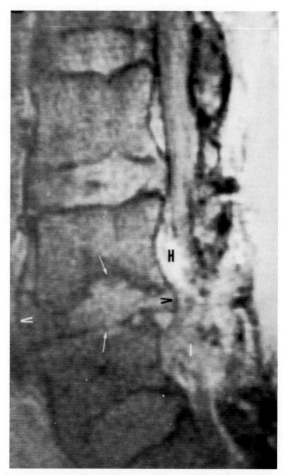

Figure 42–11. Intervertebral disc space infection. On a T2-weighted sagittal image of the lumbar spine, narrowing and bulging *(arrowheads)* of the L4–5 interspace are apparent, in association with irregular destruction of the adjacent end-plates *(arrows)*. Posterior extension of the process has resulted in an epidural abscess, characterized by mixed areas of intermediate (I) and high (H) signal intensity.

on T1-weighted images and hyperintense on T2-weighted images. The use of Gd-DTPA–enhanced MR imaging greatly improves the sensitivity for the diagnosis of such abscesses. Viable inflammatory tissue enhances on T1-weighted images after administration of contrast material.

Bone Marrow

Bone marrow historically has been poorly evaluated with conventional imaging techniques. Although CT represented a strong improvement in the investigation of the bone marrow, MR now is regarded as the state-of-the-art imaging method for this purpose. Pathologic processes involving the bone marrow can be broadly classified into five groups[98]: (1) reconversion; (2) infiltration by neoplasia, infection, or other processes; (3) myeloid depletion; (4) edema (Fig. 42–12); and (5) ischemia (Figs. 42–13 and 42–14). Normal bone marrow provides a continuous supply of red and white blood cells, platelets, and other cells to

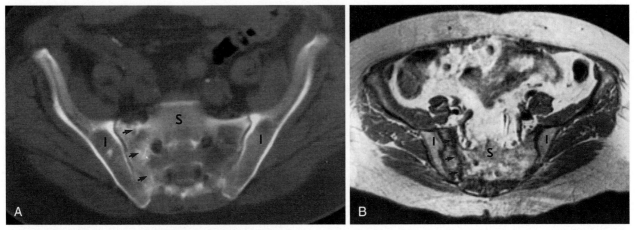

Figure 42–12. Insufficiency fracture of the sacrum. *A*, A CT image of the pelvis demonstrates an abnormal linear area of sclerosis *(arrows)* and disruption of the trabeculae in the right sacral ala. *B*, On a proton-density weighted transaxial MR image, the insufficiency fracture of the right sacrum is more conspicuous and appears as a linear area of low signal intensity *(arrows)*. Acutely, the fracture may be surrounded by diminished bone marrow signal intensity consistent with bone marrow edema (not present in this case). S, sacrum; I, ilium.

meet the body's demand for oxygenation, immunity, and coagulation. It also plays a role in bone biomechanics in terms of mechanical support and mineral deposit. Nerves, fat cells, and blood and lymphatic vessels are also part of the bone marrow. At birth, red marrow is present almost throughout the bones of the body, but it will progressively be converted to yellow marrow. In the adult, the largest red marrow reservoirs reside in the axial skeleton (spine, pelvis, and ribs), skull, and proximal portions of the humeri and femora. Other bones have yellow marrow. Normal yellow marrow has a signal that is isointense to subcutaneous fat on T1-weighted and T2-weighted images. Normal red marrow has a low signal intensity on T1-weighted images compared with subcutaneous fat, although it has a higher signal intensity than that of muscle. On T2-weighted images, red marrow remains of relatively low signal intensity.

Reconversion is a response to the depletion of the body's red marrow related to a number of different causes, such as anemia and myelofibrosis. The reconversion process will involve successively the spine, the flat bones, and, finally, the long bones. With MR imaging, marrow appears focally or diffusely hypointense on T1-weighted images, depending on the extent of the disease process. On T2-weighted images, the appearance varies depending on the water content of the process; it may appear hypointense, isointense, or hyperintense in comparison with yellow marrow.[99] Bone marrow infiltration or replacement by infection, leukemia, lymphoma, metastasis, or primary bone tumors may occur throughout the body according to the relative prevalence of red and yellow marrow. Certain infiltrating conditions of bone marrow have a low signal intensity on T1-weighted images, but signal intensity varies greatly on T2-weighted images

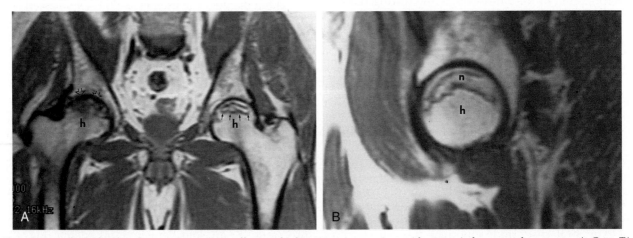

Figure 42–13. Steroid-induced avascular necrosis affecting the hip joints in a patient with systemic lupus erythematosus. *A*, On a T1-weighted coronal MR image, a heterogeneous ring-like pattern *(solid arrows)* is present in the weight-bearing aspects of the left femoral head (h), whereas the right femoral head (h) demonstrates greater surface area involvement and early collapse *(open arrows)*. *B*, A T1-weighted sagittal image reveals the full extent of surface involvement by avascular necrosis (n). h, left femoral head.

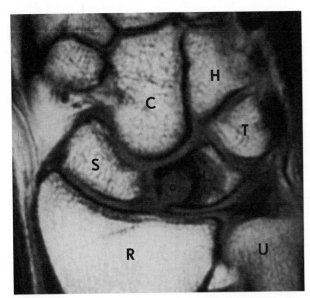

Figure 42–14. Kienböck's disease (idiopathic avascular necrosis of the lunate). On a T1-weighted coronal image, the lunate bone (L) is abnormal in signal intensity on its radial aspect. The heterogeneous decrease in signal intensity is characteristic of osteonecrosis (o) of the lunate bone. S, scaphoid; C, capitate; H, hamate; T, triquetrum; R, radius; U, ulna. (From Yu JS, Kursunoglu-Brahme S, Resnick D: MR imaging of the wrist. *In* Weissman BN (ed): Categorical Course in Musculoskeletal Radiology. Oak Brook, Ill, RSNA Publishing, 1993, pp 87–96.)

(i.e., high signal intensity for most primary tumors and infection, low signal intensity for leukemia, lymphoma, myelofibrosis, and Gaucher's disease).[100] Thus, MR imaging is extremely sensitive in the diagnosis of bone marrow involvement, but it is not specific.[101] Once a histologic diagnosis is made, MR imaging is useful in determining the extent and the response to treatment for many pathologic processes that involve the bone marrow.

Disorders resulting in myeloid depletion (e.g., irradiation) involve red marrow in such a way that the signal pattern of the diseased areas is transformed to that of yellow marrow on both T1- and T2-weighted images.[102]

Several conditions, including trauma (Fig. 42–15) and the reflex sympathetic dystrophy syndrome, can induce bone marrow edema. This edema is thought to be secondary to hypervascularity causing a regional increase in the concentration of extracellular fluid. This increase in water content appears as a lower signal intensity on T1-weighted images and an increase in signal intensity on T2-weighted images.[103, 104]

The sensitivity of MR imaging for bone marrow ischemia is extremely high. In this condition the marrow reveals a low signal intensity on T1-weighted images and variable signal intensity on T2-weighted images, probably depending on the stage of the disease.[105]

Temporomandibular Joint

The MR examination of TMJ usually includes sagittal closed- and open-mouth T1-weighted images. Be-

cause of the relatively high frequency (26 percent) of lateral or medial displacement of the meniscus, many authors also advocate coronal MR images.[106] The normal TMJ meniscus is a biconcave structure of low signal intensity with a thinner central portion. With the mouth closed, the posterior band is in contact with the mandibular condyle, and with the mouth open, the intermediate zone of the meniscus is in contact with the condyle. During motion, a complex movement of anterior translation and rotation occurs. MR abnormalities include abnormal position of the mandibular condyle or the meniscus, or both, in relation to the temporal eminence.[107]

MR is considered the best imaging method for analysis of the TMJ. It depicts, with great precision, the meniscus and the rest of the articulation, and it allows the visualization of the surrounding muscular apparatus, notably the mastication muscles (Fig. 42–16). Multiplanar views and the use of surface coils allow detection of anterior, medial, or lateral displacement of the meniscus, detection of which is not possible by simple arthrography. MR imaging also allows assessment of the underlying bone, joint effusion, and postoperative complications. Because of the functional similarity of this joint and the femoropatellar joint, real-time assessment of joint mechanics with MR imaging can be useful and is accomplished by scanning during incremental opening and closing of the mouth.[108]

Shoulder

MR imaging has had a great impact in the evaluation of the shoulder owing to the possibility of studying soft tissue and osseous anatomy (muscles, tendons, cartilage, and bones) with a multiplanar approach.[109] With its contrast sensitivity, MR can be used to assess a whole spectrum of disorders commonly leading to shoulder pain: rotator cuff pathology, impingement syndrome, bicipital tendon abnormalities, bone marrow disease, and intra-articular osteochondral bodies. CT in combination with arthrography, however, has proved to be as accurate as MR imaging in the evaluation of shoulder instability.

The impingement syndrome is a well-recognized clinical entity that is defined as the entrapment of soft tissues in the subacromial space between the humeral head and the coracoacromial arch; these soft tissues include the rotator cuff (particularly the supraspinatus muscle), the tendon of the long head of the biceps, and the subacromial bursa. Most rotator cuff problems are secondary to chronic impingement of tendons by a prominent coracoacromial ligament, abnormal slope or shape of the acromion, the presence of enthesophytes at the tip of the acromion, or degenerative changes of the acromioclavicular joint. MR findings of impingement include thickening of the subacromial bursa and decreased thickness of the supraspinatus tendon with an increased signal intensity within the tendon indicative of tendinopathy.[110] Fur-

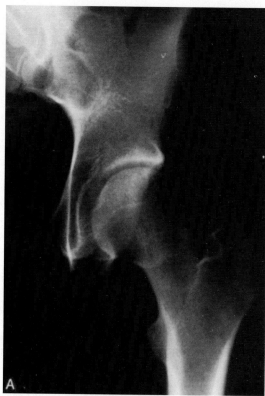

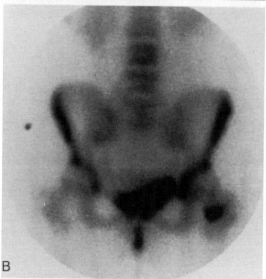

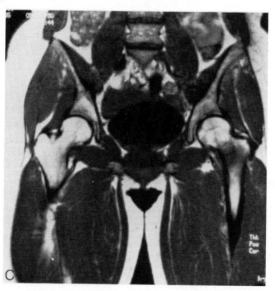

Figure 42–15. Stress fracture. *A,* Anteroposterior radiograph of the left hip showing a horizontal band of sclerosis at the medial aspect of the left femoral neck. *B,* Bone scan: abnormal radionuclide uptake at the same area. *C,* MR imaging: T1-weighted coronal image, with a band of low signal intensity along the femoral neck suggesting bone marrow edema.

ther damage to the tendon is manifested by a partial tear involving only the articular or bursal surface. Partial tears are often mistaken for full-thickness tears or tendinopathy with MR imaging. Direct MR findings of rotator cuff tears consist of focal discontinuity, tendon retraction, and abnormally increased signal intensity within the tendon.[111, 112] Chronic tears are more difficult to discern owing to replacement with fibrous or granulation tissue, although attenuation of the tendon and surface irregularity are suggestive findings. Indirect findings of rotator cuff pathology include a high-riding humeral head, fluid in the sub-

acromial-subdeltoid bursa, obliteration of the peribursal fat stripe, and joint effusion in the glenohumeral joint.[113]

MR arthrography, with Gd-DTPA as the intra-articular contrast medium, has been introduced as an additional tool for the evaluation of partial tears, with encouraging results.[114] This technique is particularly helpful in the evaluation of partial tears of the undersurface of the cuff and also in the evaluation of the glenoid labrum (Fig. 42–17) and the search for intra-articular bodies. The rationale for using an intra-articular contrast medium in cases of shoulder instability

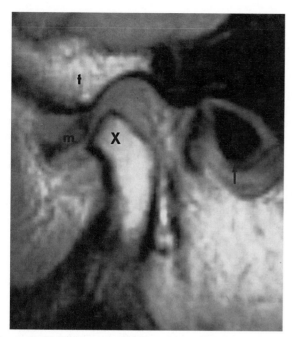

Figure 42–16. Dislocation of the temporomandibular joint meniscus. On a T1-weighted open-mouth sagittal image, the fibrocartilaginous disc (m) of low signal intensity is displaced anterior to the mandibular condyle (X), limiting the range of forward excursion. t, temporal eminentia; *arrow,* external auditory canal.

relates to the fact that labral morphology is hard to depict when the glenohumeral joint is free of fluid. Studies have emphasized the "many faces" of the normal labrum. Indeed, the normal labrum can be triangular in shape, rounded, or bifid. The best MR images are those in the transaxial plane, in which the labrum is depicted as a structure devoid of signal

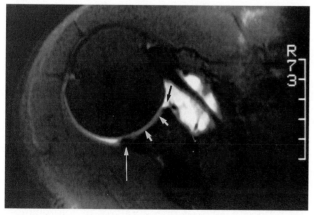

Figure 42–17. A fat-saturated T1-weighted transaxial image from an MR arthrogram of the shoulder demonstrates a torn anterior labrum *(black arrow).* The normal triangular-shaped structure is absent. The gadolinium–diethylenetetraminepenta-acetic acid (Gd-DTPA) is the paramagnetic contrast material injected into the glenohumeral joint and appears bright. The articular cartilage *(small white arrows)* has intermediate signal intensity, resulting in nice contrast between the bone and the contrast material in the joint. The posterior labrum *(long white arrow)* is low in signal intensity and may have a more rounded appearance.

because of its fibrocartilaginous nature. Labral tears may appear as regions of increased signal intensity extending to the labral surface. The region of increased signal intensity can be diffuse in nature, and the labrum may appear blunted or frayed.

Wrist

High image quality is required for optimal visualization of the small structures about the wrist.[115] In carpal tunnel syndrome, the median nerve can be damaged by compression or entrapment as it passes through the carpal tunnel, which is delineated dorsally by the carpal bones, volarly by the flexor retinaculum, ulnarly by the hook of the hamate and the pisiform, and radially by the scaphoid and the trapezium. A variety of causes of carpal tunnel syndrome can be depicted by MR imaging, including fluid collections (synovitis), fibrosis, and space-occupying lesions (e.g., neuroma and ganglion). Compression of the median nerve induces nerve edema that will be reflected by an increase in the size of the nerve on T1-weighted images and a bright signal intensity within the nerve on T2-weighted images. Other findings include distortion of the normal ovoid shape of the nerve, swelling of the flexor tendon sheaths, and palmar convexity of the flexor retinaculum.[116] Failure of surgery to relieve carpal tunnel syndrome also can be studied with MR imaging.

Other causes of wrist pain that can be demonstrated by MR include joint effusions, synovial inflammatory processes,[117, 118] and bone marrow abnormalities, such as ischemic necrosis of the proximal pole of the scaphoid and Kienböck's disease.[119] Although T1-weighted MR images reveal great anatomic detail, this technique has not yet supplanted the use of wrist arthrography in the assessment of intracarpal ligamentous pathology. The triangular fibrocartilage, however, is usually well demonstrated with coronal T1-weighted images, and both the normal and the pathologic appearance of the triangular fibrocartilage with MR imaging have been well documented.[120]

Foot and Ankle

Direct multiplanar images of the foot and ankle are obtainable with both CT and MR. MR is an efficient imaging technique for the evaluation of muscles and tendons; it depicts their anatomy with great precision and documents the presence of tenosynovial fluid or intratendinous fluid collections.[121] Normal tendons appear as smooth, well-defined, hypointense structures on T1- and T2-weighted images. In addition, a recent partial tear of a tendon is typically diagnosed with MR imaging by the presence of fluid within the tendon and tendon sheath, creating a bright signal on T2-weighted images. A complete tear manifests itself by tendon discontinuity secondary to its retraction.[122] Chronic tendon tears or chronic tendinitis appears as a diffusely thickened tendon that has low signal intensity on both T1- and T2-weighted images. Associated tenosynovial fluid collections are seen as areas of intermediate signal intensity on T1-weighted images and of high signal intensity on T2-weighted images. Morphologic alterations may be dramatic in chronic tendinopathy and may be accompanied by intratendinous ossification.[123]

Posterior tibial tendon rupture[124] and Achilles tendinitis[125] are two entities that can be specifically studied with MR. The posterior tibial tendon is one of the main stabilizers of the hindfoot. Chronic inflammation involving this tendon may lead to a complete tear. Plain-film signs of tenosynovitis or rupture of the posterior tibial tendon are subtle and include periostitis of the medial aspect of the distal tibia. The normal posterior tibial tendon appears on MR images as a dark, homogeneous, ovoid to round structure passing posterior to the medial malleolus. It is twice as large as the adjacent flexor digitorum longus or flexor hallucis longus tendon. Classification of posterior tibial tendon tears using MR imaging correlates well with surgical findings. In type I tears, the tendon appears enlarged in comparison with the normal contralateral side (both ankles are usually studied at the same time for comparison). Type I tears may also reveal foci of high signal intensity on proton-density–weighted images and of somewhat lesser signal intensity on T2-weighted images. In type II tears, the tendon appears atrophic and its size approaches that of the adjacent flexor digitorum longus tendon. Also, hypertrophy of the tendon segments above and below the ruptured area may be evident. Type III tears are manifested by a gap in the tendon itself and retraction of the proximal muscle-tendon complex.

Causes of Achilles tendinitis are multiple: strenuous athletic training, gout, rheumatoid arthritis, systemic or local use of glucocorticoids, and chronic renal failure. All of these conditions eventually can lead to rupture of this tendon. MR imaging provides important information about this tendon and the surrounding structures. The actual site of rupture generally is located 3 to 5 cm proximal to its distal insertion on the posterior aspect of the calcaneus. It is at this point that the anterior and posterior fibers cross, in a region of relative hypovascularity. Achilles tendon rupture is clinically misdiagnosed in approximately 25 percent of cases. MR imaging, therefore, plays an important role as a diagnostic tool. The optimal images are those in the transaxial plane. The normal tendon has a crescentic shape, with the concave aspect projected anteriorly; it reveals a signal void on all MR imaging sequences. A complete tear is seen as an area of increased signal intensity on T2-weighted images, discontinuity of the tendon, and retraction of the muscle-tendon junction. Tendinitis appears as a small focus of increased signal intensity within an enlarged tendon without any tendon discontinuity. Surrounding edema is seen as a brightening of the loose connective tissue anterior to the tendon. Partial tears are difficult to differentiate from tendinitis with MR imaging.

Arthrography allows accurate assessment of ligamentous integrity about the ankle. Indeed, specific patterns of contrast extravasation permit differentiation among injuries of the anterior inferior tibiofibular, anterior and posterior talofibular, calcaneofibular, and deltoid ligaments. Experience with MR imaging in the evaluation of these ligaments is limited, but findings strongly suggestive of disruption of the anterior inferior tibiofibular ligament have been described, consisting of disorganization of the soft tissues between the tibia and fibula, fluid above the expected syndesmosis, and slight subluxation of the fibula.

MR imaging is useful in the detection of radiographically occult lesions, in the assessment of the integrity of the overlying cartilage, in the detection of intra-articular bodies, in the definition of the exact location and extension of the process, and in the prediction of the stability of the osteochondral fragment. As is the case with all synovial articulations, inflammatory diseases and other synovial disorders that may involve the ankle, such as rheumatoid arthritis, juvenile rheumatoid arthritis,[126] hemophilic arthropathy,[127] or pigmented villonodular synovitis, can be studied with MR imaging. In patients with plantar fasciitis, the plantar aponeurosis becomes thickened and may be associated with a focus of increased signal intensity at its insertion into the calcaneus on T2-weighted images.[128]

Knee

MR imaging has been used increasingly in the investigation of many disorders involving the knee. A standard MR examination of the knee requires about 30 to 45 minutes and includes coronal and sagittal T1- and T2-weighted images. The protocol permits an extensive evaluation of the ligaments, menisci, articular surfaces, and bone marrow.[129] Transaxial views also are frequently obtained.

The normal signal intensity for ligaments, tendons, and menisci is low on all pulse sequences. Menisci normally have a triangular shape on sagittal and coronal planes and a C shape in the transaxial plane. The posterior horn of the medial meniscus is larger than the anterior horn. Also, the height of the meniscus is greater at the periphery than at its central part.[130] Abnormalities in the menisci are depicted as foci of increased signal intensity. Various attempts to classify abnormal signals within the meniscus have been recorded in recent literature.[131, 132] Grade I and II changes represent foci of bright signal in the meniscus that represent sites of degenerative myxoid changes without tear. Grade III changes represent abnormally increased signal that extends to the articular surface, indicative of meniscal tear. Meniscal tears can be classified according to their morphology. Chronic degenerative tears are frequently horizontal in configuration, whereas acute tears tend to be vertical or oblique. Acute tears, however, also may be radial, transverse, or complex in appearance. The bucket-handle tear represents a vertical tear in which the inner portion of the damaged meniscus is displaced into the intercondylar notch, thus causing locking of the knee. The accuracy and specificity of MR in the analysis of internal derangement of the knee are highly dependent on the experience of the interpreter. If performed preoperatively, MR imaging can facilitate the detection or treatment, or both, of some lesions. In patients with residual or recurrent symptoms after a previous menisccectomy, MR also is useful in detecting incompletely excised meniscal tears or fragments and in disclosing a new tear in the residual meniscus.

With MR imaging, ligaments are depicted as structures of low signal intensity on all imaging sequences. Anterior and posterior cruciate and collateral ligaments are well studied with MR imaging. A finding suggestive of tears is an abnormal signal within these structures or nonvisualization. The anterior cruciate ligament extends from the medial aspect of the lateral femoral condyle to the anterior tibial spine. Because of this oblique course, sagittal images spaced each 3 mm through the intercondylar notch with 10 degrees of external rotation of the knee are often necessary for better visualization of this structure.[130] An acute complete tear often appears as an area of discontinuity in the normal course of the anterior cruciate ligament, and the ligament appears globular with an intermediate to high signal intensity on T2-weighted images.[129, 130] Edema and hemorrhage within and about the ligament are responsible for the foci of increased signal intensity. Secondary signs of anterior cruciate ligament tear are related to knee instability and include bowing of the posterior cruciate ligament, anterior translation of the tibia, bone marrow contusions in the lateral femoral condyle and posterolateral tibia, and exposure of the posterior horn of the lateral meniscus.[133–135] Ninety percent of the tears typically occur in the midportion of the ligament or near its proximal femoral insertion. Avulsion of the ligament is less commonly seen (7 percent from its femoral attachment and 3 percent from its tibial attachment). MR imaging has a 95 percent accuracy in the diagnosis of anterior cruciate ligament tears and a negative predictive value of up to 100 percent.[129–132] Tears of the posterior cruciate ligament often lead to significant clinical instability of the knee. MR findings of posterior cruciate ligament tear most commonly consist of foci of increased signal intensity on T2-weighted images, similar to the appearance of anterior cruciate ligament tears. Because the posterior cruciate ligament is thicker than its anterior counterpart, this ligament may appear widened in the area of the tear but is less likely to have a masslike appearance. Posterior cruciate ligament tears are associated with other serious intra-articular injuries, including detachment of the posterior horn of the medial meniscus, disruption of the medial and lateral capsular ligaments, tears of the medial and lateral collateral ligaments, and avulsion of the tibial insertion site.[129]

Tears of the lateral and medial collateral ligaments

of the knee are well studied by MR imaging. They appear as disruptions of the normal low signal intensity of the ligament on T1-weighted images with infiltration of the surrounding area by edema and blood, resulting in a high signal intensity on T2-weighted images. Ligamentous sprain results in surrounding edema without ligamentous discontinuity. Complete dislocation of the knee is an unusual but severe injury that causes disruption of multiple ligaments that support the knee. In a recent series, nearly all patients had torn both cruciate ligaments, and a majority had torn one or both collateral ligaments.[136] Injuries to the popliteal tendon, medial and lateral menisci, peroneal nerve, and popliteal artery were common complications of this injury.[136]

MR evaluation of the articular cartilage has not yet been perfected. The transaxial plane is the preferred one for studying the patellar cartilage, which is often poorly visualized in the sagittal plane. Fat suppression images are helpful if an effusion is present because with this technique, hyaline cartilage appears gray and fluid appears white, allowing distinction between the two. Newer techniques utilizing three-dimensional gradient-echo sequences have enabled acquisition of images at thinner intervals without significant alteration of signal-to-noise ratio while providing excellent soft tissue contrast.[137]

MR imaging is preferred over other imaging methods for evaluation of pathologic processes involving the extensor mechanism.[138] Partial or complete quadriceps or patellar tendon tears as well as acute (Fig. 42–18) and chronic tendinitis are easily detected, whereas clinically these entities may not be as apparent. Patellofemoral joint malalignment also can be detected by obtaining multiple sequential transaxial images while the knee is positioned at various increments of flexion from 0 to 30 degrees, the range of flexion over which subluxation or dislocation of the patella most commonly appears. These images can be

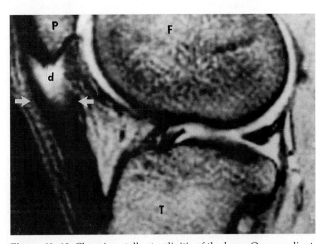

Figure 42–18. Chronic patellar tendinitis of the knee. On a gradient-recalled-echo sagittal image, the proximal patellar tendon (arrows) is thickened and contains an intratendinous focus (d) of increased signal intensity consistent with degeneration. P, patella; F, femur; T, tibia.

displayed in a cine-loop fashion to obtain a dynamic evaluation of the patellofemoral joint.[139]

MR imaging is well established as a sensitive means of evaluation of the bone marrow of the knee. It can detect abnormalities before they can be visualized on radiographs or even scintigraphy. MR is particularly sensitive in the detection of osteonecrosis, osteochondritis dissecans (Fig. 42–19), occult bone fractures, or bone contusion.[140] Osteochondritis dissecans usually involves the lateral aspect of the non–weight-bearing articular surface of the medial femoral condyle and is usually unilateral in distribution. A Segond fracture represents traumatic detachment of the lateral capsule.[141] The resulting fragment of bone is usually small and minimally displaced.

MR imaging can aid in the investigation of patients with arthritis. Although early bone erosions can be depicted with MR imaging, the main application of this technique lies in the demonstration of the inflammatory pannus, which is depicted as a thickened, irregular synovium of intermediate signal intensity on T1-weighted images. Acutely inflamed synovium has an increased signal intensity on T2-weighted images, rendering it difficult to distinguish from an adjacent joint effusion. In chronically inflamed synovium, the pannus may appear as an area of low or intermediate signal intensity on T2-weighted images, whereas the adjacent effusion appears brighter on the same imaging sequence.[142] Recent literature suggests that the intravenous injection of Gd-DTPA in patients with rheumatoid arthritis enhances the inflamed synovium, thereby helping in the detection of acute synovitis and its distinction from accompanying effusion.[143] This procedure also can allow monitoring of the inflammatory process, as well as of the response to therapy.

MR imaging allows the detection of cysts about the knee. Three types of cysts are commonly found: popliteal, meniscal, and ganglionic. Popliteal cysts are synovial cysts arising in the medial aspect of the popliteal fossa. They are caused by a communication between the posterior portion of the joint capsule and the normal gastrocnemiosemimembranous bursa. Any condition associated with increased intra-articular pressure (such as knee effusion) can result in a popliteal cyst. These conditions include rheumatoid arthritis, degenerative joint disease, gout, pigmented villonodular synovitis (Fig. 42–20), and idiopathic synovial chondromatosis. Meniscal cysts are common. They are associated with an underlying meniscal abnormality. The proposed pathogenesis relates to the intrusion of synovial fluid through a horizontal tear of the meniscus.[144] Lateral meniscal cysts occur more frequently than medial cysts. Ganglionic cysts usually contain a gelatinous material that has a high protein content. They may appear isointense to muscle on T1-weighted images but bright on T2-weighted images.[144] They most commonly appear as masses close to a joint, with which they may have a fibrous connection. They are not associated with meniscal tears.

RHEUMATOID ARTHRITIS

General Radiographic Features

Symmetry

The symmetry of rheumatoid arthritis constitutes an important diagnostic criterion for this disease.

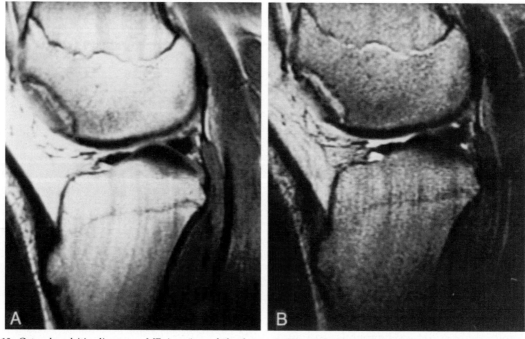

Figure 42–19. Osteochondritis dissecans. MR imaging of the knee: *A,* T1-weighted sagittal image revealing an ovoid lesion, whose marginal zone has decreased signal intensity. *B,* T2-weighted sagittal image with increase in signal intensity compatible with fluid or granulation tissue.

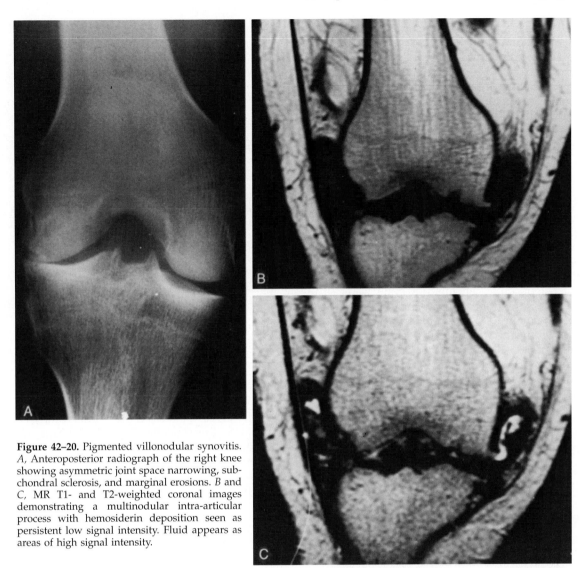

Figure 42–20. Pigmented villonodular synovitis. *A,* Anteroposterior radiograph of the right knee showing asymmetric joint space narrowing, subchondral sclerosis, and marginal erosions. *B* and *C,* MR T1- and T2-weighted coronal images demonstrating a multinodular intra-articular process with hemosiderin deposition seen as persistent low signal intensity. Fluid appears as areas of high signal intensity.

Asymmetric involvement may be noted in male patients and in men and women with early disease or neurologic deficit.[145]

Osteoporosis

Osteoporosis is a characteristic feature of rheumatoid arthritis. Early in the course of the disease, it tends to be localized to the juxta-articular region of the small peripheral joints. Later, generalized osteoporosis may be present in the axial and appendicular skeleton, often exacerbated by medications (i.e., salicylates, glucocorticoids) and disuse or immobilization. In a few patients with rheumatoid arthritis, osteomalacia may be observed.[146]

Soft Tissue Changes

Radiographic changes in the soft tissues can be of diagnostic importance in the patient with rheumatoid arthritis. Diffuse (fusiform) periarticular soft tissue swelling (Fig. 42–21) is an early finding about the small joints of the hands and feet. Intra-articular effusions are common radiographic findings in the knees, elbows, and ankles, producing characteristic displacements of adjacent fat planes. Occasionally, similar effusions in the small joints of the hand may lead to mild joint space widening. Bursal involvement can be identified as asymmetric soft tissue prominence, particularly in the knee (prepatellar bursa), elbow (olecranon bursa), heel (retrocalcaneal bursa), and shoulder (subacromia bursa). Tendinitis and tenosynovitis are most frequently identified in the wrist when involvement of the extensor carpi ulnaris tendon and its synovial sheath causes prominent soft tissue swelling adjacent to the ulnar styloid process. Rheumatoid nodules may occasionally be observed on radiographs as noncalcified, eccentric, lobular soft tissue masses, which may cause pressure erosion of adjacent bones.

Joint Space Narrowing

Progressive joint space narrowing due to destruction of articular cartilage by pannus is another hallmark of rheumatoid arthritis, which may allow its differentiation from gout, a disease in which preservation of joint width is typical. In rheumatoid arthritis, the diffuse cartilaginous loss and the tendency toward pancompartmental involvement of complex joints, such as the knee and the wrist, limit additional diagnostic possibilities. Bony ankylosis is common only in the wrist and in the midfoot; it is distinctly unusual at other sites.

Bony Erosions

Three types of bony erosions may be identified in rheumatoid arthritis. *Marginal erosions* occur at intra-articular sites that are not protected by overlying cartilage. Typically, these "bare" areas are the initial points of attack by the proliferating synovial tissue (see Fig. 42–21). *Compressive erosions* occur when collapse of osteoporotic subchondral bone leads to invagination of one bone into another. These changes occur at articulations exposed to strong muscular actions or significant weight-bearing forces. The most characteristic site of compressive erosion is the hip, where protrusio acetabuli may be identified (Fig. 42–22). Other important sites are at the metacarpophalangeal joints, where collapse of the base of a proximal phalanx by a metacarpal head produces a ball-in-socket–type articulation, and the radiocarpal joint of the wrist, where the scaphoid may appear to be "countersunk" into the distal radius. The third type of erosion seen in rheumatoid arthritis is *surface re-*

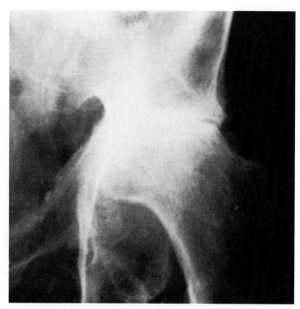

Figure 42–22. Rheumatoid arthritis. Symmetric destruction of the cartilaginous surface has resulted in axial migration of the femoral head. The femoral head has become small and flattened. Sclerosis is apparent.

sorption, usually related to inflammation of an adjacent tendon sheath (Fig. 42–23). This is an important finding in the wrist, where a characteristic erosion of the outer margin of the ulnar styloid process, due to extensor carpi ulnaris tenosynovitis, provides an early radiographic sign of rheumatoid arthritis.

Bony Cysts

Subchondral cystic lesions are frequent in rheumatoid arthritis and have been described as cysts, pseudocysts, geodes, and granulomas. Most commonly, multiple small, ill-defined subchondral radiolucencies are identified at any articulation involved in rheumatoid arthritis. The identification of larger cystic areas, especially in the hands and wrists of physically active men, has been termed *rheumatoid arthritis of the robust reaction pattern.*[147] Occasionally, very large cystic lesions may be encountered in the elbow (olecranon process of ulna, distal humerus), femoral neck, or knee (distal femur, proximal tibia, patella) and have been described as *pseudocystic rheumatoid arthritis* (Fig. 42–24).[148] These large lesions may subsequently fracture.

Deformities and Instabilities

Many types of articular deformity and instability are observed in rheumatoid arthritis (Fig. 42–25). Most of these relate to tendinous or ligamentous laxity or disruption, with alteration of the normal muscle pull across one or more articulations (e.g., boutonnière or swan-neck deformity of the fingers, ulnar

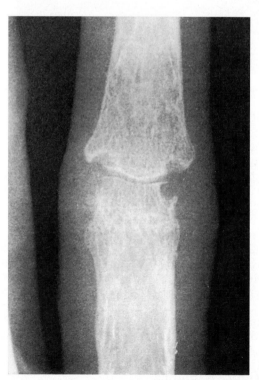

Figure 42–21. Rheumatoid arthritis. Marginal erosions are present on both sides of the interphalangeal joint. Joint space narrowing and fusiform soft tissue swelling are also evident.

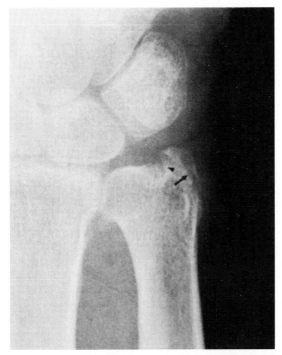

Figure 42–23. Rheumatoid arthritis. An osseous erosion is present in the outer margin of the ulnar styloid (surface erosion) *(arrow)* owing to synovitis of the extensor carpi ulnaris tendon sheath. A second erosion is present at the point of insertion of the triangular fibrocartilage on the ulnar head *(arrowhead)*. (From Resnick D, Niwayama G: Diagnosis of Bone and Joint Disorders. Philadelphia, WB Saunders, 1988.)

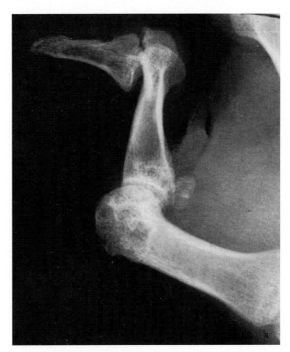

Figure 42–25. Rheumatoid arthritis. In this patient, note the prominent thumb deformity with flexion at the metacarpophalangeal joint and extension of the interphalangeal joint. This constitutes the boutonnière deformity.

deviation at the metacarpophalangeal joints, fibular deviation at the metatarsophalangeal joints, or atlantoaxial subluxation). In some cases, however, the abnormality may relate directly to bone or cartilage destruction (e.g., protrusion acetabuli). These characteristic deformities and instabilities are summarized in Table 42–3.

Abnormalities at Specific Sites

Hand

The target areas of rheumatoid arthritis in the hands are the metacarpophalangeal and proximal interphalangeal joints. The earliest changes consist of fusiform soft tissue swelling, juxta-articular osteoporosis, diffuse joint space loss, and marginal bony erosions (see Fig. 42–21). A particularly characteristic finding is indistinctness and focal loss of continuity of the dorsoradial subchondral bone plate (dot-dash pattern) of the metacarpal head.[149] In general, these radiographic findings appear initially at the second and third metacarpophalangeal joints and third proximal interphalangeal joint. The marginal osseous erosions tend to be more prominent on the proximal bone of the articulation, which tends to have a larger bare area. With progression of the disease, large erosions, complete joint space obliteration, and finger deformities appear. The end stage is usually fibrous ankylosis of the articular cavity; bony ankylosis is rare in the hand but, when present, almost exclusively involves the proximal interphalangeal joints.[145]

Wrist

The wrist is a complex articulation that should properly be viewed as a series of distinct synovial

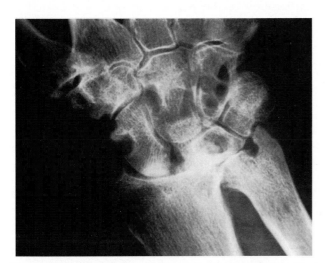

Figure 42–24. Pseudocystic rheumatoid arthritis. In this patient, large cystic erosions are present, giving the appearance of "hollow" carpal bones. Also note the narrowing of the radiocarpal joint with ulnar translocation of the carpus. (From Resnick D, Niwayama G: Diagnosis of Bone and Joint Disorders. Philadelphia, WB Saunders, 1988.)

Table 42–3. INSTABILITIES AND DEFORMITIES IN RHEUMATOID ARTHRITIS

Site	Name	Abnormality
Hand		
DIP joint	Mallet finger	Flexion DIP
PIP and DIP joints	Boutonnière deformity	Flexion PIP, extension DIP
	Swan-neck deformity	Extension PIP, flexion DIP
MCP joint		Ulnar deviation
		Volar subluxation
Wrist		
Distal radioulnar joint	Caput ulna	Subluxation/dislocation of distal radioulnar joint
Radiocarpal joint		Radial deviation
		Ulnar translocation
Intercarpal joints	Scapholunate dissociation	Scapholunate space >2 mm
	Dorsal intercalary segment instability	Dorsiflexion lunate, volar flexion scaphoid
	Volar intercalary segment instability	Volar flexion lunate, dorsiflexion scaphoid
		Subluxation of extensor carpi ulnaris tendon
Hip	Protrusio acetabuli	Acetabular wall medial to ilioischial line
		>3 mm in male
		>6 mm in female
Knee	Genu varus	Inward deviation of tibia
	Genu valgus	Outward deviation of tibia
Foot		
First MTP joint	Hallux valgus (bunion)	Lateral deviation of first MTP joint
MTP (all)		Lateral deviation of MTP joints (I–IV)
		Plantar subluxation of MTP joints
	Cock-up toe	Hyperextension and dorsal subluxation of MTP
PIP and DIP	Hammer toe	Hyperflexion PIP or DIP
Cervical spine		
Atlantoaxial joint	Atlantoaxial subluxation	Atlanto-odontoid space >3 mm
	Vertical atlantoaxial subluxation	Superior displacement odontoid
All levels	Stair-step deformity	Subluxation of apophyseal joints

Abbreviations: DIP, distal interphalangeal; PIP, proximal interphalangeal; MCP, metacarpophalangeal; MTP, metatarsophalangeal.

compartments: (1) radiocarpal, (2) inferior radioulnar, (3) midcarpal, (4) pisotriquetral, (5) common carpometacarpal, and (6) first carpometacarpal. Rheumatoid arthritis demonstrates distinctive pancompartmental involvement of the wrist, which helps to differentiate it from other arthropathies.[150] The least commonly involved area is the first carpometacarpal compartment, which may be spared even in the presence of advanced disease elsewhere in the wrist.

The distal ulna, being bounded by three important sites of synovial proliferation, occupies a prominent role as a target area in rheumatoid arthritis[151] (see Fig. 42–23). Erosions along the outer margin of the ulnar styloid are related to tenosynovitis of the extensor carpi ulnaris tendon, erosions of the styloid tip are related to involvement of the prestyloid recess of the radiocarpal compartment, and erosions of the base and juxta-articular area of the distal ulna indicate inferior radioulnar compartment involvement.

Early erosions may involve any bone in the wrist; in addition to the distal ulna, some of the more characteristic sites[152, 153] include the radial styloid, lateral scaphoid waist, triquetrum, and pisiform. These changes may be manifested as distinct erosions or as cystic lesions that give the radiographic appearance of hollow carpal bones. With time, the characteristic pancompartmental involvement becomes evident with loss of articular spaces. Bony ankylosis of the carpus is a relatively common end result of advanced

rheumatoid arthritis. In some cases diffuse carpal destruction may occur, culminating in complete disintegration of the wrist.

Numerous deformities related to soft tissue destruction and muscular imbalances may be seen. The most characteristic wrist deformities consist of ulnar translocation of the proximal carpal row, related to destruction of the triangular fibrocartilage–meniscus homolog complex, and radial deviation at the radiocarpal joint (Fig. 42–26).[154]

Elbow

The elbow is a frequent site of abnormality, particularly in patients with advanced disease. In this area a common radiographic finding consists of a positive "fat pad" sign, representing displacement of the fat pads anterior and posterior to the distal humerus owing to intra-articular effusion or synovial hypertrophy.[155, 156] Soft tissue swelling over the ulnar olecranon, related to olecranon bursitis, and about the proximal ulna, related to rheumatoid nodules, is another frequent finding. Eventually, extensive osteolysis of the humerus, radius, and ulna may resemble the findings in neuroarthropathy. Large medullary cystic lesions of the distal humerus and ulnar olecranon may be the sites of pathologic fracture.[157]

Shoulder

Two main anatomic sites are frequently involved in rheumatoid arthritis of the shoulder: the glenohumeral and acromioclavicular joints. In the former location, changes of rheumatoid arthritis are prominent joint space narrowing, bony sclerosis, and cyst formation.[152] Osseous erosions are most prominent along the superolateral margin of the humerus, adjacent to the greater tuberosity, and may resemble the Hill-Sachs fracture associated with anterior shoulder dislocation. Erosions may be present at other sites on the proximal humerus and glenoid region of the scapula. Subacromial bursitis, bicipital tendinitis, and rotator cuff tears are frequent complications.

At the acromioclavicular joint, soft tissue swelling and erosions, which tend to be more prominent on the clavicular side of the joint, are early findings.[146] Later, destruction of a large portion of the distal clavicle may be seen.

Foot

Sites of foot involvement in rheumatoid arthritis may be divided into the forefoot, the midfoot, and the heel. The forefoot is very commonly affected (80 to 90 percent) in rheumatoid arthritis, especially the metatarsophalangeal joints.[158–160] The earliest changes involve the metatarsal heads at the first and fifth metatarsophalangeal articulations (Fig. 42–27).[145] At the fifth metatarsophalangeal joint, an early and characteristic erosion occurs on the dorsolateral aspect of the metatarsal head and may be visualized only on

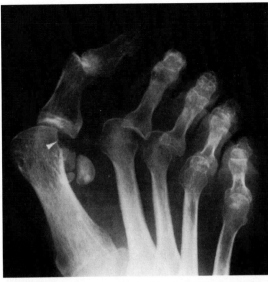

Figure 42–27. Rheumatoid arthritis. The classic forefoot deformities are well illustrated in this patient. Note the subluxation and fibular deviation at the metatarsophalangeal joints and the prominent marginal erosions of the first metatarsal head *(arrowhead)*. (From Resnick D, Niwayama G: Diagnosis of Bone and Joint Disorders. Philadelphia, WB Saunders, 1988.)

oblique radiographs. At the first metatarsophalangeal joint, the earliest involvement is along the medial aspect of the metatarsal head, with later erosions involving the adjacent sesamoid bones. With progression, diffuse joint space loss and larger erosions may be seen. Forefoot deformities in rheumatoid arthritis include hallux valgus, hammer toes, and "cock-up" toes, as well as fibular deviation of the digits and plantar subluxation of the metatarsal heads.

In the midfoot, rheumatoid arthritis is characterized by diffuse joint space loss, bony sclerosis, and osteophytosis, with osseous erosions being uncommon.[145] Osseous fusion in longstanding disease is relatively common. Differentiation of this disease from degenerative, post-traumatic, or neuropathic disorders may be difficult in this region.

In the heel, abnormalities of rheumatoid arthritis are related to involvement of the retrocalcaneal bursa, Achilles tendon, and plantar fascia. With the utilization of soft tissue–enhancing radiographic techniques, swelling of the Achilles tendon (>1 cm in diameter at the level of the posterosuperior margin of the calcaneus) or soft tissue masses adjacent to the posterosuperior margin of the calcaneus as the result of an engorged retrocalcaneal bursa may be early findings.[145, 161, 162] Osseous erosions at the posterosuperior margin of the calcaneus (Fig. 42–28) are subsequently noted. Well-defined plantar calcaneal enthesophytes, which are identical to those seen in "normal" persons, can be distinguished from the fluffy, proliferative calcaneal excrescences seen in the seronegative spondyloarthropathies.

Ankle

Although the ankle may be the site of radiographically identifiable joint effusions in the patient with

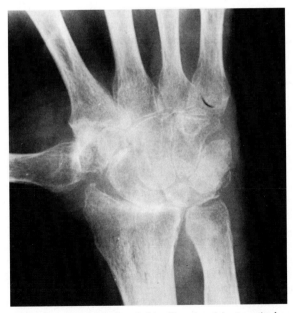

Figure 42–26. Rheumatoid arthritis. Prominent juxta-articular osteoporosis is present with radial deviation of the radiocarpal joint and ulnar translocation of the carpus. Extensive erosive changes of the radial and ulnar styloid processes and multiple carpal bones are also present. (From Resnick D, Niwayama G: Diagnosis of Bone and Joint Disorders. Philadelphia, WB Saunders, 1988.)

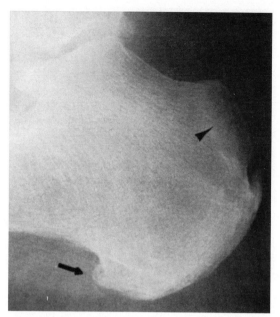

Figure 42–28. Rheumatoid arthritis. Erosions are present on the posterior *(arrowhead)* calcaneal surface. A plantar calcaneal spur is evident *(arrow)*.

rheumatoid arthritis, bony changes at this site are relatively uncommon. In some cases, diffuse osteoporosis and joint space narrowing as well as marginal and central bony erosions may be seen.[163] Rarely, with severe disease, loss of integrity of the ankle mortise may occur.

Knee

The knee is commonly affected in rheumatoid arthritis. Engorgement of the suprapatellar space of the knee joint by effusion or synovial hypertrophy is noted on the lateral radiographic projection. Small erosions along the medial and lateral margins of the tibia and femur are the earliest bony changes and are followed by joint space loss involving the medial femorotibial, lateral femorotibial, and patellofemoral compartments.[145] Subchondral cysts may be seen in the femoral condyles or proximal tibia, and subchondral sclerosis due to bony collapse may be prominent.[164] Varus or valgus deformity of the knee joint or patellar instability may be present. Rupture of the quadriceps or patellar tendon may occur with corresponding abnormalities of the soft tissue shadows about the knee. The knee is also a common site of large synovial cysts, especially in the popliteal region.[165] These synovial cysts may extend along fascial planes for a considerable distance in a proximal or distal direction.

Hip

Hip involvement in rheumatoid arthritis is less common than knee involvement. A characteristic radiographic abnormality is diffuse concentric loss of articular space, with migration of the femoral head along the plane of the axis of the femoral neck.[166] Radiolucent zones at the bone-cartilage junction of the femoral head are related to circumferential marginal erosions.[145] Central erosions of the femoral head and, less commonly, of the acetabulum may be seen. Occasionally, large pseudocystic lesions of the femoral neck occur and are liable to pathologic fracture. Acetabular protrusion is present if the inner margin of the acetabulum is medial to the ilioischial line by 3 mm or more in men or 6 mm or more in women. Mild sclerosis and small osteophytes may be noted, related to secondary degenerative disease (osteoarthritis). Osteonecrosis of the femoral heads may be encountered in rheumatoid arthritis, usually in association with glucocorticoid therapy.[167]

Sacroiliac Joints

Asymptomatic sacroiliac joint changes are common in rheumatoid arthritis of long duration.[168] In general, the findings consist of bilateral but asymmetric bony erosions that primarily involve the iliac side of the synovial articulation.

Spine

The cervical spine is one of the more common and important areas of involvement in rheumatoid arthritis. The apophyseal joints of the cervical spine are diffusely affected with bony erosion, joint space narrowing, and, eventually, subluxation that leads to a "stair-step" type of deformity (Fig. 42–29), with contiguous vertebral bodies being offset like the steps of a staircase.[169] Erosions and destruction involving the uncovertebral joints (Luschka) as well as the discovertebral junctions are also common. Between the spinous processes, the formation of adventitious bursae and their subsequent inflammation lead to characteristic erosions and a "sharpened" appearance of these processes on lateral radiographs of the cervical spine.

The most important site of cervical spine abnormality is the craniocervical junction. Erosions involving the anterior or posterior margins of the odontoid process as well as joint space narrowing and marginal osseous erosions involving the lateral occipito-atlantoaxial articulations are early findings.[169] Subsequently, laxity or destruction of the transverse atlantoaxial ligament can lead to horizontal (in the sagittal plane) atlantoaxial subluxation with encroachment of the odontoid process on the vertebral canal during flexion of the neck.[170, 171] The diagnosis of this complication is based on the identification of an abnormally wide space (>3 mm in the adult) between the posterior margin of the anterior arch of the atlas and the anterior surface of the odontoid process on lateral radiographs of the cervical spine exposed during flexion of the patient's neck. Large odontoid erosions may predispose to pathologic fracture. A second, less common but potentially fatal, pattern of cervical in-

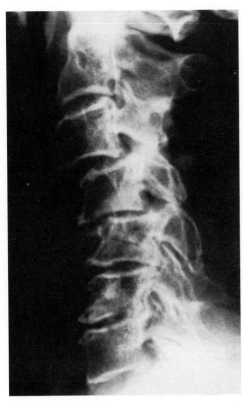

Figure 42–29. Rheumatoid arthritis. The "stair-step" deformity of the cervical spine is present with subluxation at multiple contiguous levels. Diffuse loss of intervertebral disc height and erosion of articular surfaces of the apophyseal joints are also present. (From Resnick D, Niwayama G: Diagnosis of Bone and Joint Disorders. Philadelphia, WB Saunders, 1988.)

stability in rheumatoid arthritis is vertical atlantoaxial subluxation in which compression of the lateral masses of the atlas in association with disease of the lateral atlantoaxial and atlanto-occipital joints allows the odontoid process to be elevated vertically, becoming intimate with the brainstem.[171, 172] Furthermore, occipito-atlantoaxial instability in the coronal plane can lead to lateral tilting of the head.

In contrast to the frequency of cervical spine involvement, changes in the thoracic and lumbar spine are uncommon in rheumatoid arthritis. However, erosive and destructive abnormalities about the lumbar apophyseal joints are well documented, as are irregularity, erosion, and loss of definition of the bony vertebral end-plates.[145] Synovial cysts arising from the apophyseal joints are rare causes of neurologic symptoms and signs.[173]

Other Locations

Other synovial joints that may be involved in rheumatoid arthritis include the temporomandibular and sternoclavicular joints. Not infrequently, cartilaginous articulations, such as the sternomanubrial joint and symphysis pubis, may show erosive change and narrowing.

JUVENILE CHRONIC ARTHRITIS

General Radiographic Features

Juvenile chronic arthritis (JCA) is a generic term used to describe a group of childhood articular disorders that share, to a variable degree, certain clinical, laboratory, and radiologic features. Each specific subgroup of JCA has its own distinctive radiographic appearance. However, many of the changes are nonspecific and related to effects of the disorder on growth and development of the immature skeleton. It is useful to first consider these general features of childhood arthritis prior to considering abnormalities in specific subgroups of disease.

Growth Disturbances[174–176]

Epiphyseal enlargement is a common feature of JCA and is related to growth stimulation associated with epiphyseal hyperemia. The changes occur diffusely but often are most marked at the femoral condyles, humeral condyles, and radial head. Epiphyseal overgrowth is combined with subnormal growth of the diaphyseal portion of the bone, resulting in a constricted appearance to the diaphysis with "ballooning" of the epiphysis (Fig. 42–30). The time of appearance and the size of individual bones in the wrist and midfoot may be increased. In some cases,

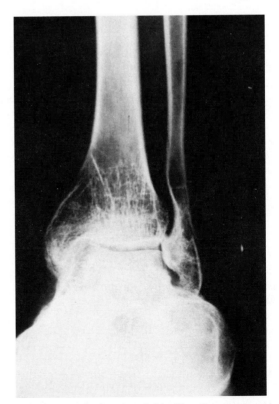

Figure 42–30. Juvenile chronic arthritis. Note the prominent juxta-articular osteoporosis with "ballooning" of the distal tibial and fibular epiphyses and a constricted appearance to the bone shafts.

overall bone length may be diminished owing to premature closure of the physis or, in other cases, increased owing to hyperemia.

Periostitis[176]

Periostitis is a common and nonspecific component of virtually all forms of JCA. This is in contrast to the specificity of periostitis in the differential diagnosis of adult arthropathies. In childhood the periosteum is relatively loosely attached to the underlying bone, a situation that allows it to be easily lifted and stimulated to produce new bone in response to inflammation. Periostitis is most common in the phalanges, metacarpals, and metatarsals but may occasionally be seen in the metaphyses and diaphyses of long tubular bones. In the small bones of the hands and feet, exuberant periosteal new bone formation may result in a "squared" appearance.

Epiphyseal Compression Fractures[176]

Flattening and deformity of the epiphyseal centers in weight-bearing articulations are common in JCA. Cupping of the epiphyseal centers of the proximal phalanges is also frequent. These changes are related to the abnormal stresses associated with joint contracture and subluxation acting on the osteoporotic epiphyses.

Osteopenia

Osteopenia, representing increased skeletal radiolucency, is generally most striking in the metaphyseal region of a bone, resulting in the formation of horizontally oriented radiolucent metaphyseal bands.[176] These lucent bands are commonly noted in the femur, tibia, fibula, and radius and are identical to those seen in childhood leukemia, metastatic neuroblastoma, and congenital infections. With time, diffuse osteoporosis can develop. Growth recovery lines (Fig. 42–31) are thin, horizontally oriented radiodense bands visualized in the diametaphyseal region of tubular bones in children with chronic illness. Presumably they are manifestations of accelerated bone growth in the intervals following exacerbations of disease. Occasionally, widespread metaphyseal sclerosis is seen (see Fig. 42–31).

Juvenile-Onset Adult-Type (Seropositive) Rheumatoid Arthritis

Soft tissue swelling, juxta-articular osteoporosis, and marginal erosions may be present in JCA, as in the typical adult case.[174] However, two features help differentiate this disorder from adult-onset rheumatoid arthritis: the presence of periostitis, especially of the small bones of the hands and feet, and the frequent occurrence of prominent marginal erosions without associated joint space narrowing.[177, 178]

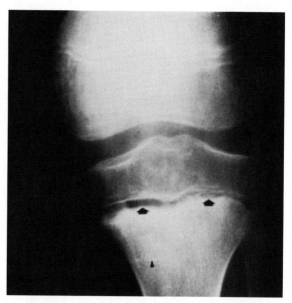

Figure 42–31. Juvenile chronic arthritis. There is overgrowth of the epiphyses about the knee. Juxta-articular osteoporosis is evident, with several horizontally oriented growth recovery lines (arrowhead). Metaphyseal sclerosis (arrows) can be visualized in the proximal tibia.

Seronegative Chronic Arthritis (Still's Disease)[179]

Classic systemic Still's disease is an acute systemic illness that rarely manifests radiographic articular changes.

Polyarticular disease may occur in the presence or absence of classic Still's disease. Symmetric involvement of the hands, wrists, knees, ankles, feet, and cervical spine is common. In the hands and feet, osteoporosis is associated with joint space narrowing, and the small bones assume a "squared" shape as a result of new bone formation. Osseous erosions are unusual in this disorder and, when present, are usually of small size. Intra-articular bony ankylosis (Fig. 42–32) is a common late complication in the small joints, in contrast to its rarity in adult-onset rheumatoid arthritis. In the larger articulations such as the knee and the hip, osteoporosis and epiphyseal overgrowth are the most typical manifestations, often occurring without joint space narrowing or bony erosions. The cervical spine is frequently the only spinal level involved in this disorder (Fig. 42–33); abnormalities predominate in the upper cervical region. The growth disturbance results in a constriction of vertebral body width and depth with relatively normal height, resulting in a slender, gracile appearance. Apophyseal joint space narrowing, bony ankylosis, and osseous erosions occur with hypoplasia of the intervertebral discs and bony ankylosis of vertebral bodies. As in adults, atlantoaxial subluxation is a frequent complication in children.

Pauciarticular and monoarticular forms of seronegative chronic arthritis are occasionally seen.[178, 180] Changes are generally confined to the larger articulations such as the knee, hip, ankle, elbow, and wrist; the small joints of the hands and feet are spared. Radiographic abnormalities are the same as those in the polyarticular pattern of disease.

Juvenile-Onset Ankylosing Spondylitis

Juvenile-onset ankylosing spondylitis is generally first manifest in the articulations of the lower extremity, particularly the hips, knees, ankles, and small joints of the feet.[174] The joints of the upper extremities are relatively spared. Sacroiliitis and spondylitis occur but are usually identified later in the course of the disease, in contrast to adult-onset ankylosing spondylitis. In the spine, thoracic and lumbar involvement is common, with involvement of the cervical spine distinctly unusual.

Radiographic changes in the peripheral skeleton consist of joint space narrowing, bony erosions and proliferation, and intra-articular osseous fusion.[181] Osteoporosis is frequently not prominent. In the sacroiliac articulations and the thoracolumbar spine, the radiographic changes are identical to those of adult-onset ankylosing spondylitis.[182] Useful features in differentiating this disorder from other types of JCA include the absence of diffuse osteoporosis, relative sparing of the articulations of the upper extremity and cervical spine, and sacroiliitis and spondylitis.

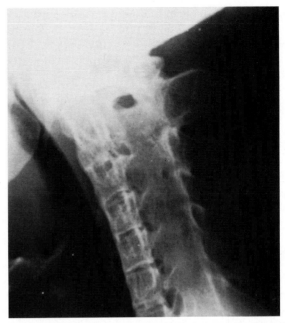

Figure 42–33. Juvenile chronic arthritis. Intervertebral and apophyseal joint bony ankylosis is present at multiple levels. The overall appearance of the cervical spine is gracile, owing to the relatively normal height of the vertebral bodies and the diminished anteroposterior vertebral diameter. (From Resnick D, Niwayama G: Diagnosis of Bone and Joint Disorders. Philadelphia, WB Saunders, 1981.)

Juvenile-Onset Psoriatic Arthritis

Juvenile-onset psoriatic arthritis is occasionally encountered. Radiographic changes simulate those in adults. Hand involvement is characterized by resorption of the terminal tufts of the distal phalanges and interphalangeal joint destruction.[179] Although sacroiliitis is common in this disorder, the normal indistinct appearance of the sacroiliac articulations in children and adolescents makes accurate radiographic diagnosis of sacroiliitis difficult.

Adult-Onset Still's Disease

Rarely, an adult patient may be encountered with a febrile illness identical to classic Still's disease.[183] When present, radiographic changes involve the wrists, knees, and fingers. Bony erosions are unusual. A peculiar tendency toward narrowing or ankylosis of the common carpometacarpal joint, especially that portion at the level of the second and third metacarpal bases, and the intercarpal joint in a pericapitate distribution has been reported.[184]

Others

Enteropathic arthropathy may be identified in childhood accompanying regional enteritis, ulcerative colitis, or bowel infections (*Salmonella, Shigella*). Its

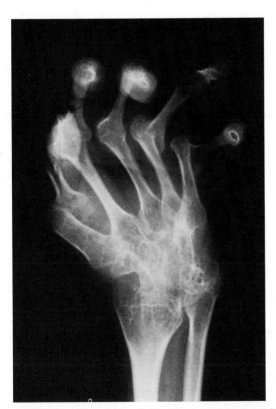

Figure 42–32. Juvenile chronic arthritis. There are prominent finger deformities, osteoporosis, and bony ankylosis, especially in the carpus. Note the elongated, slender appearance of the tubular bones, which is related to growth disturbance.

appearance is identical to that of juvenile-onset ankylosing spondylitis. Other rare causes of childhood arthropathy include systemic lupus erythematosus and familial Mediterranean fever.

SERONEGATIVE SPONDYLOARTHROPATHIES

Ankylosing Spondylitis

Synovial and cartilaginous joints as well as sites of tendon and ligament insertion (entheses) may be involved in ankylosing spondylitis and the other seronegative spondyloarthropathies.[185, 186] Axial skeletal involvement is characteristic, with a predilection for the sacroiliac, apophyseal, discovertebral, and costovertebral articulations. The initial sites of involvement are the sacroiliac joints and lumbosacral and thoracolumbar vertebral junctions. Subsequently, ascending and descending spinal disease may be encountered.[187, 188] Peripheral joint involvement, although frequent (50 percent), is usually mild.[182] The hips and glenohumeral joints are the most common extraspinal locations of disease.

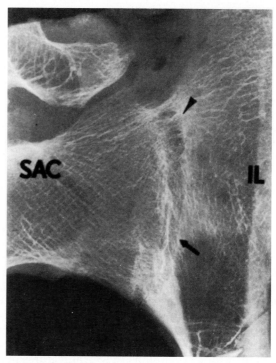

Figure 42–35. Ankylosing spondylitis. A specimen radiograph from a cadaver with the disease demonstrates complete intra-articular ankylosis of the ligamentous *(arrowhead)* and synovial *(arrow)* portions of the joint. SAC, sacrum; IL, ilium.

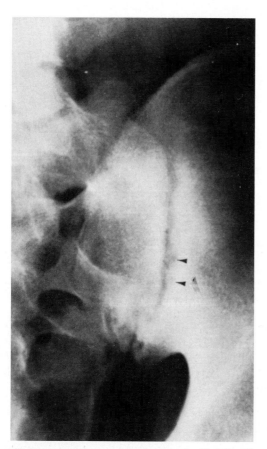

Figure 42–34. Ankylosing spondylitis. Note the ill-defined band of sclerosis and prominent erosions of the subchondral bone plate *(arrowheads)*, which are most conspicuous on the iliac side of the articulation.

Sacroiliac Joints

Involvement of the sacroiliac joint is the hallmark of ankylosing spondylitis. It is difficult to verify the diagnosis of this disease in the absence of such involvement. Rarely, spinal disease occurs in the absence of significant sacroiliac joint abnormality. Sacroiliitis occurs early in the course of ankylosing spondylitis and is characteristically bilateral and symmetric in its distribution.[187–190] On rare occasions, initial unilateral or asymmetric sacroiliac joint changes are observed. Changes occur in both the synovial and the ligamentous portions of the joint, with the abnormalities being more prominent on the iliac side of the articulation.[186] Osteoporosis, subchondral bony resorption with loss of definition of the articular margins, and superficial osseous erosions are interspersed with focal areas of bony sclerosis. Radiographically, in this stage, the articulation may appear widened. With progression of the disease, a wide, ill-defined band of sclerosis is seen on the iliac side of the joint with larger subchondral erosions (Fig. 42–34). In the late proliferative stage, bony bridges traverse the joint space, initially isolating islands of intact cartilage. Such segmental ankylosis may be followed by complete intra-articular bony fusion (Fig. 42–35) and disappearance of the periarticular sclerosis. The ligamentous (syndesmotic) portions of the sacroiliac joint may also be affected, leading to bony erosions and proliferation. In general, involvement of the ligamentous portion of the articulation is less prominent in ankylosing spondylitis than in psoriatic arthritis and Reiter's syndrome.

Spine

The initial sites of spinal involvement, especially in men, are the lumbosacral and thoracolumbar junctions. In women, the cervical spine may be affected at an early stage of disease. "Osteitis" is an initial finding, related to inflammation of the anterior portion of the discovertebral junction.[186] A focal erosive lesion at the anterosuperior and anteroinferior vertebral margins leads to loss of the normal concavity of the anterior aspect of the vertebral body, resulting in a "squared" configuration of the vertebral body in the lateral radiographic projection. This appearance is more easily identified in the lumbar spine, as the thoracic vertebral bodies may normally have a squared appearance. In ankylosing spondylitis, bony sclerosis adjacent to the sites of erosion produces a "shiny corner" sign on radiographs.

Syndesmophytes are vertically oriented bony excrescences that represent ossification of the outer fibers of the annulus fibrosus of the intervertebral disc.[191] They predominate on the anterior and lateral aspects of the spine and eventually bridge the intervertebral disc (Fig. 42–36A). In the late stages of the disease, extensive syndesmophytic formation produces a smooth, undulating spinal contour—the "bamboo spine."

It is of critical importance that the syndesmophytes that characterize ankylosing spondylitis (and enteropathic spondyloarthritis) be differentiated from other spinal and paraspinal bony excrescences (see Fig. 42–36; also see Figs. 42–43, 42–58, and 42–59). Vertebral excrescences in spondylosis deformans arise several millimeters from the discovertebral junction, are triangular in shape, and demonstrate a horizontally oriented segment of variable length at their point of origin. In diffuse idiopathic skeletal hyperostosis (DISH), bone formation in the anterior longitudinal ligament results in a flowing pattern of ossification, thicker than that seen in ankylosing spondylitis. Such ossification is best demonstrated on lateral spine radiographs. Furthermore, in DISH there is absence of erosion or widespread bony ankylosis in the sacroiliac joints. The paravertebral ossifications that characterize psoriatic arthritis and Reiter's syndrome arise in an asymmetric fashion in the soft tissues adjacent to the outer layer of the annulus fibrosus. They are initially unattached to the vertebral body but, with time, fuse with the margins of the vertebral body at a point several millimeters from the discovertebral junction.

Erosions at one or more discovertebral junctions can be prominent radiographic findings in ankylosing spondylitis. These may be classified as focal or diffuse.[192] Focal lesions may relate to intraosseous displacement of disc material (cartilaginous or Schmorl's node) or enthesitis. Diffuse destruction of the discovertebral junction may be related to a pseudarthrosis following fracture. Discal calcification is common and usually seen in association with apophyseal joint ankylosis at the same spinal level.

Early alterations in the apophyseal joints in the

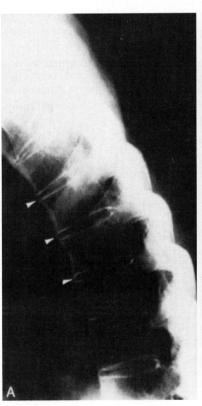
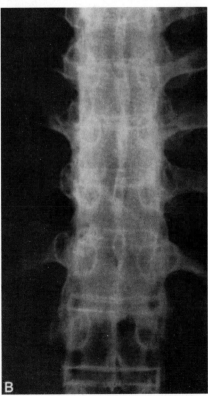

Figure 42–36. Ankylosing spondylitis. Lateral (A) and frontal (B) radiographs of the spine demonstrate complete intervertebral ankylosis, which produces the characteristic "bamboo spine" appearance. Note the thin, vertically oriented syndesmophytes (arrowheads) arising from the discovertebral junction, owing to ossification in the outermost layer of the annulus fibrosus.

lumbar, thoracic, and cervical segments consist of ill-defined erosions accompanied by reactive sclerosis. Capsular ossification or intra-articular bony ankylosis may subsequently occur. On frontal radiographs of the spine, such ossification produces vertically oriented, parallel, radiodense bands, which, when combined with a central radiodense band related to ossification of the interspinous and supraspinous ligaments, lead to the "trolley-track" sign (see Fig. 42–36B).[186]

Erosions of the odontoid process and atlantoaxial subluxation may be observed in ankylosing spondylitis, although with less frequency than in rheumatoid arthritis.[171, 187] Ankylosis of the atlantoaxial articulation, either in its normal position or in a position of subluxation, may occasionally be noted. At other levels in the cervical spine, the changes, when present, are identical to those in the thoracolumbar spine.

Extraspinal Locations

The hip is the most commonly involved peripheral articulation in ankylosing spondylitis, with the changes most frequently being bilateral and symmetric in distribution.[193] Concentric joint space narrowing with axial migration of the femoral head and marginal osteophyte formation characterizes the hip disease of ankylosing spondylitis (Fig. 42–37). Osteophytes are first observed at the lateral margin of the femoral head-neck junction and, with progression, proliferate circumferentially to produce a characteristic "ring osteophyte."[193, 194] Subchondral cysts and erosions as well as intra-articular bony ankylosis may be seen in some cases. Such hip disease can lead to signficant clinical manifestations requiring surgical intervention. However, patients with ankylosing spon-

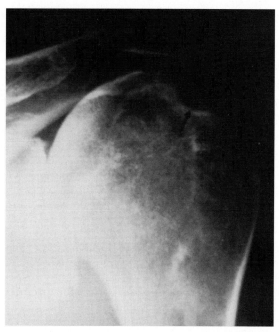

Figure 42–38. Ankylosing spondylitis. There is disruption of the musculotendinous rotator cuff with superior migration of the humeral head. The large erosion *(arrow)* of the superolateral aspect of the humeral head ("hatchet deformity") is a characteristic radiographic sign of the disease.

dylitis who undergo hip surgery, including total joint replacement, are prone to develop exuberant deposits of juxta-articular heterotopic bone, which may severely restrict postoperative hip motion.[195]

The shoulder is the second most common peripheral site of involvement in ankylosing spondylitis.[182] Bilateral involvement is common; changes are osteoporosis, joint space narrowing, bony erosions, and rotator cuff disruption. A characteristic large destructive abnormality involving the superolateral aspect of the humeral head in this disease has been termed the *hatchet* sign (Fig. 42–38).[196]

Changes in other peripheral joints occur with variable frequency. In general, these changes, which are similar to but less extensive than those in the other seronegative spondyloarthropathies, include soft tissue swelling, mild osteoporosis, joint space narrowing, bony erosions, and osseous proliferation.[186] The erosions tend to be less prominent than in rheumatoid arthritis. The presence of bone proliferation (whiskering) and periostitis in ankylosing spondylitis (and the other seronegative spondyloarthropathies) is another helpful diagnostic feature.

Inflammation with bony proliferation at sites of tendon and ligament insertion (enthesopathy), especially those of the pelvis, patella, and calcaneus, is prominent in ankylosing spondylitis (as well as in the other seronegative spondyloarthropathies). Plantar and posterior calcaneal spurs are common and may be either well defined or indistinct with feathery margins, representing the combination of erosive and proliferative change. Erosions of the posterior calcaneal

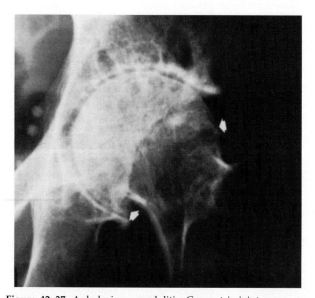

Figure 42–37. Ankylosing spondylitis. Concentric joint space narrowing with axial migration of the femoral head is present. Osteophytes *(arrows)* are present at the medial and lateral margins of the femoral head.

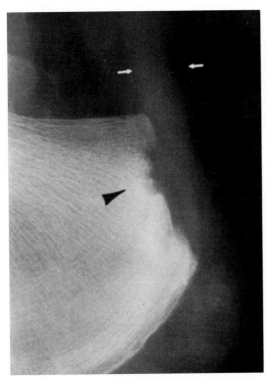

Figure 42–39. Ankylosing spondylitis. Erosive change of the posterior calcaneal margin is present *(arrowhead)* as well as thickening of the Achilles tendon *(between arrows)*.

margin due to inflammation in the retrocalcaneal bursa and thickening of the Achilles tendon may be present (Fig. 42–39).[161] The inflammatory enthesopathy of the seronegative spondyloarthropathies[186, 197] differs from the degenerative enthesopathy seen in DISH (see Fig. 42–61). In the latter disease, bony outgrowths (enthesophytes) are sharply marginated and well defined.

Other sites of involvement in ankylosing spondylitis[186] include the symphysis pubis and manubriosternal, temporomandibular, and sternoclavicular joints.

Psoriatic Arthritis

In general, psoriatic arthritis is asymmetric or unilateral with involvement of synovial and cartilaginous joints as well as entheses.[198] The most common sites of involvement are the interphalangeal joints of the hands and feet, metatarsophalangeal joints, metacarpophalangeal joints, sacroiliac joints, and the spine. Changes in the knees, ankles, elbows, and wrists and manubriosternal, acromioclavicular, and sternoclavicular joints, as well as pelvic entheses, are not uncommon. Hip or glenohumeral joint involvement is rare.

The arthritis of psoriasis is associated with periarticular soft tissue swelling, which in some cases may be manifested by diffuse, sausage-like enlargement of an entire digit.[199] The absence of osteoporosis is remarkable in many cases of psoriatic arthritis and is

an important consideration in the differential diagnosis. However, osteoporosis may occasionally be evident; thus, its presence does not exclude the diagnosis of psoriatic arthritis. Joint space narrowing or widening may be encountered, the latter being more common in the small joints of the hands and feet. Erosions progress from marginal areas in a central direction, often resulting in a "whittled" or "pencil-in-cup" deformity of the involved articulation.[200] In cases in which this severe destructive change is predominant, in combination with marked joint deformity, the term *arthritis mutilans* is frequently used. Bony proliferation is a striking feature of psoriatic arthritis and the other seronegative spondyloarthropathies (Fig. 42–40).[201] Proliferation around erosions produces a "whiskered" appearance. Diaphyseal and metaphyseal periostitis is also common.[202] In fact, osseous proliferation involving the distal phalanges may produce diffuse increased radiodensity, termed the *ivory phalanx*.[203] Intra-articular bony fusion, especially involving the proximal and distal interphalangeal joints of the hands and feet, is a common finding. An inflammatory enthesopathy consisting of fine, feathery, bony proliferation at sites of tendon and ligament insertion is also prominent in many cases.

Hands

In the hands, involvement of the distal interphalangeal joints is frequent and may be unilateral or bilateral, symmetric or asymmetric in distribution (see

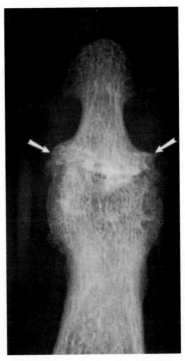

Figure 42–40. Psoriatic arthritis. The distal interphalangeal joint is narrowed, with proliferative bony erosions *(arrows)*. Also note the prominent soft tissue swelling and the abnormality of the fingernail.

Fig. 42–40). Erosions occur at the joint margins and progress centrally, with irregular destructive changes. Protrusion of one joint surface into its articular counterpart produces the pencil-in-cup deformity. Resorption of the terminal tufts of the distal phalanges may be seen. Psoriatic arthritis can lead to intra-articular bony ankylosis, a finding that is rare in rheumatoid arthritis.

Feet

Psoriatic arthritis involves two major areas in the foot: the forefoot and the calcaneus.[198] In the forefoot, changes are usually bilateral and asymmetric, predominating at the interphalangeal and metatarsophalangeal articulations. Marginal erosion, joint space narrowing (or widening), and bony proliferation are present, characteristically without significant osteoporosis. Severe destruction of the interphalangeal articulation of the great toe can be seen in psoriatic arthritis (and in Reiter's syndrome). Sesamoid involvement is also common in the foot as well as in the hand.

As in the other seronegative spondyloarthropathies, the combination of proliferative and erosive changes in the posterior and inferior surfaces of the calcaneus is an important radiographic finding of psoriatic arthritis. Erosions of the posterior surface of the calcaneus with surrounding proliferation adjacent to the retrocalcaneal bursa are common. Irregular and poorly defined spurs are typically present at the insertion of the plantar aponeurosis (Fig. 42–41), although in time, such spurs may become relatively well defined.

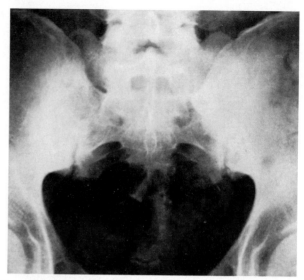

Figure 42–42. Psoriatic arthritis. Bilateral and asymmetric changes of the sacroiliac joints are present with erosions and sclerosis of the subchondral bone plate.

Sacroiliac Joints

A bilateral and symmetric distribution constitutes the most common radiographic pattern of sacroiliac joint abnormalities in psoriatic arthritis, although asymmetric involvement is not rare (Fig. 42–42).[197, 204] Initially, subchondral bony erosions and ill-defined sclerosis with apparent joint space widening are noted, abnormalities identical to those in ankylosing spondylitis. However, the frequency of intra-articular bony ankylosis in psoriatic arthritis is less than that in ankylosing spondylitis or the spondyloarthritis associated with inflammatory bowel diseases. Furthermore, in psoriatic arthritis (as in Reiter's syndrome), blurring and eburnation of apposing sacral and iliac surfaces within the ligamentous portion of the sacroiliac joint are more common than in ankylosing spondylitis.

Spine

The characteristic spinal lesion of psoriatic arthritis (as well as Reiter's syndrome) is paravertebral ossification.[205] These ossifications initially appear as either thick and irregular or thin and curvilinear densities, asymmetrically distributed parallel to the lateral surface of the intervertebral disc and vertebral body (Fig. 42–43). At this stage, the outgrowths are not attached to the vertebral body, although in later stages, the ossific densities merge with the lateral margins of the vertebral body several millimeters distal to the discovertebral junction. Occasionally, syndesmophytes identical to those in ankylosing spondylitis do occur in psoriatic arthritis[198] and Reiter's syndrome; however, in the great majority of cases, they are interspersed with the more characteristic paravertebral ossifications. "Corner osteitis," vertebral body "squar-

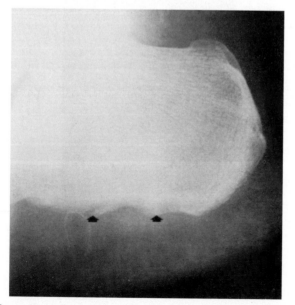

Figure 42–41. Psoriatic arthritis. The inferior surface of the calcaneus reveals the characteristic combination of erosive and proliferative changes *(arrows)* that is the hallmark of the seronegative spondyloarthropathies.

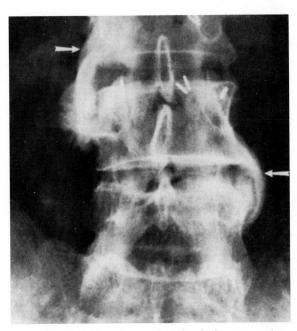

Figure 42–43. Psoriatic arthritis. Note the thick asymmetric paravertebral ossifications *(arrows)* arising from the vertebral margins in this patient with psoriatic spondylitis. These lesions, which are best visualized in the anteroposterior projection of the spine, are characteristic of psoriatic arthritis and Reiter's syndrome.

ing," and apophyseal joint ankylosis are less common than in ankylosing spondylitis.

Cervical spine changes in psoriatic arthritis may be dramatic, even in patients with minimal thoracolumbar spinal involvement.[204, 206] Discovertebral joint irregularity with extensive bony proliferation about the anterior aspect of the vertebra and extensive apophyseal joint erosion and narrowing may be seen. Atlantoaxial subluxation is common.[204]

Other Locations

In longstanding or severe disease, virtually any articulation may be involved. In most sites, the characteristic combination of erosive and proliferative change is present.

Reiter's Syndrome

Radiographic alterations occur in approximately 60 to 80 percent of patients with Reiter's syndrome.[207] These radiographic changes demonstrate morphologic characteristics that are virtually indistinguishable from those in the other seronegative spondyloarthropathies, especially psoriatic arthritis; differentiation is usually possible only by means of the distribution of abnormalities and the clinical history. Synovial joints, cartilaginous joints, and entheses may be affected. Characteristically, these changes are bilateral and asymmetric, with a predilection for involvement of the lower extremity.[207]

The most common sites of involvement are the small joints of the foot and the posterior and inferior calcaneal surfaces, followed in order of frequency by the ankle and the knee. Involvement of the hip and upper extremity is considerably less common. In the axial skeleton, the sacroiliac joints, spine, symphysis pubis, and manubriosternal joints are the most common sites of alteration.

The general radiographic features of Reiter's syndrome are soft tissue swelling, joint space narrowing, and bony erosion and proliferation. Osteoporosis is variable in frequency and extent but may be present during acute exacerbations of arthritis. Osseous proliferation at insertions of tendons and ligaments is a frequent finding, especially in the pelvis and the calcaneus.

Feet and Ankles

Asymmetric abnormalities of the metatarsophalangeal and interphalangeal joints of the forefoot are the most common manifestations of Reiter's syndrome (Fig. 42–44).[208] Frequently, effusions in the retrocalcaneal bursa may be identified as radiodense shadows obliterating the normal fat plane between the posterosuperior aspect of the calcaneus and the Achilles tendon.[162] Thickening of this tendon may also be evident. Ill-defined plantar calcaneal enthesophytes are characteristic, but as in the other seronega-

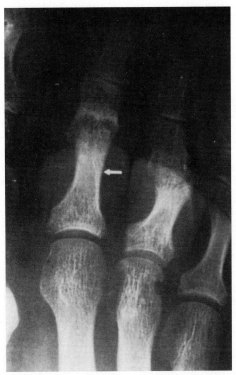

Figure 42–44. Reiter's syndrome. There is destructive change in the second and third proximal interphalangeal joints with subperiosteal proliferative reaction along the phalangeal shafts *(arrow).* Marginal erosions of the metatarsal heads and proximal phalanges are also evident.

tive spondyloarthropathies, the outgrowths may be relatively well defined in the later stages of the disease. Marginal erosions are somewhat uncommon about the ankle, but joint space narrowing, with adjacent soft tissue swelling, and fluffy periostitis of the distal tibia and fibula are seen.[207]

Knee

The most common abnormality in the knee in Reiter's syndrome is the presence of a joint effusion, which in some instances becomes massive. Osteoporosis, joint space narrowing, and periostitis of the patella and distal femoral shaft also occur. Bony erosions in the femur or tibia are rare.

Sacroiliac Joints

Sacroiliac joint abnormalities are common and may be bilateral and asymmetric or unilateral in distribution. These abnormalities are identical to those of psoriatic arthritis.

Spine

Spinal involvement is less frequent in Reiter's syndrome than in ankylosing spondylitis and psoriatic arthritis. Although in some instances the changes may be identical to those of ankylosing spondylitis, a more characteristic finding consists of asymmetrically distributed paravertebral ossifications involving the thoracolumbar spine.[209] Cervical spine involvement is unusual, and atlantoaxial subluxation is rare.

Other Locations

In the cartilaginous manubriosternal and pubic symphyseal articulations, the changes of Reiter's syndrome consist of erosions of the articular surfaces with adjacent bony proliferation and sclerosis.[206]

Severe and diffuse involvement of joints of the upper extremity is rare in Reiter's syndrome,[207] although scattered lesions, particularly in the proximal interphalangeal joints of the hands, may occasionally be seen. Distal interphalangeal or metacarpophalangeal joint alterations are less frequent. Fusiform or "sausage-like" soft tissue swelling, joint space narrowing, periarticular osteoporosis, and bony erosion and proliferation are observed.

Enteropathic Arthropathies and Related Conditions

The frequency of peripheral joint involvement in enteropathic arthritis is variable. Several types of involvement are seen[210-214]: a mild, inflammatory, self-limited peripheral arthritis in which the radiographic changes consist principally of soft tissue swelling and juxta-articular osteoporosis; a progressive, destructive peripheral arthropathy characterized by soft tissue

swelling, variable osteoporosis, joint space narrowing, osseous erosions, and bony proliferation; and sacroiliitis or spondylitis. In patients with spondyloarthritis, the changes are identical to those in ankylosing spondylitis, although the male predominance of ankylosing spondylitis is less marked in this group of disorders and isolated sacroiliitis without spinal involvement is more common.

In primary biliary cirrhosis, a severe destructive arthropathy of the hands has been described,[215] characterized by the asymmetric distribution of well-defined marginal erosions primarily involving the proximal and distal interphalangeal joints with relative sparing of the metacarpophalangeal joints. Chondrocalcinosis may be present in some patients, and occasionally, severe involvement of the hips and shoulders resembling osteonecrosis has been noted.[216]

A number of pancreatic diseases, including carcinoma, inflammation, and pancreatic duct calculi, may be associated with a syndrome characterized by subcutaneous nodules, polyarthritis, and medullary fat necrosis.[217, 218] The polyarthritis is radiographically nonspecific, with osteoporosis and soft tissue swelling being most commonly encountered. The radiographic appearance of medullary fat necrosis consists of diffuse osteolytic lesions with a "moth-eaten" appearance and periostitis. These changes closely resemble those of osteomyelitis and osteonecrosis.

OTHER CONNECTIVE TISSUE DISEASES

A number of other connective tissue disorders, including systemic lupus erythematosus, progressive

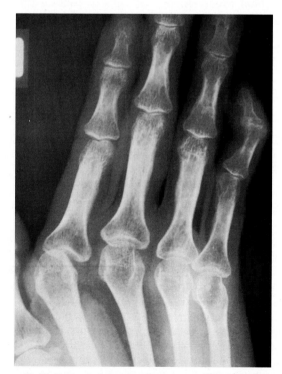

Figure 42–45. Systemic lupus erythematosus. This patient demonstrates juxta-articular osteoporosis with ulnar deviation at the metacarpophalangeal joints. No erosions are present.

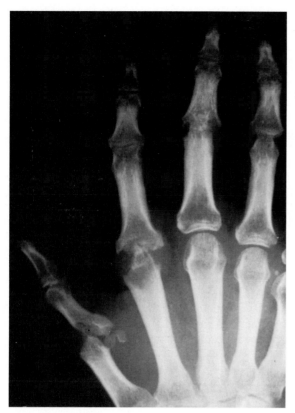

Figure 42–46. Systemic lupus erythematosus. An unusual pattern of involvement is seen. Severe erosive changes are present in the first and second metacarpophalangeal joints and third proximal interphalangeal joint. Juxta-articular osteoporosis is prominent.

systemic sclerosis, dermatomyositis, polymyositis, periarteritis nodosa, and mixed connective tissue disease, may be associated with musculoskeletal radiographic abnormalities.

Systemic Lupus Erythematosus

The roentgenographic changes of systemic lupus erythematosus (SLE) include symmetric polyarthritis, deforming nonerosive arthropathy, spontaneous tendon rupture, osteonecrosis, soft tissue calcification, infection, acrosclerosis, and tuftal resorption.[219–228] With the polyarthritis, the radiographic changes are nonspecific and consist of soft tissue swelling and periarticular osteoporosis.[219, 220]

Joint space narrowing and bony erosions are unusual. Deforming nonerosive arthropathy is seen in 5 to 40 percent of patients with SLE.[220] Symmetric involvement of the hands is typical. The specific type of deformity is variable.[219–221] Swan-neck or boutonnière deformity can be evident. Other deformities include hyperextension of the interphalangeal joint of the thumb, ulnar drift at the metacarpophalangeal joints, and subluxation of the first carpometacarpal joint (Fig. 42–45). It is the prominent thumb deformity that is especially characteristic of lupus arthropathy.

Although bony and cartilaginous abnormalities are generally not present, joint space narrowing, "hook-like" erosions of the radial and volar aspects of the metacarpal heads, and subchondral cyst formation are occasionally encountered (Fig. 42–46).[223] The radiographic findings of osteonecrosis in patients with SLE include transchondral fractures, subchondral sclerosis with cyst formation, and osseous collapse. Secondary osteoarthritis may eventually be prominent.

Linear or nodular calcific deposits in the subcutaneous tissues, particularly in the lower extremities, may occasionally be seen in SLE.[225] Sclerosis (acrosclerosis) or resorption of the tufts of the terminal phalanges also is occasionally evident in SLE.[228]

Progressive Systemic Sclerosis (Scleroderma)

Soft tissue or bony involvement in progressive systemic sclerosis (PSS) is common. The radiographic abnormalities can be divided into four main categories[228]: (1) soft tissue resorption, (2) soft tissue calcification, (3) osteolysis, and (4) erosive articular disease.

Soft tissue resorption is most commonly noted in the fingertips in association with Raynaud's phenomenon (Fig. 42–47). Early changes can be identified by

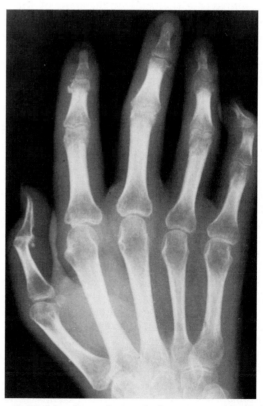

Figure 42–47. Scleroderma. Juxta-articular osteoporosis, soft tissue calcification, and resorption of the terminal tufts of the distal phalanges are present. Also note the tapered appearance of the soft tissues of the second finger and a hook-like erosion in the radial aspect of the third metacarpal head.

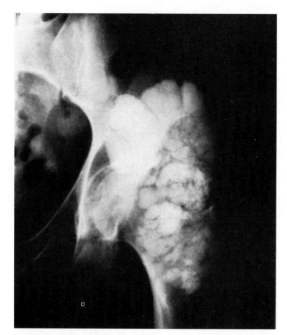

Figure 42–48. Scleroderma. A large tumoral calcific collection is present adjacent to the hip.

noting a reduction in the normal distance between the phalangeal tips and the skin (normal ≥20 percent of the transverse diameter of the base of the same distal phalanx).[229] In time, the fingertip assumes a conical shape and soft tissue calcification is often present.

Soft tissue calcification is most common in the hand but may occur at virtually any site.[230, 231] Calcification may be present in subcutaneous tissue, joint capsule, tendons, or ligaments (Fig. 42–48). The calcification typically is composed of hydroxyapatite crystals and has a soft, cloudlike radiographic appearance. Occasionally, large tumoral collections may be present adjacent to a joint. Intra-articular or intraosseous calcification may also be noted (Fig. 42–49).

Extra-articular osteolysis is a frequent manifestation of PSS. The most common site is the tuft of the distal phalanx of the hand or occasionally the foot, usually in association with Raynaud's phenomenon and soft tissue calcification. The earliest change is in the volar aspect of the tuft with continuing resorption, leading to a "sharpened" appearance of the phalanx (Fig. 42–50).[228] Elsewhere, thickening of the periodontal membrane about the roots of the teeth[232] or localized mandibular osteolysis may be seen, the latter predisposing to pathologic fracture.[233] Localized osteolysis involving the ribs, acromion, clavicle, radius, ulna, and cervical spine has also been reported.[233–236]

A severe articular disease consisting of joint space narrowing, marginal and central osseous erosions, and deformity may occur.[237] There is a distinctive tendency toward involvement of the first carpometacarpal joint (see Fig. 42–49).[238] Indeed, bilateral destructive changes of the first carpometacarpal articu-

lation with joint subluxation should arouse suspicion of PSS. Other relatively common sites of joint involvement in PSS include the distal interphalangeal, proximal interphalangeal, inferior radioulnar, and metatarsophalangeal joints.[239]

Dermatomyositis and Polymyositis

Articular abnormalities in dermatomyositis and polymyositis are usually without radiographic manifestations, although periarticular soft tissue swelling and osteoporosis may occasionally be noted.[240] More dramatic roentgenographic changes occur in the skeletal musculature, especially the large proximal muscle groups of the thorax, arm, forearm, thigh, and calf. Initial inflammation produces increased bulk and radiodensity of muscles with loss of the normal intermuscular fat planes.[241] In later stages, muscle atrophy or contractures may be prominent. The most characteristic soft tissue abnormality is calcification[242] in subcutaneous tissue, intermuscular fascia, tendons, or fat (Fig. 42–51). Subcutaneous calcific deposits simulate those of progressive systemic sclerosis, but the presence of marked linear calcific collections favors the diagnosis of polymyositis or dermatomyositis.

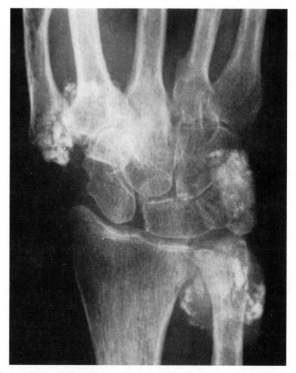

Figure 42–49. Scleroderma. Prominent soft tissue calcification and intra-articular calcification are present as well as severe erosive change of the first carpometacarpal joint. This is a characteristic "target" area of scleroderma. (From Resnick D, Niwayama G: Diagnosis of Bone and Joint Disorders. Philadelphia, WB Saunders, 1981.)

Periarteritis Nodosa

Plain-film radiographic findings are unusual in periarteritis nodosa, although joint effusions or periostitis of the tubular bones identical to that of hypertrophic osteoarthropathy may occasionally be seen.[243] Angiography is an important diagnostic modality in evaluating the extent of vascular damage in this disease.

Mixed Connective Tissue Disease and "Overlap" Syndromes

A broad spectrum of radiographic abnormalities may be present in mixed connective tissue disease (MCTD),[244, 245] including soft tissue swelling and calcification, osteoporosis, joint space narrowing, bony erosions, and joint deformity. Useful radiographic clues include (1) a radiographic pattern suggestive of more than one collagen vascular disease, (2) an erosive arthropathy with an asymmetric distribution or with prominent involvement of the distal interphalangeal joints, and (3) sausage-like soft tissue swelling of a digit. However, none of these changes is specific for MCTD.

There is a group of patients with clinical and radiographic features of more than one collagen vascular disease in whom serologic testing fails to document the presence of MCTD. Such patients are considered to have an "overlap" syndrome. Roentgenographic alterations generally indicate findings of rheumatoid arthritis, SLE, PSS, and dermatomyositis in various combinations.

DEGENERATIVE JOINT DISEASE

The most characteristic sites of osteoarthritis (OA) include the proximal and distal interphalangeal joints

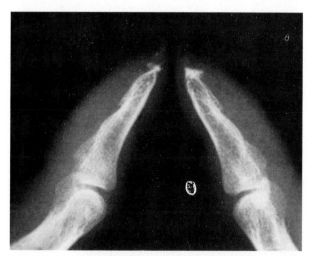

Figure 42–50. Scleroderma. There is osteolysis of the volar aspect of the distal phalanges of the thumbs with adjacent soft tissue calcification. Also note the tapered appearance of the adjacent soft tissues.

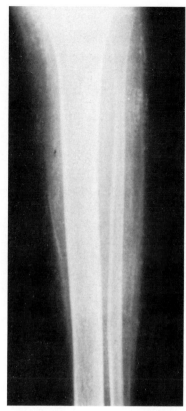

Figure 42–51. Dermatomyositis. There is prominent calcification of the subcutaneous tissue and the muscle in the leg.

of the hand, first carpometacarpal and trapezioscaphoid joints of the wrist, acromioclavicular and sacroiliac joints, hip, knee, and first metatarsophalangeal joint of the foot. Degenerative joint disease may also affect cartilaginous joints (such as the manubriosternal joint and symphysis pubis) and tendinous and ligamentous attachments to bone or entheses (such as in the pelvis, patella, and calcaneus). Degenerative disease of the spine is a separate subject and will be discussed later.

Osteoarthritis

In spite of a diversity of etiologies of OA, certain common radiographic characteristics allow a confident diagnosis in most instances. Joint space narrowing is a key diagnostic feature of the disease (Fig. 42–52).[246] In contrast to the inflammatory arthropathies, in which diffuse joint space narrowing of an involved articulation is expected, the joint space loss in OA tends to involve the portion of the joint exposed to the greatest stress (i.e., the lateral aspect of the hip, the medial compartment of the knee). Subchondral bone abnormalities are also characteristic of OA and include sclerosis (eburnation) and cyst formation, both of which predominate in the stressed area of the articulation. Subchondral eburnation results from cartilage denudation with subsequent

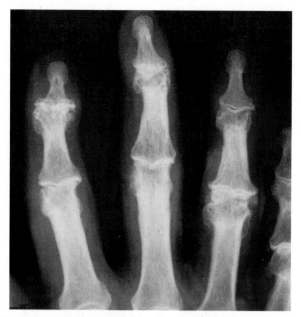

Figure 42–52. Osteoarthritis. There is narrowing of multiple interphalangeal joints with interdigitating osteophytes.

bone-to-bone contact. The origin of subchondral cysts remains in debate.[247, 248]

Osteophytes are the single most characteristic radiographic and pathologic abnormality in OA.[246] They tend to arise from endochondral ossification in areas of low stress where islands of cartilage are preserved, most commonly at joint margins. In some cases, osteophytes may arise from the synovium or joint capsule.

Hand and Wrist

The interphalangeal joints of the hand are frequent target areas of OA (see Fig. 42–52). The appearance of articular space narrowing with closely apposed interdigitating bony surfaces and marginal osteophytes is characteristic. Metacarpophalangeal joint involvement may also occur but not as an isolated event; rather, such involvement is associated with alterations at interphalangeal articulations. At the metacarpophalangeal joints, it is interosseous space narrowing that is the predominant abnormality. Osseous erosions are not apparent. The first carpometacarpal (trapeziometacarpal) joint is the characteristic site of degenerative abnormalities in the wrist (Fig. 42–53). Joint space narrowing with bony eburnation, subchondral cysts, and osteophyte formation is typical. Radial subluxation of the first metacarpal base is common. The trapezioscaphoid space is the only other common site of OA in the wrist; involvement at this site is generally combined with that at the first carpometacarpal joint. Trapezioscaphoid joint disease in the absence of first carpometacarpal joint involvement should suggest another diagnosis, especially CPPD crystal deposition disease. Similarly, a degenerative

disease–like arthropathy elsewhere in the wrist, especially at the radiocarpal joint, in the absence of significant occupational or accidental trauma is generally related to a disease other than OA.

Sacroiliac Joint

OA of the sacroiliac joint is extremely common in the older age group. Joint space narrowing with a thin, well-defined band of subchondral sclerosis, especially in the ilium, is typically present. Osteophyte formation is most common at the superior and inferior margins of the synovium-lined portion of the joint. At the former location, these osteophytes may appear as localized radiodensities projected over the joint in the anteroposterior radiographic projection. Bony erosion and intra-articular osseous fusion are not features of OA of the sacroiliac joint.

Hip

OA of the hip is exceedingly common and may lead to significant patient disability. In the typical case, cartilage loss is focal, involves the superolateral aspect of the joint, and leads to upward migration of the femoral head[249] (Fig. 42–54). Osteophyte formation is most prominent at the lateral acetabular and medial femoral margins, often in combination with thickening (buttressing) of the cortex in the medial aspect of the femoral neck. Subchondral sclerosis and cyst formation on both sides of the joint space may be marked. Focal loss of cartilage on the medial aspect of the articulation occurs in approximately 20 percent

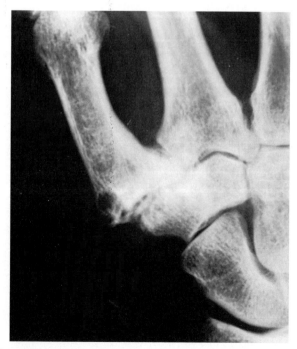

Figure 42–53. Osteoarthritis. Narrowing of the articular space and subchondral sclerosis about the first carpometacarpal joint are apparent.

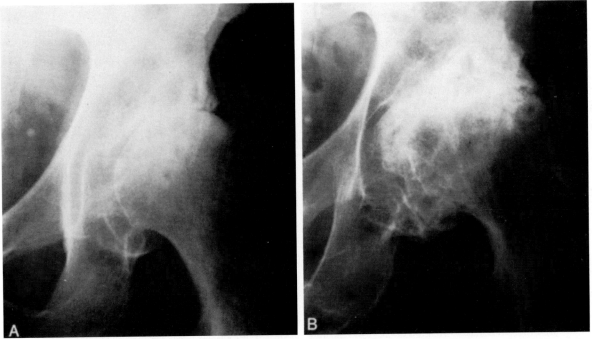

Figure 42–54. Osteoarthritis. *A,* Moderately advanced osteoarthritic changes are present, with asymmetric joint space narrowing and superior migration of the femoral head. Eburnation and cystic changes are seen in the subchondral region. *B,* Advanced changes have occurred, with collapse of the superior articular surface and the formation of large marginal osteophytes.

of patients with OA. Diffuse loss of cartilage with axial migration of the femoral head (along the axis of the femoral neck) is rare in OA. This latter feature is important in the differentiation of OA from inflammatory arthropathies such as rheumatoid arthritis.

Knee

The knee is a common site of OA. The most characteristic pattern of disease consists of involvement of the medial femorotibial compartment with joint space narrowing, osseous eburnation, subchondral cysts, and marginal osteophytes.[250] Sharpening of the tibial spines or the presence of osteophytes arising from the intercondylar notch of the femur may also be observed. A true assessment of cartilage destruction may not be possible on standard anteroposterior radiographs (obtained with the patient supine) but is better provided by radiographs obtained either in the "tunnel" projection (Fig. 42–55) or with the patient in a weight-bearing position.[251] Varus angulation of the knee is the most common deformity in OA, reflecting the more severe involvement of the medial femorotibial compartment compared with the lateral one. Symmetric medial and lateral femorotibial compartment disease is unusual. Osteoarthritic changes in the patellofemoral compartment are also common, either in isolation or accompanying medial femorotibial compartment disease.

Osseous or cartilaginous debris may be present as intra-articular bodies ("joint mice"), either free within the joint cavity or embedded in the synovial membrane. Degeneration of the fibrocartilaginous menisci is a typical feature of advanced OA.

Foot

OA in the foot typically affects the first metatarsophalangeal joint. Articular space narrowing, bony eburnation, osteophyte formation, and subchondral cysts are common. Hallux rigidus is a specific pattern of OA, which may be seen in adolescents or young adults; there is painful restriction of dorsiflexion at the first metatarsophalangeal joint.[252] Hallux valgus is another common pattern of OA about this joint, with lateral angulation of the first toe and prominent sclerosis, cyst formation, and osteophytosis on the medial aspect of the first metatarsal head.

Other Locations

Typical osteoarthritic changes in the elbows, acromioclavicular and glenohumeral joints, and ankles may be encountered, usually in patients with a history of trauma or pre-existing disease. In general, without such a history, a radiographic pattern consistent with OA[246] at an unusual site should suggest another disease process, such as acromegaly, CPPD crystal deposition disease, ochronosis, or epiphyseal dysplasia.

Inflammatory Osteoarthritis

Inflammatory osteoarthritis is a disease most common in middle-aged women. It is characterized by

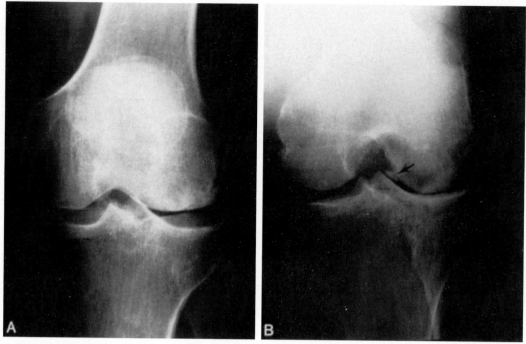

Figure 42–55. Osteoarthritis. Anteroposterior *(A)* and tunnel *(B)* projections reveal osteoarthritic changes of the knee. Note the asymmetric involvement with subchondral eburnation of the lateral articular surfaces. In this case, the actual degree of joint space narrowing is much more apparent in the tunnel projection. An osteophyte arising from the intercondylar notch is identified *(arrow in B)*.

acute episodic inflammation of the interphalangeal joints of the hand.[253] On roentgenograms, typical marginal osteophytes with or without bony erosions are seen. The erosions are first evident in the central portion of the subchondral bone, appearing as sharply marginated defects (Fig. 42–56).[246] Intra-articular ankylosis may subsequently result.[254] It must be emphasized that the clinical syndrome of inflammatory osteoarthritis can occur in the absence of radiographically demonstrable bony erosions; therefore,

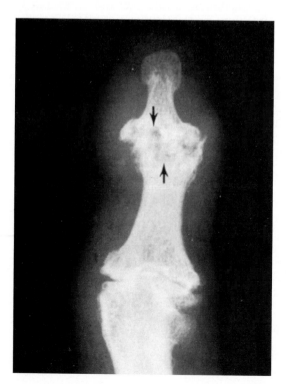

Figure 42–56. Inflammatory osteoarthritis. The combination of interphalangeal joint involvement, prominent marginal osteophytes, and central erosions of the articular surfaces *(arrows)* is characteristic of this disease. (From Resnick D, Niwayama G: Diagnosis of Bone and Joint Disorders. Philadelphia, WB Saunders, 1981.)

the term *erosive osteoarthritis* is not an ideal one for this disorder.

Degenerative Enthesopathy

Coarse, bony proliferation at sites of ligamentous and tendinous attachment is a manifestation of a degenerative enthesopathy. This is most commonly observed in the pelvis, patella, ulnar olecranon, and calcaneus. The resulting bony excrescences are identical to those encountered in diffuse idiopathic skeletal hyperostosis. They are usually coarser and better defined than the outgrowths accompanying the inflammatory enthesopathy of the seronegative spondyloarthropathies.

Degenerative Disease of the Spine

The vertebral column is composed of a complex series of synovial, cartilaginous, and fibrous articulations. Degenerative diseases of the spine can involve any of these articulations as well as ligamentous insertions (entheses).[255, 256] Many distinct degenerative processes can be identified.

Intervertebral (Osteo)chondrosis

Primary degenerative disease of the nucleus pulposus of the intervertebral disc, termed *intervertebral (osteo)chondrosis*, is a common disorder, especially in the elderly. It may occur at any spinal level but is more commonly identified in the lumbar and cervical regions.[1]

The earliest radiographic change consists of linear or circular collections of gas ("vacuum phenomena") within the disc substance (Fig. 42–57).[257] These gas collections are more prominent on radiographs obtained with the spine in extension and may disappear in flexion. The presence of a vacuum phenomenon is a useful observation, because it virtually excludes the possibility of infection.[258] Progressive narrowing of the intervertebral disc and sclerosis beneath the subchondral bone plate are additional manifestations of intervertebral (osteo)chondrosis. Herniation of portions of the intervertebral disc into the adjacent vertebral body (Schmorl's node, cartilaginous node) is a further radiographic sign. Small triangular osteophytes at the discovertebral junction are also seen (see Fig. 42–57).

Spondylosis Deformans

Spondylosis deformans[255] refers to the formation of multiple large osteophytes predominantly along the anterior and lateral aspects of the vertebral bodies (Fig. 42–58).[259] These osteophytes may occur at any level; in the thoracic spine, they predominate on the right side, presumably because their formation is inhibited on the left side by the constant pulsation of the descending thoracic aorta.[260] Narrowing of the

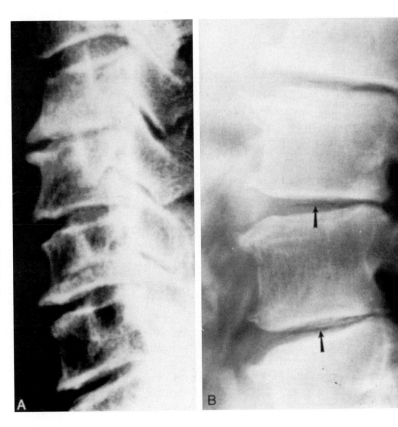

Figure 42–57. Intervertebral (osteo)chondrosis. Lateral projections of the cervical spine (A) and lumbar spine (B) reveal typical abnormalities of intervertebral (osteo)chondrosis. Intervertebral disc space narrowing with sclerosis of the vertebral end-plates and the formation of small triangular osteophytes from the anterior vertebral margins are evident. Prominent vacuum phenomena (arrows in B) are present in the lumbar spine. (From Resnick D, Niwayama G: Diagnosis of Bone and Joint Disorders. Philadelphia, WB Saunders, 1981.)

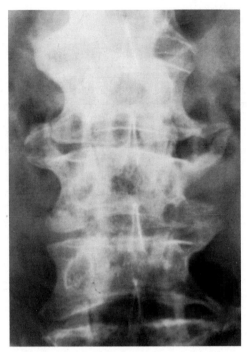

Figure 42–58. Spondylosis deformans. The frontal projection of the spine reveals multiple, large interdigitating osteophytes arising from the lateral margins of the vertebral bodies. Note that the initial portion of the osteophytes has a horizontal orientation.

intervertebral disc space, vacuum phenomena, and end-plate bony sclerosis are not features of spondylosis deformans. The differentiation of the osteophytes of spondylosis deformans from the vertebral lesions of the seronegative spondyloarthropathies has been discussed previously.

Apophyseal Joint Osteoarthritis

The synovium-lined apophyseal joint is a frequent site of degenerative disease.[256] Changes are most common in the mid- and lower cervical spine, the midthoracic spine, and the lower lumbar spine. The radiographic changes are identical to those of OA in peripheral articulations,[261] with joint space narrowing, osseous eburnation, and marginal osteophyte formation. Capsular laxity may result in apophyseal joint malalignment. In this setting or with large osteophytes arising from the joint margins, impingement of a spinal nerve root within the neural foramen may occur.

Uncovertebral Arthrosis

Degenerative changes in the cervical uncovertebral articulations (Luschka) are often identified on the frontal radiograph of the cervical spine. The nature of this process is debated, because these articulations have been shown to represent intervertebral disc extensions in early life and to contain synovium-like tissue in later life. Radiographic changes consist of

osseous sclerosis, joint space loss, and osteophyte formation.

Costovertebral Osteoarthritis

Osteoarthritic changes of the synovium-lined costovertebral joints are extremely common, especially at the level of the 11th and 12th ribs.[256] Radiographic demonstration of these abnormalities (joint space narrowing, bony sclerosis, osteophytes) is frequently difficult, owing to the superimposition of ribs and vertebral bodies over the articulations on conventional radiographic studies. Hypertrophy of adjacent ribs may accompany this disease.

Diffuse Idiopathic Skeletal Hyperostosis

DISH is a common degenerative enthesopathy and has been described under a variety of terms,[262–264] including *Forestier's disease, spondylitis ossificans ligamentosa, spondylosis hyperostotica,* and *ankylosing hyperostosis of the spine.* Although radiographic changes are evident in both the axial and the appendicular skeleton, the diagnosis of DISH is based on the presence of characteristic spinal alterations. In fact, the radiographic change in the vertebral column must fulfill three criteria before a diagnosis of DISH can be made: (1) the presence of flowing calcification or ossification along the anterolateral aspects of at least four contiguous vertebral levels; (2) relative preservation of intervertebral disc height in the involved vertebral segments without the extensive changes of primary degenerative disc disease; and (3) the absence of apophyseal joint ankylosis or sacroiliac joint erosions, sclerosis, or intra-articular bony ankylosis.

The most characteristic radiographic abnormality of DISH is calcification and ossification of the anterior longitudinal ligament of the spine.[265] This is most commonly identified in the midthoracic spine but is also evident in the cervical and lumbar levels. Early in the disease, an undulating radiodense band forms along the anterolateral aspect of the spine separated from the anterior aspect of the vertebral body by a thin radiolucent line (Fig. 42–59); with progression of the disease, the lucency may disappear. These changes, which are best demonstrated in the lateral radiographic projection of the thoracic spine, may resemble the "bamboo spine" of ankylosing spondylitis, but several important diagnostic features exist. Syndesmophytes arise from the anterosuperior and anteroinferior margins of the vertebral body, whereas the ossification in DISH attaches to the vertebral body several millimeters from these margins. In addition, syndesmophytes may be best seen in the frontal radiographic projection, in contrast to DISH, in which changes are most prominent on the lateral radiographic projection. The presence of sacroiliac joint erosions and extensive intra-articular bony ankylosis of the sacroiliac or apophyseal joints in ankylosing spondylitis constitutes another important differential diagnostic point.

In the cervical spine, bony outgrowths characteristically appear at the anteroinferior margin of the vertebral body and extend inferiorly around the disc space. With progression, a thick, armor-like mass of bone bridges the intervertebral disc, leading to markedly diminished cervical motion and, in some cases, dysphagia (Fig. 42–60).[266] Linear or Y-shaped radiolucencies in the bony mass may be noted at the level of the intervertebral disc space owing to displacement of disc material into the ossific mass. Ossification adjacent to the inferior margin of the anterior arch of the atlas is common and may be confused with traumatic changes. Ossification of the posterior longitudinal ligament may be seen as a distinct entity but occurs with increased frequency in patients with DISH (see Fig. 42–60).[267] DISH may also be associated with a rare syndrome, sternocostoclavicular hyperostosis,[267, 268] in which extensive ossification of the soft tissues between the anterior ribs, medial clavicle, and sternum is evident.

In the lumbar spine, changes of DISH resemble those in the cervical region; osteophytes are present.

Extraspinal manifestations of DISH[269] are especially common in the pelvis. Bony proliferation at sites of ligamentous and tendinous attachment (enthesopathy) results in the formation of coarse, well-marginated bony excrescences, in contrast to the finely spiculated, ill-defined bony proliferative changes of the

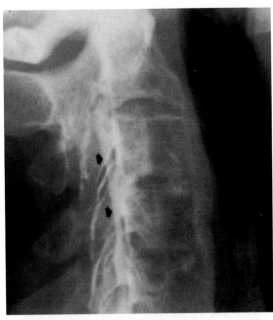

Figure 42–60. Diffuse idiopathic skeletal hyperostosis (DISH). The lateral view of the cervical spine in this patient demonstrates thick, flowing ossification along the anterior margins of the vertebral bodies. Ossification of the posterior longitudinal ligament (PLL) is also present (*arrows*).

seronegative spondyloarthropathies (Fig. 42–61). Calcification of the iliolumbar and sacrotuberous ligaments is an additional characteristic feature (Fig. 42–62). Para-articular osteophytes are commonly noted about the hip and along the inferior aspect of the sacroiliac joints.

Other extraspinal sites of prominent bony proliferation include the patellar poles, calcaneus, and olecranon process of the ulna. The "spurs" that form at these sites may be identical in appearance to localized degenerative changes in otherwise normal persons, but they demonstrate a tendency toward increased size and multiplicity. In the hand, hyperostotic changes of the metacarpal and phalangeal heads, with proliferation in the terminal tufts, may be noted. Irregular excrescences may also be seen at the femoral trochanters, deltoid tuberosity of the humerus, and anterior tibial tuberosity, and about the interosseous membranes of the forearm and leg.

NEUROARTHROPATHY

Neuroarthropathy (Charcot joint) refers to destructive and productive articular abnormalities occurring in association with loss of pain or proprioceptive sensation, or both. Although debate exists as to the precise pathogenesis of neuroarthropathy, it is believed that the cumulative effect of trauma and joint laxity due to relaxation of periarticular supporting structures is contributory.

One of the early radiographic changes of neuroarthropathy is the presence of a joint effusion,

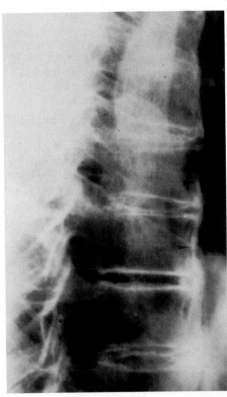

Figure 42–59. Diffuse idiopathic skeletal hyperostosis (DISH). The lateral view of the thoracic spine in this patient with DISH demonstrates ossification of the anterior longitudinal ligament (ALL). Note the characteristic lucencies between the ossified ALL and the anterior vertebral margin (*arrowheads*).

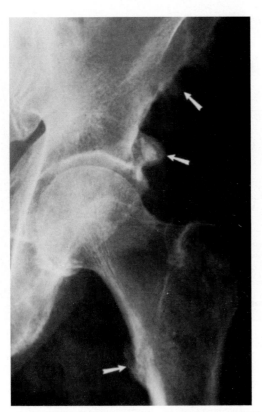

Figure 42–61. Diffuse idiopathic skeletal hyperostosis (DISH). The degenerative enthesopathy of DISH is well demonstrated with coarse bony excrescences arising from sites of ligament and tendon insertion along the lateral aspect of the ilium, superior acetabular margin, and lesser trochanter *(arrows)*. This appearance differs from that of the finely spiculated inflammatory enthesopathy of the seronegative spondyloarthropathies.

which may become large. Mild joint subluxation may then appear.[270] Subsequently, fragmentation of the articular surface occurs with eburnation of bony surfaces, leading, in time, to complete joint disorganization. These radiographic abnormalities have been subdivided into hypertrophic and atrophic types. The hypertrophic reaction is more common in central le-

sions, as in tabes dorsalis and syringomyelia. There is prominent periosteal new bone formation as well as metaplasia of the synovium with the formation of bone and cartilage within its deeper layers. Large osteocartilaginous bodies of synovial origin, in combination with fragments originating from the articular surfaces, result in a fragmented, disorganized articulation with a great deal of osseous debris (Fig. 42–63). The atrophic reaction occurs more commonly with diseases, such as diabetes mellitus, in which the abnormality involves the peripheral nerve (Fig. 42–64). Fragmentation occurs, but the osteocartilaginous debris is resorbed, resulting in disappearance of the articular surfaces. It should be emphasized that hypertrophic and atrophic patterns are not completely reliable in identifying the level of neurologic abnormality, because exceptions to these rules are common.

A great number of disorders lead to neuropathic changes. In general, the morphologic aberrations produced by these disorders are similar; however, differences in articular distribution provide clues to the specific diagnosis.

Tabes Dorsalis[270–272]

Five to 10 percent of patients with tabes dorsalis demonstrate neuroarthropathy. The articulations of the lower extremity are most commonly affected, with the knee and the hip being the most frequent target sites (see Fig. 42–63). Other sites include the ankle and the articulations in both the upper extremity and the spinal column. In peripheral joints, typical radiographic features are large effusions, bony eburnation, and fragmentation. Bilateral and symmetric changes are not uncommon. In the axial skeleton, intervertebral disc space narrowing, vertebral body sclerosis, and formation of large osteophytes may resemble the changes of unusually severe degenerative disease.

Syringomyelia[273]

Approximately 20 to 50 percent of patients with syringomyelia develop neuroarthropathy. There is a

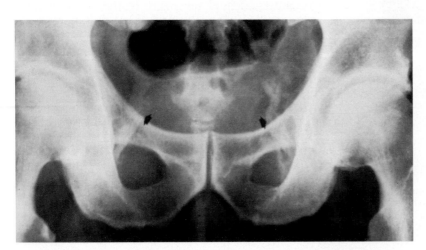

Figure 42–62. Diffuse idiopathic skeletal hyperostosis (DISH). Calcification of the sacrotuberous ligaments *(arrows)* has occurred.

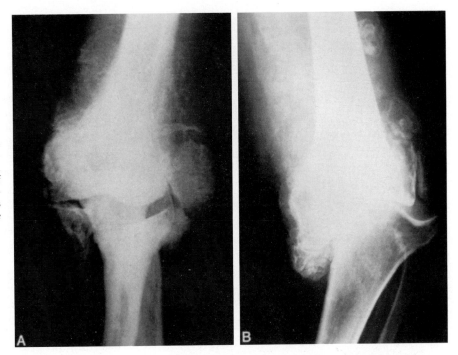

Figure 42–63. Tabes dorsalis with neuroarthropathy. Radiographs of the elbow *(A)* and knee *(B)* in patients with tabes dorsalis demonstrate changes of neuroarthropathy. Bony sclerosis, fragmentation, and instability of the joints are present with dramatic soft tissue swelling.

distinct predilection for upper extremity involvement, especially the glenohumeral joint, elbow, and wrist. Lower extremity or spinal alterations may occur in some cases. Bilateral and symmetric involvement is less frequent in syringomyelia than in tabes dorsalis.

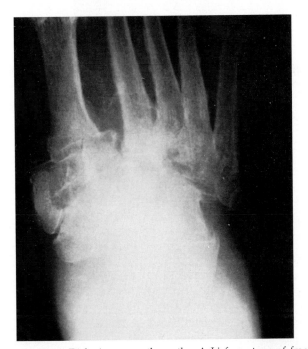

Figure 42–64. Diabetic neuroarthropathy. A Lisfranc type of fracture-dislocation has occurred as a complication of neuroarthropathy in this diabetic patient. Note the lateral displacement of the second through fifth metatarsal bases with sclerosis and fragmentation of the adjacent tarsal bones.

Diabetes Mellitus[274–276]

Diabetes mellitus is probably the most common cause of neuroarthropathy, although less than 1 percent of patients with this disease develop such changes. The articulations of the foot are affected in the majority of cases, although the ankle, knee, spine, and joints of the upper extremity may occasionally be affected. Abnormalities predominate in the tarsal and tarsometatarsal articulations, consisting of bony eburnation and fragmentation. Spontaneous fractures are common, and a Lisfranc fracture-dislocation pattern may be seen (see Fig. 42–64). In the forefoot, a resorptive pattern is most typical, with tapering or "sharpening" of metatarsal and phalangeal shafts. Concurrent or superimposed infection is a common problem in the diabetic patient. There is great difficulty in differentiating the radiographic changes of neuroarthropathy from those of infection; however, the indistinctness of bony margins in infection compared with the sharp margins in neuroarthropathy aids in correct diagnosis.

Other Disorders

Although peripheral neuropathy is common in the alcoholic patient, neuroarthropathy is rare. It resembles that in diabetes mellitus with characteristic involvement of the articulations of the foot.[277] In amyloidosis, knee and ankle involvement is most typical.[278] Neuropathic changes in childhood should suggest the possibility of congenital indifference to pain or meningomyelocele.[269] In both of these disorders, involvement of the ankle and tarsal articulations is

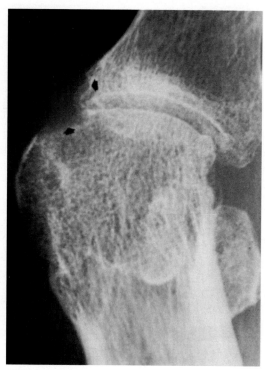

Figure 42–65. Gout. Typical erosions of the metatarsal head and proximal phalangeal base *(arrows)* are present in this patient with gouty arthritis of the first metatarsophalangeal joint.

erosions are common in long-standing gout and may be intra-articular or extra-articular in location. Intra-articular erosions most commonly involve the joint margins and proceed centrally (Fig. 42–65). Extra-articular erosions involve the cortex of the bone, frequently in association with a soft tissue mass (tophus) (Fig. 42–66). These erosions are usually round or oval, often with a sclerotic border and a "punched-out" appearance.[281] The presence of an "overhanging lip" of bone at the margin of an erosion is a characteristic feature of gout. Occasionally, a more extensive proliferative bony reaction, presumably due to a reparative process, may be noted, typically at the first metatarsophalangeal joint, intertarsal joints, and the knee.[282, 283] The joint space is usually preserved in gouty arthritis until the late stages of the disease. In fact, the presence of prominent intra-articular osseous erosions with relative preservation of the joint space suggests the diagnosis of gout. Intra-articular bony ankylosis is occasionally seen, especially involving the interphalangeal joints of the hands and feet as well as the carpal region.[282] Although transient localized osteoporosis may be present during an acute gouty attack, extensive osteoporosis is not a feature of this disease.

The general radiographic features of gout are similar at all sites; however, involvement at several specific areas may be of diagnostic importance.[279] The

seen, and changes may appear at the physis, or growth plate, with osseous irregularity, sclerosis, epiphyseal separation, and periostitis. An idiopathic form of neuroarthropathy of the elbow has been described, and neuroarthropathic changes have been observed following intra-articular administration of steroids.

CRYSTAL-RELATED ARTHROPATHIES

Several types of articular disease are related to abnormal deposition or accumulation of crystalline material in and about articulations. These include gout, CPPD crystal deposition disease, hemochromatosis, and hydroxyapatite crystal deposition disease (HADD).[279] Two other entities that may be included in this group are Wilson's disease and ochronosis (alkaptonuria).

Gout

The earliest radiographic change in gout consists of reversible soft tissue swelling about the involved articulation during an acute gouty attack. With chronicity of disease, tophi lead to nodular, lobulated soft tissue densities, especially in the feet, ankles, knees, elbows, and hands. Calcification within a tophus may be evident, particularly in patients with gouty nephritis, whereas ossification of a tophus is rare.[279, 280] Bony

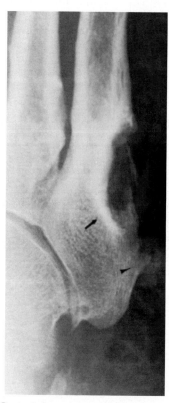

Figure 42–66. Gout. A large extra-articular erosion of the lateral aspect of the fifth metatarsal shaft is bordered by reactive bony sclerosis *(arrow)*. A smaller erosion is present more proximally *(arrowhead)* with an adjacent calcified soft tissue tophus. (From Resnick D, Niwayama G: Diagnosis of Bone and Joint Disorders. Philadelphia, WB Saunders, 1981.)

first metatarsophalangeal joint is the most characteristic site of involvement (see Fig. 42–65). Erosions are most frequent on the dorsal and medial aspects of the metatarsal head, usually in association with a hallux valgus deformity. They are best demonstrated in the oblique radiographic projection. In the hand, proximal and distal interphalangeal joint involvement is more common than metacarpophalangeal joint involvement. Wrist abnormality is frequently pancompartmental, but extensive involvement of the common carpometacarpal articulation is important, because this area is relatively spared in most other arthropathies. Erosions of the olecranon process of the elbow and the dorsal surface of the patella strongly suggest gouty bursitis.

Chondrocalcinosis is occasionally seen in patients with gout. It is usually localized to a few articulations and predominates in fibrocartilage.

Secondary gout is associated with a wide variety of situations, including glycogen storage disease (type I),[284] Lesch-Nyhan syndrome,[285] myeloproliferative disorders,[286] endocrine diseases,[287] and the administration of certain drugs.[288] In general, secondary gout resembles primary gout radiographically, although unusual sites may be affected.[284–288]

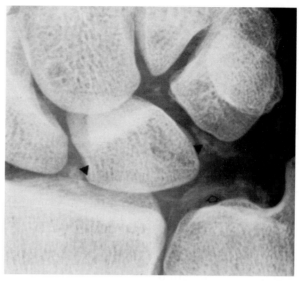

Figure 42–68. Calcium pyrophosphate crystal deposition disease (CPPD). A frontal radiograph of the wrist demonstrates calcification of the triangular fibrocartilage *(open arrow)* and several intercarpal ligaments *(arrowheads)*. (From Resnick D, Niwayama G: Diagnosis of Bone and Joint Disorders. Philadelphia, WB Saunders, 1981.)

Calcium Pyrophosphate Dihydrate Crystal Deposition Disease

CPPD crystal deposition disease is characterized by the deposition of CPPD crystals in hyaline cartilage and fibrocartilage as well as in synovium, capsule, tendons, and ligaments.[279] *CPPD crystal deposition disease* is a general term indicating the presence of CPPD crystal in or around joints. *Chondrocalcinosis* refers to calcification of hyaline cartilage or fibrocartilage, regardless of its etiology. *Pyrophosphate arthropathy* refers to a pattern of structural joint damage with or without radiographically demonstrable chondrocalcinosis. There are two main types of radiographic abnormalities in CPPD crystal deposition disease: (1) abnormal calcification and (2) destructive arthropathy. These changes may be present in combination or in isolation.

Abnormal calcification related to CPPD crystal deposition disease may be identified in articular or periarticular structures. The most common intra-articular site of calcification is within cartilage, either hyaline cartilage or fibrocartilage (Fig. 42–67). Hyaline cartilage calcification may occur in any joint but is most common in the wrist, knee, elbow, and hip. It appears as thin, curvilinear radiodensities parallel to, but distinct from, the subchondral bone plate.[279] Fibrocartilage calcification most commonly involves the menisci of the knee, triangular fibrocartilage of the wrist, symphysis pubis, annulus fibrosus of the intervertebral disc, or labra of the glenoid and acetabulum (Fig. 42–68). It appears as thick, irregular radiodensities within the involved structure. Cloudlike or speckled radiodensities, representing calcific deposits within synovium, may be seen at many locations, including bursal cavities, but are most common about the wrist. Additional sites of calcification include joint capsule, tendons, bursae, and ligaments.[289] Calcification at these sites is less frequent than within cartilage.

Pyrophosphate arthropathy exhibits a degenerative disease–type pattern of structural joint damage. Its general radiographic features include a bilateral symmetric or asymmetric distribution and changes characterized by joint space narrowing, bony sclerosis, and prominent subchondral cysts.[289] The last, repre-

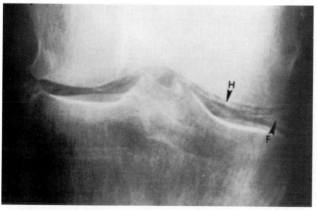

Figure 42–67. Calcium pyrophosphate crystal deposition disease (CPPD). A frontal radiograph of the knee reveals calcification of hyaline articular cartilage (H) as well as fibrocartilaginous menisci (F). (From Resnick D, Niwayama G, Goergen TG, et al: Clinical, radiographic and pathologic abnormalities in calcium pyrophosphate dihydrate deposition disease (CPPD): Pseudogout. Radiology 122:1, 1977.)

senting an important diagnostic feature of the arthropathy, are frequently numerous and large and may simulate neoplasm. These cysts may progress rapidly in size, undermining the articular surface and resulting in collapse and deformity of the joint. At times, this progression may be so rapid as to resemble infection or neuroarthropathy (Fig. 42–69). In some patients, large osteophytes may be present about involved articulations.

Pyrophosphate arthropathy is most commonly seen in the knee, wrist, and metacarpophalangeal joints, although any joint may be involved. The relatively common involvement of the wrist, elbow, and shoulder contrasts with the situation in degenerative joint disease, in which these areas are usually spared. In the hand there is a tendency toward selective involvement of the second and third metacarpophalangeal joints. In the wrist, the radioscaphoid space is frequently involved, with collapse of the proximal pole of the scaphoid into the distal radial articular surface (Fig. 42–70). Narrowing of the capitolunate space is also frequent, as is involvement of the trapezioscaphoid articulation with or without involvement of the first carpometacarpal joint. Associated calcification of the triangular fibrocartilage, intercarpal ligaments, or articular cartilage may be encountered. In the knee, the distribution of abnormalities may mimic that of osteoarthritis with involvement of the medial femorotibial and patellofemoral compartments. At times, there is isolated involvement of the patellofemoral space. In the hip, superior joint space narrowing, mimicking osteoarthritis, or axial migration of the femoral head, simulating rheumatoid arthritis, can be seen.

Calcium Hydroxyapatite Crystal Deposition Disease

HADD may be a primary idiopathic disorder or secondary to other diseases and is characterized by the deposition of calcium hydroxyapatite crystals in periarticular or, rarely, intra-articular structures. In idiopathic disease, calcification is most commonly seen about the shoulder, although involvement of the hand, wrist, hip, foot, and paraspinal tissues may be seen. Hydroxyapatite deposits appear on radiographs as soft, cloudlike densities within tendons, ligaments, joint capsules, bursae, and periarticular soft tissues. These deposits may vary in size from small collections, 1 to 2 mm in diameter, to large lobulated masses, many centimeters in diameter. On serial radiographs, deposits may enlarge, remain unchanged,

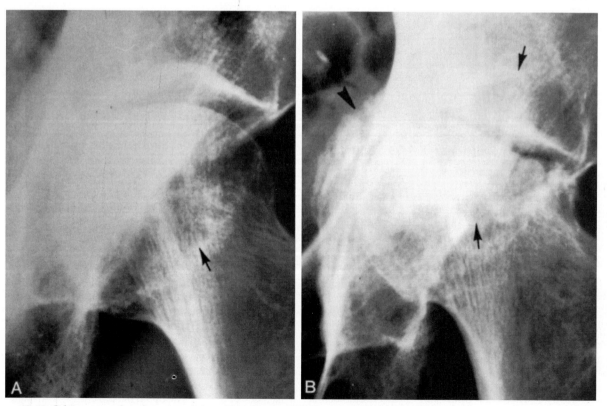

Figure 42–69. Calcium pyrophosphate crystal deposition disease (CPPD). *A* and *B* are radiographs of the hip obtained 16 months apart. *A,* There is preservation of the joint space with subtle cystic change within the femoral head *(arrow).* *B,* There is collapse of the femoral head with large cystic lesions *(arrows)* and fragmentation of the acetabulum *(arrowhead).* This rapidly progressive arthropathy is characteristic of pyrophosphate arthropathy. (From Resnick D, Niwayama G, Goergen TG, et al: Clinical, radiographic, and pathologic abnormalities in calcium pyrophosphate dihydrate deposition disease (CPPD): Pseudogout. Radiology 122:1, 1977.)

or diminish in size. They can even disappear completely.

In the shoulder, HADD is most commonly identified in the supraspinatus tendon of the fibromuscular rotator cuff. Here it is frequently referred to as *calcific tendinitis*, *peritendinitis calcarea*, or *hydroxyapatite rheumatism* (Fig. 42–71).[279] Other sites of calcification in the shoulder include the infraspinatus, teres minor, subscapularis, and bicipital tendons.[290] It should be emphasized that in most instances these deposits are not symptomatic; most patients with shoulder discomfort and periarticular calcific deposits will have another cause of pain, frequently subacromial bursitis or rotator cuff tendinitis.

Intra-articular HADD may be seen as an isolated event or in association with osteoarthritis or collagen vascular disease. Radiographically, cloudlike calcific collections within the joint are apparent. Rarely, severe articular destruction, especially in the glenohumeral joint, may be an associated feature.

Periarticular calcification, representing hydroxyapatite crystal deposition, is seen in a variety of disorders,[279] including hyperparathyroidism, renal osteodystrophy, collagen vascular diseases, hypoparathyroidism, milk-alkali syndrome, hypervitaminosis D, and sarcoidosis.

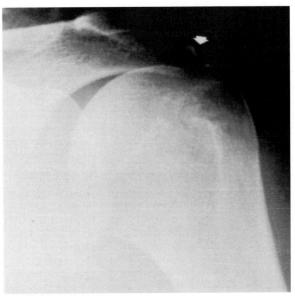

Figure 42–71. Hydroxyapatite crystal deposition disease (HADD). Calcification *(arrow)* of the supraspinatus tendon of the musculotendinous rotator cuff is present. This constitutes the single most common manifestation of this disorder. (From Resnick D, Niwayama G: Diagnosis of Bone and Joint Disease. Philadelphia, WB Saunders, 1981.)

Hemochromatosis

Radiographically, the manifestations of hemochromatosis may be divided into three major categories:

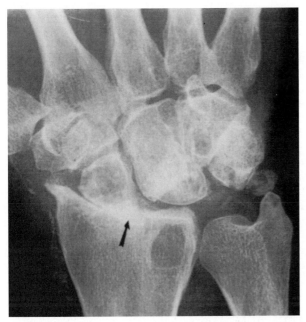

Figure 42–70. Calcium pyrophosphate crystal deposition disease (CPPD). In this patient, the changes of pyrophosphate arthropathy include narrowing of the radiocarpal joint with collapse of the scaphoid into the radial articular surface *(arrow)* as well as the presence of numerous subchondral cystic lesions. Calcification of the triangular fibrocartilage can also be noted.

(1) osteoporosis, (2) articular calcification, and (3) structural joint damage.

Diffuse osteoporosis is an important feature of hemochromatosis,[291] in contrast to idiopathic CPPD crystal deposition disease,[292] and may involve the axial and appendicular skeleton. In the spine, collapse of the vertebral end-plates leads to biconcave deformities of the vertebral body ("fish" vertebra). Osteoporosis in the appendicular skeleton tends to be diffuse, without a tendency toward a periarticular distribution.[293]

Articular calcification, related to CPPD crystal deposition (chondrocalcinosis), occurs in approximately 30 percent of patients with hemochromatosis.[279] In general, this calcification is identical to that of idiopathic CPPD crystal deposition disease, but several characteristics may help to distinguish these two disorders. In hemochromatosis, hyaline cartilage calcification tends to be more prominent and the fibrocartilage of the symphysis pubis is more commonly involved than in idiopathic CPPD crystal deposition disease.[279]

Structural articular alterations in hemochromatosis occur in slightly less than half of the cases.[294, 295] In general, the arthropathy of hemochromatosis is similar to that of idiopathic CPPD crystal deposition disease, with joint space narrowing and subchondral cyst formation being prominent features. Although the two disorders cannot be absolutely separated on a radiographic basis, several features may be useful in differential diagnosis.[279] "Hook" osteophytes are distinctive bony excrescences, most commonly identified at the radial margins of the metacarpal heads, in patients with hemochromatosis. These osteophytes tend to be small, triangular, and sharply defined (Fig. 42–72). They are not prominent in osteoarthritis or idiopathic CPPD crystal deposition disease. The distribution of abnormalities may also be a useful diagnostic feature. In both CPPD crystal deposition disease and hemochromatosis, the second and third metacarpophalangeal joints are the most commonly involved sites in the hands, but additional alterations of the fourth and fifth metacarpophalangeal joints are more frequent in hemochromatosis. In addition, the radiocarpal joint may be spared in hemochromatosis, whereas it is almost always involved in idiopathic CPPD crystal deposition disease. The arthropathy of hemochromatosis is usually slowly progressive, in contrast to idiopathic pyrophosphate arthropathy, in which a rapidly progressive arthropathy may be seen.

Wilson's Disease

Wilson's disease is a rare inherited disorder characterized by abnormal accumulation of copper in body tissues. The age of onset is typically the first through fourth decades of life. The general radiographic features consist of osteopenia and arthropathy.[279, 296] Chondrocalcinosis has been considered an important feature of this disorder, but it appears to be very rare. Osteopenia, present in approximately 50 percent of patients, is most prominent in the hands, feet, and spine. It may relate to osteoporosis or osteomalacia, or both. Changes of rickets, with Looser's zones or "pseudofractures," are prominent in some cases.[297]

The arthropathy of Wilson's disease is most commonly identified in the wrist, hand, foot, hip, shoulder, elbow, and knee. Irregularity and indistinctness of the subchondral bone plate ("paintbrush" appearance) in combination with focal radiodense excres-

cences at the central and peripheral joint margins are characteristic. Subchondral cysts and focal areas of fragmentation of the articular surface may also be observed. An additional manifestation is the occurrence of small, distinctly corticated ossicles about affected joints, especially prominent in the wrist. These structures resemble the accessory ossicles frequently seen in normal persons but are more numerous and appear in unusual locations. Joint effusions are not prominent, but spiculated bony proliferative changes are frequently noted at entheses, resembling the inflammatory enthesopathy seen in the seronegative spondyloarthropathies.

Ochronosis (Alkaptonuria)

The major radiographic features of ochronosis consist of osteoporosis, abnormal calcification and ossification, and arthropathy.[279] Osteoporosis, although generally diffuse in nature, is most evident in the spine, where it may be associated with vertebral body collapse.[298]

Abnormal calcification and ossification are most prominent in the intervertebral discs, especially those in the lumbar spine. Additional sites of calcification and ossification include the symphysis pubis, costal cartilage, helix of the ear, and peripheral tendons and ligaments.[299] The crystals are composed of calcium hydroxyapatite and demonstrate a typical "cloudlike" appearance.

In the spine, osteoporosis with wafer-like calcification of the intervertebral disc is an early radiographic finding. Intervertebral disc narrowing with the formation of radiolucent discal collections (vacuum phenomena) is also common, often obscuring the calcification.[300] Progressive discal ossification and the formation of peripheral bony bridges in the outermost layer of the annulus fibrosus may lead to the appearance of a "bamboo spine," similar to that in ankylosing spondylitis. At some levels, osteophytes may also be prominent.

In the peripheral skeleton, the knees, hips, and shoulders are most commonly involved, with relative sparing of the small joints of the hands and feet.[300] In these locations, changes resemble those of degenerative joint disease; however, osteophytes and subchondral cysts are not prominent in ochronosis. In addition, the location of abnormalities, such as the lateral femorotibial compartment of the knee, may help in differentiating ochronosis from OA. Occasionally, a rapidly progressing destructive peripheral arthropathy characterized by fragmentation of articular surfaces may be observed.

SEPTIC ARTHRITIS

Mechanisms

In general, the radiographic features of joint sepsis consist of periarticular soft tissue swelling, intra-artic-

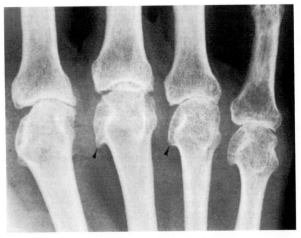

Figure 42–72. Hemochromatosis. There is joint space narrowing with erosive change about the second through fifth metacarpophalangeal joints. "Hook" osteophytes (*arrowheads*) occur at the radial margins of the metacarpal heads. (From Resnick D, Niwayama G: Diagnosis of Bone and Joint Disorders. Philadelphia, WB Saunders, 1981.)

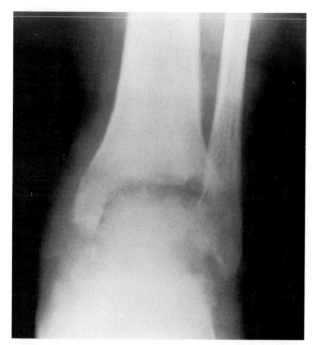

Figure 42–73. Septic arthritis. In this patient with a pyogenic arthritis of the ankle, note the soft tissue swelling, joint space loss, and large confluent subchondral erosions.

effusion, but rapid cartilage destruction results in articular space narrowing with confluent irregular erosions of the subchondral bone plate (Fig. 42–73). In children, epiphyseal centers may completely disappear as a result of the hyperemia associated with the infected joint. Diabetic patients are prone to develop indolent, slowly progressive joint infections, usually adjacent to soft tissue ulcerations. In this setting, the loss of distinctiveness of articular margins may be the only radiographic manifestation of infection (Fig. 42–74).

In contrast to bacterial infection, granulomatous infection (tuberculosis and fungal) may demonstrate a more slowly progressive pattern of joint destruction (Fig. 42–75). Osseous erosions first appear at the joint margins ("bare" areas), where synovial inflammatory tissue is in direct contact with bone. In fact, prominent juxta-articular osteoporosis and marginal bone erosions, in the absence of significant joint space loss, are characteristics of granulomatous infection. The late complications of joint sepsis include intra-articular fibrous or bony ankylosis as well as joint instability. In the spine, the latter complication may result in spinal cord or nerve root compromise.

ular effusions, cartilage destruction with joint space narrowing, and irregular erosions of the subchondral bone plate.[301–303] In the initial stage of disease, the joint may appear widened, owing to the presence of a large

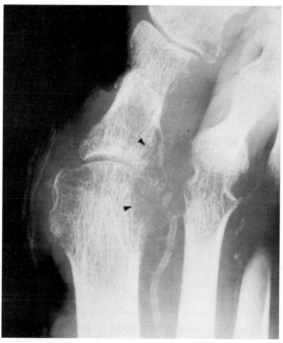

Figure 42–74. Septic arthritis. In this specimen radiograph of an infected foot in a diabetic patient, note the erosions of the lateral margins of the articular surfaces of the first metatarsal head and proximal phalanx *(arrowheads)*.

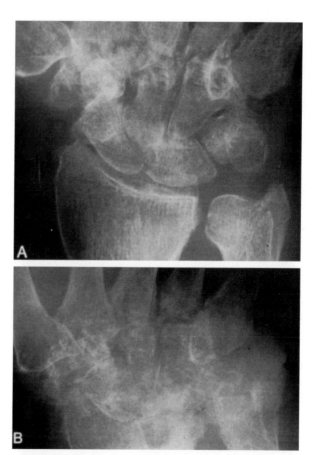

Figure 42–75. Tuberculosis. Note the gradual progression of destructive changes in radiographs obtained 18 months apart. *A,* There is prominent soft tissue swelling and osteoporosis with marginal osseous erosions at multiple sites. *B,* The process has progressed to virtually complete destruction of the carpus. A large erosion of the distal radius is also present.

The role of various imaging modalities in the diagnosis of joint sepsis should be emphasized. Early detection is important to prevent irreversible joint destruction or, in the child, significant growth disturbance. Radionuclide studies are useful in this regard, both in detecting infection early in the course of the disease and in documenting the extent of involvement. However, adjacent soft tissue or bone infections, recent surgery, or post-traumatic changes may render this important tool useless in some cases. Recognition of articular effusions and periarticular soft tissue swelling on roentgenograms is of critical importance in the early diagnosis of joint infection. Magnification radiography may provide additional diagnostic information, especially in the diabetic patient with a foot infection. Fluoroscopically guided aspiration may play an important role in the evaluation of joint sepsis, especially in deep joints such as the hip or the shoulder or in sites such as the spine, where surgical exploration may be required. Although the principal aim of this procedure is to procure a specimen for laboratory analysis, instillation of a small amount of radiopaque contrast agent may be helpful in ascertaining the extent of articular destruction and in detecting extra-articular spread of contaminated material.

MISCELLANEOUS ARTHROPATHIES

Osteonecrosis

Early in the course of epiphyseal osteonecrosis, radiographic changes are not evident. Subsequently, a

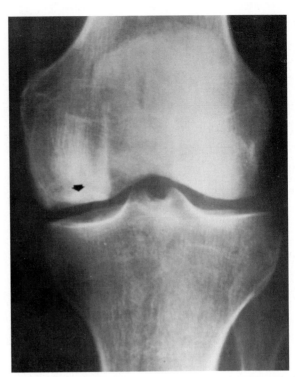

Figure 42–77. Spontaneous osteonecrosis. In this adult with the sudden onset of knee pain, the frontal radiograph demonstrates a defect in the articular surface of the medial femoral condyle *(arrow).* This is the characteristic location of this lesion. (From Resnick D, Niwayama G: Diagnosis of Bone and Joint Disorders. Philadelphia, WB Saunders, 1988.)

characteristic progression of radiographic changes will be seen. The earliest findings are a subtle, arc-like radiolucent subchondral band (crescent sign) and the formation of patchy subchondral lucent and sclerotic foci (Fig. 42–76). Fragmentation and collapse of the articular surface follow. The joint space is usually preserved until late in the course of the disease, when secondary osteoarthritis may supervene.

A peculiar form of spontaneous osteonecrosis is seen in the knee, most commonly involving the medial femoral condyle. It is manifested by the sudden appearance of pain and the radiographic changes of sclerosis, flattening, and irregularity of the femoral surface (Fig. 42–77).

Paget's Disease

Articular disease is a recognized complication of Paget's disease. Gout,[304] CPPD crystal deposition disease,[305] and rheumatoid arthritis[304] have each been observed in patients with Paget's disease. More importantly, patients with this disease demonstrate an increased incidence of OA in association with juxta-articular pagetic bony involvement.[249] This is most common in the hip and knee. Although radiographic features resemble those in idiopathic OA (Fig. 42–78), more specific changes, such as acetabular protrusion, may be seen.

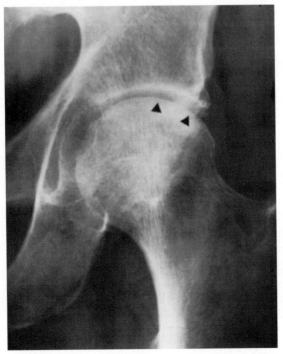

Figure 42–76. Osteonecrosis. An early radiographic change of osteonecrosis is an arc-like radiolucent band *(arrowheads)* parallel to the articular surface.

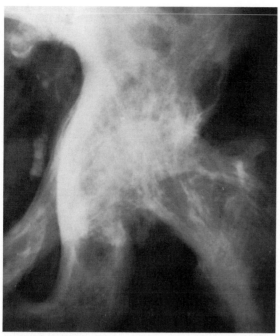

Figure 42–78. Paget's disease. Observe the prominent osteoarthritis-like changes of the hip with asymmetric joint space loss and large marginal osteophytes. The juxta-articular bone is coarsened and enlarged.

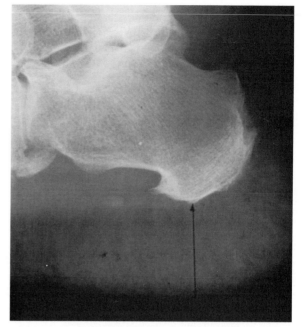

Figure 42–79. Acromegaly. Note the soft tissue prominence of the heel pad with the formation of multiple enthesophytes from the plantar and posterior surfaces of the calcaneus. (From Resnick D, Niwayama G: Diagnosis of Bone and Joint Disorders. Philadelphia, WB Saunders, 1988.)

Acromegaly

Acromegalic arthropathy most closely resembles degenerative joint disease. Some features that aid in its recognition are (1) increased soft tissue thickness (e.g., heel pad > 21 mm) (Fig. 42–79), (2) prominent phalangeal tufts and bases ("arrowhead" phalanges) (Fig. 42–80), (3) "hook-like" osteophytes in the metacarpal heads, (4) joint space widening, (5) exuberant spinal osteophytosis with widened intervertebral discs (Fig. 42–81), and (6) prominent thoracic kyphosis.[306, 307] In the later stages of the disease, loss of joint space becomes apparent. Acromegaly should be considered if a degenerative process occurs in an unusual articulation, such as the glenohumeral joint.

Hemoglobinopathies

Hemoglobinopathies may affect articular structures. The major changes in sickle cell anemia relate to vascular occlusion with osteonecrosis, which may involve epiphysis, metaphysis, or diaphysis of a tubular bone as well as flat bones. In sickle cell dactylitis (hand-foot syndrome), the changes of bone infarction are accompanied by prominent soft tissue swelling and exuberant periosteal reaction.[308] Osteomyelitis and, less commonly, septic arthritis can be seen in sickle cell anemia. *Salmonella* is frequently implicated.

Amyloidosis

Radiographically, the diagnosis of amyloidosis is suggested by the occurrence of a bilateral, symmetric ero-

sive arthropathy similar to rheumatoid arthritis but without joint space narrowing.[309, 310] Large soft tissue masses and osteolytic defects in the diaphyses of tubular bones are other prominent findings in this disorder (Fig. 42–82).

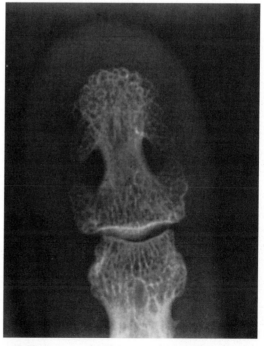

Figure 42–80. Acromegaly. There is proliferation of the margins of the base and terminal tuft of the distal phalanx, resulting in the classic "arrowhead" appearance.

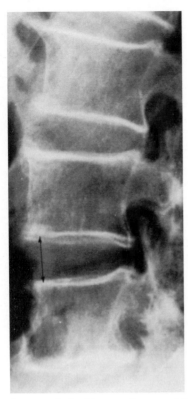

Figure 42–81. Acromegaly. In this case, the most striking finding is the abnormally increased height of the intervertebral disc spaces *(between arrowheads)*. Note posterior concavity of the vertebral bodies and degenerative changes.

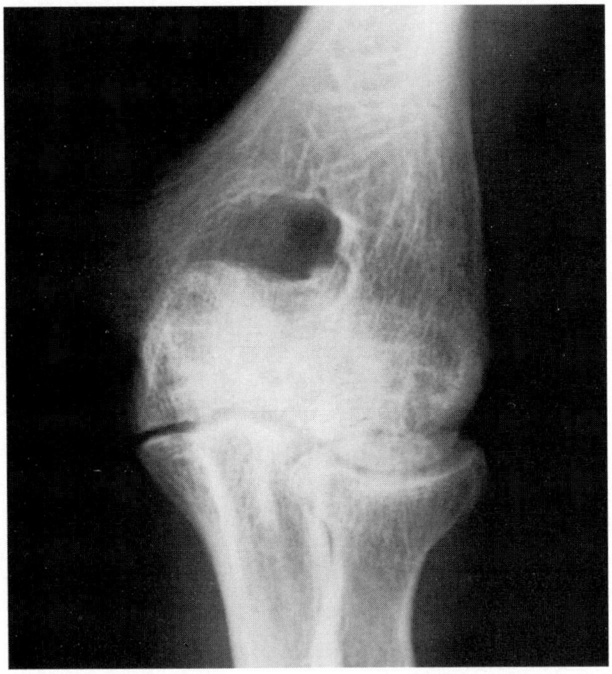

Hemophilia

The arthropathy of hemophilia is related to destructive changes associated with repeated episodes of in-

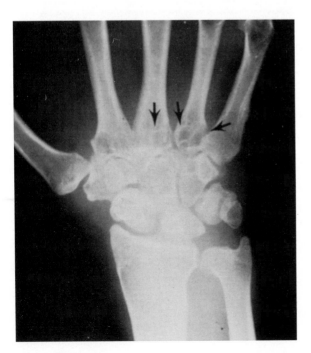

Figure 42–83. Hemophilia. There is overgrowth of the epiphyses, especially the radial head. Joint space narrowing and subchondral cysts are seen.

tra-articular hemorrhage (hemarthrosis).[311] Any joint may be involved, but changes in the knee, ankle, and elbow are most frequently identified. The earliest finding consists of juxta-articular soft tissue swelling with large intra-articular effusions. This is followed by prominent osteoporosis and, in the immature skeleton, by epiphyseal overgrowth (Fig. 42–83). Subchondral cysts and bony erosions appear, initially with

Figure 42–82. Amyloidosis. Observe the diffuse soft tissue swelling and the presence of destructive lesions in the third and fourth metacarpal bases *(arrows)*, radius, and ulna.

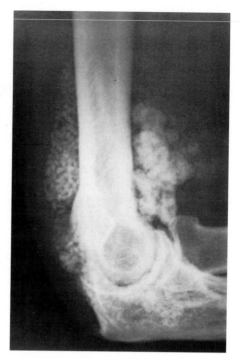

Figure 42–84. Idiopathic synovial (osteo)chondromatosis. A radiograph of the elbow reveals multiple calcified bodies of varying sizes within the confines of an enlarged joint capsule.

preservation of the cartilaginous coat, and subsequently with cartilage destruction and joint space narrowing. Late abnormalities include complete joint disorganization with obliteration of the articular space, large bony erosions, and joint instability. In the knee, radiographic features of hemophilia include widening of the intercondylar notch of the distal femur and squaring of the inferior patellar pole. The radiographic features of hemophilia may be difficult to differentiate from those of juvenile chronic arthritis.

Synovial (Osteo)chondromatosis and Pigmented Villonodular Synovitis

The typical radiographic picture of synovial (osteo)-chondromatosis is that of numerous calcific densities confined to the articular cavity (Fig. 42–84). Pressure erosions of adjacent bony surfaces may be seen. Osteoporosis and joint space narrowing are generally not prominent. In cases in which the bodies are not

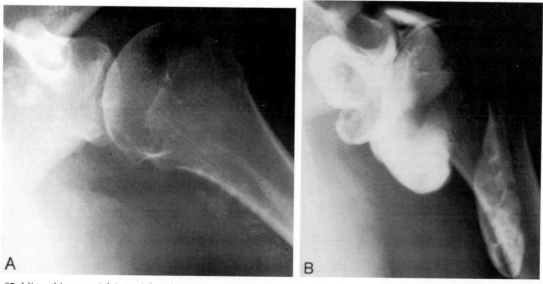

Figure 42–85. Idiopathic synovial (osteo)chondromatosis. A plain film *(A)* and arthrogram *(B)* reveal typical changes. *A*, Observe intra-articular calcified bodies along the synovial sheath of the bicipital tendons. The arthrogram defines multiple radiolucent filling defects.

calcified, arthrography may confirm the diagnosis (Fig. 42–85).

Multiple erosions and cysts on both sides of the joint are seen in pigmented villonodular synovitis. Osteoporosis and joint space narrowing are usually not prominent.[312–314] During arthrography, nodular soft tissue masses may be demonstrated, and aspiration of joint fluid will yield a characteristic "rusty" fluid. MR imaging will reveal signal characteristics diagnostic of hemosiderin deposition.

Synovial Sarcoma

The typical roentgenographic finding of a synovial sarcoma is a soft tissue mass, which contains calcification in approximately 30 percent of cases. Erosion of neighboring bone is seen in 25 to 35 percent of lesions.

References

1. Mall JC, Genant HK, Silcox DC, McCarty DJ: The efficacy of fine-detail radiography in the evaluation of patients with rheumatoid arthritis. Radiology 112:37, 1974.
2. Genant HK: Magnification radiography. In Resnick D, Niwayama G (eds.): Diagnosis of Bone and Joint Disorders. Philadelphia, WB Saunders, 1981, p 335.
3. Genant HK, Valdez Horst J, Lanzl LH, Mall JC, Doi K: Skeletal demineralization in primary hyperparathyroidism. In Mazeski RB (ed): Proceedings of the International Conference on Bone Mineral Measurement. Washington, DC, National Institute of Arthritis, Metabolism and Digestive Diseases, 1973, p 177.
4. Leach RE, Grett T, Ferris JS: Weight-bearing radiography in osteoarthritis of the knee. Radiology 97:265, 1970.
5. Resnick D, Danzig L: Arthrographic evaluation of injuries at the first metacarpophalangeal joint: Gamekeeper's thumb. AJR Am J Roentgenol 126:1046, 1976.
6. Chamberlain WE: The symphysis pubis in the roentgen evaluation of the sacroiliac joint. AJR Am J Roentgenol 24:621, 1930.
7. Martel W, Poznanski AK: The value of traction during roentgenography of the hip. Radiology 94:497, 1970.
8. Resnick D: Arthrography, tenography, and bursography. In Resnick D, Niwayama G (eds): Diagnosis of Bone and Joint Disorders. Philadelphia, WB Saunders, 1981, p 510.
9. Gelman M, Coleman RE, Stevens PM, Davey BW: Radiography, radionuclide imaging, and arthrography in evaluation of painful total hip and knee replacements. Radiology 128:677, 1978.
10. Wolfe RD, Giuliano VJ: Double-contrast arthrography in the diagnosis of pigmented villonodular synovitis of the knee. AJR Am J Roentgenol 110:793, 1970.
11. Prager RJ, Mall JC: Arthrographic diagnosis of synovial chondromatosis. AJR Am J Roentgenol 127:344, 1976.
12. Strizak AM, Danzig LA, Jackson DW, Greenway G, Resnick D, Staple T: Subacromial bursography: An anatomic and clinical study. J Bone Joint Surg 64:196, 1982.
13. Cone R, Danzig L, Resnick D: The shoulder impingement syndrome. Radiology 150:29, 1984.
14. Totty WG, Vannier MW: Complex musculoskeletal anatomy using 3-D surface reconstruction. Radiology 150:173, 1985.
15. Sartoris DJ, Pate D, Andre M, Resnick D: 3-D display of CT data. New aid to pre-op surgical planning. Diagn Imag 8:74, 1986.
16. Fishman EK, Drebin B, Magid D, Scoot WN Jr, Ney DR, Brooker AF Jr, Riley LH, et al: Volumetric rendering techniques: Applications for 3-D imaging of the hip. Radiology 163:737, 1987.
17. Cacayorin ED, Kieffer SA: Applications and limitations of CT of the spine. Radiol Clin North Am 20:185, 1982.
18. Harris JH, Edeiken-Monroe B: The Radiology of Acute Cervical Spine Trauma, 2nd ed. Baltimore, Williams & Wilkins, 1982.
19. Guerra J Jr, Garfin SR, Resnick D: Vertebral burst fractures: CT analysis of the retropulsed fragment. Radiology 153:769, 1984.
20. Daffner RH: Thoracic and lumbar vertebral trauma. Orthop Clin North Am 21:463, 1990.
21. Kaye JJ, Nance EP: Cervical spine trauma. Orthop Clin North Am 21:449, 1990.
22. Perch P, Kilgore DP, Pojima KW, Haughton VM: Cervical spine fractures: CT detection. Radiology 157:117, 1985.
23. Pitt MJ, Lund PJ, Speer DP: Imaging of the pelvis and hip. Orthop Clin North Am 21:545, 1990.
24. Fishman EK, Wyatt SH, Bluemke DA, Urban BA: Spiral CT of musculoskeletal pathology: Preliminary observations. Skeletal Radiol 22:253, 1993.
25. Burk DL Jr, Mears DC, Kennedy WH, Cooperstein LH, Herbert DL: 3-D CT of acetabular fractures. Radiology 155:183, 1985.
26. Ney DR, Fishman EK, Kawashima A, Robertson DD, Scott WW: Comparison of helical and serial CT with regard to three-dimensional imaging of musculoskeletal anatomy. Radiology 185:865, 1992.
27. Destonet JM, Gibula LA, Murphy WA, Sagel SS: CT of sternoclavicular joint and sternum. Radiology 138:123, 1981.
28. Vukich DJ, Markovichick VJ: Pulmonary and chest wall injuries. In Rosen P, Baker FJ II, Barkin RM, et al (eds): Emergency Medicine: Concepts and Clinical Practice, 2nd ed. St Louis, CV Mosby, 1988, pp 473–486.
29. Singson RD, Feldman F, Bibliani L: CT arthrographic patterns in recurrent glenohumeral instability. AJR Am J Roentgenol 149:749, 1987.
30. Beltran J: The shoulder: new approaches. Radiology 5:7, 1990.
31. Raila FA, Aitken AT, Vickers GN: Computed tomography and three-dimensional reconstruction in the evaluation of occipital condyle fractures. Skeletal Radiol 22:269, 1993.
32. Gilmer PW, Herzenberg J, Frank L, Silverman P, et al: CT analysis of acute calcaneal fractures. Foot Ankle 6:184, 1986.
33. Ramirez H Jr, Blatt ES, Cable HF, McComb BL, Zornoza J, Hibri NS: Intraosseous pneumatocysts of the ilium. Radiology 150:503, 1984.
34. Soye I, Levine E, Desmet AA, Weff JR: CT of preoperative evaluation of masses arising in or near the joints of the extremities. Radiology 143:727, 1982.
35. Heiken JP, Lee JKT, Smothers RL, Totty WG, Murphy WA: CT of benign soft tissue masses of extremities. AJR Am J Roentgenol 142:575, 1984.
36. Aisen AM, Martel W, Braumstein EM, et al: MRI and CT evaluation of primary bone and soft tissue tumors. AJR Am J Roentgenol 146:749, 1986.
37. Zimmer WD, Berquist TH, Mcload RA, Sim FH, Pritchard DJ, Shives TC, Wold LE, May GR: Bone tumors: MRI vs CT. Radiology 155:709, 1985.
38. Thompson JR, Christiansen E, Hasso AN, Hinshaw DB Jr: TMJ: High resolution CT evaluation. Radiology 150:105, 1984.
39. Thompson JR, Christiansen E, Hasso AN, Hinshaw DB Jr: Dislocation of the TMJ meniscus: Contrast arthrography vs CT. AJR Am J Roentgenol 144:171, 1985.
40. Sartoris DJ, Neumann CH, Riley RN: The TMJ: True sagittal with meniscus visualization. Radiology 150:250, 1984.
41. Simon DC, Hess MR, Similak MS, Beltran J: Direct sagittal CT of the TMJ. Radiology 157:545, 1985.
42. Manco LG, Messing SG, Busine LJ, Faculo CP, Sordill WC: Internal derangements of TMJ evaluated by direct sagittal CT: A prospective study. Radiology 157:407, 1985.
43. Dussault RG, Lander PH: Imaging of facet joints. Radiol Clin North Am 28:1033, 1990.
44. Carrera GF, Haughton VM, Syvertsen A, et al: CT of lumbar facet joints. Radiology 134:134, 1981.
45. Bjorkengren AG, Kurz LT, Resnick D, et al: Symptomatic intraspinal synovial cysts: Opacification and treatment by percutaneous injection. AJR Am J Roentgenol 149:105, 1987.
46. Hemminghytt S, Daniels DL, Williams AL, Haughton VM: Intraspinal synovial cysts: Natural history and diagnosis by CT. Radiology 145:395, 1982.
47. Russel AS, Jackson F: CT of apophyseal changes in patients with ankylosing spondylitis. J Rheumatol 13:581, 1986.
48. Forrester DM: Imaging of sacroiliac joints. Radiol Clin North Am 28:1055, 1990.
49. Durback MA, Edelstein G, Shumacher HR: Abnormalities of the sacroiliac joints in DISH: Demonstration by CT. J Rheumatol 15:1506, 1988.
50. Vantiggelen R, et al: Sacroiliitis: difficulties in the radiographic diagnosis: Advantage of CT? Preliminary report. J Belge Radiol 70:1, 1987.
51. Guyst DR, Mandi A, Kling GA: Pyogenic sacroiliitis in drug abusers. AJR Am J Roentgenol 149:1209, 1987.
52. Sartoris DJ, Resnick D, Gershumi D, Bielecki D, Meyers M: CT with multiplanar reformation and 3-D image analysis in the preoperative evaluation of ischemic necrosis of the femoral head. J Rheumatol 13:153, 1986.
53. Deutsch AL, Resnick D, Mink JH, Berman JL, Cone RO III, Resnick CS, Danzig L, Guerra J Jr: CT and conventional arthrotomography of the glenohumeral joint: Normal anatomy and clinical experience. Radiology 153:603, 1984.
54. Beltran J, Gray LA, Bools JC, et al: Rotator cuff lesions of the shoulder: Evaluation by direct sagittal CT arthrography. Radiology 160:161, 1986.
55. Gundry CR, Schils JP, Resnick D, Sartoris DJ: Arthrography in post-traumatic knee, shoulder, and wrist: Current status and future trends. Radiol Clin North Am 27:957, 1989.

56. Reikeiras O, Hoiseth A: Patellofemoral relationship in normal subjects determined by computed tomography. Skeletal Radiol 19:591, 1990.

57. Inoue M, Shino K, Hirose H, Horibe S, Ono K: Subluxation of the patella: CT of patellofemoral congruence. J Bone Joint Surg Am 70:1331, 1988.

58. Daniels DL, Grogan JP, Johansen JG, Meyer GA, Williams AL, Haughton VM: Cervical radiculopathy: Computed tomography and myelography compared. Radiology 151:109, 1984.

59. Badami JP, Norman D, Barbaro NM, Cann CE, Weinstein PR, Sobel DF: Metrizamide CT myelography in cervical myelopathy and radiculopathy: Correlation with conventional myelography and surgical findings. AJR Am J Roentgenol 144:675, 1985.

60. Penning L, Wilmink JT, van Woerden HH, Knol E: CT myelographic findings in degenerative disorders of the cervical spine: Clinical significance. AJR Am J Roentgenol 146:793, 1986.

61. Russell EJ, D'Angelo CM, Zimmermann RD, Czervionke LF, Huckman MS: Cervical disk herniation CT demonstration after contrast enhancement. Radiology 152:703, 1984.

62. Williams AL, Haughton VM, Meyer GA, Ho KC: Computed tomographic appearance of the bulging annulus. Radiology 142:403, 1982.

63. Bielecki DK, Sartoris D, Van Lom K, Resnick D, Fierer J, Haghighi P: Intraosseous and intradiscal gas in association with spinal infection: Report of three cases. AJR Am J Roentgenol 147:83, 1986.

64. Raskin SP, Keating JW: Recognition of lumbar disk disease: Comparison of myelography and computed tomography. AJR Am J Roentgenol 139:49, 1982.

65. Haughton VM, Eldevik OP, Magnaes B, Amundsen P: A prospective comparison of computed tomography and myelography in the diagnosis of herniated lumbar disks. Radiology 142:103, 1982.

66. Rosenthal DI, Stauffer AE, Davis KR, Ganott M, Taveras JM: Evaluation of multiplanar reconstruction in CT recognition of lumbar disk disease. AJR Am J Roentgenol 143:169, 1984.

67. Firooznia H, Benjamin V, Kricheff II, Rafii M, Golimbu C: CT of lumbar disk herniation: Correlation with surgical findings. AJR Am J Roentgenol 142:587, 1984.

68. Carrera GF, Williams AL, Haughton VM: Computed tomography in sciatica. Radiology 137:433, 1980.

69. Williams AL, Haughton VM, Daniels DL, Thornton RS: CT recognition of lateral lumbar disk herniation. AJR Am J Roentgenol 139:345, 1982.

70. Williams AL, Haughton VM, Daniels DL, Grogan JP: Differential CT diagnosis of extruded nucleus pulposus. Radiology 154:119, 1985.

71. Helms CA, Dorwart RH, Gray M: The CT appearance of conjoined nerve roots and differentiation from a herniated nucleus pulposus. Radiology 148:141, 1983.

72. Hoddick WK, Helms CA: Bony spinal changes that differentiate conjoined nerve roots from herniated nucleus pulposus. Radiology 154:119, 1985.

73. Teplick JG, Haskin ME: Spontaneous regression of herniated nucleus pulposus. AJR Am J Roentgenol 145:371, 1985.

74. Braun IF, Hoffman JC Jr, Davis PC, Landman JA, Tindall GT: Contrast enhancement in CT differentiation between recurrent disk herniation and postoperative scar: Prospective study. AJR Am J Roentgenol 145:371, 1985.

75. Teplick JG, Haskin ME: Intravenous contrast-enhanced CT of the postoperative lumbar spine: Improved identification of recurrent disk herniation, scar, arachnoiditis, and discitis. AJR Am J Roentgenol 143:845, 1984.

76. Brown BM, Stark EH, Dion G, Ono H: Computed tomography and chymopapain chemonucleolysis: Preliminary findings. AJR Am J Roentgenol 144:667, 1985.

77. Gentry LR, Turski PA, Strother CM, Javid MJ, Sackett JF: Chymopapain chemonucleolysis: CT changes after treatment. AJR Am J Roentgenol 145:361, 1985.

78. Konings JG, Williams FJB, Deutman R: The effects of chemonucleolysis as demonstrated by CT. J Bone Joint Surg 3:417, 1984.

79. Hernandez RJ, Taehdjian MO, Dias LS: Hip CT in congenital dislocation: Appearance of tight iliopsoas tendon and pulvinar hypertrophy. AJR Am J Roentgenol 139:335, 1982.

80. Lafferty CM, Sartoris DJ, Tyson R, Resnick D, Kursunoglu D, Pate D, Sutherland D: Acetabular alterations in untreated congenital hip dysplasia: CT with multiplanar reformation and 3-D analysis. J Comput Assist Tomogr 4:493, 1980.

81. Berquist TH: Optimizing MR imaging techniques for articular disorders. In Weissman BN (ed): RSNA Categorical Course in Musculoskeletal Radiology. Oak Brook, Ill, RSNA Publications, 1992, p 19.

82. Totterman SM, Miller R, Wasserman B, Blebea JS, Rubens DJ: Intrinsic and extrinsic carpal ligaments: Evaluation by three-dimensional Fourier transform MR imaging. AJR Am J Roentgenol 160:117, 1993.

83. Bradley WG Jr, Tsuruda JS: MR sequences parameter optimization: An algorithmic approach. AJR Am J Roentgenol 149:815, 1987.

84. Modic MT, Masaryk TJ, Ross JS, Carter JR: Imaging of degenerative disk disease. Radiology 168:177, 1988.

85. Yu S, Haughton VM, Sether LA, Wagner M: Annulus fibrosus in bulging intervertebral disks. Radiology 169:761, 1988.

86. Masaryk TJ, Ross JS, Modic MT, et al: High-resolution MR imaging of sequestered lumbar intervertebral disks. AJNR Am J Neuroradiol 9:351, 1988.

87. Lee SH, Coleman PE, Hahn FJ: Magnetic resonance imaging of degenerative disk disease of the spine. Radiol Clin North Am 26:949, 1988.

88. Grenier N, Kressel HY, Schiebler ML, et al: Normal and degenerative posterior spinal structures: MR imaging. Radiology 165:517, 1987.

89. Heithoff KB, Ray CD, Schellhas KP, Fritts HM: CT and MRI of lateral entrapment syndromes. In Genant HK (ed): Spine Update 1987. San Francisco, Radiology Research and Education Foundation, 1987, pp 203–234.

90. Burton CV: Avoiding the failed back surgery syndrome. In Cauthen JC (ed): Lumbar Spine Surgery. Baltimore, Williams & Wilkins, 1988, pp 331–341.

91. White AH, Hsu K: Failed Posterior Spine Surgery. St Louis, CV Mosby, 1987.

92. Bundschuh CV, Modic MT, Ross JS, et al: Epidural fibrosis and recurrent disk herniation in the lumbar spine: Assessment with magnetic resonance. AJNR Am J Neuroradiol 5:169, 1988.

93. Sotiropoulos S, Chafetz N, Winkler M, et al: Differentiation between postoperative scar and recurrent disk herniation: Prospective comparison of MR, CT and contrast-enhanced CT. AJNR Am J Neuroradiol 10:639, 1989.

94. Djukic S, Genant HK, Helms CA, Holt RG: Magnetic resonance imaging of the postoperative lumbar spine. Radiol Clin North Am 28:341, 1990.

95. Hueftle MG, Modic MT, Ross JS, et al: Lumbar spine: Postoperative MR imaging with Gd-DTPA. Radiology 167:817, 1988.

96. Ross JS, et al: Gadolinium-DTPA–enhanced MR imaging of the postoperative lumbar spine: Time course and mechanism of enhancement. AJR Am J Roentgenol 152:825, 1989.

97. Boden SD, Davis DO, Dina TS, et al: Contrast-enhanced MR imaging performed after successful lumbar disk surgery: Prospective study. Radiology 182:59, 1992.

98. Vogler JB III, Murphy WA: State of the art: Bone marrow imaging. Radiology 168:679, 1988.

99. Rao VM, Fishman M, Mitchell DG, et al: Painful sickle cell crisis: Bone marrow patterns observed with MR imaging. Radiology 161:211, 1986.

100. Moore SG, Gooding CA, Brasch RC, et al: Bone marrow in children with acute lymphocytic leukemia: MR relaxation times. Radiology 160:237, 1986.

101. Sugimura K, Yamasaki K, Kitagaki H, Tanaka Y, Kono M: Bone marrow diseases of the spine: Differentiation with T_1 and T_2 relaxation times in MRI. Radiology 165:541, 1987.

102. McKinstry CS, Steiner RE, Young AT, Jones L, Swirsky D, Aber V: Bone marrow in leukemia and aplastic anemia: MR imaging before, during and after treatment. Radiology 162:701, 1987.

103. Yao L, Lee JK: Occult intraosseous fracture: Detection with MRI. Radiology 167:749, 1988.

104. Bloem JL: Transient osteoporosis of the hip: MRI. Radiology 167:753, 1988.

105. Beltran J, Herman LJ, Burk JM, et al: Femoral head avascular necrosis: MRI with clinical-pathologic correlation. Radiology 166:215, 1988.

106. Katzberg RW, Westesson PL, Tallents RLH, et al: Temporomandibular joint: MR assessment of rotational and sideways disk displacements. Radiology 169:741, 1988.

107. Katzberg RW: Temporomandibular joint imaging. Radiology 170:297, 1989.

108. Conway WF, Hayes CW, Campbell RL: Dynamic MRI of the temporomandibular joint using FLASH sequences. J Oral Maxillofac Surg 46:930, 1988.

109. Huber DJ, Sauter R, Mueller E, et al: MR imaging of the normal shoulder. Radiology 158:405, 1986.

110. Seeger LL, Gold RH, Bassett LW, et al: Shoulder impingement syndrome: MR findings in 53 shoulders. AJR Am J Roentgenol 150:343, 1988.

111. Zlatkin MB, Iannotti JP, Roberts MC, et al: Rotator cuff tears: Diagnostic performance of MR imaging. Radiology 172:223, 1989.

112. Farley TE, Neumann CH, Steinbach LS, Jahnke AJ, Petersen SS: Full-thickness tears of the rotator cuff of the shoulder: Diagnosis with MR imaging. AJR Am J Roentgenol 158:347, 1992.

113. Liou JTS, Wilson AJ, Totty WG, Brown JJ: The normal shoulder: Common variations that simulate pathologic conditions at MR imaging. Radiology 186:435, 1993.

114. Flannigan B, Kursunoglu-Brahme S, Snyder S, Karzel R, et al: MR arthropathy of the shoulder: Comparison with conventional MR imaging. AJR Am J Roentgenol 155:829, 1990.

115. Yu JS: Magnetic resonance imaging of the wrist. Orthopedics 17:1041, 1994.

116. Middleton WD, Kneeland JB, Kellman GM, Cates JD, Sanger JR, Jesmanowic A, et al: MRI of carpal tunnel: Normal anatomy and preliminary findings in the carpal tunnel syndrome. AJR Am J Roentgenol 148:307, 1987.

117. Stoller DW: MRI in Orthopedics and Rheumatology. Philadelphia, JB Lippincott, 1989.

118. Gilkeson G, Polisson R, Sinclair H, Vogler J, et al: Early detection of carpal erosions in patients with rheumatoid arthritis: A pilot study of MRI. J Rheumatol 15:1361, 1988.
119. Reinus WR, Conway WF, Totty WG, Gilula LA, et al: Carpal avascular necrosis: MRI. Radiology 160:689, 1986.
120. Sugimoto H, Shinozaki T, Ohsawa T: Triangular fibrocartilage in asymptomatic subjects: Investigation of abnormal MR intensity. Radiology 191:193, 1994.
121. Beltran J, Noto AM, Herman LJ, et al: Tendons: High field-strength surface coil MRI. Radiology 162:735, 1987.
122. Daffner RH, Reimer BL, Lupetin AR, et al: MRI in acute tendon ruptures. Skeletal Radiol 15:619, 1986.
123. Yu JS, Witte D, Resnick D, Pogue W: Ossification of the Achilles tendon. Skeletal Radiol 23:127, 1994.
124. Alexander IJ, Johnson KA, Berquist TH: MRI in the diagnosis of disruption of the posterior tibial tendon. Foot Ankle 8:144, 1987.
125. Mink JH, Deutsch AL (eds): MRI of the Musculoskeletal System: A Teaching File. New York, Raven Press, 1990.
126. Yulish BS, Lieberman JM, Neuman AJ, et al: JRA: Assessment with MRI. Radiology 165:149, 1987.
127. Yulish BS, Lieberman JM, Strandjord SE, et al: Hemophilic arthropathy: Assessment with MRI. Radiology 164:759, 1987.
128. Kier R: Magnetic resonance imaging of plantar fasciitis and other causes of heel pain. Radiol Clin North Am 2:97, 1994.
129. Langer JE, Meyer SJ, Dalinka MK: Imaging of the knee. Radiol Clin North Am 28:977, 1990.
130. Mink JH, Reicher MA, Crues JV: MRI of the Knee. New York, Raven Press, 1987.
131. Stoller DW, Martin C, Crues JV, et al: Meniscal tears: Pathologic correlation with MRI. Radiology 163:731, 1987.
132. Mink JH, Levy T, Crues JV: Tears of anterior cruciate ligament and menisci of the knee: MR imaging evaluation. Radiology 167:769, 1988.
133. Jackson DW, Jennings LD, Maywood RM, et al: Magnetic resonance imaging of the knee. Am J Sports Med 16:29, 1988.
134. Mink JH, Deutsch AL (eds): MRI of Musculoskeletal System: A Teaching File. New York, Raven Press, 1990.
135. Tung GA, Davis LM, Wiggins ME, Fadale PD: Tears of the anterior cruciate ligament: Primary and secondary signs at MR imaging. Radiology 188:661, 1993.
136. Yu JS, Goodwin D, Salonen D, et al: Complete dislocation of the knee: Spectrum of associated soft-tissue injuries depicted by MR imaging. AJR Am J Roentgenol 164:135, 1995.
137. Recht MP, Resnick D: MR imaging of articular cartilage: Current status and future directions. AJR Am J Roentgenol 163:283, 1994.
138. Yu JS, Petersilge C, Sartoris D, Pathria M, Resnick D: MR imaging of injuries of the extensor mechanism of the knee. Radiographics 14:541, 1994.
139. Shellock FG, Mink JH, Fox JM: Patellofemoral joint: Kinematic MR imaging to assess tracking abnormalities. Radiology 168:551, 1988.
140. Mink JH, Deutsch AD: Occult osseous and cartilaginous injuries at the knee: MR detection, classification and assessment. Radiology 170:823, 1989.
141. Dietz GW, Wilcox DM, Montgomery JB: Second tibial condyle fracture: Lateral capsular ligament avulsion. Radiology 159:467, 1986.
142. Senac MO, Deutsch D, Bernstein BH, et al: MRI in juvenile rheumatoid arthritis. AJR Am J Roentgenol 150:843, 1988.
143. Bjorkengren AG, Geborek PL, Rydholm U, Holtas S, et al: MR imaging of the knee in acute rheumatoid arthritis: Synovial uptake of Gadolinium-DTPA. AJR Am J Roentgenol 155:329, 1990.
144. Burk DL, Dalinka MK, Kanal E, et al: Meniscal and ganglion cysts of the knee: MR evaluation. AJR Am J Roentgenol 150:331, 1988.
145. Resnick D, Niwayama G: Rheumatoid arthritis. In Resnick D, Niwayama G (eds): Diagnosis of Bone and Joint Disorders. Philadelphia, WB Saunders, 1981, p 906.
146. O'Driscoll S, O'Driscoll M: Osteomalacia in rheumatoid arthritis. Ann Rheum Dis 39:1, 1980.
147. DeHaas WHD, DeBoer W, Griffin F, Oosten-Elst P: Rheumatoid arthritis of the robust reaction type. Ann Rheum Dis 33:81, 1974.
148. Renneic C, Mainzer F, Multz CV, Genant HK: Subchondral pseudocysts in rheumatoid arthritis. AJR Am J Roentgenol 129:1069, 1977.
149. Norgaard F: Tidligste rontgenoligiske forandringer ved polyarthritis. Ugeskr Laeger 125:1312, 1963.
150. Resnick D: Rheumatoid arthritis of the wrist: The compartmental approach. Med Radiog Photog 52:50, 1976.
151. Resnick D: Rheumatoid arthritis of the wrist: Why the ulnar styloid? Radiology 112:29, 1974.
152. Berens DL, Lin RK: Roentgen Diagnosis of Rheumatoid Arthritis. Springfield, Ill, Charles C Thomas, 1969.
153. Resnick D: Early abnormalities of the pisiform and triquetrum in rheumatoid arthritis. Ann Rheum Dis 35:46, 1976.
154. Linscheid RL: The mechanical factors affecting deformity at the wrist in rheumatoid arthritis. In Proceedings of the Twenty-Fourth Annual Meeting of the American Society for Surgery of the Hand. New York, Jan. 17–18, 1969. J Bone Joint Surg 51A:790, 1969.
155. Jackman RJ, Pugh DG: The positive elbow fat pad sign in rheumatoid arthritis. Am J Roentgenol 108:812, 1970.
156. Weston WJ: The synovial changes at the elbow in rheumatoid arthritis. Aust Radiogr 15:170, 1971.
157. Rappaport AS, Sosman JL, Weissman BN: Spontaneous fractures of the olecranon process in rheumatoid arthritis. Radiology 119:83, 1976.
158. Short CL, Bauer W, Reynolds WE: Rheumatoid Arthritis. Cambridge, Mass, Harvard University Press, 1957.
159. Thould AK, Simon G: Assessment of the radiological changes in the hands and feet in rheumatoid arthritis. Ann Rheum Dis 25:220, 1966.
160. Calabro JJ: The feet as an aid in the differential diagnosis of arthritis (abstr). Arthritis Rheum 3:435, 1960.
161. Bywaters EGL: Heel lesions in rheumatoid arthritis. Ann Rheum Dis 13:42, 1954.
162. Resnick D, Feingold ML, Curd J, Niwayama G, Goergen TG: Calcaneal abnormalities in articular disorders: Rheumatoid arthritis, ankylosing spondylitis, psoriatic arthritis, and Reiter's syndrome. Radiology 125:355, 1977.
163. Kirkup JR: Ankle and tarsal joints in rheumatoid arthritis. Scand J Rheumatol 3:50, 1974.
164. Magayar E, Talerman A, Feher M, Wouters HW: Giant bone cysts in rheumatoid arthritis. J Bone Joint Surg 56B:121, 1974.
165. Genovese GR, Jayson MIJ, Dixon AS: Protective value of synovial cysts in rheumatoid knees. Ann Rheum Dis 31:179, 1972.
166. Resnick D: Patterns of migration of the femoral head in osteoarthritis of the hip: Roentgenographic-pathologic correlation and comparison with rheumatoid arthritis. AJR Am J Roentgenol 124:62, 1975.
167. Armbuster T, Guerra Jr, Resnick D, Goergen JG, Feingold ML, Niwayama G, Danzig L: The adult hip: An anatomic study: I. The bony landmarks. Radiology 128:1, 1978.
168. Sievers K, Caine V: The sacroiliac joint in rheumatoid arthritis in adult females. Acta Rheum Scand 9:222, 1963.
169. Martel W: The occipito-atlanto-axial joints in rheumatoid arthritis. In Carter ME (ed): Radiological Aspects of Rheumatoid Disease. Proceedings of an international symposium. Amsterdam, 1963. Amsterdam, Excerpta Medica, 1964, p 189.
170. Mathews JA: Atlanto-axial subluxation in rheumatoid arthritis: A 5-year follow-up study. Ann Rheum Dis 33:526, 1974.
171. Martel W: The occipito-atlanto-axial joints in rheumatoid arthritis and ankylosing spondylitis. AJR Am J Roentgenol 86:223, 1961.
172. Rana NA, Hancock DO, Taylor AR, Hill AGS: Upward translocation of the dens in rheumatoid arthritis. J Bone Joint Surg Br 55:471, 1973.
173. Linquist PR, McDonnell DE: Rheumatoid cyst causing extradural compression. J Bone Joint Surg Am 52:1235, 1970.
174. Ansell BM, Kent PA: Radiological changes in juvenile chronic polyarthritis. Skeletal Radiol 1:129, 1977.
175. Ansell BM, Bywaters EGL: Growth in Still's disease. Ann Rheum Dis 15:295, 1956.
176. Martel W, Holt JF, Cassidy JT: Roentgenologic manifestations of juvenile rheumatoid arthritis. AJR Am J Roentgenol 88:400, 1962.
177. Resnick D, Niwayama G: Juvenile chronic arthritis. In Resnick D, Niwayama G (eds): Diagnosis of Bone and Joint Disease. Philadelphia, WB Saunders, 1981, p 1008.
178. Ansell BM: Chronic arthritis in childhood. Ann Rheum Dis 37:107, 1978.
179. Schaller J, Wedgewood RJ: Juvenile rheumatoid arthritis: A review. Pediatrics 50:940, 1972.
180. Cassidy JT, Brody GL, Martel W: Monoarticular juvenile rheumatoid arthritis. J Pediatr 70:867, 1967.
181. Kleinman P, Rivelas M, Schneider R, Kaye JJ: Juvenile ankylosing spondylitis. Radiology 125:775, 1977.
182. Resnick D: Patterns of peripheral joint disease in ankylosing spondylitis. Radiology 110:523, 1977.
183. Bywaters EGL: Still's disease in the adult. Ann Rheum Dis 30:121, 1971.
184. Medsger TA Jr, Christy WC: Carpal arthritis with ankylosis in late-onset Still's disease. Arthritis Rheum 19:232, 1976.
185. Bluestone R: Histocompatibility antigens and rheumatic disease. In Current Concepts. Kalamazoo, Mich, Upjohn, 1978, p 17.
186. Resnick D, Niwayama G: Ankylosing spondylitis. In Resnick D, Niwayama G (eds): Diagnosis of Bone and Joint Disorders. Philadelphia, WB Saunders, 1981, p 1040.
187. Wilkinson M, Bywaters EGL: Clinical features and course of ankylosing spondylitis as seen in a follow-up of 222 hospital referred cases. Ann Rheum Dis 17:209, 1956.
188. Rosen PS, Graham DC: Ankylosing (Strumpell-Marie) spondylitis (A clinical review of 128 cases). AJR Am J Roentgenol 5:158, 1962.
189. Berens DL: Roentgen features of ankylosing spondylitis. Clin Orthop Rel Res 74:20, 1971.
190. Resnick D, Niwayama G, Goergen TG: Comparison of radiographic abnormalities of the sacro-iliac joint in degenerative joint disease and ankylosing spondylitis. AJR Am J Roentgenol 128:189, 1977.
191. Forestier J, Jacqueline F, Rotes-Querol J: Ankylosing Spondylitis. Springfield, Ill, Charles C Thomas, 1956.
192. Cawley MID, Chalmers TM, Kellgren JH, Ball J: Destructive lesions of

vertebral bodies in ankylosing spondylitis. Ann Rheum Dis 31:345, 1972.

193. Dwosh IL, Resnick D, Becker MP: Hip involvement in ankylosing spondylitis. Arthritis Rheum 19:683, 1976.

194. Glick EN: A radiological comparison of the hip joint in rheumatoid arthritis and ankylosing spondylitis. Proc R Soc Med 59:1229, 1976.

195. Resnick D, Dwosh IL, Goergen TG, Shapiro RF, D'Ambrosia R: Clinical and radiographic "reankylosis" following hip surgery in ankylosing spondylitis. AJR Am J Roentgenol 216:1181, 1976.

196. Rosen PS: A unique shoulder lesion in ankylosing spondylitis: Clinical comment. J Rheumatol 7:109, 1980.

197. Ball J: Enthesopathy of rheumatoid and ankylosing spondylitis. Ann Rheum Dis 30:213, 1971.

198. Resnick D, Niwayama G: Psoriatic arthritis. In Resnick D, Niwayama G (eds): Diagnosis of Bone and Joint Disorders. Philadelphia, WB Saunders, 1981, p 1103.

199. Wright V: Psoriatic arthritis. In Scott JT (ed): Copeman's Textbook of the Rheumatic Diseases, 5th ed. Edinburgh, Churchill Livingstone, 1978, p 537.

200. Zaias N: Psoriasis of the nail: A clinico-pathological study. Arch Dermatol 99:567, 1967.

201. Resnick D, Niwayama G: On the nature and significance of bony proliferation in "rheumatoid variant" disorders. AJR Am J Roentgenol 129:275, 1977.

202. Forrester DM, Kirkpatrick RW: Periostitis and pseudoperiostitis. Radiology 118:597, 1976.

203. Resnick D, Broderick RW: Bony proliferation of terminal phalanges in psoriasis: The "ivory" phalanx. J Can Assoc Radiol 28:187, 1977.

204. Killebrew K, Gold RH, Sholkoff SD: Psoriatic spondylitis. Radiology 108:9, 1973.

205. Sundaram M, Patton JT: Paravertebral ossification in psoriasis and Reiter's disease. Br J Radiol 48:628, 1975.

206. Kaplan D, Plotz CM, Nathanson L, Frank L: Cervical spine in psoriasis and psoriatic arthritis. Ann Rheum Dis 23:50, 1964.

207. Resnick D, Niwayama G: Reiter's syndrome. In Resnick D, Niwayama G (eds): Diagnosis of Bone and Joint Disorders, Philadelphia, WB Saunders, 1981, p 1130.

208. Sholkoff SD, Glickman MG, Steinback HL: Roentgenology of Reiter's syndrome. Radiology 97:497, 1970.

209. Cliff JM: Spinal bony bridging and carditis in Reiter's disease. Ann Rheum Dis 30:171, 1971.

210. Resnick D, Niwayama G: Enteropathic arthropathies. In Resnick D, Niwayama G (eds): Diagnosis of Bone and Joint Disorders. Philadelphia, WB Saunders, 1981, p 1149.

211. Jayson MIV, Salmon PR, Harrison WJ: Inflammatory bowel disease in ankylosing spondylitis. Gut 11:506, 1970.

212. McEwen C, Ditata D, Lingg C, Porini A, Good A, Rankin T: Ankylosing spondylitis and spondylitis accompanying ulcerative colitis, regional enteritis, psoriasis, and Reiter's disease. Arthritis Rheum 14:291, 1971.

213. Haslock I: Enteropathic arthritis. In Scott JT (ed): Copeman's Textbook of the Rheumatic Diseases, 5th ed. Edinburgh, Churchill Livingstone, 1978, p 567.

214. Ferguson RH: Enteropathic arthritis. In Hollander, JL, McCarty DJ (eds): Arthritis and Allied Conditions, 8th ed. Philadelphia, Lea & Febiger, 1972, p 846.

215. O'Connell DJ, Marx WJ: Hand changes in primary biliary cirrhosis. Radiology 129:31, 1978.

216. Clarke AK, Galbraith RM, Hamilton EBD, Williams R: Rheumatic disorders in primary biliary cirrhosis. Ann Rheum Dis 37:42, 1978.

217. Lucas PF, Owen TK: Subcutaneous fat necrosis, "polyarthritis," and pancreatic disease. Gut 3:146, 1962.

218. Gibson TJ, Schumacher HR, Pascual E, Brighton E, Brighton C: Arthropathy, skin and bone lesions in pancreatic disease. J Rheumatol 2:7, 1975.

219. Labowitz R, Schumacher HR Jr: Articular manifestations of systemic lupus erythematosus. Ann Intern Med 74:911, 1971.

220. Weissman BN, Rappoport AS, Sosman JL, Schur PH: Radiographic findings in the hands in patients with systemic lupus erythematosus. Radiology 126:313, 1978.

221. Bleifield CJ, Inglis AE: The hand in systemic lupus erythematosus. J Bone Joint Surg Am 56:1207, 1974.

222. Bywaters EGL: Jaccoud's syndrome: A sequel to the joint involvement in systemic lupus erythematosus. Clin Rheum Dis 1:125, 1975.

223. Twinning RH, Marcus WY, Garey JL: Tendon rupture in systemic lupus erythematosus. JAMA 189:377, 1964.

224. Klippel JH, Gerber LH, Pollack L, Decker JL: Avascular necroses in systemic lupus erythematosus: Silent symmetric osteonecrosis. Am J Med 67:83, 1979.

225. Budin JA, Feldman F: Soft tissue calcifications in systemic lupus erythematosus. AJR Am J Roentgenol 124:358, 1975.

226. Staples PJ, Gerding DN, Decker JL, Gordon RS Jr: Incidence of infection in systemic lupus erythematosus. Arthritis Rheum 17:1, 1971.

227. Goodman N: The significance of terminal phalangeal osteosclerosis. Radiology 89:709, 1967.

228. Resnick D: Scleroderma (progressive systemic sclerosis). In Resnick D, Niwayama G (eds): Diagnosis of Bone and Joint Disorders. Philadelphia, WB Saunders, 1981, p 1204.

229. Poznanski AK: The Hand in Radiologic Diagnosis. Philadelphia, WB Saunders, 1974, p 531.

230. Thibierge G, Weissenbach RJ: Concretions calcare souscutanees et sclerodermie. Ann Dermatol Syphiligr 2:129, 1911.

231. Muller SA, Brunsting LA, Winkelmann RK: Calcinosis cutis: Its relationship to scleroderma. Arch Dermatol 80:15, 1959.

232. Rowell NR, Hopper FE: The periodontal membrane in systemic lupus erythematosus. Br J Dermatol 93(suppl):23, 1975.

233. Seifert MH, Steigerwald JC, Cliff MM: Bone resorption of the mandible in progressive systemic sclerosis. Arthritis Rheum 18:507, 1977.

234. Keats TE: Rib erosions in scleroderma. AJR Am J Roentgenol 100:530, 1967.

235. Mezarsos WT: The regional manifestations of scleroderma. Radiology 70:313, 1958.

236. Kemp Harper RA, Jackson DC: Progressive systemic sclerosis. Br J Radiol 38:825, 1965.

237. Haverbush TJ, Wilde AH, Hawk WA Jr, Scherbel AL: Osteolysis of the ribs and cervical spine in progressive systemic sclerosis (scleroderma): A case report. J Bone Joint Surg 56A:637, 1974.

238. Lovell CR, Jayson MIV: Joint involvement in systemic sclerosis. Scand J Rheumatol 8:154, 1979.

239. Resnick D: Dermatomyositis and polymyositis. In Resnick D, Niwayama G (eds): Diagnosis of Bone and Joint Disorders. Philadelphia, WB Saunders, 1981, p 1230.

240. Schumacher HR, Schimmer B, Gordon GV, Bookspan MA, Brogadir S, Dorwart BB: Articular manifestations of polymyositis and dermatomyositis. Arthritis Rheum 23:491, 1980.

241. Ozonoff MB, Flynn FJ Jr: Roentgenologic features of dermatomyositis of childhood. AJR Am J Roentgenol 118:206, 1973.

242. Sewell JR, Liyanage B, Ansell BM: Calcinosis in juvenile dermatomyositis. Skeletal Radiol 3:137, 1978.

243. Resnick D: Polyarteritis nodosa and other vasculitides. In Resnick D, and Niwayama G (eds): Diagnosis of Bone and Joint Disorders. Philadelphia, WB Saunders, 1981, p 1242.

244. Bennet RM, O'Connell DJ: The arthritis of mixed connective tissue disease. Ann Rheum Dis 37:397, 1978.

245. Ramos-Niembro F, Alarcon-Segovia D, Hernandez-Ortiz J: Articular manifestations of mixed connective tissue disease. Arthritis Rheum 22:43, 1979.

246. Resnick D, Niwayama G: Degenerative disease of extraspinal locations. In Resnick D, Niwayama G (eds): Diagnosis of Bone and Joint Disorders. Philadelphia, WB Saunders, 1981, p 1270.

247. Landells JW: The bone cysts of osteoarthritis. J Bone Joint Surg Br 35:643, 1953.

248. Ferguson AB: The pathologic changes in degenerative arthritis of the hip and treatment by rotational osteotomy. J Bone Joint Surg Am 46:1337, 1964.

249. Resnick D: Patterns of migration of the femoral head in osteoarthritis of the hip: Roentgenographic-pathologic correlation and comparison with rheumatoid arthritis. AJR Am J Roentgenol 124:62, 1975.

250. Thomas RH, Resnick D, Alazraki NP, Daniel D, Greenfield R: Compartmental evaluation of osteoarthritis of the knee: a comparative study of available diagnostic modalities. Radiology 116:585, 1975.

251. Leach RE, Gregg T, Siber FJ: Weight-bearing radiography in osteoarthritis of the knee. Radiology 97:265, 1970.

252. Mann RA, Coughlin MJ, DuVries HL: Hallux rigidus: A review of the literature and a method of treatment. Clin Orthop Rel Res 142:57, 1979.

253. Crain DC: Interphalangeal osteoarthritis characterized by painful inflammatory episodes resulting in deformity of the proximal and distal articulations. JAMA 175:1049, 1961.

254. McEwen C: Osteoarthritis of the fingers with ankylosis. Arthritis Rheum 11:734, 1968.

255. Resnick D, Niwayama G: Degenerative disease of the spine. In Resnick D, Niwayama G (eds): Diagnosis of Bone and Joint Disorders. Philadelphia, WB Saunders, 1981, p 1368.

256. Schmorl G, Junghanns H: The Human Spine in Health and Disease, 2nd ed. [Translated by Besemann EF.] New York, Grune & Stratton, 1971, p 138.

257. Knutsson F: The vacuum phenomenon in the intervertebral discs. Acta Radiol 23:173, 1942.

258. Kroker P: Sichtbare Rissbildungen in den Bandscheiben der Wirbelsaule. Fortschr Geb Roentgenstr Nuklearmed 72:1, 1949.

259. Bick EM: Vertebral osteophytosis: pathologic basis of its roentgenology. AJR Am J Roentgenol 73:979, 1955.

260. Goldberg RP, Carter BL: Absence of thoracic osteophytosis in the area adjacent to the aorta: Computed tomography demonstration. J Comput Assist Tomogr 2:173, 1978.

261. Hadley LA: Anatomico-roentgenographic studies of the posterior spinal articulations. AJR Am J Roentgenol 86:270, 1961.

262. Resnick D, Niwayama G: Diffuse idiopathic skeletal hyperostosis

(DISH): Ankylosing hyperostosis of Forestier and Rotes-Querol. *In* Resnick D, Niwayama G (eds): Diagnosis of Bone and Joint Disorders. Philadelphia, WB Saunders, 1981, p 1416.

263. Forestier J, Rotes-Querol J: Senile ankylosing hyperostosis of the spine. Ann Rheum Dis 9:321, 1950.

264. Oppenheimer A: Calcification and ossification of vertebral ligaments (spondylosis ossificans ligamentosa): Roentgen study of pathogenesis and clinical significance. Radiology 38:160, 1940.

265. Resnick D, Niwayama G: Radiographic and pathologic features of spinal involvement in diffuse idiopathic skeletal hyperostosis (DISH). Radiology 119:559, 1976.

266. Bauer F: Dysphagia due to cervical spondylosis. J Laryngol Otol 67:615, 1953.

267. Resnick D, Guerra J Jr, Robinson CA, Vint VC: Association of diffuse idiopathic skeletal hyperostosis (DISH) and calcification and ossification of the posterior longitudinal ligament. AJR Am J Roentgenol 131:1049, 1978.

268. Kohler H, Uehlinger E, Kutzner J, West TB: Sternocostoclavicular hyperostosis: Painful swelling of the sternum, clavicles, and upper ribs. Ann Intern Med 87:192, 1977.

269. Resnick D, Shaul SR, Robins JM: Diffuse idiopathic skeletal hyperostosis (DISH): Forestier's disease with extraspinal manifestations. Radiology 115:513, 1975.

270. Resnick D: Neuroarthropathy. *In* Resnick D, Niwayama G (eds): Diagnosis of Bone and Joint Disorders. Philadelphia, WB Saunders, 1981, p 2422.

271. Key JA: Clinical observations on tabetic arthropathies (Charcot joints). Am J Syph 14:429, 1932.

272. Pomeranz MM, Rothberg AS: A review of 58 cases of tabetic arthropathy. Am J Syph 25:103, 1941.

273. Jaffe HL: Metabolic, Degenerative and Inflammatory Diseases of Bones and Joints. Philadelphia, Lea & Febiger, 1972, p 847.

274. Clouse ME, Gramm HF, Legg M, Flood T: Diabetic osteoarthropathy: Clinical and roentgenographic observations in 90 cases. Am J Roentgenol 121:22, 1974.

275. Gray RG, Gottlieb NL: Rheumatic disorders associated with diabetes mellitus: Literature review. Semin Arthritis Rheum 6:19, 1976.

276. Giesecke SB, Dalinka MK, Kyle GC: Lisfranc's fracture-dislocation: A manifestation of peripheral neuropathy. AJR Am J Roentgenol 131:139, 1978.

277. Thornhill HL, Richter RW, Shelton ML, Johnson CA: Neuropathic arthropathy (Charcot forefeet) in alcoholics. Orthop Clin North Am 4:7, 1973.

278. Peitzman SJ, Miller JL, Ortega L, Schumacher HR, Fernandez PC: Charcot arthropathy secondary to amyloid neuropathy. JAMA 235:1345, 1976.

279. Resnick D, Niwayama G: Crystal-induced and related diseases. *In* Resnick D, Niwayama G (eds): Diagnosis of Bone and Joint Disorders. Philadelphia, WB Saunders, 1981, p 1463.

280. Talbott JH: Gout, 3rd ed. New York, Grune & Stratton, 1967.

281. Vyhanek L, Lavicka J, Blahos J: Roentgenological findings in gout. Radiol Clin North Am 28:256, 1960.

282. Good AE, Rapp R: Bony ankylosis: A rare manifestation of gout. J Rheumatol 5:335, 1978.

283. Kawenoki-Minc E, Eyman E, Leo W, Werynska-Przybylska J: Zwyrodnienie stawow i kregoslupa u chorych na dne. Analiza 262 przypadkowdny. Reumatoligia 12:267, 1974.

284. von Hoyningen-Huene CBJ: Gout and glycogen storage disease in preadolescent brothers. Arch Intern Med 118:471, 1966.

285. Riley JD: Gout and cerebral palsy in a three-year-old boy. Arch Dis Child 35:293, 1960.

286. Gutman AB: Primary and secondary gout. Ann Intern Med 39:1062, 1953.

287. Grahme R, Sutor DJ, Mitchener MB: Crystal deposition in hyperparathyroidism. Ann Rheum Dis 30:597, 1971.

288. Dmartini FE: Hyperuricemia induced by drugs. Arthritis Rheum 8:823, 1965.

289. Resnick D, Niwayama G, Goergen TG, Utsinger PD, Shapiro RF, Hasselwood DH, Wiesner KB: Clinical, radiographic and pathologic abnormalities in calcium pyrophosphate dihydrate deposition disease (CPPD): Pseudogout Radiology 122:1, 1977.

290. Vigario DG, Keats TE: Localization of calcific deposits in the shoulder. AJR Am J Roentgenol 108:806, 1970.

291. Schumacher HR Jr: Hemochromatosis and arthritis. Arthritis Rheum 7:41, 1964.

292. Hamilton E, Williams R, Barlow KA, Smith PM: The arthropathy of hemochromatosis. Q J Med 37:171, 1968.

293. Atkins CJ, McIvor J, Smith PM, Hamilton E, Williams R: Chondrocalcinosis and arthropathy: Studies in haemochromatosis and in idiopathic chondrocalcinosis. Q J Med 39:71, 1970.

294. De Seze S, Solnica J, Mitrovic D, Miravet L, Dorfmann H: Joint and bone disorders and hypoparathyroidism in hemochromatosis. Semin Arthritis Rheum 2:71, 1972.

295. Hirsch JH, Killien C, Troupin RH: The arthropathy of hemochromatosis. Radiology 118:591, 1976.

296. Feller ER, Schumacher HR: Osteoarticular changes in Wilson's disease. Arthritis Rheum 15:259, 1972.

297. Finby N, Bearn AG: Roentgenographic abnormalities of the skeletal system in Wilson's disease (hepatolenticular degeneration). AJR Am J Roentgenol 79:603, 1958.

298. Cervenansky J, Sitaj S, Urbanek T: Alkaptonuria and ochronosis. J Bone Joint Surg Am 41:1169, 1959.

299. Mueller MN, Sorenson LB, Strandjord N, Kappas A: Alkaptonuria and ochronotic arthropathy. Med Clin North Am 49:101, 1965.

300. Martin WJ, Underahl LO, Mathieson DR, Pugh DG: Alkaptonuria: Report of 12 cases. Ann Intern Med 42:1052, 1955.

301. Resnick D, Niwayama G: Osteomyelitis, septic arthritis, and soft tissue infection: The mechanisms and situations. *In* Resnick D, Niwayama G (eds): Diagnosis of Bone and Joint Disorders. Philadelphia, WB Saunders, 1981, p 2042.

302. Chuinard RG, D'Ambrosia R: Human bite infections of the hand. J Bone Joint Surg Am 59:416, 1977.

303. Patterson FP, Brown CS: Complications of total hip replacement arthroplasty. Orthop Clin North Am 4:503, 1973.

304. Franck WA, Bress NM, Singer FR, Krane SM: Rheumatic manifestation of Paget's disease of bone. Am J Med 56:592, 1974.

305. McCarty DJ Jr: Pseudogout: articular chondrocalcinosis. *In* Hollander JL, McCarty DJ Jr (eds): Arthritis and Related Disorders, 8th ed. Philadelphia, Lea & Febiger, 1972, p 410.

306. Steinbach HL, Russell W: Measurements of the heel pad as an aid to diagnosis of acromegaly. Radiology 82:418, 1964.

307. Lang EK, Bessler WT: The roentgenologic features of acromegaly. AJR Am J Roentgenol 86:321, 1961.

308. Watson RJ, Burko H, Megas H, Robinson M: Hand-foot syndrome in sickle cell disease in young children. Pediatrics 31:975, 1963.

309. Grossman RE, Hensley GT: Bone lesions in primary amyloidosis. AJR Am J Roentgenol 101:872, 1967.

310. Weinfield A, Stern MH, Marx LH: Amyloid lesions of bone. AJR Am J Roentgenol 108:799, 1970.

311. Pettersson H, Ahlberg A, Nilsson IM: A radiologic classification of hemophilic arthropathy. Clin Orthop Rel Res 149:153, 1980.

312. Resnick D, Niwayama G (eds): Diagnosis of Bone and Joint Disorders. Philadelphia, WB Saunders, 1981, p 2638.

313. Prager RJ, Mall JC: Arthrographic diagnosis of synovial chondromatosis. AJR Am J Roentgenol 127:344, 1976.

314. Breimer CW, Freiberger RH: Bone lesions associated with villonodular synovitis. AJR Am J Roentgenol 79:618, 1958.

CHAPTER 43

Terry L. Whipple
Michael J. Duval

Arthroscopy and Synovectomy

Conventional open surgical techniques for patients with inflammatory or degenerative joint disorders involve formal arthrotomy to address intra-articular pathology. This allows direct access to joint structures, but at the expense of a large surgical exposure. Open procedures also require in-patient hospitalization and lengthy rehabilitation periods.[1,2] Loss of motion following arthrotomy that necessitates secondary procedures to restore range of motion and increased cost from hospitalization makes open procedures less attractive to both physician and patient in light of newer, less aggressive surgical techniques.[3,4]

The introduction of arthroscopic surgical technique has had a significant impact on contemporary orthopedic surgical practice. With low incidence of surgical morbidity, surgeons can obtain direct access to intra-articular structures.[5,6] Procedures can be performed on an out-patient basis with significantly shorter rehabilitation periods compared with those of conventional open techniques.[3,4,7,8]

This chapter discusses arthroscopic procedures and their role in the treatment of inflammatory arthritis. It also discusses indications and arthroscopic treatment of synovial disease and degenerative joint disorders.

HISTORICAL PERSPECTIVE

The first attempt at endoscopic visualization of intra-articular structures was undertaken by Takagi in 1918 at the University of Tokyo.[9] Initially a technique used in the knee, arthroscopy has been expanded to have applications in the shoulder, elbow, wrist, ankle, and hip joints. This application is still growing as new surgical techniques are being developed.

Knowledge of anatomic landmarks allows precise percutaneous placement of instruments into joints, avoiding damage to more superficial structures including vessels, nerves, and tendons (Fig. 43–1). Using telescopes with different lens angles, extensive visualization can be obtained in major diarthrodial joints. With the development of innovative surgical instrumentation, many procedures are now performed arthroscopically with results comparable to those of open surgery.[3,4,10] Arthroscopic synovectomy and debridement have become widely accepted techniques; however, strict surgical indications must be respected to select patients who would best benefit from such procedures.

INFLAMMATORY DISORDERS

Synovial Disorders

In inflammatory arthritis, disease progression centers around pathologic changes in the synovium that become progressive, leading to invasion and destruction of articular cartilage. One would assume removal of diseased synovium would play a central role in controlling the disease process in inflammatory arthritis. However, it remains unclear whether synovectomy actually alters the progression of disease.[11–13] It is well accepted that synovectomy can effectively reduce joint inflammation and swelling, with subjective improvement in pain and function in short-term follow-up.[8,10,14–16] In some synovial disorders, such as synovial chondromatosis and pigmented villonodular synovitis, synovectomy may even be curative. Its role still appears to be only palliative in the treatment of rheumatoid synovitis and hemophilic arthropathy.[17,18]

Initially described as an open technique for tuberculous arthropathy,[19] synovectomy gained significant popularity in the early 1900s. The technique was initially introduced in the United States by Swett, who reported on a small series of patients before the American Orthopedic Association in 1922.[20] Initially recommended as a technique for chronic infectious arthritis, open synovectomy increased in popularity, and its indications expanded to synovial diseases and inflammatory and degenerative arthritis.[20–22] Clinical series published at that time included synovectomy for multiple diagnoses, with a lack of clear indications on when to perform synovectomy. Postoperative rehabilitation was not aggressive, and many authors recommended postoperative immobilization.[23–25] After a report of 50 percent incidence of poor results in rheumatoid arthritis patients by Ghormley and Cameron in 1941, the initial enthusiasm for the procedure declined.[26] It was not until the 1960s, when a resurgence of interest in rheumatoid arthritis occurred, that open synovectomy reemerged as a popular technique.

As its popularity grew, arthroscopy emerged as a tool to both study and treat inflammatory arthritis. With its low incidence of surgical morbidity, arthroscopy became an attractive technique to perform biopsy as well as synovectomy. In 1985, Highgenboten presented his technique for arthroscopic synovectomy that addressed several pitfalls of open synovectomy.[4] Using a systematic approach and multiple portals, a complete synovectomy was possible, even in the

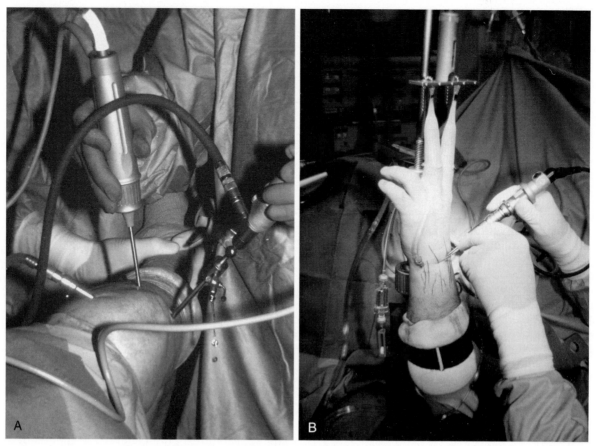

Figure 43–1. Arthroscopy. *A,* The knee. Through small stab incisions in the skin, arthroscopic sheath, shaver, and inflow cannula are placed into the knee joint. While holding the arthroscope with one hand, the surgeon uses the shaver in the opposite hand for debridement and synovectomy. Intra-articular images are projected onto a television monitor. *B,* The wrist. Preoperative identification of anatomic landmarks allows establishment of portals on the dorsum of the wrist for placement of the arthroscope, operating instruments, and inflow cannula for distention of the joint with fluid.

posterior compartment of the knee, which was previously inaccessible by an anterior arthrotomy.[27–29] Highgenboten stressed that, although not curative, arthroscopic synovectomy was beneficial in the control of pain and swelling and had a positive effect on quality of life.[4]

Salisbury and Nottage observed meniscal invasion by rheumatoid synovium prior to articular cartilage involvement (Fig. 43–2).[30]

To date, there has been no prospective study with controls that has documented the efficacy of arthroscopic synovectomy compared with medical management.[31] The largest review of arthroscopic synovectomy was published by Ogilvie-Harris and Weisleder in 1955.[32] The authors reviewed 211 arthroscopic synovectomies performed over a 10-year period. Diagnoses included rheumatoid arthritis, synovial disease, and post-traumatic synovitis. Criteria for assessment of results included pain, presence of effusion, range of motion, and overall functional capacity. The authors found good to excellent results in 80 percent of 112 cases of rheumatoid synovectomy, with an average follow-up of 4 years. The authors did not comment on radiographic progression of disease in their study. Similar findings were reported by Cleland and colleagues,[14] Klein and Jensen,[15] and Smiley and Wasilewski.[10] All agree that arthroscopic synovectomy is most efficacious when performed in the early stages of disease, which is in agreement with previous literature on open synovectomy. Poorer results were observed in patients with advanced articular cartilage destruction at the time of arthroscopy.

Although not a curative procedure, synovectomy can have a beneficial effect on quality of life in rheumatoid patients with uncontrolled synovitis. Its use should be limited to patients with chronic painful synovitis that is unresponsive to medical management. Criteria established by the American Rheumatologic Association recommend synovectomy when effusion and synovitis persist after 6 months of aggressive medical management. Patients should be in the early stages of the disease process with no significant changes on radiographs. When proper patient selection is utilized, arthroscopic synovectomy can be a useful adjunct in the management of refractive synovitis in rheumatoid arthritis.[33]

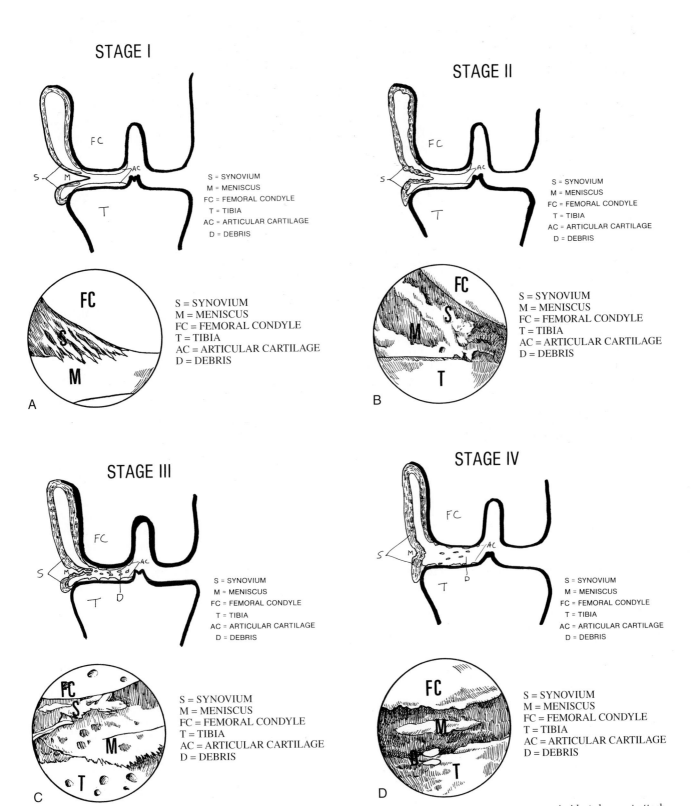

Figure 43–2. Progression of inflammatory forms of arthritis. *A*, Stage I. Synovitis only. Synovium may cover menisci but does not attach to or erode the meniscal surfaces. *B*, Stage II. Synovium erodes meniscal surfaces. *C*, Stage III. Erosion continues, producing loss of meniscal form and function, tears, and abrasive debris. *D*, Stage IV. End-stage disease with loss of meniscal integrity, load-sharing, and stability. Debris produces more debris. (From Salisbury RB, Nottage, WM: A new evaluation of gross pathologic changes and concepts of rheumatoid articular cartilage degeneration. Clin Orthop 199:242–247, 1985.)

Hemophilic Arthropathy

Patients with hemophilia develop recurrent hemarthrosis, with deposition of hemosiderin in synovial membranes.[34] Synovial proliferation within the joint cavity leads to increasing frequency of hemarthroses.[35] In uncontrolled hemophiliacs, accelerated deterioration occurs with disabling loss of motion and, in some cases, the development of bony ankylosis.[36, 37]

The technique of open synovectomy for hemophilic arthropathy was described by Storty and coworkers in 1969.[38] The authors presented 15 cases of open synovectomy of the knee with no recurrent hemarthrosis at 2-year follow-up. However, in a later report, Storty and Ascari noted that some patients in their study developed recurrent hemarthrosis after a longer follow-up period.[39] Synovectomy was beneficial by removing the fibrotic synovium, thus decreasing the frequency of recurrent hemarthrosis.[34, 40–43] A common problem after open synovectomy was difficulty in restoring range of motion.[34, 40, 44, 45]

With improvements in instrumentation, arthroscopic synovectomy has been applied to hemophilic arthropathy. Minimal joint disruption and quicker rehabilitation are attractive advantages of arthroscopy, owing to previous problems with restoration of motion after open synovectomy. Initial reports of arthroscopic synovectomy in hemophilia revealed a decreased incidence of hemarthrosis comparable with that of open techniques.[46] Klein and associates reported on a small series of patients following arthroscopic synovectomy. Their patients experienced a reduction in episodes of hemarthrosis, with minimal loss of motion following surgery.[46] In a comparison of open versus arthroscopic synovectomy by Triantafyllou and colleagues, there was an equal incidence of reduced hemarthrosis and radiographic degeneration in the two groups.[47] However, improved range of motion following synovectomy was demonstrated in the arthroscopic group.

Indications for synovectomy in hemophilic arthropathy include failure to respond to conservative protocols for a 6-month period. Best results can be obtained when intervention is taken early, before articular cartilage destruction takes place.[34, 38, 42, 46, 48, 49]

Physical therapy is begun immediately after arthroscopic synovectomy. Continuous passive motion devices have a beneficial effect on the early restoration of motion.[48, 50, 51] An excellent review of indications and perioperative considerations in hemophilia has been published by DeGnore and Wilson.[52]

Septic Arthritis

An infectious process within a diarthrodial joint can have devastating sequelae on joint function. Pathogenic organisms introduced into a joint by either direct inoculation or hematogenous spread stimulate an inflammatory response, with increased concentrations of polymorphonuclear granulocytes. Proteolytic enzymes released from granulocytes attack infectious pathogens as well as articular cartilage. Articular cartilage becomes destroyed and fibrous adhesions form within the joint cavity. The end result is joint stiffness, degeneration of articular cartilage, and impaired function. If detected and effectively treated in its early phases, the prognosis is good for return to normal joint function.[53, 54] Arthroscopic treatment of septic arthritis is an effective treatment that addresses the pitfalls of other techniques.

Jackson presented a technique for arthroscopic treatment for septic arthritis in 1985.[55] His technique involved arthroscopic irrigation and debridement along with placement of drainage tubes to allow intermittent distention and drainage of the joint.

In 1989, Thiery reviewed 46 cases of septic arthritis treated arthroscopically.[56] All patients in the series achieved flexion greater than 90 degrees in follow-up.

Similar results have been reported by Smith[57] and Ivy and Clark.[58] Both series reported excellent restoration of motion, decreased hospitalization time in comparison to open procedures, and the ability to effectively treat the infection with the use of arthroscopic techniques.

Although most of the literature regarding septic arthritis has centered around involvement of the knee, we have used arthroscopic drainage in the treatment of septic arthritis of other joints, including the shoulder, ankle, and elbow. Our technique consists of copious lavage and resection of adhesions with motorized cutting devices. Rehabilitation consists of early range of motion and the use of continuous passive-motion devices. Twenty-four hours after the initial arthroscopic drainage, the extremity is reevaluated. If the patient remains febrile, the white blood cell count remains elevated, and the clinical examination does not improve, we recommend a second irrigation and debridement. In our experience, most cases respond to a single procedure along with the use of organism-specific antibiotic therapy.

SYNOVIAL DISEASES

Synovial Chondromatosis

In synovial chondromatosis, small islands of cartilage develop from metaplasia of the synovial membrane.[29] Loose bodies eventually enlarge and become calcified.[59] Multiple loose bodies lead to mechanical interference, restricted motion, swelling, and even disruption of articular cartilage surfaces.[60]

Maurice and coworkers[60] and Dorfmann and associates[61] recommended evacuation of loose bodies with synovectomy, if indicated. Best results with lowest recurrence rates have been obtained with total synovectomy in conjunction with loose body removal. Murphy and colleagues reported a recurrence rate of only 15 percent with total synovectomy in conjunction with removal of loose bodies.[59]

Arthroscopic techniques are readily adaptable in

the surgical treatment of synovial chondromatosis.[62, 63] Maurice and coworkers recommended loose body removal alone.[60] Ogilvie-Harris and Saleh compared removal of loose bodies alone to arthroscopic synovectomy in conjunction with evacuation of loose bodies.[18] At an average follow-up of 3 years, there were no recurrences in the synovectomy group and a 60 percent recurrence rate in cases of loose body removal alone. They recommended complete synovectomy in all cases in conjunction with loose body removal.

Synovectomy performed arthroscopically is curative in most cases.

Pigmented Villonodular Synovitis

Pigmented villonodular synovitis, originally described by Jaffe and colleagues in 1941, is a proliferative synovial disease of joints, tendon sheaths, or bursae.[64] The disease was divided into two forms, localized and diffuse. These appeared to be a continuum in the stages of the disease.[64]

As the disease progresses into the diffuse form, the nodular synovium coalesces into a large mass that eventually fills the joint cavity.[64, 65]

If untreated, pigmented villonodular synovitis becomes invasive and eventually results in joint destruction. Surgical treatment involves resection of involved synovium.[66–68] Traditionally this has been performed open. Most series have reported better overall results in patients with the localized form of disease.[66, 67, 69] Schwartz and coworkers determined incomplete surgical synovectomy was associated with higher recurrence rates.[65]

The ability to perform synovectomy arthroscopically has generated interest in the role of arthroscopic resection in the treatment of pigmented villonodular synovitis.[68, 70] It is essential to have a complete preoperative work-up including a magnetic resonance imaging (MRI)-scan in order to rule out extra-articular involvement. If the disease is confined to the joint cavity, then surgical treatment can be performed arthroscopically. In localized disease, all affected synovium is resected. A complete synovectomy is recommended in diffuse cases.[17]

In 1992, Ogilvie-Harris and associates reviewed 25 patients with pigmented villonodular synovitis who underwent arthroscopic treatment.[17] All patients with localized lesions had no recurrence. Beguin and colleagues reported no recurrences in 13 patients with pigmented villonodular synovitis of the knee treated with arthroscopic resection.[71] If, at the time of synovectomy, extensive articular cartilage disease is present, then overall expectations for relief of pain will be limited.

DEGENERATIVE JOINT DISORDERS

Osteoarthritis

Proteoglycans maintain the compressive stiffness of articular cartilage.[31] With loss of proteoglycans, collagen ultrastructure is altered and articular cartilage becomes more brittle. This increases its susceptibility to injury with mechanical loading.[72] Particles break off and can become mobile within the joint (Fig. 43–3). Loose articular cartilage as well as degenerative meniscal tears are responsible for mechanical locking and pain in degenerative joints.[73] Free-floating debris within the joint invokes a secondary inflammatory response with development of synovitis.[74]

In most patients, conservative measures are very effective in controlling inflammation and pain in degenerative arthritis. Weight loss, exercise, anti-inflammatory medications, and joint injections are all effective. In patients who demonstrate mechanical symptoms, or in whom conservative treatment has

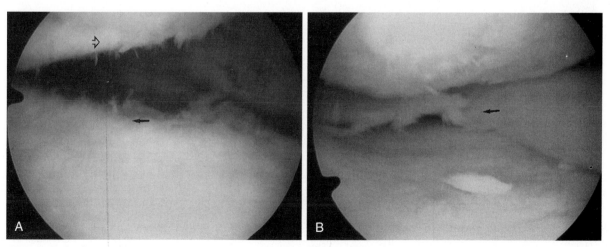

Figure 43–3. Early degenerative arthritis. *A,* Patellofemoral joint. Fissuring of the articular cartilage on the undersurface of the patella *(open arrow)* and the trochlear groove is present. *B,* Medial compartment with degenerative medial meniscus tear *(arrow).* Note fissuring of the articular cartilage on the medial femoral condyle and the medial tibial plateau. There are cartilaginous loose bodies in the foreground.

failed, consideration should be given to arthroscopic intervention.[75–78] However, several factors have been identified as poor prognostic indicators, including malalignment, tricompartmental degenerative changes on radiographs, long duration of symptoms, and loading symptoms.[75–78] Normal mechanical alignment, presence of mechanical symptoms, short duration of symptoms, and the absence of advanced degenerative changes on radiographs have all been identified as good prognostic indicators for successful pain relief from arthroscopic debridement. Patient age has not been found to be a positive or negative prognostic indicator. (Fig. 43–4).[77]

The principle of debridement in osteoarthritis was initially reported by Magnuson in 1941.[1] In his technique, articular cartilage debridement, osteophyte resection, and lavage were performed through an arthrotomy. This concept of debridement and lavage has been carried over to arthroscopic surgical procedures.[79, 80] When performing arthroscopic debridement of degenerative joints, copious lavage with irrigating fluid washes out enzyme-laden synovial fluid and articular cartilage debris and has been shown to have a beneficial effect on short-term follow-up.[81–84]

In addition to joint lavage, arthroscopy provides the opportunity to evaluate articular cartilage and meniscal pathology (Fig. 43–4). Lesions of articular cartilage are debrided to remove loose fragments (Fig. 43–5).[85] Arthroscopic debridement is a temporizing procedure with a favorable risk:benefit ratio when one considers more invasive procedures, such as osteotomy and arthroplasty.[85, 86] Options for more invasive surgery always remain. An arthroscopic debridement is an attempt to delay these until absolutely necessary.[87]

In an attempt to induce articular cartilage injuries to heal, surgeons have attempted to convert partial-

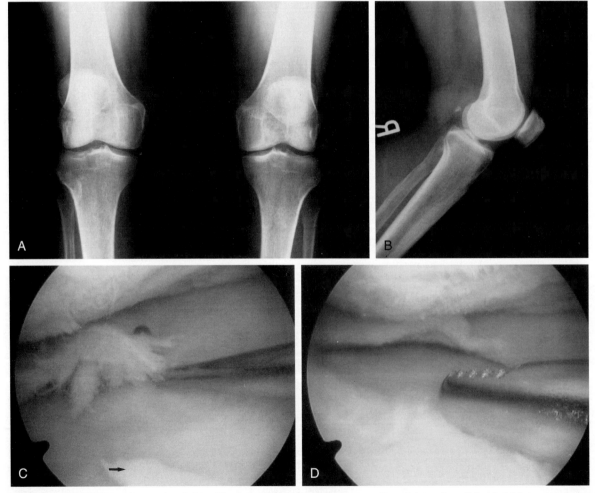

Figure 43–4. Early medial compartment arthritis of both knees in a 62-year-old man. Complaints of medial sided joint pain persisted for 6 months despite conservative treatment. *A, B,* Radiographs show no evidence of malalignment or extensive disease. *C,* Arthroscopic examination revealed degenerative tear of medial meniscus with cartilaginous loose bodies *(arrow). D,* Appearance of the medial compartment after debridement of an unstable meniscal fragment and loose articular cartilage particles. The prognosis for long-term relief of symptoms is excellent.

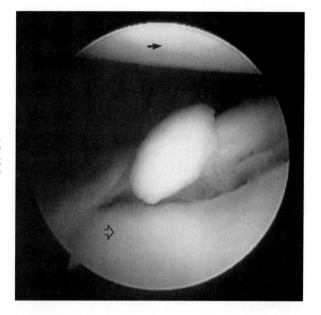

Figure 43–5. Loose body in the glenohumeral joint of a patient with previous dislocation. *Solid arrow* indicates humeral head; *open arrow* points to articular surface of glenoid. Loose bodies were free-floating within the joint and produced episodes of acute pain when they became interposed between joint surfaces.

thickness articular cartilage injuries into full-thickness injuries, initiating a healing response with formation of fibrocartilage. This concept was initially introduced by Pridie in 1959, wherein he drilled articular lesions through an open technique.[88] Although a large percentage of patients noted improvement after the operation, loss of motion following arthrotomy was present in most patients in the series.

Application of these concepts in arthroscopic surgery for arthritis was introduced by Johnson.[89] Abrasion arthroplasty, which included drilling these lesions with an arthroscopic burr, promoted formation of fibrocartilage in these defects after an 8-week period of non–weight-bearing.

Initial enthusiasm for abrasion arthroplasty has declined with reports by other authors. Bert and Maschka in 1989 compared arthroscopic debridement alone to debridement in conjunction with abrasion arthroplasty.[90] Half of the patients who underwent abrasion arthroplasty demonstrated widening of the joint space on follow-up x-rays; however, this did not correlate with improvement in level of pain. Other authors have reported similar findings with unpredictable results from abrasion arthroplasty.[91–93] It appears the best indication for abrasion arthroplasty is solitary full-thickness articular cartilage lesions involving a single compartment of a joint (Fig. 43–6). The results in patients with extensive disease are less predictable (Fig. 43–7).[76]

Rotator Cuff Disorders

In 1972, Neer described an anatomic rationale for impingement syndrome with rotator cuff compression by the coracoacromial ligament, the undersurface of the acromioclavicular joint, and the anterior inferior edge of the acromion process.[94] He described the open technique of acromioplasty with division of the coracoacromial ligament and resection of the anterior inferior acromion to decompress the rotator cuff.[95–101]

In the presence of large irreparable rotator cuff tears, good results have been reported by Rockwood and coworkers with open acromioplasty and debridement alone of torn rotator cuff tissue.[102]

Arthroscopy of the shoulder provides several advantages to surgeons in the operative approach to rotator cuff disorders.[103] Arthroscopy of the shoulder allows complete intra-articular examination of the glenohumeral joint (Fig. 43–8). This procedure also allows the surgeon to examine the undersurface of the rotator cuff, which is not possible during an open approach unless a large rotator cuff tear is present.[104] In the presence of partial rotator cuff tears, the torn portion can be debrided with a motorized shaver down to healthy-appearing tendon. Preliminary results of arthroscopic debridement of partial rotator cuff tears in conjunction with arthroscopic subacromial decompression have been encouraging.[105–107]

Ellman was the first to report on the use of arthroscopy for subacromial decompression.[108] Although the learning curve was initially steep, it is currently a well accepted technique.[105–107, 109] Several reports on arthroscopic subacromial decompression have found results comparable to those of open procedures.[105–107, 110] Prospective, randomized studies comparing arthroscopic subacromial decompression with open acromioplasty have shown overall faster rehabilitation, quicker gains in range of motion after surgery, and earlier return to work after the arthroscopic procedure, without the risks associated with detachment of the deltoid.[111–113]

OFFICE-BASED ARTHROSCOPY

At the present time, most arthroscopic procedures are performed under general anesthesia in a hospital

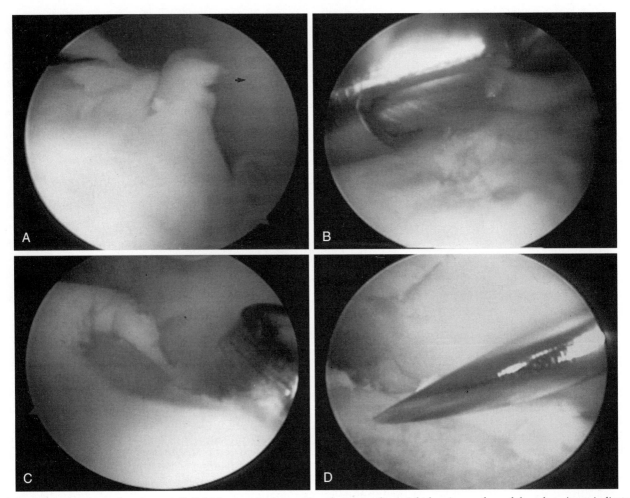

Figure 43–6. Abrasion arthroplasty. *A,* Full-thickness articular cartilage lesion on the weight-bearing surface of the talus. *Arrow* indicates medial malleolus. *B,* The arthroscopic shaver facilitates debridement of all loose articular cartilage. *C,* After complete debridement, the resulting crater has a base of subchondral bone. *D,* 2-mm drill bit is used arthroscopically to drill into subchondral bone, which facilitates bleeding with ultimate formation of fibrocartilage in the area of the defect.

setting either in a traditional operating room suite or in an outpatient surgery center. Improvement in arthroscopic equipment as well as the low incidence of complications has generated an interest in office-based arthroscopy.[5, 6]

Small and associates in 1994 reported a series of 100 patients who had undergone office arthroscopy of the knee.[114] Knee arthroscopy is performed with standard arthroscopic equipment. Procedures performed included debridement of articular cartilage disease and removal of loose bodies. Only 1 of the 100 patients had findings at the time of arthroscopy that could not be addressed under local anesthesia. The authors concluded that office-based arthroscopy of the knee is a safe, cost-effective technique with a high level of patient satisfaction in their series.

The popularity of arthroscopy along with its low incidence of complication gives it a potential for becoming an overutilized surgical technique. With adherence to strict surgical criteria in selecting patients for office-based procedures, arthroscopic surgeons can offer this procedure to patients at a lower cost with clinical results comparable with those of hospital-based procedures.

CONCLUSION

As surgical techniques and instrumentation improve, the indications for arthroscopic surgical procedures over open surgery are becoming clearer. In addition to synovectomy and debridement, arthroscopy is currently in use for ligamentous reconstruction of the knee and unstable shoulder and for fixation of intra-articular fractures. With increased experience and longer follow-up, a clear-cut understanding of when surgery is indicated should be established. As attention in health care turns toward cost containment, arthroscopic procedures offer a less expensive and less invasive approach in comparison to more costly procedures, such as total joint replacement. With a proper understanding of its applications in degenerative and inflammatory disorders, arthro-

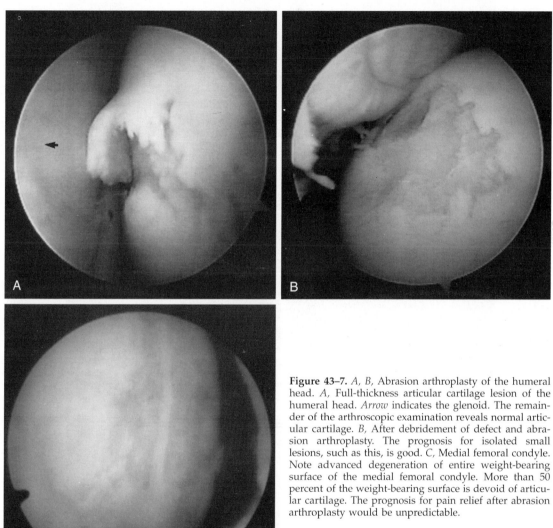

Figure 43–7. *A, B,* Abrasion arthroplasty of the humeral head. *A,* Full-thickness articular cartilage lesion of the humeral head. *Arrow* indicates the glenoid. The remainder of the arthroscopic examination reveals normal articular cartilage. *B,* After debridement of defect and abrasion arthroplasty. The prognosis for isolated small lesions, such as this, is good. *C,* Medial femoral condyle. Note advanced degeneration of entire weight-bearing surface of the medial femoral condyle. More than 50 percent of the weight-bearing surface is devoid of articular cartilage. The prognosis for pain relief after abrasion arthroplasty would be unpredictable.

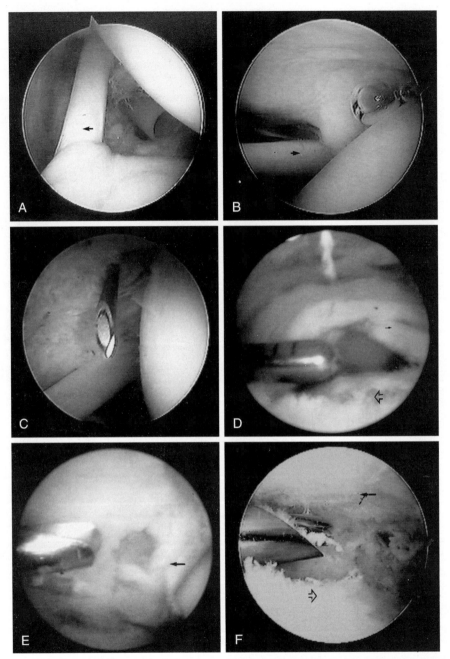

Figure 43–8. Arthroscopy in rotator cuff disease. *A,* Arthroscopy allows complete examination of the glenohumeral joint. *Solid arrow* indicates normal biceps tendon originating from superior aspect of glenoid. Note the arthroscopic cannula entering glenohumeral joint; the humeral head lies to the right. *B,* Undersurface of the rotator cuff inserting into greater tuberosity of humerus. The biceps tendon exits the glenohumeral joint. *C,* Undersurface rotator cuff tear. The needle enters glenohumeral joint through the area of undersurface fibrillation and tearing of the rotator cuff, which is debrided down to healthy tendinous tissue with the use of an arthroscopic shaver through an anterior portal. *D–F,* Subacromial bursa. *D,* Bursal view of a rotator cuff tear. The shaver facilitates debridement of the edges of the cuff and allows planning for repair prior to open surgical approach to the shoulder. *Open arrow* indicates greater tuberosity; *small arrow* indicates biceps tendon. *E,* Arthroscopic burr used for resecting undersurface of the acromion process *(arrow).* *F,* Completed subacromial decompression. Note the smooth undersurface of the acromion *(arrow)* and the bursal surface of the rotator cuff *(open arrow).*

scopic surgery can serve as a useful adjunct in the treatment of these diseases.

References

1. Magnuson PB: Joint debridement. Surgical treatment of degenerative arthritis. Surg Gynecol Obstet 73:1, 1941.
2. Ranawat CS, Ecker ML, Straub LR: Synovectomy and debridement of the knee in rheumatoid arthritis: A study of 60 knees. Arthritis Rheum 15:571–581, 1972.
3. Norlin R: Arthroscopic subacromial decompression versus open acromioplasty. Arthroscopy 5(4):321–323, 1989.
4. Highgenboten CL: Arthroscopic synovectomy. Arthroscopy 1(3):190–193, 1985.
5. Lee JC: Complications of arthroscopy in arthroscopic surgery: Results of the national survey. Arthroscopy 1(2):214–220, 1985.
6. Small NC: Complications in arthroscopy: The knee and other joints. Arthroscopy 2(4):253–258, 1986.
7. Shibata T, Shiraoka K, Takubo N: Comparison between arthroscopic and open synovectomy for the knee in rheumatoid arthritis. Arch Orthop Trauma Surg 105(5):257–262, 1986.
8. Matsui N, Taneda Y, Ohta H, et al: Arthroscopic versus open synovectomy in the rheumatoid knee. Int Orthop 13(1):17–20, 1989.
9. Watanbe M, Takeda S, Ikeuchi H: Atlas of Arthroscopy, 2nd ed. Tokyo, Igaku Shoin, 1969.
10. Smiley P, Wasilewski SA: Arthroscopic synovectomy. Arthroscopy 6(1):18–23, 1990.
11. Arthritis and Rheumatism Council and British Orthopaedic Association: Controlled trial of synovectomy of knee and metacarpophalangeal joints in rheumatoid arthritis. Ann Rheum Dis 35:437–442, 1976.
12. Arthritis Foundation Committee on Evaluation of Synovectomy: Multicenter evaluation of synovectomy in the treatment of rheumatoid arthritis: Report of results at the end of three years. Arthritis Rheum 20:765–771, 1977.
13. Doets HC, Bierman BT, von Soesbergen RM: Synovectomy of the rheumatoid knee does not prevent deterioration. Seven-year follow-up of 83 cases. Acta Orthop Scand 60(5):523–525, 1989.
14. Cleland LG, Treganza R, Dobson P: Arthroscopic synovectomy: A prospective study. J Rheumatol 13:907–910, 1986.
15. Klein W, Jensen KU: Arthroscopic synovectomy of the knee joint: Indication, technique, and follow-up results. Arthroscopy 4(2):63–71, 1988.
16. Cohen S, Jones R: An evaluation of the efficacy of arthroscopic synovectomy of the knee in rheumatoid arthritis: 12–24-month results. J Rheumatol 14:452–455, 1987.
17. Ogilvie-Harris DJ, McLean J, Zarnett ME: Pigmented villonodular synovitis of the knee. The results of total arthroscopic synovectomy, partial arthroscopic synovectomy, and arthroscopic local excision. J Bone Joint Surg Am 74(1):119–123, 1992.
18. Ogilvie-Harris DJ, Saleh K: Generalized synovial chondromatosis of the knee: A comparison of removal of the loose bodies alone with arthroscopic synovectomy. Arthroscopy 10(2):166–170, 1994.
19. Voltman R von: Cited by Hoffman R: Die Synovektomie unter Besonderer Berucksichtigung der ander Erlanger Chirurgischen Universitatsklinik erzielten Erfolge. Dissertation Erlangen, 1952.
20. Swett P: Synovectomy in chronic infectious arthritis. J Bone Joint Surg 21:110, 1923.
21. Boon-Itt SB: A study of the end results of synovectomy of the knee. J Bone Joint Surg 28:853, 1930.
22. Swett PP: A review of synovectomy. J Bone Joint Surg 36:68, 1938.
23. Henderson MS: Synovectomy for destructive arthritis of the knee joint. Surg Clin North Am 4:565–568, 1924.
24. London PS: Synovectomy of the knee in rheumatoid arthritis: An essay in surgical salvage. J Bone Joint Surg Br 37:392–399, 1955.
25. Sevill DL: Management of the rheumatoid knee. In Proceedings of the British Orthopaedic Association. J Bone Joint Surg Br 47:582, 1965.
26. Ghormley RK, Cameron DM: End results of synovectomy of the knee joint. Am J Surg 53:455–459, 1941.
27. Laurin CA, Desmarchais J, Daziano L, Gariepy R, Derome A: Long-term results of synovectomy of the knee in rheumatoid patients. J Bone Joint Surg Am 56:521–531, 1974.
28. Ishikawa H, Ohno O, Hirohata K: Long-term results of synovectomy in rheumatoid patients. J Bone Joint Surg Am 68(2):198–205, 1986.
29. Sim FH: Synovial proliferative disorders: Role of synovectomy. Arthroscopy 1(3):198–204, 1985.
30. Salisbury RB, Nottage WM: A new evaluation of gross pathologic changes and concepts of rheumatoid articular cartilage degeneration. Clin Orthop 199:242–247, 1985.
31. Harris ED Jr, Parker HG, Radin EL, Krane SM: Effects of proteolytic enzymes on structural and mechanical properties of cartilage. Arthritis Rheum 15:497–503, 1972.
32. Ogilvie-Harris DJ, Weisleder L: Arthroscopic synovectomy of the knee: Is it helpful? Arthroscopy 11(1):91–95, 1995.
33. Arnold WJ, Kalunian K: Arthroscopic synovectomy by rheumatologists: Time for a new look. Arthritis Rheum 32:108–111, 1989.
34. Arnold WD, Hilgartner MW: Hemophilic arthropathy. Current concepts of pathogenesis and management. J Bone Joint Surg Am 59(3):287–305, 1977.
35. Harris ED Jr, Evanson JM, Dibona DR, Krane SM: Collagenase in rheumatoid arthritis. Arthritis Rheum 13:83–94, 1970.
36. DePalma AF: Hemophilic arthropathy. Clin Orthop 52:145–165, 1967.
37. Stein H, Duthie RB: Pathogenesis of hemophilic arthropathy. J Bone Joint Surg Br 63:601, 1981.
38. Storty E, Traldi A, Tosatti E, et al: Synovectomy—a new approach to hemophilic arthropathy. Acta Haematol 41:193–205, 1969.
39. Storty E, Ascari E: Surgical and chemical synovectomy. Ann N Y Acad Sci 240:316–327, 1975.
40. Montane I, McCullough NC III, Lien ECY: Synovectomy of the knee for hemophilic arthropathy. J Bone Joint Surg Am 68(2):210–216, 1986.
41. Post M, Watts G, Telfer M: Synovectomy in hemophilic arthropathy: A retrospective review of 17 cases. Clin Orthop 202:139–146, 1986.
42. Canale ST, Dugdale M, Howard BC: Synovectomy of the knee in young patients with hemophilia. South Med J 81:1480, 1988.
43. Nicol RO, Menelaus MB: Synovectomy of the knee in hemophilia. J Pediatr Orthop 6:330–333, 1986.
44. Clark MW: Knee synovectomy in hemophilia. J Orthop 1:285–290, 1978.
45. Greer RB III: Operative management of hemophilic arthropathy: An overview. Orthopedics 3:135–138, 1980.
46. Klein KS, Aland CM, Kim HC, Eisele J, Saidi P: Long-term follow-up of arthroscopic synovectomy for chronic hemophilic synovitis. Arthroscopy 3(4):231–236, 1987.
47. Triantafyllou SJ, Hanks GA, Handal JA, Greer RB III: Open and arthroscopic synovectomy in hemophilic arthropathy of the knee (review). Clin Orthop 283:196–204, 1992.
48. Widel JD: Arthroscopic synovectomy for chronic hemophilic synovitis of the knee. Arthroscopy 1(3):205–209, 1985.
49. Casscells CD: Commentary: The arguments for early arthroscopic synovectomy in patients with severe hemophilia. Arthroscopy 3(2):78–79, 1987.
50. Greene WB: Use of continuous passive slow motion in the postoperative rehabilitation of difficult pediatric knee and elbow problems. J Pediatr Orthop 3:419–423, 1983.
51. Lindbird TJ, Dennis SC: Synovectomy and continuous passive motion in hemophiliac patients. Arthroscopy 3(2):74–77, 1987.
52. DeGnore LT, Wilson FC: Surgical management of hemophilic arthropathy. In American Academy of Orthopaedic Surgeons: Instructional Course Lectures, vol 38, 1989, pp 383–388.
53. Kelly PJ, Martin WJ, Conventry MB: Bacterial arthritis in the adult. J Bone Joint Surg Am 52:1595, 1970.
54. Tscherne H, Giebel G, Muhr G, Howell C: Synovectomy as treatment for purulent joint infection. Arch Orthop Trauma Surg 103:162, 1984.
55. Jackson RW: The septic knee—arthroscopic treatment. Arthroscopy 1(3):194–197, 1985.
56. Thiery JA: Arthroscopic drainage in septic arthritis of the knee. A multicenter study. Arthroscopy 5(1):65–69, 1989.
57. Smith MJ: Arthroscopic treatment of the septic knee. Arthroscopy 2:30–34, 1986.
58. Ivy M, Clark R: Arthroscopic debridement of the knee for septic arthritis. Clin Orthop 199:201–206, 1985.
59. Murphy FP, Dahlin DC, Sullivan CR: Articular synovial chondromatosis. J Bone Joint Surg Am 44:77–85, 1962.
60. Maurice H, Crone M, Watt I: Synovial chondromatosis. J Bone Joint Surg Br 70:807–811, 1988.
61. Dorfman H, Debie B, Bonvarlet JP, Boyer TH: Arthroscopic treatment of synovial chondromatosis of the knee. Arthroscopy 5(1):48–51, 1989.
62. Coolican MR, Dandy DJ: Arthroscopic management of synovial chondromatosis of the knee. Findings and results in 18 cases. J Bone Joint Surg Br 71:498–500, 1989.
63. Witwity T, Uhlmann R, Nagy MH, et al: Shoulder rheumatoid arthritis associated with chondromatosis, treated by arthroscopy. Arthroscopy 7(2):233–236, 1991.
64. Jaffe HL, Lichtenstein L, Sutro CJ: Pigmented villonodular synovitis, bursitis, and tenosynovitis—A discussion of the synovial and bursal equivalents of the tenosynovial lesion commonly denoted as xanthoma, xanthogranuloma, giant cell tumor, or myeloplexoma of the tendon sheath, with some consideration of this tendon-sheath lesion itself. Arch Pathol 31:731–765, 1941.
65. Schwartz HS, Unni KK, Pritchard DJ: Pigmented villonodular synovitis: A retrospective review of large affected joints. Clin Orthop 247:243–255, 1989.
66. Johannson JE, Ajjoub S, Coughlin LP, Wener JA, Cruess RL: Pigmented villonodular synovitis of joints. Clin Orthop 163:159–166, 1982.
67. Byers PD, Cotton RE, Deacon OW, Lowy M, Newman PH, Sissons HA, Thomson AD: The diagnosis and treatment of pigmented villonodular synovitis. J Bone Joint Surg Br 50:290–305, 1968.

68. Janssens X, Mierhaeghe JB, Verdonk R, Verjans P, Cuvelier C, Veys EM: Diagnostic arthroscopy of the hip in pigmented villonodular synovitis. Arthroscopy 3(4):283–287, 1987.
69. Granowitz SD, D'Antonio J, Mankin HJ: Pathogenesis and long-term end-results of pigmented villonodular synovitis. Clin Orthop 114:335–351, 1976.
70. Lopez-Vazquez E, Lopez-Peris JL, Vila-Donat E, Martinez-Garcia JB, Bru-Pomer A: Localized pigmented villonodular synovitis of the knee: Diagnosis and arthroscopic resection. Arthroscopy 4(2):121–123, 1988.
71. Beguin J, Locker B, Vielpeau C, Souquieres G: Pigmented villonodular synovitis of the knee. Results from 13 cases. Arthroscopy 5(1):62–64, 1989.
72. Buckwalter JA, Mow VC, Ratcliffe A: Restoration of injured or degenerated articular cartilage. J Am Acad Orthop Surg 2(4):192–201, 1994.
73. Rand JA: Arthroscopic management of degenerative meniscus tears in patients with degenerative arthritis. Arthroscopy 1:253–258, 1985.
74. Lindblad S, Hedfors E: Arthroscopic and immunohistologic characterization of knee joint synovitis in osteoarthritis. Arthritis Rheum 30(10):1313, 1987.
75. Salisbury RB, Nottage WM, Gardner V: The effect of alignment on results in arthroscopic debridement of the degenerative knee. Clin Orthop 198:268–272, 1986.
76. Ogilvie-Harris DJ, Fitsialows DP: Arthroscopic management of the degenerative knee. Arthroscopy 7(2):151–157, 1991.
77. Novak PJ, Bach BR Jr: Selection criteria for knee arthroscopy in the osteoarthritic patient (review). Orthop Rev 22(7):798–804, 1993.
78. Burks RT: Arthroscopy and degenerative arthritis of the knee: A review of the literature. Arthroscopy 6:43–47, 1990.
79. O'Connor RL: Arthroscopy in the diagnosis and treatment of acute ligament injuries of the knee. J Bone Joint Surg Am 55:1443, 1973.
80. Jackson RW: The role of arthroscopy in the management of the arthritic knee. Clin Orthop 101:28–35, 1974.
81. Arnold WJ, Mather SE, Mostello N, Tongue J: Tidal knee lavage in patients with chronic pain due to osteoarthritis of the knee. Arthritis Rheum 27:S66, 1984.
82. Ike RW, Arnold WJ, Simon CM, Eisenberg GM: Tidal knee irrigation as an intervention for chronic pain due to osteoarthritis of the knee. Arthritis Rheum 30:S17, 1987.
83. Ike RW, Arnold WJ, Rothschild EW, Shaw HL: Tidal irrigation versus conservative medical management in patients with osteoarthritis of the knee: A prospective randomized study. J Rheumatol 19:772–779, 1992.
84. Chang RW, Falconer J, Stulberg SD, et al: A randomized, controlled trial of arthroscopic surgery versus closed-needle joint lavage for patients with osteoarthritis of the knee. Arthritis Rheum 36(3):289–293, 1993.
85. McLaren AC, Blokker CP, Fowler PJ, et al: Arthroscopic debridement of the knee for osteoarthritis. Can J Surg 34(6):595–598, 1991.
86. Schonholtz GJ. Arthroscopic debridement of the knee joint (review). Orthop Clin North Am 20(2):257–263, 1989.
87. Gross DE, Brenner SL, Esformes I, et al: Arthroscopic treatment of degenerative joint disease of the knee. Orthopedics 14(12):1317–1321, 1991.
88. Insall JN: The Pridie debridement operation for osteoarthritis of the knee. Clin Orthop 101:61–67, 1974.
89. Johnson LL: Arthroscopic abrasion arthroplasty, historical and pathologic perspective: Present status. Arthroscopy 2(1):54–69, 1986.
90. Bert JM, Maschka K: The arthroscopic treatment of unicompartmental gonarthrosis: A 5-year follow-up study of abrasion arthroplasty plus arthroscopic debridement and arthroscopic debridement alone. Arthroscopy 5(1):25–32, 1989.

91. Dandy DJ: Abrasion chondroplasty. Arthroscopy 2(1):51–53, 1986.
92. Dandy DJ: Arthroscopic debridement of the knee for osteoarthritis (editorial). J Bone Joint Surg Br 73(6):877–878, 1991.
93. Rand JA: Role of arthroscopy in osteoarthritis of the knee. Arthroscopy 7(4):358–363, 1991.
94. Neer CS II: Anterior acromioplasty for chronic impingement syndrome in the shoulder. A preliminary report. J Bone Joint Surg Am 54:41, 1972.
95. Bigliani LU, D'Alessandro DF, Duralde XA, McIlveen SJ: Anterior acromioplasty for subacromial impingement in patients younger than 40 years of age. Clin Orthop 246:111–116, 1989.
96. Rosenberg PS, Clarke RP: Chronic rotator cuff tears (review). Orthop Rev 15(5):280–289, 1986.
97. Bigliani LU, Kimmel J, McCann PD, Wolfe I: Repair of rotator cuff tears in tennis players. Am J Sports Med 20(2):112–117, 1992.
98. Bjorkenheim JM, Paavolainen P, Ahovuo J, Slatis P: Subacromial impingement decompressed with anterior acromioplasty. Clin Orthop 252:150–155, 1990.
99. Daluga DJ, Dobozi W: The influence of distal clavicle resection and rotator cuff repair on the effectiveness of anterior acromioplasty. Clin Orthop 247:117–123, 1989.
100. Stuart MJ, Azevedo AJ, Cofield RH: Anterior acromioplasty for treatment of the shoulder impingement syndrome. Clin Orthop 260:195–200, 1990.
101. Rockwood CA, Lyons FR: Shoulder impingement syndrome: Diagnosis, radiographic evaluation, and treatment with a modified Neer acromioplasty. J Bone Joint Surg Am 75(3):409–424, 1993.
102. Rockwood CA Jr, Williams GR, Burkhead WZ: Debridement of irreparable degenerative lesions of the rotator cuff. Presented at the American Shoulder and Elbow Surgeons Seventh Open Meeting, Anaheim, California, March 10, 1991.
103. Paulos LE, Franklin JL, Beck CL: Arthroscopic management of rotator cuff tears. In McGinty JB, Caspari RB, Jackson RW, Poehling GG (eds): Operative Arthroscopy. New York, Raven Press, 1991, pp 529–541.
104. Adolfsson L, Lysholm J: Results of arthroscopic acromioplasty related to rotator cuff lesions. Int Orthop 17(4):228–231, 1993.
105. Andrews JR, Broussard TS, Carson WG: Arthroscopy of the shoulder in the management of partial tears of the rotator cuff: A preliminary report. Arthroscopy 1(2):117–122, 1985.
106. Snyder SJ, Pachelli AF, Del Pizzo W, et al: Partial thickness rotator cuff tears: Results of arthroscopic treatment. Arthroscopy 7(1):1–7, 1991.
107. Olsewski JM, Depew AD: Arthroscopic subacromial decompression and rotator cuff debridement for stage II and III impingement. Arthroscopy 10(1):61–68, 1994.
108. Ellman H: Arthroscopic subacromial decompression: Analysis of one-to three-year results. Arthroscopy 3:173–181, 1987.
109. Caspari RB, Thal R: Technique for arthroscopic subacromial decompression. Arthroscopy 8:23–30, 1992.
110. Altchek DW, Warren RF, Wickiewicz TL, et al: Arthroscopic acromioplasty. Technique and results. J Bone Joint Surg Am 72(8):1198–1207, 1990.
111. Watson KC, Seitz WH Jr: Open anterior acromioplasty versus arthroscopic anterior acromioplasty. Orthopedics 15(9):1099–1105, 1992.
112. Lindh M, Norlin R: Arthroscopic subacromial decompression versus open acromioplasty. A 2-year follow-up study. Clin Orthop 290:174–176, 1993.
113. Sachs RA, Stone ML, Devine S: Open versus arthroscopic acromioplasty: A prospective, randomized study. Arthroscopy 10(3):248–254, 1994.
114. Small NC, Glogau AI, Berezin MA, Farless BL: Office operative arthroscopy of the knee: Technical considerations in the preliminary analysis of the first hundred patients. Arthroscopy 10(5):534–539, 1994.

CHAPTER 44

Stanley P. Ballou
Irving Kushner

Laboratory Evaluation of Inflammation

THE CONCEPT OF INFLAMMATION

A major problem in attempting to quantitate the extent of inflammation by laboratory tests stems from the ambiguity associated with the concept of *inflammation* itself. Two points are inadequately appreciated: (1) inflammation is not a single process—different stimuli (e.g., staphylococci, schistosomes, allergens, urate crystals, myocardial infarction, and tubercle bacilli) induce different types of inflammatory responses; and (2) each type of inflammatory response represents a complex, highly orchestrated set of interactions between cells, soluble mediators, and tissue matrix. It is not reasonable to expect a single test to reflect all these processes.

A precise definition of inflammation is difficult to achieve. For centuries, it was defined primarily in clinical terms: redness, swelling, heat, pain. With the introduction of light microscopy, inflammation was defined in histologic terms, particularly infiltration by inflammatory cells. In the modern era, characteristics of inflammation have been described in terms of biochemical, ultrastructural, and molecular alterations. Because of the complexity of these events, the usual definition of inflammation has been necessarily broad and relatively imprecise: a local response elicited by injury of tissues.

Such a vague definition complicates the laboratory evaluation of inflammation in two ways. First, a single *systemic* marker (e.g., any constituent of blood) may not accurately reflect *local* inflammatory processes. Second, the varied stimuli capable of inducing different clinical types of inflammation (e.g., acute or chronic) can be associated with distinct patterns of laboratory abnormalities. Thus, acute gout and active rheumatoid arthritis each exhibit clinical findings of inflammation and are associated with elevation of the erythrocyte sedimentation rate (ESR), but leukocytosis is more frequently associated with gout, whereas the anemia of chronic disease is more characteristic of rheumatoid arthritis. Other stimuli, such as acute trauma, sometimes thought of as noninflammatory, often lead to dramatic abnormalities in many laboratory tests that are characteristic of inflammatory events.

Despite these problems, physicians have been able to exploit the *acute-phase response* to obtain objective markers that reflect the extent or degree of inflammation, albeit somewhat imperfectly. During the past 70 years, measurement of the ESR and, more recently, the serum C-reactive protein (CRP) concentration has filled this role. In recent years, several new inflammatory markers have emerged, but these have not as yet proved substantially more helpful to the clinician. This chapter focuses largely on ESR and CRP and briefly surveys newer markers.

ACUTE-PHASE RESPONSE

A large number of systemic and metabolic changes, collectively referred to as the acute-phase response, begin to occur within hours after an inflammatory stimulus.[1] Many elements of the acute-phase response appear to represent early defensive or adaptive mechanisms that precede the immune response. The acute-phase response occurs in association with a wide variety of stimuli, including bacterial infection, trauma, myocardial infarction, immunologically mediated and crystal-induced inflammatory states, and various neoplasms. A major component of the acute phase response is alteration of synthesis of a number of plasma proteins by hepatocytes. These acute phase proteins display variable changes in plasma concentration and time course of response after tissue injury (Fig. 44–1). The concentrations of some proteins, such as ceruloplasmin and several complement components, rise about 50 percent above normal; others, such as α_1-acid glycoprotein, α_1-proteinase inhibitor, haptoglobin, and fibrinogen, can increase several-fold. The two major acute-phase proteins in humans, CRP and serum amyloid A, often increase to levels several hundred times above those normally present in health and may increase more than 1000-fold in severe inflammatory states, usually infections. In contrast, concentrations of several plasma proteins, such as albumin, may fall.

Acute-phase protein synthesis by hepatocytes is induced largely by inflammation-associated cytokines, the polypeptide regulatory mediators secreted by activated monocytes, macrophages, endothelial cells, and certain other cells. Among the cytokines that contribute to acute phase protein induction are interleukin-6 (IL-6), the major inducer of acute-phase changes, as well as IL-1 and tumor necrosis factor-α. Other cytokines play more limited roles.[1] Acute-phase protein

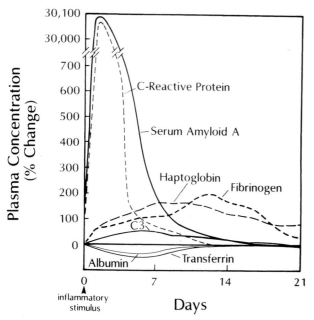

Figure 44–1. Typical plasma acute phase protein (APP) changes following a moderate inflammatory stimulus. Several patterns of response are seen: major APP, increase up to 1000-fold (e.g., C-reactive protein and serum amyloid A); moderate APP, increase two to four fold (e.g., fibrinogen, haptoglobin); minor APP, increase 50 percent to 100 percent, e.g., complement C3; and negative APP, decrease (e.g., albumin, transferrin). (Adapted from Gitlin JD, Colten HR: Molecular biology of the acute phase plasma proteins. *In* Pick E, Landy M (eds): Lymphokines, vol 14. San Diego, Academic Press, 1987, pp 123–153.)

levels do not always rise coordinately, which suggests heterogeneous and independently regulated mechanisms for induction of synthesis probably involving different combinations and interactions of cytokines and their modulators in varying circumstances. Teleologic considerations suggest that the changes in concentration of the acute-phase proteins lead to improved functional capacity to cope with the consequences of tissue injury or infection. Functional activities that have been attributed to acute-phase proteins include direct involvement in host defense (e.g., by activation of the complement pathway), proteinase inhibition, and antioxidant activity.[2] Some in vitro effects of acute-phase proteins, however, may not be relevant to in vivo phenomena, and in some cases the acute-phase response may be injurious rather than beneficial.[3] The acute-phase proteins that are of greatest value in assessing inflammation for clinical purposes are briefly discussed here.

C-Reactive Protein

C-reactive protein is present in trace concentrations in the plasma of all humans. It is a pentamer consisting of five identical noncovalently linked 23-kD subunits[4] and has been highly conserved over hundreds of millions of years of evolution; proteins bear-

ing structural and functional characteristics of CRP have been found in chickens, fish, and the ancient organism *Limulus polyphemus,* the horseshoe crab. Although the precise function of CRP during the acute-phase response is unknown, the protein does exhibit important recognition and activation capabilities.[5] Among the major biologic ligands recognized by CRP are phospholipids[6] and histone proteins,[7] which are constituents of cell membranes and nuclei, respectively, and therefore may be exposed at sites of tissue damage. The major activation functions of CRP are of two types. The best defined function is the ability of the protein to activate the classical complement pathway after interaction with many of its biologic ligands.[2] The second function relates to the ability of CRP to bind to and modulate the behavior of phagocytic cells.[8–10]

Serum levels of CRP can be accurately and reproducibly measured by a variety of methods, including radioimmunoassay, radial immunodiffusion, enzyme immunoassay, and laser nephelometry. There is no uniformity in reporting of CRP concentrations: some laboratories report CRP as mg/L or μg/ml rather than mg/dl. Clinicians must be aware of this potential pitfall in interpreting data.

Following acute inflammatory stimuli, the concentration of CRP rises dramatically and rapidly to levels that generally reflect the extent of tissue injury. Most apparently healthy adults have serum CRP levels less than 0.2 mg/dl, although concentrations up to 1 mg/dl (presumably related to minor degrees of injury that can occur during the course of everyday life) are found sufficiently often to justify regarding concentrations lower than this value as clinically insignificant.[11] Concentrations between 1 and 10 mg/dl can be considered moderate increases, and concentrations over 10 mg/dl are marked increases. Most patients with very high levels (e.g., > 15–20 mg/dl) have bacterial infections. Examples of clinical conditions associated with CRP elevations of varying degrees are shown in Table 44–1. Serum CRP levels generally reach a peak 2 or 3 days after acute stimuli and then fall relatively rapidly, with a half-life of about 18 hours.[12] Persistently elevated serum CRP concentrations are often seen in chronic inflammatory states, however, such as

Table 44–1. EXAMPLES OF CONDITIONS ASSOCIATED WITH ELEVATED C-REACTIVE PROTEIN LEVELS

Normal or Insignificant Elevation (<1 mg/dl)	Moderate Elevation (1–10 mg/dl)	Marked Elevation (>10 mg/dl)
Vigorous exercise	Myocardial infarction	Acute bacterial infection (80–85%)
Common cold	Malignancies	Major trauma
Pregnancy	Pancreatitis	Systemic vasculitis
Gingivitis	Mucosal infection (bronchitis, cystitis)	
Cerebrovascular accident		
Seizures	Most connective tissue diseases	
Angina		

active rheumatoid arthritis or pulmonary tuberculosis, or in the presence of extensive malignant disease.

Serum Amyloid A

Serum amyloid A consists of a family of proteins, some of which are constitutively expressed,[13] whereas others display acute-phase behavior even more marked than that of CRP.[14] Serum amyloid A may be associated with circulating high-density lipoproteins, but its function is not clear. Studies suggest that serum amyloid A may function as an opsonin[15] and that it may influence the movement of cholesterol between high-density lipoproteins and inflammatory cells.[16, 17] As for CRP, levels of acute-phase serum amyloid A rise within hours after tissue injury, and the magnitude of increase is probably greater than that of CRP. Relatively trivial inflammatory stimuli can lead to serum amyloid A responses.[14] Clinical studies have demonstrated correlation of serum amyloid A levels with disease activity in a variety of inflammatory disorders, including rheumatoid arthritis,[18] acute gout,[19] inflammatory bowel disease, and myocardial infarction.[20] The normal level of serum amyloid A in healthy adults is probably less than 1 mg/dl; unfortunately, reliable testing for acute-phase serum amyloid A is not yet widely available, and data about levels expected in either healthy populations or in acute and chronic disease states are limited. The recent introduction of an enzyme immunoassay[21] for quantitation of serum amyloid A may result in a greater role for measurement of this dramatic acute-phase protein in clinical situations, as will establishment by the World Health Organization of an international standard for serum amyloid A, currently underway.

Other Acute-Phase Proteins

Measurement of other acute-phase proteins has limited value for assessment of inflammation, since the response of the proteins to inflammatory stimuli is relatively slower and the magnitude of change in concentration is relatively smaller than those of CRP and serum amyloid A. The analysis of altered patterns of glycosylation of some acute-phase glycoproteins that can occur during an acute-phase response, however, is of some interest. Such glycosylation changes may occur independently of concentrations of the proteins themselves, and some studies have indicated that patterns of glycosylation heterogeneity vary according to whether the inflammatory stimulus is acute or chronic.[22] Thus, measurement of the glycosylation heterogeneity of α_1-acid glycoprotein has been used to distinguish acute infection and disease activity in rheumatoid arthritis[23] and lupus patients.[24] Although such changes are clearly of interest and potential clinical importance, the technique for measuring these changes is cumbersome and not widely available.

ERYTHROCYTE SEDIMENTATION RATE

Over the years, the ESR has been the most widely used reflector of the acute-phase response. Indeed, elevation of the ESR was recognized as a correlate of illness by the ancient Greeks.[25] In this test, anticoagulated blood is placed in a vertical tube and the rate of fall of erythrocytes is measured. The ESR is an indirect way of screening for elevated concentrations of the acute-phase plasma proteins that result in increased aggregation of erythrocytes (rouleaux formation), causing them to fall more rapidly.

The ESR can be influenced by changes in both plasma proteins and red blood cells. Two types of changes in plasma proteins commonly lead to elevation of the ESR. Because the membrane-associated charges are similar on all erythrocytes, red cells ordinarily repel each other. An increase in concentration of asymmetrically charged proteins decreases this tendency of repulsion, leading to red blood cell aggregation and rouleaux formation. Aggregated cells overcome the resistance of plasma to gravitational forces more than do single cells, and rapid red blood cell sedimentation ensues. Fibrinogen, a moderate acute-phase reactant, is the most prevalent of the asymmetric acute-phase proteins in plasma and has the greatest effect on the ESR. Second, a major increase in concentration of a single molecular species, such as the immunoglobulin elevations that occur in multiple myeloma or Waldenström's macroglobulinemia, may also lead to ESR elevation, although such changes do not reflect inflammatory states.

In addition, anemia and polycythemia may affect the ESR, and alterations in size and shape of erythrocytes may physically interfere with rouleaux formation. It is not possible to correct for alterations in size, shape, or concentration of erythrocytes.

The International Committee for Standardization in Hematology has recommended that the Westergren technique be designated as the preferred method of ESR determination, and an international panel has recently proposed some modifications.[26] The generally accepted upper limits of normal are 15 mm/hour for males and 20 mm/hour for females, but in fact the ESR progressively increases with aging, leading to great uncertainty about "normal" levels, particularly in the elderly. Values up to 40 mm/hour are not uncommon in healthy elderly people.[27] A simple formula for calculating maximum normal ESR at any age has been proposed.[28] A racial difference in ESR has also been reported.[29] Other problems with the ESR are indicated in Table 44–2. Nonetheless, the ESR retains an important place in medical practice, probably because the test is both easy to perform and inexpensive. A wealth of information about its clinical significance has accumulated over many years, so many experienced physicians believe, rightly or

Table 44–2. ADVANTAGES AND DISADVANTAGES OF ERYTHROCYTE SEDIMENTATION RATE AND C-REACTIVE PROTEIN DETERMINATION

	Erythrocyte Sedimentation Rate	C-Reactive Protein
Advantages	Inexpensive ($10–12) Much clinical information available	Rapid response to inflammatory stimulus Wide range of clinically relevant values are detectable Unaffected by age and gender Reflects value of a single acute-phase protein Can be measured on stored sera Quantitation is precise and reproducible
Disadvantages	Affected by age and gender Affected by red blood cell morphology Affected by anemia and polycythemia Reflects levels of many plasma proteins, not all of which are acute-phase proteins Responds slowly to inflammatory stimulus Requires fresh sample May be affected by drugs	Less clinical information available Relatively more expensive

wrongly, that they know how to compensate for its flaws. It remains to be seen whether the next generation of physicians will share this view.

CYTOKINES: PRODUCTS OF CONNECTIVE TISSUE OR INFLAMMATORY CELLS

With the introduction of sensitive enzyme immunoassays for quantitation of many inflammation-associated cytokines, there has been increasing interest in measuring levels of these potent inflammatory mediators in various clinical states. IL-6, in particular, may respond dramatically to inflammatory stimuli, with changes that are even more rapid in onset and greater in magnitude than those of CRP and serum amyloid A.[30] Both acute and chronic inflammation[31] and trauma[32] have been associated with increases in IL-6, and serum levels of this cytokine have been correlated with the severity and course of the disease process in rheumatoid arthritis.[33] Technical problems exist, however; there is still some uncertainty about how to reliably assay for IL-6 in body fluids.[34] Increased lev-

els of several other cytokines and circulating cytokine receptors, some of which are listed in Table 44–3, are also associated with inflammation or disease activity and sometimes behave coordinately in such conditions.[35, 36] Clinical information about these mediators is insufficient to permit definitive conclusions regarding their potential value in the objective assessment of inflammation or disease activity. It is clear that clinical application of such measurements will be limited by lack of specificity, as with measures of CRP and serum amyloid A. Nonetheless, their dramatic responsiveness and their potent biologic activities provide a powerful impetus for the continuing investigation of the role and potential clinical usefulness of measuring these polypeptide mediators in inflammatory disorders.

Serum (or synovial fluid) levels of a number of other tissue products (see Table 44–3) have been correlated with clinical measures of disease activity and disease severity.[37–41] Although the local presence of these products is undoubtedly indicative of, and perhaps contributory to, an inflammatory response, it is unclear whether measurement of these reactants will prove to be of value in the initial assessment or subsequent monitoring of disease activity. Quantitation of these molecules remains experimental, with no well-established values for normal levels.

LABORATORY EVALUATION OF INFLAMMATION IN MANAGEMENT OF RHEUMATIC DISEASES

Most clinical data have been obtained using the ESR and CRP. Accordingly, the following discussion concentrates on these tests, which serve two useful purposes. First, they are of some value in assessing the extent or severity of inflammation, thus helping to differentiate between clinical states in which substantial amounts of inflammation are present and those in which inflammation is absent or minimal. Second, repeated evaluation of these markers may be helpful for assessment of disease activity over time.

Table 44–3. RECENTLY REPORTED NON–ACUTE PHASE PROTEIN MARKERS OF INFLAMMATION

Cytokines	Products of Inflammatory and Endothelial Cells
Granulocyte-macrophage colony-stimulating factor	Calprotectin
IL-1β	von Willebrand factor
Interferon-γ	Adhesion molecules (e.g., vascular cell adhesion molecule-1)
IL-1 receptor antagonist	Hyaluronic acid
Tumor necrosis factor-α receptor	Collagen and aggrecan degradation products
IL-1 receptor	Osteocalcin

Abbreviation: IL-1, interleukin-1.

Because none of these tests possesses diagnostic specificity, results should not be used to definitely confirm any particular disease—even polymyalgia rheumatica/giant cell arteritis (see below). Furthermore, quantitation of these measures at any single point in the course of a chronic disease probably has limited prognostic value, although this continues to be a controversial issue in rheumatoid arthritis.

Rheumatoid Arthritis

Although ESR and CRP are more often and more markedly elevated in patients with early rheumatoid arthritis than in those with osteoarthritis or mild systemic lupus erythematosus (SLE), these tests cannot be reliably depended on for differential diagnosis. A careful history, physical examination, and more specific laboratory tests, such as anti-DNA and even rheumatoid factor, are clearly more helpful for diagnostic purposes. A more appropriate application of these tests is in the monitoring of disease activity in rheumatoid arthritis.[42] Although the ESR is widely used for this purpose, recent publications cast doubt on its value.[43] Several studies have suggested that CRP levels correlate better with degree of activity than does ESR.[44–46] CRP levels average about 3 to 4 mg/dl in adult rheumatoid arthritis patients with moderate disease activity, but there is considerable variation: about 7 percent of such patients have values in the normal range, whereas a few patients with severe disease activity show levels of 14 mg/dl or more. It is likely that levels of serum amyloid A have a similarly wide-ranging correlation with rheumatoid disease activity.[18]

The precise role of acute-phase reactants and to a lesser extent, other inflammatory markers, in assessment of rheumatoid arthritis progression and prognosis has been a subject of controversy. The availability of reliable predictors of disease outcome would obviously be of great benefit in decisions of which patients to treat aggressively. Some studies have suggested that high levels of acute-phase reactants at the onset of rheumatoid arthritis are associated with a relatively poor prognosis.[44, 47] Moreover, because serum CRP and ESR levels frequently fall in patients who show clinical improvement on treatment with slow-acting agents (e.g., intramuscular gold and methotrexate), while declining substantially in only a small proportion of those receiving nonsteroidal anti-inflammatory drugs, a number of clinicians regard the initial finding of moderate to marked CRP elevation as a signal to use aggressive therapy. Reports suggest that the use of repeated testing to obtain time-integrated values may provide a more valid prognostic estimate.[47, 48] Evidence is insufficient, however, to conclude with confidence that treatment that normalizes acute-phase reactants also favorably affects the array of inflammatory and biochemical processes that ultimately lead to destruction of bone, cartilage, and other connective tissues in rheumatoid arthritis. Whether these or other markers can indeed provide substantial prognostic information regarding effects of therapy on outcome in rheumatoid arthritis is an important issue that awaits more definitive study.

Systemic Lupus Erythematosus

Although serum CRP and ESR levels are elevated above normal in most patients with active SLE, a number of such patients do not show even mild elevations of CRP. In general, lupus patients with acute serositis[49] or chronic synovitis[50] are most likely to manifest substantially elevated levels of CRP, whereas those with other manifestations of lupus, such as nephritis, may have modest elevations, if any. Data are insufficient to evaluate the potential use of some of the other newer markers described earlier, but many SLE patients with normal CRP levels do show elevated IL-6 concentrations.[51]

The suggestion that CRP elevation in the course of SLE is more likely the result of superimposed infection than of activation of lupus has been directly addressed in several studies.[49, 52] Markedly elevated serum CRP levels in the hospitalized population are seen most frequently (but not exclusively) with bacterial infection.[11] Elevation of CRP levels in excess of 6 to 8 mg/dl in the course of lupus should serve as an impetus to exclude the possibility of infection, just as it should in other diseases. Such levels should not be regarded as proof of infection, however; as indicated earlier, marked CRP elevation related to active SLE can be seen in the absence of infection.

Vasculitis, Including Polymyalgia Rheumatica and Giant Cell Arteritis

The diagnosis of polymyalgia rheumatica and giant cell arteritis (PMR or GCA) is supported by an elevated ESR, often higher than 100 mm/hour. Such an elevation is no longer regarded as a *sine qua non* of these disorders; reports continue to appear describing patients with PMR or GCA who have normal ESRs.[53] Extreme elevation of the ESR in the absence of symptoms of these disorders is more likely to be related to the presence of an infection, malignancy, or renal disease than to PMR or GCA.[54]

In patients with PMR or GCA, CRP and ESR determinations are of approximately equal value in assessing disease activity. Of course, clinical manifestations of disease, even in the presence of a normal ESR or CRP level, should not be ignored. Serum IL-6 concentration also may be significantly correlated with activity in these disorders.[55] Finally, a number of markers of endothelial perturbation that, although not acute-phase reactants in the strict sense, are found in plasma in elevated concentrations in a number of inflammatory disorders of vessels, particularly PMR and GCA and other vasculitides.[56] These molecules include von Willebrand factor, thrombomodulin, some vasoactive prostanoids, and a variety of adhesion molecules, such as vascular cell adhesion molecule-1 (VCAM-1). Some patients with SLE or rheumatoid arthritis also demonstrate these abnormalities.[56]

Spondyloarthropathies

Reports suggest that levels of the cytokine IL-6[57, 58] may be correlated with clinical disease activity (and perhaps severity) in patients with ankylosing spondylitis. Most such patients also display modest elevations of ESR and CRP levels, which often bear a relation to disease activity.[59, 60] Further studies are needed to define the role of acute-phase markers, compared with evaluation of signs and symptoms, in the management of patients with spondyloarthropathies.

COST-EFFECTIVENESS OF LABORATORY EVALUATION OF INFLAMMATION

Only the ESR and serum levels of CRP are routinely measured in most clinical laboratories. The ESR is measured reliably and reproducibly by the Westergren technique at an average cost of about $10 per determination. The cost for measurement of CRP by laser nephelometry or enzyme-linked immunosorbent assay (ELISA) is somewhat greater, about $25 per determination; these results are also reproducible. An ELISA for serum amyloid A has recently been developed for experimental use.[21] Similarly, many of the cytokines listed in Table 44–3 can be measured by ELISA. In general, such assays are more expensive (up to $50 per sample) and are recommended for experimental use only at this time. Normal levels of serum amyloid A and cytokines in relation to age and gender are not well defined. Moreover, the potential influence of drugs, circulating cytokine inhibitors, and autoantibodies to cytokines might influence these measurements. Given these uncertainties and the cost of the assays, the use of such measurements for disease follow-up does not seem warranted.

References

1. Kushner I: Regulation of the acute phase response by cytokines. Perspect Biol Med 36:611, 1993.
2. Volanakis JE: Acute phase proteins. In McCarty DJ, Koopman WJ (eds): Arthritis and Allied Conditions: A Textbook of Rheumatology, 12th ed. Malvern, Pa, Lea & Febiger, 1993, pp 469–477.
3. Colten HR: Airway inflammation in cystic fibrosis. N Engl J Med 332:886, 1995.
4. Macintyre SS: C-reactive protein. In Di Sabato G (ed): Immunochemical Techniques. Part M: Chemotaxis and Inflammation. New York, Academic Press, 1988, pp 383–399.
5. Volanakis JE, Xu Y, Macon KJ: Human C-reactive protein and host defense. In Marchalonis JJ, Reinisch CL (eds): Defense Molecules. New York, Wiley-Liss, 1990, pp 161–175.
6. Volanakis JE, Kaplan MH: Specificity of C-reactive protein for choline phosphate residues of pneumococcal C-polysaccharides. Proc Soc Exp Biol Med 163:612, 1971.
7. Du Clos TW, Marnell L, Zlock LR, et al: Analysis of the binding of C-reactive protein to chromatin subunits. J Immunol 146:1220, 1991.
8. Ballou SP, Buniel J, Macintyre SS: Specific binding of human C-reactive protein to human monocytes in vitro. J Immunol 142:2708, 1989.
9. Dobrinich R, Spagnuolo PJ: Binding of C-reactive protein to human neutrophils. Arthritis Rheum 34:1031, 1991.
10. Ballou SP, Lozanski G: Induction of inflammatory cytokine release from cultured human monocytes by C-reactive protein. Cytokine 4:361, 1992.
11. Morley JJ, Kushner I: Serum C-reactive protein levels in disease. Ann N Y Acad Sci 389:406, 1982.
12. Vigushin DM, Pepys MB, Hawkins PN: Metabolic and scintigraphic studies of radioiodinated human C-reactive protein in health and disease. J Clin Invest 91:1351, 1993.
13. Whitehead AS, de Beer MC, Steel DM, et al: Identification of novel members of the serum amyloid A protein superfamily as constitutive apolipoproteins. J Biol Chem 267:3862, 1992.
14. Chambers RE, Hutton CW, Dieppe PA, et al: Comparative study of C-reactive protein and serum amyloid A protein in experimental inflammation. Ann Rheum Dis 50:677, 1991.
15. Badolato R, Wang JM, Murphy WJ, et al: Serum amyloid A is a chemoattractant: Induction of migration, adhesion, and tissue infiltration of monocytes and polymorphonuclear leukocytes. J Exp Med 180:203, 1994.
16. Shephard EG, de Beer FC, de Beer MC, et al: Neutrophil association and degradation of normal and acute-phase high-density lipoprotein 3. J Biochem 248:919, 1987.
17. Kisilevsky R, Subrahmanyan L: Serum amyloid A changes high density lipoprotein's cellular affinity. Lab Invest 66:778, 1992.
18. Grindulis KA, Scott DL, Robinson MW, et al: Serum amyloid A protein during the treatment of rheumatoid arthritis with second-line drugs. Br J Rheum 24:158, 1985.
19. Roseff R, Wohlgethan JR, Sipe JD: The acute phase response in gout. J Rheumatol 14:974, 1987.
20. Liuzzo G, Biasucci LM, Gallimore JR, et al: The prognostic value of C-reactive protein and serum amyloid A protein in severe unstable angina. N Engl J Med 331:417, 1994.
21. de Oliveira RM, Sipe JD, de Beer FC, et al: Rapid, sensitive enzyme-linked immunosorbent assays (ELISA) for serum amyloid A (apoSAA) in human plasma and tissue culture fluids. Amyloid Int J Exp Clin Invest 1:23, 1994.
22. Mackiewicz A, Gorny A: Glycoforms of α_1-acid glycoprotein as disease markers. In Mackiewicz A, Kushner I, Baumann H (eds): Acute Phase Proteins: Molecular Biology, Biochemistry, and Clinical Applications. Boca Raton, Fla, CRC Press, 1993, pp 651–661.
23. Pawlowski T, Mackiewicz S, Mackiewicz A: Microheterogeneity of alpha₁-acid glycoprotein in the detection of intercurrent infection in patients with rheumatoid arthritis. Arthritis Rheum 32:347, 1989.
24. Mackiewicz A, Marcinkowska-Pieta R, Mackiewicz S: Microheterogeneity of alpha₁-acid glycoprotein in the detection of intercurrent infection in systemic lupus erythematosus. Arthritis Rheum 30:513, 1987.
25. Kushner I: The acute phase response: From Hippocrates to cytokine biology. Eur Cytokine Net 2:75, 1991.
26. International Council for Standardization in Haematology (Expert Panel on Blood Rheology). ICSH recommendations for measurement of erythrocyte sedimentation rate. J Clin Pathol 46:198, 1993.
27. Shearn MA, Kang IY: Effect of age and sex on the erythrocyte sedimentation rate. J Rheumatol 13:297, 1986.
28. Miller A, Green M, Roberson D: Simple rule for calculating normal erythrocyte sedimentation rate. Br Med J 286:266, 1983.
29. Gillum RF: A racial difference in erythrocyte sedimentation. J Natl Med Assoc 85:47, 1993.
30. Van Snick J: Interleukin-6: An overview. Annu Rev Immunol 8:253, 1990.
31. Sehgal PB: Interleukin 6 in infection and cancer. Proc Soc Exp Biol Med 195:183, 1990.
32. Cruickshank AM, Fraser WD, Burns HJG, et al: Response of serum interleukin-6 in patients undergoing elective surgery of varying severity. Clin Sci 79:161, 1990.
33. Madhok R, Crilly A, Murphy E, et al: Gold therapy lowers serum interleukin 6 levels in rheumatoid arthritis. J Rheumatol 20:630, 1993.
34. Sehgal PB. Interleukin-6. In Mackiewicz A, Kushner I, Baumann H (eds): Acute Phase Proteins: Molecular Biology, Biochemistry, and Clinical Applications. Boca Raton, Fla, CRC Press, 1993, pp 289–308.
35. Barrera P, Boerbooms AMT, Janssen EM, et al: Circulating soluble tumor necrosis factor receptors, interleukin-2 receptors, tumor necrosis factor α, and interleukin-6 levels in rheumatoid arthritis. Arthritis Rheum 36:1070, 1993.
36. Luqmani R, Sheeran T, Robinson M, et al: Systemic cytokine measurements: Their role in monitoring the response to therapy in patients with rheumatoid arthritis. Clin Exp Rheumatol 12:503, 1994.
37. Brun JG, Jonsson R, Haga H-J: Measurement of plasma calprotectin as an indicator of arthritis and disease activity in patients with inflammatory rheumatic diseases. J Rheumatol 21:733, 1994.
38. Franck H, Ittel TH, Tasch O, et al: Osteocalcin in patients with rheumatoid arthritis: A one-year followup study. J Rheumatol 21:1256, 1994.
39. Paimela L, Leirisalo-Repo M, Risteli L, et al: Type I collagen degradation product in serum of patients with early rheumatoid arthritis: Relation-

ship to disease activity and radiological progression in a 3-year follow-up. Br J Rheum 33:1012, 1994.
40. Poole AR: Immunochemical markers of joint inflammation, skeletal damage and repair: Where are we now? Ann Rheum Dis 53:3, 1994.
41. Wollheim FA: New insight into joint damage from analysis of released biochemical markers. Br J Rheumatol 33:1, 1994.
42. Otterness IG: The value of C-reactive protein measurement in rheumatoid arthritis. Semin Arthritis Rheum 24:91, 1994.
43. Wolfe F, Michaud K: The clinical and research significance of the erythrocyte sedimentation rate. J Rheumatol 21:1227, 1994.
44. Larsen A: The relation of radiographic changes to serum acute-phase proteins and rheumatoid factor in 200 patients with rheumatoid arthritis. Scand J Rheumatol 17:123, 1988.
45. Segal R, Caspi D, Tishler M: Short term effects of low dose methotrexate on the acute phase reaction in patients with rheumatoid arthritis. J Rheumatol 16:914, 1989.
46. Cohick CB, Furst DE, Quagliata S, et al: Analysis of elevated serum interleukin-6 levels in rheumatoid arthritis: Correlation with erythrocyte sedimentation rate or C-reactive protein. J Lab Clin Med 123:721, 1994.
47. van Leeuwen MA, van der Heijde DMFM, van Rijswijk MJ, et al: Interrelationship of outcome measures and process variables in early rheumatoid arthritis: A comparison of radiologic damage, physical disability, joint counts, and acute phase reactants. J Rheumatol 21:425, 1994.
48. Hassell AB, Davis MJ, Fowler PD: The relationship between serial measures of disease activity and outcome in rheumatoid arthritis. Q J Med 86:601, 1993.
49. terBorg EJ, Horst G, Limburg PC: C-reactive protein levels during disease exacerbations and infections in systemic lupus erythematosus: A prospective longitudinal study. J Rheumatol 17:1642, 1990.
50. Moutsopoulos HM, Mavridis AK, Acritidis NC. High C-reactive protein response in lupus polyarthritis. Clin Exp Rheumatol 1:53, 1983.
51. Gabay C, Roux-Lombard P, de Moerloose P, et al. Absence of correlation between interleukin 6 and C-reactive protein blood levels in systemic lupus erythematosus compared with rheumatoid arthritis. J Rheumatol 20:815, 1993.
52. Linares LF, Gomez-Reino JJ, Carreira PE, et al: C-reactive protein (CRP) levels in systemic lupus erythematosus (SLE). Clin Rheumatol 5:66, 1986.
53. Neish PR, Sergent JS: Giant cell arteritis: A case with unusual neurologic manifestations and a normal sedimentation rate. Arch Intern Med 151:378, 1991.
54. Fincher RM, Page MI: Clinical significance of extreme elevation of the erythrocyte sedimentation rate. Arch Intern Med 146:1581, 1986.
55. Roche NE, Fulbright JW, Wagner AD, et al: Correlation of interleukin-6 production and disease activity in polymyalgia rheumatica and giant cell arteritis. Arthritis Rheum 36:1286, 1993.
56. Pearson JD: Markers of endothelial perturbation and damage. Br J Rheumatol 32:651, 1994.
57. Gratacóos J, Collado A, Filella X, et al: Serum cytokines (IL-6, TNFα, IL-β and IFN-γ) in ankylosing spondylitis: A close correlation between serum IL-6 and disease activity and severity. Br J Rheumatol 33:927, 1994.
58. Tutuncu ZN, Bilgie A, Kennedy LG, et al: Interleukin-6, acute phase reactants and clinical status in ankylosing spondylitis. Ann Rheum Dis 53:425, 1994.
59. Nashel DJ, Petrone DL, Ulmer CC, et al: C-reactive protein: A marker for disease activity in ankylosing spondylitis and Reiter's syndrome. J Rheumatol 13:364, 1986.
60. Sanders KM, Hertzman A, Escobar MR, et al: Correlation of immunoglobulin and C reactive protein levels in ankylosing spondylitis and rheumatoid arthritis. Ann Rheum Dis 46:273, 1987.

Clinical Pharmacology for Rheumatic Diseases

CHAPTER 45

Philip J. Clements
Harold E. Paulus

Nonsteroidal Antirheumatic Drugs

Nonsteroidal antirheumatic drugs reduce the signs and symptoms of established inflammation but do not in themselves eliminate the underlying causes of the inflammation. Their effects on pain, swelling, heat, erythema, and loss of function begin promptly after their absorption into the blood and become fully evident within a few weeks. Drug withdrawal is quickly followed by exacerbation of signs and symptoms of inflammation. The drugs have no effect on the course of the basic disease process and do not protect against tissue or joint injury; thus, damage to joints continues to occur during the administration of nonsteroidal antirheumatic agents to patients with chronic inflammatory arthritis.

Although these drugs have been sought and developed because of their effects on arthritis, their substantial analgesic, antipyretic, and antiprostaglandin effects have led to their widespread application in the symptomatic management of aches and pains of all types, fever, uterine cramps, closure of patent ductus arteriosus in infants, and other applications that derive from their suppression of prostaglandin synthesis. Drugs with these characteristics are generally referred to as nonsteroidal anti-inflammatory drugs (NSAIDs); examples include aspirin and the nonacetylated salicylates, phenylbutazone, indomethacin, ibuprofen, fenoprofen, ketoprofen, flurbiprofen, naproxen, tolmetin, sulindac, meclofenamate, diclofenac, ketorolac, etodolac, diflunisal, nabumetone, oxaprozin, and piroxicam.

Colchicine, also discussed in this chapter, has some of the characteristics of the NSAIDs, although it differs in its mechanism of action and its adverse effects profile. The slowly acting antirheumatic drugs, such as gold and the immunoregulatory agents, differ in their pharmacologic characteristics and clinical applications and are discussed in subsequent chapters. To some extent, the glucocorticoids resemble NSAIDs, in that they moderate established inflammation; however, they have many characteristics that clearly differentiate them from the nonsteroidal antirheumatic drugs; they are discussed in Chapter 50.

This chapter emphasizes similarities and class characteristics of the NSAIDs. The discussions of individual drugs are limited to unique characteristics, such as their pharmacokinetics, and areas in which they differ from the general characteristics of the class. Finally, a basis for clinical differentiation between the nonsteroidal antirheumatic drugs is discussed to provide some guidance in the selection of a particular drug for an individual patient.

HISTORY

Willow and poplar barks that contain salicin have been used since antiquity to treat pain, gout, and fever. Colchicine-containing extracts of the autumn crocus were used for treatment of acute gout as early as the 6th century A.D. Colchicine was isolated in 1820, and by 1900 salicylic acid and aspirin had been synthesized.[1] The term *nonsteroidal anti-inflammatory drug* was first applied to phenylbutazone, which was introduced into clinical practice in 1949, three years after the dramatic demonstration of the anti-inflammatory properties of the corticosteroids.[2] A pharmacologic breakthrough occurred when indomethacin was selected by deliberate screening of numerous chemicals for activity against inflammation induced in rat paws by injection of carrageenan. Since the introduction of indomethacin to the market in 1965, many other compounds have been found to suppress the acute development of rat paw edema following the injection of carrageenan or other irritating sub-

707

stances. Essentially all of the available NSAIDs were initially identified by their in vivo effects on this model of acute inflammation, and the model's ability to identify additional similar compounds seems limitless. Thus, the lead provided by aspirin and indomethacin has been fully exploited; the lead provided by colchicine, however, has been largely ignored.

POSSIBLE MECHANISMS OF ACTION

Inflammation is essentially a local event. Normally, the chemical mediators considered central to the inflammatory process preserve homeostasis in the microenvironment. These mediators include products of activated leukocytes and platelets, prostaglandins, leukotrienes, complement-derived products, and products of activated mast cells. If conditions within the microenvironment exceed the normal homeostatic capacity of the chemical mediators, a full inflammatory response occurs that can result in systemic manifestations if sufficiently severe.[3] The NSAIDs appear to act predominantly in this microenvironment.

Since the NSAIDs in current use were selected because of their effect on induced acute inflammation in a whole-animal model, it is apparent that they successfully moderate the general process of acute inflammation in vivo. As our knowledge of the mechanisms and pathways of inflammatory processes has become more sophisticated, various hypotheses have been advanced to explain the actions of NSAIDs. Under appropriate conditions, NSAIDs have been demonstrated to uncouple oxidative phosphorylation,[4] to displace an endogenous anti-inflammatory peptide from plasma proteins,[5] to inhibit lysosomal enzyme release,[6] to inhibit complement activation,[7] and to antagonize the generation or activity of kinins.[8] Currently favored mechanisms of NSAID action include inhibition of cyclooxygenase, inhibition of lipoxygenase, and inhibition of free radicals. None of these mechanisms completely explains the actions of NSAIDs, however, and other hypotheses are emerging. For example, Weissman estimated that in rheumatoid arthritis, arachidonic acid–derived products mediate only 25 to 30 percent of the inflammatory response[9]; if this were true, even complete suppression of arachidonic acid metabolism would have only modest benefit in this disease.

Inhibition of Arachidonic Acid Metabolites

Prostaglandin activity was discovered in seminal fluid in 1933 by Goldblatt[10] and confirmed by von Euler,[11] but it was not until 1964 that the structural identification of arachidonic acid, its metabolites, and the pertinent metabolic enzymes provided the chemical tools with which to study the interrelationships of these substances with inflammation and to characterize the effects of NSAIDs on this metabolic process.[12] This subject is discussed in detail in Chapter 19, but

is summarized briefly here because of the important effects of NSAIDs on arachidonic acid metabolism and the potential for manipulation of this process in the development of new anti-inflammatory drugs.[13]

Essentially all cells in the body have the capacity to synthesize prostaglandins (PGs) (Fig. 45–1). In response to inflammatory stimuli, arachidonic acid is cleaved from membrane phospholipids by specific phospholipases. Arachidonic acid is oxidized and cyclized by the enzyme cyclooxygenase to form a cyclic endoperoxide PGG_2. PGG_2 is converted to PGH_2 by peroxidation with concomitant production of unstable toxic oxygen radicals. The cyclic endoperoxides have a half-life of about 5 minutes, demonstrate marked effects on guinea pig and rabbit aorta, and promote the aggregation of platelets. PGH_2 is then converted to the stable prostaglandins E_2 and $F_{2\alpha}$, thromboxane, or prostacyclin by the appropriate enzymes, as shown in Figure 45–1. Thromboxane A_2 is synthesized by platelets and promotes their aggregation, but it has a half-life of only about 30 seconds before it is rapidly hydrolyzed to inactive thromboxane B_2. Prostacyclin (PGI_2) is synthesized within arterial walls, opposes the effects of thromboxane A_2 by inhibiting aggregation of platelets, and is a potent vasodilator.[12, 13]

Some of the biologic actions of the cyclic endoperoxides and their metabolites reproduce many of the signs of acute inflammation. Erythema is associated with the vasodilating activities of PGE_1, PGE_2, PGD_2, and PGI_2. Edema formation is promoted by increased vascular permeability induced by prostaglandins of the E series and their potentiation of bradykinin and histamine. Injection of PGE also causes pain and fever and promotes local bone resorption and cartilage destruction, depending on the sites of injection or application. Elevated levels of prostaglandins have been demonstrated in synovial effusions from untreated patients with inflammatory arthritis.[13]

COX-1 and COX-2

The recent discovery and characterization of two isoenzymes of cyclooxygenase have led to intense investigations that will cause the present NSAIDs to become obsolete.[14] Cyclooxygenase-1 (COX-1) is constitutively present in many tissues and is responsible for the physiologic production of homeostatic and cytoprotective prostanoids in the gastric mucosa, endothelium, platelets, and kidney. Its inhibition is linked to many of the familiar adverse effects of NSAIDs.

Cyclooxygenase-2 (COX-2) is not constitutively expressed by unstimulated cells. It is induced in leukocytes,[15] vascular smooth muscle cells,[16] human rheumatoid synoviocytes,[17] and brain neurons[18] by stimuli such as mitogens, cytokines, and endotoxin, catalyzing the synthesis of proinflammatory prostaglandins. COX-2 is associated with carrageenan-induced inflammation in experimental animals[19, 20] as well as certain aspects of inflammatory pain[20] and perhaps fever.

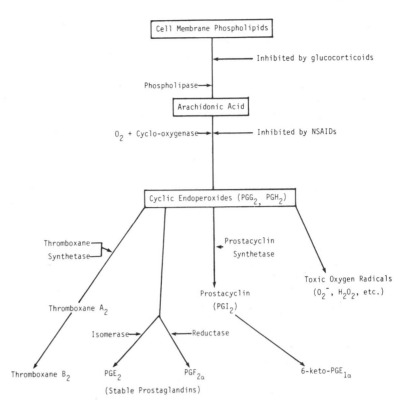

Figure 45–1. Cyclooxygenase pathway for arachidonic acid metabolism. PG, prostaglandin; NSAIDs, nonsteroidal anti-inflammatory drugs.

The complementary DNAs (cDNAs) of COX-1 and COX-2 and their respective messenger RNAs (mRNAs) have been identified, cloned, and expressed in insect cell culture, making it possible to produce pure human COX-1 and COX-2.[21] The two isoforms show only 60 percent homology of their nucleic acid and amino acid structures.[14] The availability of pure COX-1 and COX-2 makes it possible to rapidly determine the relative inhibitory potency of available and potential NSAIDs for each isoenzyme.

Using separate cell cultures that produced only COX-1 or COX-2, Mitchell and colleagues reported that it took 166 times as much aspirin (50 percent) to inhibit COX-2 as COX-1 50 percent, but only 2.8 times as much sodium salicylate for the same degree of inhibition.[22] COX-2 to COX-1 inhibitory ratios for indomethacin (60:1) and ibuprofen (15:1) were also high. Using a pure isoenzyme technique, Gierse and associates reported ratios of 9 for indomethacin, 3 for naproxen, 4 for flurbiprofen, and 11 for ibuprofen,[21] indicating that the homeostatic COX-1 isoenzyme is inhibited to a greater extent than the proinflammatory COX-2 isoenzyme when patients are treated with these standard NSAIDs. Thus, it is not surprising that their doses are limited by gastric toxicity and that their anti-inflammatory effects are modest.

The pharmaceutical industry is actively screening and developing compounds that inhibit COX-2 at concentrations much lower than those needed to inhibit COX-1. When they become available, clinically useful dosage regimens of these selective COX-2 inhibitors will permit more effective inhibition of the proinflammatory products of COX-2 without inhibiting the gastroprotective products of COX-1. This should eliminate the problem of NSAID gastropathy while allowing the determination of the full anti-inflammatory potential of a new generation of NSAIDs that can completely inhibit COX-2–associated inflammation. The only available drugs that selectively inhibit COX-2 are the corticosteroids.[17, 19] The degree to which selective COX-2–inhibiting NSAIDs will approach the anti-inflammatory efficacy of corticosteroids has not yet been determined, but the role of NSAIDs in the management of acute and chronic inflammation may be expanded.

Another pathway of arachidonic acid metabolism is catalyzed by *5-lipoxygenase* (Fig. 45–2). In contrast to cyclooxygenase, which is present in all tissues, 5-lipoxygenase appears to be limited to neutrophils, eosinophils, monocytes/macrophages, basophils, and certain mast cell populations.[13, 23] These cells—when activated and in the presence of calcium, adenosine triphosphate (ATP), and 5-lipoxygenase—enzymatically convert arachidonic acid to 5-hydroperoxyeicosatetraenoic acid (5-HPETE); this is further transformed enzymatically to form the unstable epoxide leukotriene A_4 (LTA$_4$). In neutrophils, LTA$_4$ is converted to LTB$_4$, which attracts other neutrophils to the site. LTB$_4$, in addition to thromboxane A_2, changes the adherence properties of endothelial cells, no doubt an important factor in the chemotaxis of neutrophils to the site of injury. Eosinophils do not produce LTB$_4$ but synthesize LTC$_4$, which, with its metabolites LTD$_4$ and LTE$_4$, forms the slowly reacting substance of ana-

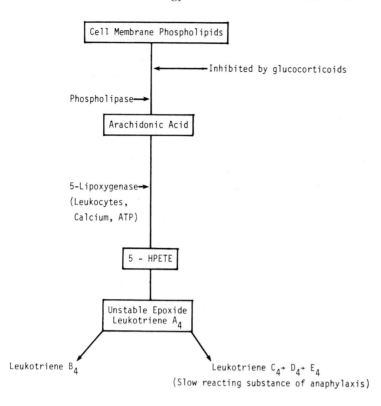

Figure 45–2. Lipoxygenase pathway for arachidonic acid metabolism; ATP, adenosine triphosphate.

phylaxis (SRSA) and profoundly increases the contractile activity of vascular and nonvascular smooth muscle, thus its relationship with anaphylaxis. Leukotriene C_4 profoundly compromises guinea pig lung function, and its intradermal injection produces a wheal and flare reaction. Monocytes can produce both LTB_4 and LTC_4. Receptor sites for LTB_4 have been found on neutrophils and monocytes, and receptors for LTD_4 are present in pulmonary tissue.[3] Neutrophils can inactivate LTB_4, and both eosinophils and neutrophils can inactivate LTC_4, LTD_4, and LTE_4.

Arachidonic acid can also be converted by 12- and 15-lipoxygenase to form 15-HPETE, which, when incubated with neutrophils, results in the formation of *lipoxin A* and *lipoxin B*. The lipoxins are reported to inhibit the cytotoxic reaction of natural killer T cells and to cause degranulation of leukocytes and contraction of bronchial smooth muscle.[12]

Lipocortins are a family of related proteins that inhibit phosphatase A_2 in vitro and that are thought to mimic the effect of corticosteroids on the arachidonic acid cascade.[24] Synthetic peptides derived from human lipocortin also inhibit phospholipase A_2, show potent anti-inflammatory activity in vivo on the carrageenan-induced rat paw edema model of acute inflammation, and inhibit neutrophil aggregation and chemotaxis induced by complement component C5A.[25]

Paradoxically, some of the stable prostaglandins can, under appropriate circumstances, exert anti-inflammatory or regulatory functions; pharmacologic doses of PGE_1 and PGE_2 have suppressed acute and chronic inflammation in several experimental mod-

els.[26] Indeed, arachidonic acid metabolites often have opposing effects on various mechanisms involved in inflammation. Thus, vessel tone is increased by $PGF_{2\alpha}$ and thromboxane A_2 and decreased by PGE_2 and PGI_2, whereas vessel permeability is increased by PGE_2, PGI_2, and LTB_4, and decreased by PGF_2. Chemotaxis is stimulated by PGE_2 and LTB_4 and is inhibited by PGI_2. It has been suggested that the generation of free radicals during arachidonic acid metabolism by cyclooxygenase may potentiate the inflammatory process.[27] The concentration of free radical oxidation products is higher in inflammatory synovial effusions and the free radical scavenger, MK-477, exerts an anti-inflammatory effect in an experimental edema model without inhibiting the production of stable prostaglandins.[13] Thus, it is evident that the effects of arachidonic acid metabolism are exceedingly local and are determined by the type of cell that is activated, by the tissue in which the activation takes place, and, probably, by other less well-defined circumstances in the microenvironment.

In 1971, Vane reported that aspirin-like drugs inhibit prostaglandin synthesis.[28] Subsequent work from many studies has established that there is good correlation between the order of potency of various NSAIDs in the suppression of prostaglandin synthesis and in the suppression of inflammation. Low concentrations of aspirin irreversibly inhibit this process by acetylating the enzyme cyclooxygenase; the other NSAIDs reversibly inhibit cyclooxygenase in a concentration related manner by competitive inhibition. Nonacetylated salicylate is much less potent than aspirin as an inhibitor of cyclooxygenase, but anti-inflammatory doses (3 g) of salicylate have been reported to reduce the urinary output of prostaglandin metabolites in humans by 85 to 95 percent,[29] perhaps because of the high concentrations of salicylate attained.

Thus, NSAIDs reduce the synthesis of prostaglandins, prostacyclin, and thromboxane but appear not to affect leukotriene production. In vitro studies show marked inhibition of lipoxygenase by benoxaprofen, moderate inhibition by diclofenac and ketoprofen, but no inhibition by indomethacin, flurbiprofen, piroxicam, or naproxen.[30] BW755C, a drug that will remain experimental because it causes hemolysis, inhibits both cyclooxygenase and 5-lipoxygenase; it suppresses leukocyte migration more effectively than indomethacin and as effectively as dexamethasone, suggesting that dual inhibition of arachidonic acid metabolism may be desirable.[29] Anti-inflammatory corticosteroids decrease arachidonic acid production from membrane phospholipids by facilitating the release of the protein lipocortin, which inhibits phospholipase A_2. Lipocortin itself has been isolated and is a potent anti-inflammatory agent.[29] Further studies with diclofenac demonstrated that it indirectly decreases leukotriene production by reducing arachidonic acid availability. In formyl-methionyl-leucyl-phenylalanine (f-MLP)–stimulated purified rat peritoneal neutrophils, diclofenac enhanced the incorporation of free arachidonic acid into triglycerides, thus decreasing the amount of arachidonic acid available for metabolism by 5-lipoxygenase or cyclooxygenase.[31] Sulfasalazine also appears to decrease both cyclooxygenase and 5-lipoxygenase pathway metabolites of arachidonic acid produced by colonic mucosa obtained from patients with inflammatory bowel disease.[32] A specific inhibitor of 5-lipoxygenase (Abbott 64077) has been reported to demonstrate some benefit in a preliminary trial in rheumatoid arthritis.[33] A combined lipoxygenase and cyclooxygenase inhibitor (tenidap) is also undergoing clinical trials in patients with rheumatoid arthritis, with reported favorable effects.[34]

Another indirect approach to regulation of leukotriene production involves the administration of dietary fish oil that contains docosahexanoic acid and eicosapentaenoic acid (EPA), which inhibit the conversion of arachidonic acid by cyclooxygenase. In addition, 5-lipoxygenase converts EPA to a pentaene rather than a tetraene series of products (LTA_5, LTB_5, LTC_5). LTB_5 is markedly less active than LTB_4 in its ability to attract human neutrophils in a chemotactic assay and to cause human leukocytes to adhere to an endothelial cell monolayer, but LTC_5 is no less active than LTC_4. Thus, induced anaphylaxis was more severe in guinea pigs fed fish oil–enriched diets than in those receiving regular diets. The biochemical effects in the neutrophils of 12 patients with rheumatoid arthritis treated with fish oil capsules for 6 weeks were selective for suppression of LTB_4 generation only. Modest clinical benefit was seen after 6 weeks but was no longer present 4 weeks after fish oil supplementation was discontinued.[35]

Other Possible Mechanisms

Other proposals for the mechanism of action of NSAIDs include their effects on proinflammatory cell functions. Under carefully controlled in vitro conditions, various investigators have demonstrated that NSAIDs inhibit phosphodiesterase; this leads to potentiation of PGE_1-mediated increased intracellular cyclic adenosine monophosphate levels and subsequent inhibition of proinflammatory cellular functions, peripheral blood lymphocyte responses to mitogen stimulation, neutrophil and monocyte migration, and various neutrophil functions.[13] Weissmann and various associates have demonstrated that NSAIDs inhibit the aggregation of human neutrophils in vitro and in vivo. They also have demonstrated this effect of NSAIDs in cells of the marine sponge, which do not contain cyclooxygenase and are unresponsive to stable prostaglandins. They suggest that NSAIDs may act by interfering with a receptor site that triggers immobilization of intracellular calcium and activation of the cell.[36]

In summary, a number of hypotheses may explain the anti-inflammatory properties of NSAIDs, and each appears to explain some of the mechanisms of NSAID action. However, the exact mode of action of this class of drugs is not yet completely understood, and clinical application of these drugs continues to be empirical.

Mechanism of Action of Colchicine

Colchicine appears to interfere with several steps of the inflammatory response in which neutrophils play a central role. Intracellular interference with the organization of labile fibrillar microtubular systems concerned with cell structure and movement may lead to microtubular disaggregation and to decreased neutrophil motility, chemotaxis, release of chemotactic factors, formation of digestive vacuoles, and lysosomal degranulation. The net effect seems to decrease the migration of neutrophils into an area of inflammation and to diminish the metabolic and phagocytic activity of the neutrophils that are already there, interrupting part of the inflammatory process of gout.[37] Colchicine binds to tubulin and prevents its polymerization into functional microtubules.[38] Lumicolchicines, photoisomers of colchicine, do not bind to microtubule proteins and have no anti-inflammatory effects.[39] Most of the in vitro effects of colchicine on neutrophils have been demonstrated at concentrations of drug that far exceeded the blood levels produced in patients treated with colchicine. However, chemotaxis of neutrophils toward bacteria, immune complex–activated serum, or endotoxin-activated serum is suppressed by colchicine in concentrations of 10^{-8} M, which are attained in neutrophils of patients treated with standard clinical doses of the drug.[37] Ehrenfeld and colleagues reported that patients on colchicine had significantly fewer neutrophils at Rebuck skin window sites 24 hours after the skin was abraded,[40] which suggests that neutrophil migration is also altered by colchicine in vivo. Neutrophils release a chemotaxic substance during phagocytosis of urate crystals; colchicine $10-6$ M inhibits the release of this substance, and $10-8$ M partially suppresses its release.[41] Colchicine has also been reported to suppress the release of chemotactic LTB$_4$ by neutrophils[42] and to have corrected suppressor T cell deficiencies in five patients with familial Mediterranean fever who were treated with 0.5 mg of colchicine twice daily.[43] The capacity for and rate of phagocytosis of yeast were significantly suppressed in neutrophils obtained from patients with acute gout after several days of treatment with oral colchicine, 1.8 mg daily, compared with baseline phagocytosis before colchicine therapy was begun.[44] Thus, investigations that focus on colchicine effects on neutrophils have shown drug-induced changes in the functions of these cells, both in humans treated with clinically tolerated doses of colchicine and in vitro with concentrations of colchicine readily attained in patients treated with the drug.

CHARACTERISTICS OF NONSTEROIDAL ANTI-INFLAMMATORY DRUGS

The NSAIDs can be classified on the basis of their chemical structure (Table 45–1). Most are organic acids with relatively low pK$_a$. This property may allow higher concentrations of active drug in in-

Table 45–1. CLASSIFICATION OF SOME NONSTEROIDAL ANTI-INFLAMMATORY DRUGS

I. **Acidic Agents**
   A. Arylcarboxylic Acids
      1. Salicylic acids: aspirin in its various forms,* diflunisal, * choline magnesium trisalicylate,* salsalate,* benorylate, sodium salicylate*
      2. Anthranilic acids (fenamates): flutenamic acid, mefenamic acid,* meclofenamic acid,* niflumic acid
   B. Arylalkanoic Acids
      1. Arylacetic acids: diclofenac,* fenclofenac, alclofenac, fentiazac
      2. Arylpropionic acids: ibuprofen,* flurbiprofen,* ketoprofen,* naproxen,* fenoprofen,* fenbufen, suprofen, indoprofen, tiaprofenic acid, benoxaprofen, pirprofen
      3. Heteroarylacetic acids: tolmetin,* zomepirac, clopirac, ketorolac tromethamine*
      4. Indole, oxazoles, and indene carboxylic acids: indomethacin,* sulindac,* etodolac,* oxaprozin,* tenidap
   C. Enolic Acids
      1. Pyrazolidinediones: phenylbutazone,* oxyphenbutazone,* azapropazone, feprazone
      2. Oxicams: piroxicam,* isoxicam, sudoxicam

II. **Nonacidic Agents**

   Proquazone, fluproquazone, tiaramide, bufexamac, flunizole, epirazole, tinoridine, nabumetone*

Modified from Dudley-Hart F, Huskisson EC: Nonsteroidal anti-inflammatory drugs: Current status and rational therapeutic use. Drugs 27:232, 1984.
*Available in the United States.

flamed tissue where the pH is lower.[45] Generally, the lower the pK$_a$, the shorter the half-life of an NSAID.[46] It is not essential that NSAIDs be acidic, however; the non-acid compounds proquazone and nabumetone have well-documented anti-inflammatory effects.[47, 48]

Almost all NSAIDs are greater than 90 percent bound to plasma proteins. If total drug concentrations are increased beyond the point where the binding sites on albumin are saturated, biologically active free drug concentrations increase disproportionately to the increasing total drug concentration. This effect is more pronounced for the less potent NSAIDs, such as salicylate and ibuprofen, for which daily doses are measured in grams, rather than for the more potent drugs, such as piroxicam, with daily doses measured in milligrams, and may help to account for apparently disproportionate increases in anti-inflammatory activity with higher doses of some NSAIDs.

The pharmacologic activities of the available NSAIDs are largely similar, although, for commercial reasons, their manufacturers have chosen to emphasize certain applications for particular drugs. For example, naproxen sodium, zomepirac, suprofen, and ketorolac were marketed as analgesics, whereas diflunisal and etodolac were initially marketed for osteoarthritis.

Anti-inflammatory Effects

Historically, plants containing salicylate and colchicine were used to treat inflammatory conditions, and the dose-response relationship of aspirin in rheumatic fever was well documented. It was not until the early 1960s, however, that aspirin was shown to have anti-inflammatory effects both in experimental models of inflammation and in clinical studies of patients with rheumatoid arthritis.[49, 50] Fremont-Smith and Bayles reported decreased ring size, increased range of motion, and increased grip strength in rheumatoid arthritis patients treated with aspirin.[50] This observation was confirmed by the American Rheumatism Association Cooperating Clinics Committee in 1965,[51] and since then innumerable clinical trials of NSAIDs in rheumatoid arthritis and other rheumatic diseases have confirmed the anti-inflammatory effects of these drugs. NSAIDs have been compared with placebo, aspirin, and each other in double-blind randomized studies using well-defined criteria for evaluation of joint inflammation. Efficacy superior to that of placebo is easily demonstrated within 1 to 2 weeks in patients with active rheumatoid arthritis who are not receiving corticosteroids or other anti-inflammatory medications. Comparisons of adequate doses of one NSAID with another or with aspirin almost always show comparable efficacy, but the newer NSAIDs are somewhat less toxic than aspirin at full dosage.[52]

The anti-inflammatory effects of NSAIDs have also been demonstrated in juvenile rheumatoid arthritis, ankylosing spondylitis, gout, and osteoarthritis. Although not as rigorously proven, their efficacy is also widely accepted in the treatment of Reiter's syndrome, psoriatic arthritis, acute and chronic bursitis, and tendonitis.

The anti-inflammatory benefit of colchicine in acute gouty arthritis is legendary. Colchicine is also used in small maintenance doses to decrease the frequency and severity of recurrent attacks of gouty arthritis.[53] Its benefit has also been shown in patients with acute episodes of pseudogout[54] and in the suppression of recurrent or chronic joint inflammation due to calcium crystal disease.[55] It is the drug of choice for prevention of attacks of familial Mediterranean fever[56] and has been used in other rheumatologic disorders, such as Behçet's disease, sarcoidosis, calcific tendonitis, amyloidosis, cutaneous necrotizing vasculitis, and Sweet's syndrome.[37]

Analgesic Effects

Colchicine has no effect on pain perception, but virtually all of the NSAIDs relieve pain when used in doses substantially smaller than those required to demonstrate suppression of inflammation. Cross-circulation experiments in 1964 by Lim and associates that induced pain by peripheral injection of bradykinin demonstrated that perfusion of the brain with aspirin does not decrease bradykinin-induced painful responses, whereas perfusion of the peripheral site with aspirin is analgesic, even when the aspirin does not circulate to the brain.[57] Because prostaglandins enhance the painful response to injections of bradykinin and other peripheral chemical or mechanical stimuli, it has been suggested that NSAID suppression of the synthesis and release of prostaglandins averts their sensitization of pain receptors to chemical mediators.[58]

Antipyretic Effects

The NSAIDs, but not colchicine, effectively suppress fever in humans and experimental animals. Injection of prostaglandin E into the lateral ventricles of cats, rabbits, and rats produces fever, and increased prostaglandin E concentrations have been reported in the cerebrospinal fluid of rabbits with fever induced by endogenous pyrogen or endotoxin, leading to the hypothesis that the antipyretic effects of NSAIDs are due to their ability to suppress prostaglandin synthesis.[59]

Other Effects

Both aspirin and NSAIDs inhibit platelet cyclooxygenase and thus markedly decrease platelet aggregation in response to various stimuli. Aspirin is commonly used as a platelet anticoagulant, but the NSAIDs have not been used in this way because their effects on platelets are only temporary. Cyclooxygenase suppression by NSAIDs has been useful in the prevention of menstrual cramping and assisting in the closure of patent ductus arteriosus in infants. Other applications are developing in the treatment of ocular inflammation, shock, periodontal disease, and sports injuries, as well as an adjunct to cancer chemotherapy.[60] Sulindac has completely suppressed colorectal polyps in three patients with familial polyposis (Gardner's syndrome).[61]

ADVERSE EFFECTS OF NONSTEROIDAL ANTI-INFLAMMATORY DRUGS

Given the widespread use of NSAIDs and their substantial pharmacologic activity, the occurrence of adverse reactions is inevitable. In general, the NSAIDs share a common spectrum of clinical toxicities, although the frequency of particular side effects varies with the compound. Both adverse effects and beneficial effects tend to be dose-related, necessitating careful evaluation of risk/benefit ratios. Important toxicities occur in the gastrointestinal (GI) tract, central nervous system, hematopoietic system, kidney, skin, and liver. A great deal of regulatory attention has been focused on the adverse effects of NSAIDs, and the package inserts (also found in the *Physician's Desk Reference*) now contain reliable information about the frequencies of specific adverse effects known to occur with each NSAID that is marketed in the United States. None of the NSAIDs is completely safe; aspirin is the most difficult to use effectively, has more frequent side effects, and is more dangerous if taken in overdose. Chronopharmacologic studies suggest that in many patients the adverse effects of NSAIDs can be minimized, and their efficacy optimized, by adjusting the time of day when drug doses are administered.[62]

Gastrointestinal Effects

Probably because of their suppression of prostaglandin synthesis, NSAIDs as a group tend to cause gastric irritation and to exacerbate peptic ulcers. In laboratory animals, prostaglandins suppress gastric acid secretion and help maintain the gastric mucosal barrier, thus providing gastrointestinal cytoprotection.[63] The administration of an exogenous PGE_2 analog, misoprostil, reduces the incidence of aspirin-induced endoscopic damage to the gastric and duodenal mucosa in humans[64] and decreases the incidence of peptic ulcer complications (i.e., bleeding, perforation, obstruction) in NSAID-treated patients with rheumatoid arthritis.[65] NSAID-related symptoms include dyspepsia, epigastric pain, indigestion, heartburn, nausea, and vomiting. They cause mucosal lesions that may range from hyperemia to diffuse gastritis, superficial erosions, or penetrating ulcer craters. Occult blood loss, especially with use of aspirin, or massive gastrointestinal bleeding may occur.[66] Indomethacin, sulindac, and meclofenamate sodium have an extensive enterohepatic recirculation, which increases gastrointestinal exposure to these drugs and enhances their gastrointestinal toxicity. A metered-release tablet of indomethacin was withdrawn from marketing in Great Britain because of its association with intestinal perforations, apparently caused by direct local irritation by the indomethacin.

Caruso and Bianchi-Porro gastroscopically evaluated the effects of 12 NSAIDs administered singly or in combination to 164 patients with rheumatoid arthritis and to 85 patients with osteoarthritis. During one year of treatment with NSAIDs, 31 percent of the patients had endoscopically confirmed gastric lesions. Lesions were present in 51 percent of patients who received concurrent multiple NSAID treatment. All of the NSAIDs caused gastric damage, the greatest offender being aspirin and the least offenders being sulindac and diflunisal.[67]

Similar findings have been reported by Lanza, who found the least mucosal injury with sulindac, enteric-coated aspirin, and low-dose ibuprofen (1200 mg daily).[68] Poor correlation has been found between subjective symptoms of dyspepsia, fecal blood loss, and endoscopic findings.[69, 70] In contrast to aspirin, the nonacetylated salicylates have not been associated with an increase in occult gastrointestinal blood loss[71] or severe gastroscopically detected mucosal injury.[72, 73]

Gastrointestinal bleeding induced by aspirin or NSAIDs tends to be severe because these drugs decrease platelet aggregation by suppressing cyclooxygenase. Thus, platelet anticoagulation is more prolonged with aspirin, which irreversibly acetylates platelet cyclooxygenase, but is also present in a concentration-related manner with the other NSAIDs, persisting as long as the platelet is exposed to adequate concentrations of the drug.

By life-table analysis of prospectively collected data from multiple NSAID submissions, the U.S. Food and Drug Administration (FDA) estimates that gastrointestinal ulcers, bleeding, and perforation occur in approximately 1 to 2 percent of patients who use NSAIDs for 3 months and approximately 2 to 5 percent of those who use them for 1 year. Based on ARAMIS (Arthritis, Rheumatism and Aging Medical Information System) data, Fries estimates that NSAID-induced gastropathy is responsible for 76,000 hospitalizations and 7600 deaths each year in the United States.[74]

The association of severe upper gastrointestinal tract disease and exposure to aspirin or NSAIDs has been evaluated in a number of case-control and cohort studies; these have been analyzed in review articles[75] and a meta-analysis.[76, 77] In a meta-analysis of nine case-control and seven cohort studies, Gabriel and colleagues reported an overall odds ratio of the risk of serious adverse gastrointestinal events associated with NSAID use (compared with controls) to be 2.74 (95 percent confidence interval [CI] 2.54–2.97).[76] The risk was higher for patients 60 years old or older (odds ratio 5.52). Concomitant corticosteroid use increased the risk of a GI event over that with use of one NSAID alone (odds ratio 1.83). The risk was

greatest during the first month of NSAID use (odds ratio 8.9), compared with 1 to 3 months of exposure (odds ratio 3.31) and more than 3 months' exposure (odds ratio 1.92). Bollini and associates reported a meta-analysis of 34 epidemiologic studies, only 12 of which were considered to be of satisfactory quality.[76] They found a higher relative risk (RR) of NSAID-associated severe GI events (RR 4.2) in studies with unsatisfactory quality than in those of satisfactory quality (RR 2.6).

Cohort studies demonstrated a lower relative risk (RR 2.0) than hospital-based (RR 4.4) and community-based (RR 3.5) case-control studies. Willett and co-workers in 1994 reviewed the epidemiology of NSAID-associated GI damage.[75] In large prospective placebo-controlled, long-term clinical trials of low-dose aspirin (75 to 1300 mg/day) for treatment or prevention of myocardial infarction or strokes, 10 to 74 excess cases of severe GI events occurred per 10,000 person-years in the aspirin-treated patients compared with the placebo-treated control patients. Savage and colleagues, in a case-control study of medication history in 494 patients hospitalized in New Zealand for GI hemorrhage or perforation and 972 hospitalized control subjects matched for age and sex, found an odds ratio of 5.1 for current NSAID use with 40 percent of index patients and 13 percent of controls taking NSAIDs.[78] Surprisingly, they found an odds ratio of 3.1 for current regular aspirin use of more than 300 mg/day and of 3.6 for current regular acetaminophen use of more than 1000 mg/day, although most other studies found no association of acetaminophen and GI toxicity.[75]

Several case-control studies that attempted to assess the risks of GI bleeding with individual NSAIDs were summarized by Langman and associates.[79] The findings are of uncertain reliability because of very small numbers of cases, controls, or both with many of the NSAIDs, as well as variations in the proportionate doses used, variable indications for the different drugs, and frequent lack of data regarding other drugs and illnesses. Nevertheless, the investigators reported that seven sets of data for ibuprofen show lower risk ratios than nine sets of data for indomethacin, naproxen, and piroxicam. Other NSAIDs were intermediate or the available data were inconclusive. Soll and coworkers observed that half of related ulcers are associated with *Helicobacter pylori*, an independent risk factor for peptic ulcer disease that has not been systematically evaluated in epidemiologic studies.[80] The effect of coexisting *H. pylori* infection and its eradication on the effectiveness of prophylaxis against NSAID-associated ulcer complications have not been determined as yet. Because some 17 million Americans take NSAIDs on a daily basis, the annual rate of 1 to 2 percent of serious upper GI complications, including death among chronic NSAID users, means that 170,000 patients are at risk each year. Although certain agents, including misoprostol, have been shown by endoscopy to decrease the rate of endoscopically proven NSAID-associated ulcers from

22 percent to 2 percent, it had not been documented until recently that healing of endoscopically proven ulcers would necessarily be associated with an improvement in serious clinical GI complications (i.e., bleeding, perforation, obstruction).

The Misoprostol Ulcer Complications Outcome Safety Assessment (MUCOSA) trial was designed to prospectively evaluate serious upper GI clinical events in a double-blind, randomized, placebo-controlled 6-month study of 8843 patients with rheumatoid arthritis ($\geq$ 52 years of age; mean age 68 years) in a protocol designed to reflect normal clinical practice.[65] All patients were taking one or more of ten specified NSAIDs. None had active peptic ulcer disease or were taking antiulcer medications. During the 6-month study, 67 events occurred that were defined as definite serious events (i.e., bleeding, perforation, or obstruction): 25 serious upper GI events (0.5 percent rate of complication) occurred in the 4404 patients taking misoprostil, 200 μg four times a day, and 42 (0.95 percent rate of complication) occurred in the 4439 patients receiving placebo, a statistically significant difference ($P = .049$ by Fisher's exact test). Thus, the misoprostol group showed a 40 percent reduction in the rate of serious complications compared with the placebo group.

Risk factors for NSAID-associated upper GI tract complications in this prospective randomized clinical trial are similar to those found in case-control and cohort studies: older age, previous peptic ulcer disease (odds ratio twice that of baseline patients), previous GI bleeding (2.5 times more common than in the baseline group), and history of cardiovascular disease (rate of cardiovascular disease history 1.84 times higher than in the baseline group). The rate of occurrence of GI adverse events over the course of the MUCOSA trial was relatively uniform in both groups, however, similar to the pattern seen in aspirin users throughout the 36-month Aspirin Myocardial Infarction study.[81] The MUCOSA trial results confirmed that it is possible to statistically isolate high-risk characteristics and that not all of the risk is carried by one or another of the subgroups. Other suspected risk factors include concomitant corticosteroid use, degree of disability, and presence of comorbidity.

The MUCOSA trial clearly demonstrated that some patients are at higher risk of GI complications from NSAIDs than others are. Misoprostol appeared to decrease the serious complications by 40 percent overall, but there was a higher protection in patients with risk factors. Therefore, when patients begin NSAID therapy, consideration should be given to including concomitant misoprostol for patients who have risk factors for potentially serious GI complications, including older age, previous peptic ulcer disease, previous GI bleeding, history of cardiovascular disease, concomitant corticosteroid use, higher degrees of disability, and presence of other significant comorbidities.

The cumulative risk of these serious events increases with the duration of therapy and is greater in patients with previous peptic ulcer disease. Fatal outcomes are more likely in elderly or debilitated patients. Higher dosages of NSAIDs probably entail greater risk than lower dosages. The patient's disease, age, and degree of inflammation need to be considered in determining the optimal dosage for each patient, and every attempt should be made to use the lowest dose that adequately controls the patient's symptoms.[82] Other strategies to minimize NSAID gastropathy include the substitution of a nonacetylated salicylate[69, 72, 73] and a supplemental gastroprotective agent, such as misoprostil, carafete, or a histamine (H2) receptor antagonist.[83]

Of even greater potential significance in preventing side effects is the recent discovery that cyclooxygenase exists in two isoforms: (1) COX-1, which is found in most tissues and is involved in the physiologic production of prostaglandins (i.e., in gut, kidneys, endothelium, and platelets); and (2) COX-2, which is cytokine-inducible and is expressed in inflammatory cells. As discussed earlier, the anti-inflammatory actions of the available NSAIDs appear to be due to inhibition of COX-2, whereas the unwanted side effects, such as gastric toxicity and nephrotoxicity, are probably due to inhibition of COX-1 (the constitutive enzyme), the products of which help to protect the stomach and kidney against damage. With few exceptions, the available NSAIDs, while inhibiting both isoforms of COX, preferentially inhibit COX-1. For example, aspirin and indomethacin are many times more potent against COX-1 than COX-2. Conversely, sodium salicylate is a weak prostaglandin inhibitor and is equally potent against both COX-1 and COX-2. The anticipated rapid development of clinically useful, potent, selective COX-2 inhibitors will markedly alter the acceptability of upper GI risks with NSAID therapy and will change the clinical paradigms for their use. Other reported GI adverse effects of NSAIDs include stomatitis and diarrhea as well as rare cases of sialoadenitis, esophageal ulceration, perforation of colonic diverticula, and pancreatitis.[84]

Hepatic Effects

During prospective clinical trials reported to the FDA, 5.4 percent of patients with rheumatoid arthritis who were treated with aspirin experienced persistent elevations of results in more than one liver function test, as did 2.9 percent of patients treated with other NSAIDs.[85] Hepatic toxicity has been reported with all NSAIDs; there appears to be a higher risk with acetaminophen, diclofenac, sulindac, and phenylbutazone and a lower risk with ibuprofen and ketoprofen.[86] Patients usually have no symptoms, and discontinuation or dose reduction generally results in normalization of the transaminase values, although rare fatal outcomes have been reported with almost all NSAIDs.[86] Advanced age, decreased renal function, multiple drug use, higher drug doses, increased duration of therapy, juvenile rheumatoid arthritis, and systemic lupus erythematosus (SLE) are considered likely to increase the risk of liver toxicity from NSAIDs.[85] Prolongation of the prothrombin time and hyperbilirubinemia are poor prognostic signs and may presage progressive liver disease and possible fatal hepatic necrosis.[87] Benoxaprofen was withdrawn because of a number of fatalities related to hepatic toxicity, mostly in elderly patients receiving high doses of the drug. Phenylbutazone-induced liver injury also has resulted in a number of fatalities; hepatocellular injury, cholestasis, and granulomatous hepatitis may occur and are more common in patients older than 60 years of age.[88] Therefore, the treatment of elderly patients with phenylbutazone is not recommended. After a patient starts or changes NSAID therapy, it is prudent to monitor liver enzyme tests during the first 4 to 6 weeks.[86]

Renal Effects

The vasodilatory prostaglandins E_2 and I_2 increase or support renal blood flow and water excretion, increase sodium chloride excretion, and stimulate renin secretion. The vasoconstrictor autocoids $PGF_{2\alpha}$ and thromboxane A_2 may decrease renal function in glomerulonephritis and transplant rejection. PGE_2 and PGI_2 produced in the glomerulus have predominant effects on glomerular blood flow and filtration rate; PGI_1 produced in renal arterioles can also regulate renal blood flow. PGE_2 is synthesized by medullary interstitial cells, helping to regulate renal blood flow to the medulla; it is also synthesized in the collecting duct, where it alters the permeability of the duct to water and its responsiveness to antidiuretic hormone.[89]

Experiments in dogs showed that reductions of renal blood flow by infusion of angiotensin II or by constriction of the main renal artery are accompanied by increased synthesis of PGE_2 followed by a compensatory increase in blood flow. Simultaneous administration of an NSAID, however, markedly augments the reduction in renal blood flow associated with angiotensin II infusion, presumably by preventing the synthesis of vasodilatory PGE_2. In healthy, well-hydrated individuals with normal kidneys, PGE_2 and PGI_2 (prostacyclin) play little or no role in controlling renal function.[90, 91] Under certain conditions of local circulatory stress often associated with elevated levels of angiotensin II and catecholamines, however, locally produced vasodilatory prostaglandins become essential to the maintenance of adequate renal function.[92, 93] Experimental induction of immune glomerulonephritis in rats, as well as ureteral obstruction and renal vein occlusion, is associated with increased production of the vasoconstrictor thromboxane A_2, which contributes to chronic renal vasoconstriction in these situations.[89, 91]

With this understanding of the role of products of the cyclooxygenase pathway of arachidonic acid metabolism and renal hemodynamics, the renal effects of NSAIDs are somewhat logical. These effects are directly related to the potency of the agents in inhibiting renal prostaglandin production, as reflected by inhibition of urinary prostaglandin excretion. In predisposed subjects, suppression of compensatory prostaglandin production may result in acute reduction in renal blood flow and glomerular filtration, associated with fluid retention, edema, and elevation of serum creatinine. Patients most at risk include those with congestive heart failure, SLE, chronic glomerulonephritis, or liver failure with ascites; premature infants; and those receiving diuretics. Marked reductions in medullary blood flow may result in papillary necrosis. Cyclooxygenase inhibition may result in hyperkalemia, most commonly in patients with diabetes mellitus or mild to moderate renal insufficiency, and patients receiving β-blockers, angiotensin converting enzyme inhibitors, or potassium-sparing diuretics. Cyclooxygenase inhibition has also been associated with blunting of antihypertensive and diuretic drug effects.[94]

Considering the huge market for aspirin and NSAIDs, there are relatively few published reports of acute nephrotoxicity associated with these drugs. The ischemic type of NSAID-induced renal insufficiency tends to occur in hospitalized patients rather than in outpatients, and NSAID-induced hyperkalemia is probably more frequent than NSAID-induced acute renal insufficiency.[94]

A meta-analysis of 50 published randomized controlled clinical trials evaluated the effects of NSAIDs on blood pressure.[95] The studies included 771 subjects and nine NSAIDs. For the pooled data, the weighted increase in mean blood pressure associated with NSAID administration was 5 mm Hg (95 percent confidence interval 1.2–8.7) and weight increased by 0.3 kg, but there were no mean changes in creatinine clearance, urinary sodium, or plasma renin activity.

Several studies have suggested that sulindac—whose active sulindac sulfide metabolite is oxidized by the kidney to the inactive sulfone metabolite or to the relatively inactive prodrug sulindac—spares the kidney and is less likely to induce renal insufficiency than other NSAIDs.[96, 97] Others, however, have demonstrated sulindac-induced impairment in renal function or renal prostaglandin synthesis, particularly in more severely hemodynamically compromised patients and with higher doses of sulindac.[98–100] Therefore, great caution should be taken in the treatment of high-risk patients with any NSAID, although sulindac or a nonacetylated salicylate (which is a weak cyclooxygenase inhibitor) probably is preferable to the more potent cyclooxygenase inhibitors, such as indomethacin.

A second type of renal adverse effect to NSAIDs involves an idiosyncratic reaction accompanied by massive proteinuria and acute interstitial nephritis. Hypersensitivity phenomena, such as fever, skin rash, and eosinophilia, are occasionally present. Renal biopsy reveals focal or diffuse interstitial nephritis with a predominance of lymphocytic infiltration, although eosinophils may be present in biopsy specimens of some patients.[89, 90, 92] This syndrome has been observed with practically all NSAIDs, but the most cases have been reported with fenoprofen.[101] After the NSAID is discontinued, complete recovery of renal function eventually occurs in almost all patients; occasionally, however, dialysis or high-dose corticosteroid therapy has been necessary for the recovery of renal function.

A third possible mechanism of NSAID-induced renal toxicity may be intratubular precipitation, of uric acid in the case of suprofen or of drug metabolite in the case of benoxaprofen. The abrupt onset of severe bilateral flank pain within 2 or 3 hours after the first or second dose of suprofen—lasting 2 or 3 days and usually associated with a rise in serum creatinine, microscopic hematuria, mild proteinuria, and polyuria—was reported to the FDA in some 300 cases during 1986. Young men were most commonly affected, and the pain resolved and renal function returned to baseline within a few days to a few weeks in all patients. This syndrome has also been observed in a few patients treated with other NSAIDs. Suprofen is a potent uricosuric, but its half-life is so short that this effect lasts for only a few hours. It has been hypothesized, however, that persons with hyperuricemia, acidic urine, and low urine flow rates may precipitate uric acid crystals and produce temporary tubular obstruction. This syndrome might be avoided if patients are well hydrated before they take the first dose of NSAID, but the manufacturer has withdrawn suprofen from the market because of this adverse effect.[82] It has also been speculated that the renal failure associated with benoxaprofen therapy may have been contributed to by a similar intratubular accumulation of a metabolite of benoxaprofen that was observed to be present in the urine as microscopic globular bodies.

It is considered to be exceedingly unusual for end-stage renal failure to develop as a complication of NSAID therapy.[94, 102] Patients starting NSAID therapy should be well hydrated. Patients with predisposing diseases or who are taking predisposing drugs should be treated with the lowest effective dose of a less potent renal cyclooxygenase inhibitor and should be observed closely. Baseline serum creatinine and electrolyte levels with repeated measurements after 5 to 7 days should be assessed.[103] Particular care should be taken with hospitalized patients, who seem to be at much greater risk.[94]

Cutaneous Effects

A wide spectrum of cutaneous reactions have been associated with NSAIDs. The spontaneous adverse reaction reporting system of the American Academy of Dermatology in 1984 reported that adverse cutaneous reactions were most frequently reported with piroxicam, zomepirac, sulindac, meclofenamate sodium, and benoxaprofen.[104] Benign morbilliform eruptions, fixed drug reactions, photosensitivity reactions, vesic-

ulobullous eruptions, serum sickness, and exfoliative erythroderma have been reported. Almost all the NSAIDs have been associated with erythema multiforme, Stevens-Johnson syndrome, or toxic epidermal necrolysis. Serious or fatal dermal reactions are most commonly reported with phenylbutazone and oxyphenbutazone.[84] NSAIDs may also cause urticaria, especially in aspirin-sensitive patients. Pseudoporphyria, a photo-induced bullous dermatitis with characteristic clinical and histopathologic features, has been reported with naproxen use.[105]

Hypersensitivity Reactions

In some patients with bronchial asthma, especially those with the triad of vasomotor rhinitis, nasal polyposis, and asthma, aspirin or NSAID ingestion may precipitate an acute asthmatic attack, probably as the result of drug-related inhibition of bronchodilating prostaglandins. It is also possible that inhibition of the cyclooxygenase metabolic pathway diverts arachidonic acid metabolism toward lipoxygenase products such as the SRSA (LTC_4 and LTD_4), which may precipitate bronchospasm.[106] Patients who exhibit this reaction generally are sensitive to all NSAIDs and should avoid them. Anaphylactoid reactions have been reported with many of the NSAIDs, especially tolmetin and zomepirac, and zomepirac has been withdrawn from the market because of this adverse effect.[84] The risk of anaphylaxis appears to be accentuated for those who use NSAIDs intermittently for relief of pain.[107]

Hematologic Effects

Aplastic anemia, agranulocytosis, and thrombocytopenia rarely are associated with NSAIDs, but are prominent among the causes of deaths attributed to these drugs. Based on Inman's estimate of 22 deaths due to blood dyscrasia per million patients[108] and FDA estimates of 16 deaths per million,[109] phenylbutazone is not recommended for initial use for any condition. The risk is about sixfold higher in women over age 60.[109] Scattered reports of blood dyscrasias associated with other NSAIDs have been published, but a large case-control study showed an association only for indomethacin and for phenylbutazone, with excess risk rates of 10.1 and 6.6 per million, respectively.[110] In view of the rarity of these problems and their unpredictable nature, monitoring for their occurrence with frequent routine blood cell counts is not mandatory, although it should be strongly considered if phenylbutazone or oxyphenbutazone is used in women older than 60 years of age.

NSAIDs reversibly impair platelet aggregation by inhibiting platelet cyclooxygenase, thereby blocking synthesis of thromboxane A_2. This effect persists only as long as the drug is present, but it can increase the severity of GI bleeding in patients taking NSAIDs.

Preoperatively, NSAIDs should be discontinued for a long enough time before surgery to permit complete excretion of the drug—generally four or five times the half-life for excretion of the drug (see Table 45–4). Thus, drugs with a short half-life, such as tolmetin or ibuprofen, can be discontinued 18 to 24 hours preoperatively, whereas drugs with a long half-life, such as piroxicam, should be discontinued about 8 days before surgery. Salsalate and nabumetone are exceptions, in that they are reported not to inhibit platelet aggregation.[111, 112] Because they may still cause GI irritation or bleeding by other mechanisms, however, they probably should still be withheld during surgery.

Central Nervous System Effects

Headaches and giddiness occur in patients taking indomethacin, and dizziness, confusion, depression, drowsiness, hallucinations, depersonalization reactions, seizures, and syncopy also have been reported. Elderly patients taking naproxen or ibuprofen have experienced cognitive dysfunction, memory loss, inability to concentrate, confusion, personality change, forgetfulness, depression, sleeplessness, irritability, light-headedness, and paranoid ideation. An acute aseptic meningitis, perhaps an unusual type of hypersensitivity reaction, has been reported in patients with SLE or mixed connective tissue disease treated with ibuprofen, sulindac, tolmetin, or naproxen.[113, 114]

Other Adverse Effects

Pulmonary edema has been reported with phenylbutazone, and pulmonary infiltrates have been reported with naproxen. Gynecomastia has been associated with sulindac, alopecia with ibuprofen, and goiter with oxyphenbutazone.

Overdoses of Nonsteroidal Anti-inflammatory Drugs

Acute overdoses of NSAIDs are much less toxic than are overdoses of aspirin or salicylate. This subject has been most carefully evaluated for ibuprofen, prompted by its approval for over-the-counter sale to the general public. Two hundred one cases of ibuprofen overdose have been reported by two poison control centers.[115, 116] Most patients did not have symptoms; those who did experienced them within 4 hours of drug ingestion. One child and one elderly woman died. Symptoms, with overdoses ranging up to 40 g, include central nervous system depression, seizures, apnea, nystagmus, blurred vision, diplopia, headache, tinnitus, bradycardia, hypotension, abdominal pain, nausea, vomiting, hematuria, abnormal renal function, coma, and cardiac arrest. Treatment includes evacuation of the stomach contents, observation, and administration of fluids. Additional information about poisoning due to specific NSAIDs is available in an encyclopedic review by Vale and Meridith.[117]

Adverse Effects of Colchicine

Colchicine does not share the adverse effects of NSAIDs that depend on the ability to suppress cyclooxygenase. About 80 percent of patients who take a full oral therapeutic dose of colchicine experience cramping abdominal pain, diarrhea, nausea, or vomiting, and these symptoms usually limit the dosage that can be given for acute gout. With chronic maintenance therapy, bone marrow depression, peripheral neuritis, hair loss, amenorrhea, dysmenorrhea, oligospermia, and azoospermia have been reported.[37] Colchicine should not be used in patients with inflammatory bowel disease or in pregnant or breast-feeding patients. It should be avoided or used with great caution and in reduced dosages in patients with hepatic or renal dysfunction because it is excreted by the liver and the kidney.

Colchicine overdoses are associated with more severe and more diffuse toxic manifestations. Gastrointestinal effects include hemorrhage, dehydration, hypokalemia, metabolic acidosis, and renal shutdown. Shock may occur as the result of profound dehydration or gram-negative septicemia associated with the GI irritation. Hepatocellular failure, seizures, myopathy, hypocalcemia, stomatitis, and coma may occur. Death has occurred with as little as 8 mg but is invariable after the ingestion of more than 40 mg. Treatment includes aspiration of the stomach, intensive support measures, and hemodialysis, although there is no evidence that colchicine can be removed by dialysis. Patients for whom colchicine is prescribed should be strongly advised to keep the medication in childproof containers and to store it in areas that are not accessible to irresponsible individuals.[37]

EFFECTS OF CONCOMITANT DRUGS, DISEASES, AGING, AND PATIENT CHARACTERISTICS

In view of the extensive use of NSAIDs under both prescription and nonprescription conditions for a wide variety of complaints and the substantial pharmacologic activity of these compounds, there are opportunities for the occurrence of almost any conceivable interaction of these drugs with other factors within the patients. Drug-drug and drug-disease interactions with NSAIDs have been reviewed in detail by Brater.[118]

Drug-Drug Interactions

Table 45–2 provides a partial list of potential interactions involving NSAIDs. The degree to which individual patients exhibit these interactions varies considerably, but the risks should be considered when one is prescribing potentially interacting drug combinations.

Table 45–2. SOME DRUG-DRUG INTERACTIONS INVOLVING NONSTEROIDAL ANTI-INFLAMMATORY DRUGS (NSAIDS)

Perturbed Drug	Perturbing Drug	Effect	Suggested Action
Salicylate	Antacids	Increased urine pH results in increased excretion with decreased salicylate levels	Review need for antacid. Select another NSAID.
Warfarin and other anticoagulants	Phenylbutazone Oxyphenbutazone	Significant prolongation of prothrombin time due to inhibition of warfarin catabolism	Beware all NSAIDS and aspirin. Avoid phenylbutazone, oxyphenbutazone, and aspirin. Ibuprofen, naproxen, and tolmetin are relatively safer.
	All NSAIDs	Increased risk of bleeding due to anticoagulant inhibition of platelet function and gastric mucosal damage	
Sulfonylurea	Phenylbutazone	Risk of hypoglycemia due to inhibition of sulfonylurea metabolism	Choose alternative NSAID.
	High-dose salicylate	Potentiation of hypoglycemia by different mechanism	Choose alternative NSAID.
β-Blocker	All prostaglandin-inhibiting NSAIDs	Blunting of hypotensive effect but not of negative chronotropic or inotropic effect	Avoid phenylbutazone, indomethacin, aspirin. Review need for, and use of, minimum dose of NSAID (especially in elderly or renally impaired patients).
Peripheral vasodilators Hydralazine Prazosin	All prostaglandin-inhibiting NSAIDs	Loss of hypotensive effect	Adjust dose of hypotensive agent for desired effect.
Angiotensin converting enzyme inhibitor	All prostaglandin-inhibiting NSAIDs	Loss of hypotensive effect	Adjust dose of hypotensive agent for desired effect.
Diuretics	All prostaglandin-inhibiting NSAIDs	Loss of natriuretic, diuretic, hypotensive effects of furosemide Loss of natriuretic effect of spironolactone Loss of hypotensive but not natriuretic or diuretic effects of thiazide	Thiazide may be preferred diuretic. Sulindac may enhance hypotensive effects of thiazide. Newer NSAIDs interact less.
Salicylate	Glucocorticoids	Increased salicylate metabolism resulting in lowered plasma salicylate level	Use minimum doses of glucocorticoids. Adjust salicylate dose or choose alternative NSAID. Check salicylate levels after changes in glucocorticoid dose.
Lithium	Many NSAIDs	Increased plasma lithium levels	Elderly and renal disease patients are more susceptible. Review need for NSAID. Use minimum dose of NSAID. Reduce lithium dose and monitor plasma lithium levels. Aspirin and sulindac may be preferred.
Methotrexate	Salicylates, phenylbutazone, other NSAIDs, probenecid	Increased methotrexate levels due to decreased renal clearance of methotrexate	Reduce dose substantially. Use another NSAID. Monitor plasma methotrexate with high doses.
Phenytoin	Phenylbutazone, oxyphenbutazone	Increased phenytoin toxicity by decreased metabolism of phenytoin	Use alternative NSAIDs. Monitor phenytoin plasma levels.
	Salicylate, ibuprofen	Displacement of active phenytoin	
Carbonic anhydrase inhibitor	Salicylate	Metabolic acidosis	Use alternative NSAID.
NSAIDs	Probenecid	Impaired or prolonged NSAID excretion; increased potential for toxicity	Adjust dose of NSAID.
Probenecid, sulfinpyrazone	Salicylate (low dose)	Inhibition of uricosuria	Choose alternative NSAID.

Table continued on following page

Table 45–2. SOME DRUG-DRUG INTERACTIONS INVOLVING NONSTEROIDAL ANTI-INFLAMMATORY DRUGS (NSAIDS) *Continued*

Perturbed Drug	Perturbing Drug	Effect	Suggested Action
NSAIDs	Aspirin	Reduced blood levels of many NSAIDs	Avoid concomitant use of aspirin with other NSAIDs.
Digoxin	Aspirin, several NSAIDs	Possibly increased digoxin levels	Monitor digoxin levels. Use minimum dose of NSAID.
NSAIDs	Omeprazole, histamine blockers	Decreased gastric acid secretion	Use cytoprotective drugs in elderly patients or those with peptic ulcer disease or dyspepsia.
	Misoprostol	Replacement of prostaglandin E in stomach	
Piroxicam	Cimetidine	Increased plasma concentrations and half-life of piroxicam	Decrease piroxicam dose.

Data from Johnson AG, Seideman P, Day RO. NSAID-related adverse drug interactions with clinical relevance: An update. Int J Clin Pharmacol Ther 32:509–532, 1994; and Gelman CR, Hess AJ, Rumack BH (eds): DRUGDEX Information System, Micromedix, Inc, Englewood, Col, 1996.

Except for nabumetone and proquazone, the NSAIDs as a group are well absorbed when administered orally. With few exceptions, concomitant food or antacid intake delays the absorption of NSAIDs but does not alter the area under the curve or overall bioavailability to any significant extent. Concomitant administration of food does, however, improve the absorption and bioavailability of nabumetone and proquazone, whereas concomitant administration of aluminum-containing antacids decreases the total absorption of diflunisal.

Because most NSAIDs bind firmly to plasma proteins, they may displace other drugs from binding sites or may themselves be displaced by other agents. Aspirin and other NSAIDs may thus increase the activity or toxicity of sulfonylurea hypoglycemic agents, oral anticoagulants, phenytoin, sulfonamides, and methotrexate by displacing these drugs from their protein binding site and increasing the free fraction of the drug in plasma.[119] Of the available NSAIDs, the ones least likely to interact with warfarin to accentuate anticoagulation include diclofenac, flurbiprofen, ibuprofen, kerotalac, tolmetin, and naproxen (see Tables 45–3 to 45–5). The NSAIDs least likely to interact with oral hypoglycemic agents to accentuate hypoglycemia are diclofenac, etodolac, fenoprofen, flurbiprofen, ibuprofen, indomethacin, ketoprofen, kerotalac, meclofenamate, tolmetin, diflunisal, naproxen, and sulindac. Caution or avoidance should be exercised if one is considering the use of other NSAIDs with warfarin or hypoglycemics. Similarly, salicylate may compete with other NSAIDs for protein binding sites, thereby decreasing their serum level when use concomitantly.[120] In most cases, however, the increase in the unbound concentration of the displaced drug is transient because increased excretion or distribution to other tissue sites results in a new steady state in which the concentration of unbound drug is the same as it was before the displacement occurred.[118]

Drug interactions also may occur if one drug interferes with the metabolism or excretion of another drug. By this mechanism, probenecid impairs the excretion of many NSAIDs, and steady-state lithium levels may increase when probenecid is given concomitantly with NSAIDs.[119] Induction of the hepatic microsomal enzyme system by phenylbutazone may induce the metabolism of digitoxin, dicumarol, and hexobarbital. Phenylbutazone also may inhibit the metabolism of carbamazepine, phenobarbital, phenytoin, tolbutamide, and warfarin.[118] As organic acids, NSAIDs may inhibit the secretion of other organic acids by the secretory pump of the proximal nephron and thus may decrease their renal clearance. This may be important with methotrexate, whose excretion is inhibited by salicylate and probenecid and is potentially inhibitable by fenoprofen, naproxen, phenylbutazone, and tolmetin.[118]

As discussed earlier, suppression of renal prostaglandins by NSAIDs during administration of a loop diuretic may result in a decrease in natriuresis by preventing prostaglandin-induced increases in renal blood flow in response to the loop diuretic. For the most part, NSAIDs do not affect the diuretic response to thiazides.[118] Reversible acute renal failure and hyperkalemia may occur, however, when indomethacin and triamterene are combined.[121]

For unclear reasons, NSAIDs may blunt the antihypertensive effects of β-blockers, angiotensin converting inhibitors, and thiazides.[118] Ethanol potentiates the GI toxicity of NSAIDs. Enhanced bleeding also may occur in patients receiving both NSAIDs and anticoagulants. The combination of NSAID-induced GI irritation and impaired hemostasis makes GI bleeding more serious.

Only a tiny fraction of the possible combinations of NSAIDs with other drugs have been examined carefully. Therefore, one should exercise caution when initiating multiple drug therapy and should carefully observe the patient for unexpected interactions.

Drug-Disease Interactions (Table 45–3)

Conditions that decrease serum albumin concentrations, decrease NSAID binding to proteins, or impair

Table 45–3. SOME DRUG-DISEASE INTERACTIONS INVOLVING NONSTEROIDAL ANTI-INFLAMMATORY DRUGS (NSAIDS)

	Interaction of NSAID with Disease States and Therapy						Dosage Adjustment of NSAID Needed for Concomitant Therapy				
	HTN*	Anti-HTN Therapy*	Renal ADR*	PUD*	Platelet Inhibition*	Aspirin Hypersensitivity*	Warfarin	Hypo-glycemia	Renal Failure	Hepatic Failure	Elderly (>70 yr)
Minimal PG inhibition											
1. Nonacetylated salicylate	0	0	0	±	0	0	Caut	Caut	Caut	Caut	None
Minimal renal PG inhibition											
1. Sulindac	0	0	±	+	+	+	Caut	None	Decr	Decr	Decr
PG inhibition short half life											
1. Aspirin	±	±	±	+ +	+ +	+ +	Caut	Caut	Caut	Caut	None
2. Diclofenac	+	+	+	+	+	+	None	None	None	None	None
3. Etodalac	+	+	+	+	+	+	ID	None	None	ID	None
4. Fenoprofen	+	+	+ +	+	+	+	Caut	None	None	ID	None
5. Flurbiprofen	+	+	+	+	+	+	None	None	None	Avoid	None
6. Ibuprofen	+	+	+	+	+	+	None	None	ID	ID	None
7. Indomethacin	+	+	+ +	+	+	+	Caut	None	None	ID	None
8. Ketoprofen	+	+	+	+	+	+	Caut	None	Decr	Decr	Decr
9. Ketoralac	+	+	+	+	+	+	None	None	Decr	ID	Decr
10. Meclofenamate	+	+	+	+	+	+	Caut	None	None	ID	None
11. Tolmetin	+	+	+	+	+	+	None	None	None	ID	ID
PG Inhibition long half life											
1. Diflunisal	+	+	+	+	+	+	Caut	None	Decr	ID	None
2. Nabumetone	+	+	+	+	0	+	ID	ID	Decr	Avoid	Decr
3. Naproxen	Min	+	±	+	+	+	None	None	Decr	Decr	Decr
4. Oxaprozin	+	+	+	+	+	+	Caut	ID	Decr	Decr	None
5. Phenylbutazone	+	+	+	+	+	+	Avoid	Avoid	Decr	Avoid	None
6. Piroxicam	+	+	+	+	+	+	Caut	ID	None	Decr	Decr
7. Tenidap	+	+	+	+	+	+	Caut	ID	ID	ID	None

Data from Gelman CR, Hess AJ, Rumack BH (eds). DRUGDEX Information System, Micromedix, Inc, Englewood, Col, 1996.
*Involves prostaglandin inhibition.
Abbreviations: Caut, cautious use; ID, insufficent data; Decr, decreased dose; none, no change in dose needed; HTN, hypertension; ADR, adverse drug reaction; PUD, peptic ulcer disease; Minimal; PG, prostaglandin.

drug metabolism or excretion by the liver or kidneys may alter the expected response of the patient to a given dose of NSAID. Most studies have shown no significant effect of rheumatoid arthritis on the clearance of NSAIDs. However, cirrhosis can both decrease serum albumin concentrations and impair hepatic metabolism of drugs.

With sulindac, the predominant effect of cirrhosis was a four-fold increase in the area under the curve of sulindac sulfide because of impairment of biliary excretion of this active metabolite; therefore, the sulindac dosage in cirrhotic patients should be only one fourth the normal dose. With naproxen, clearance of unbound drug is impaired although clearance of total drug is unchanged by cirrhosis, and patients should receive half the normal dose of naproxen.[118]

Patients with cirrhosis also may have increased susceptibility to the nephrotoxic effects of NSAIDs because maintenance of renal blood flow is more likely to depend on renal synthesis of prostaglandins in patients with portal hypertension and ascites. Thus, the changes in the pharmacokinetics of some NSAIDs in cirrhosis and the possibility of severe adverse consequences due to inhibition of prostaglandin synthesis in these patients mandate extreme caution in the use of these agents in cirrhotic patients.

Renal insufficiency is associated with a decrease in serum albumin concentrations and displacement of NSAIDs from protein binding sites by accumulated endogenous organic acids. In addition, drugs such as azapropazone and nabumetone, which to a considerable extent are excreted unchanged in urine, may have decreased drug clearance associated with decreases in creatinine clearance. Studies in patients with renal insufficiency indicate that no change in dose is necessary for diclofenac, fenoprofen, ibuprofen, indomethacin, meclofenamate, tolmetin, piroxicam, fenbufen, or etodolac. Unbound drug concentrations of naproxen and oxaprozin are doubled in patients with moderate to severe renal insufficiency, and for these drugs, doses should be half the normal amount.[118]

NSAID Use in the Elderly

Various physiologic, pharmacokinetic, and pharmacodynamic changes occur with increased age. Drug absorption is not altered, but drug distribution may be significantly changed as the result of a decrease in total body water and lean mass and an increase in body fat. In the elderly, age-related reductions in hepatic mass, blood flow, and enzymatic activity, renal plasma flow, glomerular filtration rate, and tubular function may contribute to decreased drug clearance.[113] In addition, the elderly appear to be more susceptible to the development of adverse drug reactions. They have more illnesses and take more medications compared with younger patients, and they use more over-the-counter medications; thus, they are at greater risk for drug-drug interactions. They are more likely to self-medicate and may be more likely to make mistakes in the timing or quantity of drug doses. The effect of age on the pharmacokinetics of some NSAIDs has been studied. Brater suggested that doses of naproxen, ketoprofen, and oxaprozin should be halved in the elderly but that ibuprofen and etodolac require no dosage adjustment.[118] Conclusions about the effect of aging on piroxicam disposition are conflicting,[118, 122] but discretion suggests some decrease in dosage in the elderly.

Increased attention to the aging process has emphasized the heterogeneity of older persons and the need to individualize one's approach to them. Healthy, well-nourished elderly individuals are vastly different from sick, malnourished persons for whom death is rapidly approaching. In general, greater care must be taken when treating elderly patients with NSAIDs, since increased toxicity may occur as the result of unanticipated clinically important changes in responses to drugs related to concomitant diseases, other medications, or subclinical changes in organ function.

Individual Variability in Responses to Nonsteroidal Antirheumatic Drugs

One of the most striking findings in all careful evaluations of nonsteroidal antirheumatic drugs is the wide range of responses among the patients studied, regardless of what variable is being measured. This is immediately apparent to the investigator who is dealing with the raw data but tends to be obscured in the statistical analysis and by the generalizations needed to produce a concise report. Four- to five-fold differences between subjects are frequently observed in plasma half-life and other pharmacokinetic measurements in patients who have been given the same weight-adjusted dose of the drug. In the evaluation of the efficacy of established NSAIDs, responses invariably range from marked improvement to no response or even clinical deterioration. Similarly, only rarely is one able to predict which patients will experience adverse effects to a particular drug; even when a subgroup at greater risk for an adverse effect can be identified, the adverse effect will actually occur in only a proportion of the patients at higher risk. Given the genetic, dietary, and environmental diversity of humans, this wide range of individual responses is not surprising. Genetic influences have been demonstrated in the metabolism of salicylate and phenylbutazone[123, 124] and no doubt are also factors with other drugs as well. The character and degree of inflammation being treated vary from patient to patient even when the diagnosis is the same for each patient. Concomitant drugs and environmental factors may have variable or contradictory influences on drug pharmacokinetics or pharmacodynamics. Because it is impossible to control for or even to know all of the factors impinging on the responses of a particular patient to a drug, one must be cautious in initiating treatment and increasing dosage and must maintain close communication with, and careful observation of, each patient.

DISTINCTIVE CHARACTERISTICS OF INDIVIDUAL DRUGS

The following discussion highlights important individual characteristics of selected nonsteroidal antirheumatic drugs. Characteristics that conform to the general properties of this class of drugs, as described earlier, are not repeated in the individual descriptions. As a first source for additional information about individual drugs, the reader is directed to the current package insert for that drug, or its reproduction in the *Physician's Desk Reference*. No longer a throwaway item, the package inserts for the NSAIDs have been refined to the point where they represent the most current and reliable conservative summaries of the information known about the drugs. They reflect not only published information but also all of the unpublished information in the manufacturer's files and additional information about adverse effects in the FDA's files. Especially useful are the quantitative estimates of the frequency of adverse effects associated with the drug and the advice about dosage for approved conditions. Unfortunately, there is no information about use of the drug for indications that have not yet been approved by the FDA, even though these may be well established in clinical practice.

The language of the package insert is arrived at by negotiation between representatives of the manufacturer and the FDA. Determination of this language is taken very seriously because drug company representatives are not allowed to deviate from this language in promoting the drug. Negotiations over the precise wording of the insert are, to a considerable extent, responsible for delays in the marketing of new drugs, as the manufacturer attempts to increase the flexibility of the language and the FDA attempts to preserve its accuracy.

It is useful to group the nonsteroidal antirheumatic drugs according to their half-life. Those with a long half-life can be given once or twice a day; those with a short half-life should be given every 4 to 6 hours if one wishes to obtain maximal anti-inflammatory effects.

NONSTEROIDAL ANTIRHEUMATIC DRUGS WITH A LONG HALF-LIFE

Drugs with a half-life of 12 hours or more can be administered once or twice daily (Table 45–4). Because five half-lives are required to approach steady

Table 45–4. NONSTEROIDAL ANTI-INFLAMMATORY DRUGS (NSAIDS) WITH LONG HALF-LIVES

Drug	Available Formulations (mg)	Maximal Daily Dose (mg)	Active Metabolite	% Bound	T_{max} (hr)	$T_{1/2}$ (hr)	Time to Steady State (days)	Renal Excretion Unchanged Drug (% Dose)	Changes in dose for			Influence on NSAID Efficacy by		Influence of NSAID on Toxicity of	
									Renal Failure	Hepatic Disease	Elderly	Food	Antacid	Warfarin	Hypoglycemic Agents
Diflunisal (Dolobid)	Tabs: 250, 500	1000	—	99	2–3	7–15	3–9	<3	Decrease by 50% with GFR <10 ml/min	ID	None	None	Aluminum decreases absorption	Caution	None
Nabumetone (Relafen)	Tabs: 500, 750	2000	6-Methoxy-2-naphthyl acetic acid	99	3–6	24	3–7	<1	Probably decrease	Avoid in severe	Limit to 1 g/day	Increase total absorption	None	ID	ID
Naproxen (Naprosyn, Aleve, Anaprox)	Tabs: 220, 250, 375, 500	1500	—	99	2–4	12–15	4–5	<5	Decrease dose with GFR <20 ml/min	Decrease dose by 50% with chronic liver disease	Probably decrease	None	None	None	None
Oxaprozin (Daypro)	Caplet 600	1800	—	>99 (decrease to 72–82 in renal failure)	3–6	49–60	4–7	4–5	Decrease to 600 mg daily	Decrease dose in severe liver disease	None	None	None	None	ID
Phenylbutazone (Butazolidin)	Tabs, caps: 100	400	Oxyphenbutazone	>90	2–8	29–140	7–15	5	Avoid with GFR <20 ml/min	Avoid	None	ID	ID	Avoid	Avoid
Piroxicam (Feldene)	Caps: 10, 20	20	—	99	2–5	30–86	7–21	<10	None	Decrease dose	Limit to 20 mg/day	None	None	Caution	
Sulindac (Clinoril)	Tabs: 150, 200	400	Sulfide	98	2–4	16–18 (sulfide) 7 (sulindac)	3	<7	Decrease by 50% with GFR <10 ml/min	Decrease dose	Probably decrease	None	ID	Caution	None
Tenidap	Not available	120	—	>99	0.6–5.8	12–48	11	ID	ID	ID	None	None	Decrease total absorption (Maalox)	Caution	None

Data from Gelman CR, Hess AJ, Rumack BH (eds), DRUGDEX Information System, Micromedix, Inc, Englewood, Col, 1996.
Abbreviations: T_{max}, time to maximum absorption; $T_{1/2}$, half-life; GFR, glomerular filtration rate; ID, insufficient data.

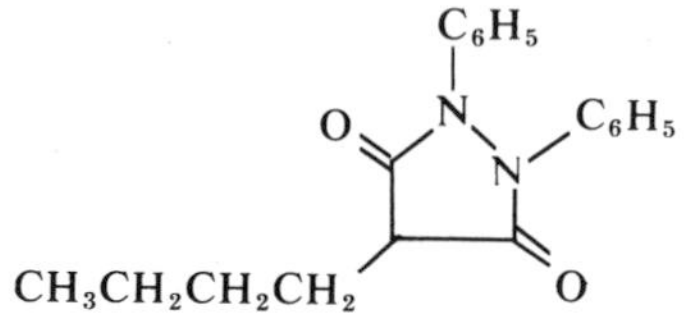

Figure 45–3. Chemical structure of phenylbutazone.

state, plasma concentrations of these drugs continue to rise for 3 days to several weeks, depending on the half-life, but thereafter tend to be fairly stable between doses. The long half-life allows ample time for equilibration of drug between plasma and synovial fluid, and synovial fluid concentrations of unbound drug usually are equal to those in plasma, whereas the sum of the bound and unbound drug concentrations is lower in synovial fluid, reflecting the lower quantity of albumin in the synovial fluid. Individual variations in drug disposition or excretion are more likely to result in excessive accumulation of drug and potentially serious side effects if the half-life is long than if it is short, although the long half-life itself does not increase the inherent toxicity of the compound. Although it might be anticipated that monitoring plasma concentrations of these drugs would be helpful in avoiding problems and although drug concentrations are easily determined, this technique has not yet been applied to routine clinical practice.

Phenylbutazone

Phenylbutazone is an exceptionally effective NSAID (Fig. 45–3) and still has a loyal following among patients who did not respond to other therapies; however, it is no longer recommended as initial therapy for any indication (and oxyphenbutazone has been withdrawn from the market by its major manufacturer) because of its well-documented serious and sometimes fatal adverse reactions, as well as the increasing availability of alternative NSAIDs.[109, 110, 125]

Naproxen

Naproxen is the active D(+) isomer of 6-methoxy-α-methyl-2-naphthaleneacetic acid (Fig. 45–4). The inactive L(−) isomer is not contained in naproxen. Naproxen is rapidly and completely absorbed after oral administration; with twice daily administration, steady-state concentrations are achieved in 4 or 5 days. It is readily absorbed rectally, but suppository preparations are not marketed in the United States. As with most NSAIDs, food and antacids do not alter the completeness of absorption but may change the rate of absorption to some extent.[126] In addition to the parent compound, naproxen is also available as naproxen sodium (Anaprox) which is more rapidly absorbed, with peak levels at 1 to 2 hours, and as

enteric-coated tablets, which are more slowly absorbed (primarily in the small intestine), with peak levels at about 4 to 6 hours. Total absorption and elimination kinetics are not different from those of naproxen itself.[127]

Protein binding of naproxen decreases with single doses greater than 500 mg; the resulting disproportionate increases in concentrations of unbound drug are associated with increases in excretion rates. Thus, single doses higher than 500 mg are not associated with proportionate increases in bioavailable naproxen. Naproxen does not accumulate in tissues; it has a low volume of distribution, and most of it remains in the plasma compartment bound to plasma proteins.

Naproxen is cleared from plasma predominantly by metabolism to glucuronide and other conjugates of naproxen, and by 6-desmethylation with subsequent conjugation of this metabolite. Almost all of the ingested drug is excreted in the urine, predominantly as inactive metabolites and conjugates.[126] Moderate renal failure has little effect on naproxen kinetics, but severe renal failure decreases naproxen protein binding, doubling unbound drug concentrations and increasing the volume of distribution. Although intrinsic clearance of the drug by hepatic metabolism increases, naproxen doses should be halved if the glomerular filtration rate is less than 20 mg/minute.[128] Patients with severe hepatic disease eliminate naproxen less rapidly because they do not metabolize it as well.[126] In one study, patients with alcoholic cirrhosis had a 60 percent decrease in clearance of unbound naproxen. Therefore, it has been suggested that naproxen doses should be halved in these patients.[129] Fluid levels of naproxen in synovial samples are lower than those in simultaneous specimens of plasma.[130]

The efficacy of naproxen has been demonstrated in rheumatoid arthritis, osteoarthritis, ankylosing spondylitis, tendonitis, bursitis, and acute gout. The drug is also effective in juvenile rheumatoid arthritis and primary dysmenorrhea, and its sodium salt has been marketed as an analgesic and for the treatment of dysmenorrhea.[131] The usual starting dose of naproxen is 250 to 500 mg every 12 hours with meals, but doses as high as 1500 mg daily have been used in patients with rheumatoid arthritis without apparent increase in toxicity. Clinical efficacy has been demonstrated to correlate with plasma naproxen concentrations in one study.[132] Seventy-six percent of patients responded when serum naproxen concentrations were greater than 50 μg/ml, whereas no patients responded to concentrations less than 18 μg/ml, when specimens

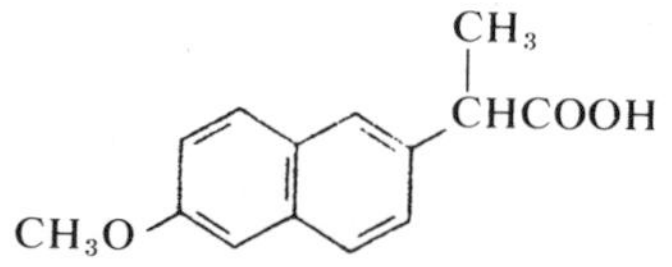

Figure 45–4. Chemical structure of naproxen.

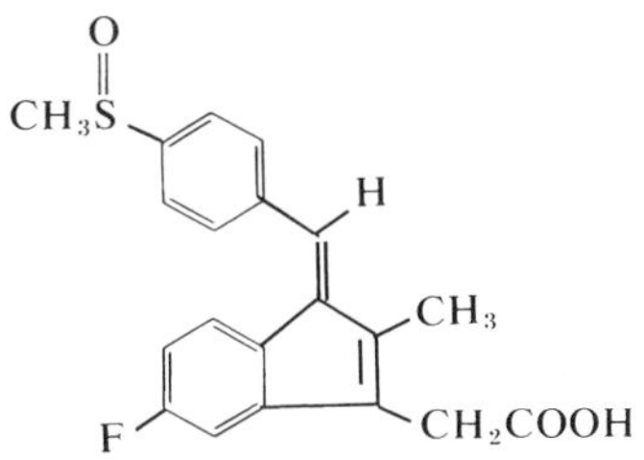

Figure 45–5. Chemical structure of sulindac.

were taken just before the next dose. Naproxen sodium has been approved as an over-the-counter analgesic (Aleve, 220-mg tablets).

The adverse effects of naproxen are typical of those described for NSAIDs. They occur less frequently than with aspirin or indomethacin, but essentially all of the class-related adverse effects have been observed with this drug. Gastric irritation is more likely to occur with higher doses.[126]

Aspirin decreases naproxen serum concentrations, probably as a result of its displacement from protein binding sites by aspirin.[126] Probenecid, 500 mg four times a day, increased the plasma half-life of a single 500-mg naproxen dose from 14 hours to 37 hours and increased steady-state naproxen concentrations by 50 percent. It decreased naproxen plasma clearance both by inhibiting naproxen glucuronide formation and by decreasing renal clearance of naproxen.[133]

Concurrent administration of naproxen, 500 mg daily, plus aspirin, 3.25 g daily, was more effective than aspirin alone in rheumatoid arthritis in one study[134]; in another study, however, the efficacy of naproxen, 1500 mg daily, was not increased by adding nonacetylated salicylate in a dose sufficient to produce average plasma salicylate concentrations of 23.5 mg/dl.[135] Indeed, naproxen, 1500 mg daily, was marginally more effective and was less toxic than this high dose of salicylate.

Sulindac

Sulindac is an indene–acetic acid derivative chemically related to indomethacin and is a prodrug (Fig. 45–5).[136] The minimally active parent drug sulindac, a sulfoxide, is reversibly metabolized to sulindac sulfide, a potent cyclooxygenase inhibitor with a half-life of 16 to 18 hours. Sulindac is also irreversibly metabolized to the inactive sulfone metabolite. Sulindac and its metabolites undergo extensive enterohepatic recirculation.[137, 138] Twenty-five to 30 percent of the dose is excreted in the stool, primarily as the sulfone and sulfide metabolites. About 50 percent of the administered dose is excreted in the urine, almost entirely as the sulfone, the sulfoxide, and sulindac glucuronide.[137] Less than 1 percent is excreted in the urine as the active sulindac sulfide. The long half-life for the biologic activity of this drug is attributed to its enterohepatic recirculation and the reversible

interconversion between the active sulfide and the parent sulfoxide. However, substantial interindividual differences have been reported in drug disposition, plasma concentrations, and areas under the plasma concentration–time curves in patients given sulindac.[139]

The adverse effects profile of sulindac is also thought to be influenced by the interrelationship of the inactive prodrug and its active metabolite. In contrast to other NSAIDs, sulindac has a relatively low incidence of gastric abnormalities in gastroscopic studies, presumably because of the lack of local cyclooxygenase suppression by the prodrug in the stomach.[67] Animal studies demonstrate that GI toxicity is proportional to the amount of sulindac sulfide in the GI tract.[140] If none of the active metabolite is present in the gut, GI toxicity should be very low. Unfortunately, significant amounts of sulfide are present in the stool, and sulindac has exhibited the usual range of GI toxicities in clinical use, including ulcers, bleeding, and diarrhea.

Similarly, absence of the active metabolite in the urine due to its conversion to sulfoxide by the kidney has been proposed as a mechanism to prevent acute renal toxicity mediated by cyclooxygenase inhibition. This was discussed in the earlier text on renal side effects of NSAIDs, but one cannot be sanguine in using sulindac in predisposed patients because acute renal toxicity has been observed in some patients taking sulindac, despite its theoretical advantages.[99]

Dimethyl sulfoxide (DMSO) decreases plasma levels of sulindac sulfide and has also been reported to cause peripheral neuropathy; it should not be used with sulindac. Salicylate and diflunisal decrease plasma levels of sulindac sulfide, and their concurrent use is not advised.[138] Clinically significant interactions do not seem to occur between sulindac and tolbutamide, warfarin, probenecid, propoxyphene, or acetaminophen.

Sulindac's clinical efficacy profile is similar to that of other NSAIDs. The maximum recommended dose is 200 mg twice daily.

Diflunisal

Difluorophenyl salicylic acid, diflunisal, differs from most other salicylic acids derivatives, in that it is not metabolized to salicylate (Fig. 45–6). It lacks an acetyl group, but it is more potent than aspirin in studies evaluating small animals, of its analgesic, antiinflammatory, and antipyretic activities.[141] Diflunisal

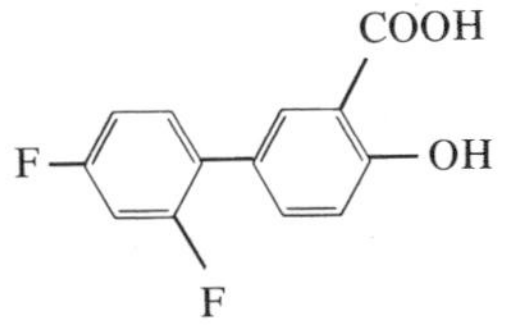

Figure 45–6. Chemical structure of diflunisal.

resembles aspirin more than salicylate in the potency of its inhibition of cyclooxygenase, but because it lacks the acetyl group, this inhibition is reversible. Nevertheless, pretreatment with diflunisal can prevent the acetylation of cyclooxygenase by aspirin. Whereas aspirin irreversibly acetylates cyclooxygenase and salicylate does not inhibit this enzyme at all in moderate concentrations, diflunisal reversibly inhibits it, as do indomethacin and most other NSAIDs. It is 99 percent bound to albumin at moderate concentrations of drug, but is displaced during renal failure when the unbound fraction can increase by as much as 370 percent.[142]

As for other salicylic acid derivatives, the pharmacokinetics of diflunisal are concentration-dependent. Thus, the plasma half-life following administration of 125 mg of diflunisal twice daily is 7 or 8 hours, but this increases to 15 hours after 500 mg twice daily. Steady-state plasma levels are achieved after 3 to 9 days and increase disproportionately as the dose is increased. Ninety-five percent of ingested drug is excreted in the urine as glucuronide metabolites.[142]

Diflunisal may prolong the prothrombin time in patients taking oral anticoagulants, but it does not interact with tolbutamide. Pharmacokinetic interactions occur with hydrochlorothiazide, acetaminophen, aspirin, sulindac, naproxen, and indomethacin, but the clinical significance of these interactions is uncertain.[142] Co-administration of diflunisal and indomethacin has been associated with fatal GI hemorrhage, and this combination should be avoided.[143] In patients with severe renal failure, total body clearance and protein binding of diflunisal were decreased and its plasma half-life was markedly increased.[144]

Diflunisal is useful for the full range of NSAID indications. Similarly, the full range of NSAID adverse effects have been observed with it. Because of the dose-related disproportionate increases in plasma concentrations and plasma half-lives and the decrease in clearance associated with renal insufficiency, one must take particular care when increasing the dose beyond the recommended maximum of 1000 mg daily, and doses should be decreased in patients with renal insufficiency.

Piroxicam

Piroxicam is a member of the oxicam family of enolic acids (Fig. 45–7). It is marketed worldwide and was first introduced in the United States in 1982. It is a potent inhibitor of cyclooxygenase but has no effect on lipoxygenase.[145] Its pharmacologic activity is similar to that of other cyclooxygenase inhibitors, but it may be a more effective inhibitor of superoxide generation in vitro by stimulated neutrophils.[146]

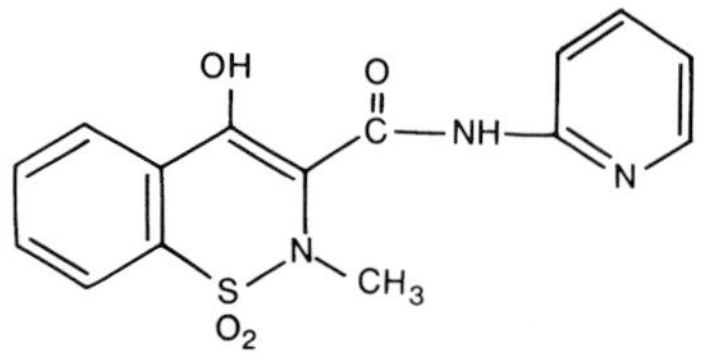

Piroxicam is slowly cleared from plasma by metabolism, with an average plasma half-life of about 38 hours and a wide range of 14 to 158 hours.[147] Steady-state plasma levels occur after 1 to 3 weeks of once daily dosage, depending on the half-life within the individual patient, and are two to four times higher than the peak levels after the first dose. Piroxicam is metabolized to at least seven inactive metabolites that are excreted in both urine and stool. It appears in breast milk at 1 to 3 percent of the maternal plasma concentration.[148] In patients with rheumatoid arthritis, synovial fluid concentrations are lower than those in plasma but the elimination half-life is the same.[149] Piroxicam levels are not elevated in patients with renal insufficiency, probably because the drug is cleared primarily by hepatic metabolism. Indeed, in one study, the elimination half-life of piroxicam was decreased in patients with renal insufficiency.[150] The effect of cirrhosis on piroxicam metabolism has not been reported, but it might be expected to increase its half-life. The co-administration of aspirin has been reported to reduce piroxicam plasma levels by about 20 percent, whereas cimetidine increases plasma piroxicam levels and half-life.[151, 152] In view of the serious toxicity of benoxaprofen encountered in some elderly patients, there has been concern about possible piroxicam accumulation in older patients. One single-dose study of healthy subjects projected that steady-state plasma levels and half-lives of piroxicam would be greater in elderly women than in young women, but that there would be no difference in these measures between young men and elderly men,[122] but other studies did not demonstrate these projected differences.[113, 153]

The toxicity of piroxicam is similar to that of other NSAIDs, as confirmed by an intensive review of the entire worldwide experience with the drug in more than 75,000 patients[154] and further review by the FDA. However, peptic ulceration is considerably more common with daily doses in excess of 20 mg, and this dose generally should not be exceeded.

Piroxicam has been approved for use in rheumatoid arthritis and osteoarthritis. It may also be effective in gout, ankylosing spondylitis, acute musculoskeletal disorders, and sports injuries.[151]

Nabumetone

Nabumetone is a 2,6-disubstituted naphthylalkanone that is not acidic and is a poor inhibitor of prostaglandin synthesis (Fig. 45–8). After absorption, it is rapidly metabolized in the liver to an acidic metabolite that is a potent inhibitor of prostaglandin synthesis. The active metabolite has a plasma half-life of about 21 hours, increasing to 29 hours in the elderly and to 39 hours in patients with creatinine

Figure 45–7. Chemical structure of piroxicam.

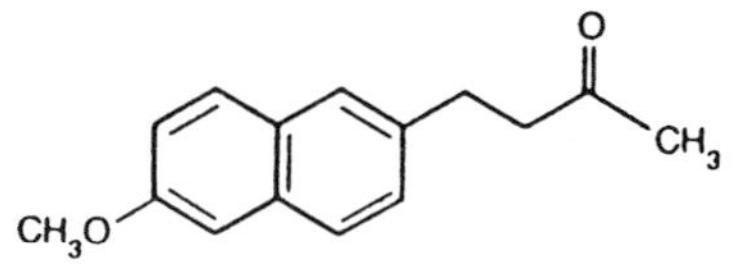

Figure 45–8. Chemical structure of nabumetone.

clearances below 30 ml/minute. It is eliminated both by direct urinary excretion (80 percent in urine and 10 percent in feces) and by metabolism to inactive metabolites. Less than 1 percent of the active metabolite appears in the urine. In animal studies, nabumetone induced less gastric damage than aspirin or comparison NSAIDs, and human studies of quantitative GI blood loss as well as endoscopic studies suggest that it is less gastrotoxic than naproxen or aspirin. Nevertheless, peptic ulcers and GI bleeding have been observed during long-term clinical trials, although perhaps less frequently than might have been anticipated with aspirin or some other NSAIDs. Oral dosing of 1 g daily for 7 days had no effect on bleeding time for healthy volunteers.[112] With doses of 1000 mg once daily at bedtime, anti-inflammatory efficacy has been demonstrated in patients with rheumatoid arthritis and osteoarthritis,[155] for which the drug is FDA-approved. Other nonapproved uses, such as treatment for soft tissue injury, have been reported.

Oxaprozin

Oxaprozin is a propionic acid derivative with a half-life of 49 to 60 hours, making once-a-day dosing feasible (Fig. 45–9).[156, 157] Although it was patented in 1969 and studied extensively in the 1980s, oxaprozin was only recently approved by the FDA for rheumatoid arthritis and osteoarthritis.

Absorption of oxaprozin from the GI tract is almost complete (95 percent).[156, 157] Peak absorption occurs 3 to 6 hours after oral ingestion. Food may delay absorption, but total absorption is not changed. Antacids have no effect on the rate or extent of oxaprozin absorption. Because of the long half-life, it may take as long as 10 to 14 days of treatment before steady-state levels are attained.

Oxaprozin itself is pharmacologically active. It is extensively metabolized in the liver to inactive metabolites (65 percent by microsomal oxidation and 35 percent by glucuronic acid conjugation).[156, 157] Only 4

to 5 percent of oxaprozin is excreted in the urine unchanged. Sixty percent of the drug and its metabolites is excreted in the urine, and 30 to 35 percent is excreted in feces. In normal subjects, oxaprozin is 99.5 percent bound to protein, but in patients who are renally impaired or on dialysis, the binding is decreased to 72 to 82 percent.[156] For this and other reasons (i.e., decreased clearance of metabolites) the manufacturer recommends that an initial dose of 600 mg daily be given and dosages increased cautiously if the desired effect is not obtained after several weeks. No dosage adjustment is required in patients with well-compensated cirrhosis, but a reduction in dose is suggested in those with severe liver disease.[156]

No significant interactions have been reported for co-administration of oxaprozin with warfarin.[156] Conversely, statistically significant inhibition of the antihypertensive effects of metoprolol by oxaprozin and inhibition of clearance of oxaprozin by cimetidine have been reported, but neither is expected to be clinically relevant.

In addition to the usual adverse effects (GI and renal especially) seen with other NSAIDs, oxaprozin has a significant incidence of photosensitivity reactions (especially vesicular eruption on sun-exposed skin areas), which were reported in 3 to 9 percent of patients.[156] Oxaprozin reversibly inhibits collagen-induced platelet aggregation and is associated with a prolongation of bleeding time, which, because of its long half-life, may persist for more than 8 days after the last dose.

Although oxaprozin has been approved by FDA for use in rheumatoid arthritis and osteoarthritis, studies also support its efficacy in juvenile rheumatoid arthritis, postoperative oral surgery pain, ankylosing spondylitis, acute gouty arthritis, and acute tendinitis and bursitis.[156]

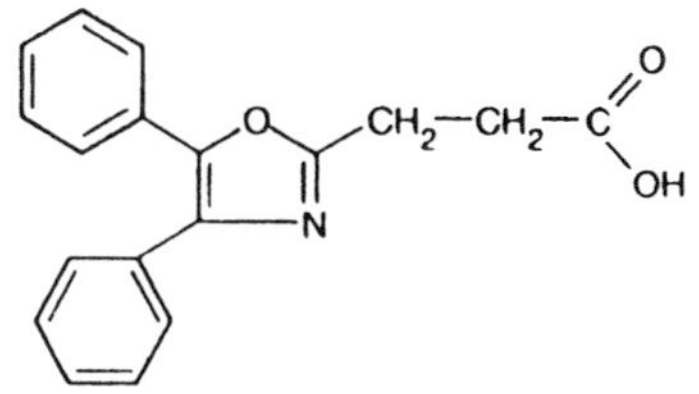

Tenidap

Tenidap sodium is a novel antirheumatic drug in a new chemical class, the oxindoles (Fig. 45–10). It is not FDA-approved in the United States. Like other NSAIDs, tenidap inhibits prostaglandin synthesis

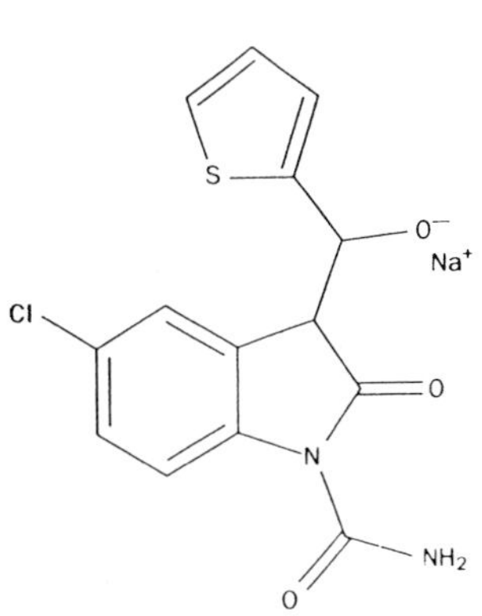

Figure 45–9. Chemical structure of oxaprozin.

Figure 45–10. Chemical structure of tenidap.

through inhibition of cyclooxygenase. Tenidap also modulates human peripheral blood monocyte production of the cytokines, interleukin-1 (IL-1), tumor necrosis factor, and interleukin-6.[162] This cytokine inhibition has been shown to induce rapid and persistent reductions in serum C-reactive protein, serum amyloid A, and erythrocyte sedimentation rate by inhibiting the production of these proteins in the liver. Significant reductions in the levels IL-1 in the synovial fluid of patients with rheumatoid arthritis have also been observed following tenidap administration.[162]

Tenidap is itself pharmacologically active. Oral tenidap is 85 percent bioavailable. The maximum serum concentration is reached within 2 or 3 hours of oral administration. Because the half-life of tenidap is 23 hours, it can be given once a day. Steady-state levels were achieved by day 11 of dosing.[162] Although it is extensively metabolized in the liver, it is not clear whether this is by means of the hepatic 450 microsomal enzyme system. Although systemic clearance was 29 percent greater on day 28 than on day 1 (suggesting that tenidap, which is subject to extensive hepatic metabolism, may induce its own metabolism), no change in dosing is recommended.[162] Although food delays tenidap absorption, total absorption is not affected. Magnesium and aluminum hydroxide antacid administration, however, decreased total absorption, but probably not to any clinically significant extent.[162] Cimetidine did not interfere in tenidap kinetics to a clinically relevant extent.[162] The effect of renal or hepatic impairment on tenidap elimination is unknown.

Tenidap affects the pharmacokinetics of lithium and phenytoin to an extent that is likely to increase their toxicity in at least some patients; careful monitoring is important when it is co-administered with either of these drugs.[162] Interactions with both angiotensin converting enzyme inhibitors and thiazide diuretics may result in reduced antihypertensive efficacy of both groups.[162] No clinically significant interaction with digoxin or warfarin occurred.

In several placebo-controlled studies, tenidap has achieved clinical efficacy in the treatment of patients with rheumatoid arthritis when administered in doses of 120 mg/day.[163, 164] It is undergoing further clinical evaluation in the United States and Europe for the treatment of patients with rheumatoid arthritis and osteoarthritis.

Several studies have reported that tenidap is clinically superior in rheumatoid arthritis to NSAIDs alone (i.e., piroxicam, diclofenac, naproxen).[164–166] These and other studies suggest that tenidap alone may be as effective as a combination of an NSAID and a weak disease-modifying antirheumatic drug (DMARD) (i.e., piroxicam plus hydroxychloroquine, auranofin plus diclofenac).[164, 167] These studies suggest that tenidap as a single drug may supplant combinations of an NSAID with a mild DMARD.[164–167]

Colchicine

Colchicine is absorbed fairly readily from the GI tract, reaching an average peak plasma level of 0.32 μg/dl 30 minutes to 2 hours after a single 1-mg dose by mouth.[158] With a half-life of less than 20 minutes, colchicine leaves the blood rapidly after intravenous (IV) administration due to rapid distribution from the plasma into cells. Peripheral blood leukocytes are known to accumulate colchicine but may not be the only tissue in which the drug is concentrated. The mean white blood cell (WBC) concentration reached a peak of 43 μg/dl 10 minutes after IV administration of 3 mg of colchicine to healthy volunteers; a plateau between 18 and 23 μg/dl was maintained during the interval from 30 minutes to 24 hours after administration. Seventy-two hours after the infusion of drug, the mean WBC concentration was 11 μg/dl, and measurable concentrations were still present in leukocytes 10 days later.[159] Thus, the elimination half-life from peripheral blood leukocytes, a probable site of drug effect, is prolonged, easily permitting once daily administration of maintenance doses of colchicine.

In a study of four patients with familial Mediterranean fever given 1 mg colchicine intravenously, the mean elimination half-life from serum was 157 minutes compared with 65 minutes in six normal subjects. Eight patients who received 1 mg of colchicine daily orally had serum concentrations of 0.3 to 2.4 ng/ml. One patient with a poor clinical response had undetectable serum levels after 2 mg daily, however, suggesting that lack of response may result from inadequate absorption or altered disposition of colchicine.[160] In another study of 13 patients with polyserositis receiving long-term colchicine therapy, plasma concentrations ranged from 0.8 to 7.8 ng/ml.[161]

Colchicine is excreted in the bile, feces, and urine. There is no evidence that colchicine is metabolized to any significant extent. The use of colchicine is well established in gout, pseudogout, and familial Mediterranean fever, but it also has been evaluated in Behçet's disease, amyloidosis, cutaneous necrotizing vasculitis, acute febrile neutrophilic dermatosis (Sweet's syndrome), and the skin manifestations of scleroderma.[37] Its toxicity has been discussed earlier in this chapter.

NSAIDs WITH A SHORT HALF-LIFE

NSAIDs with short half-lives generally have half-lives of 6 hours or less in patients and are given three or four times daily (Table 45–5). Steady state is reached within 24 to 36 hours after the drug is initially administered, but is characterized by marked fluctuations in plasma levels between peak postabsorption levels and trough levels at the time of the next dosage. Peak synovial fluid concentrations are substantially lower than peak plasma concentrations, and the half-life for disappearance from synovial fluid is usually longer than the initial half-life for disappearance from plasma, suggesting that the half-life for biologic effects may be substantially longer than the short plasma half-life. Both synovial fluid and plasma concentrations are low during this late phase

Table 45–5. NONSTEROIDAL ANTI-INFLAMMATORY DRUGS (NSAIDS) WITH SHORT HALF-LIVES

Drug	Available Formulations (mg)	Maximal Daily Dose (mg)	Active Metabolite	% Bound	T_{max} (hr)	$T_{1/2}$ (hr)	Renal Excretion Unchanged Drug (% Dose)	Changes in Dose for			Influence on NSAID Efficacy by		Influence of NSAID on Toxicity	
								Renal Failure	Hepatic Disease	Elderly Patients	Food	Antacid	Warfarin	Hypoglycemic Agents
Diclofenac (Voltaren, Cataflam)	Tabs: 25, 50, 75	200	—	99	1–3	1.2–2	<1	None	None	None	None	None	None	None
Etodolac (Lodine)	Caps: 200, 300	600	—	99	1	7.3	1	None	ID	None	None	ID	Caution	None
Fenoprofen (Nalfon)	Caps, tabs: 200, 300, 600	3200	—	99	1–2	2–3	2–5	None	ID	None	None	None	Caution	ID
Flurbiprofen (Ansaid)	Tabs: 50, 100	300	—	99	1.5–3	3–4	<15	ID	ID	None	None	None	None	ID
Ibuprofen (Motrin, Advil, Medipren, Rufen)	Tabs: 200, 300, 400, 600, 800	3600	—	99	1–2	2–2.5	<10	None	Avoid in severe disease	None	None	None	None	None
Indomethacin (Indocin)	Caps: 10, 25, 50; Sustained-release caps: 75; Oral suspension: 25 mg/5 ml; Suppositories: 50	200	—	>98	1–4	2–13	<15	None	ID	None	None	ID	Caution	ID
Ketoprofen (Orudis, Oruvail)	Caps: 25, 50, 75, 200	300	—	99	0.5–2	1–4	<10	↓ By $^{1}/_{2}$–$^{1}/_{3}$ with CrCl <10 ml/min	↓ Dose	Probably decrease	None	None	Caution	None
Ketorolac (Toradol)	Parenteral: 15, 30 mg/ml; Oral tabs: 10	IM/IV: 150 first day; 120 thereafter; p.o.: 40	—	99	0.3–1.0	4–6	60	↓ Dose by 50%	ID	↓ Dose by 50%	None	None	None	ID
Meclofenamate (Meclomen)	Caps: 50, 100	400	Hydroxy-methyl derivative	99	0.5–2.0	2–3	<4	None	ID	None	None	None	Caution (prolongs prothrombin time)	ID
Tolmetin (Tolectin)	Tabs, caps: 200, 400, 600	2000	—	99	0.5–1	1–1.5	15	None	ID	ID	None	ID	None	None

Data from Gelman CR, Hess AJ, Rumack BH (eds): DRUGDEX Information System, Micromedix, Inc, Englewood, Col, 1996.
Abbreviations: T_{max}, time to maximum absorption; $T_{1/2}$, half-life; CrCl, creatinine clearance; ID, insufficient data; p.o., by mouth.

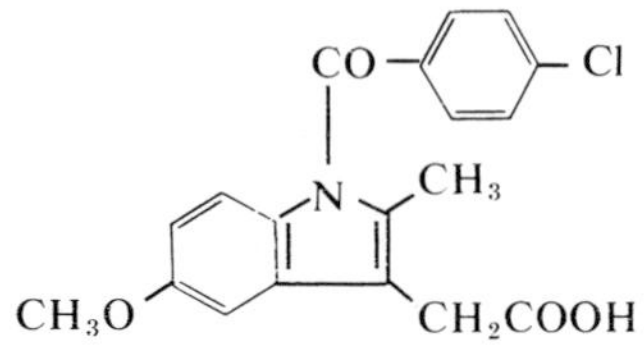

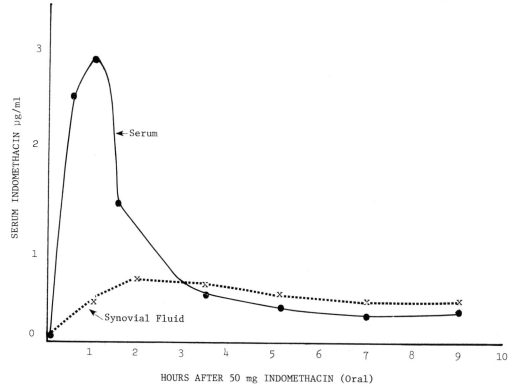

Figure 45–11. Chemical structure of indomethacin.

of delayed resorption of drug from synovial fluid and tissue stores into plasma, from which it is then excreted (Fig. 45–3). Some of these drugs with short half-lives have been marketed in delayed-release formulations to make them more convenient for patients.

Indomethacin

Indomethacin is the prototype of the short half-life NSAIDs that are potent inhibitors of cyclooxygenase (Fig. 45–11). It is an indole acetic acid, chemically related to sulindac. Indomethacin was identified by its effectiveness in suppressing the induction of edema when carrageenan was injected into rat paws.[168] It was marketed in the United States in 1965 and was observed by Vane to be an extremely potent inhibitor of prostaglandin synthesis when he originally observed that the inhibition of prostaglandin synthesis was an important mechanism of action of NSAIDs.[28]

Both the standard and the sustained-release formulations of indomethacin are well absorbed.[169] Food or antacid somewhat delays absorption but does not decrease overall bioavailability. Indomethacin crosses the placenta, with equilibrium between mother and fetus reached within 5 hours.[170] Its plasma half-life is biexponential; the initial half-life includes distribution into tissue compartments and is 1 to 2 hours in duration, whereas the terminal half-life is about 13 hours.[171] Synovial fluid indomethacin concentrations show a delayed rise and lower peak compared with plasma levels, but they then remain equal to or higher than serum levels for at least 9 hours after dosing (Fig. 45–12).[172] Indomethacin is highly metabolized to compounds that lack anti-inflammatory activity. Most of an oral indomethacin dose is excreted as metabolites.[173] Indomethacin has an extensive enterohepatic recirculation; it is estimated that greater than 43 percent of a dose is excreted in the bile.[174] The plasma half-life is prolonged in infants. In one study, the half-life was 2.2 hours in mothers but 14.7 hours in their newborn infants.[175] However, the half-life in elderly men was no different than that in younger men.[176]

Aspirin decreases indomethacin absorption, decreases its renal clearance, and increases its biliary clearance; the net effect is a slight decrease in indomethacin bioavailability when it is administered during chronic aspirin therapy.[177] In patients with rheumatoid arthritis, however, the efficacy of indomethacin alone is not detectably different from the efficacy of the same dose of indomethacin combined with

Figure 45–12. Serum and synovial fluid indomethacin concentrations in a patient after a single 50-mg oral dose. After equilibration, synovial fluid concentrations slightly exceed those in serum, a typical finding with short half-life nonsteroidal anti-inflammatory drugs.

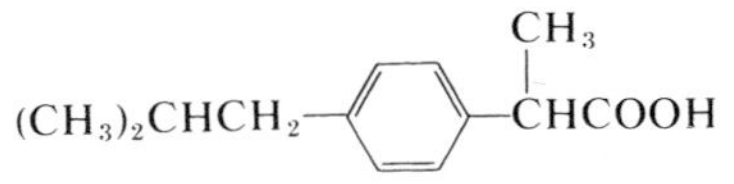

$$(CH_3)_2CHCH_2 - \underset{}{\bigcirc} - \overset{CH_3}{\underset{|}{CHCOOH}}$$

Figure 45–13. Chemical structure of ibuprofen.

therapeutic doses of aspirin.[178] Indomethacin may prevent the acetylation of platelet cyclooxygenase by aspirin.[179] Probenecid appears to decrease indomethacin biliary clearance and increases bioavailability by 63 percent[180]; when given with indomethacin, clinical improvement was also reported.[181]

As a lead compound, indomethacin has been used for all of the rheumatologic and nonrheumatologic indications for NSAIDs. In patients who tolerate it, it is generally effective, but upper GI symptoms and headaches prompt discontinuation of therapy in a substantial number of patients. The 75-mg sustained-release indomethacin capsule is designed to deliver 25 mg of drug immediately and the remaining 50 mg over the next 8 to 12 hours. Rectal suppositories, an oral suspension, and IV preparations of indomethacin are also available.

Ibuprofen

Ibuprofen is an arylpropionic acid that is present predominantly in the ionized form at physiologic pH (Fig. 45–13). Ibuprofen as well as fenoprofen and ketoprofen has an asymmetric carbon and exists as R($-$) and S($+$) optical isomers. The marketed preparations of these drugs are racemic mixtures consisting of equal parts of both isomers. The S($+$) isomer of ibuprofen is much more active than the R($-$) isomer as an inhibitor of cyclooxygenase in vitro. In vivo, however, the less potent R($-$) isomer is converted to the S($+$) isomer; consequently, it is difficult to detect differences in the pharmacologic activity of the two isomers in whole-animal studies.[182] It is greater than 98 percent bound to plasma proteins, but protein binding capacity may be exceeded with higher doses; this was reported in one study when doses exceeded 850 mg.[183] Thus, there may be disproportionate increases in biologically active unbound ibuprofen as doses increase in size. Concentrations of unbound ibuprofen are approximately equal in serum and synovial fluid; synovial fluid concentrations fluctuate less than plasma concentrations, and the drug is detectable for long periods in the synovial fluid.[184] The half-life of the active S($+$) isomer is longer than that of the R($-$) isomer, and thus a longer duration of action is possible than would be predicted by measurement of total plasma concentrations only.[185]

Ibuprofen is extensively metabolized to inactive metabolites. Enterohepatic recirculation is probably not significant in humans. Ibuprofen kinetics are not significantly different in elderly as compared with younger individuals,[186] and even severe hepatic dis-

ease with cirrhosis and ascites did not alter ibuprofen kinetics.[183]

Doses of 3600 to 4800 mg/day of ibuprofen increased the fraction of unbound warfarin by 10 to 30 percent, although lower doses do not alter warfarin-induced hypoprothrombinemia.[187] Probenecid does not increase plasma concentrations of ibuprofen, which is largely metabolized by oxidation, and ibuprofen does not interfere with the uricosuria induced by probenecid.[188] Ibuprofen appears to protect platelet cyclooxygenase from the irreversible effects of aspirin, presumably by a mechanism similar to that seen with indomethacin.[189]

Ibuprofen has been associated with all of the generic adverse effects reported with NSAIDs. It predominates in the small number of reports of NSAID-associated aseptic meningitis.[190]

Ibuprofen has been used for all of the indications for NSAIDs. Doses of 400 to 1200 mg daily are primarily analgesic; doses for rheumatoid arthritis generally are 2400 to 3600 mg daily, and doses as high as 4800 mg daily have been used for the initial treatment of acute gout.[190]

Because of its greater margin of safety, as compared with aspirin and acetaminophen, ibuprofen was approved for nonprescription sale to the public. It is recommended for use as an analgesic and for symptomatic treatment of menstrual cramps, in 200-mg doses, with a maximum recommended daily dose of 1200 mg. As discussed earlier, a number of cases of overdose of ibuprofen have been reported, but there have been very few deaths. Prospective follow-up of 43 women who were exposed to ibuprofen during pregnancy did not reveal any fetal abnormalities at delivery, but retrospective reports include one case each of anencephaly, convulsions, cerebral palsy, and microphthalmia.[191]

Fenoprofen

Fenoprofen is also a substituted arylpropionic acid whose S($+$) enantiomer is much more active than the R($-$) optical isomer as an in vitro inhibitor of cyclooxygenase from human platelets (Fig. 45–14). In vivo, the R($-$) enantiomer is stereoselectively converted to the S($+$) isomer.[192] The marketed drug is a racemic mixture of the two isomers. Its absorption has been reported to be reduced 30 percent by food.[193] Both fenoprofen and its inactive metabolite hydroxyfenoprofen are excreted in the urine as glucuronides. Its kinetics are not significantly different in elderly compared with younger patients.[194] Fenoprofen slightly decreases warfarin protein binding.[195]

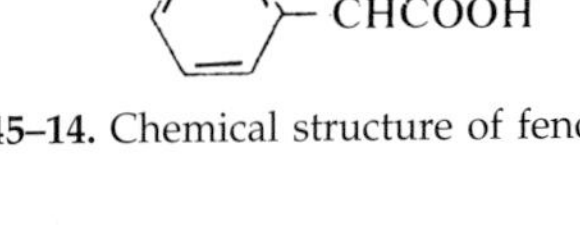

$$\underset{}{\overset{C_6H_5O}{\bigcirc}} - \overset{CH_3}{\underset{|}{CHCOOH}}$$

Figure 45–14. Chemical structure of fenoprofen.

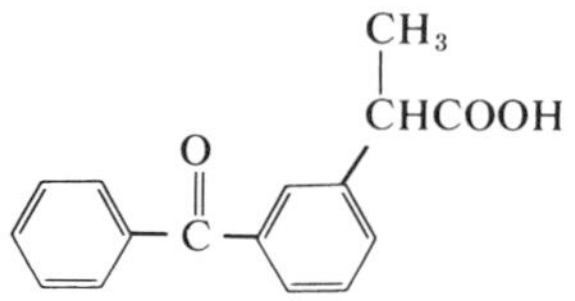

Figure 45–15. Chemical structure of ketoprofen.

For rheumatoid arthritis and osteoarthritis, fenoprofen is recommended in doses of 300 to 600 mg three or four times a day. Aspirin and fenoprofen, 900 to 1800 mg/m^2/day, were equally effective in a 3-month study of children with juvenile rheumatoid arthritis.[196] Fenoprofen has also been used in ankylosing spondylitis and gout and as an analgesic.[190] Its adverse effects are typical of drugs in its class, except that idiosyncratic nephropathy has been seen more frequently with fenoprofen than with any of the other NSAIDs.[197] Days to months after the initiation of fenoprofen therapy, patients may present with renal insufficiency, edema, and either nephrotic-range proteinuria or oliguria. Both the renal failure and the proteinuria resolve on discontinuation of the NSAID, but steroid therapy may be necessary.[190] Renal biopsy specimens have shown T lymphocyte infiltration in the renal interstitium and foot process fusion.[198] Eosinophilia is sometimes seen as part of this syndrome, and patients who have had allergic reactions to nonsteroidal drugs should be given fenoprofen only under close observation.

Ketoprofen

Ketoprofen is another arylpropionic acid that was developed about the same time as ibuprofen and fenoprofen (Fig. 45–15). It has been used extensively in Europe since 1973 and became available in the United States in 1986. Although its plasma half-life is 0.5 to 2 hours, during chronic therapy, ketoprofen-induced inhibition of platelet aggregation does not return to normal until 36 hours after the last dose, which suggests that the elimination half-life of ketoprofen from platelets (and perhaps other tissue sites of action) may be more on the order of 6 or 7 hours.[199] Consistent with this observation, the plasma disappearance curve of ketoprofen is multiexponential, with a slower terminal phase of elimination.[200] Ketoprofen also readily enters the synovial fluid, and synovial fluid PGE$_2$ concentrations remain decreased for at least 24 hours after a 100-mg dose of drug.[201] Thus, administration every 6 or 8 hours appears to be reasonable on a pharmacodynamic basis.

Both ketoprofen and its hydroxylated metabolite are extensively conjugated and excreted in the urine. Although ketoprofen is excreted in the bile, essentially all is reabsorbed and very little drug is present in the feces.[201]

Initial doses of ketoprofen should be decreased in the elderly and in patients with renal failure because of decreased clearance in both situations.[202, 203] Staffanger and associates found a direct correlation between creatinine clearance and ketoprofen clearance.[203]

A number of potential drug interactions with ketoprofen have been evaluated. Two grams of probenecid daily decreased ketoprofen protein binding by 28 percent, total ketoprofen clearance by 67 percent, renal clearance of ketoprofen conjugates by 93 percent, and clearance of unbound ketoprofen by 74 percent, resulting in increased concentrations of both free and protein-bound ketoprofen in plasma.[204] Ketoprofen plasma concentrations decrease when aspirin is added to the treatment regimen; the protein binding of ketoprofen decreases and plasma clearance increases.[205] Ketoprofen may increase plasma methotrexate concentrations with high doses of methotrexate,[206] but similar observations have not been noted with low doses of methotrexate. No interactions were seen in studies with digoxin, oral hypoglycemics, gold salts, antimalarials, or corticosteroids.[201] Ketoprofen decreases hydrochlorothiazide-induced excretion of potassium and chloride but does not alter the diuretic or antihypertensive effects of this drug.[201]

An extended-release form of Ketoprofen (Oruvail) is available as a 200-mg capsule, to be taken once daily.[207] Although absorption is delayed (peak level at 6 to 7 hours after dosing), total absorption and elimination kinetics, compared with those of the parent compound, are unchanged. Its advantage is the once-daily dosing.

Ketoprofen is usually used in doses of 100 to 300 mg daily and is effective in the treatment of rheumatoid arthritis, osteoarthritis, ankylosing spondylitis, and acute gout as well as pain management; it has also been used in juvenile arthritis.[190] The most prominent adverse effects are upper GI toxicity, but these and other adverse effects are similar to those of other NSAIDs.

Tolmetin

Tolmetin is a pyrrole acetic acid derivative with the pharmacologic characteristics of the NSAID inhibitors of prostaglandin biosynthesis (Fig. 45–16). It has a biphasic elimination half-life from plasma; the half-life of the initial phase is about 2 hours, and the half-life of the terminal phase ranges from 2 to 6.8 hours.[208] Tolmetin enters the synovial fluid and is associated with depressed concentrations of PGE$_2$ for at least 24 hours after a dose.[209] A small amount of unchanged tolmetin is excreted in the urine, but most of the drug

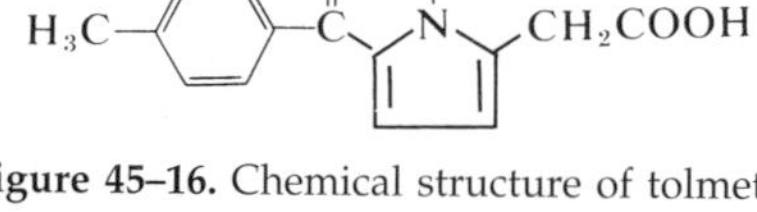

Figure 45–16. Chemical structure of tolmetin.

is excreted as the dicarboxylic acid metabolite or as glucuronide conjugates of tolmetin and its metabolite; the metabolites are inactive.[210] There does not appear to be any enterohepatic recirculation of tolmetin. No clinically significant interactions have been reported with warfarin, phenprocoumon, oral hypoglycemic agents, or aspirin.[211] There is no accumulation of tolmetin during chronic administration on a four-times-a-day schedule.[208] Doses of 600 to 2000 mg daily, in three or four divided doses, are effective in rheumatoid arthritis, osteoarthritis, and ankylosing spondylitis.[211] Tolmetin has been approved by the FDA for use in juvenile rheumatoid arthritis; the recommended starting dose for children aged 2 years and older is 20 mg/kg/day; doses greater than 30 mg/kg/day are not recommended.[211]

Gastrointestinal side effects are the most common adverse reaction and are slightly more common in elderly patients.[212] Anaphylaxis similar to that seen with zomepirac has been reported with tolmetin, and care should be exercised when the drug is reinstituted after a hiatus in treatment.[213] Pseudoproteinuria is seen if sulfasalicylic acid or other acid is used as a test for urine protein. A cloudy precipitate of tolmetin and its metabolites in the acid solution causes the appearance of marked proteinuria, but tests that do not rely on acid precipitation remain negative.

Tolmetin is particularly useful in the presurgical management of patients who require a NSAID because it is almost completely excreted within 24 hours after a dose. Therefore, discontinuation of tolmetin 36 hours before surgery avoids increased bleeding due to inhibition of platelet cyclooxygenase.

Meclofenamate Sodium and Other Fenamates

The fenamates are substituted *n*-phenyl anthranilic acids that were found to have anti-inflammatory activity in animal studies in the late 1950s and early 1960s.[214] Flufenamic acid (Fig. 45–17) and mefenamic acid (Fig. 45–18) have been marketed since then but have been used primarily as analgesics and for treatment of dysmenorrhea. They have not been popular for chronic therapy because of their associations with dose-related intestinal cramping and diarrhea in up to 25 percent of patients and with rashes in up to 16 percent. Ten to 20 percent of mefenamic acid and 36 percent of flufenamic acid is excreted in feces. Overdoses of mefenamic acid are associated with grand mal seizures. Flufenamic acid, 300 to 600 mg daily, is given in three divided doses for rheumatoid arthritis, osteoarthritis, or ankylosing spondylitis. For

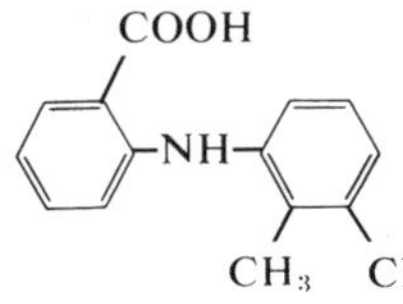

Figure 45–18. Chemical structure of mefenamic acid.

primary dysmenorrhea, mefenamic acid, 500 mg initially, is followed by 250 mg every 6 hours.[214]

The sodium salt of meclofenamic acid has been marketed in the United States since 1982. Meclofenamate is an in vitro inhibitor of both 5-lipoxygenase and cyclooxygenase pathways of arachidonic acid metabolism in human neutrophils,[215] but the clinical significance of this observation is uncertain. In addition, the major metabolite in humans has anti-inflammatory activity, although it is less active than the parent compound. After multiple doses, the mean half-life of unchanged drug in plasma is about 3 hours, but the half-life of the metabolites is about 24 hours.[216] About 25 percent of radioactivity associated with the drug was recovered from stool in a balance study in humans.[216] The remainder was excreted in the urine, primarily as glucuronides of the five major metabolites. Meclofenamic acid increases the prothrombin time of patients receiving warfarin.[217] Addition of aspirin increases GI blood loss to nearly three times that seen with either drug alone.[217] No interactions with propoxyphene or sulfinpyrazone were observed.[217]

Meclofenamate sodium is used for the treatment of rheumatoid arthritis, osteoarthritis, gout, and ankylosing spondylitis. Fifty- and 100-mg capsules are available and are usually given in three or four divided doses totaling 200 to 400 mg daily. Like the other fenamates, meclofenamate sodium causes diarrhea. This is thought to be due to the inherent laxative properties of the drug, which is a secretagogue.[214] In long-term studies, diarrhea occurred in about 15 percent of patients but drug discontinuation was required in only 7 percent.[218] The occurrence of rashes with meclofenamate sodium was not as frequent as with other fenamates.[218] Other adverse effects are those expected with NSAIDs.

Diclofenac

Diclofenac sodium is another member of the fenamate family of phenylacetic acid derivatives (Fig. 45–19). It is a potent inhibitor of platelet aggregation

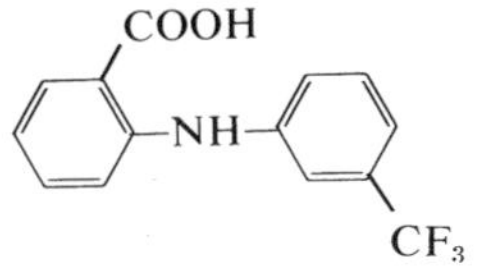

Figure 45–17. Chemical structure of flufenamic acid.

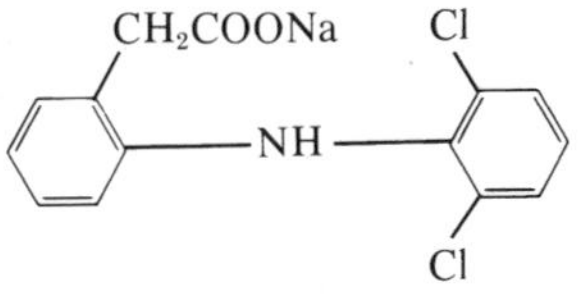

Figure 45–19. Chemical structure of diclofenac.

induced by collagen in vitro, but in doses of 75 to 100 mg daily in humans there is no effect on platelet count, platelet adhesiveness, platelet aggregation, or activated prothrombin time.[219] It suppresses prostaglandin synthesis in vitro and in vivo and decreases the production of leukotrienes by stimulating the uptake of arachidonic acid into triglycerides; the result is an inhibition of the release of intracellular arachidonic acid, although it appears to have no effect on lipoxygenase itself.[31] It is metabolized to an inactive metabolite that is excreted in both urine and bile.[220] Renal dysfunction does not influence the plasma levels of diclofenac significantly because it is cleared from plasma primarily by metabolism. Diclofenac does not accumulate during chronic use and does not displace oral anticoagulants or hypoglycemic agents.[220] Suppression of PGE_2 in synovial fluid persists for 8 to 12 hours after a dose.[221] There is no significant difference in maximum plasma concentrations or overall urinary excretion in elderly patients compared with younger subjects.[220]

Diclofenac is marketed in the United States as an enteric-coated tablet, which somewhat delays its absorption. In doses of 75 to 200 mg daily, divided into two to four doses, the drug has been reported to be effective in rheumatoid arthritis, osteoarthritis, ankylosing spondylitis, gout, nonarticular rheumatism, and pain.[220] Its toxicity is generally similar to that of other NSAIDs, although monitoring of liver enzymes is recommended for several months after treatment is initiated. The potassium salt of diclofenac (Cataflam) is more rapidly absorbed than the sodium salt (peak levels occurring at 0.33–2 hours versus 1–4 hours) and has been approved by the FDA for acute pain in addition to its use in the management of osteoarthritis, rheumatoid arthritis, and ankylosing spondylitis.[219]

Etodolac

Etodolac, an indole acetic acid, is one of a series of pyrano-carboxylic acids (Fig. 45–20). It inhibits cyclooxygenase but not lipoxygenase.[222] It is extensively metabolized and excreted in both urine and bile. The kinetics of etodolac are unchanged in the elderly and apparently are not significantly changed in renal impairment.[223] It has been approved by the FDA for treatment of osteoarthritis and pain.[223] The safety profile of etodolac is not readily distinguishable from that of other NSAIDs. The recommended dosage

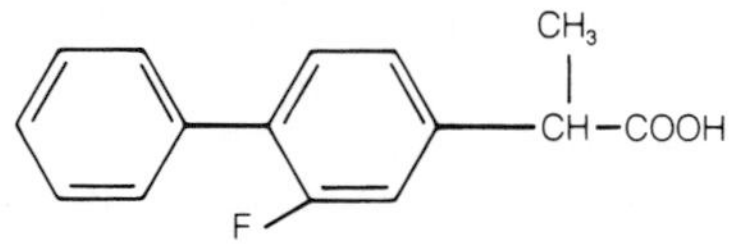

Figure 45–21. Chemical structure of flurbiprofen.

is 200 to 400 mg every 6 to 8 hours, not to exceed a total daily dose of 1200 mg.

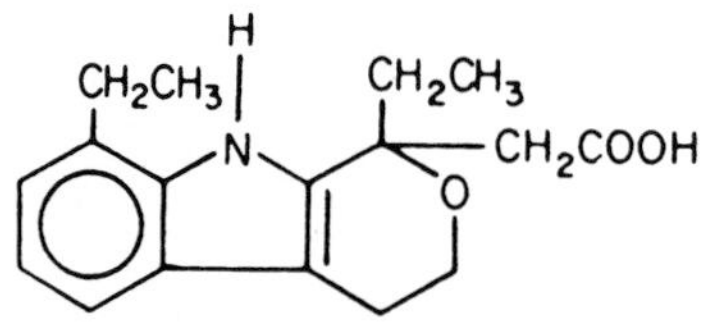

Flurbiprofen

Flurbiprofen, a biphenylpropionic acid derivative, inhibits cyclooxygenase but not lipoxygenase, and inhibits platelet aggregation in humans (Fig. 45–21). Flurbiprofen does not appear to interact with oral anticoagulants, sulfonamides, or phenytoin.[224] It is extensively metabolized, and more than 95 percent is excreted in urine as conjugates of the parent drug and its metabolites. About 5 percent of urinary excretion consists of unmetabolized flurbiprofen. One of the metabolites has minimal anti-inflammatory activity.[225] Aspirin decreases both plasma concentrations and the half-life of flurbiprofen.[226]

Flurbiprofen has been found to be effective in the treatment of rheumatoid arthritis, osteoarthritis, ankylosing spondylitis, bursitis, and acute gout. The usual doses are 100 to 300 mg daily divided into two to four doses. Acute gout is treated with 400 mg on the first day, followed by 200 mg daily. Symptoms of GI irritation have been observed in 20 to 36 percent of patients in controlled clinical trials. Other adverse effects are those expected with this class of drugs.[224]

Ketorolac

Ketorolac trimethamine is a pyrrolo-pyrrole, an acidic NSAID that was developed for intramuscular (IM) administration for the short-term management of pain (Fig. 45–22).[227] It inhibits cyclooxygenase-mediated prostaglandin production and exhibits anti-inflammatory, analgesic, and antipyretic activity in preclinical models. Peak plasma levels occur about 1 hour after IM injection, and peak analgesic effect occurs within 2 to 3 hours of administration. An oral formulation, with kinetics similar to those of the IM preparation, is also available. Ketorolac is more than 99 percent bound to plasma proteins at therapeutic concentrations and has a small volume of distribu-

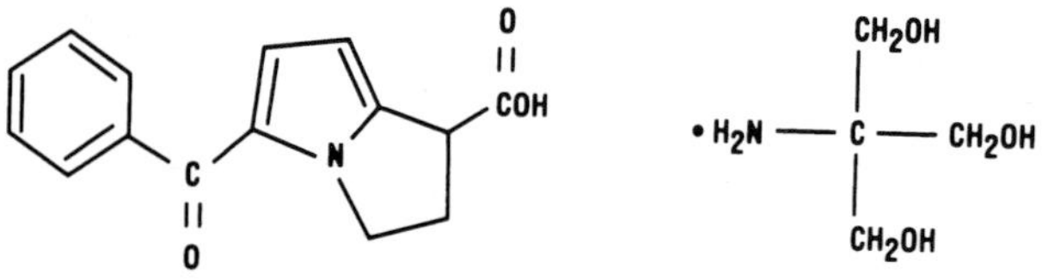

Figure 45–20. Chemical structure of etodolac.

Figure 45–22. Chemical structure of ketorolac trimethamine.

tion. The terminal plasma half-life is 4 to 6 hours in young adults and 5 to 9 hours in elderly subjects. Ketorolac is 90 percent excreted in urine as unchanged drug and metabolite; thus, the plasma half-life in patients with renal impairment was about twice as long as in normal persons.[227]

In patients with postoperative pain following orthopedic, gynecologic, abdominal, or oral surgery, ketorolac, 10mg IM, produced peak pain relief comparable to 50 mg of meperidine or 6 mg of morphine; 30 or 90 mg was comparable to 100 mg of meperidine or 12 mg of morphine, and the duration of effect was longer for ketorolac than for the narcotics.[228, 229] The maximum recommended daily dose is 120 mg, divided into four injections given every 6 hours. Ketorolac should be administered for no longer than 5 days.[229] Oral ketorolac is indicated only as continuation to parenteral therapy and the combined duration of both forms is not to exceed 5 days. Ketorolac is not a narcotic and does not depress respiration or cause constipation. Adverse effects are less frequent with short-term IM ketorolac than with chronic oral administration of aspirin or other NSAIDs, but with chronic use for persistent painful conditions, the usual adverse reactions associated with NSAIDs may occur. Ketorolac causes reversible inhibition of platelet function.[227] Its use to treat acute episodes of inflammatory arthritis, such as gout, has not been evaluated.

Because of its GI toxicity, ketorolac (oral or parenteral) is not indicated for chronic use (>5 days). The incidence of serious GI bleeding, after only 5 days of ketorolac therapy at 120 mg daily, ranges from 0.9 percent in patients with no history of GI perforation, ulcer, or bleeding to 7.8 percent in patients with such a history. Doses higher than 120 mg daily or for longer than 5 days are associated with an even higher risk of serious GI bleeding.

BASIS FOR CLINICAL DIFFERENTIATION AMONG NONSTEROIDAL ANTIRHEUMATIC DRUGS

There is little evidence to suggest that one NSAID is clearly more efficacious than another. Although the responses of individuals to different NSAIDs vary markedly, there is no way to predict which NSAID will be most effective for an individual patient.[230] Combinations of NSAIDs probably are not more beneficial than single-drug therapy. Indeed, several studies have suggested either no change or a decrease in anti-inflammatory activity when a second NSAID was added,[135, 178, 231] toxicity may well be additive,[67] and costs are certain to be increased by the second drug. Because substantial individual variability is present with respect to the pharmacology and pharmacokinetics of these drugs, it is essential to adjust the dosage to the patient's response. This is especially important in elderly patients, in whom age-related physiologic changes may further increase individual variability.[113]

One might anticipate that plasma drug concentrations would reflect efficacy and toxicity more accurately than dosage. This appears to be true in one study of naproxen[130] and was suggested in studies of carprofen in patients with rheumatoid arthritis[232] and of indomethacin in patients with juvenile rheumatoid arthritis,[233] but it has not been demonstrated with most NSAIDs.[234] Synovial fluid concentrations of NSAIDs fluctuate less than concurrent plasma concentrations[235] but have not been correlated with clinical efficacy or toxicity. Thus, clinicians receive little help from either plasma or synovial fluid drug concentration measurements in determining the optimal dose of an NSAID in an individual patient.

When prescribing a nonsteroidal antirheumatic drug, one should consider complicating illnesses and concurrent drug therapy. For example, if a patient has a history of peptic ulcer disease, one should use the lowest effective dose of NSAID and should consider using a nonacetylated salicylate (which as a class has minimal prostaglandin-inhibiting activity) instead of a more potent cyclooxygenase inhibitor. Supplemental H2 receptor antagonist, carafate, omeprozole or misoprostil may be needed in some situations. In addition, a drug with a short half-life is preferable to one that inhibits platelet aggregation for a prolonged time. If a patient is receiving warfarin or an oral hypoglycemic agent, the addition of an NSAID may require adjustment in the dose of warfarin or the oral hypoglycemic agent. In a patient with congestive heart failure, intrinsic renal disease, hepatic insufficiency, or dehydration, the potential for NSAID-induced fluid retention, electrolyte abnormalities, and renal insufficiency must be considered. Because it is impossible to know or accurately predict the effects of every possible interaction, patients should be observed closely during the introduction of an NSAID, when doses are increased, or when the patient's condition changes. With appropriate care, the benefits of NSAIDs can be achieved even in the elderly, while irreversible serious toxicity is avoided, but inattentiveness can quickly lead to trouble.

Although a number of published studies have compared two or more NSAIDs, there still is no generally accepted rank order of the desirability of individual NSAIDs for particular patients. Most studies do not show significant differences between drugs, and patient preferences vary greatly; indeed, they often vary within the same patient from time to time. Nevertheless, available evidence and clinical experience have led to some therapeutic preferences.[236]

For patients with rheumatoid arthritis who tolerate enteric-coated aspirin or a nonacetylated salicylate, plasma level–guided dosage is generally effective and relatively inexpensive. Many patients, however, are unable or unwilling to tolerate prolonged therapy with maximum salicylate dosage. When the dose is reduced to more tolerable levels, the anti-inflammatory effects decrease markedly and better results can generally be achieved with full doses of an NSAID. Patient compliance can be improved by using a once-

or twice-daily dosage regimen with an NSAID of longer half-life. If the initial dose is not sufficiently effective, it is usually better to increase the dose to the maximum permissible before trying the next drug. For specific situations, such as preoperatively, a short half-life NSAID may be preferred.

Aspirin is generally effective in juvenile rheumatoid arthritis, but serum salicylate monitoring is advisable. Tolmetin, ibuprofen, and naproxen are also approved for this disorder, and other NSAIDs have been used by pediatric rheumatologists, although they have not been approved for this indication.

Because elderly patients with osteoarthritis are more likely to experience serious adverse effects from aspirin and NSAIDs, the therapeutic approach differs from that used in rheumatoid arthritis. Generally, acetaminophen may be the agent of choice, having been shown in several studies to be as efficacious as naproxen or ibuprofen.[237, 238] Failing this, the lowest effective dose of a short half-life NSAID is used. If the NSAID is ineffective, it may be advisable to try a different one before increasing to maximal doses of the first drug. Because osteoarthritis symptoms may fluctuate, it is advisable to try to stop administration of the drug periodically to see whether the patient can get along without it. Sometimes treatment is needed only in the evening, to reduce aches and pains enough to permit a good night's sleep. When osteoarthritis is associated with acute episodes of joint inflammation, pseudogout should be considered. Even if intra-articular calcium crystals have not been documented, a trial of prophylactic colchicine, 0.6 mg twice daily, may help suppress and prevent recurrent episodes of polyarticular subacute pseudogout, and these low doses are unlikely to produce serious side effects.

Ankylosing spondylitis, Reiter's syndrome, and psoriatic arthritis are less likely to respond to salicylate than to indomethacin or to other NSAIDs. Phenylbutazone is no longer used for initial therapy of any condition but may be effective for spondyloarthropathies when all other NSAIDs have failed. High doses of an NSAID are usually preferred for the treatment of acute gout or pseudogout, although IV colchicine is also effective and well tolerated. High-dose oral colchicine is seldom used because it almost always causes diarrhea. After the acute attack subsides, maintenance prophylactic colchicine, 0.6 mg twice daily, is probably preferable to long-term maintenance with chronic NSAID therapy.

Most NSAIDs and salicylates are taken by healthy people for acute, usually self-limited musculoskeletal pain. Self-treatment with intermittent doses of aspirin, ibuprofen, ketoprofen, or naproxen sodium (over-the-counter) is used to alleviate discomfort while the condition resolves spontaneously. Similar self-treatment is fairly effective for menstrual cramps and is relatively safe in the low doses used.

Increasing understanding of the complex biochemical and cellular interactions involved in immunity and inflammation is providing many leads for the development of drugs to specifically alter certain portions of the process. These leads have not yet been translated into useful new classes of antirheumatic therapeutic agents, but they may well lead to safer and more effective treatments for certain specifically defined inflammatory conditions in the not too distant future. If such drugs with drastically different mechanisms of action become available, it may become logical to add one of these agents to one of the current cyclooxygenase inhibitors, just as gold or methotrexate is appropriately added at present.

References

1. Rodnan GP, Benedek TG: The early history of antirheumatic drugs. Arthritis Rheum 13:145, 1970.
2. Dudley-Hart F, Huskisson EC: Nonsteroidal antiinflammatory drugs: Current status and rational therapeutic use. Drugs 27:232, 1984.
3. Austen KF: The role of arachidonic acid metabolites in local and systemic inflammatory processes. Drugs 33(Suppl 1):10, 1987.
4. Adams SS, Cobb R: A possible basis for the antiinflammatory activity of salicylates and other nonhormonal antirheumatic drugs. Nature 181:773, 1958.
5. Smith MJH, Dawkins PD, McArthur JN: The relation between clinical inflammatory activity and the displacement of L-tryptophan and a dipeptide from human serum in vitro. J Pharm Pharmacol 23:451, 1971.
6. Ignarro LJ, Colombo C: Enzyme release from guinea pig polymorphonuclear leukocyte lysosomes inhibited in vitro by antiinflammatory drugs. Nature (New Biol) 239:155, 1972.
7. Harrity TW, Goldlust MB: Anticomplement effects of two antiinflammatory agents. Biochem Pharmacol 23:3107, 1974.
8. Collier HOJ: New light on how aspirin works. Nature (Lond) 223:35, 1969.
9. Weissmann G: Discussion. Drugs 33(Suppl 1):8, 1987.
10. Goldblatt MW: A depressor substance in seminal fluid. J Soc Chem Ind Lond 52:1056, 1933.
11. von Euler US: Zur kenntnis der pharmacologischen wirkungen von nativsekreten und extrakten mannlicher accessorischer Geblechtsdrusen. Naunyn Schmiedebergs Arch Exp Pathol Pharmacol 175:78, 1934.
12. Samuelsson B: An elucidation of the arachidonic acid cascade: Discovery of prostaglandins, thromboxane and leukotrienes. Drugs 33(Suppl 1):2, 1987.
13. Schlegel SI: General characteristics of nonsteroidal antiinflammatory drugs. In Paulus HE, Furst DE, Dromgoole S (eds): Drugs for Rheumatic Disease. New York, Churchill Livingstone, 1987, p 203.
14. Vane JR: Toward a better aspirin. Nature 367:215–216, 1994.
15. Lee SH, Soyoola E, Chanmugam P, Hart S, Sun W, Zhong H, Liou S, Simmons D, Hwanag D: Selective expression of mitogen-inducible cyclooxygenase in macrophages stimulated with lipopolysaccharide. J Biol Chem 267:25934–25938, 1992.
16. Pritchard KA, O'Banion MK, Miano JM, Vlasic N, Bhatia UG, Young DA, Stemerman MB: Induction of cyclooxygenase-2 in rat vascular smooth muscle cells in vitro and in vivo. J Biol Chem 269:8504–8509, 1994.
17. Crofford LJ, Wilder RL, Ristimaki AP, Sano H, Remmers EF, Epps HR, Hla T: Cyclooxygenase-1 and -2 expression in rheumatoid synovial tissues. J Clin Invest 93:1095–1101, 1994.
18. Yamagata K, Andreasson KI, Kaufman WE, Barnes CA, Worley PF: Expression of a mitogen-inducible cyclooxygenase in brain neurons: Regulation by synaptic activity and glucocorticoids. Neuron 11:371–386, 1993.
19. Masferrer JL, Zweifel BS, Manning PT, Hauser SD, Leahy KM, Smith WG, Isakson PC, Seibert K: Selective inhibition of inducible cyclooxygenase 2 in vivo is anti-inflammatory and nonulcerogenic. Proc Natl Acad Sci U S A 91:3228–3232, 1994.
20. Seibert K, Zhang Y, Leahy K, Hauser S, Masferrer J, Perkins W, Lee L, Isakson P: Pharmacological and biochemical demonstration of the role of cyclooxygenase 2 in inflammation and pain. Proc Natl Acad Sci U S A 91:12013–12017, 1994.
21. Gierse JK, Hauser SD, Creely DP, Koboldt C, Rangwala SH, Isakson PC, Seibert K: Expression and selective inhibition of the constitutive and inducible forms of human cyclooxygenase. Part 2. J Biochem 305:479–484, 1995.
22. Mitchell JA, Akarasereenont P, Thiemermann C, Flower RJ, Van JR: Selectivity of nonsteroidal anti-inflammatory drugs as inhibitors of constitutive and inducible cyclooxygenase. Proc Natl Acad Sci U S A 90:11693–11697, 1994.

23. Lewis RA, Austin KF, Soberman RJ: Leukotrienes and other products of the 5-lipoxygenase pathway. N Engl J Med 323:645–655, 1990.

24. Miele L, Cordella-Miele E, Facchiano A, Meekherjee AB: Novel antiinflammatory peptides from the region of highest similarity between uteroglobin and lipocortin I. Nature 335:726–730, 1988.

25. Camussi G, Tetta C, Bussolino F, Baglioni C: Antiinflammatory peptides (antiflammins) inhibit synthesis of platelet-activating factor, neutrophil aggregation and chemotaxis, and intradermal inflammatory reactions. J Exp Med 171:913–927, 1990.

26. Goodwin JS: Are prostaglandins proinflammatory, antiinflammatory, both or neither? J Rheumatol 18(Suppl 28):26–29, 1991.

27. Kuehl FA Jr, Humes JL, Ham FA, Egan RW, Dougherty HW: Inflammation: The role of peroxidase-derived products. In Samuelsson B, Ramwell B, Paletti R (eds): Advances in Prostaglandin and Thromboxane Research. Vol 6. New York, Raven Press, 1980, p 77.

28. Vane JR: Inhibition of prostaglandin synthesis as a mechanism of action for aspirin-like drugs. Nature (New Biol) 231:232, 1971.

29. Vane J: The evolution of non-steroidal anti-inflammatory drugs and their mechanisms of action. Drugs 33(Suppl 1):18, 1987.

30. Dawson W, Boot JR, Harvey J, Walker JR: The pharmacology of benoxaprofen with particular reference to effects on lipoxygenase product formation. Eur J Rheumatol Inflamm 5:61, 1982.

31. Ku EC, Lee W, Kothari HV, Kimble EF, Liauw L, Tjan J: The effect of diclofenac sodium on arachidonic acid metabolism. Semin Arthritis Rheum 15:36, 1985.

32. Isselbacher KJ: The role of arachidonic acid metabolites in gastrointestinal homeostasis. Biochemical, histological and clinical gastrointestinal effects. Drugs 33(Suppl 1):38, 1987.

33. Weinblatt M, Kremer J, Helfgott S, Coblyn J, Maier A, Sperling R, Petrillo G, Kesterson J, Dube L, Henson B, Teoh N, Rubin P: A 5-lipoxygenase inhibitor in rheumatoid arthritis (abstr). Arthritis Rheum 33(Suppl 9):S152, 1990.

34. Smith DM, Johnson JA, Loeser R, Turner RA: Evaluation of tenidap (CP-66, 248) on human neutrophil arachidonic acid metabolism, chemotactic potential and clinical efficacy in the treatment of rheumatoid arthritis. Agents Actions 31:102–109, 1990.

35. Sperling RI, Weinblatt M, Robin J-L, Coblyn J Fraser, P Lewis, RA Austen, KF: Effects of dietary fish oil on in vitro leukocyte function, leukotriene generation and activity of disease in rheumatoid arthritis (abstr). Arthritis Rheum 29(Suppl 4):S-18, 1986.

36. Abramson SB, Weissmann G: The mechanisms of action of nonsteroidal antiinflammatory drugs. Arthritis Rheum 32:1–9, 1989.

37. Chang Y-H, Silverman SL, Paulus HE: Colchicine. In Paulus HE, Furst DE, Dromgoole S (eds): Drugs for Rheumatic Disease. New York, Churchill Livingstone, 1987, p 431.

38. Keates RAB, Mason GB: Inhibition of microtubule polymerization by tubulin-colchicine complex: Inhibition of spontaneous assembly. Can J Biochem 59:361, 1981.

39. Malawista SE, Chang Y-H, Wilson L: Lumicolchicine, lack of antiinflammatory effect. Arthritis Rheum 15:641, 1972.

40. Ehrenfeld M, Levy M, Bar Eli M, Galliby R, Eliakim M: Effect of colchicine on polymorphonuclear leukocyte chemotaxis in human volunteers. Br J Clin Pharmacol 10:297, 1980.

41. Spilberg I, Mandell B, Mehta J, Simchowitz L, Rosenberg D: Mechanism of action of colchicine in acute urate-induced arthritis. J Clin Invest 64:775, 1979.

42. Serhan CN, Lundberg U, Weissmann G, Samuelsson B: Formation of leukotrienes and hydroxy acids by human neutrophils and platelets exposed to monosodium urate. Prostaglandins 27:563, 1984.

43. Schlesinger M, Ilfeld D, Handzel ZT, Altman Y, Kuperman O, Levin S, Netzer L, Trainin N: Effect of colchicine on immunoregulatory abnormalities in familial Mediterranean fever. Clin Exp Immunol 54:73, 1983.

44. Dellaverde E, Fan PT, Chang Y-H: Mechanisms of action of colchicine. V: Neutrophil adherence and phagocytosis in patients with acute gout treated with colchicine. J Pharmacol Exp Ther 223:197, 1982.

45. Brune K, Glatt M, Graf P: Mechanisms of action of antiinflammatory drugs. Gen Pharmacol 7:27, 1976.

46. Nuki G: Nonsteroidal analgesic and antiinflammatory agents. Br Med J 287:39, 1983.

47. Furst DE, Dromgoole S: Other nonsteroidal antiinflammatory drugs. In Paulus HE, Furst DE, Dromgoole S (eds): Drugs for Rheumatic Disease. New York, Churchill Livingstone, 1987, p 409.

48. Mangan FR: Nabumetone. In Lewis AJ, Furst DE (eds): Nonsteroidal Anti-inflammatory Drugs: Mechanisms and Clinical Use. New York, Marcel Dekker, 1987, p 439.

49. Spector WG, Willoughby DA: Antiinflammatory effects of salicylate in the rat. In Dixon A StJ, Smith MJH, Martin BK, Wood PHN (eds): Salicylates: An International Symposium. Boston, Little, Brown & Co, 1963, p 141.

50. Fremont-Smith K, Bayles B: Salicylate therapy in rheumatoid arthritis. JAMA 192:103, 1964.

51. American Rheumatism Association Cooperating Clinics Committee: Aspirin in rheumatoid arthritis: A seven-day double-blind trial preliminary report. Bull Rheum Dis 16:388, 1965.

52. Paulus HE: Pharmacological considerations. In Roth SH (ed): Handbook of Drug Therapy in Rheumatology. Littleton, Mass, PSG Publishing, 1985, p 39.

53. Paulus HE, Schlosstein LH, Godfrey RG, Klinenberg JR, Bluestone R: Prophylactic colchicine therapy of intercritical gout: A placebo-controlled study of probenecid-treated patients. Arthritis Rheum 17:609, 1974.

54. Meed SD, Spilberg I: Successful use of colchicine in acute polyarticular pseudogout. J Rheumatol 8:689, 1981.

55. Bowles C, Harrington T, Zinsmeister S, Ellman M, Reginato A, McCarty D, Ryan L, Espinosa L, Spilberg I, O'Duffy D: Colchicine prevents recurrent pseudogout: Multicenter trial. Arthritis Rheum 29:S-38, 1986.

56. Ainarello CA, Wolff SM, Goldfinger SE: Colchicine therapy for familial Mediterranean fever: A double-blind study. N Engl J Med 291:934, 1976.

57. Lim RKS, Guzman F, Rodger DW, Goto K, Brawn C, Dickerson GD, Engle RJ: Site of action of narcotic and non-narcotic analgesics determined by blocking bradykinin-evoked visceral pain. Arch Int Pharmacodyn Ther 152:25, 1964.

58. Brune K: Prostaglandins and the mode of action of antipyretic analgesic drugs. Am J Med 75:19, 1983.

59. Feldberg W, Melton AS: Prostaglandins and body temperature. In Vane JR, Ferreira SH (eds): Inflammation. New York, Springer-Verlag, 1978, p 617.

60. Lewis AJ, Furst DE (eds): Nonsteroidal Antiinflammatory Drugs: Mechanisms and Clinical Use. New York, Marcel Dekker, 1987.

61. Friend WG: Sulindac suppression of colorectal polyps in Gardner's syndrome. Am Fam Physician 41:891, 1990.

62. Reinberg A, Levi F: Clinical chronopharmacology with special reference to NSAIDs. Scand J Rheumatol (Suppl 65):118–122, 1987.

63. Miller TA, Jacobson ED: Gastrointestinal cytoprotection by prostaglandins. Gut 20:75, 1979.

64. Roth S, Agrawal M, Nahowald M, Swabb E, et al: Misoprostil heals gastroduodenal injury in patients with rheumatoid arthritis receiving aspirin. Arch Intern Med 149:775–779, 1989.

65. Silverstein FE, Graham DY, Senior JR, Davies HW, Struthers BJ, Bittman RM, Geis S: Misoprostil reduces serious gastrointestinal complications in patients with rheumatoid arthritis receiving nonsteroidal anti-inflammatory drugs. Ann Intern Med 123:241–249, 1995.

66. O'Brien WM: Pharmacology of nonsteroidal antiinflammatory drugs: Practical review for clinicians. Am J Med 75(Suppl):32, 1983.

67. Caruso I, Bianchi-Porro G: Gastroscopic evaluation of antiinflammatory agents. Br Med J 280:75, 1980.

68. Lanza FL: Endoscopic studies of gastric and duodenal injury after the use of ibuprofen, aspirin, and other nonsteroidal antiinflammatory agents. Am J Med 77(1A):19, 1984.

69. Bianchi Porro G, Petrillo M, Ardizzone S: Salsalate in the treatment of rheumatoid arthritis: A double-blind clinical and gastroscopic trial versus piroxicam: II. Endoscopic evaluation. J Int Med Res 17:320, 1989.

70. Hedenbro JL, Wetterberg P, Vallgren S, Bergqvist L: Lack of correlation between fecal blood loss and drug-induced gastric mucosal lesions. Gastrointest Endosc 34:247, 1988.

71. Cohen A: Fecal blood loss and plasma salicylate study of salicylsalicylic acid and aspirin. J Clin Pharmacol 19:242, 1979.

72. Lanza FL, Rack MF, Doucette M, Ekholm B, Goldlust B, Wilson R: An endoscopic comparison of the gastroduodenal injury seen with salsalate and naproxen. J Rheumatol 16:1570, 1989.

73. Roth S, Bennett R, Calderon P, Hartman R, Mitchell C, Doucette M, Ekholm B, Goldlust B, Lee E, Wilson R: Reduced risk of NSAID gastropathy (GI mucosal toxicity) with nonacetylated salicylate (salsalate): An endoscopic study. Semin Arthritis Rheum 19:11, 1990.

74. Fries JF: NSAID gastropathy: the second most deadly rheumatic disease? Epidemiology and risk appraisal. J Rheumatol 18(Suppl 28):6–10, 1991.

75. Willet LR, Carson JL, Strom BL: Epidemiology of gastrointestinal damage associated with nonsteroidal anti-inflammatory drugs. Drug Safety 10:170–181, 1994.

76. Gabriel SE, Jaakkimainen L, Bombardier C: Risk for serious gastrointestinal complications related to use of nonsteroidal anti-inflammatory drugs: A meta-analysis. Ann Intern Med 115:787–796, 1991.

77. Bollini P, Garcia Rodriguez LA, Perez Gutthann S, Walker AM: The impact of research quality and study design on epidemiologic estimates of the effect of nonsteroidal anti-inflammatory drugs on upper gastrointestinal tract disease. Arch Intern Med 152:1289–1295, 1992.

78. Savage RL, Moller PW, Ballantyne CL, Wells JE: Variation in the risk of peptic ulcer complications with nonsteroidal anti-inflammatory drug therapy. Arthritis Rheum 36:84–90, 1993.

79. Langman MJS, Weil J, Wainwright P, Lawson DH, Rawlins MD, Logan RFA, Murphy M, Vessey MP, Colin-Jones DG: Risks of bleeding peptic ulcer associated with individual nonsteroidal anti-inflammatory drugs. Lancet 343:1075–1078, 1994.

80. Soll AH, Weinstein WM, Kurota J, McCarthy D: Nonsteroidal anti-inflammatory drugs and peptic ulcer disease. Ann Intern Med 114:307–319, 1991.

81. Kurata JH, Abbey DE: The effect of chronic aspirin use on duodenal and gastric ulcer hospitalizations. J Clin Gastroenterol 12:260–266, 1990.

82. Paulus HE: Government affairs. FDA Arthritis Advisory Committee Meeting: Risks of agranulocytosis/aplastic anemia, flank pain, and adverse gastrointestinal effects with the use of nonsteroidal antiinflammatory drugs. Arthritis Rheum 30:593, 1987.

83. Roth SH: Prevention of NSAID-induced gastric mucosal damage and gastric ulcer: A review of clinical studies. J Drug Devel 1:255–263, 1989.

84. O'Brien WM, Bagby GF: Rare adverse reactions to nonsteroidal antiinflammatory drugs. J Rheumatol 12:13, 1985.

85. Paulus HE: Government affairs: FDA Arthritis Advisory Committee Meeting. Arthritis Rheum 25:1124, 1982.

86. Katz LM, Love PY: Hepatic dysfunction in association with NSAIDs. In Famaey JP, Paulus HE (eds): Nonsteroidal Antiinflammatory Drugs: Subpopulation Therapy and Drug Delivery Systems. New York, Marcel Dekker, 1991.

87. Benson GD: Hepatotoxicity following the therapeutic use of antipyretic analgesics. Am J Med 75(Suppl):85, 1983.

88. Benjamin SB, Ishak KG, Zimmerman HJ, Grushka A: Phenylbutazone liver injury: A clinical-pathologic survey of 23 cases and review of the literature. Hepatology 1:255, 1981.

89. Dunn M: The role of arachidonic acid metabolites in renal homeostasis. Nonsteroidal antiinflammatory drugs and renal function: Biochemical, histological and clinical effects and drug interactions. Drugs 33(Suppl 1):56, 1987.

90. Blackshear JL, Napier JS, Davidman M, Stillman MT: Renal complications of nonsteroidal antiinflammatory drugs: Identification and monitoring of those at risk. Semin Arthritis Rheum 14:163, 1985.

91. DiBona GF: Prostaglandins and nonsteroidal antiinflammatory drugs: Effects on renal hemodynamics. Am J Med 80(Suppl 1A):12, 1986.

92. Clive DM, Stoff JS: Renal syndromes associated with nonsteroidal antiinflammatory drugs. N Engl J Med 310:563, 1984.

93. Stillman MT, Napier JS, Blackshear JL: Adverse effects of nonsteroidal antiinflammatory drugs on the kidney. Med Clin North Am 68:371, 1984.

94. Zipser RD, Henrich WL: Implications of nonsteroidal antiinflammatory drug therapy. Am J Med 80(Suppl 1A):78, 1986.

95. Johnson AG, Nguyen TV, Day RO: Do nonsteroidal anti-inflammatory drugs affect blood pressure? A meta-analysis. Ann Intern Med 121:289–300, 1994.

96. Eriksson LO, Sturfelt G, Thysell H, Wollheim FA: Effects of sulindac and naproxen on prostaglandin excretion in patients with impaired renal function and rheumatoid arthritis. Am J Med 89:313–321, 1990.

97. Ciabattoni G, Cinotte GA, Pierucci A, Simonetti BM, Manzi M, Pugliese F, Barsotti P, Pecci G, Taggi F, Patrono C: Effects of sulindac and ibuprofen in patients with chronic glomerular disease. N Engl J Med 310:279, 1984.

98. Roberts DG, Gerber JG, Nies AS: Comparative effects of sulindac and indomethacin in humans. Clin Pharmacol Ther 35:269, 1984.

99. Brater DC, Anderson S, Baird B, Campbell WB: Sulindac does not spare the kidney. Clin Pharmacol Ther 35:229, 1984.

100. Svendsen G, Gerstoft J, Hansen TM, Christensen P, Lorenzen IB: The renal excretion of prostaglandins and changes in plasma renin during treatment with either sulindac or naproxen in patients with rheumatoid arthritis and thiazide-treated heart failure. J Rheumatol 11:779, 1984.

101. Abraham PA, Keane WF: Glomerular and interstitial diseases induced by nonsteroidal antiinflammatory drugs. Am J Nephrol 4:1, 1984.

102. Bennett WM, DeBroe ME: Analgesic nephropathy: A preventable renal disease. N Engl J Med 320:1269–1271, 1989.

103. Whelton A, Stout RL, Spilman PS, Klossen DK: Renal effects of ibuprofen, piroxicam and sulindac in patients with asymptomatic renal failure. Ann Intern Med 112:568, 1990.

104. Stern RS, Bigby M: An expanded profile of cutaneous reactions to nonsteroidal antiinflammatory drugs. JAMA 52:1433, 1984.

105. Suarez SM, Cohen PR, De Leo VA: Bullous photosensitivity to naproxen: "Pseudoporphyria." Arthritis Rheum 33:903, 1990.

106. Szczeklik A: Antipyretic analgesics and the allergic patient. Am J Med 75:82, 1983.

107. Strom BL, Carson JL, Morse ML, West SL, Soper KA: The effect of indication on hypersensitivity reactions associated with zomepirac sodium and other nonsteroidal antiinflammatory drugs. Arthritis Rheum 30:1142–1148, 1987.

108. Inman WH: Study of fatal bone marrow depression with special reference to phenylbutazone and oxyphenbutazone. Br Med J 1:1500, 1977.

109. Paulus HE: Government affairs: FDA Arthritis Advisory Committee Meeting. Arthritis Rheum 28:450–451, 1985.

110. The International Agranulocytosis and Aplastic Anemia Study: Risks of agranulocytosis and aplastic anemia: A first report of their relation to drug use with special reference to analgesics. JAMA 256:1749, 1986.

111. Morris H, Sherman NA, McQuain C, et al: Effects of salsalate (nonacetylated salicylate) and aspirin on serum prostaglandins in humans. Ther Drug Monit 7:435, 1985.

112. Friedel HA, Todd PA: Nabumetone. A preliminary review of its phar-

macodynamic and pharmacokinetic properties, and therapeutic efficacy in rheumatic diseases. Drugs 35:504–524, 1988.

113. Schlegel SI, Paulus HE: Nonsteroidal and analgesic therapy in the elderly. Clin Rheumat Dis 12:245, 1986.

114. Sylvia LM, Forlenza SW, Brocavick JM: Aseptic meningitis associated with naproxen. Drug Intell Clin Pharm 22:339, 1988.

115. Court H, Streete P, Volans G: Acute poisoning with ibuprofen. Hum Toxicol 2:381, 1983.

116. Hall AH, Smolinske SC, Conrad FL, Wruk KM, Kulig KW, Dwelle TL, Rumack BH: Ibuprofen overdose: 126 cases. Ann Emerg Med 15:1308, 1986.

117. Vale JA, Meridith T: Poisoning due to non-steroidal antiinflammatory drugs. In JP Famaey, Paulus HE (eds): Nonsteroidal Antiinflammatory Drugs: Subpopulation Therapy and Drug Delivery Systems. New York, Marcel Dekker, 1991.

118. Brater DC: Drug–drug and drug–disease interactions with nonsteroidal antiinflammatory drugs. Am J Med 80(Suppl 1A):62, 1986.

119. Klotz U: Interactions of analgesics with other drugs. Am J Med 75:133, 1983.

120. Grennan DM, Aarons L: Salicylate–NSAID interactions. Ann Rheum Dis 43:351, 1984.

121. Favre L, Glasson P, Vallotten MB: Reversible acute renal failure from combined triamterene and indomethacin. Ann Intern Med 96:317, 1986.

122. Richardson CJ, Blocka KLN, Ross SG, Verbeeck RK: Effects of age and sex on piroxicam disposition. Clin Pharmacol Ther 37:13, 1985.

123. Furst DE, Gupta N, Paulus HE: Salicylate metabolism in twins. J Clin Invest 60:32, 1977.

124. Vassell ES, Page JG: Genetic control of drug levels in man: Phenylbutazone. Science 154:1479, 1968.

125. Fowler PD, Faragher EB: Drug and non-drug factors influencing adverse reactions to pyrazoles. J Int Med Res 5(Suppl 2):108, 1977.

126. Dromgoole SH, Furst DE: Naproxen. In Paulus HE, Furst DE, Dromgoole SH (eds): Drugs for Rheumatic Disease. New York, Churchill Livingstone, 1987, p 347.

127. Physician's Desk Reference, 49th ed. Oradell, NJ, Medical Economics Company, 1995, Suppl A, pp A54–57.

128. Antilla M, Haataja M, Kasanen A: Pharmacokinetics of naproxen in subjects with normal and impaired renal function. Eur J Clin Pharmacol 18:263, 1980.

129. Williams RL, Upton RA, Cello JP, Jones RM, Blitstein M, Kelly J, Nierenburg D: Naproxen disposition in patients with alcoholic cirrhosis. Eur J Clin Pharmacol 27:291, 1984.

130. Jalava S, Saarimaa H, Antilla M, Sundquist H: Naproxen concentrations in serum, synovial fluid, and synovium. Scand J Rheumatol 6:155, 1977.

131. Todd PA, Clissold SP: Naproxen: A reappraisal of its pharmacology and therapeutic use in rheumatic diseases and pain states. Drugs 40:91, 1990.

132. Day RO, Furst DE, Dromgoole SH, Kamm B, Roe R, Paulus HE: Relationship of serum naproxen concentration to efficacy in rheumatoid arthritis. Clin Pharmacol Ther 31:733, 1982.

133. Runkel R, Mroszczak E, Chaplin M, Sevelius H, Segre E: Naproxen-probenecid interaction. Clin Pharmacol Ther 24:706, 1978.

134. Willkens RF, Segre EJ: Combination therapy with naproxen and aspirin in rheumatoid arthritis. Arthritis Rheum 19:677, 1975.

135. Furst DE, Blocka K, Cassell S, Harris ER, Hirschberg JM, Josephson M, Lachenbruch PA, Paulus HE, Trimble RB: A controlled study of concurrent therapy with a nonacetylated salicylate and naproxen in rheumatoid arthritis. Arthritis Rheum 38:146, 1987.

136. Duggan DE: Sulindac: Therapeutic implications of the prodrug/pharmacophore equilibrium. Drug Metab Rev 12:325, 1981.

137. Kwan KC, Duggan DE, Hucker HB: Metabolism and pharmacokinetics of sulindac. Postgraduate Medicine Communications. New York, McGraw-Hill, 1979, p 13.

138. Furst DE, Dromgoole SH: Indomethacin and sulindac. In Paulus HE, Furst DE, Dromgoole SH (eds): Drugs for Rheumatic Disease. New York, Churchill Livingstone, 1987, p 285.

139. Swanson BN, Boppano VK, Vlasses PH, Holmes CI, Monsell KC, Ferguson RK: Sulindac disposition when given once or twice daily. Clin Pharmacol Ther 32:397, 1982.

140. Duggan DE, Hooke KF, Noll RM, Hucker HB, Van Arman CG: Comparative disposition of sulindac and metabolites in five species. Biochem Pharmacol 27:2311, 1978.

141. Steelman SL, Tempero KF, Cirillo VJ: The chemistry, pharmacology, toxicology and clinical pharmacology of diflunisal. Clin Ther 1(Suppl A):1, 1978.

142. Dromgoole SH, Furst DE: Diflunisal. In Paulus HE, Furst DE, Dromgoole SH (eds): Drugs for Rheumatic Disease. New York, Churchill Livingstone, 1987, p 399.

143. Davies RO: Review of the animal in clinical pharmacology of diflunisal. Pharmacotherapy 3(Suppl 1):9S, 1983.

144. Verbeeck R, Tjandramage TB, Mullie A, Verbesselt R, Verbeckmoses R, DeSchepper PJ: Biotransformation of diflunisal and renal excretion of its glucuronides in renal insufficiency. Br J Clin Pharmacol 9:273, 1979.

145. Myers RF, Siegel MI: Differential effects of antiinflammatory drugs on

lipoxygenase and cyclooxygenase activities of neutrophils from a reverse passive Arthus reaction. Biochem Biophys Res Commun 112:586, 1983.

146. Kaplan HB, Edelson HS, Korchak HM, Given WP, Abramson S, Weissmann G: Effects of nonsteroidal antiinflammatory agents on human neutrophil functions *in vitro* and *in vivo*. Biochem Pharmacol 33:371, 1984.

147. Hobbs DC, Twomey TM: Piroxicam pharmacokinetics in man: Aspirin and antacid interaction studies. J Clin Pharmacol 19:270, 1979.

148. Ostensen M, Matheson I, Loufen H: Piroxicam in breast milk after long-term treatment. Eur J Clin Pharmacol 35:567–569, 1988.

149. Kurowski M, Dunky A: Transsynovial kinetics of piroxicam in patients with rheumatoid arthritis. Eur J Clin Pharmacol 34:401–406, 1988.

150. Dupont D, Dayer P, Balant L, Gorgia A, Fabre J: Variations intraindividuelles du comportement du piroxicam: Pharmacocinetique chez l'homme en bonne santé et chez le malade en insuffisance rénale. Pharm Acta Helv 57:20, 1982.

151. Chang Y-H, Dromgoole SH: Oxicams. *In* Paulus HE, Furst DE, Dromgoole SH (eds): Drugs for Rheumatic Disease. New York, Churchill Livingstone, 1987, p 389.

152. Said SA, Fodar AM: Influence of cimetidine on the pharmacokinetics of piroxicam in rat and man. Arzneim Forsch 39:790–792, 1989.

153. Darrugh A, Gordon AJ, Byrne HO, Hobbs D, Casey E: Single-dose and steady-state pharmacokinetics of piroxicam in elderly vs young adults. Eur J Clin Pharmacol 28:305, 1985.

154. Piroxicam Symposium: Piroxicam: a clinical perspective. Am J Med 82(Suppl 5B):1, 1986.

155. Turner RA (ed): Proceedings of a symposium: Nabumetone, a new nonsteroidal antiinflammatory drug. Am J Med 83(Suppl 4B):1–122, 1987.

156. Miller LG: Oxaprozin: A once-daily nonsteroidal anti-inflammatory drug. Clin Pharmacokinet 11:591–603, 1992.

157. Janssen FW, Jusko WJ, Chiang ST, Kirkman SK, Southgate PJ, Coleman AJ, Ruelius HW: Metabolism and kinetics of oxaprozin in normal subjects. Clin Pharmacol Ther 27:352–362, 1980.

158. Wallace SL, Ertel NH: Plasma levels of colchicine after oral administration of a single dose. Metabolism 22:749, 1973.

159. Ertel NH, Wallace SL: Measurement of colchicine in urine and peripheral leukocytes. Clin Res 19:348, 1971.

160. Halkin H, Dany S, Greenwald M, Schnaps Y, Tirosh M: Colchicine kinetics in patients with familial Mediterranean fever. Clin Pharmacol Ther 28:82, 1980.

161. Levy M, Eldor A, Zylber-Katz E, Eliakim M: The effect of long-term colchicine therapy in patients with recurrent polyserositis on the capacity of blood platelets to synthesize thromboxane A_2. Br J Clin Pharmacol 16:191, 1983.

162. Pullar T: The pharmacokinetics of tenidap sodium: Introduction. Br J Clin Pharmacol 39:(Suppl 1):1S–2S, 1995.

163. Breedveld F: Tenidap: A novel cytokine-modulating anti-rheumatic drug for the treatment of rheumatoid arthritis. Scand J Rheumatol 23(Suppl 100):31–44, 1994.

164. Madhok R: Tenidap. Lancet 346:481–485, 1995.

165. Wylie G, Appelboom T, Bolten W, Breedveld FC, Keely J. Leeming MRG, LeLoet X, Manthorpe R, Marcolongo R, Smolea J: A comparative study of tenidap, a cytokine-modulating anti-rheumatic drug, and diclofenac in rheumatoid arthritis: A 24-week analysis of a 1-year clinical trial. Br J Rheumatol 34:554–563, 1995.

166. Kirby DS, Loose LD, Weiner ES, Wilhelm FE, Shanahan WR, Ting N: Tenidap versus naproxen in the treatment of rheumatoid arthritis patients. Arthritis Rheum 36(Suppl 9):112, 1993.

167. Leeming MRG: A double-blind randomised comparison of tenidap versus auranofin plus diflofenac in early rheumatoid arthritis (RA). Arthritis Rheum 36:S111, 1993.

168. Winter CA, Risley ER, Seller RH: Anti-inflammatory activity of indomethacin and plasma corticosterone in rats. J Pharmacol Exp Ther 162:196, 1968.

169. Yeh KC, Berger ET, Breault GO, Lei BW: Effect of sustained release on the pharmacokinetic profile of indomethacin in man. Biopharm Drug Dispos 3:219, 1982.

170. Parks BR, Jordan RL, Rawson JE, Douglas BH: Indomethacin: Studies of absorption and placental transfer. Am J Obstet Gynecol 129:464, 1977.

171. Astier A, Renat B: Sensitive high performance liquid chromatographic determination of indomethacin in human plasma: Pharmacokinetic studies after a single oral dose. J Chromatogr 233:279, 1982.

172. Emori HW, Champion GD, Bluestone R, Paulus HE: Simultaneous pharmacokinetics of indomethacin in serum and synovial fluid. Ann Rheum Dis 32:433, 1973.

173. Duggan DE, Hogan AF, Kwan KC, McMahon DG: The metabolism of indomethacin in man. J Pharmacol Exp Ther 181:563, 1972.

174. Duggan DE, Kwan KC: Enterohepatic recirculation of drugs as a determinant of therapeutic ratio. Drug Metab Rev 9:21, 1979.

175. Traeger A, Noschel H, Zaumseil J: Pharmacokinetics of indomethacin in pregnant and parturient women and in their newborn infants. Zentralbl Gynakol 95:635, 1973.

176. Traeger A, Kunze M, Stein G, Ankermann M: Pharmacokinetics of indomethacin in the aged. Z Altersforsch 27:151, 1973.

177. Kwan KC, Breault GO, Davis RL, Lei BW, Czerwinski AW, Besselaar GH, Duggan DE: Effects of concomitant aspirin administration on the pharmacokinetics of indomethacin in man. J Pharmacokinet Biopharm 6:451, 1978.

178. Brooks PM, Walker JJ, Bell MA, Buchanan WW, Rhymer AR: Indomethacin-aspirin interaction: A clinical appraisal. Br Med J 11:69, 1975.

179. Livio M, Del Maschio A, Cesletti C, deGaetano G: Indomethacin prevents the long-lasting inhibitory effect of aspirin on human platelet cyclo-oxygenase activity. Prostaglandins 23:787, 1982.

180. Helleberg L: Clinical pharmacokinetics of indomethacin. Clin Pharmacokinet 6:245, 1981.

181. Brooks PM, Bell MA, Sturrock RD, Famaey JP, Dick WC: The clinical significance of indomethacin-probenecid interaction. Br J Clin Pharmacol 1:287, 1974.

182. Adams SS, Bresloff P, Mason CG: Pharmacological differences between the optical isomers of ibuprofen: Evidence for metabolic inversion of the (−) isomer. J Pharm Pharmacol 28:256, 1976.

183. Albert KS, Gernaat CM: Pharmacokinetics of ibuprofen. Am J Med 77:40, 1984.

184. Whitlam JB, Brown KF, Crooks MJ, Room JFW: Transsynovial distribution of ibuprofen in arthritic patients. Clin Pharmacol Ther 29:487, 1981.

185. Kaiser DG, Vangiessen GJ, Reischer RJ, Wechter WJ: Isomeric inversion of ibuprofen R(−) enantiomers in humans. J Pharm Sci 65:269, 1976.

186. Albert KS, Gillespie WR, Wagner JG, Pau A, Lockwood GF: Effects of age on the clinical pharmacokinetics of ibuprofen. Am J Med 77:47, 1984.

187. Slattery JT, Levy G: Effects of ibuprofen on protein-binding of warfarin in human serum. J Pharm Sci 66:1060, 1977.

188. Brooks CD, Ulrich JE: Effect of ibuprofen or aspirin on probenecid induced uricosuria. J Int Med Res 8:283, 1980.

189. Rao GHR, Johnson GG, Reddy KR, White JG: Ibuprofen protects platelet cyclo-oxygenase from irreversible inhibition by aspirin. Atherosclerosis 3:383, 1983.

190. Day R, Furst DE: Ibuprofen, fenoprofen, ketoprofen. *In* Paulus HE, Furst DE, Dromgoole S (eds): Drugs for Rheumatic Disease. New York, Churchill Livingstone, 1987, p 315.

191. Barry WS, Meinzinger MM, Howse CR: Ibuprofen overdose and exposure in utero: Results from a post marketing voluntary reporting system. Am J Med 77(Suppl 1A):35, 1984.

192. Rubin A, Knadler MP, Ho PP, Bechtol LD, Wolen RL: Stereoselective inversion of (R)− fenoprofen to (S)+ fenoprofen in humans. J Pharm Sci 74:82, 1985.

193. Chernish SM, Rubin A, Rodda BE, Ridolfo AS, Gruber CM Jr: The physiological disposition of fenoprofen in man. IV: The effects of position of subject, food ingestion and antacid ingestion on the plasma levels of orally administered fenoprofen. J Med 3:249, 1972.

194. Kamal A, Koch IM: Plasma profiles of two differing doses of fenoprofen in geriatric patients. Pharmatherapeutica 2:552, 1981.

195. Brogden RN, Pinder RM, Speight TM, Avery GS: Fenoprofen: A review of its pharmacological properties and therapeutic efficacy in rheumatic diseases. Drugs 13:241, 1977.

196. Brewer EJ, Giannini EH, Baum J, Bernstein B, Fink CW, Emery HM, Schaller JG: Aspirin and fenoprofen (Nalfon) in the treatment of juvenile rheumatoid arthritis: Results of a double-blind trial. J Rheumatol 9:123, 1982.

197. Garella S, Matarese RA: Renal effects of prostaglandins and clinical adverse effects of non-steroidal antiinflammatory agent. Medicine 63:165, 1984.

198. Stachura I, Jayakumar S, Bourke E: T and B lymphocyte subsets in fenoprofen nephropathy. Am J Med 75:9, 1983.

199. Gandini R, Cunietti E, Pappalepore V, Ferrari M, Deleo B, Locatelli E, Fasoli A: Effects of intravenous high doses of ketoprofen on blood clotting, bleeding time and platelet aggregation in man. J Int Med Res 11:243, 1983.

200. Upton RA, Williams RL, Guentert TW, Buskin JN, Reigelman S: Ketoprofen pharmacokinetics and bioavailability based on an improved and specific assay. Eur J Clin Pharmacol 20:127, 1981.

201. Vavra I: Ketoprofen. *In* Lewis AJ, Furst DE (eds): Nonsteroidal Antiinflammatory Drugs: Mechanisms and Clinical Use. New York, Marcel Dekker, 1987, p 419.

202. Advenier C, Roux A, Gobert C, Massais P, Variquax O, Flouvat B: Pharmacokinetics of ketoprofen in the elderly. Br J Clin Pharmacol 16:65, 1983.

203. Staffanger G, Larsen HW, Hansen H, Sorensen K: Pharmacokinetics of ketoprofen in patients with chronic renal failure. Scand J Rheumatol 10:189, 1981.

204. Upton RA, Williams RL, Buskin JN, Matthew-Jones R: Effects of probenecid on ketoprofen kinetics. Clin Pharmacol Ther 31:705, 1982.

205. Williams RL, Upton RA, Buskin JN, Jones RM: Ketoprofen-aspirin interactions. Clin Pharmacol Ther 30:226, 1981.

206. Thyss S, Milano G, Kubar J, Namer M, Schneider M: Clinical and

pharmacokinetic evidence of a life-threatening interaction between methotrexate and ketoprofen. Lancet 1:256, 1986.

207. Physician's Desk Reference, 49th ed. Oradell, NJ, Medical Economics, 1995, pp 2703–2706.

208. Furst DE, Dromgoole SH, Fow S, Landaw EM: Comparison of tolmetin kinetics in rheumatoid arthritis and matched healthy controls. J Clin Pharmacol 23:557, 1983.

209. Dromgoole SH, Furst DE, Desiraju RK, Nayak RK, Kirschenbaum MA, Paulus HE: Tolmetin kinetics and synovial fluid prostaglandin E levels in rheumatoid arthritis. Clin Pharmacol Ther 32:371, 1982.

210. Selley ML, Glass J, Triggs EJ, Thomas J: Pharmacokinetic studies of tolmetin in man. Clin Pharmacol Ther 17:599, 1975.

211. Dromgoole SH, Furst DE: Tolmetin. In Paulus HE, Furst DE, Dromgoole S (eds): Drugs for Rheumatic Disease. New York, Churchill Livingstone, 1987, p 365.

212. O'Brien WM: Long term efficacy and safety of tolmetin sodium in treatment of geriatric patients with rheumatoid arthritis and osteoarthritis: A retrospective study. J Clin Pharmacol 23:309, 1983.

213. Restivo C, Paulus HE: Anaphylaxis from tolmetin. JAMA 240:246, 1978.

214. Dromgoole SH, Furst DE: Fenamates. In Paulus HE, Furst DE, Dromgoole S (eds): Drugs for Rheumatic Disease. New York, Churchill Livingstone, 1987, p 379.

215. Boctor AM, Eickholt M, Pugsley TA: Meclofenamate sodium is an inhibitor of both the 5-lipoxygenase and cyclo-oxygenase pathways of the arachidonic acid cascade in vitro. Prostaglandins Leukotrienes Med 23:229, 1986.

216. Glazko AJ: Pharmacology of the fenamates. III: Metabolism and disposition. In Kendall PH (ed): Fenamates in Medicine: A Symposium. Ann Phys Med Suppl 8:23, 1966.

217. Baragar FD, Smith TC: Drug interaction studies with meclofenamate (meclomen). Curr Ther Res 23(Suppl):S51, 1978.

218. Eberl R: Long-term experience with meclofenamate sodium. Arzneimittelforschung 33:667, 1983.

219. Physician's Desk Reference, 49th ed. Oradell, NJ, Medical Economics, 1995, pp 1061–1064.

220. Brogden RN, Heel RC, Pakes GE, Speight TM, Avery GS: Diclofenac sodium: A review of its pharmacological properties and therapeutic use in rheumatic diseases and pain of varying origin. Drugs 20:24, 1980.

221. Liauw HL, Moscaritola JD, Burcher J: Diclofenac sodium (Voltaren). In Lewis AI, Furst DE (eds): Nonsteroidal Antiinflammatory Drugs: Mechanisms and Clinical Use. New York, Marcel Dekker, 1987, p 329.

222. Cayen MN, Kraml M, Fernandi ES, Gaeselin E, Dvornik D: The metabolic disposition of etodolac in rats, dogs and man. Drug Metab Dispos 12:339, 1981.

223. Sanda M, Jacob GB, Fliedner L Jr, Kennedy J, Gotz M: Etodolac. In Lewis AI, Furst DE (eds): Nonsteroidal Antiinflammatory Drugs: Mechanisms and Clinical Use. New York, Marcel Dekker, 1987, p 349.

224. Smith RJ, Lomen PL, Kaiser DG: Flurbiprofen. In Lewis AJ, Furst DE (eds): Nonsteroidal Antiinflammatory Drugs: Mechanisms and Clinical Use. New York, Marcel Dekker, 1987, p 393.

225. Kaiser DG, Brooks CD, Lomen PL: Pharmacokinetics of flurbiprofen. Am J Med 80(Suppl 3A):10, 1986.

226. Brooks PM, Khong TK: Flurbiprofen-aspirin interaction: A double-blind cross-over study. Curr Med Res Opin 5:53, 1977.

227. Ketorolac trimethamine. Med Lett 32:79–81, 1990.

228. O'Hara DA, Fragen RF, Kinzer M, Pemberton D: Ketorolac trimethamine as compared with morphine sulfate for treatment of postoperative pain. Clin Pharmacol Ther 41:556–561, 1987.

229. Physician's Desk Reference, 49th ed. Oradell, NJ, Medical Economics, 1995, pp 2492–2496.

230. Ward JR: Nonsteridal (nonsalicylate) antiinflammatory drugs. In Roth SH (ed): Rheumatic Therapeutics. New York, McGraw-Hill, 1985, p 363.

231. Miller DR: Combination use of nonsteroidal antiinflammatory drugs. Drug Intell Clin Pharmacol 15:3, 1981.

232. Furst DE, Caldwell JR, Klugman MP, Sarkissian E: Dose-response relationship for carprofen in patients with rheumatoid arthritis (RA). Arthritis Rheum 30(Suppl 4):S95, 1987.

233. Goldsmith DP, Eichenfield AH, Drott HR, Athreya BH: Plasma indomethacin levels in juvenile rheumatoid arthritis. Arthritis Rheum 30(Suppl 4):S-35, 1987.

234. Brooks PM, Day RO: Plasma concentrations and therapeutic effects of antiinflammatory and antirheumatic drugs. In Lewis AJ, Furst DE (eds): Nonsteroidal Antiinflammatory Drugs: Mechanisms and Clinical Use. New York, Marcel Dekker, 1987, p 189.

235. Famaey JP: Synovial antiinflammatory and antirheumatic drug levels: Importance in therapeutic efficacy. In Lewis AJ, Furst DE (eds): Nonsteroidal Antiinflammatory Drugs: Mechanisms and Clinical Use. New York, Marcel Dekker, 1987, p 201.

236. Schlegel SI, Paulus HE: NSAIDs, use in rheumatic disease, side effects and interactions. Bull Rheum Dis 6(36):1–7, 1986.

237. Bradley JD, Brandt KD, Katz BP, Kalasiniski LA, Ryan SI: Comparison of an antiinflammatory dose of ibuprofen, an analgesic dose of ibuprofen, and acetaminophen in the treatment of patients with osteoarthritis of the knee. N Engl J Med 325:87–91, 1991.

238. Williams HJ, Ward JR, Egger MJ, Neuner R, Brooks RH, Clegg DO, Field EH, Skosey JL, Alarcon GS, Willkens RF, Paulus HE, Russell IJ, Sharp JT: Comparison of naproxen and acetaminophen in a two-year study of treatment of osteoarthritis of the knee. Arthritis Rheum 37:1196–1206, 1993.

CHAPTER 46

Richard O. Day

Sulfasalazine

Svartz of Stockholm, believing that infection was the cause of rheumatoid disease, collaborated with the Swedish pharmaceutical company, Pharmacia, in 1938 to synthesize salicylazosulfapyridin (now known as sulfasalazine), consisting of salicylic acid (antiarthritic) and sulfapyridine (antibacterial) joined by an azo bond (Fig. 46–1). Svartz observed a 60 percent response in her chronic polyarthritic patients and good responses also occurred in ankylosing spondylitis.[1] However, in an influential but flawed study, Sinclair and Duthie (1948)[2] found sulfasalazine to be ineffective in rheumatoid arthritis. Meanwhile, the efficacy of the drug in ulcerative colitis was established. Studies by McConkey and colleagues in the late 1970s rekindled interest in sulfasalazine as a potential antirheumatic drug.[3]

CLINICAL PHARMACOLOGY

Absorption of sulfasalazine is 10 to 20 percent only, most drug reaching the colon where the azo bond is reduced by colonic bacteria, and sulfapyridine (possibly the active component in rheumatic diseases),[4] and 5-aminosalicylic acid (active in ulcerative colitis) are liberated (see Fig. 46–1).[5, 6]

Sulfapyridine appears in plasma 4 to 6 hours following a dose of sulfasalazine and is extensively metabolized in the liver by N4-acetylation and ring hydroxylation with subsequent glucuronidations (Fig. 46–2).[7] Wide intersubject variation in metabolic rates of sulfapyridine and thus blood concentrations is observed, in part due to genetically determined variation in "acetylation" and "oxidative" capacities, respectively.[7] However, there is no relationship between plasma concentrations of sulfapyridine and efficacy.[8] The pharmacokinetics, efficacy, or adverse effect rate of sulfasalazine are unaffected by age.[9, 10]

POSSIBLE MODES OF ACTION

Sulfasalazine affects various inflammatory mediators. Sulfasalazine and, to a greater extent, 5-aminosalicylic acid have been shown to scavenge reactive oxygen species and their products, which are released from activated polymorphs.[11] The drug inhibits the production of various prostanoids, including leukotriene B_4, 5-hydroxyeicosatetraenoic acid (5-HETE), and thromboxane A_2 by platelets.[12, 13]

Immunomodulatory activity of sulfasalazine is suggested by the reduction of circulating, activated lymphocytes after 12 weeks of therapy, significant falls in immunoglobulin M (IgM) and rheumatoid factor titers, an incidence of hypogammaglobulinemia of about 10 percent, inhibition of B cell activation and hyperreactivity, and restoration of normal responses of lymphocytes to various stimuli ex vivo after sulfasalazine treatment.[14, 15] Of particular interest is the finding that 16 weeks of sulfasalazine treatment altered the distribution of lymphocyte subtypes in the intestinal mucosa without producing corresponding changes in peripheral blood in rheumatoid arthritis patients.[16]

Sulfasalazine significantly reduced interleukin (IL)–1α and IL-1β and tumor necrosis factor-α in patients with rheumatoid arthritis of less than 1 year's duration in association with clinical and laboratory evidence of response to the drug, but whether the cytokine effects were primary or secondary to disease improvement was uncertain.[17] Another study has shown that sulfalsalazine reduces basal interleukin-6 production.[18]

Carlin and coworkers (1992) demonstrated that sulfasalazine and sulfapyridine inhibit the flux of second messengers, such as cytosolic calcium, diacylglycerol, and inositol triphosphate, induced by stimulation of human leukocytes in vitro. These effects may depend on drug action at the level of phospholipase C or

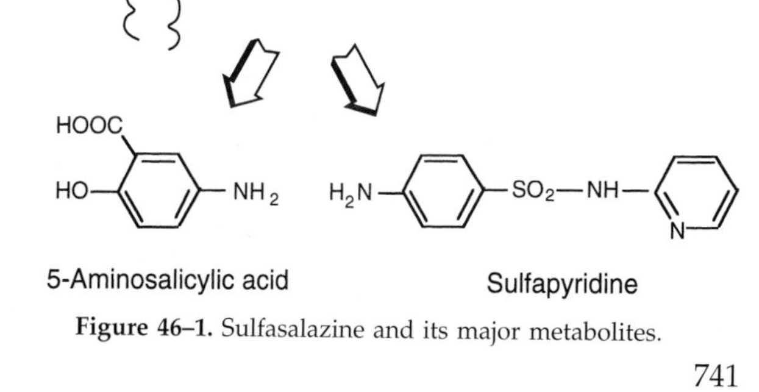

Figure 46–1. Sulfasalazine and its major metabolites.

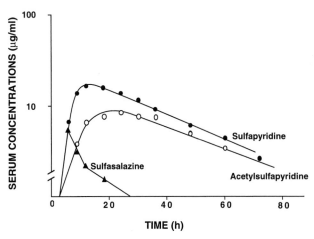

Figure 46–2. Serum concentrations of sulfasalazine, sulfapyridine, and acetylsulfapyridine after 2 g orally in a 40-year-old female. (From Taggart A, McDermott B, Delargy M, et al: The pharmacokinetics of sulphasalazine in young and elderly patients with rheumatoid arthritis. Scand J Rheumatol 64:32, 1987.)

its regulatory guanosine triphosphate (GTP)–binding protein and could explain some of the other effects of sulfasalazine on mediators of inflammation and lymphocyte function.[19]

EFFICACY

Rheumatoid Arthritis

Sulfasalazine displays antirheumatic properties and is approximately as effective as gold and penicillamine, less effective than methotrexate, but more effective than antimalarials.[20] However, sulfasalazine acts faster, effects being measurable at 4 weeks, and is better tolerated than gold or penicillamine, although the likelihood of patients continuing this drug over sustained periods is similar to that of other antirheumatic drugs[21] but less than that of methotrexate.

Two short-term, randomized, double-blind, placebo-controlled studies established the efficacy of sulfasalazine 3 g/day, but both showed relatively high rates of patient withdrawal, 28 percent in the study of Pinals and associates (1986), largely due to upper gastrointestinal adverse effects.[22, 23] In keeping with the recent trend toward earlier use of antirheumatic drugs, sulfasalazine was significantly superior to placebo in two studies in patients with rheumatoid arthritis of less than 12 months' duration[24, 25]; a trend toward fewer erosions in the sulfasalazine-treated group was observed in one of these studies.[25]

In a 48-week study comparing sulfasalazine with hydroxychloroquine in patients with early rheumatoid arthritis previously untreated with antirheumatic drugs, sulfasalazine had a faster onset of action[26] and showed significantly less radiologic progression at 24 and 48 weeks[27] and at a 3-year follow-up.[28]

Combinations with Other Antirheumatic Drugs

To date, no controlled data have led to the wide acceptance of any particular combination of antirheumatic drugs.[29] Studies of combinations of sulfasalazine with penicillamine, gold, and methotrexate, respectively, suggested marginal increases in efficacy only but, at least with gold and penicillamine, increased rates of withdrawal due to toxicity. Despite sulfasalazine and methotrexate exhibiting antifolate activity, no increased toxicity compared with that of methotrexate alone was observed.[30] The combination of sulfasalazine with hydroxychloroquine was equivalent to sulfasalazine alone but superior to hydroxychloroquine alone, thus not supporting the use of the combination.[31]

Other Inflammatory Rheumatic Diseases

Sulfasalazine has been accepted as an effective antirheumatic drug in juvenile rheumatoid arthritis,[32] although no controlled trials have been published. The drug has been used extensively in childhood inflammatory bowel disease.

Sulfasalazine is significantly superior to placebo in treating ankylosing spondylitis, the rate of onset of effect being 2 to 3 months in studies ranging from 12 to 52 weeks.[33, 34] A 3-year placebo-controlled study indicated that sulfasalazine was more effective in reducing the frequency of peripheral arthritis than in maintaining spinal mobility[35]—a finding in keeping with the drug's apparent efficacy in human leukocyte antigen (HLA)–B27–associated, asymmetric, pauciarticular arthritis.[36] Sulfasalazine is also efficacious in psoriatic arthritis without exacerbating the skin rash.[34, 37]

ADVERSE EFFECTS

Discontinuation rates for sulfasalazine are similar to those reported for gold, penicillamine, and antimalarials. One year after commencing sulfasalazine, 50 to 75 percent of subjects are still taking the drug; continuation rates decline in subsequent years to around 20 percent at 5 years. The common adverse effects with sulfasalazine are most likely in the first 2 to 3 months of therapy, are dose-related,[38] and are relatively few and less troublesome in comparison to those of parenteral gold or penicillamine, but the drug is not as well tolerated as antimalarials (Tables 46–1 and 46–2). Thus, dose reduction is a useful strategy for these adverse effects, but there appears to be no practical benefit in knowing a patient's acetylator status prior to commencing sulfasalazine.[39]

Gastroenterologic

Nausea and upper abdominal discomfort, often in association with headache and dizziness, are the most

Table 46–1. SERIOUS ADVERSE EFFECTS OF SULFASALAZINE THAT HAVE RARELY BEEN ASSOCIATED WITH DEATH

Aplastic anemia
Agranulocytosis
Fibrosing alveolitis
Hypersensitivity reactions
Irreversible neuromuscular and central nervous system effects
Renal damage
Hepatic damage

Table 46–2. MOST FREQUENT ADVERSE EFFECTS OF SULFASALAZINE

	Common Adverse Effects
Gastrointestinal tract	Nausea, vomiting, anorexia, malaise
	Abdominal pain, indigestion, dyspepsia
Central nervous system	Headache
	Fever
	Light-headedness, dizziness
	Less Common Adverse Effects
Skin	Rash (exanthem-like)
Hepatic system	Marginal enzyme elevations
Hematologic system	Leukopenia
	Hemolysis, mean corpuscular volume increased
	Methemoglobinemia

common adverse effects. Their incidence is reduced by increasing dosage gradually. These effects often are less problematic after 2 to 3 months of usage. Hepatic reactions, sometimes accompanied by fever, rash, and lymphadenopathy, are well-known adverse effects of sulfasalazine.[38]

Hematologic

The incidence of leukopenia and neutropenia varies from 1 to 5 percent, lower percentages being commoner, and the drug has to be stopped in about one third to one half of these patients. Although seen most often in the first 24 weeks of therapy, leukopenia and neutropenia can occur at any time, necessitating continued surveillance (Fig. 46–3).[40] Timely recognition is usually associated with recovery,[41] although a number of individual cases of fatal agranulocytosis have been described.[42] There are conflicting data concerning the effect of sulfasalazine on serum or red cell folate concentrations: some studies showed lowered folate levels, whereas Grindulis and McConkey (1985) found no effect.[43] Although some degree of macrocytosis and hemolysis has been common in patients taking higher doses of sulfasalazine for ulcerative colitis, frank hemolytic anemia is unusual. The latter is typically associated with methemoglobinemia, Heinz's bodies, and reticulocytosis.

Skin

Skin rashes occur in 1 to 5 percent of patients. Pruritic, maculopapular, and generalized rashes are most common, but occasional patients have urticarial reactions, and reversible and dose-dependent cases of lichen planus have been reported.[44] "Desensitization" to sulfasalazine has been successfully accomplished.[45] Some cases of alopecia have been noted. Classic serum sickness has been described,[46] and rarely, toxic epidermal necrolysis and Stevens-Johnson syndrome have been reported.

Pulmonary

A number of cases manifesting reversible pulmonary infiltrates accompanied by eosinophilia, dyspnea, fever, and weight loss have been described. Fibrosing alveolitis has been reported, with the condition slowly resolving with prednisone therapy and cessation of sulfasalazine.

Reproduction

No higher incidence of fetal abnormalities or perinatal morbidity or mortality has been observed in the

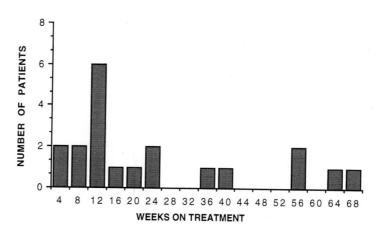

Figure 46–3. Development of leukopenia during sulfasalazine treatment, indicating that most cases occur in the first few months of therapy. (From Marabani M, Madhok R, Capell H, et al: Leucopenia during sulphasalazine treatment for rheumatoid arthritis. Ann Rheum Dis 48:506, 1989.)

offspring of males or females taking sulfasalazine at the time of conception or during pregnancy.[47] However, avoidance of antirheumatic drugs around conception and during pregnancy is always preferable. Sulfasalazine is highly protein bound and a sulfonamide, so the possibility of kernicterus suggests avoidance of the use of sulfasalazine in women near term or while breast feeding, although little sulfasalazine enters breast milk. Rapidly reversible male infertility has been observed in association with sulfasalazine and is related to the commonly observed reduction in sperm count, motility, and morphologic quality of the sperm.[48] However this effect has not been considered a contraindication to therapy in young males but the drug should be withdrawn in males wishing to sire children.

Other Adverse Effects

Changes in mood including irritability and depression are not unusual in the early months of therapy.[38] A range of central nervous system adverse effects have been documented, including aseptic meningitis.[49] Hypoimmunoglobulinemia has been described,[8] as have multiple cases of drug-induced lupus and/or induction of DNA antibodies related to sulfasalazine use.[8, 50]

DRUG INTERACTIONS

Broad-spectrum antibiotics that alter gut flora may reduce the bioavailability of sulfapyridine and 5-aminosalicylic acid as the azo link between these two metabolites of sulfasalazine is cleaved by bacterial metabolism. Concomitant cholestyramine is likely to reduce the availability of sulfapyridine as it binds sulfasalazine, rendering it unavailable for bacterial digestion. Sulfasalazine absorption is reduced if it is coadministered with oral iron preparations, but sulfapyridine concentrations are unaffected. Cimetidine does not alter the pharmacokinetics of sulfasalazine.

DOSAGE AND MONITORING

The most common adult dosage for rheumatic disease is 2 g (range, 1.5 to 3 g) of the enteric-coated formulation daily, taken as 1 g twice a day with meals. In order to minimize the risk of intolerance to the drug, starting doses of 500 mg to 1 g/day are usually employed, with dosage increments of 500 mg/day at intervals of a week or longer. Increases from 2 to 3 g/day do not seem to improve response in many patients.

Opinions vary regarding appropriate monitoring for patients taking sulfasalazine. Neutropenia, if it occurs, usually does so suddenly, so that monitoring in order to avoid this serious adverse effect is diffi-

cult. At a minimum, patients should be aware of the possibility of serious hematologic adverse effects so that they can immediately stop the drug and consult their physician should sore throat, mouth ulcers, fever, and significant malaise become apparent. Most rheumatologists request blood counts every 2 to 4 weeks during the first 3 months of therapy and reduce the frequency thereafter to every 3 months, whereas others perform the first blood count 6 weeks after commencing therapy and then every 3 months.

References

1. Svartz N: Salazopyrin, a new sulfanilamide preparation. Acta Med Scand 110:577, 1942.
2. Sinclair R, Duthie J: Salazopyin in the treatment of rheumatoid arthritis. Ann Rheum Dis 8:226, 1948.
3. McConkey B, Amos R, Durham S, et al: Sulphasalazine in rheumatoid arthritis. Br Med J 280:442, 1980.
4. Pullar T, Hunter J, Capell H: Which component of sulphasalazine is active in rheumatoid arthritis? Br Med J 290:1535, 1985.
5. Peppercorn M, Goldman P: The role of intestinal bacteria in the metabolism of salicylazosulfapyridine. J Pharmacol Exp Ther 181:555, 1972.
6. Azad Khan A, Truelove S, Aronson J: The disposition and metabolism of sulphasalazine (salicylazosulphapyridine) in man. Br J Clin Pharmacol 13:523, 1982.
7. Schroder H, Campbell D: Absorption, metabolism and excretion of salicylazo-sulfapyridine in man. Clin Pharmacol Ther 13:539, 1972.
8. Chalmers I, Sitar D, Hunter T: A one-year, open, prospective study of sulfasalazine in the treatment of rheumatoid arthritis: Adverse reactions and clinical response in relation to laboratory variables, drug and metabolite serum levels and acetylator status. J Rheumatol 17:764, 1990.
9. Taggart A, McDermott B, Delargy M, et al: The pharmacokinetics of sulphasalazine in young and elderly patients with rheumatoid arthritis. Scand J Rheumatol 64:29, 1987.
10. Wilkieson CA, Madhok R, Hunter JA, et al: Toleration, side effects and efficacy of sulfasalazine in rheumatoid arthritis patients of different ages. Q J Med 86:501, 1993.
11. Williams J, Hallett M: Effect of sulphasalazine and its active metabolite, 5-amino-salicylic acid, on toxic oxygen metabolite production by neutrophils. Gut 30:1581, 1989.
12. Stenson W, Lobos E: Inhibition of platelet thromboxane synthetase by sulfasalazine. Biochem Pharmacol 32:2205, 1983.
13. Bach M, Brashler J, Johnson M: Inhibition by sulfasalazine of LTC synthetase and of rat liver glutathione s-transferases. Biochem Pharmacol 34:2695, 1985.
14. Samanta A, Webb C, Grindulis KA, et al: Sulphasalazine therapy in rheumatoid arthritis: Qualitative changes in lymphocytes and correlation with clinical response. Br J Rheumatol 31:259, 1992.
15. Imai F, Suzuki R, Ishigashi T, et al: Effect of sulfasalazine on B cell hyperactivity in patients with rheumatoid arthritis. J Rheumatol 21:612, 1994.
16. Kanerud L, Scheynius A, Hafstrom I: Evidence of a local intestinal immunomodulatory effect of sulfasalazine in rheumatoid arthritis. Arthritis Rheum 37:1138, 1994.
17. Danis VA, Franic GM, Rathjen DA, et al: Circulating cytokine levels in patients with rheumatoid arthritis: Results of a double-blind trial with sulphasalazine. Ann Rheum Dis 51:945, 1992.
18. Crilly A, Madhok R, Watson J, et al: Production of interleukin-6 by monocytes isolated from rheumatoid arthritis patients receiving second-line drug therapy. Br J Rheumatol 33:821, 1994.
19. Carlin J, Djursater R, Smedegard G: Sulphasalazine inhibition of human granulocyte activation by inhibition of second messenger compounds. Ann Rheum Dis 51:1230, 1992.
20. Felson D, Anderson J, Meenan R: Use of short-term efficacy/toxicity tradeoffs to select second-line drugs in rheumatoid arthritis. A meta-analysis of published clinical trials. Arthritis Rheum 35:1117, 1992.
21. Situnayake R, Grindulis K, McConkey B: Long-term treatment of rheumatoid arthritis with sulphasalazine, gold or penicillamine: A comparison using life-table methods. Ann Rheum Dis 46:177, 1987.
22. Pullar T, Hunter J, Capell H: Sulphasalazine in rheumatoid arthritis: A double-blind comparison of sulphasalazine with placebo and sodium aurothiomalate. Br Med J 287:1102, 1983.
23. Pinals R, Kaplan S, Lawson J, et al: Sulphasalazine in rheumatoid arthritis: A double-blind placebo-controlled trial. Arthritis Rheum 29:1427, 1986.

24. Australian Multicentre Clinic Trial Group: Sulphasalazine in early rheumatoid arthritis. J Rheumatol 19:1672, 1992.

25. Hannonen P, Mottonen T, Hakola M, et al: Sulfasalazine in early rheumatoid arthritis. Arthritis Rheum 36:1501, 1993.

26. Nuver-Zwart I, van Riel P, van de Putte L, et al: A double-blind comparative study of sulphasalazine and hydroxychloroquine in rheumatoid arthritis: Evidence of an earlier effect of sulphasalazine. Ann Rheum Dis 48:389, 1989.

27. Van der Heijde D, van Riel P, Nuver-Zwart E, et al: Effects of hydroxychloroquine and sulphasalazine on progression of joint damage in rheumatoid arthritis. Lancet 13:1036, 1989.

28. Van der Heijde D, van Riel P, Nuver-Zwart E, et al: Sulphasalazine versus hydroxychloroquine in rheumatoid arthritis: 3-year follow-up. Lancet 335:539, 1990.

29. Felson DT, Anderson JJ, Meenan RF: The efficacy and toxicity of combination therapy in rheumatoid arthritis—a meta-analysis. Arthritis Rheum 37:10, 1994.

30. Nisar M, Carlisle L, Amos RS: Methotraxate and sulphasalazine as combination therapy in rheumatoid arthritis. Br J Rheumatol 33:651, 1994.

31. Faarvang KL, Egsmose C, Kryger P, et al: Hydroxychloroquine and sulphasalazine alone and in combination in rheumatoid arthritis: A randomised double-blind trial. Ann Rheum Dis 52:711, 1993.

32. Grondin C, Malleson P, Petty R: Slow-acting antirheumatic drugs in chronic arthritis of childhood. Semin Arthritis Rheum 18:38, 1988.

33. Ferraz M, Tugwell P, Goldsmith C, et al: Meta-analysis of sulfasalazine in ankylosing spondylitis. J Rheumatol 17:1482, 1990.

34. Dougados M, van der Linden S, Leirisalo-Repo M, et al: Sulfasalazine in the treatment of spondyloarthropathy. A randomized, multicenter, double-blind, placebo-controlled study. Arthritis Rheum 38:618, 1995.

35. Kirwan J, Edwards A, Huitfeldt B, et al: The course of established ankylosing spondylitis and the effects of sulphasalazine over 3 years. Br J Rheumatol 32:729, 1993.

36. Mielants H, Veys E: HLA-B27–related arthritis and bowel inflammation.

Part 1. Sulfasalazine (Salazopyrin) in HLA-B27–related reactive arthritis. J Rheumatol 12:287, 1985.

37. Farr M, Kitas G, Waterhouse L, et al: Sulphasalazine in psoriatic arthritis: A double-blind placebo-controlled study. Br J Rheumatol 29:46, 1990.

38. Amos R, Pullar T, Capell H: Sulphasalazine for rheumatoid arthritis: Toxicity in 774 patients monitored for 1 to 11 years. Br Med J 293:420, 1986.

39. Bax D, Greaves M, Amos R: Sulphasalazine for rheumatoid arthritis: Relationship between dose and acetylator phenotype and response to treatment. Br J Rheumatol 25:282, 1986.

40. Marabani M, Madhok R, Capell H, et al: Leucopenia during sulphasalazine treatment for rheumatoid arthritis. Ann Rheum Dis 48:505, 1989.

41. Farr M, Tunn E, Symmons D, et al: Sulphasalazine in rheumatoid arthritis: Haematological problems and changes in haematological indices associated with therapy. Br J Rheumatol 28:134, 1989.

42. Canvin JMG, El-Gabalawy HS, Chalmers IM: Fatal agranulocytosis with sulfasalazine therapy in rheumatoid arthritis. J Rheumatol 20:909, 1993.

43. Grindulis K, McConkey B: Does sulphasalazine cause folate deficiency in rheumatoid arthritis? Scand J Rheumatol 14:265, 1985.

44. Kaplan S, McDonald E, Marino C: Lichen planus in patients with rheumatoid arthritis treated with sulfasalazine. J Rheumatol 22:191, 1995.

45. Farr M, Scott D, Bacon P: Sulphasalazine desensitisation in rheumatoid arthritis. Br Med J 284:118, 1982.

46. Pettersson T, Gripenberg M, Molander G, et al: Severe immunological reaction induced by sulphasalazine. Br J Rheumatol 29:239, 1990.

47. Mogadam M, Dobbins W, Korelitz B, et al: Pregnancy in inflammatory bowel disease: Effect of sulphasalazine and corticosteroids on fetal outcome. Gastroenterology 80:72, 1981.

48. Toovey S, Hudson E, Hendry W, et al: Sulphasalazine and male infertility: Reversibility and possible mechanism. Gut 22:445, 1981.

49. Alloway JA, Mitchell SR: Sulfasalazine neurotoxicity: A report of aseptic meningitis and a review of the literature. J Rheumatol 20:409, 1993.

50. Caulier M, Dromer C, Andrieu V, et al: Sulfasalazine-induced lupus in rheumatoid arthritis. J Rheumatol 21:750, 1994.

CHAPTER 47

Richard I. Rynes

Antimalarial Drugs

HISTORICAL PERSPECTIVE

The antimalarial medications, which are also anti-rheumatic drugs, are derived from the bark of the Peruvian cinchona tree. The active agents, quinine and cinchonine, were isolated by Pelletier and Caventau in 1820.[1] In 1894, J. P. Payne, physician to St. Thomas' Hospital in London, delivered a postgraduate lecture on lupus erythematosus in which he first described the successful use of quinine for a rheumatic disease.[2] During the first half of the 20th century, extensive efforts were undertaken to synthesize antimalarial compounds with improved therapeutic/ toxicity ratios.[3] Page's seminal publication in 1951[4] provided much of the impetus for the widespread use of antimalarials to treat connective tissue diseases. He used quinacrine for patients with lupus erythematosus and reported that skin lesions improved in 17 of 18 patients. Associated "rheumatoid arthritis" also remitted in two of these patients, and systemic symptoms, including arthritis, cleared in a third, leading several groups to treat rheumatoid arthritis with antimalarials.[5, 6]

Chloroquine and hydroxychloroquine were developed in an effort to minimize antimalarial toxicity. In 1959, however, Hobbs and associates[7] recognized that long-term treatment with antimalarials might result in serious drug-induced retinal toxicity, and this led to a marked diminution in antimalarial use. More recent studies have shown that retinal toxicity is related to high daily doses and not to long-term treatment.[8] In the past several years, the spectrum of connective tissue and other immunologic diseases reported to respond to antimalarials has increased.[5, 9–14]

DEFINITION AND STRUCTURE

Only three antimalarial compounds are used to treat rheumatic diseases (Fig. 47–1). Of these, two 4-aminoquinoline derivatives, chloroquine and hydroxychloroquine, are virtually the only drugs prescribed. They differ only by the substitution of a hydroxyethyl group for an ethyl group on the tertiary aminonitrogen of the side chain of chloroquine. Hy-

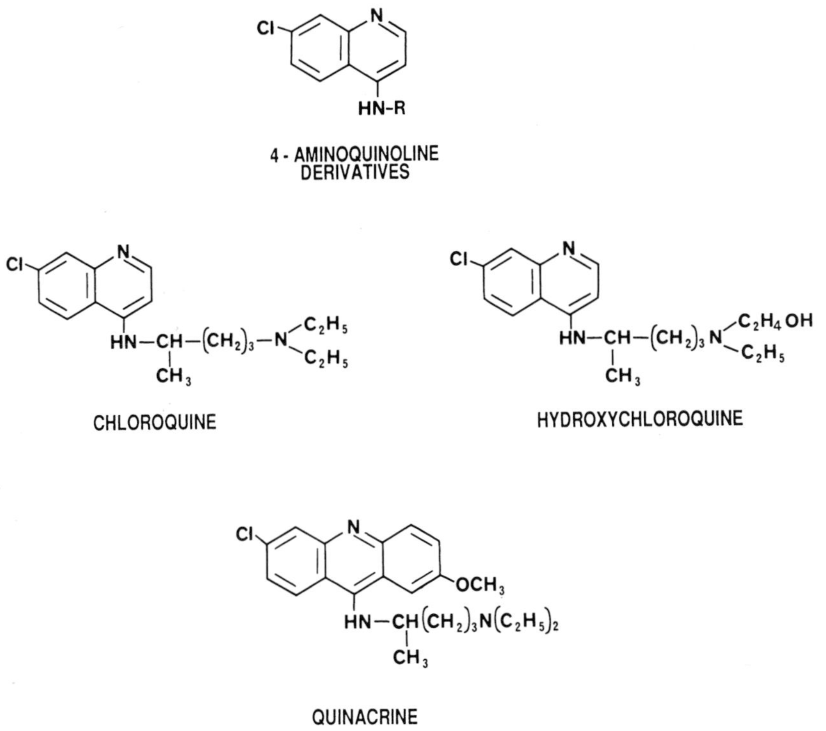

Figure 47–1. Chemical structures of antimalarial drugs used to treat rheumatic disease and the basic structure of 4-aminoquinolines. R represents the side chain.

droxychloroquine is more commonly prescribed in the United States.

Quinacrine, although not a 4-aminoquinoline, does include the chloroquine structure (see Fig. 47–1). It is occasionally used in patients with discoid lupus but may cause yellowish skin discoloration. This drug has only limited availability at this time because it is not manufactured by a United States Food and Drug Administration (FDA)–approved pharmaceutical company.

PHARMACOKINETICS

Significant difficulties have been observed in pharmacokinetic studies. Interpatient variability for most data is large.[15–19] Different daily doses affect pharmacokinetics.[16, 18] Tissue distribution affects plasma and blood drug levels to a large extent. Methodologic differences between various laboratories and the fact that studies have been conducted for 30 years may be the most important limitations in comparing various reports. On the other hand, pharmacokinetic data for comparable doses of chloroquine and hydroxychloroquine are similar.[16]

Antimalarials are rapidly absorbed after oral administration with absorption half-time for a 200-mg tablet of hydroxychloroquine ranging from 1.9 to 10 hours and the mean percent absorbed equal to 74.[17] The ratio of blood to plasma drug levels varies over a wide range but averages 7.[16] Some recent studies favor blood levels,[15] but older studies measured plasma levels. Relative values for plasma and blood become significant only if toxicity or effectiveness is related to drug levels. There is some evidence for this,[15, 20] but data are not yet firmly established and measurements are not yet useful clinically.

Drugs are quickly cleared from plasma and less rapidly from blood. The plasma and blood half-lives of antimalarials differ significantly, ranging from 3.5 days for plasma[5] to 45 days for blood.[16, 19] There is a corresponding variation in time to reach plateau levels because of blood cell distribution of drugs, ranging from 2 weeks for plasma[5] to 12 to 24 weeks for blood,[17] depending on daily dose.[17, 18] Differences in time to reach plateau levels for hydroxychloroquine have been calculated to double with 200 mg/day compared with 400 mg/day.[17] A five-fold variation in plasma levels has been reported in one series of patients treated for 2 months with chloroquine, 250 mg/day.[20]

Most of the absorbed medication is excreted in urine unchanged, but about one third is metabolized[21] to a desethyl derivative formed by alkyl degradation of a terminal amino-ethyl group in the side chain. About 8 percent can be found in feces, some of which is a result of excretion.[21] By day 77 after discontinuation of chloroquine administration, urinary daily output falls to about 1 mg.[22] At this time, about 55 percent of the total ingested dose may be accounted for by urinary excretion.[22] Small amounts of chloroquine, however, can be found in plasma, red blood cells, and urine for as long as 5 years after the last dose.[23]

Extensive tissue concentration and distribution account for this prolonged excretion time.[16, 24] Among circulating blood cells, mononuclear cells have a higher hydroxychloroquine concentration than do neutrophils in patients with rheumatoid arthritis, and monocytes have greater uptake than do lymphocytes in in vitro studies.[25] Localization of the 4-aminoquinolines in the eye assumes great importance because of retinal toxicity. High concentration is related to drug deposition in the iris and choroid.[26]

MECHANISM OF ACTION

Various drug actions that can affect rheumatic diseases are listed in Table 47–1.

The most important antimalarial action appears to interfere with cellular function in compartments in which there is an acid microenvironment, such as lysosomes, endosomes, and the Golgi complex. This basic drug action may subsequently affect pathways

Table 47–1. ANTIMALARIAL ACTIONS

Primary Actions

Interferes with intracellular function dependent on an acidic microenvironment*
Inhibits enzyme activity, including phospholipase A_2

Anti-inflammatory Activity

Stabilizes lysosomal membranes
Inhibits polymorphonuclear cell chemotaxis and phagocytosis
Affects superoxide generation
Inhibits connective tissue encapsulation
Decreases fibronectin production
Decreases histamine production
Decreases intravascular erythrocyte aggregation
Decreases platelet aggregation
Is photoprotective
Inhibits interleukin-1–induced cartilage degradation

Effects on Immune Function

Inhibits cytokine production†, ‡, §
Inhibits lymphocyte membrane receptor formation§
May decrease autoantibody production‖
Inhibits proliferative response of stimulated lymphocytes
Inhibits natural killer cell activity
Inhibits immune complex formation

Effects on Infectious Agents

Inhibits bacteria replication
Protects tissue culture from virus infection
Prevents virus replication
Induces expression of Epstein-Barr virus early antigen

Miscellaneous Actions

Forms complexes with DNA
May interfere with sulfhydryl–disulfide interchange reactions

*References not listed are cited in previous editions: Kelley et al (eds): Textbook of Rheumatology, 2nd and 4th eds. Philadelphia, WB Saunders, 1985, 1993.[3, 5]
†Data from Salmeron and Lipsky: Am J Med 75 (Suppl):19, 1983.[35]
‡Data from Sperber et al: J Rheumatol 20:803, 1993.[36]
§Data from Wallace et al: Lupus 2 (Suppl 1):S13, 1993.[40]
‖Data from Fox and Kang: Lupus 2 (Suppl 1): S9, 1993.[32]

of inflammation, the immune cascade, and enzyme activity. This effect, initially termed *lysosomotropic* action, occurs because antimalarials are weak bases that enter the lysosome, are protonated, raise the pH,[27] and interfere with enzyme activity that depends on an acid milieu. Electron micrographs of both polymorphonuclear cells and lymphocytes[28] from patients treated with chloroquine reveal abnormal lysosomal structures presumably caused by this lysosomotropic action.

Elevated intracellular pH can have a variety of other effects. Some cell surface receptors and ligands are internalized and transported by endosomes to lysosomes, where receptors are separated from ligands and returned to the cell surface. Antimalarials interfere with this receptor recycling.[29] Antimalarials also affect the Golgi complex. Chloroquine may inhibit protein secretion and the intracellular processing of proteins by blocking the proteolytic conversion of secretory protein precursors, such as the complement component precursor pro-C3.[30] These biochemical changes are associated with morphologic changes in the Golgi complex.[30]

Antimalarials affect multiple aspects of the immunologic cascade. Animal studies document that they do not inhibit antibody production to exogenous antigens.[31] Fox and Kang, however, suggest that higher pH in the endoplasmic reticulum stabilizes major histocompatability protein α- and β-chain interaction with invariant chains, preventing their displacement by low-affinity autoantigens, which thereby interferes with autoantibody production.[32] In fact, rheumatoid factor disappears in some patients with rheumatoid arthritis who are responding to antimalarials.[5]

Interference with immunologic cell function has been documented. Chloroquine inhibits the proliferative response of stimulated cultured human lymphocytes.[5] Decreased responsiveness to phytohemagglutinin has been demonstrated by lymphocytes of treated patients.[33] Natural killer cell action is inhibited both in vitro[5] and in vivo.[34] Changes in immune function are further documented by studies of cytokines and receptors on lymphocyte membranes. Salmeron and Lipsky[35] first showed inhibition of IL-1 effect by documenting suppression of lymphocyte proliferation by chloroquine in concentrations as low as 1 μg/ml. Proliferation was restored by adding a monokine, presumed to be interleukin-1 (IL-1). Drug-induced decreased production of IL-1 has been confirmed.[36] Using a chloroquine concentration that may be present in vivo, Baker's group showed inhibition of lectin binding.[37] This may be related to the inhibition of receptor recycling already described, further associating lysosomotropic action with immunologic effects. They further speculated that this inhibition of lectin binding may be a mechanism that causes diminished monokine production.[37] Antimalarials may also interfere with the action of IL-1 illustrated by hydroxychloroquine inhibition of IL-1–induced cartilage degradation.[38]

Quinacrine blocks IL-2R expression.[40] More recently, Wallace and colleagues found decreased IL-6, sCD8, and sIL-2R levels in lupus patients treated with hydroxychloroquine.[40] Another study of monocytes and T lymphocytes confirmed decreased production of IL-1 and IL-6, but not IL-2, IL-4, tumor necrosis factor-α, or interferon-γ affected. Chloroquine inhibits antigen-antibody interaction and immune complex formation.[41] Immune complex levels are reduced in treated patients who have rheumatoid arthritis.[42]

Antimalarials reduce the activity of many enzymes,[5] including phospholipase A.[43] Total prostaglandin production decreases, and in an experimental test system, leukotriene release from lung was diminished.[44] In addition to causing direct enzyme inhibition, these drugs stabilize lysosomal membranes, thereby inhibiting the release of lysosomal enzymes.[45]

Antimalarials may decrease skin inflammation by a photoprotective skin effect attributable to ultraviolet radiation absorption[46] or to a modification of an abnormal tissue response[47] to such radiation. This could account for the improvement of lupus skin lesions.

Among miscellaneous actions, antimalarials form complexes with DNA by binding of the quinoline ring to the phosphate groups and nucleotide bases and thereby interfere with nuclear events.[48, 49] Reactions between DNA and anti-DNA antibodies may be blocked.[50] This may explain the inhibition of the lupus erythematosus cell phenomenon observed by Dubois.[51]

THERAPEUTIC EFFECTIVENESS

Lupus Erythematosus

The variability of the natural course of lupus erythematosus and of the response of different manifestations of disease to various medications makes treatment evaluation difficult, but antimalarials are beneficial.

Discoid Lupus Erythematosus

Antimalarials are effective against discoid lesions. Compared with the spontaneous remissions in 15 percent, remissions or major improvements have been reported in 60 to 90 percent of treated patients.[5] Daily dosages were often much larger than those currently acceptable, however, including one placebo-controlled study.[52] Quinacrine is occasionally helpful when discoid lesions fail to respond adequately to hydroxychloroquine or chloroquine,[51, 53] but its long-term use is limited by the potential development of yellowish skin pigmentation.

The effectiveness of antimalarials in the treatment of skin lesions is often apparent within the first week, when erythematosus changes start to regress. Follicular plugging may then disappear, and after several months thickening and induration diminish or clear. Most patients who respond to antimalarial medication experience relapse after the drug is discontinued.

Winkelman and associates found that only seven of 67 patients who took quinacrine or chloroquine for 10 weeks to 4 years maintained remission for 3 years after stopping their medication.[53] Most of the 50 who experienced relapse responded to additional courses of treatment.

Systemic Lupus Erythematosus

In addition to improvement in discoid skin lesions, patients in uncontrolled studies have shown improvement in arthralgias, fever, and constitutional symptoms through antimalarial use. A placebo-controlled study found joint pain and tenderness but not joint swelling decreased on hydroxychloroquine therapy.[56] Antimalarials may have a corticosteroid-sparing effect.[57]

The strongest evidence supporting the efficacy of antimalarials in treating systemic lupus erythematosus (SLE) comes from studies in which medication was discontinued in successfully treated patients.[54, 55] A 6-month, double-blind, placebo-controlled drug discontinuation study provided substantial evidence that hydroxychloroquine prevents lupus flareups.[55] Forty-seven patients, all of whom were being treated with hydroxychloroquine, were studied. Sixteen of the 22 patients in whom placebo was substituted for hydroxychloroquine experienced flareups, whereas only nine of 25 who continued hydroxychloroquine therapy suffered a disease exacerbation ($P = .02$). Most manifestations were minor. Flares often involved abnormalities that had been present before treatment. Only one severe exacerbation occurred in the group continued on treatment, compared with five in the patients receiving placebo ($P = .06$). Three of the placebo-treated patients required hospitalization. Overall, the risk of disease flareup was increased by a factor of 2.5 for the placebo group. In a study of 43 patients who stopped taking chloroquine because of toxicity and therefore could serve as their own controls, Rudnicki and colleagues also reported fewer flareups during treatment.[54] No corticosteroid-sparing effect was seen in this study.

Antimalarials alone are not appropriate treatment for the more severe manifestations of SLE. Although one study reported substantial benefit in patients with active diffuse proliferative glomerulonephritis treated with a combination of indomethacin, 3 mg/kg/day, and hydroxychloroquine, 800 mg/day,[58] these results have not been confirmed.

Rheumatoid Arthritis

The antimalarials belong to the class termed *slow-acting antirheumatic drugs* (SAARDs). Improvement sometimes occurs within several weeks, but other patients may not benefit until months after antimalarials are started. Maximal improvement may take 6 months or even longer.[5, 6] Analogously, when antimalarial treatment is discontinued, the disease does not flare immediately but gradually worsens over weeks or months.

Hydroxychloroquine has been reported to be one half to two thirds as effective as chloroquine and one half as toxic when similar daily doses were compared.[6] On the other hand, meta-analysis of placebo-controlled studies suggests that chloroquine, 250 mg/day, is more effective than hydroxychloroquine, 400 mg/day.[60] Daily dosage may affect results, and 800 mg of hydroxychloroquine was more effective than 400 mg.[5] There was no statistically significant difference between 400 and 200 mg/day, although improvement favored patients receiving the higher dose.[5]

Older studies confirming the effectiveness of antimalarials have been extensively reviewed in previous editions of this book.[3, 5] In open studies, substantial benefit has been reported in 60 to 70 percent of patients.[6, 59] Adams and coworkers reported that 28 percent of patients had complete remission or better than 75 percent improvement.[59]

At least ten double-blind, placebo-controlled studies have confirmed the benefits of the antimalarials chloroquine and hydroxychloroquine (Table 47–2). The studies ranged from 15 weeks to 1 year and were conducted from the 1950s to 1990s. Daily dose varied, and in some was twice that currently recommended. Although the earlier studies often used parameters of efficacy no longer considered ideal, definite drug benefit was found. In these studies, mild toxicity was greater on drug therapy, but no serious adverse events occurred. In two 1-year studies measuring radiographic progression, one showed benefit for patients receiving chloroquine and the other did not.[5]

Studies preceding 1970 have been reviewed in previous textbooks.[3, 5] Three studies ranging from 6 to 12 months have been published in the 1990s.[61-63] Effectiveness was monitored by currently acceptable parameters, including the Paulus criteria in one.[63] In all three, joint index improved, as did other measurements, including global assessment. Toxicity was no greater than that with placebo.

One study assessed 104 patients with mild disease in a 1-year study.[95] Synovitis was limited to hands and feet, and the erythrocyte sedimentation rate was less than 30. All four clinical parameters assessed and erythrocyte sedimentation rate were significantly improved in the treated group compared with the baseline values, but only morning stiffness was better in the control group. Furthermore, withdrawals for lack of efficacy were significantly higher in the placebo group, 18 compared with eight ($P<.05$). Two patients receiving placebo dropped out because of early toxicity, compared with one drug-treated patient. Radiographic evaluation showed no difference in the two groups.

A 6-month study analyzed 126 patients who had rheumatoid arthritis for less than 5 years.[62] However, these patients had more widespread disease, longer duration of disease, higher erythrocyte sedimentation rates, and greater disability than those in the 1-year

Table 47–2. DOUBLE-BLIND, PLACEBO-CONTROLLED STUDIES OF CHLOROQUINE AND HYDROXYCHLOROQUINE

Drug	Dose (mg/day)	Length of Study (mo)	No. of Patients Studied	Efficacy*	Toxicity	Comments	First Author†	Year
C	200 or 300	4	69	Joint tenderness, grip strength, function tests; no change in ESR	Weight loss on C	—	Freedman	1956
HC	800	6	113	Overall assessment for function, observer assessment, individual parameters	Greater with drug; no dropouts	—	Mainland	1957
C	250	4	33	>50% on drug improved by 2 grades	Almost none in either group	50% of patients crossed over; 50% stayed on C or P	Rinehardt	1957
C	500	10	22	American Rheumatism Association rheumatoid activity—80% improved on Lansburg system indices	Greater on C, especially gastrointestinal	Crossover, 5 mo on C	Cohen	1958
C	500	12	107	Joint tenderness, joint index, walking time; dexterity improved on C and P; ESR and RF on C	Slight increase on C	Function probably improved on C; less radiographic deterioration on C	Freedman	1960
C	500 then 250	12	134	Disease activity, grip strength, functional capacity, ESR; fall in RF titer	No difference	No change in radiographic progression between C and P	Popert	1961
HC	600	6	41	Number of analgesic tablets; all parameters favored HC, but not significant at $P = .05$	2 withdrawals, P: 1 withdrawal, HC	Crossover, 3 mo on HC	Hamilton	1962
HC	400	12	104	All parameters (morning stiffness also better in P group); ESR: fever withdrawals for ineffectiveness	1 withdrawal on HC, 2 withdrawals on P	Patients had mild disease	Davis[61]	1991
HC	400	6	126	Active joints, global assessment, pain, grip strength	Mild; no discontinuations	No difference in ESR or RF	Clark[62]	1993
HC	400	9	120	Joint index, pain index, global assessment, Paulus criteria	Mild; no difference	Used current standards for efficacy; no difference in ESR or RF	HERA[63]	1995

*Efficacy refers to statistically significant improvement of patients taking antimalarial agent.
†References not cited are in previous editions: Kelley et al: Textbook of Rheumatology, 2nd and 4th eds. Philadelphia, WB Saunders, 1985, 1993.[3, 5]
Abbreviations: D, drug; HC, hydroxychloroquine; C, chloroquine; P, placebo; ESR, erythrocyte sedimentation rate; RF, rheumatoid factor.

study.[61] Significant improvement in the treated group compared with the placebo group was reported for active joints, pain, grip strength, and patient and physician global assessment, but not sedimentation rate or rheumatoid factor.[62] Toxicity was equal in the two groups and caused no drug discontinuation.

The HERA (Hydroxychloroquine Sulfate in Early Rheumatoid Arthritis) study assessed patients with less than 2 years of disease over a 9-month period.[63] Both drug- and placebo-receiving patients improved, but hydroxychloroquine was statistically superior to placebo for joint index, pain index, and physical function index. The latter two indices were better starting at 12 weeks, and joint index differed starting at 24 weeks. Using the Paulus criteria of greater than 20 percent improvement in four of six individual parameters, 54 percent of treated patients improved, compared with 36 percent of those treated with placebo ($P = .02$). There was no difference in toxicity: 39 adverse events with two withdrawals in the hydroxychloroquine group and 38 adverse events with two withdrawals in the placebo group.

Comparisons with Other Slow-Acting Antirheumatic Drugs

Studies comparing the effectiveness of antimalarials with other SAARDs are summarized in Table 47–3. Only a few were double-blind,[5, 64–66] and only one compared patients with early rheumatoid arthritis.[66]

Many of these studies suffer from methodologic problems. Two studies from one institution came to different conclusions, the first suggesting intramuscular gold was superior and the second showing equivalence to hydroxychloroquine.[5] The researchers suggested that different criteria were used for drug ineffectiveness in the two studies. In another study, no difference was observed, but the investigators still considered intramuscular gold the treatment of choice in active rheumatoid arthritis and believed that chloroquine should be considered early in disease management.[5] Studies with random assignment to one of the two drugs compared generally found no differences, although chloroquine was reported to be superior to dapsone in one study.

Three double-blind studies have been conducted. Although other investigators suggest chloroquine and hydroxychloroquine are equivalent to D-penicillamine clinically, the Mayo Clinic study showed that D-penicillamine was better at 6 and 12 months but that the two drugs were equivalent at 24 months.[64] Sulfasalazine and hydroxychloroquine were equal clinically,[65]

Table 47–3. COMPARISON OF EFFICACY OF ANTIMALARIAL AGENTS WITH OTHER SLOW-ACTING ANTIRHEUMATIC DRUGS (SAARDs)

Antimalarial*	Other SAARD	Length of Study (mo)	Type of Study	Clinical Outcome	Comment
HC	Intramuscular gold	—	Retrospective life-table analysis	Gold superior	
HC	Intramuscular gold	—	Retrospective life-table analysis	Equal	Same institution as first entry but different results
C	Intramuscular gold (gold thiomalate)	6	Random assignment of patients	Equal	See text for discussion
HC	Oral gold (auranofin)	11	Random assignment of patients	Equal	More parameters improved on HC
C	D-Penicillamine	12	Random assignment of patients	Equal	Laboratory test results and radiographic changes favored D-penicillamine
HC	D-Penicillamine	—	Retrospective life-table analysis	Equal	
HC	D-Penicillamine	24	Double-blind	D-Penicillamine superior at 6 and 12 mo, equal at 24 mo	Low daily doses of each medication; marked improvement at 24 mo: 25% for HC and 11% for D-penicillamine
HC	Sulfasalazine	11	Double-blind	Equal	Sulfasalazine more rapid improvement, greater number of parameters improved, fever withdrawals for lack of effect
C	Dapsone	6	Random assignment of patients	C superior	
C	Azathioprine	6	Random assignment of patients	Equal	
HC	Levamisole	—	Retrospective life-table analysis	HC superior	
C[66]	Cyclosporine	6	Double-blind	Equal	Slight impairment of creatinine clearance in each group

*References not cited are in previous editions: Kelley et al: Textbook of Rheumatology, 2nd and 4th eds. Philadelphia, WB Saunders, 1985, 1993.[3, 5]
Abbreviations: HC, hydroxychloroquine; C, chloroquine.

but patients who received sulfasalazine had fewer radiographic changes.[67] In uncontrolled studies, comparison of radiographic changes showed less deterioration with D-penicillamine than with chloroquine but no difference with hydroxychloroquine.[5]

Felson and colleagues[60] combined 117 treatment groups from 66 trials in a meta-analysis. Antimalarials were significantly less effective in composite treatment effect than was D-penicillamine ($P = .04$) but not other SAARDs or methotrexate. Other researchers, however, have reported that patients who fail to respond to hydroxychloroquine frequently respond to a subsequent course of methotrexate.

A recent 24-week double-blind comparison found chloroquine equivalent to cyclosporine in patients with rheumatoid arthritis who were treated within 2 years of onset.[66] In each group, 45 percent had greater than 30 percent improvement in swollen and tender joints, but erythrocyte sedimentation rates did not improve with either treatment. The drugs were equally well tolerated, although cyclosporine produced mild paresthesia in 11 patients and chloroquine did so in one. Serum creatinine levels increased in each group, with the increase on cyclosporine twice that on chloroquine, a nonsignificant difference.

Combination Therapy

Antimalarials are an attractive agent for combination treatment because their mechanism of action appears to differ from other medications and they have a high safety profile. The results of studies are mixed, unfortunately, and an improved safety record has not been established.

There is no consensus on intramuscular gold and antimalarials. Older studies[5] suggested that gold conferred therapeutic advantage when added to antimalarials, and in a controlled study, hydroxychloroquine was added to gold with increased efficacy and increased toxicity. A more recent controlled study showed no improvement or increased toxicity when hydroxychloroquine, 400 mg/day, was added to gold in 72 patients who still had significant disease after a full course of gold compared with 70 patients in whom placebo was added.[68] Antimalarials confer no additional benefit over oral gold, nor does addition of an antimalarial to D-penicillamine therapy.[5]

The combination of methotrexate and chloroquine was more effective than methotrexate and placebo in a study of 88 patients.[69] All parameters assessed except pain showed more improvement with combination therapy, but the difference was statistically significant only for joint count, grip strength, and functional ability. Adverse events were also greater in the combination group, but this was not statistically significant. Elevations of liver enzymes to less than twice normal occurred in 11 patients receiving combination treatment compared with one receiving methotrexate alone. Combinations of hydroxychloroquine and methotrexate were assessed in a multicenter study.[70] Patients who responded when both drugs were taken were subsequently assigned to continue taking hydroxychloroquine or placebo and to use methotrexate or placebo for flareups. Results were inconclusive, but the groups receiving maintainence hydroxychloroquine appeared to have fewer flares in this 38-week study.

A triple combination of hydroxychloroquine, sulfasalazine, and methotrexate has been shown to be significantly more effective than methotrexate alone or hydroxychloroquine and sulfasalazine in a 2-year study involving 100 patients.[71] Efficacy failures were only 15 percent in the triple combination compared with 60 percent in each of the other groups. All patients had failed on therapy with at least one SAARD. Toxicity was not increased in the combination group who received full dosages of each medication.

Antimalarials in combination may confer increased safety. Combination of hydroxychloroquine with either aspirin or methotrexate was less frequently associated with elevated serum levels of liver enzymes compared with methotrexate alone or with aspirin[72] in an analysis of laboratory studies in the ARAMIS (Arthritis, Rheumatism and Aging Medical Information System) data bank. Unfortunately, this was not confirmed in the clinical study discussed earlier.[69] Another study suggested that decreased liver abnormalities may be related to lower methotrexate concentrations in patients receiving hydroxychloroquine.[73] Methotrexate does not decrease hydroxychloroquine levels.[15] Hydroxychloroquine may decrease corticosteroid toxicity by lessening the hyperlipidemic effect of the steroids.[74, 90] One analysis showed that hydroxychloroquine lowered cholesterol and low-density lipoproteins.[74] Another showed no effect on cholesterol but a lowering of triglycerides and its associated apolipoprotein C.[90] Each group suggested that the changes were related to the antimalarial lysosomotropic effect.

Other Connective Tissue Diseases

Seronegative Arthropathies

The reports of response of psoriatic arthritis and of the peripheral arthritis of ankylosing spondylitis to antimalarials are anecdotal. Several investigators have reported responses similar to those seen for rheumatoid arthritis.[5, 6] Kammer and coworkers[75] reported 68-percent benefit in 50 courses of hydroxychloroquine treatment of patients with psoriatic arthritis. Exacerbation of psoriatic skin lesions may occur with antimalarial treatment.[79]

Juvenile Rheumatoid Arthritis

Several groups have found antimalarials to be efficacious in treating juvenile rheumatoid arthritis.[5] In an open, parallel study, hydroxychloroquine was equal in efficacy and was better tolerated than gold sodium thiomalate or D-penicillamine. A collaborative placebo-controlled study found neither hydroxychloroquine nor D-penicillamine to be more effective than placebo.[76]

Palindromic Rheumatism

Chloroquine and hydroxychloroquine each have been reported to be beneficial in treating palindromic rheumatism in uncontrolled studies.[5, 11] The largest series reviewed 71 patients with an average follow-up of 3.6 years.[11] Forty-seven were treated with chloroquine and four with hydroxychloroquine. Forty-one patients responded, with a 77-percent reduction in frequency and a 63-percent reduction in duration of attacks.

Eosinophilic Fasciitis

Eosinophilic fasciitis has been successfully treated with antimalarials in uncontrolled studies.[5, 12] In one series of 52 patients with this disease two of eight patients who failed to respond to prednisone and two of eight who had not received prednisone had complete resolution with hydroxychloroquine treatment, whereas six had a partial response, one had no response, and five of the 16 patients treated with hydroxychloroquine were lost to follow-up.[12] Responses occurred in 3 to 6 months on a daily dose of 200 or 400 mg.

Childhood Dermatomyositis

Hydroxychloroquine has been effective against childhood dermatomyositis in patients who had been unresponsive or partially responsive to corticosteroids.[9, 89] All seven patients in one report had improvement of skin rash, with complete clearing in three.[9] Myositis did not appear to improve, but corticosteroid dosage was tapered in two patients. A retrospective review of nine patients showed significant improvement in skin rash and in abdominal and proximal muscle strength.[89] After 6 months of treatment with hydroxychloroquine, prednisone dosage had been significantly reduced.

Erosive Osteoarthritis

A retrospective review of eight patients with erosive osteoarthritis treated with hydroxychloroquine after failure to respond to nonsteroidal anti-inflammatory drugs (NSAIDs) revealed improvement in morning stiffness, synovitis, and patient global assessment in six with a partial response in one.[13] One patient experienced a flareup after drug discontinuation and went into remission again after reinstitution of hydroxychloroquine therapy.

Calcium Pyrophosphate Crystal Deposition Disease

One controlled study of chronic calcium pyrophosphate disease lasting more than 3 months revealed a greater response rate and decreased numbers of active joints in the 17 patients treated with hydroxychloroquine compared with the placebo group.[14] These results have not yet been confirmed.

Sjögren's Syndrome

Laboratory abnormalities, including protein levels and serologic abnormalities, improved in two series of patients with Sjögren's syndrome treated with hydroxychloroquine[77, 78] one of which had a control group.[77] Sedimentation rate fell and hemoglobin rose in treated patients.[77] Clinical findings were not assessed in one study,[77] and improvement in the other could not definitely be attributed to hydroxychloroquine.[78]

SIDE EFFECTS AND TOXICITY

After it was established that antimalarials could cause loss of vision, safety became the paramount issue and the major factor limiting antimalarial use.[3] Recent studies have shown an excellent safety profile, with few discontinuations due to side effects. Comparisons with other SAARDs have consistently shown equivalent or greater safety for hydroxychloroquine or chloroquine.[5]

Meta-analysis of 71 drug placebo-controlled trials lasting at least 2 months that contained 128 treatment arms also supports the safety of antimalarials, showing less toxicity resulting in drug withdrawal than with other SAARDs or methotrexate.[60] The dropout rate for antimalarials was 8.5 percent, which was lower than that for any other treatment. The difference was statistically significant compared with intramuscular gold, sulfasalazine, or D-penicillamine, but not with oral gold or methotrexate.

Although hydroxychloroquine and chloroquine are relatively safe, the list of reported side effects is extensive (Table 47–4).

The incidence of adverse effects varies widely, depending on daily dosage. Hydroxychloroquine has been found to be half as toxic as chloroquine on a weight basis.[6] Scherbel and colleagues[6] observed reactions in 440 of 805 patients (55 percent) treated with daily doses of 250 to 500 mg of chloroquine or 400 to 600 mg of hydroxychloroquine. Sixty-seven percent were transient reactions and disappeared spontaneously. Another 26 percent responded to reductions in dosage. Only 7 percent of reactions precluded further treatment.[6]

Gastrointestinal side effects of antimalarial drugs can mimic those of NSAIDs and include epigastric burning, nausea, and vomiting. Abdominal cramps, bloating, and diarrhea are more unique to antimalarial agents.[5, 6] Antimalarials do not cause peptic ulcer disease or gastrointestinal bleeding.

Rash is the most common side effect leading to cessation of treatment.[6] These lesions may be lichenoid, urticarial, morbilliform, or maculopapular. Patients with psoriatic arthritis may experience an exacerbation of psoriatic skin lesions,[5, 79] although this was not observed in one series of 50 patients.[74] Exfoliative dermatitis has occasionally been reported.[79]

Pigmentary changes of skin or hair include either grayish hypopigmentation or blue-black hyperpigmentation.[6] Alopecia may develop[6] and must be dif-

Table 47–4. TOXIC EFFECTS OF CHLOROQUINE AND HYDROXYCHLOROQUINE*

Gastrointestinal

Anorexia*
Abdominal bloating
Abdominal cramps
Diarrhea
Heartburn
Nausea
Vomiting
Weight loss

Skin and Hair

Alopecia
Bleaching of hair
Dryness of skin
Exacerbation of psoriasis
Increased pigmentation of skin and hair
Pruritus
Rashes
  Exfoliative
  Lichenoid
  Maculopapular
  Morbilliform
  Urticarial

Neuromuscular

Convulsive seizures
Difficulty in visual accommodation
Headache
Insomnia
Involuntary movements
Lassitude
Myasthenic reaction
Mental confusion
Nervousness or irritability
Neuromyopathy
Ototoxicity

Nerve deafness
Tinnitus
Polyneuropathy
Toxic psychosis
Vestibular dysfunction
Weakness

Ocular

Corneal deposits: halos around lights
Diplopia
Defects in accommodation and convergence: various mild visual difficulties
Loss of corneal reflex
Retinopathy
  Loss of vision
  Pigment abnormalities
  Scotomata
  Visual field abnormalities

Miscellaneous

Birth defects
Blood dyscrasias
  Leukopenia
  Agranulocytosis
  Aplastic anemia
  Leukemia
Death from overdosage: peripheral circulatory collapse
Heart
  Electrocardiographic changes
  Cardiomyopathy
Precipitation of porphyria
Renal: decreased creatinine clearance†

*References are cited in previous textbook editions: Kelley et al: Textbook of Rheumatology, 2nd and 4th eds. Philadelphia, WB Saunders, 1985, 1993.[3, 5]
†Data from Landewe RBM, Vergouwen MSC, Goei HS, et al: Antimalarial drug induced decrease in creatinine clearance. J Rheumatol 22:34, 1995.[88]

ferentiated from the alopecia that is a disease manifestation of lupus erythematosus.

The more frequently seen neurologic manifestations are often of little significance because of their mildness and reversibility when the daily dosages are lowered. These include headaches, giddiness, insomnia, and nervousness.[5] A reversible myasthenic syndrome has been reported.[5] More important, but also uncommon, is a neuromuscular syndrome[5, 80] that includes proximal lower extremity muscle weakness (which may start months after treatment is begun), normal creatine phosphokinase levels, a neurogenic component, and abnormal muscle and nerve biopsy results. Biopsy changes may not be specific for drug toxicity[81] and also were present in two patients with antimalarial-induced cardiomyopathy.[82] Neuromyopathy may be confused with glococorticoid-induced muscle weakness or may be attributed to the disease being treated.

Chloroquine and hydroxychloroquine can cause three types of ocular toxicity. Defects in accommodation or convergence may cause blurred vision or difficulty in quickly changing focus and are probably due to a central neural effect, but diplopia may result from extraocular muscle palsy.[5] A second problem, corneal deposits, may be associated with halos around lights.[5] Similar symptoms caused by corticosteroid-induced glaucoma must be differentiated. These problems are benign and reversible, and may even improve with continued drug use. The third ocular problem, retinal toxicity, is potentially serious because it can cause permanent loss of vision.

Retinopathy has been extensively reviewed in previous editions of this book.[3] Hydroxychloroquine has caused fewer cases of retinopathy than has chloroquine. Only 18 cases of true visual loss with hydroxychloroquine have been published, and these were often associated with high daily doses.[8] Recent studies show that low daily dosing and regular ophthalmologic examinations using the protocol outlined in Table 47–5 can prevent visual loss even with long-term treatment.[8]

Characteristic changes of antimalarial retinopathy include pigmentary changes, clumping, and occasionally the classic bull's eye lesion. Visual acuity may be decreased in association with central scotomata, peripheral field constriction, and, later, more dense field loss.

Retinal lesions can be divided into two groups.[8] Premaculopathy is generally reversible when the medication is discontinued. True retinopathy is much more serious with more prominent pigmentary changes and visual loss even after medication is discontinued.[5]

Histologic examination shows loss of rods and cones and migration of clumps of pigment.[83] Speculation about the etiology of retinopathy centers on the binding of 4-aminoquinolines to melanin of the retinal pigment epithelium or on lysosomal dysfunction, with subsequent diminution of the protective function of the retinal pigment epithelium[83] and eventual visual loss.

Table 47–5. OPHTHALMOLOGIC SAFETY GUIDELINES FOR ANTIMALARIAL DRUGS

Drug	Daily Dose
Hydroxychloroquine	400 mg or <6.5 mg/kg
Chloroquine	250 mg or <4 mg/kg
Ophthalmologic Monitoring	
Frequency	Baseline, then every 6 months
Protocol for evaluation	Question patient about visual disturbance
	Determine best-corrected visual acuity
	Examine fundus for pigmentary abnormalities
	Assess visual fields with a 5-mm red test object; use 3-mm white test object at baseline and if red test object fields are abnormal
Adjunct methods of evaluation	Amsler grid (self-testing)
	Automated visual fields

GUIDELINES FOR USE

Antimalarials continue to have an important role in the treatment of rheumatic diseases, and the number of diseases reported to respond is increasing.[13, 14]

Although studies have shown limitations in the length of time patients continue to take antimalarials because of lack of sustained disease control, antimalarials can be used as the initial SAARD in patients with rheumatoid arthritis,[84] especially in patients with mild disease. Therapy can be started 6 to 8 weeks after NSAIDs have failed to control synovitis.[84] Advantages include high relative safety and lower cost of monitoring. Even though an ophthalmologic examination should be performed every 6 months, routine hematologic and urinary monitoring is not necessary. After the drug has been found to be well tolerated, the patient need not visit the physician more frequently than indicated by disease severity. A treatment course should not be considered to have failed until it has been tried for at least 6 months. Daily dosing is reviewed in Table 47–5. It is still unclear whether blood levels can predict effectiveness[15]; at present, they are not recommended.

The effectiveness of combination SAARD treatment including antimalarial agents has not been established, but preliminary evidence is promising. Hydroxychloroquine and methotrexate have possible advantages, such as decreased toxicity[72] and increased effectiveness,[69] and they might allow lower doses of methotrexate.[70] Hydroxychloroquine, sulfasalazine, and methotrexate may be a combination of choices.[71]

Antimalarials have an important role in the treatment of skin lesions, articular disease, fever, and malaise in patients with lupus erythematosus. More importantly, they have been shown to prevent flareups of systemic disease in patients who respond to initial treatment.[54, 55] They appear to also lower lipids, especially in patients treated with corticosteroids.[74, 90] If effective, hydroxychloroquine should be continued to prevent disease flareups.[55] Quinacrine, 100 mg/day, can be helpful in treating resistant discoid lesions.[51, 53]

Antimalarials may be used with benefit in patients with other inflammatory arthritides and rheumatic diseases, such as eosinophilic fasciitis,[12] palindromic rheumatism,[11] childhood dermatomyositis,[9, 89] and, perhaps, Sjögren's syndrome.[77, 78] Recent studies raise the possibility of benefit in erosive osteoarthritis[13] and calcium pyrophospate deposition disease.[14]

Patients with psoriatic arthritis should be warned that their skin lesions may flare, and they should be monitored carefully during the initial 3 months of treatment.[5] The potential exacerbation of skin lesions should not be considered an absolute contraindication in such patients, however.[75]

The effectiveness of antimalarial agents in juvenile chronic arthritis is under question.[76] If used, dosage must be determined on the basis of the patient's weight (see Table 47–5), because children are sensitive to antimalarial overdose. Death has resulted from ingestion of as little as 1 g (four tablets) of chloroquine.[85]

Although antimalarials are relatively safe compared with other antirheumatic medications, skin lesions, gastrointestinal symptoms, and mild central nervous system problems such as dizziness occur in a significant number of patients. Gastrointestinal and central nervous system symptoms frequently remit spontaneously or with dosage adjustment. Although uncommon, retinal toxicity cannot be excluded and ophthalmologic examinations (see Table 47–5) should be conducted regularly to detect early changes that are reversible. Medication should be stopped if funduscopic examination shows pigmentary changes, if visual fields have a 5-degree constriction compared with baseline, or if a paracentral scotoma develops, even though these rigid criteria may unnecessarily exclude some patients with non–medication-related retinal disease from treatment.

Antimalarials are not recommended for use during pregnancy because one family in which the mother was receiving treatment has been found to have birth defects involving loss of hearing.[86] It is unlikely, however, that antimalarials present great risk to the fetus. Parke[87] reviewed this subject and reported a number of succesful births with no congenital defects when the mother was treated with antimalarial agents during pregnancy.

References

1. Webster LT: Drugs used in chemotherapy of protozoal infections, malaria. *In* Gilman AG, Rall TW, Nies AS, Taylor P (eds): The Pharmacologic Basis of Therapeutics. New York, Pergamon Press, 1990, pp 978–998.
2. Payne JP: A post-graduate lecture on lupus erythematosus. Clin J 4:223, 1894.
3. Rynes RI: Antimalarials. *In* Kelley WN, Harris ED Jr, Ruddy S, Sledge CB (eds): Textbook of Rheumatology, 2nd ed. Philadelphia, WB Saunders, 1985, pp 774–785.
4. Page F: Treatment of lupus erythematosus with mepacrine. Lancet 2:755, 1951.
5. Rynes RI: Antimalarial drugs. *In* Kelley WN, Harris ED Jr, Ruddy S, Sledge CB (eds): Textbook of Rheumatology, 4th ed. Philadelphia, WB Saunders, 1993, pp 731–742.
6. Scherbel AL, Harrison JW, Atdjian M: Further observations on the use of 4-aminoquinoline compounds in patients with rheumatoid arthritis or related diseases. Cleve Clin Q 25:95, 1958.
7. Hobbs HE, Sorsby A, Freedman A: Retinopathy following chloroquine therapy. Lancet 2:478, 1959.
8. Rynes RI, Bernstein HN: Ophthalmologic safety profile of antimalarial drugs. Lupus 2(Suppl 1):S17, 1993.
9. Woo TY, Callen JP, Voorhees JJ, Bickers DR, Hanno R, Hawkins C: Cutaneous lesions of dermatomyositis are improved by hydroxychloroquine. J Am Acad Dermatol 10:592, 1984.
10. Mattingly S, Jones DW, Robinson WM, et al: Palindromic rheumatism. J R Coll Physicians Lond 15:119, 1982.
11. Youssef W, Yan A, Russell A: Palindromic rheumatism: A response to chloroquine. J Rheumatol 18:1, 1991.
12. Lakhanpal S, Ginsburg WW, Michet CJ, Doyle JA, Brenndan Moore S: Eosinophilic fasciitis: Clinical spectrum and therapeutic response in 52 cases. Semin Arthritis Rheum 17:221, 1988.
13. Bryant LR, DesRosier KF, Carpenter MT: Hydroxychloroquine in the treatment of erosive osteoarthritis. Arthritis Rheum 37(Suppl 9):S241, 1994.
14. Rothschild BM: Prospective six-month double-blind trial of Plaquenil treatment of calcium pyrophosphate deposition disease (CPPD). Arthritis Rheum 37(Suppl 9):S414, 1994.
15. Tett SE, Day RO, Cutler DJ: Concentration-effect relationship of hydroxychloroquine in rheumatoid arthritis: a cross-sectional study. J Rheumatol 20:1874, 1993.

16. Tett SE, Cutler DJ, Day RO, Brown E: A dose-ranging study of the pharmacokinetics of hydroxychloroquine following intravenous administration to healthy volunteers. Br J Clin Pharmacol 26:303, 1988.

17. Tett SE, Cutler DJ, Day RO, Brown E: Bioavailability of hydroxychloroquine table in healthy volunteers. Br J Clin Pharmacol 27:771, 1989.

18. Frisk-Holmberg M, Bergqvist Y, Termond E: Further support for changes in chloroquine disposition and metabolism between a low and high dose. Eur J Clin Pharmacol 28:721, 1985.

19. Frisk-Holmberg M, Bergqvist Y, Termond E, Domeig-Nyberg B: The single dose kinetics of chloroquine and its major metabolite desthylchloroquine in healthy subjects. Eur J Clin Pharmacol 26:521, 1984.

20. Frisk-Holmberg M, Bergqvist Y, Domeig-Nyberg B, Hellstrom L, Jansson F: Chloroquine serum concentration and side effects: Evidence of dose-dependent kinetics. Clin Pharmacol Ther 25:345, 1979.

21. McChesney EW, Conway WD, Banks WF Jr, Rogers JE, Shekosky JM: Studies on the metabolism of some compounds of the 1-amino-7-chloroquinoline series. J Pharmacol Exp Ther 151:482, 1966.

22. McChesney EW, Fasco MJ, Banks WF Jr: The metabolism of chloroquine in man during and after repeated oral dosage. J Pharmacol Exp Ther 158:323, 1967.

23. Rubin M, Bernstein HN, Zvaifler NJ: Studies on the pharmacology of chloroquine. Arch Ophthalmol 70:474, 1962.

24. Prouty RW, Kuroda K: Spectrophotometric determination and distribution of chloroquine in human tissues. J Lab Clin Med 52:477, 1958.

25. French JK, Hurst NP, O'Donnell ML, Betts WH: Uptake of chloroquine and hydroxychloroquine by human blood leucocytes in vitro: Relation to cellular concentrations during antirheumatic therapy. Ann Rheum Dis 46:42, 1987.

26. Bernstein H, Zvaifler N, Rubin M, Mansour AM: The ocular deposition of chloroquine. Invest Ophthalmol 2:384, 1963.

27. Poole B, Ohkuma S: Effect of weak bases on the intralysosomal pH in mouse peritoneal macrophages. J Cell Biol 90:665, 1984.

28. Jones CP, Jayson MIV: Chloroquine: Its effect on leukocyte auto-and heterophagocytosis. Ann Rheum Dis 43:205, 1984.

29. Gonzalez-Noriega A, Grubb JH, Talkad V, Sly WS: Chloroquine inhibits lysosomal enzyme pinocytosis and enhances lysosomal enzyme secretion by impairing receptor recycling. J Cell Biol 85:839, 1980.

30. Oda K, Koriyama Y, Yamada E, Ikehara Y: Effects of weakly basic amines on proteolytic processing and terminal glycosylation of secretory proteins in cultured rat hepatocytes. Biochem J 240:739, 1986.

31. Thompson GR, Bartholomew LE: The effect of chloroquine on antibody formation. Univ Mich Med Cent J 30:227, 1964.

32. Fox RI, Kang HI: Mechanism of action of antimalarial drugs: Inhibition of antigen processing and presentation. Lupus 2(Suppl 1):S9, 1993.

33. Panayi GS, Neill WA, Duthie J Jr, McCormick NJ: Action of chloroquine phosphate in rheumatoid arthritis. I: Immunosuppressive effect. Ann Rheum Dis 32:316, 1973.

34. Ausiello CM, Barbieri P, Spagnoli GC, Ciompi ML, Casciaru CU: In vivo effects of chloroquine treatment on spontaneous and interferon-induced natural killer activities in rheumatoid arthritis patients. Clin Exp Rheumatol 1:255, 1986.

35. Salmeron G, Lipsky PE: Immunosuppressive potential of antimalarials. Am J Med 75(Suppl):19, 1983.

36. Sperber K, Quraishi H, Kalb TH, Panja JA, Stecher V, Mayer L: Selective regulation of cytokine secretion by hydroxychloroquine: Inhibition of interleukin-1 alpha (IL-1-α) and IL-6 in human monocytes and T cells. J Rheumatol 20:803, 1993.

37. Baker DG, Baumgarten DF, Dwyer JP: Chloroquine inhibits the production of a mononuclear cell factor by inhibition of lectin binding. Arthritis Rheum 27:888, 1984.

38. Rainsford KD: Effects of anti-inflammatory drugs on catabalin-induced cartilage destruction in vitro. Int J Tissue React 7:123, 1985.

39. Ferrante A, Rowan-Kelly B, Seow WK, Thong YH: Depression of human polymorphonuclear leukocyte function by antimalarial drugs. Immunology 58:125, 1986.

40. Wallace DJ, Linker-Israeli M, Metzger AL, Stecher VJ: The relevance of antimalarial therapy with regard to thrombosis hypercholesterolemia and cytokines in SLE. Lupus 2(Suppl 1):S13, 1993.

41. Holtz G, Mantel W, Buck W: The inhibition of antigen-antibodies reactions by chloroquine and its mechanism of action. Immunitatsforsch 146:145, 1973.

42. Segal-Eiras A, Segura GM, Babini JC, Arturi AS, Fraguela MJ, Marcos JC: Effect of antimalarial treatment on circulating immune complexes in rheumatoid arthritis. J Rheumatol 12:87, 1985.

43. Wada A, Saktrai S, Kobavashi H, Yanangihara N, Izumi F: Suppression by phospholipase A2 inhibitors of secretion of catecholamines from isolated medullary cells by suppression of cellular calcium uptake. Biochem Pharmacol 32:1175, 1983.

44. Kench JG, Seale JP, Temple DM, Tennant C: The effects of nonsteroidal inhibitors of phospholipase A2 on leukotriene and histamine release from human and guinea-pig lung. Prostaglandins 20:199, 1985.

45. Weissman, G: Labilization and stabilization of lysosomes. Fed Proc 23:1038, 1984.

46. McChesney EW, Nachod FC, Tainter ML: Rationale for treatment of lupus erythematosus with antimalarials. J Invest Dermatol 29:97, 1957.

47. Shaffer B, Cahn MM, Levy EJ: Absorption of antimalarial drugs in human skin: Spectroscopic and chemical analysis in epidermis and corium. J Invest Dermatol 30:341, 1958.

48. Kurnick NB, Radcliffe EI: Reactions between DNA and quinacrine and other antimalarials. J Lab Clin Med 60:669, 1962.

49. Giak J, Hahn FE: Chloroquine: Mode of action. Science 151:347, 1966.

50. Stoller D, Levine L: Antibodies to denatured DNA in lupus erythematosus serum. V: Mechanism of DNA–anti-DNA inhibition by chloroquine. Arch Biochem 101:355, 1963.

51. Dubois EL: Effect of quinacrine (Atabrine) upon lupus erythematosus phenomenon. Arch Dermatol 71:570, 1955.

52. Kraak JH, vanKetel WG, Prakken JR, vanZwet WR: The value of hydroxychloroquine (Plaquenil) for the treatment of chronic discoid lupus erythematosus: A double-blind trial. Dermatologica 130:293, 1965.

53. Winkelman RK, Merwin CF, Brunsting LA: Antimalarial therapy of lupus erythematosus. Ann Intern Med 55:772, 1961.

54. Rudnicki RD, Gresham GE, Rothfield NF: The efficacy of antimalarials in systemic lupus erythematosus. J Rheumatol 2:323, 1975.

55. Canadian Hydroxychloroquine Study Group: A randomized study of the effects of withdrawing hydroxychloroquine sulfate in systemic lupus erythematosus. N Engl J Med 324:150, 1991.

56. Williams HJ, Egger MJ, Singer JZ, et al: Comparison of hydroxychloroquine and placebo in the treatment of the arthropathy of mild systemic lupus erythematosus. J Rheumatol 21:1457, 1994.

57. Ziff M, Esserman P, McEwen C: Observations of the course and treatment of systemic lupus erythematosus. Arthritis Rheum 1:332, 1956.

58. Conte JJ, Mignon-Conte MA, Fournie GJ: Lupus nephritis: Treatment with indomethacin-hydroxychloroquine combination and comparison with corticosteroid treatment. Nouv Presse Med 4:91, 1975.

59. Adams EM, Youcum DE, Bell CL: Hydroxychloroquine in the treatment of rheumatoid arthritis. Am J Med 75:321, 1983.

60. Felson DT, Anderson JJ, Meenan RF: The comparative efficacy and toxicity of second-line drugs in rheumatoid arthritis. Arthritis Rheum 33:1449, 1990.

61. Davis MJ, Dawes PT, Fowler PD, Clarke S, Fisher J, Shadforth MF: Should disease-modifying agents be used in mild rheumatoid arthritis? Br J Rheumatol 30:451, 1991.

62. Clark P, Cassas E, Tugwell P, et al: Hydroxychloroquine compared with placebo in rheumatoid arthritis: A randomized controlled study. Ann Intern Med 119:1067, 1993.

63. HERA Study Group: A randomized trial of hydroxychloroquine in early rheumatoid arthritis: The HERA study. Am J Med 98:156, 1996.

64. Bunch TW, O'Duffy JD, Tompkins RB, O'Fallon WM: Controlled trial of hydroxychloroquine and D-penicillamine singly and in combination in the treatment of rheumatoid arthritis. Arthritis Rheum 27:267, 1984.

65. Nuver-Swart IH, VanRiel PLCM, VanDePutte LVA, Gribnau FWJ: A double-blind comparative study of sulphasalazine and hydroxychloroquine in rheumatoid arthritis: Evidence of an earlier effect of sulphasalazine. Ann Rheum Dis 48:389, 1989.

66. Landewe RBM, Goei HS, VanRijthove AM, Breedveld FC, Dijkmans BAC: A randomized double-blind 24-week controlled study of low-dose cyclosporine versus chloroquine for early rheumatoid arthritis. Arthritis Rheum 37:637, 1994.

67. VanderHeijde DM, VanRiel PL, Zuver-Zwart IH, Gribnau FW, VanDePutte LB: Effects of hydroxychloroquine and sulphasalazine on progression of joint damage in rheumatoid arthritis. Lancet 1:1036, 1989.

68. Porter DR, Capell HA, Hunter J: Combination therapy in rheumatoid arthritis: No benefit of addition of hydroxychloroquine to patients with a suboptimal response to intramuscular gold therapy. J Rheumatol 20:645, 1993.

69. Ferraz MB, Pinheiro GRC, Helfenstein M, et al: Combination therapy with methotrexate and chloroquine in rheumatoid arthritis. Scand J Rheumatol 23:231, 1994.

70. Clegg DO: Combination hydroxychloroquine and methotrexate in the treatment of rheumatoid arthritis. Arthritis Rheum 36(Suppl 9):S53, 1993.

71. O'Dell JR, Haire CE, Erikson N, et al: Treatment of rheumatoid arthritis with methotrexate alone, sulfasalazine and hydroxychloroquine or a combination of all three medications. N Engl J Med 334:1287, 1996.

72. Fries JR, Gurkirpal S, Lenert L, Furst DE: Aspirin, hydroxychloroquine and hepatic enzyme abnormalities with methotrexate in rheumatoid arthritis. Arthritis Rheum 33:1611, 1990.

73. Seidman P, Albertone F, Beck O, Eksborg S, Peterson C: Chloroquine reduces the bioavailability of methotrexate in patients with rheumatoid arthritis. Arthritis Rheum 37:830, 1994.

74. Wallace DJ, Metzger AL, Stecher VJ, Turnbul BA, Kern PA: Cholesterol-lowering effect of hydroxychloroquine (Plaquenil) in rheumatoid disease patients: Reversal of deleterious effects of steroids on lipids. Am J Med 89:322, 1990.

75. Kammer GM, Soter NA, Gibson DJ, Schur PH: Psoriatic arthritis: A clinical, immunologic and HLA study of 100 patients. Semin Arthritis Rheum 9:75, 1979.

76. Brewer EJ, Giannini EH, Kuzima N, Alekseev L: Penicillamine and hydroxychloroquine in the treatment of severe juvenile rheumatoid arthritis. N Engl J Med 315:1269, 1986.
77. Fox FI, Chan E, Benton L, Fong S, Friedlaender M, Howel FV: Treatment of primary Sjögren's syndrome with hydroxychloroquine. Am J Med 85:62, 1988.
78. Chaouat D, Rosa DA, Aron B: Syndrome de Gougerot-Sjögren primitif: Pyrazinamide Rev Rheumatol 55:797, 1988.
79. Reed WB: Psoriatic arthritis: A complete study of 86 patients. Acta Dermatol Venereol 41:396, 1961.
80. Estes ML, Ewing-Wilson D, Chou SM, Mitsumoto H, Hanson M, Shirey E, Ratliff NB: Chloroquine neuromyotoxicity: clinical and pathological perspective. Am J Med 82:447, 1987.
81. Pearson CM, Yamazaki JN: Vacuolar myopathy in systemic lupus erythematosus. Am J Clin Pathol 29:455, 1958.
82. Ratliff NB, Estes ML, Myles JL, Shirey EK, McMahon JT: Diagnosis of chloroquine cardiomyopathy by endomyocardial biopsy. N Engl J Med 316:191, 1987.

83. Bernstein HN, Ginsberg J: The pathology of chloroquine retinopathy. Arch Ophthalmol 71:238, 1964.
84. Harris ED Jr: Hydroxychloroquine is safe and probably useful in rheumatoid arthritis. Ann Intern Med 119:1146, 1993.
85. Cann HM, Verhulst HL: Fatal acute chloroquine poisoning in children. Pediatrics 27:95, 1961.
86. Hart CW, Naunton RF: The ototoxicity of chloroquine phosphate. Arch Otolaryngol 80:407, 1964.
87. Parke AL: Antimalarial drugs in pregnancy and lactation. Lupus 2(Suppl 1):S21, 1993.
88. Landewe RBM, Vergouwen MSC, Goei HS, et al: Antimalarial drug induced decrease in creatinine clearance. J Rheumatol 22:34, 1995.
89. Olson NY, Lindlsey CB: Adjunctive use of hydroxychloroquine in childhood dermatomyositis. J Rheumatol 16:12, 1989.
90. Hodis HN, Quismorio FP Jr, Wickham E, Blankenhorn DH: The lipid, lipoprotein and apolipoprotein effects of hydroxychloroquine in patients with SLE. J Rheumatol 20:661, 1993.

CHAPTER 48

Duncan A. Gordon

Gold Compounds and Penicillamine in the Rheumatic Diseases

GOLD

Gold has been advocated for the treatment of many human diseases for centuries. After Koch, in 1890, reported the in vitro inhibition of tubercle bacilli by gold cyanide, gold compounds were used for treating tuberculous disorders.[1, 2] Forestier in 1929[3] pioneered the use of gold for the treatment of rheumatoid arthritis (RA), assuming that both conditions might have a common infectious cause. Subsequently, results of several studies confirmed this good experience.[4-7] Gold treatment is also recommended for selected patients with psoriatic arthritis or ankylosing spondylitis and for patients with juvenile rheumatoid arthritis.

Pharmacology of Gold

Gold Preparations

Numerous gold-containing compounds have been used to treat RA. Of the several oxidation states for gold compounds, only complex gold compounds are used therapeutically. Gold sodium thiomalate (GSTM), gold sodium thioglucose (GSTG), and gold thioglycoanilid are administered by intramuscular injection only.

GSTM and GSTG are the compounds used in the United States; their structural formulas are shown in Figure 48–1. They are water-soluble preparations and contain a sulfur moiety attached to the gold. Although both GSTM and GSTG are effective, GSTG may be preferred because of lesser toxicity.

An oral gold compound, auranofin (Ridaura), was the first slow-acting antirheumatic drug developed specifically for RA.[8] It is a triethylphosphine gold compound that contains 29 percent gold by weight. It is different physicochemically from the parenteral compounds.

Gold Distribution

Gold concentrations have been measured in animal and human tissue using various methods.[1] In general, the kidneys, adrenals, and reticuloendothelial system organs achieve highest gold concentrations. Intracel-

lularly, gold localizes in the nuclear, mitochondrial, and lysosomal fractions, attached to organelle membranes.

Pharmacokinetics

The details of pharmacokinetic studies of gold have been outlined previously.[1] Gold levels gradually rise

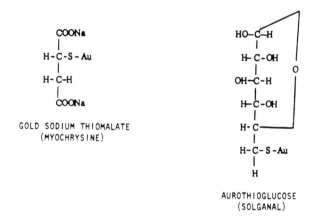

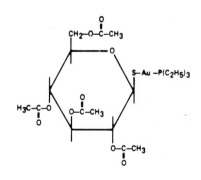

Figure 48–1. Gold sodium thiomalate and aurothioglucose, the two intramuscular gold preparations most widely used in the United States, are aurous salts, contain 50 percent gold by weight, and are attached to a sulfur moiety. Auranofin, a conjugated gold compound with two ligands, contains sulfur and is 29 percent gold by weight.

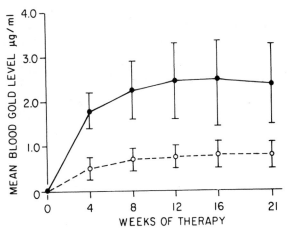

Figure 48–2. Mean whole blood gold concentrations in 59 auranofin-treated patients (○——○) and 51 gold sodium thiomalate-treated patients (●——●) after 21 weeks of therapy. Higher blood gold concentrations are achieved with conventional doses of gold sodium thiomalate than with auranofin (triethylphosphine gold). Gold levels reach a plateau after 6 to 8 weeks of injectable treatment and after 12 weeks of auranofin, reflecting the longer half-life of the oral compound. Bars show standard deviations. (Adapted from Dahl SL, et al: Lack of correlation between blood gold concentrations and clinical response in patients with definite or classic RA receiving auranofin or gold sodium thiomalate. Arthritis Rheum 28:1211, 1985. Reprinted with permission of the American College of Rheumatology.)

with treatment; a plateau is reached after 6 to 8 weeks (Fig. 48–2). Serum gold concentrations correlate with the dose of gold. About 40 percent of the dose of intramuscular gold is eliminated, 70 percent in the urine and 30 percent in the feces. Body gold retention has been measured after 20 weekly injections of 50 mg; about 300 mg of elemental gold is retained. After 20 weeks of oral gold doses of 6 mg per day, about 73 mg of gold is retained.

Mechanisms of Action

The use of gold in the treatment of RA remains empirical. Despite better knowledge of the properties of gold and the pathogenesis of RA, it is not understood exactly how gold works. Rationale for the use of gold has stemmed in part from the fact that in vitro gold compounds inhibit the growth of various microorganisms.[1] Gold compounds also affect the classical and alternative complement systems in vitro. The in vitro effects of gold on lymphocytes and monocytes have been reported.[9] Parenteral gold suppresses adjuvant-induced arthritis of rats. After passive transfer of arthritis, spleen cells from the gold-treated donor rats appeared to inhibit the development of arthritis in the recipient animals.[10] Micromolar concentrations of gold inhibit peptide-stimulated chemotactic responsiveness of human blood monocytes, but not polymorphonuclear leukocytes.[11] GSTM inhibits neutrophil chemotaxis and random migration in vitro in normal subjects and in gold-responsive patients with RA but not in gold-resistant patients.[12] Leukocyte adhesion receptors on endothelial cells ap-

pear to promote rheumatoid synovitis by recruitment of leukocytes to sites of inflammation.[13] GSTM inhibits acid phosphatase, β-glucuronidase, and malic dehydrogenase in guinea pig peritoneal macrophages; acid phosphatase, β-glucuronidase, and cathepsin in human synovial fluid cells; and several human epidermal enzymes.[14]

Clinical Applications

Patient Selection

Gold is used primarily for progressive polyarticular RA. Thus, its use should be based on a firm diagnosis. Unfortunately, in the earliest stages of RA, we lack available markers to identify progressive disease. Further, after 5 years, about 80% of patients given second-line drugs such as gold are no longer taking them because of either side effects or inefficacy. Some studies have shown that gold therapy is most effective in early, nonerosive RA,[5] and others have demonstrated its value in active disease of long duration despite joint damage.[6] Gold is not indicated for advanced RA without evidence of active synovitis, but we have found it effective in controlling monarticular or pauci-articular RA. Factors that do not apparently influence the response to chrysotherapy include patient age, sex, race, extra-articular features of RA, erythrocyte sedimentation rate, and presence or absence of rheumatoid factor.[1]

Gold compounds may be employed in patients with RA who have Felty's and Sjögren's syndromes, preexisting neutropenia, or eosinophilia.[1, 15] Available evidence suggests that with gold, neutropenia and splenomegaly improve without undue toxicity. Chronic anemia is also a feature of RA that may improve with gold. Despite earlier admonitions against gold in RA-associated Sjögren's syndrome, it is generally well tolerated.[16] Similarly, nonprogressive proteinuria or benign hematuria without renal insufficiency does not preclude gold treatment. Preexisting proteinuria and dermatitis, however, are relative contraindications to the use of gold because they could mimic toxic effects of the drug.

Parenteral therapy does not appear to affect babies born to mothers treated with gold, but any newborn exposed to maternal gold during pregnancy or lactation should be monitored closely.[17]

Efficacy

The benefit of gold treatment in RA has been well documented over the past 50 years.[1] Although past studies were mostly descriptive, they represent milestones in the evolution of better treatment for RA (Fig. 48–3).

In 1974, a 30-month, double-blind study compared a standard course of GSTM with placebo followed by a comparison of maintenance gold against placebo.[7] Twenty-seven patients with RA for less than 5 years were randomly assigned to treatment or placebo groups. Improvement required at least 3 months of

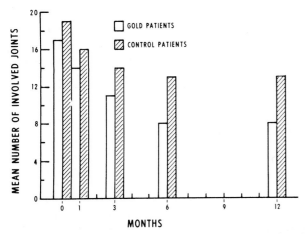

Figure 48–3. Mean number of involved joints declined significantly in gold-treated rheumatoid arthritis patients but not in control subjects. (Adapted from the Empire Rheumatism Council Study: Gold therapy in rheumatoid arthritis. Ann Rheum Dis 19:95, 1960.)

treatment and sometimes took 9 months. Good effects were maintained for a mean of 28 months. Serial radiographs of the hands and wrists revealed fewer bone erosions in the gold-treated group. A more recent study confirmed joint erosion repair in 23 percent of 29 patients followed over 18 months.[18]

Auranofin has been tested worldwide in many thousands of patients with RA.[8] Most short-term trials have shown similar efficacy with intramuscular gold, but over 1 year about half the patients taking auranofin dropped out because of inefficacy.[1]

There have also been a number of comparative studies involving other antirheumatic agents. GSTM, 50 mg/week intramuscularly; azathioprine, 1.0 to 2.0 mg/kg/day orally; or chloroquine, 250 mg/day orally, was given to 33 patients with early RA (duration, about 2 years) in a nonblinded, randomly assigned 24-week study. The azathioprine group was faring marginally better than the chloroquine group at the final evaluation (Fig. 48–4).

Two 6-month controlled trials compared sulfasalazine with GSTM and placebo. Results in 90 patients with active RA showed equal benefit for these agents.[19] A 26-week trial in 40 patients with RA compared parenteral methotrexate (MTX), 10 mg/week, with GSTM, 50 mg/week.[20] Similar efficacy was shown, but MTX side effects (20 percent) were much less than gold toxicity (50 percent).

The advantage of combining study results was shown in two meta-analyses that examined comparable controlled studies.[21, 22] Both analyses confirmed a favorable magnitude of efficacy for parenteral gold.

Another approach is the utilization of life-table analysis of treatment terminations. In one study, 80 percent of patients after 5 years were no longer using second-line medications.[23] In another report, 30 percent of patients taking gold continued to show benefit after 5 years.[24] A retrospective analysis also showed a long-term survival for patients taking gold.[25]

Although gold was previously considered a mainstay in the treatment of RA, its role in altering the long-term course of RA remains controversial. Despite the success of short-term clinical trials with gold, concern has been expressed about the disappointing long-term outcomes. Moreover, this apparent lack of long-term efficacy has led some to question the value of gold as a second-line agent.[26] This view, however, has been challenged on several grounds, including better evidence of efficacy over 1 year in a group of 98 RA patients despite a drop-out rate of 36%.[27–29] Although oral gold generates less serious toxicity than parenteral gold, its efficacy is less as well.

The foregoing lack of long-term efficacy has led to interest in the use of combinations of second-line agents for the treatment of RA. A formal overview of the topic compared the benefits and risks of combinations of agents with the same drugs used singly.[30] One study compared a combination of parenteral gold and hydroxychloroquine (52 patients) in gold and placebo (49 patients).[31] The combination group showed more rapid improvement and better overall reduction of disease activity after 12 months.

There is an association between treatment response and a rash.[32] Immunogenetic data also suggest that patients with RA possessing human leukocyte antigen (HLA)–DR3 may be both more responsive to gold treatment than patients without DR3[33] and more likely to develop certain toxicities.[39]

As noted, 6 months may be insufficient to obtain maximum benefit from chrysotherapy; treatment should be extended to 18 or more months before

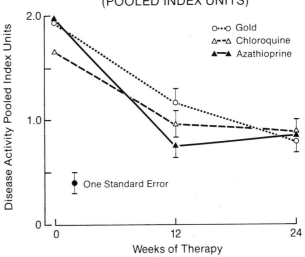

Figure 48–4. The initial disease activity was similar for all three agents in pooled index units (derived by using a combination of articular index, joint count, grip strength, morning stiffness, and erythrocyte sedimentation rate). At 12 weeks, total disease activity was significantly improved in all three groups ($P < .5$). At 24 weeks, disease activity was still significantly decreased in all three groups ($P < .001$). (Adapted from Dwosh IL, et al: Azathioprine in early RA. Arthritis Rheum 20:685, 1977. Reprinted with permission of the American College of Rheumatology.)

termination for lack of improvement.[7, 34] Although loss of efficacy may occur after long-term maintenance therapy,[23] patients whose disease exacerbates while they are receiving monthly maintenance gold injections frequently benefit from a return to weekly treatment.[35] Gold therapy can be continued indefinitely after an acceptable response if the patient and the physician are commited to long-term monitoring.

Dosage Schedules

The usual intramuscular gold dosage schedule has been derived empirically from clinical experience. At present, the standard gold schedule for adults with RA consists of test doses of 10 mg and 25 mg given 1 week apart, followed by 50 mg weekly, until the cumulative dose totals 1 g, or toxicity or major clinical improvement supervenes.

There are numerous variations in the aforementioned schedule, such as weekly injections of 25 mg rather than 50 mg of gold compound; others recommend 50 mg until 500 to 700 mg is attained, at which time the dose is reduced to 25-mg weekly. Maintenance gold therapy, which generally consists of 25 to 50 mg every 2 to 4 weeks, is advocated after completion of the initial course. Termination of gold after remission increases the probability that a second course will be ineffective.

Intermittent short-term intramuscular depot injections of corticosteroids given in conjunction with chrysotherapy have been advocated as an approach that can enhance efficacy of gold while decreasing toxicity.[36] Oral pulse corticosteroids, however, are not as effective for this induction.[37] Investigators have been unable to correlate the response to chrysotherapy with the pharmacokinetics of gold. Results of a study using atomic absorption spectrometry, however, showed that toxicity correlated with an increase in free gold over total gold levels.[38]

Cost of Gold Treatment

Administration and monitoring of the initial phase (20 weeks) of intramuscular gold treatment are expensive. Strategies to reduce costs include fewer and less frequent laboratory tests and administration of gold at home by a family member or nurse.

Toxicity of Gold

When a patient with RA does poorly despite treatment, symptoms may be related to the disease itself or to side effects from antirheumatic medications such as gold. Adverse reactions develop in about one third of patients with RA treated with intramuscular gold, varying from 5 to 30 percent (Table 48–1). Most complications are trivial, consisting primarily of localized dermatitis, stomatitis, transient hematuria, and mild proteinuria. More serious reactions involve the hematopoietic system, kidneys, liver, or other vital organs. The characteristics of complications with auranofin differ importantly from those of the injectable gold compounds (see Table 48–1). Mucocutaneous lesions and serious complications occur less commonly with auranofin than with the intramuscular preparations.[8] Gold-induced proteinuria and thrombocytopenia, representing immune-mediated reactions, are more common in patients possessing HLA-DR3.[39]

Postinjection Reactions

Reactions may be the rapid-onset vasomotor type or the slower-onset nonvasomotor type. Vasomotor (nitritoid) reactions, characterized by weakness, dizziness, nausea, vomiting, sweating, and facial flushing, may follow GSTM injections. The prevalence of this reaction has varied to as high as 34 percent. Peripheral vasodilation may cause hypotension from the action on arteriolar smooth muscle. Hypertensive patients with RA who take angiotensin converting enzyme inhibitors such as captopril or analogs may be at risk for nitritoid reactions after taking oral gold or GSTM injections.[40]

Nonvasomotor postinjection reactions, with transient arthralgia, joint swelling, fatigability, and malaise, developed in 15 percent of patients treated with GSTM. The reaction comes about 6 to 24 hours after injection but can appear within an hour or last as long as a few days. Postinjection reactions are not a reason to abandon gold treatment because a switch to GSTG can obviate them.

Mucocutaneous Effects

Dermatitis and stomatitis account for 60 to 80 percent of all adverse gold reactions. The clinical and histologic appearance of gold rash is highly variable, although most cases are pruritic, discrete, last 1 or 2 months, and are confined to the limbs or trunk. Eosinophilia, metallic taste, or proteinuria often accompanies dermatitis.

Skin punch biopsy may allow exclusion of other skin disorders, such as rheumatoid vasculitis. HLA-DR5 may be associated with increased susceptibility to these mucocutaneous reactions.[41]

When a skin eruption appears, chrysotherapy should be discontinued for a few weeks of observation until the eruption resolves. Treatment then may be reinstituted, using a reduced dosage schedule of 5 to 10 mg of gold weekly, with 5- to 10-mg increments every 1 to 4 weeks if toxicity does not recur. Reinstitution of chrysotherapy rarely results in exfoliative dermatitis.

Contact allergy to gold jewelry may develop after administration of parenteral gold,[42] and previous contact hypersensitivity to nickel may be provoked by gold injection.[43] Rarely, gray or blue discoloration of the skin, known as chrysiasis, is asymptomatic and may be associated with hyperpigmentation.[44]

Kidney

Transient proteinuria, microscopic hematuria, and nephrotic syndrome are well-described complications

Table 48–1. TOXICITY PROFILE WITH GOLD COMPOUNDS

Adverse Effects	Aurothiomalate	Aurothioglucose	Auranofin
Postinjection Reactions			
Vasomotor (nitritoid)	Uncommon*	Rare	Rare*
Anaphylaxis/syncope	Rare	Unknown	Unknown
Myalgias/arthralgias	Common	Rare	Unknown
Mucocutaneous Effects			
Dermatitis/stomatitis	Common†	Less common	Common
Pruritus	Common	Less common	Common
Alopecia	Rare	Rare	Rare
Urticaria	Rare	Rare	Uncommon
Trophic nails	Rare	Rare	Unknown
Chrysiasis/pigmentation	Rare	Rare	Unknown
Photosensitivity	Rare	Rare	Unknown
Kidney			
Proteinuria	Common‡	Less common	Rare
Hematuria	Uncommon	Less common	Rare
Nephrotic syndrome	Rare	Rare	Rare
Renal insufficiency	Rare	Rare	Unknown
Blood			
Eosinophilia	Common	Common	Rare
Thrombocytopenia	Rare‡	Rare	Rare
Granulocytopenia	Rare	Rare	Rare
Lymphocytopenia	Uncommon	Rare	Rare
Hypogammaglobulinemia	Rare	Rare	Unknown
Aplastic anemia	Rare	Rare	Unknown
Pulmonary Complications			
Diffuse infiltrates	Rare	Rare	Rare
Intestinal Effects			
Upper gastrointestinal symptoms	Rare	Rare	Uncommon
Mild enterocolitis	Rare	Rare	Common
Severe enterocolitis	Rare	Rare	Rare
Liver			
Cholestatic jaundice	Rare	Rare	Unknown
Hepatocellular effects	Rare	Rare	Uncommon
Pancreas			
Pancreatitis	Rare	Rare	Rare
Nervous System			
Peripheral/cranial			
Neuropathies	Rare	Rare	Rare
Encephalopathy	Rare	Rare	Rare
Eye			
Corneal or lens chrysiasis	Common	Common	Unknown
Conjunctivitis	Rare	Rare	Uncommon
Iritis/corneal ulcer	Rare	Rare	Unknown
Miscellaneous			
Metallic taste	Common	Common	Common
Headaches	Rare	Rare	Rare

*Reported in hypertensives on angiotensin converting enzyme inhibitors.
†HLA-DR3: possible relationship.
‡HLA-DR3: relationship proved.

of gold therapy. Urinary protein may resolve spontaneously despite continuation of chrysotherapy, but the nephrotic syndrome is the most frequent serious renal abnormality associated with gold therapy. The prognosis for gold-associated nephrotic syndrome is generally favorable; renal insufficiency is rare, with 70 percent of patients fully recovering within months to years. The HLA-DQA region genes may be the important susceptibility factor for gold-induced nephropathy.[45]

Blood

Hematologic disorders resulting from chrysotherapy include eosinophilia, leukopenia or agranulocyto-sis, thrombocytopenia, anemia, pancytopenia, and aplastic anemia. Mild eosinophilia occurs in up to 30 percent of gold-treated patients.[46]

Thrombocytopenia is a rare (1 to 3 percent) complication of gold treatment that may be serious or life-threatening.[47] It may develop shortly after gold is begun or as long as 18 months after cessation of therapy. The initial manifestations may be easy bruisability or spontaneous petechiae or purpura affecting the skin or mucous membranes. Although gold-induced thrombocytopenia may result from marrow suppression, an active marrow is usual, with peripheral destruction of platelets and platelet-associated immunoglobulin G (IgG).[47] To date, 85 percent of reported patients with gold-induced thrombocytopenia possess HLA-DR3, whereas its general frequency is 30 percent in patients with RA. Patients who develop thrombocytopenia after parenteral gold may also develop thrombocytopenia after taking other second-line agents.[48]

The prevalence of leukopenia is low, and the extent and duration of white cell reductions are variable. The most feared complication of chrysotherapy is severe pancytopenia or bone marrow aplasia.[49] The incidence of the latter is low, with a prevalence of less than 0.5 percent. In the past, the mortality rate has been high, but prognosis has been improved by aggressive therapy, including bone marrow transplantation, antithymocyte globulin,[49] or granulocyte colony-stimulating factor.[50] Gold therapy has also been associated with generalized hypogammaglobulinemia.

Other Toxicity of Gold

Acute respiratory distress associated with diffuse pulmonary infiltration characteristically causes cough productive of small amounts of sputum, shortness of breath, pleuritic chest pain, and pulmonary crackles.[51] The clinical picture develops after about 500 mg of parenteral gold. Radiographs show patchy pulmonary consolidation, and pulmonary function tests are consistent with restrictive lung disease. Bronchoalveolar lavage reveals a predominance of lymphocytes. Dramatic improvement follows withdrawal of chrysotherapy and administration of systemic glucocorticoids.

Enterocolitis is a rare but serious complication of parenteral gold, occurring primarily in middle-aged women after small total doses of gold.[52] Symptoms may include abdominal pain, bloody or nonbloody diarrhea, nausea, vomiting, and fever. Despite supportive treatment, the mortality rate approaches 50 percent. Successful treatment of gold-induced enteritis with octreotide has been reported.[53]

About 85 percent of the total dose of auranofin is eliminated in the feces. It is therefore not surprising that patients with RA taking auranofin have twice the frequency of diarrhea as patients taking parenteral gold.

Cholestatic jaundice, with hyperbilirubinemia, elevated transaminases, and high alkaline phosphatase levels, has been ascribed to gold treatment. Liver biopsy may show bile stasis and thrombi in the biliary tree or ballooning hepatocytes with sinusoidal compression and minimal cholestasis. Hepatic necrosis after gold may rarely have fatal consequences.[54] Pancreatitis may also be a rare benign complication of oral or injectable gold.[55]

Neurologic complications of chrysotherapy are rare but reversible and include peripheral neuropathy, a Guillain-Barré–type syndrome, cranial nerve palsies including ophthalmoplegia, and encephalopathy.[56] They usually arise after 3 months of weekly injections, and myokymia is a characteristic clinical sign. Recognition of the neuropathy may be difficult because it can resemble some features of RA itself. Sural nerve

biopsy, however, shows both axonal degeneration and segmental demyelination, and computed tomographic brain scan may show evidence of cerebral demyelination.

Corneal and lens chrysiasis is benign and directly related to cumulative dose, occurring in 75 percent of patients receiving more than 1500 mg of intramuscular gold.

Treatment Monitoring

Efforts to reduce untoward gold reactions have been fairly successful. The mortality rate has fallen from an estimated 4 percent in the early years of chrysotherapy to less than 0.05 percent at present. Precautionary measures do not prevent gold complications; they merely permit their recognition.

Monitoring chrysotherapy requires history about drug reactions, rash, renal disease, or proteinuria. A complete blood count with differential, platelet count, urinalysis, and biochemical profile is obtained. It is useful to have the patient keep a diary of blood counts and urinalyses as a double check to the danger signals of cytopenias or proteinuria. Blood work and urinalyses for protein are obtained every 1 to 3 weeks. Chrysotherapy is put on hold promptly should any of the aforementioned features develop.

Gold compounds should never be administered to patients with a history of prior severe gold toxicity (e.g., exfoliative dermatitis, significant depression of any blood cell type, heavy proteinuria, or chronic renal failure). Because vasomotor reactions occur within several minutes after injection, it is wise to give GSTM with the patient recumbent. Gold is not recommended for pregnant or lactating women because the safety for the fetus or newborn infant has not been established.

Treatment of Gold Toxicity

Most adverse gold reactions resolve spontaneously weeks or months after cessation of gold therapy. Most patients with symptomatic gold dermatitis benefit from antihistamines, topical corticosteroids, or other local measures. Sun and soap should be avoided. Generalized pruritic eruptions may improve with systemic glucocorticoids. Stomatitis, glossitis, cheilitis, and gingivitis may require no treatment or may require only that the patient avoid spicy foods. Stronger measures include alkaline mouthwashes or the application of lidocaine (Xylocaine Viscous) or triamcinolone (Kenalog in Orabase). We have found betamethasone (Betnesol) pellets sucked three or four times a day to be useful.

Moderate- to high-dose glucocorticoid therapy (20 to 60 mg daily in divided doses) may be beneficial in gold-induced nephrotic syndrome, thrombocytopenia, and, less often, other hematologic disorders, enterocolitis, and pulmonary infiltrates.

Dimercaprol, penicillamine, N-acetylcysteine, and other chelating agents have been employed in severe reactions unresponsive to glucocorticoid therapy or in conjunction with steroids.[1] Patients with severe thrombocytopenia associated with hemorrhage may require volume repletion and platelet transfusions. Vincristine, other potent chemotherapeutic agents, splenectomy, and, more recently, intravenous gamma globulin have been used.[47] Those patients suffering from significant granulocytopenia or agranulocytosis often improved spontaneously within 2 weeks. In unresponsive cases and in those with bone marrow aplasia, supportive measures, including androgenic hormones, bone marrow transplantation, and peritoneal dialysis, also have been used. Antithymocyte globulin has been recommended as initial treatment for gold-induced aplastic anemia.[50]

D-PENICILLAMINE

D-Penicillamine (DP) is a component of the penicillin molecule obtained by acid hydrolysis. In rheumatology, it is approved for the treatment of RA.[57] It is also used, although not labeled, for the treatment of systemic sclerosis.[58] The best effects have been seen in patients with early progressive diffuse scleroderma.[59]

Pharmacology of D-Penicillamine

Chemistry

The structural formula for DP is shown in Figure 48–5. It is a sulfhydryl (SH) amino acid that differs from the naturally occurring cysteine because of the two methyl groups that replace hydrogen in the β-carbon position. It may be made from penicillin by a semisynthetic process, or it may be made entirely synthetically. All of the DP in clinical use is the D-isomer.

Biochemistry

The biochemical and pharmacologic properties of DP in humans form the basis for certain of its clinical applications.[60] *Chelation* of divalent cations such as copper and trace metals accounts for its usefulness in the treatment of Wilson's disease and heavy metal poisoning. It forms a *thiazolidine* with pyridoxal phosphate, which may result in antagonism to vitamin B_6,

although it is much weaker in this regard than L-penicillamine.[61] A thiazolidine bond may also be formed between DP and the aldehyde groups of collagen, thereby inhibiting collagen cross-linking.[62] This is the biochemical basis for its application to the treatment of systemic sclerosis. Which, if any, of these actions is responsible for the efficacy of DP in RA is unknown.

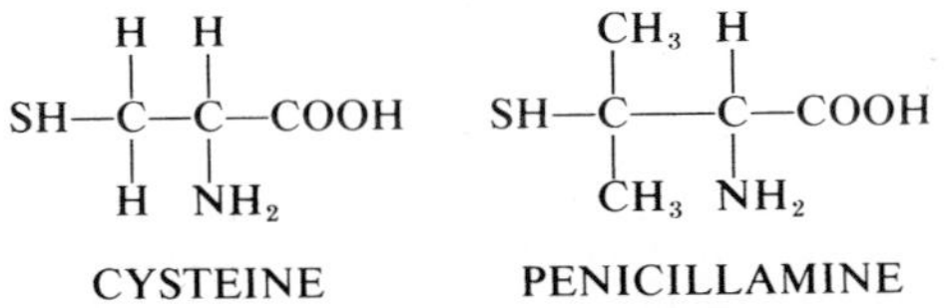

Pharmacokinetics

DP is well absorbed from the upper gastrointestinal tract when given in the postabsorptive state. About half of an orally administered dose can be accounted for in urine and feces. When DP administration is discontinued, free DP rapidly disappears from the urine, but oxidized forms can be recovered for more than 3 months.[63] Plasma binding is greatest to albumin, α-globulin, and ceruloplasmin. In tissues, radioactive DP is found in the greatest amount in collagen-containing structures, skin, and tendons.

Mechanism of Action

The mechanism of action of DP in RA is unknown. The DP molecule is so highly reactive that the demonstration of an effect in an in vitro test system cannot be extrapolated to explain its mode of action in RA. In test systems, DP is neither anti-inflammatory nor immunosuppressive, and it has no effect on animal models of arthritis.[64] After DP treatment of RA, there is a significant reduction in T lymphocytes and a disproportionate fall in the helper/inducer subset in the synovial tissue.[65] These observations suggest a selective type of immunosuppression directed against the $CD4^+$ T cells. The specificity of DP for RA is unique among the antirheumatic drugs because DP is of no benefit in any other type of inflammatory joint disease,[66] suggesting that DP acts on a pathogenetic mechanism unique to RA.

Another site of action of DP is the consistent reduction of rheumatoid factor titer and immune complexes with DP treatment. These immunoglobulins and complexes are the product of synthesis by B lymphocytes. Because DP has no direct inhibitory effect on B cell function, it is assumed that its inhibition is exerted *before* the step of antibody synthesis by B cells. In vitro, it was found that DP (with copper) produced a marked suppression of human fibroblast proliferation,[67] and perhaps inhibition of pannus formation in RA, and collagen production in scleroderma. A suppression of human endothelial production in vitro and neovascularization in vivo by DP were reported.[68]

Clinical Applications

Patient Selection

DP is indicated for the treatment of active RA and in selected patients with juvenile RA. The efficacy of

Figure 48–5. The chemical structure of penicillamine. The drug is an analog of the naturally occurring amino acid cysteine, with CH_3 groups replacing H+ at the B carbon position.

DP for RA was first established by the United Kingdom Multi-Centre Trial.[69] Subsequent studies showed it to be as effective as azathioprine, intramuscular gold, and antimalarial drugs and more effective than oral gold.[22] It has been particularly useful in some patients with RA with extra-articular manifestations, such as vasculitis, Felty's syndrome, amyloidosis, and rheumatoid lung disease.[70] It is not of value in the seronegative spondyloarthropathies,[66] psoriatic arthritis, and other types of inflammatory connective tissue disease. Because of its toxicity, it is used infrequently as an initial second-line drug in RA.

Efficacy

The pattern of improvement in a DP-responsive patient is similar to that of chrysotherapy. Objective signs of a decrease in synovitis may be found by 6 months. In responsive patients, there is a gradual improvement in the sedimentation rate and the C-reactive protein and a rise in hemoglobin. A reduction in the titer of serum rheumatoid factor is consistent and usually correlates with clinical improvement.[71]

Because of the latent period of 8 to 12 weeks before improvement is evident, analgesic and anti-inflammatory drugs must be maintained. Exacerbations in disease activity may be observed and may require an increase in maintenance dose to regain control. Antibodies to DP may develop during treatment, and this may explain the loss of efficacy in some patients.[72]

After 5 years, only about 25 percent of patients given DP continue with a satisfactory result.[73] Withdrawals are largely due to adverse reactions and less to loss of efficacy. Progression of radiologic damage has not differed between patients treated with DP for 5 years and those receiving other treatments.[74]

Dosing Schedule

DP is available as a 250- or 125-mg capsule or as a 250-mg scored tablet. Various dosage regimens have been studied in RA, and it is recommended that treatment be initiated with 125 or 250 mg/day for 4 to 8 weeks. The dosage may then be raised by a similar increment until improvement commences or a maximum of 1.0 g/day is reached. The current trend is to employ an average dose not greater than 500 mg per day.

Absorption of DP is hindered by food, antacids, and oral iron; hence, it is optimally given in the postabsorptive state.[60] It may be given in a single daily dose, 1 to 2 hours apart from food or other medicines. Both indomethacin and chloroquine have been shown to raise blood levels of DP.[75]

Contraindications and Precautions

DP is contraindicated in pregnancy. If a patient with RA becomes pregnant while receiving DP, the drug should be stopped, but termination of the pregnancy is not indicated. A history of previous allergic or hypersensitivity reaction to penicillin is *not* a contraindication to the use of DP, and no additional precautions are required.[76] Because of its potential for toxic reactions, particularly hematologic, prescriptions for DP should be written for a limited time and clearly labeled *nonrefillable*. Patients who have experienced major side effects with gold are more likely to experience toxicity with DP.[77] Intravenous pulse corticosteroids combined with DP induction showed no advantage in better efficacy or reduced toxicity of DP.[78]

Toxicity of D-Penicillamine

The adverse effects from DP administration have been the major factor limiting its usefulness. Certain of these effects can be favorably influenced by the "go low, go slow" dosage regimens, but others can occur regardless of the maximum maintenance dose or the duration of treatment.[79] Most of the side effects encountered during the first 18 months of therapy (Fig. 48-6). There is an association between HLA-B8 and HLA-DR3 and toxic reactions to both gold salts and DP, particularly with respect to nephropathy.[80-82] RA patients with Sjögren's syndrome appear more prone to DP toxicity. Antibodies to DP are also associated with a higher incidence of adverse reactions.[72]

Blood

Hematologic toxicity is certainly the most serious of the adverse reactions. Leukopenia, thrombocytopenia, and aplastic anemia have been observed. Thrombocytopenia may be dose-related, with normal numbers of megakaryocytes, and treatment can be continued, or it may be idiosyncratic and a harbinger of marrow aplasia when the megakaryocyte numbers are decreased. Complete blood counts with platelets should be done every 2 weeks for the first 6 months and

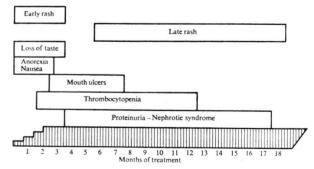

Figure 48-6. The chronopharmacology of penicillamine. This diagram depicts the peak incidence of some of the more common side effects of penicillamine during a course of therapy with a maintenance dose of 1 g per day. Most of the serious reactions will have developed during the first 18 months of treatment. Aplastic anemia was not included in this illustration, but it may occur at any time, particularly after an increment in dosage. (After Balme HW, Huskisson EC: Chronopharmacology of penicillamine and gold. Scand J Rheumatol 4[Suppl 8]:21, 1975.)

monthly thereafter. A white blood cell count below 3000 cells/mm^3 or a platelet count below 100,000 cells/mm^3 requires that the DP therapy be discontinued until the reaction can be defined.

Kidney

Nephropathy is most often of the membranous type, secondary to immune complex deposition.[83] Proteinuria may be asymptomatic or may be associated with signs of nephrotic syndrome. Urinalysis should be performed at the same time as the hematologic studies. Two groups of RA patients with DP nephropathy were compared with regard to renal function and continued DP therapy with ≤ 2.0 g protein excretion per day. In one group, DP administration was stopped after proteinuria developed, and in the other, DP therapy was continued. At the end of 1 year, renal function was the same in both groups.[84]

Microscopic hematuria is usually benign and does not require discontinuation of treatment.[85] Gross hematuria should be evaluated with regard to possible causes. If none is found, it is probably a result of the DP, and the drug should be stopped. Rapidly progressive glomerulonephritis is a rare occurrence.

Mucocutaneous Effects

Pruritus and a variety of early and late rashes are the most common side effects of the drug. Simple pruritus can often be managed by a temporary interruption of DP therapy and the addition of an antihistamine. Aphthous ulcers and stomatitis may occur, but these often resolve with a modest reduction in dosage. The appearance of bullous dermatitis might herald the development of DP-induced pemphigus. Administration of the drug must be stopped, and immunosuppressive therapy may be required.

Other Toxicity

Gastrointestinal symptoms due to penicillamine are usually not serious. Anorexia and nausea may be dose-limiting but usually disappear. There have been reports of cholestatic jaundice, but serious hepatotoxicity is extremely rare.[86]

Pulmonary complications are also rare. A Goodpasture-like syndrome has been described. There have been reports of DP-associated bronchiolitis obliterans.[87] The appearance of dyspnea associated with midinspiratory rhonchi should alert the physician to the serious event.

Neuromuscular disorders may infrequently be caused by DP. Myasthenia gravis is the most common in this category, and it is identical to the spontaneously occurring disease. There are antibodies to the acetylcholine receptor, and the patients respond to anticholesterase drugs. Myasthenia, often with ocular symptoms, is reversible after DP withdrawal, but months may be required before dependence on anticholinesterase drugs ends. Whereas spontaneous my-

asthenia is associated with HLA-DR3 and HLA-B1, DP-induced myasthenia is almost always associated with HLA-DR1 and HLA-Bw35.[88, 89]

Autoimmune syndromes have been described in the other diseases for which DP is given, such as Wilson's disease and cystinuria, indicating that they are a feature of the drug rather than an altered immune responsiveness in rheumatoid patients. Autoantibodies to insulin and the insulin receptor have been described.[72] DP-induced lupus has been well recognized, and these patients differ from those with drug-induced lupus because they have antibody to native, double-stranded DNA.[90, 91] Polymyositis and dermatomyositis also can be produced by DP.

Hypogeusia or dysgeusia-blunting taste perception is common, but self-limited. *Drug fever*, often with a morbilliform rash, usually develops shortly after treatment is begun and recurs on rechallenge.

Other Sulfhydryl Compounds

Numerous attempts have been made to find an SH compound with a DP-like beneficial effect on RA but with greater safety. Bucillamine, developed in Japan, has a molecular structure similar to that of DP, except that bucillamine has two free SH groups rather than only one. Clinical effects in patients suggest that bucillamine might suppress RA more effectively than DP. The effect of bucillamine and its metabolites on human T cells showed two types of immunosuppressive effects.[92] 5-Thiopyridoxine, pyrithioxine (pyritinol), thiopronine (-mercaptopropionyl glycine), and captopril have been studied. All were effective; captopril was the weakest. Unfortunately, they all displayed a similar and characteristic spectrum of adverse effects, including induction of autoimmune disease.[93–95]

References

1. Gordon DA: Gold compounds. In Kelley WN, Harris ED, Ruddy S, Sledge CB (eds): Textbook of Rheumatology, 4th ed. Philadelphia, WB Saunders, 1993, pp 760–766.
2. Kean WF, Forestier F, Kassam Y, Buchanan WW, Rooney PJ: The history of gold therapy in rheumatoid disease. Semin Arthritis Rheum 14:180, 1985.
3. Forestier J: Rheumatoid arthritis and its treatment by gold salts. J Lab Clin Med 20:827, 1935.
4. Hartfall SJ, Garland HG, Goldie W: Gold treatment of arthritis: A review of 900 cases. Lancet 233:838, 1937.
5. Empire Rheumatism Council: Gold therapy in rheumatoid arthritis. Final report of a multicentre controlled trial. Ann Rheum Dis 20:315, 1961.
6. The Cooperative Clinics Committee of the ARA: A controlled trial of gold salt therapy in rheumatoid arthritis. Arthritis Rheum 16:353, 1973.
7. Sigler JW, Bluhm GB, Duncan H, et al: Gold salts in the treatment of rheumatoid arthritis: A double-blind study. Ann Intern Med 80:21, 1974.
8. Abruzzo JL: Auranofin: A new drug for rheumatoid arthritis. Ann Intern Med 105:274, 1986.
9. Lipsky PE, Ziff M: Inhibition of antigen- and mitogen-induced human lymphocyte proliferation by gold compounds. J Clin Invest 59:455, 1977.
10. Cannon GW, McCall S: Inhibition of the passive transfer of adjuvant-induced arthritis by gold sodium thiomalate. J Rheumatol 17:436, 1990.
11. Ho PPK, Young AL, Southard GL: Methyl ester N-formylmethionyl-leucyl-phenylalanine. Chemotactic responses of human blood monocytes and inhibition of gold compounds. Arthritis Rheum 21:133, 1978.

12. Mowat AG: Neutrophil chemotaxis in rheumatoid arthritis. Ann Rheum Dis 37:1, 1978.
13. Corkill MM, Kirkham BW, Haskard DO, Barbatis C, Gibson T, Panayi GS: Gold treatment of rheumatoid arthritis decreases synovial expression of the endothelial leukocyte adhesion receptor ELAM-1. J Rheumatol 18:1453, 1991.
14. Penneys NS, Ziboh V, Gottlieb NL, et al: Inhibition of prostaglandin synthesis and human epidermal enzymes by aurothiomalate in vitro: Possible actions of gold in pemphigus. J Invest Dermatol 63:356, 1974.
15. Dillon AM, Luthra HS, Conn DL, Ferguson RH: Parenteral gold therapy in the Felty syndrome. Experience with 20 patients. Medicine (Baltimore) 65:107, 1986.
16. Gordon MH, Tiger LH, Ehrlich GE: Gold reactions are not more common in Sjögren's syndrome. Ann Intern Med 82:47, 1975.
17. Bennett PN, Humphries SJ, Osborne JP, Clarke AK, Taylor A: Use of sodium aurothiomalate during lactation. Br J Clin Pharmacol 29:777, 1990.
18. Buckland-Wright J, Graham S, Chikanza I, Grahame R: Quantitative microfocal radiography detects changes in erosion area in patients with early rheumatoid arthritis treated with Myocrisine. J Rheumatol 20:243, 1993.
19. Pullar T, Hunter JA, Capell AJ: Sulphasalazine in rheumatoid arthritis: A double-blind comparison of sulphasalazine with placebo and sodium aurothiomalate. Br Med J 287:1102, 1982.
20. Suarez-Almazor ME, Fitzgerald A, Grace M, Russell AS: A randomized controlled trial of parenteral methotrexate compared with sodium aurothiomalate (Myochrysine) in the treatment of rheumatoid arthritis. J Rheumatol 15:753, 1988.
21. Clark P, Tugwell P, Bennett K, Bombardier C: Meta-analysis of injectable gold in rheumatoid arthritis. J Rheumatol 16:442, 1989.
22. Felson DT, Anderson JJ, Meenan RF: The comparative efficacy and toxicity of second-line drugs in rheumatoid arthritis. Arthritis Rheum 33:1449, 1990.
23. Situnayake RD, Grindulis KA, McConkey B: Long-term treatment of rheumatoid arthritis with sulphasalazine, gold, or penicillamine: A comparison using life-table methods. Ann Rheum Dis 46:177, 1987.
24. Ferraccioli G, Salafii F, Nervetti A, Cavalieri F: Slow-acting drugs—Outcome no different than 15 years ago (letter). J Rheumatol 17:1249, 1990.
25. Lehtinen K, Isomaki H: Intramuscular gold therapy prevents premature death in patients with rheumatoid arthritis. J Rheumatol 18:524, 1991.
26. Epstein WV, Henke CJ, Yelin EH, Katz PP: Effect of parenterally administered gold therapy on the course of adult rheumatoid arthritis. Ann Intern Med 114:437, 1991.
27. Wolfe F, Hawley DJ, Cathey MA: Measurement of gold treatment effect in clinical practice: Evidence for effectiveness of intramuscular gold therapy. J Rheumatol 20:797, 1993.
28. Wolfe F: The curious case of intramuscular gold (review). Rheum Dis Clin North Am 19:173, 1993.
29. Harth M: Gold in rheumatoid arthritis: Standard, substitute or sham? J Rheumatol 20:771, 1993.
30. Boers M, Ramsden M: Long-acting drug combinations in rheumatoid arthritis: A formal overview. J Rheumatol 18:316, 1991.
31. Scott DL, Dawes PT, Tunn E, Fowler PD, Shadforth MF, Fisher J, Clarke S, Collins M, Jones P, Popert AJ, et al: Combination therapy with gold and hydroxychloroquine in rheumatoid arthritis: A prospective, randomized, placebo-controlled study. Br J Rheumatol 28:128, 1989.
32. Fremont-Smith P, Fremont-Smith K: Association between gold-induced skin rash and remission in patients with rheumatoid arthritis (letter). Ann Rheum Dis 49:271, 1990.
33. Speerstra F, Van Riel PLCM, Reekers P, Van de Putte LBA, Vanderbrouke JR, Collaborating Clinics: The influence of HLA phenotypes on the response to parenteral gold in rheumatoid arthritis. Tissue Antigens 28:1, 1987.
34. Srinivasa NR, Miller BL, Paulus HE: Long-term chrysotherapy in rheumatoid arthritis. Arthritis Rheum 22:105, 1979.
35. Sagransky DM, Greenwald RA: Efficacy and toxicity of retreatment with gold salts: A retrospective view of 25 cases. J Rheumatol 7:474, 1980.
36. Heath MJ: Measurement of "free" gold in patients receiving disodium aurothiomalate and the association of high free to total gold levels with toxicity. Ann Rheum Dis 47:18, 1988.
37. Heytman M, Ahern MJ, Smith MD, Roberts-Thomson PJ: The long-term effect of pulsed corticosteroids on the efficacy and toxicity of chrysotherapy in rheumatoid arthritis. J Rheumatol 21:435, 1994.
38. Choy EH, Kingsley GH, Corkill MM, Panayi GS: Intramuscular methyl-prednisolone is superior to pulse oral methylprednisolone during the induction phase of chrysotherapy. Br J Rheumatol 32:734, 1993.
39. Wooley PH, Griffin J, Panayi GS, Batchelor JR, Welsh KI, Gibson TJ: HLA-DR antigens and toxic reaction to sodium thiomalate and D-penicillamine in patients with rheumatoid arthritis. N Engl J Med 303:300, 1980.
40. Healey LA, Backes MB: Nitritoid reactions and angiotensin-converting-enzyme inhibitor (letter). N Engl J Med 321:763, 1989.
41. Rodriguez-Perez M, Gonzalez-Dominguez J, Mataran L, Garcia-Perez S, Salvatierra D: Association of HLA-DR5 with mucocutaneous lesions in patients with rheumatoid arthritis receiving gold sodium thiomalate. J Rheumatol 21:41, 1994.
42. Wicks IP, Wong D, McCullagh RB, Fleming A: Contact allergy to gold after systemic administration of gold for rheumatoid arthritis. Ann Rheum Dis 47:421, 1988.
43. Dijnands MJ, Perret CM, van den Hoogen FH, van de Putte LB, van Riel PL: Chrysotherapy provoking exacerbation of contact hypersensitivity to nickel (letter). Lancet 335:867, 1990.
44. Leonard PA, Moatamed F, Ward JR, Piepkorn MW, Adams EJ, Knibbe WP: Chrysiasis: The role of sun exposure in dermal hyperpigmentation secondary to gold therapy. J Rheumatol 13:58, 1986.
45. Sakkas LI, Chikanza IC, Vaughan RW, Welsh KI, Panayi GS: Gold-induced nephropathy in rheumatoid arthritis and HLA class II genes. Ann Rheum Dis 52:300, 1993.
46. Davis P, Menard H, Thompson J, Harth M, Beaudet F: One-year comparative study of gold sodium thiomalate and auranofin in the treatment of rheumatoid arthritis. J Rheumatol 12:60, 1985.
47. Adachi JD, Bensen WG, Kassam Y, et al: Gold-induced thrombocytopenia: 12 cases and a review of the literature. Semin Arthritis Rheum 16:287, 1987.
48. Wijands MJ, Allebes WA, Boerbooms AM, van de Putte LB, van Riel PL: Thrombocytopenia due to aurothioglucose sulphasalazine and hydroxychloroquine. Ann Rheum Dis 49:798, 1990.
49. Yan A, Davis P: Gold-induced marrow suppression: A review of 10 cases. J Rheumatol 17:47, 1990.
50. Collins D, Tobias J, Hill R, Bourke B: Reversal of gold-induced neutropenia with granulocyte colony-stimulating factor (G-CSF). Br J Rheumatol 32:518, 1993.
51. Gordon DA, Hyland RH, Broder I: Rheumatoid arthritis. In Cannon GW, Zimmerman GA (eds): The Lung in Rheumatic Diseases. New York, Marcel Dekker, 1990, pp 229–259.
52. Fam AG, Paton TW, Shamess CJ, Lewis AJ: Fulminant colitis complicating gold therapy. J Rheumatol 7:479, 1986.
53. Dorta G, Schnegg G, Schmied P: Treatment of gold-induced enteritis with octreotide. Lancet 342:179, 1993.
54. Watkins PB, Schade R, Mills AS, Carithers RL Jr, Van Thiel D H: Fatal hepatic necrosis associated with parenteral gold therapy. Dig Dis Sci 33:1025, 1988.
55. Eisemann AD, Backer NJ, Miner PB Jr, Fleming J: Pancreatitis and gold treatment of rheumatoid arthritis (letter). Ann Intern Med 111:860, 1989.
56. Fam AG, Gordon DA, Sarkozi J, Blair GR, Cooper PW, Harth M, Lewis AJ: Neurologic complications associated with gold therapy for rheumatoid arthritis. J Rheumatol 11:700, 1984.
57. Jaffe IA: Penicillamine. In Kelley WN, Harris ED, Ruddy S, Sledge CB (eds): Textbook of Rheumatology, 4th ed. Philadelphia, WB Saunders, 1993, pp 760–766.
58. Steen V: D-Penicillamine treatment in systemic sclerosis (editorial). J Rheumatol 18:1435, 1991.
59. Jimenez SA, Sigal SH: A 15-year prospective study of treatment of rapidly progressive systemic sclerosis with D-penicillamine. J Rheumatol 18:1496, 1991.
60. Lock HE, Lock CJ, Mewa A, Kean WF: D-Pencillamine chemistry and clinical use in rheumatoid disease. Semin Arthritis Rheum 15:261, 1986.
61. Jaffe IA, Merryman P: The antiphyridoxine effect of penicillamine in man. J Clin Invest 43:1869, 1964.
62. Nimni ME, Bavetta LA: Collagen defect induced by penicillamine. Science 15:905, 1965.
63. Joyce DA: D-Penicillamine pharmacokinetics and pharmacodynamics in man. Pharmacol Ther 42:405, 1989.
64. Lipsky PE, Ziff M: Inhibition of human helper T cell function in vitro by D-penicillamine and $CuSO_4$. J Clin Invest 65:1069, 1980.
65. Walters MT, Smith JL, Moore K, Evans PR, Cawley MID: An investigation of the action of disease-modifying antirheumatic drugs on the rheumatoid synovial membrane: Reduction in T lymphocyte subpopulations and HLA-DP and DQ antigen expression after gold or penicillamine therapy. Ann Rheum Dis 46:7, 1987.
66. Steven MM, Morrison M, Sturrock RD: Penicillamine in ankylosing spondylitis. J Rheumatol 12:735, 1985.
67. Matsubara T, Hirohata K: Suppression of human fibroblast proliferation by D-penicillamine and copper sulfate in vitro. Arthritis Rheum 31:964, 1988.
68. Tsukasa M, Saura R, Hirohata K, Ziff M: Suppression of human fibroblast proliferation by D-penicillamine and copper sulfate in vitro. Arthritis Rheum 31:964, 1988.
69. Multi-Centre Trial Group: Controlled trials of D-pencillamine in severe rheumatoid arthritis. Lancet 1:275, 1973.
70. Jones JS: Rheumatoid lung cavitation and response to penicillamine. Thorax 42:988, 1987.
71. Thoen J, Helgetveit O, Forre YH, Kass E: Effects of piroxicam on T lymphocyte subpopulations, natural killer cells, and rheumatoid factor production in rheumatoid arthritis. Scand J Rheumatol 17:91, 1988.
72. Vardi P, Brik R, Barzilai D, Lorber M, Scharf Y: Frequent induction of

insulin autoantibodies by D-penicillamine in patients with rheumatoid arthritis. J Rheumatol 19:1527, 1992.
73. Proceedings of the VIIth French Conference of Rheumatology, Paris, 1985. Rev Rhum 53:1, 1986.
74. Multi-Centre Trial Group: A prospective five-year comparison of treatment that included penicillamine with that excluding penicillamine in early rheumatoid arthritis. Br J Rheumatol 25:184, 1986.
75. Seidman P, Lindstrom B: Pharmacokinetic interactions of penicillamine in rheumatoid arthritis. J Rheumatol 16:473, 1989.
76. Bell CL, Graziano FM: The safety of administration of penicillamine to penicillin-sensitive subjects. Arthritis Rheum 26:801, 1983.
77. Kean WF, Lock CJL, Howard-Lock HE, Buchanan WW: Prior gold therapy does not influence the adverse effects of penicillamine in rheumatoid arthritis. Arthritis Rheum 25:1975, 1982.
78. Hansen TM, Kryger P, Elling H, Haar D, Kreutzfeldt M, Ingeman-Nielsen MW, Olsson AT, Pedersen C, Rahbek A, Tvede N, et al: Double-blind placebo-controlled trial of pulse treatment with methylprednisolone combined with disease-modifying drugs in rheumatoid arthritis. Br Med J 301:268, 1990.
79. Cooperative Systematic Studies of Rheumatic Disease Group: Toxicity of low-dose D-penicillamine therapy in rheumatoid arthritis. J Rheumatol 16:67, 1987.
80. Panayi GS, Wooley P, Batchelor JR: Genetic basis of rheumatoid disease: HLA antigens, disease manifestations, and toxic reactions to drugs. Br Med J 2:1326, 1978.
81. Bernolet Moens HJ, Ament BJW, Feltkamp BW, van der Korst JK: Long-term follow-up of treatment with D-penicillamine for rheumatoid arthritis: Effectivity and toxicity in relation to HLA antigens. J Rheumatol 14:1115, 1987.
82. Clarkson RWE, Sanders PA, Grennan CM: Complement C4 null alleles as a marker of gold or D-penicillamine toxicity in the treatment of rheumatoid arthritis. Br J Rheumatol 31:53, 1992.
83. Bacon PA, Tribe CR, MacKenzie JC, Verrier Jones J, Cumming RH, Amer B: Penicillamine nephropathy in rheumatoid arthritis: A clinical, pathological, and immunological study. Q J Med 45:661, 1976.
84. Hall CL, Tighe R: The effect of continuing penicillamine and gold treatment on the course of penicillamine and gold nephropathy. Br J Rheumatol 28:53, 1989.
85. Leonard PA, Bienz SR, Clegg DO, Ward JR: Hematuria in patients receiving gold and D-penicillamine. J Rheumatol 14:55, 1987.
86. Langan MN, Thomas P: Penicillamine-induced liver disease. Am J Gastroenterol 82:1318, 1987.
87. Pegg SJ, Lang BA, Mikhail EL, Hughes DM: Fatal bronchiolitis obliterans in a patient with juvenile rheumatoid arthritis receiving chrysotherapy. J Rheumatol 21:549, 1994.
88. Garlepp MJ, Dawkins RL, Christiansen F: HLA antigens and acetylcholine receptor antibodies in penicillamine-induced myasthenia gravis. Br Med J 286:338, 1983.
89. Morel E, Feuillet-Fieux MN, Vernet-der Garabedian B, Raimond F, D'Angelejan J, Bataille R, Sany H, Bach JF: D-Pencillamine–induced myasthenia gravis: A comparison with idiopathic myasthenia and rheumatoid arthritis. Clin Immunol Immunopathol 58:318, 1991.
90. Enzenauer RJ, Sterling GW, Rubin RL: D-Penicllamine–induced lupus erythematosus. Arthritis Rheum 33:1582, 1990.
91. Chin GL, Kong NCT, Lee BC, Rose IM: Penicillamine-induced lupus syndrome in a patient with classical rheumatoid arthritis. J Rheumatol 18:947, 1991.
92. Hashimoto K, Lipsky P: Immunosuppression by the disease-modifying antirheumatic drug bucillamine: Inhibition of human T lymphocyte function by bucillamine and its metabolities. J Rheumatol 20:953, 1993.
93. Jaffe IA: Adverse effects profile of sulfhydryl compounds in man. Am J Med 80:471, 1986.
94. Ehrhart A, Chicault P, Fauquert P, LeGoff P: Effets secondaires dus au traitement par la tiopronin de 74 polyarthrities rhumatoides. Rev Rhum Mal Osteoartic 58:193, 1991.
95. Lindell A, Denneberg T, Enestrom S, Fich C, Skogh T: Membranous glomerulonephritis induced by 2-mercaptopropionyl glycine (2-MPG). Clin Nephrol 34:108, 1990.

CHAPTER 49

Michael E. Weinblatt

Methotrexate

The use of methotrexate (MTX) for the treatment of systemic rheumatic diseases has evolved since the mid-1950s. MTX was initially developed as an anticancer drug; now it is being used at lower doses in a variety of diseases including rheumatoid arthritis (RA).

Farber and coworkers in 1948 reported the successful use of aminopterin, the parent compound of MTX, in the treatment of childhood leukemia.[1] Based on the observation that aminopterin was also a potent inhibitor of connective tissue proliferation, Gubner and colleagues in 1951 reported the first open study of aminopterin in patients with psoriasis, RA, and psoriatic arthritis.[2] Refinement of the aminopterin compound led to the synthesis of MTX. Dermatologists extensively studied MTX in psoriasis, and there was a natural progression to psoriatic arthritis and RA. In 1972, Hoffmeister reported a beneficial response with low-dose weekly MTX in 29 patients with active RA.[3] Several open studies and randomized trials reported efficacy with MTX in RA. In 1988, the U.S. Food and Drug Administration approved low-dose weekly MTX as a therapy for RA.

CHEMICAL STRUCTURE

The structure of folic acid (pteroylglutamic acid) consists of three elements: a multiring pteridine group linked to a para-aminobenzoic acid that is connected to a terminal glutamic acid residue (Fig. 49–1). MTX is a structural analog of folic acid with substitutions occurring in the pteridine group and para-aminobenzoic acid structure (see Fig. 49–1).

BIOCHEMICAL PHARMACOLOGY

Dietary folic acid is reduced enzymatically by the enzyme dihydrofolate reductase (DHFR) to the metabolically active reduced folates dihydrofolate and tetrahydrofolate. These reduced folates are essential in the conversion of homocysteine to methionine, in the metabolism of histidine, and in the synthesis of purines and thymidylate. DHFR is the primary enzyme responsible for the reduction of folic acid to the metabolically active reduced folates. MTX, an antimetabolite, binds and inactivates DHFR. This inhibition of DHFR results in the cessation of the synthesis of thymidylate, inosinic acid, and other purine metabo-

lites. MTX also affects protein synthesis by preventing the conversion of glycine to serine and homocysteine to methionine. Inhibition of DHFR may not be essential for the efficacy of MTX in RA. Several investigators have suggested that inhibition of other folate-dependent enzymes is as important in the drug's actions in RA.[4, 5]

Folates in the blood have a single terminal glutamate (monoglutamate) structure. Intracellular folates are metabolized from a monoglutamate to a polyglutamated compound that has a longer cellular retention and is a more efficient cofactor than the monoglutamate compound. MTX also is metabolized from a monoglutamate to a polyglutamated derivative. MTX polyglutamates have stronger cellular retention, remain within the cell in the absence of extracellular drug, and are more potent than the monoglutamate structure.[6] The synthesis of the MTX polyglutamates increases with the duration of therapy. MTX polyglutamates inhibit other folate-dependent enzymes, including thymidylate synthetase and 5-aminoimidazole-4-carboxamide ribonucleotide (AICAR) transformylase. The polyglutamated MTX is a more potent inhibitor of these enzymes than MTX, the monoglutamated compound. Thymidylate synthetase and AICAR transformylase are required for de novo purine synthesis. Partial inhibition of these enzymes could lead to inhibition of thymidylate and purine biosynthesis. Inhibition of AICAR transformylase may be one of the primary mechanisms of action of MTX in RA (Fig. 49–2).

Folinic acid (leucovorin) (see Fig. 49–1), a fully reduced metabolically active folate coenzyme, functions without the need for reduction by DHFR. Folinic acid restores thymidylate, purine, and methionine biosynthesis even in the presence of MTX. Folinic acid is used to "rescue" normal cells from the toxicity induced by MTX and is used with high-dose MTX in cancer chemotherapy and as a treatment for acute MTX overdose and hematologic toxicity. It is also used to reduce the side effects of MTX in RA.

ACTIONS OF METHOTREXATE

The mechanism of action of low-dose MTX in RA is not known. Whether its therapeutic effect is due to antifolate activity by inhibition of DHFR, inhibition of other folate-dependent enzymes, other immunomodulating or immunosuppressive properties, or

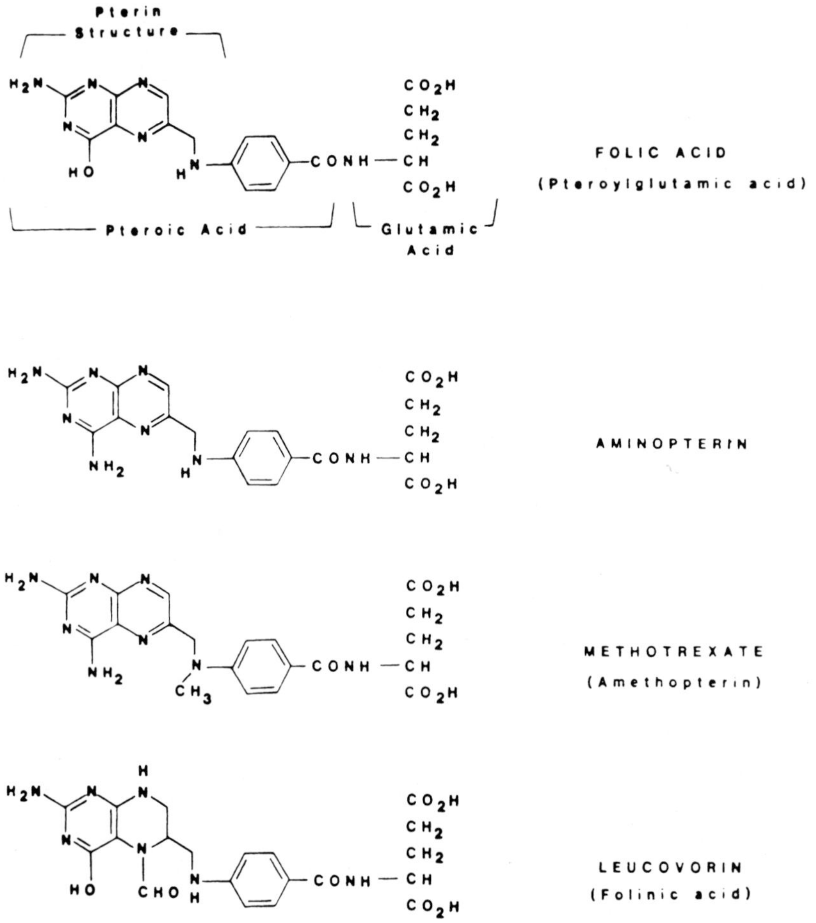

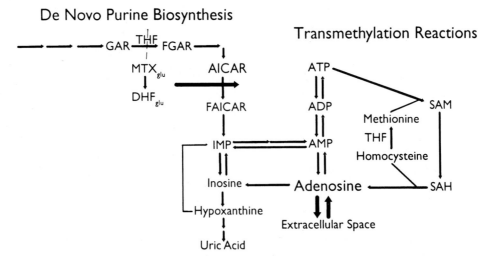

Figure 49–1. Structure of folic acid, aminopterin, methotrexate, and leucovorin.

Figure 49–2. Proposed mechanism of action of methotrexate. The major steps in purine synthesis and degradation are shown. GAR, β-glycinamide ribonucleotide; FGAR, α-*N*-formylglycinamide ribonucleotide; MTX$_{glu}$, methotrexate polyglutamate; DHF$_{glu}$, dihydrofolate polyglutamate; AICAR, 5-aminoimidazole-4-carboxamide ribonucleotide; FAICAR, formyl-AICAR; IMP, inosinic acid; THF, tetrahydrofolate (reduced); SAM, *S*-adenosylmethionine; SAH, *S*-adenosylhomocysteine. (From Cronstein BN, Naime D, Ostad E: The antiinflammatory mechanism of methotrexate. Increased adenosine release at inflamed sites diminishes leukocyte accumulation in an in vivo model of inflammation. J Clin Invest 92:2675, 1993.)

anti-inflammatory effects is under study. It is most likely that a combination of these factors accounts for its therapeutic profile in RA.

MTX inhibits DHFR and other folate-dependent enzymes. Inhibition of the enzyme AICAR transformylase by MTX also interferes with de novo purine biosynthesis.[7] Inhibition of AICAR transformylase increases the intracellular concentration of its substrate AICAR, which stimulates the release of adenosine (see Fig. 49–2). Adenosine is a potent inhibitor of stimulated neutrophil function and has potent anti-inflammatory properties. In the murine air sac model of inflammation, MTX increased intracellular accumulation of AICAR, increased adenosine concentrations in the exudates, and inhibited leukocyte accumulation, thus demonstrating anti-inflammatory effects.[4]

High-dose MTX at doses used for cancer therapy is immunosuppressive. In RA, however, a profound immunosuppressive effect has not been documented with low-dose MTX. Neither global suppression of T cell function nor phenotypes was reported in studies in RA.[8–10] Despite the lack of global immunosuppression, as measured in these studies, an immunosuppressive effect must occur owing to the reports of opportunistic infections in patients with RA receiving low-dose MTX.[11–14]

Other actions of MTX include in vitro suppression of immunoglobulin M (IgM) rheumatoid factor synthesis.[15] In clinical studies, the effect of MTX on IgM rheumatoid factor levels has been variable.[8, 9, 16] A suppression in immunoglobulin A (IgA) and IgM rheumatoid factor as measured by an enzyme-linked immunosorbent assay (ELISA) was, however, observed in one randomized trial of MTX.[17] A decrease in serum levels of immunoglobulin G (IgG), IgM, and IgA has also been noted.[9]

MTX inhibited neovascularization in a rabbit corneal model,[18] which suggested that MTX might have an antiangiogenic effect. MTX also inhibited the formation of S-adenosyl methionine, the methyl donor required for protein and lipid methylation.[19]

MTX has had multiple effects on cytokine levels, production, and activity. In vitro, an inhibitory effect of MTX on interleukin-1 (IL-1) activity but not IL-1 production or secretion was reported.[20] This inhibition of IL-1 activity was blocked by the addition of folinic acid but not folic acid.[21] No consistent effect on IL-1 levels or on stimulated IL-1 production from peripheral blood mononuclear cells was observed in one study of RA patients receiving MTX.[22] Serum[23] and synovial fluid[24] interleukin-1β (IL-1β) levels were suppressed in patients receiving MTX. A reduction in interleukin-6 (IL-6) and interleukin-8 (IL-8) levels,[25, 26] soluble tumor necrosis factor (TNF) receptor levels,[25] and soluble interleukin-2 (IL-2) receptor levels[25, 27] has been observed with MTX.

An anti-inflammatory effect with MTX has been suggested by its rapid onset of action and the flare after drug discontinuation. A decrease in C-reactive protein and erythrocyte sedimentation rate (ESR) has been noted several days after a single injection of MTX.[28] In vivo chemotaxis after stimulation with C5a or leukotriene B$_4$ (LTB$_4$) was blocked with MTX in psoriasis patients.[29, 30] Low-dose MTX decreased the generation of LTB$_4$ from stimulated neutrophils ex vivo from RA patients. This effect occurred after the initial dose of MTX[31, 32] and in patients receiving chronic MTX therapy.[33]

Lower levels of neutral metallocollagenolytic enzyme levels in synovial tissue from patients with RA treated with MTX compared with those treated with nonsteroidal anti-inflammatory drugs (NSAIDs) or corticosteroid therapy was reported.[34] After 3 months of MTX therapy, a significant decrease in collagenase gene expression but not stromelysin mRNA levels or tissue inhibitor of metalloproteinase-1 (TIMP-1) levels was also observed using in situ hybridization techniques.[35]

PHARMACOKINETICS

At low doses, MTX can be administered either orally or parenterally. The bioavailability of low-dose oral MTX is relatively high, but there is individual patient variability. In 41 RA patients who received 10 mg/m^2 of oral MTX, a mean bioavailability of 70 percent with a range of 40 to 100 percent was reported.[36] The mean absorption time was 1.2 hours, with a terminal half-life of 6 hours. Absorption is not reduced by concomitant food intake.[37] The pharmacokinetics of subcutaneous MTX is the same as intramuscular MTX[38] with the maximum serum concentration attained within 2 hours of injection. Patients not responding on oral MTX should be given a trial of parenteral MTX to ensure bioavailability. Four hours after MTX administration, synovial fluid concentrations equal serum levels.[36]

MTX distributes throughout the body, with higher concentrations found in intestinal epithelium and hepatic cells. MTX may undergo hepatic metabolism by the enzyme aldehyde oxidase to the 7-hydroxymethotrexate metabolite. Intracellular conversion of MTX from the monoglutamate to the polyglutamated derivative produces, as previously noted, potent inhibitors of DHFR, which are retained intracellularly in preference to the monoglutamated parent compound. MTX and its metabolites are excreted by the kidney by both glomerular filtration and proximal tubular secretion. Organic acids such as phenylbutazone, penicillin, sulfonamides, salicylates, and probenecid competitively inhibit tubular secretion, which may delay MTX clearance.

MTX is 50 to 60 percent bound to plasma proteins. An increase in free MTX owing to displacement from albumin by more highly protein-bound drugs such as aspirin, NSAIDs, and sulfonamides can occur. This is generally of limited clinical significance with low MTX doses, since the increase in free MTX may only be modest. A significant pharmacokinetic or clinical interaction has not been reported between low-dose MTX and a variety of NSAIDs including naproxen, sulindac, ibuprofen, and flurbiprofen.[39, 40] A decrease in MTX clearance was noted with aspirin.[41] A wide variation in the kinetics of MTX with NSAIDs has been reported in juvenile RA.[42] Administration of NSAIDs or aspirin with high MTX doses as used in cancer chemotherapy may be toxic and even fatal and must be avoided. Delayed clearance of MTX with chronic prednisolone (15 mg/day) was reported, but the clinical significance is uncertain.[43] Chloroquine decreases the concentration of MTX, and again, the clinical effect is unknown.[44]

Drugs that affect renal function should be used with great caution owing to an increased risk of toxicity. Probenecid should be avoided, since it inhibits tubular secretion of MTX. Trimethoprim/sulfamethoxazole should also be avoided owing to hematologic toxicity with MTX.[45] Possible mechanisms for this toxicity include an additive antifolate effect from trimethoprim, decreased MTX clearance owing to inhibition of tubular secretion by sulfamethoxazole and altered MTX plasma protein binding.

RHEUMATOID ARTHRITIS

Since aminopterin was a potent inhibitor of connective tissue proliferation, Gubner and colleagues,[2] in 1951, administered this drug to six patients with RA. A rapid improvement in the arthritis occurred in five of six patients, but exacerbations followed drug discontinuation. In 1972, Hoffmeister[3] reported the beneficial effect of low-dose intramuscular MTX in 29 patients. Hoffmeister expanded his series to include 78 patients, with a treatment follow-up as long as 15 years.[46] Forty-five patients (58%) had a "marked" improvement, including 28 patients who were judged to be in "complete remission." Seven patients discontinued therapy owing to adverse reactions, including elevation in liver blood tests, stomatitis, headaches, nausea, or increasing fatigue. Several other open studies noted similar improvement in arthritis activity with MTX.[47–49] In one study of 18 patients, sustained clinical response was noted after a mean of 42 months of treatment.[50] Three patients withdrew from this long-term study; 2 because of gastrointestinal toxicity and 1 owing to a planned pregnancy.

The positive results from these uncontrolled studies generated the interest in performing definitive placebo-controlled trials. Four placebo-controlled trials were performed in patients who had failed prior second-line therapies, including gold salts[8, 9, 16, 51] (Table 49–1).

Significant improvement in efficacy parameters was reported in a 35-patient, 24-week, double-blind crossover trial of low-dose (7.5 to 15 mg) weekly MTX versus placebo.[8] An improvement in clinical parameters began within 3 weeks after MTX initiation. MTX was superior to placebo in improving individual patient response (Fig. 49–3). During the crossover period, an increase in disease activity occurred within 3 weeks after MTX discontinuation. In an 18-week randomized multicenter study, 189 patients received either oral MTX (7.5 mg to 15.0 mg/week) or placebo.[16] There was a significant improvement in all clinical variables (Fig. 49–4) and in the ESR in the MTX group. Thirty patients on MTX withdrew owing to adverse reactions, including 18 because of elevated liver blood tests, 5 due to stomatitis, 3 for gastrointestinal toxicity, 2 for pancytopenia, and 2 for leukopenia. All the adverse reactions resolved with drug discontinuation.

A meta-analysis of the four randomized trials noted a significant improvement with MTX in all parameters except the 50-foot walk time.[52] Patients receiving MTX had a 46 percent greater reduction in the duration of morning stiffness, a 27 percent greater reduction in the number of painful joints, and a 26 percent greater reduction in the number of swollen joints than the patients in the placebo group. In these studies, clinical response usually developed within 4 weeks.

Two short-term crossover studies[8, 9] and two longer-term studies[53, 54] reported a flare of arthritis activity following MTX discontinuation. This flare occurred within 4 weeks of discontinuation of MTX.

Several studies have compared MTX with other second-line therapies. In patients with advanced disease who had received prior therapy with either gold salts or D-penicillamine, MTX was compared with azathioprine.[55–57] The largest trial was a 48-week randomized trial of 64 patients that compared MTX at a maximum dose of 15.0 mg/week to azathioprine at a maximum dose of 150 mg/day.[57] At week 24, significantly more improvement in the swollen joint count, pain score, disease activity score, and acute-phase reactants was noted in the MTX group than in the azathioprine group. The number of withdrawals due

Table 49–1. METHOTREXATE PLACEBO-CONTROLLED RANDOMIZED TRIALS

	Weinblatt et al[8]	Williams et al[16]	Thompson et al[51]	Anderson et al[9]
Number of patients	35	189	48	15
Design	Crossover	Parallel	Parallel	Crossover
Duration	24 weeks	18 weeks	6 weeks	26 weeks
MTX dose (mg/wk)	7.5–15.0	7.5–15.0	10.0–25.0	5.0–25.0
Administration	Oral	Oral	IM	IM
Clinical response	Improvement	Improvement	Improvement	Improvement
Withdrawal due to adverse events	1	30	2	1

Abbreviations: MTX, methotrexate; IM, intramuscular.

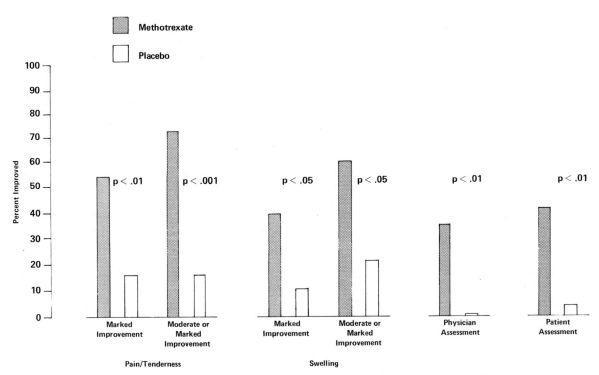

Figure 49–3. Individual patient response in a 35-patient, 24-week crossover trial. Marked improvement in the joint pain/tenderness and swelling index is defined as a decrease of 50 percent or more in their value; moderate improvement is defined as a decrease of 30 to 49 percent in these indices. Improvement in physician and patient assessments represented at least a 2-point change in a 5-point scale.

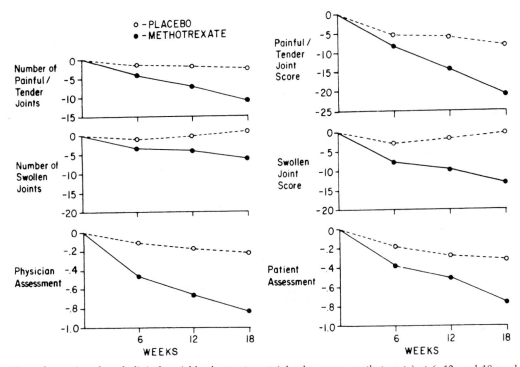

Figure 49–4. Mean change in selected clinical variables by treatment (placebo versus methotrexate) at 6, 12, and 18 weeks of therapy. (From Williams HJ, Willkens RF, Samuelson CO Jr, et al: Comparison of low dose oral pulse methotrexate and placebo in the treatment of rheumatoid arthritis: A controlled clinical trial. Arthritis Rheum 28:271, 1985. Reprinted with permission of the American College of Rheumatology.)

to side effects was also significantly higher in the azathioprine group. At week 48, only 36 percent of the patients remained in the azathioprine-treated group compared with 81 percent in the MTX-treated group.

Gold therapy, both parenteral and oral, has been compared with MTX. These studies enrolled patients with earlier and milder disease, in contrast to other studies of MTX. In small studies of 35 to 57 patients who had never received other second-line therapies, intramuscular gold therapy and MTX induced similar improvements in disease activity, but gold salts were more toxic.[58-60] A 9-month, 281-patient trial compared MTX with auranofin.[61] There was improvement in disease parameters with both drugs; however, MTX was superior to auranofin in improving disease activity parameters and individual patient response (Fig. 49-5). Auranofin was also more toxic than MTX in this study.

MTX (7.5 to 15 mg/week) was compared with cyclosporine (2.5 to 5.0 mg/day) in a 34-week, double-blind, placebo-controlled, randomized study of 264 patients who had failed at least one prior second-line therapy.[62] Both drugs were found to be statistically superior to placebo. MTX was superior to cyclosporine in improving clinical parameters, including the tender joint count, physician and patient global assessment, and functional status.

A meta-analysis of placebo-controlled and comparative clinical studies examined the relative efficacy and toxicity of standard second-line therapies.[63] MTX scored among the most efficacious of the drugs, with an extremely favorable toxicity profile.

There have been several long-term studies of MTX in RA.[64-68] Twenty-six patients completed a 24-week crossover trial[8] and enrolled in an open study of MTX.[10] In this study, the maximum dose of oral MTX was 15.0 mg/week. There was a significant improvement in disease activity, with the maximum beneficial effect being seen by month 6. After 84 months of therapy, 12 patients (46 percent) remained in the study.[64] A sustained improvement in all standard parameters was still noted. There was no difference in the degree of improvement achieved at month 12 compared with the improvement at month 84. Fifty percent of the patients were able to discontinue their prednisone therapy, and 33 percent of the patients were able to discontinue their NSAIDs. Two patients withdrew from the study owing to the development of pneumonitis.

Similar efficacy results were seen in another long-term prospective study. Twenty-nine patients enrolled in an long-term open study of MTX. Updates at 29,[69] 54,[70] and 90[65] months reported sustained clinical response with MTX. At month 90, 18 patients remained in the study.[65] A significant improvement was maintained in clinical parameters, with the maximum beneficial effect achieved by 6 months. Of the 14 patients on prednisone at baseline, 8 discontinued prednisone, with an overall reduction in the mean dose of prednisone for the entire group. Toxic reactions were as common at months 54 to 90 as during the first 53 months; however, no patient withdrew owing to toxicity between months 53 and 90.

Following completion of a 9-month randomized trial comparing MTX with auranofin,[61] 123 patients enrolled in a 5-year prospective study of MTX.[66] At year 5, 64 percent of the patients remained on drug treatment. A significant improvement in all clinical variables, ESR, and functional status was observed.

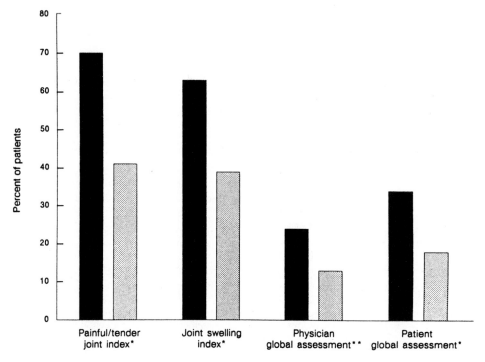

Figure 49–5. Individual patient response (methotrexate versus auranofin). Percentage of patients with marked improvement in four clinical measures of rheumatoid arthritis activity, by treatment group. Solid column = methotrexate group; shaded column = auranofin group. The significance of differences between groups was calculated by the Mantel-Haenszel chi-square test. *P = 0.01; **P = 0.03. (From Weinblatt, M, et al: Low-dose methotrexate compared with auranofin in adult rheumatoid arthritis: A 36-week, double-blind trial. Arthritis Rheum 33:330, 1990. Reprinted with permission of the American College of Rheumatology.)

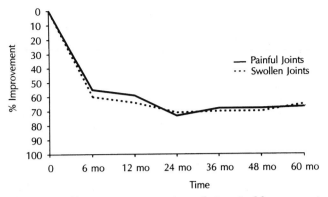

Figure 49–6. Long-term response to methotrexate. Mean percent change from baseline in the number of painful joints and the number of swollen joints in rheumatoid arthritis patients treated with methotrexate. The number of patients at each visit was as follows: 120 patients at 12 months, 109 patients at 24 months, 98 patients at 36 months, 88 patients at 48 months, and 70 patients at 60 months. (From Weinblatt ME, et al: Methotrexate in rheumatoid arthritis: A 5-year prospective multicenter study. Arthritis Rheum 37:1492, 1994. Reprinted with permission of the American College of Rheumatology.)

Sustained improvement in clinical variables including the painful and swollen joint counts was achieved during the trial (Fig. 49–6). A significant reduction in prednisone dose was achieved. Fifty-one percent of the patients with an elevated ESR at baseline normalized their ESR while on treatment. Of the 44 patients that withdrew from the study, only 8 did so owing to lack of drug efficacy. Adverse events occurred frequently and were generally mild, but 1 patient did develop cirrhosis while on therapy.

Several retrospective studies reported that a significant percentage of patients initiating MTX could be maintained on chronic therapy.[71, 72] In a study of 152 RA patients, the probability of continuing on MTX at year 1 was 71 percent, and at year 6, it was projected at 49 percent.[72] The major reason for withdrawal was drug toxicity. Studies from community-based rheumatologists reported similar high retention rates with MTX. Pincus and associates reported a study of 532 patients followed in 7 rheumatology practices.[73] The rate of MTX continuation was double that seen with other second-line therapies. In a study from a single practice of 671 patients observed over 14 years, the mean duration of MTX treatment was also approximately double that seen with other second-line therapies.[74]

The effects of MTX on radiographic activity are variable. A halting of radiographic progression has not yet been demonstrated. One study reported a healing of erosions within the first 29 months of MTX therapy[69]; however, after a mean of 54 months of therapy, new erosions were noted.[70] In another study, after a mean of 28 months of treatment, a worsening of the radiographs was noted in 6 of 14 patients.[10] An improvement in the number and size of the erosions was seen in 5 of the 14 patients, but a marked narrowing of the joint space was observed in these 5

patients. After 84 months of therapy, similar effects on the radiograph were noted.[64] In a study of 18 patients who had a significant improvement on MTX, radiographic progression continued despite 30 months of treatment.[75] In a study that compared MTX with azathioprine,[57] radiographic progression was less in the MTX group than in the azathioprine group.[76] In an MTX versus auranofin study,[61] a decrease in the rate of radiographic progression as defined by joint erosion and joint space narrowing was observed with the MTX group compared with the auranofin group.[77] In another trial comparing auranofin with MTX with the combination of MTX plus auranofin, a worsening in the joint score and joint narrowing score occurred in all treatment groups,[78] but the rate of progression was slower with MTX. A slowing in the rate of progression may occur with MTX, but cessation of radiographic progression has not yet been observed.

MTX has been used in combination with several second-line therapies. In an open study, MTX was compared with the combination of MTX plus intramuscular gold.[79] No difference was observed between groups in response or toxicity. In a 48-week prospective trial comparing MTX with auranofin with the combination of MTX and auranofin, 355 patients were studied.[80] There was no significant difference among the treatment groups with respect to response. Withdrawals owing to side effects were slightly more common in the combination therapy group. The low dose of MTX (7.5 mg/week) utilized in this study may have had an impact on the efficacy results.

In a 24-week prospective study comparing MTX with azathioprine with the combination of azathioprine plus MTX, 212 patients enrolled.[81] The maximum dose of MTX was 15.0 mg/week and the maximum dose of azathioprine was 150 mg/day. There was no difference in response between the combination of MTX plus azathioprine versus MTX, and both of these treatments were superior to azathioprine. More patients withdrew from the azathioprine group (38 percent) than from the combination group (26 percent) or the MTX group (7 percent). There was no significant advantage to the combination over MTX in this trial.

An open study suggested an advantage with the combination of MTX and sulfasalazine in patients who had an incomplete response on MTX.[82] No significant toxicities were associated with the combination. One concern with the combination of sulfasalazine and MTX would be folate deficiency. Careful monitoring of the mean corpuscular volume and red blood cell folate level and the supplemental use of folic acid or folinic acid should reduce this potential side effect.

There is also a preliminary and encouraging report on the combination of cyclosporine and MTX in patients who had an incomplete response on MTX.[83]

Several analogs of aminopterin have been developed in the attempt to develop drugs with similar efficacy but less toxicity than MTX. These analogs are potent antifolate compounds and include 10-deazaaminopterin (10-DAM) and 10-ethyl-10-deazaaminopterin (10-EDAAM). 10-DAM was compared with MTX in a 15-week, double-blind, controlled trial of 26 patients with RA.[84] Both drugs were effective with similar toxicities. Following completion of the 15-week trial, patients enrolled in a 1-year continuation study.[85] Both drugs again showed similar efficacy and tolerability.[85] Whether these analogs will be better than MTX is uncertain, but they warrant further study.

OTHER DISEASES

After the initial report[2] of the beneficial effects of aminopterin in psoriasis and psoriatic arthritis, extensive studies with MTX in psoriasis were performed. An important risk factor for toxicity was the frequency of MTX dosing. Weekly administration was less toxic than daily administration of the drug. An oral regimen based on skin kinetics was developed in which MTX was administered at 12-hour intervals for three doses once a week.[86] This regimen produced less toxicity than daily therapy and was as effective and no more toxic than weekly parenteral therapy.

In 1964, Black and coworkers reported the results of a 21-patient, randomized, placebo-controlled trial of parenteral MTX in psoriatic arthritis.[87] MTX was found to be superior to placebo in suppressing the skin manifestations and in improving joint tenderness and swelling. MTX was given as three parenteral injections at increasing doses of 1.0 to 3.0 mg/kg. Side effects were frequent with this dosing regimen and included gastrointestinal toxicity, stomatitis, and neutropenia. Willkens and colleagues performed a 12-week, double-blind, placebo-controlled trial of low-dose oral "pulse" MTX in 37 patients with psoriatic arthritis.[88] The maximum dose of MTX in this trial was 15.0 mg/week. MTX was found to be superior to placebo only in improving the physician assessment of arthritis activity and skin surface area with psoriasis. The lack of greater benefit might be attributed to the small sample size and the low dose of MTX used in the study. There is a clinical impression that higher doses of MTX are required to treat psoriatic arthritis than are needed to treat RA.

In a review of 21 patients with Reiter's syndrome, there was improvement in the mucocutaneous disease in 90 percent and an improvement in the arthritis in 75 percent of the patients.[89] Three patients discontinued therapy owing to toxicity that included stomatitis, anemia, and abnormal liver blood tests. Doses of 15 to 30 mg/week of MTX may be required for response in Reiter's syndrome.

There have been reports of the successful use of low-dose MTX in Felty's syndrome.[90, 91] Improvement in the neutrophil count generally occurred within 4 to 8 weeks of MTX initiation; however, a more delayed response has also been observed. Doses of MTX that ranged from 7.5 to 15.0 mg/week were required to improve the neutrophil count. MTX discontinuation was associated with a recurrence in the leukopenia.

Open studies in corticosteroid-resistant polymyalgia rheumatica and giant cell arteritis,[92] cutaneous vasculitis of RA,[93] adult-onset Still's disease,[94] multicentric reticulohistiocytosis,[95] scleroderma,[96] and systemic lupus erythematosus[97, 98] all report improvement with low-dose MTX. MTX (10.0 to 25.0 mg/week) has been used successfully in non–life-threatening Wegener's granulomatosus[99] and Takayasu's arteritis.[100]

Open studies reported the successful use of MTX in juvenile RA.[101, 102] A definitive randomized placebo-controlled trial was conducted by the Pediatric Rheumatology Collaborative Study Group in a multicenter trial performed in the United States and the (then) Soviet Union.[103] Enrolled in the study were 127 children. Forty-six children received MTX at a dose of 10.0 mg/m^2, 40 received a lower dose of MTX of 5.0 mg/m^2, and 41 were randomized to the placebo group. According to the composite index of several response variables, 63 percent of the children who received higher doses (10.0 mg/m^2) of MTX improved, as judged by a composite index, compared with 32 percent in the lower-dose group (5.0 mg/m^2), and 36 percent in the placebo group. The 10 mg/m^2 group had a significantly larger mean reduction in the disease parameters and ESR. Only 3 children discontinued MTX owing to mild to moderate side effects; none had severe toxicity. MTX given weekly at a dose of 10 mg/m^2 was superior to placebo. MTX is an effective treatment for children with resistant juvenile RA. MTX, as in the adult RA population, has become a widely accepted therapy for juvenile RA.

MTX has also been successfully used in polymyositis and dermatomyositis.[104] Doses between 25.0 mg and 50.0 mg/week administered parenterally may be required for clinical response.

There are also open studies on the successful use of low-dose MTX in sarcoidosis,[105] primary biliary cirrhosis,[106] and inflammatory bowel disease.[107] In sclerosing cholangitis, a small, double-blind, placebo-controlled study[108] was unable to confirm the efficacy that was originally noted in an open pilot study.[109] Open[110] and two short-term randomized studies[111, 112] reported efficacy with low-dose MTX in corticosteroid-dependent asthma. Other short-term, placebo-controlled trials reported no benefit with MTX compared with placebo in improving pulmonary function testing, corticosteroid reduction, or airway reactivity.[113, 114] The role of MTX in corticosteroid-dependent asthma remains to be defined.

DOSE AND DRUG ADMINISTRATION

MTX is given on only a *weekly basis*, since more frequent administration is associated with a greater incidence of acute and chronic toxicity. MTX is administered either orally or by parenteral injection. Oral MTX can be taken as one dose, or it can be cycled over a 24-hour period (pulse regimen). In psoriasis and psoriatic arthritis, the cycled oral "pulse" regimen is favored, whereas in RA many rheumatologists now prefer the one-dose, once-weekly regimen. The initial dose of MTX is generally 7.5 mg/week, but a lower dose may be used in patients for whom toxicity is a particular concern. If a positive response has not been noted within 4 to 8 weeks after MTX initiation and there has been no toxicity, the dose may be increased. Even though the optimum dose in RA is unknown, most studies used doses that ranged from 7.5 to 20.0 mg/week. In the randomized trial comparing auranofin to MTX, 43 percent of the MTX patients increased their MTX dose from 7.5 to 15.0 mg/week for greater efficacy.[61] A dose-response study suggested a linear dose response between placebo, 5 mg/ m^2 and 10 mg/m^2.[115] Once a satisfactory clinical response is achieved, the dose of MTX may be slowly reduced. Some patients over time may require higher doses to maintain a beneficial response. Doses above 20 mg/week should be administered parenterally owing to decreased oral bioavailability at these higher doses.

One study of 10 patients who had failed oral MTX reported efficacy and limited toxicity with intravenous MTX at an initial dose of 40 mg/m^2 and a final dose of 26 mg/m^2.[116] A pilot study of five patients with refractory disease reported efficacy and good tolerability with high-dose intravenous MTX (500 mg/m^2) and folinic acid (leucovorin) at a dose of 50 mg/m^2 administered biweekly for 8 weeks.[117] The clinical response lasted 6 to 14 weeks after completion of the infusions. In a second study, eight patients who had failed conventional MTX therapy (defined as 6 months of therapy with at least 15 mg/week of MTX) received 6 months of high-dose intravenous MTX 500 mg/mm^2 and folinic acid.[118] Five of the eight patients completed 6 months of therapy; three withdrew, one owing to lack of efficacy, one because of gastrointestinal intolerance, and one due to intercurrent medical illness. An improvement in arthritis activity was observed. A flare of arthritis occurred after completion of the 6 months of high-dose MTX and the trial was discontinued.

Despite an initial report of efficacy with intra-articular MTX,[119] subsequent trials have not demonstrated any difference between intra-articular MTX compared with saline or corticosteroid injections.[120, 121]

A depletion in the serum folate concentration and an alteration in a folate-dependent enzyme system (the C_1 index) develop with MTX therapy.[122] Supplemental folic acid at a dose of 1 mg/day did not reduce the efficacy of MTX in a 24-week, placebo-controlled trial.[123] Less toxicity was observed in the folic acid–treated group. In a second study, 5.0 mg/week of folic acid was compared with 27.5 mg/week of folic acid versus placebo in 79 patients initiating MTX therapy.[124] In this 1-year study, folic acid supplementation at either dose did not alter the efficacy of MTX. Those patients who received folic acid, however, experienced less toxicity than those who re-

ceived the placebo. There was no advantage of higher-dose versus lower-dose folic acid in reduction of side effects.

Several investigators studied the use of folinic acid (leucovorin) to reduce MTX's side effects. In one study, seven patients received folinic acid (15 mg) starting 4 to 6 hours after the MTX dose for 3 consecutive days.[125] Each patient received a total of 45 mg/week of folinic acid for 4 weeks. Nausea that was present before the study resolved on folinic acid therapy. However, a flare of arthritis occurred on folinic acid therapy and resolved with folinic acid discontinuation. Folinic acid at a dose that was equal to the MTX dose (5 to 15 mg) was administered 4 hours after the MTX in another 20-patient randomized trial.[126] There was no decrease in the efficacy of MTX; however, there was less stomatitis and nausea in the folinic acid–treated group. A randomized, placebo-controlled trial studied the effects of low-dose folinic acid (1 mg) versus placebo in patients receiving chronic MTX therapy.[127] Folinic acid was taken simultaneously with the MTX. In this 8-week study, 1 mg of folinic acid taken simultaneously with MTX did not block the efficacy of MTX. In another study, 27 patients with RA received a single oral dose of either folinic acid (15 mg) or placebo administered 2 hours after the MTX dose.[128] A flare in the arthritis occurred in all the patients treated with folinic acid, and 50 percent of the patients in the folinic acid group withdrew from the study. This study demonstrated that an exacerbation of RA is likely when higher-dose folinic acid is administered within the pharmacologic half-life of MTX. Shiroky and associates performed a 52-week, double-blind study of folinic acid (2.5 to 5.0 mg) versus placebo in patients initiating MTX.[129] Folinic acid was administered 24 hours after the dose of MTX. No difference in efficacy was noted between the two groups. There were 50 percent fewer reports of side effects and a lower withdrawal rate in the folinic acid group compared with the placebo group. It is not known whether there is any difference between folic acid and folinic acid (leucovorin) in reducing MTX toxicity. Until that study is performed, it is preferable to prescribe folic acid 1 mg/day because of its low cost as the initial therapy to offset potential side effects of MTX. In patients in whom folic acid is not adequate, a trial of folinic acid (initial dose 5 mg/week) administered 8 to 24 hours after the MTX dose is recommended. The major disadvantage of folinic acid is the cost.

TOXICITY

Adverse events occur throughout the course of MTX therapy but are most common within the first 6 months of treatment (Fig. 49–7). The most common adverse events with MTX are gastrointestinal toxicity including anorexia, nausea, vomiting, diarrhea, and weight loss.[130] In most patients, this toxicity is generally mild and usually occurs shortly after drug ad-

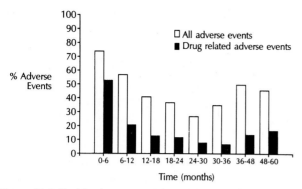

Figure 49-7. Toxicity frequency with methotrexate. (Weinblatt ME, et al: Methotrexate in rheumatoid arthritis: A 5-year prospective multicenter study. Arthritis Rheum 37:1492, 1994. Reprinted with permission of the American College of Rheumatology.)

ministration. This toxicity may improve with dose reduction, cycled oral or parenteral therapy, and folic or folinic acid therapy and may diminish with chronic exposure. In a review of 587 patients receiving therapy, gastrointestinal toxicity was noted in 10 percent; 2.5 percent of the patients had a moderate to severe reaction that led to drug withdrawal.[130] Stomatitis, consisting of erythema, painful ulcers, or erosions, may also occur, varies in severity, and may also improve with folic acid or folinic acid therapy.

Alopecia, reactivation of ultraviolet light–induced erythema, urticaria, and cutaneous vasculitis may occur with low doses of the drug. Despite an improvement in the articular disease, an increase in the number and the size of rheumatoid nodules has been observed.[10, 131] The onset of the nodules may be abrupt and tend to locate on the hands and feet, but more extensive distribution may occur. Whether MTX induces the formation of the nodules is unknown, but the nodules may reduce in size or disappear with MTX discontinuation. The nodules may return with reinstitution of MTX. The pathology is consistent with typical rheumatoid nodules.[131] Uncontrolled observations suggest that the addition of antimalarials, D-penicillamine, corticosteroids, sulfasalazine, or cyclosporine might be beneficial in reducing the nodules.

Hematologic toxicity including leukopenia, thrombocytopenia, megaloblastic anemia, and pancytopenia may occur. This toxicity was reported in less than 5 percent of patients with RA treated with MTX.[130] Risk factors for this toxicity include renal insufficiency, folic acid deficiency, dosing errors such as daily therapy, acute infections including viral illnesses, and the concomitant use of selected drugs including probenecid and trimethoprim/sulfamethoxazole.[132] An elevation in the mean corpuscular volume might be a predictor of impending hematologic toxicity.[133] Supplemental administration of folic acid is recommended to maintain adequate folate stores. Folinic acid (leucovorin) should be administered immediately for suspected MTX overdose or for hematologic toxicity. Folinic acid is generally most effective when administered within 24 to 48 hours of the dose of MTX. However, in the setting of renal insufficiency, folinic acid may still be effective even if administered after this time period. Folinic acid should be administered at a dose that is equal to the MTX dose every 4 to 6 hours until there is no longer a detectable serum level of MTX.

High-dose MTX as used in cancer chemotherapy may cause renal failure by precipitating in the renal tubules. A decline in glomerular filtration rate and renal tubular function has been reported with low-dose MTX treatment.[134] Renal insufficiency from any cause can lead to sustained and toxic levels of the drug. The drug should not be used in patients with renal failure or in patients requiring dialysis owing to poor clearance of the drug.

Transient but reversible oligospermia has been reported with high-dose MTX for cancer chemotherapy[135] and low-dose therapy in psoriasis.[136] Reversible impotence has been noted; the mechanism is unknown.[137]

Ovarian dysfunction has not been reported with the drug.[135] MTX is, however, a **definite teratogenic** agent. Aminopterin was used as a abortifacient, and its use has been associated with specific fetal abnormalities described as the "aminopterin syndrome."[138] These defects include multiple skeletal abnormalities, hydrocephalus, cleft palate, ear abnormalities,, and anacephaly. In an uncontrolled study, eight women became pregnant while receiving low-dose MTX for RA.[139] The mean duration of MTX therapy during gestation was 7.5 weeks (2 to 20 weeks). The pregnancy outcome was five full-term babies, three spontaneous abortions, and two elective abortions. Despite this report, the overwhelming evidence on the teratogenic potential of MTX supports the rigorous use of birth control in women of childbearing potential. Women should discontinue therapy at least one ovulatory cycle and males at least 90 days before attempting conception. Men and women previously treated with high-dose MTX as a therapy for childhood and adolescent malignancies have been reported to produce normal offspring.[140]

MTX has not yet been identified as a carcinogenic agent, despite concerns that relate to in vitro studies in which lymphocytes deprived of folic acid developed fragile sites. Patients receiving MTX for choriocarcinoma[141] or psoriasis[142] did not have an increased risk of malignancy. Non-Hodgkin's lymphoma has been reported in several patients receiving MTX for RA.[143, 144] Three patients with RA or dermatomyositis treated with MTX developed non-Hodgkin's lymphoma that resolved with MTX discontinuation.[14, 145] In two of these cases, an association of the lymphoma with Epstein-Barr virus was suggested, based on immunohistochemical and in situ hybridization studies.[145] The reversible nature of the lymphoma in these three cases is similar to the reversible lymphomas observed with immunosuppressive therapy in organ transplant.

Central nervous system toxicity may include headache, fatigue, mood alteration, dizziness, and depression.[146] Fever, fatigue, myalgias, and polyarthralgias have also been observed following MTX dosing.[147]

Opportunistic infections including *Nocardia, Pneumocystis carinii,* fungal infections including *Cryptococcus,* and localized and disseminated herpes zoster have been observed in RA patients receiving low-dose MTX.[11–13] Fulminant hepatitis occurring after discontinuation of MTX in a patient who was an asymptomatic carrier of hepatitis B has been reported.[148] Reactivation of quiescent infection and MTX withdrawal have been suggested as the cause.

Localized osteoporosis with severe bone pain and nontraumatic fractures has been seen in children receiving high-dose MTX treatment for acute leukemia.[149] This resolved with MTX discontinuation. High-dose MTX in animals has been associated with a reduction in trabecular bone volume and bone formation.[150] Suppression of osteoblast activity and stimulation of osteoblast recruitment have been observed in rats administered MTX at doses equivalent to those used in RA.[151]

Pulmonary toxicity, both acute and chronic, has been observed with MTX therapy. This toxicity has been reported in patients receiving MTX for malignancy, polymyositis, psoriasis, and RA.[152–154] Pulmonary reactions with MTX appear to be more common in RA patients than in those with other diseases.[154, 155] Risk factors are to date unknown, but underlying pulmonary disease, particularly interstitial fibrosis, has been suggested as a risk factor.[156, 157] Headaches and malaise are early symptoms, followed by a nonproductive cough, dyspnea, and fever. The clinical symptoms may precede the radiographic evidence of lung disease by several weeks. The chest radiograph may be initially normal, but bilateral interstitial infiltrates generally develop. Alveolar infiltrates, diffuse nodular infiltrates, hilar adenopathy, and pleural effusions have also been observed.[152] The lung pathology is indistinguishable from that of rheumatoid lung disease with inflammatory infiltrates consisting primarily of mononuclear cells, giant cells, granuloma formation, and varying degrees of bronchiolitis and fibrosis. Rarely, the fibrosis may progress, and extensive scarring of the lung with honeycomb changes may develop. Treatment includes MTX discontinuation, respiratory support, and corticosteroid administration. Infections including opportunistic organisms must be excluded. The outcome is variable but most patients have recovered; chronic dyspnea and mortality have been reported. In a patient with severely compromised lung function at baseline, other therapies for the arthritis might be considered.

Hepatic fibrosis and cirrhosis were reported shortly after the introduction of antifolate drugs for childhood leukemia and psoriasis. In 68 patients from Scandinavia who received MTX for 5 years with a mean cumulative dose of 3.9 g, fibrosis was seen in 24 percent and cirrhosis in 21 percent of the patients. Suggested risk factors for MTX-associated liver toxicity in psoriatic patients include prior arsenic therapy, insulin-dependent diabetes, renal insufficiency, mor-

bid obesity, alcohol consumption, daily or several MTX doses per week, and the cumulative dose of MTX.[158] Routine surveillance biopsies based on cumulative dose have been recommended for psoriasis patients receiving MTX. It has been reported in psoriasis that there is no correlation between liver blood test results and liver histology, but in many of the psoriasis studies, these tests were monitored only at the time of the biopsy.

The characteristic hepatic pathology associated with MTX is fibrosis or cirrhosis. A grading system developed by dermatologists to describe the histopathology is also used by rheumatologists (Table 49–2).[158] Therapy should be discontinued for marked fibrosis (IIIB) or cirrhosis (IV).

The development of serious liver disease in RA patients receiving MTX is to date uncommon. This is distinctly different than the reported experience in psoriasis. Of 295 RA patients who underwent a liver biopsy before MTX therapy, only 1 case of cirrhosis (0.3%) and 11 cases of mild fibrosis (4%) were noted.[159] Of 719 patients who underwent a liver biopsy after approximately 1.3 to 3.0 g of MTX therapy, mild fibrosis was noted in 14 percent of the patients.[159] Fibrosis was seen in many patients using only the more sensitive trichrome stain. Moderate fibrosis was noted in 6 (0.8 percent) of the patients, and 2 patients had cirrhosis. One of these patients in fact had cirrhosis on the pretreatment biopsy.

In a prospective liver biopsy study, after a mean of 52 months of therapy, mild fibrosis was noted in 52 percent of 27 patients.[160] Eighteen patients continued to undergo liver biopsies. After a mean of 81 months of therapy and a mean cumulative dose of 5.0 g, mild fibrosis was noted in 7 (38 percent) of the 18 patients.[161] In 23 RA patients who received MTX for over 10 years, there were no cases of cirrhosis.[162] There are, however, isolated reports of cirrhosis and acute decompensated liver disease with chronic active hepatitis in RA patients receiving MTX therapy.[163–165] In a case-control study that included a survey of members of the American College of Rheumatology, 24 cases of serious liver disease were identified.[166] Seri-

Table 49–2. CLASSIFICATION OF LIVER BIOPSY FINDINGS

Grade I	*Normal:* fatty infiltration; *mild:* nuclear variability—mild; portal inflammation—mild
Grade II	Fatty infiltration—moderate to severe; nuclear variability—moderate to severe; portal tract expansion, portal tract inflammation, and necrosis—moderate to severe
Grade III	*A:* Fibrosis, mild; portal fibrosis here denoted formation of fibrotic septa extending into the lobules; slight enlargement of portal tracts without disruption of limiting plates or septum formation does not put the biopsy in grade III; this distinction requires a connective tissue stain or reticular preparation *B:* Fibrosis—moderate to severe
Grade IV	Cirrhosis

ous liver disease was defined as histologic evidence of cirrhosis (7 patients) or clinical evidence of liver failure (17 patients). The estimated risk of serious liver disease at 5 years, based on these results, was projected at less than 1:1000. Independent risk factors for toxicity were age and duration of therapy. In the year prior to the development of serious liver disease, elevations in serum transaminases (aspartate aminotransferase [AST] and alanine aminotransferase [ALT]) and a decrease in serum albumin were noted more frequently in the patients who developed serious liver disease than in the control group.

Isolated elevations in serum transaminases occur frequently. These elevations are usually one to four times the normal range and generally resolve within 1 to 3 weeks after temporary drug discontinuation. The significance of an isolated enzyme elevation is uncertain. However, when monitoring is performed every 4 to 6 weeks, the number of elevations in serum AST correlated with a change in liver pathology grade.[160] A decreasing serum albumin in the setting of well-controlled arthritis may also be predictive of hepatic pathology. In an analysis of several prospective trials, it was noted that increases in serum transaminase (AST, ALT) levels occurred more frequently in the first 2 years of therapy and decreased thereafter. An abnormality of serum transaminase is defined as a level above the upper range of normal.

A committee organized by the American College of Rheumatology published guidelines for monitoring RA patients receiving MTX.[159] The commitee recommended baseline liver biopsies only in patients in whom there was a history of alcoholism or chronic hepatitis B or C infection or in those with unexplained sustained elevations in serum transaminases. Routine monitoring (every 4 to 8 weeks) of serum transaminases and albumin is recommended. Liver biopsies are recommended only in those patients in whom there are repetitive episodes of elevations in serum transaminases or the development of a low serum albumin (Table 49–3). The guidelines are of value only if routine monitoring is performed. These guidelines are distinctly different from the guidelines developed for psoriasis.[158]

PATIENT SELECTION AND MONITORING

Patients with active RA are potential candidates for MTX therapy. In patients with mild to moderate disease, we initially recommend hydroxychloroquine or sulfasalazine, owing to their safety profile. The decision about which second-line therapy to use in this type of patient is highly individualized. Considerations regarding lifestyle issues, including alcohol intake, conception timing in a young woman, timing of response and toxicity issues, must be considered. If the patient should fail these treatment options, we generally recommend MTX as the next therapy if there are no contraindications or lifestyle issues. In

Table 49–3. RECOMMENDATIONS FOR MONITORING FOR HEPATIC SAFETY IN RHEUMATOID ARTHRITIS PATIENTS RECEIVING METHOTREXATE

A. Baseline
  1. Tests for all pateints
    a. Liver blood tests (AST, alanine aminoALT, alkaline phosphatase, albumin, bilirubin), hepatitis B and C serologic studies
    b. Other standard tests, including complete blood cell count and serum creatinine
  2. Pretreatment liver biopsy (Menghini suction-type needle) only for patients with:
    a. Prior excessive alcohol consumption
    b. Persistently abnormal baseline AST values
    c. Chronic hepatitis B or C infection
B. Monitor AST, ALT, albumin at 4–8-week intervals
C. Perform liver biopsy if:
  1. Five of nine determinations of AST within a given 12-month interval (6 of 12 if tests are performed monthly) are abnormal (defined as an elevation above the upper limit of normal)
  2. There is a decrease in serum albumin below the normal range (in the setting of well-controlled rheumatoid arthritis)
D. If results of liver biopsy are:
  1. Roenigk grade I, II, or IIIA, resume MTX and monitor as in B, C1, and C2 above
  2. Roenigk grade IIIB or IV, discontinue MTX
E. Discontinue MTX in patient with persistent liver test abnormalities, as defined in C1 and C2 above, who refuses liver biopsy

From Kremer JM, Alarćon GS, Lightfoot, RW Jr, et al: Methotrexate for rheumatoid arthritis: Suggested guidelines for monitoring liver toxicity. Arthritis Rheum 37:316, 1994.
Abbreviations: AST, aspartate aminotransferase; ALT, alanine aminotransferase; MTX, methotrexate.

the patient with multiple active joints and evidence of functional impairment, we recommend MTX as the initial second-line therapy. Because of the rapid onset of action of MTX, it is the preferred drug in the patient with very active RA and functional impairment. This recommendation on the initial use of MTX is made irrespective of the duration of the disease. We also recommend folic acid, 1 mg/day, with the MTX to reduce possible adverse events. If side effects continue despite folic acid, we generally switch from folic acid to folinic acid, starting at a dose of 5 mg/week taken 8 to 12 hours after the MTX. We increase the dose of folinic acid if the 5-mg dose is not sufficient to reduce the adverse event, such as alopecia, stomatitis, headaches, fatigue, and gastrointestinal intolerance.

Patients with renal insufficiency, untreated folate deficiency, active liver disease, excessive alcohol consumption, serious concomitant medical illnesses, and noncompliance should be excluded from receiving therapy. Women of childbearing potential must use a form of birth control while receiving MTX.

Baseline laboratory parameters should include a complete blood count, platelet count, serum creatinine, and when indicated, a creatinine clearance, liver blood tests, and hepatitis B and C serologies. A chest radiograph may be recommended in a patient with suspected lung disease as a baseline prior to MTX institution. After initiation of therapy, a complete blood count is recommended monthly, and serum creatinine and liver blood tests (serum ALT, AST, and albumin) should be monitored every 4 to 8 weeks. A detailed discussion with the patient regarding the side effect profile and the rationale for monitoring including the potential need for liver biopsies is recommended. Supplemental administration of daily folic acid (1 mg) may reduce some of the adverse experiences associated with MTX, including gastrointestinal toxicity and stomatitis.

MTX should be temporarily discontinued during acute infections and for major surgical procedures. The risk of continuing MTX during the immediate postoperative period for total joint arthroplasty is unknown.[167–169] However, owing to subtle reductions in renal function in the immediate postoperative period, it is prudent to discontinue MTX for the immediate perioperative and postoperative periods.

MTX has become a major therapy in the treatment of RA. It is now regarded as one of the most significant advances since the mid-1980s in the treatment of this disease.[170]

References

1. Farber S, Diamond LK, Mercer RD, et al: Temporary remissions in acute leukemia in children produced by folic acid antagonist, 4-aminopteroyl-glutamic acid (aminopterin). N Engl J Med 238:787, 1948.
2. Gubner R, August S, Ginsberg V: Therapeutic suppression of tissue reactivity. II. Effect of aminopterin in rheumatoid arthritis and psoriasis. Am J Med Sci 22:176, 1951.
3. Hoffmeister RT: Methotrexate in rheumatoid arthritis (abstr). Arthritis Rheum 15:114, 1972.
4. Cronstein BN, Naime D, Ostad E: The antiinflammatory mechanism of methotrexate. Increased adenosine release at inflamed sites diminishes leukocyte accumulation in an in vivo model of inflammation. J Clin Invest 92:2675, 1993.
5. Baggott JE, Morgan SL, Alarcón GS, et al: Antifolates in rheumatoid arthritis: A hypothetical mechanism of action. Clin Exp Rheumatol 11(Suppl 8):S101, 1993.
6. Jolivet J, Cowan KH, Curt GA, et al: The pharmacology and clinical use of methotrexate. N Engl J Med 309:1094, 1983.
7. Cronstein BN, Eberle MA, Gruber HE, et al: Methotrexate inhibits neutrophil function by stimulating adenosine release from connective tissue cells. Proc Natl Acad Sci USA 88:2441, 1991.
8. Weinblatt ME, Coblyn JS, Fox DA, et al: Efficacy of low-dose methotrexate in rheumatoid arthritis. N Engl J Med 312:818, 1985.
9. Andersen PA, West SG, O'Dell JR, et al: Weekly pulse methotrexate in rheumatoid arthritis. Clinical and immunologic effects in a randomized, double-blind study. Ann Intern Med 103:489, 1985.
10. Weinblatt ME, Trentham DE, Fraser PA, et al: Long-term prospective trial of low-dose methotrexate in rheumatoid arthritis. Arthritis Rheum 31:167, 1988.
11. Altz-Smith M, Kendall LG Jr, Stamm AM: Cryptococcosis associated with low-dose methotrexate for arthritis. Am J Med 83:179, 1987.
12. Perruquet JL, Harrington TM, Davis DE: Pneumocystis carinii pneumonia following methotrexate therapy for rheumatoid arthritis [letter]. Arthritis Rheum 26:1291, 1983.
13. Flood DA, Chan CK, Pruzanski W: Pneumocystis carinii pneumonia associated with methotrexate therapy in rheumatoid arthritis. J Rheumatol.18:1254, 1991.
14. Shiroky JB, Frost A, Skelton JD, et al: Complications of immunosuppression associated with weekly low-dose methotrexate. J Rheumatol 18:1172, 1991.
15. Olsen NJ, Callahan LF, Pincus T: Immunologic studies of rheumatoid arthritis patients treated with methotrexate. Arthritis Rheum 30:481, 1987.
16. Williams HJ, Willkens RF, Samuelson CO Jr, et al: Comparison of low-dose oral pulse methotrexate and placebo in the treatment of rheumatoid arthritis. A controlled clinical trial. Arthritis Rheum 28:721, 1985.
17. Alarcón GS, Schrohenloher RE, Bartolucci AA, et al: Suppression of rheumatoid factor production by methotrexate in patients with rheumatoid arthritis: Evidence for differential influences of therapy and clinical status on IgM and IgA rheumatoid factor expression. Arthritis Rheum 33:1156, 1990.
18. Hirata S, Matsubara T, Saura R, et al: Inhibition of in vitro vascular endothelial cell proliferation and in vivo neovascularization by low-dose methotrexate. Arthritis Rheum 32:1065, 1989.
19. Nesher G, Moore TL: The in vitro effects of methotrexate on peripheral blood mononuclear cells: Modulation by methyl donors and spermidine. Arthritis Rheum 33:954, 1990.
20. Segal R, Mozes E, Yaron M, et al: The effects of methotrexate on the production and activity of interleukin-1. Arthritis Rheum 32:370, 1989.
21. Segal R, Yaron M, Tartakovsky B: Rescue of interleukin-1 activity by leucovorin following inhibition by methotrexate in a murine in vitro system. Arthritis Rheum 33:1745, 1990.
22. Chang D-M, Weinblatt ME, Schur PH: The effects of methotrexate on interleukin-1 in patients with rheumatoid arthritis. J Rheumatol 19:1678, 1992.
23. Kremer JM, Lawrence DA: Correlation of immune parameters with clinical and laboratory effects in prospective cohort of patients with rheumatoid arthritis receiving methotrexate (abstr). Arthritis Rheum 35:S144, 1992.
24. Thomas R, Carroll GJ: Reduction of leukocyte and interleukin-1β concentrations in the synovial fluid of rheumatoid arthritis patients treated with methotrexate. Arthritis Rheum 36:1244, 1993.
25. Barrera P, Boerbooms AMT, Janssen EM, et al: Circulating soluble tumor necrosis factor receptors, interleukin-2 receptors, tumor necrosis factor-α, and interleukin-6 levels in rheumatoid arthritis: Longitudinal evaluation during methotrexate and azathioprine therapy. Arthritis Rheum 36:1070, 1993.
26. Kremer JM, Petrillo GF, Lawrence DA: Methotrexate induces significant changes in IL-1, IL-2, IL-6 and IL-8 but not lymphocyte markers in patients with rheumatoid arthritis (abstr). Arthritis Rheum 36:S77, 1993.
27. Polisson RP, Dooley MA, Dawson DV, et al: Interleukin-2 receptor levels in the sera of rheumatoid arthritis patients treated with methotrexate. Arthritis Rheum 37:50, 1994.
28. Segal R, Caspi D, Tishler M, et al: Short-term effects of low-dose methotrexate on the acute phase reaction in patients with rheumatoid arthritis. J Rheumatol 16:914, 1989.
29. van de Kerkhof PC, Bauer FW, Maassen-de Grood RM: Methotrexate inhibits the leukotriene-B4–induced intraepidermal accumulation of polymorphonuclear leukocytes. Br J Dermatol 113:251a, 1985.
30. Ternowitz T, Bjerring P, Andersen PH, et al: Methotrexate inhibits the human C5a-induced skin response in patients with psoriasis. J Invest Dermatol 89:192, 1987.
31. Sperling RI, Benincaso AI, Anderson RJ, et al: Acute and chronic suppression of leukotriene B4 synthesis ex vivo in neutrophils from patients with rheumatoid arthritis beginning treatment with methotrexate. Arthritis Rheum 35:376, 1992.
32. Leroux JL, Damon M, Chavis C, et al: Effects of a single dose of methotrexate on 5- and 12-lipoxygenase products in patients with rheumatoid arthritis. J Rheumatol 19:863, 1992.
33. Sperling RI, Coblyn JS, Larkin JK, et al: Inhibition of leukotriene B4 synthesis in neutrophils from patients with rheumatoid arthritis by a single oral dose of methotrexate. Arthritis Rheum 33:1149, 1990.
34. Martel-Pelletier J, Cloutier J-M, Pelletier J-P: In vivo effects of antirheumatic drugs on neutral collagenolytic proteases in human rheumatoid arthritis cartilage and synovium. J Rheumatol 15:1198, 1988.
35. Firestein GS, Paine MM, Boyle DL: Mechanisms of methotrexate action in rheumatoid arthritis: Selective decrease in synovial collagenase gene expression. Arthritis Rheum 37:193, 1994.
36. Herman RA, Veng-Pedersen P, Hoffman J, et al: Pharmacokinetics of low-dose methotrexate in rheumatoid arthritis patients. J Pharm Sci 78:165, 1989.
37. Kozloski GD, De Vito JM, Kisicki JC, et al: The effect of food on the absorption of methotrexate sodium tablets in healthy volunteers. Arthritis Rheum 35:761, 1992.
38. Jundt JW, Browne BA, Fiocco GP, et al: A comparison of low-dose methotrexate bioavailability: Oral solution, oral tablet, subcutaneous and intramuscular dosing. J Rheumatol 20:1845, 1993.
39. Ahern M, Booth J, Loxton A, et al: Methotrexate kinetics in rheumatoid arthritis: Is there an interaction with nonsteroidal antiinflammatory drugs? J Rheumatol 15:1356, 1988.
40. Skeith KJ, Russell AS, Jamali F, et al: Lack of significant interaction between low-dose methotrexate and ibuprofen or flurbiprofen in patients with arthritis. J Rheumatol 17:1008, 1990.
41. Stewart CF, Fleming RA, Germain BF, et al: Aspirin alters methotrexate disposition in rheumatoid arthritis patients. Arthritis Rheum 34:1514, 1991.
42. Dupuis LL, Koren G, Shore A, et al: Methotrexate–nonsteroidal antiinflammatory drug interaction in children with arthritis. J Rheumatol 17:1469, 1990.
43. Lafforgue P, Monjanel-Mouterde S, Durand A, et al: Is there an interaction between low doses of corticosteroids and methotrexate in patients with rheumatoid arthritis? A pharmacokinetic study in 33 patients. J Rheumatol 20:263, 1993.

44. Seideman P, Albertioni F, Beck O, et al: Chloroquine reduces the bio-availability of methotrexate in patients with rheumatoid arthritis: A possible mechanism of reduced hepatotoxicity. Arthritis Rheum 37:830, 1994.
45. Thomas MH, Gutterman LA: Methotrexate toxicity in a patient receiving trimethoprim-sulfamethoxazole. J Rheumatol 13:440, 1986.
46. Hoffmeister RT: Methotrexate therapy in rheumatoid arthritis: 15 years' experience. Am J Med 75:69, 1983.
47. Willkens RF, Watson MA: Methotrexate: A perspective of its use in the treatment of rheumatic diseases. J Lab Clin Med 100:314, 1982.
48. Steinsson K, Weinstein A, Korn J, et al: Low-dose methotrexate in rheumatoid arthritis. J Rheumatol 9:860, 1982.
49. Michaels RM, Nashel DJ, Leonard A, et al: Weekly intravenous methotrexate in the treatment of rheumatoid arthritis. Arthritis Rheum 25:339, 1982.
50. Weinstein A, Marlowe S, Korn J, et al: Low-dose methotrexate treatment of rheumatoid arthritis. Long-term observations. Am J Med 79:331, 1985.
51. Thompson RN, Watts C, Edelman J, et al: A controlled two-centre trial of parenteral methotrexate therapy for refractory rheumatoid arthritis. J Rheumatol 11:760, 1984.
52. Tugwell P, Bennett K, Gent M: Methotrexate in rheumatoid arthritis. Indications, contraindications, efficacy, and safety. Ann Intern Med 107:358, 1987.
53. Kremer JM, Rynes RI, Bartholomew LE: Severe flare of rheumatoid arthritis after discontinuation of long-term methotrexate therapy. Double-blind study. Am J Med 82:781, 1987.
54. Szanto E: Low-dose methotrexate in rheumatoid arthritis: Effect and tolerance. An open trial and a double-blind randomized study. Scand J Rheumatol 15:97, 1986.
55. Hamdy H, McKendry RJ, Mierins E, et al: Low-dose methotrexate compared with azathioprine in the treatment of rheumatoid arthritis. A twenty-four-week controlled clinical trial. Arthritis Rheum 30:361, 1987.
56. Arnold MH, O'Callaghan J, McCredie M, et al: Comparative controlled trial of low-dose weekly methotrexate versus azathioprine in rheumatoid arthritis: 3-year prospective study. Br J Rheumatol 29:120, 1990.
57. Jeurissen MEC, Boerbooms AMT, van de Putte LBA, et al: Methotrexate versus azathioprine in the treatment of rheumatoid arthritis: A forty-eight-week randomized, double-blind trial. Arthritis Rheum 34:961, 1991.
58. Morassut P, Goldstein R, Cyr M, et al: Gold sodium thiomalate compared to low-dose methotrexate in the treatment of rheumatoid arthritis—a randomized, double-blind 26-week trial. J Rheumatol 16:302, 1989.
59. Suarez-Almazor ME, Fitzgerald A, Grace M, et al: A randomized controlled trial of parenteral methotrexate compared with sodium aurothiomalate (Myochrysine) in the treatment of rheumatoid arthritis. J Rheumatol 15:753, 1988.
60. Rau R, Herborn G, Karger T, et al: A double-blind randomized parallel trial of intramuscular methotrexate and gold sodium thiomalate in early erosive rheumatoid arthritis. J Rheumatol 18:328, 1991.
61. Weinblatt ME, Kaplan H, Germain BF, et al: Low-dose methotrexate compared with auranofin in adult rheumatoid arthritis. A thirty-six-week, double-blind trial. Arthritis Rheum 33:330,1990.
62. Cohen S, Rutstein J, Luggen M, et al: Comparison of the safety and efficacy of cyclosporin A and methotrexate in refractory rheumatoid arthritis: A randomized, multicentered placebo-controlled trial (abstr). Arthritis Rheum 36:S56, 1993.
63. Felson DT, Anderson JJ, Meenan RF: Use of short-term efficacy/toxicity tradeoffs to select second-line drugs in rheumatoid arthritis: A meta-analysis of published clinical trials. Arthritis Rheum 35:1117, 1992.
64. Weinblatt ME, Weissman BN, Holdsworth DE, et al: Long-term prospective study of methotrexate in the treatment of rheumatoid arthritis: Eighty-four-month update. Arthritis Rheum 35:129, 1992.
65. Kremer JM, Phelps CT: Long-term prospective study of the use of methotrexate in rheumatoid arthritis: Update after a mean of 90 months. Arthritis Rheum 35:138, 1992.
66. Weinblatt ME, Kaplan H, Germain BF, et al: Methotrexate in rheumatoid arthritis: A five-year prospective multicenter trial. Arthritis Rheum 37:1492, 1994.
67. Hanrahan PS, Scrivens GA, Russell AS: Prospective long-term follow-up of methotrexate therapy in rheumatoid arthritis: Toxicity, efficacy and radiological progression. Br J Rheumatol 28:147, 1989.
68. Sany J, Anaya JM, Lussiez V, et al: Treatment of rheumatoid arthritis with methotrexate: A prospective open long-term study of 191 cases. J Rheumatol 18:1323, 1991.
69. Kremer JM, Lee JK: The safety and efficacy of the use of methotrexate in long-term therapy for rheumatoid arthritis. Arthritis Rheum 29:822, 1986.
70. Kremer JM, Lee JK: A long-term prospective study of the use of methotrexate in rheumatoid arthritis. Update after a mean of fifty-three months. Arthritis Rheum 31:577, 1988.
71. Fehlauer CS, Carson CW, Cannon GW, et al: Methotrexate therapy in rheumatoid arthritis: 2-year retrospective follow-up study. J Rheumatol 16:307, 1989.
72. Alarcón GS, Tracy IC, Blackburn WD Jr:Methotrexate in rheumatoid arthritis. Toxic effects as the major factor in limiting long-term treatment. Arthritis Rheum 32:671, 1989.
73. Pincus T, Marcum SB, Callahan LF:Long-term drug therapy for rheumatoid arthritis in seven rheumatology private practices: II. Second-line drugs and prednisone. J Rheumatol 19:1885, 1992.
74. Wolfe F, Hawley DJ, Cathey MA: Termination of slow-acting antirheumatic therapy in rheumatoid arthritis: A 14-year prospective evaluation of 1017 consecutive starts. J Rheumatol 17:994, 1990.
75. Nordstrom DM, West SG, Andersen PA, et al: Pulse methotrexate therapy in rheumatoid arthritis. A controlled prospective roentgenographic study. Ann Intern Med 107:797, 1987.
76. Jeurissen MEC, Boerbooms AMT, van de Putte LBA, et al: Influence of methotrexate and azathioprine on radiologic progression in rheumatoid arthritis. A randomized, double-blind study. Ann Intern Med 114:999, 1991.
77. Weinblatt ME, Polisson R, Blotner SD, et al: The effects of drug therapy on radiographic progression of rheumatoid arthritis: Results of a 36-week randomized trial comparing methotrexate and auranofin. Arthritis Rheum 36:613, 1993.
78. López-Méndez A, Daniel WW, Reading JC, et al: Radiographic assessment of disease progression in rheumatoid arthritis patients enrolled in the Cooperative Systematic Studies of the Rheumatic Diseases Program randomized clinical trial of methotrexate, auranofin, or a combination of the two. Arthritis Rheum 36:1364, 1993.
79. Rau R, Herborn G, Schleusser, B, et al: Prospective open long-term observation of RA patients treated with methotrexate or MTX + gold (abstr). Arthritis Rheum 34:S92, 1991.
80. Williams HJ, Ward JR, Reading JC, et al: Comparison of auranofin, methotrexate, and the combination of both in the treatment of rheumatoid arthritis: A controlled clinical trial. Arthritis Rheum 35:259, 1992.
81. Willkens RF, Urowitz MB, Stablein DM, et al: Comparison of azathioprine, methotrexate, and the combination of both in the treatment of rheumatoid arthritis: A controlled clinical trial. Arthritis Rheum 35:849, 1992.
82. Shiroky JB, Watts CS, Neville C: Combination methotrexate and sulfasalazine in the management of rheumatoid arthritis: Case observations. Arthritis Rheum 32:1160, 1989.
83. Tugwell P, Pincus T, Yocum D, et al: A multicentre, double-blind randomized trial of low-dose cyclosporin and placebo therapy in combination with methotrexate in patients with severe rheumatoid arthritis (abstr). Arthritis Rheum 37:S361, 1994.
84. Alarcón GS, Castañeda O, Nair MG, et al: Controlled trial of methotrexate versus 10-deazaaminopterin in the treatment of rheumatoid arthritis. Ann Rheum Dis 51:600, 1992.
85. Alarcón GS, Castañeda O, Ferrándiz M, et al: Efficacy and safety of 10-deazaaminopterin in the treatment of rheumatoid arthritis: A one-year continuation, double-blind study. Arthritis Rheum 35:1318, 1992.
86. Weinstein GD, Frost P: Methotrexate for psoriasis. A new therapeutic schedule. Arch Dermatol 103:33, 1971.
87. Black RL, O'Brien WM, Van Scott EJ, et al: Methotrexate therapy in psoriatic arthritis. Double-blind study on 21 patients. JAMA 189:743, 1964.
88. Willkens RF, Williams HJ, Ward JR, et al: Randomized, double-blind, placebo-controlled trial of low-dose pulse methotrexate in psoriatic arthritis. Arthritis Rheum 27:376, 1984.
89. Lally EV, Ho G Jr: A review of methotrexate therapy in Reiter syndrome. Semin Arthritis Rheum 15:139, 1985.
90. Isasi C, Lopez-Martin JA, Angeles Trujillo M, et al: Felty's syndrome: Response to low-dose oral methotrexate. J Rheumatol 16:983, 1989.
91. Fiechtner JJ, Miller DR, Starkebaum G: Reversal of neutropenia with methotrexate treatment in patients with Felty's syndrome. Correlation of response with neutrophil-reactive IgG. Arthritis Rheum 32:194, 1989.
92. Krall PL, Mazanec DJ, Wilke WS: Methotrexate for corticosteroid-resistant polymyalgia rheumatica and giant cell arteritis. Cleve Clin J Med 56:253, 1989.
93. Espinoza LR, Espinoza CG, Vasey FB, et al: Oral methotrexate therapy for chronic rheumatoid arthritis ulcerations. J Am Acad Dermatol 15:508, 1986.
94. Aydintug AO, D'Cruz D, Cervera R, et al: Low-dose methotrexate treatment in adult Still's disease. J Rheumatol 19:431, 1992.
95. Gourmelen O, Le Loët X, Fortier-Beaulieu M, et al: Methotrexate treatment of multicentric reticulohistiocytosis. J Rheumatol 18:627, 1991.
96. van den Hoogen F, Boerbooms A, Rasker J, et al: Treatment of systemic sclerosis with methotrexate: Results of a one-year open study (abstr). Arthritis Rheum 33:S66, 1990.
97. Rothenberg RJ, Graziano FM, Grandone JT, et al: The use of methotrexate in steroid-resistant systemic lupus erythematosus. Arthritis Rheum 31:612, 1988.
98. LeBlanc BAE, Dagenais P, Urowitz MB, et al: Methotrexate in systemic lupus erythematosus. J Rheumatol 21:836, 1994.

99. Hoffman GS, Leavitt RY, Kerr GS, et al: The treatment of Wegener's granulomatosis with glucocorticoids and methotrexate. Arthritis Rheum 35:1322, 1992.

100. Hoffman GS, Leavitt RY, Kerr GS, et al: Treatment of glucocorticoid-resistant or relapsing Takayasu arteritis with methotrexate. Arthritis Rheum 37:578, 1994.

101. Truckenbrodt H, Hafner R: Methotrexate therapy in juvenile rheumatoid arthritis: A retrospective study. Arthritis Rheum 29:801, 1986.

102. Wallace CA, Bleyer WA, Sherry DD, et al: Toxicity and serum levels of methotrexate in children with juvenile rheumatoid arthritis. Arthritis Rheum 32:677, 1989.

103. Giannini EH, Brewer EJ, Kuzmina N, et al: Methotrexate in resistant juvenile rheumatoid arthritis—results of the U.S.A.–U.S.S.R. double-blind, placebo-controlled trial. N Engl J Med 326:1043, 1992.

104. Arnett FC, Whelton JC, Zizic TM, et al: Methotrexate therapy in polymyositis. Ann Rheum Dis 32:536, 1973.

105. Lower EE, Baughman RP: The use of low-dose methotrexate in refractory sarcoidosis. Am J Med Sci 299:153, 1990.

106. Kaplan, MM, Knox TA: Treatment of primary biliary cirrhosis with low-dose weekly methotrexate. Gastroenterology 101:1332, 1991.

107. Kozarek RA, Patterson DJ, Gelfand MD, et al: Methotrexate induces clinical and histologic remission in patients with refractory inflammatory bowel disease. Ann Intern Med 110:353, 1989.

108. Knox TA, Kaplan MM: A double-blind controlled trial of oral-pulse methotrexate therapy in the treatment of primary sclerosing cholangitis. Gastroenterology 106:494, 1994.

109. Kaplan MM, Arora S, Pincus SH: Primary sclerosing cholangitis and low-dose oral pulse methotrexate therapy. Clinical and histologic response. Ann Intern Med 106:231, 1987.

110. Mullarkey MF, Webb DR, Pardee NE: Methotrexate in the treatment of steroid-dependent asthma. Ann Allergy 56:347, 1986.

111. Mullarkey MF, Blumenstein BA, Andrade WP, et al: Methotrexate in the treatment of corticosteroid-dependent asthma. A double-blind crossover study. N Engl J Med 318:603, 1988.

112. Shiner RJ, Nunn AJ, Chung KF, et al: Randomised, double-blind, placebo-controlled trial of methotrexate in steroid-dependent asthma. Lancet 336:137, 1990.

113. Erzurum SC, Leff JA, Cochran JE, et al: Lack of benefit of methotrexate in severe, steroid-dependent asthma. A double-blind, placebo-controlled study. Ann Intern Med 114:353, 1991.

114. Coffey MJ, Sanders G, Eschenbacher WL, et al: The role of methotrexate in the management of steroid-dependent asthma. Chest 105:117, 1994.

115. Furst DE, Koehnke R, Burmeister LF, et al: Increasing methotrexate effect with increasing dose in the treatment of resistant rheumatoid arthritis. J Rheumatol 16:313, 1989.

116. Gabriel S, Creagan E, O'Fallon WM, et al: Treatment of rheumatoid arthritis with higher-dose intravenous methotrexate. J Rheumatol 17:460, 1990.

117. Shiroky J, Allegra C, Inghirami G, et al: High-dose intravenous methotrexate with leucovorin rescue in rheumatoid arthritis. J Rheumatol 15:251, 1988.

118. Shiroky JB, Neville C, Skelton JD: High-dose intravenous methotrexate for refractory rheumatoid arthritis. J Rheumatol 19:247, 1992.

119. Hall GH, Jones BJ, Head AC, et al: Intra-articular methotrexate. Clinical and laboratory study in rheumatoid and psoriatic arthritis. Ann Rheum Dis 37:351, 1978.

120. Marks JS, Stewart IM, Hunter JA: Intra-articular methotrexate in rheumatoid arthritis (letter). Lancet 2:857, 1976.

121. Bird HA, Ring EF, Daniel R, et al: Comparison of intra-articular methotrexate with intra-articular triamcinolone hexacetonide by thermography. Curr Med Res Opin 5:141, 1977.

122. Morgan SL, Baggott JE, Altz-Smith M: Folate status of rheumatoid arthritis patients receiving long-term, low-dose methotrexate therapy. Arthritis Rheum 30:1348, 1987.

123. Morgan SL, Baggott JE, Vaughn WH, et al: The effect of folic acid supplementation on the toxicity of low-dose methotrexate in patients with rheumatoid arthritis. Arthritis Rheum 33:9, 1990.

124. Morgan SL, Baggott JE, Vaughn WH, et al: Supplementation with folic acid during methotrexate therapy for rheumatoid arthritis. A double-blind, placebo-controlled trial. Ann Intern Med 121:833, 1994.

125. Tishler M, Caspi D, Fishel B, et al: The effects of leucovorin (folinic acid) on methotrexate therapy in rheumatoid arthritis patients. Arthritis Rheum 31:906, 1988.

126. Buckley LM, Vacek PM, Cooper SM: Administration of folinic acid after low-dose methotrexate in patients with rheumatoid arthritis. J Rheumatol 17:1158, 1990.

127. Weinblatt ME, Maier AL, Coblyn JS: Low-dose leucovorin does not interfere with the efficacy of methotrexate in rheumatoid arthritis: An 8-week randomized placebo-controlled trial. J Rheumatol 20:950, 1993.

128. Joyce DA, Will RK, Hoffman DM, et al: Exacerbation of rheumatoid arthritis in patients treated with methotrexate after administration of folinic acid. Ann Rheum Dis 50:913, 1991.

129. Shiroky JB, Neville C, Esdaile JM, et al: Low-dose methotrexate with leucovorin (folinic acid) in the management of rheumatoid arthritis: Results of a multicenter randomized, double-blind, placebo-controlled trial. Arthritis Rheum 36:795, 1993.

130. Weinblatt ME: Toxicity of low-dose methotrexate in rheumatoid arthritis. J Rheumatol 12(Suppl 12):35, 1985.

131. Kerstens PJSM, Boerbooms AMT, Jeurissen MEC, et al: Accelerated nodulosis during low-dose methotrexate therapy for rheumatoid arthritis. An analysis of ten cases. J Rheumatol 19:867, 1992.

132. MacKinnon SK, Starkebaum G, Willkens RF: Pancytopenia associated with low-dose pulse methotrexate in the treatment of rheumatoid arthritis. Semin Arthritis Rheum 15:119, 1985.

133. Weinblatt ME, Fraser P: Elevated mean corpuscular volume as a predictor of hematologic toxicity due to methotrexate therapy. Arthritis Rheum 32:1592, 1989.

134. Seideman P, Müller-Suur R, Ekman E: Renal effects of low-dose methotrexate in rheumatoid arthritis. J Rheumatol 20:1126, 1993.

135. Shamberger RC, Rosenberg SA, Seipp CA, et al: Effects of high-dose methotrexate and vincristine on ovarian and testicular functions in patients undergoing postoperative adjuvant treatment of osteosarcoma. Cancer Treat Rep 65:739, 1981.

136. Sussman A, Leonard JM: Psoriasis, methotrexate, and oligospermia. Arch Dermatol 116:215, 1980.

137. Blackburn WD Jr, Alarcón GS: Impotence in three rheumatoid arthritis patients treated with methotrexate (letter). Arthritis Rheum 32:1341, 1989.

138. Milunsky A, Graef JW, Gaynor MF Jr: Methotrexate-induced congenital malformations. J Pediatr 72:790, 1968.

139. Kozlowski RD, Steinbrunner JV, MacKenzie AH, et al: Outcome of first-trimester exposure to low-dose methotrexate in eight patients with rheumatic disease. Am J Med 88:589, 1990.

140. Green DM, Zevon MA, Lowrie G, et al: Congenital anomalies in children of patients who received chemotherapy for cancer in childhood and adolescence. N Engl J Med 325:141, 1991.

141. Rustin GJ, Rustin F, Dent J, et al: No increase in second tumors after cytotoxic chemotherapy for gestational trophoblastic tumors. N Engl J Med 308:473, 1983.

142. Stern RS, Zierler S, Parrish JA: Methotrexate used for psoriasis and the risk of noncutaneous or cutaneous malignancy. Cancer 50:869, 1982.

143. Ellman MH, Hurwitz H, Thomas C, et al: Lymphoma developing in a patient with rheumatoid arthritis taking low-dose weekly methotrexate. J Rheumatol 18:1741, 1991.

144. Kingsmore SF, Hall BD, Allen NB, et al: Association of methotrexate, rheumatoid arthritis and lymphoma: Report of 2 cases and literature review. J Rheumatol 19:1462, 1992.

145. Kamel OW, Van de Rijn M, Weiss LM, et al: Reversible lymphomas associated with Epstein-Barr virus occurring during methotrexate therapy for rheumatoid arthritis and dermatomyositis. N Engl J Med 328:1317, 1993.

146. Wernick R, Smith DL: Central nervous system toxicity associated with weekly low-dose methotrexate treatment. Arthritis Rheum 32:770, 1989.

147. Halla JT, Hardin JG: Underrecognized postdosing reactions to methotrexate in patients with rheumatoid arthritis. J Rheumatol 21:1224, 1994.

148. Flowers MA, Heathcote J, Wanless IR, et al: Fulminant hepatitis as a consequence of reactivation of hepatitis B virus infection after discontinuation of low-dose methotrexate therapy. Ann Intern Med 112:381, 1990.

149. Stanisavljevic S, Babcock AL: Fractures in children treated with methotrexate for leukemia. Clin Orthop 125:139, 1977.

150. Friedlaender GE, Tross RB, Doganis AC, et al: Effects of chemotherapeutic agents on bone. I. Short-term methotrexate and doxorubicin (Adriamycin) treatment in a rat model. J Bone Joint Surg Am 66:602, 1984.

151. May KP, West SG, McDermott MT, et al: The effect of low-dose methotrexate on bone metabolism and histomorphometry in rats. Arthritis Rheum 37:201, 1994.

152. Sostman HD, Matthay RA, Putman CE, et al: Methotrexate-induced pneumonitis. Medicine (Baltimore) 55:371, 1976.

153. Cannon GW, Ward, JR, Clegg DO, et al: Acute lung disease associated with low-dose pulse methotrexate therapy in patients with rheumatoid arthritis. Arthritis Rheum 26:1269, 1983.

154. St Clair EW, Rice JR, Snyderman R: Pneumonitis complicating low-dose methotrexate therapy in rheumatoid arthritis. Arch Intern Med 145:2035, 1985.

155. Carson CW, Cannon GW, Egger MJ, et al: Pulmonary disease during the treatment of rheumatoid arthritis with low-dose pulse methotrexate. Semin Arthritis Rheum 16:186, 1987.

156. Searles G, McKendry RJ: Methotrexate pneumonitis in rheumatoid arthritis: Potential risk factors. Four case reports and a review of the literature. J Rheumatol 14:1164, 1987.

157. Carroll GJ, Thomas R, Phatouros CC, et al: Incidence, prevalence and possible risk factors for pneumonitis in patients with rheumatoid arthritis receiving methotrexate. J Rheumatol 21:51, 1994.

158. Roenigk HH Jr, Auerbach R, Maibach HI, et al: Methotrexate in psoriasis: Revised guidelines. J Am Acad Dermatol 19:145, 1988.

159. Kremer JM, Alarcón GS, Lightfoot RW Jr, et al: Methotrexate for rheu-

matoid arthritis: Suggested guidelines for monitoring liver toxicity. Arthritis Rheum 37:316, 1994.

160. Kremer JM, Lee RG, Tolman KG: Liver histology in rheumatoid arthritis patients receiving long-term methotrexate therapy. A prospective study with baseline and sequential biopsy samples. Arthritis Rheum 32:121, 1989.

161. Kremer JM: Long-term prospective sequential liver biopsies (Bxs) in patients with rheumatoid arthritis (RA) on weekly oral methotrexate (MTX) (abstr). Arthritis Rheum 33:S40, 1990.

162. Aponte J, Petrelli M: Histopathologic findings in the liver of rheumatoid arthritis patients treated with long-term bolus methotrexate. Arthritis Rheum 31:1457, 1988.

163. Phillips CA, Cera PJ, Mangan TF, et al: Clinical liver disease in patients with rheumatoid arthritis taking methotrexate. J Rheumatol 19:229, 1992.

164. Clegg DO, Furst DE, Tolman KG, et al: Acute, reversible hepatic failure associated with methotrexate treatment of rheumatoid arthritis. J Rheumatol 16:1123, 1989.

165. Kujala GA, Shamma'a JM, Chang WL, et al: Hepatitis with bridging fibrosis and reversible hepatic insufficiency in a woman with rheumatoid arthritis taking methotrexate. Arthritis Rheum 33:1037, 1990.

166. Walker AM, Funch D, Dreyer NA, et al: Determinants of serious liver disease among patients receiving low-dose methotrexate for rheumatoid arthritis. Arthritis Rheum 36:329, 1993.

167. Perhala RS, Wilke WS, Clough JD, et al: Local infectious complications following large joint replacement in rheumatoid arthritis patients treated with methotrexate versus those not treated with methotrexate. Arthritis Rheum 34:146, 1991.

168. Bridges SL Jr, López-Méndez A, Han KH, et al: Should methotrexate be discontinued before elective orthopedic surgery in patients with rheumatoid arthritis? J Rheumatol 18:984, 1991.

169. Sany J, Anaya J-M, Canovas F, et al: Influence of methotrexate on the frequency of postoperative infectious complications in patients with rheumatoid arthritis. J Rheumatol 20:1129, 1993.

170. Fries JF: Advances in management of rheumatic disease 1965 to 1985. Arch Intern Med 149:1002, 1989.

CHAPTER 50

C. Michael Stein
Theodore Pincus

Glucocorticoids

In 1949, Hench, who with others subsequently shared a Nobel prize for their pioneering work with adrenocoriticosteroids, demonstrated the dramatic clinical effects of cortisone and adrenocorticotropic hormone (ACTH; corticotropin) in the treatment of rheumatoid arthritis.[1] Because of their adverse effects, initial enthusiasm gave way to disappointment and an aversion to the use of glucocorticoids. For many patients with inflammatory rheumatic diseases, however, glucocorticoids remain one of the most effective treatments. Despite more than 40 years of clinical usage, many controversies remain about the risks, benefits, and optimal clinical usage of one of the few therapies that result in dramatic clinical improvement in inflammatory rheumatic diseases, particularly regarding the role of glucocorticoids in the management of rheumatoid arthritis.

STRUCTURE

Glucocorticoids are 21-carbon steroid molecules. The structures of cortisol (hydrocortisone), the major endogenous biologically active glucocorticoid, and of several synthetic glucocorticoids are shown in Figure 50–1. Corticosteroids with an 11-ketone group (cortisone and prednisone) are biologically inactive until reduced to the 11-hydroxyl compound (hydrocortisone and prednisolone, respectively).[2, 3] Therefore, preparations such as cortisone and prednisone that require bioactivation in the liver are used only systemically. If a local effect, such as an intra-articular injection is desired, a biologically active compound such as methylprednisolone or triamcinolone is used.

Alteration in molecular structure has yielded preparations with useful differences in potency, mineralocorticoid activity, and pharmacokinetic profiles (Table 50–1). The goal of synthesizing a glucocorticoid that has anti-inflammatory effects without accompanying unwanted effects on protein and carbohydrate metabolism, remains elusive, however, although reports have suggested that newer preparations, such as deflazacort, may have fewer side effects than prednisone.[4]

REGULATION OF CORTISOL SECRETION

Physiology of the Hypothalamic-Pituitary-Adrenal Axis

The hypothalamic-pituitary-adrenal (HPA) axis forms a complex system that regulates basal and stress-induced glucocorticoid release.[5] The production of cortisol by the adrenal cortex is regulated by ACTH secreted from the anterior pituitary gland. This release of ACTH is in turn regulated by corticotropin-releasing hormone (CRH) released from the hypothalamus. CRH is secreted in small pulses into the local hypophyseal portal circulation and is transported to the anterior pituitary, where it stimulates the synthesis and pulsatile secretion of ACTH. ACTH, a 39–amino acid peptide, binds to specific ACTH receptors, stimulates cyclic adenosine monophosphate (cAMP) production, and through cAMP-dependent phosphorylation, stimulates cholesterol uptake and adrenal steroid synthesis.[6] Corticosteroids are not stored in the adrenal glands in significant amounts; therefore, continuing synthesis and release are required to maintain basal secretion or to increase levels during stress.

The total daily basal secretion of cortisol in humans is approximately 20 mg. Basal secretion follows a diurnal pattern, with highest levels occurring in the early morning and lowest levels in the evening.[3] Increased cortisol release may result from stimulation of the HPA axis by stressors such as cold, exercise, infection, and surgery. The HPA axis is sensitive to negative feedback, with increased levels of cortisol or synthetic glucocorticoids inhibiting the synthesis and release of both CRH and ACTH[3, 5] and thereby decreasing cortisol production. Protracted negative feedback, such as occurs with prolonged glucocorticoid therapy, results in atrophy of the adrenals and blunting of the HPA axis, and a consequent reduced capacity to produce additional glucocorticoids in response to ACTH or stress.

Hypothalamic-Pituitary-Adrenal Axis and Inflammation

Inflammatory mediators and glucocorticoid responses are linked in a complex network.[5, 7] Exogenous glucocorticoids are administered most frequently for their anti-inflammatory and immunosuppressive actions, which are achieved through multiple actions discussed in detail later. Endogenous glucocorticoids, however, previously thought to play a largely homeostatic role, may also modify inflammatory responses. Disease activity in rheumatoid arthritis fluctuates in a diurnal fashion, with lowest disease activity approximately 6 hours after natural peak cortisol levels,[8] and treatment with metyrapone, which decreases endoge-

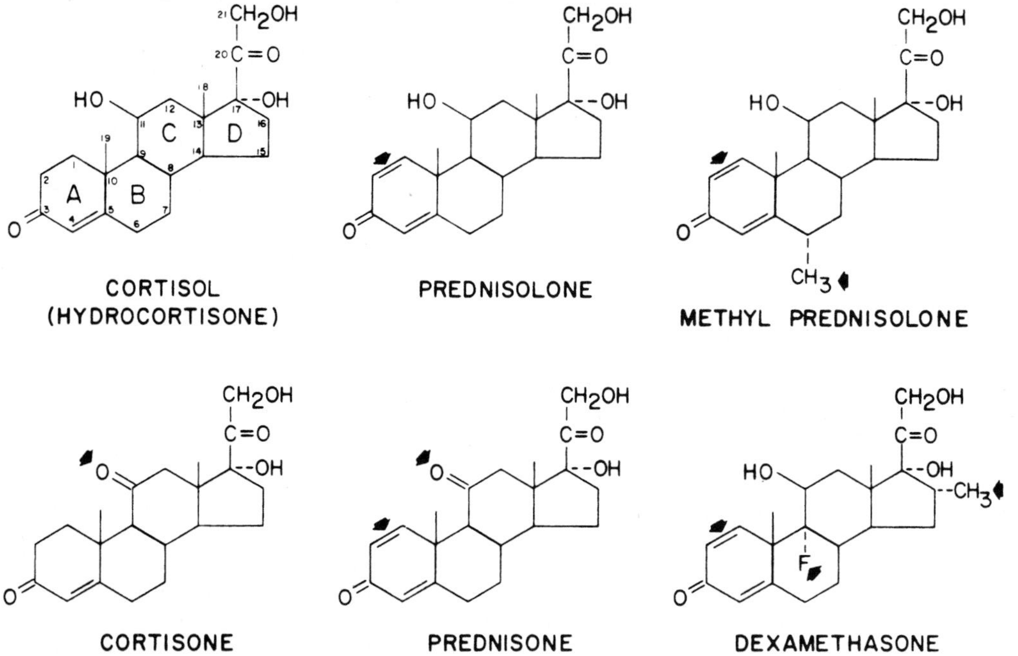

Figure 50–1. Structure of commonly used glucocorticoids. In the representation of cortisol, the 21 carbon atoms of the glucocorticoid skeleton are numbered and the four rings are designated by letters. (From Axelrod L: Glucocorticoid therapy. Medicine 55:39, 1976. By permission of Williams & Wilkins, 1979.)

nous cortisol production, results in worsening of disease activity,[9] suggesting that endogenous cortisol has an anti-inflammatory function. Further studies in animals[10] and in patients with rheumatoid arthritis[11, 12] indicate that impaired endogenous glucocorticoid responsiveness may be important in the pathogenesis or maintenance of inflammation, perhaps explaining why subphysiologic doses of glucocorticoids are often clinically effective.

In addition to the capacity of glucocorticoids to modify inflammatory mediators, these inflammatory mediators may modify glucocorticoid responses. The cytokine tumor necrosis factor-α (TNF-α), interleukin-1 (IL-1), and, in turn, IL-6 can independently or jointly stimulate CRH secretion.[5, 7]

MECHANISMS OF ACTION

Glucocorticoid Receptors

The effects of glucocorticoids are mediated through binding to cytoplasmic glucocorticoid receptors in target cells. Glucocorticoid receptors, which are expressed on almost every type of human cell, including lymphocytes, monocytes, and neutrophils,[13, 14] are members of a supergene family that includes cytosolic receptors for other steroid hormones such as estrogen and vitamin D. At least three important domains have been identified: the steroid-binding domain at the C-terminal end, the DNA-binding domain in the center of the molecule, and the N-terminal domain.[13, 14] The

Table 50–1. COMPARATIVE POTENCIES, DURATION OF ACTION, AND EQUIVALENT DOSES OF GLUCOCORTICOIDS

Drug	Duration of Action	Glucocorticoid Potency	Mineralocorticoid Potency	Equivalent Dose* (mg)
Short Acting				
Cortisol (hydrocortisone)	8–12 hr	1	1	20
Cortisone	8–12 hr	0.8	0.8	25
Intermediate Acting				
Prednisone	12–36 hr	4	0.8	5
Prednisolone	12–36 hr	4	0.8	5
Methylprednisolone	12–36 hr	5	0.5	4
Long Acting				
Dexamethasone	36–72 hr	25–30	0	0.7

Data from Axelrod L: Glucocorticoid therapy. Medicine 55:39, 1976; and Schimmer BP, Parker KL: Adrenocorticotropic hormone: adrenocortical steroids and their synthetic analogs; inhibitors of the synthesis and actions of adrenocortical hormones. *In* Hardman JG, Limbird LE, Molinoff PB, et al (eds): The Pharmacologic Basis of Therapeutics. New York, McGraw-Hill, 1966 p 1466.[3]

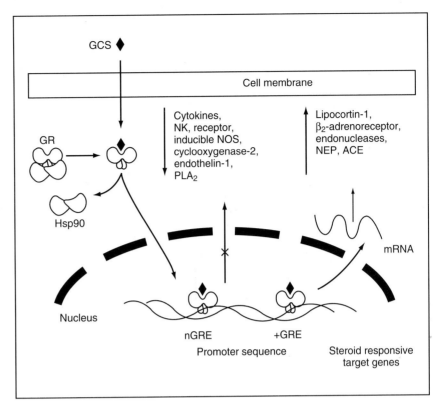

Figure 50–2. Glucocorticoid effects on gene transcription. Glucocorticoids (GCS) bind to cytosolic glucocorticoid receptors (GR), which are associated with two molecules of heat shock protein 90 (Hsp90). The GCS-GR complex translocates to the nucleus and binds to glucocorticoid response elements (GRE and nGRE) in the promoter sequence of target genes, resulting in increased (GRE) or decreased (nGRE) transcription. (Modified from Barnes PJ, Adcock I: Anti-inflammatory actions of steroids: Molecular mechanisms. Trends Pharmacol Sci 14:436, 1993.)

receptor, when not bound to glucocorticoids, is bound at the C-terminal end to a large protein complex that forms a heterohexamer composed of the receptor and a heat shock protein (Hsp) complex.[15] After glucocorticoid has bound to the receptor, the ligand-receptor complex dissociates from the Hsp complex, allowing nuclear localization of the ligand-receptor complex that binds to DNA at sites in the promoter region of target genes known as glucocorticoid response elements (GREs) (Fig. 50–2).[13] The clinical significance of glucocorticoid receptor regulation is poorly understood.[16]

Effects of Glucocorticoids on Gene Transcription

Glucocorticoids produce their effects through the hormone-receptor complex binding to the GREs and either stimulating or suppressing transcription of these target genes (Table 50–2).[17] A second mechanism is through interactions with DNA, altering the capacity of other transcription-regulating proteins to interact with their own response elements.[18] Activated glucocorticoid receptors interact directly with other transcription factors, such as c-*jun*, affecting gene transcription through interaction with the activated protein complex-1 (AP-1) site.[19] Glucocorticoids also regulate post-transcriptional events, including RNA translation, protein synthesis, and secretion, and may also have effects that do not involve direct interaction with DNA.[20, 21] Altered regulation at the molecular level, rather than pharmacologic variability, may explain the clinical observation of glucocorticoid resistance in certain patients.[7, 20, 22]

ANTI-INFLAMMATORY EFFECTS

Glucocorticoids suppress inflammation induced by a variety of immunologic, mechanical, chemical, and infectious stimuli, through multiple interacting mechanisms. Effects are seen on both immunomodulating proteins and immunomodulating cells, including decreased inflammatory exudate, decreased production and efficacy of inflammatory mediators, decreased recruitment of inflammatory cells to the site of inflammation, and decreased activation of inflamma-

Table 50–2. EFFECTS OF GLUCOCORTICOIDS ON MODULATORS OF INFLAMMATION

Inhibited by Glucocorticoids	Stimulated by Glucocorticoids
IL-1, IL-3, IL-4, IL-5, IL-6, IL-8, TNF-α, IFN-γ, GM-CSF	Lipocortin-1
Prostaglandins and leukotrienes	Neutral endopeptidase
Cyclooxygenase-2	Plasminogen activator inhibitor
Inducible nitric oxide synthase	Vasocortin
Plasminogen activator	

Abbreviations: IL, interleukin; TNF-α, tumor necrosis factor-α; IFN-γ; interferon-γ; GM-CSF, granulocyte-macrophage colony-stimulating factor.

tory cells. In general, glucocorticoids suppress cellular immunity more than humoral immunity.

Effects on Modulators of Inflammation

Lipocortin and Prostaglandins. Glucocorticoids inhibit prostaglandin synthesis[21, 23] through stimulation of a protein, lipocortin-1 (or annexin-1), which inhibits eicosanoid synthesis.[23, 24] The mechanisms of inhibition of arachidonic acid release by lipocortin are controversial and may include regulatory actions on phospholipase A_2 and on substrate phospholipids.[23, 24] In addition, lipocortin-1 has direct immunomodulatory effects that are independent of eicosanoid inhibition, including inhibitory effects on leukocyte migration.[25] Furthermore, one of the two cyclooxygenase enzymes, COX-2, is inhibited by glucocorticoids, whereas COX-1 is constitutively expressed and is not affected by glucocorticoids.[26, 27]

Cytokines. Glucocorticoids inhibit transcription of TNF-α, IL-1, IL-2, IL-3, IL-4, IL-5, IL-6, IL-8, interferon-γ (IFN-γ), and granulocyte-macrophage colony-stimulating factor (GM-CSF).[28–31] Glucocorticoids not only decrease the synthesis or release of cytokines but also blunt their actions indirectly, through counteracting the effects of activating transcription factors such as AP-1 on gene transcription.[13] Glucocorticoids may inhibit T cell activation by cytokines at several sites, including by inhibiting tyrosine phosphorylation, inhibiting calcium-modulin kinase II, and increasing messenger RNA (mRNA) degradation.[31]

Adhesion Molecules. Glucocorticoids inhibit expression of adhesion molecules, such as intercellular adhesion molecule-1 (ICAM-1) and endothelial leukocyte adhesion molecule-1 (ELAM-1), both directly[32] and indirectly through inhibitory effects on cytokines such as IL-1 and TNF-α.

Other Modulators of Inflammation. Glucocorticoids induce angiotensin converting enzyme and neutral endopeptidase, which degrade bradykinin,[33] resulting in decreased inflammatory exudate. In addition, glucocorticoids may decrease vascular permeability and inflammatory exudate through synthesis of proteins such as vasocortin[34] and direct effects on endothelial cells.[21] Other effects of glucocorticoids include inhibition of the inducible form of nitric oxide synthase[26, 27]; decreased formation of plasminogen-activating factor, platelet-activating factor (PAF), collagenase, and elastase; and inhibition of chemotactic factors.[21]

Effects on Cells That Modulate Inflammation

Glucocorticoids, through many of the mediators mentioned, have effects on particular cells important in the pathogenesis of inflammation (Table 50–3).

Neutrophils. The anti-inflammatory effects of glucocorticoids on neutrophils are not mediated through a decrease in total circulating numbers of cells, but

Table 50–3. ANTI-INFLAMMATORY EFFECTS OF GLUCOCORTICOIDS IN DIFFERENT CELLS

Cell	Effects
Neutrophils	Increased numbers, decreased trafficking, relatively unaltered neutrophil function
Macrophages and monocytes	Decreased numbers, decreased trafficking, decreased phagocytosis and bactericidal effects, inhibited antigen presentation, decreased cytokine release, decreased eicosanoid release
Lymphocytes	Decreased numbers, decreased trafficking, decreased cytokine production, decreased proliferation and impaired activation; little effect on immunoglobulin synthesis
Eosinophils	Decreased numbers, increased apoptosis
Basophils	Decreased numbers, decreased release of mediators

rather through decreased accumulation of neutrophils at sites of inflammation.[35] In fact, glucocorticoids increase circulating neutrophils. In healthy volunteers, 40 mg oral prednisone increased the neutrophil count by approximately 4000 cells/mm[3] within 4 hours[36] through release of neutrophils from the bone marrow, an increase in neutrophil life span due to glucocorticoid inhibition of programmed cell death (apoptosis),[37] reduced vascular margination of cells, and decreased trafficking of neutrophils to sites of inflammation.[36] These increases may be even greater in patients who receive glucocorticoids chronically for the treatment of inflammatory diseases.[36] Neutrophil functions such as phagocytosis and bactericidal activity are relatively unaffected by physiologic or pharmacologic concentrations of glucocorticoids.[36]

Macrophages. Monocyte and macrophage numbers are decreased by glucocorticoids,[36] as is their localization at sites of inflammation, perhaps through inhibition of macrophage migration inhibition factor.[38] Monocyte and macrophage function is inhibited, resulting in impaired phagocytosis and bactericidal activity[36] and decreased release of cytokines (IL-1, TNF-α) and eicosanoids. Glucocorticoids suppress antigen presentation and class II major histocompatibility class (MHC) antigen expression in such cells.[39] In human monocytes, however, the inhibitory effects of glucocorticoids on antigen presentation may be dissociated from inhibition of MHC class II antigen expression.[40]

Lymphocytes. The administration of a single dose of a glucocorticoid results in a decrease in the number of circulating lymphocytes, monocytes, and eosinophils that is maximal 4 to 6 hours after administration of the drug and that returns to normal within 24 hours. All lymphocyte subpopulations are affected, but T lymphocytes are affected more than B lymphocytes.[36] The mechanism of glucocorticoid lymphopenia in humans is largely due to redistribution of lymphocytes.[36] Mature human lymphocytes do not undergo lysis after exposure to glucocorticoids,[41] although certain activated lymphocyte subpopulations may be susceptible to lysis through apoptosis.[42]

Glucocorticoids inhibit lymphocyte proliferation both in vitro and ex vivo.[36, 43] Antigen binding to a T cell receptor initiates events, including the production of IL-2, which stimulates T cell proliferation. Glucocorticoids decrease both IL-2 production and IL-2 gene transcription and blunt the effects of IL-2 by inhibiting both binding of IL-2 to IL-2 receptors[44] and IL-2–dependent phosphorylation of intracellular proteins.[45] In addition, glucocorticoids decrease lymphocyte proliferation through inhibitory effects on other cytokines.

The effects of glucocorticoids on B cell function and immunoglobulins are of lesser importance and may reflect alterations in B cell function secondary to alterations in helper T cell function. In low doses, glucocorticoids have little effect on immunoglobulin levels or on antigen-stimulated antibody production.[46]

Eosinophils. Glucocorticoids result in a decrease in the number of eosinophils through cell redistribution processes,[47] as well as inhibition of cytokines, such as IL-5, which are needed for eosinophil survival and thus lead to increased apoptosis.[48]

Other Cells. Glucocorticoids decrease circulating basophil counts, inhibit basophil migration, inhibit the release of histamine and leukotrienes from basophils,[21, 49] and, in animal species, inhibit the degranulation of mast cells.[50]

Nonimmunomodulatory Effects of Glucocorticoids

Glucocorticoids have profound metabolic effects that are not directly related to their immunomodulatory activities but that may result in adverse effects. Glucocorticoids are catabolic, leading to the breakdown of protein to form carbohydrate, diminished peripheral utilization of glucose, and increased glycogen deposition—a situation that facilitates insulin resistance and impaired glucose tolerance.[51] Alterations in plasma lipid concentrations occur, and, overall, glucocorticoids may facilitate development of atherosclerosis.[52, 53]

Aldosterone, the endogenous mineralocorticoid, enhances renal tubular Na^+ reabsorption and increases urinary excretion of K^+ and H^+. Most synthetic glucocorticoids have little or no mineralocorticoid action (see Table 50–1).

PHARMACOKINETICS

The pharmacokinetics of glucocorticoids have been reviewed[54-56] and are summarized here. A two- to three-fold range in inter-individual variation in glucocorticoid disposition is seen.[55]

Absorption

Glucocorticoids are well absorbed after oral, intramuscular, intrasynovial, and topical administration. After oral administration of prednisone or prednisolone, 50 to 90 percent of a dose is absorbed.[54, 55] Administration with food may delay peak prednisolone concentrations but has no significant effect on overall bioavailability. Prednisone itself is inactive and is converted in the liver to prednisolone. Interconversion between prednisone and prednisolone is rapid and efficient. The administration of equal doses of prednisone and prednisolone results in almost identical plasma concentrations of the active drug, prednisolone (Fig. 50–3).[57, 58] Prednisone and prednisolone can be used interchangeably in most patients.

Plasma Transport Proteins

Most cortisol (80 percent) in plasma is reversibly bound to a glycoprotein, corticosteroid-binding globulin (CBG). About 10 percent of the cortisol is not bound to CBG but is bound to albumin.[59] Approximately 10 percent of cortisol is free (i.e., not bound to protein) and is physiologically active. Protein binding of prednisolone is concentration dependent. CBG has a low capacity for binding prednisolone and is saturated at low doses.[59] With higher doses, as CBG becomes saturated, more prednisolone is bound to albumin, which has a greater capacity but lower affinity than does CBG, and more prednisolone (35 to 55 percent) is in the unbound state.[58] Diurnal fluctuations in CBG concentrations and prednisolone pharmacokinetics occur,[60] but these effects are minor.[54]

Metabolism and Excretion

Elimination of glucocorticoids is largely hepatic, with initial hydroxylation, subsequent conjugation, and excretion of metabolites in the urine.[61, 62] Fecal and biliary excretion is insignificant, and small amounts of prednisone (1 to 2 percent) and prednisolone (6 to 12 percent) are eliminated unchanged in the urine after the administration of prednisone.[62] Within the usual therapeutic dosing range (<70 mg), dose-dependent increases in clearance and volume of distribution are seen with prednisolone[63] and hydrocortisone,[64] but no change in half-life occurs.[63]

Half-Life and Biologic Effect

In comparisons of the different glucocorticoid preparations, three major pharmacologic considerations are seen (see Table 50–1):

1. Elimination of half-life—the time required for the plasma concentration to decline by half
2. Potency—the dose required to obtain a given effect
3. Duration of biologic activity

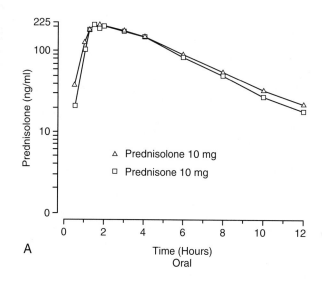

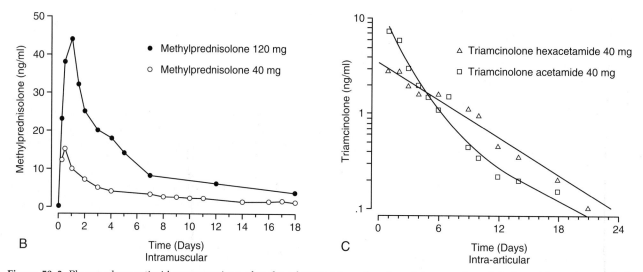

Figure 50–3. Plasma glucocorticoid concentrations after the administration of oral prednisone and prednisolone, 10 mg, intra-articular triamcinolone hexacetonide and triamcinolone acetonide, 40 mg, and intramuscular methylprednisolone, 40 and 120 mg. (Data from Ferry JJ, Horvath AM, Bekersky I, et al: Relative and absolute bioavailability of prednisone and prednisolone after separate oral and intravenous doses. J Clin Pharmacol 28:81, 1988; Dasgupta B, Gray J, Fernandes L, Ollif C: Treatment of polymyalgia rheumatica with intramuscular injections of depot methylprednisolone. Ann Rheum Dis 50:942, 1991; and Derendorf H, Mollman H, Gruner A, Haack D, Gyselby G: Pharmacokinetics and pharmacodynamics of glucocorticoid suspensions after intra-articular administration. Clin Pharmacol Ther 39:313–317, 1986.)

Approximate plasma half-lives for glucocorticoids in common use are cortisol, 90 minutes; prednisone, 3 to 4 hours; prednisolone and methylprednisolone, 2 to 3 hours; and dexamethasone, 2 to 5 hours.[2, 55] The minor differences between glucocorticoids in plasma half-life contrasts with marked differences in potency and duration of biologic activity (see Table 50–1).

Glucocorticoids can be divided into three groups according to their duration of biologic action[2, 3] (see Table 50–1).

• Short-acting (8 to 12 hours)—cortisol and cortisone
• Intermediate-acting (12 to 36 hours)—prednisone, prednisolone, methylprednisolone, and triamcinolone

• Long-acting (36 to 72 hours)—dexamethasone

The administration of depot corticosteroids results in a prolonged exposure to glucocorticoids, with elimination occurring over several weeks (see Fig. 50–3).[65, 66]

Pharmacokinetic Considerations in Special Circumstances

Liver Disease. Although liver disease can result in a slight impairment of the conversion of prednisone to prednisolone, the overall consensus is that this effect is more than balanced by reduced hepatic clearance of prednisolone. Therefore, patients with severe liver disease have higher levels of prednisolone.[54] Increased adverse effects reported in patients with hypoalbuminemia[67] may result from higher plasma concentrations of prednisolone in patients with severe liver disease rather than be due to hypoalbuminemia itself.[54]

Renal Disease. Renal excretion of unchanged prednisone or prednisolone is of relatively minor importance. Increased glucocorticoid concentrations have been reported in patients with chronic renal failure and in some studies of renal transplant patients.[54] Decreased total, but unaltered free, concentrations of prednisolone are found in patients with nephrotic syndrome and low serum albumin concentrations.[54]

Age. A significant inverse relationship between age and hepatic and renal clearance of prednisolone has been reported,[54, 68] with elderly subjects having higher free concentrations of prednisolone. Bioavailability of oral prednisone and the interconversion between prednisone and prednisolone are unaltered in elderly subjects (>65 years), however.

Hyperthyroidism. Both bound and free concentrations of prednisolone are significantly lower in hyperthyroid patients[54] as a result of decreased absorption and increased hepatic clearance.

Pregnancy and Lactation. Glucocorticoids may retard fetal growth,[69] but this is not a universal finding.[70] The fetal malformation rate is not higher than that in the background population,[71] and the increase in oral clefts reported in animal studies has not been found in humans. Overall, glucocorticoids are well tolerated during pregnancy. Prednisone and prednisolone result in a maternal to cord blood drug concentration ratio of approximately 10:1.[72] The placenta has the capacity to convert prednisolone to the inactive drug prednisone.[73] By contrast, dexamethasone crosses the placenta well and results in similar maternal and fetal drug concentrations.[74] Therefore, if the therapeutic aim is to treat the mother and not the fetus, prednisone or prednisolone should be used, whereas dexamethasone should be used if the therapeutic aim is to treat the fetus, as for fetal myocarditis[75] or to prevent respiratory distress syndrome.[76] Concentrations of prednisone and prednisolone in breast milk are low,[77] equivalent to less than 10 percent of a neonate's endogenous cortisol production, even with a dose of 80 mg/day.[78] The American Academy of Pediatrics considers treatment with prednisone or prednisolone to be compatible with breastfeeding.[79]

Drug Interactions

Hepatic Microsomal Enzyme Induction. A drug interaction of practical clinical importance involves the capacity of many drugs to rapidly induce hepatic microsomal drug metabolizing capacity, resulting in increased clearance of glucocorticoids. Enzyme-induc-

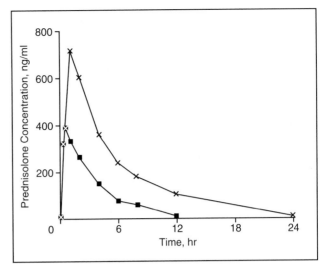

Figure 50–4. The effect of rifampin on plasma prednisolone concentrations in a patient receiving prednisone. Squares = with rifampin; x = without rifampin. (Modified from Carrie F, Roblot P, Bouquet S, et al: Rifampin-induced nonresponsiveness of giant cell arteritis to prednisone treatment. Arch Intern Med 154:1521, 1994. Copyright 1994, American Medical Association.)

ing drugs, including phenytoin, rifampin, barbiturates, and carbamazepine,[54, 61, 80] may result in a 80 to 90 percent increase in glucocorticoid clearance and a 40 to 60 percent decrease in the area under the concentration time curve (Fig. 50–4).[54, 80] When it is necessary to co-administer prednisone and rifampin in patients with temporal arteritis, it has been suggested that the dose of prednisone be doubled to 2 mg/kg/day and that this may be a situation in which the measurement of prednisolone plasma concentrations[68] could be useful,[80] although this assay is generally not needed.

Hepatic Microsomal Enzyme Inhibition. Enzyme-inhibiting drugs, such as cimetidine, macrolide antibiotics, and cyclosporine, do not inhibit the metabolism of prednisolone to a clinically significant degree.[54] Ketoconazole has been reported to inhibit the metabolism of prednisolone in some but not all studies.[54, 81] Estrogen-containing oral contraceptives decrease the metabolism of prednisone by approximately 50 percent.[54]

Effects of Glucocorticoids on Other Drugs. Co-administration of a glucocorticoid and salicylate results in decreased plasma salicylate concentrations,[82] but this is seldom clinically important. Glucocorticoids, through their metabolic effects, may indirectly alter responses to other drugs, such as increasing requirements for insulin or oral hypoglycemic agents.

ADVERSE EFFECTS

Adverse effects from therapeutic use of glucocorticoids (Table 50–4) result mainly from prolonged exposure to high doses. As a general principle, most ad-

Table 50–4. ADVERSE EFFECTS OF GLUCOCORTICOID THERAPY

Immunologic	Increased susceptibility to infection, decreased inflammatory responses, suppressed delayed hypersensitivity, neutrophilia, lymphocytopenia
Musculoskeletal	Osteoporosis complicated by fractures, avascular necrosis, myopathy
Gastrointestinal	Peptic ulceration in combination with nonsteroidal anti-inflammatory drugs, pancreatitis
Cardiovascular	Hypertension, fluid retention, accelerated atherosclerosis
Dermatologic	Acne, hirsutism, purple striae, skin fragility, ecchymoses
Neuropsychiatric	Altered mood, emotional lability, euphoria, insomnia, depression, psychosis, pseudotumor cerebri
Ophthalmologic	Posterior subcapsular cataracts, glaucoma
Endocrine and metabolic	Glucose intolerance, diabetes mellitus, diabetic coma, weight gain, hyperlipoproteinemia, fat redistribution, negative nitrogen balance, growth suppression, muscle wasting, impaired wound healing, sodium and water retention, increased potassium loss, hypokalemic alkalosis, impotence, menstrual irregularities, hypothalamic-pituitary-adrenal axis suppression, acute adrenal insufficiency (addisonian crisis)

verse effects are dose related, and a short course of corticosteroid therapy (2 weeks), even at high doses, has a low risk. By contrast, all subjects who receive substantial doses of glucocorticoids for prolonged periods, such as 30 mg of a prednisone equivalent for 3 months, suffer adverse effects, although threshold doses for adverse effects differ between individuals. Pharmacokinetic variables, such as lower clearance and increased half-life, have sometimes been associated with increased risk of adverse effects,[83] but this has not been a consistent finding, and monitoring of drug concentrations is unlikely to be useful in minimizing adverse effects in individual patients. The primary toxicities of corticosteroids[84] are discussed in the sections that follow (see Table 50–4).

Immunologic

Increased Susceptibility to Infection. The immunologic effects of glucocorticoids, discussed under their mechanisms of action, also result in the un-

wanted effect of increasing the risk of bacterial, viral, fungal, and protozoal infections.[84–87] Data about the risk of infection are complex and difficult to evaluate, since most conditions for which glucocorticoids are used themselves predispose to infection. Furthermore, patients with more severe disease tend to receive the highest doses of corticosteroids, as well as combinations of drugs that may be immunosuppressive.[88] Low doses of corticosteroids, even over prolonged periods, do not appear to increase the risks of tuberculosis or other infections,[89, 90] but continued use of high-dose corticosteroid therapy is associated with substantially increased risks of infection.[88] Estimated relative risks (RR) of infection in patients treated with corticosteroids are as follow: mean prednisone dose below 20 mg/day, RR 1.3 (95 percent confidence intervals 1.0 to 1.6); and mean prednisone dose over 20 mg/day, RR 2.1 (95 percent confidence interval 1.3 to 3.6).[88] No increased risk of infection was seen in patients with a cumulative prednisone dose below 700 mg.[88]

Other Immunologic Effects. The anti-inflammatory effects of glucocorticoids may mask the fever and inflammatory signs associated with infection and delay the diagnosis of infection. Furthermore, diagnostic confusion and inappropriate investigation can result if it is not recognized that corticosteroid therapy results in a neutrophilia and an elevated total white blood cell count.[36]

Musculoskeletal

Osteoporosis. Glucocorticoids cause osteoporosis through several suggested mechanisms, including decreased intestinal calcium absorption, increased renal calcium loss, secondary hyperparathyroidism, inhibition of osteoblast function, inhibition of growth factors, increased bone resorption, and decreased concentrations of sex hormones.[91] The estimated risk of fracture in patients taking glucocorticoids varies from 11 to 50 percent,[91, 92] and is influenced by both the underlying disease and the glucocorticoid dose. In patients with rheumatoid arthritis, for example, both functional impairment and glucocorticoid dose are risk factors for fracture.[93]

Glucocorticoid-induced bone loss is most rapid during the first 6 to 12 months of therapy, and may result in 10 to 40 percent loss of bone mass at certain sites, affecting trabecular bone more than cortical bone. This bone loss may be partially reversible after the drug is discontinued, and results in vertebral fractures more commonly than hip fractures.[93] Osteoporosis is dose dependent, but whether a threshold dose exists is controversial. It is generally agreed that doses in excess of 7.5 to 10 mg of prednisone per day result in measurable bone loss. Studies suggest that daily doses of prednisone in the 5- to 9-mg range may also be associated with bone loss in the lumbar spine but not the femoral neck,[94] but doses of 1 to 4 mg have not been associated with bone loss at either site.[93, 94]

Selection of strategies to prevent and treat glucocorticoid-induced osteoporosis is hampered by the absence of data about the effects on the fracture rate. The use of bone mineral density as a surrogate marker may be a poor substitute.[93] Appropriate prophylactic strategies to prevent corticosteroid-induced osteoporosis include using low doses, eliminating other osteoporosis risk factors such as smoking and alcohol, encouraging exercise, and ensuring an adequate intake of calcium (1000 to 1500 mg/day) and vitamin D (400 to 800 U/day).[93] Consideration of more aggressive prophylaxis depends on the individual patient's risk factors and the proposed dose and duration of therapy.

Hormone replacement therapy preserves bone mass in postmenopausal women receiving glucocorticoids[95, 96] and should be considered for every postmenopausal woman receiving glucocorticoids. Documentation of low bone density before corticosteroid therapy may strengthen the case for hormone replacement therapy.[93] Data about the efficacy of calcitriol and other vitamin D preparations in the prophylaxis of glucocorticoid-induced osteoporosis are of interest, but are incomplete.[97] Preliminary studies have suggested that calcitonin, administered by either the subcutaneous or the intranasal route, decreases corticosteroid-induced bone loss.[96, 97] The bisphosphonates etidronate and pamidronate preserve bone density in patients receiving corticosteroids,[96] but osteomalacia with etidronate and the lack of information about fracture rates limit recommending their use routinely. Additional studies are required to further define the clinical usefulness of vitamin D preparations, nasal calcitonin, newer bisphosphonates and new glucocorticoid preparations such as deflazacort, which may result in lower levels of osteoporosis.[4, 98]

Avascular Necrosis. The risk of avascular necrosis, which is increased in patients with rheumatoid arthritis and systemic lupus erythematosus, is further increased by glucocorticoid therapy.[99] The pathogenesis is unknown but several mechanisms, including fat embolism and compression of intramedullary blood vessels by hypertrophied lipocytes, have been proposed.[100] Avascular necrosis most commonly affects the hips and then the knees or shoulders; it is often bilateral. The risk added by glucocorticoids is related to dose and duration of therapy,[101] but avascular necrosis has been described occurring as rapidly as within 6 weeks of starting therapy, and has occurred both with low oral doses and high-bolus intravenous doses of glucocorticoids.

Myopathy. Glucocorticoids may induce a myopathy, most commonly in patients receiving relatively high doses (>30 mg/day) for prolonged periods. The myopathy presents as gradual onset of proximal muscle weakness without elevation of muscle enzymes.[102, 103] A more acute form has been described after short-term high-dose corticosteroid therapy. Anabolic steroids and potassium supplements are not of therapeutic benefit.[84]

Gastrointestinal

Peptic Ulceration. A possible association between peptic ulceration and glucocorticoid therapy is con-

troversial and based on small series of cases and meta-analyses of clinical trial data.[104–106] These analyses have been weakened by the inclusion of single-blind studies, and it is likely that any increased risk of peptic ulceration, if present, is small. The use of corticosteroids in combination with nonsteroidal anti-inflammatory drugs (NSAIDs), however, does appear to increase the risk of peptic ulceration and gastrointestinal hemorrhage,[107, 108] although these findings may again be confounded by use of both drugs in patients with more severe disease. Glucocorticoids may mask the symptoms and signs usually associated with the occurrence of an intra-abdominal complication, such as perforation of the intestine, and can lead to a delay in diagnosis with increased morbidity.[109]

Pancreatitis. In animal studies, corticosteroids have caused pancreatic lesions.[110] In humans who had received glucocorticoids recently before death, histologic pancreatic abnormalities were commonly seen, although these changes were largely clinically silent.[111] The increased risk of clinical pancreatitis in patients receiving glucocorticoids is difficult to quantify, but is small. Again, development of this complication in a patient with systemic lupus erythematosus may be caused by the rheumatic disease and not be causally associated with the therapy.[112]

Cardiovascular

Hypertension. Hypertension occurs in association with both excessive endogenous production and exogenous administration of glucocorticoids.[113] Because dexamethasone has no mineralocorticoid effect and prednisone has very little, the mechanisms of glucocorticoid-induced hypertension are not simply attributable to mineralocorticoid-induced sodium and water retention. Altered vascular responsiveness to endogenous pressor agents is thought to be important.[114] Low doses of prednisone (<10 mg/day) have only minor effects on blood pressure and are not an important cause of hypertension.[115]

Atherosclerosis. It is likely, based on animal studies and clinical studies in humans, that corticosteroids accelerate atherosclerosis.[52, 53, 116] In patients with systemic lupus erythematosus, prednisone treatment was found to be an independent risk factor for coronary artery disease.[117] Again, because more severely ill patients are more likely to receive higher doses of prednisone, it is difficult to eliminate the confounding factor of the underlying disease. The effects of glucocorticoids on atherosclerosis are likely to be mediated through several mechanisms, including alterations in serum lipoproteins, blood pressure, and vascular effects.[118]

Dermatologic

Many skin changes are of relatively minor clinical importance but may be disturbing to the patient.

These include acne, hirsutism, striae, skin thinning and increased fragility, and ecchymoses.[84]

Neuropsychiatric

Corticosteroids may result in a wide range of psychiatric symptoms, including altered mood, emotional lability, euphoria, insomnia, depression, and psychosis.[119–121] These have been described with most of the glucocorticoids in current rheumatologic practice, including parenteral preparations such as triamcinolone.[120] Mood changes account for 90 percent of the psychiatric side effects of corticosteroids.[121] The frequency of psychiatric adverse effects is related to dose and occurred in 1.3 percent of patients receiving less than 40 mg/day prednisone, 4.6 percent of those receiving 41 to 80 mg/day, and 18.4 percent of those receiving more than 80 mg/day.[122] There are no reliable predictors of risk other than dose[121]; however, some patients experience mood changes with prednisone doses less than 3 mg/day.

More than half the patients who experience an adverse psychiatric effect do so within the first 5 days of therapy, but delayed responses noticed only after many weeks of therapy have occurred.[121, 122] Rare patients may experience "steroid psychosis." Symptoms generally respond, in days to weeks, to a decrease in the dose of glucocorticoid.[119, 121] Treatment with phenothiazines or lithium[119–121, 123] has been reported to be effective.

Pseudotumor Cerebri. Pseudotumor cerebri, also known as benign intracranial hypertension, presents signs of raised intracranial pressure (headache, papilledema), and has rarely been described in association with corticosteroid therapy, often at a time when the dose is being reduced.[124] It is uncommon, and children appear to be at greater risk than adults.

Ophthalmologic

Cataracts and Glaucoma. The frequency of posterior subcapsular cataracts in patients receiving glucocorticoids increases with the dose and duration of therapy. They occur in 50 to 80 percent of patients who receive 5 mg prednisone or more per day for more than 1 year but are less common in patients who receive less than 10 mg/day.[84, 125] Younger patients and children may develop cataracts in a shorter time and on lower doses of corticosteroids than do older patients.[126] Posterior subcapsular cataracts are usually bilateral and may cause some glare disturbance but do not usually result in visual impairment, although occasional patients have required cataract extraction.[125] Corticosteroids may increase intraocular pressure and aggravate glaucoma.[127]

Endocrine and Metabolic

Carbohydrate Metabolism. Effects of corticosteroids on carbohydrate metabolism result in glucose intolerance, insulin resistance, occasional overt diabetes mellitus, and, rarely, diabetic coma.[84, 128] Diabetes is usually reversible when the corticosteroid treatment is discontinued, but this may take weeks or months, and some patients require treatment with insulin to control the diabetes.

Fat Metabolism. Weight gain, due to both increased appetite and metabolic alterations, is common with moderate or high doses of glucocorticoids. Fat redistribution results in the moon facies, truncal obesity, and buffalo hump typical of Cushing's syndrome.[84]

Protein Metabolism. Increased protein catabolism results in negative nitrogen balance, muscle wasting, and impaired wound healing. Growth suppression occurs in children and is mediated by effects on protein, bone, and growth hormone.[129]

Other Metabolic Effects. The mineralocorticoid effects of some glucocorticoids may result in increased potassium loss, hypokalemic alkalosis, and sodium and water retention.[84]

Suppression of the Hypothalamic-Pituitary-Adrenal Axis

Sudden discontinuation of glucocorticoid therapy may result in acute adrenal insufficiency, which can be life-threatening unless treated. The risk of HPA axis suppression is related to the dose and duration of glucocorticoid therapy. In individual patients, however, it is not possible to predict HPA axis function from the dose or duration of therapy or from the basal plasma cortisol concentration.[130] The likelihood of the same daily dose of glucocorticoid resulting in suppression of the HPA axis is increased by administration in the following ways: divided doses exceeding single daily dose; single evening dose exceeding morning dose; and single morning dose exceeding alternate-day dose.[36, 131] Suppression of the HPA axis may occur rapidly, within 5 days after administration of prednisolone, 25 mg twice daily.[132] With lower doses administered once daily, however, HPA axis suppression, if it occurs, does so more slowly. Similarly, the rapidity of recovery of the HPA axis after discontinuation of glucocorticoids is inversely related to the duration of the preceding therapy. After prolonged therapy, it may be a year before HPA responses return to normal.[133]

Other Adverse Effects

Miscellaneous other adverse effects have been described. Symptoms may occur when corticosteroid therapy is discontinued, and a steroid withdrawal syndrome (which is not due to HPA axis suppression) characterized by fatigue, arthralgia, myalgia, and occasional fever has been described.[84] Rare anaphylactoid reactions to glucocorticoids occur,[134] although they are difficult to explain.

CLINICAL CONSIDERATIONS

The clinical use of corticosteroids has been characterized by considerable controversy since their introduction. After initial enthusiasm for use of corticosteroids, it was recognized by the late 1950s that controlled studies suggested only marginal clinical benefits, and long-term use of high-dose corticosteroids was associated with substantial toxicities. Therefore, during the 1960s and 1970s, physicians were taught to avoid corticosteroids whenever possible and to use a minimal dose if needed, other than in life-threatening disease situations, in which high doses were indicated. During the 1980s and 1990s, new approaches to the use of corticosteroids, primarily rapid tapering of high doses and use of low doses in rheumatoid arthritis, have resulted in more effective clinical treatment for many patients.

Although the toxicities of corticosteroids just discussed are respected and feared, it is likely that the literature concerning corticosteroids may have underestimated efficacy and overestimated toxicity, given the following considerations:

1. Most analyses were based on exposure to relatively high doses of corticosteroids over relatively long periods, which was the practice until the 1980s. *All* people who take more than 30 mg of prednisone or equivalent for more than 3 months experience significant clinical sequelae. By contrast, during the past decade, many patients have taken doses of less than 5 mg/day for many years without any evidence of meaningful problems. The distinction of high- and low-dose corticosteroids may be analogous to the distinction of one glass of wine per day, which may prolong longevity, versus many glasses of wine per day, which may shorten the life span. Much of the literature about toxicity of corticosteroids is only marginally relevant to current clinical practices.

2. The clinical severity of inflammatory rheumatic diseases traditionally has been underestimated; rheumatoid arthritis is a leading cause of disability and historically has been associated with a shortening of life span by about 10 years.[135] Systemic lupus erythematosus and vasculitis with renal involvement or polymyositis with pulmonary involvement are among the most severe diseases recognized, with a natural history of mortality considerably higher than that of many malignant and cardiovascular diseases.[136] Therefore, the side effects of corticosteroids may have been emphasized relative to the "side effects" of the inflammatory rheumatic diseases.[137] For example, it is not questioned whether use of corticosteroids is justified in patients with Hodgkin's disease, a disease with a better prognosis than vasculitis or polymyositis.

3. The efficacy of treatment with NSAIDs and second-line drugs was overestimated until recent years. Use of second-line drugs and corticosteroids in the management of rheumatoid arthritis was often deferred for many years according to traditional approaches, and gold, hydroxychloroquine, and D-penicillamine were considered "remission-inducing drugs." Therefore, evidence of radiographic progression and development of deformities while patients were taking corticosteroids was regarded as evidence that corticosteroids were not effective. Radiographic progression, however, is now recognized in almost all patients with rheumatoid arthritis treated according to traditional approaches,[138] and sustained remission is rare.[139] Therefore, evidence of disease progression in patients who take corticosteroids (or other drugs) does not necessarily indicate the absence of a disease-modifying effect, particularly since radiographic damage is present in more than 50 percent of patients within the first 2 years of disease.[140]

4. As mentioned, patients who receive corticosteroids generally have severe clinical involvement and would be expected to be more likely to experience complications of their disease, which may be interpreted as complications of corticosteroids. For example, corticosteroids are recognized as a marker for increased mortality risk from gastrointestinal bleeding in rheumatoid arthritis. However, histamine (H_2) blockers are also recognized as a marker for increased likelihood of death due to gastrointestinal bleeding,[107] not because H_2 blockers cause gastrointestinal bleeding, but because their use is more common in patients who have had symptoms and prior ulcers. Similarly, it is not known whether corticosteroids cause all vascular events, infections, and other complications experienced by patients, or rather serve as a marker for more severe disease, even in studies that have attempted to match patients who received or did not receive corticosteroid therapy.[141]

5. The efficacy of corticosteroids has been measured primarily according to traditional laboratory data, which often do not reflect clinical improvement in patients, such as lower levels of pain, malaise, and fatigue, and increased functional capacity. Until recently, these clinical phenomena were not measured and were detectable primarily through patient questionnaires or standardized clinical forms.[142] Therefore, the potential benefits of corticosteroids in patients with systemic lupus erythematosus, polymyositis, or rheumatoid arthritis have not been documented effectively in traditional clinical practice.

These considerations have led to a reassessment of clinical use of corticosteroids at this time.

USE IN RHEUMATOID ARTHRITIS

The history of studies of corticosteroids in rheumatoid arthritis is instructive about the complexity of analyzing the results of therapies for chronic diseases. During the 1950s, several formal studies were conducted in the United Kingdom by the Medical Research Council (MRC) and Nuffield Foundation. The initial study was conducted to compare cortisone, 80 mg/day (16 mg prednisone per day equivalent) with aspirin, 4.5 g/day, in patients monitored for 1 year at 3-month intervals.[143] No differences were seen between the two groups in joint tenderness, grip strength, and patient and physician global assessments, although hemoglobin levels and erythrocyte sedimentation rates were more improved in patients treated with cortisone than in those treated with aspirin.[143] Treatments were tapered for a full week before assessments at the end of each 3-month period, however, which would likely have reduced or eliminated any potential advantage of corticosteroids.

A second study of the Empire Rheumatism Council[144] involved 100 patients monitored for 1 year, 50 receiving an average of 69 mg/day of cortisone (14 mg prednisone equivalent) and 50 receiving 4 g/day of aspirin. Although radiographic progression was greater in the aspirin-treated patients, differences from the cortisone-treated patients were not statistically significant. Furthermore, no significant clinical differences were seen between the two groups of patients, leading to the conclusion that aspirin and cortisone were equivalent.[144]

A third study was reported in 1959[145] in which 41 patients who received prednisolone beginning at 20 mg/day, which was tapered to a median of 10 mg at year 2 were compared with 36 patients who received high-dose aspirin for 2 years. Radiographs of the hands and feet at baseline, 1 year, and 2 years indicated that radiographic progression occurred in seven of 41 patients treated with prednisolone after 1 year and 17 at 2 years compared with 17 of the 36 patients treated with aspirin after 1 year and 26 after 2 years. These differences were statistically significant for both hands and feet, and they documented a clinically meaningful advantage to corticosteroids. Patients were monitored during the third year,[145] at the end of which differences between the groups were not significant. However, eight of 35 patients treated initially with aspirin were given prednisone during the third year, and differences in progression may be explained by contamination of the control group.

In a 1967 report, patients who had been included in the 1959 MRC study were reviewed over longer periods.[146] Among 39 patients who had received prednisolone, 30 did not have new erosions, including 20 of the patients whose daily dose of prednisolone was less than 11 mg/day, whereas 32 of 34 patients treated with aspirin alone had new erosions over longer periods.[146] This little-known abstract indicates substantial advantages to corticosteroids.

A report in 1961[147] indicated that radiographic progression had continued in 183 patients with rheumatoid arthritis treated with hydrocortisone in the range of 25 to 100 mg/day. Functional capacity was preserved in the corticosteroid-treated patients, despite radiographic progression[147]; 136 of the patients had been treated previously with gold salts, indicating that disease had been present at least several years.

The first study of prednisone at 5 to 7.5 mg/day indicated that these doses were well tolerated and effective.[148] It was found that patients preferred the prednisone in the evening, but the study did not compare prednisone with placebo.

A short-term, double-blind study was conducted by Harris and associates, in which 18 patients received either 5 mg of prednisolone daily or placebo for 24 weeks.[149] The slight functional improvement that was seen in prednisolone-treated patients was lost when the patients were crossed over to placebo. Hand erosions progressed in one prednisolone-treated patient and four placebo-treated patients, although these differences were not statistically significant. This exploratory study suggested an advantage to corticosteroids,[149] which could not be documented definitively because of the short time frame and small numbers of patients.[150]

A report by Kirwan and associates of a randomized double-blind study over 2 years indicated that radiographic progression was statistically significantly lower in patients who took 7.5 mg prednisolone daily than in control patients given placebo.[151] Among 147 patients who had no erosions at initiation of the study, 15 of 68 (22 percent) patients in the prednisolone group versus 36 of 79 (46 percent) in the placebo group had erosions, also a statistically significant difference. Patients in the prednisolone group had greater reductions in pain and disability scores, which were significant at several intervals. No differences were seen in levels of acute-phase reactants, indicating a disassociation in evidence of disease progression according to different clinical measures.[152, 153]

Taken together, the studies suggest that prednisolone is of value in the management of rheumatoid arthritis. All formal double-blind studies indicate some advantages to corticosteroids. These studies are limited, however, by a relatively short time frame, as is the case of all randomized controlled clinical trials on rheumatoid arthritis,[150] and the toxicity of corticosteroids may be cumulative over time.[93] Therefore, a number of experts maintain that corticosteroids should be used minimally, if at all, in patients with rheumatoid arthritis,[154] and the question, unfortunately, remains open after more than 40 years of clinical use. In 15 private rheumatology practices in the United States during the mid-1980s, 75 percent of patients with rheumatoid arthritis were taking corticosteroids, generally in doses of 7.5 mg or less,[155] whereas in Europe, less than 25 percent of patients were taking prednisone.[151]

CLINICAL CONSIDERATIONS IN OTHER SITUATIONS

Inflammatory Rheumatic Diseases Other Than Rheumatoid Arthritis

In inflammatory rheumatic diseases such as systemic lupus erythematosus, vasculitis, and polymyositis, corticosteroids in the range of 1 mg/kg/day have been a standard therapy for more than three decades. Some clinicians advocate the use of higher doses, including pulses of 1 g/day. We have not found doses higher than 60 mg/day to be necessary in almost any clinical situation. This therapy should be instituted on the basis of potentially life- or organ-threatening clinical symptoms, not on the basis of a diagnosis itself, since lower doses than 1 mg/day or no corticosteroid may be appropriate in certain patients under certain circumstances.

A major problem historically has been that high-dose corticosteroids were continued for long periods. It is our current practice to initiate therapy with a immunomodulatory drug—generally methotrexate, occasionally azathioprine, and, in vasculitis, cyclo-phosphamide—in almost all patients treated with corticosteroids over longer than 60 days. We also begin to taper high-dose corticosteroids within 2 weeks of beginning the treatment, with a goal of reaching a prednisone dose below 20 mg/day within 2 to 3 months. It is rare that the dosage cannot be reduced to these levels, and substantial problems with clinical use of prolonged high-dose corticosteroids can be avoided.

Intramuscular Depot Glucocorticoid Therapy

An intramuscular injection of a long-acting corticosteroid such as methylprednisolone acetate results in low circulating concentrations of the drug for several weeks. This is useful for flareups of inflammatory rheumatic disease as an alternative to a tapering dose pack of oral prednisone. In rheumatoid arthritis, intramuscular methylprednisolone acetate, 120 mg at weeks 0, 4, and 8 controlled symptoms better than did 500 mg oral methylprednisolone pulses in patients who began therapy with gold.[156] In the management of acute gout, oral corticosteroids (prednisone, 20 to 50 mg/day tapered over 1 to 3 weeks) are effective.[157] An alternative regimen, which we prefer, is to administer a single intramuscular injection of a depot glucocorticoid. This has the advantage of a much lower total dose of corticosteroid (equivalent to 60 to 80 mg prednisone), avoids the need for complex tapering regimens, and is as effective as indomethacin in managing acute gout.[158]

Pulse Glucocorticoid Therapy

High-dose, pulsed corticosteroid treatment, usually in combination with other immunosuppressive treatment, is used to treat serious complications of systemic lupus erythematosus or vasculitis. The data that suggest efficacy in these complex clinical situations are largely from uncontrolled observations. More controversial is the use of such pulse therapy to treat active rheumatoid arthritis. The advantages of such pulses are that they do not suppress the HPA axis and they do not appear to cause osteoporosis,[159] but it is unknown whether they are more effective or safer than low doses of oral corticosteroids or intermittent use of depot injections of glucocorticoids. Significant short-term improvement in patients with

rheumatoid arthritis has been demonstrated, but the data about efficacy, duration of efficacy, and dose-response for pulse corticosteroid therapy are controversial. Pulse therapy with 1000 mg methylprednisolone administered daily for 3 days has resulted in clinical response that lasts 4 to 12 weeks[160, 161] in some reports. The minimum effective dose is unknown, and some studies have indicated other regimens, such as intravenous pulses of 320 or 100 mg, intramuscular pulses of 320 mg, or oral pulses of 1000 mg, are as effective as 1000-mg intravenous pulses.

Intravenous pulse therapy is generally safe. Serious adverse effects, including fatal arrhythmias, are rare and have been described most often in renal transplant patients. Administering the glucocorticoid slowly, over 1 to 2 hours, may decrease the likelihood of this problem. Flushing, minor increases in blood pressure, headache, and hyperglycemia (blood glucose level >110 mg/dL) are relatively common. Avascular necrosis has occurred in patients who have received pulse therapy, and although a relatively infrequent complication in patients with rheumatoid arthritis, it remains a concern.

Intra-articular Glucocorticoids

Joint and soft tissue injections of corticosteroids provide effective relief of inflammation and are commonly performed by rheumatologists.[162] This use of corticosteroids is discussed in detail in Chapter 40.

Alternate-Day Oral Glucocorticoid Therapy

The administration of a glucocorticoid of intermediate duration, such as prednisone, every second day has been advocated since it results in fewer adverse effects than the daily administration of a similar total dose.[163] Suppression of growth, suppression of the HPA axis, and cushingoid features are lessened, but osteoporosis is not prevented by alternate-day administration. Switching from single daily dosing to alternate-day dosing should be gradual—usually over weeks. This is most easily achieved by simultaneously increasing the dose on the "on" day and decreasing the dose on the "off" day. Although alternate-day therapy may be effective in certain patients, almost all patients with inflammatory rheumatic disease have better results with daily administration of corticosteroids.

Perioperative Glucocorticoid Cover

Supplemental glucocorticoid cover should be considered for any patient who has received corticosteroids for more than a few weeks in the previous year. The integrity of the HPA axis can be tested using an ACTH stimulation test. Adrenal function can be regarded as normal if the plasma cortisol level is over 18 to 20 µg/dl 30 minutes after 250 µg of ACTH is adminstered intravenously or intramuscularly.[164] A formal test is clinically unnecessary, however, and it is pragmatic to administer supplemental corticosteroids to all patients who are taking glucocorticoids.

The dose required for perioperative glucocorticoid cover is not high. Physiologic cortisol secretion in response to major surgery is approximately 75 to 150 mg/day and returns to baseline 24 to 48 hours after surgery.[165] The doses of hydrocortisone commonly administered for perioperative corticosteroid supplementation (100 mg with anesthetic induction and every 6 hours thereafter for 72 hours) are, therefore, more than adequate. Several regimens with lower doses have been suggested. These include 100 mg hydrocortisone infused continuously over 24 hours and administration of the usual dose of oral prednisone on the day of surgery followed by hydrocortisone, 25 to 50 mg, immediately preoperatively and every 8 hours thereafter for 48 to 72 hours.[165] Glucocorticoid supplementation requirements for minor or moderate surgical procedures are even lower, and patients can return to their usual prednisone dose on the second postoperative day.[165]

GUIDELINES FOR USE IN CLINICAL PRACTICE

Clinical use of corticosteroids continues to evolve. It is hoped that further studies will become available to clarify the matter further. Some guidelines for clinicians might include the following[166, 167]:

1. It is important to recognize the difference between high-dose and low-dose corticosteroids. Doses of 50 to 80 mg prednisone are needed in certain patients but are undesirable for longer than 2 to 3 months. Doses above 7.5 mg are contraindicated in most patients with rheumatoid arthritis. At the same time, many patients with rheumatoid arthritis have experienced great benefit with doses of prednisone in the range of 2 to 4 mg/day.

2. High-dose corticosteroids in the range of 60 to 80 mg/day may be lifesaving in acute flares of diseases such as systemic lupus erythematosus, polymyositis, and vasculitis. However, the dosage should be reduced to 30 mg/day or less within 6 to 10 weeks, and maintenance therapy should be conducted at levels of 15 mg/day or lower. Most patients with these diseases should also be treated with an immunomodulatory drug, often at onset of treatment.

3. Use of low-dose corticosteroids, which are in clinical use in more than 75 percent of patients with rheumatoid arthritis treated in private practices of rheumatology in the United States, appears to be a reasonable practice, based on data about the HPA axis in patients with inflammatory rheumatic diseases. Such therapy may be associated with improved outcomes, although some experienced observers continue to advocate avoidance of all corticosteroids in patients with rheumatoid arthritis.

4. Corticosteroids alone rarely are effective in ob-

taining optimal control of *any* chronic inflammatory rheumatic disease, including rheumatoid arthritis, systemic lupus erythematosus, polymyositis, or vasculitis. An immunomodulatory drug is generally needed as an adjunct for optimal control; in rheumatoid arthritis and polymyositis, methotrexate is the preferred drug in vasculitides and in some cases of lupus nephritis or cerebritis, in which case cyclophosphamide is the cytotoxic drug of choice.

5. Once disease control has been established, the corticosteroid dose is tapered to below 15 mg/day. In patients receiving doses of corticosteroids greater than 30 mg/day, the dose can be tapered relatively rapidly at rates of 5 to 10 mg/week. When the dose is below 20 mg/day prednisone, however, the dose should be tapered by 2.5 to 5 mg every 2 to 4 weeks. When patients are taking 10 mg or less, the usual practice is to taper prednisone in 1-mg decrements each month.

6. Adverse effects of corticosteroids are largely related to dose and duration of therapy. It is reasonable to consider interventions to prevent osteoporosis in any patient who is or will be treated with prolonged corticosteroid therapy, particularly at high doses.[94, 168] The therapeutic intervention chosen may be influenced by measurement of bone density. Measurement of baseline bone density in patients likely to receive long-term low-dose corticosteroid therapy may provide useful baseline and monitoring data for making decisions regarding prevention of osteoporosis in an individual patient.

7. A practice of maintaining therapy with long-term low-dose maintenance corticosteroids, rather than discontinuing therapy entirely in patients with inflammatory rheumatic diseases, has been adapted by some rheumatologists. Most rheumatologists have experienced a situation in which the physician and patient thought that something important had been accomplished as a patient was taken off steroid therapy, but a substantial flareup occurred 1 to 6 months later. Indefinite low dosing (2–5 mg daily) of prednisone may be a reasonable practice for many patients, although this has not been proved.

8. To document these situations, it is desirable that clinicians monitor self-report questionnaires and develop data bases of the collected information, which are the *only* ways in which better information will become available about clinical use of corticosteroids in patients with rheumatic diseases.[142] Randomized, double-blind, controlled trials have many significant limitations,[150] particularly the short time frame, and are not likely to ever provide the best information about the optimal uses of corticosteroids in patients with rheumatic disease.

References

1. Hench PS: The reversibility of certain rheumatic and non-rheumatic conditions by the use of cortisone or of the pituitary adrenocorticotropic hormone. Ann Intern Med 36:1, 1952.
2. Axelrod L: Glucocorticoid therapy. Medicine 55:39, 1976.

3. Schimmer BP, Parker KL: Adrenocorticotropic hormone: Adrenocortical steroids and their synthetic analogs; inhibitors of the synthesis and actions of adrenocortical hormones. *In* Hardman JG, Limbird LE, Molinoff PB, Ruddow RW, Gilman A (eds): The Pharmacological Basis of Therapeutics. New York, McGraw-Hill, 1996, pp 1459–1485.

4. Markham A, Bryson HM: Deflazacort: A review of its pharmacological properties and therapeutic efficacy. Drugs 50:317, 1995.

5. Tsigos C, Chrousos GP: Physiology of the hypothalamic-adrenal axis in health and dysregulation in psychiatric and autoimmune diseases. Endocrinol Metab Clin North Am 23:451, 1994.

6. Chrousos GP: Regulation and dysregulation of the hypothalamic-pituitary-adrenal axis: The corticotropin-releasing hormone perspective. Endocrinol Metab Clin North Am 21:833, 1992.

7. Chrousos GP: The hypothalamic-pituitary-adrenal axis and immune-mediated inflammation. N Engl J Med 332:1351, 1995.

8. Harkness JAL, Richter MB, Panayi GS, et al: Circadian variation in disease activity in rheumatoid arthritis. Br Med J 284:551, 1982.

9. Saldahna C, Touzas G, Grace E: Evidence for the inflammatory effects of normal circulating plasma cortisol. Clin Exp Rheumatol 4:365, 1986.

10. Sternberg EM, Young WS, Bernadini R, et al: A central nervous system defect in the biosynthesis of CRH is associated with susceptibility to streptococcal cell wall–induced arthritis in Lewis rats. Proc Natl Acad Sci USA 86:4771, 1989.

11. Neeck G, Federlin K, Graek V, et al: Adrenal secretion of cortisol in patients with rheumatoid arthritis. J Rheumatol 17:24, 1990.

12. Chikanza IC, Petrou P, Kingsley G, et al: Defective hypothalamic response to immune and inflammatory stimuli in patients with rheumatoid arthritis. Arthritis Rheum 35:1281, 1992.

13. Barnes PM, Adcock I: Antiinflammatory actions of steroids: Molecular mechanisms. Trends Pharmacol Sci 14:436, 1993.

14. Evans RM: The steroid and thyroid hormone receptor superfamily. Science 240:889, 1988.

15. Pratt WB: The role of heat shock proteins in regulating the function, folding and trafficking of the glucocorticoid receptor. J Biol Chem 268:21455, 1993.

16. Schmidt TJ, Meyer AS: Autoregulation of corticosteroid receptors: How, when, where, and why? Receptor 4:229, 1994.

17. Truss M, Beato M: Steroid hormone receptors: interactions with deoxyribonucleic acid and transcription factors. Endocr Rev 14:459, 1993.

18. Akerblom IE, Slater EP, Beato M, et al: Negative regulation by glucocorticoid through interference with a cAMP responsive enhancer. Science 24:350, 1988.

19. Yang-Yen HF, Chambard JC, Sun YL, et al: Transcriptional interference between c-Jun and the glucocorticoid receptor: Mutual inhibition of DNA binding due to direct protein-protein interaction. Cell 62:1205, 1990.

20. Chrousos GP, Detera-Wadleigh SD, Karl M: Syndromes of glucocorticoid resistance. Ann Intern Med 119:1113, 1993.

21. Schleimer RP: An overview of glucocorticoid anti-inflammatory actions. Eur J Clin Pharmacol 45(Suppl 1):S3, 1993.

22. Barnes PJ, Adcock IM: Steroid resistance in asthma. Q J Med 88:455, 1995.

23. Flower RJ, Rothwell NJ: Lipocortin-1: Cellular mechanisms and clinical relevance. Trends Pharmacol Sci 15:71, 1994.

24. Bailey JM: New mechanisms for the effects of anti-inflammatory glucocorticoids. Biofactors 3:97, 1991.

25. Peretti M, Flower RJ: Modulation of IL-1–induced neutrophil migration by dexamethasone and lipocortin 1. J Immunol 150:992, 1993.

26. Masferrer JL, Seibert K, Zweifel B, et al: Endogenous glucocorticoids regulate an inducible cyclooxygenase enzyme. Proc Natl Acad Sci U S A 89:3917, 1992.

27. Radomski MW, Palmer RMJ, Moncada S: Glucocorticoids inhibit the expression of an inducible, but not the constitutive, nitric oxide synthase in vascular endothelial cells. Proc Natl Acad Sci U S A 87:10043, 1990.

28. Guyre PM, Girard MT, Morganelli PM, et al: Glucocorticoid effects on the production and actions of immune cytokines. J Steroid Biochem 30:89, 1988.

29. Paliogianni F, Raptis A, Ahuja SS, et al: Negative transcriptional regulation of the human interleukin-2 gene by glucocorticoids through interference with nuclear factors Ap-1 and NF-AT. J Clin Invest 91:1481, 1993.

30. Arya SK, Wong-Staal F, Gallo RC: Dexamethasone mediated inhibition of human T cell growth factor and gamma interferon messenger RNA. J Immunol 133:273, 1984.

31. Boumpas DT, Chrousos GP, Wilder RL, et al: Glucocorticoid therapy for immune-mediated disease: Basic and clinical correlates. Ann Intern Med 119:1198, 1993.

32. Cronstein BN, Kimmel SC, Levin RI, et al: A mechanism for the antiinflammatory effects of corticosteroids: The glucocorticoid receptor regulates leukocyte adhesion to endothelial cells and expression of endothelial-leukocyte adhesion molecule-1 and intracellular adhesion molecule-1. Proc Natl Acad Sci USA 89:9991, 1992.

33. Borson DB, Jew S, Gruenert DC: Glucocorticoids induce neutral endopeptidase in transformed human tracheal epithelial cells. Am J Physiol 260:L83, 1991.

34. Carnuccio R, Di Rosa M, Guerrasio B, et al: Vasocortin: A novel glucocorticoid-induced anti-inflammatory protein. Br J Pharmacol 90:443, 1987.

35. Dale DC, Fauci AS, Wolff SM: Alternate day prednisone. Leukocyte kinetics and susceptibility to infections. N Engl J Med 291:1154, 1974.

36. Fauci AS, Dale DC, Balow JE: Glucocorticoid therapy: Mechanisms of action and clinical considerations. Ann Intern Med 84:304, 1976.

37. Cox G: Glucocorticoid treatment inhibits apoptosis in human neutrophils: Separation of survival and activation outcomes. J Immunol 154:4719, 1995.

38. Balow JE, Rosenthal AS: Glucocorticoid suppression of macrophage migration inhibitory factor. J Exp Med 137:1031, 1973.

39. Ponzin D, Bellini F, Chizzolini C: Antigen presentation is inhibited in vivo by betamethasone. Life Sci 56:1595, 1995.

40. Gerrard TL, Cupps TR, Jurgensen CH, et al: Hydrocortisone-mediated inhibition of monocyte antigen presentation: Dissociation of inhibitory effect and expression of DR antigens. Cell Immunol 85:330, 1984.

41. Claman HN, Moorhead JW, Benner WH: Corticosteroids and lymphoid cells in vitro. I: Hydrocortisone lysis of human, guinea pig, and mouse thymus cells. J Lab Clin Med 78:499, 1971.

42. Nieto MA, Gonzalex A, Gambon F, et al: Apoptosis in human thymocytes after treatment with glucocorticoids. Clin Exp Immunol 88:341, 1992.

43. Nowell PC: Inhibition of human leukocyte mitosis by prednisone in vitro. Cancer Res 21:344, 1961.

44. Horst HJ, Flad HJ: Corticosteroid–interleukin-2 interactions: Inhibition of binding of interleukin 2 to interleukin 2 receptors. Clin Exp Immunol 68:156, 1987.

45. Paliogianni F, Ahuja FS, Balow JP, et al: Novel mechanism for inhibition of T cells by glucocorticoids (GC): GC modulate signal transduction through IL 2 receptor. J Immunol 151:4081, 1993.

46. Cupps TR, Gerrard TL, Flakoff RJ, et al: Effects of in vitro corticosteroids on B cell activation, proliferation, and differentiation. J Clin Invest 75:754, 1985.

47. Andersen V, Bro-Rasmussen F, Hougaard K: Autoradiographic studies of eosinophil kinetics: Effects of cortisol. Cell Tissue Kinet 2:139, 1969.

48. Wallen H, Kita H, Weiler D, et al: Glucocorticoids inhibit cytokine-mediated eosinophil survival. J Immunol 147:3490, 1991.

49. Schleimer RP, Derse CP, Friedman B, et al: Regulation of human basophil mediator release by cytokines. I: Interaction with antiinflammatory steroids. J Immunol 143:1310, 1989.

50. Daeron M, Sterk AR, Hirata F, et al: Biochemical analysis of glucocorticoid-induced inhibition of IgE-mediated histamine release from mouse mast cells. J Immunol 129:1212, 1982.

51. McMahon M, Gerich J, Rizza R: Effects of glucocorticoids on glucose metabolism. Diabetes Metab Rev 4:17, 1988.

52. Ettinger WH, Goldberg AP, Applebaum-Bowden D, et al: Dyslipoproteinemia in systemic lupus erythematosus: Effect of corticosteroids. Am J Med 83:503, 1987.

53. Ettinger WH, Klinefelter HF, Kwiterovitch PO: Effect of short-term, low dose corticosteroids on plasma lipoprotein lipids. Atherosclerosis 63:167, 1987.

54. Frey BM, Frey FJ: Clinical pharmacokinetics of prednisone and prednisolone. Clin Pharmacokinet 19:126, 1990.

55. Pickup ME: Clinical pharmacokinetics of prednisone and prednisolone. Clin Pharmacokinet 4:111, 1979.

56. Begg EJ, Atkinson HC, Giararakis N: The pharmacokinetics of corticosteroid agents. Med J Aust 146:37, 1987.

57. Ferry JJ, Horvath AM, Bekersky I, et al: Relative and absolute bioavailability of prednisone and prednisolone after separate oral and intravenous doses. J Clin Pharmacol 28:81, 1988.

58. Powell LW, Axelsen E: Corticosteroids in liver disease: Studies on the biological conversion of prednisone to prednisolone and plasma protein binding. Gut 13:690, 1972.

59. Brien TG: Human corticosteroid binding globulin. Rev Clin Endocrinol 14:193, 1981.

60. Meffin PJ, Brooks PM, Sallustio BC: Alterations in prednisolone disposition as a result of time of administration, gender, and dose. Br J Clin Pharmacol 17:394, 1984.

61. Stjernholm MR, Katz FH: Effects of diphenylhydantoin, phenobarbital and diazepam on the metabolism of methylprednisolone and prednisolone in man. J Clin Endocrinol Metab 41:887, 1975.

62. Garg V, Jusko WJ: Bioavailability and reversible metabolism of prednisone and prednisolone in man. Biopharm Drug Dispos 15:163, 1994.

63. Tanner A, Bochner F, Caffin J, et al: Dose-dependent prednisolone kinetics. Clin Pharmacol Ther 25:571, 1979.

64. Toothaker RD, Welling PG: Effect of dose size on the pharmacokinetics of intravenous hydrocortisone during endogenous hydrocortisone suppression. J Pharmacokinet Biopharm 10:147, 1982.

65. Dasgupta B, Gray J, Fernandes L, et al: Treatment of polymyalgia

rheumatica with intramuscular injections of depot methylprednisolone. Ann Rheum Dis 50:942, 1991.

66. Derendorf H, Mollman H, Gruner A, et al: Pharmacokinetics and pharmacodynamic of glucocorticoid suspensions after intra-articular administration. Clin Pharmacol Ther 39:313, 1986.

67. Lewis GP, Jusko WJ, Burke CW, et al: Prednisone side-effects and serum protein levels. Lancet 2:778, 1971.

68. Hill MR, Szefler SJ, Ball BD, et al: Monitoring glucocorticoid therapy: A pharmacokinetic approach. Clin Pharmacol Ther 1995.

69. Reinisch JM, Simon NG: Prenatal exposure to prednisone in humans and animals retards intra-uterine growth. Science 202:147, 1978.

70. Logaridis TE, Doran TA, Scott JG, et al: The effect of maternal steroid administration on fetal platelet count in immunologic thrombocytopenic purpura. Am J Obstet Gynecol 145:147, 1983.

71. Ostensen M: Optimization of antirheumatic drug treatment in pregnancy, Clin Pharmakokinet 27:486, 1994.

72. Beitins IZ, Bayard F, Ances IG, et al: The transplacental passage of prednisone and prednisolone in pregnancy near term. J Pediatr 81:936, 1972.

73. Levitz M, Jansen V, Dancis J: The transfer and metabolism of corticosteroids in the perfused human placenta. Am J Obstet Gynecol 132:363, 1978.

74. Osathanondh R, Tulchinsky D, Kamali H, et al: Dexamethasone levels in treated pregnant women and newborn infants. J Pediatr 90:617, 1977.

75. Rider LG, Buyon JP, Rutledge J, et al: Treatment of neonatal lupus: case report and review of the literature. J Rheumatol 20:1208, 1993.

76. Liggins GC, Howie RN: A controlled trial of antepartum glucocorticoid treatment for prevention of the respiratory distress syndrome in premature infants. Pediatrics 50:515, 1972.

77. Katz FH, Duncan BR: Entry of prednisone into human breast milk. N Engl J Med 293:1154, 1975.

78. Rayburn WF: Glucocorticoid therapy for rheumatic diseases: Maternal, fetal and breast-feeding considerations. Am J Reprod Immunol 28:138, 1992.

79. Committee on Drugs, American Academy of Pediatrics: The transfer of drugs and other chemicals into human breast milk. Pediatrics 84:924, 1989.

80. Carrie F, Roblot P, Bouquet S, et al: Rifampin-induced nonresponsiveness of giant cell arteritis to prednisone treatment. Arch Intern Med 154:1521, 1994.

81. Yamashita SK, Ludwig EA, Middleton E, et al: Lack of pharmacokinetic and pharmacodynamic interactions between ketoconazole and prednisolone. Clin Pharmacol Ther 49:558, 1991.

82. Klinenberg JR, Miller F: Effects of corticosteroids on blood salicylate concentration. JAMA 194:131, 1965.

83. Kozower M, Veatch L, Kaplan MM: Decreased clearance of prednisolone, a factor in the development of corticosteroid side effects. J Clin Endocrinol Metab 38:407, 1974.

84. Cooper C, Kirwan JR: The risks of local and systemic corticosteroid administration. Baillieres Clin Rheumatol 4:305, 1990.

85. Beisel WR, Rapoport MI: Adrenocortical function and infectious illness. N Engl J Med 280:541, 1969.

86. Dale DC, Petersdorf RG: Corticosteroids and infectious disease. Med Clin North Am 57:1277, 1973.

87. Aucott JN: Glucocorticoids and infection. Endocrinol Metab Clin North Am 23:655, 1994.

88. Stuck AE, Minder CE, Frey FJ: Risk of infectious complications in patients taking glucocorticoids. Rev Infect Dis 11:954, 1989.

89. Smyllie HC, Connoly CK: Incidence of serious complications of corticosteroid therapy in respiratory disease: A retrospective survey of patients in the Brompton Hospital. Thorax 23:571, 1968.

90. Leiberman P, Patterson RP, Kunski R: Complication of long-term steroid therapy for asthma. J Allergy Clin Immunol 49:329, 1972.

91. Lukert BP, Raisz LG: Glucocorticoid-induced osteoporosis. Rheum Dis Clin North Am 20:629, 1994.

92. Sambrook PN, Jones G: Corticosteroid osteoporosis. Br J Rheumatol 34:8, 1995.

93. Dequeker J, Westhovens R: Low dose corticosteroid associated osteoporosis in rheumatoid arthritis and its prophylaxis and treatment: Bones of contention. J Rheumatol 22:1013, 1995.

94. Buckley LM, Leib ES, Cartularo KS, et al: Effects of low dose corticosteroids on the bone mineral density of patients with rheumatoid arthritis. J Rheumatol 22:1055, 1995.

95. Hall GM, Daniels M, Doyle DV, et al: Effect of hormone replacement therapy on bone mass in rheumatoid arthritis patients treated with and without steroids. Arthritis Rheum 10:1499, 1994.

96. Joseph JC: Corticosteroid-induced osteoporosis. Am J Hosp Pharm 51:188, 1994.

97. Adachi JD, Bensen WG, Hodsman AB: Corticosteroid-induced osteoporosis. Semin Arthritis Rheum 22:375, 1993.

98. Messina OD, Barreira JC, Zanchetta JR, et al: Effect of low doses of deflazacort on bone mineral content in premenopausal rheumatoid arthritis. J Rheumatol 19:1520, 1992.

99. Mankin HJ: Nontraumatic necrosis of bone (osteonecrosis). N Engl J Med 326:1473, 1992.

100. Zizic TM: Osteonecrosis. Curr Opin Rheumatol 3:481, 1991.

101. Felson DT, Anderson JJ: A cross-study evaluation of association between steroid dose and bolus steroids and avascular necrosis of bone. Lancet 1:902, 1987.

102. Bowyer SL, LaMothe MP, Hollister JR: Steroid myopathy: Incidence and detection in a population with asthma. J Allergy Clin Immunol 76:234, 1985.

103. Dekhuizen PN, Decramer M: Steroid-induced myopathy and its significance to respiratory disease: A known disease rediscovered. Eur Respir J 5:997, 1992.

104. Conn HO, Blitzer BL: Nonassociation of adrenocorticosteroid therapy and peptic ulcer. N Engl J Med 294:473, 1976.

105. Messer J, Reitman D, Sacks HS, et al: Association of adrenocorticosteroid therapy and peptic ulcer disease. N Engl J Med 309:21, 1983.

106. Conn HO, Poynard T: Adrenocorticosteroid administration and peptic ulcer: A critical analysis. J Chronic Dis 38:457, 1985.

107. Fries JF, Williams CA, Bloch DA, et al: Nonsteroidal anti-inflammatory drug–associated gastropathy: Incidence and risk factor models. Am J Med 91:213, 1991.

108. Piper JM, Ray WA, Daugherty JR, et al: Corticosteroid use and peptic ulcer disease: Role of nonsteroidal anti-inflammatory drugs. Ann Intern Med 114:735, 1991.

109. Sterioff S, Oringer MB, Cameron JL: Colon perforation associated with steroid therapy. Surgery 75:56, 1974.

110. Stumpf HH, Wilens SL, Somoza C: Pancreatic lesions and peripancreatic fat necrosis in cortisone treated rabbits. Lab Invest 5:224, 1956.

111. Carone FA, Liebow AA: Acute pancreatitis lesions in patients treated with ACTH and adrenal corticoids. N Engl J Med 257:690, 1957.

112. Petri M: Pancreatitis in systemic lupus erythematosus: Still in search of a mechanism. J Rheumatol 19:1014, 1992.

113. Danese RD, Aron DC: Cushing's syndrome and hypertension. Endocrinol Metab Clin North Am 23:299, 1994.

114. Walker BR, Edwards CR: New mechanisms for corticosteroid-induced hypertension. Br Med Bull 50:342, 1994.

115. Jackson SHD, Beevers DG, Myers K: Does long-term, low-dose, corticosteroid therapy cause hypertension? Clin Sci 61(Suppl 7):381S, 1981.

116. Nashel DJ: Is atherosclerosis a complication of long-term corticosteroid therapy? Am J Med 80:925, 1986.

117. Petri M, Perez-Gutthan S, Spence D, et al: Risk factors for coronary artery disease in patients with systemic lupus erythematosus. Am J Med 93:513, 1992.

118. Maxwell SR, Moots RJ, Kendall MJ: Corticosteroids: Do they damage the cardiovascular system? Postgrad Med J 70:863, 1994.

119. Lewis AD, Smith RD: Steroid-induced psychiatric syndromes. J Affect Disord 5:319, 1983.

120. Ling MH, Perry PJ, Tsuang MT: Side effects of corticosteroid therapy: Psychiatric aspects. Arch Gen Psychiatry 38:471, 1981.

121. Klein JF: Adverse psychiatric effects of systemic glucocorticoid therapy. Am Fam Physician 46:1469, 1992.

122. Boston Collaborative Drug Surveillance Program: Acute adverse reactions to prednisone in relation to dose. Clin Pharmacol Ther 13:694, 1972.

123. Falk WE, Mahnke MW, Poskanzer DC: Lithium prophylaxis of corticotropin-induced psychosis. JAMA 241:1011, 1979.

124. Intracranial hypertension and steroids. (editorial). Lancet 2:1052, 1964.

125. Urban RC Jr, Cotlier E: Corticosteroid-induced cataracts. Surv Ophthalmol 31:102, 1986.

126. Loredo A, Rodriguez RS, Murillo L: Cataracts after short-term corticosteroid treatment. N Engl J Med 286:160, 1972.

127. Urban RC, Dreyer EB: Corticosteroid-induced glaucoma. Int Ophthalmol Clin 33:135, 1993.

128. Blerau R, Weingarten C: Diabetic acidosis secondary to steroid therapy. N Engl J Med 271:836, 1964.

129. Seale JP, Compton MR: Side-effects of corticosteroid agents. Med J Aust 144:139, 1986.

130. Schlagheck R, Kornely E, Santen RT, et al: The effect of long-term glucocorticoid therapy on pituitary-adrenal responses to exogenous corticotropin-releasing hormone. N Engl J Med 326:226, 1992.

131. Harter JG, Reddy WJ, Thorn GW: Studies of an intermittent corticosteroid dosage regimen. N Engl J Med 269:591, 1963.

132. Streck WF, Lockwood DH: Pituitary adrenal recovery following short-term suppression with corticosteroids. Am J Med 66:910, 1979.

133. Livanou T, Ferriman D, James VHT: Recovery of hypothalamo-pituitary adrenal function after corticosteroid therapy. Lancet 2:857, 1967.

134. Fulcher DA, Katelaris CH: Anaphylactoid reaction to intravenous hydrocortisone succinate: A case report and literature review. Med J Aust 154:210, 1991.

135. Pincus T, Wolfe F, Callahan LF: Updating a reassessment of traditional paradigms concerning rheumatoid arthritis. In Wolfe F, Pincus T (eds): Rheumatoid Arthritis: Pathogenesis, Assessment, Outcome, and Treatment. New York, Marcel Dekker, 1994, p 1.

136. Callahan LF, Pincus T: Mortality in rheumatic diseases. Arthritis Care Res 1995 8:229, 1995.
137. Pincus T, Callahan LF: The "side effects" of rheumatoid arthritis: Joint destruction, disability and early mortality. Br J Rheumatol 32(Suppl 1):28, 1993.
138. Fuchs HA, Pincus T: Radiographic damage in rheumatoid arthritis: Description by nonlinear models (editorial). J Rheumatol 19:1655, 1992.
139. Wolfe F, Hawley DJ: Remission in rheumatoid arthritis. J Rheumatol 12:245, 1985.
140. Fuchs HA, Kaye JJ, Callahan LF, et al: Evidence of significant radiographic damage in rheumatoid arthritis within the first 2 years of disease. J Rheumatol 16:585, 1989.
141. McDougall R, Sibley J, Haga M, Russell A: Outcome in patients with rheumatoid arthritis receiving prednisone compared to matched controls. J Rheumatol 21:1207–1213, 1994.
142. Pincus T: Why should rheumatologists collect patient self-report questionnaires in routine rheumatologic care? Rheum Dis Clin North Am 21:271, 1995.
143. Joint Committee of the Medical Research Council and Nuffield Foundation: A comparison of cortisone and aspirin in the treatment of early cases of rheumatoid arthritis. Br Med J 29:1223, 1954.
144. Empire Rheumatism Council: Multi-centre controlled trial comparing cortisone acetate and acetyl salicylic acid in the long-term treatment of rheumatoid arthritis. Ann Rheum Dis 14:353, 1955.
145. Joint Committee of the Medical Research Council and Nuffield Foundation: A comparison of prednisolone with aspirin or other analgesics in the treatment of rheumatoid arthritis. Ann Rheum Dis 18:173, 1959.
146. West HF: Rheumatoid arthritis: The relevance of clinical knowledge to research activities. Abstr World Med 41:401, 1967.
147. Berntsen CA, Freyberg RH: Rheumatoid patients after five or more years of corticosteroid treatment: A comparative analysis of 183 cases. Ann Intern Med 54:938, 1961.
148. deAndrade JR, McCormick JN, Hill AGS: Small doses of prednisolone in the management of rheumatoid arthritis. Ann Rheum Dis 23:158, 1964.
149. Harris ED Jr, Emkey RD, Nichols JE, et al: Low dose prednisone therapy in rheumatoid arthritis: A double blind study. J Rheumatol 10:713, 1983.
150. Pincus T, Stein M: What is the best source of useful data on the treatment of rheumatoid arthritis: Clinical trials, clinical observations, or clinical protocols? J Rheumatol 22:1611, 1995.
151. Kirwan JR, and The Arthritis and Rheumatism Council Low-Dose Glucocorticoid Study Group: The effect of glucocorticoids on joint destruction in rheumatoid arthritis. N Engl J Med 333:142, 1995.
152. Fuchs HA, Callahan LF, Kaye JJ, et al: Radiographic and joint count findings of the hand in rheumatoid arthritis: Related and unrelated findings. Arthritis Rheum 31:44, 1988.
153. Pincus T, Callahan LF: Prognostic markers of activity and damage in rheumatoid arthritis: Why clinical trials and inception cohort studies indicate more favorable outcomes than studies of patients with established disease. Br J Rheumatol 34:196, 1995.
154. Ramos-Remus C, Sibley J, Russell AS: Steroids in RA: The honeymoon revisited. J Rheumatol 19:667, 1992.
155. Pincus T, Marcum SB, Callahan LF: Long-term drug therapy for rheumatoid arthritis in seven rheumatology private practices. II: Second-line drugs and prednisone. J Rheumatol 19:1885, 1992.
156. Choy EHS, Kingsley GH, Corkhill MM, et al: Intramuscular methylprednisolone is superior to pulse oral methylprednisolone during the induction phase of chrysotherapy. Br J Rheumatol 32:734, 1993.
157. Groff GG, Franck WA, Raddatz DA: Systemic steroid therapy for acute gout: A clinical trial and review of the literature. Semin Arthritis Rheum 19:329, 1990.
158. Alloway JA, Moriarty MJ, Hoogland YT, et al: Comparison of triamcinolone acetonide with indomethacin in the treatment of acute gouty arthritis. J Rheumatol 20:111, 1993.
159. Smith MD, Bertouch JV, Smith AM, et al: The clinical and immunological effects of pulse methylprednisolone therapy in rheumatoid arthritis. I: Clinical effects. J Rheumatol 15:229, 1988.
160. Weusten BLAM, Jacobs JWG, Bijlsma JWJ: Corticosteroid pulse therapy in active rheumatoid arthritis. Semin Arthritis Rheum 23:183–192, 1993.
161. George E. Kirwan Jr: Corticosteroid therapy in rheumatoid arthritis. Baillieres Clin Rheum 4:621, 1990.
162. McCarthy GM, McCarty DJ: Intrasynovial corticosteroid therapy. Bull Rheum Dis 43:2, 1994.
163. Fauci AS: Alternate-day corticosteroid therapy. Am J Med 64:729, 1978.
164. May ME, Carey RM: Rapid adrenocorticotropin hormone test in practice. Am J Med 79:679, 1985.
165. Salem M, Tanish RE, Bromberg J, et al: Perioperative glucocorticoid coverage: A reassessment 42 years after emergence of a problem. Ann Surg 219:416, 1994.
166. Weiss MM: Corticosteroids in rheumatoid arthritis. Semin Arthritis Rheum 19:9–21, 1989.
167. Weisman MH: Should steroids be used in the management of rheumatoid arthritis? Rheum Dis Clin North Am 19:189–199, 1993.
168. Meunier PJ: Is steroid-induced osteoporosis preventable? N Engl J Med 328:1781–1782, 1993.

CHAPTER 51

Anthony S. Fauci
K. Randall Young, Jr.

Immunoregulatory Agents

Immunoregulation can be broadly defined as the complex process whereby immunologic reactivity, either cellular or humoral, is constantly modulated to result in the net expression of an appropriate or, in certain circumstances, inappropriate immune response.[1] Intensive interest and investigation in immunology, which have led to certain rather striking advances in our understanding of the complexities of immune function and regulation in animal models as well as in humans, together with the observations that many rheumatic diseases are at least associated with aberrancies of immune function including immunoregulation,[1–5] form the intellectual basis for the use of immunoregulatory agents in the treatment of certain rheumatic diseases. It should be pointed out, however, that the use of cytotoxic and other immunoregulatory agents in these diseases antedated the most recent advances in our understanding of many of the subtle complexities of immune regulation. This is particularly true of the use of glucocorticoids and cytotoxic agents in diseases whose clinicopathologic manifestations were strongly suggestive of aberrant inflammatory or immune-mediated phenomena. Because the use of these agents generally resulted in suppression of inflammation and immune function, it is not surprising that they have been extensively used in certain rheumatic, connective tissue, and autoimmune diseases.[6–10]

Unfortunately, even though advances in our understanding of immune function and regulation have allowed a greater intellectual understanding of the potential mechanisms of aberrant immune function in the diseases in question, the extraordinary complexity of the immune system, with its various inductive, regulatory effector, and feedback mechanisms, has made it clear to clinical investigators that perturbation of the system by agents used for therapeutic purposes may have multifaceted effects on the system, some of which might be unpredictable, if not unrecognized. This very complexity of the system in the face of the relatively crude and usually nonspecific modulation effected by most of the therapeutic agents in question may result in only a minor or temporary dampening of the expression of the disease process. On the other hand, the adverse effects associated with perturbation of the immune system in this manner may place the resultant therapeutic efficacy beyond the limits of the price that one is willing to pay for such an effect. Certain immunoregulatory agents have been used and are being used inappropriately in diseases whose severity or projected clinical course clearly does not warrant such an aggressive approach. Nonetheless, despite these general caveats, certain cytotoxic and other immunoregulatory agents have been successfully and appropriately employed in the treatment of a number of rheumatic diseases and in certain situations with rather impressive results.[6, 8–10]

It is the aim of this chapter to consider some of the real and potential mechanisms whereby one can feasibly and successfully modify the expression of aberrant inflammatory and immune responses. This chapter also discusses the mechanisms of action of the various categories of immunoregulatory agents as well as their proven and potential usefulness in the treatment of rheumatic diseases to better appreciate the positive and negative aspects of such a therapeutic approach.

IMMUNE SYSTEM AND ITS REGULATION

A number of models of the immune system and its regulation have been proposed, and each almost invariably has the common denominator of a cellular and humoral network of immune reactivity reflected by different cell types. The dual limbs of the immune response hypothesized years ago[11–14] and now clearly substantiated are the thymus-derived (T) lymphocyte limb and the bone marrow–derived or bursa-equivalent (B) lymphocyte limb, both of which derive from a common stem cell. Other cell types, such as the monocyte-macrophage, play a major role in the inductive, regulatory, and effector phases of the immune response.[15]

A somewhat simplified scheme of the immune system is illustrated in Figure 51–1. Despite its inherent simplification, this figure illustrates the manifold complexity and multiple interrelationships among various immune cells. As has been previously and extensively described, the expression of immune function can be conveniently looked on as a series of phases. Both T and B lymphocytes mediate a number of critical immune functions, and each of these cell types, when given the appropriate signal, passes through phases, from activation or induction through proliferation, differentiation, and ultimately effector function.[3, 5] The effector function that is expressed may be at the endpoint of a response, such as secretion of antibody by a differentiated B lymphocyte or

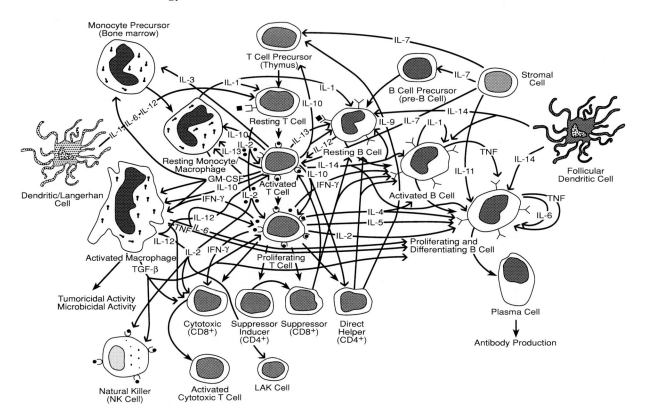

Figure 51–1. Schematic diagram of the human immunoregulatory network. IL, interleukin; IFN, interferon; LAK, lymphokine-activated killer cell; TGF-β, transforming growth factor-β; TNF, tumor necrosis factor; GM-CSF, granulocyte-macrophage colony-stimulating factor. See text.

plasma cell, or it might serve a regulatory function that modulates other end-stage functions, as is seen with inducer or suppressor T lymphocytes that modulate the function of B lymphocytes, T lymphocytes, other lymphoid cells, or even certain nonlymphoid cell types. Briefly, in addition to induction and suppression, T lymphocytes in cooperation with other mononuclear cells mediate a number of other important immune functions, such as specific cell-mediated cytotoxicity, certain types of graft rejection, graft-versus-host phenomena, delayed-type hypersensitivity, and the production and release of a broad range of soluble mediators termed *cytokines*, which have profound effects on virtually all phases of the immune response.[1]

On the other hand, B lymphocytes subserve a much more uniform function. They are the precursors of antibody-forming cells, and when appropriately stimulated, they proliferate and differentiate into cells that secrete antibody of the various classes and subclasses. Natural killer (NK) cells are lymphoid cells. They are of neither B lymphocyte nor T lymphocyte lineage, although they share some, but not all, phenotypic characteristics of T lymphocytes.[16] These cells are believed to be involved in immune surveillance against neoplastically transformed cells as well as in the elimination of virus-infected target cells.[17]

The monocyte-macrophage system, which is represented by monocytes in the peripheral blood and by

macrophages in various tissues, plays a major role in the expression of immune reactivity by mediating a number of important functions, such as the presentation of antigen to lymphocytes and the secretion of factors such as interleukin-1 (IL-1), that are involved in the activation of lymphocytes. In addition, they directly mediate certain effector functions, such as the destruction of antibody-coated bacteria, tumor cells, or even normal cells such as hematologic elements in certain types of autoimmune cytopenias.[15, 18] Furthermore, activated macrophages can directly eliminate various cell types even in the absence of antibody.

Finally, nonlymphoid cells such as neutrophils, eosinophils, and basophils play a major role in the inflammation that results from certain immune-mediated reactions and, as such, must be considered in the scheme of immune function despite their not being classically viewed as part of the immune system.

The net expression of immune function, be it a specific or nonspecific effector function, is the result of a balance between positive and negative influences mediated by immunoregulatory populations of cells alluded to previously.[1, 3, 5] They may exert their influence either directly or via the release of soluble immunoregulatory molecules. In addition to the classic cellular regulation of immune reactivity, the idiotypic network has been proposed as a potentially important mechanism of immunoregulation. Elaborate and complex schemes have been proposed for the mechanisms of such immunoregulation,[19] with secreted idiotype and anti-idiotype antibodies as well as idiotype-bearing and anti–idiotype-bearing cells having been demonstrated as playing a major role in the regulation of immune function in the murine system.[20] The demonstration of regulation of human immune function by idiotype–anti-idiotype reactions has been reported[21] and awaits further delineation before its role in the regulation of normal and abnormal lymphocyte physiology can be fully appreciated.

ABERRANCIES OF IMMUNE REACTIVITY

The established and potential mechanisms of disease activity in the broad range of rheumatic diseases are discussed in the individual chapters dealing with these disorders. It is clear that there are a number of potential mechanisms for the expression of aberrant immune reactivity related to the occurrence of even slight perturbations of the delicate balance in the cellular or humoral immunoregulatory network. In addition to imbalances in immunoregulation, one can have primary hyperreactivity of certain effector functions such as B lymphocyte reactivity.[1] Under these circumstances, it is conceivable that even a normally functioning immunoregulatory network might not successfully dampen the aberrant B lymphocyte hyperreactivity. Even more likely, there may be a combination of hyperactive effector cell function such as hyperreactivity at the B lymphocyte level together with abnormalities of immunoregulatory T lymphocyte function. The immunopathogenic processes in systemic lupus erythematosus (SLE) typifies the extraordinary complexity of immunoregulatory abnormalities in chronic autoimmune diseases. Active SLE is characterized by an overproduction of pathogenic autoantibodies, whereas the latent or preclinical state is characterized by multiclonal B cell and T cell activation. This leads to the secretion of an array of cytokines by these activated lymphocytes that facilitate anti-self immune responses.[22]

In this regard, the net expression of immune function in most of the rheumatic diseases appears to be one of aberrant hyperreactivity. As such, we generally distinguish these disorders from immunodeficiency diseases in which the net expression of immune function is usually that of hypoactivity. Given the balance between positive and negative influences in the immune network, however, one can easily appreciate that a deficiency of immune function such as suppressor cell activity (hence, strictly speaking an immunodeficiency state) can actually result in hyperactive effector immune function.[1, 23] This point is not trivial and has important implications in appreciating the basis of certain of the therapeutic strategies that are described later. Thus, although we commonly refer to the therapeutic strategy of immunosuppression for diseases of inflammation or immunologic hyperreactivity, we would more correctly think in terms of therapeutic immunoregulation either by dampening hyperactive responses or by directly or indirectly enhancing defective negative immunoregulatory influences.

POTENTIAL AREAS OF MODIFICATION OF IMMUNE RESPONSES BY THERAPEUTIC AGENTS

Suppression

Abnormally hyperactive immune responses at either the T or the B lymphocyte level can be theoretically as well as practically eliminated or at least dampened by nonspecifically suppressing the entire immune system. Clearly, sufficient amounts of cytotoxic agents, irradiation, antilymphocyte sera, and other immunosuppressive agents can be administered to eliminate virtually any immune response. These therapeutic modalities are truly nonspecific in that they do not selectively eliminate abnormally active lymphoid cells, nor do they spare normal lymphoid cells. Thus, although the desired effect can ultimately be obtained, the inevitable toxic side effects render such an approach infeasible in the treatment of nonneoplastic diseases. Within the realm of nonspecific suppression of immune function, therapeutic strategies are employed that strike a balance between the desired effect of suppression of aberrant immune reactivity and the maintenance of sufficient immune function as well as phagocyte, particularly neutrophil, cell number and function to maintain the integrity of the host defense system as well as the level of inflammatory and immune function required to maintain immunologic homeostasis.

This approach usually takes the form of administration of cytotoxic drugs in dosage regimens that, although still nonspecific, would relatively more selectively dampen the ongoing aberrant immune response. An example is the use of chronically administered cyclophosphamide in doses of 2 mg/kg/day in certain of the severe systemic vasculitis syndromes.[24, 25] These disorders are characterized by hyperreactivity of B lymphocyte responses with hypergammaglobulinemia, immune complex deposition, and spontaneous secretion of polyclonal immunoglobulin (Ig) by activated B lymphocytes.[26] Administration of cyclophosphamide in the regimen just discussed results in a selective suppression of B lymphocyte responses despite the fact that a total lymphocytopenia inevitably results from such long-term therapy.[27] Thus, although all B lymphocyte function is suppressed, rendering such an approach nonspecific, there appears to be a selective suppression of the hyperactive B lymphocyte function more than other lymphoid cell function.[27]

Other nonspecific but less globally immunosuppressive modalities include thoracic duct drainage, plasmapheresis, leukopheresis, the use of antilymphocyte globulin or monoclonal antibodies directed against lymphocyte subsets, irradiation of groups of regional lymph nodes, and the use of agents such as cyclosporine, which relatively selectively suppresses T lymphocyte function while sparing other lymphoid and nonlymphoid cells. Each of these approaches represents an attempt within the realm of a fundamentally nonspecific immunosuppressive regimen to render the approach somewhat more selective.

Despite these attempts at introducing varying degrees of selectivity into nonspecific immunosuppressive regimens, the extraordinary complexity of the immune system, with its multiple levels of regulation and feedback mechanisms, adds a considerable degree of uncertainty to such approaches. Nonetheless, despite the limitations of such an approach, nonspecific immunosuppression has resulted in favorable therapeutic results in a number of rheumatic diseases. Given the state of the art at present, however, realization of these limitations is essential for proper application of such regimens as well as for providing an impetus to continue the search for more specific and less toxic forms of immunosuppression.

Enhancement

As already mentioned, even disorders that express a net hyperactive immune response may have components that are hypoactive. In this regard, immune enhancement should theoretically be beneficial, provided that the defective element can be selectively enhanced. Because virtually all of the immune-enhancing drugs or agents that are discussed subsequently are indeed nonspecific, they suffer from the same limitations as immunosuppressive agents in the modulation of aberrant immune reactivity in disease states. Nonetheless, certain drugs that enhance immune responses have been used with limited success in certain immunologically mediated diseases and are mentioned subsequently.

The ultimate enhancement of the immune response would be complete replacement, as with ablation and bone marrow transplantation. Despite the dramatic advances being made in bone marrow transplantation, however, such an approach is not feasible at present for rheumatic diseases. Transfer of mature immune-competent lymphoid cells has the theoretical potential of reversing the imbalance of immunoregulatory lymphocyte subsets. Again, logistical constraints, with regard to histocompatibility requirements and restrictions, make such an approach untenable. Of particular interest, however, has been the availability of purified preparations of lymphokines such as interleukin-2 (IL-2) and the various interferons. These factors, particularly IL-2, are capable of exerting profound enhancing effects on the immune response in vitro,[28] and the therapeutic use of such factors holds at least theoretical promise for the future.

CYTOTOXIC AGENTS

General Considerations

Of all the immunoregulatory agents that are used in the treatment of rheumatic diseases, the cytotoxic drugs pose perhaps the greatest difficulty for the clinician from both theoretical and practical standpoints. This stems largely from the fine line between risk and benefit, which exists for virtually all such agents used in the treatment of these diseases. Unfortunately, the terminology that is frequently employed with regard to the cytotoxic agents is somewhat misleading, in that the term *cytotoxic agent* is often misused synonymously with the term *immunosuppressive agent*. Indeed, cytotoxic agents can be and frequently are immunosuppressive; however, a number of other drugs discussed in this chapter as well as the glucocorticoids (see Chapter 50) can be potent immunosuppressive agents. The cytotoxic agents differ from many of these other agents in that the common denominator of their effect is that they destroy cells, hence the derivation of the term *cytotoxic*, which means simply that the drugs are directly toxic or damaging to cells. It is the ability to kill cells that distinguishes the cytotoxic immunosuppressive agents from the other categories of immunosuppressive drugs and explains their extensive use in the treatment of a variety of neoplastic diseases. Indeed, their use as antineoplastic agents long antedates their use as immunosuppressive agents in non-neoplastic inflammatory and immune-mediated diseases. Only when the profound immunosuppressive effects of these agents as used in the treatment of neoplastic diseases became apparent did clinical investigators conceive of their use in diseases that manifested marked inflammatory responses and apparent immune-mediated mechanisms. Certain of the mechanisms of action of cytotoxic agents on inflammatory and immunologic responses are listed in Table 51–1.

It cannot be emphasized too strongly that the rationale for the use of cytotoxic agents as well as the goals that one wishes to achieve by therapy are for the most part quite different depending on whether one uses these agents in the treatment of non-neoplastic, immune-mediated diseases or of neoplastic diseases. The rationale and goal for the use of cytotoxic agents in the treatment of neoplastic diseases are sim-

Table 51–1. PRINCIPAL MECHANISMS OF ACTION OF CYTOTOXIC AGENTS ON INFLAMMATORY AND IMMUNOLOGIC REACTIONS

Elimination of sensitized and immunologically committed lymphoid cells
Elimination of nonsensitized lymphoid cells secondarily engaged in aberrant immunologic reactivity
Elimination of nonlymphoid cells engaged in nonspecific inflammatory responses to aberrant immunologic reactions
Suppression of functional capabilities of surviving lymphoid cells

ply to eliminate, where possible, every tumor cell. This approach is almost invariably associated with significant destruction of the normal elements of host defense mechanisms, such that a life-threatening or near life-threatening state exists for variable periods of time during and after chemotherapy until the normal cellular elements can recover. If the tumor is sensitive to the chemotherapeutic agents used, such that a reasonable chance of remission or cure exists, the attendant risks are clearly justifiable, since the malignant neoplasm will otherwise inevitably result in the death of the patient. Under such circumstances, the goals are rather clear-cut, and the options are few.

The situation is quite different when using these agents to treat non-neoplastic diseases. Because there are no recognizable malignant clones in the immune-mediated diseases, the rationale and goal are usually to suppress the aberrant inflammatory and immune-mediated reactions that are responsible for the tissue damage without markedly suppressing the normal host defense mechanisms, which would put the patient at significant risk for either an infection or a neoplasm resulting from the suppression of normal immune surveillance mechanisms.[24, 25] Unfortunately, maintaining this balance between risk and benefit is not an easy task because, as mentioned previously, the agents employed are almost always nonspecific in their suppressive effects, and suppression of normal immune mechanisms will variably accompany suppression of the aberrant reactions. It is hoped that suppression of these abnormal immune mechanisms occurs, so the patient will not be at a significant risk.

Of equal if not greater importance than the suppression of normal immunologic mechanisms is the suppression of normal nonspecific mechanisms of host defenses in the form of circulating polymorphonuclear neutrophils. Owing to the relatively rapid turnover of the neutrophil series in the bone marrow, cytotoxic agents are particularly effective in causing a neutropenia, which becomes one of the major limiting factors in the use of these agents. In this regard, another important difference in the use of these agents in neoplastic versus non-neoplastic diseases is that in non-neoplastic diseases the drugs are usually administered chronically over extended periods of time, ranging from months to years, and so the risk of a host defense defect is a relatively persistent problem, as opposed to the relatively brief (albeit usually more severe) periods of defect seen following the intermittent courses of chemotherapy usually administered for neoplastic diseases.

Finally, the major difference in the use of these agents in the treatment of neoplastic versus non-neoplastic diseases lies in the exercise of clinical judgment as to when to employ such an aggressive chemotherapeutic approach in a non-neoplastic disease that might not be invariably fatal. The clinical course of most neoplastic diseases that are left untreated or that are not aggressively treated is usually rather clear, which makes the decision to initiate aggressive therapy relatively easy. In contrast, many

of the rheumatic diseases, such as SLE, rheumatoid arthritis, the systemic vasculitides, scleroderma, and dermatomyositis/polymyositis, as well as several of the organ-specific autoimmune diseases in which cytotoxic agents have been used have variable clinical courses. Only when the disease seems to be progressing with irreversible organ system dysfunction that is not responsive to more conventional therapy, such as nonsteroidal anti-inflammatory agents or glucocorticoids, does one consider employing a cytotoxic agent. This is often a difficult decision because the efficacy of these agents in many of these diseases has not been conclusively proved by appropriately controlled studies. Furthermore, the chronicity of most of these diseases dictates that even though a cytotoxic agent may be effective in suppressing disease activity, the agent cannot be used indefinitely. Thus, it is essential to set reasonable goals for the use of cytotoxic agents in the treatment of rheumatic diseases.

Therapeutic Goals

Few situations exist in which the use of cytotoxic agents can be expected to effect a true and long-term "cure" of a non-neoplastic disease. One such situation is the use of these agents, particularly cyclophosphamide, in the treatment of certain vasculitic syndromes. Paramount among these syndromes is Wegener's granulomatosis, in which long-term remissions have been effected in as many as 90 percent of patients treated with cyclophosphamide, 2 mg/kg/day, together with prednisone, 1 mg/kg/day, administered first daily and then on an alternate-day schedule.[24, 25] Similar results have been obtained with other vasculitic syndromes, particularly the polyarteritis nodosa group of the systemic necrotizing vasculitides.[29] Before the institution of this therapy, virtually all patients with Wegener's granulomatosis died of the disease, as did most patients with the polyarteritis nodosa–type of systemic necrotizing vasculitis.[24, 25] It is likely that the drug does not in fact "cure" the disease but merely suppresses the inflammatory and aberrant immune-mediated mechanisms long enough for the disease to run its course spontaneously and remit permanently. Therefore, given these reported therapeutic results, a reasonable goal for the use of cytotoxic agents (in this case, cyclophosphamide) in these vasculitic syndromes is a true permanent remission. One can hope that a single course of therapy, which is usually administered for over a year, will result in a situation in which the drug would not have to be used again in the patient. At worst, it may be necessary to treat relapses with additional courses of therapy. In this regard, relapses in patients with Wegener's granulomatosis were seen in up to 50 percent of patients treated with immunosuppressive regimens, and these patients could usually be put back into remission by reinstitution of therapy.[30]

The goals for the use of cytotoxic agents in most

of the other immune-mediated rheumatic diseases, particularly the classic connective tissue diseases, are somewhat different from those of the vasculitic syndromes. Because the connective tissue diseases usually run waxing and waning courses, which are characterized by exacerbations and remissions, the use of cytotoxic agents should be reserved for treatment of flares of disease in which there is a clear-cut danger of irreversible organ system dysfunction. Even though cytotoxic agents have been used for several years in the treatment of the severe manifestations of the connective tissue and other rheumatic diseases, there are unfortunately few controlled studies that definitively document the efficacy of such an approach.[6, 8, 9] A few controlled trials of cytotoxic agents have been carried out, and they have documented short-term benefits in flares of disease activity. In this regard, Austin and colleagues[31] compared intravenous cyclophosphamide plus low-dose prednisone with prednisone alone in the treatment of lupus nephritis and concluded that cyclophosphamide, when used in this manner, reduced the risk of end-stage renal disease. There is, however, still little information available regarding long-term effects of these agents on the ultimate course of the disease. Thus, given the present state of knowledge in this area, a reasonable goal for the use of cytotoxic agents in the connective tissue diseases would be to suppress flares of disease activity that are serious enough to be organ system–threatening or life-threatening until such a point that the disease goes into remission and the drug can be withdrawn. Under such circumstances, the drug can be used again for a limited course should another relapse occur.

If it is necessary to continue the cytotoxic agent indefinitely to effect a sustained remission or even a partial remission, one must carefully examine the risks of such long-term treatment with a drug whose potential adverse side effects are so substantial.[10, 32] A classic example of this latter point would be the use of chronic cytotoxic therapy in a patient with rheumatoid arthritis. Given the normal life expectancy in patients with rheumatoid arthritis (see Chapters 54 and 56), it may be inappropriate to risk a serious and even fatal complication of therapy to suppress disease activity that is rarely life-threatening. On the other hand, the patient's life situation may be such that he or she feels that the risk is worth the benefit of suppressing certain unacceptable manifestations of disease activity. Thus, the goals and analysis of risks versus benefits may differ depending on the individual patient.

Individual Cytotoxic Agents

Although a wide variety of cytotoxic agents of various classes have been used in the chemotherapy of neoplastic diseases, only a limited number of these have been regularly employed in the treatment of non-neoplastic, inflammatory, and immune-mediated diseases. The three major categories of cytotoxic drugs employed in the latter disease are the alkylating agents and two groups of antimetabolites—the purine analogs and the folic acid antagonists. The mechanisms of action of these cytotoxic agents are outlined in Table 51–2, and their structures are illustrated in Figure 51–2. Other cytotoxic agents that are used almost exclusively in the treatment of neoplastic diseases are covered in detail elsewhere[33] and include other antimetabolites such as the pyrimidine analogs in the form of 5-fluorouracil, cytosine arabinoside, and triacetyl-6-azauridine. In addition, natural products used in the treatment of neoplastic diseases include the *Vinca* alkaloids (vinblastine and vincristine) and antibiotics (actinomycin D, daunomycin, rubidomycin, adroblastina, bleomycin, mithramycin, and mitomycin C). Finally, miscellaneous cytotoxic agents include cisplatin, hydroxyurea, procarbazine, and mitotane. The list is surely not complete, as newer agents are constantly being developed. Within this group of agents used predominantly in neoplastic processes are some that have also been used in certain non-neoplastic diseases. For example, as is discussed later, vincristine has been successfully employed as a

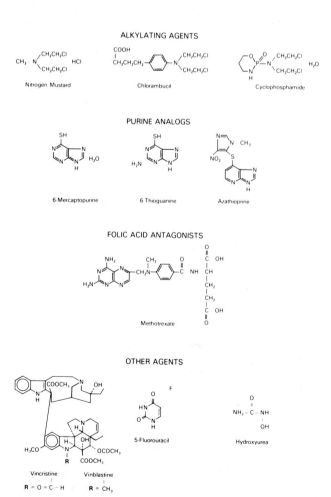

Figure 51–2. Structure of cytotoxic agents used in the treatment of certain rheumatic diseases.

Table 51–2. MECHANISMS OF ACTION OF CLASSES OF CYTOTOXIC AGENTS COMMONLY EMPLOYED IN TREATMENT OF INFLAMMATORY AND IMMUNE-MEDIATED NON-NEOPLASTIC DISEASES

Class	Typical Agent	Mechanisms of Action
Alkylating agents	Nitrogen mustard Cyclophosphamide Chlorambucil	Under physiologic conditions, the drug reacts chemically with biologically vital macromolecules such as DNA by contributing alkyl groups to the molecule, resulting in cross-linkage.
Purine analogs	6-Mercaptopurine Thioguanine Azathioprine	Although incorporation of the analog into cellular DNA with subsequent inhibition of nucleic acid synthesis is generally considered the basic mechanism of action of these agents, they likely exert their cytotoxic effects by one or more of multiple mechanisms, including effects on purine nucleotide synthesis and metabolism as well as alterations in the synthesis and function of RNA and DNA.
Folic acid antagonists	Methotrexate	The drug with high affinity to dihydrofolate reductase, preventing the formation of tetrahydrofolate and thus causing an acute intracellular deficiency of folate coenzymes. Consequently, one-carbon transfer reactions critical for de novo synthesis of purine nucleotides and thymidylate cease, with resulting interruption of the synthesis of DNA and RNA.

therapeutic modality in idiopathic thrombocytopenic purpura,[34] and hydroxyurea has been employed in the treatment of the idiopathic hypereosinophilic syndrome.[35]

Alkylating Agents

Alkylating agents are chemicals that can substitute alkyl radicals into other molecules. Biologically effective alkylating agents are usually bifunctional or polyfunctional in that each molecule has two or more alkylating groups.[33] Thus, each molecule of the alkylating agent can covalently bind with two or more molecules of other substances. In this manner, two or more molecules may be linked to each other, i.e., in cross-linkage. By virtue of the induction of these structural changes at the molecular level, alkylating agents can potentially alter the function of proteins and nucleic acids. For example, when the DNA of a cell such as a lymphocyte is cross-linked by the agent, replication of its strands is blocked and the cell cannot divide properly, leading ultimately to cell death.[36]

Nitrogen Mustard

Mechlorethamine was the first of the nitrogen mustards to be used clinically. The drug is administered intravenously, and its clearance from the blood is extremely rapid. Following administration, the drug rapidly undergoes chemical transformation and combines with either water or reactive compounds of cells such that the drug is no longer present in its active form after only a few minutes.[33] Nitrogen mustard has been virtually replaced by cyclophosphamide as the alkylating agent of choice in the treatment of nonneoplastic diseases. The former has the disadvantage of requiring intravenous administration, it has significant potential toxic side effects, and its therapeutic index in experimental animals has been shown to be much lower than that of cyclophosphamide with

respect to immunosuppressive effects. Historically, however, nitrogen mustard is an important agent that led the way for the use of cyclophosphamide in the treatment of immune-mediated diseases. For example, the early success in treatment of a patient with Wegener's granulomatosis with nitrogen mustard in 1954[37] laid the rational basis for the use of cyclophosphamide in the successful induction of remission in large numbers of patients with that disease.[25, 30]

Cyclophosphamide

Cyclophosphamide is well absorbed orally and thus has the advantage of administration by either the oral or the intravenous route. The drug is inert and is activated by metabolism in the liver by the mixed-function oxidase system of the smooth endoplasmic reticulum.[38] The plasma half-life of cyclophosphamide is 6 to 7 hours; this may be significantly prolonged by prior treatment with allopurinol.[39] Maximum concentrations are reached in plasma 1 hour after administration, and urinary recovery of unmetabolized drug is approximately 14 percent with negligible fecal recovery after intravenous administration.[33] Because approximately 60 percent of the drug is excreted through the kidney in the form of active metabolites, renal failure may result in impaired excretion of these active metabolites, with a resulting relative increase in immunosuppressive effect as well as in toxicity of a given dose of drug. Because certain enzymes of the mixed-function oxidase system can be induced by drugs such as barbiturates and glucocorticoids, these agents can influence the metabolism of cyclophosphamide from its inert to its active form.[40] The biologic actions of cyclophosphamide, however, seem to be more substantially affected by alterations in the rates of detoxification and elimination than by changes in the rate of generation of the active metabolites.[33] Indeed, the antitumor and therapeutic index of cyclophosphamide was shown not to be significantly modified by pretreatment of animals with phenobarbital.[41]

Although cyclophosphamide acts primarily during the S phase of the cell cycle and so has a profound effect on rapidly dividing cells, it also affects cells at all phases of the cell cycle including resting (G_0) cells.[8] A large amount of literature has accumulated, particularly using the mouse and other animal models, demonstrating the effects of cyclophosphamide on virtually all components of the cellular and humoral immune responses.[42, 43] Of particular note is the ability of cyclophosphamide to inhibit antibody production. Although this has been shown to occur most dramatically when the drug is administered before the antigen,[43, 44] for practical purposes, cyclophosphamide inhibits antibody production when given at the same time or even after the antigen. Cyclophosphamide has been shown to inhibit suppressor T lymphocytes selectively as opposed to inducer or helper T lymphocytes.[45, 46] In the therapeutic protocols in which cyclophosphamide is administered to patients with rheumatic diseases, however, a more global rather than a selective suppression of T lymphocyte function is seen. The immunosuppressive effects of chronically administered cyclosphosphamide therapy in humans[27, 47–49] are summarized in Table 51–3. The most consistent finding in cyclophosphamide-treated patients is a lymphocytopenia of both T and B lymphocytes. B lymphocyte function is clearly more profoundly suppressed than T lymphocyte function, and this is reflected at the cellular level as well as in the suppression of Ig production and serum levels of Ig in patients treated chronically with cyclophosphamide.

Cyclophosphamide is generally administered to patients with non-neoplastic diseases in a dosage regimen of 2 mg/kg/day orally. Immunosuppressive and clinical effects are usually seen within 2 to 3 weeks after initiation of therapy. An alternative regimen is the administration of single large intravenous bolus doses of 750 to 1000 mg/m². This latter regimen is usually reserved for patients with neoplastic diseases but has been used for the treatment of rheumatic

Table 51–3. IMMUNOSUPPRESSIVE EFFECTS OF CHRONICALLY ADMINISTERED CYCLOPHOSPHAMIDE THERAPY IN HUMANS

Absolute lymphocytopenia of both T and B lymphocytes, with early preferential depletion of B lymphocytes
Significant suppression of in vitro lymphocyte blastogenic responses to specific antigenic stimuli, with only mild suppression of responses to mitogenic stimuli
Suppression of antibody response and cutaneous delayed hypersensitivity to a new antigen, with relative sparing of established cutaneous delayed hypersensitivity
Reduction of elevated serum immunoglobulin levels as well as occurrence of hypogammaglobulinemia in patients treated for extended periods of time (years)
Selective suppression of in vitro B lymphocyte function, with diminution of increased spontaneous immunoglobulin production of individual B lymphocytes as well as suppression of mitogen-induced immunoglobulin production

Table 51–4. TOXIC SIDE EFFECTS OF CHRONICALLY ADMINISTERED LOW-DOSE* CYCLOPHOSPHAMIDE THERAPY

Marrow suppression—predominantly neutropenia
Gonadal suppression—oligospermia, ovarian dysfunction
Alopecia
Gastrointestinal intolerance
Hemorrhagic cystitis
Hypogammaglobulinemia after extended use
Pulmonary interstitial fibrosis
Oncogenesis

*2 mg/kg/day.

diseases such as SLE. In a study by Austin and colleagues,[31] bolus cyclophosphamide combined with oral prednisone was determined to be effective in reducing the incidence of end-stage renal disease in patients with SLE and nephritis. Hoffman and co-workers[50] examined the use of intermittent high-dose intravenous cyclophosphamide in the treatment of 14 patients with Wegener's granulomatosis. Initial response rates were high, but responses were not maintained or patients failed to tolerate continued treatment, leading the authors to conclude that daily low-dose cyclophosphamide remains the treatment of choice for this disorder. As with the use of any cytotoxic and potentially myelosuppressive agent, the dosage must be modified throughout the therapeutic course in accordance with the degree of myelosuppression that occurs (see later in this chapter).

Although cyclophosphamide has proved to be an extremely effective immunosuppressive agent in the treatment of non-neoplastic diseases, its potential toxic side effects are considerable, and the physician must be aware of them whenever she or he undertakes the treatment of a patient with this agent[31, 32] (Table 51–4). Although suppression of all marrow elements is seen with cyclophosphamide therapy, neutropenia is clearly the most important hematologic effect of the drug with regard to factors limiting its use. It should be appreciated that chronically administered cyclophosphamide will have a cumulative effect on the bone marrow reserve, such that a dose that is well tolerated at one point in time may produce significant neutropenia after 1 or more years of therapy. This will necessitate frequent monitoring of the white blood cell (WBC) count and appropriate adjustment of dosage. Gonadal suppression is almost an invariable effect of long-term administration of cyclophosphamide and is due to the damaging effects of the drug on the germinal epithelium.[51, 52] The oligomenorrhea and amenorrhea in premenopausal women[51] may be permanent if treatment is continued for a year or longer. Although prepubertal testes are damaged, return of spermatogenesis after drug withdrawal occurs more frequently in this younger age bracket.[53, 54]

Although significant alopecia occurs quite frequently after high doses of cyclophosphamide, only minor degrees occur during long-term low-dose therapy; in both cases, it is reversible on cessation of the drug. Gastrointestinal intolerance is unpredictable and can be quite severe in certain patients. Although treated with antiemetics, gastric discomfort may be refractory to the usual therapeutic modalities. The latter complication not infrequently disappears on continuation of the drug.

Hemorrhagic cystitis is seen in between 15 and 30 percent of patients and can be a most difficult complication.[25] Although the cystitis usually clears on cessation of the drug, bladder fibrosis, intractable hemorrhage, and bladder carcinoma have been reported.[55] Under most circumstances, the onset of hemorrhage cystitis is an absolute indication for discontinuation of the drug. If the cystitis is severe, the drug must be stopped regardless of the circumstances. If lack of an adequate substitute makes it necessary to continue the drug in a patient with only mild cystitis, however, the dosage should be decreased and the patient followed with urinary cytologic studies and intermittent cystoscopies. If the cystitis persists or worsens on the lower dose, the drug must be discontinued even though the alternative drug for the disease in question is inferior to cyclophosphamide. Patients should be instructed to take cyclophosphamide early in the day, to avoid leaving the drug and its metabolites in the urine overnight, and to drink plenty of fluids to maximize excretion.

The authors have noted a few patients who have developed hypogammaglobulinemia during chronically administered cyclophosphamide therapy. This is of potential importance because of the synergistic host defense defects created by neutropenia and hypogammaglobulinemia. Although pulmonary and cardiac toxicity are generally seen only at high doses of the drug,[56, 57] interstitial pulmonary fibrosis can occur with chronically administered low-dose cyclophosphamide, and the physician should be alert to this possibility. In addition, an antidiuretic hormone effect has been reported with large doses of cyclophosphamide but not with lower doses.[58, 59] Finally, neoplastic diseases, particularly lymphomas and leukemias, may occur as a result of cyclophosphamide therapy.[60]

Chlorambucil

Chlorambucil is available for oral administration, and absorption is adequate and reliable. The drug is related to nitrogen mustard in that the methyl group of the mustard is replaced by phenylbutyric acid. The drug is metabolized by β oxidation of the butyric acid.[61] The drug is almost completely metabolized and has a plasma half-life of approximately 90 minutes. At recommended doses, chlorambucil is the slowest-acting nitrogen mustard in clinical use.[33]

The mechanism of action of chlorambucil is similar to that of other alkylating agents. At high doses, it suppresses all myeloid elements, and the therapeutic strategy is to suppress immune function mediated by lymphocytes before the suppression of other bone marrow elements.[62] In this regard, it has been reported that at lower does, chlorambucil exerts a more selective effect on lymphopoiesis than on granulopoiesis. Clearly, chlorambucil has not been as extensively studied as cyclophosphamide with regard to its immunosuppressive effects. It is generally believed, however, that it is not as potent an immunosuppressive agent as cyclophosphamide, and although its toxic side effects may be somewhat less than those of cyclophosphamide, its efficacy in suppressing disease activity in the non-neoplastic diseases is probably less than that of cyclophosphamide. An example of this is the greater efficacy of cyclophosphamide compared with chlorambucil in suppressing disease activity in generalized Wegener's granulomatosis.[63] Nonetheless, chlorambucil has been used with some success in certain of the connective tissue diseases.[8]

Chlorambucil is generally administered to patients with non-neoplastic diseases in a dosage regimen of 0.1 or 0.2 mg/kg/day orally. The dose is adjusted according to the degree of nonlymphocytic myelosuppression that is encountered, i.e., neutropenia and thrombocytopenia. When severe myelosuppression occurs, the drug should be discontinued. Marrow function usually recovers rapidly; however, irreversible marrow failure has been reported in a number of patients treated with chlorambucil for non-neoplastic diseases.[64] Such complications highlight the inherent danger in the treatment of non-neoplastic diseases with cytotoxic agents of any class. Other side effects include gastrointestinal discomfort with nausea and vomiting, hepatotoxicity, dermatitis, and infertility.[33] Oncogenesis is a particularly disturbing potential complication of chlorambucil therapy, and a marked increase in the incidence of leukemia and other tumors has been associated with the use of this agent.[65, 66]

Purine Analogs

The two major purine analogs that have been used clinically are 6-mercaptopurine (6-MP) and azathioprine, which is the purine analog currently used almost exclusively; 6-MP is an analog of hypoxanthine in which the 6-OH radical is replaced by a thiol group. When an imidazole group is attached to the S of 6-MP, azathioprine is formed. In vivo, azathioprine is metabolized to 6-MP, which is the active drug. The ultimate mechanism of action of 6-MP is the inhibition of nucleic acid synthesis. Despite extensive studies in this area, however, the precise mechanism of action whereby these purine analogs cause cell death or cytotoxicity remains unclear. Certain potential mechanisms of action have been proposed, including the conversion of 6-MP to its ribonucleotide, which inhibits the enzymes necessary for the conversion of inosinic acid to xanthylic acid as well as for the conversion of adenylosuccinic acid to adenylic acid, leading to the inhibition of DNA synthesis.[67] In addition, feedback inhibition of 5-phosphoribosylamine occurs with reduction of de novo purine biosynthesis and resulting inhibition of DNA synthesis and cell death.

Azathioprine and 6-MP are available for oral administration, and absorption is quite good. Because azathioprine is converted in vivo to 6-MP, which is the active drug, their pharmacokinetics can be considered together. About one half of an oral dose of drug is found excreted in the urine within the first 24 hours.[33] After an intravenous dose, the half-life of the drug is 60 to 90 minutes, with clearance from the blood resulting from uptake by cells, renal excretion, and metabolic degradation. There are two major pathways for the metabolism of 6-MP. The first is the methylation of the sulfhydryl group and oxidation of the methylated derivatives. The second is the oxidation of 6-MP to 6-thiouric acid by the enzyme xanthine oxidase.[33] Because allopurinol inhibits xanthine oxidase, this drug decreases the metabolism of 6-MP and so accounts for the increase in toxicity of azathioprine and 6-MP when allopurinol is simultaneously administered.

Azathioprine and 6-MP inhibit both cell-mediated and humoral immunity. Because of the diversity of studies that have been carried out in animal models and humans, there have been certain disagreements with regard to the type and extent of immunosuppression that occurs during azathioprine and 6-MP therapy.[42, 67] Despite this, there have been some rather consistent findings with regard to the effects of azathioprine and 6-MP on immune and inflammatory responses. Azathioprine and 6-MP cause a total lymphocytopenia of both T and B lymphocytes.[68] Gamma globulin synthesis is suppressed by azathioprine therapy,[69] as is the antibody response (particularly the secondary response) to vaccination.[70] In addition, B lymphocyte proliferation is suppressed by azathioprine.[71] There has been some controversy with regard to the effects of these agents on T lymphocytes, including inhibition of sheep red blood cell rosette formation.[72] Other studies, however, claim no selective effect on T lymphocytes and in fact demonstrate that treatment with azathioprine has little suppressive effect on mitogen-induced blastogenesis of human T lymphocytes.[73, 74] In this regard, there seems to be little question that azathioprine is not as effective as cyclophosphamide in the suppression of lymphocyte function. Azathioprine and 6-MP can suppress the induction of de novo delayed hypersensitivity; however, it is generally agreed that established delayed hypersensitivity remains intact during drug therapy.[70, 74] Azathioprine has potent anti-inflammatory effects, which are probably related to its ability to reduce the number of monocytes in an inflammatory site by inhibition of monocyte production.[75] This suppression of monocyte function may also explain the effects of these drugs on the induction of delayed hypersensitivity.[76]

Azathioprine and 6-MP are generally administered in doses of approximately 2 mg/kg/day. As with the other cytotoxic agents, the dosage must be adjusted according to the degree of resulting myelosuppres-

Table 51–5. TOXIC SIDE EFFECTS OF CHRONICALLY ADMINISTERED AZATHIOPRINE AND 6-MERCAPTOPURINE THERAPY

Marrow suppression—predominantly neutropenia
Hepatotoxicity—probably on an allergic basis
Infectious disease complications—not necessarily correlated with neutropenia
Gastrointestinal intolerance
Oncogenesis—particularly lymphoid malignancies

sion. Immunosuppressive and clinical effects are usually seen within 3 or 4 weeks after initiation of therapy. Patients with impaired renal function may have reduced clearance of the drug and its metabolites, with a resulting cumulative effect and increased toxicity unless the dosage is appropriately adjusted downward.

The major toxicity of both 6-MP and azathioprine is bone marrow suppression, with leukopenia rather than thrombocytopenia and anemia being the major manifestations. The major toxic side effects of chronically administered azathioprine or 6-MP therapy[77] are listed in Table 51–5. Of note with regard to the neutropenia associated with these agents is the fact that a rapid fall in WBC within a week of starting therapy has been reported and resembles an idiosyncratic reaction. In addition, the peripheral WBC cannot always be an accurate measure of the host defense defect, since infections may occur in individuals with normal neutrophil counts, suggesting a functional impairment of immune-competent cells involved in host defense, most likely at the T lymphocyte–monocyte axis. The suppression of delayed hypersensitivity by these agents[75, 76] as well as the fact that neutrophil function is generally normal in individuals receiving azathioprine[78] adds credence to this hypothesis. This point should be fully appreciated, since infectious disease complications cannot be totally predicted regardless of the level of the WBC. Finally, although the effects on gonadal function have not been fully evaluated with regard to azathioprine, it is clear that sterility is not the invariable rule, since several normal pregnancies have been reported in patients who had been receiving azathioprine. Fetal abnormalities do not appear to be a problem.[32]

Other Agents

Methotrexate

Methotrexate is discussed in detail in Chapter 49.[79]

Vinca Alkaloids

The commonly used *Vinca* alkaloids, vincristine and vinblastine, are cell cycle–specific agents that block mitosis by interfering with protein assembly of the mitotic spindle, leading to metaphase arrest.[33] Vincristine is administered intravenously in doses of 2 mg/ m² of body surface area weekly. After intravenous injection, vincristine is cleared almost entirely from the blood in approximately 30 minutes. The drug is excreted primarily by the liver into the bile, with less than 5 percent of the drug appearing in the urine.

Immunosuppression with these compounds has been negligible, and antibody formation in rabbits was shown not to be significantly affected by administration of *Vinca* alkaloids.[42] Vinblastine has been employed in a unique immunosuppression protocol in the treatment of idiopathic thrombocytopenia, in which the drug was bound to platelets for the purposes of delivering the toxic drug directly and selectively to the cells that were removing and killing the platelets.[80]

The major toxic side effect of the *Vinca* alkaloids is neurotoxicity. This is usually manifested by peripheral neuropathy in the form of paresthesias, loss of deep tendon reflexes, neuritic pain, muscle weakness, and wasting. Other toxicities include hoarseness owing to vocal cord paralysis, diplopia, severe constipation, bladder atony, alopecia, cytopenias, pyuria, dysuria, fever, gastrointestinal symptoms, mutagenicity, local inflammation at sites of venous extravasation, and inappropriate secretion of antidiuretic hormone.

5-Fluorouracil

5-Fluorouracil (5-FU) is a pyrimidine analog that competes with uracil in various metabolic pathways but cannot be converted to thymidine. Thus, it ultimately blocks DNA synthesis. In addition, it inhibits enzymes such as thymidylate synthetase required for the synthesis of ribonucleotides and deoxyribonucleotides. The drug has been used predominantly in the treatment of neoplastic diseases, and its precise immunosuppressive properties are not well studied in humans.[33] The drug works throughout the cell cycle, and it is metabolized almost exclusively in the liver. It is usually administered intravenously, since absorption after oral ingestion is unpredictable and incomplete. The major toxic side effects result from the inevitable myelosuppression, particularly leukopenia. Other side effects include nausea and vomiting, alopecia, dermatitis, nail changes, atrophy of the skin, ulcerative stomatitis and gastroenteritis, and neurologic manifestations such as cerebellar ataxia.[33]

Hydroxyurea

Hydroxyurea inhibits the enzyme ribonucleotide diphosphate reductase, which catalyzes the reductive conversion of ribonucleotides to deoxyribonucleotides and is a crucial step in the synthesis of DNA. The drug is specific for the S phase of the cell cycle.[33] It is readily absorbed from the gastrointestinal tract, and peak plasma concentrations are reached within 2 hours of administration of an oral dose. Within 24 hours, it is undetectable in the blood, with approximately 80 percent of the drug recovered in the urine within 12 hours after oral or intravenous administration. The drug is administered orally in doses of 20 to 30 mg/kg/day as a single dose. Although the drug has been used predominantly in the management of chronic myelogenous leukemia, it has also been used in the treatment of the idiopathic hypereosinophilic syndrome.[35] Toxic side effects include myelosuppression, nausea and vomiting, gastrointestinal ulcerations, and mild skin rashes.

Hydroxyurea has attracted substantial attention as a therapeutic modality for sickle cell anemia, in which it appears to act not as an immunosuppressive agent but rather influences the production of fetal hemoglobin.[81–83]

THEORETIC AND PRACTICAL CONSIDERATIONS IN THE USE OF CYTOTOXIC AGENTS FOR TREATMENT OF NON-NEOPLASTIC DISEASES

As already mentioned, one of the major goals in the use of cytotoxic agents for the treatment of non-neoplastic diseases is to achieve a degree of immunosuppression that results in suppression of the aberrant inflammatory and immune reactivity in a disease state without seriously compromising host defense mechanisms, which would lead to an increased incidence of infectious disease complications. For reasons that are not entirely clear, in those inflammatory and immune-mediated diseases for which cytotoxic agents have proved to be beneficial, it appears that disease activity can indeed be suppressed without the invariable occurrence of a serious defect in clinically relevant host defense mechanisms.

Although the cytotoxic agents have a number of immediate and long-term toxic side effects that must be considered in the decision to employ such agents in a given patient, once the decision has been made to use a cytotoxic agent, awareness and recognition of these side effects become of paramount importance in the successful management of the patient. In this regard, although the different classes of cytotoxic agents used in the treatment of non-neoplastic diseases differ somewhat in their mechanisms of action, the major immediate limiting side effect common to virtually all of them is myelosuppression, particularly neutropenia and, to a lesser extent, thrombocytopenia and anemia.

When the physician undertakes the treatment of non-neoplastic diseases with these agents, it is essential to appreciate the necessity for careful and continuous monitoring of the WBC, with appropriate modification of the dosage regimen to maintain the WBC above the neutropenic range. It has been consistently observed that if the WBC is maintained above 3000 to 3500 cells/mm³, which usually results in a neutrophil count of 1000 to 1500/mm³, there is little chance of opportunistic infections as a result of drug-induced host defense defects, particularly when the agent employed is an alkylating agent such as cyclophosphamide or chlorambucil. For example, this has clearly been shown to be the case with the use of cyclophosphamide in the treatment of Wegener's granulomatosis[25] and other of the severe systemic vasculitic syndromes.[24, 26] This observation holds true provided there is no concomitant and synergistic cause of host defense defects, such as daily glucocorticoid therapy. For this reason, it is suggested that glucocorticoids be administered on an alternate-day basis, when possible, in patients receiving cytotoxic agents together with glucocorticoids for the treatment of non-neoplastic diseases.[24–26] Using such a regimen of chronically administered cyclophosphamide at a dose of 2 mg/kg/day, with frequent adjustments of dosage to maintain the WBC above 3000 cells/mm³, together with prednisone 60 mg/day or less, with conversion to alternate-day prednisone within 1 to 2 months of initiating therapy and maintenance of alternate-day prednisone together with the cyclophosphamide, there has been virtually no increased incidence of opportunistic infections in a large series of patients.[25] The exception to this was an increased incidence of herpes zoster infections in patients receiving long-term cyclophosphamide therapy.[84] The zoster did not disseminate viscerally in any patient, and there were no serious sequelae of the infection.

Maintaining the WBC above the neutropenic level while effecting remission of disease activity requires continuous monitoring of the WBC as well as appreciation that as patients receive a cytotoxic agent for extended periods of time, their tolerance for a given dose will decrease, necessitating downward adjustment of the dose. It should also be pointed out that an appreciation of the slope of the curve of the WBC is important, in that the effect of a given dose of drug on one day may be reflected several days later. Therefore, one should not wait until the patient is already seriously neutropenic before decreasing the dose of cytotoxic agent but should decrease the dose based on the projection of the downward slope of the WBC curve. In this way, a smooth plateauing of the WBC can be maintained and infectious disease complications largely avoided. This phenomenon is illustrated in Figure 51–3.

The preceding principles of the relationship between neutropenia and infection generally hold true except under certain circumstances, such as the concomitant use of other agents, which cause a host defense defect but do not cause neutropenia. As mentioned, this is the case with the use of daily glucocorticoids, which negates the ability to use the WBC as an accurate gauge of the degree of host defense defect. Further, agents such as azathioprine can result in an increased incidence of infectious disease complications even without neutropenia. When using such agents, it is still important to monitor the WBC; however, the danger of the occurrence of unpredicted infectious disease complications must be appreciated. In addition, the gradual dropping of the WBC on a constant dose of cytotoxic agent is the rule, but certain drugs such as azathioprine can give an idiosyncratic, precipitous drop in WBC. All of these possibilities

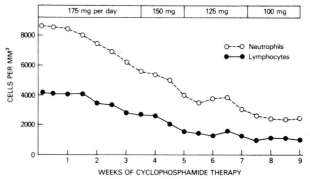

Figure 51–3. Schematic diagram of the use and modification of cyclophosphamide therapy according to the white blood cell count in a patient with Wegener's granulomatosis. The major goal in the treatment of non-neoplastic diseases with cytotoxic agents such as cyclophosphamide is the suppression of disease activity and avoidance of toxic side effects such as significant neutropenia. As shown with the patient indicated in this figure, the dose of drug must be continually modified in accordance with the white blood cell count so as to allow the total white blood cell count to remain above 3000 to 3500 cells/mm³, which generally results in a neutrophil count above 1000 to 1500 cells/mm.³ It is essential to realize that the dosage must be decreased as the slope of the white blood cell count declines, since a given dose of drug will be reflected by the white blood cell count several days later. One must anticipate this and modify the dosage so as to arrive smoothly at a maintenance dose of cyclophosphamide, which is almost always lower than the initial induction dose. Once the maintenance dose is reached, the patient will usually be able to tolerate it for several months. However, usually even this dose must ultimately be decreased, as the bone marrow is less able to tolerate the drug over a period of time. Again, this requires frequent and consistent monitoring of the counts throughout the period of drug administration.

must be taken into consideration in the use of these agents.

It should be pointed out that under certain circumstances, the bone marrow reserve of a given patient may be suppressed to a point at which the dosage of cyclophosphamide must be reduced even though the disease is still active. In these situations, the addition of or increase in the dose of alternate-day prednisone may allow one to administer higher doses of cyclophosphamide with a lesser degree of leukopenia. It is thought that the mechanism of this marrow-sparing effect of glucocorticoid in patients treated with cyclophosphamide is the result of a beneficial effect on marrow regeneration, most likely caused by an altering of cell cycle characteristics of granulocyte progenitor cells.[25]

Once disease remission has been achieved and maintained for an adequate period of time with the use of cytotoxic agents, it is important to attempt to taper the dosage of drug continually with the ultimate goal of discontinuation. The time for maintenance of remission on cytotoxic agents varies with each disease. The general principle stands, however, that the physician should always have the ultimate discontinuation of the cytotoxic agent as a goal of the regimen.

Finally, a thorough familiarization with all of the other immediate as well as long-term potential side effects of these agents should be undertaken by the physician who prescribes them, and careful following of the patient during and after use of these agents is essential to detect the onset of these complications as early as possible.

THERAPEUTIC APHERESIS

The word *apheresis* is a Greek derivative meaning withdrawal. Therapeutic apheresis implies withdrawal of a substance from a patient, ultimately leading to clinical improvement in a disease state. Although the original aphereses were solely confined to the removal of plasma for hyperviscosity states such as Waldenström's macroglobulinemia, the development of sophisticated equipment for removal of plasma as well as selected cellular components has led to an acceleration of the use of apheresis in a number of different disease states, including hematologic, connective tissue, neurologic, and even neoplastic disorders.[85] Plasmapheresis is the removal of plasma without significant removal of cellular elements. Cytapheresis is the removal of cells without significant removal of noncellular elements such as plasma. For example, lymphocytapheresis is the selective removal of mononuclear cells, especially lymphocytes, without significant removal of either plasma or nonlymphoid cellular elements. Selective lymphocyte removal can be accomplished either by thoracic duct drainage (which, strictly speaking, is lymphocytapheresis) or by continuous-flow cell separators via venous access. Lymphoplasmapheresis is the removal of both plasma and lymphocytes with sparing of nonlymphoid cellular elements.

In addition to the removal of the hyperviscous macroglobulin in Waldenström's macroglobulinemia, plasmapheresis has the theoretical and practical effect of removing pathogenic autoantibodies in diseases such as Goodpasture's syndrome, immune thrombocytopenia, autoimmune hemolytic anemia, myasthenia gravis, and severe Rh disease.[85–89] Plasmapheresis has been used in the treatment of connective tissue diseases, particularly rheumatoid arthritis and SLE, and to a lesser degree in the treatment of certain of the vasculitic syndromes.[89–93] Given the evidence that lymphocytes appear to be involved in both the initiation and the propagation of the inflammatory responses in rheumatoid arthritis, lymphocytapheresis and lymphoplasmapheresis have been performed in the treatment of this disease.[94, 95] Finally, evidence has indicated that a form of plasmapheresis in which plasma is perfused over immobilized protein A may be effective in inducing tumor rejection in patients with malignant neoplasms by removing serum factors that inhibit rejection.[96] In this regard, the area of selective removal of potentially harmful components of plasma by extracorporeal modification of plasma either by selective absorption, cryogelation, and membrane filtration or by chemical and physical precipitation is under intensive study.[97, 98]

The major rationale for the use of plasmapheresis in the treatment of immune complex–mediated disease such as SLE is the physical removal of the immune complexes from the circulation, making them unavailable for deposition in tissue. A further rationale, however, may relate to abnormalities in reticuloendothelial system (RES) function seen in certain immune complex–mediated diseases such as SLE.[99] A study has demonstrated that plasmapheresis reestablished previously abnormal splenic reticuloendothelial system function, and this did not necessarily correlate with immune complex levels.[92] In addition, studies have demonstrated that defective monocyte function improved following plasmapheresis.[100] Hence, the therapeutic efficacy of plasmapheresis may well extend beyond the mere removal of a substance that is directly toxic to tissues.

Plasmapheresis carries with it the potential problem of a rebound in production of antibodies to higher levels than those before treatment by removal of either feedback inhibitory mechanisms or actual suppressor factors.[86] This difficulty, however, is generally obviated because most protocols employing plasmapheresis also call for the simultaneous administration of immunosuppressive agents, which not only synergize with the effects of the plasmapheresis but also blunt any potential rebound phenomena that might occur.[101]

Plasmapheresis protocols vary considerably in the specific details of the procedure. Current uses of plasmapheresis, however, are usually true plasma exchanges, in that large amounts of plasma are removed and replaced by various types of replacement fluids. A commonly used protocol is the performance of plasma exchanges three times per week over a 2- to 6-week period. Each procedure usually lasts from 2 to 4 hours. At each procedure, variable amounts of plasma may be removed, but a relatively standard amount is 40 ml of plasma/kg of body weight or up to 3 L per exchange. Plasma volume is usually replaced by a combination of albumin and normal saline solution with or without other fluids such as acid citrate dextrose.[90] Replacement of plasma volume and oncotic pressure are accomplished by these materials.

Theoretically, however, one must at least consider the replacement of other factors, such as Ig, clotting factors, and other proteins. It has been reported that a prolongation of prothrombin, partial thromboplastin, and thrombin times as well as a reduction in fibrinogen, clotting factors, and platelet counts occurred 4 hours after plasmapheresis; however, these all cleared up by 24 hours.[102] The effect of plasmapheresis with albumin replacement on normal plasma constituents was also studied.[103] All plasma constituents were shown to have recovered within 48 hours except fibrinogen, C3, cholesterol, IgG, and IgM. Although fresh frozen plasma is the most physiologic replacement fluid available, as it supplies Ig, coagulation factors, complement, and possibly other factors that might be beneficial to and lacking in the patient, it does carry the risk of transmission of viral disease.

Thus, albumin and normal saline solution remain the standard replacement fluids.

Sakamoto and associates[104] examined the effects of apheresis on a small number of patients with rheumatoid vasculitis and found beneficial responses in a majority of individuals.

Lymphapheresis, like plasmapheresis, has been carried out under a variety of protocols. In one study, lymphapheresis was carried out in a group of patients with rheumatoid arthritis, and each procedure was repeated two to three times per week for a total of 13 to 16 procedures over a 5-week period.[94] A mean of 13.7×10^{10} lymphocytes were removed per patient during the study, and every patient became lymphopenic. Although short periods of lymphapheresis resulted in equal losses of T and B lymphocytes, this extended 5-week course resulted in a disproportionate fall in circulating T lymphocytes by 26 to 58 percent. In addition, serum IgM fell by 30 percent. Clearly, significant lymphodepletion with resulting immunosuppression can be achieved with repeated lymphocytapheresis using continuous-flow centrifugation.[105] In a double-blind controlled trial of lymphoplasmapheresis versus sham apheresis in patients with rheumatoid arthritis, by the ninth treatment, treated patients had significant reductions in absolute lymphocyte counts; total serum protein; $\alpha\beta\gamma$ globulins; IgG, IgM, IgA; C3; and circulating immune complexes; there were no significant changes in WBC, serum sodium, potassium, or albumin.[95] Of note is the fact that Westergren sedimentation rates fell significantly, as did rheumatoid factor titers.

Lymphapheresis has for the most part replaced thoracic duct drainage as a modality for removing lymphocytes largely because of the ease, convenience, and relative lack of complications of the former. Significantly favorable and sometimes dramatic clinical responses, however, have been reported in a study of the effects of long-term thoracic duct drainage in a group of patients with autoimmune diseases.[106] Significant degrees of immunosuppression, particularly of T lymphocyte–mediated responses, were noted in the treated patients,[106, 107] and disease was transiently exacerbated in three patients in whom autologous lymphocytes were reinfused.[107]

Detrimental side effects and complications of apheresis include depletion of platelets as well as important components of plasma, such as clotting factors, with resulting bleeding diatheses, hypotension, fluid and electrolyte imbalance, and complications relating to access sites. The potential long-term complications of these procedures are unclear at present.

The long-term therapeutic benefits from apheresis are uncertain, and a number of controlled and uncontrolled studies are being conducted to determine the precise immediate and long-term benefits of this approach in several rheumatic diseases. Several studies have indicated at least a significant short-term clinical improvement in patients with rheumatoid arthritis treated with various apheresis protocols.[85, 94, 95, 104] The situation is less clear in SLE, and a review of the available data indicates no significant benefit of plasmapheresis in the treatment of SLE.[91]

IONIZING RADIATION

Ionizing radiation exerts its effects on tissues by inducing the ionization of atoms, leading to the formation of highly reactive free radicals. These free radicals interact with biologically relevant macromolecules such as DNA.[108] Rapidly dividing cells such as those of bone marrow, intestinal epithelium, and certain types of lymphocytes appear to be selectively affected by irradiation. However, irradiation may also impair cell function and viability by mechanisms unrelated to the mitotic event.[108]

Ionizing radiation can have profound effects on lymphoid cells, including those involved in the initiation and propagation of immune-mediated connective tissue diseases. The ultimate effect of irradiation on the immune system of the host is highly dependent on the dose delivered. Although this may vary according to the protocol employed, there is generally a gradation of sensitivity of lymphoid subsets as well as of lymphoid cells at various stages of differentiation to increasing doses of irradiation.[109] Precursor cells are usually exquisitely sensitive to irradiation. Low doses of irradiation may selectively kill certain subpopulations of T and B lymphocytes while sparing others. Resting or undifferentiated B lymphocytes are quite sensitive to irradiation, whereas fully differentiated plasma cells are rather resistant to the effects of radiation.[110] Among immunoregulatory T lymphocyte subsets, suppressor T lymphocytes are generally more sensitive to irradiation than are helper T lymphocytes.[110] It should be pointed out that the net effect of irradiation on lymphocyte subpopulations in particular and on immune function in general is usually highly dependent on the total dosage and the dosage schedule employed. For example, total body irradiation is profoundly immunosuppressive and is designed to eliminate as extensively as possible the immune competence of the host. The side effects of this modality are extreme and may be fatal. Therefore, this type of radiation protocol is reserved for special clinical circumstances such as preparation for bone marrow transplantation. For this reason, we do not discuss this modality in the present setting.

Total Lymph Node Irradiation

A potentially important advance in the use of radiation therapy for non-neoplastic disease has been made with the introduction of the use of fractionated total lymph node irradiation in the treatment of rheumatoid arthritis. The rationale for this approach is similar to that described for the use of lymphapheresis in that evidence indicates that lymphocytes, particularly T lymphocytes, appear to be involved in the immunopathogenic expression of rheumatoid arthritis. Total lymph node irradiation has been used since the early 1970s in the treatment of Hodgkin's disease and non-Hodgkin's lymphoma.[111–113] Of note is the fact that there have been no serious long-term sequelae such as leukemia, second tumors, or serious host defense defects leading to infectious disease complications. Nonetheless, cell-mediated immunity was shown to be suppressed for several years following treatment. Thus, this approach has been employed in the treatment of intractable rheumatoid arthritis as an alternative to the use of cytotoxic agents such as cyclophosphamide and azathioprine.

The results of several studies, including randomized double-blind trials, have demonstrated substantial efficacy in patients with rheumatoid arthritis, employing doses ranging between 750 and 3000 cGy administered over 1 to 4 months.[114–121] Significant side effects were noted, however, especially at higher doses; these adverse effects included viral and bacterial infections, cytopenias, xerostomia, hypothyroidism, cutaneous vasculitis, and pericarditis. Controlled comparisons of irradiation with immunosuppressive therapy are needed to better define the precise role this modality should play in the treatment of advanced rheumatoid arthritis.

Although the usefulness of total lymphoid irradiation in treating other autoimmune disorders has been less well studied, Strober and colleagues[122] reported improvement in each of ten patients who received irradiation for the treatment of intractable lupus nephritis.

Total lymphoid irradiation has recently been used as an immunosuppressive maneuver in the prevention and treatment of rejection in patients receiving solid organ transplants.[123–126] When administered before organ transplantation in experimental models, it appears to induce a state of partial tolerance, and clinical studies have demonstrated efficacy in cardiac and renal transplantation. The mechanism has not been fully elucidated, but increases in CD8 suppressor T lymphocyte populations and decreases in B lymphocyte populations have been observed. Side effects appear to be few, but leukopenia, thrombocytopenia, and activation of cytomegalovirus infection have been observed.

GLUCOCORTICOIDS

Glucocorticoids are used extensively in the treatment of rheumatic diseases. These agents manifest both anti-inflammatory and immunosuppressive effects.[7] Although virtually any function of an inflammatory or immune-competent cell can be suppressed by a high enough concentration of a glucocorticoid in vitro, in the dosages of drug that are generally employed in the treatment of rheumatic diseases, the effects of the drug are somewhat selective for one or another of the components of the inflammatory or immune response.[7, 127] For example, the inductive phase of the immune response is clearly more sensi-

tive to the immunosuppressive effects of glucocorticoids than is the effector phase.[7] Furthermore, the T lymphocyte or cell-mediated limb of immunity is clearly more sensitive to glucocorticoids than is the B lymphocyte or humoral limb. In addition, within the T lymphocyte fraction, certain subsets are selectively more sensitive to the drug than are others.[128, 129]

Of particular importance in the understanding of the effects of glucocorticoids on inflammatory and immune-competent cells is an appreciation that the drugs can affect the inflammatory and immune responses by a number of mechanisms. For example, administration of a glucocorticoid may affect the circulatory kinetics of a given cell type such as a neutrophil, monocyte, or lymphocyte subset and thus block the availability of these cells to the inflammatory site without directly suppressing the functional capability of the cell. On the other hand, the drug may directly affect the functional capability of a cell in a situation in which circulatory kinetics are not relevant.[7] In general, lower concentrations of the drug are required to affect circulatory kinetics, whereas higher concentrations are needed to directly suppress a functional capability of a cell.[7] Finally, the effects of glucocorticoids on a given cell type may vary, depending on the state of activation of the cell in question. Understanding these concepts is important in the proper design of therapeutic protocols for the use of glucocorticoids in the treatment of non-neoplastic diseases. A detailed discussion of the use of glucocorticoid therapy is contained in Chapter 50. Nonglucocorticoid hormones, including androgens, estrogens, growth hormone, thyroxine, and insulin, may also exert potent effects on immunoregulation.[130]

CYCLOSPORINE, FK506, AND RAPAMYCIN

The fungal products cyclosporine and FK506 have received considerable attention as immunosuppressive agents for use in preventing and treating rejection in transplant recipients and for the treatment of autoimmune disease. As noted subsequently, these two compounds, although differing in structure, share similarities in their mechanism of action and thus are considered together. The structures of these two molecules are illustrated in Figure 51–4.

Cyclosporine

Cyclosporine was discovered in 1972 during a search for biologically produced antifungal agents. It is a 1200-dalton fungal metabolite, which proved to be only mildly active as an antifungal agent but did manifest certain profound effects on the immune response. Cyclosporine is a cyclic endecapeptide of original chemical structure in which some amino acids are unconventional or modified (N-methylated).[131] This latter property is responsible for the drug's effectiveness by oral administration in that pH

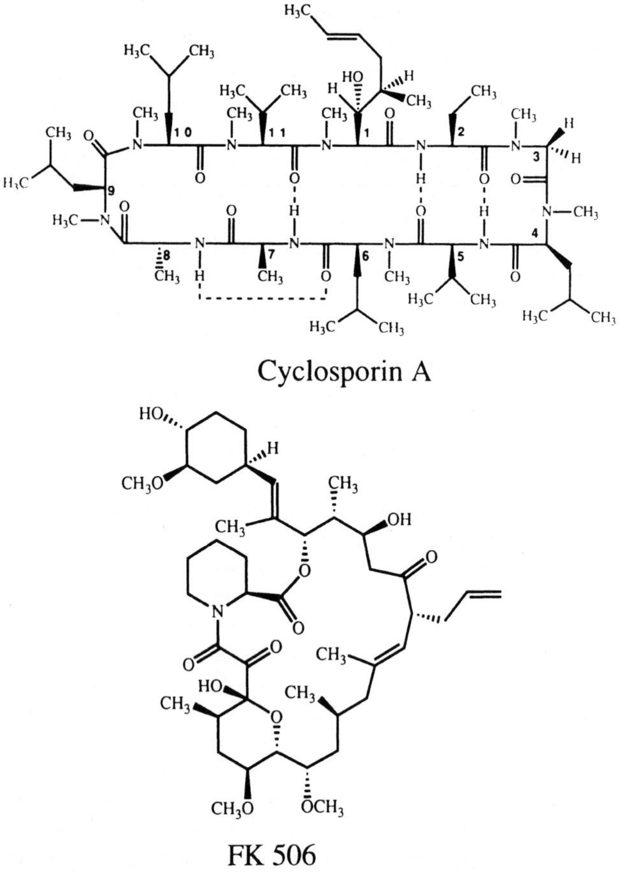

Figure 51–4. Structures of the immunosuppressant molecules cyclosporin A (cyclosporine) and FK506. (Adapted from Sigal NH, Siekierka JJ, Dumont FJ: Observations on the mechanism of action of FK 506. Biochem Pharmacol 40:2201, 1990. Copyright 1990, Pergamon Press Ltd.)

and enzymes of the gastrointestinal tract do not seem to inactivate it. It can be administered by both parenteral and oral routes, it exhibits poor water solubility, and it does not need to be activated in vivo, as witnessed by the fact that it is directly active in vitro. The drug has been employed extensively as an immunosuppressive agent for organ transplantation.[132] It is administered either as the sole immunosuppressive agent or together with glucocorticoids and other compounds. The optimum dose with regard to efficacy balanced against toxic side effects has not been precisely determined, but most protocols employ doses of 3 to 5 mg/kg/day, with close monitoring of cyclosporine blood levels. Because of its nephrotoxicity, cyclosporine is being used in some transplant protocols mainly in the induction phase and to treat acute rejection, whereas conventional immunosuppressive therapy is employed in long-term maintenance.[132–135]

The availability of cyclosporine and the consequent ability of transplant protocols to rely less heavily on other immunosuppressive drugs have virtually revolutionized the field of organ transplantation. The implications of this experience are extraordinary for the use of organ transplantation in a wide variety of clinical situations. In this regard, studies have demonstrated the efficacy of cyclosporine in suppressing graft-versus-host reactions in bone marrow transplants.[132, 136]

The major constraint in the use of cyclosporine, as with other immunosuppressive agents, lies in its toxicity. Although it has few myelotoxic effects, use of the agent is not without risks. By far the most serious toxic side effect of the drug is its nephrotoxicity.[132, 137–140] This toxic side effect is particularly serious in a renal transplantation program, since it is often unclear whether a deterioration in renal function is due to insufficient drug, allowing rejection to occur, or to too much cyclosporine, causing nephrotoxicity.

Feutren and Mihatsch examined risk factors for cyclosporine-induced nephropathy in patients with autoimmune disease[141] and concluded that allowing a dose no higher than 5 mg/kg/day and avoiding increases in serum creatinine of more than 30 percent above the patient's baseline value would minimize the development of cyclosporine-induced renal toxicity.

Other toxic side effects include abnormalities of liver function tests, transient hirsutism, and gum hypertrophy. Bacterial infection has not been a problem with the use of this drug. Reactivation of certain viral infections, however, particularly Epstein-Barr virus, has occurred sporadically. Of note is the fact that lymphomas have occurred in patients treated with cyclosporine that were believed to result from the immunosuppressive effects rather than from any carcinogenicity of the drug.[142]

Of particular interest for the present discussion is the potential for the use of cyclosporine in the treatment of rheumatic diseases characterized by hyperreactivity or aberrant immune function at the T lymphocyte level. A number of studies have extended the potential role of cyclosporine to the treatment of autoimmune diseases. Nussenblatt and coworkers[143–145] have been successful in treating uveitis with cyclosporine in patients whose ocular disease had been resistant to glucocorticoids and cytotoxic agents. Van Rijthoven and associates[146] examined the effect of cyclosporine in 36 patients with rheumatoid arthritis in a double-blind, placebo-controlled trial. They noted that treated patients experienced significant improvement in joint disease compared with their condition on entering the study and in comparison to the placebo group. In subsequent studies, Dougados and Amor[147] and other investigators[148] confirmed the efficacy of cyclosporine in refractory rheumatoid arthritis. In all of these investigations, use of the drug was frequently limited by toxicity.

Additionally, more limited investigations have suggested that cyclosporine may be useful in the treatment of diverse immune-mediated disorders such as autoimmune chronic active hepatitis,[149] pulmonary sarcoidosis,[150] inflammatory bowel disease,[151–153] bullous pemphigoid,[154] psoriasis,[155, 156] asthma,[157] Graves' ophthalmopathy,[158] and primary biliary cirrhosis.[159]

Significant interest has focused on the use of cyclosporine in the treatment of type 1 diabetes mellitus, in which an autoimmune component is frequently present.[160]

Although the need for additional carefully controlled trials of cyclosporine in the treatment of inflammatory disorders is clear, it is evident that this potent drug will likely prove to be extremely useful in certain patients with rheumatic and autoimmune diseases.

FK506

FK506 is a macrolide produced by the fungus *Streptomyces tsukubaensis*.[161, 162] In vitro and in vivo studies have suggested that FK506 has immunosuppressant effects comparable with those of cyclosporine but at doses 10 to 100 times lower.[163] Studies of organ transplantation in a variety of animal models have demonstrated that this compound is extremely effective in preventing rejection, although these studies have been hampered by the development of toxicities that may be unique to the species studied, including the interesting finding in dogs of arteritis and lymphocytic infiltration of organs.[164] These toxicities have not been observed in primates or in human studies.

Clinical studies of FK506 in human liver transplantation were begun in 1989, and the Pittsburgh group has reported remarkable success in their early trials.[165] Additional trials are ongoing at a number of medical centers around the world.

Toxicities of FK506 in human transplant recipients have been remarkably few. In one study of 31 liver transplant recipients, 87 percent of patients reported no side effects.[166] Some individuals experienced headache and insomnia. Other investigators, however, have noted the occurrence of nephrotoxicity and hyperglycemia[167] in individuals receiving FK506.

Information has begun to appear in the literature regarding the potential efficacy of FK506 in inflammatory disorders. In animal studies, the compound has proved effective in treating collagen-induced arthritis,[168] nephrotoxic serum glomerulonephritis,[169] autoimmune uveoretinitis,[170] autoimmune encephalomyelitis,[171] and autoimmune disease in MRL/lpr and (NZB x NZW) F1 mice.[172]

Data on the use of FK506 in the treatment of human autoimmune disease are more limited, but case reports suggesting efficacy in the treatment of cyclosporine-induced hemolytic uremic syndrome following organ transplantation[173] and in steroid-resistant focal sclerosing glomerulonephritis[174] have been published.

Thomson and colleagues at Pittsburgh summarized their experience with FK506 in the treatment of autoimmune diseases.[175] Beneficial effects have been observed in a variety of inflammatory disorders, including uveitis, multiple sclerosis, ulcerative colitis, Crohn's disease, autoimmune chronic active hepatitis, primary biliary cirrhosis, psoriasis and new-onset type 1 diabetes. In several patients, FK506 therapy produced efficacious results after cyclosporine treatment had failed.

Molecular Mechanism of Action of Cyclosporine and FK506

These two compounds and related ones such as rapamycin appear to function via binding to novel cellular proteins with specific binding properties.[176] The binding proteins, termed *immunophilins*, have been described, and insights into the biology of these proteins and their ligands have significantly advanced our understanding of the activation of immune cells.

Cyclosporine and FK506 share the feature of being potent inhibitors of T cell activation, and in particular they inhibit the transcription of early T cell activation genes.[177, 178] These genes include IL-2, IL-3, IL-4, granulocyte-macrophage colony-stimulating factor (GM-CSF), tumor necrosis factor-α (TNF-α), and interferon-γ (IFN-γ).

The mechanism of action of these two immunosuppressive agents has been studied in great detail. The major cyclosporine-binding protein cyclophilin and the predominant FK506-binding protein (FKBP) are enzymes with peptidyl-prolyl isomerase activity, important in catalyzing the interconversion of *cis*-rotamers and *trans*-rotamers of amide bonds in cellular peptides and proteins.[176] Several lines of evidence, however, suggest that inhibition of this isomerase or rotamase activity is not sufficient to explain the drugs' immunosuppressive action.[179] It has been further demonstrated that a central step in the activity of these drugs is the binding of drug-immunophilin complex to calcineurin, a serine-threonine phosphatase.[180] Calcineurin phosphatase activity appears to be an important if not critical component of calcium-dependent cell-triggering events. Blockade of calcineurin activity by cyclosporine or FK506 inhibits the nuclear translocation of a transcription factor NF-AT that is crucial for the activation of T lymphocytes.[181]

The immunologic effects of cyclosporine and FK506 are complex but appear to be specific for lymphocytes. Numerous studies have demonstrated the ability of cyclosporine to block the activation of T lymphocytes,[182] and effects on B cells are also likely.[183]

Rapamycin

Rapamycin is a structural homolog of FK506 and binds to FKBP but acts at a later point in the cell cycle to inhibit cell cycle progression. In several animal models of autoimmune disease, including arthritis, uveoretinitis, and experimental allergic encephalomyelitis, rapamycin has shown promising immunosuppressive effects.[184–186]

OTHER AGENTS

Levamisole

Levamisole is a three-ring molecule with the extremely low molecular weight of 241. It was introduced into veterinary practice in 1966 as a nematocidal agent and was subsequently used in humans. It is highly active against a wide range of nematodes and is particularly effective in ascariasis. It has, however, received attention as an immunoenhancing agent in humans. Levamisole is absorbed rapidly from the gastrointestinal tract. Following administration of a 150-mg dose in humans, peak blood levels of 5 g/ml are reached at 2 hours.[187] The plasma half-life is approximately 4 hours, and the drug is metabolized predominantly in the liver, with excretion of the breakdown products via the kidney and to a lesser extent in the feces.

The mechanism of action of levamisole remains in doubt, but it has a number of well-recognized immunologic effects. These include correction of chemotactic defects of monocytes[188] and neutrophils[189] from patients with viral infections or the hyperimmunoglobulin E syndrome,[190] enhancement of delayed-type hypersensitivity,[191] and enhancement of a variety of lymphocyte functions.[192]

Levamisole has been used in malignant diseases as an adjuvant agent, most notably gastrointestinal carcinomas,[193] and it has been approved by the U.S. Food and Drug Administration for this purpose. It has also been used in a number of nonmalignant diseases. Of particular interest has been its use in the treatment of rheumatoid arthritis in which rather favorable clinical responses have been reported.[194, 195] The drug is generally administered in doses of 150 mg orally on a daily basis for periods up to 16 weeks. The major constraint of its use clinically is the incidence and severity of the toxic side effects, which have included gastrointestinal disturbances, fatigue, fever, and skin rash. The most severe and limiting toxic side effect, however, is granulocytopenia, which seems to be disproportionately more frequent in patients with rheumatic diseases. It is of particular interest that agranulocytosis owing to levamisole is particularly common in patients with human leukocyte antigen (HLA)–B27.[196, 197] In a study of the treatment of 20 rheumatoid arthritis patients with levamisole, agranulocytosis or neutropenia occurred at some time in 4 patients. Despite the favorable clinical results with regard to the activity of rheumatoid arthritis in that study, the toxicity clearly renders the drug unacceptable for routine use in rheumatoid arthritis.

Other Immune Enhancers and Adjuvants

Clearly the most extensive employed adjuvant in experimental animals is complete Freud's adjuvant (CFA), which is composed of paraffin oil and an emulsifying agent to which killed mycobacteria have been added. Injection of emulsions of antigens in CFA into experimental animals results in markedly augmented antibody responses as well as delayed hypersensitivity.[198] Unfortunately, the severe local and systemic toxic side effects of CFA render it unacceptable for use in humans. Preparations of adjuvants such as the synthetic N-acetylmuramyl-L-alanyl-D-isoglutamine have been shown to be effective enhancers of antibody production without appreciable toxic side effects.[199] Such studies may prove extremely fruitful in the ultimate development of a clinically acceptable adjuvant, which could be used in the enhancement of immune function in the absence of significant toxic effects.

Dapsone

Dapsone is a sulfone (4,4'-diaminodiphenyl sulfone) that first gained attention as an agent effective in the treatment of *Mycobacterium leprae*. It has been recognized as an effective agent in the treatment of dermatitis herpetiformis[200] and erythema elevatum diutinum[201] as well as the bullous eruptions of SLE.[202] Dapsone is available for oral administration and is slowly and nearly completely absorbed from the gastrointestinal tract. Peak concentrations of dapsone are reached in plasma 1 to 3 hours after oral administration, and its half-life ranges from 10 to 50 hours, with a mean of 28 hours.[203] Twenty-four hours after an oral dose of 100 mg, plasma concentrations range from 0.4 to 1.2 μg/ml. The sulfones are distributed throughout the total body water and are present in all tissues. They tend to be retained in skin, muscle, liver, and kidney, with traces of the drug present in these organs up to 3 weeks after cessation of administration. Dapsone is acetylated in the liver, and about 70 to 80 percent of a dose is excreted in the urine.

The drug is administered orally in doses of 50 to 100 mg/day. The effect is seen within days, and particularly with erythema elevatum diutinum, relapses occur almost immediately after cessation of the drug,[201] which is somewhat paradoxical given that the drug is present in organs for weeks after cessation of therapy. The sudden relapses following cessation might be explained by a need for a critical concentration of drug in plasma below which a dramatic deterioration in clinical condition is seen.

The limiting factor in the use of dapsone is its toxicity, which includes hemolysis and methemoglobinemia and which occurs relatively frequently. Other side effects include anorexia, nausea, and vomiting. Rarely, headache, nervousness, insomnia, and peripheral neuropathy have been reported.

CONCLUSIONS

The use of cytotoxic and other immunoregulatory agents has played a major role in the treatment of non-neoplastic, immune-mediated disease. Most of these agents are nonspecific, however, and are invariably associated with a variety of toxic side effects (Table 51–6). Because most of the rheumatic diseases in which these agents are used are chronic in nature and are rarely curable, the physician must establish the clear-cut goals of a given therapeutic regimen and must be aware of the actual as well as the potential and the immediate as well as the long-term toxic side effects of these agents. Insightful use of these agents under appropriate clinical circumstances can often lead to dramatic improvements in lifestyle. Under other circumstances, the effects may even be lifesaving. Use of these agents, however, should be avoided in circumstances in which a less aggressive approach

Table 51–6. PHARMACOLOGIC PROPERTIES OF IMMUNOREGULATORY AGENTS

Agent	Administration	Dosage	Gastrointestinal Absorption	Plasma Half-life	Major Side Effects
Cytotoxic Agents					
Nitrogen mustard	IV	0.4 mg/kg q 3–4 weeks	—	Few minutes	Leukopenia, thrombocytopenia, nausea, vomiting, local reactions at injection site
Cyclophosphamide	IV or oral	2 mg/kg/day orally or IV; 750 mg/m² IV bolus	Excellent	6–7 hours	Neutropenia, gonadal suppression, cystitis, alopecia, oncogenesis, pulmonary fibrosis, gastrointestinal intolerance
Chlorambucil	IV or oral	0.1–0.2 mg/kg/day orally	Good	90 minutes	Leukopenia, thrombocytopenia, oncogenesis, gonadal suppression, gastrointestinal intolerance, hepatotoxicity, dermatitis
Azathioprine and 6-mercaptopurine	IV or oral	2 mg/kg/day orally	Excellent	60–90 minutes	Leukopenia, hepatotoxicity, gastrointestinal intolerance, oncogenesis, host defense defect
Methotrexate	IV or oral	5–50 mg/week as single IV dose or orally in 3 divided doses (q 12 hours) or orally daily for 5 days of the week	Intermittent to good	2 hours	Leukopenia, thrombocytopenia, oral mucositis, gastrointestinal intolerance, hepatotoxicity, fetal intolerance in first trimester of pregnancy
Vinca alkaloids (vincristine and vinblastine)	IV	2 mg/m²	—	Less than 30 minutes	Neurotoxicity
5-Fluorouracil	IV	12 mg/kg/day for 4 days followed by 6 mg/kg on alternate days for 2–4 doses; repeat monthly with adjustment of dose according to response	Unpredictable	10–20 minutes	Leukopenia, gastrointestinal intolerance, alopecia, dermatitis, mucositis
Hydroxyurea	IV or oral	20–30 mg/kg/day orally	Good	6–8 hours	Myelosuppression, gastrointestinal intolerance and ulcerations, mild skin rashes
Other Agents					
Levamisole	Oral	Up to 150 mg/day	Excellent	4 hours	Granulocytopenia, gastrointestinal intolerance, fever, skin rash, fatigue
Cyclosporine	IV or oral	5–8 mg/kg/day	Fair to good	2–24 hours	Nephrotoxicity, hepatotoxicity, reactivation of viral infections, oncogenesis, transient hirsutism, gum hypertrophy
FK506	IV, SC, oral	~0.3 mg/kg/day	Good		Headache, insomnia, nephrotoxicity, hyperglycemia
Dapsone	Oral	50–100 mg/day	Good	10–50 hours	Hemolysis, methemoglobinemia, gastrointestinal intolerance

Abbreviations: IV, intravenous; SC, subcutaneous.

would be more appropriate given the nature of the illness and the projected balance between clinical results and toxic side effects. The treating physician should be acquainted as much as possible with the established results of controlled trials as they appear in the literature and should critically evaluate uncontrolled trials, which may represent a true advance in therapy but which may also give a false sense of security that a particular agent will be beneficial. All things considered, sound clinical judgment applied to each individual patient with regard to the choice and actual usage of an immunoregulatory agent is indispensable.

As our understanding of the immunopathology of the various rheumatic and autoimmune disorders advances, it is highly likely that more specific and less toxic immunoregulatory regimens will be devised, carrying with them the hope for even better patient outcomes.

References

1. Haynes BF, Fauci AS: Cellular and molecular basis of immunity. *In* Isselbacher KJ, Braunwald E, Wilson JW, Martin JB, Fauci AS, Kasper DL (eds): Harrison's Principles of Internal Medicine, 13th ed. New York, McGraw-Hill, 1994.
2. Report of the NIAID Task Force on Immunology and Allergy. U.S. Department of Health and Human Services, Public Health Service, National Institutes of Health, NIH Publication No. 91–2414, 1990.
3. Paul WE: The immune system: An introduction. *In* Paul WE (ed): Fundamental Immunology, 3rd ed. New York, Raven Press, 1993.
4. Fauci AS: The revolution in clinical immunology. JAMA 246:2567, 1981.
5. Fauci AS, Lane HC, Volkman DJ: Activation and regulation of human immune responses: Implications in normal and disease states. Ann Intern Med 98:76, 1983.
6. Steinberg AD, Plotz PH, Wolff SM, Wong VG, Agus SG, Decker JL: Cytotoxic drugs in treatment of nonmalignant diseases. Ann Intern Med 76:619, 1972.
7. Fauci AS, Dale DC, Balow JE: Glucocorticosteroid therapy: Mechanisms of action and clinical considerations. Ann Intern Med 84:304, 1976.
8. Gerber NL, Steinberg AD: Clinical use of immunosuppressive drugs. Part I. Drugs 11:36, 1976.
9. Gerber NL, Steinberg AD: Clinical use of immunosuppressive drugs. Part II. Drugs 11:90, 1976.
10. Handschumacher RE: Immunosuppressive agents. *In* Gilman AG, Rall TW, Nies AS, Taylor PL (eds): Goodman and Gilman's The Pharmacologic Basis of Therapeutics, 8th ed. New York, Pergamon Press, 1990.
11. Cooper MD, Peterson RDA, South MA, Good RA: The functions of the thymus system and the bursa system in the chicken. Nature 205:143, 1965.
12. Cooper MD, Peterson RDA South MA, Good RA: The functions of the thymus system and the bursa system in the chicken. J Exp Med 123:75, 1966.
13. Claman HN, Chaperon EA, Triplett RF: Thymus-marrow cell combinations. Synergism in antibody production. Proc Soc Exp Biol Med 12:1167, 1966.
14. Miller JFAP, Mitchell GF: Cell-cell interactions in immune response. I. Hemolysin-forming cells in neonatally thymectomized mice reconstituted with thymus or thoracic duct lymphocytes. J Exp Med 128:801, 1968.
15. Unanue ER: Macrophages, antigen-presenting cells, and the phenomena of antigen handling and presentation. *In* Paul WE (ed): Fundamental Immunology, 3rd ed. New York, Raven Press, 1993.
16. Möller G (ed): Natural killer cells. Immunol Rev 44:1, 1979.
17. Herberman RB, Ortaldo JR: Natural killer cells: Their role in defenses against disease. Science 214:24, 1981.
18. Gallin JI, Fauci AS (eds): Advances in Host Defense Mechanisms. Vol 1. New York, Raven Press, 1982.
19. Jerne NK: Towards a network theory of the immune system. Ann Immunol (Inst Pasteur) 125:373, 1974.
20. Möller G (ed): Immune networks. Immunol Rev 110:1, 1989.
21. Geha RS: Presence of auto–anti-idiotypic during the normal human immune response to tetanus toxoid antigen. J Immunol 129:139, 1982.
22. Klinman DM, Steinberg AD: Inquiry into murine and human lupus. Immunol Rev 144:157, 1995.
23. Fitch FW, Lanchi DW, Gajewski TF: T-cell-mediated regulation: Help and suppression. *In* Paul WE (ed): Fundamental Immunology, 3rd ed. New York, Raven Press, 1993.
24. Fauci AS, Haynes BF, Katz P: The spectrum of vasculitis: Clinical, pathologic, immunologic, and therapeutic considerations. Ann Intern Med 89:660, 1978.
25. Fauci AS, Haynes BF, Katz P, Wolff SM: Wegener's granulomatosis: Prospective clinical and therapeutic experience with 85 patients over 21 years. Ann Intern Med 98:76, 1983.
26. Fauci AS: The vasculitis syndromes. *In* Isselbacher KI, Braunwald E, Wilson JW, Martin JB, Fauci AS, Kasper DK (eds): Harrison's Principles of Internal Medicine, 13th ed. New York, McGraw-Hill, 1994.
27. Cupps TR, Edgar LC, Fauci AS: Suppression of human B lymphocyte function by cyclophosphamide. J Immunol 1289:2453, 1982.
28. Howard MD, Miyajima A, Coffman R: T-cell–derived cytokines and their receptors. *In* Paul WE (ed): Fundamental Immunology, 3rd ed, New York, Raven Press, 1993.
29. Fauci AS, Katz P, Haynes FF, Wolff SM: Cyclophosphamide therapy of severe necrotizing vasculitis. N Engl J Med 301:235, 1979.
30. Hoffman GS, Kerr GS, Leavitt RY, Hallahan CW, Lebovics RS, Travis WD, Rottem M, Fauci AS: Wegener's granulomatosis: An analysis of 158 partients. Ann Intern Med 116:488, 1992.
31. Austin HA III, Klippel HH, Balow JE, le Riche NG, Steinberg AD: Therapy of lupus nephritis: Controlled trial of prednisone and cytotoxic drugs. N Engl J Med 301:235, 1979.
32. Schein PS, Winokur ST: Immunosuppressive and cytotoxic chemotherapy: Long-term complications. Ann Intern Med 82:84, 1975.
33. Calabresi P, Chabner BA: Antineoplastic agents. *In* Gilman AG, Rall TW, Nies AS, Taylor P (eds): Goodman and Gilman's The Pharmacologic Basis of Therapeutics, 8th ed. New York, Pergamon Press, 1990.
34. Ahn YS, Harrington WJ, Seelman RC, Eytel CS: Vincristine therapy of idiopathic and secondary thrombocytopenias. N Engl J Med 291:376, 1974.
35. Fauci AS, Harley JB, Roberts WC, Ferrans VJ, Gralnick HR, Bjornson BJ: The idiopathic hypereosinophilic syndrome: Clinical, pathologic and therapeutic considerations. Ann Intern Med 97:78, 1982.
36. Roberts JJ, Brent TP, Crathorn AR: Evidence for the inactivation and repair of the mammalian DNA template after alkylation by mustard gas and half mustard gas. Eur J Cancer 7:515, 1971.
37. Fahey JL, Leonard E, Churg J, Godman G: Wegener's granulomatosis. Am J Med 17:168, 1954.
38. Brock N: Pharmacologic characterization of cyclophosphamide (NSC-26271) and cyclophosphamide metabolites. Cancer Chemother Rep 51:315, 1967.
39. Bagley CM, Bostick FW, DeVita VT Jr: Clinical pharmacology of cyclophosphamide. Cancer Res 33:226, 1973.
40. Gershwin ME, Goetzel EJ, Steinberg AD: Cyclophosphamide: Use in practice. Ann Intern Med 80:531, 1974.
41. Sladek NE: Therapeutic efficacy of cyclophosphamide as a function of its metabolism. Cancer Res 32:535, 1972.
42. Makinodan T, Santos GW, Quinn RP: Immunosuppressive drugs. Pharmacol Rev 22:189, 1970.
43. Shand FL: The immunopharmacology of cyclophosphamide. Int J Pharmacol 1:165, 1979.
44. Berenbaum MC, Brown IN: Dose-response relationships for agents inhibiting the immune response. Immunology 7:65, 1964.
45. Askenase PW, Hayden BJ, Gershon RK: Augmentation of delayed-type hypersensitivity by doses of cyclophosphamide which do not effect antibody responses. J Exp Med 141:697, 1965.
46. Sy MS, Miller SD, Claman HN: Immune suppression with supraoptimal doses of antigen in contact sensitivity. I. Demonstration of suppressor cells and their sensitivity to cyclophosphamide. J Immunol 119:240, 1977.
47. Fauci AS, Wolff SM, Johnson JS: Effect of cyclophosphamide upon the immune response in Wegener's granulomatosis. N Engl J Med 285:1493, 1972.
48. Fauci AS, Dale DC, Wolff SM: Cyclophosphamide and lymphocyte subpopulations in Wegener's granulomatosis. Arthritis Rheum 17:355, 1974.
49. Dale DC, Fauci AS, Wolff SM: The effect of cyclophosphamide on leukocyte kinetics and susceptibility to infection in patients with Wegener's granulomatosis. Arthritis Rheum 16:657, 1973.
50. Hoffman GS, Leavitt RU, Fleisher TA, Minor JR, Fauci AS: Treatment of Wegener's granulomatosis with intermittent high-dose intravenous cyclophosphamide. Am J Med 89:403, 1990.
51. Warne GL, Fairley KF, Hobbs JB, Martin FIR: Cyclophosphamide-induced ovarian failure. N Engl J Med 289:1159, 1973.
52. Schilsky RL, Lewis BJ, Sherins RJ, Young RC: Gonadal dysfunction in patients receiving chemotherapy for cancer. Ann Intern Med 93:109, 1980.
53. Trompeter RS, Evans PR, Barratt TM: Gonadal function in boys with steroid-responsive nephrotic syndrome treated with cyclosphamide for short periods. Lancet 1:1177, 1981.

54. Fairley KF, Barrie JU, Johnson W: Sterility and testicular atrophy related to cyclophosphamide therapy. Lancet 1:568, 1972.

55. Plotz PH, Klippel JH, Decker JL, et al: Bladder complications in patients receiving cyclophosphamide for systemic lupus erythematosus or rheumatoid arthritis. Ann Intern Med 91:221, 1979.

56. Cooper JAD Jr, White DA, Matthay RA: State of the art: Drug-induced pulmonary disease. Am Rev Respir Dis 133:321, 1986.

57. Appelbaum FR, Strauchen JA, Graw RG Jr, et al: Acute lethal carditis caused by high-dose combination chemotherapy. A unique clinical and pathological entity. Lancet 1:58, 1976.

58. De Fronzo RA, Braine H, Colvin OM, Davis PJ: Water intoxication in man after cyclophosphamide therapy. Time course and relation to drug activation. Ann Intern Med 78:861, 1973.

59. Bressler RB, Huston DT: Water intoxication following moderate-dose intravenous cyclophosphamide. Arch Intern Med 145:548, 1985.

60. Penn I: Depressed immunity and the development of cancer. Clin Exp Immunol 45:459, 1981.

61. McLean A, Newell D, Baker G: The metabolism of chlorambucil. Biochem Pharmacol 25:2331, 1976.

62. Stukov AN: Experimental study of the combined effect of leukoran, degranol, and prednisolone. Neoplasma 22:181, 1976.

63. Israel H, Patchefsky AS: Treatment of Wegener's granulomatosis of lung. Am J Med 58:671, 1975.

64. Rudd P, Fried JF, Epstein WV: Irreversible bone marrow failure with chlorambucil. J Rheumatol 2:421, 1975.

65. Cameron S: Chlorambucil and leukemia. N Engl J Med 296:1065, 1977.

66. Lerner HJ: Acute myelogenous leukemia in patients receiving chlorambucil as long-term adjuvant chemotherapy for Stage II breast cancer. Cancer Treat Rep 60:1431, 1978.

67. Gabrielsen AE, Good RA: Chemical suppression of adaptive immunity. Adv Immunol 6:91, 1967.

68. Yu DT, Clements PJ, Peter JB, Levy J, Paulus HE, Barnett EV: Lymphocyte characteristics in rheumatic patients and the effect of azathioprine therapy. Arthritis Rheum 17:37, 1974.

69. Levy J, Barnett EV, MacDonald NS, Klinenberg JR, Pearson CM: The effect of azathioprine on gammaglobulin synthesis in man. J Clin Invest 51:2233, 1972.

70. Maibach HI, Epstein WL: Immunologic responses of healthy volunteers receiving azathioprine (Imuran). Int Arch Allergy 27:102, 1965.

71. Abdou NI, Zweiman B, Casella SR: Effects of azathioprine therapy on bone marrow–dependent and thymus-dependent cells in man. Clin Exp Immunol 13:55, 1973.

72. Fournier C, Bach MA, Dardenne M, Bach JF: Selective action of azathioprine on T cells. Transplant Proc 5:523, 1973.

73. Campbell AC, Skinner JM, Hersey P, Roberts-Thompson P, MacLennan ICM, Truelove SC: Immunosuppression in the treatment of inflammatory bowel disease. I. Changes in lymphoid subpopulations in the blood and rectal mucosa following cessation of treatment with azathioprine. Clin Exp Immunol 16:521, 1974.

74. Sharbaugh RJ, Ainsworth SK, Fitts CT: Lack of effect of azathioprine on phytohemagglutinin-induced lymphocyte transformation and established delayed cutaneous hypersensitivity. Int Arch Allergy Appl Immunol 51:681, 1976.

75. Gassman AE, van Furth R: The effect of azathioprine (Imuran) on the kinetics of monocytes and macrophages during the normal steady state and an acute inflammatory reaction. Blood 46:51, 1975.

76. Phillips SM, Zweiman B: Mechanisms in the suppression of delayed hypersensitivity in the guinea pig by 6-mercaptopurine. J Exp Med 137:1494, 1973.

77. Rosman M, Bertino JR: Azathioprine. Ann Intern Med 79:694, 1973.

78. Losito A, Williams DG, Harris L: The effects on polymorphonuclear leukocyte function of prednisolone and azathioprine in vivo and prednisolone, azathioprine and 6-mercaptopurine in vitro. Clin Exp Immunol 32:423, 1978.

79. Henderson FS, Adamson RH, Oliverio VT: The metabolic rate of tritiated methotrexate. II. Absorption and excretion in man. Cancer Res 25:1018, 1965.

80. Ahn YS, Byrnes JJ, Harrington WJ, et al: The treatment of idiopathic thrombocytopenia with vinblastine-loaded platelets. N Engl J Med 298:1101, 1978.

81. Rodgers GP, Dover GJ, Noguchi CT, Schecter AN, Nienhuis AW: Augmentation by erythropoietin of the fetal-hemoglobin response to hydroxyurea in sickle cell disease. N Engl J Med 328:73, 1993.

82. Yarbro JW: Mechanism of action of hydroxyurea. Semin Oncol 19:1, 1992.

83. Rodgers GP, Dover GJ, Uyesaka N, Noguchi CT, Schecter AN, Nienhuis AW: Hematologic responses of patients with sickle cell disease to treatment with hydroxyurea. N Engl J Med 322:1037, 1990.

84. Cupps TR, Silverman GJ, Fauci, AS: Herpes zoster in patients with treated Wegener's granulomatosis. A possible role for cyclophosphamide. Am J Med 69:881, 1980.

85. Tindall RSA (ed.): Therapeutic Apheresis and Plasma Perfusion. New York, AR Liss, 1980.

86. Branda RF, Molodow CF, McCollough JJ, Jacob HS: Plasma exchange in the treatment of immune disease. Transfusion 5:570, 1975.

87. Lockwood CM, Pearson TA, Rees AJ, Evans DJ, Peters DK, Wilson CB: Immunosuppression and plasma exchange in the treatment of Goodpasture's syndrome. Lancet 1:711, 1976.

88. Pinching AJ, Peters DK, Newsom Davis J: Remission of myasthenia gravis following plasma-exchange. Lancet 2:1373, 1976.

89. Vogler WR: Therapeutic apheresis: Where we've been and where we are going. In Tindall RSA (ed): Therapeutic Apheresis and Plasma Perfusion. New York, AR Liss, 1980.

90. Wallace DJ, Goldfinger D, Gatti R, et al: Plasmapheresis and lymphoplasmapheresis in the management of rheumatoid arthritis. Arthritis Rheum 22:703, 1979.

91. Balow JE, Tsokos GC: Plasmapheresis in systemic lupus erythematosus: Facts and perspectives. Int J Artif Organs 5:286, 1982.

92. Lockwood CM, Worlledge S, Nicholas A, Cotton D, Peters DK: Reversal of impaired splenic function in patients with nephritis or vasculitis (or both) by plasma exchange. N Engl J Med 300:524, 1979.

93. Kauffmann RH, Houwert DA: Plasmapheresis in rapidly progressive Henoch-Schoenlein glomerulonephritis and the effect on circulating IgA immune complexes. Clin Nephrol 16:155, 1982.

94. Karsh J, Klippel JH, Plotz PH, Decker JL, Wright DG, Flye MW: Lymphapheresis in rheumatoid arthritis. A randomized trial. Arthritis Rheum 24:867, 1981.

95. Wallace D, Goldfinger D, Lowe C, et al: A double-blind controlled study of lymphoplasmapheresis versus sham apheresis in rheumatoid arthritis. N Engl J Med 306:1406, 1982.

96. Terman DS, Young JB, Shearer WT, et al: Preliminary observations of the effects on breast adenocarcinoma of plasma perfused over immobilized protein A. N Engl J Med 305:1195, 1981.

97. Saal SD, Gordon BR: Extracorporeal modification of plasma and whole blood. In Tindall RSA (ed): Therapeutic Apheresis and Plasma Perfusion. New York, AR Liss, 1980.

98. Pineda AA: Methods for selective removal of plasma constituents. In Tindall RSA (ed): Therapeutic Apheresis and Plasma Perfusion. New York, AR Liss, 1980.

99. Hamburger MI, Lawley TJ, Kimberly RP, Plotz PH, Frank MM: A serial study of splenic reticuloendothelial system Fc receptor functional activity in systemic lupus erythematosus. Arthritis Rheum 25:48, 1982.

100. Steven MM, Tanner AR, Holdstock TJ, Wright R: Effect of plasma exchange on the in vitro monocyte function of patients with immune complex diseases. Clin Exp Immunol 45:240, 1981.

101. Lockwood CM, Rees AJ, Pearson TA, Evans DJ, Peters DK, Wilson CB: Immunosuppression and plasma exchange in the treatment of Goodpasture's syndrome. Lancet 1:711, 1976.

102. Flaum MA, Cuneo RA, Appelbaum FA, Deisseroth AB, Engel WK, Gralnick HR: The hemostatic imbalance of plasma-exchange transfusion. Blood 54:694, 1979.

103. Orlin JB, Berkman EM: Partial plasma exchange using albumin replacement: Removal and recovery of normal constituents. Blood 56:1055, 1980.

104. Sakamoto H, Takaoka T, Usami M, et al: Apheresis: Clinical response of patients unresponsive to conventional therapy. Trans Am Soc Artif Intern Organs 31:704, 1985.

105. Wright DG, Karsh J, Fauci AS, et al: Lymphocyte depletion and immunosuppression with repeated leukapheresis by continuous flow centrifugation. Blood 58:451, 1981.

106. Machleder HI, Paulus H: Clinical and immunological alterations observed in patients undergoing long-term thoracic duct drainage. Surgery 84:157, 1978.

107. Paulus HE, Machleder HI, Levine S, Yu DTY, Macdonald NS: Lymphocyte involvement in rheumatoid arthritis. Studies during thoracic duct drainage. Arthritis Rheum 20:1249, 1977.

108. Hutchinson F: The molecular basis for radiation effects on cells. Cancer Res 26:2045, 1966.

109. Anderson RE, Warner NL: Ionizing radiation and the immune response. Adv Immunol 24:215, 1976.

110. Fauci AS, Pratt KR, Whalen G: Activation of human B lymphocytes. VIII. Differential radiosensitivity of subpopulations of lymphoid cells involved in the polyclonally induced PFC responses of peripheral blood B lymphocytes. Immunology 35:715, 1978.

111. Kaplan HS: Hodgkin's Disease 2nd ed. Cambridge, Harvard University Press, 1980.

112. Hellman S, Mauch P, Goodman RL, Rosenthal DS, Moloney WC: The place of radiation in the treatment of Hodgkin's disease. Cancer 42:971, 1978.

113. Fuks Z, Strober S, Bobrove AM, Sasazuki T, McMichael A, Kaplan HS: Long-term effects of radiation on T and B lymphocytes in peripheral blood of patients with Hodgkin's disease. J Clin Invest 58:803, 1976.

114. Kotzin BL, Strober S, Engleman EG, et al: Treatment of intractable rheumatoid arthritis with total lymphoid irradiation. N Engl J Med 305:969, 1981.

115. Trentham DE, Belli JA, Anderson RJ, et al: Clinical and immunologic

effects of fractionated total lymphoid irradiation in refractory rheumatoid arthritis. N Engl J Med 305:976, 1981.

116. Strober S, Slavin S, Gottlieb M, et al: Allograft tolerance after total lymphoid irradiation (TLI). Immunol Rev 46:87, 1979.

117. Strober S, Tanay A, Field E, et al: Efficacy of total lymphoid irradiation in intractable rheumatoid arthritis. A double-blind, randomized trial. Ann Intern Med 102:441, 1985.

118. Hanly JG, Hassan J, Moriarty M, et al: Lymphoid irradiation in intractable rheumatoid arthritis. A double-blind, randomized study comparing 750-rad treatment with 2,000-rad treatment. Arthritis Rheum 29:16, 1986.

119. Brahn E, Helfgott SM, Belli JA, et al: Total lymphoid irradiation therapy in refractory rheumatoid arthritis. Arthritis Rheum 27:481, 1984.

120. Nusslein HG, Herbst M, Manger BJ, et al: Total lymphoid irradiation in patients with refractory rheumatoid arthritis. Arthritis Rheum 28:1205, 1985.

121. Tanay A, Field EH, Hoppe RT, Strober S: Long-term follow-up of rheumatoid arthritis patients treated with total lymphoid irradiation. Arthritis Rheum 30:1, 1987.

122. Strober S, Field E, Hoppe RT, et al: Treatment of intractable lupus nephritis with total lymphoid irradiation. Ann Intern Med 102:450, 1985.

123. Kirklin JK, George JF, McGiffin DC, Naftel DC, Salter MM, Bourge RC: Total lymphoid irradiation: Is there a role in pediatric heart transplantation? J Heart Lung Transplant 12:S293, 1993.

124. Salter MM, Kirklin JK, Bourge RC, Naftel DC, White-Williams C, Tarkka M, Waits E, Bucy RP: Total lymphoid irradiation in the treatment of early or recurrent heart rejection. J Heart Lung Transplant 11:902, 1992.

125. Evans MA, Schomberg PJ, Rodeheffer RJ, et al: Total lymphoid irradiation: A novel and successful therapy for resistant cardiac allograft rejection. Mayo Clin Proc 67:785, 1992.

126. Myburgh JA, Meyers AM, Margolius L, et al: Total lymphoid irradiation in clinical renal transplantation—results in 73 patients. Transplant Proc 23:2033, 1991.

127. Cupps TR, Fauci AS: Corticosteroid-mediated immunoregulation in man. Immunol Rev 65:133, 1982.

128. Fauci AS, Dale DC: The effect of in vivo hydrocortisone on subpopulations of human lymphocytes. J Clin Invest 53:240, 1974.

129. Haynes BF, Fauci AS: The differential effect of in vivo hydrocortisone on kinetics of subpopulations of human peripheral blood thymus-derived lymphocytes. J Clin Invest 61:703, 1978.

130. Stevenson HC, Fauci AS: The effect of glucocorticosteroids and other hormones on inflammatory and immune responses. In Oppenheim JJ, Rosenstreich DL, Potter M (eds): Cellular Functions in Immunity and Inflammation. New York, Elsevier/North Holland, 1981.

131. Borel JF, Feurer C, Gubler HU, Stahelin H: Biological effects of cyclosporin A: A new antilymphocytic agent. Agents Actions 6:468, 1976.

132. Cohen DJ, Loertscher R, Rubin MF, Tilney NL, Carpenter CB, Strom TB: Cyclosporine: A new immunosuppressive agent for organ transplantation. Ann Intern Med 101:667, 1984.

133. Preliminary Results of a European Trial: Cyclosporin A as a sole immunosuppressive agent in recipients of kidney allografts from cadaver donors. Lancet 2:57, 1982.

134. Starzl TE, Klintmalm GBG, Weil R III, et al: Cyclosporin A and steroid therapy in sixty-six cadaver kidney recipients. Surg Gynecol Obstet 153:486, 1982.

135. Morris PJ, Chapman JR, Allen RD, et al: Cyclosporin conversion versus conventional immunosuppressive agents for organ transplantation. Ann Intern Med 101:667, 1984.

136. Powles RL, Clink HM, Spence D, et al: Cyclosporin A to prevent graft-versus-host disease in man after allogenic bone-marrow transplantation. Lancet 1:327, 1980.

137. Palestine AG, Austin HA III, Balow JE, et al: Renal histopathologic alterations in patients treated with cyclosporine for uveitis. N Engl J Med 314:1293, 1986.

138. Palestine AG, Austin HA III, Nussenblatt RB: Renal tubular function in cyclosporine-treated patients. Am J Med 81:419, 1986.

139. Dijkmans BA, van Rijthoven AW, Goei The HS, Montnor-Beckers ZL, Jacobs PC, Cats A: Effect of cyclosporin on serum creatinine in patients with rheumatoid arthritis. Eur J Clin Pharmacol 31:541, 1987.

140. Kolkin S, Nahman NS Jr, Mendell JR: Chronic nephrotoxicity complicating cyclosporine treatment of chronic inflammatory demyelinating polyradiculoneuropathy. Neurology 37:147, 1987.

141. Feutren G, Mihatsch MJ: Risk factors for cyclosporine-induced nephropathy in patients with autoimmune diseases. N Engl J Med 326:1654, 1992.

142. Beveridge T, Krupp P, McKibbin C: Lymphoma and lymphoproliferative lesions developing under cyclosporin therapy. Lancet 1:788, 1984.

143. Nussenblatt RB, Palestine AG, Chan CC, Mochizuki M, Yancey K: Effectiveness of cyclosporin therapy for Behçet's disease. Arthritis Rheum 28:671, 1985.

144. Nussenblatt RB, Palestine AG, Rook AH, Scher I, Wacker WC, Gery I: Treatment of intraocular inflammatory disease with cyclosporin A. Lancet 2:235, 1983.

145. Nussenblatt RB, Palestine AG, Chan CC: Cyclosporin A in the treatment of intraocular inflammatory disease resistant to systemic corticosteroids and cytotoxic agents. Am J Ophthalmol 96:275, 1983.

146. van Rijthoven AW, Dijkmans BA, Goei The HS, et al: Cyclosporin treatment for rheumatoid arthritis: A placebo-controlled, double-blind, multicentre study. Ann Rheum Dis 45:726, 1986.

147. Dougados M, Amor B: Cyclosporin A in rheumatoid arthritis: Preliminary clinical results of an open trial. Arthritis Rheum 30:83, 1987.

148. Panayi GS, Tugwell P: The use of cyclosporin A in rheumatoid arthritis: Conclusions of an international review. Br J Rheumatol 33:967, 1994.

149. Mistilis SP, Vickers CR, Darroch MH, McCarthy SW: Cyclosporin, a new treatment for autoimmune chronic active hepatitis. Med J Aust 143:463, 1985.

150. Rebuck AS, Stiller CR, Braude AC, Laupacis A, Cohen RD, Chapman KR: Cyclosporin for pulmonary sarcoidosis. Lancet 1:1174, 1984.

151. Allison MC, Pounder RE: Cyclosporin for Crohn's disease. Lancet 1:902, 1984.

152. Bianchi PA, Mondelli M, Quarto-di-Palo R, Ranzi T: Cyclosporin for Crohn's disease. Lancet 1:1242, 1984.

153. Choi PM, Targan SR: Immunomodulator therapy in inflammatory bowel disease. Dig Dis Sci 39:1885, 1994.

154. Thivolet J, Barthelmy H, Rigot-Muller G, Bendelac A: Effects of cyclosporin on bullous pemphigoid and pemphigus. Lancet 1:334, 1985.

155. Mueller W, Hermann B: Cyclosporin A for psoriasis. N Engl J Med 301:555, 1984.

156. Garcovich A, Gatti M, Pompili A, Olivetti G, Catamo F: Short-term treatment with cyclosporin in severe psoriasis: Four years of experience. Acta Derm Venereol Suppl (Stockh) 186:92, 1994.

157. Kay AB: Immunosuppressive agents in chronic severe asthma. Allergy Proc 15:147, 1994.

158. Weetman AP, McGregor AM, Ludgate M, et al: Cyclosporin improves Graves' ophthalmopathy. Lancet 2:486, 1983.

159. Routhier G, Epskin O, Janossy G, et al: Effects of cyclosporin A on suppressor and inducer T lymphocytes in primary biliary cirrhosis. Lancet 2:1223, 1980.

160. Cyclosporin in autoimmune disease. Lancet 1:909, 1985.

161. Kino T, Hatanaka H, Hashimoto M, et al: FK506, a novel immunosuppressant isolated from a Streptomyces. I. Fermentation, isolation, and physicochemical and biological characteristics. J Antibiot (Tokyo) 40:1249, 1987.

162. Kino T, Hatanaka H, Miyata S, et al: FK506, a novel immunosuppressant isolated from a Streptomyces. II. Immunosuppressive effect of FK506 in vitro. J Antibiot (Tokyo) 41:1256, 1988.

163. Thomson AW: FK506—How much potential? Immunol Today 10:6, 1989.

164. Collier DStJ, Calne RY, Thiru S, Friend PJ, Lim SML, White DJG: FR-900506 (FK 506) in experimental renal allografts in dogs and primates. Transplant Proc 20:226, 1988.

165. Starzl TE, Todo S, Fung J: FK 506 for liver, kidney, and pancreas transplantation. Lancet 2:1000, 1989.

166. Shapiro R, Fung JJ, Jain A: The side effects of FK 506 in humans. Transplant Proc 22:35, 1990.

167. White DJG: FK506: The promise and the paradox. Clin Exp Immunol 83:1, 1991.

168. Arita C, Hotokebuchi T, Miyahara H, Arai K, Sugioka Y, Kaibara N: Inhibition by FK 506 of established lesions of collagen-induced arthritis in rats. Clin Exp Immunol 82:456, 1990.

169. Hara S, Fukatsu A, Suzuki N, Sakamoto N, Matsuo S: The effects of a new immunosuppressive agent, FK506, on the glomerular injury in rats with accelerated nephrotoxic serum glomerulonephritis. Clin. Immunol Immunopathol 57:351, 1990.

170. Kawashima H, Fujino Y, Mochizuki M: Effects of a new immunosuppressive agent, FK-506, on experimental autoimmune uveoretinitis in rats. Invest Ophthalmol Vis Sci 29:1265, 1988.

171. Inamura N, Hashimoto M, Nakahara K, et al: Immunosuppressive effect of FK-506 on experimental allergic encephalomyelitis in rats. Int J Immunopharmacol 10:991, 1988.

172. Takabayashi K, Koike T, Kurasawa K, et al: Effect of FK-506, a novel immunosuppressive drug, on murine systemic lupus erythematosus. Clin Immunol Immunopathol 51:110, 1989.

173. McCauley J, Bronsther O, Fung J, Todo S, Starzl TE: Treatment of cyclosporin-induced haemolytic uraemic syndrome with FK 506. Lancet 2:1516, 1989.

174. McCauley J, Tzakis AG, Fung JJ, Todo S, Starzl TE: FK 506 in steroid-resistant focal sclerosing glomerulonephritis of childhood. Lancet 1:674, 1990.

175. Thomson AW, Carroll PB, McCauley J, et al: FK 506: A novel immunosuppressant for treatment of autoimmune disease. Springer Semin Immunopathol 14:323, 1993.

176. Schreiber SL: Chemistry and biology of the immunophilins and their immunosuppressive ligands. Science 251:283, 1991.

177. Tocci MJ, Matkovich DA, Collier KA, et al: The immunosuppressant FK-506 selectively inhibits expression of early T cell activation genes. J Immunol 143:718, 1989.

178. Emmel EA, Verweij CL, Durand DB, Higgins KM, Lacy E, Crabtree GR: Cyclosporin-A specifically inhibits function of nuclear proteins involved in T-cell activation. Science 246:1617, 1989.
179. Bierer BE, Hollander G, Fruman D, Burakoff SJ: Cyclosporin A and FK506: Molecular mechanisms of immunosuppression and probes for transplantation biology. Curr Opin Immunol 5:763, 1993.
180. Fruman DA, Klee CB, Bierer BE, Burakoff SJ: Calcineurin phosphatase activity in T lymphocytes is inhibited by FK506 and cyclosporin A. Proc Natl Acad Sci U S A 89:3686, 1992.
181. McCaffrey PG, Perrino BA, Soderling TR, Rao A: NF-ATp: A T lymphocyte DNA-binding protein that is a target for calcineurin and immunosuppressive drugs. J Biol Chem 268:3747, 1993.
182. Shevach EM: The effects of cyclosporin A on the immune system. Annu Rev Immunol 3:397, 1985.
183. Muraguchi A, Butler JL, Kehrl JH, Falkoff RJM, Fauci AS: Selective suppression of an early step in human B-cell activation by cyclosporin A. J Exp Med 158:690, 1983.
184. Carlson RP, Baeder WL, Caccese RG, Warner LM, Sehgal SN: Effects of orally administered rapamycin in animal models of arthritis and other autoimmune diseases. Ann N Y Acad Sci 685:86, 1993.
185. Roberge FG, Xu D, Chan CC, deSmet MD, Nussenblatt RB, Chen H: Treatment of autoimmune uveoretinitis in the rat with rapamycin, an inhibitor of lymphocyte growth factor signal transduction. Curr Eye Res 12:197, 1993.
186. Carlson RP, Hartman DA, Tomchek LA, Walter TL, Lugay JR, Calhoun W, Sehgal SN, Chang JY: Rapamycin, a potential disease-modifying antiarthritic drug. J Pharmacol Exp Ther 266:1125, 1993.
187. Symoens J, Rosenthal M: Levamisole in the modulation of the immune response: The current experimental and clinical state. J Reticuloendothel Soc 21:175, 1977.
188. Snyderman R, Pike MC: Pathophysiologic aspects of leukocyte chemotaxis: Identification of a specific chemotactic factor binding site on human granulocytes and defects of macrophage function associated with neoplasia. In Gallin JI, Quie PG (eds): Leukocyte Chemotaxis: Methods, Physiology and Clinical Implications. New York, Raven Press, 1978.
189. Rabson AR, Whiting DA, Anderson R, Glover A, Koornhof HJ: Depressed neutrophil motility in patients with recurrent herpes simplex virus infections: In vitro restoration with levamisole. J Infect Dis 135:113, 1977.
190. Wright DG, Kirkpatrick CH, Gallin JI: Effects of levamisole on normal and abnormal leukocyte locomotion. J Clin Invest 59:941, 1977.
191. Tripodi D, Parks LC, Brugmans J: Drug-induced restoration of cutaneous delayed hypersensitivity in anergic patients with cancer. N Engl J Med 289:354, 1973.
192. Sampson D, Lui A: The effect of levamisole on cell-mediated immunity and suppressor cell function. Cancer Res 36:952, 1976.
193. Moertel CG, Fleming TR, Macdonald JS, et al: Levamisole and fluorouracil for adjuvant therapy of resected colon carcinoma. N Engl J Med 322:352, 1990.
194. Miller R, DeMerieux P, Srinivasan R, et al: Double-blind placebo-controlled crossover evaluation of levamisole in rheumatoid arthritis. Arthritis Rheum 23:172, 1980.
195. Runge LA, Pinals RS, Lourie SH, Tomar RH: Treatment of rheumatoid arthritis with levamisole. A controlled trial. Arthritis Rheum 20:1445, 1977.
196. Schmidt KL, Mueller-Eckhardt C: Agranulocytosis, levamisole and HLA-B27–positive rheumatoid arthritis. Lancet 1:148, 1978.
197. Veys EM, Mielants H, Verbruggen G: Levamisole-induced adverse reactions in HLA-B27–positive rheumatoid arthritis. Lancet 1:148, 1978.
198. Freund J: Some aspects of active immunization. Annu Rev Microbiol 1:291, 1947.
199. Chedid L, Audibert F, LeFrancier P, Chory J, Lederer E: Modulation of the immune response by a synthetic adjuvant and analogs. Proc Natl Acad Sci U S A 73:2472, 1976.
200. Katz SI, Hall RP, Lawley TJ, Strober W: Dermatitis herpetiformis: The skin and the gut. Ann Intern Med 93:857, 1980.
201. Katz SI, Gallin JI, Hertz KC, Fauci AS, Lawley TJ: Erythema elevatum diutinum: Skin and systemic manifestations, immunologic studies and successful treatment with dapsone. Medicine 56:443, 1977.
202. Hall RP, Lawley TJ, Smith HR, Katz SI: Bullous eruption of systemic lupus erythematosus. Ann Intern Med 97:165, 1982.
203. Mandell GL, Sande MA: Drugs used in the chemotherapy of tuberculosis and leprosy. In Gilman AG, Rall TW, Nies AS, Taylor P (eds): Goodman and Gilman's The Pharmacologic Basis of Therapeutics, 8th ed. New York, Pergamon Press, 1990.

CHAPTER 52

H. Ralph Schumacher, Jr.
Irving H. Fox

Antihyperuricemic Drugs

The existence of hyperuricemia, a common biochemical abnormality, requires investigation to discern the cause. Treatment is usually appropriate only for symptomatic hyperuricemia, including gout and renal calculi associated with hyperuricemia or hyperuricaciduria, as well as for the prevention of acute uric acid nephropathy. Cost-effectiveness of urate-lowering therapy in gout has been studied, with the conclusion that therapy *is* cost-saving in patients who have two or more attacks a year.[1]

There are two major causes of hyperuricemia— increased production of uric acid and decreased excretion of uric acid. The two major therapeutic approaches to antihyperuricemic therapy oppose these mechanisms of hyperuricemia. One approach involves the inhibition of urate synthesis with allopurinol. The other approach is to increase the excretion of urate through the use of uricosuric drugs such as sulfinpyrazone and probenecid. A third rarely used therapeutic approach involves increasing the destruction of urate by the use of the enzyme uricase, which destroys urate. Uricase is being used experimentally, but it is difficult to use and is not available in the United States.

On the rare occasions when one therapy is not effective alone, these therapies are combined. Most commonly, a combination involving inhibition of urate synthesis and stimulation of uric acid excretion is used. This is only rarely necessary, however.

INHIBITION OF URATE SYNTHESIS

Allopurinol

Allopurinol, the classic inhibitor of urate synthesis, is a drug usually used for the treatment of gout.

Mechanism of Action

In the final steps of urate synthesis, hypoxanthine is oxidized to xanthine and xanthine is oxidized to uric acid. This reaction is catalyzed by a single enzyme, xanthine dehydrogenase.

Allopurinol decreases urate synthesis by inhibiting xanthine dehydrogenase (Fig. 52–1). Allopurinol is itself a substrate for xanthine dehydrogenase and is oxidized to oxipurinol. In fact, 6 hours after administration of a single dose of allopurinol, it is no longer

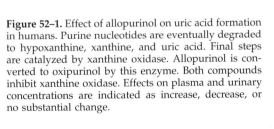

Figure 52–1. Effect of allopurinol on uric acid formation in humans. Purine nucleotides are eventually degraded to hypoxanthine, xanthine, and uric acid. Final steps are catalyzed by xanthine oxidase. Allopurinol is converted to oxipurinol by this enzyme. Both compounds inhibit xanthine oxidase. Effects on plasma and urinary concentrations are indicated as increase, decrease, or no substantial change.

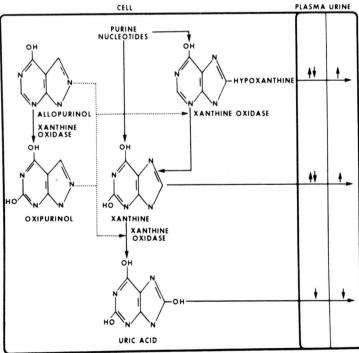

detectable in the plasma and only oxipurinol is present.[2] Oxipurinol actively inhibits xanthine dehydrogenase.

Allopurinol (4-hydroxypyrazolo[3,4-d]pyrimidine) and its major metabolic product oxipurinol (4,6-dihydroxypyrazolo[3,4-d]pyrimidine) are analogs of hypoxanthine and xanthine, respectively. Both are potent inhibitors of xanthine dehydrogenase.[3-5] The Michaelis constant of allopurinol for this enzyme is one twentieth the Michaelis constant of xanthine. In contrast, oxipurinol and xanthine have similar Michaelis constants. Allopurinol is a competitive inhibitor of xanthine dehydrogenase. Both allopurinol and oxipurinol produce pseudoirreversible inactivation of

xanthine dehydrogenase. Inactivation results from the incubation of allopurinol and enzyme without substrate. Oxipurinol inactivates the enzyme with the addition of xanthine and molecular oxygen as the hydrogen acceptor.

Allopurinol and its derivatives have additional actions on purine and pyrimidine metabolism that are explained by its own complex metabolism (Fig. 52–2).[6,7] As a result of inhibition of xanthine dehydrogenase, there is a build-up of hypoxanthine and xanthine in body fluids. Xanthinuria results from this activity. Orotic aciduria and orotidinuria also occur during allopurinol therapy. This is related to inhibition of de novo pyrimidine synthesis at orotidylic

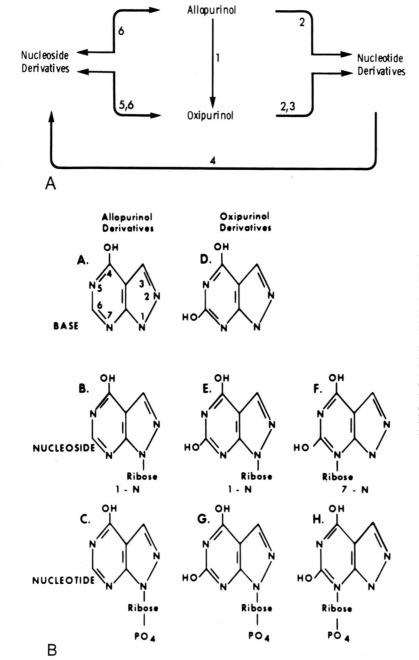

Figure 52–2. Allopurinol metabolism in humans. A, Allopurinol undergoes a complex series of metabolic alterations. It is oxidized to oxipurinol. Small quantities of these compounds are converted to the nucleoside and nucleotide derivatives. The reactions are catalyzed by the enzymes indicated: 1 = xanthine dehydrogenase; 2 = hypoxanthine-guanine phosphoribosyltransferase; 3 = orotate phosphoribosyltransferase; 4 = 5'-nucleotidase; 5 = pyrimidine nucleoside phosphorylase; 6 = purine nucleoside phosphorylase. B, The structures of the allopurinol metabolites are outlined. Oxipurinol has two types of derivatives, the 7-N or 1-N, depending on whether metabolism occurred by orotate phosphoribosyltransferase or hypoxanthine-guanine phosphoribosyltransferase, respectively.

decarboxylase by allopurinol ribonucleotide and oxipurinol ribonucleotide.

Allopurinol therapy also decreases total urinary purine excretion. This decrease in total urinary purine excretion requires hypoxanthine-guanine phosphoribosyltransferase and is not observed with a deficiency of this enzyme.[6] The decreased urinary purine excretion is associated with inhibition of de novo purine synthesis. This inhibition results from nucleotide derivatives of allopurinol and oxipurinol[6, 7] or from enhanced reutilization of hypoxanthine.[8]

Metabolism and Pharmacokinetics

By virtue of its being a structural analog of hypoxanthine, allopurinol undergoes complex interconversions (see Fig. 52–2).[6, 7] There are three pathways of metabolism. Allopurinol can be converted to a nucleoside 5'-monophosphate derivative (1-N[5'-ribosyl]allopurinol) monophosphate. This can be dephosphorylated to a nucleoside derivative (1-N[5'-ribosyl]allopurinol). The latter compound can also be formed directly from allopurinol by the reaction of purine nucleoside phosphorylase. The major pathway of allopurinol metabolism is oxidation to oxipurinol.

Oxipurinol is a structural analog of xanthine and has four distinct pathways of metabolism. In parallel to allopurinol, xanthine is a substrate for hypoxanthine-guanine phosphoribosyltransferase and purine nucleoside phosphorylase. The purine nucleotide and nucleoside derivatives are similarly formed. In contrast to allopurinol, oxipurinol is also a substrate for orotate phosphoribosyltransferase and pyrimidine nucleoside phosphorylase. The compounds formed are 7-N(5'-phosphoribosyl)oxipurinol and 7-N(5'-ribosyl)oxipurinol derivatives.

Allopurinol is completely absorbed from the gastrointestinal tract. Parenteral and rectal administration can be used for patients unable to ingest oral medication. However, drug absorption is limited by poor solubility.[2] A prodrug approach has been recommended to overcome this problem, including the use of N_1 acyclomethyl derivatives of allopurinol.[9] Allopurinol has a half-life in vivo of 39 to 180 minutes. Forty-five to 65 percent of allopurinol is rapidly oxidized to oxipurinol in vivo. Allopurinol is cleared by the kidney at a rate of 14 to 20 ml/minute.[3, 5, 10]

Oxipurinol is only poorly absorbed from the gastrointestinal tract.[3, 11] It is excreted by a monoexponential decay, with a half-life ranging from 12 to 17 hours.[12] The half-life can be markedly increased to 50 hours with a low-protein diet.[12] Therefore, in protein-malnourished patients, the dose of allopurinol should be reduced. Oxipurinol is cleared by the kidney at a rate of 23 to 31 ml/minute.

There are important therapeutic implications for the metabolism and excretion of allopurinol and oxipurinol.[3] Because of its prolonged half-life, oxipurinol is primarily responsible for xanthine dehydrogenase inhibition in vivo when allopurinol is administered. In addition, factors that change uric acid excretion generally alter oxipurinol excretion in a similar direction.[13] For example, uricosuric agents increase the renal excretion of oxipurinol and uric acid, and renal insufficiency reduces the excretion of both compounds. Therefore, dose adjustments are required to compensate for these clinical considerations. Uncontrolled hyperglycemia may also increase excretion of oxipurinol.[14]

Because allopurinol and uricosuric drugs are occasionally used together, their interaction needs to be considered. Allopurinol lengthens the biologic half-life of probenecid and thus potentiates its uricosuric effect. Conversely, uricosuric drugs increase the clearance of oxipurinol in humans[13] and thus diminish the degree of xanthine dehydrogenase inhibition. The net effect of these drug interactions suggests that lower than usual doses of probenecid and greater than usual doses of allopurinol would be indicated when the drugs are used concurrently. Clinically, however, the drugs are tolerated so well that they can be used together without altering the usual dosages of either.

Therapeutic Actions

The administration of allopurinol to patients with normal renal function is followed by a decrease in serum and urinary uric acid values within 24 to 48 hours. Maximum reductions are achieved in 4 to 14 days. Serum urate values then remain relatively constant over prolonged periods[3, 5] (Fig. 52–3). Withdrawal of allopurinol usually results in a return to pretreatment serum urate levels within a few days. After 3 to 6 months of normouricemia, a reduction in the frequency of gouty attacks may be expected. This probably varies, depending on the amount of tophi to be mobilized, but this requires further study.

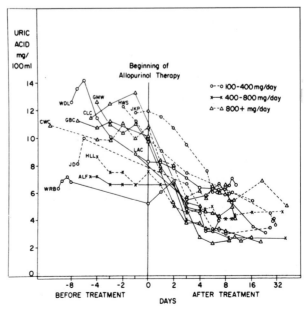

Figure 52–3. Effect of allopurinol on serum uric acid in 12 patients with gout.

Allopurinol has proved to be a highly effective drug for the treatment of hyperuricemia and gout after use for more than 25 years.[15] Normal serum urate values can be achieved in most patients with normal renal function using a dose of 300 mg/day.[16] The optimal endpoint of antihyperuricemic therapy is the reduction of serum urate concentration to a level at which the urate concentration is no longer saturating (i.e., less than 6 mg/dl). A single 300-mg tablet can be used once each day because of the long biologic half-life of oxipurinol. For some patients, a dose higher than 300 mg/day is needed. The maximum dose is 800 mg.

In some patients with frequent episodes of gout, beginning with a low dose, such as 100 mg, may decrease the probability of precipitating a series of incapacitating attacks. In all patients being treated with allopurinol or any antihyperuricemic agent, the drug dosage should be adjusted to the individual's need through monitoring the serum urate concentration. In individuals with lowered glomerular filtration rates, it may be advisable to reduce the maintenance dose of allopurinol because of the prolonged half-life of oxipurinol in patients with renal failure. In patients with renal impairment, the creatinine clearance is highly correlated to the plasma oxipurinol concentrations.[13, 17] Table 52–1 lists suggested doses for allopurinol in patients with different glomerular filtration rates. Parenteral and rectal administration can be tried for patients unable to ingest oral medication.

Tophi resolve in 6 to 12 months with maintenance of normal serum urate levels.[3] Destructive arthritis improves in most patients. In an occasional patient with rapid resolution of tophi, bony lesions do not heal and telescoped digits may result.[18] Slower improvement can be anticipated in patients with renal insufficiency. However, the progression of gouty nephropathy appears to halt in most patients.

Once antihyperuricemic therapy is instituted for firm medical indications, it should be continued indefinitely if possible. Intermittent administration of allopurinol is less effective than continuous therapy in controlling the symptoms of gout.[19] If allopurinol is stopped after a few years of control of hyperuricemia, the patient may reenter an asymptomatic phase.[20] Ultimately, acute attacks then recur.

Uricosuric agents are occasionally used together with allopurinol to hasten mobilization of urate deposits in tophaceous gout.[3, 4] The administration of allopurinol and a uricosuric agent to a patient with good renal function usually increases urinary uric acid excretion and further decreases the serum urate level.

Despite the availability of allopurinol for many years, the clinical use of the drug is not always appropriate. In one study, less than 20 percent of physicians diagnosed gout definitely before prescribing allopurinol.[21] In another study, many physicians did not cover the introduction of allopurinol with anti-inflammatory agents, titrate the dose against the uric acid, or adjust the dose according to the serum creatinine level.[17, 22] The possibility that allopurinol has other beneficial effects also needs consideration. For example, allopurinol can inhibit the generation of superoxide radicals.[23, 24]

Tolerability and Adverse Reactions

Acute Attacks of Gout. There is a relatively high frequency of gouty attacks on initiation of therapy.[23] Typical attacks have occurred with serum urate levels as low as 2 mg/dl and comparably low urinary urate excretions. Daily colchicine is generally given during at least the first months of therapy with allopurinol to minimize the likelihood of acute attacks. Recent reviews have raised the question of whether such prophylaxis is needed, and for how long, as there have been no controlled studies on prevention of these attacks.[26, 27]

Xanthine Stones. The urinary excretion of xanthine, a poorly soluble compound, increases during full-dose allopurinol therapy to the level of xanthine excretion observed in hereditary xanthinuria.[3, 4] In this disorder associated with deficient xanthine oxidase activity, the major disorder is the formation of urinary calculi composed of xanthine. Development of xanthine crystalluria or lithiasis as a complication of allopurinol therapy has been observed rarely during the treatment of gout or uric acid stones,[3] usually in patients with partial deficiency of hypoxanthine-guanine phosphoribosyl-transferase.[3]

In addition, xanthine stone formation induced by allopurinol therapy has been reported in children with Lesch-Nyhan syndrome[28] and patients with lymphosarcoma or Burkitt's lymphoma.[29] Allopurinol should be given cautiously and in minimal doses to patients with extraordinarily great uric acid excretion values, particularly those with an inability to reutilize hypoxanthine and xanthine because of hypoxanthine-guanine phosphoribosyltransferase deficiency.

Acute xanthine nephropathy has been observed in the acute tumor lysis syndrome during allopurinol therapy.[30] The mechanism for this is the same as for xanthine calculi.

Formation of oxipurinol sludge and stones in the urinary tract has been reported rarely.

Toxicity. Serious toxicity of allopurinol therapy occurs but is unusual. Some adverse reactions may represent hypersensitivity to cell-mediated allopurinol, oxipurinol, or both.[31]

Table 52–1. RECOMMENDED MAINTENANCE DOSE OF ALLOPURINOL BASED ON THE GLOMERULAR FILTRATION RATE (GFR)

GFR (ml/min)	Dose (mg)
100	300
80	250
60	200
40	150
20	100
10	100 q2d
0	100 q3d

About 5 percent of patients find it necessary to discontinue therapy with the drug. Allopurinol may lead to the development of gastrointestinal intolerance, skin rashes (sometimes with fever), occasionally toxic epidermal necrolysis, alopecia, bone marrow suppression with leukopenia and thrombocytopenia, agranulocytosis, aplastic anemia,[32] granulomatous hepatitis, severe jaundice, sarcoidlike reaction, and vasculitis.[3, 32] The incidence of side effects of all kinds is about 20 percent.[3, 4] Most side effects appear to occur in patients given excessive doses, often for asymptomatic hyperuricemia.[33]

Skin rashes occur in about 2 percent of patients receiving allopurinol. This increases ten-fold in patients receiving allopurinol and ampicillin.[34] The occurrence of skin rash in a patient receiving allopurinol does not necessarily require that the drug be discontinued. The rash of allopurinol often involves the hands and feet alone, or at least chiefly. There may be swelling and intense itching, and the body and face may be involved. Provided there is no laryngeal edema, it may suffice to administer large doses of diphenhydramine or other antihistaminic agent to control the itching. A minimal amount of swelling of the hands and feet then is often well tolerated. After a few weeks, it may be possible to stop the antihistaminic therapy without recurrence of the rash. Reduction of the dose of allopurinol may also reduce the severity of the skin lesions, especially in patients with renal insufficiency. Desensitization has apparently been effective in patients allergic to allopurinol by initiating therapy with a very low dose of allopurinol (e.g., 0.05 mg/day) and gradually increasing the amount given over 30 days.[35, 36]

Toxic effects occur more often in the presence of renal insufficiency and thiazide therapy. The allopurinol hypersensitivity syndrome consists of a constellation of findings, including fever, skin rash, progressive renal insufficiency, eosinophilia, and hepatitis. In a group of 78 patients with this putative syndrome, the following abnormalities were observed: skin rash, 92 percent; fever, 87 percent; worsening renal function, 85 percent; eosinophilia, 73 percent; hepatitis, 68 percent; and leukocytosis, 39 percent.[38] Twenty-one percent of these patients died. Diffuse vasculitis involving multiple organ systems was observed at postmortem examination. The median dose of allopurinol was 300 mg/day, and the mean duration of therapy was 3 weeks. Prior renal insufficiency was recorded in 81 percent of these patients, and 49 percent received concomitant diuretic therapy.[39] Despite the rarity of allopurinol hypersensitivity syndrome, its potential severity emphasizes (1) the need for restricting allopurinol therapy to those hyperuricemic patients who have specific indications for antihyperuricemic therapy, and (2) the need to reduce the dose of allopurinol in patients with renal insufficiency (see Table 52–1).

Interactions with Other Drugs

Several drug–drug interactions involving allopurinol are important clinically. The use of allopurinol and a uricosuric drug together was described earlier. The effects of compounds that are inactivated by xanthine dehydrogenase, such as 6-mercaptopurine and azathioprine, are potentiated by allopurinol administration. An increased incidence of bone marrow suppression has been observed in patients taking allopurinol who are also receiving cyclophosphamide.[6, 40] Allopurinol has been shown to reduce the activity of hepatic microsomal drug-metabolizing enzymes and thus to prolong the half-lives of anti-pyrine, aminophenazene, dicumarol, warfarin sodium, and theophylline.[41]

Oxipurinol

The therapeutic effects of allopurinol are mediated by its metabolic product oxipurinol, whose half-life is about eight times longer than that of allopurinol. A direct comparison of the two agents given orally indicates that allopurinol is the more effective because of the relatively poor absorption of oxipurinol from the gastrointestinal tract.[3] Nevertheless, oxipurinol has been effectively used therapeutically in some patients who are sensitive to allopurinol. In most patients allergic to allopurinol, hyperuricemia can be controlled with oxipurinol without evidence of toxicity.[35, 36] However, toxic reactions identical to those observed with allopurinol were observed in 30 percent of the patients treated with oxipurinol. Cross-sensitivity to the two drugs is expected on the basis of their structural similarities. Oxipurinol is not marketed in the United States but is available through the manufacturer for compassionate use and is marketed in Europe and Japan.

Other Xanthine Oxidase Inhibitors

Experimental work in chimpanzees has been reported with a novel inhibitor.[37]

ENHANCEMENT OF URIC ACID EXCRETION

Uricosuric Drugs and Mechanism of Action

Uricosuric therapy has been used to treat hyperuricemia and gout for about 40 years. A uricosuric drug increases the rate of excretion of uric acid.[42] Uric acid is normally handled in the human kidney by filtration at the glomerulus and by secretion and reabsorption mechanisms in the renal tubules. Uricosuric drugs modify the tubular transport mechanisms of uric acid and have their pharmacologic activity in the renal tubule. Uric acid and other drugs handled by these transport mechanisms are organic anions.

There are separate transport systems for the secretion and reabsorption of organic anions, including uric acid.[42] Because urate is reabsorbed by a renal tubular brush border transporter, this reabsorption of urate can be inhibited when uricosuric drugs such as probenecid are present in the lumen and compete

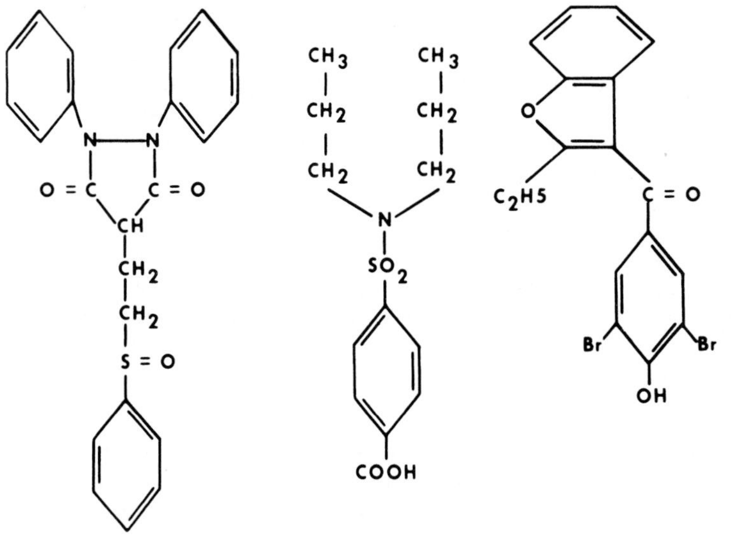

Figure 52–4. Structure of sulfinpyrazone, probenecid, and benzbromarone.

with urate for the brush border transporter. In this way, uricosuric drugs inhibit urate reabsorption. The secretory transport system is quantitatively much smaller than reabsorption and is located at the basolateral membrane of the renal tubule. When uricosuric drugs are given in very low doses, they actually decrease the renal excretion of uric acid by inhibiting this secretory transport system. Decreased excretion usually occurs at low dose, and increased excretion is observed at a higher dose of uricosuric drugs, with inhibition of the reabsorptive anion transporter. This higher dose is usually the dose recommended for uricosuric therapy.

The fact that uric acid and other organic anions are secreted in the tubule is of importance clinically, because it may lead to interactions between uricosuric drugs and other organic anionic drugs secreted in the tubule. This is responsible for some of the interactions of uricosuric drugs with other drugs that are described later.

Thus, the pharmacologic action of uricosuric drugs such as probenecid is to inhibit the transport of organic acids across epithelial barriers.[43, 44] Uric acid is the only important endogenous compound whose excretion is known to be increased by probenecid. This results from inhibition of uric acid resorption. Probenecid and sulfinpyrazone (Fig. 52–4) are most widely used for this purpose in the United States. In Europe, benzbromarone and zoxazolamine are used as well.

The uricosuric action of probenecid and sulfinpyrazone is blunted by the concomitant administration of salicylate, which is an organic anion. Probenecid inhibits the tubular secretion of a number of other drugs (Table 52–2). In addition, probenecid inhibits the transport of 5-hydroxyindoleacetic acid and other acid metabolites of cerebral monoamines from the subarachnoid space to the plasma. Furthermore, probenecid is secreted into the bile and depresses the

biliary secretion of other compounds. This ability to inhibit biliary secretion allows probenecid to increase plasma levels of rifampin during the treatment of tuberculosis.

Many drugs with diverse chemical structures decrease the serum urate concentration in humans by enhancing the renal excretion of uric acid (see Table 52–2).[3]

Metabolism and Pharmacokinetics

Probenecid

Probenecid is readily absorbed from the gastrointestinal tract. The half-life of probenecid in plasma is

Table 52–2. DRUGS SHOWN TO BE URICOSURIC IN HUMANS

Acetoheximide	Halofenate (MK 185)
Adrenocorticotropic hormone	Iodopyracet
Amflutizole	Iopanoic acid
Ascorbic acid	Meclofenamic acid
Azapropazone	Meglumine iodipamide
Azauridine	Mersalyl
Benzbromarone	Metiazininic acid
Benziodarone	Niridazole
Calcitonin	Orotic acid
Calcium ipodate	Outdated tetracyclines
Carinamide	Phenolsulfonphthalein
Chlorprothixene	Phenylbutazone
Cinchophen	Phenylindandione
Citrate	Phenoxyisobutyric acid
Dicumarol	Probenecid and metabolites
Difumidone	Salicylates
Diflunisal	Sodium diatrizoate
Estrogens	Sulfaethylthiadiazole
Ethyl biscoumacetate	Sulfinpyrazone
Ethyl p-chlorophenoxyisobutyric acid	Ticrynafen
Glyceryl guaiacholate	W 2354 (5-chlorosalicylic acid)
Glycine	Zoxazolamine
Glycopyrrolate	

dose dependent,[45] and ranges from 6 to 12 hours. This may be prolonged by the concomitant administration of allopurinol. Probenecid is extensively bound to plasma proteins (89 to 94 percent of drug) and is largely confined to the extracellular fluid. The maintenance dose of probenecid ranges from 500 mg/day to 3 g/day given in three or four divided doses.[3, 4]

Probenecid is rapidly metabolized in vivo. Less than 5 percent of the administered dose is recovered in the urine within 24 hours. The major urinary metabolite, probenecid acyl monoglucuronide, accounts for 41 percent of the administered compound within 48 hours. The rest of the metabolites result from oxidation of the n-propyl side chain.[3] These side chain metabolites possess uricosuric activity in animals.[46]

Sulfinpyrazone

Sulfinpyrazone is rapidly and completely adsorbed from the gastrointestinal tract.[3] The peak concentration is reached in the serum 1 hour after its oral administration, and the half-life is 1 to 3 hours. The drug is bound to plasma proteins and as a result it is largely confined to the extracellular fluid. Most of the drug is excreted in the urine as the parahydroxyl metabolite, which is also uricosuric in humans. Some 20 to 45 percent of the drug is excreted unchanged in 24 hours.

Sulfinpyrazone is three to six times more potent than probenecid on a weight basis.[44] The usual daily dose is 300 to 400 mg/day given in three or four divided doses.

Benziodarone and Benzbromarone

Benziodarone and benzbromarone are potent uricosuric agents in humans.[3, 4] Benziodarone contains iodine, and benzbromarone contains bromide (see Fig. 52–4). The former compound has found limited clinical use, in part because of its effect on thyroid function. The latter drug has been well tolerated during clinical uses.[46]

Benzbromarone is bound to plasma proteins. It undergoes successive oxidation of the ethyl side chain and one- and two-fold hydroxylation of the benzofuran ring followed by methylation of one of the hydroxyl groups.[48, 49] The two main metabolites are 1'-hydroxybenzbromarone and aryl hydroxybenzbromarone of unknown structure.[48, 49]

Therapeutic Action

Therapy with uricosuric drugs is started at a low dose to minimize the risk of renal calculi associated with the transient increase in uric acid excretion. In patients with normal renal function, a full therapeutic dose of probenecid may cause a brisk and pronounced uricosuria (Fig. 52–5). Because uric acid is relatively insoluble, especially in acid urine, this sudden increase in uric acid excretion can lead to the

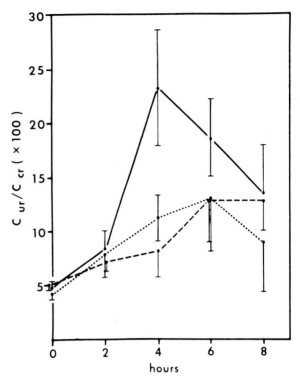

Figure 52–5. Uricosuric effects of sulfinpyrazone and benzbromarone. Sulfinpyrazone, 300 mg (••••••), benzbromarone 160 mg (—), or both drugs together (––––) were given to four, six, and four patients, respectively. Each point represents the mean percentage of Curate: Creatinine plus or minus the standard error of the means. Sulfinpyrazone had its peak effect at 4 to 6 hours, whereas benzbromarone had its peak effect at 2 to 4 hours but continued its uricosuria beyond 8 hours, up to 24 hours. With sulfinpyrazone, the mean serum urate diminished from a control value of 7.0 to 6.0 after 8 hours and to 6.6 mg/dl after 24 hours. With benzbromarone, the mean serum urate concentration decreased from a control value of 7.8 to 6.1 after 8 hours and to 4.3 mg/dl after 24 hours. Administration of both drugs resembled the sulfinpyrazone effect for the first 6 hours. (From Sinclair DS, Fox IH: The pharmacology of hypouricemic effect of benzbromarone. J Rheumatol 2:437, 1975.)

precipitation of uric acid crystals in the collecting ducts of the kidney or ureters or, more commonly, to the development of uric acid stones in 9 percent of the patients treated.[50]

Uric acid precipitation with initiation of uricosuric therapy is unusual in the normal producer of uric acid. The maintenance of adequate urine flow and alkalinization of the urine with oral sodium bicarbonate (2 to 6 g/day) or sodium citrate (Scholl's solution, 20 to 60 ml/day) further diminish the possibility of uric acid stone formation, but use of these drugs is probably unnecessary in most patients.

Sulfinpyrazone administration is started at a dose of 50 mg twice per day, increasing in a few days to 100 mg three or four times each day. The maximum effective dose is 800 mg/day. Probenecid therapy is started at a dose of 250 mg twice per day, increasing after several weeks to 500 to 1000 mg two or three times each day. The maximum effective dose is 3 g/day.

Probenecid and sulfinpyrazone are effective for

most gouty patients. Some 75 to 80 percent of patients with tophaceous gout have improved. In the remaining 20 percent of patients whose conditions are not brought under ideal control, failure is a result of drug intolerance, concomitant salicylate ingestion, or impaired renal function. Salicylate ingestion at any dose blocks the uricosuric effect of probenecid and sulfinpyrazone. When the glomerular filtration rate is below 20 to 30 ml/minute, most uricosuric drugs are ineffective.

An extensive clinical experience attests to the usefulness of sulfinpyrazone.[3] Tolerance for sulfinpyrazone is somewhat better than that for probenecid.[50, 51] Nevertheless, almost one quarter of patients stop therapy with the drug for one reason or another. The leading causes of failure of control, as with probenecid, are concomitant salicylate ingestion and renal insufficiency.

Benzbromarone is a potent uricosuric drug during clinical use. It is more effective than other uricosuric agents in patients with renal insufficiency. It has been well tolerated and effective in cyclosporine-treated renal transplant patients as long as their creatinine clearance is over 25 ml/min.[52]

Tolerability and Adverse Reactions

The major side effects of uricosuric drugs are skin rash, precipitation of acute gouty arthritis, gastrointestinal intolerance, and uric acid calculus formation. Probenecid has a calciuric action in gouty patients.[3, 4] The complication of urinary uric acid crystal or stone formation is preventable by forcing fluids and urinary alkalinization as described earlier. This complication of probenecid therapy reinforces the contraindication for use in gouty patients with nephrolithiasis or with overproduction of uric acid. In addition, probenecid should not be used in hyperuricemic cystinuric patients because of increased cystine and decreased cysteine–penicillamine mixed disulfide and penicillamine disulfide metabolites.[3, 4]

A potential complication of all forms of antihyperuricemic drug therapy is the precipitation of an attack of acute gouty arthritis during the initial days or weeks of therapy, at a time when serum urate levels are being lowered. This complication occurs in 10 to 20 percent of patients started on probenecid therapy alone.[50] The incidence can be greatly reduced by concomitant administration of colchicine or indomethacin.

The frequency of side effects of probenecid has been extensively documented[54] as follows: hypersensitivity reactions, 0.3 percent; drug fever, 0.4 percent; skin rash, 1.4 percent; and gastrointestinal disturbances, 3.1 percent. In longer-term studies of gouty patients, there was an 8 to 18 percent incidence of gastrointestinal complaints and a 5 percent incidence of hypersensitivity and rash.[55]

Serious toxicity of probenecid is rare. Hepatic necrosis has been reported in one patient and the nephrotic syndrome in at least two.[3] Autoimmune hemolytic anemia has been reported with probenecid therapy.[56] About one third of patients eventually become intolerant of probenecid and discontinue its use.[52] The experience with sulfinpyrazone is similar.

Interaction with Other Drugs

Uricosuric drugs alter the transport of other organic acids across cell membranes, resulting in numerous drug interactions (Table 52–3).[3, 4, 42]

Because of these interactions, certain drugs should be used with caution in patients receiving probenecid. Dapsone and indomethacin, for example, should be used at a lower dose in patients receiving probenecid.[3] Not only does probenecid delay the renal excretion of salicylic acid, diflunisal,[58] and many of their glucuronide derivatives, but acetylsalicylate completely blocks the uricosuric effect of probenecid and most other uricosuric agents. Diuretics, on the other hand, do not block the uricosuric effect of probenecid. Subtherapeutic doses of heparin may have profound anticoagulant effects in patients receiving probenecid.[59]

The effect of probenecid on the metabolism of some drugs has been used to enhance their clinical activity. The renal excretion of penicillin and ampicillin is decreased by probenecid, and thus the half-life of these antibiotics is prolonged. Therefore, probenecid has been used, for example, to enhance the blood levels of ampicillin and penicillin. In addition, the half-life of rifampin is also prolonged because the hepatic uptake of rifampin is impaired by probenecid.

Table 52–3. EFFECTS OF PROBENECID ON METABOLISM OF OTHER DRUGS

Decreased Renal Excretion

p-Aminohippuric acid
Phenolsulfonphthalein
Salicylic acid and its acyl and phenolic glucuronides
Phlorizin and its glucuronide
Acetazolamide
Dapsone and its metabolites
Sulfinpyrazone and its parahydroxyl metabolite
Indomethacin
Ampicillin
Penicillin
Cephradine

Reduced Volume of Distribution

Ampicillin
Ancillin
Nafcillin
Cephaloridine

Impairment of Hepatic Uptake

Bromsulfonphthalein
Indocyanin green
Rifampicin

Delayed Metabolism

Heparin

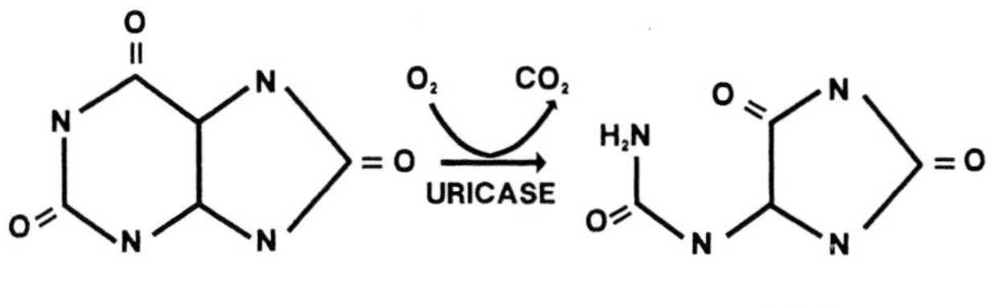

Figure 52–6. Uricase degrades uric acid to allantoin.

The prolonged half-lives of rifampin[60] and cephradine[61] in the presence of probenecid may be therapeutically useful. Probenecid reduces the volume of distribution of several antibiotics, including ampicillin, ancillin, nafcillin, and cephaloridine.[61] If the concentration of these antibiotics is significantly reduced in body fluids in the presence of probenecid, the net effect could be detrimental. Probenecid has also recently been shown to inhibit renal excretion of the acquired immunodeficiency syndrome drug 3'-azido-3' deoxythymide (AZT) in rats and to raise plasma levels of AZT.[62]

The interaction of uricosuric drugs with allopurinol was described earlier.

DESTRUCTION OF URATE

The enzymatic destruction of urate provides a novel experimental approach to treat hyperuricemia and the related disorders. Urate oxidase degrades uric acid to allantoin and carbon dioxide (Fig. 52–6). The administration of urate oxidase is especially promising in prophylaxis against acute uric acid nephropathy.[6, 63, 64] Polyethylene glycol–conjugated uricase may be particularly useful, since it has a prolonged half-life and appears to be non-antigenic.[63] After intermuscular injection of uricase, activity appears in the plasma rapidly, peaks within 24 hours, and persists for about 5 days.[65]

In patients with non-Hodgkin's lymphoma, uricase at 3 units/kg of body weight administered during the first 30 hours lowered the serum urate concentration from 15.3 to 3.2 mg/dl.[65] A dose of 2 units/kg every 5 to 6 days maintained the serum urate level at 9 mg/dl or lower.

Urate oxidase given intramuscularly or intravenously at 1000 units/day, 7 days per month, has decreased tophi in three heart transplant recipients.[66]

References

1. Ferraz MB, O'Brien B: A cost effective analysis of urate lowering drugs in non-tophaceous recurrent gouty arthritis. J Rheumatol 22:908, 1995.
2. Appelbaum SJ, Mayersohn M, Dorr RT, Perrier D: Allopurinol kinetics and bioavailability: Intravenous, oral and rectal administration. Cancer Chemother Pharmacol 8:93, 1982.
3. Kelley WN, Fox IH: Antihyperuricemic drugs. In Kelley WN, Harris ED Jr, Ruddy S, Sledge CB (eds): Textbook of Rheumatology, 3rd ed. Philadelphia, WB Saunders, 1989, p 889.
4. Palella TD, and Fox IH: Hyperuricemia and gout. In Scriver CR, Beaudet AL, Sly WS, Valle D (eds): The Metabolic Basis of Inherited Disease, 6th ed. New York, McGraw-Hill, 1989, p 965.
5. Rundles RW, Wyngaarden JB, Hitchings GH: Drugs and uric acid. Annu Rev Pharmacol 9:345, 1969.
6. Wyngaarden JB, Kelley WN: Gout. In Stanbury JB, Wyngaarden JB, Frederickson DS, Goldstein JL, Brown MS (eds): The Metabolic Basis of Inherited Disease, 5th ed. New York, McGraw-Hill, 1983, p 1043.
7. Rundles RW: The development of allopurinol. Arch Intern Med 145:1492, 1985.
8. Edwards NL, Recker D, Airozo D, Fox IH: Enhanced purine salvage during allopurinol therapy: An important pharmacologic property in humans. J Lab Clin Med 98:673, 1981.
9. Bundgaard H, Falch E: Improved rectal and parenteral delivery of allopurinol using the prodrug approach. Arch Pharm Chem Sci Ed 13:39, 1985.
10. Hande K, Reed E, Chabner B: Allopurinol kinetics. Clin Pharmacol Ther 23:598, 1978.
11. Chalmers RA, Kromer H, Scott JT: A comparative study of the xanthine oxidase inhibitors, allopurinol and oxipurinol in man. Clin Sci 35:353, 1968.
12. Berlinger WG, Park GD, Spector R: The effect of dietary protein on the clearance of allopurinol and oxypurinol. N Engl J Med 313:771, 1985.
13. Elion GB, Yu TF, Gutman AB: Renal clearance of oxipurinol, the chief metabolite of allopurinol. Am J Med 45:69, 1968.
14. Moriwaki Y, Yamamoto T, Takahashi S, Suda M, Higashino K: Effects of glucose infusion on the renal transport of purine bases and oxypurinol. Nephron 69:424, 1995.
15. Rundles RW: The development of allopurinol. Arch Intern Med 145:1492, 1985.
16. Yu TF: The effect of allopurinol in primary and secondary gout. Arthritis Rheum 8:907, 1965.
17. Day RO, Miners JO, Birkett DJ: Allopurinol dosage selection: Relationships between dose and plasma oxipurinol and urate concentrations and urinary urate excretion. Br J Clin Pharmacol 26:423, 1988.
18. Gottlieb NL, Gray RG: Allopurinol-associated hand and foot deformities in chronic tophaceous gout. JAMA 238:1663, 1977.
19. Bull PW, Scott JT: Intermittent control of hyperuricemia in the treatment of gout. J Rheumatol 16:1246, 1989.
20. Loebl WY, Scott JT: Withdrawal of allopurinol in patients with gout. Ann Rheum Dis 33:304, 1974.
21. Zell SC, Carmichael JM: Evaluation of allopurinol use in patients with gout. Am J Hosp Pharm 46:1813, 1989.
22. Bellamy N, Gilbert JR, Brooks PM: A survey of current prescribing practices of antiinflammatory and urate lowering drugs in gouty arthritis in the province of Ontario. J Rheumatol 15:1841, 1988.
23. Miesel R, Zuber M, Sanocka D, Graetz R, Kroeger H: Effects of allopurinol on in vivo suppression of arthritis in mice and ex vivo modulation of phagocytic production of oxygen radicals in whole human blood. Inflammation 18:577, 1994.
24. Singh D, Nazhat NB, Fairburn R, Sahinoglu T, Blake DR, Jones P: Electron spin resonance spectroscopic demonstration of the generation of reactive oxygen species by diseased human synovial tissue following ex vivo hypoxia-reoxygenation. Ann Rheum Dis 54:94, 1995.
25. Yu TF, Gutman AB: Effects of allopurinol [4-hydroxypyrazolo (3,4-d) pyrimidine] on serum and urinary uric acid in primary and secondary gout. Am J Med 37:885, 1964.
26. Ferraz MB: An evidence based reappraisal of the management of nontophaceous interval gout. J Rheumatol 22:1618, 1995.
27. Fam AG: Should patients with interval gout be treated with urate lowering drugs? J Rheumatol 22:1621, 1995.
28. Greene ML, Fujimoto WY, Seegmiller JE: Urinary xanthine stones: A rare complication of allopurinol therapy. N Engl J Med 280:426, 1969.
29. Band PR, Silverberg DS, Henderson JF: Xanthine nephropathy in a patient with lymphosanoma treated with allopurinol. N Engl J Med 283:254, 1970.
30. Hande KR, Hixson CB, Chabner BA: Postchemotherapy purine excretion in lymphoma patients receiving allopurinol. Cancer Res 41:2273, 1981.
31. Braden GL, Warzynski MJ, Golighty M, Ballow M: Cell-mediated immunity in allopurinol-induced hypersensitivity. Clin Immunol Immunopathol 70:145–151, 1994.
32. Okafuji K, Shinohara K: Aplastic anemia probably induced by allopurinol in a patient with renal insufficiency. Rinsho Ketsueki 31:89, 1990.
33. Arellano F, Sacritan JA: Allopurinol hypersensitivity syndrome: A review. Ann Pharmacother 27:337, 1993.
34. Boston Collaborative Drug Surveillance Program: Excess of ampicillin rashes associated with allopurinol or hyperuricemia. N Engl J Med 286:505, 1972.
35. Fam AG, Paton TW, Chaiton A: Reinstitution of allopurinol therapy for gouty arthritis after cutaneous reactions. Can Med Assoc J 123:128, 1980.
36. Meyrier A: Desensitization in a patient with chronic renal disease and severe allergy to allopurinol. Br Med J 2:458, 1976.
37. Komoriya K, Osada Y, Hasegawa M, Honuchi H, Kondo S, Couch RC, Griffin TB. Hypouricemic effect of allopurinol and the novel exsanthine

oxidase inhibitor TEI 6729 in chimpanzees. Eur J Pharmacol 250:455, 1993.

38. Hande KR, Noone RM, Stone WJ: Severe allopurinol toxicity: Description and guidelines for prevention in patients with renal insufficiency. Am J Med 76:47, 1984.

39. Singer JZ, Wallace SL: The allopurinol hypersensitivity syndrome: Unnecessary morbidity and mortality. Arthritis Rheum 29:82, 1986.

40. Fox IH, Kelly WN: Management of gout. JAMA 242:361, 1979.

41. Barry M, Feely J: Allopurinol influences aminophenazone elimination. Clin Pharmacokinet 19:167, 1990.

42. Weiner IM, Mudge GH: Inhibitors of tubular transport of organic compounds. In Gilman AG, Rall TW, Nies AS, Taylor P (eds): The Pharmacologic Basis of Therapeutics, 8th ed. New York, Pergamon Press, 1990, p 920.

43. Diamond HS: Uricosuric drugs. In Kelley WN, Weiner IM (eds): Uric Acid. Berlin, Springer-Verlag, 1978, p 459.

44. Weiner IM, Blanchard KC, Mudge GH: Factors influencing renal excretion of foreign organic acids. Am J Physiol 207:953, 1964.

45. Dayton PG, Yu TF, Chen W: The physiological disposition of probenecid, including renal clearance in man, studied by an improved method for its estimation in biological material. J Pharmacol Exp Ther 140:278, 1963.

46. Israeli ZA, Perel JM, Cunningham RF: Metabolites of probenecid: Chemical, physical and pharmacological studies. J Med Chem 15:709, 1972.

47. de Gery A, Auscher C, Saporta L: Treatment of gout and hyperuricemia by benzbromarone, ethyl 2 (dibromo-3,5-hydroxy-4-benzoyl)-3 benzofuran. In Sperling O, de Vries A, Wyngaarden JB (eds): Purine Metabolism in Man. New York, Plenum Press, 1974, p 683.

48. Maurer H, Wollenberg P: Urinary metabolites of benzbromarone in man. Arzneimittelforschung 40:460, 1990.

49. De Vries JX, Walter-Sack I, Voss A, Forster W, Ilisistegui Pons P, Stoetzer F, Spraul M, Ackermann M, Moyna G: Metabolism of benzbromarone in man: Structures of new oxidative metabolites, 6-hydroxy- and 1'-oxo-benzbromarone, and the enantioselective formation and elimination of 1'-hydroxybenzbromarone. Xenobiotica 23:1435–1450, 1993.

51. Persellin RH, Schmid FR: The use of sulfinpyrazone in the treatment of gout reduces serum uric acid levels and diminishes severity of arthritis attacks, with freedom from significant toxicity. JAMA 175:971, 1961.

52. Zurcher RM, Bock HA, Thiel G: Excellent uricosuric efficacy of benzbromarone in cyclosporin A treated renal transplant patients: A prospective study. Nephrol Dial Transplant 9:548, 1994.

53. Emmerson BT: A comparison of uricosuric agents in gout, with special reference to sulphinpyrazone. Med J Aust 1:839, 1963.

54. Boger WP, Strickland SC: Probenecid (Benemid): Its use and side-effects in 2502 patients. Arch Intern Med 95:83, 1955.

55. Gutman AB, Yu TF: Protracted uricosuric therapy in tophaceous gout. Lancet 2:1258, 1957.

56. Kickler TS, Buck S, Ness P, Shirley RS, Sholar PW: Probenecid-induced immune hemolytic anemia. J Rheumatol 13:208, 1986.

57. de Seze S, Ryckewaert A, d'Anglejan G: The treatment of gout by probenecid (a study based on 156 cases, 68 of which were treated from 1 to 9 years). Rev Rhum Mal Osteoartic 30:93, 1963.

58. MacDonald JF, Wallace SM, Herman RJ, Verbeeck RK: Effect of probenecid on the formation and elimination kinetics of the sulfate and glucuronide conjugates of diflurisal. Eur J Clin Pharmacol 47:519, 1995.

59. Sanchez G: Enhancement of heparin effect by probenecid. N Engl J Med 292:48, 1975.

60. Kenwright S, Levi AJ: Impairment of hepatic uptake of rifamycin antibiotics by probenecid, and its therapeutic implications. Lancet 2:1401, 1973.

61. Gibaldi M, Schwartz MA: Apparent effect of probenecid on distribution of penicillin in man. Clin Pharmacol Ther 9:345, 1968.

62. Aiba T, Sakurai Y, Tsukada S, Koizumi T: Effects of probenecid and cimetidine on the renal excretion of 3'-azido-3' deoxythymidine in rats. J Pharmacol Exp Ther 272:94, 1995.

63. Davis S, Park YK: Hypouricaemic effect of polyethyleneglycol modified urate oxidase. Lancet 1:281, 1981.

64. Masera G, Jankovic M, Zurlo MG, Locasciulli A, Rossi MR, Uderzo C, Recchia M: Urate-oxidase prophylaxis of uric acid–induced renal damage in childhood leukemia. J Pediatr 100:152, 1982.

65. Chua CC, Greenberg ML, Viau AT: Use of polyethylene glycol-modified uricase (PEG-uricase) to treat hyperuricemia in a patient with non-Hodgkin lymphoma. Ann Intern Med 109:114, 1988.

66. Rozenberg S, Roche B, Dorent R, Koeger AC, Borget C, Wrona N, Bourgeois P: Urate oxidase for the treatment of tophaceous gout in heart transplant recipients. A report of 3 cases. Rev Rhum (English) 62:392, 1995.

CHAPTER 53

Vibeke Strand
Edward C. Keystone

Biologic Agents in the Treatment of Rheumatoid Arthritis

Advances in biotechnology and an understanding of basic immunologic mechanisms have led to the development of biologic agents capable of selectively targeting elements of the immunopathologic processes underlying autoimmune disorders such as rheumatoid arthritis (RA). The use of recombinant and hybridoma technology has enabled the synthesis of a diverse array of monoclonal antibodies, cytokine antagonists, and other molecules for targeted immunotherapy. Many of these are patterned after regulatory elements of the normally functioning immune system.

Although the pathophysiologic mechanisms underlying the disease process in RA and other autoimmune conditions have not been fully elucidated, our knowledge has prompted a variety of therapeutic approaches designed to interfere with specific elements of the inflammatory process. These include the recruitment of inflammatory cells into sites of inflammation; lymphocyte activation and collaboration; and secretion and action of proinflammatory cytokines such as interleukin-1 (IL-1), interleukin-6 (IL-6), and tumor necrosis factor-α (TNF-α) (Fig. 53–1).

INFLAMMATORY CELL RECRUITMENT AS A THERAPEUTIC TARGET

The inflammatory response observed in the synovium and other tissues depends on the recruitment of polymorphonuclear cells (PMNs), lymphocytes, and monocytes from the circulation. Cell adhesion molecules (CAMs) expressed on the surface of endothelial cells and their ligands present on white blood cells in the circulation determine the type of cell affected and the site to which it migrates. Evidence suggests that vascular cell adhesion molecule-1 (VCAM-1) and its ligand vascular leukocyte antigen-4 (VLA-4) play a major role in mediating the adhesion of T cells to endothelial cells through the action of IL-1, IL-4, and TNF-α.[1] Interactions between intercellular adhesion molecule-1 (ICAM-1) and its ligand by leukocyte function-associated antigen-1 (LFA-1) appear to mediate transendothelial trafficking of T cells into the joints through the action of IL-1 and TNF-α. In addi-

tion, interactions between matrix molecule ligands and their respective T cell integrins influence T cell activation and function.

A variety of biologic products are currently under development to interrupt the interaction between CAMs and their cell surface ligands. These include monoclonal antibodies to ICAM-1, VLA-4, and E-selectin; soluble ICAM-1 receptors; soluble VCAM-1; oligosaccharide analogs of E- and L-selectins to block binding; and antisense molecules to block transcription and/or translation and subsequent surface expression (Table 53–1). Murine monoclonal antibodies (mAbs) to ICAM-1 and LFA-1 have ameliorated manifestations of antigen-induced arthritis in rabbits,[2] adjuvant arthritis in rats,[3] and collagen- and proteoglycan-induced arthritis in mice.[4, 5] Preliminary studies have shown delay in the development of lupus-like disease in parental mice injected at birth with F_1 hybrid spleen cells.[6] A preliminary report suggests that combination therapy with mAbs to several cell adhesion molecules may offer additional benefit.[5]

A murine IgG2a mAb against ICAM-1 has been evaluated in an open-label protocol in 32 patients with longstanding refractory RA.[7] Improvement was observed in some patients for as long as 3 months. A preliminary report in 10 patients with early RA suggested that the duration of clinical benefit was greater than for patients with refractory disease.[8] Adverse effects included fever, nausea and/or vomiting, and headache in the majority of patients. Two observations suggested that administration of the mAb altered peripheral lymphocyte recruitment and activation: an increase in peripheral putatively activated interleukin-2 receptor (IL-2R)–expressing T cells (CD25+ cells), and an increase in peripheral CD4 T cell numbers. In addition, the anergy observed in several patients during therapy resolved after treatment was completed.[7, 9] An increased incidence of infections was not reported. As a result of these preliminary positive data, further clinical work is expected utilizing a humanized mAb.

Another potential therapeutic strategy is the inhibition of VLA-4/VCAM-1 interactions. A recombinant human adenovirus encoding a soluble form of VCAM-1 has been constructed that, if successfully introduced, would interfere with VLA-4 binding to VCAM-1 on the surface of synoviocytes, thereby inhibiting lymphocyte migration. A preliminary communication demonstrated that, in vitro, virally encoded VCAM-1 secreted by transfected human synoviocytes blocked the adhesion of human peripheral blood T cells.[10]

Binding of the LFA-1 ligand to the ICAM-1 receptor plays a substantial role in stabilizing the cell-cell contact involved in binding the T cell receptor to the antigen–1 major histocompatibility complex (MHC) on antigen-presenting cells.[11] Interventions designed to block this interaction would be expected to interfere with a variety of complex lymphocyte functions necessary for the inflammatory response.[11, 12] The recently observed inhibition of TNF-α and IL-1 production by mAb to ICAM-1 supports its potential therapeutic role in the treatment of inflammatory arthritidies such as RA.[13]

T CELL SURFACE ANTIGENS AS A THERAPEUTIC TARGET

Antigen-driven T cells are thought to be central to the pathogenesis of RA.[14] Antigen-presenting cells (APCs) such as macrophages, dendritic cells, or B cells present antigen in the form of peptides in association with MHC class II molecules to arthritogenic T cells.[15] These T cells bind to the peptide-MHC complex and are thereby activated. This T cell–MHC–

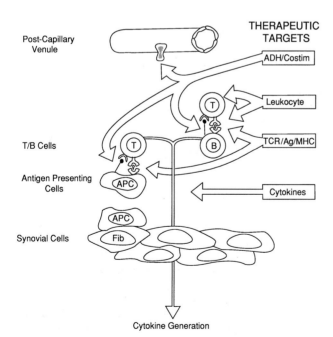

Figure 53–1. Targets for selective immunomodulation. (1) Adhesion/costimulatory (ADH/Costim) molecules to inhibit cell recruitment into the synovium and block cell-cell interaction. (2) Immune cells to deplete or inhibit function. (3) T cell receptor (TCR)/antigen (Ag)/major histocompatibility complex (MHC) to block antigen specific TCR activation. (4) Cytokines to inhibit proinflammatory effect of molecules. APC, antigen-presenting cell; Fib, fibrinogen.

Table 53–1. CURRENT THERAPEUTIC APPROACHES USING BIOLOGIC AGENTS

Non–Antigen-Specific Techniques	Examples
Inflammatory Cell Recruitment as a Therapeutic Target	
mAb to adhesion molecules	Anti-ICAM-1/LFA-1
Soluble adhesion molecules	sVCAM-1
T Cell Surface Antigens as a Therapeutic Target	
CD4	Anti-CD4 mAbs
Other structural antigens	CD5 IC, CAMPATH-1H mAb
Activation antigens	Anti-TAC, anti–IL-2R, anti-CD7 mAbs
	DAB IL-2 fusion toxin
T and B Cell Collaboration as a Therapeutic Target	
Blockade of gp39-CD40 interaction	Anti-gp39 mAb
Blockade of CD28-B7 interaction	CTLA-4 immunoglobulin
Monocytes/Macrophages as a Therapeutic Target	
Cytokines as a Therapeutic Target	
Cytokine receptor antagonist proteins	IL-1ra (IRAP)
Soluble receptors	sIL-1RI, sTNF-α RI and II
mAb to cytokines	Anti–IL-1, anti–TNF-α, anti–IL-6
"Anti-inflammatory" cytokines	IFN-γ, IL-4, IL-10
Potential Antigen-Specific Techniques	
Ag-MHC-TCR Interactions as a Therapeutic Target	
T cell vaccination	
T cell receptor Vβ peptides	Vβ-14, -17 peptides
MHC blockade	HLA-DR4/1 peptide
Oral tolerance	Oral collagen
Anti-idiotypic mAb to autoantibody	Anti-DNA idiotypic mAb

Abbreviations: mAb, monoclonal antibody; ICAM, intercellular adhesion molecule; LFA, leukocyte function-associated antigen; VCAM, vascular cell adhesion molecule; CD, cluster of differentiation; IC, immunoconjugate; IL, interleukin; R, receptor; S, soluble; TNF-α, tumor necrosis factor-α; IFN, interferon; Ag, antigen; MHC, major histocompatibility complex; TCR, T cell receptor; V, variable-region; HLA, human leukocyte antigen; DNA, deoxyribonucleic acid.

peptide interaction, with other costimulatory signals, leads to activation of macrophages, synoviocytes, and chondrocytes resulting in the release of proinflammatory mediators including cytokines and degradative lysosomal enzymes that cause cartilage and bone destruction.[16] Activation of T cell–driven autoreactive B cells results in autoantibody production with subsequent immune complex formation and further release of proinflammatory mediators.

The central role of T cells in the initiation and perpetuation of disease has been shown in a number of murine models of autoimmunity, including the New Zealand black/white (NZB/W) model of lupus[17, 18] and the collagen-induced arthritis model of

RA.[19] Substantial evidence implicates T cells in the pathogenesis of RA in humans: the T cell is the predominant mononuclear cell infiltrating the synovium[20]; synovial T cells express cell surface activation antigens[21]; there is a striking association of MHC class II alleles (HLA-DR4) with RA[22]; immunotherapy with thoracic duct drainage,[23] total lymphoid irradiation (TLI),[24] and lymphopheresis[25] has effectively mediated disease activity in some patients; and patients with RA who develop acquired immunodeficiency syndrome (AIDS) may experience a complete remission of their arthritis.[26]

Although implicated in the pathogenesis of RA, the particular T cells that are reactive to the inciting antigen have not been identified, nor is the nature of the antigens inciting and/or perpetuating the inflammatory process known. As a consequence, therapeutic approaches to date have largely been non–antigen specific, directed at the T cell population as a whole or its specific subsets.

CD4 Surface Antigen as a Target

One of the first biologic approaches to the treatment of RA was the use of mAbs directed at the CD4 antigen. CD4 T cells provide help in the generation of cell-mediated and humoral immunity. The CD4 antigen is an integral membrane glycoprotein that functions as a co-receptor of the T cell antigen receptor complex,[27] acting as an adhesion molecule to stabilize the cellular contact of T cells with MHC class II–bearing APCs.[28] Involvement of CD4 T cells in the pathogenesis of RA is suggested by their predominance in the T cell infiltrate in the synovial membrane and the association of RA with the HLA-DR4 antigen.[29] Improvement in a variety of murine models of autoimmunity has followed treatment with the rat anti-mouse L3T4 mAb, GK 1.5 (analogous to human anti-CD4).[30]

The mAbs initially studied in humans were murine in origin, of differing isotypes and targeting different epitopes on the CD4 molecule. Results from open-label clinical trials have been reported in approximately 75 patients with RA.[27, 31–33] Most patients had longstanding disease and had failed multiple second-line agents. Clinical responses were observed in 60 to 75 percent of patients, with generally 3 to 6 months of benefit. No correlation between the observed biologic effects and clinical responses were noted with any of the mAbs. Adverse events, predominantly constitutional symptoms, were mild and attributed to cytokine release.

Several mechanisms have been considered to account for the depleting effects of anti-CD4 mAb. Possibilities include trapping of antibody-coated CD4 T cells in the reticuloendothelial system through Fc or complement-mediated mechanisms, and depletion by direct killing via antibody-dependent cell-mediated cytotoxicity (ADCC), complement-dependent cytotoxicity (CDC), or apoptosis.[34–36] Binding of the anti-CD4 mAb may block the interaction of CD4 cells with MHC class II APCs or inhibit coaggregation of the CD4 antigen with T cell receptor with (TCR)–CD3 structures after cell activation.[37, 38] Anti-CD4 mAb may modulate surface antigen expression, thereby transmitting inhibitory signals to CD4-bearing cells.[39]

Although pilot studies with murine mAbs showed benefit, concern was expressed that the generation of a human immune response against the murine protein would prevent retreatment. Murine mAbs were unlikely to mediate ADCC or CDC in humans and would be expected to be less effective. Therefore, chimeric or hybrid murine-human and subsequently humanized mAb were generated to decrease immunogenicity, increase effectiveness, and prolong the serum half-life. The murine portion of these engineered chimeric and humanized antibodies constituted the complementarity-determining region of the antigen-binding Fab portion of the molecule.

Despite promising results in open-label studies of the chimeric anti-CD4 mAb (cMT412), two randomized control trials (RCTs) demonstrated no benefit. One study comprised 64 patients with longstanding RA who were taking methotrexate[40] and the other, 60 patients with RA of less than 1 year's duration.[41] Neither showed significant clinical responses compared with placebo, despite effective and persistent CD4 T cell depletion for as long as 30 months.[42, 43] Nonetheless, infection suggestive of immunosuppression was rare. Adverse events were mild and well tolerated.

Studies utilizing IgG4 isotype anti-CD4 mAbs that do not mediate CDC are currently in progress. A primatized anti-CD4 mAb (CE 9.1) was developed utilizing macaque variable and human constant regions and is expected to result in little immunogenicity. A preliminary report of an open-label phase I trial indicated it to be well tolerated and to cause only transient depletion of peripheral CD4 T cells with early evidence of clinical benefit.[44]

Other Structural Antigens as Targets

Cell surface antigens other than CD4 have been targeted by mAbs, including CD5 and CDw52.

An early biologic agent used in RA was an immunoconjugate (IC) of murine IgG1 mAb against CD5 (CD5 IC) coupled to the ricin A chain (a ribosomal inhibitory protein). CD5 is a cell surface antigen expressed on most human T cells, as well as a B cell subset, and is believed to function as a receptor for a "second signal" in T cell activation.[45] Although open-label phase I studies in 76 patients demonstrated clinical benefit in a majority,[46] a subsequent RCT in 104 patients with early disease did not show therapeutic efficacy. Of significance in this study was that responses in the placebo group exceeded the active treatment groups and persisted for 60 to 90 days. In all studies, transient peripheral T and CD5 + B cell depletion occurred with normalization to 50 percent or more of pretreatment levels within 30 to 45 days, regardless of clinical response. Administration of the CD5 IC was associated with constitutional symptoms, pedal edema, and myalgias.

CAMPATH-1H, a humanized mAb that targets a surface antigen (CDw52) expressed on most human peripheral monocytes and lymphocytes, was developed by inserting the hypervariable region genes of the rat mAb into human immunoglobulin genes.[47] Although clinical benefit was observed in open-label studies in approximately 106 patients, profound depletion of peripheral T cell counts occurred, with persistent CD4 cytopenia for up to 32 months.[33] In a blinded randomized study comparing higher doses of CAMPATH-1H in 41 patients,[48] profound lymphopenia immediately following treatment was frequently associated with infection. Adverse events were significant, including high fevers associated with rigor, nausea, and hypotension attributed to lympholysis and resultant cytokine release. Anti-idiotype host immune responses occurred in 90 percent of patients.

The initial positive open-label data following administration of selected mAbs directed against T cell surface antigens were not confirmed in placebo RCTs. Nor was there correlation between biologic effects and clinical benefit. The profound and prolonged CD4 cytopenia observed with the chimeric anti-CD4 and CAMPATH-1H mAbs has led to the development of "nondepleting" IgG4 isotype anti-CD4 mAbs, which are still under evaluation.

T Cell Activation Antigens as Targets

Monoclonal Antibody to Activation Antigens

Peripheral T cells are activated in RA, as evidenced by the presence of the high-affinity IL-2R (CD25), which is not expressed on the surface of resting T cells.[49] A rat IgG2β mAb to IL-2R has been administered to three RA patients with transient benefit.[50] A humanized mAb to the CD25-antigen, anti-TAC, is currently under evaluation in autoimmune disorders.[51]

Treatment with both murine and chimeric mAbs targeting the T cell activation antigen CD7 has been evaluated in ten patients with active RA.[52] This surface-activation antigen is up-regulated on a majority of synovial T cells. Despite modulation of antigen expression, only transient and mild clinical improvement was observed.

Fusion Toxins

Another approach to target activated T cells is the use of a fusion protein consisting of IL-2 and an enzymatically active fragment of diphtheria toxin, DAB_{389} IL-2. It binds specifically to the high-affinity IL-2R and is rapidly internalized, resulting in cell death as a consequence of protein synthesis inhibi-

tion.[53] In two short-term RCTs in patients with refractory RA, no significant clinical benefit was seen in the active groups compared with placebo.[54, 55] Adverse events included nausea, fever, headache, elevated liver transaminases, and rash. Despite a host immune response, retreatment was beneficial and associated with less incidence of transaminase elevations.

T AND B CELL COLLABORATION AS A THERAPEUTIC TARGET

gp39-CD40 Interaction

Collaboration between activated T cells and B cells is mediated by contact-dependent cell surface receptor-ligand interactions and cytokines. Combinations of these signals determine antibody production and isotype switching. Among the variety of cell surface molecules involved, interactions between the CD40 antigen on B cells and its ligand gp39 on activated T cells have recently been shown to be critically important.[56] An mAb specific to murine gp39 blocks its binding to CD40, thereby inhibiting T helper cell–dependent B cell activation in vitro. Administration of anti-gp39 prevented the development of collagen-induced arthritis in rodents and serum antibody titers to collagen.[57] A preliminary report has also shown that anti-CD40 ligand mAb reduced the incidence or delayed the onset of nephritis in NZB/W female mice.[58] No studies in human disease have been reported.

CTLA-4 Immunoglobulin

The CD28 receptor on T cells and its counter-receptor, B7 (expressed on activated B cells, dendritic cells, and macrophages), mediate another cell surface receptor-ligand interaction required for B cell responses to T cell–dependent antigens as well as T cell antigen responses.[59] The CD28 receptor is stimulated during contact of T cells with APCs. The B7 molecule also binds to CTLA-4, a receptor structurally related to CD28, which is expressed in low numbers on T cells after activation but binds with higher affinity than CD28.[60] Recently, a soluble hybrid of the extracellular domain of human CTLA-4 and immunoglobulin constant region, CTLA-4 Ig, was constructed that blocks the binding of B7 to CD28.[61] Selective inhibition of the B7-CD28 interactions with CTLA-4 Ig produces antigen-specific T cell unresponsiveness in vitro and suppresses immune function in vivo, including T cell–dependent B cell responsiveness.[62] A murine CTLA-4 Ig was effective in both prevention and treatment of disease in NZB/W mice by blocking autoantibody production and prolonging life even when therapy was delayed until the late stages of renal disease.[63]

Monocytes and Macrophages as a Therapeutic Target

Recent data suggest that the monocyte and macrophage cell populations are more important in the perpetuation of RA than previously thought. Although T cell–derived cytokines are expressed at low levels in rheumatoid synovial tissue, there are high levels of expression of monocyte cytokine, protein, and gene products.[64] Moreover, monocytes and macrophages constitute a substantial proportion of the rheumatoid synovial cell population.

To date, no studies of therapy have been specifically directed at monocytes in RA. Circumstantial evidence has implicated monocyte depletion as a mechanism for an anti-CD4 antibody effect. Trials of both murine and chimeric anti-CD4 therapy in RA have demonstrated reductions in circulating monocytes, including neopterin and CD14.[38, 65, 66] Of significance, a striking correlation was observed between monocytopenia and therapeutic response in one study.[63]

CYTOKINES AS A THERAPEUTIC TARGET

IL-1, TNF-α, and IL-6 are cytokines that share many proinflammatory properties and have been implicated in the pathogenesis of inflammatory disorders such as RA. They may activate and thereby trigger proliferation of synovial cells, inducing collagenase production, inhibiting proteoglycan synthesis, and stimulating bone resorption.[67] They induce the expression of adhesion molecules, resulting in further cell recruitment and release of cytokines. Of significance, deregulated production of TNF-α in transgenic mice results in the development of a chronic polyarthritis resembling RA that is rapidly fatal.[68] Together, these data suggest IL-1 and TNF-α to be key targets for downregulation in RA.

Several techniques have been developed to inhibit the effector functions of cytokines. These include receptor antagonist proteins,[69] soluble receptor antagonists,[70] and mAbs to cytokines or their receptors (Fig. 53–2; see also Table 53–1). Receptor-binding antagonist proteins are biologically inactive proteins that compete with the cytokine for binding to the membrane receptor. To be effective, receptor antagonist proteins must bind to more than 90 percent of the receptors on the cell surface. Since large doses are required for such an effect, these proteins have low efficiency despite high specificity. Soluble receptors are truncated forms of the cell surface receptor devoid of the transmembrane and intracytoplasmic domains, although they retain binding affinity comparable to the full-length membrane-bound receptors. In contrast to receptor antagonist proteins, soluble receptor molecules bind to free cytokine, inhibiting its binding to cell surface receptors. To be effective, they must be retained within the circulation, although a lower dose is needed than for receptor antagonist proteins. Compared with anti-cytokine mAbs, soluble receptors

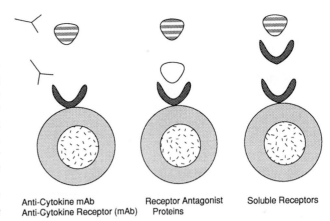

Figure 53–2. Selective inhibition of cytokine action by (1) monoclonal antibodies (mAb) that recognize either cytokine or cytokine receptor; (2) receptor antagonist proteins that are biologically inactive proteins competing with cytokine for binding to membrane receptor; (3) soluble receptors that are truncated forms of the cell receptor capable of binding to the cytokine without generating a cell signal.

have much higher (1000-fold) affinity and are smaller, possibly enabling a wider distribution.

IL-1 as a Therapeutic Target

IL-1ra

The IL-1 receptor antagonist protein (IL-1ra) is a naturally occurring antagonist of IL-1. IL-1ra binds to the two receptor forms of human IL-1, type I and type II,[71] and specifically inhibits binding of both IL-1α and IL-1β without stimulating the cells to which it binds. Although IL-1ra binds to type I IL-1 receptors with the same affinity as IL-1α and IL-1β, 10- to 100-fold amounts are required to substantially inhibit the biologic responses to IL-1α or β in vitro. Large doses are also required to inhibit IL-1α or β effects in vivo. The affinity of IL-1ra for the type II IL-1 receptor is lower than for IL-1β, which may be relevant, as IL-1β is the predominant form of IL-1 produced in the inflamed synovium.

In vitro, IL-1ra blocks IL-1α- or β-induced synthesis of collagenase and prostaglandin E_2 in chondrocytes and synovial cells, and inhibits the IL-1α- or β-induced breakdown of proteoglycans and inhibition of glycosaminoglycan synthesis.[72, 73] In vivo, IL-1ra has effectively reduced joint inflammation in adjuvant, streptococcal cell wall, and collagen II–induced arthritis models in the rat.[74, 75]

Recently, IL-1ra protein (IRAP) was successfully delivered by gene transfer ex vivo into the synovium of joints in rabbits; subsequent intra-articular injection of IL-1β failed to induce synovitis in those joints.[76] A preliminary report also demonstrated the suppression of antigen-induced arthritis in rabbits utilizing ex vivo gene therapy introduction of the IL-1ra gene.[77] These experiments demonstrate the feasibility of treating arthritis with gene transfer technology, although expression of the introduced gene product may be transient. Preliminary work is under way in humans.

A randomized, blinded study compared a number of dosing regimens of subcutaneously administered recombinant IL-1ra in 175 patients with RA.[78] Although of short duration, clinical improvement was observed in patients receiving the most intensive initial treatment courses. Serum C-reactive protein (CRP) levels declined during the weeks when multiple doses were administered. No biologic marker of drug effect was observed; in vitro measures of T cell proliferation remained unchanged. Serious infections (soft tissue infections, urinary tract infection, prostatitis) were reported in 4 percent of patients; injection site reactions caused discontinuation of therapy in 5%. A large 6-month, placebo-controlled randomized trial is currently under way.

Soluble IL-1 Receptor

A naturally occurring form of soluble IL-1R (sIL-1R) exists as the soluble type II IL-1R. Although both soluble type I and II receptors completely abrogate binding of IL-1α or IL-1β at sufficiently high concentrations, type I IL-1R is a better inhibitor of IL-1α and type II IL-1R is a better inhibitor of IL-1β.

A type I IL-1R fused to the Fc portion of IgG1 (rhu IL-1R) was recombinantly produced. It has shown benefit in several animal models of autoimmune disease, including experimental allergic encephalomyelitis (EAE) and antigen-induced arthritis.[79] Even when treatment was initiated after the establishment of arthritis, it suppressed adjuvant arthritis. It also prevented autoantibody expression and development of lupus-like disease in MRL/lpr mice. A phase 1 dose-ranging placebo-controlled study involving intra-articular administration of recombinant human type I sIL-1R in patients with active RA produced only modest benefit, possibly because of its lesser effect on IL-1β.[80] Preliminary data from an RCT dose-ranging study using subcutaneous administration produced similar effects with minimal toxicity.[81]

Recently, a type II IL-1 soluble receptor–immunoglobulin fusion protein was developed for therapeutic use because of its higher affinity for IL-1β and lower affinity for IL-1ra. A preliminary report of an in vitro study showed that it inhibited IL-1β effects on cultured chondrocytes.[82]

Anti–IL-1 Monoclonal Antibody

A neutralizing murine mAb against (murine) IL-1β was shown effective in preventing the development of collagen-induced arthritis in mice despite an absence of effect on anti-collagen antibody titers.[83] To date, no studies have been performed in humans.

TNF-α as a Therapeutic Target

Considerable evidence has accumulated implicating TNF-α in the pathogenesis of arthritis.[60] The biologic activity of TNF-α is dependent on binding to either p55 or p75 cell surface TNF-α receptors on macrophages, fibroblasts, chondrocytes, or endothelial cells.

Anti–TNF-α Monoclonal Antibodies

Administration of a chimeric (human/murine) IgG1 mAb to TNF-α (cA2) abrogated the severe arthritis observed in transgenic mice with constitutive TNF-α production, and prolonged survival.[84] A combination of anti–TNF-α and anti-CD4 mAb therapy suppressed collagen type II arthritis in mice more profoundly than did anti–TNF-α alone.[85] Moreover, a preliminary report indicated that the duration of benefit with the combination was significantly longer than with anti–IL-1R alone, anti–TNF-α alone, or anti–IL-1R in combination with anti–TNF-α.[86] These data underscore the importance of the synergistic effects of IL-1 and TNF-α in inflammatory arthritis and support the concept of combination biologic therapy.

An initial phase 1 open-label clinical trial of the chimeric anti–TNF-α (cA2) mAb in 20 patients with refractory RA demonstrated significant clinical response with concordant reductions in serum CRP and IL-6 levels.[87] Onset of effect was rapid. Marked improvement in the malaise and fatigue as well as in arthritis was reported. Median duration of response was 3 months; all patients eventually relapsed. Repetitive treatment with the mAb after disease relapse resulted in continued reduction in disease activity, although the magnitude and duration of the response lessened with each successive administration.[88] An RCT in 73 patients confirmed these original observations, with significant improvement noted at 4 weeks in the active treatment groups compared with placebo.[89] Adverse effects of fever, rash, and nausea were mild and well tolerated.

A preliminary report of a RCT ascending-dose trial of a humanized IgG4 mAb to TNF-α (CDP571) in 36 RA patients indicated similar rapid onset of benefit with good tolerability.[90]

Soluble TNF-α Receptors

A preliminary report has shown that a recombinant form of two human soluble p75 (type II) TNF-α receptors conjugated to the Fc portion of IgG1 (rhu TNFR:Fc) was effective in inhibiting streptococcal cell wall–induced arthritis in rats, either alone or in combination with rhu IL-1R.[91] Currently, several soluble TNF-α receptor proteins are under evaluation in patients with RA. A preliminary report from a phase I placebo-controlled dose-escalation study of (the type II) rhu TNFR:Fc administered intravenously and subcutaneously in 16 patients showed clinical benefit with good tolerability.[92]

IL-6 as a Therapeutic Target

A murine IgG1 anti–IL-6 mAb was evaluated in a small, open-label, phase I study of five patients with refractory RA.[93] Transient improvement in clinical and biologic measures of disease was reported.

Together, these preliminary results suggest that cytokine antagonists may be an effective modality in the treatment of inflammatory arthropathies. The data suggest that combination therapy, or products designed to inhibit the effects of both IL-1β and TNF-α, may offer additional benefit.

"Anti-inflammatory" Cytokines

Cytokines such as interferon-γ (IFN-γ), transforming growth factor-β (TGF-β), interleukin-4 (IL-4), and interleukin-10 (IL-10) may act to suppress the inflammatory process.

IFN-γ has the capacity to suppress the inflammatory response by antagonizing the effects of other proinflammatory cytokines. It blocks IL-1– and TNF-α–mediated induction of synoviocyte proliferation, and collagenase release[94]; it inhibits IL-1–mediated prostaglandin generation and TNF-α–mediated granulocyte-monocyte colony stimulating factor (GM-CSF) production; and it has been shown to inhibit B cell activation and immunoglobulin synthesis. These findings, together with the paucity of IFN-γ detected in RA synovium, provide a rationale for its therapeutic use in RA. In murine models of collagen-induced and adjuvant arthritis, data are conflicting as to the efficacy of IFN-γ possibly owing to differences in doses and timing of administration.[95, 96]

In patients with RA, six randomized placebo-controlled trials have demonstrated modest beneficial effects with mild adverse reactions.[33] Statistically significant improvement was observed in the IFN-γ–treated patients compared with placebo in two of the studies.

Distinct subpopulations of CD4 T cells, termed *Th1* and *Th2*, mediate cellular and humoral immune responses, respectively. Th1 cells synthesize IFN-γ, TNF-α, TNF-β, and IL-2; Th1 cells generate IL-4, IL-5, IL-6, and IL-10 but not IFN-γ or IL-2.[97] Recent data indicate that the products of Th1 and Th2 cells negatively regulate each other's functions.[98] IL-10 and IL-4 have been shown to suppress Th1 responses in a synergistic manner.[99] Evidence implicates Th1 cells in the pathogenesis of RA,[100] although a role for Th2 cells is also likely. IL-10 can up-regulate IL-1ra production. IL-4 and IL-10 may therefore be useful therapeutic agents in RA.

In several animal models of autoimmunity, IL-4 administration has ameliorated clinical disease. In animals with EAE, IL-4 treatment improved symptomatology and induced myelin basic protein (MBP)–specific (regulatory) Th2 cells.[101] In nonobese diabetic mice, IL-4 reversed T cell proliferative anergy and delayed the onset of clinical diabetes.[102] However, in autoimmune disorders with differing underlying pathophysiologic mechanisms, these cytokines may have opposing effects. For example, administration of IL-10 accelerated the onset of disease in the NZB/W murine model of lupus, whereas treatment with anti–IL-10 mAbs delayed the onset of glomerulonephritis and increased survival.[103]

POTENTIAL ANTIGEN-SPECIFIC THERAPIES

Although the antigen putatively inciting and/or perpetuating the inflammatory process has yet to be identified in human disease, techniques have been developed to interfere with the trimolecular complexes of antigen-MHC-TCR through recognition of the TCR or MHC involved in the complex (Fig. 53–3; see also Table 53–1).

T Cell Vaccination

Inoculation of attenuated T cell clones recognizing the inciting autoantigen has been shown to specifi-

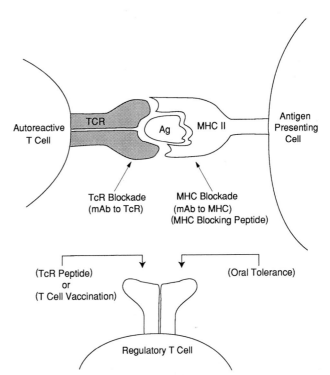

Figure 53–3. Selective antigen-specific immunosuppression by (1) inhibition of T cell receptor (TCR; TcR) activation by blocking the major histocompatibility complex [MHC]–binding site to any antigenic peptide including autoantigen by monoclonal antibody (mAb) to MHC or MHC-blocking peptides; (2) depletion or functional inactivation of Vβ T cells by specific anti-Vβ mAb; (3) functional inactivation of autoreactive T cells by administration of autoantigen, i.e., peptide in tolerogenic form; (4) induction or enhancement of regulatory T cells able to control the activity of pathogenic autoreactive T cells by vaccination-like treatments. The first two strategies inhibit the response of a fraction of the T cell repertoire; the last two specifically target autoreactive T cells. (Adapted from Adorini L, Guéry J-C, Trembleau S: Approaches toward peptide-based immunotherapy of autoimmune diseases. Springer Semin Immunopathol 14:187, 1992.)

cally prevent the induction of experimental autoimmune disease models, including adjuvant[104, 105] and collagen II–induced arthritis.[106] This T cell vaccination is thought to protect by generation of short-lived anti-activated T cell responses and long-lived anti-clonotypic T cell responses. Based on these results, a phase I study was conducted in 13 RA patients utilizing subcutaneous inoculation of attenuated autologous T cell clones or lines isolated from synovial tissue or fluid.[107] A mild decrease in disease activity was most marked at 8 weeks after injection. Specific immune reactivity against the injected T cells was not detected. No adverse events were observed.

T Cell Receptor Vβ Peptide Therapy

Another approach to selective targeting of autoreactive T cells involves TCR gene products. A direct contribution of TCRs to autoimmune disease is suggested by the conservation of TCR structure among T cells mediating inflammation in the experimental models of EAE and collagen II–induced arthritis. Utilization of a limited number of TCR-β variable-region (Vβ) families allows for selective targeting of T cells through the TCR either by passive infusion of anti-TCR mAbs or by active immunization with TCR Vβ peptides. Immunization with TCR Vβ peptides is a refinement of the T cell vaccination approach. In the collagen II–induced arthritis model, arthritis was suppressed by administration of mAbs to specific Vβs, namely, Vβ-2, Vβ-5, and Vβ-8; mAbs to other Vβ regions were ineffective.[108] Vaccination with a synthetic peptide of the encephalitogenic TCR in the EAE model of multiple sclerosis has resulted in protection from the MBP-induced EAE.[109] TCR peptide vaccination is more attractive than antibody treatment because it generates an immunoregulatory response after vaccination.

Although no consensus has been reached regarding which particular TCR variable-region gene families may be overexpressed in RA synovium, biased Vβ gene family usage has been amply demonstrated in different peripheral tissue compartments. A number of studies have reported an overrepresentation of Vβ-14 and Vβ-17 among unselected or activated IL-2R+ synovial T cell populations in RA.[110, 111] These data prompted a study of the safety and biologic effects of immunization with a 17–amino acid sequence derived from the human TCR Vβ-17 with incomplete Freund's adjuvant. A preliminary report of a phase I study in RA patients demonstrated a modest clinical effect in patients as well as significant T cell proliferation in response to the immunizing Vβ-17 peptide.[112]

MHC-Antigen Interaction

Monoclonal antibodies directed against disease-related MHC class II antigens have been therapeutically effective in collagen II–induced and antigen arthritis models.[113, 114] An open-label trial of murine anti-idiotypic mAb to the MHC class II HLA-DR4 susceptibility gene product in nine patients with RA resulted in mild clinical benefit.[115]

An alternative approach to MHC class II blockade is the use of peptides that compete for MHC binding, resulting in selective inhibition of autoreactive T cell activation.[116] Studies in the EAE model demonstrated that immunization of mice simultaneously with the analog blocking peptide and the encephalitogenic peptide suppressed paralysis.[117] However, the peptide to block MHC recognition must be continually supplied to be effective, making this form of therapy much less feasible in human disease. A trial utilizing vaccination with HLA-DR4/1 peptides in RA is currently under way.

Oral Tolerance

Oral administration of antigen has been shown to induce a state of specific immunologic unresponsiveness (to the antigen alone) called oral tolerance. However, the mechanisms behind this phenomenon remain unclear. Oral administration of native type II collagen was effective in suppressing arthritis in type II collagen–induced and adjuvant arthritis[118, 119]; both T cell and anti-collagen antibody responses were inhibited in the tolerant mice. An RCT examined administration of oral chicken collagen to patients with RA.[120] Results of this short-term study revealed a modest reduction in arthritis in collagen-treated patients without apparent toxicity.

Anti-idiotypic/Anti-clonotypic Therapy

Immunoglobulin molecules serve as antigen receptors on the surface of B cells. They carry unique determinants termed *idiotypes* that are themselves immunogenic. Monoclonal antibodies directed against these idiotypes may be therapeutic if they are capable of generating a response that interferes with binding of a pathogenic antibody. An anti-idiotype mAb directed to anti-collagen antibody inhibited the development of collagen 2II–induced arthritis in mice.[121] In addition, an anti-idiotype mAb to anti-DNA has been demonstrated to retard the onset of nephritis and prolong survival in NZB/NZW mice.[122] Recently, a lupus-related murine anti-DNA autoantibody from MRL/lpr autoimmune mice was identified and cloned. The idiotype of this antibody has also been demonstrated in sera of patients with systemic lupus erythematosus (SLE). A phase 1 clinical study of vaccination utilizing this idiotype was conducted in a small number of patients with SLE.[123] Generation of an appropriate anti-idiotypic response with reduction in anti–double-stranded DNA titers occurred in some patients.

An analogous therapeutic approach utilized anti-clonotypic mAbs specific for three distinct T cell clones demonstrated to be arthritogenic in collagen II–induced arthritis. Administration of these mAbs decreased the incidence of arthritis when given prophylactically and reduced manifestations of arthritis when initiated at the onset of disease.[124]

CONCLUSIONS

Recent experience with biologic agents has substantially contributed to our knowledge of RA (and autoimmune diseases in general) in a number of areas: (1) pathophysiology of the underlying disease, (2) current paradigms of research, and (3) new directions for future therapy.

The use of biologic agents has confirmed the roles of a number of immunopathologic elements in the initiation and perpetuation of disease. For example, in RA the role of adhesion molecules in recruitment of lymphocytes into the synovium is supported by the clinical and biologic effects of mAbs directed against ICAM-1. The substantial role played by cytokines in the inflammatory process in RA is supported by the marked effect of anti–TNF-α mAb therapy on CRP and IL-6 levels with concomitant improvement in the malaise and fatigue associated with the disease. These and other data provide ample evidence for the use of selective targeting of immunopathologic elements not only as a therapeutic tool but also as a method for dissecting the underlying process of disease.

Insight into the research paradigms in relation to human disease has come from these studies as well. A striking example is the profound and prolonged depletion of T cells following administration to humans of the chimeric anti-CD4 and CAMPATH-1H mAbs, in contrast to the transient T cell depletion following use of anti-L3T4 mAbs in rodent models. This finding underscores the concern that species specificity may limit the usefulness of animal models in preclinical studies and emphasizes the need for preclinical studies that accurately mirror the human situation. Initial human studies often require the dose of a new biologic agent to be well below the expected therapeutic range. More extensive dose escalation and dosing schedule studies are usually required to determine the optimal therapeutic regimen.

Experience with biologic agents also has confirmed the importance of the synovium as a window for monitoring the effects of therapeutic interventions. Effects on blood cells and synovium of anti-CD4 and CAMPATH-1H mAbs emphasize this; even with profound peripheral CD4 T cell cytopenia, sufficient T cells remain to perpetuate the inflammatory process in affected joints.

Finally, the critical importance of well-designed randomized placebo-controlled trials has been particularly demonstrated with biologic agents. Although most products tested have demonstrated benefit in open-label studies, few have been shown effective in RCTs. Reasons for such discrepancies include the observed higher placebo response in trials of parenterally administered products, as well as differences in expectations by both patient and physician when "exciting new immunologically based therapies" are utilized.

The experience accumulated to date with these newer biologic agents suggests that clinical effects are of relatively short duration, necessitating repetitive administration for long-term effect. Limitations on repeated courses of treatment may be imposed by the required parenteral route, cost of administration, injection site reactions, and patient (as well as physician) acceptance. In this day and age, the cost of treatment cannot be overemphasized. It may be difficult to rationalize treatment with many of these newer agents until clinical benefit of at least 6 to 12 months' duration can be demonstrated.

References

1. Oppenheimer-Marks N, Lipsky P: Transendothelial migration of T cells in chronic inflammation. Immunologist 2:58, 1994.
2. Jasen HE, Lightfoot E, Davis LS, et al: Amelioration of antigen-induced arthritis in rabbits treated with monoclonal antibodies to leukocyte adhesion molecules. Arthritis Rheum 35:541, 1992.
3. Iigo Y, Takashi T, Tamatani T, et al: ICAM-1 dependent pathway is critically involved in the pathogenesis of adjuvant arthritis in rats. J Immunol 147:4167, 1991.
4. Kakimoto K, Nakamura T, Ishii K, et al: The effect of anti-adhesion molecule antibody on the development of collagen-induced arthritis. Cell Immunol 142:326, 1992.
5. Milkacz K, Brennan FR, Kim JH, et al: Immunotherapy with antibodies to cell adhesion molecules in proteoglycan-induced arthritis. Arthritis Rheum 37:S397, 1994.
6. Merino J, Revilla C, Conde C, et al: The effects of the treatment with anti-LFA-1a or anti-ICAM-1 mAb on the tolerance and autoimmunity in mice injected at birth with F_1 hybrid cells depends on the saturation of these molecules in different lymphoid organs. Arthritis Rheum 37:S390, 1994.
7. Kavanaugh AF, Davis LS, Nichols LA, et al: Treatment of refractory rheumatoid arthritis with a monoclonal antibody to intercellular adhesion molecule-1 (ICAM-1). Arthritis Rheum 37:992, 1994.
8. Kavanaugh A, Jain R, McFarlin J, et al: Anti-CD54 (intercellular adhesion molecule-1; ICAM-1) monoclonal antibody therapy in early rheumatoid arthritis. Arthritis Rheum 37:S220, 1994.
9. Davis L, Kavanaugh AF, Lipsky P: T cell hyporesponsiveness after treatment of rheumatoid arthritis patients with anti–ICAM-1 antibody. Arthritis Rheum 37:S340, 1994.
10. Valiance D, Davidson B, Roessler B: Transgenic expression of soluble VCAM-1 by synoviocytes inhibits lymphocyte binding in vitro. Arthritis Rheum 37:S220, 1994.
11. Springer T, Dustin M, Kishimoto T, et al: The lymphocyte function-associated LFA-1, CD2 and LFA-3 molecules: Cell adhesion receptors of the immune system. Annu Rev Immunol 5:233, 1987.
12. Patarroyo M, Makagoba MW: Leukocyte adhesion to cells: molecular basis, physiological relevance, and abnormalities. Scand J Immunol 30:129, 1989.
13. Geissler D, Gaggl S, Most J, et al: A monoclonal antibody directed against the human intercellular adhesion molecule (ICAM-1) modulates the release of tumor necrosis factor-α, interferon-γ, and interleukin-1. Eur J Immunol 20:2591, 1990.
14. Panayi GS, Lanchbury JS, Kingsley GW: The importance of the T cell in initiating and maintaining the chronic synovitis of rheumatoid arthritis. Arthritis Rheum 35:729, 1992.
15. Winchester RF, Gregersen PK: The molecular basis of susceptibility to rheumatoid arthritis: The confirmational equivalence hypothesis. Springer Semin Immunopathol 10:119, 1988.
16. Gay S, Gay RE, Koopman WJ: Molecular and cellular mechanisms of joint destruction in rheumatoid arthritis: Two cellular mechanisms explain joint destruction? Ann Rheum Dis 52:S39, 1993.
17. Wofsy D, Seaman W: Successful treatment of autoimmunity in NZB/NZW F_1 mice with monoclonal antibody to L3T4. J Exp Med 161:378, 1985.
18. Wofsy D, Seaman W: Reversal of advanced murine lupus in NZB/W

F₁ mice by treatment with monoclonal antibody to L3T4. J Immunol 138:3247, 1987.

19. Rauges GE, Sriram S, Cooper SM: Prevention of type II collagen–induced arthritis by *in vivo* treatment with anti-L3T4. J Exp Med 162:1105, 1985.

20. van Boxel JA, Paget SA: Predominantly T cell infiltrate in rheumatoid synovial membrane. N Engl J Med 293:517, 1975.

21. Cush JJ, Lipsky PE: Phenotypic analysis of synovial tissue and peripheral blood lymphocytes isolated from patients with rheumatoid arthritis. Arthritis Rheum 31:1230, 1988.

22. Gregersen PK, Silver J, Winchester RJ: The shared epitope hypothesis: An approach to understanding the molecular genetics of susceptibility to rheumatoid arthritis. Arthritis Rheum 30:1205, 1987.

23. Paulus HE, Machleder HI, Levine S, et al: Lymphocyte involvement in rheumatoid arthritis: Studies during thoracic duct drainage. Arthritis Rheum 20:1249, 1977.

24. Strober S, Tanay A, Field E, et al: Efficacy of total lymphoid irradiation in intractable rheumatoid arthritis: A double-blind, randomized trial. Ann Intern Med 102:441, 1985.

25. Karsh J, Klippel JH, Plotz PH, et al: Lymphopheresis in rheumatoid arthritis. A randomized trial. Arthritis Rheum 24:867, 1981.

26. Calabrese LH, Wilke WS, Parkins AD, et al: Rheumatoid arthritis complicated by infection with immunodeficiency virus and the development of Sjögren's syndrome. Arthritis Rheum 32:1453, 1989.

27. Barber EK, Dasgupta JD, Schlossman SF, Trevillyan JM, Rudd CE: The CD4 and CD8 antigens are coupled to a protein-tyrosine kinase (p56) that phosphorylates the CD3 complex. Proc Natl Acad Sci U S A 86:3277, 1989.

28. Doyle C, Strominger JL: Interaction between CD4 and class II MHC molecules mediates cell adhesion. Nature 330:256, 1987.

29. Panayi GS, Lanchbury JS, Kingsley GH: The importance of the T cell in initiating and maintaining the chronic synovitis of rheumatoid arthritis. Arthritis Rheum 35:729, 1992.

30. Steinman L: The use of monoclonal antibodies for treatment of autoimmune disease. J Clin Immunol 10:30S, 1990.

31. Elliot MJ, Maini RN: New directions for biological therapy in rheumatoid arthritis. Int Arch Allergy Immunol 104:112, 1994.

32. Delafuente JC, Resman-Targoff BH: Monoclonal antibodies in the treatment of rheumatoid arthritis. Ann Pharmacother 28:650, 1994.

33. Strand V, Keystone EC: Biologic intervention in rheumatoid arthritis: Part 1. J Biotech Healthcare 1:283, 1995.

34. Dalesandro MR, Kinney CS, Happ MP, et al: An investigation of the mechanism of depletion of CD4 cells by a mouse/human chimeric CD4 mAb. J Cell Biochem 17B:53, 1993.

35. Alters S, Steinman L, Oi V: Comparison of rat and rat-mouse chimeric anti-murine CD4 antibodies *in vitro.* J Immunol 142:2018, 1989.

36. Choy EHS, Adjaye J, Forrest L, et al: Chimaeric anti-CD4 monoclonal antibody cross-linked by monocyte Fcγ receptor mediates apoptosis of human CD4 lymphocytes. Eur J Immunol 23:2676, 1993.

37. Carteron NL, Schimenti CL, Wofsy D: Treatment of murine lupus with F(ab')2 fragments of monoclonal antibody to L3T4. J Immunol 142:1470, 1989.

38. Saizawa K, Rojo J, Janeway CA Jr: Evidence for a physical association of CD4 and the CD3: a b T cell receptor. Nature 328:260, 1987.

39. Wassmer PJ, Chan C, Lögdberg L, Shevack EM: Role of the L3T4-antigen in T cell activation: II. Inhibition of T cell activation by monoclonal anti-L3T4 antibodies in the absence of accessory cells. J Immunol 135:2237, 1985.

40. Moreland LW, Pratt P, Mayes M, et al: Minimal efficacy of a depleting chimeric anti-CD4 (CM-T412) in treatment of patients with refractory rheumatoid arthritis (RA) receiving concomitant methotrexate (MTX). Arthritis Rheum 36:S39, 1993.

41. van der Lubbe PA, Dykmans BAC, Markusse HM, et al: Lack of clinical effect of CD4 monoclonal antibody therapy in early rheumatoid arthritis: A placebo-controlled trial. Arthritis Rheum 37:S294, 1994.

42. Moreland LW, Pratt PW, Bucy RP, et al: Treatment of refractory rheumatoid arthritis with a chimeric anti-CD4 monoclonal antibody: Long-term followup of CD4+ T cell counts. Arthritis Rheum 37:834, 1994.

43. Van der Lubbe P, Reiter C, Breedvelt FC: Chimeric CD4 monoclonal antibody cM-T412 as a therapeutic approach to rheumatoid arthritis. Arthritis Rheum 36:1375, 1993.

44. Solinger AM, Yocum DE, Tesser J: Clinical activity in an early phase 1 trial of promitized IDEC-CE9.1-anti-CD4 monoclonal antibody in RA. Arthritis Rheum 37:S337, 1994.

45. Ceuppens JL, Baraja MR: Monoclonal antibodies to the CD5 antigen can provide the necessary second signal for activation of isolated resting T cells by solid phase bound OKT3. J Immunol 137:1816, 1986.

46. Doyle C, Strominger JL: Interaction between CD4 and class II MHC molecules mediates cell adhesion. Nature 330:256, 1987.

47. Xia M-Q, Tone M, Packman L, et al: Characterization of the CAMPATH-1 antigen: Biochemical analysis and cDNA cloning revealing an unusually small peptide backbone. Eur J Immunol 21:1677, 1991.

48. Isaacs JD, Mann VK, Hazelman BL, et al: CAMPATH 1H in RA—A study of multiple i.v. dosing. Arthritis Rheum 36:S40, 1993.

49. Akasu F, Poplonski L, Snow K, et al: Impaired generation of high-affinity interleukin-2 receptors in the autologous mixed lymphocyte reaction in rheumatoid arthritis. Clin Immunol Immunopathol 63:142, 1992.

50. Kyle V, Coughlan RJ, Tighe H, et al: Beneficial effect of monoclonal antibody to interleukin 2 receptor on activated T cells in rheumatoid arthritis. Ann Rheum Dis 48:428, 1989.

51. Junghans RP, Waldmann TA, Landolfi NF, et al: Anti-Tac-H: A humanized antibody to the interleukin 2 receptor with new features for immunotherapy in malignant and immune disorders. Cancer Res 50:1495, 1990.

52. Kirkham BW, Thien F, Pelton B, et al: Chimeric CD7 monoclonal antibody therapy in rheumatoid arthritis. J Rheumatol 19:1348, 1992.

53. Williams D, Parker K, Bacha P, et al: Diphtheria toxin receptor binding domain with interleukin-2: Genetic construction and properties of a diptheria toxin–related interleukin-2 fusion protein. Protein Eng 1:493, 1992.

54. Sewell KL, Moreland LW, Cush JJ, et al: Phase I/II double blind dose response trial of a second fusion toxin, DAB 389 IL-2 in rheumatoid arthritis. Arthritis Rheum 3:S130, 1993.

55. Sewell KL, Parker KC, Woodworth TG, et al: DAB486 IL-2 fusion toxin in refractory rheumatoid arthritis. Arthritis Rheum 36:1223, 1993.

56. Noelle RJ, Ledbetter JA, Aruffo A: CD40 and its ligand, an essential ligand-receptor pair for thymus-dependent B cell activation. Immunol Today 13:431, 1992.

57. Durie FH, Fava RA, Roy TM, et al: Prevention of collagen-induced arthritis with an antibody to gp39, the ligand of CD40. Science 261:1328, 1993.

58. Mohan C, Shi Y, Ion D, et al: Long-term benefits of a brief anti-gp39 therapy in murine lupus. Arthritis Rheum 37:S369, 1994.

59. June CH, Ledbetter JA, Linsley PS, et al: The role of the CD28 receptor in T-cell activation. Immunol Today 11:211, 1990.

60. Schwartz RH: Costimulation of T lymphocytes: The role of CD28, CTLA-4 and B7/BB1 in interleukin production and immunotherapy. Cell 71:1065, 1992.

61. Lipsky PS, Ledbetter JA: The role of the CD28 receptor during T cell responses to antigen. Ann Rev Immunol 11:191, 1993.

62. Tarutani S: Collagen-induced arthritis suppressed with monoclonal anti-idiotypic antibody. Microbiol Immunol 37:135, 1993.

63. Finck MK, Bonomo A, Scott DE, et al: Cytokine-induced immune deviation as a therapy for inflammatory autoimmune disease. J Exp Med 180:1961, 1994.

64. Firestein GC, Zvaifler NJ: How important are T cells in chronic rheumatoid synovitis? Arthritis Rheum 33:768, 1990.

65. Horneff G, Sack U, Kalden JR, et al: Reduction of monocyte macrophage activation markers upon anti-CD4 treatment. Decreased levels of IL-1, IL-6, neopterim and soluble CD14 in patients with rheumatoid arthritis. Clin Exp Immunol 91:207, 1993.

66. Choy EHS, Chikanza IC, Kingley EH, et al: Treatment of rheumatoid arthritis with single dose or weekly pulses of chimaeric anti-CD4 monoclonal antibody. Scand J Immunol 36:291, 1992.

67. Keffer J, Probert L, Cazlaris A, Georgopoulos S, Kaslaris E, Kioussis D, Kollias G: Transgenic mice express human tumor necrosis factor, a predictive genetic model of arthritis. EMBO J 10:4025, 1991.

68. Keffer J, Probert L, Cazlaris H, et al: Transgenic mice-expressing human tumor necrosis factor: A predictive genetic model of arthritis. EMBO J 10:4025, 1991.

69. Arend WP: Interleukin-1 receptor antagonist: A new member of the interleukin family. J Clin Invest 88:1445, 1991.

70. Fernandez-Botran R: Soluble cytokine receptors: Their role in immunoregulation. FASEB J 5:2567, 1991.

71. Arend WP, Joslin RG, Thompson RC, et al: An IL-1 inhibitor from human monocytes: Production and characterization of biologic properties. J Immunol 142:1851, 1989.

72. Smith RJ, Chin JE, Sam LM, et al: Biologic effects of an interleukin-1 receptor antagonist protein of interleukin-1 stimulated cartilage erosion and chondrocyte responsiveness. Arthritis Rheum 34:78, 1991.

73. Henderson BRC, Thompson T, Hardingham T, et al: Inhibitor of interleukin-1 induced synovites and articular cartilage proteoglycan loss in the rabbit knee by recombinant human interleukin-receptor antagonist. Cytokine 3:246, 1991.

74. Schwab JH, Anderle SK, Brown RR, et al: Pro- and anti-inflammatory roles of interleukin in recurrence of bacterial cell wall–induced arthritis in rats. Infect Immunol 59:4436, 1991.

75. Wooley PH, Whalen JD, Chapman DL, et al: The effect of an interleukin-1 receptor antagonist protein on type II collagen and antigen-induced arthritis in mice. Arthritis Rheum 33:S20, 1990.

76. Bandara G, Mueller GM, Galea-Lauri J, et al: Intra-articular expression of biologically active interleukin-1 receptor antagonist protein by *ex vivo* gene transfer. Proc Natl Acad Sci 90:10764, 1993.

77. Ohtani K, Nita I, MacAulay W: Suppression of antigen-induced arthritis in rabbits by ex vivo gene therapy. Arthritis Rheum 37:S295, 1994.

78. Lebsack ME, Paul CC, Martindale JJ, et al: A dose and regimen ranging

study of IL-1 receptor antagonist in patients with rheumatoid arthritis. Arthritis Rheum 36:S39, 1993.

79. Schorlemmer HV, Kanzy EJ, Langner KD, et al: Immunomodulatory activity of recombinant IL-1 receptor (IL-1-R) on models of experimental rheumatoid arthritis. Agents Actions 39:C113, 1993.

80. Drevlow B, Capezio J, Lovis R, et al: Phase 1 study of recombinant human interleukin-1 receptor (RHU-IL-1R) administered intraarticularly in active rheumatoid arthritis. Arthritis Rheum 36:S39, 1993.

81. Drevlow B, Lovis R, Haag MA: Phase 1 study of recombinant human interleukin-1 receptor (RHU IL-1R) administered subcutaneously in patients with active rheumatoid arthritis. Arthritis Rheum 37:S339, 1994.

82. Dudler J, Raz E, Lotz M: Inhibition of IL-1 effects by a soluble II-1 receptor/IG fusion protein. Arthritis Rheum 37:S340, 1994.

83. Joosten LAB, Helsen MMA, van de Loo FAJ, et al: Amelioration of established collagen-induced arthritis (CIA) with anti–IL-1. Agents Actions C174, 1994.

84. Williams RO, Feldmann M, Maini RN: Anti–tumor necrosis factor ameliorates joint disease in murine collagen-induced arthritis. Proc Natl Acad Sci U S A 89:9785, 1992.

85. Williams RO, Mason LJ, Feldmann M, et al: Synergy between anti-CD4 and anti–tumor necrosis factor in the amelioration of established collagen-induced arthritis. Proc Natl Acad Sci U S A 91:2762, 1994.

86. Williams RO, Feldmann M, Main RN: Evaluation of anti–IL-1R and anti-TNF therapy in murine collagen arthritis and comparison with combined anti-TNF/anti-CD4 therapy. Arthritis Rheum 37:S279, 1994.

87. Elliott MJ, Maini RN, Feldmann M, et al: Treatment of rheumatoid arthritis with chimeric monoclonal antibodies to tumor necrosis factor α. Arthritis Rheum 36:1681, 1993.

88. Elliott MJ, Maini RN, Feldmann M, et al: Repeated therapy with monoclonal antibody to tumor necrosis factor α (cA2) in patients with rheumatoid arthritis. Lancet 344:1127, 1994.

89. Elliott MJ, Maini RN, Feldmann M, et al: Randomized double-blind comparison of chimeric monoclonal antibody to tumor necrosis factor α (cA2) versus placebo in rheumatoid arthritis. Lancet 344:1105, 1994.

90. Rankin ECC, Choy EHS, Kassumos D, et al: A double-blind, placebo-controlled ascending dose trial of the recombinant humanized anti-TNF α antibody CDP 571 in patients with rheumatoid arthritis. Arthritis Rheum 37:S295, 1994.

91. Russell D, Tugker K, Konno H, et al: Inhibition of tumor necrosis factor (TNF) is effective alone or in combination with inhibition of interleukin-1 (IL-1) in reducing joint swelling in rodent bacterial cell wall–induced arthritis. Arthritis Rheum 37:S279, 1994.

92. Moreland LW, Margolies GR, Heck IW, et al: Soluble tumor necrosis factor receptor (sTNFR): Results of a phase I dose-escalation study in patients with rheumatoid arthritis. Arthritis Rheum 37:S295, 1994.

93. Wendling D, Racadote E, Wijdenes J: Treatment of severe rheumatoid arthritis by anti–interleukin 6 monoclonal antibody. J Rheumatol 20:259, 1993.

94. Taylor DJ, Feldmann M, Evanson JM, et al: Comparative and combined effects of transforming growth factor α and β interleukin-1 and interferon γ on rheumatoid synovial cell proliferation, glycolysis and prostaglandin E production. Rheumatol Int 9:65, 1989.

95. Nakajima H, Takamori H, Hiyama Y, et al: The effect of treatment with interferon γ on type II collagen–induced arthritis. Clin Exp Immunol 81:441, 1990.

96. Mauritz NJ, Holmdahl R, Jousson R, et al: Treatment with γ interferon triggers the onset of collagen arthritis in mice. Arthritis Rheum 31:297, 1988.

97. Mosemann TR, Coffman RL: TH1 and TH2 cells: Different patterns of lymphokine secretion lead to different functional properties. Annu Rev Immunol 7:145, 1989.

98. Mosemann TR, Moore KW: The role of IL-10 in crossregulation of TH1 and TH2 responses. Immunol Today 12:A49, 1991.

99. Pourie F, Menon S, Coffman RL: Interleukin 4 and interleukin 10 are synergistic to inhibit cell-mediated immunity in vivo. Eur J Immunol 23:2223, 1993.

100. Quayle AJ, Chromart P, Miossec P, et al: Rheumatoid inflammatory T cell clones express TH1 but also TH2 and mixed (TH0-like) cytokine patterns. Scand J Immunol 38:75, 1993.

101. Racke MK, Bonomo A, Scott DE, et al: Cytokine-induced immune deviation as a therapy for inflammatory autoimmune disease. J Exp Med 180:1961, 1994.

102. Rapoport MJ, Jaramillo A, Zipris D, et al: Interleukin 4 reverses T cell proliferative unresponsiveness and prevents the onset of diabetes in nonobese diabetic mice. J Exp Med 178:87, 1993.

103. Ishida H, Muchammuel T, Sakaguchi S, et al: Continous administration of anti-interleukin 10 antibodies delays onset of autoimmunity in NZB/WF1 mice. J Exp Med 179:305, 1994.

104. Lider O, Karin N, Shinitsky M, et al: Therapeutic vaccination against adjuvant arthritis using autoimmune T cells treated with hydrostatic pressure. Proc Natl Acad Sci U S A. 84:4577, 1987.

105. Mor F, Lohse AW, Karin N, et al: Clinical modeling of T cell vaccination against autoimmune diseases in rats: Selection of antigen-specific T cells using a mitogen. J Clin Invest 85:1594, 1990.

106. Kakimoto K, Katsuki M, Huofuji T, et al: Isolation of T-cell line capable of protecting mice against collagen-induced arthritis. J Immunol 140:78–83, 1988.

107. van Laar JM, Miltenburg AMM, Verdonk MJA, Leow A, Elferink BG, Daha MR, Cohen IR, de Vries RRP, Breedveld FC: Effects of inoculation with attenuated autologous T cells in patients with rheumatoid arthritis. J Autoimmun 6:159, 1993.

108. Chiocchia G, Boissier MC, Fournier C: Therapy against murine collagen-induced arthritis with T cell receptor Vβ specific antibodies. Eur J Immunol 21:2899, 1991.

109. Vandenbark AA, Hashim G, Offner W: Immunization with a synthetic T cell receptor V region peptide protects against experimental autoimmune encephalomyelitis. Nature 341:S41, 1989.

110. Paliard X, West SG, Lafferty JA, et al: Evidence for the effects of a superantigen in rheumatoid arthritis. Science 253:325, 1991.

111. Howell MD, Divelfy JP, Lundean KA, et al: Limited T cell receptor β chain heterogeneity among interleukin-2 receptor positive synovial T cells suggests a role for superantigen in rheumatoid arthritis. Proc Natl Acad Sci U S A 88:10921, 1991.

112. Moreland LW, Heck IW Jr, Koopman WJ, et al: Vβ17 T cell receptor peptide vaccine: results of a phase 1 dose-finding study in patients with rheumatoid arthritis. Arthritis Rheum 37:S337, 1994.

113. Wooley PH, Luthra HS, Lafuse WP, et al: Type II collagen-induced arthritis in mice III. Suppression of arthritis by using monoclonal and polyclonal anti-Ia antisera. Immunol 134:2366, 1985.

114. van de Brock MF, van de Berg WB, van de Rutte LBA: Monoclonal anti-Ia antibodies suppress the flare-up reaction of antigen induced arthritis in mice. Clin Exp Immunol 66:320, 1986.

115. Quaghata F, Schenkelaars EJ, Ferrone S: Immunotherapeutic approach to rheumatoid arthritis with anti-idiotypic antibodies to HLA-DR4. Isr J Med 29:154, 1993.

116. Gaur A and Fathman CG: Immunotherapeutic strategies directed at the trimolecular complex. Adv Immunol 56:219, 1994.

117. Lamot AG, Sette A, Fujinami R, et al: Inhibition of experimental autoimmune encephalomyelitis induction in SJL/J mice by using peptide with high affinity for IA molecules. J Immunol 145:1687, 1990.

118. Nagler-Anderson C, Bober LA, Robinson ME, et al: Suppression of type II collagen–induced arthritis by intragastric administration of soluble type II collagen. Proc Natl Acad Sci U S A 83:7443, 1986.

119. Zang ZJ, Lee CS, Lider O, et al: Suppression of adjuvant arthritis in Lewis rats by oral administration of type II collagen. J Immunol 145:2489, 1990.

120. Trentham DE, Dynesius-Trentham RA, Orav EJ, et al: Effects of oral administration of type II collagen on rheumatoid arthritis. Science 261:1727, 1993.

121. Tartutani S: Collagen-induced arthritis suppressed with monoclonal anti-idiotypic antibody. Microbiol Immunol 37:135, 1993.

122. Hahn B, Ebling FM: Suppression of murine lupus nephritis by administration of an anti-idiotypic antibody to anti-DNA. J Immunol 132:187, 1984.

123. Lee ML, Spertini F, Leimgruber A, et al: Phase 1 clinical results with an idiotype vaccine (3E10) for systemic lupus erythematosus (SLE). Arthritis Rheum 37:S368, 1994.

124. Peacock DJ, Ku E, Banquerigo ML, et al: Suppression of collagen arthritis with antibodies to an arthritogenic oligoclonal T cell line. Cell Immunol 140:444, 1992.

Gary S. Firestein

Etiology and Pathogenesis of Rheumatoid Arthritis

Rheumatoid arthritis (RA) is the most common inflammatory arthritis, affecting about 1 percent of the general population worldwide.[1] Although the incidence is surprisingly constant across the globe, regardless of geographic location and race, there are some exceptions. For instance, the incidence in China is somewhat lower (about 0.3 percent), whereas it is substantially higher in other groups, such as the Pima Indians, in North America (about 5 percent). Because of its prevalence and the ready accessibility of joint samples for laboratory investigation, RA has, in many ways, served as a model for the study of inflammatory and immune-mediated diseases.

Although RA is properly considered a disease of the joints, it is important to recognize that it can exhibit a variety of extra-articular manifestations. These manifestations clearly show that RA has features of a systemic disease, capable of involving a variety of major organ systems. Moreover, one of the great mysteries of RA is why the synovium is the primary target. Keys to understanding these phenomena lie in comprehension of arthrotropism of antigens and inflammatory cells and in learning what specific receptors and chemotactic gradients exist to focus the inflammation within joints.

To explain the tissue specificity, a number of hypotheses are found. One possibility is that the disease localizes to the joint owing to its abundant blood supply and rich capillary network. As with immune-complex glomerulonephritis, immune complexes of a specific size, electrostatic charge, or composition might be concentrated in the synovium based on the physical properties of blood vessels. The very fact that diarthrodial joints are designed to move suggests a possible relation. For instance, it has been recognized for decades that immobilization (either by bedrest, splinting, or due to a cerebrovascular accident) can ameliorate joint inflammation in RA. Another

difference between joints and other spaces in the body is that the joint lining has no epithelial tissue. Many synovial lining cells are mesenchymal in origin; the lining itself is discontinuous and lacks a formal basement membrane. The intimal lining cells are loosely associated with each other, and there are occasional gaps resulting in direct contact between the "sub-lining" tissue and the synovial fluid. The joint contains some cell types (like synoviocytes or chondrocytes) that are unique and could serve as a source of privileged antigens or targets for an infectious agent, which might explain the restricted inflammation in the majority of RA patients. Whether or not these obvious differences between joints and other organs have relevance to why the chronic inflammation of RA occurs in joints is not known, but these differences must be encompassed in any set of hypotheses.

The first criteria for classification (not diagnosis) of RA were published in 1958. These were used heavily, but criticized, for 30 years[2] and were revised in 1988.[3] They are listed in Chapter 55.

Rheumatologists in previous decades have defined very well the clinical manifestations of RA. Although clues have been provided by detailed studies of immunogenetics of the class II major histocompatibility (MHC) loci and the usage of specific rheumatoid factor genes, the plain truth is that we still do not know what causes RA. The area of pathogenesis has shown the most progress in the last 10 years, where the role of small molecule mediators of inflammation (e.g., arachidonic acid metabolites), cytokines, growth factors, chemokines, adhesion molecules, and metalloproteinases have been carefully defined. These products attract and activate cells from the peripheral blood and evoke proliferation and activation of synoviocytes. The proteases can subsequently lead to behavior similar to a localized tumor, invading and destroying articular cartilage, subchondral bone, tendons, and ligaments (Fig. 54–1). New appreciation of these pathogenic mechanisms has increased awareness that irreversible loss of articular cartilage begins relatively early in the course of RA and that therapies to suppress the synovitis must be effective early if joint destruction is to be avoided.

In order to improve treatment strategies and target novel therapies at key inflammatory or immune pathways, it is also essential to realize that different stages of the disease can have very distinct pathogenetic mechanisms. When the disease has progressed to late phases, therapy is unlikely to reverse or retard destruction of articular cartilage. Therapeutic approaches to early disease should be targeted to specific immune cells (e.g., T cells) involved in the initiation process of RA because the mechanisms of late disease could be independent of this original stimulus. The recognition that RA is a heterogeneous disease with many pathogenic mechanisms at its various stages is bedeviling to the clinical investigator, yet the recognition offers the best chance for ultimately defining specific therapies.

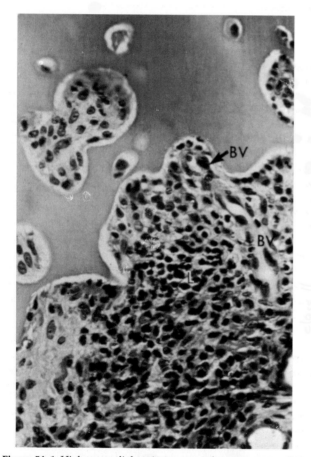

Figure 54–1. High-power light microscopy at the pannus-synovium junction. The space between them is shrinkage artifact. Tongues of proliferating tissue have invaded the residual cartilage shown at the upper left. Small blood vessels (BV) are seen just below the cartilage-pannus junction. Small, darkly staining cells, probably lymphocytes (L) or primitive mesenchymal cells, are just below the invading surface.

SUSCEPTIBILITY TO DEVELOPMENT OF RHEUMATOID ARTHRITIS

The etiology of RA remains a mystery, but a variety of studies suggest that a blend of environmental and genetic factors is responsible; a contribution of either one is necessary but not sufficient for full expression of the disease. The most compelling example is in monozygotic twins, where the concordance rate is perhaps 30 to 50 percent when one twin is affected, compared to 1 percent for the general population. The risk for a fraternal twin of a patient with RA is also high (about 2 to 5 percent), but this is not more than the rate for other first-degree relatives.

Immunogenetic and Other Heritable Predisposing Factors

Evidence is accumulating that the structure of class II surface molecules on antigen-presenting cells is of great importance at the initiation of the immune response in RA. Chapter 14 presents a detailed discussion of class I and class II major histocompatibility complex (MHC) antigens and of the insights provided by intensive study of the molecular genetics of RA. Initiation of certain T cell immune responses is dependent, in part, on the presence or absence of particular MHC (in this case, DR) allelic products. The MHC also helps determine the T cell repertoire in a given individual; those T cells that cannot recognize the endogenous MHC antigens are eliminated in fetal development through thymic deletion. At the same time, autoreactive T cells are eliminated. The end result in the thymus is a fine balance in discrimination between self and nonself; it is not surprising in light of the complexity of this process that autoantibodies can occur to various antigens, to a variable extent, in all of us. The role of the MHC in shaping T cell receptor gene usage is not a trivial point because, as will be discussed later, characterizing specific T cell repertoires in the joint or blood of RA patients has been a subject of intense scrutiny, and a bias in the usage of T cell receptor genes has been assumed to be de facto evidence of ongoing T cell activation. Since HLA-DR haplotypes are not randomly distributed among RA patients compared to normal controls, it is only natural to expect that the T cell repertoire in these patients will be skewed as well.

In the 1970s, Stastny provided evidence that RA was associated with an antigen of the HLA-D locus.[4] HLA-Dw4, identified by the mixed lymphocyte reaction, was shown to be the D locus antigen associated with RA, as well as with more severe forms of the disease.[5] The finding of B cell alloantigens closely related to HLA-D enabled investigators to demonstrate that the B lymphocyte alloantigen HLA-DR4 occurred in 70 percent of patients compared with 28 percent of controls, giving a relative risk of having RA to those with HLA-DR4 of approximately 4 to 5.[6]

Later, careful study of the MHC using cDNA

probes directed against specific α and β chains of the DR loci have revealed "susceptibility cassettes" or shared epitopes on the β chains of DR that predispose to development of RA. HLA-DR4 can be divided into at least five subtypes: Dw4, Dw10, Dw13, Dw14, and Dw15. The susceptibility to RA is associated with the third hypervariable region of DR β chains, from amino acid 70 through 74.[7, 8] The susceptibility epitope is glutamine-leucine-arginine-alanine-alanine (QKRAA), a sequence found in Dw4 and Dw14 (in which RA is more prevalent) in addition to some DR1 β chains. Current nomenclature attempts to clarify these ambiguities by including information on the specific DR β sequences. For instance, the DR4 β chain with the greatest association with RA are referred to as DRB*0401, DRB*0404, DRB*0101 and DRB*1402 (Table 54–1). Individuals with DR β-chains exhibiting other substitutions in this region (e.g., Dw10) have no increased susceptibility to RA. Once the structure of this sequence is considered, up to 96 percent of patients with RA exhibit the appropriate HLA-DR locus.[9] In some ethnic and racial groups, the association with DR4 positivity is not nearly as prominent.[10]

The QKRAA epitope might also predict for the severity of RA once it is established.[9, 11] In one study, 100 percent of patients who inherited two DRB*04 genes had rheumatoid nodules compared to 59 percent of patients with only one gene. Major organ system involvement was observed in 61 percent and 11 percent of these patients, respectively. These data suggest a "dose response" effect of the HLA genes and imply that severity, rather than susceptibility, is the major contribution of HLA-DR to the disease. This notion is not universally accepted and the interpretation depends greatly on the inclusion of patients with transient, self-limited arthritis. If such patients (who frequently lack HLA-DR4) are included in the

analysis, then the correlations between DR4 and RA susceptibility are significantly weakened.[10, 12]

What is special about the susceptibility cassette? The crystal structure of HLA-DR1 has been solved and one can infer the three-dimensional structure of other HLA-DR alleles.[13] The region that is so carefully associated with RA (QKRAA) lies adjacent to the antigen-binding cleft of the DR molecule and might determine the specificity of peptides that bind the DR molecule and can be presented to CD4+ helper T cells. This corresponds nicely with the notion that antigen presentation (and a specific arthrotropic etiologic agent) is responsible for RA, since only individuals with the appropriate antigen-binding groove would be able to mount an immune response that ultimately leads to arthritis. There are (at least) two caveats: (1) other factors clearly must be involved because many normal individuals carry the QKRAA motif and do not develop RA; and (2) the converse hypothesis is also plausible; i.e., QKRAA might create a "hole" in the immune response as a result of a DR topography that prevents an arthrotropic agent from binding. This could, in turn, prevent an appropriate T cell–mediated response that would, under normal circumstances, clear the etiologic agent.

The class II MHC associations described earlier primarily implicate cellular immune responses. However, there are some associations noted in the humoral system, albeit not as striking. For example, a particular immunoglobulin *kappa* genotype appears to confer risk of RA.[14] Although it cannot be considered an immunogenetic determinant, strictly speaking, information is accumulating that deficient galactosylation of immunoglobulin may be a risk factor for development of autoimmune diseases, including RA.[15] The IgG glycosylation defect has been demonstrated to exist prior to the onset of RA[16] and is especially prominent on the IgG1, 2, and 4 isotypes of rheumatoid factor.[17] The cause might be reduced galactosyl transferase activity in RA B cells.[18] Deficient galactosylation is also thought to be predictive in some settings for patients with early synovitis who will progress ultimately to full-blown RA.[19] Passive transfer of arthritis in T cell–primed mice is exacerbated by infusions of IgG fractions that lack galactose, whereas the galactosylated fraction is nonpathogenic.[20]

Given the importance of cytokines in the perpetuation phase of RA (discussed later), it would not be surprising that some cytokine genotypes might be associated with RA. The most intriguing evidence relates to TNF-α production in chronic inflammatory diseases. This proinflammatory factor is thought to be a major cytokine in the pathogenesis of RA, and the TNF genes are located in the MHC locus on chromosome 6 in humans. There are high- and low-TNF–producing strains of mice associated with specific restriction fragment polymorphisms, and the low-TNF phenotype correlates with susceptibility to lupus-like disease.[21] The low-TNF phenotype also appears to be associated with nephritis in human systemic lupus erythematosus.[22] In light of other known

Table 54–1. NOMENCLATURE FOR HLA-DR ALLELES AND ASSOCIATIONS WITH RHEUMATOID ARTHRITIS

Old Nomenclature	New Nomenclature (HLA-DRB1* Alleles)	Association with Rheumatoid Arthritis
HLA-DR1	0101	+
HLA-DR4 Dw4	0401	+
HLA-DR4 Dw14	0404/0408	+
HLA-DRw14 Dw16	1402	+
HLA-DR4 Dw10	0402	−
HLA-DR2	1501, 1502, 1601, 1602	−
HLA-DR3	0301, 0302	−
HLA-DR5	1101–1104, 1201, 1202	−
HLA-DR7	0701, 0702	−
HLA-DRw8	0801, 0803	−
HLA-DR9	0901	−
HLA-DRw10	1001	−
HLA-DRw13	1301–1304	−
HLA-DRw14 Dw9	1401	−

From Weyand CM, Hicok KC, Conn DL, Goronzy JJ: The influence of HLA-DRB1 genes on disease severity in rheumatoid arthritis. Ann Intern Med 177:801, 1992.

associations within the MHC locus in RA, it would clearly be of great interest to know the molecular basis of such phenotypes and whether they confer susceptibility to RA. With regard to other cytokines, allelic variations were recently described for IL-1α[23] and IL-1ra,[24] a naturally occurring IL-1 antagonist.

Another genetic possibility, intriguing but unproved, is that certain individuals have a deficient hypothalamic response to acute inflammation. Experiments showed that defects in the hypothalamic–pituitary axis contribute to susceptibility in the streptococcal cell wall (SCW) arthritis model in Lewis rats. This strain has markedly impaired plasma corticotropin and corticosterone responses to SCW or to other phlogistic compounds, and corticotropin-releasing hormone mRNA is not generated in the hypothalamus of these animals.[25] Other strains of rats with a normal axis do not develop arthritis after SCW injection, and administration of replacement doses of corticosteroids to Lewis rats prevents the development of disease. It is tempting to develop the hypothesis that a genetic impairment in hypothalamic–pituitary–adrenal responsiveness to inflammation would be sufficient to permit symmetrical synovitis to develop and proliferate, and eventually to become a self-sustaining process that we diagnose as RA. Although the clinical studies are difficult to perform owing to the number of medications and presence of a chronic disease, patients with RA appear to have lower circulating levels of cortisol and an abnormal hypothalamic–pituitary axis.[26] Perhaps this confers susceptibility to RA, which is consistent with the observation that low doses of prednisone that approximate simple replacement therapy (as opposed to pharmacologic doses) can effectively ameliorate many symptoms.

Gender

Rheumatoid arthritis is one of many chronic inflammatory diseases that predominates in women. The ratio of female to male patients (2:1 to 4:1) is significant yet not nearly as high as that found in Hashimoto's thyroiditis (25:1 to 50:1), systemic lupus erythematosus (SLE) (9:1), or even autoimmune diabetes mellitus (type I, 5:1).[27] The basis of the gender differences is not known, but presumably it is related to the hormonal milieu. Moreover, estrogens have multiple effects on T lymphocytes and may inhibit neutrophil activation.[28]

Still incompletely understood are the mechanisms underlying the effect of pregnancy on RA. Pregnancy usually is associated with remission of the disease in the last trimester.[29, 30] More than 75 percent of pregnant patients with RA improve, starting in the first or second trimester; but 90 percent of these will experience a flare of disease associated with a rise in rheumatoid factor titers in the weeks or months after delivery.[31]

The mechanism of protection might be related to the production of large amounts of the suppressive cytokines like IL-10 during pregnancy or alterations in cell-mediated immunity.[32] In murine proteoglycan-induced synovitis, for example, the development of arthritis is related to the production of anti-proteoglycan antibodies. Pregnancy decreases clinical arthritis in these animals even though titers of pathogenic antibody are unchanged.[33] A possible relationship between alleviation of RA symptoms during the last trimester of pregnancy and immunogenetics may be supported by the observation that alloantibodies in the maternal circulation develop during pregnancy against paternal HLA antigens.[34] More recently, maternal–fetal disparity in HLA class II phenotypes was correlated with pregnancy-induced remission. Over three fourths of pregnant women with maternal–fetal disparity of HLA-DRB1, DQA, and DQB haplotypes had significant improvement, whereas disparity was observed in only one fourth of women whose pregnancy was characterized by continuous active arthritis.[35] This also suggested that suppression of maternal immune responses to paternal HLA haplotypes might be protective.

Consonant with the relief of RA during pregnancy are the data indicating a decreased risk of RA in women who had been pregnant[36]; in this study the relative risk was 0.49 compared with that of women never pregnant and was a factor independent of oral contraceptive use, measurable immunogenetic factors, or family history of RA. These data are at odds with an older study suggesting that pregnancy might increase the risk of RA.[37] In either case, though, the magnitude of the effects is relatively small and of uncertain clinical relevance.

In 1978 it was reported that oral contraceptives protected against the development of RA.[38] A similar negative association was found between the onset of RA and the previous use of noncontraceptive hormones; this negative association persisted with univariant and multivariant control of potentially confounding variables, as well as with the subgroup analysis.[39, 40] A decrease in the incidence of RA noted in Rochester, Minnesota, after 1960 was ascribed to the availability of oral contraceptives and postmenopausal estrogens.[41] However, two subsequent case studies by the Mayo Clinic group in this same population failed to confirm any protection from RA of prior or current oral contraceptive use.[42, 43]

POSSIBLE DIRECT CAUSES OF RHEUMATOID ARTHRITIS

As reviewed earlier, one or multiple genetic factors may predispose an individual to develop rheumatoid arthritis. However, no direct causative factor has consistently been implicated. A "best guess" is that several environmental stimuli, possibly viruses or retroviruses, infect an individual who has the appropriate genetic background and through some mechanism the inflammatory response is focused in joints (Table

Table 54–2. ETIOLOGY OF RA: POSSIBLE INFECTIOUS CAUSES

Infectious Agent	Potential Pathogenic Mechanisms
Mycoplasma	Direct synovial infection; superantigens
Parvovirus B19	Direct synovial infection
Retroviruses	Direct synovial infection
Enteric bacteria	Molecular mimicry (QKRAA)
Mycobacteria	Molecular mimicry (proteoglycans, QKRAA)
Epstein-Barr virus	Molecular mimicry (QKRAA)

54–2). After getting a start there, the synovitis will persist even in the absence of the offending agent because of local autoimmunity and the cyclic automaticity that enables the disease to become self-perpetuating.

Infectious Agents

Bacteria, Mycobacteria, Mycoplasma, and Their Components

There is no good evidence that a pyogenic bacterium or mycobacterium causes rheumatoid arthritis, although animal models of arthritis in which immunization with bacterial cell walls (e.g., SCW arthritis in Lewis rats) or killed mycobacteria (e.g., adjuvant arthritis in Lewis rats) exhibit many clinical and histologic features of RA. Extensive searches for such organisms in synovial tissue or joint effusions have been negative. Similarly, considerable attention has been directed at a potential role for mycoplasma in arthritis. Mycoplasma-derived superantigens, such as from mycoplasma arthritides, can directly induce T cell–independent cytokine production by macrophages[44] and can exacerbate or trigger arthritis in mice immunized with type II collagen.[45] Treatment of RA with tetracycline-like drugs might ameliorate the disease, consistent with a mycoplasma infection.[46] Furthermore, some mycoplasma infections are known to cause arthritis in animals. Despite this and other circumstantial evidence, serious efforts to identify mycoplasma organisms or DNA in joint samples have been essentially negative, and there is no direct evidence to name these organisms as etiologic agents.[47]

The striking similarity of histopathologic changes in RA and in joints of occasional patients with Lyme disease, caused by the spirochete *Borrelia burgdorferi*, leaves open the possibility that an as yet unappreciated or unknown organism is causative. Lyme disease is different from RA in its immunogenetic background. When HLA-DR4–positive patients are excluded from consideration, a secondary association with HLA-DR2 is noted to be an independent, dominant marker for Lyme disease.[48] The hypothesis is that a spirochetal antigen can be presented by DR2 much like a rheumatoid agent could bind to DR4 (and QKRAA). The role of class II molecules and cellular immunity in the pathogenesis of Lyme arthri-

tis, however, is unclear since SCID mice develop a progressive tenosynovitis after *Borrelia* infection despite the virtual absence of T cell function.[49] However, Lyme arthritis provides a clear example of an infectious arthritis caused by an organism that can be very difficult to detect or grow from joint tissue. It is not known if chronic Lyme arthritis requires continued antigen exposure or whether, as might occur in RA, the inciting organism can be eradicated without necessarily curing the synovitis.[50]

Epstein-Barr Virus, Escherichia coli, and Molecular Mimicry

In 1975, an antibody was described in the sera of patients with rheumatoid arthritis that reacted with an antigen extracted from a lymphoblastic cell line carrying Epstein-Barr virus (EBV).[51] These antibodies, named *rheumatoid arthritis precipitin* (RAP), were indeed directed against EBV-specific antigens. Although it was demonstrated that there was an abnormally elevated frequency of EBV-infected B cells in blood of patients with RA,[52] it also was shown that in patients with early RA, titers of antibody to EBV-associated nuclear antigen or to viral capsid antigen were not elevated, suggesting that EBV infection was a sequel to, and not the cause of, RA.[53] Sophisticated techniques to look for the EBV genome in rheumatoid synovial tissue have been unsuccessful.[54, 55]

Despite these data, there are still reasons to implicate EBV in the pathogenesis, if not the etiology, of RA. The EBV receptor on human B lymphocytes is actually the complement receptor type 2 (CR2) and the virus gains access to the cell at this site. The EBV is a polyclonal activator of B lymphocytes, which could result in the production of rheumatoid factor, and, as will be reiterated later in detail, rheumatoid macrophages and T cells combine to generate a defect in suppression of EBV proliferation in human B cells. Rheumatoid patients appear to have higher levels of EBV shedding in throat washings, an increased number of virus-infected B cells in the circulating blood, higher levels of antibodies to the EBV antigens, and abnormal EBV-specific cytotoxic T cell responsiveness compared with controls.[56] Patients with RA have problems with the control and elimination of EBV-transformed lymphocytes[57]; this has helped fuel speculation that a lymphocyte defect is the principal triggering event in this disease and that abnormal control of EBV is pathogenic.

Additional intriguing data implicating EBV in RA are derived from sequence homology between the susceptibility cassette in HLA-DR4 and DR1 and the EBV glycoprotein gp110, which like DRB*0401, contains the QKRAA motif, and patients with serologic evidence of a previous EBV infection have antibodies against this epitope.[58, 59] An inference from these data is that T cell recognition of EBV epitopes in some patients with HLA-DR4, -DR14, or -DR1 may cause an immune response directed at innocent bystander cells through "molecular mimicry," whereas in those with other class II MHC alleles, no cross-reactivity with EBV proteins would exist. This hypothesis could potentially account for disease perpetuation in the absence of active infection in patients with a specific MHC genotype, a scenario that is consistent with many observations in the chronic rheumatoid joint. However, the data are primarily circumstantial, and gp110 is only one of many xenoproteins that contains QKRAA. The *E. coli* dnaJ protein, which is a bacterial heat shock protein, also expresses the cassette and might represent a potential link between gut bacteria and chronic arthritis. T cells in RA, especially synovial fluid T cells but not normal peripheral blood cells, have increased proliferative responses to this protein, perhaps supporting the molecular mimicry link between any of a variety of QKRAA-containing proteins and arthritis.[60]

Parvovirus

Small particles resembling parvoviruses in morphologic and physicochemical properties have been derived from rheumatoid synovial tissue.[61] Polyclonal antibodies developed against this putative virus were able to detect reactive antigen and synovial cells from different rheumatoid arthritis patients but not from individuals with osteoarthritis. Additional evidence supports an etiologic role for parvovirus B19. Some patients with early rheumatoid arthritis have serologic evidence of a recent infection with B19.[62] Anti-human parvovirus immunoglobulin G (IgG) levels later declined but were still present 8 months or more after the onset of symptoms. Patients with acute parvoviral infections developed transient rheumatoid factor in the blood.[63] Despite these cases, it is important to point out that very few rheumatoid patients have evidence of such a coincident infection; in a total of 69 patients with RA, only 4 acquired the parvovirus infection near the time of onset of their RA.[63] Using sensitive PCR methods to detect B19 genes in synovial tissue, however, 75 percent of RA synovium were positive compared to 17 percent of non-RA controls.[64] Many of the B19-positive RA patients did not have serum anti-B19 antibodies. In another study, however, there was no evidence of the B19 genome in synovial fluid or synovial fluid cells.[65] Of interest, the presence of B19 antibody in peripheral blood was not predictive of disease in discordant monozygotic or fraternal twins in which one twin had RA.[66] How is one to interpret these disparate data at this point? Unfortunately, a final conclusion cannot be drawn regarding the role of B19 in RA. This virus clearly causes a distinctive arthritis in children and might be responsible for a subset of patients with an RA-like disease. This probably represents a relatively small proportion of patients.

Other Viruses

Lentiviruses are a subfamily of retroviruses that derive their name from the slow time course of the infections they cause in humans and animals. Pathologic changes in lentivirus infections are, for the most part, indirectly mediated by the immune and inflammatory responses of the host. Finding cells infected by virus is often extremely difficult. An epidemic deforming arthritis in goats and sheep is caused by lentiviruses, which are difficult to detect although known to be the cause of the disease.[67] The pathogenesis of the disease appears to be infection of monocytes that migrate to the synovium; resultant cytokine production leads to the accumulation of lymphocytes and other cells.[68] Hence, a "Trojan horse" mechanism can be invoked; the viral genome can be concealed within monocytes and transported without detection to other sites. Restricted viral gene expression is the underlying mechanism in the persistence and spread of lentiviruses and the slow evolution of the disease that they produce. Although similar retroviral infections have been suggested many times as the etiology of RA,[69] extensive searches for potential agents have not been fruitful.[70] This does not rule out the possibility that difficult-to-detect agents might be present, or even that endogenous retroviruses play a role. Some indirect studies are suggestive of retroviral infection, such as the demonstration of zinc-finger transcription factors in cultured synoviocytes.[71] In addition, the pX domain of one human retrovirus, HTLV-1, causes synovitis in transgenic mice[72] and synoviocytes from patients infected with HTLV-1 express some features of a transformed phenotype, with increased proliferation and cytokine production.[73]

Because rubella virus and the rubella vaccine can cause synovitis in humans, there is interest in this virus as a triggering agent. In one series, 21 instances were reported in which live rubella virus was isolated from synovial fluid obtained from 6 patients with inflammatory oligoarthritis or polyarthritis over a period of 2 years in the absence of firm clinical evidence of rubella.[74] However, none of these patients had the classic polyarticular involvement seen so often in RA; most had an oligoarthritis involving large joints. As with B19 infection, it is possible that a subset of patients with chronic polyarthritis have disease that is due to direct infection with wild-type or attenuated rubella virus.

In summary, the hypothesis that one or more viral infections may serve as a triggering agent in the genetically susceptible host is both appealing and intellectually satisfying. Qualities of candidate viruses should be similar to those of the lentivirus, which has a restricted expression within cells and can remain hidden from defense mechanisms in the host. It is possible that just a small alteration in T cell reactivity or responsiveness induced by a viral infection, or generation of a neoantigen by insertion of a viral genome into the host itself, could be sufficient to trigger the disease. Alternatively, certain specific HLA-DR haplotypes associated with RA might not permit efficient presentation of pathogenic viral/retroviral antigens and a subsequent infection of synovial cells might lead to autonomous activation (as observed with HTLV-1–infected synoviocytes in humans or lentivirus-infected macrophages in goats) and an inability to mount an appropriate immune response that would clear infected cells. It is also possible that subsequent infection by a ubiquitous second virus (such as EBV) capable of generating polyclonal B cell stimulation would be sufficient to amplify the immune response and, in the immunogenetically appropriate host, enable it to become self-perpetuating through cross-reactivity of epitopes.

Heat Shock Proteins—Ubiquitous and Cross-Reactive

There appears to be a link between heat shock proteins (HSP) and RA. The HSP are a family of mainly medium-sized (60–90 kD) proteins produced by cells of all species in response to stress. These proteins have conserved amino acid sequences; for example, certain HSP of *Myobacterium tuberculosis* have a 65 percent sequence homology with HSP of humans.[75, 76] The HSP may facilitate intracellular folding and translocation of proteins as they protect from insults induced by heat, bacteria, host cell attack (in the case of bacteria), oxygen radicals, and nutrient depletion. T lymphocytes from animals with adjuvant arthritis recognize an epitope of mycobacteria HSP 65 (amino acids 180 to 188). Some of these cells also recognize cartilage proteoglycan epitopes,[77] perhaps explaining the targeting to the joint. Experimental arthritis can be transferred to naïve animals by such reactive T cells, and protection is conferred on rats by preimmunization with mycobacterial HSP.

Some patients with RA have elevated levels of antibodies to mycobacterial HSP, especially in synovial fluid.[78, 79] The majority of T cell clones isolated from RA synovial fluid with specificity to mycobacterial components have the γδ T cell receptor (instead of the more common αβ form) and express neither CD4 nor CD8 surface antigens. Freshly isolated synovial fluid T cells from patients with RA demonstrate a brisk proliferative response to both the acetone-precipitable fraction of MTB and recombinant 65-kD HSP.[80, 81] However, proliferation in response to other recall antigens, like tetanus toxoid, is not increased. Synovial fluid mononuclear cells activated by 60-kD mycobacterial HSP inhibit proteoglycan production by human cartilage explants.[82] This effect is dependent on the generation of cytokines like IL-1 and TNF-α by the activated cells. Human 60-kD HSP is expressed in the synovium, although the amount expressed per cell appears to be similar in OA, RA, and normal tissue.[83]

How could HSP be related to the cause of RA? As noted earlier, the possibility exists of cross-reactive epitopes; HSP from bacteria display "molecular mimicry" (i.e., similar amino acid sequences) with numerous human proteins and proteoglycans. More interesting, yet more complex, is the hypothesis that antibodies and T cells exist that recognize epitopes shared by HSP of both infectious agents and host

cells; in inflammation of the joints, synovial cells could express HSP, and these could then be recognized by cross-reactive T cells and antibodies. Given the preservation of various HSP sequences between eukaryotes and prokaryotes, this is certainly within the realm of possibility. Moreover, the fact that at least one HSP, the *E. coli* dnaJ protein, contains the QKRAA motif raises additional questions about the relationship between HSP and immunity directed against the HLA-DR molecule vis-à-vis an autologous mixed lymphocyte reaction. Within this paradigm, the identity of a specific etiologic agent could vary among patients; the critical step required to initiate RA would reside in the combination of an appropriate class II MHC haplotype and a pathogen that expresses cross-reactive HSPs. Alternatively, the HSP might function as a superantigen, reactive with T cells in virtually all species and tissues. In that context it is of interest that staphylococcal enterotoxin B superantigen, which directly stimulates T cells and macrophages in an antigen-independent manner, can cause arthritis in susceptible mice.[84]

Arthritis Induced by Collagen—Is There Relevance for Rheumatoid Arthritis?

The discoveries that immunization with type II collagen can cause arthritis in rats and mice and that the disease can be passively transferred by IgG fractions containing anticollagen antibodies[85] or by transfer of lymphocytes from affected animals[86] have spawned extensive experiments that illustrate the antigenicity of collagen, the arthrotropic nature of the disease produced, and the dependence of experimental animals on immune-response genes for reactivity. In these rodents, it is clear that (1) functional T cells are necessary to initiate a collagen-induced arthritis, (2) a major immunogenic and arthritogenic epitope on type II collagen resides in a restricted area of the type II collagen chains,[87] and (3) susceptibility to collagen-induced arthritis is directly linked to the class II MHC locus.[88] One provocative study demonstrated that spleen cells from mice immunized with immune complexes containing both native type II collagen and a monoclonal anticollagen type II antibody produce lymphocyte clones that secrete monoclonal IgG rheumatoid factors, at least one of which also appeared to be an anti-idiotype of anticollagen II antibodies.[89]

Most data on humans are consistent with the hypothesis that rheumatoid arthritis is not caused by development of antibodies to type II collagen but that the inflammatory response is amplified by production of these antibodies. Systemic immunity to type II collagen (the major species in hyaline cartilage) as a primary pathogenic event is more likely in a disease like relapsing polychondritis with more generalized pathology in cartilage than in RA. Nevertheless, these antibodies can produce ancillary destruction in a joint that is already inflamed. Monoclonal antibodies to native type II collagen react with cells within the invasive synovium at the pannus–cartilage junction in material taken from rheumatoid joints.[90] These antibodies are directed only against type II collagen and are not found in cartilage of patients with osteoarthritis.[91] Sera from patients with RA contain antibody titers to denatured bovine type II collagen that are significantly higher than those found in control sera[92]; however, there is no difference in antibody titers to native collagen, suggesting that the denatured form generated after breakdown of connective tissue might serve as the immunogen. It has been suggested that antibodies against collagen have pathogenic capability in RA, especially among the IgG3 subclass of anti-type II collagen antibodies.[93] It was also demonstrated that the anti-collagen antibodies purified from the sera of patients with RA had the capability to activate complement, generating—among other products—C5a when these antibodies became bound to cartilage. This has relevance to the observations that anti-collagen antibodies can be eluted from rheumatoid articular cartilage.[94] In addition, isolated synovial tissue B lymphocytes actively secrete anti-type II collagen antibodies in almost all patients with seropositive RA, whereas articular B cells from non-RA patients do not.[95] The anti-collagen antibody in these RA patients cannot always be detected in the serum, indicating that local, rather than systemic, immunity is probably more important. Some of the biologic details relating to collagen as an immunogen are included in Chapter 10.

Rheumatoid Factor: Cause or Effect in Rheumatoid Arthritis?

The identification and characterization of rheumatoid factor (RF) as an autoantibody was the first direct evidence that autoimmunity might play a role in RA. For many years, immune complexes made up of RF and other immunoglobulins were thought to contribute mightily to RA as a primary pathogen. One piece of indirect evidence suggesting that this is not necessarily the case, documented in 1957, was that rheumatoid arthritis and agammaglobulinemia caused by inactive B lymphocytes occurred simultaneously in a number of patients.[96] Thus, B cells are not essential in development of RA. More recent paradigms of RA posit that cellular immune processes predominate while RFs amplify rheumatoid synovitis through activation of complement and formation of immune complexes that are ingested by neutrophils in synovial fluid. This acute inflammatory response can ultimately recruit additional cells to the joint. Even so, one can learn a great deal about RA by examining its most characteristic and reproducible laboratory abnormality: the presence of RF in blood and synovial fluid.

The chemistry and biology of rheumatoid factors are discussed in detail in Chapter 16, and their clinical relevance is detailed in Chapter 55. As reviewed in these chapters, it has been shown by use of archived serum samples that, although some patients have rheumatoid factor present in their sera prior to the onset of any symptoms of arthritis, this does not usually occur. However, the report in 1973 of cross-reactive idiotypes among monoclonal IgM proteins with anti-IgG activity[97]—and the possible implications of expression of this germline by many individuals—has continued to stimulate interest in the possibility that antibodies against IgG might contribute to the triggering event. Some patients who are seronegative but otherwise have a clinical diagnosis consistent with RA have "hidden" rheumatoid factors in their 19S or 7S serum fractions and these can be identified by antibody specific for the major rheumatoid factor cross-reactive idiotype.[98]

The rheumatoid factors produced by RA B cells differ from those produced by B cells from normal individuals.[99] The germline-derived rheumatoid factors are produced by immature CD5 positive B cells, and many paraproteins produced by malignant B cells (like Waldenström's macroglobulinemia) are derived from the germline. Rheumatoid factors produced by RA B cells are distinct in that these proteins are often not encoded by germline sequences. Instead, their sequence appears to be derived through rearrangements and somatic mutations that occur during life. Rheumatoid factor analysis in synovial membrane cultures from patients with a variety of diseases has indicated that only cells from patients with seropositive RA synthesize RF spontaneously.[100] IgM RF represents about 7 percent of total IgM produced by cells, and IgG RF represents 3 percent of IgG synthesized in those cultures. Significantly, no IgG or IgM RFs are detectable in seronegative patients, accentuating the growing appreciation that seronegative RA might be a different disease from its seropositive counterpart.

Expression of any particular idiotype on rheumatoid factors (or other immunoglobulins, for that matter) is under genetic control. This limited response is related to restriction of the number of relevant or expressible V genes available in the germline.[101, 102] The kappa light chain repertoire expressed in RF-producing cells isolated from a patient with chronic RA revealed enrichment for two specific V kappa genes, known as Humvk325 and Humvk328, which are also frequently associated with RF factor paraproteins.[103] However, the kappa variable domains contained many somatic mutations and non-germline-encoded nucleotides. Based on the extent of substitutions, it was concluded that selection and production of these specific RFs was due to antigenic drive rather than a derivation directly from the germline as is the case with many paraproteins. Additional RFs have been identified with characteristics similar to an antigen-driven response, although some examples of germline RFs have also been isolated from RA synovium.

THE INFLAMMATORY AND IMMUNE RESPONSE IN RHEUMATOID ARTHRITIS

For several decades, it has generally been assumed that T lymphocytes, particularly the CD4+ helper/

inducer cells, are a crucial component of the early rheumatoid response. Although these conclusions are based largely on circumstantial evidence, the data are, in some cases, persuasive. This section is designed to explore some of the cell-mediated immune responses in RA that might establish and perpetuate rheumatoid synovitis.

Antigen Presentation to T Lymphocytes

In the subsynovial areas around the small capillaries and high endothelial venules in synovium, tissue macrophages and dendritic-like cells are available to process and present antigen to T lymphocytes (Fig. 54–2). Many different types of cells in chronically inflamed tissues, including rheumatoid synovium, bear HLA-DR antigens on their surfaces, although this does not always correlate with antigen-presenting function. Normal synovial lining cells can mediate T lymphocyte proliferation, but their activating ability appears to be lower than that of epidermal Langerhans cells, which stand as barriers to entrance of antigen through the skin. Rheumatoid synovial dendritic cells, however, are extremely efficient in allogeneic T cell activation.[104] The microheterogeneity of the rheumatoid synovial tissue, with different numbers and proportions of cell lineages in each area, suggests not only variations in function within the synovium (i.e., some areas would be involved in active T cell activation, other areas might not) but also that the proper ratio of antigen-presenting cells, T lymphocytes, and other accessory cells and factors necessary for amplification of the immune response would be present in some areas but not in others.

At many sites in the synovium, the histopathologic findings resemble those of a classic delayed-type hypersensitivity reaction.[105] Large, strongly HLA-DR–positive macrophages or dendritic-like cells form close contact with lymphocytes bearing CD4 markers. B cells also express class II MHC antigens and can present antigen and produce activating cytokines. Using standard light microscopy and immunohistochemistry, the majority of synovial T cells are of the small memory type that express activation antigens like HLA-DR, transferrin receptors, and LFA-1 on their surface. This should not necessarily be construed as a priori evidence that they were activated within the articular cavity, because this is precisely the phenotype of cells that is preferentially recruited from peripheral blood by the activated endothelium of RA synovium. In some areas, especially in the "transitional zones" between lymphocyte-enriched regions, ultrastructural studies show direct contact between antigen-presenting cells and blast-like cells, with long processes enveloping the latter.[106] Although the antigen remains undefined, this presumably results in helper cell activation.[107] When antigen, DR molecules, and IL-1 are available, the CD4-positive T cell generates a cascade of activation steps that includes secretion of products such as interferonγ (IFN-γ) and interleukin-2 (IL-2) that can feed back on the mononuclear phagocyte system (although, as described later, functional sequelae of such activation is actually quite difficult to detect in RA and might be very limited).[108]

T Lymphocyte Activation in Rheumatoid Arthritis

A specific etiologic agent has not been identified in RA, but it is often assumed that the initiation phase

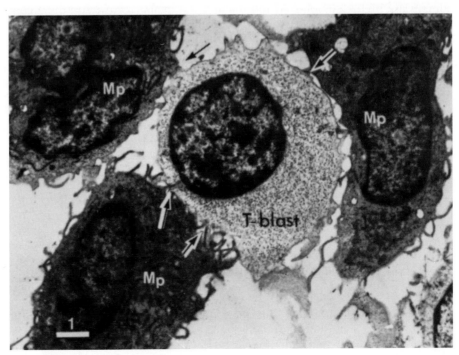

Figure 54–2. T lymphoblast in rheumatoid synovial tissue surrounded by three macrophages (Mp). The *arrows* point to probable intercellular bridging. This may be the morphologic manifestation of presentation of antigen to the helper T cell by the antigen-presenting cells. (Courtesy of H. Ishikawa and M. Ziff, University of Texas Southwestern Medical Center, Dallas, Tex.)

of the disease is marked by localization of an arthrotropic agent in the joint followed by antigen presentation and specific T cell activation. Stimulated T cells would subsequently generate a panoply of cytokines, including IFN-γ, that activate macrophages, other T cells, B cells (which produce rheumatoid factor), and endothelial cells. Activation of the vascular endothelium by cytokines induces adhesion molecules and recruits new cells that express the appropriate counterreceptors into the joint. The accumulation of T cells would ultimately result from nonspecific infiltration of the synovium with cells from the blood as well as local proliferation of lymphocytes in the synovium that recognize their specific antigen in the context of MHC molecules.

The primacy of T cells in the pathogenesis of RA is based on a number of histologic, experimental, and therapeutic observations. First and most persuasive, as discussed in some detail earlier, are the MHC associations with RA. The conclusion that this association is due to the presentation of a specific pathogenic antigen, though logical, is still speculative; one could also surmise that the specific HLA associations result in defective responses against an arthritogenic agent. The histopathology of RA, with exuberant infiltration of the synovium with T lymphocytes, is often pointed to as evidence of a T cell–mediated disease because this is characteristic of antigen-specific responses. However, the synovium can only respond to inflammation in a limited number of ways; in fact, the histology of chronic arthritides that are clearly not mediated by T cells (e.g., chronic tophaceous gout) exhibits many of the same features as RA. Many animal models of arthritis, like collagen-induced arthritis, adjuvant arthritis, and SCW arthritis are clearly T cell–dependent. The relevance of these models to RA is not always clear, given that the clinical courses are highly compressed in time and the inciting agents are thought not to be specifically related to RA. Some animal models have also been developed that are relatively independent of T cells, such as Lyme arthritis in SCID mice that lack T cell function, or transgenic mice that overexpress TNF-α or oncogenes like c-fos.[109] Much has been made of the observation that RA appears to improve after HIV infection or development of AIDS. To date, however, the data remain anecdotal. There are no controlled studies to determine the true rate of remission, and recent case reports actually contradict this notion. In addition, it is naïve to think that T cells are the only immune cells infected with HIV; monocytes and macrophages express small amounts of CD4 on their surface, and their function is also profoundly depressed in AIDS.[110]

More direct evidence for T cell involvement is often cited from experimental therapeutics. A fistula of the thoracic duct that removes T lymphocytes from the body was shown in 1970 to have some efficacy in RA,[111] and leukapheresis has been associated with brief improvement associated with the return toward normal in vitro anergy of peripheral blood mononuclear cells.[112] Total nodal irradiation is a very effective means of suppressing systemic helper T cell function. In clinical studies, this procedure did offer some benefit, although symptoms could return despite persistent suppression of delayed-type hypersensitivity.[113, 114] Treatment with antibodies that deplete T cells, including anti-CD4, anti-CD5, and anti-CD52, have been reported at various times.[115–117] The responses, if any, were usually very modest and transient despite profound and sometimes prolonged lymphopenia and immunosuppression. Interpretation of such studies needs to take into account the fact that some anti-T cell therapies (e.g., anti-T cell receptor antibody) can prevent arthritis in T cell–dependent animal models; however, if treatment is delayed until after the onset of clinical signs the results are less impressive and the therapy can sometimes worsen the disease. The stage of disease might therefore be an important determinant of the clinical response after T cell depletion. However, a recent report showed that even treatment of early RA with anti-CD4 antibody was ineffective.[118] In addition, the degree of peripheral lymphopenia does not necessarily correlate with depletion of the synovial T cell population.[119] Potent immunosuppressive drugs like cyclosporine have also shown efficacy in RA. Yet, this agent, which can suppress allograft rejection, results in clinically significant responses in only a minority of patients.[120] IL-2–diphtheria toxin fusion protein designed to kill IL-2 receptor–bearing T cells has not been effective in a controlled trial.[121] A variety of more specific treatments, like anti–T cell receptor antibodies or vaccines, will hopefully provide more definitive evidence (either pro or con) regarding the potential efficacy of suppressing T cell function in RA.

The questions to be answered about T lymphocytes in RA include: What is the level of activation of these cells? Is there oligoclonal proliferation of lymphocytes? Are there common epitopes recognized by different patients? The presentation of counter-arguments regarding the major evidence of T cell involvement should remind people that the pathogenesis of RA might vary depending on the stage of disease. It is important to recognize that alternative explanations exist for each of these observations and that continued experimentation is needed before definitive conclusions can be reached.

Peripheral Blood T Lymphocytes in Rheumatoid Arthritis

The numbers of CD4+ helper T cells are mildly increased in the peripheral blood of patients with RA, with a concomitant decrease in cytotoxic (CD8) lymphocytes (and an increased CD4:CD8 ratio).[122, 123] The surface phenotype of circulating T cells in RA suggests activation in some studies, but not in others. For instance, an increased percentage of cells express HLA-DR and the adhesion protein VLA-4 (α4/β1 integrin).[124, 125] The latter is especially critical in that VLA-4 plays an important role in the recruitment of cells to the synovium through interactions with counterreceptors VCAM-1 and CS1 fibronectin on endothelial cells. Increased HLA-DR is present on γδ T cell receptor–bearing lymphocytes as well as αβ cells.[126] Surface CD4 is lower on RA peripheral T cells compared to normal controls, a phenomenon observed after lymphocyte activation. The decreased surface CD4 is not matched by an increase in circulating soluble CD4 protein.[127] Other markers of activation are not necessarily elevated on RA T cells, including IL-2 receptors, the costimulatory molecule B7, and VLA-1[128, 129] (Table 54–3). Elevated levels of soluble IL-2 receptors, which are shed by activated T cells, are found both in sera and synovial fluid of rheumatoid patients, and the levels appear to correlate with disease activity.[130] In summary, these studies suggest that peripheral blood T cells express phenotypic characteristics of partial activation. It is not clear whether this process occurs in the periphery or whether cells are activated in the synovium and reenter the circulation via the synovial lymphatics.

Another approach to assessing T cell activation and proliferation in peripheral blood is to perform detailed analysis of T cell receptor (TcR) expression. The vast majority of peripheral blood T cells express an α/β heterodimer. In theory, the TcR repertoire in immune-mediated diseases should lead to expansion of cells with similar α and β chains. Typically, studies are performed to assess TcR gene expression at the protein level using monoclonal antibodies (which is probably the least likely to suffer from artifacts) or at the level of DNA or mRNA using Southern blots or reverse transcriptase-polymerase chain reaction (RT-PCR), respectively. It is also important to recognize that the HLA-DR haplotype of an individual is important in shaping the T cell repertoire. When trying to evaluate data on the TcR bias, it is critical that the controls be appropriately matched for class II MHC genes, taking into account the potential role of the susceptibility cassette as a determinant of TcR gene usage.

Table 54–3. LYMPHOCYTE PHENOTYPES IN RA[124]

	Peripheral Blood*		RA Synovium*
	RA	*Control*	
Activation antigens			
HLA-DR	760	326	1804
IL-2 receptor	212	91	100
Adhesion antigens			
LFA-1	2332	1680	3220
VLA-1	383	62	1217
T cell differentiation antigens			
CD3	4077	7367	3642
CD4	1941	2459	1578
CD8	3321	4121	2290

*Data are presented as total lymphocyte expression for each antigen as determined by flow cytometry (i.e., percentage of cells positive × mean fluorescence channel).
Data from Cush JJ, Lipsky PE: Phenotypic analysis of synovial tissue and peripheral blood lymphocytes isolated from patients with rheumatoid arthritis. Arthritis Rheum 31:1230, 1988.

A number of studies have examined the T cell repertoire in peripheral blood in RA, although most appropriately focused on differences between blood and joint samples (see later in this chapter). Some studies suggest a preponderance of one or another gene, but no specific T cell receptor genes are consistently overexpressed in RA peripheral blood compared to normal individuals.

In 1981 the first suggestions of an interesting immunoregulatory dysfunction in RA were noted.[131, 132] It was observed that the outgrowth of EBV-infected B lymphocytes was inadequately suppressed by lymphoid cells from rheumatoid patients. This was related to a defect in suppressor T cell function. The deficient T cell response could be correlated somewhat with disease activity, but it was noted also that the abnormality was present in T cells of patients with inflammatory arthropathies other than RA.[133] A more specific defect was also apparent in the autologous mixed lymphocyte reaction (AMLR), in which T cells proliferate and produce cytokines in response to class II MHC antigens expressed on autologous antigen–presenting cells.[134] IFN-γ production is significantly suppressed in RA cultures, and the abnormality is corrected by the addition of indomethacin. Additional studies suggest that IFN-γ production is low because of a heightened sensitivity of RA cells to prostaglandin E. Peripheral blood T lymphocytes from rheumatoid patients also demonstrate defective IL-2 production.[135] Indomethacin can partially reverse this abnormality in the presence of mononuclear cells, again implicating prostaglandin sensitivity. Unlike lymphocytes from control patients, recombinant IL-2 has minimal effect on IFN-γ production by peripheral blood lymphocytes from patients with active RA.[136]

Synovial Fluid Lymphocytes in Rheumatoid Arthritis

The cell mix in synovial fluid differs from peripheral blood as well as synovial tissue. Therefore, analysis of synovial fluid cells is not necessarily an accurate reflection of the synovium. Even though synovial effusions contain an abundance of T cells, the CD4:CD8 ratio is actually reversed compared to blood or synovial tissue, with an excess of CD8+ suppressor cells relative to CD4+ lymphocytes. In addition, synovial tissue is nearly devoid of neutrophils, which often constitute 50 to 75 percent of synovial fluid cells. Hence, synovial fluid does not contain a random distribution of cells shed from synovial tissue, and data regarding T cell receptor usage or the state of activation should be interpreted with this in mind (see later in this chapter). The signals that induce a cell to leave the synovium and enter the intra-articular cavity are not established but presumably involve chemotactic gradients that enable certain cell types to overcome interactions with adhesion receptors on synovial cells and with extracellular matrix proteins and then migrate through the intimal lining.

Synovial fluid, like peripheral blood, contains activated T cells based on the presence of surface HLA-DR antigens.[137] Other activation antigens that are not increased on peripheral blood cells, however, are increased on synovial fluid lymphocytes, including VLA-1.[128] Surprisingly, IL-2 receptor expression is not increased. Of CD4$^+$ cells in rheumatoid synovial fluid, most are memory cells and express CD45RO on their surface.[138, 139] Despite the phenotypic appearance of activation, synovial fluid T cell function is rather deficient when compared to peripheral blood cells. For instance, synovial fluid lymphocyte proliferation in response to mitogens or most recall antigens, like tetanus toxoid, is significantly lower than paired blood T lymphocytes.[81] Mycobacterial antigens and the 60-kD heat shock protein appear to be exceptions, where proliferation is greater in cells isolated from rheumatoid effusions. Cytokine production by synovial fluid T cells in vitro is also low. IFN-γ release after stimulation by mitogens like phytohemagglutinin is defective.[135] The amount of IL-2 produced by synovial fluid lymphocytes is significantly less than that produced by the corresponding blood cells.[140]

A possible mechanism that might contribute to defective T cell responses among synovial fluid mononuclear cells from rheumatoid patients is the presence of local inhibitors of cell activation. For example, an IL-1 receptor antagonist (IL-1ra) produced by macrophages has been purified, and its gene cloned and expressed.[141, 142] Recent data specifically point to IL-1ra and TGF-β as possible T cell suppressants in the joint because both have been identified as components of synovial effusions that can inhibit thymocyte proliferation.[143, 144] Because IL-1 plays a critical role in enhancing and facilitating activation of T lymphocytes, an inhibitor of IL-1 could impair T lymphocyte function in the joint. This might further decrease the expected amplification of suppressor cell proliferation, leading to unrestricted polyclonal B cell proliferation and diminished NK cell and LAK cell activity. Nonspecific components of joint effusions like hyaluronic acid can be toxic to cells and can indirectly suppress T cell activation.

The data on TcR rearrangements in RA are very controversial. TcR gene usage has been examined in synovial fluid, synovial tissue, and, as previously noted, in peripheral blood. Studies of articular cells are probably the most relevant because the joint is the site of the disease and antigen-driven paradigms of RA imply that in situ T cell activation and expansion are pivotal steps. Several dozen studies have been published in the last few years purporting to find one or another gene overexpressed in the joint (either synovial fluid or tissue) compared to the blood. In some cases, a pattern appears to be emerging that suggests an increased number of T cells expressing Vβ3, 14, and 17, especially in synovial tissue.[145–148] These particular Vβ genes are structurally related and are particularly susceptible to activation by superantigens. This supports the hypothesis that specific T cells can be activated by bacterial or mycoplasmal

superantigens, leading to oligoclonal expansion and release of cytokines.

The final answer to the question of T cell oligoclonality is still open, and other studies have either not found evidence for the restricted clonality of T cells in RA synovial fluid, synovial tissue, and blood or identified expansion of different Vβ or α chains.[149–155] The reasons that various groups arrive at such contradictory conclusions might involve differences in study populations, probe selection, techniques for assessing TcR abundance, and methods of handling cells prior to examination. For instance, there were marked differences in how the cells were processed, including whether the cells were expanded with cytokines, anti-CD3 monoclonal antibodies, or mitogens. In some cases, only subpopulations of cells (e.g., IL-2 receptor positive) were studied. Unfortunately, very few studies include non-RA controls, and, when they have, their T cell repertoire does not look very different from RA patients. Many studies rely heavily on quantitative analysis of RT-PCR amplification of TcR genes. This procedure, though elegant, is fraught with considerable risk of artifacts owing to nonspecific hybridization, nonlinear amplification, and variable primer efficiency. It is also important to appreciate the challenge of interpreting an expanded population even if it is found. Although it would be nice to believe that "oligoclonal expansion" results from exposure to a primary pathogenic antigen, secondary antigens like proteoglycans or type II collagen that do not initiate RA but could elicit a T cell response might be responsible. Therapeutic interventions designed to target a specific Vβ gene (if one were convincingly shown) might not eliminate pathogenic clones but instead delete less important T cells involved in secondary responses. Furthermore, if RA is caused by an infectious pathogen that is partially controlled by expanded T cells in the joint, one runs the risk of exacerbating disease.

The best opportunity for detecting the appropriate pathogenic T cell clones in RA would be to study very early RA because disease chronicity causes T cells to accumulate in an antigen-independent manner. This is best exemplified in the experimental allergic encephalitis model in rats, which is caused by autoimmunity against myelin basic protein. In the earliest phases, there is a strong bias in the central nervous system for a few antigen-specific pathogenic TcR genes.[156] As the disease progresses, this bias is rapidly overwhelmed by the continued influx of nonspecific cells recruited into the brain by chemokines and adhesion molecules, not by antigen. The same situation likely occurs in RA and other chronic inflammatory arthritides, and the study of TcRs in chronic disease might not give accurate information on the inciting populations.

There is another population of lymphocytes in rheumatoid synovial fluid that may contribute to the synovitis.[157] These are the "double negative" $\gamma\delta$ cells without CD4 or CD8 surface proteins and T cell receptors distinct from the $\alpha\beta$-bearing cells. These $\gamma\delta$ cells are not MHC restricted and therefore may respond by proliferation to many stimulators, including "superantigens" and heat shock proteins. There is a suggestion of a bias toward use of the δ1 or δ2 gene among this population in RA synovial fluid.[158]

Lymphocyte Infiltration within the Synovial Membrane

The synovium in early rheumatoid arthritis is marked by endothelial cell injury, tissue edema, and a very modest infiltration of the sublining region with mononuclear cells and, on occasion, with neutrophils.[159] As the disease progresses, the continued influx of cells, especially T lymphocytes, perhaps in association with local proliferation, leads to an organizational structure that often resembles a lymph node.[160] The distribution of lymphocytes in the tissue varies from discrete lymphoid aggregates to diffuse sheets of mononuclear cells, with the most prominent location for T cells being the perivascular region. These collections consist of small, CD4-positive memory T cells (CD45RO positive) with scant cytoplasm. Peripheral to these foci is a transitional zone with a heterogeneous mixture of cells, including lymphocytes, occasional undifferentiated blast cells, plasma cells, and macrophages (see Fig. 54–2). It is likely that much intercellular communication by mediators takes place here, and it has been shown that activated T cells bind to synovial cells in vitro, a process mediated by their lymphocyte function–associated antigen.[161] Immunoelectron microscopic study of the distribution of T cell subsets has shown that the majority of lymphocytes present in the lymphocyte-rich areas near blood vessels have CD4 surface proteins, indicating that they are helper/inducer cells. The transitional areas of cellular heterogeneity show a mixture of both CD4+ and CD8+ cells amidst the macrophages.

Normally, one would expect antigen presentation and T cell activation to be accompanied by the production of T cell cytokines like IL-2, IFN-γ, and IL-4. This is a natural sequela of T cell activation in both in vitro and in vivo models. Surprisingly, as will be discussed in detail later, such T lymphocyte products are difficult to detect in RA. There are a number of potential explanations for this observation, including: (1) T cells are anergized; (2) suppressive factors, like TGF-β, IL-1ra, or IL-10, suppress T cell cytokine production; (3) the cytokines are produced in the microenvironment and are present in functionally active concentrations that are too low to detect; (4) cell-to-cell contact delivers membrane-bound cytokines directly to target cells; (5) T cell activation is intermittent and transient; or (6) chronic RA is relatively independent of T cells and their products are not as important in the chronic phase of the disease. Evidence exists for each of these possibilities, although it is not currently possible to state with certainty which (or how many) are true.

Overall, within the synovium, T cells predominate over B cells.[162] T cells make up about 50 percent or more of cells in most RA synovia, whereas only 5 percent or less of cells are B lymphocytes. The B cells are located primarily within reactive lymphoid centers, whereas plasma cells and macrophages are often found outside these centers. This arrangement is consistent with T cell–dependent B lymphocyte activation; plasma cells, the main immunoglobulin producers, migrate away from the germinal centers after differentiation.[163] CD4+ cells in RA synovium are intimately related to B lymphocytes and to HLA-DR–positive cells,[164, 165] which resemble morphologically the interdigitating cells of lymph nodes.

In contrast to peripheral blood in RA, synovial lymphocytes bear a more activated phenotype, with fewer CD8+ cells and high expression of DR antigens (see Table 54–3).[166] Synovial lymphocytes also bear adhesion molecules of the VLA and LFA superfamily of integrins, which may enable the inflammatory response to localize and persist within the synovium.[124, 167, 168] However, T cell activation and induction of adhesion molecules probably does not occur within the joint; rather, the reason that T cells enter the synovium in the first place and then remain within the joint is their armamentarium of adhesion molecules. The cytokine milieu of the joint induces adhesion molecules like ICAM-1, VCAM-1, and CS1 fibronectin on vascular endothelium, and these, in conjunction with chemokines and other chemoattractants, call the cells to the joint based precisely on this phenotype. Hence, this antigen-independent process is responsible for the mononuclear cell infiltrate, not antigen-specific local expansion. T cells that might respond to a specific "RA pathogen" likely amount to a small percentage of cells, perhaps less than 1 percent. Local proliferation and activation probably accounts for only a very small percentage of T cells in the synovium. The few T cells that proliferate are primarily CD8+, not CD4+.[169]

CYTOKINES: THE ROLE OF MACROPHAGE AND FIBROBLAST PRODUCTS IN DISEASE PERPETUATION

Cytokines are hormone-like proteins that enable immune cells to communicate. In addition to playing a critical role in normal immune responses, an explosion of information in the last decade has indicated that they play an integral role in the initiation and perpetuation of synovitis. The cytokine milieu in RA is not random, although early studies suggested an unrestricted abundance of cytokines. However, increasing evidence shows that factors produced by T lymphocytes are actually diminished in RA, whereas those generated by macrophages and by synovial fibroblasts are increased (Table 54–4).[170] In this section, the function of cytokines and other soluble mediators will be reviewed, with an emphasis on the prevalence of macrophage and fibroblast products as dominant driving forces during the perpetuation phase of RA. Basic and general aspects of cytokines are covered in

Table 54–4. LEVEL OF PRODUCTION OF SYNOVIAL CYTOKINES IN RHEUMATOID ARTHRITIS ACCORDING TO CELLULAR SOURCE

Cellular Source	Level of Production in RA Synovium
T cells	
Interleukin-2	−
Interleukin-3	−
Interleukin-4	−
Interleukin-6	±
Interferon-γ	−
TNF-α	−
TNF-β	−
GM-CSF	−
Macrophages*/Fibroblasts†	
Interleukin-1	+
IL-1ra	+
Interleukin-6	+
Interleukin-10	+
TNF-α	+
M-CSF (CSF-1)	+
GM-CSF	+
TGF-β	+
Interferon-α	±
Chemokines (IL-8, MCP-1, etc.)	+
Fibroblast growth factor	+

Adapted from Firestein GS, Zvaifler NJ: How important are T cells in chronic rheumatoid synovitis? Arthritis Rheum 33:768, 1990; with permission.
*Tissue macrophages or type A synoviocytes.
†Tissue fibroblasts or type B synoviocytes.
−, absent or very low concentrations.
+, present.
Abbreviations: M-CSF, macrophage colony-stimulating factor; GM, granulocyte-macrophage; TNF, tumor necrosis factor; TGF, transforming growth factor.

Chapter 18. Macrophages, in particular, are the most vigorous producers of intercellular mediators. These cells, which are present in small numbers in normal synovium, increase in number by migration from extrasynovial sites (e.g., the bone marrow) after inflammation begins. Their responses include secretion of more than 100 substances (see Chapter 8) and cover a biological array of activity from induction of cell growth to cell death.[171]

Cell-cell communication is generally based on either direct contact or release of soluble mediators that diffuse to a target cell. An example of cell–cell contact is the display on cell surfaces, of lymphotoxin (LT) which is made up of LT-α and LT-β chains that are anchored to the cell through a transmembrane domain.[172] Surface LT can bind directly to LT (or TNF) receptors on target cells in the vicinity without any measurable cytokine released into the environment. The role that this direct method of communication plays in RA is not known and is difficult to quantify. Other methods include immunologic localization and mRNA analyses; they are discussed in Chapter 18.

T Cell Cytokines

Gamma Interferon (IFN-γ)

IFN-γ is the most potent inducer of MHC class II antigen mononuclear cells. It concurrently activates synthetic and secretory activity in the monocytes/macrophages. After incubation with IFN-γ, monocytes show morphologic, metabolic, and phenotypic changes consistent with activation to vigorous macrophages; they also begin to express class II MHC antigens and Fc receptors while down-regulating expression of CD14, the LPS receptor.[173] Endothelial cells, as well as a host of other cells, also express class II MHC antigens after stimulation with IFN-γ. It is important to remember, however, that although multiple cell types in RA can be demonstrated to express class II antigens on their surface membranes, this is not synonymous with their ability to act as antigen-presenting cells. Also, the increased DR expression on the cell surface does not in and of itself mean enhanced antigen-presenting capacity in macrophages. IFN-γ induces adhesion molecules like VCAM-1 and ICAM-1 on the surface of endothelial cells and can help recruit inflammatory cell accumulation at sites of injury.[174, 175]

Early studies of rheumatoid cytokine levels in synovial fluid focused on IFN-γ. This was due, in large part, to the expression of massive amounts of HLA-DR on synovial cells. Because IFN-γ was the only known DR-inducing agent at the time, it was only natural to assume that IFN was the responsible cytokine. Viral cytopathic inhibition assays, which take advantage of the fact that the interferons (α, β, and γ) protect cells from viral infections, demonstrated IFN-like activity in synovial fluid.[176] Surprisingly, when studies were later repeated using sensitive and specific immunoassays, only very low concentrations of IFN-γ were detected.[177] Synovial fluid levels of the lymphokine were far below the amounts needed to induce HLA-DR expression on monocytes. Furthermore, neutralizing antibodies to IFN-γ did not block the ability of synovial fluid to induce HLA-DR expression on cultured monocytes. The relative lack of IFN-γ in rheumatoid joints has since been confirmed, including studies employing RT-PCR to detect specific RNA transcripts.[178] The deficiency in IFN-γ production is even more striking if one considers that peripheral blood monocytes from patients with RA also have defective HLA-DR and HLA-DQ induction by IFN-γ compared with normal cells.[179] The difficulty detecting IFN-γ in RA does not appear to be due to methodological problems since it is easily measured in other diseases known to be mediated by T cells, such as tuberculous pleuritis. IFN-γ mRNA was detected in tuberculous pleura by in situ hybridization[180] but RA synovial tissue was negative using similar techniques.

One of the most important functions for IFN-γ, and one that may be used therapeutically in the future, is its capacity to alter the balance of extracellular matrix synthesis and degradation. IFN-γ inhibits collagen synthesis both in vitro[181] and in vivo[182] and has been shown to decrease levels of type I and type III procollagen mRNAs in rheumatoid synovial fibroblast-like cells.[183] IFN-γ also inhibits metalloproteinase production by cultured fibroblast-like synoviocytes that have been stimulated with IL-1 or TNF-α.[184, 185] In the case of IL-1, IFN-γ specifically decreases stromelysin gene expression and protein production. This indirectly decreases collagenase activity in culture supernatants because stromelysin, at least in vitro, is required to activate procollagenase protein through limited proteolysis. The mechanism by which IFN-γ blocks TNF-α–mediated collagenase production is not as well worked out. However, it is clear that IFN-γ inhibits a variety of TNF-α–mediated activities of synoviocytes, including GM-CSF production, collagenase activity, and proliferation. This is not due to down-regulation of TNF receptors on synoviocytes, since IFN-γ paradoxically increases expression of the TNF receptors.[186] Of interest, IFN-γ antagonism of TNF-α on synoviocytes is selective, since the two factors are synergistic in some other assays, such as induction of the adhesion molecules ICAM-1 and VCAM-1.[187, 188] TNF-α also can block IFN-γ–mediated induction of HLA-DR on synoviocytes. The inverse effects of these two cytokines on many aspects of synoviocyte function has been termed *mutual antagonism*.

The antagonism between TNF-α and IFN-γ raises the interesting possibility that the relative *lack* of T cell factors like IFN-γ might actually contribute to the perpetuation of chronic RA. Longstanding disease should, of course, be distinguished from the initiation stages of RA, because there is no information on the expression of this cytokine at the earliest time points where it might be more important. Furthermore, its role as an inducer of HLA-DR in chronic disease appears to have been supplanted by other cytokines, especially GM-CSF.[189] The rather heretical notion that the absence of T cell factors might actually exacerbate RA is supported by clinical studies demonstrating that pharmacologic doses of IFN-γ systemically have mild beneficial effects.[190] Further still, intra-articular administration of very large amounts of recombinant IFN-γ does not exacerbate the disease (unpublished observation). Other T cell factors that are low in chronic RA, like IL-4, can inhibit rheumatoid factor and metalloproteinase production by RA synovial explants, and their absence from the joint could also contribute to RA activity. The inhibitory action of IL-4 might be mediated by decreased c-*jun* and c-*fos* expression, which is required for efficient production of metalloproteinases and cytokines.[191] IL-4 also inhibits IL-8 production by synovial fluid mononuclear cells.[192] To incorporate this novel hypothesis into current models of RA, some recent paradigms have shifted from a purely T cell–driven process to a complex process involving macrophage and fibroblast cytokine networks in combination with defective T cell responses.

Other T Cell Products

The situation for other T cell factors is similar to that of IFN-γ; i.e., the amounts detected in synovial fluid or in synovial tissue are usually quite small. For example, interleukin-2 (IL-2), which is a T cell–derived cytokine that serves as a major autocrine or paracrine T cell growth factor, was originally reported to be present in synovial fluid using biological assays.[193] However, specific monoclonal antibodies that block the IL-2 receptor do not interfere with this activity.[194] More specific assays showed that IL-2 was found in only a small percentage of RA synovial effusions and, when detected, was present in low concentrations.[195] An immunofluorescence study of RA synovium also demonstrated only trace amounts of immunoreactive protein in frozen sections of RA synovium.[196] Studies of IL-2 gene expression in synovial tissue (ST) are mixed, and some studies detect specific IL-2 mRNA and others do not. Moreover, the possible presence of IL-2 mRNA without protein production could suggest that the T cells are anergic.

Many laboratories have attempted to measure other T cell products in articular samples. Usually the concentrations have been rather low. As just noted, IL-4 was not detected in RA synovial fluid; TNF-β (lymphotoxin) and IL-3 were also not found.[194, 195] Many of these same factors, like IFN-γ, have been easily detected in other inflammatory diseases. For instance, IL-2 and GM-CSF are abundant in cutaneous allergic reactions and in allergen-induced asthma.[197, 198] This suggests that the relative deficiency of T cell products in RA is not strictly an artifact of insensitive methods; rather, the pathogenesis of RA (and the role of T cells) must be very different compared with other chronic inflammatory conditions known to be antigen specific. Also note that if one uses sensitive enough techniques, such as RT-PCR, it is possible to detect some T cell cytokine mRNA, especially from the Th1 subset of helper cells.[199] These data should be considered in the context of the extraordinary sensitivity of this method. TNF-α, GM-CSF, and IL-6 can be made by T cells under some circumstances and are present in synovial fluid, but the primary sources of these cytokines in the rheumatoid joint are not T cells.

Why Are T Cell Lymphokines Difficult to Detect?

As noted earlier, many potential explanations exist for the relative absence of T cell products in the synovium, although the final answer is not known. A trivial explanation is that the methods are too insensitive or that cytokines are delivered in the microenvironment and cannot be detected using current technology. This possibility is supported by the observation that islet cells isolated from the non-obese diabetic mouse model of diabetes also produce little IFN-γ even though systemic administration of anti–IFN-γ antibodies to the animals improves the disease.[200] Alternatively, a number of immunosuppressive factors known to be present in synovial fluid could be responsible, including TGF-β, IL-10, and IL-1ra. For some cytokines, especially IFN-γ, RA patients have a specific defect that might contribute to deficient expression. Other cytokines might be bound to extracellular matrix proteins. This provides a form of depot cytokine release that might not be detected in culture supernatants or in synovial effusions. It is possible that some cytokines escape detection after being bound to the extracellular matrix in this manner. The absence of mRNA for some lymphokines makes this and membrane-bound cytokines less likely explanations. T cell anergy is another potential mechanism for suppressing cytokine production and can result, in some cases, with either lower mRNA levels or low protein production despite the presence of mRNA. Finally, it is possible that the T cells in the synovium have not received the appropriate activation signal (i.e., antigen) and that the chronic disease is perpetuated through other mechanisms.

Macrophage and Fibroblast Products

Although detection of T cell factors has been a problem in RA, the same is not true for products of macrophages and fibroblasts. A reductionist view would state that virtually every macrophage/fibroblast mediator that has been sought in the RA synovium has been detected. This is obviously a simplification, but it is not far from the truth. In this section, some of the major cytokines and effectors produced in the joint will be enumerated.

Interleukin-1

IL-1 is a ubiquitous family of polypeptides with a wide range of biologic activity. Its actions make it a candidate for the major amplification factor and translator of the inflammatory response of RA into a proliferative one. IL-1, including its properties and its actions in comparison with those of other active factors, is discussed in Chapter 18. The potential for a major role for IL-1 in the initiation of inflammatory and proliferative responses is great. It has been demonstrated, for example, that recombinant IL-1β injected into rabbit knee joints induces the accumulation of polymorphonuclear and mononuclear leukocytes in the joint space and the loss of proteoglycan from articular cartilage.[201] Leukocytes alone did not explain the depletion of proteoglycans, and there was no measurable increase of production of prostaglandins or leukotrienes in this process. It was inferred that IL-1 was inducing chondrocytes or synovial cells, or both, to generate enzymes that degrade proteoglycans in this relatively simple model. IL-1 activity—produced by peripheral blood mononuclear cells that are adherent to surfaces and have macrophage function—was much greater when cells were collected from rheumatoid patients who had recent onset or an exacerbation than from patients with stable arthritis or from controls.[202] IL-1 activity sufficient to stimulate collagenase and PGE$_2$ production from synovial lining fibroblasts has been shown to be generated by monocytes/macrophages isolated from synovial fluid of patients with RA.[203] High-affinity receptors for IL-1α and IL-1β have been identified on cultured human rheumatoid synovial cells.[204] Even PMNs stimulated by phagocytosis or by other activating substances produce IL-1.[205] Thus, the macrophages, synovial fibroblasts, PMNs, and endothelial cells[206] can be induced to generate this powerful mediator.

In terms of cytokine mRNA production, the synovial macrophage is the most prolific cell in the joint, and nearly half of all CD11b-positive macrophages from the RA synovium contain significant amounts of IL-1β mRNA.[207] Immunohistologic studies confirm this, with especially abundant IL-1 protein in synovial lining macrophages adjacent to type B synoviocytes, as well as in sublining macrophages in and about blood vessels. The IL-1 in the lining can subsequently activate type B synoviocytes to proliferate and secrete a variety of mediators, including metalloproteinases. IL-1 activity has been detected in culture supernatants of rheumatoid synovial biopsies; and, in one study, the amount produced correlated with joint destruction found on roentgenograms.[208] A broad range of substances are capable of inducing IL-1 production; for example, immunoglobulin Fc fragments and, to a lesser extent, immune complexes can generate IL-1 production by rheumatoid synovial monocytes/macrophages.[209] Collagen fragments can induce IL-1 production, and it is intriguing that type IX collagen, which has been found only in articular cartilage and localized into intersections of collagen fibrils, is a potent inducer of interleukin-1 by human monocytes/macrophages.[210] Signals from T cells can also enhance IL-1 production during antigen presentation. Early studies showed that production of mononuclear cell factor (later shown to be identical to IL-1) was produced by mononuclear cells with help from T lymphocytes.[211] This has been confirmed in many subsequent studies.[212] IFN-γ enhances the production of IL-1 by endothelial cells that have been activated.[206] GM-CSF, which is produced by RA synovial cells, can also increase IL-1 release by activated macrophages.[213]

Within the rheumatoid joint, IL-1 has activities besides inducing prostaglandin and collagenase formation. It induces fibroblast proliferation, stimulates biosynthesis of IL-6 and GM-CSF by synovial cells, and enhances collagen production.[214] IL-1 stimulates glycosaminoglycan (GAG) production in human synovial fibroblast cultures,[215] although the effect of IL-1 on production of intact proteoglycan molecules by articular cartilage in some models seems to be inhibitory,[216] indicating that production of components of the GAG complex by IL-1 may be altered. Additionally, IL-1 stimulates human synovial cells to increase both cell-associated and extracellular plasminogen activator activity,[217] and it has been demonstrated that the cytokine osteoclast-activating factor (OAF) that is capable of stimulating bone resorption is identical to IL-1β.[218] Another activity of interleukin-1, that of chemotactic activity for B and T cells, can be found in rheumatoid synovial fluids; a proportion of the chemotactic activity can be removed by specific antibody to IL-1.[219] IL-1 induces a number of adhesion molecules on fibroblast-like synoviocytes and endothelial cells, including VCAM-1 and ICAM-1.[188]

Tumor Necrosis Factor-α

This activity was named of the capability of a purified polypeptide to cause necrosis in certain tumors in mice. Extensive purification and cloning of the factor have revealed that there are at least two forms, TNF-α and TNF-β (lymphotoxin [LT]), that have similar cytotoxic effects on neoplastic cell lines. As noted above, LT is not a single gene product, but is a heterotrimer composed of distinct α and β chains. Two TNF receptors from the nerve growth factor family of receptors have been identified (p55 and p75). Both receptor types bind TNF-α and can be shed from activated cell surfaces by proteolytic cleavage. The shed receptors can still bind TNF-α and represent a potential counterregulatory mechanism for antagonizing cytokine action (see "Suppressive Cytokines and Cytokine Antagonists"). TNF-α has been detected in rheumatoid synovial fluid and serum, but not TNF-β (which is primarily a T cell–derived lymphokine).[195] Levels of TNF-α correlate with erythrocyte sedimentation rates and synovial fluid leukocyte counts. Of great interest is that, except for the failure of TNF to facilitate T cell activation by antigen or mitogen, IL-1 and TNF have similar activities (see Chapter 18), including the ability to enhance cytokine production, adhesion molecule expression, proliferation, and metalloproteinase production by cultured synoviocytes. In some systems, the effects of these two agents are more than additive, suggesting synergism. If this were true, inhibition of one might drastically minimize the effects of the other and provide a useful therapy. TNF-α stimulates collagenase and PGE$_2$ production by human synovial cells and dermal fibroblasts,[220] induces bone resorption, inhibits bone formation in vitro,[221] and stimulates resorption of proteoglycan and inhibits its biosynthesis in explants of cartilage.[222] In situ hybridization and immunohistochemistry suggest that TNF-α, like IL-1, is primarily a product of synovial macrophages in RA. TNF blockade has demonstrated some efficacy in animal models of arthritis, like collagen-induced arthritis in mice,[223] and preliminary studies using monoclonal antibodies suggest that this approach might also be useful in RA.[224]

Interleukin-6

Interleukin-6 is an IL-1–inducible protein produced by T cells, monocytes, and fibroblasts that is also spontaneously produced by cultured fibroblast-like synoviocytes.[225] It can induce immunoglobulin synthesis in B cell lines, is involved in differentiation of cytotoxic T lymphocytes, and is the major factor in regulation of acute-phase response proteins by the liver.[226] In patients with RA, a striking correlation between serum IL-6 activity and serum levels of C-reactive protein, α$_1$-antitrypsin, fibrinogen, and haptoglobin was found.[227] Very high levels of IL-6 are present in RA synovial fluid, and synovial cells in culture from diverse inflammatory arthropathies produce IL-6.[228] In situ hybridization of frozen sections of ST also show IL-6 mRNA in the intimal lining and immunoperoxidase studies show IL-6 in protein lining and sublining regions.[207, 229] Although many synovial macrophages express the IL-6 gene, the majority of IL-6 appears to be produced by type B synoviocytes. T cells might contribute to synovial IL-6 production, but the amount is quantitatively small.

Granulocyte-Macrophage Colony-Stimulating Factor (GM-CSF)

GM-CSF has the ability to support differentiation of bone marrow precursor cells to mature granulocytes and macrophages. As with other major colony-stimulating factors (e.g., macrophage-CSF, granulocyte-CSF, and IL-3), GM-CSF also participates in normal immune responses. It is a potent macrophage activator, including the induction of HLA-DR expression, tumoricidal activity, IL-1 secretion, intracellular parasite killing, and priming for enhanced release of TNF-α and PGE$_2$. Neutrophil function is also regulated by GM-CSF, which enhances antibody-dependent cytotoxicity, phagocytosis, chemotaxis, and production of oxygen radicals.

GM-CSF is present in RA synovial fluid (SF) and is produced by RA ST cells.[207, 230] The major source in the synovium appears to be macrophages, although IL-1 or TNF-α–stimulated fibroblast-like synoviocytes also express the GM-CSF gene.[231] In situ hybridization studies show little or no GM-CSF mRNA in synovial T cells. Its ability to induce HLA-DR gene expression on macrophages might be of particular importance in RA: GM-CSF, not IFN-γ, is the major DR-inducing cytokine in RA synovial fluid and in supernatants of cultured synovial tissue cells.[189]

Chemokines

Chemokines are a family of related chemoattractant peptides that, with the assistance of adhesion molecules, summon cells into inflammatory sites. Chemokines, which generally are relatively small proteins (8 to 10 kD), are divided into two major families, known as C-C or C-X-C based on the position of characteristic cysteine residues (Table 54–5). Each individual factor has the ability to attract specific lineages of cells after interacting with specific cell surface receptors. A host of chemokines have been identified in the rheumatoid joint. IL-8, a C-X-C chemokine that was originally characterized as a potent chemoattractant for neutrophils (although it is now known to also attract monocytes and other cells), along with immune complexes and other chemotactic peptides like C5a, contributes to the large influx of polymorphonuclear leukocytes into the joint. Immunohistochemical analysis of ST demonstrates IL-8 protein in sublining

Table 54–5. CLASSIFICATION OF CHEMOKINES

	C-X-C Subfamily	C-C Subfamily
Chromosome	4 (q12–21)	17 (q11–32)
Chemokine	IL-8	Monocyte chemoattractant protein 1, 2, 3, and 4
	GRO α, β, and γ	Monocyte inhibitory protein 1α and 1β
	Platelet factor 4	RANTES
	Epithelial neutrophil activating peptide-78	
	Interferon-inducible protein-10	
	Granulocyte attractant protein-2	
	Platelet basic protein and derivatives (βTG, NAP-2, CTAP III)	

perivascular macrophages as well as in scattered lining cells.[232] Cultured ST macrophages constitutively produce IL-8, and fibroblast-like synoviocytes express the gene if they are stimulated with IL-1 or TNF-α. Although proinflammatory cytokines IL-1 and TNF-α are capable of inducing expression of a large number of chemokines by cultured synoviocytes, IL-8 accounts for the majority of neutrophil-attracting activity. Addition of anti–IL-8 neutralizing antibodies eliminates about 40 percent of the neutrophil chemoattractant activity in synovial fluid. IL-8 has a number of other activities: it activates neutrophils through G-protein–coupled receptors and is a potent angiogenesis factor.[233]

Macrophage inhibitory protein-1α (MIP-1α), MIP-1β, macrophage chemoattractant protein-1 (MCP-1), and RANTES (all members of the C-C subfamily) are produced by RA synovium.[234, 235] Epithelial neutrophil activating peptide-78 (ENA-78), which is a C-X-C chemokine, is also abundant.[236] ENA-78 accounts for about 40 percent of the chemotactic activity for neutrophils in RA synovial fluid. In each case, as one might expect, the source of the chemokine appears to be synovial macrophages or cytokine-stimulated type B synoviocytes. The regulation of each chemokine appears to be distinct in fibroblast-like synoviocytes. For instance, IL-8 production is inhibited by IFN-γ and enhanced by IL-4, whereas the opposite is true for RANTES.[237] The concentrations of chemokines are higher in RA synovial effusions compared to samples from noninflammatory arthritides like osteoarthritis. Although the chemokines can also be detected in the blood, the levels are considerably lower than in the joint, thereby providing a gradient that signals cells to migrate into the synovium.

Transforming Growth Factor

Transforming growth factor (TGF) is a family of proteins that stimulate cells to lose contact inhibition. Two major forms have been isolated and characterized, TGF-α and TGF-β (see Chapter 18). Although TGF-β alone has a modest effect on the expression of genes for collagenase and collagenase inhibitor, in the presence of other growth factors (such as EGF) it not only represses the production of collagenase (in contrast to IL-1 or TNF-α, which stimulates it) but can superinduce expression of tissue inhibitor of

metalloproteinases.[238] TGF-β also inhibits mast cell proliferation but not mast cell differentiation or mediator release.[239] It accelerates healing of incisional wounds,[240] and this is consistent with its ability to induce both fibrosis and angiogenesis in experimental animals.[241] It would appear, therefore, that TGF-β is an important mediator of tissue repair and, like IFN-γ, can alter the balance between extracellular production and destruction.

Large amounts of TGF-β are present in synovial fluid (although it is mainly found in an inactive latent form) and the mRNA can be detected in RA synovial tissue.[242, 243] Although typically thought of as an immunosuppressive cytokine with wound-healing properties, the role of TGF-β in RA is quite complex as demonstrated by its conflicting results in various animal models. When it is injected directly into the knees of animals, cellular infiltration and massive synovial lining hyperplasia develops.[244] In streptococcal cell wall arthritis, parenteral administration of the protein ameliorates the disease.[245] Intra-articular administration of anti–TGF-β antibody decreases arthritis in the injected joint but not in the contralateral joint in the same model.[246]

Platelet-Derived Growth Factor

One of the most potent growth factors yet isolated is platelet-derived growth factor (PDGF).[247] PDGF is both chemoattractant and mitogenic for fibroblasts, and it induces collagenase expression.[248] Given the presence of new blood vessels and the frequency of formation of vascular microthrombi in RA, PDGF may play a major role in generating proliferation of these synovial cells as the progression of rheumatoid synovitis continues in a given individual (see Chapter 18).

In a study of comparative effects of numerous cytokines (e.g., PDGF, fibroblast growth factor, epidermal growth factor, TGF-β, IL-1, TNF-α, and IFN-α), PDGF was clearly the most potent stimulator of long-term growth of synovial cells in culture.[249] In these experiments, the strong mitogenic activity of rheumatoid synovial fluids was inhibited by an anti-PDGF antibody; TGF-β antagonized these proliferative effects of PDGF (although other studies suggest that TGF-β can serve as an autocrine growth factor for cultured synovial fibroblasts[250]). PDGF is overexpressed in vascular endothelial cells in other synovial sublining cells in the rheumatoid compared to the normal synovium.[251] The PDGF receptor also is expressed in the same regions of RA synovium, suggesting the presence of an autocrine or paracrine system.[252]

Fibroblast Growth Factors

Fibroblast growth factors (FGF) are a family of peptide growth factors with pleotropic activities. In rheumatoid patients, it is likely that heparin binding growth factor (HBGF-1), the precursor of acidic fibroblast growth factor (aFGF), is a major mitogen for many cell types, and stimulates angiogenesis.[253, 254] The interaction between FGF and proteoglycans might be required for biological activity.[255] Unbound FGF does not appear to recognize FGF receptors. The interaction between bFGF and heparin causes either a conformational change or oligomerization that subsequently activates the growth factor. FGF induces capillary endothelial cells to invade a three-dimensional collagen matrix, organizing themselves to form characteristic tubules that resemble blood capillaries.[256] This invasive quality of endothelial cells is mediated by their capacity to produce plasminogen activator and metalloproteinases, as well as inhibitors of these proteinases,[257] in response to angiogenic stimuli. These are the same enzymes that are involved subsequently in destruction of cartilage, tendon, ligament, and bone. Immunostaining of rheumatoid synovial tissue has revealed HBGF-1, and mRNA for HBGF-1 is present in the same tissue samples in rough proportion to the mononuclear cell infiltrate within the tissues.[258] FGF is present in RA synovial fluid, and the genes are expressed by synovial cells.[259] Synovial fibroblasts express FGF receptors and proliferate after exposure to the growth factor. Hence, FGF might serve as an autocrine stimulus that contributes to synovial lining hyperplasia.

Connective Tissue–Activating Peptides

One set of factors with clear anabolic capability and a potential for involvement in synovial inflammation are the connective tissue–activating peptides (CTAP). Synovial cells in culture are activated by CTAP I from lymphoid cells; CTAP III and IV from human platelets; and CTAP V, from endothelial cells. The actions on these cells include increased glucose transport, glycolysis, PGE_2 formation, cyclic adenosine monophosphate (cAMP) accumulation, increased hyaluronic acid and proteoglycan synthesis, and, in some instances, mitogenesis.[260] CTAP III has common antigenic determinants with platelet factor IV and β-thromboglobulin. Amino terminal sequence data suggest that CTAP III, platelet factor IV, and β-thromboglobulin have remarkable sequence homology. What remains to be determined is how these peptides interact with other factors mentioned above within inflamed connective tissue.

Leukemia Inhibitory Factor (LIF)

LIF is a potent macrophage product present in high concentrations in synovial fluid.[261, 262] The gene is expressed by chondrocytes and RA synovium. Depending on the culture conditions and the cell line selected, LIF can either induce differentiation in myeloid leukemic cell lines or prevent differentiation in normal pluripotential embryonic stem cells.[263] Among its many activities, LIF might contribute to bone resorption in RA through its ability to activate osteoclasts.[264] Exogenous IL-4 is able to markedly suppress LIF production by RA synovial tissue explants, and the relative absence of IL-4 in RA might accelerate osteoporosis or bone destruction.[265]

Alternative Models: The Role of Macrophage/Fibroblast Cytokine Networks

To incorporate new information on the cytokine profile into current concepts of rheumatoid arthritis, a variety of alternative models have been proposed.[170] A central theme of these paradigms is that the chronic inflammatory process might achieve a certain degree of autonomy that permits inflammation to persist after a T cell response has been down-regulated. This could occur if the inflammation is sustained by factors produced by neighboring macrophages and synovial fibroblasts in the joint lining in paracrine or autocrine networks. Several cytokines that have been identified in the synovium or synovial fluid can participate in this system and might explain lining cell hyperplasia, HLA-DR and adhesion molecule induction, and synovial angiogenesis. The list of potential candidates in this highly redundant system is very long. For the sake of example, one can assume that at least two—IL-1 and TNF-α—play particularly central roles. Both are produced by synovial macrophages and stimulate synovial fibroblast proliferation and secretion of IL-6, GM-CSF, and chemokines as well as effector molecules like metalloproteinases and prostaglandins. GM-CSF, which is produced by both synovial macrophages and IL-1β–or TNF-α–stimulated synovial fibroblasts, can in turn, induce IL-1 secretion to form a positive feedback loop. GM-CSF, especially in combination with TNF-α, also increases HLA-DR expression on macrophages. Macrophage and fibroblast cytokines could also indirectly contribute to the evidence for local T cell and B cell activation, including rheumatoid factor production.

This model for the perpetuation of RA clearly does not eliminate the likelihood that synovitis is initiated by a specific arthritogenic antigen. In fact, unless RA is truly caused by transformed cells, it requires an external stimulus to initiate the process, with periodic restimulation possibly required. T cell–mediated responses, either directed against an inciting antigen or a secondary target like type II collagen or proteoglycans can occur along with this macrophage/fibroblast cytokine network and might enhance the local inflammatory response. The factors released by macrophages and fibroblasts are reasonably well defined; however, the precise function of synovial T cells remains unknown. The role of T cells and antigen-specific stimulation might even change during various phases of the disease. In early RA, antigen-specific T cell activation might be most important. As the disease progresses, the cytokine networks become established and antigen-independent processes might assume a central position.

Neuropeptides

Evidence is accumulating that implicates neuropeptides, substance P in particular, in the pathogenesis of rheumatoid arthritis. Pain is a common symptom of RA. Kinins, prostaglandins, and leukotrienes lower the activation threshold of peripheral unmyelinated afferent fibers.[266] These same fibers generate inflammatory mediators when the neurons are activated, thus contributing to inflammation. Substance P, the best studied of these, is a nine-amino-acid peptide that can stimulate the release of other mediators, such as leukotrienes; can stimulate lymphocyte proliferation; can support proliferation of synovial cells; can induce the biosynthesis of matrix metalloproteinases by these cells[267]; and can induce release of IL-1, TNF-α, and interleukin-6 from monocytes.[268] Elevated synovial fluid levels of substance P are found in RA as well as other forms of inflammatory, traumatic, and degenerative arthritis. It is intriguing to postulate that the centrally directed release of neuropeptides at terminal efferent nerve endings in joints may explain the symmetry of rheumatoid arthritis.

Enkephalins are endogenous neuropeptides that bind to opiate receptors and regulate nociception. One of the enkephalin peptides, met-enkephalin, can also modulate the immune system. Met-enkephalin enhances B cell antibody production and macrophage oxygen radical generation and is a chemotactic factor. Like substance P, immunoreactive met-enkephalin is present in synovial fluid. The source of met-enkephalin in the joint is not fully established. Although it certainly could be produced by the local nerves,[269] monocytes and chondrocytes are other possible sources.[270]

Suppressive Cytokines and Cytokine Antagonists

The proinflammatory cytokine network described earlier is balanced by a variety of suppressive factors that attempt to reestablish homeostasis. Underproduction of these suppressive cytokines could potentially contribute to the perpetuation of the RA. As described, relative deficiency of IFN-γ or IL-4 might lead to unopposed activation of synoviocytes by TNF-α or other cytokines. However, in addition to these, there are many other cytokine antagonists or natural immunosuppressives that represent potential therapeutic targets for the treatment of inflammatory diseases (see Chapter 18).

IL-1 Receptor Antagonist (IL-1ra)

IL-1ra is a naturally occurring IL-1 inhibitor that binds directly to type I and II IL-1 receptors (IL-1R) and competes with IL-1 for the ligand binding site.[271, 272] Even though IL-1ra has high affinity for IL-1R, it is a relatively weak inhibitor because IL-1 can activate cells even if only a small percentage of IL-1Rs are occupied. Because of this, a large excess of the inhibitor is needed to saturate the receptor and thereby block IL-1–mediated stimulation (usually 10- to 100-fold excess of IL-1ra).[142] Recombinant IL-1ra inhibits a variety of IL-1–mediated events in cultured cells derived from the joint, including the induction of metalloproteinase and prostaglandin production by chondrocytes and synoviocytes. It can block synovitis in rabbits induced by direct intra-articular injection of recombinant IL-1 but not antigen-induced arthritis.[273, 274] Two structural variants of IL-1ra have been described: (1) secretory IL-1ra, or sIL-1ra, which is synthesized with a signal peptide that allows it to be transported out of cells; and (2) intracellular IL-1ra, or icIL-1ra, which lacks a leader peptide as a result of alternative splicing of mRNA and therefore remains intracellular.[275] sIL-1ra is a major product of mononuclear phagocytes, particularly mature tissue macrophages; and icIL-1ra is the dominant form in cultured fibroblast-like synoviocytes as well as keratinocytes and epithelial cells. IL-1 and IL-1ra production are often closely linked, although they clearly have distinct regulatory controls.[276] Cell maturity is one important determinant, with IL-1 predominating in immature monocytes, whereas IL-1ra is more prevalent in mature macrophages.

High concentrations of the IL-1ra (up to 50 ng/mL) are present in rheumatoid synovial effusions.[277] Neutrophils are a major source of the protein in synovial fluid.[278] Immunohistochemical studies of rheumatoid synovium reveal abundant IL-1ra protein especially in perivascular mononuclear cells and the synovial intimal lining.[279, 280] The IL-1ra protein and mRNA can be detected in synovial macrophages and, to a lesser extent, in type B synoviocytes (Fig. 54–3). The presence of IL-1ra in synovium is not specific to RA, since osteoarthritis synovial tissue also contains IL-1ra, albeit in lesser amounts; normal synovium contains little, if any, IL-1ra protein. Despite the presence of significant amounts of IL-1ra in synovial tissue, its importance as an IL-1 antagonist can be evaluated only in the context of the IL-1/IL-1ra ratio. Although it is impossible to measure the amounts of IL-1 and IL-1ra directly in the synovial microenvironment, studies of synovial cell culture supernatants show that the amount of IL-1ra is insufficient to antagonize synovial IL-1.[281] There are two reasons for the relatively low levels of IL-1ra released by synovial cells: (1) fibroblast-like synoviocytes, which account for much of the immunoreactive IL-1ra in the synovial

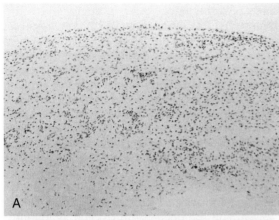

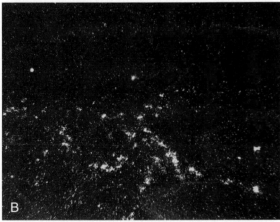

Figure 54–3. Localization of interleukin-1 receptor antagonist (IL-1ra) messenger RNA (mRNA) in rheumatoid arthritis (RA) synovial tissue by in situ hybridization. The specific RNA transcript was detected in perivascular cells, especially macrophages. Panel *A* shows the bright field view, and panel *B* shows the same area using a darkfield filter. Silver grains in the darkfield view show the location of IL-1ra positive cells. (Courtesy of Dr. G. S. Firestein, University of California, San Diego, School of Medicine, La Jolla, Calif.)

intimal lining, selectively produce the intracellular form of IL-1ra; and (2) synovial macrophages appear to have defective IL-1ra production compared to macrophages isolated from other sites, secreting only about 1 percent as much as alveolar macrophages or monocyte-derived macrophages.

Interleukin-10

IL-10 is a major immunosuppressive cytokine that was originally characterized as a cytokine synthesis inhibitory factor based on its ability to block T cell cytokine production by deactivating macrophages.[282] Its immunosuppressive actions might be important in pregnancy to suppress an immune response directed against paternal MHC antigens, and it might regulate susceptibility to some parasitic infections.[283] An interesting relationship exists between EBV and human IL-10; an EBV protein with strong structural homology to human IL-10 might contribute to EBV-induced

immunosuppression.[284] IL-10 protein is present in RA synovial fluid, and the gene is expressed by synovial tissue cells.[285, 286] Synovial macrophages are the major source of IL-10 in RA.

TGF-β

In addition to its tissue repair activities described earlier, TGFβ also has immunosuppressive actions that might be important. For instance, synovial fluid is known to inhibit IL-1–mediated thymocyte proliferation. This activity is neutralized by anti–TGF-β antibody.[143] TGF-β also down-regulates IL-1 receptor expression on chondrocytes.[287]

Soluble Cytokine Receptors

Soluble cytokine receptors and binding proteins can absorb free cytokines and prevent them from engaging functional receptors on cells. These obviously could inhibit cytokine action, but it should be kept in mind that they also could act as carrier proteins that protect cytokines from proteolytic degradation and/or deliver them directly to cells. A 47-kD soluble IL-1 binding protein has been identified in supernatants of a human B cell line and in RA synovial fluid.[288] The protein is released after proteolytic cleavage from the cell surface by serine proteases. Both the biologically active 17-kD form of IL-1β and the inactive 31-kD precursor bind to the protein. Recent studies suggest that the binding protein might be a soluble form of the type II IL-1R. Moreover, specific immunoassays now clearly show that the type II receptor is present in RA synovial fluid, along with lesser amounts of the type I receptor.[289] These soluble receptors can bind to IL-1 or IL-1ra in synovial effusions and can interfere with standard immunoassays, especially for IL-1β and IL-1ra.

Soluble TNF-receptors (TNF-R) have also been detected in RA synovial fluid.[290] Both the p55 and p75 receptors are present, sometimes in very high concentrations (>50 ng/mL). This is considerably higher than the concentration of TNF-α in blood or synovial fluid and probably explains why biologically active TNF is difficult to detect in RA synovial fluid despite the presence of immunoreactive protein. Synovial membrane mononuclear cells have increased surface expression and mRNA levels for both TNF-Rs compared to osteoarthritis or peripheral blood cells.[291] Cultured fibroblast-like synoviocytes express TNF receptors and constitutively shed them into culture supernatants.[186] It is not clear how TNF-α functions in RA in the presence of such an enormous excess of soluble receptor.

BLOOD VESSELS IN ARTHRITIS: ADHESION MOLECULES AND ANGIOGENESIS

Blood vessels used to be thought of as passive conduits through which red cells and leukocytes circulated while en route to an inflammatory site. This is now known to be far from the truth: the microvasculature plays an extremely active role in such processes, not only as the means of selecting which cells should enter the tissue but also as a determinant of tissue growth and nutrition through the proliferation of new capillaries.

Angiogenesis in Rheumatoid Arthritis: The Basis for Synovitis

From the vantage of the proliferation of new blood vessels in the synovium, synovitis in rheumatoid arthritis resembles both tumor growth and wound healing. The importance of luxurious new capillary growth early in the development of synovitis was emphasized by Kulka and associates many years ago[292] (Fig. 54–4). Decades later, Folkman and colleagues demonstrated the first soluble factors responsible for inducing an endothelial cell with the capability to proliferate and develop new capillaries. The importance of new blood vessel formation in inflammatory arthritis has been elegantly demonstrated in the collagen-induced arthritis model. The disease was markedly attenuated in animals pretreated with an angiostatic compound similar to fumagillin, which is derived from aspergillus.[293] This compound is cytotoxic to proliferating but not resting endothelial cells. In addition, there was regression of established arthritis if treatment was initiated well into the course of the disease. Hence, angiogenesis is essential for the establishment and progression of inflammatory arthritis, either because of the need for blood vessels to recruit leukocytes or to provide nutrients and oxygen to starved tissue.

Most observers feel that the absolute number of blood vessels is increased in RA synovium, with a rich network of sublining capillaries and postcapillary venules in histologic sections stained with endothelial-specific antibodies. However, it is possible that the mass of tissue might outstrip angiogenesis in RA as determined by the number of blood vessels per unit area.[294] This could result in local tissue ischemia, a situation that has been amply documented in vivo. Synovial fluid oxygen tensions can be remarkably low, lactate measurements are frequently high, and pH as low as 6.8 has been found.[295] Mean rheumatoid synovial fluid PO_2 in 85 samples from rheumatoid knees was 27 mm Hg,[296] and, in a subsequent study, a PO_2 of less than 15 mm Hg was measured in a quarter of fluids examined.[297] Another cause of diminished blood flow may be the increased positive pressure exerted by synovial effusions within the joint, a process that could effectively obliterate capillary flow and exacerbate the decrease in oxygen availability to these tissues while producing ischemia-reperfusion injury in the joint.[298, 299] Physiologic determinations by Simkin and colleagues have supported this[300]; clearance values generated by kinetics of iodine-123 removal from synovial fluid have shown that small solute clearance from rheumatoid synovial effusions is less than in normal individuals or in patients with other rheumatic diseases. Patients with the lowest synovial iodide clearance have the lowest synovial fluid pH, the lowest synovial fluid to serum glucose ratios, the lowest synovial fluid temperatures, the highest synovial fluid lactate levels, and the highest numbers of synovial fluid neutrophils. Thus, the most seriously affected rheumatoid joints may be both hypoperfused and ischemic. Diminished blood flow relative to need may be decreased further by high intrasynovial pressure from effusions, as well as the existence of abnormal microvascular structures.[159, 301] Altered vascular flow may not be the only cause of hypoxia in joints. It has been estimated that the oxygen consumption of the rheumatoid synovium (per gram of tissue) is 20 times normal.[302]

Hypoxic drive is a potent stimulus for angiogenesis. One of the mechanisms by which this occurs is through the production of angiogenic factors like

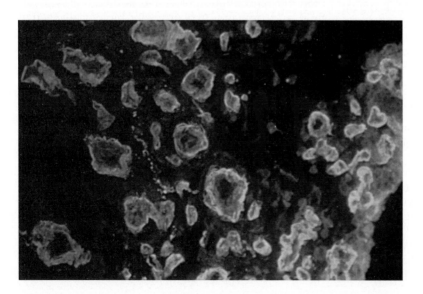

Figure 54–4. Human rheumatoid synovial membrane (4-µm thickness) stained with rabbit anti-human type IV collagen. This gives precise definition in blood vessels, the only structures in synovium that contain type IV collagen. Virtually all of these blood vessels have formed in response to angiogenic stimuli after the rheumatoid process had been initiated. (Courtesy of Drs. S. and R. Gay, University of Alabama Medical Center, Birmingham, Ala.)

vascular endothelial growth factor (VEGF).[303] VEGF, which is also known as *vascular permeability factor*, is a specific endothelial cell mitogen that also possesses some chemotactic activity. It is present in high concentrations in synovial fluid, and immunoreactive VEGF is readily detected in the synovium in and about blood vessels.[304, 305] VEGF is able to stimulate the expression of collagenase, which can degrade the extracellular matrix to make room for advancing pannus.[306] The VEGF receptor is also present in the same area. In addition to the hypoxia-driven stimulus for blood vessel growth, the inflammatory cytokine milieu of the joint also encourages angiogenesis. Several cytokines known to be produced in the joint, including IL-8, FGF, and TNF-α, are known to be angiogenic factors. Some factors that inhibit capillary proliferation, such as platelet factor-4 and thrombospondin, are also produced by the joint.[307, 308]

Blood vessels also control the rate that various proteins leave the circulation and enter the joint. It has been known for many years that there is an inverse relationship between the molecular weight of proteins and their concentrations in minimally inflamed synovial fluid; the high-molecular-weight serum proteins gain access more easily to synovial fluid in inflamed joints, and the relatively high concentration of IgG in RA synovial fluid is good evidence for local (synovial) synthesis of IgG.[309] In recent studies, "protein traffic" in human synovial effusion has been measured by determining clearance of albumin and other proteins from synovial fluid. This gives a useful measure of afferent synovial lymph flow. An increased "permeance" of proteins in rheumatoid patients was found to be more than seven times greater than that suggested by ratios of synovial fluid to serum and underscores the severity of the microvascular lesion in rheumatoid synovitis.[310]

Adhesion Molecule Regulation and Arthritis

Formation of new capillaries is only one aspect of blood vessel involvement in the rheumatoid process. Endothelial cells are also activated by cytokines to express adhesion proteins that bind to counterreceptors on leukocytes from the circulation and facilitate their transfer from the circulation into the subsynovial tissue (see Chapter 20). When activated, some endothelial cells in postcapillary venules take on a tall, plump appearance, which in the aggregate are referred to as *high endothelial venules* (HEVs). The HEV are a major site of blood cell adhesion and subsequent migration into the tissue, a process mediated by adhesion proteins. There are several categories of adhesion molecules. The selectins (E-, L-, and P-selectin) are a family of adhesion molecules whose primary ligands are carbohydrates, especially sialyl Lewis$_x$ and related oligosaccharides.[311] The integrin family is complex and is described in Chapter 20. These adhesion proteins are heterodimers made up of α and β chains. The counterreceptors depend on the specific combination of these chains and frequently are proteins in the immunoglobulin supergene family (e.g., the combination of ICAM-1 and αM/β2) or extracellular matrix proteins (e.g., the combination of fibronectin and α5/β1). The currently accepted paradigm for leukocyte recruitment into inflammatory sites is a sequential cascade[312] and is detailed in Chapter 20.

As one might expect, adhesion molecule expression is increased in the RA synovium (Table 54–6). This is almost certainly due to exposure of the vasculature to the rich cytokine milieu, especially IL-1 and TNF-α. IFN-γ and IL-4 are also known to increase adhesion molecule expression, but their role is uncertain due to the relatively low production in RA. High levels of ICAM-1 are expressed in the rheumatoid synovium.[313] Immunohistochemistry techniques have localized ICAM-1 to sublining macrophages, macrophage-like synovial lining cells, and fibroblasts in greater amounts than normal tissue. Significant amounts are also present on the majority of vascular endothelial cells, although the ICAM-1 levels are quantitatively similar to vessels in normal endothelium. Cultured fibroblast-like synoviocytes constitutively express ICAM-1. TNF-α, IL-1, and IFN-γ dramatically increase synoviocyte ICAM-1 expression.[187, 188] Maintenance of ICAM-1 expression requires continuous cytokine exposure, and ICAM-1 levels decrease to baseline within a couple of days if the cytokine is removed. The function of ICAM-1 on nonendothelial cells like synoviocytes is not known. It might serve as a counterreceptor to leukocyte integrins and act as a barrier to cells trying to migrate through the tissue to the synovial fluid space. Alternatively, integrin counterreceptors are costimulatory molecules that participate in the activation of T lymphocytes through αL/β2 (LFA-1).

The role of α4/β1 in cell trafficking and adhesion is well documented.[314] Adhesion to cytokine-activated

Table 54–6. MAJOR ADHESION MOLECULE INTERACTIONS WITH RA SYNOVIAL ENDOTHELIUM

Endothelial Cell Adhesion Molecule	Leukocyte Counterreceptors	Leukocytes Expressing Counterreceptor
ICAM family	β$_2$ integrins	Neutrophils, lymphocytes, monocytes
VCAM-1	α$_4$β$_1$(VLA-4); α$_4$β$_7$	Lymphocytes, monocytes
CS1 fibronectin	α$_4$β$_1$(VLA-4), α$_4$β$_7$	Lymphocytes, monocytes
E-selectin, P-selectin	L-selectin	Neutrophils, lymphocytes, monocytes

ECs can be mediated by vascular cell adhesion molecule-1 (VCAM-1). Under some culture conditions, VLA-4 mediates CD18-independent monocyte transendothelial migration.[315] VLA-4, which is predominantly expressed on lymphocytes, monocytes, and eosinophils, but not on neutrophils,[316] serves as a receptor for both the 6- and 7-domain forms of VCAM-1 and a 25 amino acid sequence in an alternatively spliced region of fibronectin known as *CS1*.[317, 318] The binding sites for CS1 and VCAM-1 on VLA-4 are either very close to each other or physically overlap.[319]

A role for VLA-4 in arthritis has been suggested by a number of experimental observations. In adjuvant arthritis in rats, anti-α4 antibody decreased lymphocyte accumulation in the joint but not lymph nodes, suggesting that VLA-4 is more important in recruitment to inflamed sites than to noninflamed sites.[320] In streptococcal cell wall arthritis, intravenous injection of CS1 peptide decreased the severity of acute and chronic arthritis.[321] T lymphocytes isolated from the synovial fluid and synovial membrane of RA patients exhibit increased VLA-4–mediated adherence to both CS1 and VCAM-1 relative to autologous peripheral blood lymphocytes.[322, 168] These studies also suggest that leukocytes expressing functionally activated VLA-4 are selectively recruited to inflammatory sites in RA.

Moderate amounts of VCAM-1 are expressed in RA synovial blood vessels.[188] Surprisingly, the intimal lining is the location of the most intense staining with anti–VCAM-1 antibodies on histologic sections of synovium. Even normal synovial tissue expresses VCAM-1 in the lining, albeit less than in RA tissue. Cultured fibroblast-like synoviocytes constitutively express small amounts of VCAM-1, and the level can be increased by IL-1, TNF-α, IFN-γ, and IL-4. VCAM-1 on synoviocytes is functionally active and can support T cell binding. VCAM-1 also contributes to T cell adhesion to high endothelial venules in frozen sections of RA synovium.[323]

The expression and functional significance of CS1-containing forms of fibronectin (FN) generated by alternative splicing have also been studied in RA.[324] Unlike most molecular forms of FN typically found in the extracellular matrix, CS1 expression is restricted to inflamed RA vascular endothelium and the synovial intimal lining (Fig. 54–5). Normal synovial tissue contains little, if any, CS1 fibronectin. Ultrastructural studies show that CS1-expressing fibronectin molecules decorate the lumen of RA endothelial cells but not the abluminal side of the endothelium. RA synovial endothelium binds activated T lymphocytes; this can be blocked by anti-α4 antibody and synthetic CS1 peptide but not anti–VCAM-1 antibody suggesting that the CS1-VLA-4 interaction is critical to lymphocyte homing to the joint. Immunoelectron microscopy also showed that CS1 fibronectin is expressed on the surface of fibroblast-like synoviocytes in the synovial intimal lining. Binding studies confirmed this in vitro since a portion of VLA-4–mediated T cell adhesion to cultured synoviocytes is blocked by CS1 peptides.[188]

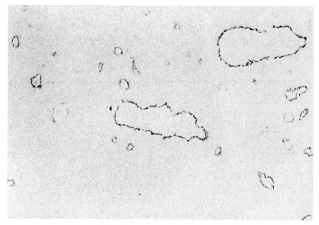

Figure 54–5. CS1 fibronectin is expressed by rheumatoid arthritis synovial vascular endothelium. This immunoperoxidase study was performed using a specific anti-CS1 antibody to identify alternatively spliced fibronectin. The interstitial regions are negative for CS1, although other forms of fibronectin are abundant throughout the tissue (not shown). (From Elices MJ, Tsai V, Strahl D, Goel A, Tollefson V, Arrhenius T, Wayner E, Gaeta F, Fikes J, Firestein GS: Expression and functional significance of alternatively spliced CS1 fibronectin in rheumatoid arthritis microvasculature. Reproduced from The Journal of Clinical Investigation, 1994, vol 93, p 405, by copyright permission of the American Society for Clinical Investigation.)

The integrin α4/β7, which can also bind to VCAM-1, is analogous to LPAM-1, a specific adhesion molecule involved in lymphocyte homing to Peyer's patches. Nearly all intraepithelial and 40 percent of lamina propria lymphocytes express α4/β7; this molecule is rarely identified in other lymphoid tissues.[325] A recently published study found that α4/β7 expression on peripheral blood lymphocytes of patients with RA was similar to controls (7.3 percent), and 25.4 percent of synovial fluid lymphocytes express this adhesion molecule.[326] Moreover, 62 percent of the α4/β7 positive cells in synovial fluid lymphocytes were of the CD8 subtype. Why this occurs when other lymphoid tissues do not express α4/β7 is undefined. It does suggest, however, another potential linkage between the gastrointestinal epithelium and the joint, which has been a source of much discussion in several inflammatory joint diseases.

E-selectin expression has also been described in rheumatoid synovium, although the levels are much lower than those of the integrins.[327] This might be due, in part, to the kinetics of E-selectin expression on endothelial cells. The protein is not found on resting endothelial cells and peaks after about 3 hours of cytokine stimulation. However, even in the continued presence of cytokine, E-selectin expression then declines to near basal levels after about 6 hours. This might explain the relatively low amounts of this protein in chronically inflamed tissue. In one study, E-selectin expression was decreased in synovial biopsy specimens after patients were treated with injectable gold and corticosteroids.[328]

B CELL ACTIVATION AND RHEUMATOID FACTOR

Activated B lymphocytes are present in peripheral blood as well as in the rheumatoid synovium. Using flow cytometry, it has been demonstrated that many RA patients with normal circulating numbers of lymphocytes show an abnormal κ chain to λ chain analysis compared with controls. This implies oligoclonal B cell proliferation.[329] It is not known whether this reflects expansion of the restricted number of clones capable of producing rheumatoid factor or whether the inciting antigen is something other than IgG and related specifically to RA.

The process of B cell activation and the mediators controlling it are detailed elsewhere (see reference[330] and Chapter 7), but it is useful to review this in the context of rheumatoid arthritis. As with other activation systems in this disease (as well as in normal physiology), cytokines play a major role in antibody production and isotype switching. The B cell subset that is enriched in autoantibody production is characterized by a surface determinant CD5.[331, 332] In humans, IL-2 plays a leading role in inducing all immunoglobulin isotypes; although other cells can enhance this response, none affects lymphocyte responses of activation, proliferation, or differentiation in the absence of IL-2. IL-4 has growth-promoting effects on human B cells and induces class II MHC expression on B cells. IL-4 directly enhances both T cell proliferation and IL-2 production[333] and is responsible for isotype switching to IgE antibodies.[334]

The driving force behind rheumatoid factor production has not been elucidated. Enhanced helper T cell function has been correlated with the spontaneous production of rheumatoid factor, although only for the IgM isotype.[335] The NK cells and the cytokine profile of the joint (especially IL-6), can also support nonspecific B cell activation.[336]

Although no data clearly implicate rheumatoid factor (RF) as a principal causative agent in RA, the role of antiglobulins in the amplification and perpetuation of the process is well supported:

1. Although some patients with virtually no circulating IgG develop RA,[96] it is known that patients with a positive test for rheumatoid factor in blood have more severe clinical disease and complications[337] than do seronegative patients.

2. Polyclonal IgM RF is able to fix and activate complement by the classical pathway.[338]

3. IgG RF produced in large quantity in rheumatoid synovial tissue can form large complexes of itself through self-association,[339] because these molecules have a much higher frequency of double valent Fc binding regions than do most normal IgG molecules. It appears that these large complexes fix complement and can bind to IgM RF.

4. Immune complexes containing rheumatoid factor have been localized within synovial tissues by immunofluorescent techniques.[340, 341]

5. Increased levels of IgG RF have been associated with a high frequency of subcutaneous nodules, vasculitis, elevated erythrocyte sedimentation rate (ESR), decreased complement levels, and increased number of involved joints.[342, 343]

6. In experiments performed on patients with RA, a marked inflammatory response was elicited when rheumatoid factor from the patient was injected into a joint, but not when normal IgG was given.[344] Rheumatoid factor becomes involved in pathogenesis when it forms immune complexes sufficiently large to activate complement and/or be phagocytized by macrophages or PMNs.

Several hypotheses have been advanced to explain how IgG could become immunogenic. First, new determinants on IgG might be exposed following polymerization among molecules to form aggregates or as IgG complexes with specific non-IgG antigens.[345] Second, structural anomalies in the IgG of rheumatoid patients may render it immunogenic, such as a possible defect in the hinge region of rheumatoid IgG that could increase the binding affinity to membrane Fc receptors on B lymphocytes.[346] Alternatively, depletion of suppressor T lymphocytes might allow B lymphocytes to produce autoantibodies against certain determinants on IgG. Finally, autoantigenic reactivity of IgG could be related to demonstrated changes in the relative extent of galactosylation. A deficiency of the galactosylation enzyme machinery may increase the relative risk of developing RA.[15]

In addition to rheumatoid factors of the mu (μ) and gamma (γ) isotypes in RA, epsilon (ε) isotypes also have been demonstrated in certain patients.[347, 348] Of 13 sera containing IgE immune complexes, 11 were from patients with extra-articular manifestations. It has been suggested that IgE RF could complex with aggregated (self-associating) IgG in synovial tissue and that the IgG–IgE complexes could then activate mast cells and basophils in the synovium. This is of particular interest in light of reports that there are numerous mast cells in rheumatoid synovium and that these may release factors capable of stimulating collagenase production by synovial cells.[349]

Considering the restricted number of idiotypes of rheumatoid factor, it is interesting that the four major classes of immunoglobulins (IgM, IgG, IgA, and IgE) are all produced in rheumatoid arthritis. It has been shown that, whereas only 73 percent of patients with RA were seropositive by standard tests for RF, 92 percent were positive for IgM RF using enzyme-linked immunosorbent assays (ELISA).[350] This study is significant because it lowers the numbers of "seronegative" rheumatoid arthritis in this and presumably other populations. In the same group, 65 percent, 68 percent, and 66 percent were positive for IgA, IgE, and IgG rheumatoid factor, respectively. Disease activity correlated with IgM RF and IgA RF, as did levels of circulating immune complexes. Extra-articular features correlated positively with levels of IgA and IgE rheumatoid factor.

METALLOPROTEINASES: MEDIATORS OF TISSUE DESTRUCTION

The metalloproteinases are a family of enzymes that participate in extracellular matrix degradation and remodeling. Although the substrate specificity for individual members of the family differs, they have several structural and functional similarities. For instance, metalloproteinases are usually secreted as inactive proenzymes. Their proteolytic activity requires limited cleavage or denaturation to reveal a zinc cation at the core that is normally chelated to a cysteine residue in the latent form (see Chapter 21).

Many different families of proteinases are found in the joint (Table 54–7), but the metalloproteinases are thought to play a pivotal role in joint destruction. Nevertheless, other proteases can potentially contribute. Serine proteases and cysteine protease, though less well characterized in RA, are likely to be important. In fact, cysteine protease inhibitors significantly decrease joint damage in the rat adjuvant arthritis model.[351] The relative importance of each type of enzyme as either a primary effector or as an activator of other enzymes is not yet known.

The cytokine milieu has the capacity to induce biosynthesis of metalloproteinases by synovial cells and alter the balance between extracellular matrix production and degradation. PDGF directly induces proteinase production by mesenchymal cells, as well as being both a chemoattractant and a mitogen for these cells.[248] It is likely that PDGF is released into rheumatoid tissues in large quantities as platelet activation in the presence of angiogenesis and clot formation occurs. IL-1 and TNF-α also directly induce metalloproteinase gene expression by many cells, including fibroblast-like synoviocytes.[184] These two cytokines are additive or synergistic when used in combination. In models in vitro it has been shown that, though culture medium from rheumatoid synovium stimulates cartilage degradation, this can be inhibited by an antibody against IL-1; these data implicate rheumatoid synovium as a source of IL-1 that activates chondrocytes to produce proteases.[352] IL-6 does not induce metalloproteinase production by synovial cells but instead increases production of TIMP-1, a naturally occurring inhibitor of metalloproteinases.[353]

Table 54–7. KEY PROTEASES AND INHIBITORS IN RHEUMATOID SYNOVIUM

Protease	Inhibitor
Metalloproteinases Collagenase Stromelysin 92-kD gelatinase	TIMP family; α₂-macroglobulin
Serine proteases	SERPINs α₂-macroglobulin
Cathepsins	α₂-macroglobulin

Abbreviations: TIMP, tissue inhibitor of metalloproteinases; SERPIN, serine proteinase inhibitor.

In contrast to cytokines that induce production of enzymes that degrade connective tissue, there are several that inhibit biosynthesis of proteolytic enzymes. One of these, TGF-β, inhibits collagenase synthesis in vitro and enhances production of TIMP by fibroblasts and chondrocytes.[354, 355] TGF-β also increases collagen production,[356] apparently shifting the balance to matrix production and preservation.

Substances other than cytokines are capable of inducing synovial cells to produce metalloproteinases in vitro, and it is probable that many have a role in vivo as well. It is not known for many whether their effects are mediated through cytokines such as PDGF. Proteinases,[357] phagocytosable debris,[358] soluble iron,[359] collagens,[360] crystals of monosodium urate monohydrate,[361] and various calcium crystals[362] are found in joints at one time or another and stimulate collagenase biosynthesis. The crystals, and perhaps other substances in this group, stimulate metalloproteinase production by triggering IL-1 (and possibly other cytokine) production. Some proteases, such as the 92-kD gelatinase, are made constitutively by early passage RA synoviocytes.[363] These factors operate, it is presumed, by activating receptors that, in turn, enhance expression of trans-acting factors that bind to *cis*-element in the 5' flanking region of the metalloproteinase genes. One of these, AP-1, is a complex of proteins expressed by the cellular *jun* and *fos* proto-oncogenes (Jun and Fos, respectively) that are held together by a leucine "zipper," in which residues of leucine in a portion of the protein that is an α-helix project out and interact with homologous residues on another protein. This combination of Jun and Fos juxtaposes the DNA-binding domains of Jun and Fos and enables them to attach (as AP-1) to specific *cis*-elements on the DNA, enhancing expression of metalloproteinase mRNA.[364] Glucocorticoid-mediated inhibition of collagenase gene expression is due to interference with the Fos–Jun complex by the glucocorticoid receptor.[365]

Collagenase and Stromelysin

Collagenase and stromelysin have, between them, the capacity to degrade all the important structural proteins in the extracellular tissues within joints[366–368] (see Chapter 21). The temperature of the interaction between collagenase and collagen is a crucial determinant of rate of lysis; an increase of only a few degrees (as one would expect within an inflamed joint) may increase the rate of collagenolysis manyfold, a fact that has led some investigators to question the benefit of applying deep heat (e.g., microwave) to inflamed arthritic joints.

The collagenase gene is expressed by RA synovial tissue as well as by cartilage. In situ hybridization studies show that the primary location of collagenase gene expression is the intimal lining, especially in fibroblast-like cells.[369, 370] Collagenase protein cannot be readily detected in frozen sections by immunostaining unless synovial explants are first cultured briefly in the presence of monensin, which interferes with protein transport,[371] indicating that collagenase protein is not stored intracellularly but is secreted very rapidly after synthesis. Increased metalloproteinase gene expression is an early feature of RA and occurs during the first few weeks or months of disease.[372] This underscores the need for early therapy to prevent joint destruction.

Stromelysin (or matrix metalloproteinase 3; MMP3) was described first from rheumatoid synovial cells in 1986[373] as a metalloproteinase of similar molecular weight to collagenase and having the same pH range for activity. It has no activity against interstitial collagens but effectively degrades type IV collagen, fibronectin, laminin, proteoglycan core protein and type IX collagen.[374] Stromelysin removes the NH2-terminal propeptides from type I procollagen, thereby producing products similar to those produced by procollagen N-proteinase, the enzyme believed responsible in vivo for performing this function. Stromelysin is integrally involved in activation of procollagenase. Like collagenase, stromelysin gene expression is almost exclusively in the intimal lining (Fig. 54–6).[375]

Most data indicate that there is a cascade of activation of the matrix metalloproteinases. Prostromelysin is activated and the presence of stromelysin is essential for subsequent activation of procollagenase. Prostromelysin from human synovial cells can be activated by other proteases, including cysteine proteases (the cathepsins), trypsin, chymotrypsin, plasma kallikrein, plasmin, and mast cell tryptase.

Inhibitors of Metalloproteinase Activity

It was demonstrated many years ago that α_2-macroglobulin (α_2M) accounted for more than 95 percent of collagenase inhibitory capacity in serum.[376] The mechanism of inhibition by α_2M involves hydrolysis by the proteinase of a susceptible region in one of the four polypeptide chains of α_2M (sometimes called the "bait") with subsequent trapping of the proteins within the interstices of the α_2M. Ultimately, the protease is covalently linked to a portion of the α_2M molecule. The SERPINs, or serine protease inhibitors, are also abundant in synovial effusions and plasma and can serve a dual purpose of directly blocking serine protease function and indirectly decreasing metalloproteinase activity by preventing serine proteases from activating metalloproteinase proenzymes. One SERPIN, α_1-antitrypsin, has been well characterized in synovial fluid and is frequently in an inactivated state after oxidation by reactive oxygen species.[377]

The first inhibitor of mammalian collagenase to be isolated and purified from human tissues was a protein of 25 kD produced by cells in explants of human tendons. This inhibitor blocked trypsin-activated rheumatoid synovial collagenase as well as the collagenase obtained from polymorphonuclear leukocytes.[378] The same protein was subsequently purified

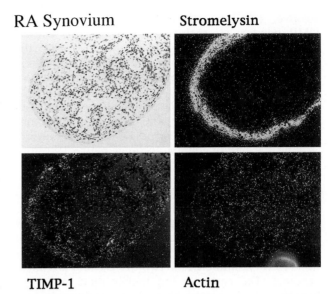

RA Synovium   **Stromelysin**

TIMP-1   **Actin**

Figure 54–6. Localization of stromelysin, TIMP-1, and actin messenger RNA (mRNA) in RA synovial tissue by in situ hybridization. Stromelysin and, to a lesser extent, TIMP-1 are mainly expressed in the synovial intimal lining, presumably by cytokine-stimulated type B synoviocytes. Actin mRNA is evenly distributed throughout the synovium. Bright field *(top left)* and darkfield views *(top right and bottom)* are shown. (Courtesy of D. Boyle, Gensia, Inc., San Diego, Calif.)

from skin; the primary structure has been determined and the gene cloned[379]; the protein is known as *tissue inhibitor of metalloproteinases (TIMP)*. Since then, additional members of TIMP family have been cloned and characterized, each of which has distinctive patterns of affinity for each metalloproteinase.[380] The TIMP proteins block proteinase activity by binding directly to metalloproteinases in a 1:1 molar ratio. TIMP generally binds only to the active enzyme; there are some exceptions, such as TIMP-2, which can interact with type IV procollagenase. The inhibitors bind to metalloproteinases with extremely high avidity and, though the interaction does not result in new covalent bonds, it is essentially irreversible. TIMP is present in RA synovial fluid in excess. It is, in fact, very difficult to detect free active collagenase or stromelysin, and they are usually complexed with TIMP.[381] The majority of metalloproteinase is not complexed and is in the proenzyme form. This suggests that metalloproteinase activation in the joint is slow and, when it occurs, the enzyme is rapidly inactivated by TIMP. Active matrix degradation must occur at a privileged site where TIMP does not have ready access. Immunohistochemical studies have localized the inhibitor in hyperplastic synovial lining cells in rheumatoid synovium but not in the cells of normal synovium.[371] TIMP gene expression is not significantly altered by IL-1 or TNF-α but is increased by IL-6.[353]

TIMP mRNA, like metalloproteinases, is primarily localized to the synovial intimal lining. Using doublelabel in situ hybridization, three phenotypes of cells could be detected in the intimal lining and among cultured synoviocytes: TIMP negative/stromelysin positive, TIMP negative/stromelysin positive, and TIMP positive/stromelysin positive.[382] This underscores the differential regulation of TIMP and the metalloproteinases and shows that some "confused" cells simultaneously seek matrix destruction and protection.

Given the important role of metalloproteinases in tissue destruction, it follows that the relative balance between metalloproteinases and TIMPs ultimately determine the fate of the extracellular matrix. Presumably, RA with its more destructive potential would have a ratio that favors degradation, whereas osteoarthritis (OA) might have a more destructive ratio. This has been examined directly using quantitative in situ hybridization to study synovial mRNA levels, and it appears that the metalloproteinse:TIMP ratio is, indeed, higher in RA.[369] The levels of TIMP gene expression are very similar in the two disease and are likely maximal. The cause of the higher ratio in RA is, therefore, the increased amount of metalloproteinase mRNA. The differences between OA and RA are not dramatic, and it may be that rather subtle changes in the balance can have profound effects over years (or decades) of disease. Perhaps more important is the question of whether drug treatment can alter this balance. This possibility has been investigated using in situ hybridization to quantify synovial gene expression (Table 54–8): Intra-articular corticosteroid injections markedly decreased synovial collagenase, stromelysin, and TIMP gene expression. In contrast, chronic low dose methotrexate therapy specifically decreased collagenase mRNA (by about two thirds) but not stromelysin or TIMP-1.[383] The specificity for collagenase but not stromelysin gene expression is a bit unusual, but other studies have shown discoordinate expression of these two genes.[384] The selective decrease in collagenase gene expression suggests that a decreased collagenase:TIMP ratio is a mechanism of decreased bone destruction observed in some patients treated with methotrexate. In another study, tenidap significantly decreased stromelysin gene expression.[385]

SYNOVIAL PATHOLOGY

There are many dimensions to rheumatoid arthritis. Gross changes have been correlated with disease ac-

Table 54–8. EFFECT OF ANTIRHEUMATIC DRUGS ON IN VIVO RHEUMATOID SYNOVIAL GENE EXPRESSION*

	Collagenase	Stromelysin	TIMP-1
Intra-articular corticosteroid	↓	↓	↓
Methotrexate	↓	↔	↔
Tenidap	↔	↓	↔
Piroxicam	↔	↔	↔

*Gene expression was determined by quantitative in situ hybridization in serial synovial biopsies.[369, 383, 385]
↓ = decreased by drug.
↔ = no change.

tivity, as have the findings at microscopic and electron microscopic levels, but geographic differences of disease within individual joints are of major importance as well.

Gross Pathologic Changes

In considering gross pathologic findings, one must account for the change from the relatively acellular lining of mesenchymal cells (one to two layers deep with relatively few blood vessels) to the bulky, hyperplastic, hypervascular, proliferative lesion resembling a tumor. All of the synovium in a normal knee joint may weigh less than 5 g; synovial tissue taken from a rheumatoid knee joint can weigh more than 10 times as much.

The built-in redundancy of the joint space permits this proliferative growth; there is room for tissue accumulation within diarthrodial joints without immediate increase in pressure or displacement of other tissue. The geometry of synovial proliferation enables an enormous surface area of cells to maintain contact with synovial fluid. Synovium does not proliferate as a tumorous mass within a capsule. There is an intricate system of villus fronds that proliferate as would branches of ferns from a common stalk. At times, distal portions of villi become necrotic, as blood supply cannot keep pace with cellular proliferation. These dead areas may consolidate into acellular fibrinous masses, be auto-amputated, and accumulate in the synovial fluid. The loss of the terminal vasculature can produce arteriovenous shunting and synovial hypoxia as discussed earlier.

What are the associations between gross pathologic changes and invasiveness between rheumatoid synovium? There appears to be some correlation between the location of synovial involvement and joint destruction. A detailed study using double contrast arthrography in patients with classic rheumatoid arthritis has provided geographic patterns of synovium within rheumatoid knee joints.[386, 387] Panarticular disease involved all the surfaces of the joint space, including the suprapatellar pouch. Joint destruction was rapid and severe in these patients, which is not surprising. Interestingly, highly proliferative synovium confined to the suprapatellar pouch was not destructive, nor was disease localized in the posterior pouches of the knee. "Burnt-out" disease characterized by fibrotic and relatively avascular synovium was not observed in patients who have any remaining cartilage.

The increasing use of arthroscopy has enabled investigators to look for correlations of joint destruction with the appearance of synovium. One series of observations of 51 knees in 32 patients has identified four distinct stages of disease progression.[388]

Stage I. Visible evidence of joint pathologic changes was restricted to the synovial lining and, although villus proliferation had taken place, there was no invasion of meniscal or articular cartilage. Radiographic examination was normal in most of these patients.

Stage II. Proliferative pannus extended over meniscal surfaces, and erosions and fissuring of the menisci were visible, but articular cartilage appeared normal by observation and radiographs.

Stage III. Full-thickness meniscal tears and free-floating debris were observed, as was articular cartilage erosion associated with invasive, full-thickness craters containing proliferative tissue. Radiographic appearance was normal in 75 percent of these patients, and in the remaining 25 percent there was minimal joint-line narrowing.

Stage IV. Only when articular cartilage was severely eroded and menisci were often missing in their entirety were significant numbers of patients shown to have radiographic defects.

The importance of this classification is that invasion of meniscal cartilage appears to occur earlier than that of articular cartilage. It is now recognized that magnetic resonance imaging (MRI) can provide early evidence of meniscal cartilage disease and give, therefore, a fair warning before articular cartilage invasion by synovitis begins[388] and, in some instances, visualize pannus as it begins to spread over articular cartilage. It is not clear if the advent of miniarthroscopy will provide significant prognostic information, including detection of early cartilage erosions or staging the degree or extent of synovial hypertrophy. There is also high hope that some features of early biopsies using the miniarthroscope (e.g., histology, cytokine gene expression, metalloproteinase gene expression) will offer a guide to determine which patients warrant more aggressive therapy.

The Synovium in Rheumatoid Arthritis: A Heterogenous Mixture of Cells

Perhaps the major effector region of the synovium is the intimal lining, which is the loosely organized collection of cells that form an interface between the synovium and the synovial fluid space. Two major cell types are found in the lining: a macrophage-like cell known as a *type A synoviocyte* and a fibroblast-like cell called a *type B synoviocyte*. The former is derived from the bone marrow, expresses macrophage surface markers and abundant HLA-DR, and the latter expresses little if any class II MHC antigens, is devoid of macrophage markers, and has a scant endoplasmic reticulum. The numbers of type A and B cells are relatively equal in normal synovium. There is an absolute increase in both cell types in RA, although the percentage increase in macrophage-like cells appears to be greater.[389] In addition, the type A synoviocytes tend to accumulate in the more superficial regions of the intimal lining. However, some studies using immunolocalization of metalloproteinases have shown that as many as 60 percent of "synovial lining cells" have morphologic and immunostaining characteristics of type B cells, and the remainder were cells that did not stain for metalloproteinases and had the ultrastructural appearance of macrophages.[390]

The synovial intimal lining cells are loosely associated with each other and lack tight junctions and a definite basement membrane. The increase in cell number can be quite substantial. In the normal joint, the lining is only 1 to 2 cell layers deep, whereas in RA it is usually 4 to 10 cells deep (and sometimes over 20). Although macrophages are terminally differentiated cells that presumably do not divide in the joint, it is presumed that the mesenchymally derived type B synoviocytes divide locally in response to the proliferative factors generated by the activated immune response. It is logical to assume that PDGF, TNF-α, and IL-1 produced by many different cells combine with products of arachidonic acid metabolism to generate proliferation of these cells presumed to be synovial fibroblasts. One problem with this hypothesis is that studies attempting to quantify active cell division in the rheumatoid synovium rarely show mitotic figures, and thymidine uptake occurs in only a small percentage of synovial cells.[391] Using a monoclonal antibody that recognizes dividing cells, an even lower rate of cell division (~0.05 percent) was found.[392] More recently, however, a much higher percentage of cells that express the cell cycle–specific antigen PCNA were identified in RA lining and the nuclear rearrangement apparatus (associated with cell division) compared with osteoarthritis.[393] This correlated with the expression of the proto-oncogene c-myc by lining cells, a gene that is intimately linked with fibroblast proliferation.[394] The reason for the differences with earlier studies is not clear, although it is possibly related to variations in the stage of the disease or the location within the joint. When all of the data are considered, it is likely that type B cell proliferation is modestly increased in RA and contributes to lining hyperplasia.

Using enzymatically dissociated rheumatoid cells, adherent cells from rheumatoid synovial tissue can be divided into three types using monoclonal antibodies.[395] As might be expected from studies of intact tissue, one type of cell is macrophage-like; these cells have DR antigens, Fc receptors, and monocyte lineage differentiation antigens and are capable of phagocytosis. They have a limited life span in vitro, rarely surviving more than a few weeks even in the presence of exogenous growth factors or colony-stimulating factors. A second distinctive cell population is nonphagocytic and has abundant DR antigens, but lacks IgG Fc receptors, monocyte lineage antigens, or fibroblast-associated antigens. Many cells in this group have a dendritic morphology. A third type is defined by the presence of antigens expressed primarily on fibroblasts and by the absence of phagocytic capability, demonstrable DR antigens, or antigens of the monocytic lineage. When the enzymatically dispersed cells are cultured for several passages, it is this last cell type that ultimately survives and proliferates, resulting in a relatively homogeneous population of fibroblast-like cells that are presumed (but not proven) to be derived from the type B synoviocytes in the intimal lining. A successful attempt to clone dissociated rheumatoid synovial cells and place them in long-term culture has supported this classification.[396] Each type of cell could be cloned, but the macrophage-like and fibroblast-like cells grew slowly, with a doubling time of 5 to 7 days. The dendritic cells had a doubling time of 1 to 2 days. Fibroblast-like cells generated a dendritic appearance when they were incubated with PGE_2.[397] After removal of the prostaglandin, the cells reverted to normal appearance, unlike the dendritic-like cells that maintained the stellate appearance through their slow doubling times. A study on cloned synovial cells indicated that the dendritic-like cells produced significant amounts of IL-1.[396]

The fibroblast-like cells that can be grown from the dispersed cells can be passaged for several months in vitro. Their doubling time is rapid at first, perhaps due to the presence of cytokines produced by contaminating macrophages in the culture or due to a carry-over effect from the synovial milieu. Over time, the rate of proliferation slows and after 12 to 15 passages the cells gradually become senescent and ultimately cease to grow. Synovial fibroblasts from RA have some characteristics reminiscent of tumors or transformed cells, a notion that seems to fit well with the concept of RA as a locally invasive mesenchymal tumor. As noted above, synoviocytes express oncogenes like c-myc and c-fos that are associated with cell activation and proliferation. Although the fibroblast-like cells normally grow in monolayers and are restrained by contact inhibition, under some culture conditions (e.g., in the presence of PDGF in a semisolid culture medium) they develop anchorage-independent growth patterns; this phenotype is characteristic of transformed cells and can be readily inhibited by TGFβ.[398] The concentrations of both TGFβ and PDGF in rheumatoid synovial fluid are well above that needed for synovial cell stimulation or suppression.

There are many ways to link mitogenic and proliferative factors released by macrophages and the profusion of synovial cells that develop in this disease. However, it is also worth observing that the arthritis that develops in MRL/1pr mice, even though caused by a specific defect in T lymphocytes, is associated with a synovial pannus tissue that consists largely of transformed mesenchymal cells and few T cells.[399, 400] The lymphocyte defect is due to an abnormal fas protein, which normally controls the process of apoptosis (i.e., programmed cell death).[401] Hence, autoimmunity in this model appears to be due to defective T cell death. This has also led to the suggestion that the accumulation of cells in the RA lining might be partly due to defective apoptosis. However, using techniques designed to detect apoptotic cells within the synovium, a surprisingly high percentage of cells in RA synovium contained fragmented DNA that is characteristic of programmed cell death.[402] This was especially true of macrophages and suggests that re-

plenishment of the intimal lining macrophage population is an active process. Fibroblast-like cells also exhibit evidence of apoptosis, which, on first glance, is surprising given the active proliferation in this population as well. Perhaps these observations can be explained by the fact that c-myc, which is expressed by synoviocytes, regulates apoptosis as well as proliferation by acting, in a sense, like a control switch to prevent overgrowth of cells owing to excessive proliferation. Of interest, the cells in the synovium with the least evidence of apoptosis are lymphocytes in lymphoid aggregates. These cells (but not intimal lining cells) express bcl-2, which protects cells from programmed cell death, perhaps explaining the persistence of memory T cells in the rheumatoid synovium.

Previous discussion has emphasized the different types of synovial cells and their membrane antigens, the presence of new blood vessels, the diverse types of lymphocytes and their microscopic distribution, and the relative paucity of polymorphonuclear leukocytes in the synovial lesion. Indeed, although rare PMNs have been described in the pannus, existing either as small microabscesses or as isolated cells,[403] there are remarkably few PMNs in the synovium when one considers the enormous numbers that are frequently present in synovial fluid and that they must have traversed the synovium en route to the joint space. NK cells have also been identified in RA synovium, especially in early disease.[404] The NK cells contain large amounts of granzymes, which are serine proteases produced by activated cytotoxic NK cells. One potentially important immunoregulatory role of NK cells is that they can stimulate B cells to produce rheumatoid factors.[405]

The mast cells are present in the synovial membranes of patients with rheumatoid arthritis[406] and may be localized in some patients at sites of cartilage erosion.[407] In one study, rheumatoid synovial membranes contained over ten times as many mast cells in histologic sections than control synovial samples from patients undergoing surgery for meniscectomy. Patients with high numbers of mast cells had more intense clinical synovitis in the affected joints.[349] Mast cells also have been prominent in intraosseous invasive tissue. Mast cells can be found in a majority of synovial fluid specimens from inflammatory synovitis, and there is measurable histamine content in these synovial fluids.[408] Rheumatoid synovial fluids contained higher levels of histamine than did corresponding plasma samples.[409] A detailed analysis of several indicators of proliferation and the enumeration of synovial mast cells[410] has demonstrated strong positive correlations between the number of mast cells per cubic millimeter of synovial tissue and the degree of lymphocyte infiltration (the number of helper T lymphocytes and plasma cells). Glucocorticoid injections into joints decreased the number of synovial tissue mast cells by 70 to 90 percent.

What could be the contribution of mast cells to rheumatoid synovitis? On the one hand, they could be responding to cytokines that stimulate mast cell growth and chemotaxis, such as a mast cell growth factor that was identified in RA synovial fluid.[194] Extracts of mast cells can induce adherent rheumatoid synovial cells to increase production of PGE_2 and collagenase; the stimulatory factor was neither histamine nor heparin.[411] Heparin, however, does have significant effects on connective tissue. In particular, it may modulate the effects of bone hormones on osseous cells and thereby alter the balance of bone synthesis toward degradation. Heparin increases basal cAMP levels in both bone cells and adherent rheumatoid synovial cells; the significance of these changes to cartilage or bone destruction must be determined.[412]

Cartilage Destruction and the Pannus–Cartilage Junction

Multiple different types of histopathologic findings have been seen at the pannus–cartilage junction (Fig. 54–7). In RA, the cartilage is often covered by a layer of tissue composed of fibroblast-like cells and that might represent the progenitor of the aggressive mature pannus. In the established lesion, numerous areas are seen in which "aggressive cell clusters" of mesenchymal cells, both macrophage-like and fibroblast-like, appear to have a leading edge of penetration into cartilage matrix far from blood vessels and lymphocytes.[413] However, some areas show relatively acellular pannus tissue, suggesting that there is little if any enzyme action in these areas,[414] whereas other sections show microfoci of one particular cell type, including microabscesses of polymorphonuclear leukocytes, mast cells, or dendritic or "stellate" cells. Macrophagic and fibroblastic foci were three to five times more common than those containing mast cells or PMNs.[415] Rarely, proliferating small blood vessels surrounded by cellular infiltrates penetrate deeply into the cartilage.[416] Multinucleate giant cells are particularly common at the erosive front when penetration is from the subchondral side of cartilage. Both osteoclasts and giant cells named *chondroclasts* have been observed degrading bone and mineralized cartilage, as well as areas of unmineralized (hyaline) articular cartilage.[417] These multinucleate cells stain brightly for acid phosphatase. It should be remembered that experimental production of multinucleate cells in cultures of synovial fibroblasts is associated with enormous increase in production in these cultures of collagenase and, presumably, other matrix metalloproteinases.[418] It may be that bradykinin released by the proliferating cells has a significant effect on bone resorption at the pannus–cartilage junction; it appears to stimulate osteoclast-mediated bone degradation by a process that is dependent on endogenous prostaglandin formation.[419]

There may be consistent variations in the histopathology of the cartilage–pannus junction between different joints. Invasive pannus is more commonly found in histologic sections from involved metatarsophalangeal joints as compared with hip and knee joints in which a layer of resting fibroblasts appeared to separate pannus from cartilage.[420] This may explain the fact that erosions are seen more often around small joints such as metatarsophalangeal joints, whereas joint space narrowing without erosions is more common in knees. A more primitive cell type might play a role in RA, especially at the cartilage–pannus junction. This less differentiated cell type could, then, be responsible for the aggressive degradation of the extracellular matrix and help drive the destructive phase of the disease. Recently, a cell type with phenotypic and functional features that appear to be distinct from fibroblast-like synoviocytes and chondrocytes has been isolated from pannus tissue in RA.[421] This cell has the ability to grow in culture for a prolonged time without becoming senescent and expresses very high amounts of the adhesion molecule VCAM-1. It remains to be seen if this represents a separate lineage of cells or if it is derived from other more differentiated cell types at the cartilage–pannus junction.

Cartilage is destroyed in RA by both enzymatic and mechanical processes. The enzymes induced by factors such as IL-1, TNF-α, phagocytosis of debris by synovial cells, and both free and bound iron cause the joint destruction. Early in synovitis, proteoglycans are depleted from the tissue, most likely due to the catabolic effect of cytokines like IL-1 on chondrocytes, and this leads to mechanical weakening of cartilage. As proteoglycans are depleted from cartilage (Fig. 54–8), it loses the ability to rebound from a deforming load and thereby becomes susceptible to mechanical fragmentation and fibrillation and eventually loss of functional integrity concurrent with its complete dissolution by collagenase and stromelysin.[422] There is also increasing evidence that the metalloproteinases responsible for this process are also derived from the chondrocytes themselves. Both stromelysin and collagenase mRNA levels are increased in RA cartilage by northern blot analysis, and in situ hybridization studies confirm the presence of the specific RNA transcripts within chondrocytes.[423, 424] Hence, the cartilage is under attack from a multitude of sources: not only is it being bathed in protease-rich synovial fluid and under extrinsic attack from the invasive pannus, but the chondrocytes themselves contribute to destruction from within.

Although many studies have focused on the pannus–cartilage junction, enzyme release from polymorphonuclear leukocytes in synovial fluid could also have an effect on loss of cartilage. Consistent with the findings of immune complexes in superficial layers of cartilage, electron microscopic examinations of articular cartilage in RA have revealed amorphous-appearing material and evidence of breakdown of collagen and proteoglycan consistent with superficial diffuse activity of joint fluid enzymes (Fig. 54–9).[425] However, in a rabbit model of arthritis in which IL-1 was injected directly into the joint, the degree of cartilage damage as measured by proteoglycan levels in

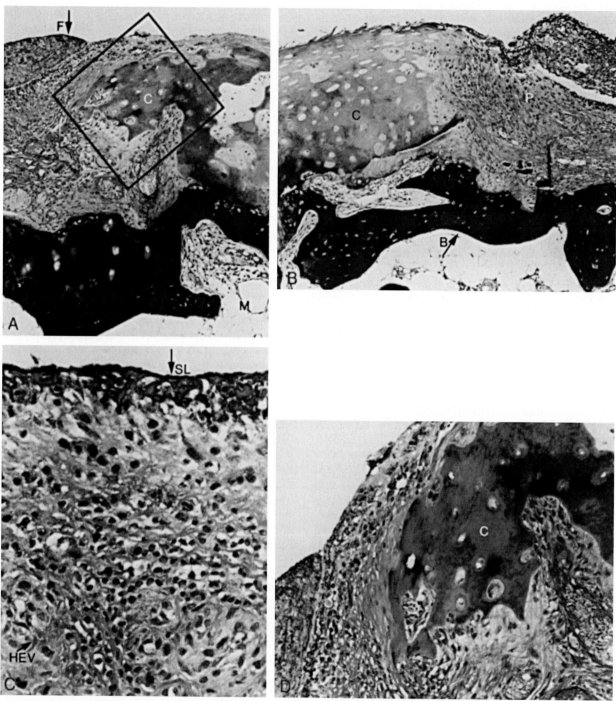

Figure 54–7. Four microscopic views of a rheumatoid metatarsal head removed at time of arthroplasty and stained as a trichrome preparation. In *A* and *B,* the black areas represent subchondral bone. M, marrow; P, pannus; C, cartilage. *D* is the square from *A* enlarged. *A,* The heterogeneity of the invasive pannus is shown. Whorls of proliferative synovial tissue become relatively avascular as they abut against the remaining cartilage, destroying it by proteases. The rheumatoid process in the marrow is capable of destroying bone as well. *B,* A similar picture to *A.* In the invasive pannus, there are numerous lymphocytes (left of P) but these are relatively rare at the invasive front. Several large lacunae are seen in the cartilage, probably representing tongues of invasive pannus, but other areas show enlarged areas without matrix surrounding individual chondrocytes that have been activated to produce proteases by cytokines. B, subchondral bone. *C,* A section through synovial tissue near the invasive front. The synovial cells on the surface (SL) in continuity with synovial fluid always develop a distinct morphology from sublining cells, even though they are, presumably, the same cell (macrophage or fibroblast). One small capillary, HEV, shows plump, tall endothelium. Lymphocytes here are not organized into a follicular pattern but distribute irregularly throughout the synovium. *D,* Different patterns of cells surrounding cartilage being destroyed. (*A–D,* Photomicrographs courtesy of Donald Regula, M.D., Department of Pathology, Stanford University Medical Center. Tissue samples provided from surgery by Gordon Brody, M.D.)

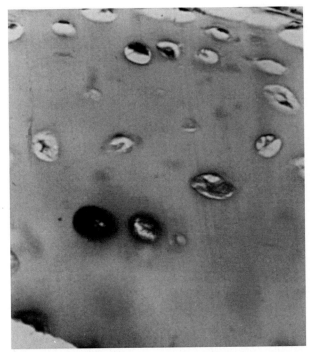

Figure 54–8. Human articular cartilage from active RA removed at joint arthroplasty and stained for metachromasia. The only metachromatic stain surrounds a few chrondrocytes that, presumably, are actively making proteoglycan only to have it broken down by proteinases derived from synovial fluid, chondrocytes, or synovial tissue. The form of this depleted cartilage is normal; however, its functional capacity to rebound from a deforming load is seriously impaired.

of extracellular matrix, suggesting that synovium-derived metalloproteases were more important.

The rate-limiting step in cartilage loss is degradation of collagen, because proteoglycans are degraded very soon after inflammation begins. Metalloproteinases, released into the extracellular space and active at neutral pH, are probably responsible for the majority of effective proteolysis of articular cartilage proteins, but other classes of enzymes may play a role in joint destruction. Enzymes such as cathepsins B, D, G, L, and H may play a role within and outside of cells in degrading noncollagenous matrix proteins. Serine proteinases (e.g., elastase and plasmin) are doubtless involved as well.

SYNOVIAL FLUID IN RHEUMATOID ARTHRITIS

It would be advisable to examine synovial tissue from each patient with rheumatoid arthritis to compare histologic changes with those from previous specimens and perhaps assay for T cell subsets, rheumatoid factor production, and cytokine production by synovial cells, but this is impractical (although mini-arthroscopy might some day permit one to "stage" RA in this manner to determine prognosis and appropriate therapy). As stressed earlier, blood is far removed from the site of disease and the focus of inflammatory activity. Despite some clear reservations, synovial fluid is a reasonable compromise; by examination of its characteristics one can gain a good appreciation for the extent of inflammation, and by using synovial fluid investigators can learn much about events within the synovium itself. Chapter 41 describes techniques for analysis of synovial fluid. Components of the inflammatory and proliferative

synovial fluid correlated best with the stromelysin concentrations in synovial effusions (presumably derived from synoviocytes).[426] Neutrophil depletion of animals did not interfere with subsequent destruction

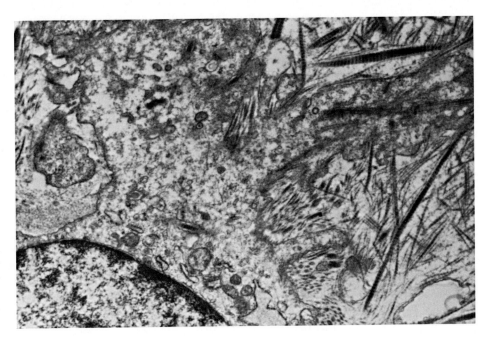

Figure 54–9. The leading edge of a pannus cell extends diffusely into cartilage. Collagen fibers, characterized by 69 nm periodicity, can be seen about to be or actually engulfed by the cell. This close contact of synovium and cartilage is found in less than 10 percent of patients but is the type of process associated with phagocytosis of collagen by this leading edge of cells (30,000×). (Electron photomicrograph by Andrey M. Glauert. From Harris ED Jr, Glauert AM, Murley AH: Intracellular collagen fibers at the pannus-cartilage junction in rheumatoid arthritis. Arthritis Rheum 20:657, 1977.)

response that can be dissected by examination of synovial fluid from patients will be discussed next.

Polymorphonuclear Leukocytes

The number of PMNs remains one of the most accurate indices of inflammation within a particular joint. These are cells that truly amplify inflammatory responses and, although it is unlikely that they destroy much cartilage directly, their role in amplification and, thereby, perpetuation of the inflammation within joints, is probably significant.

The joint space serves as a depository for PMNs[427]; they enter the synovial fluid by direct passage from postcapillary venules in the synovium. Neutrophils adhere to activate synovial microvasculature owing to the action of selectins and the β2 integrins. After adherence, however, agents such as IL-8 produced by endothelium and fibroblasts may facilitate egress through the capillaries into the chemoattractant gradients of the synovium. Once they arrive in the joint space they have no way to leave. Thus, considering the survival time of PMNs in synovial fluid, it has been estimated that the breakdown with an average (30 mL) rheumatoid effusion containing 25,000 PMNs per mm^3 may well exceed a billion cells each day (Fig. 54–10).[427] The ultimate fate of many of these cells is programmed cell death.[428]

The physiology of granulocytes is discussed in detail in Chapter 9. As described there, the strong attraction of chemotactic agents within the synovial fluid in RA is responsible for the large number of cells found there (occasionally up to 100,000 per mm^3). Few PMNs are seen in the pannus itself and subsynovial tissue; once in the synovium they move rapidly to the synovial fluid, drawn by the activated component of cleavage of the fifth component of complement (C5a), leukotriene B$_4$ (LTB$_4$), platelet-activating factor, and chemokines. The reason that neutrophils can move into the articular cavity without resistance and mononuclear cells collect in the sublining is not clear. It might be related to the fact that neutrophils do not express VLA-4 and therefore are unimpeded by the VCAM-1 and CS1 fibronectin-rich intimal lining. In the synovial fluid PMNs come in contact with immune complexes and particulate material (i.e., fibrin, cell membranes, cartilage fragments). Phagocytosis occurs, particularly to particles coated with IgG. After phagocytosis begins, the PMN is activated. Through a complex set of changes in the membrane potential of the cell involving calcium flux and both phospholipid metabolism and cyclic nucleotide activation, the neutrophil begins to degranulate, to generate products of oxygen metabolism, to metabolize arachidonic acid, and to develop the capacity for aggregation.[429] In addition, PMNs from synovial fluid in RA release de novo synthesized proteins, including fibronectin,[430] neutral proteinases, and IL-1.[205] Neutrophils also secrete IL-1ra as a major product.[431] Although the

amount of IL-1ra that each neutrophil produces is low compared to macrophages, the sheer number of PMNs allows them to produce massive amounts in synovial effusions.

Immune Complexes in Rheumatoid Arthritis

The significance of gamma globulin complexes circulating in blood and in synovial fluid was appreciated several decades ago.[432] However, it was not until more reliable assays for immune complexes were available that broad studies correlating disease activity and immune complexes could be generated.

As with studies of lymphocytes, studies of synovial fluid have generated data more relevant to the pathophysiology of the disease than the same studies in blood of the same patients, because the disease process is initiated and perpetuated in the synovium. Findings in blood may reflect only what "spills out" from the synovial fluid and synovial tissue. Levels of IgM-containing circulating immune complexes are elevated in both RA and SLE, although levels of IgG immune complexes are not.[433] In all assays for circulating immune complexes, the possibility of in vitro formation of IgM and IgG complexes giving false positive tests must be considered.[434] Assays such as the C1q binding assay overestimate the concentration of immune complexes. False positive results are also found in the Raji cell test. In studies designed to identify the components of immune complexes in the circulation of rheumatoid patients, most data have found no specific antigen other than IgG complexed with RF. Using more sensitive techniques, it has been found that circulating immune complexes in RA are composed of as many as 20 polypeptides, including albumin, immunoglobulin, complement, and acute phase reactants.

Most relevant to the pathogenesis of joint destruction in RA has been the identification of immunoglobulins and complement in articular collagenous tissues from rheumatoid arthritis. Ninety-two percent of cartilage and meniscal samples from rheumatoid patients had evidence of these components in the avascular connective tissue.[425] Electron microscopic morphology of immunoglobulin aggregates showed that there were pathologic changes in the matrix of cartilage in the microenvironment of the aggregates themselves.[435] Immune complexes were absent under areas in cartilage invaded actively by synovial pannus, suggesting that phagocytic cells in the invasive synovium had perhaps ingested the immune complexes,[436] lending credence to the possibility that immune complexes deposited in the avascular superficial layers of cartilage in the joint may serve as chemoattractants for the pannus and be an explanation for the centripetal orientation of the rheumatoid lesion. Immune complexes have been extracted from cartilage of rheumatoid and osteoarthritic patients.[94] Rheumatoid cartilage contained 37 times more IgM and 14 times more IgG than did normal cartilage extracts. IgM RF was found in 13 of 16 rheumatoid cartilage extracts and in none of 11 osteoarthritic or 6 normal control extracts. In addition, more than 60 percent of the rheumatoid cartilage extracts were positive for native and denatured collagen type II antibody, as were osteoarthritic specimens.

These observations help support the hypothesis that the presence of cartilage itself, and perhaps these complexes, contribute to the chronicity and persistence of rheumatoid inflammation. Orthopedic surgeons have noted many times that joints from which all cartilage is removed do not participate in general flares of rheumatoid disease following surgery. "Burnt out" RA may mean that with the combination of loss of motion and loss of cartilage in a joint there is nothing to sustain continued inflammation.

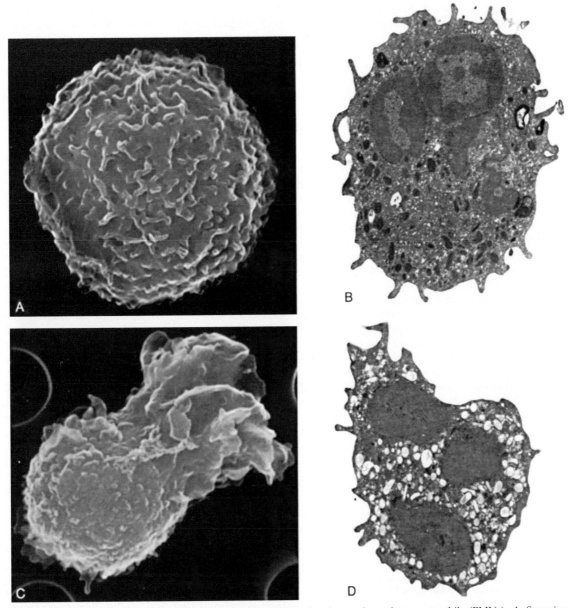

Figure 54–10. Normal and rheumatoid arthritis (RA) peripheral blood polymorphonuclear neutrophils (PMNs). *A,* Scanning electron micrograph (SEM) of a PMN from peripheral blood of a normal 73-year-old man (30,000×). It is characteristically apolar and spherical with surfaces completely covered by plasma membrane elaborated into irregular ridges or small ruffles. *B,* Transmission electron micrograph (TEM) of PMN from a normal man. The apolar cell has few phagocytic vacuoles but many undischarged electron-dense granules (19,800×). *C,* SEM of a PMN from peripheral blood of a 78-year-old woman with RA. This striking polarized appearance is much more common in rheumatoids than in normal individuals and suggests that the cells have been activated (19,200×). *D,* TEM of a PMN from peripheral blood of a 59-year-old woman with RA. This cell has many phagocytic vacuoles but relatively few undischarged electron-dense granules (17,500×). (From McCarthy DA, Holburn CM, Pell BK, et al: Scanning electron microscopy of rheumatoid arthritis peripheral blood polymorphonuclear leucocytes. Ann Rheum Dis 45:899, 1986. Courtesy of the publisher and the authors.)

Oxygen Radicals in Rheumatoid Arthritis

Because of the chemoattractant agents in synovial fluid and perhaps the lack of VLA-4, the polymorphonuclear leukocytes accumulate there rather than in the synovium itself. Among the other consequences of phagocytosis by these cells and their subsequent activation is production of free radicals of oxygen, including hypochlorite (OCl), superoxide anion, hydroxyl radical, and chloramines. Phagocytosis triggers a "respiratory burst" characterized by increased oxygen consumption, increased anaerobic glycolysis, and the generation of these oxygen radicals. Using chemiluminescence assays, it has been demonstrated that activation of the neutrophil myeloperoxidase-H_2O_2 system takes place at a vigorous rate in synovial fluids from patients with RA.[437] This oxidant stress may contribute to the cyclic, self-perpetuating nature of rheumatoid inflammation.

There could also be an important role for the oxygen radicals, especially when considering possible alterations in matrix and the enzymes that degrade it. It has been demonstrated that enzymatically generated superoxide radicals, reacting with hydrogen peroxide in vitro to produce hypochlorite (i.e., bleach), can depolymerize purified hyaluronic acid[438] and damage protease inhibitors allowing certain proteinases to act unabated.[377, 439] Reactive oxygen species can also cause DNA nicks and apoptosis, perhaps accounting for some of the evidence for DNA fragmentation observed in RA synovium.

There are many checks and balances in a system in which such potentially toxic elements are released in sites of inflammation. Oxygen radical scavengers should be protective in inflammation. Superoxide dismutase is a ubiquitous and important intracellular enzyme. It is protective against oxygen radical-mediated damage. Catalase, found in the cytoplasm of cells, reduces H_2O_2 to water. Glutathione peroxidase also detoxifies H_2O_2. Ceruloplasmin, a major copper-containing protein in serum, chemically scavenges superoxide radicals[440]; an acute phase reactant, it is found in elevated levels in rheumatoid arthritis. Sodium urate may have significant antioxidant properties. Copper-penicillamine complexes can reduce superoxide concentrations, and vitamin E can terminate free radical lipid peroxidative reactions affecting cell membranes.

Arachidonate Metabolites in Rheumatoid Arthritis

Accompanying activation of PMNs is the increased mobilization of membrane phospholipids in these cells to arachidonic acid and its subsequent oxidation by cyclooxygenase to prostaglandins and thromboxanes, or by lipoxygenases to leukotrienes. Although the stable prostaglandins (PGs), especially PGE_2, do produce vasodilation, cause increased vascular permeability, and are involved centrally in fever production, there is increasing evidence that they have significant anti-inflammatory activities as well. For example, stable PG can retard development of adjuvant arthritis,[441] and the drug misoprostol, a prostaglandin analogue, may have significant anti-inflammatory or immunomodulatory effects.[442] Physiologic concentrations of PGE_2 inhibit IFN-γ production by T cells, HLA-DR expression by macrophages, and T cell proliferation.[443, 177] Of course, the clinical improvement noted in patients treated with cyclooxygenase inhibitors implicates prostaglandins in the acute inflammatory responses in RA. The fact that many patients require second-line agents and that the bone destruction continues unabated despite near ablation of cyclooxygenase activity indicate that many other mediators are involved. Much of the data being generated about the effect of nonsteroid anti-inflammatory drugs (NSAIDs) on arachidonic acid metabolism and neutrophil function suggest that the principal mode of action of these drugs may be to inhibit neutrophil function through an effect on early events critical to activation of PMNs.[444]

As detailed in Chapter 19, leukotriene B_4 (LTB$_4$), rather than the prostaglandins, is currently receiving considerable attention as a proinflammatory product of neutrophil activation. It is chemotactic for neutrophils, eosinophils, and macrophages; it promotes neutrophil aggregation; it enhances neutrophil adherence to endothelium; and it enhances NK cell cytotoxic activity. Neutrophils become apoptotic or necrotic in the abyss of synovial fluid, having no means of easy exit from the joint. Metabolism of arachidonic acid into the pathway mediated by lipoxygenase is directly proportional to breakdown of these cells in the joint cavity; cell breakdown facilitates access of arachidonic acid to lipoxygenase from the cytosol.[445] It is of interest that peripheral blood PMNs from rheumatoid patients have an enhanced capacity for production of LTB$_4$ compared with similar cells from control groups.[446] No mechanism for this has been elucidated, and it is not known whether synovial fluid leukocytes have the same enhanced capacity for LTB$_4$ release. In murine collagen–induced arthritis, a specific LTB$_4$ antagonist significantly decreased paw swelling and joint destruction, suggesting a pivotal role for this potent chemoattractant.[447]

Therapeutic studies have given indirect support for the role of arachidonic acid metabolites in promoting the inflammation in rheumatoid arthritis. In a study from Boston and London, 12 patients with active RA supplemented their usual diet with 20 g of eicosapentaenoic acid (EPA) and docosahexaenoic acid, both found in fish oils.[448] Following this supplementation, the ratio of arachidonic acid to eicosapentaenoic acid in the patients' neutrophil cellular lipids decreased from 8:1 to 3:1, and the capacity of these cells to generate LTB$_4$ declined by one third. In addition, there was a significant decline in platelet-activating factor generation by mononuclear cells. Of interest, chemotactic response of the rheumatoid patients' neutrophils to agents such as LTB$_4$ was diminished before the study. It increased substantially during dietary supplementation with fish oil.

Complement in Rheumatoid Arthritis

The components and pathways involved in complement activation are described in Chapter 15. As in studies of lymphocyte function and in measures of inflammation, synovial fluid serves as a better index of complement metabolism in RA than does peripheral blood. The liver is the major source of complement synthesis in humans and passive transfer of serum proteins into effusions can account for some of the complement proteins found there. The synovial tissue also actively produces complement proteins.[449] Macrophages and fibroblasts can produce complement proteins under the influence of cytokines. IFN-γ induces C2,[450] whereas IL-1 and TNF-α increase C3 production.[451] In situ hybridization shows that C2 is expressed in the synovial intimal lining, whereas C3 appears to be produced by synovial sublining macrophages.[369] Northern blot analysis of synovial tissue shows that all complement genes from the classical pathway are expressed in RA synovium as well as normal synovium.[452] Despite local production of complement components, the activities of C4, C2, and C3 and total hemolytic complement in rheumatoid (seropositive) synovial effusions are lower than in synovial fluids from patients with other joint diseases.[453, 454] A low synovial fluid C3 level might be modestly predictive of more erosive disease.[455]

Using a sensitive solid phase radioimmunoassay to quantify the activation of the classical pathway of complement by rheumatoid factor, it has been demonstrated that IgM RF is a much more important determinant of complement activation than IgG RF in both sera and synovial fluids.[456] Combined with other data showing that there is an accelerated catabolism of C4 in RA, and that the presence of C4 fragments in the plasma of rheumatoid patients correlates with titers of IgM RF, the weight of evidence indicates a role in vivo for IgM RF in complement activation.[457]

The biologically active products of complement activation are probably the most important consequence of intra-articular complement consumption. Like proteinases from PMNs, these inflammatory components may build up in synovial fluid during acute inflammation. The potential for interaction between PMNs and the complement system is substantial. Neutrophil lysosomal lysates contain enzymatic activity capable of generating chemotactic activity (probably C5a) from fresh serum.[458] C5a, in addition to being a principal chemotactic factor in inflammatory effusions, is capable of mediating lysosomal release from human PMNs. This sets up one of many amplification loops in inflammatory synovial fluid.

Other Synovial Fluid Manifestations of Rheumatoid Inflammation

A number of diverse biologic activities and proteins have been assayed in rheumatoid synovial fluid. These include the following:

Enzymes

Both polymorphonuclear leukocytes and synovial lining cells contribute to the proteolytic activity found in synovial fluid. Neutral proteinases, collagenase, and elastase are present.[459–461] As with other active substances, there is an equilibrium between enzymes and their inhibitors. The net effect biologically or pathologically is the sum of these. For instance, it has been demonstrated that in rheumatoid synovial fluid free collagenolytic activity is not generally measurable unless the PMN count is greater than 50,000/mm^3. This might be related to the fact that in the higher cell counts seen in severe rheumatoid disease, inflammation from sepsis, or crystal synovitis, the protease inhibitors in synovial fluid (principally α2-macroglobulin and TIMP) are saturated and free enzyme activity can act on articular connective tissue.[459, 462] The direct effect of these enzymes on articular cartilage may be substantial and may augment the proteoglycan depletion in cartilage that is manifested early in rheumatoid inflammation.

Coagulation and Kinin System Activation

The role of the clotting system in fibrinolysis is well known, but it is also important to remember the interrelationships among the soluble mediators in synovial infusions. For example, activation of Hageman factor can be an initial step in kinin formation. Rheumatoid factor–IgG complexes activate kininogens, although RF and unaltered, nonassociated IgG do not.[463] Kallikrein activator and kininase are both present in human granulocytes, and kallikrein itself is a potent and versatile proteinase that can activate plasminogen to plasma, precursor to active Hageman factor, and latent to active synovial collagenase. Plasminogen-derived peptides also can have profound effects on angiogenesis; one recently described 38-kD plasminogen fragment called *angiostatin* is a potent inhibitor of blood vessel proliferation.[464]

The endpoint of activation of the clotting sequence is the formation of fibrin. The accumulation of fibrin is one of the most striking pathologic features of rheumatoid synovitis. Fibrin accumulates on the synovial surface, on cartilage surfaces, in areas of subsynovial hemorrhage or infarction, and as particulate aggregates in synovial fluid. At the final stages of fibrin formation, fibrinopeptides are formed (released from fibrinogen by the action of thrombin during clotting), which may have the capacity to increase vascular permeability. What initiates the clotting sequence? It has not been demonstrated that immune complexes of RF and IgG can do this,[465] but plasmin (activated by plasminogen activator from plasminogen) has the capability, as (possibly) does collagen. Production of procoagulant activity by mononuclear cells in culture is stimulated by immune complexes.[466]

The presence of fibrin on synovium and cartilage may impede normal nutrition to these tissues and may amplify conditions that lead to hypoxia and acidosis in synovial fluid. It is possible that, in addition to being entrapped in the collagen matrix, immune complexes may be caught up in fibrin clots within the joint space, a phenomenon that would perpetuate the inflammatory and proliferative disease. Like the build-up of other components of the inflammatory reaction, the accumulation of fibrin in joints reflects an imbalance caused by the inability of the joint lining to clear the large quantities of by-products of inflammation. In some rheumatoid joints a strong inhibition of fibrinolysis by plasmin has been observed, as well as diminished activity of plasminogen activator.[467]

References

1. Wolfe AM: The epidemiology of rheumatoid arthritis: A review. Bull Rheum Dis 19:518, 1968.
2. Mitchell DM, Fries JF: An analysis of the American Rheumatism Association criteria for rheumatoid arthritis. Arthritis Rheum 25:481, 1982.
3. Arnett FC, and committee: The American Rheumatism Association 1987 revised criteria for the classification of rheumatoid arthritis. Arthritis Rheum 31:315, 1988.
4. Stastny P: Mixed lymphocyte cultures in rheumatoid arthritis. J Clin Invest 57:1148, 1976.
5. McMichael AJ, Sasazuki T, McDevitt HO, Payne RO: Increased frequency of HLA-Cw3 and HLA-Dw4 in rheumatoid arthritis. Arthritis Rheum 30:1037, 1977.
6. Stastny P: Association of the B-cell alloantigen DRw4 with rheumatoid arthritis. N Engl J Med 298:869, 1978.
7. Gregersen PK, Shen M, Song QL, et al: Molecular diversity of HLA-DR4 haplotypes. Proc Natl Acad Sci U S A 83:2642, 1986.
8. Nepom GT, Byers P, Seyfried C, et al: HLA genes associated with rheumatoid arthritis: Identification of susceptibility alleles using specific oligonucleotide probes. Arthritis Rheum 32:15, 1989.
9. Weyand CM, Hicok KC, Conn DL, Goronzy JJ: The influence of HLA-DRB1 genes on disease severity in rheumatoid arthritis. Ann Intern Med 117:801, 1992.
10. Boki KA, Drosis AA, Tzioufas GA, Lanchbury JS, Panayi GS, Moutsopoulos HM: Examination of HLA-DR4 as a severity marker for rheumatoid arthritis in Greek patients. Ann Rheum Dis 52:517, 1993.
11. Calin A, Elswood J, Klouda PT: Destructive arthritis, rheumatoid factor, and HLA-DR4: Susceptibility versus severity, a case control study. Arthritis Rheum 32:1221, 1989.
12. Thomson W, Pepper L, Payton A, Carthy D, Scott D, Ollier W, Silman A, Symmons D: Absence of an association between HLA-DRB1*04 and rheumatoid arthritis in newly diagnosed cases from the community. Ann Rheum Dis 52:539, 1993.
13. Brown JH, Jardetzky TS, Gorga JC, Stern LJ, Urban RG, Strominger JL, Wiley DC: Three dimensional structure of the human class II histocompatability antigen HLA-DR1. Nature 364:33, 1993.
14. Moxley G: DNA polymorphism of immunoglobulin kappa confers risk of rheumatoid arthritis. Arthritis Rheum 32:634, 1989.
15. Parekh RB, Dwek RA, Sutton BJ, Fernandes DL, Leung A, Stanworth D, Rodemacher TW: Association of rheumatoid arthritis and primary osteoarthritis with changes in the glycosylation pattern of total serum IgG. Nature 316:452, 1985.
16. Schrohenloher RE, Tomana M, Koopman WJ, del Puente A, Bennett PH: Occurrence of IgG galactosylation deficiency prior to the onset of rheumatoid arthritis. Abstracts for Southeast region, American College of Rheumatology, April 1991.
17. Tsuchiya N, Endo T, Shiota M, Kochibe N, Ito K, Kobata A: Distribution of glycosylation abnormality among serum IgG subclasses from patients with rheumatoid arthritis. Clin Immunol Immunopathol 70:47, 1994.
18. Axford JS, Lydyard PM, Isenberg DA, MacKenzie L, Hay FC, Roitt IM: Reduced B-cell galactosyltransferase activity in rheumatoid arthritis. Lancet 2:1486, 1987.
19. Young A, Sumar N, Bodman K, Goyal S, Sinclair H, Roitt I, Isenberg D: Agalactosyl IgG: An aid to differential diagnosis in early synovitis. Arthritis Rheum 34:1425, 1991.
20. Rademacher TW, Williams P, Dwek RA: Agalactosyl glycoforms of IgG autoantibodies are pathogenic. Proc Natl Acad Sci U S A 91:6123, 1994.
21. Jacob CO, McDevitt HO: Tumour necrosis factor-alpha in murine auto-immune 'lupus' nephritis. Nature 331:356, 1988.
22. Jacob CO, Fronek Z, Lewis GD, Koo M, Hansen JA, McDevitt HO: Heritable major histocompatibility complex class II-associated differences in production of tumor necrosis factor alpha: Relevance to genetic predisposition to systemic lupus erythematosus. Proc Natl Acad Sci U S A 87:1233, 1990.
23. McDowell TL, Symons JA, Ploski R, Forre O, Duff G: A genetic association between juvenile rheumatoid arthritis and a novel interleukin-1α polymorphism. Arthritis Rheum 38:221, 1995.
24. Tarlow JK, Blakemore AI, Lennard A, Solari R, Hughes HN, Steinkasserer A, Duff GW: Polymorphism in human IL-1 receptor antagonist gene intron 2 is caused by variable numbers of an 86-bp tandem repeat. Hum Gen 91:403, 1993.
25. Sternberg EM, Hill JM, Chrousos GP, Kamilaris T, Listwak SJ, Gold PW, Wilder RL: Inflammatory mediator-induced hypothalamic-pituitary-adrenal axis activation is defective in streptococcal cell wall arthritis-susceptible Lewis rats. Proc Natl Acad Sci U S A 86:2374, 1989.
26. Chikanza IC, Petrou P, Kingsley G, Chrousos G, Panayi GS: Defective hypothalamic response to immune and inflammatory stimuli in patients with rheumatoid arthritis. Arthritis Rheum 35:1281, 1992.
27. Ahmed SA, Penhale WJ, Talal IN: Sex hormones, immune responses, and autoimmune diseases. Am J Pathol 121:431, 1985.
28. Buyon JP, Korchak HM, Rutherford LE, Ganguly M, Weissmann G: Female hormones reduce neutrophil responsiveness in vitro. Arthritis Rheum 27:623,1984.
29. Persellin RH: The effect of pregnancy on rheumatoid arthritis. Bull Rheum Dis 27:922, 1977.
30. Hench PS: The ameliorating effect of pregnancy on chronic atrophic (infectious rheumatoid) arthritis, fibrositis, and intermittent hydrarthrosis. Mayo Clin Proc 13:161, 1938.
31. Quinn C, Mulpeter K, Casey EB, Feighery CF: Changes in levels of IgM RF and alpha 2 PAG correlate with increased disease activity in rheumatoid arthritis during the puerperium. Scand J Rheumatol 22:273, 1993.
32. Lin H, Mosmann TR, Guilbert L, Tuntipopipat S, Wegmann TG: Synthesis of T helper 2–type cytokines at the maternal-fetal interface. J Immunol 151:4562, 1993.
33. Buzas EI, Hollo K, Rubliczky L, Garzo M, Nyirkos P, Glant TT: Effect of pregnancy on proteoglycan-induced progressive polyarthritis in BALB/c mice: Remission of disease activity. Clin Exp Immunol 94:252, 1993.
34. Combe B, Cosso B, Clot J, Bonneau M, Sany J: Human placenta-eluted gamma globulins in immunomodulating treatment of rheumatoid arthritis. Am J Med 78:920, 1985.
35. Nelson JL, Hughes KA, Smith AG, Nisperos BB, Branchaud AM, Hansen JA: Maternal-fetal disparity in HLA class II alloantigens and the pregnancy-induced amelioration of rheumatoid arthritis. N Eng J Med 329:466, 1993.
36. Hazes JM, Dijkmans BA, Vandenbroucke JP, de Vries RR, Cats A: Pregnancy and the risk of developing rheumatoid arthritis. Arthritis Rheum 33:1770, 1990.
37. Oka M: Effect of pregnancy on the onset and course of rheumatoid arthritis. Ann Rheum Dis 12:227, 1953.
38. Wingrave SJ, Kay CR: Reduction in incidence of rheumatoid arthritis associated with oral contraceptives. Lancet 1:569, 1978.
39. Vandenbroucke JP, Witteman JCM, Valkenburg HA, Boersma JW, Cats A, Festen JJM, Hartman AP, Huber-Bruning O, Rasker JJ, Weber J: Noncontraceptive hormones and rheumatoid arthritis in perimenopausal and postmenopausal women. JAMA 255:1299, 1986.
40. Hazes JM, Dijkmans BC, Vendenbroucke JP, de Vries RR, Cats A: Reduction of the risk of rheumatoid arthritis among women who take oral contraceptives. Arthritis Rheum 33:173, 1990.
41. Linos A, Worthington JW, O'Fallon WM, Kurland LT: The epidemiology of rheumatoid arthritis in Rochester, Minnesota: A study of incidence, prevalence, and mortality. Am J Epidemiol 111:87, 1980.
42. Linos A, Worthington JW, O'Fallon WM, Kurland LT: Case-control study of rheumatoid arthritis and prior use of oral contraceptives. Lancet 1:1299, 1983.
43. del Junco DJ, Annegers JF, Luthra HS, Coulam CB, Kurland LT: Do oral contraceptives prevent rheumatoid arthritis? JAMA 254:1938, 1985.
44. al-Daccak R, Mehindate K, Hebert J, Rink L, Mecheri S, Mourad W: Mycoplasma arthritidis-derived superantigen induces proinflammatory monokine gene expression in the THP-1 human monocytic cell line. Infect Immun 62:2409, 1994.
45. Cole BC, Griffiths MM: Triggering and exacerbation of autoimmune arthritis by the Mycoplasma arthritidis superantigen MAM. Arthritis Rheum 36:994, 1993.

46. Kloppenburg M, Breedveld FC, Terwiel JP, Mallee C, Dijkmans BA: Minocycline in active rheumatoid arthritis. A double-blind, placebo-controlled trial. Arthritis Rheum 37:629, 1994.

47. Barile MF, Yoshida H, Roth H: Rheumatoid arthritis: new findings on the failure to isolate or detect mycoplasmas by multiple cultivation or serologic procedures and a review of the literature. Rev Infect Dis 13:571, 1991.

48. Steere AC, Dwyer E, Winchester R: Association of chronic Lyme arthritis with HLA-DR4 and HLA-DR2 alleles. N Engl J Med 323:219, 1990.

49. Barthold SW, Sidman CL, Smith AL: Lyme borreliosis in genetically resistant and susceptible mice with severe combined immunodeficiency. Am J Trop Med Hyg 47:605, 1992.

50. Asch ES, Bujak DI, Weiss M, Peterson MG, Weinstein A: Lyme disease: An infectious and postinfectious syndrome. J Rheumatol 21:454, 1994.

51. Alspaugh MA, Tan EM: Antibodies to cellular antigens in Sjögren's syndrome. J Clin Invest 55:1067, 1975.

52. Tosato G, Steinberg AD, Yarchoan R, Heilman CA, Pike SE, De Seau V, Blaese RM: Abnormally elevated frequency of Epstein-Barr virus–infected B cells in the blood of patients with rheumatoid arthritis. J Clin Invest 73:1789, 1984.

53. Silverman SL, Schumacher HR: Antibodies to Epstein-Barr viral antigens in early rheumatoid arthritis. Arthritis Rheum 24:1465, 1981.

54. Alspaugh MA, Shoji H, Nonoyama M: A search for rheumatoid arthritis-associated nuclear antigen and Epstein-Barr virus specific antigens or genomes in tissues and cells from patients with rheumatoid arthritis. Arthritis Rheum 26:712, 1983.

55. Fox RI, Chilton T, Rhodes G, Vaughan JH: Lack of reactivity of rheumatoid arthritis synovial membrane DNA with cloned Epstein-Barr virus DNA probes. J Immunol 137:498, 1986.

56. Depper JM, Zvaifler NJ: Epstein-Barr virus. Its relationship to the pathogenesis of rheumatoid arthritis. Arthritis Rheum 24:755, 1981.

57. Slaughter L, Carson DA, Jensen FC, Holbrook TL, Vaughan JH: In vitro effects of Epstein-Barr virus on peripheral blood mononuclear cells from patients with rheumatoid arthritis and normal subjects. J Exp Med 148:1429, 1978.

58. Roudier J, Rhodes G, Petersen J, Vaughan JH, Carson DA: The Epstein-Barr virus glycoprotein gp110, a molecular link between HLA DR4, HLA DR1, and rheumatoid arthritis. Scand J Immunol 27:367, 1988.

59. Roudier J, Petersen J, Rhodes GH, et al: Susceptibility to rheumatoid arthritis maps to a T-cell epitope shared by the HLA-Dw4 DR beta-1 chain and the Epstein-Barr virus glycoprotein gp110. Proc Natl Acad Sci U S A 86:5104, 1989.

60. Albani S, Ravelli A, Massa M, De Benedetti F, Andree G, Roudier J, Martini A, Carson DA: Immune responses to the Escherichia coli dnaJ heat shock protein in juvenile rheumatoid arthritis and their correlation with disease activity. J Pediatr 124:561, 1994.

61. Simpson RW, McGinty L, Simon L, Smith DA, Godzeski CA, Boyd RJ: Assocation of parvoviruses with rheumatoid arthritis of humans. Science 223:1425, 1984.

62. Cohen BJ, Buckley MM, Clewley JP, Jones VE, Puttick AH, Jacoby RK: Human parvovirus infection in early rheumatoid and inflammatory arthritis. Ann Rheum Dis 45–832, 1986.

63. Naides SJ, Field EH: Transient rheumatoid factor positivity in acute human parvovirus B19 infection. Arch Intern Med 148:2587, 1988.

64. Saal JG, Steidle M, Einsele H, Muller CA, Fritz P, Zacher J: Persistence of B19 paravovirus in synovial membranes of patients with rheumatoid arthritis. Rheumatol Int 12:147, 1992.

65. Nikkari S, Luukkainen R, Mottonen T, Meurman O, Hannonen P, Skurnik M, Toivanen P: Does parvovirus B19 have a role in rheumatoid arthritis? Ann Rheum Dis 53:137, 1994.

66. Hajeer AH, MacGregor AJ, Rigby AS, Ollier WE, Carthy D, Silman AJ: Influence of previous exposure to human parvovirus B19 infection in explaining susceptibility to rheumatoid arthritis: An analysis of disease discordant twin pairs. Ann Rheum Dis 53:137, 1994.

67. Haase AT: Pathogenesis of lentivirus infections. Nature 322:130, 1986.

68. Narayan O, Sheffer D, Clements JE, Tennekoon G: Restricted replication of lentiviruses. Visna viruses induce a unique interferon during interaction between lymphocytes and infected macrophages. J Exp Med 162:1954, 1985.

69. Wilder RL: Hypothesis for retroviral causation of rheumatoid arthritis. Curr Opin Rheumatol 6:295, 1994.

70. di Giovine FS, Bailly S, Bootman J, Almond N, Duff GW: Absence of lentiviral and human T cell leukemia viral sequences in patients with rheumatoid arthritis. Arthritis Rheum 37:349, 1994.

71. Aicher WK, Heer AH, Trabandt A, Bridges SL Jr, Schroeder HW Jr, Gay RE, Eibel H, Peter HH, Siebenlist U, Koopman WJ, et al: Overexpression of zinc-finger transcription factor Z-225/Egr-1 in synoviocytes from rheumatoid arthritis patients. J Immunol 152:5940, 1994.

72. Yamamoto H, Sekiguchi T, Yamamoto I: Histopathological observation of joint lesions of extremities in mice transferred genome. Exp Toxicol Pathol 45:233, 1993.

73. Nakajima T, Aono H, Hasunuma T, Yamamoto K, Maruyama I, Nosaka T, Hatanaka M, Nishioka K: Overgrowth of human synovial cells driven by the human T cell leukemia virus type I tax gene. J Clin Invest 92:186, 1993.

74. Grahame R, Armstrong R, Simmons N, Wilton JMA, Dyson M, Laurent R, Millis R, Mims CA: Chronic arthritis associated with the presence of intrasynovial rubella virus. Ann Rheum Dis 42:2, 1983.

75. Kaufmann SHE: Heat-shock proteins: A link between rheumatoid arthritis and infection? Curr Opin Rheumatol 2:420, 1990.

76. van Eden W, Thole JE, van der Zee R, Noordzij A, van Embden JD, Hensen EJ: Cloning of the mycobacterial epitope recognized by T lymphocytes in adjuvant arthritis. Nature 331:171, 1988.

77. van Eden W, Holoshitz J, Nevo Z, Frenkel A, Klajman A, Cohen IR: Arthritis induced by a T-lymphocyte clone that responds to Mycobacterium tuberculosis and to cartilage proteoglycans. Proc Natl Acad Sci U S A 82:5117, 1985.

78. Tsoulfa G, Rook GA, Van-Embden JD, Young DB, Mehler A, Isenberg DA, Hay FC: Raised serum IgG and IgA antibodies to mycobacterial antigens in rheumatoid arthritis. Ann Rheum Dis 48:118, 1989.

79. Oda A, Miyata M, Kodama E, Satoh H, Sato Y, Nishimaki T, Nomaguchi H, Kasukawa R: Antibodies to 65 kD heat-shock protein were elevated in rheumatoid arthritis. Clin Rheumatol 13:261, 1994.

80. Gaston JSH, Life PF, Bailey LC, Bacon PA: In vitro responses to a 65-kilodalton mycobacterial protein by synovial T cells from inflammatory arthritis patients. J Immunol 143:2494, 1989.

81. Pope RM, Lovis RM, Gupta RS: Activation of synovial fluid T lymphocytes by 60-kd heat-shock proteins in patients with inflammatory synovitis. Arthritis Rheum 35:43, 1992.

82. Wilbrink B, Holewijn M, Bijlsma JW, van Roy JL, den Otter W, van Eden W: Suppression of human cartilage proteoglycan synthesis by rheumatoid synovial fluid mononuclear cells activated with mycobacterial 60-kd heat-shock protein. Arthritis Rheum 36:514, 1993.

83. Sharif M, Worrall JG, Singh B, Gupta RS, Lydyard PM, Lambert C, McCulloch J, Rook GA: The development of monoclonal antibodies to the human mitochondrial 60-kd heat-shock protein, and their use in studying the expression of the protein in rheumatoid arthritis. Arthritis Rheum 35:1427, 1992.

84. Mountz JD, Zhou T, Gay RE, Gay S, Blüthmann H, Edwards CK: T cell influence on superantigen-induced arthritis in MRL-lpr/lpr mice. Arthritis Rheum 37:113–24, 1994.

85. Stuart JM, Cremer MA, Townes AS, Kang AH: Type II collagen-induced arthritis in rats: Transfer with serum. J Exp Med 155:1, 1982.

86. Trentham DE, Dynesius RA, David JR: Passive transfer by cells of type II collagen–induced arthritis in rats. J Clin Invest 62:359, 1978.

87. Terato K, Hasty KA, Cremer MA, Stuart JM, Townes AS, Kang AH: Collagen-induced arthritis in mice: Localization of an arthritogenic determinant to a fragment of the type II collagen molecule. J Exp Med 162:637, 1985.

88. Wooley PH, Luthra HS, Stuart JM, David CS: Type II collagen–induced arthritis in mice: I. Major histocompatibility complex (I region) linkage and antibody correlates. J Exp Med 154:688, 1981.

89. Holmdahl R, Nordling C, Rubin K, Tarkowski A, Klareskog L: Generation of monoclonal rheumatoid factors after immunization with collagen II-anti-collagen immune complexes: An anti-idiotype antibody to anti-collagen II is also a rheumatoid factor. Scand J Immunol 24:197, 1986.

90. Klareskog L, Johnell O, Hulth A, Holmdahl R, Rubin K: Reactivity of monoclonal anti–idiotype II collagen antibodies with cartilage and synovial tissue in rheumatoid arthritis and osteoarthritis. Arthritis Rheum 29:1, 1986.

91. Terato K, Shimozuru Y, Katayama K, Takemitsu Y, Yamashita I, Miyatsu M, Fujii K, Sagara M, Kobayashi S, Goto M, Nishioka K, Miyasaka N, Nagai Y: Specificity of antibodies to type II collagen in rheumatoid arthritis. Arthritis Rheum 33:1493, 1990.

92. Rowley M, Tait B, Mackay IR, Cunningham T, Phillips B: Collagen antibodies in rheumatoid arthritis. Significance of antibodies to denatured collagen and their association with HLA-DR4. Arthritis Rheum 29:174, 1986.

93. Watson WC, Cremer MA, Wooley PH, Townes AS: Assessment of the potential pathogenicity of type II collagen autoantibodies in patients with rheumatoid arthritis. Arthritis Rheum 29:1316, 1986.

94. Jasin HE; Autoantibody specificities of immune complexes sequestered in articular cartilage of patients with rheumatoid arthritis and osteoarthritis. Arthritis Rheum 28:241, 1985.

95. Tarkowski A, Klareskog L, Carlsten H, Herberts P, Koopman WJ: Secretion of antibodies to types I and II collagen by synovial tissue cells in patients with rheumatoid arthritis. Arthritis Rheum 32:1087, 1989.

96. Good RA, Rotstein J, Mazzitello WF: The simultaneous occurrence of rheumatoid arthritis and agammaglobulinemia. J Lab Clin Med 49:343, 1957.

97. Kunkel HG, Agnello V, Jaslin FG, Winchester RJ, Capra JD: Cross-idiotypic specificity among monoclonal IgM proteins with anti-IgG activity. J Exp Med 137:331, 1973.

98. Bonagura VR, Wedgwood JF, Agostino N, Hatam L, Mendez L, Jaffe I, Pernis B: Seronegative rheumatoid arthritis, rheumatoid factor cross

reactive idiotype expression, and hidden rheumatoid factors. Ann Rheum Dis 48:488, 1989.

99. Carson DA, Chen PP, Kipps TJ: New roles for rheumatoid factor. J Ciln Invest 87:379, 1991.

100. Wernick RM, Lipsky PE, Marban-Arcos E, Maliakkal JJ, Edelbaum D, Ziff M: IgG and IgM rheumatoid factor synthesis in rheumatoid synovial membrane cell cultures. Arthritis Rheum 28:742, 1985.

101. Fong S, Chen PP, Gilbertson TA, Weber JR, Fox RI, Carson DA: Expression of three cross-reactive idiotypes on rheumatoid factor autoantibodies from patients with autoimmune diseases and seropositive adults. J Immunol 137:122, 1986.

102. Bouvet JP, Xin WJ, Pillot J: Restricted heterogeneity of polyclonal rheumatoid factor. Arthritis Rheum 30:998, 1987.

103. Lee SK, Bridges SL Jr, Koopman WJ, Schroeder HW Jr: The immunoglobulin kappa light chain repertoire expressed in the synovium of a patient with rheumatoid arthritis. Arthritis Rheum 35:905, 1992.

104. Poulter LW, Janossy G: The involvement of dendritic cells in chronic inflammatory disease. Scand J Immunol 21:401, 1985

105. Klareskog L, Forsum U, Scheynius A, Kabelitz D, Wigzell H: Evidence in support of a self-perpetuating HLA-DR-dependent delayed-type cell reaction in rheumatoid arthritis. Proc Natl Acad Sci U S A 79:3632, 1982.

106. Kurosaka M, Ziff J: Immunoelectron microscopic study of the distribution of T cell subsets in rheumatoid synovium. J Exp Med 158:1191, 1983.

107. Janossy G, Panayi GS, Duke O, Bofill M, Poulter LW, Goldstein G: Rheumatoid arthritis: A disease of T-lymphocyte/macrophage immunoregulation. Lancet 1:839, 1981.

108. Unanue ER, Allen PM: The basis for the immunoregulatory role of macrophanges and other accessory cells. Science 236:551, 1987.

109. Shiozawa S, Tanaka Y, Fujita T, Tokuhisa T: Destructive arthritis without lymphocyte infiltration in H2-c-fos transgenic mice. J Immunol 148:3100, 1992.

110. Ho WZ, Cherukuri R, Douglas SD: The macrophage and HIV-1. Immunol Ser 60:569–87, 1994.

111. Wegelius O, Laine V, Lindstrom B, Klockars M: Fistula of the thoracic duct as immunosuppressive treatment in rheumatoid arthritis. Acta Med Scand 187:539, 1970.

112. Wahl SM, Wilder RL, Katona IM, Wahl LM, Allen JB, Scher I, Decker JL: Leukapheresis in rheumatoid arthritis: Association of clinical improvement with reversal of anergy. Arthritis Rheum 26:1076, 1983.

113. Zvaifler NJ: Fractionated total lymphoid irradiation: A promising new treatment for rheumatoid arthritis? Yes, no, maybe. Arthritis Rheum 30:109, 1987.

114. Tanay A, Field EH, Hoppe RT, Strober S: Long-term followup of rheumatoid arthritis patients treated with total lymphoid irradiation. Arthritis Rheum 30:1, 1987.

115. Watts RA, Isaacs JD, Hale G, Hazleman BL, Waldmann H: CAMPATH-1H in inflammatory arthritis. Clin Exp Rheumatol 11 Suppl 8:S165, 1993.

116. Strand V, Lipsky PE, Cannon GW, Calabrese LH, Wiesenhutter C, Cohen SB, Olsen NJ, Lee ML, Lorenz TJ, Nelson B: Effects of administration of an anti-CD5 plus immunoconjugate in rheumatoid arthritis. Results of two phase II studies. The CD5 Plus Rheumatoid Arthritis Investigators Group. Arthritis Rheum 36:620, 1993.

117. Moreland LW, Pratt PW, Bucy RP, Jackson BS, Feldman JW, Koopman WJ: Treatment of refractory rheumatoid arthritis with a chimeric anti-CD4 monoclonal antibody. Long-term followup of CD4+ T cell counts. Arthritis Rheum 37:834, 1994.

118. van der Lubbe B, Dijkmans AC, Markusse HM, Nassander U, Breedveld FC: A randomized, double-blind, placebo-controlled study of CD4 monoclonal antibody treatment in early rheumatoid arthritis. Arthritis Rheum 38:1097, 1995.

119. Ruderman EM, Weinblatt ME, Thurmond LM, Pinkus GS, Gravallese EM: Synovial tissue response to treatment with CAMPATH-1H. Arthritis Rheum 38:254, 1995.

120. Wells G, Tugwell P: Cyclosporin A in rheumatoid arthritis: Overview of efficacy. Brit J Rheum 32(suppl 1):51, 1993.

121. Sewell KL, Parker KC, Woodworth TG, Reuben J, Swartz W, Trentham DE: DAB486IL-2 fusion toxin in refractory rheumatoid arthritis. Arthritis Rheum 36:1223, 1993.

122. Luyten F, Suykens S, Veys EM, Van Lerbeirghe J, Ackerman C, Mielants H, Verbruggen G: Peripheral blood T lymphocyte subpopulations determined by monoclonal antibodies in active rheumatoid arthritis. J Rheumatol 13:864, 1986.

123. Goto M, Miyamoto T, Nishioka K, Okumura KO: Selective loss of suppressor T cells in rheumatoid arthritis patients: Analysis of peripheral blood lymphocytes by 2-dimensional flow cytometry. J Rheumatol 13:853, 1986.

124. Cush JJ, Lipsky PE: Phenotypic analysis of synovial tissue and peripheral blood lymphocytes isolated from patients with rheumatoid arthritis. Arthritis Rheum 31:1230, 1988.

125. Laffon A, Garcia-Vicuna R, Humbria A, Postigo AA, Corbi AL, de Landazuri MO, Sanchez-Madrid F: Upregulated expression and function of VLA-4 fibronectin receptors on human activated T cells in rheumatoid arthritis. J Clin Invest 88:546, 1991.

126. Lamour A, Jouen-Beades F, Lees O, Gilbert D, Le Loet X, Tron F: Analysis of T cell receptors in rheumatoid arthritis: The increased expression of HLA-DR antigen on circulating gamma delta+ T cells is correlated with disease activity. Clin Exp Immunol 89:217, 1992.

127. Dooley RM, Cush JJ, Lipsky PE, Dawson DV, Pisetsky DS: The effects of nonsteroidal antiinflammatory drug therapy in early rheumatoid arthritis on serum levels of soluble interleukin 2 receptor, CD4, and CD8. J Rheumatol 20:1857, 1993.

128. Hemler ME, Glass D, Coblyn JS, Jacobson JG: Very late activation antigens on rheumatoid synovial fluid T lymphocytes. Association with stages of T cell activation. J Clin Invest 78:696, 1986.

129. Verwilghen J, Lovis R, De Boer M, Linsley PS, Haines GK, Koch AE, Pope RM: Expression of functional B7 and CTLA4 on rheumatoid synovial T cells. J Immunol 153:1378, 1994.

130. Keystone EC, Snow KM, Bombardier C, Chang CH, Nelson DL, Rubin LA: Elevated soluble interleukin-2 receptor levels in the sera and synovial fluids of patients with rheumatoid arthritis. Arthritis Rheum 31:844, 1988.

131. Tosato G, Steinberg AD, Blaese RM: Defective EBV-specific suppressor T-cell function in rheumatoid arthritis. N Engl J Med 305:1238, 1981.

132. Depper JM, Bluestein HG, Zvaifler NJ: Impaired regulation of Epstein-Barr virus-induced lymphocyte proliferation in rheumatoid arthritis is due to a T cell defect. J Immunol 127:1899, 1981.

133. Gaston JSH, Rickinson AB, Yao QY, Epstein MA: The abnormal cytotoxic T cell response to Epstein-Barr virus in rheumatoid arthritis is correlated with disease activity and occurs in other arthropaties. Ann Rheum Dis 45:932, 1986.

134. Hasler F, Bluestein HG, Zvaifler NJ, Epstein LB: Analysis of the defects responsible for the impaired regulation of EBV-induced B cell proliferation by rheumatoid arthritis lymphocytes: II. Role of monocytes and the increased sensitivity of rheumatoid arthritis lymphocytes to prostaglandin E. J Immunol 131:768, 1983.

135. Combe B, Pope RM, Fischbach M, Darnell B, Baron S, Talal N: Interleukin 2 in rheumatoid arthritis: Production of and response to interleukin 2 in rheumatoid synovial fluid, synovial tissue, and peripheral blood. Clin Exp Immunol 59:520, 1985.

136. Hasler F, Dayer JM: Diminished IL-2-induced gamma-interferon production by unstimulated peripheral-blood lymphocytes in rheumatoid arthritis. B J Rheumatol 27:15, 1988.

137. Fox RI, Fong S, Sabharwal N, Carstens SA, Kung PC, Vaughan JH: Synovial fluid lymphocytes differ from peripheral blood lymphocytes in patients with rheumatoid arthritis. J Immunol 128:351, 1982.

138. Lasky HP, Bauer K, Pope RM: Increased helper inducer and decreased suppressor inducer phenotypes in the rheumatoid joint. Arthritis Rheum 31:52, 1988.

139. Pitzalis C, Kingsley G, Murphy J, Panayi G: Abnormal distribution of the helper-inducer and suppressor-inducer T-lymphocyte subsets in the rheumatoid joint. Clin Immunol Immunopathol 45:252, 1987.

140. Nouri AME, Panayi GS: Cytokines and the chronic inflammation of rheumatic disease: III. Deficient interleukin-2 production in rheumatoid arthritis is not due to suppressor mechanisms. J Rheumatol 14:902, 1987.

141. Eisenberg SP, Evans RJ, Arend WP, Verderber E, Brewer MT, Hannum CH, Thompson RC: Primary structure and functional expression from complementary DNA of a human interleukin-1 receptor antagonist. Nature 343:341, 1990.

142. Arend WP, Welgus HG, Thompson RC, Eisenberg SP: Biological properties of recombinant human monocyte-derived interleukin 1 receptor antagonist. J Clin Invest 85:1694, 1990.

143. Wahl SM, Allen JB, Wong HL, Dougherty SF, Ellingsworth LR: Antagonistic and agonistic effects of transforming growth factor-beta and IL-1 in rheumatoid synovium. J Immunol 145:2514, 1990.

144. Firestein GS, Berger AE, Tracey DE, Chosay JG, Chapman DL, Paine MM, Yu C, Zvaifler NJ: IL-1 receptor antagonist protein production and gene expression in rheumatoid arthritis and osteoarthritis synovium. J Immunol 149:1054, 1992.

145. Grom AA, Thompson SD, Luyrink L, Passo M, Choi E, Glass DN: Dominant T-cell-receptor beta chain variable region V beta 14+ clones in juvenile rheumatoid arthritis. Proc Natl Acad Sci U S A 90:11104, 1993.

146. Paliard X, West SG, Lafferty JA, Clements JR, Kappler JW, Marrack P, Kotzin BL: Evidence for the effects of a superantigen in rheumatoid arthritis. Science 253:325, 1991.

147. Howell MD, Diveley JP, Lundeen KA, Esty A, Winters ST, Carlo DJ, Brostoff SW: Limited T-cell receptor beta-chain heterogeneity among interleukin 2 receptor-positive synovial T cells suggests a role for superantigen in rheumatoid arthritis. Proc Natl Acad Sci U S A 88:10921, 1991.

148. Jenkins RN, Nikaein A, Zimmermann A, Meek K, Lipsky PE: T cell receptor V beta gene bias in rheumatoid arthritis. J Clin Invest 92:2688, 1993.

149. Keystone EC, Minden M, Klock R, Poplonski L, Zalcberg J, Takadera T, Mak TW: Structure of T cell antigen receptor beta chain in synovial fluid cells from patients with rheumatoid arthritis. Arthritis Rheum 31:1555, 1988.

150. Brennan FM, Allard S, Londei M, Savill C, Boylston A, Carrel S, Maini RN, Feldmann M: Heterogeneity of T cell receptor idiotypes in rheumatoid arthritis. Clin Exper Immunol 73:417, 1988.

151. Savill CM, Delves PJ, Kioussis D, Walker P, Lydyard PM, Colaco B, Shipley M, Roitt IM: A minority of patients with rheumatoid arthritis show a dominant rearrangement of T-cell receptor beta chain genes in synovial lymphocytes. Scand J Immunol 25:629, 1987.

152. Duby AD, Sinclair AK, Osborne-Lawrence SL, Zeldes W, Kan L, Fox DA: Clonal heterogeneity of synovial fluid T lymphocytes in patients with rheumatoid arthritis. Proc Natl Acad Sci U S A. 86:6206, 1989.

153. Uematsu Y, Wege H, Straus A, Ott M, Bannwarth W, Lanchbury J, Panayi G, Steinmetz M: The T-cell-receptor repertoire in the synovial fluid of a patient with rheumatoid arthritis is polyclonal. Proc Natl Acad Sci U S A. 88:8534, 1991.

154. Pluschke G, Ricken G, Taube H, Kroninger S, Melchers I, Peter HH, Eichmann K, Krawinkel U: Biased T cell receptor V alpha region repertoire in the synovial fluid of rheumatoid arthritis patients. Eur J Immunol 21:2749, 1991.

155. Olive C, Gatenby PA, Serjeantson SW: Analysis of T cell receptor V alpha and V beta gene usage in synovia of patients with rheumatoid arthritis. Immunol Cell Biol 69:349, 1991.

156. Karin N, Szafer F, Mitchell D, Gold DP, Steinman L: Selective and nonselective stages in homing of T lymphocytes to the central nervous system during experimental allergic encephalomyelitis. J Immunol 150:4116, 1993.

157. Holoshitz J, Koning F, Coligan JE, DeBruyn J, Strober S: Isolation of CD4- CD8-mycobacteria-reactive T lymphocyte clones from rheumatoid arthritis synovial fluid. Nature 339:226, 1989.

158. Olive C, Gatenby PA, Serjeantson SW: Evidence for oligoclonality of T cell receptor delta chain transcripts expressed in rheumatoid arthritis patients. Eur J Immunol 22:2587, 1992.

159. Schumacher HR, Kitridou RC: Synovitis of recent onset. A clinicopathological study during the first month of disease. Arthritis Rheum 15:465, 1972.

160. Ziff M: Relation of cellular infiltration of rheumatoid synovial membrane to its immune response. Arthritis Rheum 17:313, 1974.

161. Haynes BF, Grover BJ, Whichard LP, Hale LP, Nunley JA, McCollum DE, Singer KH: Synovial microenvironment-T cell interactions: Human T cells bind to fibroblast-like synovial cells in vitro. Arthritis Rheum 31:947, 1988.

162. van Boxel JJ, Paget SA: Predominantly T-cell infiltrate in rheumatoid synovial membranes. N Engl J Med 293:517, 1975.

163. Konttinen YT, Reitamo S, Ranki A, Hayry P, Kankaanpaa U, Wegelius O: Characterization of the immunocompetent cells of rheumatoid synovium from tissue sections and eluates. Arthritis Rheum 24:71, 1981.

164. Duke O, Panayi GS, Janossy G, Poulter LW: An immunohistological analysis of lymphocyte subpopulations and their microenvironment in the synovial membranes of patients with rheumatoid arthritis using monoclonal antibodies. Clin Exp Immunol 49:22, 1982.

165. Poulter LW, Duke O, Panayi GS, Hobbs S, Raftery MJ, Janossy G: Activated T lymphocytes of the synovial membrane in rheumatoid arthritis and other arthropathies. Scand J Immunol 22:683, 1985.

166. Nakao H, Eguchi K, Kawakami A, Migita K, Otsubo T, Ueki Y, Shimomura C, Tezuka H, Matsunaga M, Maeda K, Nagataki S: Phenotypic characterization of lymphocytes infiltrating synovial tissue from patients with rheumatoid arthritis: Analysis of lymphocytes isolated from minced synovial tissue by dual immunofluorescent staining. J Rheumatol 17:142, 1990.

167. Laffon A, Garcia-Vicuna R, Humbria A, Postigo AA, Corbi AL, de Landazuri MO, Sanchez-Madrid F: Upregulated expression and function of VLA-4 fibronectin receptors on human activated T cells in rheumatoid arthritis. J Clin Invest 88:546, 1991.

168. Postigo AA, Garcia-Vicuna R, Diaz-Gonzalez F, Arroyo AG, De Landazuri MO, Chi-Rosso G, Lobb RR, Laffon A, Sanchez-Madrid F: Increased binding of synovial T lymphocytes from rheumatoid arthritis to endothelial-leukocyte adhesion molecule-1 (ELAM-1) and vascular cell adhesion molecule-1 (VCAM-1). J Clin Invest 89:1445, 1992.

169. Nykanen P, Bergroth V, Raunio P, Nordstrom D, Konttinen VT: Phenotypic characterization of 3H-thymidine incorporating cells in rheumatoid arthritis synovial membrane. Rheumatol Intl 6:269, 1986.

170. Firestein GS, Zvaifler NJ: How important are T cells in chronic rheumatoid synovitis? Arthritis Rheum 33:768, 1990.

171. Nathan CF: Secretory products of macrophages. J Clin Invest 79:319, 1987.

172. Crowe PD, VanArsdale TL, Walter BN, Ware CF, Hession C, Ehrenfels B, Browning JL, Din WS, Goodwin RG, Smith CA: A lymphotoxin-beta-specific receptor. Science 264:707, 1994.

173. Firestein GS, Zvaifler NJ: Down regulation of human monocyte differentiation antigens by gamma interferon. Cell Immunol 104:343, 1987.

174. Thornhill MH, Kyan-Aung U, Lee TH, Haskard DO: T cells and neutrophils exhibit differential adhesion to cytokine-stimulated endothelial cells. Immunol 69:287, 1990.

175. Thornhill MH, Haskard DO: IL-4 regulates endothelial cell activation by IL-1, tumor necrosis factor, or IFN-gamma. J Immunol 145:865, 1990.

176. Hooks JJ, Moutsopoulos HM, Geis SA, Stahl NI, Decker JL, Notkins AL: Immune interferon in the circulation of patients with autoimmune diseases. N Engl J Med 301:5, 1985.

177. Firestein GS, Zvaifler NJ: Peripheral blood and synovial fluid monocyte activation in inflammatory arthritis: II. Low levels of synovial fluid and synovial tissue interferon suggest that γ-interferon is not the primary macrophage activating factor. Arthritis Rheum 30:864, 1987.

178. Chen E, Keystone EC, Fish EN: Restricted cytokine expression in rheumatoid arthritis. Arthritis Rheum 36:901, 1993.

179. Bergroth V, Zvaifler NJ, Firestein GS: Cytokines in chronic inflammatory arthritis: III. Rheumatoid arthritis monocytes are not unusually sensitive to γ-interferon, but have defective γ-interferon-mediated HLA-DQ and HLA-DR induction. Arthritis Rheum 32:1074, 1989.

180. Barnes PF, Fong SJ, Brennan PJ, Twomey PE, Mazumder A, Modin RL: Local production of tumor necrosis factor and IFN-γ in tuberculous pleuritis. J Immunol 145:149, 1990.

181. Duncan MR, Berman B: γ Interferon is the lymphokine and β interferon the monokine responsible for inhibition of fibroblast collagen production and late but not early fibroblast proliferation. J Exp Med 162:516, 1985.

182. Granstein RD, Murphy GF, Margolis RJ, Byrne MH, Amento EP: Gamma-interferon inhibits collagen synthesis in vivo in the mouse. J Clin Invest 79:1254, 1987.

183. Stephenson ML, Krane SM, Amento EP, McCroskery PA, Byrne M: Immune interferon inhibits collagen synthesis by rheumatoid synovial cells associated with decreased levels of the procollagen mRNAs. FEBS Lett 180:43, 1985.

184. Alvaro-Gracia JM, Zvaifler NJ, Firestein GS: Cytokines in chronic inflammatory arthritis. V. Mutual antagonism between interferon-gamma and tumor necrosis factor-alpha on HLA-DR expression, proliferation, collagenase production, and granulocyte macrophage colony-stimulating factor production by rheumatoid arthritis synoviocytes. J Clin Invest 86:1790, 1990.

185. Unemori EN, Bair MJ, Bauer EA, Amento EP: Stromelysin expression regulates collagenase activation in human fibroblasts: Dissociable control of two metalloproteinases by interferon-gamma. J Biol Chem 266:23477, 1991.

186. Alvaro-Gracia JM, Yu C, Zvaifler NJ, Firestein GS: Mutual antagonism between interferon-gamma and tumor necrosis factor-alpha on fibroblast-like synoviocytes: Paradoxal induction of IFN-gamma and TNF-alpha receptor expression. J Clin Immunol 13:212, 1993.

187. Chin JE, Winterrowd GE, Krzesicki RF, Sanders ME: Role of cytokines in inflammatory synovitis: The coordinate regulation of intercellular adhesion molecule 1 and HLA class I and class II antigens in rheumatoid synovial fibroblasts. Arthritis Rheum 33:1776, 1990.

188. Morales-Ducret J, Wayner E, Elices MJ, Alvaro-Gracia JM, Zvaifler NJ, Firestein GS: Alpha 4/beta 1 integrin (VLA-4) ligands in arthritis: Vascular cell adhesion molecule expression in synovium and on fibroblast-like synoviocytes. J Immunol 149:1424, 1992.

189. Alvaro-Gracia JM, Zvaifler NJ, Firestein GS: Cytokines in chronic inflammatory arthritis: IV. Granulocyte/macrophage colony-stimulating factor-mediated induction of class II MHC antigen on human monocytes: A possible role in rheumatoid arthritis. J Exp Med 170:865, 1989.

190. Cannon GW, Emkey RD, Denes A, Cohen SA, Saway PA, Wolfe F, Jaffer AM, Weaver AL, Manaster BJ, McCarthy KA: Prospective 5-year followup of recombinant interferon-gamma in rheumatoid arthritis. J Rheumatol 20:1867, 1993.

191. Doketer WH, Esselink MT, Halie MR, Vellenga E: Interleukin-4 inhibits the lipopolysaccharide-induced expression of c-jun and c-fos messenger RNA and activator protein-1 binding activity in human monocytes. Blood 81:337, 1993.

192. Deleuran B, Iversen L, Kristensen M, Field M, Kragballe K, Thestrup-Pedersen K, Stengaard-Pedersen K: Interleukin-8 secretion and 15-lipoxygenase activity in rheumatoid arthritis: in vitro anti-inflammatory effects by interleukin-4 and interleukin-10, but not by interleukin-1 receptor antagonist protein. Br J Rheumatol 33:520, 1994.

193. Ruschen S, Lemm G, Warnatz H: Interleukin-2 secretion by synovial fluid lymphocytes in rheumatoid arthritis. Br J Rheumatol 27:350, 1988.

194. Firestein GS, Xu WD, Townsend K, Broide D, Alvaro-Gracia J, Glasebrook A, Zvaifler NJ: Cytokines in chronic inflammatory arthritis: I. Failure to detect T cell lymphokines (interleukin 2 and interleukin 3) and presence of macrophage colony-stimulating factor (CSF-1) and a novel mast cell growth factor in rheumatoid synovitis. J Exp Med 168:1573, 1988.

195. Miossec P, Navillat M, Dupuy d'Angeac A, Sany J, Banchereau J: Low levels of interleukin-4 and high levels of transforming growth factor beta in rheumatoid arthritis. Arthritis Rheum 145:2514, 1990.

196. Husby G, Williams RC Jr: Immunohistochemical studies of interleukin-2 and interferon-γ in rheumatoid arthritis. Arthritis Rheum 28:174, 1985.

197. Broide DH, Lotz M, Cuomo AJ, Coburn DA, Federman EC, Wasserman SI: Cytokines in symptomatic asthma airways. J Allergy Clin Immunol 89:958, 1992.

198. Broide DH, Firestein GS: Endobronchial allergen challenge in asthma:

Demonstration of cellular source of granulocyte macrophage colony-stimulating factor by in situ hybridization. J Clin Invest 88:1048, 1991.

199. Simon AK, Seipelt E, Sieper J: Divergent T-cell cytokine patterns in inflammatory arthritis. Proc Natl Acad Sci U S A 91:8562, 1994.

200. Cambell IL, Kay TWH, Oxbrow L, Harrision LC: Essential role for interferon-gamma and interleukin 6 in autoimmune insulin-dependent diabetes in NOD/WEHI mice. J Clin Invest 87:739, 1991.

201. Pettipher ER, Higgs GA, Henderson B: Interleukin 1 induces leukocyte infiltration and cartilage proteoglycan degradation in the synovial joint. Proc Natl Acad Sci U S A 83:8749, 1986.

202. Shore A, Jaglal S, Keystone EC: Enhanced interleukin 1 generation by monocytes in vitro is temporally linked to an early event in the onset or exacerbation of rheumatoid arthritis. Clin Exp Immunol 65:293, 1986.

203. Poubelle P, Damon M, Blotman F, Dayer J-M: Production of mononuclear cell factor by mononuclear phagocytes from rheumatoid synovial fluid. J Rheumatol 12:412, 1985.

204. Chin J, Rupp E, Cameron PM, MacNaul KL, Lotke PA, Tocci MJ, Schmidt JA, Bayne EK: Identification of a high-affinity receptor for interleukin 1α and interleukin 1β on cultured human rheumatoid synovial cells. J Clin Invest 82:420, 1988.

205. Tiku K, Tiku MS, Skosey JL: Interleukin 1 production by human polymorphonuclear neutrophils. J Immunol 136:3677, 1986.

206. Miossec P, Ziff M: Immune interferon enhances the production of interleukin 1 by human endothelial cells stimulated with lipopolysaccharide. J Immunol 137:2848, 1986.

207. Firestein GS, Alvaro-Gracia JM, Maki R: Quantitative analysis of cytokine gene expression in rheumatoid arthritis. J Immunol 144:3347, 1990.

208. Miyasaka N, Sato K, Goto M, Sasano M, Natsuyama M, Inoue K, Nishioka K: Augmented interleukin-1 production and HLA-DR expression in the synovium of rheumatoid arthritis patients: Possible involvement in joint destruction. Arthritis Rheum 31:480, 1988.

209. Dayer J-M, Passwell HJ, Schneeberger EE, Krane SM: Interactions among rheumatoid synovial cells and monocyte-macrophhages: Production of collagenase-stimulating factor by human monocytes exposed to concanavalin A or immunoglobulin Fc fragments. J Immunol 124:1712, 1980.

210. Dayer JM, Ricard-Blum S, Kaufman MT, Herbage D: Type IX collagen is a potent inducer of PGE$_2$ and interleukin 1 production by human monocyte macrophages. FEBS Lett 198:208, 1986.

211. Dayer JM, Goldring SR, Robinson DR, et al: Cell-cell interactions and collagenase production. In Wooley DE, Evanson JM (eds): Collagenase in Normal and Pathological Connective Tissues. New York, John Wiley & Sons 1980, p. 873.

212. Wood DD, Ihrie EJ, Hamerman D: Release of interleukin-1 from human synovial tissue in vitro. Arthritis Rheum 28:853, 1985.

213. Morrissey PJ, Bressler L, Park LS, Alpert A, Gillis S: Granulocyte-macrophage colony-stimulating factor augments the primary antibody response by enhancing the function of antigen-presenting cells. J Immunol 139:1113, 1987.

214. Postlethwaite AE, Lachman LB, Kang AH: Induction of fibroblast proliferation by interleukin-1 derived from human monocytic leukemia cells. Arthritis Rheum 27:995, 1984.

215. Yaron I, Meyer FA, Dayer JM, Yaron M: Human recombinant interleukin-1β stimulates glycosaminoglycan production in human synovial fibroblast cultures. Arthritis Rheum 30:424, 1987.

216. Tyler JA: Articular cartilage cultured with catabolin (pig interleukin 1) synthesizes a decreased number of normal proteoglycan molecules. Biochem J 227:869, 1985.

217. Mochan E, Uhl J, Newton R: Interleukin 1 stimulation of synovial cell plasminogen activator production. J Rheumatol 13:15, 1986.

218. Dewhirst FE, Stashenko PP, Mole JE, Tsurumachi T: Purification and particle sequence of human osteoclast-activating factor: Identify with interleukin 1β. J Immunol 135:2562, 1985.

219. Miossec P, Dinarello CA, Ziff M: Interleukin-1 lymphocyte chemotactic activity in rheumatoid arthritis synovial fluid. Arthritis Rheum 29:461, 1986.

220. Dayer JM, Beutler B, Cerami A: Cachectin/tumor necrosis factor stimulates collagenase and prostaglandin E$_2$ production by human synovial cells and dermal fibroblasts. J Exp Med 162:2163, 1985.

221. Bertolini DR, Nedwin GE, Bringman TS, Smith DD, Mundy GR: Stimulation of bone resorption and inhibition of bone formation in vitro by human tumour necrosis factors. Nature 319:516, 1986.

222. Saklatvala J: Tumour necrosis factor α stimulates resorption and inhibits synthesis of proteoglycan in cartilage. Nature 322:547, 1986.

223. Williams RO, Mason LJ, Feldmann M, Maini RN: Synergy between anti-CD4 and anti-tumor necrosis factor in the amelioration of established collagen-induced arthritis. Proc Natl Acad Sci U S A 91:2762, 1994.

224. Elliott MJ, Maini RN, Feldmann M, Long-Fox A, Charles P, Bijl H, Woody JN: Repeated therapy with monoclonal antibody to tumour necrosis factor alpha (cA2) in patients with rheumatoid arthritis. Lancet 344:1125, 1994.

225. Guerne PA, Zuraw BL, Vaughan JH, Carson DA, Lotz M: Synovium as a source of interleukin 6 in vitro: Contribution to local and systemic manifestations of arthritis. J Clin Invest 83:585, 1989.

226. Gauldie J, Richards C, Harnish D, Landsdorp P, Baumann H: Interferon β$_2$/BSF-2 shares identity with monocyte derived hepatocyte stimulating factor (HSF) and regulates the major acute phase protein response in liver cells. Proc Natl Acad Sci U S A 84:7251, 1987.

227. Houssiau FA, Devogelaer J-P, van Damme J, Nagant de Deuxchaisnes C, van Snick J: Interleukin-6 in synovial fluid and serum of patients with rheumatoid arthritis and other inflammatory arthritides. Arthritis Rheum 31:784, 1988.

228. Guerne PA, Zuraw BL, Vaughan JH, Carson DA, Lotz M: Synovium as a source of interleukin 6 in vitro: Contribution to local and systemic manifestations of arthritis. J Clin Invest 83:585, 1989.

229. Field M, Chu C, Feldman M, Maini RN: Interleukin-6 localisation in the synovial membrane in rheumatoid arthritis. Rheumatol Intl 11:45, 1991.

230. Xu WD, Firestein GS, Taetle R, Kaushansky K, Zvaifler NJ: Cytokines in chronic inflammatory arthritis: II. Granulocyte-macrophage colony-stimulating factor in rheumatoid synovial effusions. J Clin Invest 83:876, 1989.

231. Alvaro-Gracia JM, Zvaifler NJ, Brown CB, Kaushansky K, Firestein GS: Cytokines in chronic inflammatory arthritis: VI. Analysis of the synovial cells involved in granulocyte-macrophage colony-stimulating factor production and gene expression in rheumatoid arthritis and its regulation by IL-1 and tumor necrosis factor-alpha. J Immunol 146:3365, 1991.

232. Koch AE, Kunkel SL, Burrows JC, Evanoff HL, Haines GK, Pope RM, Strieter RM: Synovial tissue macrophage as a source of the chemotactic cytokine IL-8. J Immunol 147:2187, 1991.

233. Koch AE, Polverini PJ, Kunkel SL, Harlow LA, DiPietro LA, Elner VM, Elner SG, Strieter RM: Interleukin-8 as a macrophage-derived mediator of angiogenesis. Science 258:1798, 1992.

234. Koch AE, Kunkel SL, Harlow LA, Johnson B, Evanoff HL, Haines GK, Burdick MD, Pope RM, Strieter RM: Enhanced production of monocyte chemoattractant protein-1 in rheumatoid arthritis. J Clin Invest 90:772, 1992.

235. Hosaka S, Akahoshi T, Wada C, Kondo H: Expression of the chemokine superfamily in rheumatoid arthritis. Clin Exper Immunol 97:451, 1994.

236. Koch AE, Kunkel SL, Harlow LA, Mazarakis DD, Haines GK, Burdick MD, Pope RM, Walz A, Strieter RM: Epithelial neutrophil activating peptide-78: A novel chemotactic cytokine for neutrophils in arthritis. J Clin Invest 94:1012, 1994.

237. Rathanaswami P, Hachicha M, Sadick M, Schall TJ, McColl SR: Expression of the cytokine RANTES in human rheumatoid arthritis synovial fibroblasts: Differential regulation of RANTES and interleukin-8 genes by inflammatory cytokines. J Biol Chem 268:5834, 1993.

238. Edwards DR, Murphy G, Reynolds JJ, Whitham SE, Docherty AJP, Angel P, Heath JK: Transforming growth factor beta modulates the expression of collagenase and metalloproteinase inhibitor. EMBO J 6:1899, 1987.

239. Broide DH, Wasserman SI, Alvaro-Gracia J, Zvaifler NJ, Firestein GS: Transforming growth factor-beta 1 selectively inhibits IL-3-dependent mast cell proliferation without affecting mast cell function or differentiation. J Immunol 143:1591, 1989.

240. Mustoe TA, Pierce GF, Thomason A, Gramates P, Sporn MB, Deuel TF: Accelerated healing of incisional wounds in rats induced by transforming growth factor-β. Science 237:1333, 1987.

241. Roberts AB, Sporn MB, Assoian RK, Smith JM, Roche NS, Wakefield LM, Heine UI, Liotta LA, Falanga V, Kehrl JH, Fauci AS: Transforming growth factor type β: Rapid induction of fibrosis and angiogenesis in vivo and stimulation of collagen formation in vitro. Proc Natl Acad Sci U S A 83:4167, 1986.

242. Lafyatis R, Thompson NL, Remmers EF, Flanders KC, Roche NS, Kim SJ, Case JP, Sporn MB, Roberts AB, Wilder RL: Transforming growth factor-beta production by synovial tissues from rheumatoid patients and streptococcal cell wall arthritic rats: Studies on secretion by synovial fibroblast-like cells and immunohistologic localization. J Immunol 143:1142, 1989.

243. Fava R, Olsen N, Keski-Oja J, Moses H, Pincus T: Active and latent forms of transforming growth factor beta activity in synovial effusions. J Exp Med 169:291, 1989.

244. Allen JB, Manthey CL, Hand AR, Ohura K, Ellingsworth L, Wahl SM: Rapid onset synovial inflammation and hyperplasia induced by transforming growth factor beta. J Exp Med 171:231, 1990.

245. Brandes ME, Allen JB, Ogawa Y, Wahl SM: Transforming growth factor beta 1 suppresses acute and chronic arthritis in experimental animals. J Clin Invest 87:1108, 1991.

246. Wahl SM, Allen JB, Costa GL, Wong HL, Dasch JR: Reversal of acute and chronic synovial inflammation by anti-transforming growth factor beta. J Exp Med 177:225, 1993.

247. Doolittle RF, Hunkapiller MW, Hood LE, Devare SG, Robbins SA, Antoniades HN: Simian sarcoma virus oncogene, v-sis, is derived from the gene (or genes) encoding a platelet-derived growth factor. Science 221:275, 1983.

248. Bauer EA, Cooper TW, Huang JS, Altman J, Deuel TF: Stimulation of in vitro human skin collagenase expression by platelet-derived growth factor. Proc Natl Acad Sci U S A 82:4132, 1985.

249. Remmers EF, Lafyatis R, Kumkumian GK, Case JP, Roberts AB, Sporn MB, Wilder RL: Cytokines and growth regulation of synoviocytes from patients with rheumatoid arthritis and rats with streptococcal cell wall arthritis. Growth Factors 2:179, 1990.

250. Goddard DH, Grossman SL, Williams WV, Weiner DB, Gross JL, Eidsvoog K, Dasc JR: Regulation of synovial cell growth: Coexpression of transforming growth factor beta and basic fibroblast growth factor by cultured synovial cells. Arthritis Rheum 35:1296, 1992.

251. Remmers EF, Sano H, Lafyatis R, Case JP, Kumkumian GK, Hla T, Maciag T, Wilder RL: Production of platelet derived growth factor B chain (PDGF-B/c-sis) mRNA and immunoreactive PDGF B-like polypeptide by rheumatoid synovium: Coexpression with heparin binding acidic fibroblast growth factor-1. J Rheumatol 18:7, 1991.

252. Reuterdahl C, Tingstrom A, Terracio L, Funa K, Heldin CH, Rubin K: Characterization of platelet-derived growth factor beta-receptor expressing cells in the vasculature of human rheumatoid synovium. Lab Invest 64:321, 1991.

253. Folkman J, Klagsbrun M: Angiogenic factors. Science 235:442, 1987.

254. Thompson JA, Anderson KD, DiPietro JM, Zwiebel JA, Zametta M, Anderson WF, Maciag T: Site-directed neovessel formation in vivo. Science 241:1349, 1988.

255. Yayon A, Klagsbrun M, Esko JD, Leder P, Ornitz DM: Cell surface, heparin-like molecules are required for binding of basic fibroblast growth factor to its high affinity receptor. Cell 64:841, 1991.

256. Montesano R, Vassalli JD, Baird A, Guillemin R, Orci L: Basic fibroblast growth factor induces angiogenesis in vitro. Proc Natl Acad Sci U S A 83:7297, 1986.

257. Herron GS, Banda MJ, Clark EJ, Gavrilovic J, Werb Z: Secretion of metalloproteinases by stimulated capillary endothelial cells: II. Expression of collagenase and stromelysin activities is regulated by endogenous inhibitors. J Biol Chem 261:2814, 1986.

258. Sano H, Forough R, Maier JAM, Case JP, Jackson A, Engleka K, Maciag T, Wilder RL: Detection of high levels of heparin binding growth factor-1 (acidic fibroblast growth factor) in inflammatory arthritic joints. J Cell Biol 110:1417, 1990.

259. Melnyk VO, Shipley GD, Sternfeld MD, Sherman L, Rosenbaum JT: Synoviocytes synthesize, bind, and respond to basic fibroblast growth factor. Arthritis Rheum 33:493, 1990.

260. Castor CW, Miller JW, Waltz DA: Structural and biological characteristics of connective tissue activating peptide (CTAP-III): A major human platelet-derived growth factor. Proc Natl Acad Sci U S A 80:765, 1983.

261. Lotz M, Moats T, Villiger PM: Leukemia inhibitory factor is expressed in cartilage and synovium and can contribute to the pathogenesis of arthritis. J Clin Invest 90:888, 1992.

262. Waring PM, Carroll GJ, Kandiah DA, Buirski G, Metcalf D: Increased levels of leukemia inhibitory factor in synovial fluid from patients with rheumatoid arthritis and other inflammatory arthritides. Arthritis Rheum 36:911, 1993.

263. Metcalf D: The induction and inhibition of differentiation in normal and leukaemic cells. Philos Trans R Soc Lond B Biol Sci 327:99, 1990.

264. Cornish J, Callon K, King A, Edgar S, Reid IR: The effect of leukemia inhibitory factor on bone in vivo. Endocrinology 132:1359, 1993.

265. Miossec P, Chomarat P, Dechanet J, Moreau JF, Roux JP, Delmas P, Bancherau J: Interleukin-4 inhibits bone resorption through an effect on osteoclasts and proinflammatory cytokines in an ex vivo model of bone resorption in rheumatoid arthritis. Arthritis Rheum 37:1715, 1994.

266. Levine JD, Goetzl EJ, Basbaum AI: Contribution of the nervous system to the pathophysiology of rheumatoid arthritis and other polyarthritides. Rheum Dis Clin N Amer 13:369, 1987.

267. Lotz M, Carson DA, Vaughan JH: Substance P activation of rheumatoid synoviocytes: Neural pathway in pathogenesis of arthritis. Science 235:893, 1987.

268. Lotz M, Vaughan JH, Carson DA: Effect of neuropeptides on production of inflammatory cytokines by human monocytes. Science 241:1218, 1988.

269. Gronblad M, Konttinen VT, Korkala O, Liesi P, Hukkanen M, Polak JM: Neuropeptides in synovium of patients with rheumatoid arthritis and osteoarthritis. J Rheumatol 15:1807, 1988.

270. Kuis W, Villiger PM, Leser HG, Lotz M: Differential processing of proenkephalin-A by human peripheral blood monocytes and T lymphocytes. J Clin Invest 88:817, 1991.

271. Arend WP: Interleukin 1 receptor antagonist: A new member of the interleukin 1 family. J Clin Invest 88:1445, 1991.

272. Dripps DJ, Brandhuber BJ, Thompson RC, Eisenberg SP: Interleukin-1 (IL-1) receptor antagonist binds to the 80-kDa IL-1 receptor but does not initiate IL-1 signal transduction. J Biol Chem 266:10331, 1991.

273. Henderson B, Thompson RC, Hardingham T, Lewthwaite J: Inhibition of interleukin-1-induced synovitis and articular cartilage proteoglycan loss in the rabbit knee by recombinant human interleukin-1 receptor antagonist. Cytokine 3:246, 1991.

274. Lewthwaite J, Blake SM, Hardingham TE, Warden PJ, Henderson B: The effect of recombinant human interleukin 1 receptor antagonist on the induction phase of antigen induced arthritis in the rabbit. J Rheumatol 21:467, 1994.

275. Haskill S, Martin G, Van Le L, Morris J, Peace A, Bigler CF, Jaffe GJ, Hammerberg C, Sporn SA, Fong S, et al: cDNA cloning of an intracellular form of the human interleukin 1 receptor antagonist associated with epithelium. Proc Natl Acad Sci U S A 88:3681, 1991.

276. Arend WP, Smith MF Jr, Janson RW, Joslin FG: IL-1 receptor antagonist and IL-1 beta production in human monocytes are regulated differently. J Immunol 147:1530, 1991.

277. Malyak M, Swaney RE, Arend WP: Levels of synovial fluid interleukin-1 receptor antagonist in rheumatoid arthritis and other arthropathies. Potential contribution from synovial fluid neutrophils. Arthritis Rheum 36:781, 1993.

278. Malyak M, Smith MF Jr, Abel AA, Arend WP: Peripheral blood neutrophil production of interleukin-1 receptor antagonist and interleukin-1 beta. J Clin Immunol 14:20, 1994.

279. Firestein GS, Berger AE, Tracey DE, Chosay JG, Chapman DL, Paine MM, Yu C, Zvaifler NJ: IL-1 receptor antagonist protein production and gene expression in rheumatoid arthritis and osteoarthritis synovium. J Immunol 149:1054, 1992.

280. Deleuran BW, Chu CQ, Field M, Brennan FM, Katsikis P, Feldmann M, Maini RN: Localization of interleukin-1 alpha, type 1 interleukin-1 receptor and interleukin-1 receptor antagonist in the synovial membrane and cartilage/pannus junction in rheumatoid arthritis. Br J Rheum 31:801, 1992.

281. Firestein GS, Boyle DL, Yu C, Paine MM, Whisenand TD, Zvaifler NJ, Arend WP: Synovial interleukin-1 receptor antagonist and interleukin-1 balance in rheumatoid arthritis. Arthritis Rheum 37:644, 1994.

282. Moore KW, O'Garra A, de Waal Malefyt R, Vieira P, Mosmann TR: Interleukin-10. Annu Rev Immunol 11:165, 1993.

283. Holaday BJ, Pompeu MM, Jeronimo S, Texeira MJ, Sousa A de A, Vasconcelos AW, Pearson RD, Abrams JS, Locksley RM: Potential role for interleukin-10 in the immunosuppression associated with kala azar. J Clin Invest 92:2626, 1993.

284. Vieira P, de Waal-Malefyt R, Dang MN, Johnson KE, Kastelein R, Fiorentino DF, deVries JE, Roncarolo MG, Mosmann TR, Moore KW: Isolation and expression of human cytokine synthesis inhibitory factor cDNA clones: Homology to Epstein-Barr virus open reading frame BCRFI. Proc Natl Acad Sci U S A 88:1172, 1991.

285. Katsikis KD, Chu CQ, Brennan FM, Maini RN, Feldmann M: Immunoregulatory role of interleukin 10 in rheumatoid arthritis. J Exp Med 179:1517, 1994.

286. Cush JJ, Splawski JB, Ranjeny T, McFarlin JE, Schulze-Koops H, Davis LS, Fujita K, Lipsky PE: Elevated interleukin-10 levels in patients with rheumatoid arthritis. Arthritis Rheum 38:96, 1995.

287. Harvey AK, Hrubey PS, Chandrasekhar S: Transforming growth factor-beta inhibition of interleukin-1 activity involves down-regulation of interleukin-1 receptors on chondrocytes. Exp Cell Res 195:376, 1991.

288. Symons JA, Eastgate JA, Duff GW: Purification and characterization of a novel soluble receptor for interleukin 1. J Exp Med 174:1251, 1991.

289. Arend WP, Malyak M, Smith MF Jr, Whisenand TD, Slack JL, Sims JE, Giri JG, Dower SK: Binding of IL-1 alpha, IL-1 beta, and IL-1 receptor antagonist by soluble IL-1 receptors and levels of soluble IL-1 receptors in synovial fluids. J Immunol 153:4766, 1994.

290. Cope AP, Aderka D, Doherty M, Engelmann H, Gibbons D, Jones AC, Brennan FM, Maini RN, Wallach D, Feldmann M: Increased levels of soluble tumor necrosis factor receptors in the sera and synovial fluid of patients with rheumatic diseases. Arthritis Rheum 35:1160, 1992.

291. Brennan FM, Gibbons DL, Mitchell T, Cope AP, Maini RN, Feldmann M: Enhanced expression of tumor necrosis factor receptor mRNA and protein in mononuclear cells insolated from rheumatoid arthritis synovial joints. Eur J Immunol 22:1907, 1992.

292. Kulka JP, Blocking D, Ropes MW, Bauer W: Early joint lesions of rheumatoid arthritis. Arch Pathol 59:129, 1955.

293. Peacock DJ, Banquerigo ML, Brahn E: Angiogenesis inhibition suppresses collagen arthritis. J Exp Med 175:1135, 1992.

294. Stevens CR, Blake DR, Merry P, Revell PA, Levick JR: A comparative study by morphometry of the microvasculature in normal and rheumatoid synovium. Arthritis Rheum 34:1508, 1991.

295. Falchuk H, Goetzl J, Kulka P: Respiratory gases of synovial fluids. Am J Med 49:223, 1970.

296. Lund-Olesen K: Oxygen tension in synovial fluids. Arthritis Rheum 13:769, 1970.

297. Treuhaft PS, McCarty DJ: Synovial fluid pH, lactate, oxygen and carbon dioxide partial pressures in various joint diseases. Arthritis Rheum 14:475, 1971.

298. Jayson MIV, Dixon AStJ: Intra-articular pressure in rheumatoid arthritis of the knee. Ann Rheum Dis 29:261, 1970.

299. Jayson MIV, Dixon AStJ: Intra-articular pressure in rheumatoid arthritis of the knee: II. Effect of intra-articular pressure on blood circulation to the synovium. Ann Rheum Dis 29:266, 1970.

300. Wallis WJ, Simkin PA, Nelp WB: Low synovial clearance of iodide provides evidence of hypoperfusion in chronic rheumatoid synovitis. Arthritis Rheum 28:1096, 1985.

301. Kulka JP: Vascular derangement in rheumatoid arthritis. In Hill AGS

(ed): Modern Trends in Rheumatology. London, Butterworths, 1961, p 49.

302. Dingle JTM, Page-Thomas DP: In vitro studies in human synovial membrane: A metabolic comparison of normal and rheumatoid disease. Br J Exp Pathol 37:318, 1956.

303. Shweiki D, Itin A, Soffer D, Keshet E: Vascular endothelial growth factor induced by hypoxia may mediate hypoxia-initiated angiogenesis. Nature 359:843, 1992.

304. Fava RA, Olsen NJ, Spencer-Green G, Yeo KT, Berse B, Jackman RW, Senger DR, Dvorak HF, Brown LF: Vascular permeability factor/endothelial growth factor (VPF/VEGF): accumulation and expression in human synovial fluids and rheumatoid synovial tissue. J Exp Med 180:341, 1994.

305. Koch AE, Harlow LA, Haines GK, Amento EP, Unemori EN, Wong WL, Pope RM, Ferrara N: Vascular endothelial growth factor: A cytokine modulating endothelial function in rheumatoid arthritis. J Immunol 152:4149, 1994.

306. Unemori EN, Ferrara N, Bauer EA, Amento EP: Vascular endothelial growth factor induces interstitial collagenase expression in human endothelial cells. J Cell Physiol 153:557, 1992.

307. Maione TE, Gray GS, Petro J, Hunt AJ, Donner AL, Bauer SI, Carson HF, Sharpe RJ: Inhibition of angiogenesis by recombinant human platelet factor-4 and related peptides. Science 247:77, 1990.

308. Koch AE, Friedman J, Burrows JC, Haines GK, Bouck NP: Localization of the angiogenesis inhibitor thrombospondin in human synovial tissues. Pathobiology, 61:1, 1993.

309. Kushner I, Somerville JA: Permeability of human synovial membrane to plasma proteins: Relationship to molecular size and inflammation. Arthritis Rheum 14:560, 1971.

310. Wallis WJ, Simkin PA, Nelp WB: Protein traffic in human synovial effusions. Arthritis Rheum 30:57, 1987.

311. Picker LJ, Warnock RA, Burns AR, Doerschuk CM, Berg EL, Butcher EC: The neutrophil selectin LECAM-1 presents carbohydrate ligands to the vascular selectins ELAM-1 and GMP-140. Cell 66:921, 1991.

312. Butcher EC: Leukocyte-endothelial cell recognition: three (or more) steps to specificity and diversity. Cell 67:1033, 1991.

313. Hale LP, Martin ME, McCollum DE, Nunley JA, Springer TA, Singer KH, Haynes BF: Immunohistologic analysis of the distribution of cell adhesion molecules within the inflammatory synovial microenvironment. Arthritis Rheum 32:22, 1989.

314. Tuckwell DS, Weston SA, Humphries MJ: Integrins: A review of their structure and mechanisms of ligand binding. Symp Soc Exp Biol 47:107, 1993.

315. Chuluyan HE, Issekutz AC: VLA-4 integrin can mediate CD11/CD18-independent transendothelial migration of human monocytes. J Clin Invest 92:2768, 1993.

316. Hemler ME: VLA proteins in the integrin family: Structures, functions, and their role on leukocytes. Annu Rev Immunol 8:365, 1990.

317. Elices MJ, Osborn L, Takada Y, Crouse C, Lubowskyj S, Hemler ME, Lobb R: VCAM-1 on activated endothelium interacts with the leukocyte integrin VLA-4 at a site distinct from the VLA-4/fibronectin binding site. Cell 60:577, 1990.

318. Guan JL, Hynes RO: Lymphoid cells recognize an alternatively spliced segment of fibronectin via the integrin receptor α4β1. Cell 60:53, 1990.

319. Masumoto A, Hemler ME: Multiple activation states of VLA-4: Mechanistic differences between adhesion to CS1/fibronectin and to vascular cell adhesion molecule-1. J Biol Chem 268:228, 1993.

320. Issekutz TB, Issekutz AC: T lymphocyte migration to arthritic joints and dermal inflammation in the rat: Differing migration patterns and the involvement of VLA-4. Clin Immunol Immunopathol 61:436, 1991.

321. Wahl SM, Allen JB, Hines KL, Imamichi T, Wahl AM, Furcht LT, McCarthy JB: Synthetic fibronectin peptides suppress arthritis in rats by interrupting leukocyte adhesion and recruitment. J Clin Invest 94:655, 1994.

322. Laffon A, Garcia-Vicuna R, Humbria A, Postigo AA, Corbi AL, de Landazuri MO, Sanchez-Madrid F: Upregulated expression and function of VLA-4 fibronectin receptors on human activated T cells in rheumatoid arthritis. J Clin Invest 88:546, 1992.

323. van Dinther-Janssen AC, Pals ST, Scheper RJ, Meijer CJ: Role of the CS1 adhesion motif of fibronectin in T cell adhesion to synovial membrane and peripheral lymph node endothelium. Ann Rheum Dis 52:672, 1993.

324. Elices MJ, Tsai V, Strahl D, Goel A, Tollefson V, Arrhenius T, Wayner E, Gaeta F, Fikes J, Firestein GS: Expression and functional significance of alternatively spliced CS1 fibronectin in rheumatoid arthritis microvasculature. J Clin Invest 93:405, 1994.

325. Berg EL, Goldstein LA, Jutila MA, Nakache M, Picker LJ, Streeter PR, Butcher EI: Human receptor and vascular adressins: Cell surface molecules that direct lymphocyte traffic. Immunol Rev 108:5, 1989.

326. Jorgensen C, Travaglio-Encinoza A, Bologna C: Human mucosal lymphocyte marker expression in synovial fluid lymphocytes of patients with rheumatoid arthritis. J Rheumatol 21:1602, 1994.

327. Koch AE, Burrows JC, Haines GK, Carlos TM, Harlan JM, Leibovich SJ: Immunolocalization of endothelial and leukocyte adhesion molecules

in human rheumatoid and osteoarthritic synovial tissues. Lab Invest 64:313, 1991.

328. Corkill MM, Kirkham BW, Haskard DO, Barbatis C, Gibson T, Panayi GS: Gold treatment of rheumatoid arthritis decreases synovial expression of the endothelial leukocyte adhesion receptor ELAM-1. J Rheumatol 18:1453, 1991.

329. Fox DA, Smith BR: Evidence for oligoclonal B cell expansion in the peripheral blood of patients with rheumatoid arthritis. Ann Rheum Dis 45:991, 1986.

330. Lipsky PE: The control of antibody production by immunomodulatory molecules. Arthritis Rheum 32:1345, 1989.

331. Burastero SE, Casali P, Wilder RL, Notkins AL: Monoreactive high affinity and polyreactive low affinity rheumatoid factors are produced by CD5+ B cells from patients with rheumatoid arthritis. J Exp Med 168:1979, 1988.

332. Hardy RR, Hayakawa K, Shimizu M, Yamasaki K, Kishimoto T: Rheumatoid factor secretion from human Leu-1+ B cells. Science 236:81, 1987.

333. Mitchell LC, Davis LS, Lipsky PE: Promotion of human T lymphocyte proliferation by IL-4. J Immunol 142:1548, 1989.

334. Thyphronitis G, Tsokos GC, June CH, Levine AD, Finkelman FD: IgE secretion by Epstein-Barr virus-infected purified human B lymphocytes is stimulated by interleukin 4 and suppressed by interferon gamma. Proc Natl Acad Sci U S A, 86:5580, 1989.

335. Patel V, Panayi GS: Enhanced T helper cell function for the spontaneous production of IgM rheumatoid factor in vitro in rheumatoid arthritis. Clin Exp Immunol 57:584, 1984.

336. Poupart P, Vandenabeele P, Cayphas S, Van Snick J, Haegeman G, Kruys V, Fiers W, Content J: B cell growth modulating and differentiating activity of recombinant human 26-kd protein (BSF-2, HuIFN-beta 2, HPGF). EMBO J 6:1219, 1987.

337. Cats A, Hazevoet HM: Significance of positive tests for rheumatoid factor in the prognosis of rheumatoid arthritis. Ann Rheum Dis 29:254, 1970.

338. Tanimoto K, Cooper NR, Johnson JS, Vaughan JH: Complement fixation by rheumatoid factor. J Clin Invest 55:437, 1975.

339. Pope RM, Teller DC, Mannik M: The molecular basis of self-association of antibodies to IgG (rheumatoid factor) in rheumatoid arthritis. Proc Natl Acad Sci U S A 71:517, 1974.

340. Rodman WS, Williams RC Jr, Bilka PJ, Muller-Eberhard HJ: Immunofluorescent localization of the third and fourth component of complement in synovial tissues from patients with rheumatoid arthritis. J Lab Clin Med 69:141, 1967.

341. Zvaifler NJ: Immunopathology of joint inflammation in rheumatoid arthritis. Immunology 16:265, 1973.

342. Theofilopoulos AN, Burtonboy G, LoSpalluto JJ, Ziff M: IgM rheumatoid factor and low molecular weight IgM: An association with vasculitis. Arthritis Rheum 17:272, 1977.

343. Allen C, Elson CJ, Scott DGI, Bacon PA, Bucknall RC: IgG antiglobulins in rheumatoid arthritis and other arthritides: Relationship with clinical features and other parameters. Ann Rheum Dis 40:127, 1981.

344. Rawson AJ, Hollander JL, Quismorio FP, Abelson NM: Experimental arthritis in man and rabbit dependent upon serum anti-immunoglobulin factors. Ann N Y Acad Sci 168:188, 1969.

345. Henney CS, Stanworth DR, Gell PGH: Demonstration of the exposure of new antigenic determinants following antigen-antibody combination. Nature 205:1079, 1965.

346. Johnson PM, Watkins J, Scopes PM, Tracey BM: Differences in serum IgG structures in health and rheumatoid disease. Ann Rheum Dis 33:366, 1974.

347. Zuran BL, O'Hair CH, Vaughan JH, Mathison DA, Curd JG, Katz DH: Immunoglobulin E-rheumatoid factor in the serum of patients with rheumatoid arthritis, asthma, and other diseases. J Clin Invest 68:1610, 1981.

348. Metetey K, Falus A, Erhardt CC, Maini RN: IgE and IgE-rheumatoid factors in circulating immune complexes in rheumatoid arthritis. Ann Rheum Dis 41:405, 1982.

349. Crisp AJ, Chapman CM, Kirkhan S, Schiller AL, Krane SM: Synovial mastocytosis in adult rheumatoid arthritis. Arthritis Rheum 26:552, 1983.

350. Paquet-Gioud M, Auvinet M, Raffin T, Girard P, Bouvier M, Lejeune E, Monier JC: IgG rheumatoid factor (RF), IgA RF, IgE RF, and IgG RF detected by ELISA in rheumatoid arthritis. Ann Rheum Dis 46:65, 1987.

351. Esser RE, Angelo RA, Murphey MD, Watts LM, Thornburg LP, Palmer JT, Talhouk JW, Smith RE: Cysteine proteinase inhibitors decrease articular cartilage and bone destruction in chronic inflammatory arthritis. Arthritis Rheum 37:236, 1994.

352. Yodlowski ML, Hubbard JR, Kispert J, Keller K, Sledge CB, Steinberg JJ: Antibody to interleukin 1 inhibits the cartilage degradative and thymocyte proliferative actions of rheumatoid synovial culture medium. J Rheumatol 17:1600, 1990.

353. Lotz M, Guerne PA: Interleukin-6 induces the synthesis of tissue inhibitor of metalloproteinases-1/erythroid potentiating activity (TIMP-1/EPA). J Biol Chem 266:2017, 1991.

354. Overall CM, Wrana JL, Sodek J: Independent regulation of collagenase, 72-kDa progelatinase, and metalloendoproteinase inhibitor expression in human fibroblasts by transforming growth factor-beta. J Biol Chem 264:1860, 1989.

355. Gunther M, Haubeck HD, van de Leur E, Blaser J, Bender S, Gutgemann I, Fischer DC, Tschesche H, Greiling H, Heinrich PC, et al: Transforming growth factor beta 1 regulates tissue inhibitor of metalloproteinases-1 expression in differentiated human articular chondrocytes. Arthritis Rheum 37:395, 1994.

356. Raghu G, Masta S, Meyers D, Narayanan AS: Collagen synthesis by normal and fibrotic human lung fibroblasts and the effect of transforming growth factor-beta. Am Rev Resp Dis 140:95, 1989.

357. Werb Z, Aggeler J: Proteases induce secretion of collagenase and plasminogen activator by fibroblasts. Proc Natl Acad Sci U S A 75:1839, 1978.

358. Werb Z, Reynolds JJ: Stimulation by endocytosis of the secretion of collagenase and neutral proteinase from rabbit synovial fibroblasts. J Exp Med 140:1482, 1974.

359. Okazaki I, Brinckerhoff CE, Sinclaire JF, Sinclaire PR, Bonkowsky HL, Harris ED Jr: Iron increases collagenase production by rabbit synovial fibroblasts. J Lab Clin Med 97:396, 1981.

360. Fisher WD, Golds EE, van der Rest M, Cooke TD, Lyons HE, Poole AR: Stimulation of collagenase secretion from rheumatoid synovial tissue by human collagen peptides. J Bone Joint Surg Am 64:546, 1982.

361. Hasselbacher P, McMillan RM, Vater CA, Hahn J, Harris ED Jr: Stimulation of secretion of collagenase and prostaglandin E_2 by synovial fibroblasts in response to crystals of monosodium urate monohydrate: A model for joint destruction in gout. Trans Assoc Am Physicians 94:243, 1981.

362. Cheung HS, Halverson PB, McCarty DJ: Release of collagenase, neutral proteinase, and prostaglandins from cultured mammalian synovial cells by hydroxyapatite and calcium pyrophosphate dihydrate crystals. Arthritis Rheum 24:1338, 1981.

363. Unemori EN, Hibbs MS, Amento EP: Constitutive expression of a 92-kD gelatinase (type V collagenase) by rheumatoid synovial fibroblasts and its induction in normal human fibroblasts by inflammatory cytokines. J Clin Invest 88:1656, 1991.

364. Bohmann D, Bos TJ, Admon A, Nishimura T, Vogt PK, Tjian R: Human proto-oncogene c-jun encodes a DNA binding protein with structural and functional properties of transcription factor AP-1. Science 238:1386, 1987.

365. Yang-Yen HF, Chambard JC, Sun VL, Smeal T, Schmidt TJ, Drouin J, Karin M: Transcriptional interference between c-Jun and the glucocorticoid receptor: Mutual inhibition of DNA binding due to direct protein-protein interaction. Cell 62:1205, 1990.

366. Evanson JM, Jeffrey JJ, Krane SM: Human collagenase: Identification and characterization of an enzyme from rheumatoid synovium in culture. Science 158:499, 1967.

367. McCroskery PA, Wood S Jr, Harris ED Jr: Gelatin: A poor substrate for a mammalian collagenase. Science 182:70, 1973.

368. Welgus HG, Jeffrey JJ, Stricklin GP, Roswit WT, Eisen AZ: Characteristics of the action of human skin fibroblast collagenase on fibrillar collagen. J Biol Chem 255:6806, 1980.

369. Firestein GS, Paine MM, Littman BH: Gene expression (collagenase, tissue inhibitor of metalloproteinases, complement, and HLA-DR) in rheumatoid arthritis and osteoarthritis synovium: Quantitative analysis and effect of intraarticular corticosteroids. Arthritis Rheum 34:1094, 1991.

370. McCachren SS, Haynes BF, Niedel JE: Localization of collagenase mRNA in rheumatoid arthritis synovium by in situ hybridization histochemistry. J Clin Immunol 10:19, 1990.

371. Okada Y, Gonoji Y, Nakanishi I, Nagase H, Hayakawa T: Immunohistochemical demonstration of collagenase and tissue inhibitor of metalloproteinases (TIMP) in synovial lining cells of rheumatoid synovium. Virchows Arch 59:305, 1990.

372. Zvaifler NJ, Boyle D, Firestein GS: Early synovitis—Synoviocytes and mononuclear cells. Semin Arthritis Rheum 23 (Suppl 2):11–16, 1994.

373. Okada Y, Nagase H, Harris ED Jr: A metalloproteinase from human rheumatoid synovial fibroblasts that digests connective tissue matrix components: Purification and characterization. J Biol Chem 261:14245, 1986.

374. Okada Y, Konomi H, Yada T, Kimata K, Nagase H: Degradation of type IX collagen by matrix metalloproteinase 3 (stromelysin) from human rheumatoid synovial cells. FEBS Lett 244:473, 1989.

375. Gravallese EM, Darling JM, Ladd AL, Katz JN, Glimcher LH: In situ hybridization studies of stromelysin and collagenase messenger RNA expression in rheumatoid synovium. Arthritis Rheum 34:1076, 1991.

376. Eisen AA, Bauer EA, Stricklin GP, Seltzer JL, Koob TJ, Jeffrey JJ: Control of human skin collagenase activity. In McCabe BF, Sade J, Abramson M (eds): Cholesteatoma: First International Conference. Birmingham, Aesculapius, 1977, p 115.

377. Abbink JJ, Kamp AM, Nuijens JH, Swaak TJ, Hack CE: Proteolytic inactivation of alpha 1-antitrypsin and alpha 1-antichymotrypsin by neutrophils in arthritic joints. Arthritis Rheum 36:168, 1993.

378. Vater CA, Mainardi CL, Harris ED Jr: An inhibitor of mammalian collagenases from cultures in vitro of human tendon. J Biol Chem 254:3045, 1979.

379. Carmichael DF, Sommer A, Thompson RC, Anderson DC, Smith CG, Welgus HG, Stricklin GP: Primary structure and cDNA cloning of human fibroblast collagenase inhibitor. Proc Natl Acad Sci U S A 83:2407, 1986.

380. Stetler-Stevenson WG, Krutzsch HC, Liotta LA: Tissue inhibitor of metalloproteinase (TIMP-2). A new member of the metalloproteinase inhibitor family. J Biol Chem 264:17374, 1989.

381. Clark IM, Powell LK, Ramsey S, Hazleman BL, Cawston TE: The measurement of collagenase, tissue inhibitor of metalloproteinases (TIMP), and collagenase-TIMP complex in synovial fluids from patients with osteoarthritis and rheumatoid arthritis. Arthritis Rheum 36:372, 1993.

382. Firestein GS, Paine MM: Stromelysin and tissue inhibitor of metalloproteinases gene expression in rheumatoid arthritis synovium. Am J Pathology 140:1309–14, 1992.

383. Firestein GS, Paine MM, Boyle DL: Mechanisms of methotrexate action in rheumatoid arthritis. Selective decrease in synovial collagenase gene expression. Arthritis Rheum 37:193, 1994.

384. MacNaul KL, Chartrain N, Lark M, Tocci MJ, Hutchinson NI: Discoordinate expression of stromelysin, collagenase, and tissue inhibitor of metalloproteinases-1 in rheumatoid human synovial fibroblasts: Synergistic effects of interleukin-1 and tumor necrosis factor-alpha on stromelysin expression. J Biol Chem 265:17238, 1990.

385. Littman BH, Drury CE, Schumacher R, Boyle D, Weisman M, Firestein GS: In vivo reduction of RA synovial tissue metalloproteinase mRNA levels by tenidap. Arthritis Rheum 37:S420, 1994.

386. Fujikawa K: Arthrographic study of the rheumatoid knee. Part 1. Synovial proliferation. Ann Rheum Dis 40:332, 1981.

387. Fujikawa K, Tanaka Y, Matsubayashi T, Iseki F: Arthrographic study of the rheumatoid knee: 2. Articular cartilage and menisci. Ann Rheum Dis 40:344, 1981.

388. Salisbury MD, Nottage WM: A new evaluation of gross pathologic changes and concepts of rheumatoid articular cartilage degeneration. Clin Orthop 199:243, 1985.

389. Hogg N, Palmer DG, Revell PA: Mononuclear phagocytes of normal and rheumatoid synovial membrane identified by monoclonal antibodies. Immunol 56:673, 1985.

390. Okada Y, Takeuchi N, Tomita K, Nakanishi I, Nagase H: Immunolocalisation of matrix metalloproteinase 3 (stromelysin) in rheumatoid synovioblasts (B cells): Correlation with rheumatoid arthritis. Ann Rheum Dis 48:645, 1989.

391. Nykanen P, Helve T, Kankaanpaa U, Larsen A: Characterisation of the DNA-synthesizing cells in rheumatoid synovial tissue. Scand J Rheumatol 7:118, 1978.

392. Revell PA, Mapp PI, Lalor PA, Hall PA: Proliferative activity of cells in the synovium as demonstrated by a monoclonal antibody, Ki67. Rheumatol Int 7:183, 1987.

393. Qu Z, Garcia CH, O'Rourke LM, Planck SR, Kohli M, Rosenbaum JT: Local proliferation of fibroblast-like synoviocytes contributes to synovial hyperplasia: Results of proliferating cell nuclear antigen/cyclin, c-myc, and nucleolar organizer region staining. Arthritis Rheum 37:212, 1994.

394. Ritchlin C, Dwyer E, Bucala R, Winchester R: Sustained and distinctive patterns of gene activation in synovial fibroblasts and whole synovial tissue obtained from inflammatory synovitis. Scand J Immunol 40:292, 1994.

395. Burmester GR, Dimitriu-Bona A, Waters SJ, Winchester RJ: Identification of three major synovial lining cell populations by monoclonal antibodies directed to Ia antigens and antigens associated with monocytes/macrophages and fibroblasts. Scand J Immunol 17:69, 1983.

396. Goto M, Sasano M, Yamanaka H, Miyasaka N, Kamatani N, Inove K, Nishka K, Miyamoto T: Spontaneous production of an interleukin 1–like factor by cloned rheumatoid synovial cells in long-term culture. J Clin Invest 80:786, 1987.

397. Baker DG, Dayer JM, Roelke M, Schumacher HR, Krane SM: Rheumatoid synovial cell morphologic changes induced by a mononuclear cell factor in culture. Arthritis Rheum 26:8, 1983.

398. Lafyatis R, Remmers EF, Roberts AB, Yocum DE, Sporn MB, Wilder RL: Anchorage-independent growth of synoviocytes from arthritic and normal joints: Stimulation by exogenous platelet-derived growth factor and inhibition by transforming growth factor-beta and retinoids. J Clin Invest 83:1267, 1989.

399. Tarkowski A, Johnsson R, Holmdahl R, Klareskog L: Immunohistochemical characterization of synovial cells in arthritis in MRL-lpr/lpr mice. Arthritis Rheum 30:75, 1987.

400. Gay RE, Snider C, Gay S, et al: Cellular composition of proliferating synovial tissue involved in the destructive arthritis of MRL/l mice. Clin Res 33:788, 1985.

401. Wu J, Zhou T, He J, Mountz JD: Autoimmune disease in mice due to integration of an endogenous retrovirus in an apoptosis gene. J Exper Med 178:461, 1993.

402. Firestein GS, Yeo M, Zvaifler NJ: Apoptosis in rheumatoid arthritis synovium. J Clin Invest 96:1631, 1995.

403. Mohr W, Wessinghage D: The relationship between polymorphonuclear granulocytes and cartilage destruction in rheumatoid arthritis. J Rheumatol 37:81, 1978.

404. Tak PP, Kummer JA, Hack CE, Daha MR, Smeets TJM, Erkelens WE, Meinders AE, Kluin PM, Breedveld FC: Granzyme-positive cytotoxic cells are specifically increased in early rheumatoid synovial tissue. Arthritis Rheum 37:1735–1743, 1994.

405. Santiago Schwartz F, Kay C, Panagiotopoulos C, Carsons SE: Rheumatoid arthritis serum or synovial fluid and interleukin 2 abnormally expand natural killer–like cells that are potent stimulators of IgM rheumatoid factors. J Rheumatol 19:223, 1992.

406. Crisp AJ, Chapman CM, Kirkham SE, Schiller AL, Krane SM: Articular mastocytosis in rheumatoid arthritis. Arthritis Rheum 27:845, 1984.

407. Bromley M, Fisher WD, Woolley DE: Mast cells at sites of cartilage erosion in the rheumatoid joint. Ann Rheum Dis 43:76, 1984.

408. Malone DG, Irani AM, Schwartz LB, Barrett KE, Metcalfe DD: Mast cell numbers and histamine levels in synovial fluids from patients with diverse arthritides. Arthritis Rheum 29:956, 1986.

409. Frewin DB, Cleland LG, Johnsson JR, Robertson PW: Histamine levels in human synovial fluid. J Rheumatol 13:13, 1986.

410. Malone DG, Wilder RL, Saavedra-Delgado AM, Metcalfe DD: Mast cell numbers in rheumatoid synovial tissues. Arthritis Rheum 30:130, 1987.

411. Yoffe JR, Taylor DJ, Woolley DE: Mast cell products stimulate collagenase and prostaglandin E production by cultures of adherent rheumatoid synovial cells. Biochem Biophys Res Commun 122:270, 1984.

412. Crisp AJ, Roelke MS, Goldring SR, Krane SM: Heparin modulates intracellular cyclic AMP in human trabecular bone cells and adherent rheumatoid synovial cells. Ann Rheum Dis 43:628, 1984.

413. Annefeld M: The potential aggressiveness of synovial tissue in rheumatoid arthritis. J Pathol 139:399, 1983.

414. Shiozawa S, Shiozawa K, Fujita T: Morphologic observations in the early phase of the cartilage-pannus junction. Arthritis Rheum 26:472, 1983.

415. Bromley M, Woolley DE: Histopathology of the rheumatoid lesion. Arthritis Rheum 27:857, 1984.

416. Kobayashi I, Ziff M: Electron microscopic studies of the cartilage-pannus junction in rheumatoid arthritis. Arthritis Rheum 18:475, 1975.

417. Bromley M, Woolley DE: Chondroclasts and osteoclasts at subchondral sites of erosion in the rheumatoid joint. Arthritis Rheum 27:968, 1984.

418. Brinckerhoff CE, Harris ED Jr: Collagenase production by cultures containing multinucleated cells derived from synovial fibroblasts. Arthritis Rheum 21:745, 1978.

419. Lerner UH, Jones IL, Gustafson GT: Bradykinin, a new potential mediator of inflammation-induced bone resorption. Arthritis Rheum 30:530, 1987.

420. Allard SA, Muirden KD, Maini RN: Correlation of histopathological features of pannus with patterns of damage in different joints in rheumatoid arthritis. Ann Rheum Dis 50:278, 1991.

421. Zvaifler NJ, Firestein GS: Pannus and pannocytes: Alternative models of joint destruction in rheumatoid arthritis. Arthritis Rheum 37:783, 1994.

422. Harris ED Jr, Parker HG, Radin EL, Krane SM: Effects of proteolytic enzymes on structural and mechanical properties of cartilage. Arthritis Rheum 15:497, 1972.

423. Wolfe GC, MacNaul KL, Buechel FF, McDonnell J, Hoerrner LA, Lark MW, Moore VL, Hutchinson NI: Differential in vivo expression of collagenase messenger RNA in synovium and cartilage: Quantitative comparison with stromelysin messenger RNA levels in human rheumatoid and osteoarthritis patients and in two animal models of acute inflammatory arthritis. Arthritis Rheum 36:1540, 1993.

424. Nguyen Q, Mort JS, Roughley PJ: Preferential mRNA expression of prostromelysin relative to procollagenase and in situ localization in human articular cartilage. J Clin Invest 89:1189, 1992.

425. Cooke TD, Hurd ER, Jasin HE, Bienenstock J, Ziff M: Identification of immunoglobulins and complement in rheumatoid articular collagenous tissues. Arthritis Rheum 18:541, 1975.

426. McDonnell J, Hoerrner LA, Lark MW, Harper C, Dey T, Lobner J, Eiermann G, Kazazis D, Singer II, Moore VL: Recombinant human interleukin-1 beta-induced increase in levels of proteoglycans, stromelysin, and leukocytes in rabbit synovial fluid. Arthritis Rheum 35:799, 1992.

427. Hollingsworth JW, Siegel ER, Creasey WA: Granulocyte survival in synovial exudate of patients with rheumatoid arthritis and other inflammatory joint diseases. Yale J Biol Med 39:289, 1967.

428. Jones ST, Denton J, Holt PJ, Freemont AJ: Possible clearance of effete polymorphonuclear leucocytes from synovial fluid by cytophagocytic mononuclear cells: Implications for pathogenesis and chronicity in inflammatory arthritis. Ann Rheum Dis 52:121, 1993.

429. Korchak HM, Vienne K, Rutherford LE, Weissmann G: Neutrophil stimulation: Receptor, membrane, and metabolic events. Fed Proc 43:2749, 1984.

430. Beaulieu AD, Lang F, Belles-Isles M, Poubelle P: Protein biosynthetic activity of polymorphonuclear leukocytes in inflammatory arthropathies: Increased synthesis and release of fibronectin. J Rheumatol 14:656, 1987.

431. McColl SR, Paquin R, Menard C, Beaulieu AD: Human neutrophils produce high levels of the interleukin 1 receptor antagonist in response to granulocyte/macrophage colony-stimulating factor and tumor necrosis factor alpha. J Exper Med 176:593, 1992.

432. Winchester RJ, Agnello V, Kunkel HG: Gamma globulin complexes in synovial fluids of patients with rheumatoid arthritis. Clin Exp Immunol 6:689, 1970.

433. Panush RS, Katz P, Longley S, Yonker RA: Detection and quantitation of circulating immune complexes in arterial blood of patients with rheumatic disease. Clin Immunol Pathol 36:217, 1985.

434. Faaber P, Truus PM, Schilder R, Capel PJA, Koene RAP: Circulating immune complexes and rheumatoid arthritis. J Rheumatol 12:849, 1985.

435. Ohno O, Cooke TD: Electron microscopic morphology of immunoglobulin aggregates and their interactions in rheumatoid articular collagenous tissues. Arthritis Rheum 21:516, 1978.

436. Shiozawa S, Jasin HE, Ziff M: Absence of immunoglobulins in rheumatoid cartilage-pannus junctions. Arthritis Rheum 23:816, 1980.

437. Nurcombe HL, Bucknall RC, Edwards SW: Activation of the neutrophil myeloperoxidase-H_2O_2 system by synovial fluid isolated from patients with rheumatoid arthritis. Ann Rheum Dis 50:237, 1991.

438. McCord JM: Free radicals and inflammation: Protection of synovial fluid by superoxide dismutase. Science 185:529, 1974.

439. Davis P, Johnston C, Bertouch J, Starkebaum G: Depressed superoxide radical generation by neutrophils from patients with rheumatoid arthritis and neutropenia: Correlation with neutrophil reactive IgG. Ann Rheum Dis 45:51, 1987.

440. Goldstein I, Edelson HS, Kaplan MB, Weissman G: Ceruloplasmin: A scavenger of superoxide union radicals. J Biol Chem 254:4040, 1979.

441. Zurier RB, Quagliata F: Effect of prostaglandin E_1 on adjuvant arthritis. Nature 234:304, 1971.

442. Nicholson PA: Recent advances in defining the role of misoprostol in rheumatology. J Rheumatol 17:50, 1990.

443. Nakajima H, Hiyama Y, Tsukada W, Warabi H, Uchida S, Hirose S: Effects of interferon gamma on cultured synovial cells from patients with rheumatoid arthritis: Inhibition of cell growth, prostaglandin E_2, and collagenase release. Ann Rheum Dis 49:312, 1990.

444. Abramson S, Korchak H, Ludewig R, Edelson H, Haines K, Levin RI, Herman R: The modes of action of aspirin-like drugs. Proc Natl Acad Sci U S A 82:7227, 1985.

445. McGuire J, McGee J, Crittenden N, Fitzpatrick F: Cell damage unmasks 15-lipoxygenase activity in human neutrophils. J Biol Chem 260:8316, 1985.

446. Elmgreen J, Haagen N, Ahnfelt-Ronne I: Enhanced capacity for release of leucotriene B_4 by neutrophils in rheumatoid arthritis. Ann Rheum Dis 46:501, 1987.

447. Griffiths RJ, Pettipher ER, Koch K, Farrell CA, Breslow R, Conklyn MJ, Smith MA, Hackman BC, Wimberly DJ, Milici AJ, Scampoli DN, Cheng JB, Pillar JS, Pazoles CJ, Doherty NS, Melvin LS, Reiter LA, Biggars MS, Falkner FC, Mitchell DY, Liston TE, Showell HJ: Leukotriene B4 plays a critical role in the progression of collagen-induced arthritis. Proc Natl Acad Sci U S A 92:517, 1995.

448. Sperling RI, Weinblatt M, Robin JL, Ravalese J III, Hoover RL, House F, Coblyn JS, Fraser PA, Spur BW, Robinson DR, Lewis RA, Austen KF: Effects of dietary supplementation with marine fish oil on leukocyte lipid mediator generation and function in rheumatoid arthritis. Arthritis Rheum 30:988, 1987.

449. Ruddy S, Colten HR: Rheumatoid arthritis. Biosynthesis of complement proteins by synovial tissues. N Engl J Med 290:1284, 1974.

450. Littman BH, Dastvan FF, Carlson PL, Sanders KM: Regulation of monocyte/macrophage C2 production and HLA-DR expression by IL-4 (BSF-1) and IFN-gamma. J Immunol 142:520, 1989.

451. Perlmutter DH, Goldberger G, Dinarello CA, Mizel SB, Colten HR: Regulation of class III major histocompatibility complex gene products by interleukin-1. Science 232:850, 1986.

452. Gulati P, Guc D, Lemercier C, Lappin D, Whaley K: Expression of the components and regulatory proteins of the classical pathway of complement in normal and diseased synovium. Rheumatol Int 14:13, 1994.

453. Ruddy S, Austen KF: The complement system in rheumatoid synovitis: I. An analysis of complement component activities in rheumatoid synovial fluids. Arthritis Rheum 13:713, 1970.

454. Pekin TJ Jr, Zvaifler NJ: Hemolytic complement in synovial fluid. J Clin Invest 43:1372, 1964.

455. Luukkainen R, Alanaatu A, Kaarela K, Huhtala H: Predictive value of synovial fluid analysis in rheumatoid arthritis: A 7.5-year follow-up study. Eur J Med 2:284, 1993.

456. Sabharwal UK, Vaughan JH, Fong S, Bennett PH, Carson DA, Curd JG: Activation of the classical pathway of complement by rheumatoid factors: Assessment by radioimmunoassay for C4. Arthritis Rheum 25:161, 1982.

457. Elmgren J, Hansen TM: Subnormal sensitivity of neutrophils to complement split-product C5a in rheumatoid arthritis: Relation to complement catabolism and disease extent. Ann Rheum Dis 44:514, 1985.

458. Goldstein IM, Weissmann G: Generation of C5-derived lysosomal enzyme-releasing activity (C5a) by lysates of leukocyte lysosomes. J Immunol 113:1583, 1974.

459. Harris ED Jr, Faulkner CS II, Brown FE: Collagenolytic systems in rheumatoid arthritis. Clin Orthop 110:303, 1975.

460. Gysen P, Malaise M, Gaspar S, Franchimont P: Measurement of proteoglycans, elastase, collagenase and protein in synovial fluid in inflammatory and degenerative arthropathies. Clin Rheumatol 4:39, 1985.

461. Al-Haik N, Lewis DA, Struthers G: Neutral protease, collagenase and elastase activities in synovial fluid in inflammatory and degenerative arthropathies. Clin Rheumatol 4:39, 1985.

462. Harris ED Jr, DiBona DR, Krane SM: Collagenases in human synovial fluid. J Clin Invest 48:2104, 1969.

463. Melmon KL, Cline MJ: Kallikrein activator and kininase in human granulocytes: A model of inflammation. *In* Rocha E, Silva M (eds): Symposium on Vasoactive Polypeptides: Bradykinin and Related Kinins. Oxford, Pergamon Press, 1967.

464. O'Reilly MS, Holmgren L, Shing Y, Chen C, Rosenthal RA, Moses M, Lane WS, Cao Y, Sage EH, Folkman J: Angiostatin: A novel angiogenesis inhibitor that mediates the suppression of metastases by a Lewis lung carcinoma. Cell 79:315, 1994.

465. Cochrane CG, et al: The interaction of Hageman factor and immune complexes. J Clin Invest 51:2736, 1972.

466. Rothberger H, Zimmerman TS, Spiegelberg HL, Vaughan JH: Leucocyte procoagulant activity: Enhancement of production in vitro by IgG and antigen-antibody complexes. J Clin Invest 59:549, 1977.

467. Van de Putte LBA, Hegt VN, Overbeek TE: Activators and inhibitors of fibrinolysis in rheumatoid and non-rheumatoid synovial membranes. Arthritis Rheum 20:671, 1977.

CHAPTER 55

Clinical Features of Rheumatoid Arthritis

Edward D. Harris, Jr.

Medical historians disagree as to the first references to rheumatoid arthritis (RA) in lay and medical writings.[1-6] Some have concluded that RA developed only recently as a clear-cut entity, whereas others interpret writings of Soranus in the second century as referring to a patient with RA.

Regardless of its recorded history, RA has become an important cause of disability and morbidity and a drain on human and monetary resources. In 1985 the average annual costs for inpatient and outpatient care of a rheumatoid patient seen only by a rheumatologist were over $2000[7]; by 1994 costs had increased to $2500. RA is a chronic and progressive disease; once it is active and chronic in a given individual, it will likely become progressively worse. If active disease has been present for 1 year in a particular joint, cartilage loss is probably irreversible.

CRITERIA FOR DIAGNOSIS

The diagnosis of RA is primarily based on clinical grounds. Despite the usefulness of tests for rheumatoid factor (RF) in both diagnosis and understanding of the pathophysiology of the disease, neither the presence of anti-IgG nor any other laboratory variable is specific for RA. For epidemiologic studies, several sets of criteria have been developed for classification of adult RA by the American Rheumatism Association (ARA). The most recent criteria were published in 1988 and were constructed using data from 262 RA patients and 262 controls representing a cross-section of rheumatic diseases.[8] Table 55-1 lists the 1988 ARA criteria.

EPIDEMIOLOGY

Wolfe[9] summarized the results of 14 studies of population samples, including the National Health Survey[10]; the survey of Tecumseh, Michigan[11]; various Native American groups[12]; and representative atomic bomb survivors from Hiroshima and Nagasaki.[13] Using 1958 ARA criteria for definite RA, the prevalence rate varied from 0.3 to 1.5 percent. In 1994 an estimate of 5 million cases of RA in the United States is reasonable; an estimate of prevalence of a little less than 1 percent in the adult population is appropriate. A conservative estimate is that 170,000 new cases of definite or classic RA developed in the United States in 1994. The lifetime costs of RA, including medical expenses and costs associated with illness-related work loss, can be estimated to exceed $32,000 per case in 1994 dollars, as great as the costs for stroke or coronary artery disease.[14]

Regional variations from these incidence and prevalence data are unusual, and this indicates that specific genetic and environmental influences on the development of RA, if significant, are widespread in the world. These are primarily related to heritable variables in the human leukocyte antigen (HLA) class II major histocompatibility complex (MHC) DRB1 chains.

Since 1948, when the studies of Rose and colleagues[15] confirmed the findings of Waaler[16] linking a factor in sera of patients with RA to agglutination of normal and sensitized sheep red blood cells, the presence or absence of RF in serum has occupied the attention of epidemiologists in this field. RF is found more frequently (3 to 5 percent) than RA in population studies; in the general population the prevalence of seropositivity is approximately equal between men and women.[17, 18] Frequently, patients appear to have RA yet are seronegative.[19] These individuals probably have a distinct disease.[20] The assay for RF itself may explain false-positive results, because when an enzyme-linked immunosorbent assay (ELISA) is used instead of the usual agglutination tests, almost complete specificity for RA (99 percent) has been demonstrated.[21]

Evidence that genetic factors are predisposing for RA using twin studies is variable. The data have ranged from evidence for discordance[22] to findings of almost 50 percent concordance.[23] In another study, the risk of erosive arthritis in monozygotic twins was found to be about 30 times that in the reference population, while in dizygotic twins and in nontwin siblings the risk was about 6 times that of control groups.[24, 25] Relative risk in a nationwide Finnish study was less impressive[26]; a series of 4137 monozygotic and 9162 dizygotic twins showed a relative risk of 8.2 for monozygotic and 3.4 for dizygotic twins. Functionally incapacitating (grade 3 or 4) RA has been found to occur at four times the expected rate in first-degree relatives of probands with seropositive disease; erosive radiographic changes were found at

Table 55–1. 1988 REVISED ARA CRITERIA FOR CLASSIFICATION OF RHEUMATOID ARTHRITIS*

Criterion	Definition
1. Morning stiffness	Morning stiffness in and around the joints lasting at least 1 hour before maximal improvement
2. Arthritis of three or more joint areas	At least three joint areas simultaneously having soft tissue swelling or fluid (not bony overgrowth alone) observed by a physician (the 14 possible joint areas are [right or left] PIP, MCP, wrist, elbow, knee, ankle, and MTP joints)
3. Arthritis of hand joints	At least one joint area swollen as above in wrist, MCP, or PIP joint
4. Symmetric arthritis	Simultaneous involvement of the same joint areas (as in criterion 2) on both sides of the body (bilateral involvement of PIP, MCP, or MTP joints is acceptable without absolute symmetry)
5. Rheumatoid nodules	Subcutaneous nodules over bony prominences or extensor surfaces, or in juxta-articular regions, observed by a physician
6. Serum rheumatoid factor	Demonstration of abnormal amounts of serum "rheumatoid factor" by any method that has been positive in less than 5 percent of normal control subjects
7. Radiographic changes	Changes typical of RA on PA hand and wrist radiographs, which must include erosions or unequivocal bony decalcification localized to or most marked adjacent to the involved joints (osteoarthritis changes alone do not qualify)

*For classification purposes, a patient is said to have RA if he or she has satisfied at least four of the seven criteria. Criteria 1 through 4 must be present for at least 6 weeks. Patients with two clinical diagnoses are not excluded. Designation as classic, definite, or probable rheumatoid arthritis is *not* to be made.

Abbreviations: ARA, American Rheumatism Association; PIP, proximal interphalangeal; MCP, metacarpophalangeal; MTP, metatarsophalangeal; RA, rheumatoid arthritis; PA, posteroanterior.

three times the expected rate. Serologic study in first-degree relatives of patients with RA has revealed no higher frequency of RF than in relatives of matched controls.[27]

Still inadequately understood is the apparent negative association between gout and rheumatoid arthritis. In 1979 it was estimated that there should be 1000 cases of coexistent gout and RA in the United States rather than the 7 cases reported.[28] In a subsequent study, 12 of 160 seropositive RA patients were found to have hyperuricemia. Eleven of the 12 had quiet

disease; indeed, the onset of hyperuricemia and improvement of RA appeared to coincide. In patients with fluctuations in uric acid levels, there was a statistically significant correlation ($r = -.66$, $P \leq .01$) between an increase in serum uric acid concentration and improvement in disease activity.[29] Thus, the hypothesis stands: the hyperuricemic state may be anti-inflammatory.

CLINICAL SYNDROME OF EARLY RHEUMATOID ARTHRITIS

In the Northern Hemisphere, the onset of RA is more frequent in winter than in summer. In several series, the onset of RA from October to March was found to be twice as frequent as in the other 6 months,[30, 31] and exacerbations of the disease are more common in winter.[32] Comparable data from the Southern Hemisphere are not available.

Recent data suggest that the appearance of RF may be more likely to precede symptoms of arthritis in patients than was previously recognized. In 30 patients whose frozen sera were available from a time before symptoms of RA began, half had a positive latex fixation test,[33] and many more of these were men than women.

Much more diffuse, subjective, and difficult to study are the precipitating factors of arthritis. There is no evidence that any of these factors has a direct cause-and-effect relationship. Trauma is one of the most common preludes to arthritis; this can include surgery. Other stimuli, including infections, vaccine inoculations, and emotional trauma, have been implicated by many patients as causes of their problems.

Patterns of Onset

Insidious Onset

RA usually has an insidious, slow onset over weeks to months (Table 55–2). Fifty-five to 70 percent of cases begin this way.[30, 34] The initial symptoms may

Table 55–2. ONSET OF RHEUMATOID ARTHRITIS IN 300 PATIENTS WITH DEFINITE OR CLASSIC DISEASE

Characteristic		Percentage
Mode of onset	Rapid* (days or weeks)	46
	Insidious	54
Site of onset	Small joints	32
	Medium-sized joints	16
	Large joints	29
	Combined	26
Pattern of onset	Monarticular	21
	Oligoarticular	44
	Polyarticular	35

From Fallahi S, Halla JT, Hardin JG: Clin Res 31:650A, 1983.
*This time frame includes patients described in other studies as having "intermediate" onset.

be systematic or articular. In some patients, fatigue, malaise, or diffuse musculoskeletal pain may be the first nonspecific complaint, with joints becoming involved later. Although symmetric involvement is common, asymmetric presentation (often with more symmetry developing later in the course of disease) is not unusual. The reason for symmetry of joint involvement may be related to the release of phlogistic neuropeptides at terminal nerve endings in joints.

Morning stiffness may be the first symptom, appearing even before pain. This phenomenon is probably related to accumulation of edema fluid within inflamed tissues during sleep, and it clears as edema and products of inflammation are absorbed by lymphatics and venules and returned to the circulation by motion accompanying the use of muscles. Pain and stiffness may develop in other joints, but it is rare for symptoms to remit completely in one set of joints while developing in another. This quality of arthritis sets RA apart from rheumatic fever, in which a true migratory pattern of arthritis is common.

A subtle, early change in RA is development of muscle atrophy around affected joints. This decreases efficiency and strength, and weakness develops that is out of proportion to pain. Opening doors, climbing stairs, and doing repetitive work become more demanding. A low-grade fever without chills is not uncommon. Depression and both focused and nonspecific anxiety affect the patient and accentuate symptoms. Weight loss is common and is exacerbated by anorexia.

Acute Onset

Eight to 15 percent of patients have acute onset of symptoms, occurring within a few days. Rarely, a patient will pinpoint the onset of disease to a specific time or activity, such as opening a door or driving a golf ball. Symptoms mount, with pain developing in other joints, often in a less symmetric pattern than in patients who have an insidious type of onset. Pain in muscles can be severe and mimic that accompanying muscle necrosis from ischemia. Diagnosis of acute-onset RA is difficult to make, and sepsis or vasculitis must be ruled out.

Intermediate Onset

Fifteen to 20 percent of patients have an intermediate type of onset, in which symptoms develop over days or weeks. Systemic complaints are more noticeable than in the insidious type of onset.

Joint Involvement in Early Rheumatoid Arthritis

The joints most commonly involved first in RA are the metacarpophalangeal (MCP) joints, proximal interphalangeal (PIP) joints, and wrists.[35] Larger joints generally become symptomatic after small joints. This raises the question of whether early disease in large

joints remains asymptomatic for a longer time. Researchers in one study sought the answer by performing xenon clearances on clinically normal knees of patients with early RA.[36] Seven of 22 had abnormally high perfusion, supporting this hypothesis. A recent anatomic study correlated the area, in square centimeters, of synovial membrane with that of hyaline cartilage in each joint. The joints with the highest ratio of synovium to articular cartilage correlated positively with the joints most frequently involved in the disease.[37]

Unusual Patterns of Early Disease

Adult-Onset Still's Disease

Still's disease appears in adults, usually in the third or fourth decade, as a syndrome similar to that seen in children with the acute, febrile onset of juvenile arthritis. Still's disease was first described in 14 patients by Bywaters.[38] Women are more commonly affected than men. Serologic studies (RF and antinuclear antibody) are negative, and patients do not have subcutaneous nodules.[39] Most are febrile. Fever patterns in these patients are usually quotidian (i.e., reaching normal levels at least once each day). The disease is often characterized by the appearance of salmon-colored or pink macules that are evanescent and become more prominent when patients are febrile. The cervical spine is involved, and loss of neck motion may be striking. Pericarditis, pleural effusions, and severe abdominal pain may be present and confound attempts at diagnosis.[40] Unlike the case in systemic lupus erythematosus (SLE), serum complement level is normal or high.[41]

In one series, 11 patients (all of whom were white women), followed for a mean of 20.2 years after disease onset, had the following characteristics:[42]

- Ten had a polycyclic pattern (characterized by remissions and exacerbations).
- Patterns of exacerbations were similar to but less severe than the original presentations.
- Loss of wrist extension was the most common clinical abnormality, and carpal ankylosis was present in 10 patients.
- Five of 11 patients had distal interphalangeal (DIP) joint involvement.
- Biopsy of the characteristic skin rash of Still's disease and juvenile rheumatoid arthritis (JRA) showed perivascular infiltrate of neutrophils in the superficial dermis.

In another group,[43] 20 percent showed significant functional deterioration from erosive joint disease. Functional class III/IV (Steinbrocker's classification) was usually related to hip disease. As in classic RA in adults, polyarticular disease was more often associated with a poor functional outcome than was oligoarticular disease. Individuals with monocyclic or polycyclic systemic disease, no arthritis at presentation, or oligoarticular presentation and progression tended to have a considerably better functional outcome. The incidence of amyloidosis may be as high as 30 percent within 10 years of onset of the illness.[44]

Palindromic Pattern of Onset

Palindromic rheumatism was described by Hench and Rosenberg in 1941.[45] Like many other clinical complexes in rheumatology, it should be considered a syndrome that can be the initial manifestation of many different organic processes or one that never evolves into anything more. Pain usually begins in one joint; symptoms worsen for several hours and are associated with swelling and erythema. Joints involved in a series of 227 patients are listed in Table 55–3.

An intercritical period, as in gout, is asymptomatic. It is likely that 20 to 40 percent of patients with palindromic rheumatism go on to develop RA, particularly those with HLA-DR4. It is significant that in a compilation of 653 patients from nine series, only 15 percent became asymptomatic after at least 5 years with a palindromic syndrome (Table 55–4).[46] In these, multiple joints become involved, swelling does not subside completely between attacks, and tests become positive for RF. Neither the characteristics of joint fluid nor the pathologic findings of synovial biopsies allows the prediction that RA will evolve from palindromic rheumatism.[47] Of 51 patients with palindromic rheumatism, 41 experienced marked improvement in frequency and duration of attacks during treatment with antimalarials.[48]

Effect of Age on Onset

RA developing in older persons (60 years of age and older), more often men than women, is often dominated by stiffness, limb girdle pain, and diffuse boggy swelling of the hands, wrists, and forearms.

Table 55–3. DISTRIBUTION OF JOINTS INVOLVED IN ATTACKS BASED UPON A CUMULATIVE EXPERIENCE WITH 227 PATIENTS

Joint Involvement	Mean % of Patients	Range of % of Patients
MCP, PIP	91	74–100
Wrists	78	54–82
Knees	64	41–94
Shoulders	65	33–75
Ankles	50	10–67
Feet	43	15–73
Elbows	38	13–60
Hips	17	0–40
Temporomandibular	8	0–28
Spine	4	0–11
Sternoclavicular	2	0–6
Para-articular sites	27	20–29

Modified from Guerne P-A, Weisman MH: Palindromic rheumatism: Part of or apart from the spectrum of rheumatoid arthritis. Am J Med 16:451–460, 1992.[46]

Table 55–4. EVOLUTION OF PATIENTS WITH PALINDROMIC RHEUMATISM (PR) IN NINE SERIES TOTALING 653 PATIENTS*

Series of Patients	Number of Cases	Remission or Cure (%)	Persistent PR (%)	PR-RA (%)	Other Diseases (%)
[1]	34	15	85	0	0
[2]	140	8	52	36	4
[3]	179	10	47	38	5
[4]	39	0	56	44	0
[5]	70	24	34	30	12
[6]	38	8	66	15	11
[7]	43	23	23	49	5
[8]	50	0	46	54	0
[9]	60	43	21	35	2
Total/average	653	15	48	33	4

Modified from Guerne P-A, Weisman MH: Palindromic rheumatism: Part of or apart from the spectrum of rheumatoid arthritis. Am J Med 16:451–460, 1992.[46]

*In each series, the number of patients undergoing a remission or a cure, remaining palindromic, evolving toward rheumatoid arthritis (PR-RA), or developing another disease is expressed as a percentage.

One study has emphasized that an initial clinical onset resembling polymyalgia rheumatica occurs four times more frequently in the elderly than in younger patients.[49] Those with onset at age 60 or later are less likely to have subcutaneous nodules or RF at the onset of disease, despite the high prevalence of RF in the general population in this age group. In general, elderly individuals who develop RA tend to have a more benign course than younger patients; there is a lower frequency of positive tests for RF, but there is a strong association with HLA-DR4.[50] Onset is slow, but the stiffness often is incapacitating. In other respects, the disease is similar to other forms of adult RA, but the therapy should not be the same. Nonsteroidal anti-inflammatory drugs (NSAIDs) are rarely effective, but low-dose glucocorticoids (<7.5 mg prednisone per day) may be helpful in reducing edema and increasing motion and function.

Rheumatoid Arthritis and Paralysis: Asymmetric Disease

Being relatively common, RA is likely to occur with many other types of chronic disease. A striking asymmetry or even unilateral involvement has been described in patients with poliomyelitis, meningioma, encephalitis, neurovascular syphilis, strokes, and cerebral palsy.[51, 52] Joints are spared on the paralyzed side, and the degree of protection demonstrates a rough correlation with the extent of paralysis.[53] The protective effect on the affected side is less if a neurologic deficit develops in a patient who already has RA.[54]

Arthritis Robustus

Arthritis robustus is not so much an unusual presentation of disease as an unusual reaction of patients to the disease.[55, 56] Men dominate this group. Their disease is characterized by proliferative synovitis that appears to cause little pain and even less disability.

Patients are athletic and invariably keep working (often at physical labor). Osteopenia is less severe, and new bone proliferation at joint margins is common. Bulky subcutaneous nodules develop. Subchondral cysts also develop, presumably from the excessive pressure developed from synovial fluid within a thick joint capsule during muscular effort.

COURSE OF RHEUMATOID ARTHRITIS

Intermittent Course (15 to 20 percent)

Intermittent-course RA is marked by partial to complete remissions without the need for continuous therapy. It is a mild disease initially, and only a few joints are involved. Insidious return of disease is often marked by involvement of more joints than were involved during the first episode.[57, 58] Of this group it is reported that approximately half had remissions lasting more than a year, and for the entire group remissions lasted longer than exacerbations.

Long Clinical Remissions (10 percent)

In one study of 250 patients receiving only simple medical and orthopedic treatment, almost 10 percent were in clinical remission for 12 to 31 years (mean 22 years).[32] Many of these patients had acute onset of symptoms with marked fever and severe joint pain and inflammation, raising the question (in retrospect) of whether they indeed had RA. Nevertheless, some sign of disease activity (e.g., an elevated erythrocyte sedimentation rate [ESR]) persisted in many throughout the "clinical remission," and a few patients had brief but true flares of disease in one or a few joints.

Progressive Disease (65 to 70 percent)

Progressive RA may follow a rapid or slow course, but the end result may be the same: disabling, destructive disease. In assessing symptoms in RA, both patients and their physicians must be aware of environmental factors that may accentuate symptoms. One of these, the weather, has a strong basis in folklore as a major determinant of symptom severity in RA and other rheumatic diseases. Using a climate-controlled chamber for patients, early data suggested that symptoms worsened if humidity was raised and barometric pressure lowered simultaneously,[59] and another study showed that pain in patients with RA increased significantly as temperature and vapor pressure increased.[60] The folklore may be accurate: a consistently dry and temperate climate appears to alleviate symptoms in RA.

DIAGNOSIS OF RHEUMATOID ARTHRITIS

Diagnosis of RA must be by established criteria that are based on effective clinical history and examination, laboratory tests, and diagnoses that exclude it. No single feature allows a definite diagnosis. The ARA criteria for classification need not be used in individual cases for diagnosis; however, the requirement that objective evidence for synovitis must be present for at least 6 weeks is an important one. A physician should not make a premature diagnosis of RA in a patient who may have a self-limited synovitis; on the other hand, to prevent irreversible damage to joints, the diagnosis of RA should be confirmed or ruled out within 2 months after the onset of synovitis.

The characteristic patient with RA complains of pain and stiffness in multiple joints. The joint swelling is boggy and includes both soft tissue and synovial fluid. These joints are tender to the touch, especially the small joints of the hands and feet. Palmar erythema and prominent veins on the dorsum of the hand and wrist indicate increased blood flow to the joint areas. Distal interphalangeal joints rarely are involved. Temperature over the involved joints (except the hip) is elevated, but the joints are not usually red. Range of motion is limited, and muscle strength and function around inflamed joints are diminished. Soft, poorly delineated subcutaneous nodules are often found in the extensor surface of the forearm. Findings on general physical examination are normal, except for a possible low-grade fever (38°C); soft, small lymph nodes are found occasionally in epitracheal, axillary, and cervical areas. Movement is guarded, and apprehension often dominates facial expression. Initial laboratory tests often show the following:

- Slight leukocytosis with normal differential white blood cell (WBC) count
- Thrombocytosis
- Slight anemia (hemoglobin ≥ 10 g/dl), normochromic and either normocytic or microcytic
- Normal urinalysis
- ESR of 30 mm or more per hour (Westergren's method)
- Normal renal, hepatic, and metabolic function
- Normal serum uric acid level (before initiation of salicylate therapy)
- Positive RF test and negative antinuclear antibody (ANA) test
- Elevated levels of α_2- and α_1-globulins
- Normal or elevated serum complement level

A "typical" arthrocentesis in early RA reveals the following: Joint fluid is straw-colored and slightly cloudy and contains many flecks of fibrin. A clot forms in the fluid on standing at room temperature. There are 5000 to 25,000 WBCs per cubic millimeter, and at least 85 percent of these are polymorphonuclear leukocytes (PMNs). Some large PMNs with granules staining positively for immunoglobulins (IgG and IgM) and complement C3 are found. No crystals are present. The mucin clot is fair. Complement C4 and C2 levels are slightly depressed, but C3 is normal. IgG in synovial fluid may approach serum concentrations. Synovial fluid glucose level is depressed, occasionally to less than 25 mg/dl. Cultures are negative.

Differential Diagnosis of Rheumatoid Arthritis

Other diseases must be excluded before the diagnosis of RA is made.[61] One of the most difficult challenges is the patient with polyarthritis and fever; for this patient a full work-up may be required to define the underlying cause, which may be more life-threatening than RA itself.[62] The following diseases are listed in alphabetical order and their relative frequency specified as common, uncommon, or rare.

Angioimmunoblastic Lymphadenopathy (Rare)

Nonerosive, symmetric, seronegative polyarthritis involving large joints can be an initial complaint in angioimmunoblastic lymphadenopathy.[63] Typical clinical features are lymphadenopathy, hepatosplenomegaly, rash, and hypergammaglobulinemia. It can resemble Still's disease in adults if the arthritis precedes other manifestations. Diagnosis is based on the characteristic appearance of a lymph node or skin biopsy specimen, which includes effacement of lymph node architecture, proliferation of small vessels, and a cellular infiltrate (immunoblasts, plasma cells, T lymphocytes, and histiocytes) within amorphous acidophilic interstitial material. It is believed that symptoms may be related to excessive production of interleukin-2 by T helper cells in this process.

Ankylosing Spondylitis, Seronegative Spondyloarthropathy, and Reactive Arthritis (Common)

Ankylosing spondylitis, seronegative spondyloarthropathy, and reactive arthritis are often referred to as the "B27-associated diseases." The problem in differentiating them from RA arises with the patient (particularly a woman) who has minimal back pain and definite peripheral joint involvement. Indications against RA include noninvolvement of small joints, asymmetric joint disease, and lumbar spine involvement. (See Chapter 59.)

In some cases, the conclusion is inescapable that RA and ankylosing spondylitis are present in the same patient. In one series, nine patients with RF in serum had spinal ankylosis and symmetric erosive polyarthritis; eight of the nine carried HLA-B27.[64] If these two diseases occur completely independently of each other, simultaneous appearance in the same patient should occur once in every 50,000 to 200,000 adults.

In distinguishing patients with *Reiter's syndrome* from those with RA, a careful search for heel pain or tenderness and ocular or urethral symptoms is of great importance. Polyarthritis persists chronically in over 80 percent of patients with Reiter's syndrome. The characteristics of enthesopathy in patients with Reiter's syndrome (i.e., "sausage" digits indicating periarticular soft tissue inflammation, insertional tendinitis, periostitis, and peri-insertional osteoporosis or erosions) may point to the diagnosis.

The differential diagnosis between RA with psoriasis and psoriatic arthritis may be artificial (see Chapter 61). Some patients with DIP joint involvement and severe skin involvement obviously have a disease other than RA. Others, however, have a seropositive symmetric polyarthritis that appears to be RA, yet they also have psoriasis. These patients can be treated with the same disease-modifying drugs as those with progressive RA.

A syndrome described extensively in the French literature, *acne-pustulosis-hyperostosis-osteitis,*[65] may resemble psoriatic arthritis and, occasionally, when peripheral arthritis is present, RA. As the name implies, these patients variably express severe acne, palmar and plantar pustules, hyperostotic reactions (particularly in the clavicles and sternum), sacroiliitis, and peripheral inflammatory arthritis.

Inflammatory bowel disease (IBD) (ulcerative colitis and Crohn's disease) is associated with arthritis in 20 percent of cases[66] (see Chapter 62). Peripheral arthritis occurs more commonly than spondylitis in many series.[67] Ankles, knees, and elbows are the most typically involved peripheral joints, with PIP joints and wrists next in frequency. Simultaneous attacks of arthritis and development of erythema nodosum are not uncommon. Only two or three joints are affected at once. Involvement is usually asymmetric, and erosions are uncommon. The occurrence of peripheral arthritis in IBD is not related to HLA-B27.

Behçet's syndrome is marked by asymmetric polyarthritis in 50 to 60 percent of cases (see Chapter 68).[68] It is rare, with a prevalence of less than 1 in 25,000 in the United States. In more than half of the cases, the attacks of arthritis are monarticular.[69] Knees, ankles, and wrists are affected most often; synovial fluid usually contains more than 5000 but less than 30,000 WBCs/mm³. Joint deformity is unusual. Painful oral and genital ulcers and central nervous system (CNS) involvement are characteristic. Uveal tract involvement in Behçet's syndrome must be differentiated from scleritis characteristic of RA in patients with ocular and joint disease. Methotrexate and cyclosporine are the preferred therapy for this debilitating syndrome.[48]

Enteric infections are complicated occasionally by inflammatory joint disease resembling RA. The joint disease associated with *Yersinia enterocolitica* infections occurs several weeks after the gastrointestinal illness.[70] Knees and ankles are the joints most commonly involved, and the majority of patients (even those with peripheral arthritis and no spondylitis) have HLA-B27.[71] Reactive arthritis also has been reported after *Salmonella, Shigella,* and *Campylobacter (Helicobacter) jejuni.*

Arthropathy may precede other findings of Whipple's disease (see Chapter 62). The pattern is that of a migratory poly- or oligoarthritis involving ankles, knees, shoulders, elbows, and fingers, as with IBD. Remission may occur when diarrhea begins. Joint destruction in Whipple's disease is rare,[72] presumably because the synovitis lacks sustained chronicity.

Arthritis Associated with Oral Contraceptives (Uncommon)

A syndrome of persistent arthralgias, myalgias, and morning stiffness with occasional development of polyarticular synovitis has been described in women, usually in their 20s, who have been taking oral contraceptives (estrogens and progestins).[73] Positive tests for ANA are common, and patients may have circulating RF. Symptoms resolve after the contraceptive is discontinued.

Arthritis of Thyroid Disease (Uncommon)

In hypothyroidism, synovial effusions and synovial thickening simulating RA have been described.[74] The ESR may be elevated because of hypergammaglobulinemia. Joint fluid is noninflammatory and may have increased viscosity. Knees, wrists, hands, and feet are involved most often, and coexisting calcium pyrophosphate dihydrate (CPPD) deposition disease is not infrequently found. (See Chapter 96.)

The syndrome of thyroid acropachy complicates less than 1 percent of cases of hyperthyroidism.[75] This represents periosteal new bone formation, which may be associated with a low-grade synovitis similar to hypertrophic osteoarthropathy. Patients with coexisting RA and hyperthyroidism have pain from their arthritis that, although impossible to quantitate, appears to exceed that expected from the degree of inflammation.

Bacterial Endocarditis (Uncommon)

Arthralgias, arthritis, and myalgias occur in approximately 30 percent of patients with subacute bacterial endocarditis (SBE).[76] Symptoms typically occur in one or several joints, usually large proximal ones. This synovitis is probably caused by circulating immune complexes.[77] Fever out of proportion to joint findings in the setting of leukocytosis should lead to consideration of infective endocarditis as a diagnostic possibility, even in the absence of a significant heart murmur. It is wise to obtain blood cultures in all patients with polyarthritis and significant fever. Embolic phenomena with constitutional symptoms, including arthralgias, can be presenting symptoms of atrial myxoma, but this process usually mimics systemic vasculitis or SBE more than it does RA.[78]

Calcium Pyrophosphate Dihydrate Deposition Disease (Common)

CPPD deposition disease is a crystal-induced synovitis that takes many different forms, ranging from a syndrome of indolent osteoarthrosis to that of an acute, hot joint. About 5 percent of patients have a chronic polyarthritis (sometimes referred to as pseudorheumatoid arthritis) associated with proliferative erosions at subchondral bone.[79] Although radiographs are of great help when chondrocalcinosis is present, CPPD deposition may be present in the absence of calcification on radiographs.[80] Diagnosis then can be made only by arthrocentesis. One of the radiographic signs of CPPD deposition that helps to differentiate it from RA is the presence of unicompartmental disease in the wrists. (See Chapter 81.)

Diffuse Connective Tissue Disease: Systemic Lupus Erythematosus, Scleroderma, Dermatomyositis/Polymyositis, Vasculitis, Mixed Connective Tissue Disease (Common)

The entities comprised in diffuse connective tissue disease, discussed in depth in other chapters, may begin with a syndrome of mild systemic symptoms and minimal polyarthritis involving the PIP and MCP joints. It is not uncommon for one of these illnesses to evolve into another as years go by. The following list contains rules of thumb for characterizing joint disease of the various entities:

1. In systemic lupus erythematosus (SLE), an organized synovitis that causes erosions is rare. Soft tissue and muscle inflammation may lead to dislocation of normal tendon alignment, resulting in ulnar deviation similar to Jaccoud's arthropathy.
2. Limitation of joint motion in scleroderma is due to taut skin bound to underlying fascia. The same holds for dermatomyositis and polymyositis; proliferative synovitis is rarely sustained in these processes.
3. In reports of mixed connective tissue disease (MCTD) (i.e., patients with arthralgias, arthritis, hand swelling, sclerodactyly, Raynaud's phenomenon, esophageal hypomotility, and myositis with circulating antibody to ribonucleoprotein) 60 to 70 percent of patients have arthritis. Although few have significant titers in serum of RF, many are given an initial diagnosis of RA. Numerous studies of MCTD have revealed deforming, erosive arthritis. In one series, for example, 8 of 17 patients had presentation similar to that of RA.[81] Articular and periarticular osteopenia alone was found in 8. Six had loss of joint space, and 5 had erosions typical of RA. (See Chapters 64, 66 to 68, 70, and 73.)

Amyloidosis (Rare)

Deposits of amyloid can be found in synovial and periarticular tissues[82] and are presumably responsible for the joint complaints of some patients. The synovial fluid in amyloid arthropathy is noninflammatory, and particulate material with apple-green fluorescence after Congo red staining may be found in the fluid. Amyloid formed of β_2-microglobulin is found in joints of patients with chronic renal failure, usually those who are on dialysis. (See Chapter 86.)

Chronic Fatigue Syndrome (Common)

Numerous physicians prefer to separate chronic fatigue syndrome from fibromyalgia because of the possibility that it is caused by a slow virus infection (e.g.,

Epstein-Barr virus). However, because of the great overlap between the two, the best approach is to consider both as forms of "generalized rheumatism" and manage them in the same way. The finding of true synovitis essentially rules out the diagnosis of either chronic fatigue syndrome (perhaps caused by hypomagnesemia) or fibromyalgia. (See Chapter 34.)

Calcific Periarthritis (Uncommon)

Although usually involving single joints, calcific periarthritis can be confused with polyarthritis.[83] The skin is red over and around the affected joints; the tissues are boggy and tender, but no joint effusion is present. Passive motion is easier than active motion. Periarticular calcification is visible on radiographs. Unless the periarthritis can be differentiated from true arthritis, the findings may mimic palindromic rheumatism or early monarticular RA.

Congenital Camptodactyly and Arthropathy (Rare)

Congenital campodactyly and arthropathy is a deformity that begins in utero and produces synovial cell hypertrophy and hyperplasia without inflammatory cells.[84] Clinical manifestations include contractures of the fingers, flattening of the metacarpals, and short, thick femoral necks. This can present as oligoarticular seronegative RA.

Familial Mediterranean Fever (Uncommon)

The articular syndrome in familial Mediterranean fever is an episodic monarthritis or oligoarthritis of the large joints that appears in childhood or adolescence, mimicking oligoarthritic forms of juvenile RA (JRA).[85] Sephardic Jews account for up to 60% of reported cases. Episodes of arthritis come on acutely with fever and other signs of inflammation (e.g., peritonitis or pleuritis) and can precede other manifestations of the disease. Although usually limited to days or weeks, attacks occasionally last for months and are associated with radiographic changes of periarticular osteopenia without erosions. The abdominal pain that these patients experience can be a key to diagnosis. Amyloidosis (type AA) is a late complication of this syndrome in a number of patients. Regular doses of colchicine (0.5 to 2.0 mg/day) have been effective in decreasing the frequency of attacks and also prevent development of amyloidosis.

Fibromyalgia (Fibrositis) (Common)

In fibromyalgia there is rarely evidence of synovitis. Although no specific diagnostic tests define fibrositis, certain nonarticular locations for pain are common to different patients. In an analysis contrasting the pain properties with those of RA,[86] the fibromyalgia patients used diverse adjectives to describe their pain, the most common being pricking, pressing, shooting,

gnawing, cramping, splitting, and crushing. A majority in both groups defined the pain as aching and exhausting. Evidence is accumulating that patients with RA may develop a superimposed fibromyalgia. Rheumatoid patients have fewer psychologic disturbances than patients with primary fibrositis, but patients with both syndromes score higher on testing scales for hypochondriasis, depression, and hysteria than those with RA who do not have fibrositis. (See Chapter 34.)

Glucocorticoid Withdrawal Syndrome (Common)

Often confused with RA are the symptoms of glucocorticoid withdrawal. Patients on glucocorticoids who are being treated for nonrheumatic diseases may have diffuse polyarticular pain, particularly in the hands, if the glucocorticoid dose is tapered too rapidly. Although glucocorticoids suppress inflammation and pain, there is an arthropathy associated with their use[87] that resembles avascular necrosis.

Gout (Common)

Before a diagnosis of chronic erosive RA is made, chronic tophaceous gout must be ruled out. The reverse applies as well. Features of gouty arthritis that can mimic those of RA include polyarthritis, symmetric involvement, fusiform swelling of joints, subcutaneous nodules, and subacute presentation of attacks. Conversely, certain aspects of RA that suggest gouty arthritis include hyperuricemia (after treatment with low doses of aspirin), periarticular nodules, and seronegative disease (particularly in men).[88] Radiographic findings may be similar, with the appearance of the subcortical erosions of RA resembling small osseous tophi in gout.[89] Although large asymmetric erosions with ballooning of the cortex are more likely to be caused by gout than by RA, this is not always the case.[90] Serologic test results may be misleading as well; RF has been found in as many as 30 percent of patients with chronic tophaceous gout[91] with no clinical or radiographic signs of RA.

The coexistence of RA and gout is rare, and curiously so. Only 10 cases of gout coexisting with RA have been reported in the medical literature since 1881. Wallace and associates have calculated that, considering the prevalence of the two diseases, gout and RA should be anticipated to coexist in 10,617 cases in the United States.[28] In several patients with definite RA and persistent hyperuricemia, flares of the rheumatoid process coincided with normalization of the uric acid level.[29] Several other case reports have noted this and, as mentioned earlier in the chapter, the possibility that the hyperuricemic state is anti-inflammatory must be investigated further. (See Chapter 80.)

Hemochromatosis (Uncommon)

The characteristic articular feature of hemochromatosis that is almost diagnostic is firm bony enlargement of the MCP joints, particularly the second and third, with associated cystic degenerative disease on radiographs and, not infrequently, chondrocalcinosis.[92] Marginal erosions, juxta-articular osteoporosis, synovial proliferation, and ulnar deviation are not seen in the arthropathy of hemochromatosis but are common in RA. Wrists, shoulders, elbows, hips, and knees are involved less often than the MCP joints. More than one third of patients with this iron overload syndrome have an arthropathy.[93] (See Chapter 88.)

Hemoglobinopathies (Uncommon)

In homozygous (SS) sickle cell disease, the most common arthropathy is associated with crises and is believed to be a result of microvascular occlusion in articular tissues or gout.[94] However, in some cases a destructive arthritis with loss of articular cartilage has been reported[95] that resembles severe RA. In most patients with sickle cell disease and joint complaints, periosteal elevation, bone infarcts, fishmouth vertebrae, and avascular necrosis can be found on radiographs.[94] In a series of 37 patients with SS disease from which those with gout or avascular necrosis of the femoral head were excluded, 12 complained of a monarthritis or oligoarthritis associated with painful crises; tenderness was most marked over the epiphyses rather than the joint space, and synovial fluid was noninflammatory. Another 12 patients had arthritis of the ankle associated with a malleolar ulcer; this arthritis was chronic and resolved with improvement of the leg ulcer.[96] Episodic polyarthritis and noninflammatory synovial effusions are also found in sickle cell–beta-thalassemia.[97] (See Chapter 95.)

Hemophilic Arthropathy (Uncommon)

A deficiency of factor VIII or, less frequently, factor IX sufficient to produce clinical bleeding frequently results in hemarthroses. The iron overload in the joint generates a proliferative synovitis that often leads to joint destruction. The clotting abnormality is rarely overlooked, however, and it is unlikely that a diagnosis of RA would be made in the setting of hemophilia A or B. (See Chapter 94.)

HIV Infection (Common)

Several types of arthropathy have been described in association with human immunodeficiency virus (HIV) infection[62]:

- Brief, acute arthralgias concurrent with the initial HIV viremia
- AIDS-associated arthritis, lower extremity oligoarthritis, or a persistent polyarthritis[98]
- Seronegative spondyloarthropathy, resembling Reiter's syndrome, psoriatic arthritis, or reactive arthritis, often more severe than in patients without HIV infection[99]

The importance of ruling out HIV in any patient with an acute polyarthritis and fever is crucial: HIV-positive patients do not do well on immunosuppressive drugs! (See Chapter 93.)

Hyperlipoproteinemia (Uncommon)

Achilles tendinitis and tenosynovitis can be presenting symptoms in familial type II hyperlipoproteinemia and may be accompanied by arthritis.[100] Synovial fluid findings may resemble those of mild RA, and the tendon xanthomas may be mistaken for rheumatoid nodules or gouty tophi. Similarly, bilateral pseudoxanthomatous rheumatoid nodules have been described.[101] Asymmetric and oligoarticular synovitis has been described in type IV hyperlipoproteinemia.[102] The absence of morning stiffness in the presence of noninflammatory synovial effusions helps rule out RA. The treatment of hyperlipoproteinemia with clofibrate may cause an acute muscular syndrome[103] that resembles myositis or polymyalgia rheumatica more than RA.

Hypertrophic Osteoarthropathy (Uncommon)

Hypertrophic osteoarthropathy may present as oligoarthritis involving the knees, ankles, or wrists. The synovial inflammation accompanies periosteal new bone formation that can be seen on radiographs. Correction of the inciting factor (e.g., cure of pneumonia in a child with cystic fibrosis) will likely alleviate the synovitis. The synovium is characterized primarily by an increased blood supply and synovial cell proliferation. Little infiltration by mononuclear cells is seen.[104] Pain, which increases when extremities are dependent, is characteristic, although not always present. If clubbing is not present or is not noticed, this entity is easily confused with RA. (See Chapter 97.)

Idiopathic Hypereosinophilic Syndrome with Arthritis (Rare)

The poorly defined idiopathic hypereosinophilic syndrome often includes myalgias and arthralgias and evolves into a clinical picture of hepatomegaly with or without pericarditis, pulmonary hypertension, subcutaneous nodules, and cardiomyopathy. Synovitis, characterized by inflammatory joint fluid, rarely is erosive or deforming.[105] The similarities between this and toxic oil syndrome and eosinophilia-myalgia syndrome, both of which are caused by ingestion of toxic substances, suggests a basic hypersensitivity reaction.

Infectious Arthritis (Common)

Bacterial sepsis may be superimposed on RA. Viral infections, however, may present as arthritis, with many characteristics of RA. Rubella arthritis occurs more often in adults than in children and may affect small joints of the hands.[106] Lymphocytes predominate in synovial effusions.

Arthritis often precedes viral hepatitis and is associated with the presence of circulating hepatitis B surface antigen (HBsAg) and hypocomplementemia.[107] HBsAg has been found in synovial tissues using direct immunofluorescence, and this supports the concept that this synovitis is mediated by immune complexes.[108] A relatively acute onset of diffuse polyarthritis with small joint effusions and minimal synovial swelling should prompt the physician to obtain liver function tests in the patient with a history of exposure to hepatitis. With the onset of icterus, the arthritis usually resolves without a trace.

Fever, sore throat, and cervical adenopathy followed by symmetric polyarthritis are compatible with infection due to hepatitis B, rubella, adenovirus type 7, echovirus type 9, *Mycoplasma pneumoniae,* or Epstein-Barr virus,[109] as well as acute rheumatic fever or adult-onset Still's disease.

A chronic polyarthritis resembling RA has been described following serologic proof of parvovirus infection. Usually the process is self-limited and does not progress to a destructive synovitis. (See Chapter 90.)

Intermittent Hydrarthrosis (Common)

Intermittent hydrarthrosis is a syndrome of periodic attacks of benign synovitis in one or few joints, usually the knee, beginning in adolescence.[110] The difference between this and oligoarticular JRA or RA is one of degree, not kind. In contrast to palindromic rheumatism, in which acute synovitis may occur in different joints during successive attacks,[111] the same joint or joints are affected during each attack in intermittent hydrarthrosis.[112] Joint destruction does not occur because there is no proliferative synovitis.

Lyme Disease (Common in Some Areas)

Lyme disease can closely simulate RA in adults or children because of its intermittent course with development of chronic synovitis.[113] A proliferative, erosive synovitis necessitating synovectomy has evolved in several cases. Histopathology of the prolif- erative synovium is not different from that of RA. (See Chapter 92.)

Malignancy (Common)

Direct involvement by cancer of synovium usually presents as a monarthritis.[114] However, non-Hodgkin's lymphoma can present as seronegative polyarthritis without hepatomegaly or lymphadenopathy.[115] In children, acute lymphocytic leukemia can present as a polyarticular arthritis.[116] T lymphocyte malignancy has been associated with arthritis; several patients with a seronegative, erosive arthritis have been described who developed mycosis fungoides more than 4 years after the presentations of synovitis.[117] (See Chapter 98.)

Multicentric Reticulohistiocytosis (Rare)

Multicentric reticulohistiocytosis is particularly interesting because it causes severe arthritis mutilans with an opera-glass hand *(main en lorgnette).*[118] Other causes of arthritis mutilans are RA, psoriatic arthritis, erosive osteoarthritis treated with glucocorticoids, and gout (after treatment with allopurinol). The cell that effects damage to tissues is the multinucleate lipid-laden histiocyte, which appears to release degradative enzymes sufficient to destroy connective tissue. (See Chapter 89.)

Osteoarthritis (Common)

Although osteoarthritis begins as a degeneration of articular cartilage and RA begins as inflammation in the synovium, each process approaches the other as the diseases progress (Table 55–5). In osteoarthritis, as cartilage deteriorates and joint congruence is altered and stressed, a reactive synovitis often develops. Conversely, as the rheumatoid pannus erodes cartilage, secondary osteoarthritic changes in bone and cartilage develop. In end-stages of both degenerative joint dis-

Table 55–5. FACTORS USEFUL FOR DIFFERENTIATING EARLY RHEUMATOID ARTHRITIS FROM OSTEOARTHROSIS (OSTEOARTHRITIS)

	Rheumatoid Arthritis	Osteoarthritis
Age at onset	Childhood and adults, peak incidence in 50s	Increases with age
Predisposing factors	HLA-DR4, -DR1	Trauma, congenital abnormalities (e.g., shallow acetabulum)
Symptoms, early	Morning stiffness	Pain increases through the day and with use
Joints involved	Metacarpophalangeal joints, wrists, proximal interphalangeal joints most often; distal interphalangeal joints almost never	Distal interphalangeal joints (Heberden's nodes), weight-bearing joints (hips, knees)
Physical findings	Soft tissue swelling, warmth	Bony osteophytes, minimal soft tissue swelling early
Radiologic findings	Periarticular osteopenia, marginal erosions	Subchondral sclerosis, osteophytes
Laboratory findings	Increased erythrocyte sedimentation rate, rheumatoid factor, anemia, leukocytosis	Normal

ease and RA, the involved joints appear the same. To differentiate clearly between the two, therefore, the physician must delve into the early history and functional abnormalities of the disease. Erosive osteoarthritis occurs frequently in middle-aged women (more frequently than in men) and is characterized by inflammatory changes in PIP joints with destruction and functional ankylosis of the joints. The PIP joints can be red and hot, yet there is almost no synovial proliferation or effusion. Joint swelling involves hard, bony tissue and not synovium. The ESR may be slightly elevated, but RF is not found.[119] (See Chapter 83.)

Parkinson's Disease (Common)

Although the tremor or rigidity of Parkinson's disease is rarely confused with symptoms of rheumatoid arthritis, Parkinson's patients have a predilection for developing swan neck deformities of the hands, a phenomenon generally unappreciated by rheumatologists. This abnormality was first described in 1864,[120] and its pathogenesis is still unknown (Fig. 55–1).

Pigmented Villonodular Synovitis (Rare)

Pigmented villonodular synovitis is a nonmalignant but proliferative disease of synovial tissue that

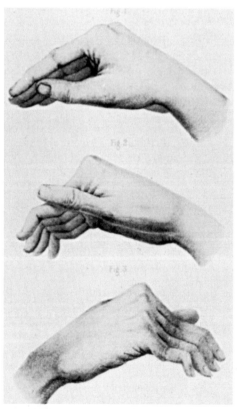

Figure 55–1. These swan neck deformities are a result of Parkinson's disease, not rheumatoid arthritis. (From Ordenstein L.: Sur la Paralysie Agitante et la Sclérose en Plaques Generalisée. Paris, Imprimerie de E. Martinet, 1864.)

has many functional characteristics similar to those of RA and usually involves only one joint. The histopathology is characterized by proliferation of histiocytes, multinucleate giant cells, and hemosiderin and lipid-laden macrophages. Clinically, this is a relatively painless chronic synovitis (most often of the knee) with joint effusions and greatly thickened synovium.[121] Subchondral bone cysts and cartilage erosion may be associated with the bulky tissue. It is not clear whether this should be classified as an inflammation or neoplasm of synovium. (See Chapter 102.)

Polychondritis (Uncommon)

Polychondritis can mimic infectious processes, vasculitis, granulomatous disease, or RA. Patients with RA and ocular inflammation (e.g., scleritis) usually have active joint disease before ocular problems develop; the reverse is true in polychondritis. In addition, polychondritis is not associated with rheumatoid factor. The joint disease is usually episodic. Nevertheless, erosions can develop that are not unlike those of RA. In affecting cartilage of the external ears, nose, larynx, trachea, and costochondral areas, this disease may represent a true immune response against cartilage. (See Chapter 85.)

Polymyalgia Rheumatica and Giant Cell Arteritis (Common)

Although joint radionuclide imaging studies have indicated increased vascular flow in the synovium of patients with classic polymyalgia rheumatica (PR), it remains appropriate to exclude PR as a diagnosis if significant synovitis (soft tissue proliferation or effusions) is detected. Otherwise, many patients who actually have RA would be diagnosed as having PR and treated with potentially harmful doses of glucocorticoids. A careful history can usually differentiate shoulder or hip girdle muscle pain from shoulder or hip joint pain. Examination of synovial biopsy specimens from PR patients indicates that the synovitis is more mild than that found in RA.[122] RA and PR probably coexist in numerous patients, but careful descriptions of such patients are rare.

Several patients have been described whose initial symptom of giant cell arteritis (GCA) was a peripheral polyarthritis clinically indistinguishable from RA.[123] In 19 such patients in a group of 522 with biopsy-proven GCA, however, only 3 were positive for RF. The interval between the onsets of each set of symptoms was 3 years or less in 15 of the 19, which also suggests a relationship between the two. (See Chapter 69.)

Rheumatic Fever (Uncommon)

Rheumatic fever is much less common than it once was but still must be considered in adults with polyarthritis. In adults, the arthritis is the most prominent clinical finding of rheumatic fever; carditis is less common than in children, and erythema marginatum, subcutaneous nodules, and chorea are rare.[124, 125] The presentation is often that of an additive, symmetric, large joint polyarthritis (involving lower extremities in 85 percent of patients), developing within a week and associated with a severe tenosynovitis.[124] This extremely painful process is dramatically responsive to salicylates.[126] Unlike Still's disease in the adult, rheumatic fever generally has no remittent or quotidian fevers and shows evidence of antecedent streptococcal infection. It also has a less protracted course than Still's disease. There are many similarities between rheumatic fever in adults and "reactive" postinfectious synovitis developing from *Shigella, Salmonella, Brucella, Neisseria,* or *Yersinia* infections. The latter processes do not respond well to salicylates, however. As rheumatic fever becomes less common and as penicillin prophylaxis effectively prevents recurrence of the disease, Jaccoud's arthritis (chronic post–rheumatic fever arthritis) is becoming rare. This entity, described first by Bywaters in 1950,[127] results from severe and repeated bouts of rheumatic fever and synovitis, which stretches joint capsules and produces ulnar deformity of the hands without erosions.[128] The same deformity can develop in SLE characterized by recurrent synovitis and soft tissue inflammation or in Parkinson's disease. Differentiating rheumatic fever from RA is particularly difficult when subcutaneous nodules are present with rheumatic fever.[129] (See Chapter 75.)

Sarcoidosis (Uncommon)

The two most common forms of sarcoid arthritis are usually easily differentiated from RA. In the acute form with erythema nodosum and hilar adenopathy (Lofgren's syndrome), the articular complaints are usually related to periarthritis affecting large joints of the lower extremities. Differential diagnosis may be complicated because many of these patients have RF in serum.[130] Joint erosions and proliferative synovitis do not occur in this form of sarcoidosis.

In chronic granulomatous sarcoidosis, cyst-like areas of bone destruction, mottled rarefaction of bone, and a reticular pattern of bone destruction with a lacelike appearance on radiographs may simulate destructive RA. This form of sarcoidosis is often polyarticular, and biopsy of bone or synovium for diagnosis may be essential, because there is often no correlation between joint disease and clinical evidence for sarcoid involvement of other organ systems.[131] It is likely that Poncet's disease or tuberculous rheumatism[132] actually represents granulomatous "idiopathic" arthritis (i.e., sarcoidosis). (See Chapter 87.)

Sweet's Syndrome (Rare)

Sweet's syndrome is also called acute febrile neutrophilic dermatosis.[133, 134] It has been described in adults, often following an influenza-like illness. The three major features are an acute illness with fever,

leukocytosis, and raised, painful plaques on the skin that show neutrophilic infiltration of the dermis on biopsy. Joint disease occurs in 20 to 25 percent of cases and is characterized by acute, self-limited polyarthritis. Because of the skin lesions, Sweet's syndrome is confused with SLE, erythema nodosum, and erythema elevatum diutinum more often than with RA. It has been treated effectively with indomethacin[134] and glucocorticoids.

Thiemann's Disease (Rare)

Thiemann's disease is a rare form of idiopathic vascular necrosis of the PIP joints of the hands with occasional involvement of other joints.[135, 136] Bony enlargement begins relatively painlessly, and the digits (one or more may be involved) become fixed in flexion. The primary lesion is in the region of the epiphysis and generally begins before puberty, distinguishing it from erosive osteoarthritis, which it resembles radiographically. It is clearly a heritable disease, but the genetic factors have not been defined.

COURSE AND COMPLICATIONS OF ESTABLISHED RHEUMATOID ARTHRITIS

Involvement of Specific Joints: Effects of Disease on Form and Function

The effects of rheumatoid synovitis on joints are a complex function of the intensity of the underlying disease, its chronicity, and the stress put on individual joints by the patient.

Cervical Spine

Unlike other nonsynovial joints, such as the sternomanubrial joint or symphysis pubis, the discovertebral joints in the cervical spine often manifest osteochondral destruction in RA[137, 138] and on lateral radiographs may be found to be narrowed to less than 5 mm. (See Chapter 27.) There is significant pain, but passive range of motion in the absence of muscle spasm may be normal. There are two possible mechanisms for this process: (1) extension of the inflammatory process from adjacent neurocentral joints, the joints of Luschka, which are lined by synovium, into the discovertebral area,[137, 138] and (2) chronic cervical instability initiated by apophyseal joint destruction leading to vertebral malalignment or subluxation.[139] This may produce microfractures of the vertebral endplates, disc herniation, and degeneration of disc cartilage.

The atlantoaxial joint is prone to subluxation in several directions:

1. The atlas moves *anteriorly* on the axis (most common). This results from laxity of the ligaments induced by proliferative synovial tissue developing in adjacent synovial bursa or from fracture or erosion of the odontoid process.

2. The atlas moves *posteriorly* on the axis. This can occur only if the odontoid peg has been fractured from the axis or destroyed.

3. The atlas is *vertically* subluxated in relation to the axis (least common). This results from destruction of the lateral atlantoaxial joints or of bone around the foramen magnum. It is apparent now that vertical (superior) migration of the odontoid can develop from unattended anterior or posterior subluxation.

The earliest and most common symptom of cervical subluxation is pain radiating up into the occiput.[140] Two other, less common clinical patterns are as follows:

1. Slowly progressive spastic quadriparesis, frequently with painless sensory loss in the hands.

2. Transient episodes of medullary dysfunction associated with vertical penetration of the dens and probable vertebral artery compression.[141] Paresthesias in the shoulders or arms may occur during movement of the head.

Physical findings suggestive of atlantoaxial subluxation include loss of occipitocervical lordosis, resistance to passive spine motion, and abnormal protrusion of the axial arch felt by the examining finger on the posterior pharyngeal wall. Radiographic views (lateral, with the neck in flexion) reveal more than 3 mm of separation between the odontoid peg and the axial arch.[141, 142] In symptomatic patients, the films in flexion should be taken only after radiographs (including an open-mouth posteroanterior view) have ruled out an odontoid fracture or severe atlantoaxial subluxation. Studies have indicated that computed tomography (CT) is useful for demonstrating spinal cord compression by loss of posterior subarachnoid space in patients with C1–C2 subluxation.[143] Magnetic resonance imaging (MRI) will prove valuable in the future in determining pathologic anatomy in this syndrome.[144]

Neurologic symptoms often have little relationship to the degree of subluxation and may be related to individual variations in the diameter of the spinal canal. Symptoms of spinal cord compression that demand intervention include[145]:

• A sensation of the head falling forward on flexion of the cervical spine
• Changes in level of consciousness
• "Drop" attacks
• Loss of sphincter control
• Dysphagia, vertigo, convulsions, hemiplegia, dysarthria, or nystagmus
• Peripheral paresthesias without evidence of peripheral nerve disease or compression

Some of these symptoms may be related to compression of the vertebral arteries, which must wind through foramina in the transverse processes of C1 and C2, rather than to compression of the spinal cord.

The progression of peripheral joint erosions parallels cervical spine disease in RA. The two coincide in severity and timing; development of cervical subluxation is more likely in patients with erosion of the hands and feet.[146] In a series of 113 patients with RA referred for hip or knee arthroplasty, 61 percent had roentgenographic evidence of cervical spine instability.[147]

Is mortality increased in patients with atlantoaxial subluxation? It was shown in a 5-year follow-up that neurologic signs do not inevitably develop in patients with large subluxations.[148] On the other hand, when signs of cervical cord compression do appear, myelopathy progresses rapidly, and 50 percent of these patients die within a year.[149, 150] In one series of 104 consecutive autopsies of patients with RA, 11 cases of severe dislocation were found.[151] In all 11 cases the odontoid protruded posterosuperiorly and impinged on the medulla within the foramen magnum. In 5 spinal cord compression was determined to be the only cause of death. These patients are at risk from even small falls, whiplash injuries, and general anesthesia with intubation. Cervical collars should be prescribed for stability. Operative stabilization may be considered if symptoms are progressive. In a series of 84 patients with some form of subluxation but without cord or brainstem lesions, one fourth worsened and one fourth improved without surgery over 5 to 14 years of follow-up.[152] Some data support the hypothesis that early C1–C2 fusion for atlantoaxial subluxation before the development of superior migration of the odontoid decreases the risk of further progression of cervical spine instability.[153] However, the incidence of sustained neurologic deterioration related to surgery may be as high as 6 percent,[154] and this emphasizes the importance of a skilled surgical team and the careful assessment of each patient.

Vertical atlantoaxial subluxation is important and may follow anterior or posterior subluxation. It was noted in 13 of 476 (3.7 percent) hospitalized patients with RA in one study.[155] Symptoms associated with this collapse of the lateral support system of the atlas occur in patients with severe erosive disease. Neurologic findings have included decreased sensation in the distribution of cranial nerve V and sensory loss in the C2 area, nystagmus, and pyramidal lesions. Vertical subluxations are believed to have a worse prognosis than the other varieties.[150]

Bywaters has demonstrated the existence of bursal spaces between the cervical interspinous processes in autopsies of patients without joint disease; in rheumatoid patients, bursal proliferation led in several cases to radiographically demonstrated destruction of the spinous processes.[156]

MRI is particularly valuable in the assessment of cervical spine disease in RA because the spinal cord as well as bone can be visualized.[144] This technology has enabled new diagnoses, including rheumatoid pannus–induced syringomyelia, to be made.[157]

Thoracic, Lumbar, and Sacral Spine

The thoracic, lumbar, and sacral portions of the spine usually are spared in RA. The exceptions are the apophyseal joints; rarely, synovial cysts at the apophyseal joint can impinge as an epidural mass on the spinal cord, causing pain and/or neurologic deficits.[158]

Temporomandibular Joints

The temporomandibular joint (TMJ) is commonly involved in RA. Histories reveal that 55 percent of patients have jaw symptoms at some time during the course of their disease.[159] Radiographic examination reveals structural alterations in 78 percent of the joints examined. An overbite may develop[160] as the mandibular condyle and the corresponding surface of the temporal bone, the eminentia articularis, are eroded. Physical examination of the rheumatoid patient should include palpation for tenderness and auscultation for crepitus. Occasionally, patients have acute pain and an inability to close the mouth, necessitating intra-articular glucocorticoids to suppress the acute process. It is important to remember that TMJ abnormalities are very common in non-rheumatoid populations. The only specific findings for RA in the TMJ are erosions and cysts of the mandibular condyle detected by CT or MRI, and there is no correlation between clinical and CT findings of the TMJ in RA.[161]

Cricoarytenoid Joints

The cricoarytenoid joints are small diarthrodial joints with an important function: They rotate with the vocal cords as they abduct and adduct to vary pitch and tone of the voice. Careful histories may reveal hoarseness in up to 30 percent of rheumatoid patients.[162] This is not disabling in itself, but there is a danger that the cricoarytenoid joints may become inflamed and immobilized, with the vocal cords adducted to the midline, causing inspiratory stridor.[163] Autopsy examinations have demonstrated cricoarytenoid arthritis in almost half the patients with RA, suggesting that much significant disease of the larynx may be asymptomatic.[164] This is borne out by the finding that although CT scans detected laryngeal abnormalities in 54 percent of patients with moderately severe RA, no symptoms suggested these abnormalities.[165] In contrast, findings with indirect laryngoscopy, which detected mucosal and gross functional abnormalities (including rheumatoid nodules), were abnormal in 32 percent of the same patients and correlated with symptoms of sore throat and difficult inspiration. It follows that the latter examination should be obtained in symptomatic rheumatoid patients. Asymptomatic cricoarytenoid synovitis may occasionally lead to aspiration of pharyngeal contents, particularly at night.

Ossicles of the Ear

Many rheumatoid patients experience a decrease in hearing. In general, this has been ascribed to salicylate toxicity, and it is believed to be reversible when the drug is discontinued. On the other hand, conductive hearing loss in patients not taking salicylates was reported by Copeman.[166] Studies using otoadmittance measurements have been carried out in patients with RA in an attempt to determine whether the interossicle joints were involved.[167] The data showed that 38 percent of "rheumatoid ears" and only 8 percent of controls demonstrated a pattern characteristic of increased flaccidity of a clinically normal tympanic membrane. This is consistent with erosions and shortening of the ossicles produced by the erosive synovitis, not with ankylosis.

Sternoclavicular and Manubriosternal Joints

Sternoclavicular and manubriosternal joints, both possessing synovium and a large cartilaginous disc, are often involved in RA.[168] Because of their relative immobility, there are few symptoms; however, patients occasionally complain of experiencing pain in sternoclavicular joints while lying on their sides in bed. When symptoms do occur, the physician must be concerned about superimposed sepsis. CT or MRI is useful for careful delineation of the sternoclavicular joint.

Manubriosternal involvement is almost never clinically important, although by tomographic criteria it is common in RA.[169] Some patients experience manubriosternal joint subluxation.

Shoulder

RA of the shoulder not only affects synovium within the glenohumeral joint but also involves the distal third of the clavicle, various bursae and the rotator cuff, and multiple muscles around the neck and chest wall.

Involvement of the rotator cuff in RA has been recognized as a principal cause of morbidity. The function of the rotator cuff is to stabilize the humeral head in the glenoid. Weakness of the cuff results in superior subluxation. Rotator cuff tears or insufficiency from other causes can be demonstrated by shoulder arthrogram. In a series of 200 consecutive patients with RA studied by arthrography, 21 percent had rotator cuff tears and an additional 24 percent had evidence of frayed tendons.[170] One likely mechanism behind tears is that the rotator cuff tendon insertion into the greater tuberosity is vulnerable to erosion by the proliferative synovitis that develops there.[171] Previous injury and aging may predispose to the development of tears.[172] Sudden tears may be accompanied by pain and inflammation so great as to suggest sepsis.

Standard radiographic examinations of the shoulder in RA reveal erosions (69 percent) and superior subluxation (31 percent).[173] Arthrograms, in addition to showing tears of the rotator cuff, can demonstrate diffuse nodular filling defects, irregular capsular attachment, bursal filling defects, adhesive capsulitis, and dilation of the biceps tendon sheath (perhaps unique to RA).[174] High-resolution CT or MRI may provide much of this information without invasive techniques. Marked soft tissue swelling of the antero-lateral aspect of the shoulders in RA may be caused by chronic subacromial bursitis rather than by gleno-humeral joint effusions.[175] In contrast to rotator cuff tears, bursal swelling is not necessarily associated with decreased range of motion or pain. Synovial proliferation within the subdeltoid bursa may explain the resorption of the undersurface of the distal clavicle seen in this disease.[176] Rarely, the shoulder joint may rupture, with symptoms resembling those of obstruction of venous return from the arm.[177]

Elbow

Severe pain in the elbow, perhaps because it is a stable hinge joint, rarely is manifest in RA. Nevertheless, involvement of the elbow is common, and if lateral stability at the elbow is lost as the disease progresses, disability can be severe.

The frequency of elbow involvement varies from 20 to 65 percent, depending on the severity of disease in the patient populations studied. One of the earliest findings, often unnoticed by the patient, is loss of full extension. Because the elbow is principally a connecting joint between the hand and trunk, the shoulder and wrists can compensate for the loss of elbow motion.[178]

Hand and Wrist

The hand and wrist should be considered together because they form a functional unit. There are data, for example, linking disease of the wrist to ulnar deviation of the MCP joints.[179, 180] The hypothesis is that weakening of the extensor carpi ulnaris muscle leads to radial deviation of the wrist as the carpal bones rotate (the proximal row in an ulnar direction, the distal ones in a radial direction).[179] In response to this, ulnar deviation of the fingers (a "zigzag" deformity) occurs to keep the tendons to the phalanges in a normal line with the radius. Other factors, including the tendency for power grasp to pull the fingers into an ulnar attitude[181] and inappropriate intrinsic muscle action,[182] are involved (Fig. 55–2).[183–187] It is important to note that erosion of bone or articular cartilage is not essential for the development of ulnar deviation. Significant although reducible ulnar deviation can result from repeated synovitis or muscle weakness in the hands (e.g., in SLE).

Dorsal swelling on the wrist within the tendon sheaths of the extensor muscles is one of the earliest signs of disease. Typically, the extensor carpi ulnaris and extensor digitorum communis sheaths are involved. Rarely, cystic structures resembling ganglia are early findings of RA.[188, 189]

As the synovial proliferation develops within the wrist, pressure increases within the relatively nondistensible joint spaces. Proliferative synovium develops enzymatic machinery sufficient to destroy ligaments,

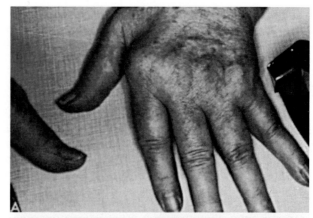

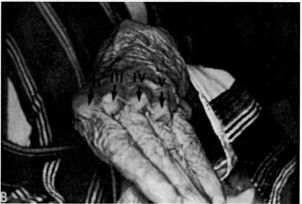

Figure 55–2. *A,* Early ulnar deviation of the metacarpophalangeal joints without subluxation. Extensor tendons have slipped to the ulnar side. The fifth finger, in particular, is compromised with weak flexion, causing loss of power grip. *B,* Complete subluxation with marked ulnar deviation at the metacarpophalangeal joints of a 90-year-old woman with rheumatoid arthritis. *Arrows* mark the heads of the metacarpals, now in direct contact with the joint capsule instead of the proximal phalanges. (Courtesy of James L. McGuire, M. D.)

tendons, and the articular disc distal to the ulnar head. Pressure and enzymes combine to produce communications among radiocarpal, radioulnar, and midcarpal joints.[160, 190] Integrity of the distal radioulnar joint is lost. The ulnar collateral ligament, stretched by the proliferative synovium of the radioulnar joint, finally either ruptures or is destroyed, and the ulnar head springs up into dorsal prominence, where it "floats" and is easily depressed by the examiner's fingers.

On the volar side of the wrist, synovial protrusion cysts develop; they can be palpated, and their origins can be confirmed by arthrography.[191] The thick transverse carpal ligament prevents significant resistance to decompression, however, and the hyperplastic synovium compressing the median nerve can cause carpal tunnel syndrome.

Progression of disease in the wrist is characterized either by loss of joint space and loss of bone or by ankylosis. Disintegration of the carpus has been quantitated in terms of a carpal to metacarpal (C:MC) ratio (length of the carpus divided by that of the third

Table 55–6. FACTORS DIMINISHING HAND GRASP STRENGTH IN RHEUMATOID ARTHRITIS

Synovitis in joints
Reflex inhibition of muscular contraction secondary to pain
Altered kinesiology; distorted relation of joint, bones, and tendons during motion
Flexor tenosynovitis, with or without rheumatoid nodules on tendons
Vascular ischemia → pain, from altered sympathetic tone
Edema of all structures, from inflammation and perhaps altered lymphatic drainage
Intrinsic muscle atrophy and/or fibrosis

metacarpal). There is a linear decrease in the C:MC ratio with progressive disease.[192] This is caused by compaction of bone at the radiolunate, lunate-capitate, and capitate–third metacarpal joints, which usually accompanies severe disease. One study has confirmed the usefulness of the C:MC ratio for quantitating joint destruction and making correlations with anatomic progression over time.[193] Early detection of carpal bone involvement by RA is possible using MRI,[163] which reveals early synovial proliferation and carpal bone erosions. Bony ankylosis is associated with both the duration and the severity of disease[194] and probably is found in joints that have been relatively immobilized by pain, inflammation, treatment, or all of these.

The hand may have many joints involved in RA. A sensitive index of hand involvement is grip strength (Table 55–6). The act of squeezing puts stress on all hand joints. Muscular contraction causes ligamentous tightening around joints, compressing inflamed synovium. The immediate result is weakness, with or without pain; the reflex inhibition of muscular contraction due to pain may be a primary factor in this weakness. Quantitative radiographic scores for joint space narrowing, erosion, and malalignment correlate well with loss of motion but do not correlate with joint count tenderness scores[195]; these data support the

concept that inflammatory synovitis and the erosive/destructive potential of proliferative synovitis in RA are not one and the same, but rather reflect different aspects of the same disease.

The *swan neck deformity* is one of flexion of the DIP and MCP joints with hyperextension of the PIP joint. The lesion probably begins with shortening of the interosseous muscles and tendons. Shortening of the intrinsic muscles exerts tension on the dorsal tendon sheath, leading to hyperextension of the PIP joint (Fig. 55–3).[196] Deep tendon contracture or, rarely, DIP joint involvement with RA leads to the DIP joint flexion.[197] Rupture of the sublimis tendon, which reduces capacity to flex the PIP joint, can lead to the same deformity.[198] Marginal erosive changes in the DIP joints occur more often in patients with RA who have coexisting osteoarthritis.[199]

If, during chronic inflammation of a PIP joint, the extensor hood stretches or is avulsed, the joint may pop up in flexion, producing a *boutonnière deformity* (Fig. 55–4).[184, 198] The DIP joint remains in hyperextension. Without either of these deformities, limitation of movement develops at the PIP and DIP joints. Limitation of full flexion of the DIP joint is common

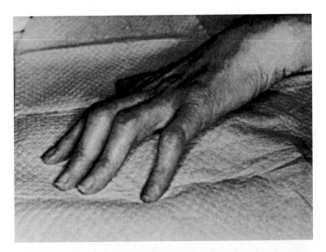

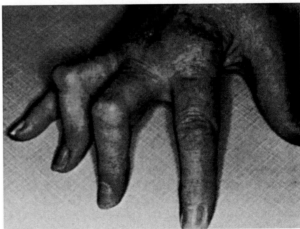

Figure 55–3. Early swan neck deformity in RA. Synovial proliferation and early subluxation of the metacarpophalangeal joints are present as well. (Courtesy of G. Uribarri and the Ministerio de Sanidad y Consuma, Madrid, Spain.)

Figure 55–4. Early *(top)* and late *(bottom)* "boutonnière" deformity of the phalanges in RA. *Bottom,* Moderate soft tissue swellings at the second and third metacarpophalangeal joints are visible.

in RA and represents incomplete profundus contraction. Similarly, tight intrinsic muscles may prevent full flexion of PIP joints when the MCP joints are in full extension.

The most serious result of rheumatoid involvement of the hand is resorptive arthropathy, defined as severe resorption of bone that begins at the articular cartilage and spreads along the diaphysis of the involved phalanges. Digits appear shortened, excess skin folds are present, and phalanges can be retracted (telescoped) into one another and then pulled out into abnormally long extension, often without pain. It occurs in about 5 percent of rheumatoid patients[167] and is associated with longer duration of aggressive synovitis.

Three types of deformity have been described for the thumb[167]:

1. Type I: Metacarpophalangeal inflammation leads to stretching of the joint capsule and a boutonnière-like deformity.

2. Type II: Inflammation of the carpometacarpal (CMC) joint leads to volar subluxation during contracture of the adductor hallucis.

3. Type III: After prolonged disease of both MCP joints, exaggerated adduction of the first metacarpus, flexion of the MCP joint, and hyperextension of the DIP joint result from the patient's need to provide a means to pinch.

The DIP joints have less synovial membrane than PIP joints; perhaps because of this and lower intra-articular temperatures protecting them, DIP joints are less often involved in RA. However, in one study using DIP joints as a primary focus, radiographic abnormalities (surface erosions and joint space narrowing) were observed in 37 percent of 62 RA patients and only in 14 percent of control patients. The DIP joint changes were not related to the duration or overall severity of the RA.[200]

One of the most common manifestations of RA in hands is tenosynovitis in flexor tendon sheaths, and this can be a major cause of hand weakness.[169] This is manifested on the volar surfaces of the phalanges as diffuse swelling between joints or a palpable grating within flexor tendon sheaths in the palm, and may occur in up to 55 percent of patients.[201] Although hand flexor tenosynovitis has not been found to be associated with more prolonged or severe disease, an association has been revealed with a number of para-articular manifestations (distinct from extra-articular manifestations).[202] It is particularly important to diagnose *de Quervain's tenosynovitis* because it causes severe discomfort and yet is relatively easily treated; it represents tenosynovitis in the extensors of the thumb. Pain originating from these sheaths can be demonstrated by Finklestein's test: ulnar flexion at the wrist after the thumb is maximally flexed and adducted.

Not infrequently, rheumatoid nodules develop within tendon sheaths and may "lock" the finger painfully into flexion, necessitating surgical excision or glucocorticoid injections when they become chronic and recurrent.

Hip

The hip is less frequently involved early in RA than in JRA. Hip joint involvement must be ascertained by a careful clinical examination. Pain on the lateral aspect of the hip is often a manifestation of trochanteric bursitis rather than synovitis.

About half of the patients with established RA have radiographic evidence of hip disease.[203] The femoral head may collapse and be resorbed, and the acetabulum is often re-formed as it is pushed medially, leading to protrusio acetabuli. Significant protrusion occurs in about 5 percent of all patients with RA.[204] Loss of internal rotation on physical examination correlates best with radiographic findings. Similar to the situation in other weight-bearing joints, the femoral head may develop cystic lesions. Communication of these with the joint space can often be demonstrated on surgically resected femoral heads.[205]

Knees

In contrast to the hips, in the knees synovial inflammation and proliferation are readily demonstrated. Early in knee disease, often within a week after the onset of symptoms, quadriceps atrophy is noticeable and leads to the application of more force than usual through the patella to the femoral surface. Another early manifestation of knee disease in RA is loss of full extension, a functional loss that can become a fixed flexion contracture unless corrective measures are undertaken.[206]

Flexion of the knee markedly increases the intra-articular pressure and may produce an outpouching of posterior components of the joint space, a popliteal or Baker's cyst. Jayson and Dixon have demonstrated that fluid from the anterior compartments of the knee may enter the popliteal portion but does not readily return.[207] This one-way valve may produce pressures so high in the popliteal space that it may rupture down into the calf or, rarely, superiorly into the posterior thigh. Rupture occurs posteriorly between the medial head of the gastrocnemius and the tendinous insertion of the biceps. Clinically, popliteal cysts and their complications have several manifestations (Table 55–7). The intact popliteal cyst may compress superficial venous flow to the upper part of the leg, producing dilation of superficial veins and/or edema.[208]

Table 55–7. DIFFERENTIAL DIAGNOSIS OF POPLITEAL CYSTS

Lipoma	Hemangioma
Xanthoma	Lymphadenopathy
Fibrosarcoma	Charcot's joint
Vascular tumor	Thrombophlebitis
Varicose veins	

Rupture of the joint posteriorly with dissection of joint fluid into the calf may resemble acute thrombophlebitis with swelling and tenderness, as well as systemic signs of fever and leukocytosis.[209, 210] One helpful sign in identifying joint rupture may be the appearance of a crescentic hematoma beneath one of the malleoli.[211] Although arthrography will clearly define the abnormal anatomy of a Baker's cyst, this invasive procedure has been replaced by ultrasound[212] and, when necessary, MRI.

It has been well documented that high-resolution MRI accurately portrays the gross state of articular cartilage in the knee, including its precise thickness, erosions or thinning, and irregularities.[213]

Ankle and Foot

The ankle rarely is involved in mild or oligoarticular RA but often is damaged in severe progressive forms of the disease. Clinical evidence for ankle involvement is a cystic swelling anterior and posterior to the malleoli. Much of the stability of the ankle depends on the integrity of the ligaments holding the fibula to the tibia and these two bones of the talus. In RA, inflammatory and proliferative disease may loosen these connections by stretching and eroding the collagenous ligaments. The result is incongruity, which progresses to pronation deformities and eversion of the foot

The Achilles tendon is a major structural component and kinetic force in the foot and ankle. Rheumatoid nodules develop in this collagenous structure, and spontaneous rupture of the tendon has been reported when diffuse granulomatous inflammation is present.[214] The subtalar joint controls eversion and inversion of the foot on the talus; patients with RA invariably have more pain while walking on uneven ground, and this is related to the relatively common subtalar joint involvement in RA.[215]

More than one third of patients with RA have significant disease in the feet (Fig. 55–5).[216] Metatarsophalangeal (MTP) joints are often involved, and gait is altered as pain develops during push-off in striding. It is of interest that downward subluxation of the metatarsal heads occurs soon after the MTP joints become involved, producing "cock-up" toe deformities of the PIP joints. Hallux valgus and bunion or callus formation appear if disease continues. Cystic collections representing outpouchings of flexor tendon sheaths often develop under the MTP joints.[217] Patients with subluxation of metatarsal heads to the subcutaneous area may develop pressure necrosis. Alternatively, patients who have subluxation of MTP joints often develop pressure necrosis over the PIP joints that protrude dorsally (hammer toes).

The sequence of changes as disease progresses in the foot is as follows[215, 218]:

1. Intermetatarsal joint ligaments stretch.
2. Spread of the forefoot occurs.
3. The fibrofatty cushion on the plantar surface migrates anteriorly.
4. Subluxation of toes occurs dorsally, and extensor tendons shorten.
5. Subluxation of metatarsal heads to a subcutaneous site on the plantar surface occurs.
6. Development of hallux valgus results in "stacking" of the second and third toes on top of the great toe.

It is important to note that DIP joints of the foot rarely are affected in RA. A functional rigid hallux caused by muscle spasm of the great toe intrinsic

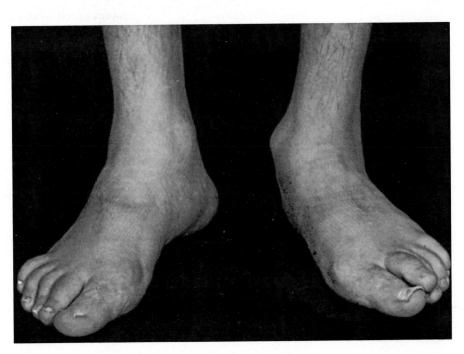

Figure 55–5. Valgus of ankle, pes planus, and forefoot varus deformity of the left foot related to painful synovitis of the ankle, forefoot, and metatarsophalangeal joint in a 24-year-old man with severe rheumatoid arthritis.

muscles in an effort to relieve pressure on the lesser metatarsal heads can be very painful and require surgical intervention.[219]

Another cause of foot pain in rheumatoid patients is the tarsal tunnel syndrome. In a group of 30 patients with RA, radiographically demonstrated erosions in the feet, and foot pain, 4 (13 percent) were shown by electrodiagnostic techniques to have slowing of medial and/or lateral plantar nerve latency.[220]

Involvement of the Skeleton

The skeleton has two anatomically and functionally separate components, cortical and trabecular bone, which respond differently to systemic and local diseases and to drugs. Three questions about bones are of great interest to those studying and caring for patients with RA: Does RA produce a generalized osteopenia? What are the influences of sex and age on the skeleton in patients with RA? What are the effects of low-dose glucocorticoids on bone in RA and, if deleterious, can they be prevented or treated? The available data on these topics have been reviewed in the discussions of glucocorticoid therapy (see Chapters 50, 56, 100, and 101).

The diffuse loss of bone in RA, whether or not it is related to glucocorticoid therapy, leads to the high incidence of stress fractures of long bones in RA.[221, 222] The fibula is the most common fracture site. Acute leg pain in the thin, elderly rheumatoid patient, even without a history of trauma, should generate suspicion of a stress fracture. Geodes (i.e., subchondral cysts developed by synovial penetration of the cortex or subchondral plate and subsequent proliferation) weaken bone and can predispose bone to fracture, even in phalanges.[223]

Muscle Involvement

Clinical weakness is common in RA, but is it caused by muscle involvement in the rheumatoid inflammation or is it a reflex weakness response to pain? Most rheumatoid patients have muscle weakness, but few have muscle tenderness. An exception to this is the occasional patient with a severe flare of activity disease; such a patient may cry out in severe pain, unable to move either muscles or joints. These symptoms resemble those of vascular insufficiency (ischemic pain) in their intensity.

In an early autopsy series, focal accumulations of lymphocytes and plasma cells with some contiguous degeneration of muscle fibers were found in all rheumatoid patients, a condition termed *nodular myositis*.[224] More recent studies have pointed to at least five different stages of muscle disease in RA[225, 226]:

- Diminution of muscle bulk with atrophy of type II fibers
- Peripheral neuromyopathy, usually due to mononeuritis multiplex

- Steroid myopathy
- Active myositis and muscle necrosis with foci of endomysial mononuclear cell infiltration
- Chronic myopathy resembling a dystrophic process, probably the end-stage of inflammatory myositis.

Atrophy of type II fibers is most common. Active myositis and focal necrosis is not uncommonly noted on biopsy specimens of patients with active disease, particularly in an interesting subset with mild synovitis and a disproportionately high ESR.[226] Emphasizing the systemic nature of RA, in some patients the lymphocytes in biopsied muscle have been shown to synthesize IgM rheumatic factor. Thus, the "nodules of myositis" contain plasma cells as well as lymphocytes. Unlike polymyositis/dermatomyositis, myositis in RA is patchy, and the weakness experienced by these patients responds readily to low-dose prednisone.

Involvement of Skin

The most frequently recognized skin lesion in RA is the rheumatoid nodule (discussed on the next page), but there are several other manifestations as well. Perhaps related to the underlying synovitis, skin—particularly over the hands and fingers—becomes thin and atrophic. Palmar erythema is common, but Raynaud's syndrome is rarely found. Manifestations of vasculitis can range from occasional nail fold infarcts to a deep, erosive, scarring pyoderma gangrenosa. Palpable purpura in rheumatoid patients often is related to a reaction to a drug that the patient is taking, but can be primary and a direct function of the severity of articular disease.[227]

Involvement of the Eye

Virtually all ocular manifestations of rheumatoid arthritis can be considered complications of the disease. *Keratoconjunctivitis sicca* is a component of Sjögren's syndrome and is discussed in Chapter 58. More directly related to the rheumatoid process seen in the synovium and within rheumatoid nodules are scleritis and episcleritis. The highly differentiated connective tissues in the eye make rheumatoid manifestations particularly interesting and, when they occur in aggressive form, very serious.[228]

The episclera of the eye is highly vascular compared with the dense sclera. Either scleritis or episcleritis or both occur in fewer than 1 percent of rheumatoid patients.[229] In episcleritis, the eye becomes red within minutes. Unlike conjunctivitis, there is no discharge other than tearing in response to the gritty discomfort. Loss of vision does not occur as a direct result of the episcleritis, but a keratitis or cataract developing secondarily can cause visual loss. Scleritis causes severe ocular pain and a dark red discoloration (Fig 55–6). No discharge is present. Depending on the

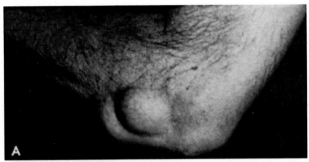

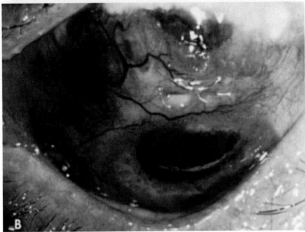

Figure 55–6. Manifestations of increased reactivity of mesenchymal tissue in rheumatoid arthritis appearing *(A)* as nodules on the elbow and *(B)* within the sclera of the eye. The eye lesion represents scleral perforation associated with a granulomatous scleral reaction. Treatment was placement of a scleral patch graft. Note the increase in vascularity of the sclera. The dark areas represent scleral thinning with exposure of uveal pigment. (Patient of Drs. S. Arthur Bouchoff and G. N. Fouhls. Photograph courtesy of Marty Schener.)

intensity of the process, scleritis can be localized and superficial or generalized, with or without granulomatous resorption of the sclera down to the uveal layer, a complication known as scleromalacia perforans.

EXTRA-ARTICULAR COMPLICATIONS OF RHEUMATOID ARTHRITIS

The complications of RA may be fatal. In general, the number and severity of extra-articular features vary with the duration and severity[230, 231] of the disease. A number of these features may be related to extra-articular foci of an immune response,[232] based on evidence of independent and qualitatively different production of RF in the pleural space, pericardium, muscle, and even meninges. These patients with "spill-over" immune responses have true rheumatoid disease, not just rheumatoid arthritis.

Rheumatoid Nodules

The pathologic findings in rheumatoid nodules are well documented.[233, 234] The well-formed nodule has a

central area of necrosis rimmed by a corona of palisading fibroblasts that is surrounded by a collagenous capsule with perivascular collections of chronic inflammatory cells. The earliest nodules, a nest of granulation tissue, have been identified at a size of less than 4 mm.[235] The nodules grow by accumulating cells that expand centrifugally, leaving behind central necrosis initiated by vasculopathy and compounded by protease destruction of the connective tissue matrix.

Careful histologic study of early lesions[236] suggests that development of the nodule is mediated through affected small arterioles and resulting complement activation and terminal vasculitis.[237] This immunologic response is linked to proliferation of resident histiocytes and fibroblasts, as well as an influx of macrophages from circulation. Both the proliferation of cells and the supporting scaffold of connective tissue are mediated by cytokines.[235] However, the precipitating event may be local trauma. Thus, nodules appear at pressure points such as the olecranon process and, in bedridden patients, even on the occiput that rests against the bed.

Data from studies using monoclonal antibodies against receptors for complement C3b and C3bi, monocytes, activated macrophages, and HLA-DR molecules suggest that mononuclear phagocytes that are constantly being recruited into the peripheral layers subsequently migrate into the palisade layer and make up most of the cell population in this area.[238] Other studies, using cytochemical markers (nonspecific esterase and CD68—a protein associated with lysosomes—for macrophages, and prolyl hydroxylase for fibroblasts), indicate that a mixture of macrophages and non–synoviocyte fibroblasts make up the cellular content of nodules.[239] This evidence fits with data from nodule tissue in organ culture. The cells have the capacity to produce collagenase and protease in large quantity, similar to synovial tissue.[240] It has been suggested that these enzymes released by the palisading layer of cells may be sufficient to result in destruction of the extracellular matrix collagen around the cells, leading to their death and to the centrifugally expanding central necrosis commonly found in these nodules.

Occurring in 20 to 35 percent of patients with definite or classic RA, nodules are found most easily on extensor surfaces such as the olecranon process and the proximal ulna. They are subcutaneous and vary in consistency from a soft, amorphous, entirely mobile mass to a hard, rubbery mass attached firmly to the periosteum.

RF is almost always found in the serum of patients with rheumatoid nodules. Rarely, such nodules are present in the absence of obvious arthritis.[241] The presence of multiple nodules on the hands and a positive test for RF associated with episodes of acute intermittent synovitis and subchondral cystic lesions of small bones of the hands and feet represent a condition that has been called *rheumatoid nodulosis*.[242, 243] Aggressive therapy with second-line drugs helped induce complete resolution of all nodules in one patient.[244]

The differential diagnosis of rheumatoid nodules includes the following:

1. *"Benign" nodules.* These usually are found in healthy children without RF or arthritis. They are nontender; appear often on the pretibial regions, feet, and scalp; increase rapidly in size; and are histologically identical to rheumatoid nodules.[245] They usually resolve spontaneously, although in one case classic RA developed 50 years after the first appearance of "benign" olecranon nodules.[246]

2. *Granuloma annulare.* These nodules are intracutaneous but histologically identical to rheumatoid nodules. They slowly resolve and are not associated with other disease.[247]

3. *Xanthomatosis.* These nodules usually have a yellow tinge, and patients have abnormally high plasma lipoprotein and cholesterol levels. There is no underlying bone involvement.[101]

4. *Tophi.* These collections of monosodium urate crystals in patients with gout are associated with small, punched-out bone lesions and are rarely found in patients with a normal serum urate concentration. A search for crystals with a polarizing microscope will reveal the classic needle-shaped, negatively birefringent crystals.

5. *Miscellaneous nodules.* The nodules of multicentric reticulohistiocytosis have been described. Numerous proliferative disorders that affect cutaneous tissue, including erythema elevatum diutinum, acrodermatitis chronica atrophicans, bejel, yaws, pinta, and leprosy, can resemble rheumatoid nodules. A rheumatoid nodule, particularly when it occurs on the face, may simulate basal cell carcinoma.[248]

The appearance of nodules in unusual sites may lead to confusion in diagnosis. Sacral nodules may be mistaken for bedsores if the overlying skin breaks down.[249] Occipital nodules also occur in bedridden patients. In the larynx, rheumatoid nodules on the vocal cords may cause progressive hoarseness.[250] Nodules found in the heart and lungs will be discussed later. Nodules on the sclera can produce perforation of this collagenous tissue. There have been at least 14 reports of rheumatoid nodule formation within the CNS,[251] involving leptomeninges more than parenchyma. Some patients develop rheumatoid nodules within vertebral bodies, resulting in bone destruction and signs of myelopathy.[252]

Fistula Development

Cutaneous sinuses near joints develop rarely in seropositive patients with long-standing disease and positive tests for RF.[253] These fistulas can be either sterile or septic and connect the skin surface with a joint, with a para-articular cyst in bone or soft tissues,[254] or with a bursa.[255] The pathogenesis of fistulas without a septic origin is particularly difficult to understand because the rheumatoid process usually is so clearly centripetal (that is, progressing toward the center of the joint) rather than centrifugal in nature.

Infection

There have been no reports of a higher frequency of genitourinary or bronchopulmonary infections either before or after the onset of joint disease in rheumatoid patients compared with osteoarthritic patients.[256] Thus, the increased mortality in RA from infection appears related to factors that evolve during the course (and treatment) of the disease and not to any predisposition to infection. The incidence of infections as a complication of RA has paralleled the use of glucocorticoids and immunosuppressive agents.[257] Pulmonary infections, skin sepsis, and pyarthrosis are most common.[258, 259] In addition to the presence of drugs that suppress host resistance, the phagocytic capacity of leukocytes in RA may be less than normal.[260] Difficulty in diagnosis is accentuated by the similarity of aggressive RA to infection, particularly in joints; a "pseudoseptic" arthritis in rheumatoid patients, associated with fever, chills, and grossly purulent synovial fluid, can be part of a severe exacerbation of RA and clearly must be distinguished from infection.[261]

Cancer

It is very difficult to distinguish the influence of RA associations with malignancy because of the strong oncogenic influences from the immunosuppressive treatments used in the disease, each of which can be shown to lead to neoplasms of the immune system. Indeed, there is justified debate about whether cancer occurring in rheumatoid patients should be viewed as a complication or an association. There appears to be an increased risk for malignancy in all RA patients, with a markedly increased risk in certain patient subsets.[262] The exception to this is cancer of the gastrointestinal tract, for which there appears to be a reduced risk for RA patients.[263] It is possible that NSAIDs lower the risk of this form of cancer, as supported by evidence that these drugs can diminish the occurrence and numbers of colonic polyps.

RA patients confront a risk of Hodgkin's disease, non-Hodgkin's lymphoma, and leukemia two to three times that of the normal population; this is independent of immunosuppressive therapy.[264, 265] Of the lymphomas arising in RA, about half are low-grade and half high-grade; most of these are B cell lymphomas, although there is no evidence that these originated from clonally proliferated lymphocytes associated with RA. In contrast, although the relative risk for total cancer in patients with Felty's syndrome is only 2, the relative risk for non-Hodgkin's lymphoma is near 13,[266] similar to that associated with Sjögren's syndrome.[267]

Hematologic Abnormalities

The majority of patients with RA have a mild normocytic hypochromic anemia that correlates with the ESR elevation and with activity of the disease.[268, 269]

Anemia is often of mixed causes in RA. One deficiency may mask evidence of others, resulting in ineffective therapy. In a European series[270] of 25 patients, iron deficiency (assessed by bone marrow iron content) was present in 52 percent, vitamin B_{12} deficiency in 29 percent, and folate deficiency in 21 percent. All these patients are likely to have anemia of chronic disease. The following guidelines may be helpful in distinguishing anemia in the rheumatoid patient:

1. Anemia of chronic disease is associated with significantly higher serum ferritin concentration than is iron deficiency.

2. Folate and B_{12} deficiency may mask iron deficiency by increasing the mean cell volume and mean cell hemoglobin of erythrocytes.

3. The ESR correlates inversely with hemoglobin in RA, as expected in anemia of chronic disease.[271]

4. Erythropoietin levels are elevated more in patients with iron deficiency anemia than in those with anemia of chronic disease; rheumatoid patients also have a diminished response to erythropoietin.[270]

In patients with the anemia of chronic disease, total erythroid heme turnover is slightly reduced, and ineffective erythropoiesis accounts for a much higher than normal percentage of total heme turnover.[272–274] These patients also may demonstrate a diminished ability to absorb iron through the gastrointestinal tract, a condition usually related to the irritative presence of an anti-inflammatory medication.[275] In contrast to anemia associated with blood loss, the ineffective erythropoiesis will return to normal in RA if remission can be induced.[276] Red blood cell aplasia, immunologically mediated, is a rare finding in RA. However, because erythropoiesis in animals has been shown to be dependent on T lymphocytes, it is logical to search for immunologic factors that can induce anemia in RA. Serum from RA patients profoundly suppresses erythroid colony formation,[277] but T lymphocytes from bone marrow of rheumatoid patients have not been shown to inhibit erythroid development in vitro, as do T cells from certain patients with aplastic anemia or pure red blood cell aplasia.[278]

Eosinophilia and *thrombocytosis* are often associated with RA. Eosinophilia (≥ 5 percent of total WBC count) was observed in 40 percent of patients with severe seropositive disease.[279] Similarly, there is a significant relationship between thrombocytosis and extra-articular manifestations of rheumatoid disease[280] and disease activity.[281]

An interesting subset of patients with RA have increased numbers of large granular lymphocytes (LGLs) in the peripheral blood, bone marrow, and liver. The lymphocytes contain many azurophilic granules in the cytoplasm and may account for more than 90 percent of mononuclear cells in blood. They are increased in certain viral infections. The cells are E rosette–positive, are Fc receptor–positive, do not produce interleukin-2, respond poorly to mitogens, and have either antibody-dependent cell-mediated cytotoxicity activity (expressing CD3, CD8, and CD57) or natural killer (NK) cells (expressing CD16 and CD56).[282, 283] Of previously described patients with LGL proliferation, almost one third have had RA.[284] Because the *LGL syndrome* in patients with RA has the same HLA-DR4 association seen in Felty's syndrome, the proposal has been made that both Felty's and the LGL syndrome represent different variants of a broader syndrome comprising RA, neutropenia, LGL expansions, HLA-DR4 positivity, and variable splenomegaly.[282]

Vasculitis

In one sense, it is redundant to think of vasculitis as a complication of RA, as the initial pathologic change in RA is believed to occur in small blood vessels. However, it is useful to use the term *vasculitis* to group those extra-articular complications related not to proliferative granulomas but rather to inflammatory vascular disease.

Clinical vasculitis usually takes one of the following forms:

- Distal arteritis (ranging from splinter hemorrhages to gangrene)
- Cutaneous ulceration (including pyoderma gangrenosum)
- Peripheral neuropathy
- Pericarditis
- Arteritis of viscera, including heart, lungs, bowel, kidney, liver, spleen, pancreas, lymph nodes, and testis
- Palpable purpura

The pathologic finding in rheumatoid vasculitis is that of a panarteritis. All layers of the vessel wall are infiltrated with mononuclear cells. Fibrinoid necrosis is seen in active lesions. Intimal proliferation may predispose to thrombosis. Obliterative endarteritis of the finger is one of the most common manifestations of vasculitis, and immune complex deposits have been demonstrated in those vessels.[285, 286] When larger vessels are involved, the pathologic changes resemble those of polyarteritis nodosa.[287] In addition, a venulitis associated with RA has been described.[288, 289] In patients with hypocomplementemia, the cellular infiltrate around the vessels contains neutrophils; in normocomplementemic patients, lymphocytes predominate. Uninvolved skin from rheumatoid patients is positive for immunoglobulin and complement when sections for histopathology are stained with fluorescein-labeled antibodies to these components. The presence of IgG correlates directly with circulating immune complexes, vasculitic skin lesions, subcutaneous nodules, and a high titer of RF.[290]

It is unusual for vasculitis to be active in any but

the sickest patients, those with severe deforming arthritis and high RF titers; this subgroup represents fewer than 1 percent of patients with RA. Although RA is more common in women than in men, vasculitis is more often seen in men with RA. Supporting the hypothesis that vascular injury is mediated by deposition of circulating immune complexes are (1) depressed levels of C2 and C4,[291] (2) hypercatabolism of C3,[292] (3) deposition of IgG, IgM, and C3 in involved arteries,[293] and (4) the presence of large amounts of cryoimmunoglobulin in serum of patients with vasculitis.[294]

Neurovascular disease may be the only manifestation of vasculitis. The two common clinical patterns are a mild distal sensory neuropathy and a severe sensorimotor neuropathy (mononeuritis multiplex).[295] The latter form is characterized by severe arterial damage on nerve biopsy specimens. Symptoms of the milder form may be paresthesias or "burning feet" in association with decreased touch and pin sensation distally. Patients with mononeuritis multiplex have weakness (e.g., footdrop) in addition to sensory abnormalities. Symptoms and signs are identical to those found in polyarteritis. Rheumatoid pachymeningitis is a rare complication of RA; confined to the dura and pia mater, this process may be limited to certain areas (e.g., lumbar cord or cisternae).[296] Elevated levels of IgG (including IgM and IgG rheumatoid factors and low-molecular-weight IgM) and immune complexes are found in the cerebrospinal fluid. Although there is a possible negative association between psychosis and RA, organic brain syndromes may be related to RA in patients not taking glucocorticoids or indomethacin,[297] and it is presumed that these manifestations are caused by small-vessel disease. In addition, there appears to be a real entity of autonomic nervous system disease in RA that is isolated from other peripheral or central nervous system damage.[298]

Visceral lesions occur generally as claudication or infarction of the organ supplied by the involved arteries. Intestinal involvement with vasculitis presents as abdominal pain, at first intermittent and progressing often to continuous pain and a tender, quiet belly on examination. If infarction develops, resection must be accomplished promptly.[299] The presence of gangrene of digits and extremities, the development of intestinal lesions with bleeding or perforation, cardiac or renal involvement, and mononeuritis multiplex indicate extensive vasculitis and are associated with a poor prognosis.[300, 301]

Renal Disease

The kidney is an example of an organ that is rarely involved directly in RA but often is compromised indirectly. Amyloidosis is a complication of chronic RA and particularly of Still's disease. Another indirect cause of renal disease is toxicity from therapy. Phenacetin abuse causes renal papillary necrosis, and salicylates and other NSAIDs may cause abnormalities as well.[302] A membranous nephropathy is the pathologic lesion related to therapy with gold salts and D-penicillamine. Rarely, a focal necrotizing glomerulitis is seen in patients dying with RA and disseminated vasculitis.[303]

Pulmonary Disease

There are at least six forms of lung disease in RA:

- Pleural disease
- Interstitial fibrosis
- Nodular lung disease
- Bronchiolitis
- Arteritis, with pulmonary hypertension
- Small airways disease

Pleural Disease

Pleuritis is commonly found on autopsy of patients with RA, but clinical disease during life is seen less frequently.[304] In about 20 percent of patients it develops concurrently with onset of the arthritis. Pleuritic pain is not usually major, perhaps because effusions can be large, sometimes enough to cause dyspnea. Characteristics of the exudative rheumatoid effusions are as follows: glucose, 10 to 50 mg/dl; protein, >4 g/dl; cells, 100 to 3500 (mononuclear) per mm³; lactic dehydrogenase, elevated; and CH_{50}, depressed. The low glucose concentrations are of interest. Sepsis (particularly tuberculosis) is the only other condition that commonly has such a low pleural fluid glucose level. An impaired transport of glucose into the pleural space appears to be the cause.[305]

Interstitial Fibrosis

The increased reactivity of mesenchymal cells in RA is believed to be the cause of pulmonary fibrosis in this disease. Similar to findings in scleroderma, physical findings are of fine, diffuse dry rales. Radiographs show a diffuse reticular (interstitial) or reticulonodular pattern in both lung fields;[306, 307] these progress to a honeycomb appearance on plain radiographs and a characteristic lattice net on high-resolution CT. The pathologic findings are those of diffuse fibrosis in the midst of a mononuclear cell infiltrate.[306] The principal functional defect is impairment of alveolocapillary gas exchange with decreased diffusion capacity, best measured utilizing single-breath carbon monoxide diffusion capacities.[308, 309] It is likely that RA patients who smoke are at a higher risk for fibrotic complications in the lungs than are those in the general population. It has been reported that bronchoalveolar lavage may reveal increased numbers of lymphocytes, even in those with only mildly abnormal chest radiographs and normal pulmonary function test results.[310]

Nodular Lung Disease

Pulmonary nodules may appear singly or in clusters that coalesce. Single ones appear as a coin lesion and, when significant peripheral arthritis and nodules are present, can be diagnosed by needle biopsy without thoracotomy. Caplan's syndrome,[311] in which pneumoconiosis and RA are synergistic and produce a violent fibroblastic reaction with obliterative granulomatous fibrosis, has become a rare occurrence as the respiratory environment in mining operations has improved. Nodules may cavitate and create a bronchopleural fistula[312] and may precede arthritis.[313] In several cases, solitary pulmonary nodules in RA patients have proved to be a rheumatoid nodule and a coexistent bronchogenic carcinoma,[314] a finding that suggests caution in interpreting "benign" results from fine needle aspiration biopsy in such patients.

Bronchiolitis

A rare finding is an interstitial pneumonitis that progresses to alveolar involvement and bronchiolitis, respiratory insufficiency, and death. Pathologic studies show a cellular loose fibrosis and proteinaceous exudate in bronchioles and alveoli; interstitial infiltrations of lymphocytes attest to the immunogenic aspects of the disease (Fig. 55–7).

Arteritis

Pulmonary hypertension from arteritis of the pulmonary vasculature is rare and is occasionally associated with digital arteritis.[315] One patient with pleurities, interstitial lymphocytic infiltrate, arterial hypertension, and venous sclerosis has been described.[316]

Small Airways Disease

Defined by a reduced maximal mid-expiratory flow rate and maximal expiratory flow rate at 50 percent of functional vital capacity, small airways disease was observed in 50 percent of 30 RA patients, compared with 22 percent of a control population.[317] The study was adjusted for pulmonary infections, α_1-antitrypsin deficiency, penicillamine treatment, environmental pollution, and smoking. Other investigations have not found small airways dysfunction in RA and have suggested that, if present, it probably is related to factors other than RA.[318] If real, this phenomenon may be part of a generalized exocrinopathic process in the disease, expressed most flagrantly, of course, in Sjögren's syndrome.

Cardiac Complications

Cardiac disease in RA can take many forms related to granulomatous proliferation or vasculitis. Advances in echocardiography have made diagnosis of pericarditis and endocardial inflammation easier and more specific.[319] Myocardial biopsy through vascular catheters has facilitated diagnosis and classification of myocarditis.

Pericarditis

Infrequently diagnosed on the basis of history and physical examination in RA, pericarditis is present in up to 50 percent of patients at autopsy.[320, 321] In one study, 31 percent of patients with RA had echocardiographic evidence of pericardial effusion. The same study revealed only rare evidence of impaired left ventricular function in prospectively studied outpatients with RA.[322] Although unusual, cardiac tamponade with constrictive pericarditis develops in RA and may require pericardectomy.[323, 324] Most patients have a positive test for RF, and half have nodules.

Myocarditis

Myocarditis can take the form of either granulomatous disease or interstitial myocarditis. The granulomatous process resembles subcutaneous nodules and could be considered specific for the disease. Diffuse infiltration of the myocardium by mononuclear cells, on the other hand, may involve the entire myocardium and yet have no clinical manifestations.[324]

Endocardial Inflammation

Echocardiographic studies have reported evidence of previously unrecognized mitral valve disease diagnosed by a reduced E–F slope of the anterior leaflet of the mitral valve.[325, 326] Although aortic valve disease and arthritis are generally associated through ankylosing spondylitis, a number of granulomatous nodules in the valve have been reported.[327]

Conduction Defects

Atrioventricular (AV) block is unusual in RA but is probably related to direct granulomatous involvement. Pathologic examination may reveal proliferative lesions[328, 329] or healed scars.[330] Complete heart block has been described in more than 30 patients with RA. It generally occurs in patients with established erosive nodular disease.[330] It usually is permanent and is caused by rheumatoid granulomas in or near the AV node or bundle of His. Rarely, amyloidosis is responsible for heart block.

Coronary Arteritis

Patients with severe RA and active vasculitis who develop a myocardial infarction are likely to have coronary arteritis as a basis for the process.[331]

Granulomatous Aortitis or Valvular Disease

In severe rheumatoid heart disease, granulomatous disease can spread to involve even the base of the

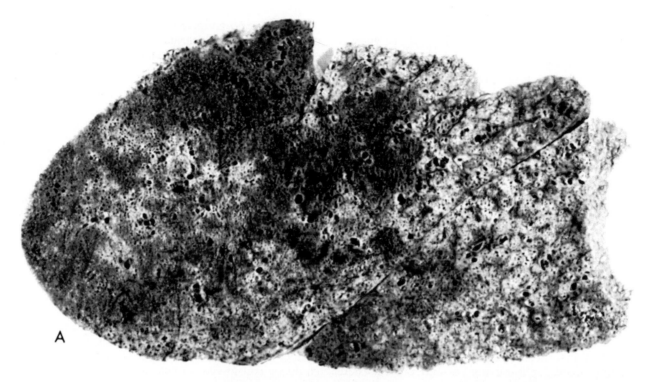

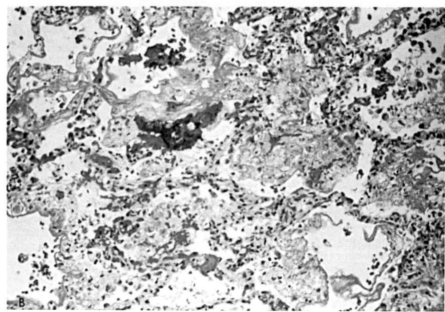

Figure 55–7. Severe, subacute interstitial pneumonitis in rheumatoid arthritis (RA). This complication proved fatal in 5 weeks in this 66-year-old woman with severe, active seropositive RA. *A,* The gross photograph of the left lung shows dense interalveolar thickening by a fibrofibrinous exudate. Air sacs are becoming obliterated. Lungs were heavy and incompressible, but there was only a trace of excess fluid. *B,* Microscopic sections showed thickened alveolar septa with a rich fibrinous exudate present. (Courtesy of Charles Faulkner III, M.D.)

aorta.[332] Occasionally, granulomatous disease associated with RA necessitates urgent valve replacement for aortic incompetence.[333]

PROGNOSIS IN RHEUMATOID ARTHRITIS

Natural History

Epidemiologists have pointed out the multiple difficulties in attempting to establish change in patterns of RA in different time periods or different communities. The best data suggest that patients currently admitted to the hospital for RA are likely to have fewer joint contractures and less ankylosis of peripheral joints at admission than patients admitted 20 years ago, whereas the prevalence of RF and subcutaneous nodules and the mean number of affected joints have, if anything, increased slightly.[334] These and other findings suggest that the disease is not changing, but that earlier, more effective treatment has perhaps diminished the morbidity. As with other chronic diseases, both physicians and patients are eager to know the prospects for remission and are anxious about the threat of severe morbidity or death.

There are now well-tested criteria for a clinical remission.[335] Six have yielded optimal discrimination (Table 55–8). Few patients achieve five of six of these criteria, and most fail to achieve a true remission. On the basis of these criteria in an analysis of 450 patients with RA followed prospectively for 6 years, 18 percent had at least one remission.[336] In the aggregate, the remission periods represented 35 percent of the duration of follow-up of those entering remission; the mean length of the remission was 10 months. Being male or developing RA after age 60 years increased chances of remission. Early development of erosions decreased chances of remission. Not definitively determined in this study is whether drug treatment increases the likelihood of remission.

In well-established RA, median life expectancy is less than in control populations.[337] In one study, a 25-year prospective follow-up of 208 patients, median life expectancy was shortened by 7 years in males and 3 years in females.[338] Infection, renal disease, and respiratory failure are the primary factors contributing to excess mortality in RA patients.[339] A more recent study revealed that of 100 patients with RA followed for 25 years, 63 had died—an excess mortality of approximately 40 percent.[340]

The challenge to rheumatologists is to predict which patients will do well and which will not. In an attempt to identify initial factors that might predict subsequent disability, 39 potentially predictive variables were studied over 11.9 years in 681 consecutive patients[341] diagnosed as having definite or classic RA. Initially, 48 percent were without disability; at the end of the study, the proportion had declined to 17 percent. Similarly, only 3 percent were completely disabled at onset of the study, compared with 16 percent at the conclusion. Disability developed most rapidly during the first 2 years of the disease and progressed slowly in subsequent years, especially in older women with decreased function. Absent from the list of valuable predictors were factors previously thought to correlate with disease outcome; thus, there was no evidence that disease with an acute, explosive onset had a better prognosis.[341, 342] The reason that patients with large proximal joint involvement do worse than those with disease limited to hands[35] may be related to the larger area of these involved joints; the correlation of surface area of involved joints with the C-reactive protein (CRP) and of CRP with joint destruction may provide a basis for this observation.

Death associated with RA generally is due to the complications (both articular and extra-articular) of RA and to side effects of therapy. The probability of death varies directly with the severity of complications. Potentially morbid articular complications include the various forms of atlantoaxial subluxation, cricoarytenoid synovitis, and sepsis of involved joints. Extra-articular complications directly causing a higher mortality include Felty's syndrome, Sjögren's syndrome, cardiopulmonary complications, diffuse vasculitis, gastrointestinal complications of therapy, amyloidosis, and infection.[257, 343, 344]

One of the largest and best-documented studies of survival, prognosis, and causes of death in rheumatoid arthritis was published by Mitchell and associates.[345] In this prospective study of 805 patients including 12 years of observation, 233 died during the course of the study; survivorship was only 50 percent of that in population controls. As reinforced by other studies,[346] the increased mortality associated with RA is impressive and equals that of all patients with Hodgkin's disease, diabetes mellitus, and stroke (age-adjusted). In another group of 107 patients followed for 8 years, each of whom had extra-articular disease or needed hospitalization for some aspect of the disease,[347] those with cutaneous ulcers, vasculitic rash, neuropathy, and scleritis had a higher mortality than those whose disease was confined to joints. Of great concern to all health care workers is the correlation of lack of formal education with increased mortality in RA.[346, 348] Total mortality from cancer does not appear to differ between patients with RA and controls, although more patients with RA die of lymphoma compared with control patients.[349]

Variables Related to Prognosis

Rheumatoid Factor

Many studies have confirmed that seropositivity is associated with a poorer prognosis in RA. One series of 60 patients with active disease revealed this association.[350] Patients with RF have more involved joints when they visit a physician for the first time, and more erosions and ligamentous instability develop.[30, 351] As mentioned previously, an increasing number of individuals with a diagnosis of seronegative RA[352] are being recognized as having other classifiable entities.

Of all the RF isotypes, IgA RF correlates best with ESR and grip strength, and its presence may indicate patients likely to develop aggressive, erosive disease.[353]

Table 55–8. CRITERIA FOR COMPLETE CLINICAL REMISSION IN RHEUMATOID ARTHRITIS (RA)

A minimum of five of the following requirements must be fulfilled for at least 2 consecutive months in a patient with definite or classic RA:
1. Morning stiffness not exceeding 15 minutes
2. No fatigue
3. No joint pain
4. No joint tenderness or pain on motion
5. No soft tissue swelling in joints or tendon sheaths
6. ESR (Westergren) less then 30 mm/hr (females) or 20 mm/hr (males)

Exclusions: Clinical manifestations of active vasculitis, pericarditis, pleuritis, or myositis and/or unexplained recent weight loss or fever secondary to RA prohibit a designation of complete clinical remission.

From Pinals RS, Masi AT, Larsen RA: Preliminary criteria for clinical remission in rheumatoid arthritis. Arthritis Rheum 24:1308–1315, 1981.

Rheumatoid Nodules

Rheumatoid nodules occur almost always in patients with RF, although there is no correlation with titer of RF.[30, 343, 351] Therefore, similar to those patients with RF alone, patients with subcutaneous nodules have a poorer outcome and a higher incidence of bone erosions.[343, 354, 355]

Sex

In young adults with RA, females generally have a worse outcome with more swollen and tender joints and erosions than males.[351]

Synovial Histopathology

Although it is generally agreed that the persistence and intensity of synovial inflammation are related to joint destruction, no single feature or group of features demonstrable by routine histopathologic examinations of synovium have been correlated with destructive lesions in RA.[356, 357] In part, this may be related to the major histologic variations from area to area within the synovium.[358] A finding of cartilage erosion associated with synovial lining cell proliferation and few subsynovial lymphocytes[359] has not been confirmed.[356, 357] The finding of meniscal cartilage erosions using MRI may be the earliest sign of potentially destructive disease of articular cartilage of the knee (see Chapter 42).

Synovial Fluid Analysis

Chemotactic factors in synovial fluid in RA attract PMNs, which accumulate and eventually are lysed within the joint space. It has been demonstrated that when the joint fluid leukocyte count exceeds 50,000 to 60,000 per mm³, protease inhibitors in the fluid can be saturated or inhibitors can be damaged or rendered effete, so that protease activity is manifest.[360] It is probable that at times such as these, proteases (e.g., collagenase and stromelysin) act unopposed on cartilage components. Acidosis of synovial fluid correlates with leukocyte counts in synovial fluid[361] and with radiographic evidence of joint destruction.[362] Depression of glucose and complement components in synovial fluid can be roughly correlated with the intensity of inflammation in the fluid and levels of IgG with the degree of subsynovial lymphocyte accumulation.[363] (See Chapter 36.)

CLASSIFICATION AND ASSESSMENT OF RHEUMATOID ARTHRITIS

The inflammatory lesion in RA is reflected reasonably well by heat, pain, swelling, and tenderness. Joint destruction can occur with minimal inflammation, however, and means to assess cartilage destruction are limited to radiographic determination of ap-

parent joint space narrowing and erosions. MRI may, as it evolves, provide a way to visualize pannus development and loss of cartilage (Fig. 55–8), but this procedure is too expensive for routine use.

While the Steinbrocker criteria appear to correlate hand radiographs very poorly with functional health status of rheumatoid patients,[364] the more recently developed Larsen grading system[365] appears to be a more sensitive and reproducible index of disease progression.[366] To emphasize the differences between the inflammatory and the proliferative/destructive components of RA, Sharp makes a good case for having radiographic assessment incorporated into clinical trials of all new drugs developed for treatment of RA.[367]

The availability of computer technology for comparison of articular indices in RA has made objective assessment of these indices possible. Traditionally, three indices have been used in most studies (Table 55–9).[368–372]

For office practice, clinical studies, and epidemiologic surveys, a *reduced joint survey* (RJS)[373] was developed as a compromise between laborious redundancy and superficial evaluation. The RJS indices were developed using statistical and clinical approaches. The data suggest that five chief groups of joints improved or deteriorated together: MCP joints of hands, interphalangeal joints of the hand, MTP joints of feet, interphalangeal joints of feet, and large joints. The data suggested that RJS indices can be utilized reason-

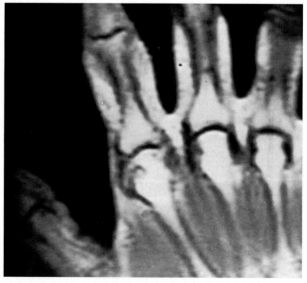

Figure 55–8. Magnetic resonance (MR) image of the right hand of a 35-year-old woman with a 6-year history of rheumatoid arthritis. Physical examination revealed soft tissue swelling of the metacarpophalangeal joint. Radiographs showed some narrowing of the second metacarpophalangeal joint, without bone erosions. The MR image shows bone in white, articular capsule in black, and pannus as gray mottled areas on the medial portion of the second and third metacarpal heads. (These T2-weighted [T_R2000 m; T_E34 ms] images are provided courtesy of Reuben Mesrich, M.D., and James Seibold, M.D.)

Table 55–9. ARTICULAR INDICES

Ritchie Articular Index[368]

This index sums grades of tenderness.

Single Joints

Elbows
Wrists
Hips
Knees
Ankles
Talocalcaneal joints
Midtarsal joints

Units

Temporomandibular joint
Cervical spine (assayed by passive motion)
Sternoclavicular joint
Acromioclavicular joint
MCP joint
PIP joint
MTP joint

American Rheumatism Association Index[369]

"Clinically active" joints are defined as tenderness *and/or* pain,
   and/or soft tissue swelling, of the following joints examined
   individually or bilaterally:
   Temporomandibular joint
   Sternoclavicular joint
   Acromioclavicular joint
   Shoulder
   IP of the thumb
   Hip
   Knee
   Ankle (mortise)
   Tarsus
   IP of great toe
and of the following joints as units and bilaterally:

Wrist	1 unit
MCP joints	5 units
PIP and DIP joints of fingers	8 units
MTP joints	5 units
PIP and DIP joints of toes	4 units

Lansbury Articular Index[370–372]

"Severity of inflammation" for each joint is weighted by joint
   surface area. Joints examined bilaterally are the same as for
   the ARA index, but the following joints are examined
   separately:
   Carpometacarpal
   Transverse carpal
   PIP and DIP of toes
   Transverse intertarsal
   Tarsometatarsal
   Talonavicular-calcaneocuboid
   Talocalcaneal

---

ably by both the clinician and the researcher in quantifying the status of joint disease in RA.

Computer technology has opened the possibility of comparing great numbers of indices. The problem has been, however, to determine what standard to measure indices against. Radiographic and functional indices over time are affected by factors other than joint inflammation. Thompson and associates make a case for measuring effectiveness of indices against levels of CRP.[374] The CRP shows a fast response, short half-life, large incremental change, and a constant catabolic rate (see Chapter 44), and has been shown to have predictive value for development of erosion.

Thompson and coworkers studied 66 combinations of indices, including the Ritchie,[368] ARA,[369] and Lansbury,[370–372] and found the best correlations with CRP in an index that is relatively simple to use. It links joint surface area to joints with *simultaneous* tenderness and swelling that can readily be assessed. It incorporates three changes from previous indices:

- Weighting of the index by surface area of the joint (e.g., PIP = 1×; wrist = 6×; elbow = 10×; knee = 19×)
- Requiring that joints identified as inflamed exhibit *simultaneous* tenderness and swelling, not one or the other
- Exclusion of joints that are difficult to examine for true synovitis (i.e., TMJ, cervical spine, shoulders, and hips)

This system is shown in Table 55–10. Until better information is available, this method for scoring activity of RA should be considered first by clinicians, as well as those planning controlled therapeutic trials.

Classification of RA also can be achieved by functional analysis.[375] It also is appropriate to correlate functional class with an anatomic radiographic staging system.[375] Functional assays determined by self-report questionnaires issued to patients appear to be cost-effective in assessing and monitoring the status

Table 55–10. WEIGHTED AND SELECTIVE INDEX FOR ACTIVITY OF SYNOVITIS

Joint	Weighted Factor (Related to Joint Surface Area)	Degree of Tenderness *and* Swelling (Scale: 0 to 3)	Joint Score
Elbow			
R	48	_____	_____
L	48	_____	_____
Wrist			
R	32	_____	_____
L	32	_____	_____
MCP (separately)			
R	5	_____	_____
L	5	_____	_____
PIP (separately)			
R	5	_____	_____
L	5	_____	_____
Knee			
R	95	_____	_____
L	95	_____	_____
Ankle (mortise)			
R	32	_____	_____
L	32	_____	_____
First MTP			
R	8	_____	_____
L	8	_____	_____
Second to fifth MTP (separately)			
R	5	_____	_____
L	5	_____	_____
Total			_____

From Thompson PW, Silman AJ, Kirwan JR, et al: Articular indices of joint inflammation in rheumatoid arthritis: Correlation with the acute-phase response. Arthritis Rheum 30:618–623, 1987.

Table 55–11. ACTIVITIES OF DAILY LIVING AND VISUAL ANALOG QUESTIONNAIRE

A. How often is it *painful* for you to:

	Never	Sometimes	Most of the Time	Always
Dress yourself?	_____	_____	_____	_____
Get in and out of bed?	_____	_____	_____	_____
Lift a cup or glass to your lips?	_____	_____	_____	_____
Walk outdoors on flat ground?	_____	_____	_____	_____
Wash and dry your entire body?	_____	_____	_____	_____
Bend down to pick up clothing from the floor?	_____	_____	_____	_____
Turn faucets on or off?	_____	_____	_____	_____
Get in and out of a car?	_____	_____	_____	_____

B. How much pain have you had in the *past week* (mark the scale):
   No pain _____ Pain as bad as it could be
          0   100

From Callahan LF, Brooks RH, Summey JA, et al: Quantitative pain assessment for routine care of rheumatoid arthritis patients, using a pain scale based on activities of daily living and a visual analog pain scale. Arthritis Rheum 30:630–636, 1987.

of RA in an individual patient.[376] In evaluating the status of a particular patient, the physician can use, as a rough guide, the radiographic staging system as an index of whether the functional status of that individual is appropriate. For instance, if a functional grade III patient has only grade II radiographic changes, it is likely that aggressive physical therapy and/or attention to care of nonarticular complications of the disease may improve functional status.

Patients can take an active role in assessing disease activity. A pain scale (Table 55–11) based on activities of daily living and a visual analog scale required less than 5 minutes to complete and was simple for patients to fill out.[377] The results correlated moderately well with joint counts and some other objective measurements of disease activity.

Care of the rheumatoid patient should include a careful record of the physical examination and functional and radiographic assessment. This permits care of patients in a prospective fashion and provides a systematic assessment of disease activity. With proper assessment, effective therapy (as outlined in Chapter 56) can be initiated, evaluated, and changed if necessary.

References

1. Snorrason E: Landre-Beauvais and his goutte asthenique primitive. Acta Med Scand 142(Suppl 266):115, 1952.
2. Boyle JA, Buchanan WW: Clinical Rheumatology. Philadelphia, FA Davis, 1971.
3. Short CL: The antiquity of rheumatoid arthritis. Arthritis Rheum 17:193–205, 1974.
4. Copeman WSC: A Short History of the Gout and the Rheumatic Diseases. Berkeley, University of California Press, 1964.
5. Soranus of Ephesus: On Acute Diseases and on Chronic Diseases. Trans-lated into Latin by Caelius Aurelianus (5th century). English translation by Drabkin IE. Chicago, University of Chicago Press, 1950.
6. Ruffer MA, Rietti A: On osseous lesions in ancient Egyptians. J Pathol Bacteriol 16:439, 1912.
7. Lubeck DP, Spitz PW, Fries JF, et al: A multicenter study of annual health service utilization and costs in rheumatoid arthritis. Arthritis Rheum 29:488–493, 1986.
8. Arnett FC, Edworthy SM, Bloch DA, et al: The American Rheumatism Association 1987 revised criteria for the classification of rheumatoid arthritis. Arthritis Rheum 31:315–324, 1988.
9. Wolfe AM: The epidemiology of rheumatoid arthritis: A review. I. Surveys. Bull Rheum Dis 19:518–523, 1968.
10. Engel A, Roberts J, Burch TA: Rheumatoid arthritis in adults in the United States, 1960–1962. In Vital and Health Statistics, Series 11, Data from the National Health Survey, Number 17. Washington, DC, National Center for Health Statistics, 1966.
11. Mikkelsen WM, Dodge HJ, Duff IF, et al: Estimates of the prevalence of rheumatic disease in the population of Tecumseh, Michigan, 1959–1960. J Chronic Dis 20:351–369, 1967.
12. O'Brien WM, Bennett PH, Burch TA, et al: A genetic study of rheumatoid arthritis and rheumatoid factor in Blackfeet and Pima Indians. Arthritis Rheum 10:163–179, 1967.
13. Wood WJ, Kato H, Johnson KG, et al: Rheumatoid arthritis in Hiroshima and Nagasaki, Japan. Arthritis Rheum 10:21, 1967.
14. Stone CE: The lifetime economic costs of rheumatoid arthritis. J Rheumatol 11:819–827, 1984.
15. Rose HM, Ragan C, Pearce E, et al: Differential agglutination of normal and sensitized sheep erythrocytes by sera of patients with rheumatoid arthritis. Proc Soc Exp Biol Med 68:1, 1948.
16. Waaler E: On the occurrence of a factor in human serum activating the specific agglutination of sheep blood corpuscles. Acta Pathol Microbiol Scand 17:172, 1940.
17. Lawrence JS: Prevalence of rheumatoid arthritis. Ann Rheum Dis 20:11, 1961.
18. Lawrence JS, Laine VAI, DeGraaff R: The epidemiology of rheumatoid arthritis in northern Europe. Proc R Soc Med 54:454, 1961.
19. Plotz CM, Singer JM: The latex fixation test: II. Results in rheumatoid arthritis. Am J Med 21:893, 1956.
20. Alarcon GS, Koopman WJ, Acton RT, et al: Seronegative rheumatoid arthritis. A distinct immunogenetic disease? Arthritis Rheum 25:502–507, 1982.
21. Noritake DT, Colburn KK, Chan G, et al: Rheumatoid factors specific for active rheumatoid arthritis. Ann Rheum Dis 49:910–915, 1990.
22. Meyerowitz S, Jacox RF, Hess DW: Monozygotic twins discordant for rheumatoid arthritis: A genetic, clinical and psychological study of 8 sets. Arthritis Rheum 11:1–21, 1968.
23. Harvald B, Hauge M: Genetics and the Epidemiology of Chronic Diseases. Washington, DC: US Government Printing Office, 1965, p 61.

24. Lawrence JS: Genetics of rheumatoid factor and rheumatoid arthritis. Clin Exp Immunol S2:769–783, 1967.

25. Lawrence JS: Heberden Oration, 1969. Rheumatoid arthritis—Nature or nurture? Ann Rheum Dis 29:357–379, 1970.

26. Aho K, Koskenvuo M, Tuominen J, et al: Occurrence of rheumatoid arthritis in a nation-wide series of twins. J Rheumatol 13:899–902, 1986.

27. Siegel M, Lee SL, Widelock D, et al: A comparative family study of rheumatoid arthritis and systemic lupus erythematosus. N Engl J Med 273:893, 1965.

28. Wallace DJ, Klinenberg JR, Morham D, et al: Coexistent gout and rheumatoid arthritis. Case report and literature review. Arthritis Rheum 22:81–86, 1979.

29. Agudelo CA, Turner RA, Panetti M, et al: Does hyperuricemia protect from rheumatoid inflammation? A clinical study. Arthritis Rheum 27:443–448, 1984.

30. Jacoby RK, Jayson MI, Cosh JA: Onset, early stages, and prognosis of rheumatoid arthritis: A clinical study of 100 patients with 11-year follow-up. Br Med J 2:96–100, 1973.

31. Lawrence JS: Surveys of rheumatic complaints in the population. In Dixon A St J (ed): Progress in Clinical Rheumatology. London: Churchill Livingstone, 1965, p 1.

32. Short CL, Bauer W: The course of rheumatoid arthritis in patients receiving simple medical and orthopedic measures. N Engl J Med 238:142, 1948.

33. Aho K, Palosuo T, Raunio V, et al: When does rheumatoid disease start? Arthritis Rheum 28:485–489, 1985.

34. Fleming A, Crown JM, Corbett M: Early rheumatoid disease: 1. Onset. Ann Rheum Dis 35:357–360, 1976.

35. Fleming A, Benn RT, Corbett M, et al: Early rheumatoid disease: II. Patterns of joint involvement. Ann Rheum Dis 35:361–364, 1976.

36. Dick WC, Grayson MF, Woodburn A, et al: Indices of inflammatory activity: Relationship between isotope studies and clinical methods. Ann Rheum Dis 29:643–648, 1970.

37. Mens JM: Correlation of joint involvement in rheumatoid arthritis and in ankylosing spondylitis with the synovial:cartilagenous surface ratio of various joints (letter). Arthritis Rheum 30:359–360, 1987.

38. Bywaters EGL: Still's disease in the adult. Ann Rheum Dis 30:121–133, 1971.

39. Gupta RC, Mills DM: Still's disease in an adult: A link between juvenile and adult rheumatoid arthritis. Am J Med Sci 269:137–144, 1975.

40. Aptekar RG, Decker JL, Bujak JS, et al: Adult onset juvenile rheumatoid arthritis. Arthritis Rheum 16:715–718, 1973.

41. Stramp IJ, Lozar JD: Adult-onset Still's disease. Variant of rheumatoid arthritis. Postgrad Med 58:175, 1975.

42. Elkon KB, Hughes GR, Bywaters EG, et al: Adult-onset Still's disease: Twenty-year followup and further studies of patients with active disease. Arthritis Rheum 25:647–654, 1982.

43. Cush JJ, Medsger TA Jr, Christy WC, et al: Adult-onset Still's disease: Clinical course and outcome. Arthritis Rheum 30:186–194, 1987.

44. Cabane J, Michon A, Ziza JM, et al: Comparison of long-term evolution of adult onset and juvenile onset Still's disease, both followed up for more than 10 years. Ann Rheum Dis 49:283–285, 1990.

45. Hench PS, Rosenberg EF: Palindromic rheumatism: New oft-recurring disease of joints (arthritis, periarthritis, para-arthritis) apparently producing no articular residues: Report of 34 cases. Proc. Mayo Clin. 16:808, 1942.

46. Guerne P-A, Weisman MH: Palindromic rheumatism: Part of or apart from the spectrum of rheumatoid arthritis. Am J Med 93:451–460, 1992.

47. Schumacher HR: Palindromic onset of rheumatoid arthritis: Clinical, synovial fluid, and biopsy studies. Arthritis Rheum 25:361–369, 1982.

48. Youssef W, Yan A, Russell AS: Palindromic rheumatism: A response to chloroquine. J Rheumatol 18(1):35–37, 1991.

49. Deal CL, Meenan RF, Goldenberg DL, et al: The clinical features of elderly-onset rheumatoid arthritis: A comparison with younger-onset disease of similar duration. Arthritis Rheum 28:987–994, 1985.

50. Terkeltaub R, Decary F, Esdaile J: An immunogenetic study of older age onset rheumatoid arthritis. J Rheumatol 11:147–149, 1984.

51. Yoghmai I, Rooholamini SM, Faunce HF: Unilateral rheumatoid arthritis: Protective effects of neurologic deficits. Am J Roentgenol 128:299–301, 1977.

52. Bland J, Eddy W: Hemiplegia and rheumatoid hemiarthritis. Arthritis Rheum 11:72–80, 1968.

53. Glick EN: Asymmetrical rheumatoid arthritis after poliomyelitis. Br Med J 3(556):26–28, 1967.

54. Thompson M, Bywaters EGL: Unilateral rheumatoid arthritis following hemiplegia. Ann Rheum Dis 21:370, 1961.

55. Bywaters EGL: The hand. In Radiological Aspects of Rheumatoid Arthritis. Amsterdam, Excerpta Medica Foundation, No. 64, 1964, p 43.

56. de Haas WHD, de Boer W, Griffioen F, et al: Rheumatoid arthritis of the robust reaction type. Ann Rheum Dis 33:81–85, 1974.

57. Short CL, Bauer W, Reynolds WE: Rheumatoid Arthritis: A Definition of the Disease and a Clinical Description Based on a Numerical Study of 293 Patients and Controls. Cambridge, Mass, Harvard University Press, 1957.

58. Short CL: Rheumatoid arthritis: Types of course and prognosis. Med Clin North Am 52:549–557, 1968.

59. Hollander JL, Yeostros SJ: The effects of simultaneous variations of humidity and barometric pressure on arthritis. Bull Am Meteorol Soc 44:389, 1963.

60. Patberg WR, Nienhuis RL, Veringa F: Relation between meteorological factors and pain in rheumatoid arthritis in a marine climate. J Rheumatol 12:711–715, 1985.

61. Hoffman GS: Polyarthritis: The differential diagnosis of rheumatoid arthritis. Semin Arthritis Rheum 8:115–141, 1978.

62. Pinals RS: Polyarthritis and fever. N Engl J Med 330:769–774, 1994.

63. Davies PG, Fordham JN: Arthritis and angioimmunoblastic lymphadenopathy. Ann Rheum Dis 42:516–518, 1983.

64. Fallet GH, Mason M, Berry H, et al: Rheumatoid arthritis and ankylosing spondylitis occurring together. Br Med J 1(6013):804–807, 1976.

65. Chamot AM, Benhamou CL, Kahn MF, et al: Le syndrome acne pustulose hyperostose osteite (SAPHO)—85 observations. Rev Rhum Mal Osteoartic 54:187–196, 1987.

66. Morris RI, Metzger AL, Bluestone R, et al: HLA B27—A useful discriminator in arthropathies of inflammatory bowel disease. N Engl J Med 290:1117–1119, 1974.

67. McEwen C, Lingg C, Kirsner JB: Arthritis accompanying ulcerative colitis. Am J Med 33:923, 1962.

68. Zizic TM, Stevens MB: The arthropathy of Behçet's disease. Johns Hopkins Med J 136:243–250, 1975.

69. Yurdakul S, Yazici H, Tuzuir Y, et al: The arthritis of Behçet's disease: A prospective study. In press.

70. Ahvonen P, Sievers K, Ano K: Arthritis associated with Yersinia enterocolitica infection. Acta Rheumatol Scand 15:232–253, 1969.

71. Aho K, Ahvonen P, Lassus A, et al: HLA-B27 in reactive arthritis: A study of Yersinia arthritis and Reiter's disease. Arthritis Rheum 17:521–526, 1974.

72. Hawkins CF, Farr M, Morris CJ, et al: Detection by electron microscope of rod-shaped organisms in synovial membrane from a patient with the arthritis of Whipple's disease. Ann Rheum Dis 35:502–509, 1976.

73. Bole GG Jr, Friedlaender MH, Smith CK: Rheumatic symptoms and serological abnormalities induced by oral contraceptives. Lancet 1(590):323–326, 1969.

74. Bland JH, Frymoyer JW: Rheumatic syndromes of myxedema. N Engl J Med 282:1171–1174, 1970.

75. Gimlette TMD: Thyroid acropachy. Lancet 1:22, 1960.

76. Churchill MD Jr, Geraci JE, Hunder GG: Musculoskeletal manifestations of bacterial endocarditis. Ann Intern Med 87:754–759, 1977.

77. Bayer AS, Theofilopoulos AN, Eisenberg R, et al: Circulating immune complexes in infective endocarditis. N Engl J Med 295:1500–1505, 1976.

78. Bulkley BH, Hutchins GM: Atrial myxomas: A fifty-year review. Am Heart J 97:639–643, 1979.

79. McCarty DJ: Diagnostic mimicry in arthritis—Patterns of joint involvement associated with calcium pyrophosphate dihydrate crystal deposits. Bull Rheum Dis 25:804, 1975.

80. Utsinger PD, Zvaifler NJ, Resnick D: Calcium pyrophosphate dihydrate deposition disease without chondrocalcinosis. J Rheumatol 2:258–264, 1975.

81. Halla JT, Hardin JG: Clinical features of the arthritis of mixed connective tissue disease. Arthritis Rheum 21:497–503, 1978.

82. Gordon DA, Pruzanski W, Ogryzlo MA, et al: Amyloid arthritis simulating rheumatoid disease in five patients with multiple myeloma. Am J Med 45:142–154, 1973.

83. Pinals RS, Short CL: Calcific periarthritis involving multiple sites. Arthritis Rheum 9:566, 1966.

84. Martin JR, Huang SN, Lacson A, et al: Congenital contractural deformities of the fingers and arthropathy. Ann Rheum Dis 44:826–830, 1985.

85. Heller H, Gafni J, Michaeli D, et al: Arthritis of familial Mediterranean fever (FMF). Arthritis Rheum 9:1–17, 1966.

86. Wolfe F, Cathey MA, Kleinkeksel SM, et al: Psychological status in primary fibrositis and fibrositis associated with rheumatoid arthritis. J Rheumatol 11:500–506, 1984.

87. Velayos EE, Leidholt JD, Smyth CJ, et al: Arthropathy associated with steroid therapy. Ann Intern Med 64:759, 1966.

88. Talbott JH, Altman RD, Yu TF: Gouty arthritis masquerading as rheumatoid arthritis or vice versa. Semin Arthritis Rheum 8:77–114, 1978.

89. Resnick D: Gout-like lesions in rheumatoid arthritis. AJR Am J Roentgenol 127:1062, 1976.

90. Rappoport AS, Sosman JL, Weissman BN: Lesions resembling gout in patients with rheumatoid arthritis. Am J Roentgenol 126:41–45, 1976.

91. Kozin F, McCarty DJ: Rheumatoid factor in the serum of gouty patients. Arthritis Rheum 20:1559–1560, 1977.

92. Hirsch JH, Killien FC, Troupin RH: The arthropathy of hemochromatosis. Radiology 118:591–596, 1976.

93. Dymock IW, Hamilton EBD, Laws JW, et al: Arthropathy of hemochromatosis: Clinical and radiological analysis of 63 patients with iron overload. Ann Rheum Dis 29:469–476, 1970.

94. Schumacher HR, Andrews R, McLaughlin G: Arthropathy in sickle-cell disease. Ann Intern Med 78:203–211, 1973.

95. Schumacher HR, Dorwart BB, Bond J, et al: Chronic synovitis with early cartilage destruction in sickle cell disease. Ann Rheum Dis 36:413–419, 1977.

96. deCeulaer K, Forbes M, Roper D, et al: Non-gouty arthritis in sickle cell disease: Report of 37 consecutive cases. Ann Rheum Dis 43:599–603, 1984.

97. Crout JE, McKenna CH, Petitt RM: Symptomatic joint effusions in sickle cell–beta-thalassemia disease: report of a case. JAMA 235:1878–1879, 1976.

98. Calabrese LH: Human immunodeficiency virus infection and arthritis. Rheum Dis Clin North Am 19:477–488, 1993.

99. Solomon G, Brancato L, Winchester R: An approach to the human immunodeficiency virus–positive patient with a spondyloarthropathic disease. Rheum Dis Clin North Am 17:43–58, 1991.

100. Glueck CJ, Levy RI, Frederickson DS: Acute tendinitis and arthritis: A presenting symptom of familial type II hyperlipoproteinemia. JAMA 206:2895–2897, 1968.

101. Watt TL, Baumann RR: Pseudoxanthomatous rheumatoid nodules. Arch Dermatol 95:156–160, 1967.

102. Buckingham RB, Bole GG, Bassett DR: Polyarthritis associated with type IV hyperlipoproteinemia. Arch Intern Med 135:286–290, 1975.

103. Langer T, Levy RI: Acute muscular syndrome associated with administration of clofibrate. N Engl J Med 279:856–858, 1968.

104. Schumacher HR Jr: Articular manifestations of hypertropic pulmonary osteoarthropathy in bronchogenic carcinoma. Arthritis Rheum 19:629–636, 1976.

105. Brogadir SP, Goldwein MI, Schumacher HR: A hypereosinophilic syndrome mimicking rheumatoid arthritis. Am J Med 69:799–802, 1980.

106. Yanez JE, Thompson GR, Mikkelsen WM, et al: Rubella arthritis. Ann Intern Med 64:772, 1966.

107. Alpert E, Isselbacher KJ, Schur PH: The pathogenesis of arthritis associated with viral hepatitis: Complement component studies. N Engl J Med 285:185–189, 1971.

108. Schumacher HR, Gall EP: Arthritis in acute hepatitis and chronic active hepatitis: Pathology of the synovial membrane with evidence for the presence of Australia antigen in synovial membranes. Am J Med 57:655–664, 1974.

109. Sigal LH, Steere AC, Niederman JC: Symmetric polyarthritis associated with heterophile-negative infectious mononucleosis. Arthritis Rheum 26:553–556, 1983.

110. Weiner AD, Ghormley RK: Periodic benign synovitis: Idiopathic intermittent hydrarthrosis. J Bone Joint Surg Am 38:1039, 1956.

111. Williams MH, Sheldon PJ, Torrigiani G, et al: Palindromic rheumatism: Clinical and immunological studies. Ann Rheum Dis 30:375–380, 1971.

112. Ehrlich GE: Intermittent and periodic rheumatic syndromes. Bull Rheum Dis 24:746, 1974.

113. Steere AC, Malawista SE, Hardin JA, et al: Erythema chronicum migrans and Lyme arthritis: The enlarging clinical spectrum. Ann Intern Med 86:685–698, 1977.

114. Moutsopoulos HM, Fye KH, Pugay PI, et al: Monarthritic arthritis caused by metastatic breast carcinoma: Value of cytologic study of synovial fluid. JAMA 234:75–76, 1975.

115. Dorfman HD, Siegel HL, Perry MC, et al: Non-Hodgkin's lymphoma of the synovium simulating rheumatoid arthritis. Arthritis Rheum 30:155–161, 1987.

116. Emkey RD, Ragsdale BD, Ropes MW, et al: A case of lymphoproliferative disease presenting as juvenile rheumatoid arthritis: Diagnosis by synovial fluid examination. Am J Med 54:825–828, 1973.

117. Schapira D, Kerner H, Scharf Y: Erosive arthritis in a patient with mycosis fungoides. J R Soc Med 86:176–177, 1993.

118. Gold RH, Metzger AL, Mirra JM, et al: Multicentric reticulohistiocytosis (lipoid dermato-arthritis): An erosive polyarthritis with distinctive clinical, roentgenographic and pathological features. Am J Roentgenol 124:610–624, 1975.

119. Ehrlich GE: Inflammatory osteoarthritis: I. The clinical syndrome. J Chronic Dis 25:317–328, 1972.

120. Ordenstein L: Sur la Paralysie Agitante et la Sclérose en Plaques Generalisée. Paris, Imprimerie de E. Martinet, 1864.

121. Granowitz SP, Mankin HJ: Localized pigmented villonodular synovitis of knee: Report of five cases. J Bone Joint Surg Am 49:122–128, 1967.

122. Chou C-T, Schumacher HR Jr: Clinical and pathological studies of synovitis in polymyalgia rheumatica. Arthritis Rheum 27:1107–1117, 1984.

123. Ginsburg WW, Cohen MD, Hall SB, et al: Seronegative polyarthritis in giant cell arteritis. Arthritis Rheum 28:1362–1366, 1985.

124. McDanald EC, Weisman MH: Articular manifestations of rheumatic fever in adults. Ann Intern Med 89:917–920, 1978.

125. Barnett AL, Terry EE, Persellin RH: Acute rheumatic fever in adults. JAMA 232:925–928, 1975.

126. Stollerman GH, Markowitz M, Tarania A, et al: Jones' criteria (revised) for guidance in the diagnosis of rheumatic fever. Circulation 32:664, 1965.

127. Bywaters EGL: Relation between heart and joint disease including "rheumatoid heart disease" and chronic post-rheumatic arthritis (type Jaccoud). Br Heart J 12:101, 1950.

128. Zvaifler NJ: Chronic postrheumatic-fever (Jaccoud's) arthritis. N Engl J Med 267:10, 1962.

129. Ruderman JE, Abruzzo JL: Chronic post rheumatic-fever arthritis (Jaccoud's): Report of a case with subcutaneous nodules. Arthritis Rheum 9:640, 1966.

130. Spilberg I, Siltzbach LE, McEwen C: The arthritis of sarcoidosis. Arthritis Rheum 12:126–137, 1969.

131. Kaplan H: Sarcoid arthritis: A review. Arch Intern Med 112:162, 1963.

132. Poncet A: Address to the Congress Français de Chirurgie, 1897. Bull Acad Med Paris 46:194, 1901.

133. Krauser RE, Schumacher HR: The arthritis of Sweet's syndrome. Arthritis Rheum 18:35–41, 1975.

134. Hoffman GS: Treatment of Sweet's syndrome (acute febrile neutrophilic dermatosis) with indomethacin. J Rheumatol 4:201–206, 1977.

135. Thiemann H: Juvenile epiphysenstorungen. Fortschr Geb Rontgenstr Nuklearmed 14:79, 1909–10.

136. Rubinstein HM: Thiemann's disease: A brief reminder. Arthritis Rheum 18:357–360, 1975.

137. Bland J: Rheumatoid arthritis of the cervical spine. J Rheumatol 1:319, 1974.

138. Ball J: Enthesopathy of rheumatoid and ankylosing spondylitis. Ann Rheum Dis 30:213–223, 1971.

139. Martel W: Pathogenesis of cervical discovertebral destruction in rheumatoid arthritis. Arthritis Rheum 20:1217–1225, 1977.

140. Stevens JC, Cartlidge NE, Saunders M, et al: Atlanto-axial subluxation and cervical myelopathy in rheumatoid arthritis. Q J Med 40:391–408, 1971.

141. Nakano KK, Schoene WC, Baker RA, et al: The cervical myelopathy associated with rheumatoid arthritis: Analysis of patients, with 2 postmortem cases. Ann Neurol 3:144–151, 1978.

142. Martel W: The occipito-atlanto-axial joints in rheumatoid arthritis and ankylosing spondylitis. Am J Roentgenol 86:223, 1961.

143. Raskin RJ, Schnapf DJ, Wolf CR, et al: Computerized tomography in evaluation of atlantoaxial subluxation in rheumatoid arthritis. J Rheumatol 10:33–41, 1983.

144. Breedveld FC, Algra PR, Veilvoye CJ, et al: Magnetic resonance imaging in the evaluation of patients with rheumatoid arthritis and subluxations of the cervical spine. Arthritis Rheum 30:624–629, 1987.

145. Mayer JW, Messner RP, Kaplan RJ: Brain stem compression in rheumatoid arthritis. JAMA 236:2094–2095, 1976.

146. Winfield J, Young A, Williams P, et al: Prospective study of the radiological changes in hands, feet, and cervical spine in adult rheumatoid disease. Ann Rheum Dis 42:613–618, 1983.

147. Collins DN, Barnes CL, FitzRandolph RL: Cervical spine instability in rheumatoid patients having total hip or knee arthroplasty. Clin Orthop 272:127–135, 1991.

148. Pellicci PM, Ranawat CS, Tsairis P, et al: A prospective study of the progression of rheumatoid arthritis of the cervical spine. J Bone Joint Surg 65:342–350, 1981.

149. Meijers KA, Cats A, Kremer HPH, et al: Cervical myelopathy in rheumatoid arthritis. Clin Exp Rheumatol 2:239–245, 1984.

150. Davidson RC, Horn JR, Herndon JH, et al: Brain-stem compression in rheumatoid arthritis. JAMA 238:2633–2634, 1977.

151. Mikulowski P, Wollheim FA, Rotmil P, et al: Sudden death in rheumatoid arthritis with atlanto-axial dislocation. Acta Med Scand 198:445–451, 1975.

152. Smith PH, Benn RT, Sharp J: Natural history of rheumatoid cervical luxations. Ann Rheum Dis 31:431–439, 1972.

153. Agarwal AK, Peppelman WC, Kraus DR, et al: Recurrence of cervical spine instability in rheumatoid arthritis following previous fusion: Can disease progression be prevented by early surgery? J Rheumatol 19(9):1364–1370, 1992.

154. Yonenobu K, Hosono N, Iwasaki M, et al: Neurologic complications of surgery for cervical compression myelopathy. Spine 16(11):1277–1282, 1991.

155. Henderson DR: Vertical atlanto-axial subluxation in rheumatoid arthritis. Rheumatol Rehab 14:31–38, 1975.

156. Bywaters EG: Rheumatoid and other diseases of the cervical interspinous bursae, and changes in the spinous process. Ann Rheum Dis 41:360–370, 1982.

157. Tumiati B, Casoli P: Syringomyelia in a patient with rheumatoid subluxation of the cervical spine. J Rheumatol 18(9):1403–1405, 1991.

158. Jacob JR, Weisman MH, Mink JH, et al: Reversible cause of back pain and sciatica in rheumatoid arthritis: An apophyseal joint cyst. Arthritis Rheum 29:431–435, 1986.

159. Ericson S, Lundberg M: Alterations in the temporomandibular joint at various stages of rheumatoid arthritis. Acta Rheumatol Scand 13:257–274, 1967.

160. Marbach JJ, Spiera H: Rheumatoid arthritis of the temporomandibular joints. Ann Rheum Dis 26:538–543, 1967.

161. Goupille P, Fouquet B, Cotty P, et al: The temporomandibular joint

in rheumatoid arthritis: Correlations between clinical and computed tomography features. J Rheumatol 17:1285–1291, 1990.

162. Lofgren RH, Montgomery WW: Incidence of laryngeal involvement in rheumatoid arthritis. N Engl J Med 267:193, 1962.

163. Polisar IA, Burbank B, Levitt LM, et al: Bilateral midline fixation of cricoarytenoid joints as serious medical emergency. JAMA 172:901, 1960.

164. Bienenstock H, Ehrich GE, Freyberg RH: Rheumatoid arthritis of the cricoarytenoid joint: A clinicopathologic study. Arthritis Rheum 6:48, 1963.

165. Lawry GV, Finerman ML, Hanafee WN, et al: Laryngeal involvement in rheumatoid arthritis: A clinical, laryngoscopic, and computerized tomographic study. Arthritis Rheum 27:873–882, 1984.

166. Copeman WSC: Rheumatoid oto-arthritis. Br Med J 2:1536, 1963.

167. Moffat DA, Ramsden RT, Rosenberg JN, et al: Otoadmittance measurements in patients with rheumatoid arthritis. J Laryngol Otol 91:917–927, 1977.

168. Kalliomaki JL, Viitanen SM, Virtama P: Radiological findings of sterno-clavicular joints in rheumatoid arthritis. Acta Rheumatol Scand 14:233–240, 1968.

169. Kormano M: A microradiographic and histological study of the manu-briosternal joint in rheumatoid arthritis. Acta Rheumatol Scand 16:47–59, 1970.

170. Ennevaara K: Painful shoulder joint in rheumatoid arthritis: A clinical and radiological study of 200 cases, with special reference to arthrography of the glenohumeral joint. Acta Rheumatol Scand 11:1–116, 1967.

171. Weiss JJ, Thompson GR, Doust V, et al: Rotator cuff tears in rheumatoid arthritis. Arch Intern Med 135:521–525, 1975.

172. Mosley HF: Ruptures of the Rotator Cuff—Shoulder Lesions, 3rd ed. Edinburgh: E & S Livingston, 1969, p 73.

173. Edeiken J, Hodes PJ: Roentgen Diagnosis of Disease of Bone, 2nd ed. Baltimore: Williams & Wilkins, 1978, p 690–709.

174. DeSmet AA, Ting YM, Weis JJ: Shoulder arthrography in rheumatoid arthritis. Radiology 116:601–605, 1975.

175. Huston KA, Nelson AM, Hunder GG: Shoulder swelling in rheumatoid arthritis secondary to subacromial bursitis. Arthritis Rheum 21:145–147, 1978.

176. Resnick D, Niwayama G: Resorption of the undersurface of the distal clavicle in rheumatoid arthritis. Radiology 120:75–77, 1976.

177. deJager JP, Fleming A: Shoulder joint rupture and pseudothrombosis in rheumatoid arthritis. Ann Rheum Dis 43:503–504, 1984.

178. Peterson LF, Janes JM: Surgery of the rheumatoid elbow. Orthop Clin North Am 2:667–677, 1971.

179. Shapiro JS: A new factor in the etiology of ulnar drift. Clin Orthop 68:32–43, 1970.

180. Hastings DE, Evans JA: Rheumatoid wrist deformities and their relation to ulnar drift. J Bone Joint Surg Am 57:930–934, 1975.

181. Inglis AE: Rheumatoid arthritis in the hand. Am J Surg 109:368, 1965.

182. Swezey RL, Fiegenberg DS: Inappropriate intrinsic muscle action in the rheumatoid hand. Ann Rheum Dis 30:619–625, 1971.

183. Fearnley GR: Ulnar deviation of the fingers. Ann Rheum Dis 10:126, 1951.

184. Flatt AE: Surgical rehabilitation of the arthritic hand. Arthritis Rheum 11:278, 1959.

185. Hakstian RW, Tubiana R: Ulnar deviation of the fingers: The role of joint structure and function. J Bone Joint Surg Am 49:299–316, 1967.

186. Snorrason E: The problem of ulnar deviation of the fingers in rheumatoid arthritis. Acta Med Scand 140:359, 1951.

187. Vainio K, Oka M: Ulnar deviation of the fingers. Ann Rheum Dis 12:122, 1953.

188. Martin LF, Bensen WG: An unusual synovial cyst in rheumatoid arthritis. J Rheumatol 14:139–141, 1987.

189. Croft JD Jr: Rheumatoid "ganglion" as an unusual presenting sign of rheumatoid arthritis. JAMA 203:144–146, 1968.

190. Harrison MO, Freiberger RH, Ranawat CS: Arthrography of the rheumatoid wrist joint. AJR Am J Roentgenol 112:480–486, 1971.

191. Iveson JM, Hill AG, Wright V: Wrist cysts and fistulae: An arthrographic study of the rheumatoid wrist. Ann Rheum Dis 34:388–394, 1975.

192. Trentham DE, Masi AT: Carpo:metacarpal ratio: A new quantitative measure of radiologic progression of wrist involvement in rheumatoid arthritis. Arthritis Rheum 19:939–944, 1976.

193. Alarcon GS, Koopman WJ: The carpometacarpal ratio: A useful method for assessing disease progression in rheumatoid arthritis. J Rheumatol 12:846–848, 1985.

194. Kaye JJ, Callahan LF, Nance EP Jr, et al: Bony ankylosis in rheumatoid arthritis: Associations with longer duration and greater severity of disease. Invest Radiol 22(4):303–309, 1987.

195. Fuchs HA, Callahan LF, Kaye JJ, et al: Radiographic and joint count findings of the hand in rheumatoid arthritis: Related and unrelated findings. Arthritis Rheum 31:44–51, 1988.

196. Brewerton DA: Hand deformities in rheumatoid disease. Ann Rheum Dis 16:183, 1957.

197. McCarty DJ, Gatter RA: A study of distal interphalangeal joint tenderness in rheumatoid arthritis. Arthritis Rheum 9:325, 1966.

198. Vaughan-Jackson OJ: Rheumatoid hand deformities considered in the light of tendon imbalance. J Bone Joint Surg Br 44:764, 1962.

199. Abbott GT, Bucknall RC, Whitehouse GH: Osteoarthritis associated with distal interphalangeal joint involvement in rheumatoid arthritis. Skeletal Radiol 20:495–497, 1991.

200. Jacob J, Sartoris D, Kursunoglu S, et al: Distal interphalangeal joint involvement in rheumatoid arthritis. Arthritis Rheum 29:10–15, 1986.

201. Kellgren JH, Ball J: Tendon lesions in rheumatoid arthritis. A clinico-pathological study. Ann Rheum Dis 9:48, 1950.

202. Gray RG, Gottlieb NL: Hand flexor tenosynovitis in rheumatoid arthritis: Prevalence, distribution, and associated rheumatic features. Arthritis Rheum 20:1003–1008, 1977.

203. Duthie RB, Harris CM. A radiographic and clinical survey of the hip joint in sero-positive rheumatoid arthritis. Acta Orthop Scand 40:346–364, 1969.

204. Hastings DE, Parker SM: Protrusio acetabuli in rheumatoid arthritis. Clin Orthop 108:76–83, 1975.

205. Colton C, Darby A: Giant granulomatous lesions of the femoral head and neck in rheumatoid arthritis. Ann Rheum Dis 29:626–633, 1970.

206. Gupta PJ: Physical examination of the arthritis patient. Bull Rheum Dis 20:596, 1970.

207. Jayson MIV, Dixon A St J: Valvular mechanisms in juxta-articular cysts. Ann Rheum Dis 29:415–420, 1970.

208. Hench PK, Reid RT, Reames PM: Dissecting popliteal cyst stimulating thrombophlebitis. Ann Intern Med 64:1259–1264, 1966.

209. Hall AP, Scott JT: Synovial cysts and rupture of the knee joint in rheumatoid arthritis. Ann Rheum Dis 25:32–41, 1966.

210. Tait GBW, Bach F, Dixon A St J: Acute synovial rupture. Ann Rheum Dis 24:273, 1965.

211. Kraag G, Thevathasan EM, Gordon DA, et al: The hemorrhagic crescent sign of acute synovial rupture (letter). Ann Intern Med 85:477–478, 1976.

212. Gordon GV, Edell S: Ultrasound evaluation of popliteal cysts. Arch Intern Med 140:1453–1455, 1980.

213. Karvonen RL, Negendank WG, Fraser SM, et al: Articular cartilage defects of the knee: Correlation between magnetic resonance imaging and gross pathology. Ann Rheum Dis 49:672–675, 1990.

214. Rask MR: Achilles tendon rupture owing to rheumatoid disease: Case report with a nine-year follow-up. JAMA 239:435–436, 1978.

215. Dixon A St J: The rheumatoid foot. In Hill AGS (ed): Modern Trends in Rheumatology. London, Butterworths, 1971, pp 158–173.

216. Vidigal E, Jacoby R, Dixon A St J, et al: The foot in chronic rheumatoid arthritis. Ann Rheum Dis 34:292–297, 1975.

217. Bienenstock H: Rheumatoid plantar synovial cysts. Ann Rheum Dis. 34:98–99, 1975.

218. Calabro JJ: A critical evaluation of the diagnostic features of the feet in rheumatoid arthritis. Arthritis Rheum 5:19, 1962.

219. Clayton ML, Ries MD: Functional hallux rigidus in the rheumatoid foot. Clin Orthop 271:233–238, 1991.

220. McGuigan L, Burke D, Fleming A: Tarsal tunnel syndrome and peripheral neuropathy in rheumatoid disease. Ann Rheum Dis 42:128–131, 1983.

221. Maddison PJ, Bacon PA: Vitamin D deficiency, spontaneous fractures and osteopenia in rheumatoid arthritis. Br Med J 4:433–435, 1974.

222. Schneider R, Kaye JJ: Insufficiency and stress fractures of the long bones occurring in patients with rheumatoid arthritis. Radiology 116:595–599, 1975.

223. Lowthian PJ, Calin A: Geode development and multiple fractures in rheumatoid arthritis. Ann Rheum Dis 44:130–133, 1985.

224. Steiner G, Freund HA, Leichtentritt B, et al: Lesion of skeletal muscles in rheumatoid arthritis. Am J Pathol 22:103, 1946.

225. Haslock DI, Wright V, Harriman DGF: Neuromuscular disorders in rheumatoid arthritis: A motor-point muscle biopsy study. Q J Med 39:335–358, 1970.

226. Halla JT, Koopman WJ, Fallahi S, et al: Rheumatoid myositis: Clinical and histologic features and possible pathogenesis. Arthritis Rheum 27:737–743, 1984.

227. Soter NA, Franks AG Jr: The skin and rheumatic diseases. In Kelley WN, Harris ED Jr, Ruddy S, Sledge CB (eds): The Textbook of Rheumatology, 4th ed. Philadelphia, WB Saunders, 1993, pp 519–534.

228. Ferry AP: The eye and rheumatic diseases. In Kelley WN, Harris ED Jr, Ruddy S, Sledge CB (eds): The Textbook of Rheumatology, 4th ed. Philadelphia: WB Saunders, 1993, pp 507–518.

229. Watson PG, Hayreh SS: Scleritis and episcleritis. Br J Ophthalmol 60:163–191, 1976.

230. Hurd ER: Extra-articular manifestations of rheumatoid arthritis. Semin Arthritis Rheum 8:151–176, 1979.

231. Hart FD: Rheumatoid arthritis: Extra-articular manifestations. Br Med J 3:131–136, 1969.

232. Halla JT, Schrohenloher RE, Koopman WJ: Local immune responses in certain extra-articular manifestations of rheumatoid arthritis. Ann Rheum Dis 51:698–701, 1992.

233. Collins DH: The subcutaneous nodule of rheumatoid arthritis. J Pathol Bacteriol 45:97, 1937.

234. Bennett GA, Zeller JW, Bauer W: Subcutaneous nodules of rheumatoid arthritis and rheumatic fever: A pathologic study. Arch Pathol 30:70, 1940.

235. Ziff M: The rheumatoid nodule. Arthritis Rheum 33(6):761–767, 1990.

236. Sokoloff L: The pathophysiology of peripheral blood vessels in collagen diseases. *In* Orbison JL, Smith DE (eds): The Peripheral Blood Vessels. Baltimore: Williams & Wilkins, 1963, p 297.

237. Mellbye OJ, Førre Ø, Mollnes TE, et al: Immunopathology of subcutaneous rheumatoid nodules. Ann Rheum Dis 50:909–912, 1991.

238. Palmer DG, Hogg N, Highton J, et al: Macrophage migration and maturation within rheumatoid nodules. Arthritis Rheum 30:728–736, 1987.

239. Edwards JCW, Wilkinson LS, Pitsillides AA: Palisading cells of rheumatoid nodules: Comparison with synovial intimal cells. Ann Rheum Dis 52:801–805, 1993.

240. Harris ED Jr: A collagenolytic system produced by primary cultures of rheumatoid nodule tissue. J Clin Invest 51:2973–2976, 1972.

241. Ganda OP, Caplan HI: Rheumatoid disease without joint involvement. JAMA 2281:338–339, 1974.

242. Ginsberg MH, Genant HK, Yu TF, et al: Rheumatoid nodulosis: An unusual variant of rheumatoid disease. Arthritis Rheum 18:49–58, 1975.

243. Brower AC, NaPombejara C, Stechschulte DJ, et al: Rheumatoid nodulosis: Another cause of juxta-articular nodules. Radiology 125:669–670, 1977.

244. McCarty DJ: Complete reversal of rheumatoid nodulosis. J Rheumatol 18(5):736–737, 1991.

245. Simons FE, Schaller JG: Benign rheumatoid nodules. Pediatrics 56:29–33, 1975.

246. Olive A, Maymo J, Lloreta J, et al: Evolution of benign rheumatoid nodules into rheumatoid arthritis after 50 years. Ann Rheum Dis 46:624–625, 1987.

247. Wood MG, Beerman H: Necrosiosis lipoidica, granuloma annulare: Report of a case with lesions in the galea aponeurotica of a child. Am J Dis Child 96:720, 1958.

248. Healey LA, Wilske KR, Sagebiel RW: Rheumatoid nodules simulating basal-cell carcinoma. N Engl J Med 277:7–9, 1967.

249. Sturrock RD, Cowden EA, Howie E, et al: The forgotten nodule: Complications of sacral nodules in rheumatoid arthritis. Br Med J 4:92–93, 1975.

250. Friedman BA: Rheumatoid nodules of the larynx. Arch Otolaryngol 101:361–363, 1975.

251. Jackson CG, Chess RL, Ward JR: A case of rheumatoid nodule formation within the central nervous system and review of the literature. J Rheumatol 11:237–240, 1984.

252. Pearson ME, Kosco M, Huffer W, et al: Rheumatoid nodules of the spine: Case report and review of the literature. Arthritis Rheum 30:709–713, 1987.

253. Bywaters EGL: Fistulous rheumatism: A manifestation of rheumatoid arthritis. Ann Rheum Dis 12:114, 1953.

254. Shapiro RF, Resnick D, Castles JJ, et al: Fistulization of rheumatoid joints: Spectrum of identifiable syndromes. Ann Rheum Dis 34:489–498, 1975.

255. Bassett LW, Gold RH, Mirra JM: Rheumatoid bursitis extending into the clavicle and to the skin surface. Ann Rheum Dis 44:336–340, 1985.

256. Vandenbroucke JP, Kaaks R, Valkenburg HA, et al: Frequency of infections among rheumatoid arthritis patients, before and after disease onset. Arthritis Rheum 30:810–813, 1987.

257. Baum J: Infection in rheumatoid arthritis. Arthritis Rheum 14:135–137, 1971.

258. Gaulhofer de Klerch EH, Van Dam G: Septic complications in rheumatoid arthritis. Acta Rheumatol Scand 9:254, 1963.

259. Huskisson EC, Hart FD: Severe, unusual and recurrent infections in rheumatoid arthritis. Ann Rheum Dis 31:118–121, 1972.

260. Bodel PT, Hollingsworth JW: Comparative morphology, respiration, and phagocytic function of leukocytes from blood and joint fluid in rheumatoid arthritis. J Clin Invest 45:580, 1966.

261. Singleton JD, West SG, Nordstrom DM: "Pseudoseptic" arthritis complicating rheumatoid arthritis: A report of six cases. J Rheumatol 18:1319–1322, 1991.

262. Cash JM, Klippel JH: Second-line drug therapy for rheumatoid arthritis. N Engl J Med 330:1368–1375, 1994.

263. Gridley G, McLaughlin JK, Ekbom A, et al: Incidence of cancer among patients with rheumatoid arthritis. J Natl Cancer Inst 85:307–311, 1993.

264. Hakulinen T, Isomaki H, Knekt P: Rheumatoid arthritis and cancer studies based on linking nationwide registries in Finland. Am J Med 78(1A):29–32, 1985.

265. Prior P, Symmons DP, Hawkins CF, et al: Cancer morbidity in rheumatoid arthritis. Ann Rheum Dis 43:128–131, 1984.

266. Gridley G, Klippel JH, Hoover RN, et al: Incidence of cancer among men with the Felty syndrome. Ann Intern Med 120(1):35–39, 1994.

267. Kassan SS, Thomas TL, Moutsopoulos HM, et al: Increased risk of lymphoma in sicca syndrome. Ann Intern Med 89:888–892, 1978.

268. Mowat AG: Hematologic abnormalities in rheumatoid arthritis. Semin Arthritis Rheum 1:195–219, 1971.

269. Engstedt L, Strandberg O: Haematological data and clinical activity of the rheumatoid diseases. Acta Med Scand 180:13, 1966.

270. Vreugdenhil G, Wognum AW, van Eijk HG, et al: Anaemia in rheumatoid arthritis: The role of iron, vitamin B_{12}, and folic acid deficiency, and erythropoietin responsiveness. Ann Rheum Dis 49:93–98, 1990.

271. Beck JR, Cornwell GG, Rawnsley HM: Multivariate approach to predictive diagnosis of bone-marrow iron stores. Am J Clin Pathol 70:665–670, 1978.

272. Samson D, Halliday D, Gumpel JM: Role of ineffective erythropoiesis in the anaemia of rheumatoid arthritis. Ann Rheum Dis 36:181–185, 1977.

273. Cartwright GE: The anemia of chronic disorders. Semin Hematol 3:351–375, 1966.

274. Raymond FD, Bowie MA, Dugan A: Iron metabolism in rheumatoid arthritis. Arthritis Rheum 8:233, 1965.

275. Ridolfo AS, Rubin A, Crabtree RE, et al: Effects of fenoprofen and aspirin on gastrointestinal microbleeding in man. Clin Pharmacol Ther 14:226–230, 1973.

276. Williams RA, Samson D, Tikerpae J, et al: In-vitro studies of ineffective erythropoiesis in rheumatoid arthritis. Am J Rheum Dis 41:502–507, 1982.

277. Reid CD, Prouse PJ, Baptista LC, et al: The mechanism of anaemia in rheumatoid arthritis: Effects of bone marrow adherent cells and of serum on *in vivo* erythropoiesis. Br J Haematol 58:607–615, 1984.

278. Prouse PJ, Bonner B, Gumpel JM, et al: Stimulation of bone marrow erythropoiesis by T lymphocytes of anaemic patients with rheumatoid arthritis. Ann Rheum Dis 44:220–223, 1985.

279. Winchester RJ, Koffler D, Litwin SD, et al: Observations on the eosinophilia of certain patients with rheumatoid arthritis. Arthritis Rheum 14:650–665, 1971.

280. Hutchinson RM, Davis P, Jayson MI: Thrombocytosis in rheumatoid arthritis. Ann Rheum Dis 35:138–142, 1976.

281. Farr M, Scott DL, Constable TJ, et al: Thrombocytosis of active rheumatoid disease. Ann Rheum Dis 42:545–549, 1983.

282. Bowman SJ, Sivakumaran M, Snowden N, et al: The large granular lymphocyte syndrome with rheumatoid arthritis: Immunogenetic evidence for a broader definition of Felty's syndrome. Arthritis Rheum 37(9):1326–1330, 1994.

283. Combe B, Andary M, Caraux J, et al: Characterization of an expanded subpopulation of large granular lymphocytes in a patient with rheumatoid arthritis. Arthritis Rheum 29:675–679, 1986.

284. Loughran TP Jr: Clonal diseases of large granular lymphocytes. Blood 82:1–14, 1993.

285. Wittenborg A, Gille J, Ostertag H, et al: Die dugitalartritis bei chronischer polyarthritis. Folia Angiol 22:409, 1974.

286. Fischer M, Mielke H, Glaefke S, et al: Generalized vasculopathy and finger blood flow abnormalities in rheumatoid arthritis. J Rheumatol 11:33–37, 1984.

287. Sokoloff L, Bunin JJ: Vascular lesions in rheumatoid arthritis. J Chronic Dis 5:668, 1957.

288. Kulka JP, Bocking D, Ropes MW, et al: Early joint lesions of rheumatoid arthritis: Report of 8 cases with knee biopsies of less than one year's duration. Arch Pathol 59:129, 1955.

289. Soter NA, Mihm MC Jr, Gigli I, et al: Two distinct cellular patterns in cutaneous necrotizing angiitis. J Invest Dermatol 66:344–350, 1976.

290. Rapoport RJ, Kozin F, Mackel SE, et al: Cutaneous vascular immunofluorescence in rheumatoid arthritis. Am J Med 68:344, 1976.

291. Mongan ES, Cass RM, Jacox RF, et al: A study of the relation of seronegative and seropositive rheumatoid arthritis to each other and to necrotizing vasculitis. Am J Med 47:23–25, 1969.

292. Weinstein A, Peters K, Brown D, et al: Metabolism of the third component of complement (C3) in patients with rheumatoid arthritis. Arthritis Rheum 15:49–56, 1972.

293. Conn DL, McDuffie FC, Dyck PJ: Immunopathologic study of sural nerves in rheumatoid arthritis. Arthritis Rheum 15:135–143, 1972.

294. Weisman M, Zvaifler N: Cryoimmunoglobulinemia in rheumatoid arthritis: Significance in serum of patients with rheumatoid vasculitis. J Clin Invest 56:725–739, 1975.

295. Schmid FR, Cooper NS, Ziff M, et al: Arteritis in rheumatoid arthritis. Am J Med 30:56, 1961.

296. Markenson JA, McDougal JS, Tsairis P, et al: Rheumatoid meningitis: A localized immune process. Ann Intern Med 119:359, 1967.

297. Siomopoulus V, Shah N: Acute organic brain syndrome associated with rheumatoid arthritis. J Clin Psychol 40:46, 1979.

298. Toussirot E, Serratrice G, Valentin P: Autonomic nervous system involvement in rheumatoid arthritis: 50 cases. J Rheumatol 20(9):1508–1514, 1993.

299. Bienenstock H, Minick CR, Rogoff B: Mesenteric arteritis and intestinal infarction in rheumatoid disease. Arch Intern Med 119:359–364, 1967.

300. Geirsson AJ, Sturfelt G, Truedsson L: Clinical and serological features of severe vasculitis in rheumatoid arthritis: Prognostic implications. Ann Rheum Dis 46:727–733, 1987.

301. Scott DG, Bacon PA, Elliott PJ, et al: Systemic vasculitis in a district general hospital 1972–80: Clinical and laboratory features, classification and prognosis of 80 cases. Q J Med 51:292–311, 1982.

302. Lawson AA, MacLean N: Renal disease and drug therapy in rheumatoid arthritis. Ann Rheum Dis 25:441–449, 1966.
303. Via CS, Hasbargen JA, Moore J Jr, et al: Rheumatoid arthritis and membranous glomerulonephritis: A role for immune complex dissociative techniques. J Rheumatol 11:342–347, 1984.
304. Walker WC, Wright V: Pulmonary lesions and rheumatoid arthritis. Medicine 47:501–520, 1968.
305. Dodson WH, Hollingsworth JW: Pleural effusion in rheumatoid arthritis: Impaired transport of glucose. N Engl J Med 275:1337–1342, 1966.
306. Walker WC, Wright V: Diffuse interstitial pulmonary fibrosis and rheumatoid arthritis. Ann Rheum Dis 28:252–259, 1969.
307. Dixon A St J, Ball J: Honeycomb lung and chronic rheumatoid arthritis: A case report. Ann Rheum Dis 16:241, 1957.
308. Stack BHR, Grant IWB: Rheumatoid interstitial lung disease. Br J Dis Chest 59:202, 1965.
309. Frank ST, Weg JG, Harkleroad LE, et al: Pulmonary dysfunction in rheumatoid disease. Chest 63:27–34, 1973.
310. Tishler M, Grief J, Fireman E, et al: Bronchoalveolar lavage—A sensitive tool for early diagnosis of pulmonary involvement in rheumatoid arthritis. J Rheumatol 13:547–550, 1986.
311. Caplan A: Certain unusual radiographic appearances in the chest of coal miners suffering from RA. Thorax 8:29, 1953.
312. Portner MM, Gracie WA, Jr: Rheumatoid lung disease with cavitary nodules, pneumothorax and eosinophilia. N Engl J Med 275:697–700, 1966.
313. Hull S, Mathews JA: Pulmonary necrobiotic nodules as a presenting feature of rheumatoid arthritis. Ann Rheum 41:21–24, 1982.
314. Shenberger KN, Schned AR, Taylor TH: Rheumatoid disease and bronchogenic carcinoma—Case report and review of the literature. J Rheumatol 11:226–228, 1984.
315. Gardner DL, Duthie JR, MacLeod J, et al: Pulmonary hypertension in RA: Report of a case study with intimal sclerosis of pulmonary and digital arteries. Scott Med J 2:183, 1957.
316. Scully RE, Mark EJ, McNeely WF, et al: Case 37-1992: Presentation of case. N Engl J Med 327(12):873–880, 1992.
317. Radoux V, Menard HA, Begin R, et al: Airways disease in rheumatoid arthritis patients: One element of a general exocrine dysfunction. Arthritis Rheum 30:249–259, 1987.
318. Sassoon CS, McAlpine SW, Tashkin DP, et al: Small airways function in non-smokers with rheumatoid arthritis. Arthritis Rheum 27:1218–1226, 1984.
319. Popp RL: Echocardiography (first of two parts). N Engl J Med 323:101–109, 1990.
320. Bonfiglio TA, Atwater EC: Heart disease in patients with seropositive rheumatoid arthritis: A controlled autopsy study and review. Arch Intern Med 124:714–719, 1969.
321. Lebowitz WB: The heart in rheumatoid arthritis: A clinical and pathological study of 62 cases. Ann Intern Med 58:102, 1963.
322. MacDonald WJ Jr, Crawford MH, Klippel JH, et al: Echocardiographic assessment of cardiac structure and function in patients with rheumatoid arthritis. Am J Med 63:890–896, 1977.
323. Lange RK, Weiss TE, Ochsner JL: Rheumatoid arthritis and constrictive pericarditis: A patient benefited by pericardectomy. Arthritis Rheum 8:403, 1965.
324. Thadini U, Iveson JM, Wright V: Cardiac tamponade, constrictive pericarditis and pericardial resection in rheumatoid arthritis. Medicine 54:261–270, 1975.
325. Prakash R, Atassi A, Poske R, et al: Prevalence of pericardial effusion and mitral-valve involvement in patients with rheumatoid arthritis without cardiac symptoms. N Engl J Med 289:597, 1975.
326. Weintraub AM, Zvaifler NJ: The occurrence of valvular and myocardial disease in patients with chronic joint disease. Am J Med 35:145, 1963.
327. Iveson JM, Thadani U, Ionescu M, et al: Aortic valve incompetence and replacement in rheumatoid arthritis. Ann Rheum Dis 34:312–320, 1975.
328. Gowans JDC: Complete heart block with Stokes-Adams syndrome due to rheumatoid heart disease. N Engl J Med 262:1012, 1960.
329. Lev M, Bharati S, Hoffman FG, et al: The conduction system in rheumatoid arthritis with complete atrioventricular block. Am Heart J 90:78–83, 1975.
330. Ahern M, Lever JV, Cosh J: Complete heart block in rheumatoid arthritis. Ann Rheum Dis 42:389–397, 1983.
331. Swezey RL: Myocardial infarction due to rheumatoid arteritis: An antemortem diagnosis. JAMA 199: 855–857, 1967.
332. Reimer KA, Rodgers RF, Oyasu R: Rheumatoid arthritis with rheumatoid heart disease and granulomatous aortitis. JAMA 235:2510–2512, 1976.
333. Camilleri JP, Douglas-Jones AG, Pritchard MH: Rapidly progressive aortic valve incompetence in a patient with rheumatoid arthritis. Br J Rheumatol 30:379–381, 1991.
334. Valkenburg HA: Pattern of rheumatoid disease in society: Change or disappearance? Scand J Rheumatol 5(Suppl 12):89–95, 1975.
335. Pinals RS, Masi AT, Larsen RA: Preliminary criteria for clinical remission in rheumatoid arthritis. Arthritis Rheum 24:1308–1315, 1981.
336. Wolfe F, Hawley DJ: Remission in rheumatoid arthritis. J Rheumatol 12:245–252, 1985.
337. Pinals RS: Survival in rheumatoid arthritis. Arthritis Rheum 30:473–475, 1987.
338. Vandenbroucke JP, Hazevoet HM, Cats A: Survival and cause of death in rheumatoid arthritis: A 25-year prospective followup. J Rheumatol 11:158–161, 1984.
339. Harris ED Jr: The challenge of therapy for rheumatoid arthritis. Eur J Int Med 1:325–330, 1990.
340. Reilly PA, Cosh JA, Maddison PJ, et al: Mortality and survival in rheumatoid arthritis. A 25-year prospective study of 100 patients. Ann Rheum Dis 49:363–369, 1990.
341. Sherrer YS, Block DA, Mitchell DM, et ai: The development of disability in rheumatoid arthritis. Arthritis Rheum 29:494–500, 1986.
342. Luukkainen R, Isomaki H, Kajander A: Prognostic value of the type of onset of rheumatoid arthritis. Ann Rheum Dis 42:274–275, 1983.
343. Sharp JT, Calkins E, Cohen AS, et al: Observations on the clinical, chemical, and serological manifestations of rheumatoid arthritis, based on the course of 154 cases. Medicine 43:41, 1964.
344. Cobb S, Anderson F, Baurer W: Length of life and cause of death in rheumatoid arthritis. N Engl J Med 249:553, 1953.
345. Mitchell DM, Spitz PW, Young DY, et al: Survival, prognosis, and causes of death in rheumatoid arthritis. Arthritis Rheum 29:706–714, 1986.
346. Pincus T, Callahan LF, Sale WG, et al: Severe functional declines, work disability, and increased mortality in seventy-five rheumatoid arthritis patients studied over nine years. Arthritis Rheum 27:864–872, 1984.
347. Erhardt CC, Mumford PA, Venables PJ, et al : Factors predicting a poor life prognosis in rheumatoid arthritis: An eight-year prospective study. Ann Rheum Dis 48:7–13, 1989.
348. Pincus T, Callahan LF: Taking mortality in rheumatoid arthritis seriously—Predictive markers, socioeconomic status and comorbidity. J Rheumatol 13:841–845, 1986.
349. Laakso M, Mutru O, Isomaki H, et al: Cancer mortality in patients with rheumatoid arthritis. J Rheumatol 13:522–526, 1986.
350. Kellgren JH, O'Brien WM: On the natural history of rheumatoid arthritis in relation to the sheep cell agglutination test (SCAT). Arthritis Rheum 5:115, 1962.
351. Masi AT, Maldonado-Cocco JA, Kaplan SB, et al: Prospective study of the early course of rheumatoid arthritis in young adults: Comparison of patients with and without rheumatoid factor positivity at entry and identification of variables correlating with outcome. Semin Arthritis Rheum 4:299–326, 1976.
352. Dixon A St J: "Rheumatoid arthritis" with negative serological reaction. Ann Rheum Dis 19:209, 1960.
353. Withrington RH, Teitsson I, Valdimarsson H, et al: Prospective study of early rheumatoid arthritis: II. Association of rheumatoid factor isotypes with fluctuations in disease activity. Ann Rheum Dis 43:679–685, 1984.
354. Duthie JJR, Brown PE, Truelove LH, et al: Course and prognosis in rheumatoid arthritis: A further report. Ann Rheum Dis 23:193, 1964.
355. Ragan C, Farrington E: The clinical features of rheumatoid arthritis. JAMA 181:663, 1962.
356. Henderson DR, Jayson MI, Tribe CB: Lack of correlation of synovial histology with joint damage in rheumatoid arthritis. Ann Rheum Dis 34:7–11, 1975.
357. Yates DB, Scott JT: Rheumatoid synovitis and joint disease: Relationship between arthroscopic and histological changes. Ann Rheum Dis 34:1–6, 1975.
358. Cruickshank B: Interpretation of multiple biopsies of synovial tissue in rheumatic diseases. Ann Rheum Dis 11:137, 1952.
359. Muirden KD, Mills KW: Do lymphocytes protect the rheumatoid joint? Br Med J 4:219–221, 1971.
360. Harris ED Jr, Faulkner CS II, Brown FE: Collagenolytic systems in rheumatoid arthritis. Clin Orthop Rel Res 140:303–316, 1975.
361. Ward TT, Steigbigel RT: Acidosis of synovial fluid correlates with synovial fluid leukocytosis. Am J Med 64:933–936, 1978.
362. Geborek P, Saxne T, Pettersson H, et al : Synovial fluid acidosis correlates with radiological joint destruction in rheumatoid arthritis knee joints. J Rheumatol 16:468–472, 1989.
363. Ruddy S: Synovial fluid: Mirror of the inflammatory lesion in rheumatoid arthritis. In Harris ED Jr (ed): Rheumatoid Arthritis. New York, Medcom Press, 1974, p 75.
364. Regan-Smith MG, O'Connor GT, Kwoh CK, et al: Lack of correlation between the Steinbrocker staging of hand radiographs and the functional health status of individuals with rheumatoid arthritis. Arthritis Rheum 32:128–133, 1989.
365. Larsen A, Dale K, Eek M: Radiographic evaluation of rheumatoid arthritis and related conditions by standard reference films. Acta Radiol 18:481–491, 1977.
366. O'Sullivan MM, Lewis PA, Newcombe RG, et al: Precision of Larsen grading of radiographs in assessing progression of rheumatoid arthritis in individual patients. Ann Rheum Dis 49:286–289, 1990.
367. Sharp JT: Radiologic assessment as an outcome measure in rheumatoid arthritis. Arthritis Rheum 32:221–229, 1989.

368. Ritchie DM, Boyle JA, McInnes JM, et al: Clinical studies with an articular index for the assessment of joint tenderness in patients with rheumatoid arthritis. Q J Med 37:393–406, 1968.
369. Cooperating Clinics Committee of the ARA: A seven-day variability study of 499 patients with peripheral rheumatoid arthritis. Arthritis Rheum 8:302, 1965.
370. Lansbury J: Report of a three-year study on the systemic and articular indexes in rheumatoid arthritis: Theoretic and clinical considerations. Arthritis Rheum 1:505, 1958.
371. Lansbury J, Haut DD: Quantitation of the manifestations of rheumatoid arthritis: Area of joint surfaces as an index to total joint inflammation and deformity. Am J Med Sci 232: 150, 1956.
372. Lansbury J: Quantitation of activity of rheumatoid arthritis: Method for summation of systemic indices of rheumatoid activity. Am J Med Sci 232:300, 1956.
373. Egger MJ, Huth DA, Ward JR, et al: Reduced joint count indices in the evaluation of rheumatoid arthritis. Arthritis Rheum 28:613–619, 1985.
374. Thompson PW, Silman AJ, Kirwan JR, et al: Articular indices of joint inflammation in rheumatoid arthritis: correlation with the acute-phase response. Arthritis Rheum 30:618–623, 1987.
375. Steinbrocker O, Traeger CH, Batterman RC: Therapeutic criteria in rheumatoid arthritis. JAMA 140:659, 1949.
376. Pincus T, Callahan LF, Brooks RH, et al: Self-report questionnaire scores in rheumatoid arthritis compared with traditional, physical, radiographic, and laboratory measures. Ann Intern Med 110:259–266, 1989.
377. Callahan LF, Brooks RH, Summey JA, et al: Quantitative pain assessment for routine care of rheumatoid arthritis patients, using a pain scale based on activities of daily living and a visual analog pain scale. Arthritis Rheum 30:630–636, 1987.

CHAPTER 56

Edward D. Harris, Jr.

Treatment of Rheumatoid Arthritis

Several important truths have emerged from outcome studies of patients with rheumatoid arthritis observed over many years and exposed to diverse regimens of therapy:

- No single therapeutic regimen or combination of therapies has been consistently associated with marked and sustained improvement, or with a halt in progression of loss of joint structure and function.[1]
- In many cases, irreversible loss of articular cartilage begins within months of the onset of disease, and in most cases within a year of onset of continuously active disease. Analysis of radiographic data from several studies suggests that 50 percent of the maximum damage to joints happens within the first 5 years of the disease.[2, 3] The use of magnetic resonance imaging (MRI) has enabled clinicians to detect erosions early in the course of disease, long before they are visible on plain films.[4]
- Side effects or complications of therapy lead all too often to increased morbidity or even death.
- The only parameter that accurately identifies patients destined to develop severe erosive or extra-articular disease is the amino acid sequence in the third hypervariable region of the major histocompatibility complex (MHC) class II human leukocyte antigen (HLA)–DRB1 chain.
- Clinically available and effective assessments of prognosis include the Health Assessment Questionnaire (HAQ) and its modifications, functional tests, acute-phase reactants, and the presence of and titer of rheumatoid factor.
- Patients treated early in their disease course by rheumatologists tend to have a better long-term outcome than those treated by physicians who are not specialists in rheumatology, perhaps because rheumatologists are more likely to treat patients early and more aggressively. One study has confirmed the reluctance of primary care physicians to prescribe disease-modifying drugs; although 73 percent had heard of them and were aware of their value, only 14 percent used them in clinical practice.[5]
- Homeopathy is no more effective than placebo,[6] although rheumatologists have long recognized the extraordinary power of placebo in clinical trials.

Two criteria are available for which needed data must be collected at several points in time for each patient:

- The degree of sustained synovitis
- The intensity of synovitis

Accurate assessment of these two parameters gives the physician a crude index of the degree of urgency for instituting more aggressive therapy. Thus, the patient with intermittent flares of synovitis who is relatively symptom-free during partial remissions is less likely to go on to loss of joint function or severe extra-articular disease than the patient with continuously active synovitis. Similarly, the intensity of disease activity, measured by clinical examination and laboratory tests as well as the patient's own assessment, is a useful predictor of which patient will face a higher risk of death or disability.

The challenge for treating rheumatoid arthritis, therefore, is to begin early with therapy that is likely to down-regulate the disease process without causing morbidity or death from side effects.

There are a few reasons to be optimistic that an earlier, more aggressive therapeutic approach may be beneficial. One is that we know much more about the risk of long-term side effects of drugs than previously, and therefore we should be able to use them more carefully and effectively. Another is that we are at the threshold of potential availability of biologic therapies targeting specificity within the pathophysiologic mechanisms that generate and sustain rheumatoid arthritis. These should involve less risk than the shotgun-like therapies we often are forced to use now.

A reason for discouragement, or at worst, therapeutic nihilism, in the treatment of rheumatoid arthritis is that the drugs we use are toxic. It is rare for second-line drugs to be continued for more than 2 or 3 years in any one patient—either because of lack of efficacy or because of unacceptable side effects.[2, 7–9] Another discouraging reality is that no long-term analysis of radiographic progression of joint disease shows significant breaks in the curve toward joint destruction, regardless of therapy. The most optimistic interpretation of all this is the principle, mentioned earlier, that the only path available to effectively delay or cancel joint destruction in rheumatoid arthritis is to begin therapy early enough to prevent the amplified cycle of destructive elements from becoming self-sustaining.

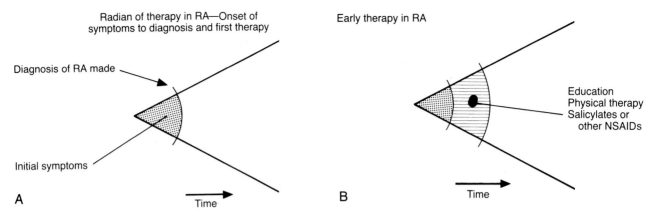

Figure 56–1. *A*, Rheumatoid arthritis (RA) begins before the diagnosis is made. In the interval between onset of the disease and diagnosis, a variable amount of both reversible and irreversible damage occurs in each patient. In this figure and the next, RA is beginning at the intersection of the two lines. With time, and at a variable rate that is unique to each patient, the disease progresses. Schematically, patients with primarily systemic involvement will be progressing along the upper line, and those with disease marked primarily by joint destruction along the lower line. *B*, Phase I of therapy is nonspecific. It would be appropriate for any form of inflammatory arthritis. Education must be emphasized; without it, the patient's attitudes about himself or herself and the disease will be inadequate, and the compliance with therapy will be variable. Now, not later, is the time to emphasize principles of joint protection and exercise.

The American College of Rheumatology has recently published two manuscripts on the management of rheumatoid arthritis. One provides useful algorithms to help evaluate disease activity, time consultations, and revise treatment plans.[9a] A second tabulates the usefulness of virtually all drugs mentioned in this chapter, enumerates their toxicities, and provides a logical sequence for their use in this disease.[9b]

STAGES OF RHEUMATOID ARTHRITIS AND IMPLICATIONS FOR THERAPY (Fig. 56–1)

Although patients with rheumatoid arthritis may be similar, no two are identical. In management of individuals, it is the subtleties of the particular disease pace and process, matched with elements of personality, that make each therapeutic challenge unique.

To provide a framework within which to focus on special qualities of each person's illness, a staging system has been developed using concepts partially developed previously.[10, 11] The pace of the process, the extent to which the synovitis is continuous, and the functional class can be matched with the pathology at the time that treatment options are presented.

The four stages of rheumatoid arthritis and rough correlations with available therapies are detailed in Table 56–1.

EDUCATION ABOUT ARTHRITIS: A MAINSTAY OF THERAPY

One of the most interesting findings that relates various subsets of rheumatoid patients to poor outcome is the inverse correlation of formal education status and mortality: those patients with fewer years of schooling are more likely to die earlier than a well-educated patient, all other variables being relatively equal. Thus, it is notable that an alternative to formal education (i.e., education in the clinic about what rheumatoid arthritis is, how it affects a person, and how it should be treated) has a positive effect on outcome of the disease. For example, arthritis self-management teaches patients and, equally important, enables them to be involved in therapy and therapeutic decisions from the beginning of physician-supervised treatment.[12, 13]

In one study of 70 randomly selected patients with rheumatoid arthritis, 62 percent knew that the cause of rheumatoid arthritis is as yet unknown, but 27 percent thought it could be caused by injury and 11 percent by cold, damp weather. Fifty-two percent had no idea why they were given blood tests. Concerning the logic of, use of, and side effects of disease-modifying drugs, knowledge was abysmally inadequate.[14]

Physicians themselves may be the patients' teachers; another option is the wise use of nonphysician health professionals. The trained nurse practitioner or physician's assistant has more than sufficient knowledge to give a full education about the disease. Patients in whom it is too early to make a diagnosis should nevertheless be given education about self-management of synovitis and trials of anti-inflammatory medication.

REST, EXERCISE, AND OTHER MODALITIES

As recently as the 1980s, patients with rheumatoid arthritis who had flares of disease activity were often admitted to general medical units or arthritis centers in hospitals, primarily for rest and supervised exercise. Although long-term outcome may not have been changed by these interludes in hospital, the short-term benefits were positive.[15, 16] Close work with physical therapists and occupational therapists and a

Table 56-1. RHEUMATOID ARTHRITIS: STAGING AND THERAPY*

Stage of Disease	Time After Onset of Synovitis	Clinical Characteristics	Laboratory Findings	Pathologic Process	Biopathology	Management
1	*Days to several weeks*	Onset may be relatively acute or have a gradual onset over several weeks. Morning stiffness and fatigue are often first symptoms. Pain and swelling are variable. Wrists, MCP, PIP, and MTP joints are usually affected first. Anxiety is at a high level. Joints are tender and grip strength slightly less than normal. Skin temperature over joints may be normal or warm. Fluid may be detectable in MCP joints, PIP joints, or knees. Hips are rarely involved now. Venous pattern may be prominent on skin over joints.	ESR/CRP usually a function of the severity, but rarely highly abnormal. RF helpful if positive. Platelet count, WBC count, eosinophils may be increased. Radiographs are normal. Fever, occasionally.	In synovium, new capillaries begin to form near mononuclear cells; tissue is edematous and cells are scattered without a pattern. Synovial lining two to four cell layers deep. Electron micrographs could show antigen-presenting cells in contact with lymphocytes near capillaries. Macrophages begin to proliferate.	Antigen presented by class II MHC-bearing cells to CD4 + cells that have migrated to joints. Adhesion molecules in tall endothelium stop and fix rolling lymphocytes. Polymorphonuclear leukocytes begin to accumulate within increased amounts of synovial fluid produced by transudation from capillaries with added protein and hyaluronan from synovial cells. In response to angiogenic factors such as FGF, new capillaries sprout from existing ones.	Too early for a definite diagnosis. Nonsteroidal anti-inflammatory drugs or, in selected cases, salicylates. Education about self-management. Physical therapy to keep muscle tone and full range of motion. Instruction in joint protection. *Tests:* CBC RF Anti-nuclear antibody ESR and/or CRP DRB1 sequence at third hypervariable region, if available, in a research setting Arthrocentesis if fluid is palpable
2	*Approximately 6 weeks to 6 months*	Nodules rarely are present. Although the symptoms may wax and wane, the overall course is one of continued joint swelling, morning stiffness, pain on motion, and fatigue. New joints, knees, and elbows especially may become symptomatic. Nodules may appear in active, aggressive disease with positive RF. Definite diagnosis possible at this time.	70% will have positive test for rheumatoid factor by 3 months. ESR/CRP elevated. WBC and platelets increased. Radiographs may show early juxta-articular demineralization. Arthrocentesis will give additional useful information about the level of inflammation in the joint.	Synovial lining cells proliferate. Lymphocytes accumulate in foci around proliferating capillaries. Plasma cells appear. Monocytes/macrophages begin to phagocytose debris. At insertion of synovium into subchondral bone, proliferating synovium begins to invade bone and to encroach on peripheral surface of cartilage. Synovial effusions are often large, and contain from 5,000 to 100,000 WBC/mm³.	Lymphokines from activated CD4 + cells and cytokines from macrophages generate synovial cell proliferation and activation. B cells are activated and begin synthesis of RF. Synovium may have 20 to 100 times the weight and volume of normal synovium. Early chondrocyte activation results in protease release and local degradation of proteoglycans. TNF-α is the driving cytokine for IL-1β production.	*Crucial Stage of Therapy* With a definite diagnosis made, a carefully designed, aggressive therapeutic regimen is indicated to halt the progressive synovial inflammation. Nonsteroidal drugs or salicylates should be continued at maximal dose. In selected patients, prednisone, 5 mg/day, may be added. Hydroxychloroquine or—in particularly aggressive disease—methotrexate is appropriate. Appropriate exercise and protocols for joint protection, and continued education about the disease are important.

Table continued on following page

935

Table 56-1. RHEUMATOID ARTHRITIS: STAGING AND THERAPY *Continued*

Response of patients at this stage of disease is crucial if joint destruction is to be avoided. Although the process has a different rate of progression in each patient, the pathologic process in the synovium is well on its way to becoming cyclic and self-sustaining. Using the best predictors possible, the physician must weigh the possible side effects of medications against the risk of cartilage and bone loss. A complete remission is not a realistic goal, but a significant decrease in joint swelling, tenderness, and pain are appropriate objectives. Hydroxychloroquine or methotrexate can be given a full 2-month trial. Many would advocate their combination. If the therapy is not efficacious, it is appropriate to try additional second line drugs or, alternatively, to enlist the patient to join in a trial of biologic agents.

Stage of Disease	Time After Onset of Synovitis	Clinical Characteristics	Laboratory Findings	Pathologic Process	Biopathology	Management
3	*6 to 9 months to 2 years*	If the synovitis has not subsided in response to therapy by this time, it has undergone substantial polarization and proliferation. Although it would be early for deformity to develop, loss of range of motion from soft tissue contracture is common, especially in knees and elbows. Muscle mass is diminished from disuse from pain. Functional tests reveal loss of dexterity and an increased time to accomplish simple tasks. Particular joints may cause special problems (e.g., loss of shoulder abduction or extension, very tender MTP joint). As a function of the degree of inflammation, generalized weakness and debilitation can be prominent. Extra-articular disease such as vasculitis, Sjögren's syndrome, or Felty's syndrome may develop. Special problems such as cervical spine subluxation, fractures, flexion contractures, dysfunctional grasp, and severe pain from foot and ankle involvement may dominate the clinical picture.	Lab tests are more often needed to monitor therapy rather than to assess the disease process. Tests to monitor the activity of RA should be those found empirically that vary with clinical symptoms. RF is not likely to be an indicated test. Routine hemoglobins are needed to assess possible GI blood loss from nonsteroidal drugs.	The polarized synovitis has achieved a mass sufficient to invade subchondral bone, the periphery of cartilage, and the surface. Loss of proteoglycans from cartilage leaves the tissue susceptible to damage from weight bearing.	The proliferating synovial cells release stromelysin, gelatinase, and collagenase in large quantities, particularly at the cartilage/pannus junction. IgG deposits with antigen and complement components in the superficial layers of cartilage may serve as chemoattractants for this polarized, invasive pannus. Natural inhibitors in synovial fluid (e.g., $\alpha_2 M_1$) may be saturated, and TIMP levels may be inadequate to retard joint destruction. Depending on the degree to which the process expands beyond joints, lymphocytic infiltration may be found in the spleen (Felty's syndrome) or salivary and lacrimal glands (Sjögren's syndrome). IgG complexes in small arterioles can generate a vasculitis and be symptomatic in nerves, heart, lung, or GI tract.	When the disease has progressed this far, it is apparent that response to even aggressive therapy has been minimally effective. Before joint deformity develops, it is appropriate to use joint injections with a glucocorticoid such as triamcinolone hexacetonide. Gold or penicillamine should have been tried, and continued if efficacious. Methotrexate, and combinations of methotrexate with other drugs, should be used. *These patients are candidates for trials of biologic agents.* Orthopedic consultation should be retained earlier rather than later to prevent, as much as possible, loss of function.

4   *2 years to >25 years with active disease*

These patients have developed deformity and have substantial loss of function. It is likely that side effects of medications have limited options for therapy or have produced anemia, kidney disease, leukopenia, or other problems. Risk for fracture and tendon rupture is high.

Complications of therapy often dominate any panels of abnormal laboratory tests. Radiographs show loss of cartilage, subluxed joints, erosions of bone, fractures, and osteopenia. Tolerance to therapy is known, and there are few surprises in laboratory tests. Anemia, hypoalbuminemia, hyperglobulinemia, or hypocemia can be caused by the disease itself. Proteinuria and bone marrow aplasias may reflex toxicity of therapy.

The changes here are extensions of stage 3. As all cartilage is lost from a particular joint, the synovitis may become less proliferative and luxuriant, and synovial effusions decrease. Granulomas invade bone that has become osteopenic. Fibrosis often increases over cellularity in the synovium. Tendon rupture may occur. Changes of osteoarthritis increase as the cellular synovitis diminishes.

The findings are an extension of those in stage 3. The downstream effects of TNF-α dominate, producing cachexia as well as helping to accelerate destruction of cartilage, ligaments, and bone. "Reparative" cytokines (e.g., TGF-β) have only a mild effect.

Specific medications for arthritis should not be used unless a particular one is demonstrated to be effective; this is not likely considering that the disease has progressed so far. New compounds should be used with caution. Major emphasis should be on functional restoration through careful arthroplasty, osteotomy, tendon repairs, etc.

---

*Response of patients at this stage of disease is crucial if joint destruction is to be avoided. Although the process has a different rate of progression in each patient, the pathologic process in the synovium is well on its way to becoming cyclic and self-sustaining. Using the best predictors possible, the physician must weigh the possible side effects of medications against the risk of cartilage and bone loss. A complete remission is not a realistic goal, but a significant decrease in joint swelling, tenderness, and pain are appropriate objectives. Many would advocate their combination. If the therapy is not efficacious, it is appropriate to try additional cytotoxic drugs or, alternatively, The hydroxychloroquine or methotrexate can be given a full 2-month trial. Many would advocate their combination. If the therapy is not efficacious, it is appropriate to try additional cytotoxic drugs or, alternatively, to enlist the patient to join in a trial of biologic agents.

Abbreviations: MCP, metacarpophalangeal; PIP, proximal interphalangeal; MTP, metatarsophalangeal; ESR, erythrocyte sedimentation rate; CRP, C-reactive protein; RF, rheumatoid factor; MHC, major histocompatibility complex; FGF, fibroblast growth factor; CBC, complete blood count; WBC, white blood cells; RBC, red blood cells; TNF, tumor necrosis factor; RA, rheumatoid arthritis; GI, gastrointestinal; TIMP, tissue inhibitor of metalloproteinase; TGF, transforming growth factor.

"vacation" from home or the workplace was a tonic of encouragement for patients. It also was an ideal time for physicians to reassess drug therapy regimens and check laboratory values to assay for disease activity and for early toxicity of medications.

These hospitalizations were often prolonged and, of course, very expensive, and data appear to indicate that short-term benefit could accrue from hospital stays as short as 2 weeks.[17] Despite this and other evidence[18] that inpatient therapy of rheumatoid arthritis can be cost-effective, insurance companies and managed care health plans currently deny coverage for many if not most admissions for rest and therapy of rheumatoid patients unless there is a concurrent co-morbid acute process. Rest and exercise are modalities of therapy that must be managed and directed outside the hospital.

Rest

Determining the proper amount of rest for a rheumatoid patient is a substantial challenge. Patients enter the disease process with different baselines of activity. Some are vigorous athletes or manual laborers. Others have had a lifestyle that never involves running or perspiring. An additional variable is individual sensitivity to pain; some patients are made almost catatonic by their disease, whereas others either do not sense or ignore the pain of inflammatory synovitis, resulting in destruction of joints with few expressed symptoms. The challenge is to down-regulate the activity of the athletes and vigorous workers and to up-regulate the activity of the slothful patients. Lack of mobility can generate loss of self-confidence, and this can spiral down into a pseudo-catatonic depression for the hurting patient with polyarticular synovitis.

Exercise for the Patient with Inflammatory Synovitis

Long before the diagnosis is definitive for a patient with polyarthritis, much can be accomplished toward instructing him or her about exercise. For assessing the needs of patients by non-rheumatologists, it has been shown that the standardized HAQ results correlate significantly with formal tests of muscle function.[19] Compliance is likely, however, only if the exercise produces minimal discomfort during the exercise and virtually none following it; indeed, pain control is the primary consideration in any rehabilitative program.[20] For this reason, variable-resistance isotonic exercise is rarely appropriate for a patient with acutely inflamed joints. Isometric exercise has been shown to cause the least joint inflammation, increase in intra-articular pressure, and periarticular bone destruction.[21] The technique does produce an increase in blood pressure and demand on cardiac output,

so it must be used with caution in patients with cardiovascular disease.

For the patient with acutely and severely inflamed joints, either at the onset or during the course of rheumatoid arthritis, actual splinting to produce immobilization with twice-daily full and slow passive range of motion to prevent soft tissue contracture may be all that is tolerated. The more typical patient with moderate synovitis requires a prescribed isometric program for the involved joints, progressing to well-supervised variable-resistance programs when the synovitis subsides.[22, 23]

Fortunate is the patient who has no foot, ankle, or knee involvement early in the disease process; this individual can engage in active walking that maintains general muscle tone and emotional well-being.

Instruction in the Manner of Performing the Activities of Daily Living

The early phases of synovitis are important for defining for the patient how to use joints so as not to contribute to subsequent joint destruction. The basic principle underlying instruction in activities of daily living (ADL) supervised by occupational therapists should be to avoid, as much as possible, application of excessive force across both weight-bearing and non–weight-bearing joints. The concept is simple in the weight-bearing joints: avoid jarring impact (e.g., running on hard surfaces) or forceful and repetitive quadriceps contracture during weight bearing (e.g., mountain climbing, heavy lifting, or skiing moguls). For the non–weight-bearing joints the key is to avoid powerful muscle contractions. For example, since it requires more force to grasp a small handle than a larger one, pots, pans, and utensils with larger-circumference handles are better for the patient with active synovitis, and it is better to lift with two hands rather than one. Another basic guideline is to avoid, as much as possible, repetitive motion that accentuates the force of gravity normally working on joints. Principles of rehabilitation are discussed in detail in Chapter 103.

Temperature Modalities

The rationale for using heat or cold is simple: to relieve pain.[20] There are many ways to apply heat, including hot soaks, warm towels, heating pads, and more expensive methods such as diathermy or ultrasound. The latter techniques, aside from being more expensive, may do more harm than good.[24]

Debate centers on the use of heat therapy, prompted by evidence that collagen type II, the major structural protein of articular cartilage, is degraded significantly more rapidly by synovial collagenase at 37 to 39°C than at 33 to 36°C, the measured temperature of noninflamed joints.[25] Hot paraffin coating has been found to increase skin surface temperature by 8 to 9°C and the temperature within the underlying joint by 3 to 5°C.[26] The one study attempting to evaluate the progression of erosions in 16 patients, each with one hand heated by an electric mitten and the contralateral hand left at room temperature, showed no difference in hand radiographs after the study;[27] thus, based on the current state of knowledge, there is no confirmed contraindication to the use of daily or twice-daily heat therapy on rheumatoid joints.

Diet

Few modalities of treatment for rheumatoid arthritis involve more different options than food. The lists of "arthritis diets" and "arthritis cookbooks" are staggeringly long, and have been for many years. Are there any data supporting the claim that diet can beneficially affect rheumatoid arthritis?

The most obvious and most important dietary factor is the quantity of food eaten and the weight of the patient eating it. Obesity is very harmful for arthritis in weight-bearing joints. Added weight magnifies the degradative potential of weight bearing in patients with active synovitis.

There is a scientific rationale for eliminating precursors of arachidonic acid from the diet: prostaglandins and leukotrienes are proinflammatory. Eicosapentaenoic acid and docosahexaenoic acid supplements[28] in the diet exert measurable suppression of several inflammatory mediators produced by rheumatoid patients.[29] Improvement with these supplements has been demonstrated in several trials. Dietary manipulation, however, is difficult to comply with. Except for those who easily accept vegetarian regimens and fish oil supplements, a balanced diet, daily multivitamin supplements, and achievement of ideal weight constitute a good approach for all patients.

NONSTEROIDAL ANTI-INFLAMMATORY DRUGS

An estimated 30,000,000 people worldwide take nonsteroidal anti-inflammatory drugs (NSAIDs).[30] These certainly are among the most frequently prescribed medicines in the United States. If, as calculated in one study, 100 million prescriptions are written each year[31] and the average 30-day supply costs $50, the total price tag for these drugs is between $3 and $4 billion per year. (See Chapter 45.)

An NSAID ought to be a staple of therapy at the first visit of the patient with arthritis, even before a diagnosis is possible. Prescribing an NSAID for the first time should be a teaching exercise for the physician, and an opportunity for the patient to learn some basic concepts about what joint inflammation is and how the NSAID may work to alleviate it. Equally important, however, is an honest accounting of the possible side effects.

At a minimum, the patient should be warned about

gastrointestinal (GI) distress, interaction with antihypertensive medications and other cardiac drugs, and central nervous system (CNS) changes (e.g., depression, disorientation, headaches) and should be encouraged to contact the physician or nurse when an abnormal sensation of any kind appears that did not predate initiation of the NSAID. In selected patients who very much need NSAIDs but who are at risk for peptic ulceration, misoprostol (100-200 μg/day) may help reduce the incidence of serious GI complications.[118]

The details of therapy with aspirin and other NSAIDs are found in Chapter 45.

THE ROLE OF GLUCOCORTICOIDS

The following indications apply for glucocorticoid therapy (almost always using prednisone) in rheumatoid arthritis:

- *Vasculitis*, presenting as skin ulcers, mononeuritis multiplex, rapidly progressive pulmonary interstitial fibrosis, coronary arteritis, or severe systemic toxicity with fever and intense pain. Doses used (prednisone equivalents) are in the range of 40 to 120 mg daily; the initial dose used should be whatever is needed to suppress the process.
- As a *bridge therapy* when NSAID therapy is insufficient to control the process, and second-line drugs have not yet had an effect (Fig. 56–2). Doses used should be less than 7.0 mg given each day in the morning.
- To blunt the manifestations of *drug toxicity*, such as skin rash in D-penicillamine therapy.

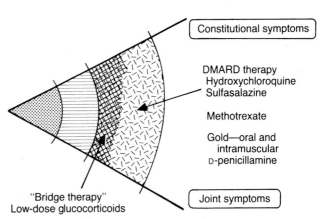

Figure 56–2. Phases I and II of therapy. "Bridge therapy" of glucocorticoids may not be necessary if the decision to initiate therapy with second-line drugs is made relatively early so their effect begins before a phase of intolerable pain or functional impairment. As shown in the figure by the *shaded* area within disease-modifying antirheumatic drug (DMARD) therapy, glucocorticoid bridge therapy may have to be continued longer in patients with more constitutional symptoms than in those primarily with joint symptoms. More and more, methotrexate is being used as a second-line drug; in some instances, it may be justified to use it before, or instead of, gold and/or D-penicillamine.

- As short courses in doses greater than 60 mg/day for *severe flares of arthritis* or systemic complications.
- As *intra-articular injections* using a long-acting compound such as triamcinolone hexacetonide. This is particularly useful when a few joints are involved in a flare of disease.

More than any drug used for arthritis, glucocorticoids are a two-edged sword. The immediate effect of their use is gratifying, and yet the long-term toxicity can be very discouraging. For these reasons it is not surprising that health care analysts have found great variation among rheumatologists in the usage patterns of these drugs in rheumatoid arthritis.[32]

Any glucocorticoid dose that provides symptomatic relief of active rheumatoid synovitis within 24 to 36 hours will, within a month, be associated with chronic and deleterious toxicity. In contrast, there rarely is immediate change in rheumatoid arthritis after the institution of 5.0 mg prednisone given each day, but this dose is sufficient to produce some additive suppressive effects on both inflammation and synovial proliferation after many weeks. This was demonstrated in a 24-week double-blind controlled study of 5 mg of prednisone given daily to patients already taking NSAIDs but not second-line drugs.[33]

If patients on second-line therapy, NSAIDs, and a good physical and occupational therapy regime have a sudden and aggressive flare of synovitis, it is better to give a short intravenous "mini-pulse" of methylprednisolone rather than increase the daily dose over weeks or months. A randomized double-blind study of 36 patients with flared synovitis showed that 100 mg of methylprednisolone daily for 3 days was as efficacious as the "conventional" 1000 mg daily for 3 days in producing a prompt and sustained benefit.[34]

It is an unproven hypothesis that glucocorticoid pulsing can augment the efficacy or decrease the toxicity of gold salt or D-penicillamine therapy.[35]

The use of glucocorticoids for intrasynovial therapy and long-term therapy are detailed in Chapter 50.

Prednisone and Fractures in Rheumatoid Arthritis

There is no doubt that factors other than prednisone use in rheumatoid patients put them at risk for fracture.[36, 37] These include:

- Postmenopausal state
- Previous diagnosis of osteoporosis
- Disability
- Age
- Lack of physical activity
- Female sex
- Family history of osteoporosis
- Disease duration
- Impaired grip strength
- Low body mass
- Fair complexion
- Cigarette smoking

Nevertheless, glucocorticoids do produce osteopenia in rheumatoid patients, damaging trabecular bone more than cortical bone.

What are the options for preserving bone in patients being treated with glucocorticoids? In the postmenopausal woman, *estrogens* should be used whenever possible. When estrogen is inappropriate, the antiresorptive *bisphosphonates* can produce modest increases in bone mass; although these effects level off after a few years, bisphosphonates are appropriate adjuncts in patients in whom the risk and danger of developing more osteopenia is high. Intermittent etidronate therapy given for 6 months to postmenopausal women receiving prednisone for temporal arteritis has been shown to prevent vertebral bone loss.[38] Aledronate, a bisphosphonate, recently approved by the U.S. Food and Drug Administration (FDA) to use in osteoporosis, can be given continuously at a dose of 10 mg/day. In a study of 103 patients starting long-term glucocorticoid therapy, it was found that the use of *calcitriol* (1,25-dihydroxycalciferol), 0.6 µg/day, and *calcium*, 1000 mg/day, with or without calcitonin, 400 I.U./day, was more effective in preventing bone loss from the lumbar spine than calcium alone.[39]

Complications from administering *sodium fluoride* for the treatment or prevention of osteoporosis have been frequent and sometimes serious, including gastric bleeding and microfractures. However, with the use of slow-release preparations, new fractures were inhibited over a 2.5-year period, the mean spinal bone mass increased without loss of cortical bone, and there were no significant side effects.[40]

Although co-administration of *human growth hormone* prevents the protein catabolic effects of prednisone,[41] it is not cost-effective or practical to use in the great majority of rheumatoid patients.

An alternative to prednisone in treatment of rheumatoid arthritis may be *deflazacort*, an oxazoline derivative of prednisone that causes less suppression of intestinal absorption of calcium than does prednisone and induces less hypercalciuria.[42]

SECOND-LINE TREATMENT OF RHEUMATOID ARTHRITIS

The drugs used when it has become apparent that a rheumatoid patient's arthritis has become established and is not responding adequately to NSAIDs or low-dose glucocorticoids are most fairly named "second-line drugs."

Perhaps the greatest differences among the second-line drugs are the patterns of toxicity. In a study of 2479 patients from five centers in the ARAMIS system, the toxicity profile for each was different:[43]

- Oral gold (auranofin) produced substantial lower GI toxicity (i.e., 399 diarrhea "events"/1000 patient-years).
- Methotrexate generated hepatotoxicity and mucosal

ulcers but had the lowest discontinuation rate in the first 6 months.

- D-penicillamine altered taste.
- Skin rash was seen more frequently with gold and D-penicillamine.

Hydroxychloroquine

Hydroxychloroquine is an antimalarial drug that has been used for decades in rheumatoid arthritis. However, studies linking an irreversible retinopathy with chloroquine therapy precipitated a distinct decline in the use of these drugs for rheumatoid arthritis.[44] The use of dosage schedules not exceeding 400 mg of hydroxychloroquine each day and the fact that less than 20 cases of true retinopathy leading to visual loss have been reported[45] have reassured clinicians that hydroxychloroquine is safer than most other drugs and, in a subset of patients, efficacious. In most double-blind controlled studies, antimalarials have clinical efficacy equal to that of gold salts or D-penicillamine.[46]

Meta-analysis of 66 short-term trials of second-line drugs showed that intramuscular gold was the most toxic and antimalarials and methotrexate the least toxic.[47] The relative benignity of hydroxychloroquine was confirmed in an analysis of a large cohort of patients over a long period.[48]

Skin rash and stomach pain have been the most bothersome side effects. The dropout rate for antimalarials in these studies averages less than 8 percent,[47] or about twice that for placebo therapy.

The ocular toxicities of concern are a "bull's-eye" retinal pigmentation around the macula and pigmentary stippling of the macula as the drug is deposited; the appearance of these is an indication to stop the drug. Although the risk of maculopathy is low, patients with a visual field loss or decreased visual acuity should not be started on antimalarial drugs. An ophthalmologic examination every 6 months after the drug is started is a reasonable course[49] for all patients taking antimalarials.

Sulfasalazine

Several studies have suggested that sulfasalazine has the ability to slow progression of erosive disease, even chronically active and destructive disease.[50, 51] In one study 80 patients with the diagnosis of rheumatoid arthritis for less than a year were randomized to placebo (plus NSAIDs and low-dose glucocorticoids) or sulfasalazine (500 mg increasing to 2000 mg, when tolerated, in 4 weeks).[52] The sulfasalazine-treated group improved modestly more than the control group, and seronegative rheumatoid arthritis patients improved more than seropositive patients. There were fewer erosive changes in the sulfasalazine-treated group, but not significantly so.

One intriguing study that measured gastrointestinal (GI) blood loss and examined gastroduodenal endoscopic biopsies suggested that sulfasalazine reduces the intestinal inflammation and blood loss induced by NSAIDs, whereas gold, D-penicillamine, and hydroxychloroquine do not.[53] This offers a rationale for the use of sulfasalazine relatively early in rheumatoid arthritis in conjunction with baseline NSAIDs.

If the annoying nausea and vomiting generated by sulfasalazine could be prevented or minimized by different preparations for oral administration, the demonstrated efficacy of the drug could be exploited effectively, and it could be used early in the disease course.

Gold Salts

In the early 1960s, drug therapy for rheumatoid arthritis was limited to salicylates, phenylbutazone, hydroxychloroquine, and gold salts. The last appeared to be the most potent, and a study of gold salt therapy carried out by the Empire Rheumatism Council[54] supported use of injectable gold salts as an effective therapy in rheumatoid arthritis. This double-blind study was one of the first well-controlled trials in rheumatology. A growing cadre of rheumatologists in Europe, Great Britain, and the United States began using aurothiomalate or aurothioglucose with enthusiasm. Although the use of gold salts required patients to come to the physicians' offices or clinics once a week for checks of blood and urine and for the weekly injection, this system was remarkably well tolerated by both patients and the health insurance companies.

The bothersome need for injections stimulated development of an oral preparation of gold, and auranofin—the first drug developed specifically for use in rheumatoid arthritis—was introduced in the mid-1980s.[55] Although auranofin is associated with significantly less of the serious toxicity of injectable preparations, it also has less efficacy. In a meta-analysis including 66 clinical trials and 117 treatment groups,[47] in each outcome auranofin tended to have less efficacy than methotrexate, injectable gold, D-penicillamine, or sulfasalazine.

The side effects of injectable gold salts and of auranofin are very different. Whereas the injectable preparations often cause the more serious problems of thrombocytopenia and proteinuria, a reversible but annoying syndrome of loose stools related to a mild enterocolitis is common with auranofin. Indeed, although the toxicity index for auranofin was quite high in one large study,[48] the poor showing was almost entirely due to high incidences of relatively minor symptoms (e.g., diarrhea, nausea, and skin rash).

Despite the serious but uncommon toxicities of parenteral gold, in a study in Finland of 573 patients with rheumatoid arthritis treated first during the period of 1961 to 1966 gold therapy did not appear to be associated with premature death in these patients. To the contrary, long-term gold therapy was associated with improved survival.[56] The details of use of both injectable and oral gold preparations are presented in Chapter 48.

Does Gold Therapy Really Help?

The difficulty of evaluating therapy in a chronic disease such as rheumatoid arthritis was highlighted by a prospective observational study of patients over a 5-year period under the care of community rheumatologists in the San Francisco Bay area.[57] A total of 822 patients with rheumatoid arthritis entered the study. Outcomes were compared between those receiving gold therapy for no less than 2 years and patients who did not receive parenteral gold at any time during the 5 years of study. At the end of the study, 574 patients were still participating, and there were no differences at enrollment between those who remained and those who dropped out.

The data showed that functional disability as assessed by the HAQ and the number of painful joints in the 574 patients was, on average, unchanged over 5 years and was unaffected by use of gold therapy. Although the average duration of disease exceeded 10 years, there were no differences in the function score and report of painful joints in those patients whose disease duration was less than 2 years, whether or not gold therapy was given.

These data are different from those of other studies in two important respects: gold was not efficacious, and there was no deterioration of function in any group of patients. In contrast, most studies demonstrate a relentless deterioration of patients with rheumatoid arthritis over time. The data in this study attest more to the effective treatment or relatively benign course of disease in *all* patients in this group than to the failure of gold therapy.[58]

Guidelines for Usage

The following specific points about the use of gold salts are useful for any physician considering use of these drugs:

- In patients with early but active synovitis who are intolerant to methotrexate (with or without concomitant hydroxychloroquine therapy) or in whom methotrexate is contraindicated because of liver disease or alcoholism, parenteral gold is the best choice for a second-line drug.
- "Bridge" therapy with prednisone (<7 mg/day) during the weeks to months required for gold to have demonstrable efficacy is appropriate.
- Gold can be used in patients with neutropenia from Felty's syndrome or eosinophilia associated with active disease.
- Because pre-existing proteinuria or dermatitis can mimic side effects of gold therapy, they are relative contraindications to initiation of gold therapy.
- If improvement achieved with a 6-month course of

weekly injections of 50 mg is not maintained by monthly injections, re-establishment of benefit may be achieved by returning to weekly therapy.[59]
- Four times as many patients (20 percent) withdraw because of intolerance from intramuscular gold than from oral gold.
- A "nitritoid" reaction (weakness, dizziness, nausea, sweating, and facial flushing) is not uncommon with gold thiomalate but is rare with gold thioglucose.
- Although most patients who develop the nephrotic syndrome on parenteral gold recover completely, auranofin is a better choice for patients with proteinuria or chronic renal failure.
- HLA-DR3 is found in 85 percent of patients who develop thrombocytopenia on intramuscular gold, whereas it is found in only 30 percent of the general population.[60] HLA-DR3 may be associated with a better response to gold therapy.[61]
- Consistent monitoring of white blood count, peripheral blood smear, and urinalysis during gold therapy does not prevent toxicity but allows early detection, enabling a better outcome.
- Rare but disturbing side effects of gold therapy include a pulmonary hypersensitivity presenting as acute respiratory distress, enterocolitis (particularly in older women), and neurologic complications resembling encephalopathy, Guillain-Barré syndrome, or cranial nerve palsies.[62]

D-Penicillamine

The niche for D-penicillamine in the treatment of rheumatoid arthritis is in patients who have failed hydroxycholoroquine and methotrexate, or gold salts, or a combination of these, and in whom disease is still active. In patients with active vasculitis involving skin or internal organs, it often is used as primary therapy. The same applies to rheumatoid patients with manifestations that are fibrotic in nature (e.g., pulmonary interstitial fibrosis or soft tissue contractures); the rationale for this use is that D-penicillamine inhibits collagen cross-links and could slow collagen deposition in fibrotic processes.[63, 64]

There are many similarities between D-penicillamine and gold salts in terms of response patterns and toxicity. D-penicillamine must be taken each day for 2 to 4 months before a beneficial response is obtained. The recommended dose is 750 to 1000 mg/day, but development of toxicity can often be prevented if therapy is started with only 125 mg/day and gradually increased to 750 to 1000 mg/day over a period of 6 to 8 weeks.

Meta-analysis showed that in a composite-treatment-effect analysis D-penicillamine is as effective as intramuscular gold, methotrexate, and sulfasalazine; slightly more efficacious than hydroxychloroquine; and significantly more effective than oral gold.[47] Progression of joint space narrowing or bone erosions is not retarded,[65] but this could be related to the fact that once synovitis has been active for 2 years or more, irreversible changes are set in motion that inexorably destroy connective tissue. In patients who respond clinically, acute-phase reactants decrease and hemoglobin increases, implying a definite suppression of disease activity.[66]

The toxicity of D-penicillamine is at once disturbing and fascinating. Certain side effects are similar to those with gold therapy:

- Urticarial, macular, or papular eruptions are the most common causes of skin toxicity.
- Excretion of 0.5 g/day of protein in the urine occurs in approximately 9 percent of patients,[67] and uncommonly the nephrotic syndrome develops. Previous proteinuria during gold therapy and the presence of HLA-B8 increase the risk of this complication;[67] a membranous glomerulonephritis is usually present and generally resolves after cessation of the drug.
- Thrombocytopenia and neutropenia can occur at any time, perhaps due to a suppressive effect on stem cell maturation. Neutropenia is the most common fatal complication of D-penicillamine therapy.[68]

The other class of side effects includes unusual ones that probably are related to the reactive thiol group in D-penicillamine. One, a taste disturbance characterized by a metallic flavor and diminished ability to taste food, is related to chelation of zinc within enzymes essential for taste perception. Others, fortunately rare, are autoimmune in their presentation and often serious:

- *Myasthenia gravis*, which may take over a year to resolve
- *Dermatomyositis/polymyositis*, which usually resolves rapidly after cessation of the drug
- *Systemic lupus erythematosus* (SLE), in a form resembling that occurring secondary to procainamide more than the idiopathic form, although glomerulonephritis or neurologic involvement occasionally is seen
- *Pemphigus*, a complication associated with significant mortality secondary to infection of exposed dermis and to fluid and electrolyte disturbances; serious cases may require plasmapheresis and systemic glucocorticoid therapy

Methotrexate

The use of oral methotrexate in a low dose, once weekly, has become the mainstay of therapy for advancing and sustained rheumatoid arthritis for which a second-line drug is indicated. There are a number of reasons for this ascendancy:

- The drug is inexpensive, and monitoring for routine toxicity is less expensive than for gold, D-penicillamine, or the other cytotoxic drugs.
- Compared with other drugs, patients are more likely to be taking methotrexate 2 to 5 years after it is first given.

- Methotrexate is believed less likely to be a cause of malignancy than any of the other cytotoxic drugs (e.g., cytoxan or azathioprine).
- Methotrexate acts relatively quickly after initiation, often within several weeks.
- Concerns about toxicity of methotrexate have lessened over the years, not increased.
- Most important, methotrexate appears to have genuine efficacy.

Physicians first used the folic acid antagonist aminopterin for treatment of rheumatoid arthritis after observing amelioration of joint symptoms when the drug was used for severe psoriasis. The more stable and better-tolerated N-10-methylaminopterin, or methotrexate, gradually was introduced in low-dose treatment regimens for rheumatoid arthritis. Four randomized, short-term, placebo-controlled studies confirmed the efficacy of methotrexate.[69–72] The U.S. Food and Drug Administration approved methotrexate for the treatment of rheumatoid arthritis in 1988.

Meta-analysis of these four trials showed the following:[73]

- Joint pain and swelling improved 25 percent.
- Morning stiffness improved 46 percent.
- The erythrocyte sedimentation rate fell by 15 percent.

Studies involving longer use also showed improvement and a satisfactory tolerance of the drug by most patients over more than four years:

1. Willkens and Watson studied 67 patients for up to 10 years.[74] Although 16 patients did not respond to therapy, 49 had demonstrable benefit.

2. In a prospective study designed to study the effects of methotrexate on liver function and histology,[75] clinical improvement was noted in the joint count, morning stiffness, grip strength, and walking time. Improvement was also reflected in assessments of both physicians and patients that began within a month after beginning therapy and were sustained over more than 2 years. In an extension of the study,[76] after a mean of 53 months of therapy, 25 of 29 patients remained in the study, the overall efficacy was good, and side effects were minimal.

3. In an open study Weinblatt studied 26 patients,[77, 78] first evaluated at 36 weeks. The oral dose was no more than 15 mg/week. Patients were withdrawn from the study for the following reasons: 1 died after open-heart surgery; 8 failed to, or did not want to, adhere to protocol; and 1 had no efficacy from methotrexate.

As in other studies, the maximal effect was noted after 6 months. Sixty percent had improvement in joint counts. Of 14 patients taking prednisone at baseline, reduction from 7.1 mg/day to 2.9 mg/day was accomplished. Radiographic analyses showed worsening in 6, no change in 3, and an improvement in erosion size but continued loss of joint space in 5. Sixty-two percent had adverse side effects, but toxicity was not the reason for withdrawal from the study for any patient. An increase in the size of rheumatoid nodules was seen in 3 patients. Liver biopsies of 17 patients at 24 months showed no evidence of fibrosis or cirrhosis.

After 45 months of therapy in this same cohort (16 remained in the study), sustained improvement continued[79] after a mean cumulative dose of 2.1 g. One patient biopsied had mild fibrosis in the liver.

4. Results in community practices with methotrexate are not quite as optimistic as those from university clinics but are still encouraging considering that the same assiduous attention to patients is more difficult in practice than in the university. In a life-table analysis of 587 patients in eight rheumatologic practices in Australia, 75 percent of patients assessed 70 months from commencement of therapy were still taking methotrexate.[80]

5. In a meta-analysis of 558 patients in 11 studies involving quantitation of bone erosions at joint margins, methotrexate-treated patients had slower rates of disease progression than those treated with azathioprine, but not those treated with gold salts.[81] The problem in this analysis, consistent with the hypothesis that early treatment is the key to cartilage protection, is that some methotrexate and gold-treated patients had been ill at baseline for less than 2 years, whereas no azathioprine-treated patient had had rheumatoid arthritis for less than 8.7 years at the start of therapy. The challenge is to have a cohort of methotrexate-treated and "other" patients enrolled in a radiographic progression study after less than a year of active disease.

The side effects and toxicity of methotrexate are outlined in Chapter 49. One additional caveat about therapy should be noted. Many rheumatologists are advocating the use of pentamidine prophylaxis against *Pneumocystis carinii* in rheumatoid patients who are given even the smaller doses of methotrexate on a weekly basis.

CYTOTOXIC AND IMMUNOSUPPRESSIVE THERAPY FOR RHEUMATOID ARTHRITIS

Cytotoxic and immunosuppressive rheumatoid arthritis therapy represents the broad class of drugs and biologic compounds that are attracting the most interest by physicians, clinical investigators, and biotech/pharmaceutical corporations. The drugs initially used were cytotoxic, borrowed from medical oncology because they effectively destroyed many types of cells that were in a relatively rapid phase of division and multiplication. Among the cells killed were immunocytes. More recently the lymphocytes and their function have been targeted more specifically, both by drugs with more focused action and by monoclonal antibodies and products of recombinant DNA technology. In addition, the increased understanding of the pathogenic pathways involved in am-

plification of the immune and proliferative responses in rheumatoid arthritis have brought into play biologic substances that act to blunt effects of cytokines driving these pathways.

Azathioprine, Cyclophosphamide, and Chlorambucil

Although azathioprine and cyclophosphamide have traditionally been used much more than chlorambucil, with the advent of increased and earlier use of methotrexate, the use of all three is declining. Specificity is lacking with these agents, and the short- and long-term toxicities are significant. Details of their pharmacology, toxicity, and general use in rheumatic diseases is presented in Chapter 51.

Azathioprine is a purine analog that interferes with the synthesis of adenosine and guanine in the construction of nucleic acids. Used in doses of 1.5 to 2.5 mg/kg per day, it has been used singly and in combination in rheumatoid arthritis. It has an established benefit of enabling glucocorticoid doses to be tapered in patients who are developing side effects of glucocorticoids.[82, 83] It is not effective in doses less than 1.0 mg/kg per day. Although it has no more early toxicity than gold or D-penicillamine, it is not measurably more efficacious than either of these. There are as yet no convincing data to implicate azathioprine given as treatment for rheumatoid arthritis in the pathogenesis of lymphoma.[84] Monitoring during therapy of the circulating white blood count is essential; marrow suppression with neutropenia is the most common complication.

Cyclophosphamide is an alkylating agent that cross-links DNA, affecting cells in all phases of their growth cycle. The usual dose is 2 mg/kg orally. Intravenous pulse therapy with doses of 750 to 1000 mg/m^2 are being used frequently in aggressive SLE, Wegener's granulomatosis, and systemic vasculitis. No benefit for severe synovitis in rheumatoid arthritis was found in one study.[85] In general, the toxicity of cyclophosphamide is greater than most patients with rheumatoid synovitis and their physicians are willing to accept. The major side effects are:[86]

- Marrow suppression—predominantly neutropenia
- Gonadal suppression—oligospermia, ovarian dysfunction
- Alopecia
- GI intolerance

A link between cyclophosphamide therapy of rheumatoid patients and subsequent development of malignancy is fairly strong, particularly for hematologic, skin, and bladder tumors.[87, 88] Bladder toxicity caused by acrolein, a metabolite of cyclophosphamide, is counteracted by mesna, a sulfhydryl-containing compound, but data are not available to indicate whether the protective effect applies to daily oral dosing as well as to intravenous administration.

Chlorambucil is a bifunctional alkylating agent, as

is cyclophosphamide. Except for a period of popularity in France in the 1960s,[89] it has been used infrequently in rheumatoid arthritis. The unavailability of intravenous preparation rules out the possibility of pulse therapy. Delay in onset of action was as long as 2 to 3 months in the French series.

In summary, although intravenous cyclophosphamide may be indicated in an aggressive case of rheumatoid vasculitis, and although azathioprine is appropriately used as a "steroid-sparing agent" in selected cases, the short-term toxicity as well as the possibility of a malignancy developing with use of these cytotoxic drugs with broad action makes them poor choices for rheumatoid arthritis.

Cyclosporine

Cyclosporine acts more specifically on the immune system than the other cytotoxic/immunosuppressive drugs just discussed. It is a fungal peptide and is used widely in organ transplantation to prevent graft rejection.

The use of cyclosporine for rheumatoid arthritis was popularized in Europe. In an early double-blind study[90] from Paris, the treatment with 5 mg/kg per day was considered "good or very good" by 14 of 26 treated patients compared with only 2 of 26 placebo-treated patients. In treated patients, five of seven clinical assessment criteria improved. A similar study from the National Institutes of Health and Georgetown University used daily doses of 10 mg/kg versus 1 mg/kg; after 6 months, 10 of 15 high-dose and 4 of 16 low-dose patients experienced improvement by subjective and objective criteria.[91] Although the numbers were small, anergic patients appeared to respond better than non-anergic patients to cyclosporine.

The major problem with cyclosporine is renal toxicity.[91] By aggressive lowering of the dose the loss of function can be kept to less than 20 precent elevation of serum creatinine. Glomerular filtration and renal plasma flow decrease concomitantly, probably driven by an increase in renal vascular resistance.[91–93] Loss of renal function was greater in patients given cyclosporine and NSAIDs.[94] In a trial of 6 months using 5 mg/kg/day there was an irreversible loss of about 15 percent of renal function;[95] results such as these led to trials using 2.5 mg/kg/day.[96]

By beginning therapy with this lower dose it has been possible to use the drug earlier in the disease, to compare cyclosporine against other second-line drugs, and to combine it with drugs that act at other sites. For example, a randomized, double-blind study compared cyclosporine (2.5 mg/kg initially, increased to a median dose of 3.6 mg/kg/day) against chloroquine (300 mg/day, decreasing to 100 mg/day) in 44 patients with a mean disease duration of 6 months.[97] Both drugs were efficacious, one no more than the other, and lowering the cyclosporine dose made the toxicity of the two similar. In a study of patients only partially responsive to either gold or methotrexate, cyclosporine was added at a dose of 2.5 mg/kg/day. All measures of efficacy showed statistically and clinically significant improvements; and after cyclosporine was tapered off at 6 months, all had clinical flares of arthritis and a return of rheumatoid nodules that had diminished or disappeared while on the combination therapy.[98]

The immunosuppressant FK 506 has a mode of action similar to that of cyclosporine. It may be as much as 100 times more potent than cyclosporine in selective inhibition of IL-2, IL-3, and IL-4 production. It has been very successful in liver transplantation.[99] The degrees of its renal toxicity and other side effects, in comparison with cyclosporine, have not yet been clarified in patients who are not recipients of organ transplants.

Targeted Immunotherapy: Possible Therapies for the Future

Objectives for targeted immunotherapeutic agents are to focus on immunologic events specific for rheumatoid arthritis while minimizing effects on unrelated immunologic activity preceding or following the use of these substances. Details of most available biologic modifiers are presented in Chapter 53.

None of the biologic modifiers evaluated in clinical trials have been able to down-regulate the rheumatoid processes sufficiently to produce remissions. The knowledge gained from them, however, has been invaluable in preparing both for development of modifiers for future use and for design of trials in years to come.

Some important inferences taken from these trials are summarized as follows:

1. Lymphocyte precursors in the marrow are easily damaged by antibodies against T cell surface glycoproteins. Therefore, repopulation of lymphocyte reservoirs may be slowed or even stopped, leading to the risk of opportunistic infections.

2. The most promising modifier studied in clinical trials has been anti–tumor necrosis factor-α (anti–TNF-α). Sustained clinical benefit, a decrease in acute-phase reactants, and minimal toxicity has been reported. These observations are consistent with the data implicating TNF-α as a crucial initiator of inflammatory and proliferative cascades in this disease.

3. Combinations of biologic modifiers aimed at different components of the pathogenic process may be synergistic in efficacy. Thus, there is increasing support for using a compound (e.g., soluble TNF-α receptors) aimed at the cytokine pathways and another directed against adhesion molecules that facilitate emigration of leukocytes from the circulation into the synovium.

4. In the spectrum of biologic modifiers developed to date, only substances used in attempt to "tolerize" patients are suitable for oral administration. Their use is based on the premise that down-regulating

a secondary, "bystander" immune response against endogenous proteins (e.g., collagen type II) may be sufficient to alleviate much of the inflammation.

5. Monoclonal antibodies used in therapy should be "humanized" chimeric proteins that produce minimal, if any, immunogenic stimulus of their own.

A major problem confronting rheumatologists involved in clinical trials of biologic agents will be finding a sufficient population of patients with early disease to produce well-controlled trials of the many promising biologic modifiers that will be coming out of development in laboratories. There is also the threat that decisions about which modifiers to be put into trials will be based on the financial resources of various corporations rather than on objective analyses of which agent, or combinations, would be most efficacious and least toxic.

Therapeutic Regulation of Autoimmunity by Intravenous Immunoglobulin

Intravenous (IV) immunoglobulin used for treatment of many different diseases, most of which have an apparent autoimmune component of pathogenesis. In addition to evidence that IgG down-regulates autoantibody production or binding to antigen, T cell–mediated disease has been alleviated as well; the number of exacerbations of multiple sclerosis was reported to decrease in patients given long-term infusions of IgG.[100] The same investigators published data showing that IV IgG inhibited the active induction of adjuvant arthritis.[100] It also was effective when given just at the onset of clinical disease. A diminished production of TNF-α by spleen cells from treated animals was noted.

In rheumatoid arthritis, placenta-eluted gamma globulins (PEGG) have been used for therapy based on the hypothesis that alloantibodies to class II HLA antigens in the PEGG would down-regulate disease,[101] and naturally occurring antibodies to inflammatory cytokines are found in normal individuals.

COMBINATION THERAPY

One rationale for combining drugs is based on the evidence that rheumatoid arthritis becomes destructive and entrenched more rapidly than previously appreciated. In an effort to reassess therapeutic approaches, the concept of "inverting the pyramid" by using more potent therapy early in the disease and combining more than one therapy in an effort to induce a long-lasting remission has been embraced by a number of investigators. Additional support for the idea is scientifically based: if two drugs target different arms of the inflammatory-immune response that is rheumatoid arthritis, is it not logical to try to cut off both arms at the same time?

After a 10-year observation period, McCarty and

Carrera reported in 1982 results of a personal series using cyclophosphamide, azathioprine, and hydroxychloroquine in combination.[102] Good results were blunted by the unacceptable toxicity of even the low dose used (30 mg/day) of cyclophosphamide, leading to substitution of methotrexate for cyclophosphamide. Results of treating 169 patients with three different regimens for at least 1 year (mean for the entire group, 7 years) have been published.[103] Improvement in 80 percent of the variables leading to remission in 69 percent of the methotrexate-azathioprine-hydroxychloroquine cohort was recorded, although the disease flared in patients when the therapies were tapered or stopped. Survival was no different from that in the general population. Herpes zoster flared in 17 patients.

As noted by the authors, the general principle of the multidrug regimen was to use "whatever it takes" to produce disease remission, including intrasynovial glucocorticoid injections, the use of D-penicillamine in patients taking methotrexate in whom multiple rheumatoid nodules appeared, and, when necessary, prescription of 2 to 3 g/day of sulfasalazine or 500 mg/day hydroxyurea. Prednisone requirements dropped from a mean daily dose of 9.3 to 5.9 mg.

One of the most important lessons from this study is that patients respond to a physician as well as to a drug. Caring optimism linked with judgment, skill, and experience can help greatly in the care of a chronic disease such as rheumatoid arthritis. In addition, this study emphasizes the difficulties involved in duplicating encouraging results such as these in rigorously controlled double-blind studies in which the drugs used and doses prescribed are fixed.

In this context, five trials of combination therapy have been found that met inclusion criteria for meta-analysis.[104] In all, 749 entering and 516 completing patients were found. Differences in efficacy between combination and single-drug therapy were clinically marginal, and 9 percent more combination-therapy patients experienced side effect–related discontinuation of therapy than patients on single-drug therapy. In reviews of combination therapy, one trend is clear: nonblinded, nonrandomized studies are likely to be enthusiastically positive about the use of combination therapy, whereas the double-blind, randomized control studies seldom suggest the efficacy or comparative safety of combination therapy.

Are there combinations for which data suggest that the effects of two or more drugs might be additive, or even synergistic?

One lead is the use of misoprostol for potential immunosuppressive effects in addition to gastric cytoprotection. It has been reported that misoprostol improves renal function and decreases the incidence of acute rejection in renal transplant patients.

It is apparent that the most impressive data have involved using methotrexate in combination with other second-line and immunosuppressive drugs. In one randomized and double-blind trial, cyclosporine 92.5 to 5 mg/kg was added to methotrexate given at the maximal tolerated dose to patients who had had only a partial response to methotrexate.[106] Forty-eight percent of the cyclosporine/MTX group met the criteria of the American College of Rheumatology for improvement, whereas only 16 percent of those given methotrexate and placebo improved significantly. In another study,[105] rheumatoid patients were randomized to (1) methotrexate alone, (2) sulfasalazine and hydroxychloroquine, or (3) all three drugs. Fifty of the 102 patients experienced a 50 percent improvement that was maintained for 2 years without evidence of major toxicity; those improving represented 24 of 31 treated with all three drugs, 12 of 36 treated with methotrexate alone, and 14 of 35 given the other two drugs. Especially interesting was the lack of additive toxicity in these regimens, which gives added hope that combinations of drugs that attack different pathways of the inflammation and proliferative lesions of rheumatoid arthritis will be useful in treating the disease.

OTHER NEW THERAPIES FOR RHEUMATOID ARTHRITIS

No data have directly linked mycoplasma to rheumatoid arthritis, but in recent years data have accumulated that *tetracyclines* might have benefit for rheumatoid patients for other reasons. Most relevant is their capacity to inhibit biosynthesis and activity of matrix metalloproteinases by mechanisms unrelated to their antibiotic capabilities.[107] In addition to preventing cartilage matrix resorption by metalloproteinase inhibition, doxycycline stimulates cartilage growth and disrupts the terminal differentiation of chondrocytes.[108] Bone resorption is similarly repressed in various models.[109] Somewhat surprisingly, tetracyclines can suppress human neutrophil function[110] and T cell proliferation after exposure to activation stimuli.[111]

Two double-blind, placebo-controlled trials of minocycline in rheumatoid arthritis have been reported.[112, 113] From the Netherlands came the report of 80 patients with active rheumatoid arthritis randomized to placebo or minocycline, 100 mg twice daily. Concurrent use of second-line drugs and prednisone (10 mg/day) was permitted. Sixty-five patients completed the study. Although no patients in either group had a decrease in progression of radiographic abnormalities, there were 15 responders in the minocycline group and 7 in the placebo group. There were no failures in the minocycline group, and nine failures in the placebo group. No improvement in either group was found in the following parameters: pain, fatigue, morning stiffness, and grip strength. The laboratory test changes, similar to the findings in the studies testing anti–TNF-α, were most interesting: the ESR, C-reactive protein, hemoglobin, and IgM rheumatoid factor titers all improved significantly.

In a larger, multicenter trial of 219 patients[111, 113] with a similar profile and concomitant therapeutic regimen including second-line drugs, similar results were obtained: significant changes in laboratory tests for the better in the minocycline group, a 50 percent or greater improvement in joint swelling and tenderness, and annoying toxicity of dizziness. A remarkable improvement of 39 percent and 41 percent in joint swelling and tenderness, respectively, was noted in the placebo group. Clinical evaluations were improved in the treatment group only at the $P<.023$ level, but laboratory tests (e.g., hematocrit, ESR, and rheumatoid factor) improved more.

The obvious unanswered question about minocycline treatment is, What would be the results from a blinded and controlled trial if patients early in disease who were being treated only with NSAIDs were the cohort randomized and tested?

Radiation Synovectomy with Dysprosium 165–Ferric Hydroxide Macroaggregates

Dysprosium 165–ferric hydroxide macroaggregate radiation synovectomy has been tailor-made to provide beta emissions with a short half-life and tissue penetration of less than 6 mm. After a single injection into the knees of 270 mCi, an 86 percent improvement in patients with relatively early radiographic changes was noted after 1 year.[114] In a subsequent study, 13 patients who failed to respond to an initial injection had a repeat injection, and of these 54 percent of the knees were better 1 year later.[115] Limited to centers with an adjacent source of short-lived isotopes, this therapy is useful for patients with one or two severely active joints.

Total Lymphoid Irradiation

In 1981, two studies treated intractable and severe rheumatoid arthritis with total lymphoid irradiation, using fields and dosages introduced for treatment of Hodgkin's disease.[116, 117] The results from both centers were very good after one year, but then remissions and complications occurred. Rheumatoid patients, many of them frail, were susceptible to infections by bacteria and viruses and were bothered by xerostomia, pericarditis, cutaneous vasculitis, and other annoying problems. Evolution of amyloidosis may have been accelerated in some patients, and the specter of delayed lymphoid malignancy still exists as a feared possibility. Although total lymphoid irradiation is no longer appropriate therapy in rheumatoid arthritis for any but the most desperate situations, its legacy is one of an effective treatment too toxic for general use.

SUMMARY

In summary, there are numerous exciting possibilities for effective therapy on the horizon. For now, careful use of one or several of the currently available options for treatment outlined here will be beneficial to patients. The key is beginning with broad therapy early in the disease, adding more patent and focused medications relatively soon if the process remains resistant, and constantly monitoring the balance between efficacy and toxicity of the treatments used.

References

1. Ferraccioli G, Salaffi F, Nervetti A, et al: Slow-acting drugs—Outcome is no different than 15 years ago. J Rheumatol 117:1249, 1990.
2. Pincus T, Callahan LF: The "side effects" of rheumatoid arthritis: Joint destruction, disability and early mortality. Br J Rheumatol 32(Suppl 1):28–37, 1993.
3. Fuchs HA, Pincus T: Radiographic damage in rheumatoid arthritis: Description by nonlinear models. J Rheumatol 19(11):1655–1658, 1992.
4. Gilkeson G, Polisson R, Sinclair H, et al: Early detection of carpal erosions in patients with rheumatoid arthritis: A pilot study of magnetic resonance imaging. J Rheumatol 15:1361, 1988.
5. Stross JK: Relationships between knowledge and experience in the use of disease-modifying antirheumatic agents: A study of primary care practitioners. JAMA 262:2721, 1989.
6. Andrade LEC, Ferraz MB, Atra E, et al: A randomized controlled trial to evaluate the effectiveness of homeopathy in rheumatoid arthritis. Scand J Rheumatol 20:204–208, 1991.
7. Pincus T, Marcum SB, Callahan LF, et al: Long-term drug therapy for rheumatoid arthritis in seven rheumatology private practices: I. Nonsteroidal antiinflammatory drugs. J Rheumatol 19:1874–1884, 1992.
8. Pincus T: The case for early intervention in rheumatoid arthritis. J Autoimmun 5(Suppl A):209–226, 1992.
9. Wolfe F, Hawley DJ, Cathey MA: Termination of slow-acting antirheumatic therapy in rheumatoid arthritis: A 14-year prospective evaluation of 1017 consecutive starts. J Rheumatol 17:994–1002, 1990.
9a. American College of Rheumatology and Ad Hoc Committee on Clinical Guidelines: Guidelines for the management of rheumatoid arthritis. Arthritis Rheum 39:713–722, 1996.
9b. American College of Rheumatology and Ad Hoc Committee on Clinical Guidelines: Guidelines for monitoring drug therapy in rheumatoid arthritis. Arthritis Rheum 39:723–731, 1996.
10. Harris ED Jr: Rheumatoid arthritis: Pathophysiology and implications for therapy. N Engl J Med 322:1277–1289, 1990.
11. Willkens RF: Prognostic staging for therapy of rheumatoid arthritis. Semin Arthritis Rheum 21(Suppl 1):40–43, 1991.
12. Lorig KR, Lubeck D, Kraines RG, et al: Outcomes of self-help education for patients with arthritis. Arthritis Rheum 28:680, 1985.
13. Lorig K: Development and dissemination of an arthritis patient education course. Fam Community Health 9:23, 1986.
14. Hill J, Bird HA, Lawton RH, et al: The development and use of a patient knowledge questionnaire in rheumatoid arthritis. Br J Rheumatol 30:45–49, 1991.
15. Mills JA, Pinals RS, Ropes MW, et al: Value of bed rest in patients with rheumatoid arthritis. N Engl J Med 284:453–458, 1971.
16. Lee P, Kennedy AC, Anderson J, et al: Benefits of hospitalization in rheumatoid arthritis. Q J Med 43:205–214, 1974.
17. Spiegel JS, Spiegel TM, Ward NB, et al: Rehabilitation for rheumatoid arthritis patients: A controlled trial. Arthritis Rheum 29:628–637, 1986.
18. Helewa A, Bombardier C, Goldsmith CH, et al: Cost-effectiveness of inpatient and intensive outpatient treatment of rheumatoid arthritis: A randomized, controlled trial. Arthritis Rheum 32:1505–1514, 1989.
19. Ekdahl C, Broman G: Muscle strength, endurance, and aerobic capacity in rheumatoid arthritis: A comparative study with healthy subjects. Ann Rheum Dis 51:35–40, 1992.
20. Swezey RL: Rheumatoid arthritis: The role of the kinder and gentler therapies. J Rheumatol 17(Suppl 25):8–13, 1990.
21. Jason M IV, Dixon ASJ: Intra-articular pressure in rheumatoid arthritis of the knee: III. Pressure changes during joint use. Ann Rheum Dis 29:401, 1970.
22. Nordemar R, Edstrom L, Ekblom B: Changes in muscle fibre size and physical performance in patients with rheumatoid arthritis after short-term physical training. Scand J Rheumatol 5:70–76, 1976.
23. Nordemar R, Berg U, Ekblom B, et al: Changes in muscle fibre size and physical performance in patients with rheumatoid arthritis after 7 months physical training. Scand J Rheumatol 5:233–238, 1976.
24. Goddard DH, Revell PA, Cason J, et al: Ultrasound has no anti-inflammatory effect. Ann Rheum Dis 42:582–584, 1983.
25. Harris ED, McCroskery PA: The influence of temperature and fibril stability on degradation of cartilage collagen by rheumatoid synovial collagenase. N Engl J Med 290:1–6, 1974.
26. Oosterveld FGJ, Rasker JJ, Jacobs JWG, et al: The effect of local heat and cold therapy on the intraarticular and skin surface temperature of the knee. Arthritis Rheum 35:146–151, 1992.
27. Mainardi CL, Walter JM, Spiegel PK, et al: Rheumatoid arthritis: Failure of daily heat therapy to affect its progression. Arch Phys Med Rehabil 60:390–393, 1968.
28. Kremer JM, Jubiz W, Michalek A, et al: Fish-oil fatty acid supplementation in active rheumatoid arthritis: A double-blinded, controlled, crossover study. Ann Intern Med 106:497, 1987.
29. Harris ED Jr. Treatment of rheumatoid arthritis. In Kelley WN, Harris ED Jr, Ruddy S, Sledge CB (Eds): Textbook of Rheumatology. Philadelphia, WB Saunders, 1993, pp 912–923.
30. Gibson T: Nonsteroidal anti-inflammatory drugs: Another look. Br J Rheumatol 27:87, 1988.
31. Brooks PM, Day RO: Nonsteroidal antiinflammatory drugs—Differences and similarities. N Engl J Med 324:1716–1725, 1991.
32. Criswell LA, Redfearn WJ: Variation among rheumatologists in the use of prednisone and second-line agents for the treatment of rheumatoid arthritis. Arthritis Rheum 37:476–480, 1994.
33. Harris ED Jr, Emkey RD, Nichols JE: Low-dose prednisone therapy in rheumatoid arthritis: A double-blind study. J Rheumatol 10:713, 1983.
34. Iglehart IW III, Sutton JD, Bender JC, et al: Intravenous pulsed steroids in rheumatoid arthritis: A comparative dose study. J Rheumatol 17:159–162, 1990.
35. Wong CS, Champion G, Smith MD, et al: Does steroid pulsing influence the efficacy and toxicity of chrysotherapy? A double-blind, placebo-controlled study. Ann Rheum Dis 49:370–372, 1990.
36. Michel BA, Bloch DA, Wolfe F, et al: Fractures in rheumatoid arthritis: An evaluation of associated risk factors. J Rheumatol 20:1666–1669, 1993.
37. Dequeker J, Geusens P: Osteoporosis and arthritis. Ann Rheum Dis 49:276–280, 1990.
38. Mulder H, Shelder HAA: Effect of cyclical etidronate regimen on prophylaxis of bone loss of glucocorticoid therapy in postmenopausal women. Bone Miner Res 17(Suppl 1):168, 1992.
39. Sambrook P, Birmingham J, Kelly P, et al: Prevention of corticosteroid osteoporosis: A comparison of calcium, calcitriol, and calcitonin. N Engl J Med 328:1747–1752, 1993.
40. Pak CYC, Sakhaee K, Piziak V, et al: Slow-release sodium fluoride in the management of postmenopausal osteoporosis: A randomized controlled trial. Ann Intern Med 120:625–632, 1994.
41. Horber FF, Haymond MW: Human growth hormone prevents the protein catabolic side effects of prednisone in humans. J Clin Invest 86:265–272, 1990.
42. Gennari C, Imbimbo B, Montagniani M: Effect of prednisone and deflazacort on mineral metabolism and parathyroid hormone activity in humans. Calcif Tissue Int 36:245, 1984.
43. Singh G, Fries JF, Williams CA, et al: Toxicity profiles of disease modifying antirheumatic drugs in rheumatoid arthritis. J Rheumatol 18:188–194, 1991.
44. Hobbes HE, Sorsby A, Freedman A: Retinopathy following chloroquine therapy. Lancet 2:478, 1959.
45. Bernstein HN: Ocular safety of hydroxychloroquine. Ann Ophthalmol 23:292, 1991.
46. Rynes RI: Antimalarial drugs. In Kelley WN, Harris ED Jr, Ruddy S, Sledge CB (eds): Textbook of Rheumatology. Philadelphia, WB Saunders, 1993, pp 731–742.
47. Felson DT, Anderson JJ, Meenan RF: The comparative efficacy and toxicity of second-line drugs in rheumatoid arthritis: Results of two metaanalyses. Arthritis Rheum 33:1449–1461, 1990.
48. Fries JF, Williams CA, Ramey D, et al: The relative toxicity of disease-modifying antirheumatic drugs. Arthritis Rheum 36:297–306, 1993.
49. Mazzuca SA, Yung R, Brandt KD, et al: Current practices for monitoring ocular toxicity related to hydroxychloroquine (Plaquenil) therapy. J Rheumatol 21:59–63, 1994.
50. van der Heijde D, van Riel P, Nuver-Zwart E, et al: Sulphasalazine versus hydroxychloroquine in rheumatoid arthritis: 3-year follow-up. Lancet 335:539, 1990.
51. Pullar T, Hunter J, Capell H: Effect of sulphasalazine on the radiological progression of rheumatoid arthritis. Ann Rheum Dis 46:398, 1987.
52. Hannonen P, Mottonen T, Hakola M, Oka M: Sulfasalazine in early rheumatoid arthritis: A 48-week double-blind, prospective, placebo-controlled study. Arthritis Rheum 36:1501, 1993.
53. Haylar T, Smith T, MacPherson A, et al: Nonsteroidal antiinflammatory drug–induced small intestinal inflammation and blood loss. Arthritis Rheum 37:1146, 1994.
54. Research Sub-committee of the Empire Rheumatism Council: Gold therapy in rheumatoid arthritis: Report of a multi-centre controlled trial. Ann Rheum Dis 19:95, 1960.
55. Abruzzo JL: Auranofin: A new drug for rheumatoid arthritis. Ann Intern Med 105:274, 1986.

56. Lehtinen K, Isomäki H: Intramuscular gold therapy is associated with long survival in patients with rheumatoid arthritis. J Rheumatol 18:524–529, 1991.

57. Epstein WV, Henke CJ, Yelin EH, et al: Effect of parenterally administered gold therapy on the course of adult rheumatoid arthritis. Ann Intern Med 114:437–444, 1991.

58. Pincus T, Wolfe F: Treatment of rheumatoid arthritis: Challenges to traditional paradigms. Ann Intern Med 115:825–826, 1991.

59. Sagransky DM, Greenwald RA: Efficacy and toxicity of retreatment with gold salts: A retrospective view of 25 cases. J Rheumatol 7:474, 1980.

60. Gordon DA: Gold compounds in the rheumatic diseases. In Kelley WN, Harris ED Jr, Ruddy S, Sledge CB (eds): Textbook of Rheumatology. Philadelphia, WB Saunders, 1993, pp 743–759.

61. Speerstra F, van Riel PLCM, Reekers P, et al: The influence of HLA phenotypes on the response to parenteral gold in rheumatoid arthritis. Tissue Antigens 28:1, 1987.

62. Fam AG, Gordon DA, Sarkozi J, et al: Neurologic complications associated with gold therapy for rheumatoid arthritis. J Rheumatol 11:700, 1984.

63. Nimni ME, Bavetta LA: Collagen defect induced by penicillamine. Science 150:905, 1965.

64. Harris ED Jr: Effect of penicillamine on human collagen and its possible application to treatment of scleroderma. Lancet 2:996, 1966.

65. Scott DL, Greenwood A, Bryans R, et al: Progressive joint damage during penicillamine therapy for rheumatoid arthritis. Rheumatol Int 8:135, 1988.

66. Dixon ASTJ, Pickup ME, Lowe JR, et al: Discriminatory indices of response in patients with rheumatoid arthritis treated with D-penicillamine. Ann Rheum Dis 34:416, 1980.

67. Stein HB, Schroder ML, Dillon AM: Penicillamine-induced proteinuria: Risk factors. Semin Arthritis Rheum 15:282, 1986.

68. Kay A: Myelotoxicity of D-penicillamine. Ann Rheum Dis 38:232, 1979.

69. Williams H, Willkens RF, Samuelson CO Jr, et al: Comparison of low-dose oral pulse methotrexate and placebo in the treatment of rheumatoid arthritis: A controlled clinical trial. Arthritis Rheum 28:721–730, 1985.

70. Weinblatt ME, Coblyn JS, Fox DA, et al: Efficacy of low-dose methotrexate in rheumatoid arthritis. N Engl J Med 312:818–822, 1985.

71. Andersen PA, West SG, O'Dell JR, et al: Weekly pulse methotrexate in rheumatoid arthritis: Clinical and immunologic effects in a randomized double-blind study. Ann Intern Med 103:489–496, 1985.

72. Thompson RN, Watts C, Edelman J, et al: A controlled two-center trial of parenteral methotrexate therapy for refractory rheumatoid arthritis. J Rheumatol 11:760–763, 1984.

73. Tugwell P, Bennett K, Gent M: Methotrexate in rheumatoid arthritis: Indications, contraindications, efficacy and safety. Ann Intern Med 197:358–366, 1987.

74. Willkens RF, Watson MA: Methotrexate: A perspective of its use in the treatment of rheumatic disease. J Lab Clin Med 100:314–321, 1982.

75. Kremer JM, Lee JK: The safety and efficacy of the use of methotrexate in long-term therapy for rheumatoid arthritis. Arthritis Rheum 29:822–831, 1986.

76. Kremer JM, Lee JK: A long-term prospective study of the use of methotrexate in rheumatoid arthritis: Update after a mean of fifty-three months. Arthritis Rheum 31:577–584, 1988.

77. Weinblatt ME, Trentham DE, Fraser PA, et al: Long-term prospective trial of low-dose methotrexate in rheumatoid arthritis. Arthritis Rheum 31:167–175, 1988.

78. Weinblatt ME, Maier AL: Long-term experience with low-dose weekly methotrexate in rheumatoid arthritis. J Rheumatol 17(Suppl 22):33–38, 1990.

79. Weinblatt ME, Fraser PA, Holdsworth DE, et al: Long-term prospective study of methotrexate in rheumatoid arthritis: 45 month update (abstr). Arthritis Rheum 31:S115, 1988.

80. Buchbinder R, Hall S, Sambrook PN, et al: Methotrexate therapy in rheumatoid arthritis: A life table review of 587 patients treated in community practice. J Rheumatol 20(4):639–644, 1993.

81. Whiting-O'Keefe QE, Fye KH, Sack KD: Methotrexate and histologic hepatic abnormalities: A meta-analysis. Am J Med 90:711–716, 1991.

82. Luqmani RA, Palmer RG, Bacon PA: Azathioprine, cyclophosphamide and chlorambucil. Baillieres Clin Rheumatol 4:595–619, 1990.

83. Mason M, Currey HLF, Barnes CG, et al: Azathioprine in rheumatoid arthritis. Br Med J 1:420–422, 1969.

84. Cash JM, Klippel JH: Malignancy and rheumatoid arthritis. Clin Exp Rheumatol 9:109–112, 1991.

85. Walters MT, Cawley MID: Combined suppressive drug treatment in severe refractory rheumatoid disease: An analysis of the relative effects of parenteral methylprednisolone and cyclophosphamide. Ann Rheum Dis 47:924, 1988.

86. Fauci AS, Young KR Jr: Immunoregulatory agents. In Kelley WN, Harris ED Jr, Ruddy S, Sledge CB (eds): Textbook of Rheumatology. Philadelphia, WB Saunders, 1993, pp 797–821.

87. Baker GL, Kahl LE, Zee BC, et al: Malignancy following treatment of rheumatoid arthritis with cyclophosphamide: Long-term case-control follow-up study. Am J Med 83:1–9, 1987.

88. Radis CD, Kahl LE, Baker GL, et al: Effects of cyclophosphamide on the development of malignancy and on long-term survival of patients with rheumatoid arthritis: A 20-year follow-up study. Arthritis Rheum 38:1120–1127, 1995.

89. Kahn MF, Bedoisear M, de Seze S: Immunosuppressive drugs in the management of malignant and severe rheumatoid arthritis. Proc R Soc Med 60:130, 1967.

90. Dougados M, Awada H, Amor B: Cyclosporin in rheumatoid arthritis: A double-blind, placebo-controlled study in 52 patients. Ann Rheum Dis 47:127–133, 1988.

91. Yocum DE, Klippel JH, Wilder RL, et al: Cyclosporin A in severe, treatment-refractory rheumatoid arthritis. Ann Intern Med 109:863–869, 1988.

92. Curtis JJ, Luke RG, Dubovsky E, et al: Cyclosporin in therapeutic doses increases renal allograft vascular resistance. Lancet 2:477–479, 1986.

93. Dougados M, Duchesne L, Awada H, et al: Assessment of efficacy and acceptability of low-dose cyclosporin in patients with rheumatoid arthritis. Ann Rheum Dis 48:550–556, 1989.

94. Altman RD, Perez GO, Sfakianakis GN: Interaction of cyclosporine A and nonsteroidal anti-inflammatory drugs on renal function in patients with rheumatoid arthritis. Am J Med 93:396–402, 1992.

95. van Rijthoven AWAM, Dijkmans BAC, Thè HSG, et al: Long-term cyclosporine therapy in rheumatoid arthritis. J Rheumatol 18:19–23, 1991.

96. Dijkmans BAC, Landewé RBM, van Rijthoven AWAM, et al: Cyclosporine in rheumatoid arthritis (RA): State of the art, with emphasis on the treatment of early RA. Reumatismo 44(Suppl 2):35–42, 1992.

97. Landewé RBM, Thè HSG, van Rijthoven AWAM, et al: A randomized, double-blind, 24-week controlled study of low-dose cyclosporine versus chloroquine for early rheumatoid arthritis. Arthritis Rheum 37(5):637, 1994.

98. Bensen W, Tugwell P, Roberts RM, et al: Combination therapy of cyclosporine with methotrexate and gold in rheumatoid arthritis (2 pilot studies). J Rheumatol 31:2034–2038, 1994.

99. Macleod AM, Thomson AW: FK 506: An immunosuppressant for the 1990s? Lancet 337:25–27, 1991.

100. Achiron A, Pras E, Gilad R, et al: Open controlled therapeutic trial of intravenous immune globulin in relapsing-remitting multiple sclerosis. Arch Neurol 49:1233–1236, 1992.

101. Moynier M, Cosso B, Brochier J, et al: Identification of class II HLA alloantibodies in placenta-eluted gamma globulins used for treating rheumatoid arthritis. Arthritis Rheum 30:375–381, 1987.

102. McCarty DJ, Carrera GF: Treatment of intractable rheumatoid arthritis with combined cyclophosphamide, azathioprine and hydroxychloroquine. JAMA 255:2215–2219, 1982.

103. McCarty DJ, Harman JG, Grassanovich JL, et al: Combination drug therapy of seropositive rheumatoid arthritis. J Rheumatol 22:1636–1645, 1995.

104. Felson DT, Anderson JJ, Meenan RF: The efficacy and toxicity of combination therapy in rheumatoid arthritis: A metaanalysis. Arthritis Rheum 37:1487–1491, 1994.

105. O'Dell JR, Haire CE, Erikson N: Treatment of rheumatoid arthritis with methotrexate alone, sulfasalazine and hydroxychloroquine, or a combination of all three medications. N Engl J Med 334:1287–1294, 1996.

106. Tugwell P, Pincus T, Yocum D, et al: Combination therapy with cyclosporine and methotrexate in severe rheumatoid arthritis: The Methotrexate-Cyclosporine Combination Study Group. N Engl J Med 333:137–141, 1995.

107. Greenwald RA, Golub LM, Lavietes B, et al: Tetracyclines inhibit synovial collagenase in vivo and in vitro. J Rheumatol 14:28–32, 1987.

108. Cole AA, Chubinskaya S, Luchene LJ, et al: Doxycycline disrupts chondrocyte differentiation and inhibits cartilage matrix degradation. Arthritis Rheum 37:1727–1734, 1994.

109. Yu LP Jr, Smith GN, Hasty KA, et al: Doxycycline inhibits type XI collagenolytic activity of extracts from human osteoarthritic cartilage and of gelatinase. J Rheumatol 18:1450–1452, 1991.

110. Gabler WL, Creamer HR: Suppression of human neutrophil function by tetracyclines. J Periodontol Res 26:52–58, 1991.

111. Kloppenburg M, Miltenburg AMM, Verdonk MJA, et al: Minocycline inhibits T cell proliferation and interferon gamma (IFN-gamma) production after stimulation with anti-CD3 monoclonal antibodies. Br J Rheumatol 31(Suppl 2):41, 1992.

112. Kloppenburg M, Breedveld FC, Terwiel JP, et al: Minocycline in active rheumatoid arthritis: A double-blind, placebo-controlled trial. Arthritis Rheum 37:629–636, 1994.

113. Tilley B, Alarcon G, Heyse S, et al: Minocycline in rheumatoid arthritis. A 48-week, double-blind, placebo-controlled trial: MIRA Trial Group. Ann Intern Med 122:81, 1995.

114. Sledge CB, Zuckerman JD, Zalutsky MR, et al: Treatment of rheumatoid synovitis of the knee with intraarticular injection of dysprosium 165–ferric hydroxide macroaggregates. Arthritis Rheum 29:153–159, 1986.

115. Vella M, Zuckerman JD, Shortkroff S, et al: Repeat radiation synovectomy with dysprosium 165–ferric hydroxide macroaggregates in rheumatoid knees unresponsive to initial injection. Arthritis Rheum 31:789–792, 1988.

116. Kotzin BL, Strober S, Engleman EG, et al: Treatment of intractable rheumatoid arthritis with total lymphoid irradiation. N Engl J Med 305:969–976, 1981.

117. Trentham DE, Belli JA, Anderson RJ, et al: Clinical and immunologic effects of fractionated total lymphoid irradiation in refractory rheumatoid arthritis. N Engl J Med 305:976–982, 1981.

118. Silverstein FE, Graham DY, Senior JR, et al: Misoprostol reduces serious gastrointestinal complications in patients with rheumatoid arthritis receiving nonsteroidal anti-inflammatory drugs. Ann Intern Med 123:241–249, 1995.

CHAPTER 57

Robert S. Pinals

Felty's Syndrome

In 1924, Felty[1] described the triad of chronic arthritis, splenomegaly, and leukopenia. Felty's syndrome represents one of many systemic complications of seropositive rheumatoid arthritis occurring in a group of patients with unusually severe extra-articular disease and immunologic abnormalities.[2] The term "hypersplenism" was derived from the observation that splenectomy usually results in partial or complete resolution of the granulocytopenia, but the role of the spleen in pathogenesis has been a subject of considerable controversy for many years. There is evidence for its participation both in the removal of granulocytes from the circulating pool and in the suppression of granulopoiesis. With a complex pathogenesis that varies from case to case, Felty's syndrome must be still defined in descriptive terms as a variant of seropositive rheumatoid arthritis with splenomegaly and granulocytopenia (<2000/mm³). Although the complete triad is required for a diagnosis of Felty's syndrome, some rheumatoid arthritis patients may be encountered at a time when only granulocytopenia is present. Such individuals resemble patients with full-blown Felty's syndrome in most clinical and serologic features. The true prevalence of Felty's syndrome is unknown, but it may be found in more than 3 percent of rheumatoid arthritis patients.[3] Splenomegaly alone is more common, but the majority of these patients never develop neutropenia.

DIFFERENTIAL DIAGNOSIS

Patients with rheumatoid arthritis may also develop superimposed illnesses that result in splenomegaly or granulocytopenia. Drug reactions, myeloproliferative disorders, reticuloendothelial malignancies, hepatic cirrhosis, amyloidosis, sarcoidosis, tuberculosis, and other chronic infections must be considered and excluded with reasonable clinical certainty before the diagnosis of Felty's syndrome is accepted. A syndrome of neutropenia and large granular lymphocytosis has been associated with rheumatoid arthritis.[4, 5] Large granular lymphocytes may be found rarely in normal human blood (Fig. 57–1). Cells with natural-killer and antibody-dependent cell-mediated cytotoxic activity are found in this population. Among patients with an abnormal proliferation of these cells, neutropenia, splenomegaly, and susceptibility to infections are common. In some cases, there is a progressive course of malignant proliferation, but most are stable over a period of several years. Chronic inflammatory arthritis, usually seropositive and often fulfilling criteria for rheumatoid arthritis, is also commonly associated with large granular lymphocytosis, and these patients have a high frequency of human leukocyte antigen (HLA)–DR4. In one series, 23 percent of patients with large granular lymphocytosis identified in a large referral center over a 10-year

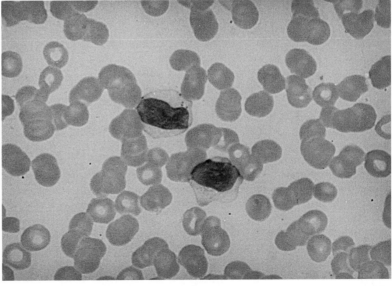

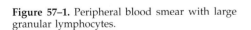
Figure 57–1. Peripheral blood smear with large granular lymphocytes.

period had rheumatoid arthritis, and most would have been classified as having Felty's syndrome if not for the discovery of typical cells in the bone marrow or peripheral blood, or both.[4] In this report, the prevalence of true Felty's syndrome was twice that of large granular lymphocytosis in rheumatoid arthritis patients with neutropenia. However, other evidence suggests that occult clonal expansions of large granular lymphocytes may occur in classic Felty's syndrome.[5] The simultaneous appearance of arthritis and neutropenia, the absence of deformity, and the finding of lymphocytosis on peripheral blood smears may provide clues to the presence of large granular lymphocytosis. This condition is often relatively benign and may require no specific therapy. However, splenectomy, which corrects neutropenia in most Felty's syndrome patients, may be unsuccessful.

CLINICAL FEATURES

About two thirds of patients with Felty's syndrome are women. HLA-DR4 is found in 95 percent of patients with Felty's syndrome.[2] This may account for the rarity of Felty's syndrome in blacks, who are known to have a low frequency of DR4.[6] The condition is usually recognized in the fifth through the seventh decades of life in patients who have had rheumatoid arthritis for 10 years or more.[3] Splenomegaly and granulocytopenia may be present before symptoms or signs of arthritis in rare instances.[7] The articular disease is usually severe[8, 9] but not more so than in seropositive rheumatoid arthritis of comparable duration.[3] About one third of the patients have relatively inactive synovitis, as judged by signs and symptoms, but even these patients continue to have an elevated erythrocyte sedimentation rate (ESR).[8] In one large series, the mean ESR was 85 mm/hour.[9]

The spleen size is variable. In 5 to 10 percent of patients, it is not large enough to be palpable, but occasionally there is massive splenomegaly.[10] The median splenic weight in Felty's syndrome is about four times normal.[10] There is no correlation between spleen size and the degree of granulocytopenia.[8, 9]

Patients with Felty's syndrome tend to have more extra-articular manifestations than others with rheumatoid arthritis (Table 57–1). Weight loss may be striking and unexplained, often occurring for several months before the diagnosis of Felty's syndrome is made. Brown pigmentation over exposed surfaces of the extremities, especially over the tibia, may be related to stasis and to extravasation of red blood cells secondary to disease of small vessels.[8] Leg ulcers are frequent but do not seem to differ from those in other rheumatoid arthritis patients in terms of chronicity, recurrence, and presumed relationship to vasculitis.

Felty's syndrome patients have a 20-fold increase in frequency of infections compared with matched rheumatoid arthritis controls.[2] The degree of granulocytopenia correlates poorly with the number and severity of infections until the granulocyte count falls

Table 57–1. FREQUENCY OF EXTRA-ARTICULAR MANIFESTATIONS IN FELTY'S SYNDROME*

Rheumatoid nodules	76%
Weight loss	68%
Sjögren's syndrome†	56%
Lymphadenopathy	34%
Leg ulcers	25%
Pleuritis	19%
Skin pigmentation	17%
Neuropathy	17%
Episcleritis	8%

*From a review of 10 reports since 1962.
†Determined by positive Schirmer's test.

below 1000/mm³. Other risk factors for infection include skin ulcers, corticosteroids, severity of the underlying rheumatoid process, and resulting disability.[11, 12] Sepsis is the principal factor in the reduced survival of Felty's syndrome patients compared with that of rheumatoid arthritis controls.[2] Most of the infections are caused by common bacteria, such as staphylococcus, streptococcus, and gram-negative bacilli,[9] and involve common sites, particularly the skin and respiratory tract. In spite of the granulocytopenia, pus may accumulate in an appropriate fashion, suggesting that the site of infection is capable of competing successfully with the spleen for available granulocytes. The response to antibiotic therapy is usually adequate.[9]

Mild hepatomegaly is common in Felty's syndrome, and elevations of alkaline phosphatase and the transaminases are described in about a quarter of the patients.[2, 9] An unusual type of liver involvement may be associated with Felty's syndrome but occurs rarely in other rheumatoid arthritis patients.[13] Histologically, the picture is described as nodular regenerative hyperplasia.[14] Although there is mild portal fibrosis or infiltration with lymphocytes and plasma cells, the appearance is not characteristic of cirrhosis. Obliteration of portal venules may compromise portal blood flow, leading to atrophy and regenerative nodule formation, portal hypertension, and gastrointestinal hemorrhage.

Patients with Felty's syndrome are at increased risk for the development of malignancies, particularly non-Hodgkin's lymphoma.[15]

HEMATOLOGIC AND SEROLOGIC FEATURES

The leukopenia in Felty's syndrome is relative and absolute granulocytopenia, in contrast to systemic lupus erythematosus, in which lymphopenia is a more prominent feature. There is often considerable spontaneous variation in the granulocyte count. Patients with mild lowering may return to the normal range, but this is rarely seen when depression is severe. Thus, spontaneous remissions have been observed[8, 16] but are uncommon. During infections or other stressful episodes, the granulocyte count often returns to the normal range but is seldom elevated. This may conceal the diagnosis temporarily, since blood counts may be ordered mainly in the setting of an infection or other acute illness. The bone marrow may show no abnormality, but in most cases, there is a myeloid hyperplasia, with a relative excess of immature forms, often described as "maturation arrest." Although this might reflect an impaired myelopoietic response, early release of mature forms would result in the same appearance.[8, 9] Rarely, the marrow suggests a depression in myeloid activity or shows an increased lymphocytic infiltration. A mild to moderate anemia is found in most patients, representing the anemia of chronic disease with an additional component of shortened red blood cell survival, which is corrected by splenectomy. Thrombocytopenia is seldom severe enough to cause purpura.

The alterations in immune response commonly found in rheumatoid arthritis are amplified in patients with Felty's syndrome. Rheumatoid factor is present in 98 percent of the patients, generally in high titer,[9] and antinuclear antibodies are found in 67 percent. Anti-nDNA is elevated occasionally.[2] Antihistone antibodies are present in 83 percent,[17] and anti-neutrophil cytoplasmic antibodies in 77 percent. Most of the latter are reactive against lactoferrin.[18] Immunoglobulin levels are higher than in other rheumatoid arthritis patients, and complement levels are lower,[8, 9] although most patients have levels within the normal range. Immune complexes have been detected by various techniques in the majority of Felty's syndrome patients, always in much higher frequency than in rheumatoid controls.[19]

PATHOGENESIS

The hematologic improvement resulting from splenectomy led some to postulate that the spleen had been producing a humoral inhibitor of granulocyte production,[20] and others to support splenic sequestration and destruction of granulocytes as the principal mechanism.[21] The debate appeared to be settled in favor of the latter proposal when granulocyte counts were shown to be lower in the splenic vein than in the artery.[21] However, more recent studies suggest that the two viewpoints are not mutually exclusive and that a number of factors may contribute to the development of granulocytopenia. Ingestion and surface-coating of immune complexes leads to impaired granulocyte function and facilitates their removal by the reticuloendothelial system.[22, 23] Specific antibodies directed against granulocyte cell surface antigens may also be involved.[24] Sequestration or margination of granulocytes in the spleen and venules in the lungs and elsewhere results in a diminished circulating pool.[25] In some patients, the marrow does not respond appropriately to granulocytopenia because of the action of a humoral inhibitor[26, 27] and/or T lymphocytes that suppress myelopoiesis.[28, 29] There may be different subsets of Felty's syndrome, as illustrated by one report in which both humoral and cell-mediated mechanisms were investigated. About two thirds of the patients had high levels of neutrophil-bound immunoglobulin G (IgG). In the remaining patients, peripheral blood mononuclear cells inhibited colony growth in normal marrow.[30] In another study, T cell marrow suppression was found to be a more frequent mechanism than serum anti–precursor cell activity.[28] More than one mechanism may account for neutropenia in an individual patient.

The increased susceptibility to infection is probably related to several factors in addition to granulocytopenia. Granulocyte reserves are diminished, and defective function of granulocytes in phagocytosis,[31] chemotaxis,[32] and superoxide production[33] has been demonstrated.

The familial occurrence of Felty's syndrome suggests that immunogenetic factors are operative.[34] HLA-DR4 is present more frequently than in other rheumatoid arthritis patients, and there also appear to be a DQ β–linked susceptibility gene and a C4B-null allele that increase the risk of Felty's syndrome in HLA-DR4–positive rheumatoid arthritis patients.[2, 35, 36]

MANAGEMENT

Splenectomy

Since splenectomy usually reverses the hematologic abnormalities in Felty's syndrome, it was advocated in the past as the treatment of choice, either in all cases or in those patients with very low granulocyte counts or serious infections.[10, 11] A prompt hematologic response is observed within minutes or hours after splenectomy,[11] but granulocytopenia recurs and persists in about one quarter of these patients. Continuing immune-mediated granulocyte sequestration may be responsible for these secondary failures. Recurrent or persistent infection was noted in only 26 percent of patients in one large series[10] but in 60 percent in four others.[11] Patients who did not experience infection prior to splenectomy usually continued to be free of infection afterward, whereas those with the most severe infections had variable and inconsistent responses to splenectomy, suggesting that functional defects in granulocytes and disease severity variables may be as important as granulocytopenia in determining susceptibility to infection.[11, 12]

Thrombocytopenia usually improves after splenectomy, as does anemia, to the extent that it is due to a hemolytic component. Although dramatic improvement in synovitis has been observed, it is often temporary and does not occur in most cases. Leg ulcers may also respond, even those that are not significantly infected,[10] but the variability in etiology and natural course makes these reports difficult to interpret.

In recent years, granulocytopenia has been shown to respond to various nonsurgical measures. Splenectomy should probably be reserved for patients who are unresponsive to these therapies.

Other Treatments

Frequently granulocytopenia may improve during treatment with the second-line antirheumatic drugs.[11] Gold salt injections resulted in a complete hematologic response in 60 percent of patients and partial response in 20 percent in the largest reported series.[37] Penicillamine appeared to be both less efficacious than gold and more likely to produce serious toxicity. Limited experience with methotrexate suggests that it is also effective.[38, 39] Low doses of corticosteroids do not produce consistent improvement in granulocytopenia and also predispose to infection.[8, 9] The mechanisms whereby these second-line agents raise granulocyte counts are undetermined, as are their response rates and relative efficacy. In one series, most patients failed to increase neutrophil counts by 50 percent on second-line drug treatment, and several untreated patients improved spontaneously.[2] Therefore, these agents may not be justified in patients without synovitis, unless serious infections have occurred.

Other therapies may be directed specifically at the granulocytopenia. High-dose parenteral testosterone may stimulate granulopoiesis but is not suitable for women. Lithium salts also increase granulopoiesis by augmenting colony-stimulating activity, but long-term benefit has not yet been demonstrated, and the treatment has been unsuccessful in the experience of some investigators.[2] Recombinant granulocyte colony-stimulating factor (G-CSF) raises granulocyte counts, but its use is limited by cost, adverse reactions, and exacerbation of arthritis.[40] G-CSF may be most useful as adjunctive therapy during serious infections or in preparation for surgery. Splenic embolization has been investigated as an alternative to splenectomy.[41]

References

1. Felty AR: Chronic arthritis in the adult, associated with splenomegaly and leucopenia. Johns Hopkins Hosp Bull 35:16, 1924.
2. Campion G, Maddison PJ, Goulding N, et al: The Felty syndrome: A case-matched study of clinical manifestations and outcome, serologic features, and immunogenetic association. Medicine 69:69, 1990.
3. Sibley JT, Haga M, Visram DA, et al: The clinical course of Felty's syndrome compared to matched controls. J Rheumatol 18:1163, 1991.
4. Saway PA, Prasthofer EF, Barton JC: Prevalence of granular lymphocyte proliferation in patients with rheumatoid arthritis and neutropenia. Am J Med 86:303, 1989.
5. Bowman SJ, Sivakumaran M, Snowden N, et al: The large granular lymphocyte syndrome with rheumatoid arthritis. Immunogenic evidence for a broader definition of Felty's syndrome. Arthritis Rheum 37:1326, 1994.
6. Termini TE, Biundo JJ, Ziff M: The rarity of Felty's syndrome in blacks. Arthritis Rheum 22:999, 1979.
7. Bradley JD, Pinals RS: Felty's syndrome presenting without arthritis. Clin Exp Rheumatol 1:257, 1983.
8. Ruderman M, Miller LM, Pinals RS: Clinical and serologic observations on 27 patients with Felty's syndrome. Arthritis Rheum 11:377, 1968.
9. Sienknecht CW, Urowitz MB, Pruzanski W, Stein HG: Felty's syndrome. Clinical and serological analysis of 34 cases. Ann Rheum Dis 36:500, 1977.
10. Laszlo J, Jones R, Silberman HR, Banks PM: Splenectomy for Felty's syndrome: Clinicopathological study of 27 patients. Arch Intern Med 138:597, 1978.
11. Breedveld FC, Fibbe WE, Cats A: Neutropenia and infections in Felty's syndrome. Br J Rheumatol 27:191, 1988.
12. Breedveld FC, Fibbe WE, Hermans J, et al: Factors influencing the incidence of infections in Felty's syndrome. Arch Intern Med 147:915, 1987.
13. Thorne C, Urowitz MB, Wanless IR, Roberts E, Blendis LM: Liver disease in Felty's syndrome. Am J Med 73:35, 1982.
14. Wanless IR, Godwin TA, Allen F, Feder A: Nodular regenerative hyperplasia of the liver in hematologic disorders: A possible response to obliterative portal venopathy. Medicine 59:367, 1980.
15. Gridley G, Klippel JH, Hoover RN, et al: Incidence of cancer among men with the Felty syndrome. Ann Intern Med 120:35, 1994.
16. Luthra HS, Hunder GG: Spontaneous remission of Felty's syndrome. Arthritis Rheum 18:515, 1975.
17. Cohen MG, Webb J: Antihistone antibodies in rheumatoid arthritis and Felty's syndrome. Arthritis Rheum 32:1319, 1989.
18. Coremans IEM, Hagen EC, van der Voort EAM, et al: Autoantibodies to neutrophil cytoplasmic enzymes in Felty's syndrome. Clin Exp Rheumatol 11:255, 1993.
19. Andreis M, Hurd ER, Lospalluto J, Ziff M: Comparison of the presence of immune complexes in Felty's syndrome and rheumatoid arthritis. Arthritis Rheum 21:310, 1978.
20. Dameshek W: Hypersplenism. Bull N Y Acad Sci 31:113, 1955.
21. Wright CS, Doan CA, Bouroncle BA, Zollinger RM: Direct splenic arterial and venous blood studies in the hypersplenic syndromes before and after epinephrine. Blood 6:195, 1951.
22. Hurd ER: Presence of leucocyte inclusions in spleen and bone marrow of patients with Felty's syndrome. J Rheumatol 5:26, 1978.
23. Goldschmeding R, Breedveld FC, Engelfriet CP, et al: Lack of evidence for the presence of neutrophil autoantibodies in the serum of patients with Felty's syndrome. Br J Haematol 68:37, 1988.
24. Starkebaum FG, Arend WP, Nardella FA, Gavin SE: Characterization of immune complexes and immunoglobulin G antibodies reactive with neutrophils in the sera of patients with Felty's syndrome. J Lab Clin Med 96:238, 1980.
25. Hashimoto Y, Ziff M, Hurd ER: Increased endothelial cell adherence, aggregation and superoxide generation by neutrophils incubated in systemic lupus erythematosus and Felty's syndrome sera. Arthritis Rheum 12:1409, 1982.
26. Gupta R, Robinson WA, Albrecht D: Granulopoietic activity in Felty's syndrome. Ann Rheum Dis 34:156, 1975.
27. Goldberg LS, Bacon PA, Bucknall RC, Fitchen J, Cline MJ: Inhibition of human bone marrow–granulocyte precursors by serum from patients with Felty's syndrome. J Rheumatol 7:275, 1980.
28. Abdou NL: Heterogeneity of bone marrow–directed immune mechanisms in the pathogenesis of neutropenia of Felty's syndrome. Arthritis Rheum 26:947, 1983.
29. Bagby GC Jr, Gabourel JD: Neutropenia in three patients with rheumatic disorders: Suppression of granulocytes by cortisol-sensitive thymus-dependent lymphocytes. J Clin Invest 64:72, 1979.
30. Starkebaum G, Singer JW, Arend WP: Humoral and cellular immune mechanisms of neutropenia in patients with Felty's syndrome. Clin Exp Immunol 39:307, 1980.
31. Breedveld FC, van den Barselaar MT, Leijh PCJ, et al: Phagocytosis and intracellular killing by polymorphonuclear cells from patients with rheumatoid arthritis and Felty's syndrome. Arthritis Rheum 28:395, 1985.
32. Howe GB, Fordham JN, Brown KA, Currey HLF: Polymorphonuclear cell function in rheumatoid arthritis and in Felty's syndrome. Ann Rheum Dis 40:370, 1981.
33. Davis P, Johnston C, Bertouch J, Starkebaum G: Depressed superoxide radical generation by neutrophils from patients with rheumatoid arthritis and neutropenia: Correlation with neutrophil reactive IgG. Ann Rheum Dis 46:51, 1987.
34. Runge LA, Davey FR, Goldberg J, Boyd PR: The inheritance of Felty's syndrome in a family with several affected members. J Rheumatol 13:39, 1986.
35. Thomson W, Sanders PA, Davis M, et al: Complement C4B-null alleles in Felty's syndrome. Arthritis Rheum 31:984, 1988.
36. So AKL, Warner CA, Sanson D, Walport MJ: DQ B polymorphism and genetic susceptibility to Felty's syndrome. Arthritis Rheum 31:990, 1988.
37. Dillon AM, Luthra HS, Conn DL, Ferguson RH: Parenteral gold therapy in the Felty syndrome. Medicine 65:107, 1986.
38. Fiechtner JJ, Miller DR, Starkebaum G: Reversal of neutropenia with methotrexate treatment in patients with Felty's syndrome. Arthritis Rheum 32:194, 1989.
39. Tan N, Grisanti MW, Grisanti JM: Oral methotrexate in the treatment of Felty's syndrome. J Rheumatol 20:599, 1993.
40. Yasuda M, Kihara T, Wada T, et al: Granulocyte colony-stimulating factor induction of improved leukocytopenia with inflammatory flare in a Felty's syndrome patient. Arthritis Rheum 37:145, 1994.
41. Nakamura H, Ohishi A, Asano K, et al: Partial splenic embolization for Felty's syndrome: A 10-year follow-up. J Rheumatol 21:1964, 1994.

CHAPTER 58

Robert I. Fox

Sjögren's Syndrome

Sjögren's syndrome (SS) refers to the combination of a particular form of dry eyes (keratoconjunctivitis sicca [KCS]) and a dry mouth due to infiltration of these glands by lymphocytes. These "sicca" symptoms result from a systemic autoimmune process that also may affect other organs, including central and peripheral neural systems, skin, mucosal surfaces such as upper airways and vagina, lungs, and kidneys. In addition, SS patients have an increased risk of developing non-Hodgkin's lymphoma compared with their age- and sex-matched controls and with patients with most other systemic autoimmune diseases. Physicians who provide "primary" care to SS patients should be familiar with the treatments used by ophthalmologists, dermatologists, gynecologists, and dentists. The medications used by other health care specialists may exacerbate the sicca symptoms, and SS patients also have particular needs at the time of surgery that must be conveyed to the surgeon and anesthesiologist. SS is divided into primary and secondary forms, where the sicca symptoms are associated with other well-defined autoimmune diseases such as rheumatoid arthritis (RA), systemic lupus erythematosus (SLE), or progressive systemic sclerosis (PSS). Since the diagnosis and treatment of the associated diseases are covered elsewhere in this text, this chapter will concentrate on the current issues of diagnosis and treatment of primary SS.

BACKGROUND

In 1888 Johan van Mikulicz Radecki described a 42-year-old Prussian farmer with enlargement of lacrimal and salivary glands "consisting of small round cells."[1] In 1933 Henrik Sjögren described the association of KCS, dry mouth (xerostomia), and RA.[2] Although this association of symptoms is generally known as Sjögren's syndrome, it is occasionally referred to as *Gougerout-Sjögren syndrome* to acknowledge the earlier report by Gougerout in 1925.[3] In 1953 Morgan and Castleman[4] demonstrated that a histologically similar infiltrate was present in both SS and Mikulicz's disease. Block and colleagues[5] suggested that SS be subdivided into primary SS and secondary SS. Secondary SS was defined as that form occurring in patients with sicca symptoms in association with particular diseases such as RA, SLE, PSS, and dermatomyositis; primary SS patients lacked these particular diseases. A wide spectrum of extra-glandular features, including pulmonary, lung, renal, and neurologic involvement, have been reported in primary SS patients.

EPIDEMIOLOGY

The frequency of primary SS in the general population has been an issue of considerable debate. The specific criteria for inclusion obviously dictate the frequency. The referral pattern to a specific medical center of a patient with an "unusual" condition will further influence estimates of disease prevalence. Although the ophthalmic component (i.e., KCS) is well defined, the criteria for classifying the oral component remains controversial, and no uniform diagnostic criteria for SS exist. On the one hand, the San Diego criteria (Table 58–1) require objective evidence of KCS, xerostomia, characteristic lymphocytic infiltrate on minor salivary gland biopsy, and presence of autoantibodies.[6] A classification system based on a characteristic minor salivary gland biopsy with a focal lymphocytic infiltrate has very close agreement with the San Diego criteria.[7] On the other hand, the European preliminary criteria for SS can be fulfilled in the absence of biopsy or autoantibodies.[7, 8] A comparison of these criteria systems has recently been published.[9] Only approximately 15 percent of the patients with a diagnosis of SS using the European Economic Community (EEC) criteria[8] fulfill the San Diego criteria.[9]

We favor stringent criteria for the diagnosis of SS (see Table 58–1). These become important in assessing the frequency of extraglandular symptoms and signs associated with SS. For example, symptoms of dryness of eyes or mouth, myalgias, and fatigue are extremely common in the general population. They are associated with anxiety, depression, medications with anticholinergic side effects, and many diseases associated with disruption of the autonomic neural system.[9] If stringent criteria for SS are not utilized, then misapplication of the label "SS" may prevent a diligent search for other, treatable causes of the dryness symptoms.

One approach to determining the frequency of SS in the general population has been the evaluation of consecutive blood donor samples for the presence of anti–SS-B antibody in random female blood donors;[10] this criterion yielded a frequency of approximately 1 in 2500. Retrospective studies have shown a high association of anti–SS-B antibody with clinical sicca symptoms and positive minor salivary gland biopsies.[11] Because antibodies against SS-B have been found in about 40 to 50 percent of primary SS patients

Table 58–1. CRITERIA FOR DIAGNOSIS OF PRIMARY AND SECONDARY SJÖGREN'S SYNDROME

I. **Primary SS**
  A. Symptoms and objective signs of ocular dryness
    1. Schirmer's test: less than 8 mm wetting per 5 minutes
    2. Positive rose bengal or fluorescein staining of cornea and conjunctiva to demonstrate keratoconjunctivitis sicca
  B. Symptoms and objective signs of dry mouth
    1. Decreased parotid flow rate using Lashley cups or other methods
    2. Abnormal biopsy of minor salivary gland (focus score of ≥2 based on average of 4 evaluable lobules)
  C. Evidence of a systemic autoimmune disorder
    1. Elevated rheumatoid factor >1:160
    2. Elevated antinuclear antibody >1:160
    3. Presence of anti–SS-A (Ro) or anti–SS-B (La) antibodies
II. **Secondary SS**
  A. Characteristic signs and symptoms of SS (described above) plus clinical features sufficient to allow a diagnosis of RA, SLE, polymyositis, or scleroderma
  B. Exclusions: sarcoidosis, pre-existent lymphoma, acquired immunodeficiency disease, hepatitis, other known causes of keratitis sicca, salivary gland enlargement, or autonomic neuropathy

Modified from Fox RI, Robinson C, Curd J, et al: First international symposium on Sjögren's syndrome: suggested criteria for classification. Scand J Rheumatol 562:28, 1986.

Diagnosis of definite primary SS requires the presence of item I,A,1,2; item I,B,1,2; item I,C,1 or 2; and lack of exclusions in item II. Probable SS can be diagnosed if other criteria are fulfilled but in the absence of a minor salivary gland biopsy (item I,B,2).

Abbreviations: SS, Sjögren's syndrome; RA, rheumatoid arthritis; SLE, systemic lupus erythematosus.

meeting the strict criteria for diagnosis,[8] an estimate of primary SS incidence of about 1 in 1250 females may serve as an approximation. When patients with RA and secondary SS are included, a much higher prevalence may result; these would not be included in the aforementioned estimate because secondary SS patients with RA frequently lack anti–SS-B antibody.

OCULAR MANIFESTATIONS OF SJÖGREN'S SYNDROME

Patients with the ocular manifestations of SS (i.e., KCS) suffer from a decrease in the aqueous component of tears.[12] This results from destruction of the serous glands and from interruption of their neurovascular innervation.[13, 14] The imbalance in aqueous and mucinous tear secretions leads to a relative increase in tenacious secretions, which are clinically noted as long mucinous threads that can be extracted from the patient's eyes. The decrease in aqueous tear flow leads to decreased tear film stability, manifested by a rapid tear breakup time and increased debris in the tear film. As a result, defects in visual acuity and discomfort may occur.[15] The most characteristic symptom is a burning sensation that increases as the day progresses and that is relieved by instillation of artificial tears. Severe eye dryness leads to filamentary keratitis (fine filaments on the anterior surface of the cornea) in SS patients. The filaments are composed primarily of mucus (mucoproteins and mucopolysaccharides) that binds to the cornea and conjunctiva.

The mucoproteins likely bind to specific receptors on the epithelium that have been exposed by a deficiency in the tear film.[16, 17] These filaments cause a severe foreign-body sensation and may be associated with photophobia and blepharospasm. Corneal edema and conjunctivitis may also occur. These changes are not specific for SS and may also be seen in wearers of contact lenses; in patients who have undergone intraocular surgery; and in patients with diabetes, ectodermal dysplasia, neurotrophic keratitis, trachoma, ocular pemphigoid, and sarcoidosis.

Other ocular symptoms in SS patients include an increased frequency of inflammation of the eyelids (blepharitis), due in part to abnormalities affecting the meibomian glands. Irritating side effects from the preservatives in artificial tears and obstruction of the glands by ocular lubricants (discussed later), however, contribute to some cases of ocular irritation and blepharitis.

Patients meeting stringent criteria for SS manifest a variety of ocular symptoms (Table 58–2). The most characteristic complaint is a foreign-body sensation that often became more severe as the day progressed. Although patients also complain of dry eye, red eye, or painful eye, these manifestations are also prevalent in the general population.[10, 18] Photosensitivity is not a common complaint unless the keratoconjunctivitis is quite severe.[19] The presence of this symptom suggests anterior uveitis rather than SS. Causes of keratitis other than SS, listed in Table 58–3, include pemphigoid, sarcoidosis, trauma infection, vitamin deficiency, neuropathy, and allergy.[17]

It is worth emphasizing that only a small proportion of patients with "painful" eyes have SS. The majority of patients with the tear film abnormalities of KCS are unlikely to have any other manifestations of a systemic autoimmune disease such as SS, and they need to be reassured in this regard.[15] Decreases in ocular tear production occur as a consequence of aging,[20] as do decreases in saliva production. This decrease in tearing with age appears to occur more

Table 58–2. CLINICAL FEATURES OF KERATOCONJUNCTIVITIS SICCA

Clinical Features	Sjögren's Syndrome Patients (%)	Control Patients (%)
Symptoms		
Foreign-body sensation that is worse in the evening	85	6
"Dry eye" or "painful eye"	98	22
Dry eye feeling that improves after use of artificial tears	75	7
Itching of the eyes	27	19
Signs		
Dilation of the bulbar conjunctival vessels (usually interpalpebral)	31	7
Dullness of the conjuctiva and/or cornea	27	0
Schirmer's test: ≤9 mm/5 min	95	10
Abnormal rose bengal and/or fluorescein	100	5

Table 58–3. CAUSES OF KERATITIS AND
SALIVARY GLAND ENLARGEMENT
OTHER THAN SJÖGREN'S SYNDROME

Keratitis

Mucous membrane pemphigoid
Sarcoidosis
Infections: virus (adenovirus, herpes, vaccinia), bacteria, or
   Chlamydia (i.e., trachoma)
Trauma (i.e., from contact lens) and environmental irritants,
   including chemical burns, exposure to ultraviolet lights, or
   roentgenograms
Neuropathy, including neurotropic keratitis (i.e., damage to fifth
   cranial nerve) and familial dysautonomia (Riley-Day syndrome)
Hypovitaminosis A
Erythema multiforme (Stevens-Johnson syndrome)

Salivary Gland Enlargement

Sarcoidosis, amyloidosis
Bacterial (including gonococci and syphilis) and viral infections
   (i.e., infectious mononucleosis, mumps)
Tuberculosis, actinomycosis, histoplasmosis, trachoma, leprosy
Iodide, lead, or copper hypersensitivity
Hyperlipemic states, especially types IV and V
Tumors (usually unilateral), including cysts (Warthin's tumor),
   epithelial (adenoma, adenocarcinoma), lymphoma, and mixed
   salivary gland tumors
Excessive alcohol consumption
Human immunodeficiency virus

frequently in women and to intensify after menopause. It may manifest suddenly in patients who
receive medications with anticholinergic side effects,
such as antidepressants, cold remedies, and certain
cardiac medications.

From the diagnostic point of view, the rheumatologist needs to determine if the patient's history of
ocular dryness symptoms corresponds to objective
findings on physical examination.[18] Indeed, in today's
environment of increased managed care, the need for
and timing of an ophthalmology consultation often
is determined on the basis of the rheumatologist's
evaluation. Several key points in the history are relevant. Since many patients complain of ocular dryness
at night and upon awakening in the morning, these
symptoms have relatively little specificity for diagno-

sis. Although the best evaluation of KCS requires
the use of a slit lamp, rheumatologists can detect
significant abnormalities in a rapid, cost-effective
manner in their outpatient clinics with readily available equipment and supplies. For example, the traditional Schirmer I test involves the measurement of
tear flow in 5 minutes using paper strips placed in
the lower conjunctival sac (with normal values usually >6 mm/5 min). In addition, the Schirmer II test
involves measuring the rate of tearing that occurs
after stimulation of the nasolacrimal gland reflex by
insertion of a cotton swab gently into the nose. The
resulting stimulation is analogous to a "stress test" to
measure stimulated tear flow and correlates well with
KCS.[18] An additional useful test is the rose bengal
test. A small drop of this dye is put into the lower
conjunctival sac and rinsed out with an artificial tear
solution. Areas of devitalized conjunctiva and corneal
epithelia retain the dye, giving a "raccoon" appearance (Fig. 58–1), which initially occurs in the regions
where tear film evaporation is not prevented by the
eyelids.[21] In addition, areas of corneal abrasion are
rapidly exposed and indicate the need for early referral to an ophthalmologist. The presence of symptoms
such as severe ocular pain and photophobia in the
absence of abnormal rose bengal staining indicates
that KCS is not the responsible process.

Another cause of eye discomfort in patients is
blepharitis (i.e., irritation of the lids and conjunctiva),
which results from blockage or infection of the meibomian glands that line the eyelids. The use of viscous
eye drops and ocular lubricants (particularly at night)
may lead to this complication, which exacerbates
symptoms in dry eye patients. Other causes of ocular
discomfort include eye strain (poor refraction), blepharospasm (uncontrolled blinking due to an increased
local neural reflex circuit), defects of the mucus-pro-
ducing cells of the conjunctiva (e.g., pemphigoid, Stevens-Johnson syndrome), uveitis, retinitis, and symptoms due to anxiety or depression.

ORAL FEATURES

The second cardinal feature of SS is oral dryness
(xerostomia). Symptoms of dry mouth at night and in

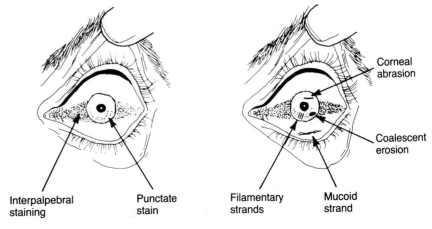

Figure 58–1. Schematic illustration of increased interpalpebral staining with rose
bengal. Since eyelids normally retard evaporation, disruption in the epithelial lining
and tear film is most marked in the interpalpebral region *(A)*, leading to increased
risk of corneal abrasions *(B)*.

Interpalpebral
staining

Punctate
stain

Filamentary
strands

Mucoid
strand

Corneal
abrasion

Coalescent
erosion

the morning are extremely common in the general population and thus lack specificity for the diagnosis of SS. Symptoms of night and morning dryness reflect the normal diurnal variation in autonomic neural stimulation that maintains basal secretion of the glands. A history of a patient's need to take water in order to swallow food is more closely correlated with objective sicca complex.[8] A dry mouth is not necessarily a painful mouth. For example, it is common for an SS patient with chronic dry mouth to seek medical attention when he or she experiences a painful mouth after developing oral candidiasis (discussed later). A common scenario is the use of steroids and/or antibiotics for an upper respiratory tract infection resulting in persistent mouth discomfort. Another common finding is the precipitation of increased mouth discomfort with medications possessing anticholinergic side effects (discussed later).

On examination of the mouth, the SS patient is found to lack the normal salivary pooling under the tongue and may have rapidly progressive caries. The mouth frequently exhibits macular erythema of the hard palate and other areas of the oral mucosa. Also common in SS patients is evidence of chronic erythematosus oral candidiasis on the mucosal surfaces and angular cheilitis at the angles of the lips. In contrast, it is unusual to find the plaquelike lesions of pseudomembranous candidiasis that are present in severely immunocompromised patients. In examining the patient with dentures, it is important that these be removed since oral irritation and even ulcerations are common on the underlying mucosal surfaces.

Dental caries in SS patients occur at the gum line and incisor surfaces. The loss of teeth and requirement for dentures at any age may have significant emotional and economic consequences. Patients with dentures may change their patterns of interpersonal interaction. For example, social life frequently involves eating meals with friends, and patients with dentures may feel uncomfortable about not being able to eat the same foods. In addition, the patient's diet may be shifted to the "preprocessed" foods, which are often higher in sugars, and this accelerates the rate of caries progression.

Measurement of saliva from the parotid glands can be performed using a Lashley cup that fits over the opening of Stensen's duct.[10] Particularly in research studies, this prevents the contamination of parotid saliva with fluid emanating from the gingival tissue, which may be highly inflammatory because of carious teeth or periodontal disease. Multiple methods are available for quantitating total salivary flow, including placement of a cotton sponge under the tongue for 3 minutes and comparing the dry weight to the wet weight.[22] A simpler method is to give the patient a sugarless candy and estimate the decrease in size over a 3-minute period. Variables that significantly influence total salivary flow include medications with anticholinergic side effects, times since last meal and last tooth brushing, and ingestion of caffeine or nicotine (i.e., smoking).

Because there are so many different causes of decreased salivary gland flow, a minor salivary gland specimen may be obtained and examined for the presence of focal lymphocytic infiltrates.[7, 23] Although the specimens will be interpreted by the pathologist, it is important for the rheumatologist to verify the adequacy of the specimen and to confirm the diagnosis. Figure 58–2 shows examples of a minor salivary gland specimen from a primary SS patient (A) and from a normal individual (B). The key feature in this biopsy is that the lymphocytes occur in a focal infiltrate. In contrast, specimens from non-SS patients frequently have scattered infiltrates consisting of a few lymphocytes (often perivascular) and granulocytic infiltrates (surrounded ruptured ducts) that are nonspecific and not characteristic of SS.[23] The site of the specimen (through histologically normal oral mucosa) and the size of the specimen (at least four evaluable salivary gland lobules) are important for the results to be interpretable.

Several methods for evaluating biopsy specimens have been proposed. We use the system of Daniels,[23] in which the average number of lymphocytic foci (a focus is defined as a cluster of 50 or more lymphocytes) per 4 mm^2 is determined. The focus score for the entire biopsy is expressed based on the average of at least four evaluable salivary gland lobules. For example, Figure 58–2A shows a portion of the minor salivary gland specimen with a focus score of 4. Incorrect methods of biopsy (especially biopsy through an area of oral mucositis) and failure to record the average focus score are common causes of misdiagnosis of SS. Also, rheumatologists must be aware that different scoring methods are used by different pathologists. For example, a grade IV biopsy specimen on the Chisholm-Mason scale (from normal = I to abnormal = IV)[24] is not equivalent to a focus score of 4 on the Daniels scale.[14] Since the Chisholm-Mason score is more heavily weighted toward infiltrates with a focus score <1, the scoring method of Daniels[23] is preferred.

Other methods are used to evaluate salivary gland function and size.[25] The use of sialograms using oil-based contrast materials introduced through Stensen's or Wharton's duct has been reported, but this procedure has been discontinued because of the risk of inflammatory reactions provoked by the viscous contrast materials. Complications of oil-based sialograms can include severe chronic granulomatous reactions that can persist for many years and mimic development of parotid infections and lymphomas. Water-based contrast materials may also be used in sialograms,[26] and this is more common in Europe. Rheumatologists need to be cautioned that these studies should never be performed during an acute episode of salivary gland swelling. Also, they should be performed only by radiologists experienced in sialograms to prevent perforation of the parotid duct by the cannula and to ensure that scanning equipment is positioned in a manner that will allow a reproducible quantitative evaluation of secretory rates.

Potential tumors in the salivary glands and other

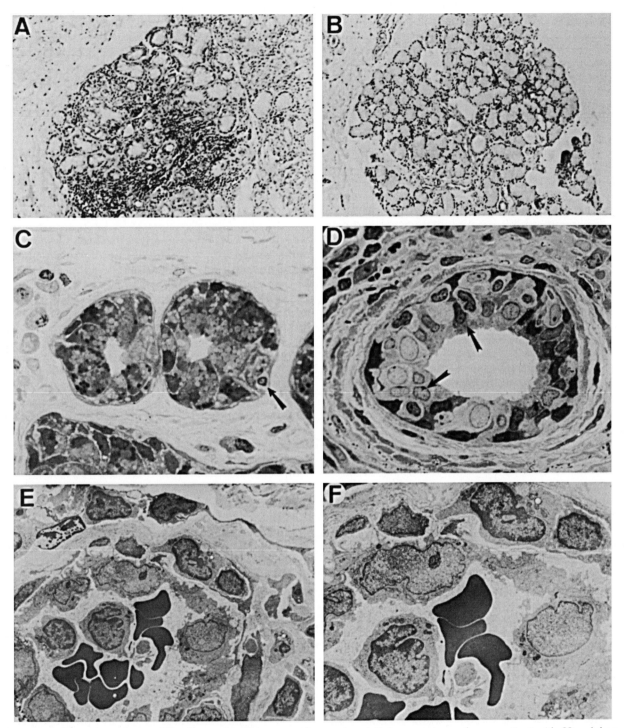

Figure 58–2. Sjögren's syndrome (SS) salivary gland biopsy specimens. *A* and *B* show specimens from a patient with SS and from a normal individual, respectively. The initial appearance of lymphocytic infiltrates in the central portion of the salivary gland *(A)* is similar to that noted in the minor salivary gland specimens of SS patients. Under higher magnification, the location of lymphocytes adjacent to salivary gland epithelial cells (i.e., beneath the basement membrane enclosing acini and ducts) can be seen. Under electron microscopy *(C, D)*, the appearance of high endothelial venules (containing red blood cells and lymphocytes adherent to the vascular endothelium) as well as the absence of electron-dense immune complexes near the basement membrane *(E, F)* can be noted.

neck masses are best evaluated using magnetic resonance imaging (MRI) methods. Attention to cervical lymph nodes as well as to the parotid/submandibular areas is important. Salivary gland imaging by sonography has been suggested,[26, 27] but lack of uniform methods of grading this noninvasive method have hindered its widespread application.[25]

Salivary gland enlargement can occur in diseases other than SS (see Table 58–3). Diseases such as sarcoidosis, amyloidosis, and infection (bacterial, fungal, or viral) or the presence of a tumor must be considered. The finding of elevated angiotensin-converting enzyme (ACE) is a helpful indication of sarcoidosis, because this enzyme is rarely elevated in glandular swelling due to SS. An unusual presentation of sarcoidosis is uveoparotid fever (Heerfordt's disease), in which patients exhibit parotid enlargement and ocular symptoms but lack other features of sarcoidosis (hilar lymphadenopathy, diffuse lung infiltrates, skin sarcoid, or hepatosplenomegaly). A sudden increase in salivary gland pain or size suggests the possibility of infection, which is more frequent in SS patients owing to inadequate salivary flow rate. The most common offending organisms are *Staphylococcus, Streptococcus viridans, Streptococcus hemolyticus,* and *Pneumococcus,* all normal flora of the oral cavity. Cultures must be taken of the pus escaping from Stensen's or Wharton's duct. Salivary gland infections must be treated promptly to prevent formation of abscesses.

INVOLVEMENT OF EXTRAGLANDULAR SITES

Pulmonary Sites

Involvement in SS of exocrine glands in the upper respiratory tract frequently leads to dryness of the nasal passages and bronchi. Hunninghake and Fauci[28] emphasized the high incidence of pulmonary abnormalities in patients with SS, including pleurisy with or without effusion, interstitial fibrosis, desiccation of tracheobronchial mucous membrane, and lymphoid interstitial disease (Table 58–4). In our clinic, the development of respiratory problems associated with mucus plug inspissation is a relatively common problem. This often occurs in the setting of an upper respiratory tract infection, resulting in increased tenacious secretions that cannot be adequately mobilized from the small airways.[29] This problem may be compounded by the patient taking cold remedies containing compounds with anticholinergic side effects. It may also occur in the postoperative setting when the anesthesiologist gives the SS patient an anticholinergic drug to control upper respiratory tract secretions during surgery, resulting in the inspissation of the patient's secretions. These problems can be minimized by the use of smaller doses of anticholinergic medicines, the use of humidified oxygen in the operating room, and attention to respiratory therapy during the postoperative period.

Clinical studies of pulmonary function in primary SS patients have yielded conflicting results. Newball and Brahim[30] and Siegal and colleagues[31] found evidence of mild to moderate obstructive airway disease in almost 50 percent of their primary SS patients. In another study, Oxholm and associates[32] did not find obstructive changes in any of 43 patients with primary SS, but did note decreased diffusing capacity and suggested that interstitial pneumonitis was relatively common. During a 7-year follow-up study, these SS patients did not undergo significant deterioration of their diffusing capacity.[33]

Gastrointestinal Sites

Difficulty in swallowing is a frequent occurrence in primary SS patients, primarily as a result of decreased saliva production.[34] The patient describes difficulty in deglutition (i.e., food gets stuck in the upper throat) as opposed to the subjective feeling of obstruction at the substernal level reported by scleroderma patients. Abnormal esophageal motility (particularly in the upper third of the esophagus) may also contribute to dysphagia in some primary SS patients.[35] Increased symptoms of heartburn and discomfort in distal esophageal structures may be due in part to reflux of gastric acid into the esophagus, where it is not adequately neutralized by the diminished amount of saliva. Gastric biopsy specimens show an increased frequency of chronic atrophic gastritis[36] and lymphocytic infiltrates.[34] Patients with marked gastric involvement can be identified by their decreased serum pepsinogen levels[37] and increased gastrin levels.[38] Investigation of pancreatic function has shown impaired response to secretin and pancreozymin, suggesting subclinical pancreatic disease.[39] Overt pancreatic insufficiency manifesting as diabetes mellitus or malabsorption, however, does not appear to be significantly increased in frequency. Antibodies against pancreatic duct antigen have been found in some patients, but antibodies to pancreatic islet cells have not been detected.[40]

Clinical or biochemical evidence of liver disease is found in 5 to 10 percent of primary SS patients.[41] The elevations found in liver function tests are generally mild (less than twice normal) and without clinical significance. When higher levels of liver enzymes are noted, possibilities such as viral hepatitis and drug toxicity (including nonsteroidal anti-inflammatory drugs [NSAIDs] and aspirin) should be investigated. In a small proportion of SS patients, the presence of antimitochondrial antibodies indicates coexistent primary biliary cirrhosis (PBC). It is relatively common for PBC patients to develop sicca symptoms late in their disease. Salivary gland biopsy specimens from these patients show lymphoid infiltrates. These findings suggest that a similar pathogenic process may be responsible for salivary gland destruction and damage to the exocrine hepatic apparatus. It is uncommon, however, for PBC patients to exhibit anti-

Table 58–4. EXTRAGLANDULAR MANIFESTATIONS IN PATIENTS WITH PRIMARY SJÖGREN'S SYNDROME

Respiratory	Endocrine, Neurologic, and Muscular
Chronic bronchitis secondary to dryness of upper and lower airway with mucous plugging	Thyroiditis
Lymphocytic interstitial pneumonitis	Peripheral neuropathy—symmetric involvement of hands and/or feet
Pseudolymphoma with nodular infiltrates	Mononeuritis multiplex
Lymphoma	Myalgias
Pleural effusions	**Hematologic**
Pulmonary hypertension, especially with associated scleroderma	Neutropenia, anemia, thrombocytopenia
Gastrointestinal	Pseudolymphoma
Dysphagia associated with xerostomia	Angioblastic lymphadenopathy
Atrophic gastritis	Lymphoma and myeloma
Liver disease, including biliary cirrhosis and sclerosing cholangitis	**Renal**
Skin	Tubulointerstitial nephritis
Vaginal dryness	Glomerulonephritis—in absence of antibodies to DNA
Hyperglobulinemic purpura—nonthrombocytopenic	Mixed cryoglobulinemia
Raynaud's phenomenon	Amyloidosis
Vasculitis	Obstructive nephropathy due to enlarged periaortic lymph nodes
	Lymphoma
	Renal artery vasculitis

bodies against SS-B antigen,[42] and thus the PBC-associated sicca complex probably represents a form of secondary SS.

Elevated serum amylase levels may derive from the salivary glands and lead to potential confusion with evaluation of potential pancreatic problems.

Cutaneous Sites

Dryness of the skin has been attributed to a decrease in the secretory capacity of the sebaceous glands in some patients. Oral candidiasis, particularly angular cheilitis, is extremely common in these patients and is a typical contributing factor in their increased mouth pain and decreased sensation of taste. It is particularly common in SS patients who are receiving glucocorticoids, and the onset of symptoms can frequently be traced to the use of antibiotics for another reason.

Vasculitis in SS patients may take various forms. The most common "vasculitis" reported in our clinic is hypergammaglobulinemic purpura that occurs symmetrically in the lower extremities.[43] This is found in patients with IgG levels higher than 2000 mg/dl, and the earliest stage of the rash exhibits multiple nonpalpable petechial lesions 2 to 3 mm in size. As these acute lesions fade, they are replaced by hyperpigmentation that may persist from months to years. In addition to nonpalpable purpura, SS patients may develop a palpable purpura due to leukocytoclastic vasculitis and skin lesions of erythema multiforma.[44, 45] Periungual telangiectasis may be detected in these patients, and the presence of these lesions in large numbers suggests an increased chance of later development of scleroderma.

Endocrine Sites

Clinically apparent hypothyroidism has been reported in 10 to 15 percent of SS patients[46, 47] and occurs in a similar proportion of our patients.[10] Antibody to thyroglobulin and thyroid microsomal antigen levels may be elevated in an additional 4 to 5 percent of patients,[46] suggesting that subclinical thyroid damage may be relatively common in SS patients. Thus, endocrine as well as exocrine glandular cells may be targets for immune attack in primary SS. Insulin-dependent diabetes mellitus[47] and pernicious anemia[46] occur with a frequency in primary SS similar to their frequency in the general population.

Renal Manifestations

Renal tubular function is not a routine clinical measurement, and renal functional evaluation in primary SS remains incomplete, with the available data perhaps not truly representative. The most common functional renal abnormality noted in SS patients is the inability to acidify the urine in response to an administered acid load, such as ammonium chloride.[48–53] This is generally believed to be due to dysfunction of the distal nephron and may be present in 20 to 40 percent of SS patients in a latent form.[48, 52] Talal and coworkers[54] demonstrated impairment of urinary acidification in 6 of 12 patients with SS who also had marked hypergammaglobulinemia. This defect may lead to a higher incidence of nephrocalcinosis.[50, 52]

Proteinuria is uncommon in patients with SS. Only 2 of 36 patients in one series had proteinuria higher than 3.5 g.[51] Glomerulonephritis in primary SS is unusual,[54–57] and its occurrence suggests an associated disease process such as SLE, amyloidosis, vasculitis, or mixed cryoglobulinemia.[58–60] Membranoproliferative and membranous forms of glomerulonephritis have been described, and immunopathologic studies suggest that the glomerular lesions are associated with accumulation of immune complex material.

In considering SS as part of the differential diagnosis of interstitial nephritis, it must be remembered that a wide group of diseases may affect the interstitium and tubules while sparing the glomeruli.[61] The renal abnormalities of interstitial nephritis can occur in virtually any autoimmune disease and are most frequently found in association with hypergammaglobulinemia.[62–65] Of particular importance are the side effects of drugs (antibiotics, NSAIDs) associated with nephropathy, because SS patients frequently receive these medications.

Hematologic Abnormalities

Leukopenia (total white blood cell [WBC] count <4000/mm³) is present in 20 percent of our SS patients; previous reports have noted leukopenia in 6 to 33 percent of patients.[5, 46] The mechanism of this leukopenia remains unclear but may involve antibodies to leukocytes, splenic sequestration, or abnormal bone marrow maturation of leukocytes in certain patients.[66]

SS patients have increased levels of serum and urinary paraproteins.[67, 68] They also exhibit increased levels of cryoglobulins, particularly in association with hypergammaglobulinemic purpura.[42] The cryoglobulin is frequently a type II mixed cryoglobulin containing an IgM-κ monoclonal rheumatoid factor similar to that found in Waldenström's macroglobulinemia.[67] Among Japanese SS patients, an increased incidence of non-IgM paraproteins has been reported.[69]

The relative risk for development of lymphoma in patients with primary SS has been estimated to be approximately 40-fold higher than for age-matched, sex-matched control subjects by investigators at the National Institutes of Health.[70] Whaley and colleagues[46] in Glasgow, however, did not find such an increased prevalence. This discrepancy may be attributed to several factors, including the relatively small number of patients reported with lymphoma and ascertainment bias in patient referral patterns. It also may reflect the difficulty in distinguishing lymphoma from extensive infiltrates due to "benign" SS or pseudolymphoma (Fig. 58–3).[71] The lymphomas are predominantly non-Hodgkin's B cell (IgM-κ) tumors that arise in the salivary gland and cervical lymph nodes. Although the finding of myoepithelial islands (i.e., a degenerating tubule surrounded by lymphocytes) is often interpreted as an indication that the tumor is "benign," malignant lymphomas can be found in the same biopsy specimen that contains myoepithelial islands.[72] Distinguishing malignant lymphoma from pseudolymphoma in SS patients is often quite difficult, even when recombinant DNA methods are used.[73–76] Other forms of nonmalignant lymphoid proliferation in primary SS patients include thymoma[45] and angioimmunoblastic lymphadenopathy.[77] Both pseudolymphoma and angioblastic lymphadenopathy appear to be associated with a high frequency of progression to frank lymphoma.[70, 78] To allow earlier

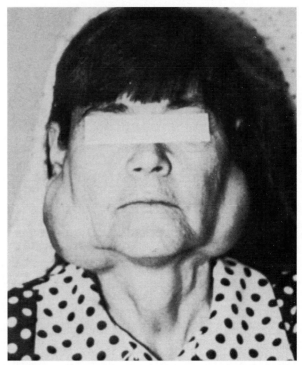

Figure 58–3. Massive bilateral parotid gland enlargement in a patient with pseudolymphoma and Sjögren's syndrome. (From Fox RI, Adamson TC III, Fong S, et al: Lymphocyte phenotype and function of pseudolymphomas associated with Sjögren's syndrome. Reproduced from the Journal of Clinical Investigation, 1983, vol 72, p 52 by copyright permission of the American Society for Clinical Investigation.)

detection of lymphomas, methods of in situ hybridization[79] and polymerase chain reaction[80] have been described. However, these methods are limited by the observation that clonal expansion as detected by Southern blotting methods[73, 75] are found in biopsies without overt lymphomas.[81]

Neurologic Manifestations

SS patients may exhibit both central and peripheral nervous system manifestations. The frequency of these complications varies among reported series. Alexander and coworkers[82] found central nervous system abnormalities in approximately 20 percent of their primary SS patients. In particular, they found a multiple sclerosis–like symptom with the use of abnormal cerebrospinal fluid analysis and MRI of the brain.[83] The central nervous system symptoms were associated with cutaneous vasculitis.[43] In comparison, Metz and associates[84] and Sandberg-Wollheim and colleagues[85] did not find increased frequency of autoantibodies or abnormal labial biopsies among patients with multiple sclerosis; an increased frequency of sicca symptoms was noted among the multiple sclerosis patients but was attributed to anticholinergic side effects of medicines and perhaps to underlying neurologic dysfunction. Peripheral neuropathies in primary

SS include symmetric peripheral neuropathies and mononeuritis multiplex. The symmetric neuropathies frequently present as a sensory neuropathy involving the feet in patients with hypergammaglobulinemic purpura. Mononeuritis multiplex with sensory and motor components occurs less frequently and is often associated with leukocytoclastic vasculitis.[6]

AUTOANTIBODIES

The frequency of antinuclear antibodies (ANAs) in SS patients depends strongly on the classification criteria used. Using immunofluorescence assays and Hep-2 cells, a homogeneous or fine speckled pattern is most commonly noted. Based on immunodiffusion assays, SS sera were found to contain antibodies directed against SS-A (also termed Ro) antigen, as well as against SS-B (also termed La) antigen. The antibodies against SS-A are not specific for SS, since they are also found in SLE patients lacking SS. The antibodies against SS-B have a higher association with SS.[11] However, the association of anti–SS-A and anti–SS-B antibodies is probably higher with specific HLA class II antigens (to be discussed) than with specific clinical manifestations of autoimmune disease.[86, 87]

Antibodies against SS-A and SS-B are predominantly IgG, with preferential utilization of IgG1 subclass.[88] Although the antibodies may cross the placenta and participate in neonatal SLE syndromes and congenital heart block,[89] the role of anti–SS-A/B antibodies in the pathogenesis of SS is unclear, particularly since the target antigens have a ubiquitous distribution in all nucleated cells. False-negative ANA results were found to occur in some laboratories due to "overfixation" of slides in alcohol, because the SS-A antigen is relatively soluble in alcohol.[90] Indeed, many cases of "subacute SLE associated with a negative ANA but with presence of an anti–SS-A antibody" are probably the result of laboratory artifacts that used "overpreserved" substrate to measure the ANA. Conversely, the new "commercial" enzyme-linked immunosorbent assay (ELISA) tests using either cell extracts enriched for SS-A/B or recombinant SS-A/B products have become so exquisitely sensitive that the clinical correlations with SS have become unclear.

Immunoblotting and immunoprecipitation techniques have demonstrated that anti–SS-A antibodies react with at least two distinct proteins with molecular masses of 60 and 52 kD; these proteins are associated with an abundant class of small cellular RNAs termed *hYRNAs*.[91] Some sera from SS patients react predominantly with the 60-kD antigen or with the 52-kD antigen, whereas most SS sera react with both proteins.[91–93] The anti–SS-B antibodies reacted with a 48-kD phosphoprotein that is complexed with recent RNA polymerase III transcripts. The association of SS-A and SS-B with Epstein-Barr virus early RNA (EBER) transcripts induced by Epstein-Barr virus has led to speculation about a role in pathogenesis.[94]

The location and tissue-specific expression of SS-A and SS-B proteins has been the subject of significant controversy. The SS-A and SS-B proteins are expressed in all nucleated cells and may also be expressed in red blood cells and platelets.[95] The SS-A 60- and 52-kD proteins are found predominantly in the nucleus; the relative proportion of 60-kD and 52-kD proteins varies in different tissues in some species.[96, 97] Further, alternative splicing or post-translational modification gives rise to different sizes of SS-A antigens in different tissues, as demonstrated by blotting.[98] In a similar manner, the SS-B 48-kD protein is found predominantly in the nucleus, where it can be detected in the nucleolus during the G_1 and early S phases of the cell cycle. This location corresponds to the functional ability of SS-B binding to precursors of 5s RNA and transfer RNA, but not to corresponding mature transcripts. This ability to bind to RNA precursors suggests an important role for SS-B in the regulation of transcription by RNA polymerase III; these processes occur in the nucleolus. It has been suggested that SS-B also may shuttle back and forth to the cytoplasm.[99] Further, Baboonian and coworkers[100] reported that viral infection may induce redistribution of the nuclear antigen to the cell membrane and that this may contribute to the autoimmune process.

Molecular cloning of the SS-A 60-kD protein indicates an RNA binding domain and a zinc finger motif, structures thought to facilitate recognition (and thus regulation) of DNA or RNA molecules. The cloning of the SS-A 52-kD protein demonstrated a homology to *rfp* (a cellular homolog of the human transforming protein *ret*) and to the mouse *rpt-2* (a T cell regulatory protein that down-regulates the IL-2 receptor and the long terminal report promoter of HIV). Also, the SS-A 52-kD protein contains a zipper finger motif, which also suggests a role in regulation of gene expression.[101] An additional structural homology of the SS-A 52-kD protein is butyrophilin, a glycoprotein that is expressed on the apical surfaces of secretory cells in lactating mammary tissues but is absent in virgin cows. The age- and sex-related control of gene expression in an exocrine gland may have importance in the early stages of pathogenesis of SS. An additional 60-kD molecule was originally thought to be part of the SS-A complex; this protein had homology to calreticulin,[102] but more recent studies indicate that it is probably not closely associated with SS.[103]

DNA sequence has shown RNA binding domains in SS-B. Also, alternative splicing of the SS-B gene has been shown to give rise to two different-sized transcripts.[104] Of importance, only the longer transcript contains an exon with transcription factor binding sites, including a nuclear factor (NF)-κ B element. This suggests that the transcriptional differences of the SS-B gene may contribute to pathogenesis of SS. SS-B expression is up-regulated 15-fold after herpesvirus infection in vitro,[105] indicating a possible link to induction of autoimmune reaction and putative viral infection in SS (discussed later).

GENETICS

The occurrence of anti–SS-A and anti–SS-B antibodies in SS patients and in some SLE patients is closely associated with particular major histocompatibility complex (MHC) class II antigens. In the old terminology based on serologic typing, this extended haplotype in Caucasian SS patients includes the HLA-B8-DR3-Dw52a genes that are often associated with complement C4 null deletion.[106] Also, an important role for heterozygosity of specific HLA-DQ alleles was noted.[87] Using DNA restriction mapping and polymerase chain reaction, the extended haplotype is called HLA-DRB1*0301-DRB3*0101-DQA1*0305-DQB1*0204.[107] Of importance, a different haplotype is found in non-Caucasian patients such as Chinese and Japanese SS patients[108] and black patients.[109, 110] In each population, one or more extended haplotypes were found to be increased in the SS patients compared with local controls. However, the particular haplotype was distinct for each ethnic group. The finding of different "risk" genes in different ethnic populations of SS patients is different from the common "epitopes" found in patients with rheumatoid arthritis or insulin-dependent diabetes of different ethnic background. It indicates that multiple different class II antigens can participate in the pathogenesis of SS.

PATHOGENESIS

The specific etiology of SS remains unknown. It likely involves both genetic and environmental features. Theories of pathogenesis should include the following features:

1. The lacrimal and salivary glands become infiltrated with CD4+ T cells and, to a lesser extent, B cells.[111, 112]

2. The salivary epithelial cells express high levels of HLA-DR in comparison with normal salivary gland epithelial cells.[113, 114]

3. Antibodies made within the gland are directed against rheumatoid factor (Fc region of IgG)[67] and antinuclear antigens (SS-A, SS-B),[90] which are not specific to salivary or lacrimal glands.

4. Although antibodies against salivary ductal antigens are occasionally detected, they are relatively uncommon and unlikely to play a primary role in pathogenesis.[115]

5. Genetic predisposition in Caucasians is linked to HLA-DR3[106, 107] and to heterozygosity of HLA-DQ,[87] whereas different genetic markers appear to be important in other ethnic groups.

6. SS patients have increased risk of lymphoma due to IgM-κ B cells, and these lymphomas generally originate in the lacrimal/salivary glands or cervical lymph nodes.

At the DNA level, expansion of one or more B cell clones within salivary gland specimens of SS patients has been demonstrated by Southern blot methods.[73, 75]

Because these biopsy specimens did not fulfill histologic criteria for malignancy, this suggested that proliferation of certain "autoimmune" clones was responsible for the observed clonal expansion of cells corresponding to the 5 to 10 percent of B cells within the biopsy specimen. It is likely that such clonal expansions of B cells are the source of oligoclonal proteins frequently found in the sera or urine of these patients.[68]

Studies on cytokine production using complementary DNA (cDNA) produced from SS biopsies (and amplified using polymerase chain reaction methods) have indicated the presence of IL-2 and interferon-γ.[116] Also present in the SS biopsies were IL-1 and IL-10, produced predominantly by the salivary gland epithelial cells. Surprisingly, no transcripts for IL-4 and IL-5 transcription were noted in the cDNA produced by the SS gland in situ, but lymphocytes eluted from the SS gland could be stimulated in vitro to produce IL-4 and IL-5 mRNAs. These results suggest that T-lymphocytes in the SS gland express predominantly a "Th1-like" activity (i.e., interferon-γ, which may act to "suppress" the "Th2-like" cells (i.e., IL-4, IL-5) that are present in the gland.

The presence of interferon-γ and IL-1 may play a role in induction of HLA-DR antigens[113] and in the up-regulation of cell adhesive molecules (including integrins, selectins, and cadherins) in the SS gland.[117–119] The increased expression of these molecules on the endothelial cells and epithelial cells in SS biopsies may play an important role in antigen presentation and regulation of the lymphocytic repertoire.[120–122] For example, it may be possible to "break" tolerance to autoantigens when the relevant peptide is "presented" by MHC class II cells expressed on glandular epithelial cells. Cofactors that may contribute to the emergence of T cell autoimmune clones[123, 124] include "cross-priming" by other antigens (such as viral antigens), up-regulation of cellular adhesion molecules, and growth factors normally present in the salivary glands.

The initial inciting lesion in SS remains unknown. One candidate is Epstein-Barr virus (EBV).[125] In normal individuals, primary infection with EBV (infectious mononucleosis) involves the salivary glands, and EBV has a normal site of latency and reactivation in the salivary gland.[126, 127] Further, EBV can stimulate production of polyclonal antibodies and autoantibodies such as rheumatoid factor.[128] In biopsies of SS patients, an increased frequency of salivary gland epithelial cells expressing EBV-associated antigens and EBV DNA can be detected.[125] Increased EBV DNA can also be detected in SS biopsies by polymerase chain reaction[129] and by in situ hybridization methods.[130] Increased antibody responses to EBV early antigens can be detected in SS patients.[131] Taken together, these findings suggest a potential role for EBV in the pathogenesis of SS. The antibody titers, however, become progressively elevated late in the course of SS and suggest that viral reactivation could occur as a consequence of immune dysregulation in the salivary gland.[132] Because EBV is a strong stimulator of immune T cell responses,[133] reactivation of EBV within the SS salivary gland may serve as a perpetuating factor in salivary gland distribution.

Retroviruses have been suggested as a candidate in some SS patients. Talal and colleagues[134] found increased reactivity with retroviral protein p24 in a majority of SS sera, and a type A intracisternal particle was subsequently isolated from two salivary gland biopsies by Garry and associates.[135] Further studies are required to extend and confirm these interesting results.

CLINICAL MANAGEMENT OF THE PATIENT WITH SJÖGREN'S SYNDROME

The goals of SS treatment are to decrease symptoms and to prevent progression. Many SS patients have only mild, stable symptoms of dryness of eyes and mouth, whereas other patients have systemic manifestations including arthritis, myositis, nephritis, and vasculitis. Therefore, careful diagnosis of the "extent" and activity of the systemic autoimmune component of SS is crucial. In this regard, the overall diagnostic and therapeutic approach to the SS patient must be similar to that for the SLE or scleroderma patient. In addition, the rheumatologist must coordinate the clinical management of the SS patient with other specialists, including dentists, ophthalmologists, and anesthesiologists to prevent medical complications due to their sicca symptoms.

Treatment of Dry Eyes

A wide variety of artificial tear preparations are commercially available that differ in their preservatives and their viscosity. In evaluating the response to an artificial tear preparation, the key questions to the patient are: (1) How often is it administered? (2) Does it "burn" immediately after instillation into the eyes? (3) How long does relief last?

In some patients, the use of a particular artificial tear formula may lead to a burning sensation in the eye. This may be due to topical irritation resulting from the preservative used.[136] Thus, all preparations of artificial tears are not identical and interchangeable. Recognition of this problem can lead to the choice of another preparation with a different preservative. Also, several types of preservative-free artificial tears have been developed. If an artificial tear preparation is helpful but relief does not last long enough (e.g., drops must be instilled every hour), a preparation with greater viscosity might be introduced. In some patients, punctal occlusion might be employed by the ophthalmologist. A variety of different types of "plugs" can be tested to determine whether permanent punctal occlusion would be beneficial.

It is worth emphasizing that SS patients are at increased risk for corneal abrasions during anesthesia owing to the use of anticholinergic agents and the low humidity of the operating room. Therefore, ocular lubricants should be used in all SS patients during surgery and in the postoperative recovery room. The use of humidifiers is also helpful. In areas where the water is hard, distilled water should be used to prevent aerosolization of excessive minerals that may prove irritating to eyes and upper airways.

Treatment of Dry Mouth

Special toothpastes and oral gels introduced for the patient with dry mouth have proven helpful. In parts of the United States where the water supply is not fluoridated, the topical use of a neutral fluoride may help strengthen dental enamel and retard dental deterioration. A common problem in the SS patient is oral candidiasis, which may contribute to symptoms of painful mouth and decreased sense of taste. Treatment with topical nystatin or clotrimazole for 4 to 6 weeks may be required to alleviate symptoms and prevent recurrences. The onset of oral candidiasis often occurs during treatment with antibiotics for another indication. Angular cheilitis, also due to *Candida,* must be treated with a topical antifungal agent to prevent recurrence.

Treatment of Myalgias and Fatigue

It is always important to rule out hypothyroidism (which is relatively common in this population)[10] and to look for disordered sleep patterns, especially when the patient arises from bed in the morning with significant fatigue. Such sleep disorders may be due to polydipsia/polyuria or nocturnal myoclonus. The component of fatigue caused by active autoimmune disease is often difficult to assess. The elevation of erythrocyte sedimentation rate and total IgG, however, both provide an index of the activity of the disease process. In patients with objective evidence of a systemic inflammatory process (i.e., elevated acute-phase reactants) and subjective symptoms of arthralgias and myalgias, we have used hydroxychloroquine at a dose of 5 to 7 mg/kg.[137] Treated patients exhibited decreased acute-phase reactants, decreased symptoms, and little toxicity.

For arthralgias, NSAIDs may be used with particular caution, since they may precipitate renal or liver abnormalities. In addition, these agents may provoke esophageal injury[101] by adhering to the dryer walls of the esophagus in the absence of the normal salivary flow. To minimize this problem, the patient should take all medicines with a large amount of water while sitting upright.

Treatment of Other Systemic Manifestations

Systemic steroids are generally reserved for life-threatening vasculitis, hemolytic anemia, and pleuropericarditis resistant to NSAIDs.[93] As in SLE patients, other drugs may be used to help lower the dosage of steroids, including hydroxychloroquine (5 to 7 mg/kg/day) and azathioprine (50 to 150 mg/day). In some patients, chlorambucil (4 to 8 mg/day) has proved helpful. We have tried to avoid daily cyclophosphamide in SS patients because of its potential risk of carcinogenesis. When the use of cyclophosphamide is necessary for the treatment of vasculitis, we have administered this medication as an intravenous pulse (250 to 750 mg) at 1- to 3-month intervals.

SUMMARY

SS is a systemic autoimmune disease characterized by lymphocytic infiltrations of lacrimal and salivary glands. Extraglandular organs including skin, nerve, lung, and kidney may also be involved. These patients produce a variety of autoantibodies, including rheumatoid factor and antinuclear antibodies. In particular, they produce autoantibodies against ribonuclear proteins SS-A (Ro) and SS-B (La), which are involved in the transport and post-transcriptional modification of mRNA. Genetic factors, including HLA-DR3 and HLA-DQ, are predisposing to SS.

The precipitating cause of SS remains unknown, although viruses have been suggested as a potential cofactor in pathogenesis. The salivary gland and lacrimal gland are infiltrated by CD4[+] T cells. The ductal epithelial cells express HLA-DR[+] and DQ[+] antigens, thus permitting these epithelial cells to interact with CD4[+] T cells. The infiltrating T cells release cytokines that can perpetuate the immune process by altering blood vessels to become high endothelial venules, stimulating B cells to produce autoantibodies and promoting further influx of T cells.

At the present time, a great deal of confusion remains regarding the precise definition of SS. As a result, both patients and clinicians frequently have difficulty making a specific diagnosis and instituting a specific plan of therapy. Regardless of the diagnostic label, all patients with significant eye and mouth dryness should receive conservative therapy of tear replacement and intensive oral hygiene. Based on the evidence of systemic autoimmunity, additional therapies may prove beneficial in controlling the symptoms and progression of SS.

References

1. Mikulicz JH: Uber eine eigenartige symmetrische Erkrankung der Tranen und Mundspeicheldrusen. Beitr Chir Fortschr, 1892.
2. Sjögren HS: Zur kenntnis der keratoconjunctivitis sicca (Keratitis folliformis bei hypofunktion der tranendrusen). Acta Ophthalmol 2:1, 1933.
3. Gougerout A: Insuffisance progressive et atrophie des glandes salivaires et muqueuses de la bouche, des conjonctives (et parfois des muqueuses, nasale, laryngee, vulvaire). "Secheresse" de la bouche, des conjonctives, etc. Bull Soc Fr Derm Syph 32:376, 1925.
4. Morgan W, Castleman B: A clinicopathologic study of Mikulicz's disease. Am J Pathol 29:471, 1953.
5. Block KJ, Buchanan WW, Woho MJ, et al: Sjögren's syndrome: A clinical,

pathological and serological study of 62 cases. Medicine (Baltimore) 44:187, 1956.
6. Fox RI, Robinson CA, Curd JC, et al: Sjögren's syndrome: Proposed criteria for classification. Arthritis Rheum 29:577, 1986.
7. Daniels TE, Whitcher JP: Association of patterns of labial salivary gland inflammation with keratoconjunctivitis sicca: Analysis of 618 patients with suspected Sjögren's syndrome. Arthritis Rheum 37:869, 1994.
8. Vitali C, Bombardieri S, Moutsopoulos HM, et al: Preliminary criteria for the classification of Sjögren's syndrome—results of a prospective concerted action supported by the European community. Arthritis Rheum 36:340, 1993.
9. Fox R: Classification criteria for Sjögren's syndrome. Rheum Dis Clin North Am. 20:391, 1994.
10. Fritzler MJ, Pauls JD, Kinsella TD, et al: Antinuclear, anticytoplasmic, and anti-Sjögren's syndrome antigen A (SS-A/Ro) antibodies in female blood donors. Clin Immunol Immunopathol 36:120, 1985.
11. Martinez-Lavin M, Vaughan J, Tan E: Autoantibodies and the spectrum of Sjögren's syndrome. Ann Intern Med 91:185, 1979.
12. Pflugfelder SC, Wilhelmus KR, Osato MS, et al: The autoimmune nature of aqueous tear deficiency. Ophthalmology 93:1513, 1986.
13. Kontinen Y, Sorsa T, Kukkanen M, et al: Topology of innervation of labial salivary glands. J Rheumatol 19:30, 1992.
14. Konttinen YT, Hukkanen M, Kemppinen P, et al: Peptide-containing nerves in labial salivary glands in Sjögren's syndrome. Arthritis Rheum 35:815, 1992.
15. Lemp MA: Lacrimal hyposecretions. In Fraunfelder FT, Roy FH (eds): Current Ocular Therapy. Vol 2. Philadelphia, WB Saunders, 1985, p 429.
16. Lemp MA, Hamill JR Jr: Factors affecting tear film breakup in normal eyes. Arch Ophthalmol 89:103, 1973.
17. Holly FJ, Lemp MA: Tear physiology and dry eyes. Surv Ophthalmol 22:69, 1977.
18. Tsubota K: The importance of Schirmer test with nasal stimulation. Am J Ophthalmol 11:106, 1991.
19. Bridges A, Burns R: Acute iritis associated with Sjögren's syndrome. Arthritis Rheum 35:560, 1992.
20. Whaley K, Williamson J, Chisholm D, et al: Sjögren's syndrome: I. Sicca components. Q J Med 66:279, 1973.
21. Fox RI, Howell FV, Bone RC, et al: Primary Sjögren's syndrome: Clinical and immunopathologic features. Semin Arthritis Rheum 14:77, 1984.
22. Stevens WJ, Swartele FE, Empsten FA, et al: Use of the Saxon test as a measure of saliva production in a reference population of schoolchildren. Am J Dis Child 144:570, 1990.
23. Daniels TE: Labial salivary gland biopsy in Sjögren's syndrome. Arthritis Rheum 27:147, 1984.
24. Chisholm D, Waterhouse J, Mason D: Lymphocytic sialadenitis in the major and minor glands: A correlation in postmortem subjects. J Clin Pathol 23:690, 1970.
25. Daniels TE, Powell MR, Sylvester RA, et al: An evaluation of salivary scintigraphy in Sjögren's syndrome: Comparison with parotid sialography. Arthritis Rheum 22:809, 1979.
26. De Clerck LS, Corthouts R, Francx L, et al: Ultrasonography and computer tomography of the salivary glands in the evaluation of Sjögren's syndrome: Comparison with parotid sialography. J Rheumatol 15:1777, 1988.
27. Kawamura J, Taniguchi N, Itoh K, et al: Salivary gland echography in patients with Sjögren's syndrome. Arthritis Rheum 33:505, 1990.
28. Hunninghake G, Fauci A: Pulmonary involvement in the collagen vascular diseases. Am Rev Respir Dis 119:471, 1979.
29. Fairfax A, Haslam P, Pavia D, et al: Pulmonary disorders associated with Sjögren's syndrome. Q J Med 50:279, 1981.
30. Newball H, Brahim S: Chronic obstructive airway disease in patients with Sjögren's syndrome. Am Rev Respir Dis 115:295, 1977.
31. Siegal I, Fink G, Machtey I, et al: Pulmonary abnormalities in Sjögren's syndrome. Thorax 36:286, 1981.
32. Oxholm P, Bundgaard A, Madsen E, et al: Pulmonary function in patients with primary Sjögren's syndrome. Rheumatol Int 2:179, 1982.
33. Linstow M, Kriegbaum NJ, Backer V, et al: A follow-up study of pulmonary function in patients with primary Sjögren's syndrome. Rheumatol Int 10:47, 1990.
34. Kjellén G, Fransson SG, Lindström F, et al: Esophageal function, radiography, and dysphagia in Sjögren's syndrome. Dig Dis Sci 31:225, 1986.
35. Ramirez-Mata M, Pena-Acir F, Alarcon-Segovia D: Abnormal esophageal motility in Sjögren's syndrome. J Rheumatol 3:63, 1976.
36. Maury CPJ, Törnroth T, Teppo A-M: Arthropic gastritis in Sjögren's syndrome. Arthritis Rheum 28:388, 1985.
37. Jebavy M, Hradsky M, Herout V: Gastric biopsy in patients with Sjögren's syndrome. Z Med 16:930, 1961.
38. Maury C, Rasaneu V, Teppo A, et al: Serum pepsinogen I in rheumatic diseases: Reduced levels in Sjögren's syndrome. Arthritis Rheum 25:1059, 1982.
39. Fenster L, Buchanan W, Laster L, et al: Studies of pancreatic function in Sjögren's syndrome. Ann Intern Med 61:498, 1964.
40. Sundkvist G, Lindahl G, Koskinen P, et al: Pancreatic autoantibodies

and pancreatic function in Sjögren's syndrome. J Intern Med 229:61, 1991.

41. Webb J, Whaley K, MacSween R, et al: Liver disease in rheumatoid arthritis and Sjögren's syndrome. Ann Rheum Dis 34:70, 1975.

42. Fujikura S, Davis PA, Fox R, et al: Autoantibodies to purified mitochondrial 2 OXO acid dehydrogenases in patients with Sjögren's syndrome. J Rheumatol 17:1453, 1990.

43. Kyle R, Gleich G, Baynd E, et al: Benign hyperglobulemic purpura of Waldenström. Medicine (Baltimore) 50:113, 1971.

44. Alexander E, Provost TT: Sjögren's syndrome: Association of cutaneous vasculitis with central nervous system disease. Arch Dermatol 123:801, 1987.

45. Alexander EL, Arnett FC, Provost TT, et al: Sjögren's syndrome: Association of anti-Ro(SS-A) antibodies with vasculitis, hematologic abnormalities, and serologic hyperactivity. Ann Intern Med 98:155, 1983.

46. Whaley K, Webb J, McAvoy B, et al: Sjögren's syndrome: 2. Clinical associations and immunological phenomena. Q J Med 66:513, 1973.

47. Karsh J, Paulidis N, Weintraub B, et al: Thyroid disease in Sjögren's syndrome. Arthritis Rheum 23:1326, 1980.

48. Bailey RR, Swainson CP: Renal involvement in Sjögren's syndrome. N Z Med J 99:579, 1986.

49. Kahnm M, Merritt A, Orloff J: Renal concentrating defect in Sjögren's syndrome. Ann Intern Med 56:883, 1962.

50. Shioji R, Furuyama T, Onodera S, et al: Sjögren's syndrome and renal tubular acidosis. Am J Med 48:456, 1970.

51. Siamopoulos KC, Mavridis AK, Elisaf M, et al: Kidney involvement in primary Sjögren's syndrome. Scand J Rheumatol Suppl 43:156, 1986.

52. Tu W, Shearn M: Interstitial nephritis in Sjögren's syndrome. Ann Intern Med 69:1163, 1968.

53. Winer RL, Cohen AH, Sawhney AS, et al: Sjögren's syndrome with immune-complex tubulointerstitial renal disease. Clin Immunol Immunopathol 8:494, 1977.

54. Talal N, Zisman E, Schur P: Renal tubular acidosis, glomerulonephritis and immunologic factors in Sjögren's syndrome. Arthritis Rheum 11:774, 1968.

55. Kahn MA, Akhtar M, Taher SM: Membranoproliferative glomerulonephritis in a patient with primary Sjögren's syndrome: Report of a case with review of the literature. Am J Nephrol 8:235, 1988.

56. Moutosoupoulos HM, Balow JE, Lawley TJ, et al: Immune complex glomerulonephritis in sicca syndrome. Am J Med 64:955, 1978.

57. Moutsopoulos HM, Fauci AS: Immunoregulation in Sjögren's syndrome. J Clin Invest 65:519, 1980.

58. Aizawa H, Zawadzki ZA, Micolonghi TS, et al: Vasculitis and Sjögren's syndrome with IgA-IgG cryoglobulinemia terminating in immunoblastic sarcoma. Am J Med 67:160, 1979.

59. Palcoux JB, Janin-Mercier A, Campagne D, et al: Sjögren's syndrome and lupus erythematosus nephritis. Arch Dis Child 59:175, 1984.

60. Schwartzberg M, Burnstein SL, Calabro JJ, et al: The development of membranous glomerulonephritis in a patient with rheumatoid arthritis and Sjögren's syndrome. J Rheumatol 6:65, 1979.

61. Harrington TM, Bunch TW, Van Den Berg CJ: Renal tubular acidosis: A new look at treatment of musculoskeletal and renal disease. Mayo Clin Proc 58:354, 1983.

62. McCurdy RC, Cornwell GG III, DePratti VJ: Hyperglobulinemic renal tubular acidosis. Ann Intern Med 67:110, 1967.

63. Morris RC, Fudenberg HH: Impaired renal acidification in patients with hypergammaglobulinemia. Medicine (Baltimore) 46:57, 1967.

64. Runeberg L, Lahdevirta J, Collan Y, et al: Renal tubular dysfunction and hypergammaglobulinaemia: Electrolyte balance, electron microscopic and immunohistochemical studies. Acta Med Scand 189:341, 1971.

65. Wilson ID, Williams RC, Tobian L Jr: Renal tubular acidosis: Three cases with immunoglobulin abnormalities in the patients and their kindreds. Am J Med 43:356, 1967.

66. Starkebaum G, Dancey J, Arend W: Chronic neutropenia: Possible association with Sjögren's syndrome. J Rheumatol 8:679, 1982.

67. Fox RI, Chen PP, Carson DA, et al: Expression of a cross-reactive idiotype on rheumatoid factor in patients with Sjögren's syndrome. J Immunol 136:477, 1986.

68. Moutsopoulos HM, Costel R, Drosos AA, et al: Demonstration and identification of monoclonal proteins in the urine of patients with Sjögren's syndrome. Ann Rheum Dis 44:109, 1985.

69. Sugai T, Konda T, Shirasaka T, et al: Non-IgM monoclonal gammopathy in patients with Sjögren's syndrome. Am J Med 68:861, 1980.

70. Kassan SS, Thomas TL, Moutsopoulos HM, et al: Increased risk of lymphoma in sicca syndrome. Ann Intern Med 89:888, 1978.

71. Fox RI, Adamson TC III, Fong S, et al: Lymphocyte phenotype and function of pseudolymphomas associated with Sjögren's syndrome. J Clin Invest 72:52, 1983.

72. Schmid U, Helbron D, Lennert K: Development of malignant lymphoma in myoepithelial sialadenitis (Sjögren's syndrome). Virchows Arch 395:11, 1982.

73. Fishleder A, Tubbs R, Hesse B, et al: Immunoglobulin-gene re-

74. arrangement in benign lymphoepithelial lesions. N Engl J Med 316:1118, 1987.

74. Freimark B, Fox RI: Immunoglobulin gene rearrangements in Sjögren's syndrome (letter). N Engl J Med 317:1158, 1987.

75. Freimark B, Fantozzi R, Bone R, et al: Detection of clonally expanded salivary gland lymphocytes in Sjögren's syndrome. Arthritis Rheum 32:859, 1989.

76. Pisa E, Pisa P, Kang H, et al: High frequency of t(14;18) translocation in salivary gland lymphomas from Sjögren's syndrome patients. J Exp Med 174:1245, 1991.

77. Pierce P, Stern R, Jaffee R, et al: Immunoblastic sarcoma with features of Sjögren's syndrome and SLE in a patient with immunoblastic lymphadenopathy. Arthritis Rheum 22:911, 1979.

78. Lukes R, Tindle B: Immunoblastic lymphadenopathy. A hyperimmune entity resembling Hodgkin's disease. N Engl J Med 292:1, 1975.

79. Speight PM, Jordan R, Colloby P, et al: Early detection of lymphomas in Sjögren's syndrome by in situ hybridization for kappa and lambda light chain mRNA in labial salivary glands. Eur J Cancer B Oral Oncol 4:244, 1994.

80. Pablos JL, Carreira PE, Morillas L, et al: Clonally expanded lymphocytes in the minor salivary glands of Sjögren's syndrome patients without lymphoproliferative disease. Arthritis Rheum 37:1441, 1994.

81. Cruickshank AH: Benign lymphoepithelial salivary lesion to be distinguished from adenolymphoma. J Clin Pathol 18:391, 1965.

82. Alexander EL, Malinow K, Lejewski JE, et al: Primary Sjögren's syndrome with central nervous system disease mimicking multiple sclerosis. Ann Intern Med 104:323, 1986.

83. Alexander EL, Beall SS, Gordon B, et al: Magnetic resonance imaging of cerebral lesions in patients with the Sjögren's syndrome. Ann Intern Med 108:815, 1988.

84. Metz LM, Seland TP, Fritzler MJ: An analysis of the frequency of Sjögren's syndrome in a population of multiple sclerosis patients. J Clin Lab Immunol 30:121, 1989.

85. Sandberg-Wollheim M, Axell T, Hansen B, et al: Primary Sjögren's syndrome in patients with multiple sclerosis. Neurology 42:845, 1992.

86. Harley JB, Sestalk AL, Willia LG, et al: A model for disease heterogenecity in systemic lupus erythematosus. Arthritis Rheum 32:826, 1989.

87. Harley J, Reichlin M, Arnett F, et al: Gene interaction at HLA-DQ enhances autoantibody production in primary Sjögren's syndrome. Science 232:1145, 1986.

88. Lindstrom FD, Eriksson P, Tejle K, et al: IgG subclasses of anti-SS-A/Ro in patients with primary Sjögren's syndrome. Clin Immunol Immunopathol 73:358, 1994.

89. Scott J, Maddison P, Taylor P: Connective tissue disease, antibodies to ribonucleoprotein and congenital heart block. N Engl J Med 309:209, 1983.

90. Tan EM: Antinuclear antibodies: Diagnostic markers for autoimmune diseases and probes for cell biology. Adv Immunol 44:93, 1989.

91. Chan EKL, Pollard KM: Autoantibodies to ribonucleoprotein particles by immunoblotting. In Rose NR, Friedman H, Fahey JL (eds): Manual of Clinical Laboratory Immunology. American Society of Microbiology, 1992, p 755.

92. Ben-Chetrit E, Fox RI, Tan EM: Dissociation of immune responses to the SS-A (Ro) 52-kd and 60-kd polypeptides in systemic lupus erythematosus and Sjögren's syndrome. Arthritis Rheum 33:349, 1990.

93. Rader MD, Codding C, Reichlin M: Differences in the fine specificity of anti-Ro(SS-A) in relation to the presence of other precipitating autoantibodies. Arthritis Rheum 32:1563, 1989.

94. St Clair W, Burch J, Saitta M: Specificity of autoantibodies for recombinant 60-kd and 52-kd Ro autoantigens. Arthritis Rheum 37:1373, 1994.

95. Wolin SL, Steitz JA: The Ro small cytoplasmic ribonucleoproteins: Identification of the antigenic protein and its binding site on the Ro RNAs. Proc Natl Acad Sci U S A 81:1996, 1984.

96. Rader M, O'Brien C, Liu Y, et al: Heterogeneity of the Ro/SS antigen: Different molecular forms in lymphocytes and red blood cells. J Clin Invest 83:1293, 1989.

97. Itoh Y, Itoh K, Frank M: Protein heterogeneity in the human Ro/SS ribonucleoprotein. J Clin Invest 87:177, 1991.

98. Itoh Y, Kriett J, Reichlin M: Organ distribution of SS-A ribonuclear protein. Arthritis Rheum 33:1815, 1990.

99. Bachmann M, Pfeifer K, Schröder HC, et al: The nucleocytoplasmic shuttling of the La antigen in CV-1 cells. Mol Biol Rep 12:239, 1987.

100. Baboonian C, Venables PJW, Booth P, et al: Virus infection induces redistribution and membrane localization of the nuclear antigen La (SS-B): A possible mechanism for autoimmunity. Clin Exp Immunol 78:454, 1989.

101. Chan E, Andrade L: Antinuclear antibodies in Sjögren's syndrome. Rheum Clin North Am 18:561, 1992.

102. McCauliffe DP, Zappi E, Lieu T-S, et al: A human Ro/SS-A autoantigen is the homologue of calreticulin and is highly homologous with onchocercal RAL-1 antigen and an aplysia "memory molecule." J Clin Invest 86:332, 1990.

103. Rokeach L, Haselby J, Meilof J: Characterization of the autoantigen calreticulin. J Immunol 147:3031, 1991.

104. Troster H, Metzger TE, Semsei I, et al: One gene, two transcripts: Isolation of an alternative transcript encoding for the autoantigen La/SS-B from a cDNA library of a patient with primary Sjögren's syndrome. J Exp Med 180:2059, 1994.

105. Bachmann M, Falk D, Preuhs J: Occurrence of novel small RNAs with concomitant inhibition of cellular U small nuclear RNA synthesis in Vero cells infected with herpes simplex virus. J Gen Virol 67:2587, 1986.

106. Mann D, Moutsopoulos H: HLA-DR alloantigens in different subsets of patients with Sjögren's syndrome and in family members. Ann Rheum Dis 42:533, 1983.

107. Fei HM, Kang H-I, Scharf S, et al: Specific HLA-DQA and HLA-DRB1 alleles confer susceptibility to Sjögren's syndrome and autoantibody SS-B production. J Clin Lab Anal 5:382, 1991.

108. Kang H-I, Fei HM, Saito I, et al: Comparison of HLA class II genes in Caucasoid, Chinese, and Japanese patients with primary Sjögren's syndrome. J Immunol 150:3615, 1993.

109. Reveille JD: Molecular genetics of systemic lupus erythematosus and Sjögren's syndrome. Curr Opin Rheumatol 2:733, 1990.

110. Reveille JD, Macleod MJ, Whittington K, et al: Specific amino acid residues in the second hypervariable region of HLA-DQB1 chain genes promote the Ro (SS-A)/La (SS-B) autoantibody responses. J Immunol 146:3871, 1991.

111. Adamson TC III, Fox RI, Frisman DM, et al: Immunohistologic analysis of lymphoid infiltrates in primary Sjögren's syndrome using monoclonal antibodies. J Immunol 130:203, 1983.

112. Fox RI, Hugli TE, Lanier LL, et al: Salivary gland lymphocytes in primary Sjögren's syndrome lack lymphocyte subsets defined by Leu 7 and Leu 11 antigens. J Immunol 135:207, 1985.

113. Fox RI, Bumol T, Fantozzi R, et al: Expression of histocompatibility antigen HLA-DR by salivary gland epithelial cells in Sjögren's syndrome. Arthritis Rheum 29:1105, 1986.

114. Lindahl G, Hedfors E, Klöreskog L, et al: Epithelial HLA-DR expression and T-cell subsets in salivary glands in Sjögren's syndrome. Clin Exp Immunol 61:475, 1985.

115. MacSween RNM, Goudie RB, Anderson JR, et al: Occurrence of antibody to salivary duct epithelium in Sjögren's disease, rheumatoid arthritis, and other arthritides. Ann Rheum Dis 26:402, 1967.

116. Fox R, Kang H, Pisa E: Cytokine transcription in salivary gland biopsies of Sjögren's syndrome. J Immunol 151:132, 1994.

117. St Clair EW, Angellilo JC, Singer KH: Expression of cell-adhesion molecules in the salivary gland microenvironment of Sjögren's syndrome. Arthritis Rheum 35:62, 1992.

118. Edwards JC, Wilkinson LS, Speight P, et al: Vascular cell adhesion molecule 1 and alpha 4 and beta 1 integrins in lymphocyte aggregates in Sjögren's syndrome and rheumatoid arthritis. Ann Rheum Dis 52:806, 1993.

119. Aziz KE, Montanaro A, McCluskey P, et al: Vascular endothelial and lymphocyte adhesion molecules in minor salivary glands in Sjögren's syndrome. Clin Lab Immunol 37:39, 1992.

120. Springer TA: Adhesion receptors of the immune system. Nature 346:425, 1990.

121. Belmont M, Buyon J, Giorno R, et al: Upregulation of endothelial cell adhesion molecules characterizes disease activity in SLE. Arthritis Rheum 37:376, 1994.

122. Cyster J, Hartley S, Goodnow C: Competition for follicular niches excludes self-reactive cells from the recirculating B-cell repertoire. Nature 371:389, 1994.

123. Fatenejad S, Mamula MJ, Craft J: Role of intermolecular/intrastructural B- and T-cell determinants in the diversification of autoantibodies to ribonucleoprotein particles. Proc Natl Acad Sci U S A 90:12010, 1993.

124. Mamula M, Fatenejad S, Craft J: B cells process and present lupus autoantigens that initiate autoimmune T cell responses. J Immunol 152:1453, 1994.

125. Fox RI, Pearson G, Vaughan JH: Detection of Epstein-Barr virus–associated antigens and DNA in salivary gland biopsies from patients with Sjögren's syndrome. J Immunol 137:3162, 1986.

126. Zur Hausen H: Biochemical detection of the virus genome. In Epstein M, Achong B (eds): The Epstein-Barr Virus. New York, Springer-Verlag, 1979.

127. Miller G: Biology of Epstein-Barr virus. In Klein G (ed): Viral Oncology. New York, Raven Press, 1980.

128. Slaughter L, Carson DA, Jensen F, et al: In vitro effects of Epstein-Barr virus on peripheral blood mononuclear cells from patients with rheumatoid arthritis and normal subjects. J Exp Med 148:1429, 1978.

129. Saito I, Servenius B, Compton T, et al: Detection of Epstein-Barr virus DNA by polymerase chain reaction in blood and tissue biopsies from patients with Sjögren's syndrome. J Exp Med 169:2191, 1989.

130. Mariette X, Gozlan J, Clerc D, et al: Detection of Epstein-Barr virus DNA by in situ hybridization and polymerase chain reaction in salivary gland biopsy specimens from patients with Sjögren's syndrome. Am J Med 90:286, 1991.

131. Fox RI, Scott S, Houghton R, et al: Synthetic peptide derived from the Epstein-Barr virus encoded early diffuse antigen (EA-D) reactive with human antibodies. J Clin Lab Anal 1:140, 1987.

132. Fox RI: Epstein-Barr virus and human autoimmune diseases: Possibilities and pitfalls. J Virol Methods 241:1218, 1988.

133. Rickinson A, Moss D, Wallace L: Long-term T-cell-mediated immunity to EBV. Cancer Res 41:4216, 1981.

134. Talal N, Dauphinée M, Dang H, et al: Detection of serum antibodies to retroviral proteins in patients with primary Sjögren's syndrome. Arthritis Rheum 33:774, 1990.

135. Garry RF, Fermin CD, Hart DJ, et al: Detection of a human intracisternal A-type retroviral particle antigenically related to HIV. Science 250:1127, 1990.

136. Fox RI, Chan R, Michelson JB, et al: Beneficial effect of artificial tears made with autologous serum in patients with keratoconjunctivitis sicca. Arthritis Rheum 27:459, 1984.

137. Fox RI, Chan E, Benton L, et al: Treatment of primary Sjögren's syndrome with hydroxychloroquine. Am J Med 85:62, 1988.

Index

Note: Page numbers in *italics* refer to illustrations; page numbers followed by t indicate tables. Plate numbers refer to color plates at the beginning of each volume.

A band, in skeletal muscle, 78, *80*

Abbott 64077, anti-inflammatory effect of, 711

Abdomen, pain in, in rheumatic fever, 1232
  in systemic lupus erythematosus, 1036
  wall of, muscles of, reflex testing of, 406t

Abrasion arthroplasty, for osteoarthritis, 693, *694, 695*

Abscess, of skeletal muscle, tuberculous, 1454
  of spine, postsurgical, magnetic resonance imaging of, *637, 637*
  tuberculous, 1451

Absorptiometry, in osteoporosis, 1565–1566, *1566*, 1567t

Accessory nerve, disorders of, muscle tests for, 399t

Acetabulum. See also *Hip.*
  bone grafting to, in hip replacement, 1797, *1798*
  in resistance to compression, 91, *91*
  labrum of, disorders of, and pain, 470
  positioning of, in radiography, after arthroplasty, 1785–1788, *1785–1788*
  protrusion of, in rheumatoid arthritis, 1724, *1725*

Acetaminophen, for osteoarthritis, 1398
  of hip, 1852, *1852*
  toxicity of, to liver, 715

Acetylcholine, in skeletal muscle contraction, 81
  receptors of, aggregation of, agrin and, 44
  in skeletal muscle, 79t

Achilles bursitis, and pain, 486
  glucocorticoid injection for, 598, 606

Achilles tendon, in ankylosing spondylitis, imaging of, *657, 657*
  inflammation of, and pain, 486
  glucocorticoid injection for, 598, 606
  magnetic resonance imaging of, 642
  tophi of, in gout, 1316, *1318*

Achondroplasia, 1555

Acid maltase deficiency, and myopathy, 1192

Acne-pustulosis-hyperostosis-osteitis syndrome, vs. rheumatoid arthritis, 903

Acquired immunodeficiency syndrome, 1265–1278. See also *Human immunodeficiency virus (HIV) infection.*

Acrodermatitis enteropathica, in Lyme disease, 1466

Acromegaly, 1506–1508, *1507*, 1507t
  imaging of, 679, *679, 680*
  osteoarthritis with, 385

Acromioclavicular joint. See also *Shoulder.*

Acromioclavicular joint *(Continued)*
  arthritis of, 358, 428
  disorders of, in sports medicine, 548–549, *549*
  examination of, 358

Acromioplasty, for rotator cuff impingement, 424, *425*

Acropachy, thyroid, 1504, *1504*
  with hypertrophic osteoarthropathy, 1516

Actin, in neutrophil activation, 177
  in neutrophil migration, 150
  in skeletal muscle, 78, 79, 79t, *81*, Plate 1

α-Actinin, in skeletal muscle, 79t

Actinomycosis, spinal, and low back pain, 451

Activities of daily living, in rheumatic disease, in assessment, 1619–1620
  in rheumatoid arthritis, in assessment, 926, 926t
  instruction in, 938

Acute-phase response, in inflammation, 699–701, *700*, 700t
  cytokines in, 273–274

Acyl-CoA dehydrogenase deficiency, and hyperuricemia, 1338

Addison's disease, 1506

Addressins, in lymphocyte homing, in inflammatory response, 191–192

Adductor muscles, of thigh, reflex testing of, 406t

Adenosine, in neutrophil function, 149

Adenosine deaminase, deficiency of, in severe combined immunodeficiency, 1295
  intrauterine diagnosis of, 1299

Adenosine diphosphate, in skeletal muscle contraction, 82, *82*

Adenosine triphosphatase, in skeletal muscle, 79t

Adenosine triphosphate, degradation of, in hyperuricemia, *1337*, 1337–1338
  in skeletal muscle contraction, 82, *82*

Adenovirus infection, and arthritis, 1480–1481

Adhesion molecules, 303–317. See also specific types, e.g., *Selectins.*
  expression of, cytokines and, 268–269
  extracellular matrix components as, 43
  in inflammation, in leukocyte homing, 314–316
  therapeutic targeting of, 316–317
  in rheumatoid arthritis, 873t, 873–874, *874*
  in synovial lining, 12, *13*
  in synovial vasculature, *14*, 14–15
  inhibition of, glucocorticoids and, 790
  on myeloid cells, 135t

Adhesion molecules *(Continued)*
  types of, 303, *304, 305*, Plate 2

Adhesion receptors, in lymphocyte migration, 120t, 120–121, 121t

Adhesive capsulitis, and pain, 431–432
  arthrography of, 417, *417*
  glucocorticoids for, 596
  in hyperthyroidism, 1505
  with calcific tendinitis, 425, *426*

Adrenal gland, disorders of, in antiphospholipid syndrome, 1061
  in Addison's disease, 1506
  in cortisol secretion, 787–788
  suppression of, exogenous glucocorticoids and, 796
  in Cushing's syndrome, 1506

β-Adrenergic blockers, interactions of, with nonsteroidal anti-inflammatory drugs, 719t, 720

Adrenocorticotropic hormone, for gout, with acute arthritis, 1343–1344
  in cortisol secretion, 787

Adult respiratory distress syndrome, leukotrienes in, 297t

Advil. See *Ibuprofen.*

Agammaglobulinemia, X-linked, 1284t, 1285t, 1286–1288, *1287*

Aggrecan, in extracellular matrix, *39, 42*, 45

Aging. See also *Elderly.*
  and osteoarthritis, 1376
  and osteoporosis, 1563–1564
  of articular cartilage, 10–11
  rheumatic disease in, *541*, 541–544, 543t

Agrin, in extracellular matrix, 44

AIDS, 1265–1278. See also *Human immunodeficiency virus (HIV) infection.*

Alanine aminotransferase, blood level of, after methotrexate therapy, for rheumatoid arthritis, 1864t, 1864–1866, 1865t

Albright's hereditary osteodystrophy, 1499, 1502–1503, *1503*

Albumin, in inflammation, in acute-phase response, 699, *700*
  in renal disorders, and binding of nonsteroidal anti-inflammatory drugs, 721

Alcohol, use of, and gout, 1319, 1346
  and osteonecrosis, 1584

Alendronate, for osteoporosis, 1569t, 1570
  for Paget's disease of bone, 1577

Aleve. See *Naproxen.*

Alkaline phosphatase, blood level of, after methotrexate therapy, for rheumatoid arthritis, 1864t, 1864–1866, 1865t
  in bone mineralization, 64
  in Paget's disease, of bone, 1575

Alkaptonuria (ochronosis), imaging in, 676
  synovial biopsy in, 622, *622*, Plate 10
  synovial fluid analysis in, 612, *613*,
    Plate 7
Alkylating agents, in immunosuppression,
    for non-neoplastic diseases, *810*,
    810–813, 811t, 812t, 823t
Alleles. See *Genetics.*
Allergic angiitis, with granulomatosis
    (Churg-Strauss syndrome),
    1097–1099
  in children, 1261
  in human immunodeficiency virus in-
    fection, 1278
  pathogenesis of, 1081–1082, *1084*
  skin lesions in, 503
Allergic granulomatosis, in children, 1261
Allergic purpura (Henoch-Schönlein
    purpura), 503, *1105*, 1105–1106
  in children, 1242t, *1258*, 1258–1259
  in human immunodeficiency virus infec-
    tion, 1278
Allergic rhinitis, leukotrienes in, 297t
Allergy, to food, and arthritis, 531–532
Allopurinol, for hyperuricemia, *829–831*,
    829–833, 832t, *1344*, 1344–1346, 1345t
Alopecia, antimalarial drugs and, 754–755
  cyclophosphamide and, 812–813
  in common variable immunodeficiency,
    1288, *1288*
  in lupus erythematosus, 500, 1036
Alpha-actinin, in skeletal muscle, 79t
Alpha$_1$-antichymotrypsin, 328, 329t
Alpha$_1$-antiplasmin, as protease inhibitor,
    328, 329t
Alpha$_2$-antiplasmin, 328, 329t
Alpha$_1$-antitrypsin, deficiency of, and
    emphysema, 34–35
Alpha-granules, in platelets, 176, 177t
Alphavirus infection, and arthritis,
    1478–1479
Alport's syndrome, 1556
  collagen gene defect in, 31
ALT, blood level of, after methotrexate
    therapy, for rheumatoid arthritis,
    1864t, 1864–1866, 1865t
Alveolar cell carcinoma, scleroderma and,
    1529, 1531t
Alzheimer's disease, amyloid fibrils in,
    1410
American Rheumatism Association index,
    in rheumatoid arthritis, 925, 925t
Amethopterin. See *Methotrexate.*
Amino acids, in collagen synthesis, *24*,
    25–28
  in glycine substition, 28, *29, 30*
  in elastin, 31–33, *34*
5-Aminoimidazole-4-carboxamide
    ribonucleotide transformylase,
    methotrexate inhibition of, 771, *772*,
    773
Aminopterin, structure of, 771, *772*
4-Aminoquinolines. See *Antimalarial drugs.*
5-Aminosalicylic acid, 741, *741*
Amitriptyline, for neuropathy, in
    amyloidosis, 1416t
Amoxicillin, for Lyme disease, 1469, 1469t
  with clavulanic acid, for *Neisseria* infec-
    tion, 1446
  with dental procedures, after hip
    arthroplasty, 1730–1731
Ampicillin, for *Neisseria* infection, 1446
  metabolism of, probenecid and, 836
Amyloid A, serum, in inflammation, 699,
    700, 701

Amyloid A *(Continued)*
  production of, cytokines and, 273
Amyloidosis, 1409–1415
  classification of, 1409, 1410t
  clinical features of, 1412–1415, *1413, 1414*
  diagnosis of, 1411, *1412, 1413*
  imaging of, 679, *680*
  of endocrine glands, 1510
  pathology of, 1411
  pauciarticular arthropathy in, 384
  precursor proteins in, 1409–1411, 1410t,
    1411
  skin lesions in, 507–508, *508*
  synovial biopsy in, 622, *622*, Plate 10
  treatment of, 1412–1415, 1415t, 1416t
  vs. rheumatoid arthritis, 904
Amyotrophic lateral sclerosis, vs.
    inflammatory muscle disease, 1190
Analgesia, postoperative, 1644–1645
Anaphylactoid purpura (Henoch-Schönlein
    purpura), 503, *1105*, 1105–1106
  in children, 1242t, *1258*, 1258–1259
  in human immunodeficiency virus infec-
    tion, 1278
Anaphylaxis, nonsteroidal anti-
    inflammatory drugs and, 717
Anaprox. See *Naproxen.*
Androgens, for systemic lupus
    erythematosus, 1054
  in bone cell metabolism, 60–61
  in musculoskeletal disorders, 1509–1510
Anemia, hemolytic, in systemic lupus
    erythematosus, 1030t, 1035
  in juvenile rheumatoid arthritis, 1212–
    1213
  in mixed connective tissue disease, 1073
  in rheumatic fever, 1233
  in rheumatoid arthritis, 919
  sickle cell, 1493–1497. See also *Sickle cell
    anemia.*
Anesthesia, 1640–1645
  airway management in, 1640–1641,
    1641t, *1642*
  extubation after, 1641–1642, *1642*
  in arthroplasty, in juvenile rheumatoid
    arthritis, 1781
    of hip, 1729–1730
      postoperative injection for, with
        arthrographic contrast agent,
        1810
  in rheumatic disease, comorbid condi-
    tions with, 1640, 1641t
  in shoulder pain, in diagnosis, 420–422
  intraoperative management of, 1643–
    1644
  local, intra-articular injection for, with
    glucocorticoids, 594–595, 599
  regional, 1642–1643
Aneurysms, aortic, collagen gene defect
    and, 31, 33t
  in giant cell arteritis, 1127
  retroperitoneal fibrosis with, 1166
  in Kawasaki disease, in children, 1256,
    1257
Angiitis, allergic, with granulomatosis
    (Churg-Strauss syndrome),
    1097–1099
  in children, 1261
  in human immunodeficiency virus
    infection, 1278
  pathogenesis of, 1081–1082, *1084*
  skin lesions in, 503
  necrotizing, paraneoplastic, 1524, 1527t
    skin lesions in, 502t, 502–504, *503*,
      Plate 5

Angiitis *(Continued)*
  of central nervous system, in human im-
    munodeficiency virus infection, 1278
    isolated, 1090–1091
Angina, and shoulder pain, 435
Angiogenesis, cytokines in, 274
  in inflammatory response, 184
    endothelial cells and, 183–184, 193–
      194, 194t
  in rheumatoid arthritis, 869, *872*, 872–
    873
Angiography, in giant cell arteritis, 1127,
    1127, 1129
  in Takayasu's arteritis, 1089, *1090*
  in vasculitis, 1086, 1086t, 1087
Angioimmunoblastic lymphadenopathy,
    vs. rheumatoid arthritis, 903
Angioplasty, coronary, restenosis after, in
    antiphospholipid syndrome,
    1060–1061
Angiotensin, in synovial vasculature, 13,
    14, *14*
Angiotensin-converting enzyme, in
    sarcoidosis, 1418
  inhibitors of, for hypertension, in
    Takayasu's arteritis, 1090
  interactions of, with nonsteroidal anti-
    inflammatory drugs, 719t, 720
Ankle, anatomy of, *369*, 369–370
  arthritis in, monoarticular, differential di-
    agnosis of, 373t
  arthrocentesis of, 600–601, *601*
  arthrodesis of, 1761–1763, *1762*
  arthroplasty of, 1761, 1763–1766
    radiography of, 1836, *1838–1840*
  Charcot's arthropathy of, in diabetes,
    1500, 1501
  computed tomography of, *629*, 630, *630*
  debridement of, 1761, 1763, *1763–1765*
  disorders of, causes of, 1759–1760, *1760*
  diagnosis of, 1760
  in ankylosing spondylitis, imaging of,
    656–657, *657*
  in Reiter's syndrome, imaging of, 660
    with human immunodeficiency virus
      infection, 1269
  in rheumatoid arthritis, 481–483, *915*,
    915–916, 1760
    imaging of, 649–650
  injuries of, in sports medicine, 560, *561*
  magnetic resonance imaging of, 481,
    641–642
  motion of, in lifting, 92, *93*
  orthoses for, *1626, 1627*, 1760–1761
  osteoarthritis of, arthroscopic surgery in,
    694
  pain in, 479–487
    gout and, 484–485
    imaging in, 481
    neuropathic osteoarthropathy and, 485
    osteoarthritis and, 483, 484
    physical examination in, 480–481
    rheumatoid arthritis and, 481–483
    spondyloarthropathy and, 486
    tendinitis and, 486
  physical examination of, 370
Ankylosing hyperostosis (diffuse
    idiopathic skeletal hyperostosis), and
    low back pain, 450
  imaging of, 668–669, *669, 670*
  in diabetes mellitus, 1501
  vs. ankylosing spondylitis, 655, 657
  vs. osteoarthritis, 1391–1392
Ankylosing spondylitis, 969–981
  and bone loss, 1565

Ankylosing spondylitis (Continued)
  and low back pain, 450, 973, 973t
  arthroplasty in, evaluation for, 1635–1636
  clinical features of, 973t, 973–975, 975
  diagnosis of, 970, 971t, 977, 977–978, 978
  diclofenac for, 734
  epidemiology of, 971–973, 972, 972t, 973t
  fenamates for, 733
  gender differences in, 978
  gout with, 1320
  historical aspects of, 969
  human leukocyte antigens in, 217t, 217–218, 218t, 224, 224t
  imaging of, 654–657, 654–657, 975, 975–977, 976t
  juvenile-onset, imaging of, 653
    psychosocial impact of, 536
  management of, 979–981, 980t
  monitoring of, 979, 979t
  nonsteroidal anti-inflammatory drugs for, 736, 980
  ocular disorders in, 494, 974
  of cervical spine, 1718–1720, 1719, 1720
  of foot, 486
  pathology of, 973
  physical examination in, 975–976
  polyarthritis with, 384
  prognosis of, 978–979
  rehabilitation in, exercise in, 1622–1623
  surgery for, anesthesia in, 1643
  synovial biopsy in, 620–621
  tolmetin for, 733
  vs. rheumatoid arthritis, 903
Anlage, in bone development, 63–64
Annexin I, in neutrophilic secretion, 151
Annulus fibrosus, of intervertebral discs, development of, 5
Ansaid (flurbiprofen), 729t, 734, 734
  in cyclooxygenase pathway inhibition, 709
Anserine bursitis, glucocorticoids for, 597, 605
Anterior interosseous nerve syndrome, 571–572, 572
Anterior tarsal tunnel syndrome, 579
Antibiotic(s), for bacterial arthritis, 1443, 1443–1444
  for knee infection, after arthroplasty, 1754
  for Lyme disease, 1468–1470, 1469t
    with fatigue and fibromyalgia, 1872–1878, 1874t–1877t
  for postenteritic reactive arthritis, 1010, 1010
  for Reiter's syndrome, 994–995, 995t
  prophylactic use of, with prosthetic joint replacement, 1440, 1441t
  with hip arthroplasty, 1730–1731
Antibiotic proteins, in neutrophils, 147
Antibodies. See also specific types, e.g., Antinuclear antibodies.
  deficiency disorders of, and immunodeficiency, 1285t, 1285–1292, 1287, 1288
    treatment of, 1300–1301
    with near-normal immunoglobulins, 1285t, 1291–1292
Anticardiolipin syndrome. See Antiphospholipid syndrome.
Anti-CD18 antibodies, in anti-inflammatory treatment, 317
Anti-CD54 antibodies, in anti-inflammatory treatment, 317
Anti-centromere antibodies, in scleroderma, 258, 258t, 1143

α_1-Antichymotrypsin, 328, 329t
Anticoagulant(s), aspirin as, 713
  for thrombosis, in antiphospholipid syndrome, 1062
    in systemic lupus erythematosus, 1051
  interactions of, with nonsteroidal anti-inflammatory drugs, 719t, 720
  with arthroplasty, of hip, 1730
    of knee, 1751
Anti-DNA antibodies, in systemic lupus erythematosus, 255t, 255–256, 1021, 1022, 1023, 1024, 1024t, 1031, 1031t
  tests for, 254–255
Anti-DNA topoisomerase I, in scleroderma, 258t, 258–259, 1143
Antiendothelial antibodies, in vasculitis, 1081, 1081
Anti-fibrillarin antibodies, in inflammatory muscle diseases, 261
  in scleroderma, 258t, 259
Antigen-presenting cells, in T cell activation, 114–117, 115
  in rheumatoid arthritis, 859, 859
  mononuclear phagocytes as, 141–143, 142
Antigens, recognition of, by B cells, 106–112, 108, 109
  by T cells, 112
Antihistamines, interaction of, with nonsteroidal anti-inflammatory drugs, 720t
Anti-histone antibodies, in systemic lupus erythematosus, 255t, 256
Anti-hUBF antibodies, in scleroderma, 258t, 259
Antihyperuricemic drugs, 829–837. See also Gout and Hyperuricemia.
Anti-inflammatory drugs, nonsteroidal. See Nonsteroidal anti-inflammatory drugs.
Anti-kinetochore (anti-centromere) antibodies, in scleroderma, 258, 258t, 1143
Anti-Ku antibodies, in systemic lupus erythematosus, 255t, 256
Anti-La antibodies, in Sjögren's syndrome, 261, 261t
  in systemic lupus erythematosus, 255t, 257
Anti-MA-I antibodies, in Sjögren's syndrome, 261, 261t
Antimalarial drugs. See also specific agents, e.g., Hydroxychloroquine.
  adverse effects of, 754–755, 755t
  for calcium pyrophosphate deposition disease, 754
  for dermatomyositis, in children, 754
  for eosinophilic fasciitis, 754
  for lupus erythematosus, discoid, 749–750
    systemic, 749–750, 1042–1043, 1043t
  for osteoarthritis, erosive, 754
  for palindromic rheumatism, 754
  for psoriatic arthritis, 753, 756
  for rheumatic disease, 747–756
    historical aspects of, 747
    mechanisms of action of, 748t, 748–749
    pharmacokinetics of, 748
    structure of, 747, 747–748
  for rheumatoid arthritis, 750–753, 751t, 752t, 941, 946, 947
    vs. gold, 761, 761
  for Sjögren's syndrome, 754
  guidelines for use of, 756
Anti-Mi-2 antibodies, in inflammatory muscle diseases, 260, 260t

Antineutrophil cytoplasmic antibodies, in vasculitis, 1081, 1081–1083
  in Wegener's granulomatosis, 1099, 1101–1102
Anti-NOR 90 antibodies, in scleroderma, 258t, 259
Antinuclear antibodies, 250–262
  diagnostic characteristics of, 250, 251t
  diseases associated with, 250, 250t, 255–262
  historical aspects of, 250
  in clinical evaluation, 262, 262
  in inflammatory muscle diseases, 259–261, 260t
  in juvenile rheumatoid arthritis, 1213
  in scleroderma, 258t, 258–259
  in Sjögren's syndrome, 963
  in synovial fluid analysis, 617
  in systemic lupus erythematosus, 255t, 255–258, 1031t, 1031–1032
    in children, 1242
    in diagnosis, 347, 348
  testing for, 1885
    anti-DNA antibodies in, 254–255
    counterimmunoelectrophoresis in, 253
    enzyme-linked immunosorbent assay in, 253
    immunoblotting in, 254
    immunodiffusion in, 252–253, 253, 253t
    immunofluorescence in, 250–252, 252
    immunoprecipitation in, 253–254, 254
Antioxidants, trace metals as, 524–526
  vitamins as, 523–524
Anti-PCNA antibodies, in systemic lupus erythematosus, 255t, 256
Anti-p80-coilin antibodies, in Sjögren's syndrome, 261, 261t
Antiphospholipid antibodies, in pregnancy, and fetal loss, 1051, 1052t, 1061–1063
Antiphospholipid syndrome, 1057–1063
  antibodies in, detection of, 1057–1058
    mechanism of action of, 1058
  classification of, 1057, 1057t, 1058
  clinical features of, 1058–1062, 1059, 1060
  eicosanoid pathway inhibition in, 298
  genetics in, 1058
  historical aspects of, 1057
  management of, 1062–1063
  pathology of, 1058
  with cancer, 1526, 1527t
α_2-Antiplasmin, 328, 329t
Antiplatelet drugs, with glucocorticoids, for polyarteritis, 1096
Anti-PM-Scl antibodies, in inflammatory muscle diseases, 260t, 260–261
  in scleroderma, 258t, 259
Antiribonucleoprotein antibodies, in inflammatory muscle diseases, 260, 260t
  in mixed connective tissue disease, 1067–1068, 1069
  in Sjögren's syndrome, 257, 261, 261t
  in systemic lupus erythematosus, 255, 255t, 257–258
Anti-ribosome antibodies, in systemic lupus erythematosus, 255t, 257–258
Anti-RNA antibodies, in systemic lupus erythematosus, 258
Anti-RNAP antibodies, in scleroderma, 258t, 259
  in systemic lupus erythematosus, 256
Anti-Ro antibodies, in Sjögren's syndrome, 261, 261t
  in systemic lupus erythematosus, 255t, 257

Anti-Scl-70 antibodies, in scleroderma, 258t, 258–259, 1143
Anti-snRNP antibodies, in inflammatory muscle diseases, 260, 260t
Anti-SRP antibodies, in inflammatory muscle diseases, 260
Anti-synthetase antibodies, in inflammatory muscle diseases, 259–260, 260t
Anti–T cell antibodies, for rheumatoid arthritis, 860
Anti-Th snoRNP antibodies, in scleroderma, 258t, 259
Anti-topoisomerase I antibodies, in scleroderma, 258t, 258–259, 1143
α_1-Antitrypsin, as proteinase inhibitor, 328, 329t
    deficiency of, and emphysema, 34–35
Anti–tumor necrosis factor-α, for rheumatoid arthritis, 945
Anti-U3 snoRNP antibodies, in inflammatory muscle diseases, 261
    in scleroderma, 258t, 259
Aorta, aneurysms of, collagen gene defect and, 31, 33t
    in giant cell arteritis, 1127
    in Kawasaki disease, 1256, 1257
    retroperitoneal fibrosis with, 1166
    constitutents of, 23t, 24
    in Marfan syndrome, 1552–1553
    in relapsing polychondritis, 1406, 1407
Aortic arch, in Takayasu's arteritis, 1088–1090, 1090
Aortic regurgitation, in Reiter's syndrome, 990
Aortic stenosis, supravalvular, 1554
Aortic valve, lesions of, granulomatous, in rheumatoid arthritis, 922
    in antiphospholipid syndrome, 1060, 1060
Aortitis, granulomatous, in rheumatoid arthritis, 921–922
    in Cogan's syndrome, 1112, 1113
    retroperitoneal fibrosis with, 1166
Apatite. See Hydroxyapatite.
Apheresis, for scleroderma, 1152
    for systemic lupus erythematosus, 1053
    in antiphospholipid syndrome, 1062
    therapeutic, 817–818
Aply grind test, for meniscal tears, 368
Apnea, in sleep, in fibromyalgia syndrome, 516, 517
Apophyseal joints, osteoarthritis of, imaging of, 668
Apprehension test, in shoulder examination, in sports medicine, 548
Aprotinin, 329, 329t
Arachidonic acid, in eicosanoid synthesis, 287–288, 527, 527, 528, 529
    in cyclooxygenase pathways, 288, 289
    in lipoxygenase pathways, 291, 292, 292, 294, 295
    in mast cell mediation, 169, 169
    in neutrophil function, 149, 149
    in neutrophil metabolism, 153–154
    metabolites of, in synovial fluid, in rheumatoid arthritis, 886–887
        inhibition of, nonsteroidal anti-inflammatory drugs in, 708–711, 709, 710
Arachnodactyly, in Marfan syndrome, 1552, 1553
Aredia (pamidronate), for osteoporosis, 1571
    for Paget's disease of bone, 1576–1577

Arginine vasopressin, for hemophilia, 1489
Aristospan. See Triamcinolone.
Arrowhead phalanges, in acromegaly, 679, 679
Arteries, rupture of, in Ehlers-Danlos syndrome, 1550
Arteriography, in polyarteritis, 1095, 1095
Arteriosclerosis, glucocorticoids and, 795
    gout with, 1319
Arteriovenous malformation, synovial, 1598, 1599
Arteritis, and pulmonary hypertension, in rheumatoid arthritis, 921
    coronary, in rheumatoid arthritis, 921
    giant cell, 1123–1130. See also Giant cell arteritis.
    granulomatous, in children, 1260–1261
    paraneoplastic, 1525, 1527t
    polyarteritis, 1091–1097. See also Polyarteritis.
    Takayasu's, 1088–1090, 1090
        in children, 1260
        pathogenesis of, 1084, 1084
Arthralgia, causes of, 1882–1883
    in systemic lupus erythematosus, conservative management of, 1040–1041
    vs. arthritis, polyarticular, 386
Arthritis. See also specific joints, e.g., Knee.
    and disability, prevalence of, 1619
    apatite deposition and, acute, 1363, 1364
        familial, 1364–1365
    bacterial, 1435–1447. See also Bacterial arthritis.
    calcium pyrophosphate deposition in, 1352–1362. See also Calcium pyrophosphate deposition disease.
    collagen-induced, vs. rheumatoid arthritis, 857–858
    degenerative, 1369–1401. See also Osteoarthritis.
    enteropathic, 1006–1013. See also Enteropathic arthritis.
    extracellular matrix degradation in, proteinases in, 331–333, 332t
    food allergy and, 531–532
    in common variable immunodeficiency, 1288, 1288
    in gout, acute, 1314–1315, 1338–1340
        management of, 1342–1344
        colchicine for, 713
    in Henoch-Schönlein purpura, 1258–1259
    in mixed connective tissue disease, 1069, 1069, 1070
    in polychondritis, relapsing, 1406
    in Reiter's syndrome. See Reiter's syndrome.
    in rheumatic fever, 992, 1230–1231, 1234
    in systemic lupus erythematosus, 1030t, 1032, 1040–1041
    in X-linked agammaglobulinemia, 1287
    infectious, 1435–1482
        vs. rheumatoid arthritis, 906–907
    interleukins in, 275–276, 279
    juvenile rheumatoid, 1207–1222. See also Juvenile rheumatoid arthritis.
    mast cells in, 171–172
    monarticular, 371–379
        acute, 376–378
        chronic inflammatory, 378
        crystal-induced, 377
        diagnosis of, 378–379
            differential, 371–373, 372t, 373t
        enteropathic, 377
        history in, 373–376, 374t–375t
        noninflammatory, 378

Arthritis (Continued)
    pauciarticular, peripheral, causes of, 383–384, 384
    plain radiographic series in, 626, 627t
    polyarticular. See Polyarthritis.
    psoriatic, 999–1004. See also Psoriatic arthritis.
    psychosocial impact of, in adolescents, 535–536
        in children, 535
    pyogenic, paraneoplastic, 1526, 1527t
    reactive, vs. rheumatoid arthritis, 903
    rehabilitation in, 1619–1630. See also Rehabilitation.
    rheumatoid, 851–966. See also Rheumatoid arthritis.
    septic. See Septic arthritis.
    signs of, in physical examination, 355–356
    surgery for, evaluation for, 1634–1637
        goals of, 1633–1634
        management after, 1637–1638
        patient selection for, 1637
    synovectomy in, arthroscopic, 687–688, 689
    tumor necrosis factor-α in, 276
    viral, 1473–1482. See also Viral infection, and arthritis.
Arthritis mutilans, 361, 657, 1000, 1000, 1002t
    arthrodesis in, 1661
Arthritis robustus, 901–902
Arthrocentesis, in rheumatoid arthritis, early, 902
    of ankle, 600–601, 601
    of elbow, 602, 602
    of first carpometacarpal joint, 601, 602
    of hip, 602–603, 603
    of interphalangeal joints, of fingers, 601–602, 602
    of knee, 600, 600
    of metacarpophalangeal joints, 601–602, 602
    of metatarsophalangeal joints, 602
    of shoulder, 600, 601
    of temporomandibular joint, 603, 603
    of toes, 602
    of wrist, 601, 602
    precautions in, 593
    technique of, 599–600
        for synovial fluid analysis, 609–610
Arthrochalasis multiplex congenita, 1549, 1549–1550
Arthrodesis, in arthritis mutilans, 1661
    of ankle, 1761–1763, 1762
    of foot, 1767, 1768, 1769, 1769, 1770
    of hip, 1727
    of knee, in osteoarthritis, 1739
    of shoulder, 1707
    of wrist, in rheumatoid arthritis, 1654
Arthrofibrosis, and knee pain, 464
Arthrography, indications for, 627
    of hip, 468
        after arthroplasty, anesthetic injection with, 1810
        infection in, 1805–1807, 1807t
        loosening in, 1805–1809, 1806, 1807t, 1808, 1808t, 1809
    of knee, 460, 460
        after arthroplasty, loosening in, 1824–1826
    of rotator cuff, in sports medicine, 551, 551
    of shoulder, painful, 416, 416–417, 417, 422, 422t

Arthroplasty, intra-articular glucocorticoid injection after, 599
  of ankle, 1761, 1763–1766
    radiography of, 1836, *1838–1840*
  of elbow, 1682–1690. See also *Elbow.*
  of femoral head, for osteonecrosis, 1588–1589
  of fingers, in rheumatoid arthritis, 1658–1661, *1659*
  of hip, 1727–1737, 1782–1816. See also *Hip.*
  of knee, 1743–1755, 1816–1833. See also *Knee.*
  of metacarpophalangeal joints, in rheumatoid arthritis, 1655–1658, *1657*
  of shoulder, 1707–1709, *1708*, 1709t
    imaging of, 1833–1835, *1834, 1835*
    in juvenile rheumatoid arthritis, 1775, 1780
    resection, 1707
  of wrist, in rheumatoid arthritis, 1654–1655
  patient selection for, 1637
Arthroscopy, 687–697
  for synovial biopsy, 619
  in osteoarthritis, 1388
  in surgery, for osteroarthritis, 1401
    in synovectomy, 687–697. See also *Synovectomy.*
      of hip, 1727
      of rotator cuff, 424–425, 693, *696*
  of hip, 469
  of knee, 457, *458*, 460–461
    with lavage, for osteoarthritis, 1857–1858
  of shoulder, in pain assessment, 419–420, 422
  office-based, 693–694
  technique of, 687, *688*
Arthus reaction, immune complexes in, 229
Articular cartilage, aging of, 10–11
  composition of, 1369–1370, 1370t
  in joint development, 4–5
  in minimization of frictional forces, 89
  in resistance to compression, 90, 90–91
  mechanical properties of, 9–10, *10*
  metabolism in, 1370–1371
  nutrition of, 9
  organization of, 7–9, *8*
  osteoarthritic changes in, arthroscopic management of, 692–693, *694, 695*
    etiology of, 1376–1379
    mechanisms of, *1372*, 1372–1375, *1373*
    nonsteroidal anti-inflammatory drugs and, 1398
  repair of, 10
Aschoff's nodules, in rheumatic fever, 1229
Ascorbic acid (vitamin C), antioxidant effect of, 524
  deficiency of, and scurvy, synovial biopsy in, 623
  in collagen synthesis, 26
Aspartate aminotransferase, blood level of, after methotrexate therapy, for rheumatoid arthritis, 1864t–1866t, 1864–1867, *1866*
Aspartic proteinases, in extracellular matrix degradation, 323, 324t, 325t
Aspergillosis, 1458–1459, 1459t
Aspirin, adverse effects of, gastrointestinal, 713–715
  and hematoma, after foot surgery, 1771
  for headache, in mixed connective tissue disease, 1074t

Aspirin *(Continued)*
  for juvenile rheumatoid arthritis, 1216–1217
  for Kawasaki disease, 1256
  for rheumatic fever, 1236
  for rheumatoid arthritis, in pregnancy and lactation, 1902t
  in antiphospholipid syndrome, in pregnancy, 1062
    in thrombocytopenia, 1063
  in cyclooxygenase pathway inhibition, 709, 710
  in eicosanoid pathway inhibition, 298
  in management of pregnancy, in systemic lupus erythematosus, 1051, 1052t
  in osteoarthritis, of hip, 1853
  interactions of, with indomethacin, 730–731
    with naproxen, 725
    with other drugs, 719t, 720, 720t
Assistive devices, in rehabilitative medicine, 1627, *1628*
AST, blood level of, after methotrexate therapy, for rheumatoid arthritis, 1864t–1866t, 1864–1867, *1866*
Asthma, leukotrienes in, 297t, 298–299
  nonsteroidal anti-inflammatory drugs and, 717
Ataxia telangiectasia, 1286t, 1297
  genetics of, 1284, 1284t
Atheroma, of vertebral artery, 400
Atherosclerosis, glucocorticoids and, 795
  gout with, 1319
Athletes. See *Sports medicine.*
Atlantoaxial joint, anatomy of, 396, *396*
  in ankylosing spondylitis, displacement of, 1720, *1720*
  in juvenile rheumatoid arthritis, subluxation of, radiography of, 1214, *1214*
  in rheumatoid arthritis, 909–910
    cervical spinal, fusion of, 1718
    subluxation of, 1713–1715, *1714–1716*
Atrioventricular block, in rheumatoid arthritis, 921
Atrophie blanche, 504
Auranofin. See *Gold.*
Auricle, in relapsing polychondritis, 1404–1405, *1405, 1407*
  tophi of, in gout, 1316, *1317*
Aurothioglucose. See *Gold.*
Autoimmunity. See also specific disorders, e.g., *Systemic lupus erythematosus.*
  genetic predisposition to, 209–210
  human leukocyte antigens in, class II, 218
  in inflammatory muscle disease, 1178, 1178t, 1186–1187, 1196, 1196t
  in rheumatic fever, 1226
  syndromes of, D-penicillamine and, 767
Avascular necrosis, glucocorticoids and, 795
  in antiphospholipid syndrome, 1061
  in osteoarthritis, 1390
  in sickle cell disease, 1496–1497
  in systemic lupus erythematosus, 1032
  magnetic resonance imaging of, 637–638, *638, 639*
  of hip, 1724
Axillary arteries, inflammation of, giant cell, 1127, *1127*
Axillary nerve, disorders of, muscle testing for, 399t
  entrapment of, 578
    and shoulder pain, *433*, 433–434

Axillary nerve *(Continued)*
  reflex testing of, 406t
Axis, articulation of, with atlas. See *Atlantoaxial joint.*
  dens of, anatomy of, 396, *396*, 397
    calcification of, and pain, 409
    in juvenile rheumatoid arthritis, 1214, *1214*
Axons, in peripheral nerve anatomy, 564–565, *565, 566*
Axonotmesis, definition of, 565–566
Azathioprine, and cancer, 1530
  for gout, after organ transplantation, 1346
  for inflammatory muscle disease, 1201
  for Reiter's syndrome, 994, 995t
  for rheumatoid arthritis, 944, 946, 1898t, 1901
    in pregnancy and lactation, 1902t
    vs. antimalarial drugs, 752t
    vs. gold, 761, *761*
    vs. methotrexate, 774–777
  for systemic lupus erythematosus, 1046, 1048t, 1048–1050, 1050t
    with thrombocytopenia, 1052–1053
  for Wegener's granulomatosis, 1102
  in immunosuppression, for non-neoplastic diseases, 810, 811t, 813–814, 814t, 823t
  in Sjögren's syndrome, 966
AZT (zidovudine), excretion of, probenecid inhibiting, 837
  for human immunodeficiency virus infection, and myopathy, 1277
    with diffuse infiltrative lymphocytosis, 1276
    with psoriatic skin disease, 1272
Azurocidin, in neutrophils, 147
Azurophil granules, of neutrophils, 146t, 146–147

B12 capture, in mast cell assessment, 171
B cell stimulatory factor-2. See *Interleukin-6.*
B cell(s), 95–97, 96t
  activation of, 118–119, *119*
  development of, 113–114
  free radical damage to, vitamin E and, 524
  in antigen-specific recognition, 106–112, *108, 109*
  in common variable immunodeficiency, 1289
  in immune response, 805–806, *806*
    to silicone, 1171
  in rheumatoid arthritis, 875
    in synovial membrane, 863
  in rheumatoid factor synthesis, 244
  in selective immunoglobulin M deficiency, 1291
  in systemic lupus erythematosus, 1019–1022, 1020t
  interaction of, with T cells, 119, *119*, 121–122
    therapy targeting, for rheumatoid arthritis, 840t, 842–843
      for systemic lupus erythematosus, 1054
  memory in, 114
    immune complexes and, 228
  migration of, to inflammatory sites, 119–121, 120t
  subsets of, 96–97

B cell(s) (Continued)
  suppression of, purine analogs and, 814
  surface markers of, 95–96, 96t
  testing for, in recurrent infection, 1283–1284
Bacille Calmette-Guérin, and rheumatic syndromes, 1455
Bacilli, gram-negative, in arthritis, 1442
Back, disorders of, glucocorticoid injection for, 597t, 598, 606
  low, pain in, 439–454. See also *Low back pain*.
Bacteremia, as contraindication to glucocorticoid injection, intra-articular, 593, 598, 599
Bacterial arthritis, 1435–1447
  Charcot's arthropathy with, 1439, 1439t
  crystal-induced arthritis with, 1438–1439, 1439t
  diagnosis of, 1436t, 1436–1438, *1437, 1438*
  hemarthrosis with, 1439, 1439t
  human immunodeficiency virus infection with, 1441
  in children, 1441
  in elderly, 1441
  in sacroiliitis, 1443
  intra-articular injection and, 1439, 1439t
  intravenous drug use and, 1439, 1439t
  monarticular, 376
  Neisseria infection and, *1445*, 1445–1447, *1446*
  osteoarthritis with, 1439, 1439t
  paraneoplastic, 1526, 1527t
  pathophysiology of, 1435–1436
  prosthetic joint infection and, 1439–1440, *1440*, 1440t, 1441t
  rheumatoid arthritis with, 1438, 1439t
  specific infective agents in, 1441–1443
  sternoclavicular, 1443
  synovial biopsy in, 621, *621*
  systemic illness with, 1441
  treatment of, *1443*, 1443–1445
  vs. rheumatoid arthritis, 906, 907
Bacterial infection, after hip arthroplasty, 1731
  and endocarditis, arthritis with, pauciarticular, 384
    rheumatoid factors in, 244
    vs. rheumatoid arthritis, 904
  and myopathy, 1191, 1191t
  and rheumatoid arthritis, 855, 855t, 856
  and vasculitis, 1086, 1086t
  gastrointestinal, and reactive arthritis, 1008–1010, 1009t, *1010*
  immune complex assays in, 232t
  in psoriatic arthritis, 1000
  in Reiter's syndrome, 983–985
  in X-linked agammaglobulinemia, 1286
  of knee, after arthroplasty, 1753–1754
  resistance to, mononuclear phagocytes in, 139
  rheumatoid factors in, 242, 242t, 244
  spinal, and low back pain, 451–452
  vs. juvenile rheumatoid arthritis, 1215
  with cytotoxic drug therapy, for systemic lupus erythematosus, 1049, 1050, 1050t
Bactericidal/permeability-increasing protein, in neutrophils, 147
Baker's cyst, 366, 466, 1593
  in osteoarthritis, 1388
  in rheumatoid arthritis, 914t, 914–915
  ultrasonography of, 460, *460*
Balance, disorders of, cervical spinal disorders and, 403

Balance (Continued)
  in Cogan's syndrome, 1112
Balanitis circinata, in Reiter's syndrome, 988, *989*, 993
Bamboo spine, in ankylosing spondylitis, 655, *655*
Band keratopathy, in juvenile rheumatoid arthritis, 492, *492*
Bankart lesion, magnetic resonance imaging of, *422*
Basement membrane, 37–40
Basophils, activation of, 162–163, 170, *170*
  growth of, 164
  mediator(s) of, 161, 162t
    histamine as, 164–166, *165, 166*
  secretion by, 170–171
  structure of, 161, *162*
Bateman hip prosthesis, 1782, *1783*
Bayles' test, 481, *481*
Bed rest, and bone remodeling, 71
Behçet's disease, *1114*, 1114t, 1114–1116, *1115*, Plate 12
  and arthritis, pauciarticular, 384
  English walnut extract sensitivity in, 531
  ocular disorders in, 494, *494*, Plate 4
  vs. rheumatoid arthritis, 903
Bennett's lesion, of rotator cuff, 423
Benoxaprofen, toxicity of, to kidney, 717
  to liver, 716
Benzathine penicillin G, in prevention of rheumatic fever, 1236–1238, 1237t, 1238t
Benzbromarone, for hyperuricemia, *834*, 834–836, 1344
Benziodarone, for hyperuricemia, 835
Beta-blockers, interactions of, with nonsteroidal anti-inflammatory drugs, 719t, 720
Beta-carotene, antioxidant effect of, 523–524
Betaglycan, in extracellular matrix, 37, *38, 39, 42, 44, 45*
Betamethasone. See also *Glucocorticoids*.
  contraindication to, in pregnancy, 1051
  intra-articular injection of, 594, 594t
Biceps brachii muscle, reflex testing of, 406t
Biceps brachii tendon, dislocation of, magnetic resonance imaging of, *422*
  disorders of, with rotator cuff tears, ultrasonography of, 418–419, *419*
  inflammation of, 427–428
    calcific, 426
    glucocorticoid injection for, into tendon sheath, 603–604, *604*
  rupture of, 428
Biceps femoris muscle, reflex testing of, 406t
Biglycan, in extracellular matrix, *39, 42*, 45
Bile, in peritonitis, liver biopsy and, 1867, 1871t
Biliary cirrhosis, primary, 1165
  arthropathy with, imaging of, 660
  in scleroderma, 1147
  in Sjögren's syndrome, 960–961
Biliary tract, disorders of, gold therapy and, 764
Bilirubin, blood level of, after methotrexate therapy, for rheumatoid arthritis, 1864, 1864t, 1865t
Biopsy, in amyloidosis, 1411, *1412, 1413*
  in angiitis, of central nervous system, 1091
  in arthritis, monarticular, 379
  in collagenous colitis, 1012, *1012*

Biopsy (Continued)
  in dermatomyositis, 1182, *1182*
    in children, 1246, 1247, *1247*
  in giant cell arteritis, 1129, 1130t
  in inflammatory muscle disease, 1197–1199, *1198*
  in polyarteritis, 1095
  in polychondritis, relapsing, 1406, *1407*
  in polymyositis, *1180*, 1181, *1181*
  in pulmonary fibrosis, 1164
  in reticulohistiocytosis, multicentric, 1430, 1432, *1432*
  in sarcoidosis, 1419, *1419*
    ocular, 493–494
  in scleroderma, 1138, *1138*
  in Sjögren's syndrome, 958, *959*
  in vasculitis, 1086t, 1086–1087
    cutaneous, 1104
    hypocomplementemic, 1106
  in Wegener's granulomatosis, 1102
  of forearm nodules, technique of, 604, *606*
  of kidney, in systemic lupus erythematosus, 1033, 1033t
  of liver, in iron storage disease, 1427
    in methotrexate toxicity, 1860–1863, 1862t, 1863t
    costs of, 1867, 1867t, 1871t
    risks of, 1867, 1867t, 1871t
  of synovium, 617–623
    findings in, 620–623, *620–623*, Plates 9 and 10
    tissue acquisition in, *618*, 618–619
    tissue handling in, *619*, 619–620, *620*
  spinal, in infection, with low back pain, 451
Birth. See also *Pregnancy*.
  peripheral nerve injury in, to mother, 586
Bisphosphonates, for osteoporosis, 1569t, 1569–1570
  for Paget's disease of bone, 1576–1577
Bladder, cancer of, treatment of, bacille Calmette-Guérin in, and rheumatic syndromes, 1455
  toxicity to, cyclophosphamide and, 813, 944
Blastema, in joint development, 2, *2, 3*
Blastomycosis, 1457, 1459, 1459t
  spinal, and low back pain, 451
Bleeding, and edema, acute, 504
  from nose, in rheumatic fever, 1232
  gastrointestinal, ketorolac and, 735
    nonsteroidal anti-inflammatory drugs and, 350–351, 713–715, 1852–1853
  in cystitis, cyclophosphamide and, 813
  liver biopsy and, 1867, 1871t
  pulmonary, in antiphospholipid syndrome, 1061
  therapeutic, for iron storage diseases, 1428
Blepharitis, in Sjögren's syndrome, 957
Blindness, in juvenile rheumatoid arthritis, 1220–1222
Blood, apheresis of, 817–818
    for scleroderma, 1152
    for systemic lupus erythematosus, 1053
  conservation of, in surgery, 1644
  disorders of, gold and, 763t, 763–764
    in amyloidosis, familial, 1414, *1414*, 1416t
    in antiphospholipid syndrome, 1062
    in eosinophilic fasciitis, 1529–1530, 1531t

Blood (Continued)
   in Felty's syndrome, *951*, 951–954
   in juvenile rheumatoid arthritis, 1212–1213
   in mixed connective tissue disease, 1073
   in Sjögren's syndrome, 961t, 962
   in systemic lupus erythematosus, 1030t, 1035–1036, 1052–1053
   methotrexate and, 780
   nonsteroidal anti-inflammatory drugs and, 717–718
   D-penicillamine and, 766–767, 943
   sulfasalazine and, 743, *743*, 743t, 744
   with rheumatoid arthritis, 919
Blood pressure, elevated. See *Hypertension.*
Blood vessels. See also specific vessels, e.g., *Aorta*, and disorders, e.g., *Raynaud's phenomenon.*
   disorders of, and polyarticular pain, 386
      paraneoplastic, 1524–1525, 1527t
   endothelium of, in inflammatory response, dilatation of, 184–185
      increased permeability of, 185–186
   of synovium, 13–15, *14, 15*
   tumors of, *1598*, 1598–1599, *1599*
BM-40 (osteonectin), in bone matrix, 62–63
   in extracellular matrix, 49–50
Bone(s). See also *Osteo-* and specific structures, e.g., *Tibia*, and disorders, e.g., *Avascular necrosis.*
   architecture of, 65–69, *66, 67, 69*
   blood supply of, 68–69, *69*
   composition of, 62–63
   constitutents of, 23, 23t
   cortical drifts in, 67
   development of, 63–64
   disorders of, and polyarticular pain, 386–387
   erosion of, in rheumatoid arthritis, imaging of, 646, *646, 647*
   grafting of, in knee replacement, 1823
      to acetabulum, in hip replacement, 1797, *1797*
      to femur, for osteonecrosis, 1588, *1588*
      in hip replacement, 1797, *1798*
   lamellar, 66, *67*
   metabolism of, diseases of, 1563–1577
      systemic regulation of, 60–62, *61*
   metaphyseal reshaping in, 68
   mineralization of, 64–65, *65*
   pain in, vs. arthritis, monarticular, 371
   remodeling of, 55–60, *56–59*, 57t
      haversian, 68
   strength of, 69–70
   structural adaptation in, 70–72
   subchondral, effect of, on articular cartilage, 11
   toughness of, 70
   woven, 66, *66*
Bone marrow, hyperplasia of, in Felty's syndrome, 953
   in osteonecrosis, 1581. See also *Osteonecrosis.*
   in sickle cell disease, 1493, *1494*
   magnetic resonance imaging of, 637–639, *638–640*, 644
   mononuclear phagocyte maturation in, 131t, 131–134, 132t, *133*, 135t
   toxicity to, chlorambucil and, 813
      cyclophosphamide and, 812
      methotrexate and, 1898t, 1900
      sulfasalazine and, in rheumatoid arthritis, 1898t, 1900
   transplantation of, for cellular immunodeficiency, *1300, 1301*, 1301–1302

Bone marrow (Continued)
      graft-versus-host disease after, 1525
   in Wiskott-Aldrich syndrome, 1296–1297
Bone morphogenetic proteins, 2, 27–28, 56
Bone scans. See *Radionuclide imaging.*
Bone sialoprotein, in extracellular matrix, 42, 49
Borrelia burgdorferi infection, 1462–1470. See also *Lyme disease.*
Bouchard's nodes, 361, *362*
   in osteoarthritis, 1389
Boutonnière deformity, examination for, 361
   imaging of, 646, *647*
   in rheumatoid arthritis, 913, *913*
Bowel. See also *Gastrointestinal tract.*
   cancer of, Sjögren's syndrome and, 1528, 1531t
   disorders of, and arthritis. See *Enteropathic arthritis.*
   in scleroderma, 1147
   inflammatory disease of, leukotrienes in, 297t, 299
Braces, in rehabilitative medicine, 1625, 1626
Brachial plexus, disorders of, 397
   muscle tests for, 399t
   in thoracic outlet syndromes, 577
   injury to, in surgery, 586
   neuritis of, and shoulder pain, 433
Brachialis muscle, reflex testing of, 406t
Brachioradialis muscle, reflex testing of, 406t
Breast(s), cancer of, scleroderma and, 1529, 1531t
   silicone implants in, and rheumatic disease, 1169t, 1169–1174, 1172t
Breast-feeding, after silicone breast implantation, 1173–1174
   glucocorticoid use in, 793
   in rheumatoid arthritis, drug treatment in, 1902t, 1903
   sulfasalazine use in, 744
Brevican, in extracellular matrix, 45–46
Bronchiolitis, in rheumatoid arthritis, 921, *922*
Bronchoalveolar lavage, in pulmonary fibrosis, 1163–1164
   in sarcoidosis, 1418
Brooks atlantoaxial fusion, 1718
Brucellosis, and arthritis, 1442–1443
   spinal, and low back pain, 451
Bruton's agammaglobulinemia, 1284t, 1285t, 1286–1288, *1287*
Bucillamine, for rheumatoid arthritis, 767
Buerger's disease, 1113–1114
Bulbocavernosus muscle, reflex testing of, 405, 406t
Bulge sign, in knee examination, 366, *367*
Bullae, in epidermolysis bullosa, 1556–1557
Bunions, in osteoarthritis, *483*, 483–484
Bupivacaine, injection of, with arthrographic contrast agent, after hip arthroplasty, 1810
   with glucocorticoids, for rotator cuff impingement, 424
Bursa(e), in synovial joints, 6
   olecranon, tophi of, in gout, 1316, *1317*
Bursitis, apatite deposition and, 1363
   glucocorticoid injection for, 597–598, 604–606
   iliopsoas, examination for, 364
   of foot, and pain, 486
   of hip, and pain, 474–475

Bursitis (Continued)
   of knee, and pain, 462, 465–466
      examination for, 366–367
   olecranon, examination for, 358
      in sports medicine, 552–553
   septic, 1447
   trochanteric, examination for, 364
   vs. arthritis, monarticular, 372, 373t
Bursography, indications for, 627
Buschke-Ollendorff syndrome, genetic defect in, 34
BW755C, anti-inflammatory effects of, 711
Bypass surgery, coronary, occlusion after, in antiphospholipid syndrome, 1060–1061
   intestinal, arthritis-dermatitis syndrome after, 1010–1011, *1011*

Cachectin. See *Tumor necrosis factor-α.*
Cadherins, 303–306, *304, 305*, Plate 2
Calcaneal bursitis, glucocorticoid injection for, 598, 606
Calcaneocuboid joint, anatomy of, 480, *480*
Calcaneofibular ligament, injury of, 560
Calcaneus, erosion of, in rheumatoid arthritis, 649, *650*
   fracture of, arthrosis after, 1759–1760, *1760*
   in acromegaly, 679, *679*
   in psoriatic arthritis, 1002, *1002*
   in Reiter's syndrome, 988, *988*, 991
Calcific periarthritis, vs. rheumatoid arthritis, 905
Calcification, in scleroderma, radiography of, *661, 662*, 662
Calcineurin, effect of, on cytokine production, 105
Calcinosis, in dermatomyositis, 504–505, *506*
   in children, *1248*, 1248–1249, *1249*
   in scleroderma, 1146, *1146*
   of hand, 1669, *1670*
Calcitonin, for adhesive capsulitis, 432
   for osteoporosis, 1569, 1571
   for Paget's disease of bone, 61, 1576
   in bone cell metabolism, 61
   receptors for, in osteoclasts, in bone remodeling, 59, *59*
Calcitriol. See *Vitamin D.*
   in mononuclear phagocyte regulation, 136
Calcium, deposition of, in knee, and meniscal tears, 464
   in scleroderma, in children, 1250, *1250*
   in tendinitis, of shoulder, 425–426
   for osteoporosis, 1568, 1568t, 1570, 1571, 1571t
   in bone remodeling, 57, 59
   in neutrophilic metabolism, 153
   in skeletal muscle contraction, 81, 82
   metabolism of, disorders of, and myopathy, 1194, 1194t
   supplemental, with glucocorticoids, 795
      in rheumatoid arthritis, 940
      in systemic lupus erythematosus, 1050, 1050t
Calcium channel blockers, for Raynaud's phenomenon, in scleroderma, 1153
Calcium hydroxyapatite deposition disease, 1362t, 1362–1365, *1364*
   imaging of, 674–675, *675*
   with hemochromatosis, 1424
Calcium pyrophosphate deposition disease, 1352–1362

Calcium pyrophosphate deposition disease (Continued)
and osteoarthritis, 385, 1377, 1379, 1391
bacterial arthritis with, 1438–1439, 1439t
clinical features of, 1355–1356, 1356
conditions associated with, 1352, 1352t, 1354–1355
epidemiology of, 1352–1355, 1354t
follow-up studies in, 1357
glucocorticoids for, intra-articular injection of, 596
hand in, surgery of, 1671
historical aspects of, 1352
hydroxychloroquine for, 754
imaging of, 673–674, 673–675
laboratory diagnosis of, 1356–1357, 1357t
management of, 1362
monarticular arthritis in, 377
pathology of, 1353, 1358–1362
pauciarticular arthritis in, 384
radiography of, 1357, 1358–1361
synovial biopsy in, 622, 622, Plate 9
synovial fluid analysis in, 614, 614, 615, Plate 7
vs. rheumatoid arthritis, 904
with hemochromatosis, 1424–1426
imaging of, 675
Calculi, renal, in gout, 1322, 1345
Calmette-Guérin bacillus, and rheumatic syndromes, 1455
Calpains, in extracellular matrix degradation, 324, 324t, 325t
Calpastatin, 329t, 330
Calsequestrin, in sarcoplasmic reticulum, 78
CAMPATH-1H, for rheumatoid arthritis, 842
Camptodactyly, arthropathy with, vs. rheumatoid arthritis, 905
Campylobacter infection, gastrointestinal, and reactive arthritis, 1009, 1009t, 1010
Canalicular system, open, in platelets, 176, 177t
Cancer, and low back pain, 453
chemotherapy for, and rheumatic disorders, 1530
cyclophosphamide and, 944, 945
hypercalcemia with, calcitonin for, 61
immunosuppressive therapy and, 1530
joint involvement in, vs. rheumatoid arthritis, 907
mastectomy for, silicone breast implants after, and rheumatic disease, 1169t, 1169–1174, 1172t
metastatic, to musculoskeletal system, 1521–1522, 1522t
methotrexate and, 780
musculoskeletal syndromes with, 1521–1532
as preexisting conditions, 1528t, 1528–1530, 1531t
directly associated, 1521–1523, 1522t
indirectly associated, 1523t, 1523–1526, 1527t
myositis with, 1183
of bladder, treatment of, bacille Calmette-Guérin in, and rheumatic syndromes, 1455
of bone, synovial reaction to, 1523
of joints, primary, 1610–1615, 1611, 1613–1615
secondary, 1615–1616
orthopedic implants and, 1530–1532
radiation therapy and, 1530
synovial, imaging of, 682

Cancer (Continued)
vasculitis with, 1086, 1112
skin lesions in, 503
vs. inflammatory muscle disease, 1190
with reticulohistiocytosis, multicentric, 1431–1432, 1524
with rheumatoid arthritis, 918, 923
with scleroderma, 1150, 1525, 1527t, 1529, 1531t
Candida albicans extract, in skin testing, of T cell function, 1283
Candidiasis, 1458, 1459t
Canes, in hip disorders, biomechanics of, 1723, 1723–1724
in rehabilitative medicine, 1628–1629
Capillaries, in dermatomyositis, in children, 1246, 1246
in joint development, 4
Capsaicin, for osteoarthritis, 1399
Capsulitis, adhesive, and pain, 431–432
arthrography of, 417, 417
glucocorticoids for, 596
in hyperthyroidism, 1505
with calcific tendinitis, 425, 426
Carbidopa, for sleep disturbances, in fibromyalgia syndrome, 517
Carbohydrates, in extracellular matrix, 43
metabolism of, disorders of, glucocorticoids and, 796
Carbon monoxide, diffusion of, in systemic lupus erythematosus, 1035
Carbonic anhydrase, deficiency of, and osteoporosis, 59–60
inhibitors of, interaction of, with nonsteroidal anti-inflammatory drugs, 719t
Carboxypeptidase, in mast cell mediation, 167
Carcinoid tumors, fibrosis with, 1166
Carcinoma. See also Cancer.
alveolar cell, scleroderma and, 1529, 1531t
metastatic, to joints, 1616
polyarthritis with, 1523t, 1523–1524
squamous cell, osteomyelitis and, 1529, 1531t
Cardiomyopathy, in antiphospholipid syndrome, 1060
Carditis, in rheumatic fever, clinical features of, 1231
pathology of, 1229
prognosis of, 1235, 1235
Carey-Coombs murmur, in rheumatic fever, 1231
Caries, dental, in Sjögren's syndrome, 958
Carnitine deficiency, and myopathy, 1192–1193
Carotenoids, antioxidant effect of, 523–524
Carpal joints. See Wrist.
Carpal tunnel, anatomy of, 359
Carpal tunnel syndrome, 567–571, 568, 569, 569t
amyloidosis and, 1415
glucocorticoid injection for, 593, 604–605
in acromegaly, 1507
in hypothyroidism, 1505–1506
in pregnancy, 1508
magnetic resonance imaging of, 641
Carpometacarpal joint(s), in scleroderma, imaging of, 662, 662
in systemic lupus erythematosus, surgery of, 1665–1667, 1666–1667
of thumb, arthrocentesis of, 601, 602
osteoarthritis of, surgery for, 1672–1673
Cartilage. See also Chondro-.

Cartilage (Continued)
articular. See Articular cartilage.
constituents of, 23, 23t, 24
destruction of, in rheumatoid arthritis, 881–883, 882, 883
in bone development, 63–64
keratan sulfate in, in extracellular matrix, 41
transplantation of, to knee, in osteoarthritis, 1740
Cartilage matrix protein, in extracellular matrix, 42, 46
Cartilage-hair hypoplasia, 1285t, 1297
Cataflam, 734
Cataracts, glucocorticoids and, 796
Cathepsins, in extracellular matrix degradation, 323–324, 324t, 325t
in mast cell mediation, 167
in neutrophils, 147
regulation of, cellular, 334
Catheters, entrapment of, after knee arthroplasty, 1830
Cauda equina syndrome, 449
in ankylosing spondylitis, 975, 975, 977
Causalgia, and shoulder pain, 434–435
Cavitation, in joint development, 4, 4, 5
Cavities, dental, in Sjögren's syndrome, 958
CD1, expression of, 113
CD2, expression of, 97t, 98, 99t, 113
in T cell activation, 117
CD3, deficiency of, and immunodeficiency, 1285t, 1299
expression of, 97t, 97–98, 99t
in T cell activation, 115
CD4, expression of, 97, 97t, 98, 99t, 113
in diffuse infiltrative lymphocytosis, in human immunodeficiency virus infection, 1275, 1276
in human immunodeficiency virus infection, 1265–1266
in Reiter's syndrome, 1270–1271
in rheumatoid arthritis, 860–863, 861t
therapy targeting, 841
in T cell activation, 115
CD5, expression of, 96t, 96–97
in rheumatoid arthritis, therapy targeting, 841–842
CD7, expression of, 97, 97t, 99t, 113
CD8, expression of, 97t, 98, 99t, 113
in diffuse infiltrative lymphocytosis, in human immunodeficiency virus infection, 1275, 1276
in lymphocytopenia, and immunodeficiency, 1285t, 1299
genetics of, 1284, 1284t
in T cell activation, 115
CD9, expression of, 96t
CD11/CD18, 307, 307
in lymphocyte migration, 120, 120t, 121, 121t
in monocyte adhesion, to endothelial cells, 129
CD18, monoclonal antibodies to, in anti-inflammatory treatment, 317
CD19, expression of, 96, 96t, 114
CD20, expression of, 96, 96t, 114
CD21, expression of, 96, 96t, 114
CD22, expression of, 96, 96t
CD23, expression of, 96, 96t
CD24, expression of, 96t
CD28, in rheumatoid arthritis, therapy targeting, 842
in T cell activation, 117–118
CD34, L-selectin binding to, 310–312

CD40, expression of, 96, 96t
in B cell activation, 119
in endothelial cell activation, 192
in immunoglobulin M deficiency, selective, 1291
in rheumatoid arthritis, therapy targeting, 842
CD41/CD61, 307, 308, *308*
CD44, *304*, 313
in extracellular matrix, *38*, *39*, *42*, 44, 46
in lymphocyte migration, 120, 120t
CD45, in T cell activation, 116
CD49/CD29, 309
CD49d/β7, in lymphocyte migration, 120, 120t, 121, 121t
CD51/CD61, 307, 308, *308*
CD54. See *Intercellular adhesion molecule-1 (CD54)*.
CD62. See *Selectins*.
CD72, expression of, 96, 96t
CD80, expression of, 96t
CD86, expression of, 96t
CDw52, in rheumatoid arthritis, therapy targeting, 842
Ceftizoxime, for *Neisseria* infection, in arthritis, 1446
Ceftriaxone, for Lyme disease, 1469, 1469t
for *Neisseria* infection, in arthritis, *1445*, 1446
side effects of, 1874–1875, 1875t
Cefuroxime, for Lyme disease, 1469, 1469t
Celestone Soluspan (betamethasone). See also *Glucocorticoids*.
contraindication to, in pregnancy, 1051
intra-articular injection of, 594, 594t
Celiac disease, and arthritis, 1011
Cell adhesion molecule(s), 303–317. See also *Adhesion molecules* and specific types, e.g., *Integrins*.
Cell adhesion molecule-1, glycosylated, in leukocyte homing, 315
L-selectin binding to, 310–312
Cement, in arthroplasty. See *Methyl methacrylate*.
Cement line, in bone remodeling, *57*, 62
Central nervous system. See *Nervous system, central*.
Centromere, antibodies to, in scleroderma, 258, 258t, 1143
Cerebral venous sinus, thrombosis of, in antiphospholipid syndrome, 1060
Cerebroglycan, in extracellular matrix, 47
Cerebrovascular accident, in systemic lupus erythematosus, 1034, 1053
thrombotic, in antiphospholipid syndrome, 1059
Cerebrum, amyloid angiopathy of, 1410
Cervical spine. See *Spine*.
Cervicobrachial syndrome, occupational, 394
Charcot joint, bacterial arthritis with, 1439, 1439t
imaging of, 669–672, *671*
in diabetes, *1500*, 1501
knee arthroplasty for, 1747, *1748*
monarticular, 377
Charcot-Leyden crystal protein, in eosinophils, 155, *155*
Chemical sensitivity, multiple, vs. fibromyalgia syndrome, 514
Chemokines, in cell migration, 269, 269t, 270t
in cell recruitment, 269, 269t, 270t
in monocyte adhesion, to endothelial cells, 130

Chemokines (*Continued*)
in rheumatoid arthritis, 867–868, 868t
Chemonucleolysis, of intervertebral discs, computed tomography after, 634
in back pain, with spinal stenosis, 449
Chemotherapy, for cancer, and rheumatic disorders, 1530
Chest, in ankylosing spondylitis, limited expansion of, 976
pain in, 974
Chiari malformation, and headache, 409
Chickenpox, and arthritis, 1481
Chikungunya virus infection, and arthritis, 1478–1479
Childbirth. See also *Pregnancy*.
peripheral nerve injury in, to mother, 586
Children. See also *Infants*.
bacterial arthritis in, 1441
dermatomyositis in, 1245t, 1245–1249, *1246–1249*, 1249t
antimalarial drugs for, 754
clinical features of, 1182
psoriatic arthritis in, imaging of, 653
rheumatic fever in, 1225–1238. See also *Rheumatic fever*.
rheumatoid arthritis in, 1207–1222. See also *Juvenile rheumatoid arthritis*.
scleroderma in, 1242t, 1249–1253, 1250t, *1250–1253*
systemic lupus erythematosus in, 1241–1245, 1242t, *1244*
vasculitis in, 1242t, 1253–1261
in giant cell arteritis, 1259–1260, *1260*
in granulomatous arteritis, 1260–1261
necrotizing, 1242t, *1254*, 1254t, 1254–1259, 1255t, *1256–1258*
Chlamydia infection, in Reiter's syndrome, 984, 986, 989–995
Chlorambucil, for Behçet's disease, 1116
for reticulohistiocytosis, multicentric, 1433
for rheumatoid arthritis, 944–945, 1899t, 1903
in pregnancy and lactation, 1902t
in immunosuppression, for non-neoplastic diseases, *810*, 811t, 813, 823t
in Sjögren's syndrome, 966
Chloroquine, adverse effects of, 754–755, 755t
for lupus erythematosus, 749–750, 1042, 1043t
for rheumatoid arthritis, 750–753, 751t, 752t
vs. gold, 761, *761*
guidelines for use of, 756
mechanisms of action of, 748t, 748–749
pharmacokinetics of, 748
structure of, 747, *747*
Cholangitis, sclerosing, 1165
Cholecalciferol. See *Vitamin D*.
Cholestasis, with jaundice, gold therapy and, 764
Cholesterol crystals, in synovial fluid analysis, 614, *615*, Plate 8
Chondrification, in joint development, 2, *2*, *3*
Chondrocalcinosis, and meniscal tears, 464
in calcium pyrophosphate deposition disease, epidemiology of, 1352–1353
imaging of, 673, *673*
radiography of, 1357, *1358*, *1359*
with hemochromatosis, 1424–1426
in hemochromatosis, imaging of, 675
in hyperparathyroidism, 1502

Chondrocytes, in articular cartilage, 7–9
in bone development, 63
metabolism in, in osteoarthritis, 1377, 1378
Chondrodysplasia, genetic defects in, 30, 31, *32*, *33*
Chondrodystrophy, 1554–1556
lethal, genetic mutation in, 1540–1541
Chondroitin sulfate, in extracellular matrix, *41*, *42*, 43
in mast cell mediation, 167–169, *168*
Chondrolysis, and knee pain, 465
Chondroma, of tendon sheath, 1603–1604
periarticular, 1604, *1604*
Chondromalacia, osteoarthritis with, 385
Chondromatosis, synovial, 1600–1603, *1601–1603*
arthroscopic synovectomy in, 690–691
imaging of, *681*, 681–682
in osteoarthritis, 1390–1391
Chondrosarcoma, 1610–1612, *1611*
Chorea, in antiphospholipid syndrome, 1060
in rheumatic fever, 1229–1230, 1232
Choroiditis, 490
Christmas disease, arthropathy with, 1485–1491. See also *Hemophilia*.
Chromatin, antigens associated with, in systemic lupus erythematosus, 255t, 255–256
in antigen-specific recognition, by B cells, 110
Chronic fatigue syndrome, vs. fibromyalgia syndrome, 513–514
vs. Lyme disease, 1468
vs. rheumatoid arthritis, 904–905
Chronic granulomatous disease, neutrophilic metabolism in, 154
Chronic obstructive pulmonary disease, leukotrienes in, 297t
Chrysotherapy. See *Gold*.
Churg-Strauss syndrome, 1097–1099
in children, 1261
in human immunodeficiency virus infection, 1278
pathogenesis of, 1081–1082, *1084*
skin lesions in, 503
Chymase, in extracellular matrix degradation, 324t, 325, 325t
in mast cell mediation, 167, 167t
Chymopapain, in chemonucleolysis, of intervertebral discs, computed tomography after, 634
in back pain, with spinal stenosis, 449
Cigarette smoking, and Buerger's disease, 1113–1114
and osteoporosis, 1564
Cimetidine, interaction of, with piroxicam, 720t
Cirrhosis. See also *Liver*.
methotrexate and, 781t, 781–782, 782t
nonsteroidal anti-inflammatory drug use in, 722
primary biliary, 1165
arthropathy with, imaging of, 660
in scleroderma, 1147
in Sjögren's syndrome, 960–961
Claudication, in giant cell arteritis, 1126
with lumbar spinal stenosis, 450
Clavicle, articulation of, with acromion. See also *Shoulder*.
arthritis of, 358, 428
disorders of, in sports medicine, 548–549, *549*

Clavicle *(Continued)*
  examination of, 358
Clavulanic acid, with amoxicillin, for
  Neisseria infection, 1446
Clioril (sulindac), 723t, 725, *725*
  adverse effects of, gastrointestinal, 713–
    714
  in systemic lupus erythematosus, 1041
  on kidney, 716
  on liver, 715, 721
Clonazepam, for sleep disturbances, in
  fibromyalgia syndrome, 517
Clonotypes, monoclonal antibodies to, for
  rheumatoid arthritis, 846–847
Clotting. See *Coagulation.*
Clubbing, of digits, in hypertrophic
  osteoarthropathy, 1514–1516, *1515*,
  1518
  of foot, in sarcoidosis, 1420–1421
Clusters of differentiation. See *CD-.*
Coagulation, disorders of, as
  contraindication to intra-articular
  glucocorticoid injection, 599
  in hemophilia. See *Hemophilia.*
  in rheumatoid arthritis, 887–888
  in systemic lupus erythematosus, 1030t,
    1035–1036
  inhibition of. See *Anticoagulant(s).*
Coagulation factors, secretion of, by
  macrophages, 137t
Coccidioidomycosis, 1456–1457, 1459t
  spinal, and low back pain, 451
Coenzyme Q_{10} deficiency, and myopathy,
  1193
Cogan's syndrome, 1112–1113
Colchicine, 728
  adverse effects of, 718
  anti-inflammatory effect of, 713
  for amyloidosis, 1412–1414, 1415t
  for calcium pyrophosphate deposition
    disease, 1362
  for familiar Mediterranean fever, 905
  for gout, with arthritis, 713, 1342–1344
  for spondyloarthropathy, 736
  history of, 707
  mechanism of action of, 711–712
Cold, in rehabilitative medicine, 1623,
  1624, 1624t
  in therapy, for rheumatoid arthritis, 938
  sensitivity to, in Raynaud's phenome-
    non, in scleroderma, 1140–1142
Colitis, collagenous, arthritis with,
  1011–1012, *1012*
  ulcerative, arthritis with, *1007*, 1007–
    1008, 1008t
    monarticular, 377
    vs. rheumatoid arthritis, 903
Collagen, arthritis induced by, vs.
  rheumatoid arthritis, 857–858
  biosynthesis of, 26–28, *27*
    nucleated growth in, 28–29, *29*, *30*
  fibrillar structure of, *24*, 24t, 25–26
  genes for, mutations of, and disease, 29–
    31, *30*, 31t, *32*, *33*, 33t
  structure of, 26
  in aorta, 23t, 24
  in articular cartilage, 7, 1370, 1371
    in aging, 10–11
    in load carriage, 10
    in osteoarthritis, 1372–1374
    in resistance to compression, 90, *90*
  in bone, 23, 23t, 62
    in remodeling, 56, 57t
  in cartilage, 23, 23t, 24
  in dermis, 23, 23t

Collagen *(Continued)*
  in extracellular matrix, *39*, 40, *41*, *42*
    degradation of, by proteinases, 330–
      331, *331*
      with fibroblast proliferation, 203–
        204
    synthesis of, defects of, 1536–1540,
      1537, 1537t, 1540t
    types of, 1535–1536, 1536t
  in ligaments, 23t, 23–24
  in menisci, 6–7
  in scleroderma, 1138–1139, 1139t
  in tendons, 23t, 23–24
  metabolic turnover of, 28
  type I, 23t, 23–25, *24*, 24t
    disorders of, and aortic stenosis, supra-
      valvular, 1554
      and cutis laxa, 1553–1554
        X-linked, 1551
      and Ehlers-Danlos syndrome, 1546–
        1551, *1547–1549*, 1548t, *1551*
      and Marfan syndrome, 1552–1553
      and osteogenesis imperfecta, 1542–
        1546, 1543t, *1545*
      and pseudoxanthoma elasticum,
        1554
      and Williams' syndrome, 1554
  type II, 23t, 24, 24t
    disorders of, 1554–1556
  type III, 23t, 24, 24t, 25
  type IV, 23t, 24t, 25, *25*
    disorders of, 1556–1557
  type V, 23t, 24t, 25
  type VII, 23t, 24t, 25
  type VIII, 24t, 25
  type IX, 23t, 24t, 25
  type X, 23t, 24t, 25
  type XI, 23t, 24t, 25
  type XII, 24t
  type XIV, 25
Collagenase, in extracellular matrix
  degradation, 324t, 325t, 326, 327t, *328*
  in rheumatoid arthritis, 876t, 876–878
Collagenous colitis, arthritis with,
  1011–1012, *1012*
Collateral ligaments, of knee, injury of, in
  sports medicine, 557–558, *559*
  tears of, magnetic resonance imaging
    of, 643
Colon. See also *Gastrointestinal tract.*
  cancer of, Sjögren's syndrome and, 1528,
    1531t
  disorders of, and arthritis. See *Entero-
    pathic arthritis.*
    in scleroderma, 1147
  inflammatory disease of, leukotrienes in,
    297t, 299
Colony-stimulating factors, in mononuclear phagocyte maturation, in bone
  marrow, 131t, 131–133, *133*
Combined immunodeficiency disease,
  mast cells in, 164
  partial, 1286t, 1296–1299
  severe, 1286t, *1294*, 1294–1295
Common variable immunodeficiency,
  1285t, *1288*, 1288–1289
Compartment syndromes, 582–584, *583*,
  584
Complement, activation of, 232–235, 233t,
  234
  alternative pathway of, 232–234, 233t,
    234
  biologic consequences of, 235, 235t,
    236t
  classical pathway of, 232–233, *234*

Complement *(Continued)*
  immune complexes in, 228–229
  termination sequence in, 234–235
  assays for, 236–237
  components of, secretion of, by macro-
    phages, 137t
  deficiencies of, and rheumatic disease,
    1305–1310, *1306*, 1308t
    and vasculitis, *1106*, 1106–1107
  genetic control of, 1305–1306, *1306*
  in immune complex assays, 230t, 231t,
    231–233
  in synovial fluid, 617
    in rheumatoid arthritis, 887
  interaction of, with platelets, 179
  metabolism of, 235–236
    hypercatabolism in, 237t, 237–238
  receptors of, on mononuclear phago-
    cytes, 134
    on myeloid cells, 135t
    on neutrophil surface, in phagocyto-
      sis, 150, 151, 151t
  synthesis of, 235–236
    excessive, 237
Complement receptors, in vasculitis,
  1080–1081
Compression, in joint biomechanics,
  resistance to, 90, 90–91, *91*
Compression fractures, of epiphyses, in
  juvenile chronic arthritis, imaging of,
  652
Compression syndromes, 564–582. See also
  Entrapment syndrome(s) and specific
  disorders, e.g., *Tarsal tunnel syndrome.*
Computed tomography, 628–635
  after trauma, 629–630, *630*
  in inflammatory muscle disease, 1199
  in low back pain, 445–446, *447*
  in osteoarthritis, 1387–1388
  of ankylosing spondylitis, 977
  of articular sepsis, 634
  of bone infection, 630
  of congenital diseases, 634–635
  of hip, 468, 632, 1726
  of knee, 460, *460*, 632–633
  of sacroiliac joint, 631–632
  of shoulder, 632, *632*
    in evaluation of pain, 417, *418*, 422,
      422t
    preoperative, 1698
  of spine, *629*, 631–635, *632*, *634*
    cervical, 408
      in rheumatoid arthritis, 1717
    lumbar facet joints in, 631, *632*
  of sternoclavicular joint, 631, *631*
  of temporomandibular joint, 630–631
  of tumors, 630
  technical aspects of, 628, *628*
Condensation, in joint development, 2, *2*
Conglutinin, in immune complex assays,
  230t, 231t
Conjunctiva, in sarcoidosis, 493–494
Conjunctivitis, in Reiter's syndrome, 989,
  993–994
  with keratitis, 488–489, *489*, 489t, Plate 3
  in Sjögren's syndrome, 956t, 956–957,
    957, 957t, 965
Connective tissue, constituents of, 23t,
  23–24
  disease of. See also specific diseases,
    e.g., *Scleroderma.*
  mixed, 1067–1075. See also *Mixed con-
    nective tissue disease.*
Connective tissue–activating peptides, in
  rheumatoid arthritis, 869

Contraceptives, and arthritis, vs. rheumatoid arthritis, 904
   effects of, on osteoarticular disorders, 1509
   in systemic lupus erythematosus, 1037
Contracture, Dupuytren's, 359, 1165–1166
Contrast agents, in arthrography, of hip arthroplasty, with loosening, 1807–1808, *1808*
Coonrad elbow prosthesis, Mayo modification of, 1686, *1688–1689, 1691,* 1691–1692, *1835*
Copper, in immune response, *523,* 526
   metabolism of, Wilson's disease of, arthropathy in, 676
Cornea, disorders of, in Cogan's syndrome, 1112
   in juvenile rheumatoid arthritis, 492, *492*
   in Wegener's granulomatosis, 493, *493,* Plate 4
   inflammation of, 488–489, *489,* 489t, Plate 3
   in Sjögren's syndrome, 956t, 956–957, *957,* 957t, 965
   keratan sulfate in, in extracellular matrix, *41*
   toxicity to, gold therapy and, 764
Coronary arteries, inflammation of, in rheumatoid arthritis, 921
   surgery of, occlusion after, in antiphospholipid syndrome, 1060–1061
Cortical drifts, in bone, 67
Corticosteroids. See *Glucocorticoids.*
Corticotropin-releasing hormone, 787
Cortisol. See also *Hydrocortisone.*
   secretion of, regulation of, 787–788
   structure of, 787, *788*
Cortisone. See also *Glucocorticoids.*
   for rheumatoid arthritis, 798
   potency of, 788t
   structure of, 787, *788*
Costovertebral osteoarthritis, imaging of, 668
Cotton-wool spots, in systemic lupus erythematosus, 492, *493*
Counterimmunoelectrophoresis, in antinuclear antibody detection, 253
Coxsackievirus infection, and arthritis, 1480
Cramping, menstrual, nonsteroidal anti-inflammatory drugs for, 713, 731
Cranial nerves, in systemic lupus erythematosus, 1034
Craniosynostosis, genetic mutation in, 1539
C-reactive protein, in inflammation, 699–701, *700,* 700t, 702t, 703, 704
   production of, cytokines and, 273
Creatine kinase, in inflammatory muscle disease, 1195
   in polymyositis, 1180–1181
   in skeletal muscle, in contraction, 82
Creatine phosphokinase, in skeletal muscle, 78, 79t
Cremaster muscle, reflex testing of, 406t
Crepitation, in physical examination, 355, 1882
CREST syndrome, 505–506, *506,* 1066, *1066,* 1134–1135
   hand surgery in, 1669
   in children, 1249, 1251
Cricoarytenoid joint, examination of, 357
   in rheumatoid arthritis, 911
Crithidia luciliae test, for antinuclear antibodies, 255

Crohn's disease, arthritis with, 1007–1008, 1008t
   vs. rheumatoid arthritis, 903
Cruciate ligament(s), injury of, in sports medicine, 555–557, *556, 557*
   posterior, in arthroplasty, 1742–1746, *1743, 1744, 1747*
   tears of, magnetic resonance imaging of, 643
Crutches, in rehabilitative medicine, 1629–1630
Cryoglobulinemia, and vasculitis, 1108–1110
   mixed, rheumatoid factors in, 242, 244–246
   with malignancy, 1524–1525, 1527t
Cryopheresis, for systemic lupus erythematosus, 1053
Cryoproteins, in vascular injury, with malignancy, 1524–1525, 1527t
Cryptococcosis, *1457,* 1457–1458, 1459t
   spinal, and low back pain, 451
Crystal deposition disease. See *Calcium hydroxyapatite deposition disease; Calcium pyrophosphate deposition disease;* and *Gout.*
Crystal-induced arthritis, monarticular, 377
CS1 fibronectin, in rheumatoid arthritis, 874, *874*
CTLA-4 immunoglobulin, for rheumatoid arthritis, 842
Cubital tunnel syndrome, *573,* 573–574
   glucocorticoids for, 597
Cumulative trauma, 584–585, 585t
   and carpal tunnel syndrome, 571
   and medial tibial stress syndrome, 558–559
   to rotator cuff, in sports medicine, 550–551, *551*
   vs. fibromyalgia syndrome, 514
Cushing's syndrome, 1506
Cutis laxa, 34, 1553–1554
   X-linked, 1551
Cyclooxygenase pathways, in eicosanoid synthesis, 288–291, *289,* 289t, 290t
   inhibition of, by nonsteroidal anti-inflammatory drugs, 708–711, *709*
      side effects of, 715, 716
      for inflammatory diseases, 298
Cyclophosphamide, and cancer, 1530
   for reticulohistiocytosis, multicentric, 1433
   for rheumatoid arthritis, 944–946, 1899t, 1903
      in pregnancy and lactation, 1902t
   for systemic lupus erythematosus, 812, 1046–1050, 1048t, 1050t
      in children, 1243–1244
      with thrombocytopenia, 1052–1053
   for Wegener's granulomatosis, 809, 812, 815–816, *816,* 1102–1103
   in immunosuppression, 807
      for non-neoplastic diseases, *810,* 811t, 811–813, 812t, 823t
   in Sjögren's syndrome, 966
   side effects of, 812t, 812–813, 823t, 944, 945
Cyclosporine, and bone loss, 1565
   effect of, on cytokine production, 105
   for Behçet's disease, 1116
   for inflammatory muscle disease, 1201
   for rheumatoid arthritis, 860, 945–947, 1899t, 1903
      in pregnancy and lactation, 1902t
      vs. antimalarial drugs, 752t

Cyclosporine *(Continued)*
      vs. methotrexate, 776
   for systemic lupus erythematosus, 1053–1054
   in immunosuppression, 819–821, *820,* 823t
   in inhibition of histamine release, 163
   toxicity of, and gout, 1323
Cyst(s), ganglion, 1593–1595, *1594, 1595*
   of wrist, aspiration of, 597, 604
      physical examination for, 360
   of knee, 1593
      and pain, 466
      examination for, 366
      in rheumatoid arthritis, 914t, 914–915
      magnetic resonance imaging of, 644, *645*
      ultrasonography of, 460, *460*
   subchondral, in rheumatoid arthritis, imaging of, 646, *647*
   synovial, 1593–1594, *1594*
      of hip, computed tomography of, *628*
Cystatins, 329t, 330
Cysteine, in activation of metalloproteins, 335, *336*
   in collagen gene mutations, 31, 31t
Cysteine proteinases, in extracellular matrix degradation, 323–324, 324t, 325t
   inhibitors of, 329t, 330
Cystic fibrosis, leukotrienes in, 297t
Cystitis, cyclophosphamide and, 813, 944
Cytapheresis, therapeutic, 817, 818
Cytochrome, in neutrophilic metabolism, 152–153
Cytokine(s), 101–105, 102t–103t, 267–282, 806, *806.* See also specific types, e.g., *Interleukin-2.*
   and adhesion molecule expression, 268–269
   and vascular permeability, in inflammatory response, 185
   effects of, regulation of, 278t, 278–282
   in angiogenesis, 274
   in B cell development, 114
   in B cell regulation, 122
   in bone remodeling, 59
   in cell migration, 269, 269t, 270t
   in cell recruitment, 269, 269t, 270t
   in fibroblast activation, 199, 201t, 201–205, 202t, 204t
   in immune cell development, 270–272, *272*
   in inflammation, chronic, 275–278, *277*
      in acute-phase response, 273–274, 699–700
      laboratory measurement of, 702, 702t
   in inflammatory cell development, 272–273
   in inflammatory myopathy, 1188
   in lymphocyte migration, 121
   in mast cell mediation, 162t, 170
   in rheumatoid arthritis, 863–871, 864t
      and metalloproteinase synthesis, 876
      therapy targeting, 839, 840t, *843,* 843–845
   in Sjögren's syndrome, 964
   in synovial fluid analysis, 617
   in T cell activation, 193
   inhibition of, glucocorticoids in, 790
      macrophage secretions in, 137t, 138
      methotrexate in, 773
   production of, deficiency of, and immunodeficiency, 1285t, 1299
      replacement therapy for, *1301,* 1302

Cytokine(s) (Continued)
　　induction of, 267–268, 268t
　　macrophages in, 137t
　　T cells in, 101–105, 102t–103t
　　receptors of, on mononuclear phago-
　　　cytes, 136
　　types of, 267
Cytokine response modifier A, 329t, 330
Cytomegalovirus infection, and arthritis,
　　1481–1482
Cytotoxic drugs, for lupus erythematosus,
　　1046–1050, 1048t, 1050t
　　　with thrombocytopenia, 1052–1053
　　for polyarteritis, 1096
　　for reticulohistiocytosis, multicentric,
　　　1433
　　for rheumatoid arthritis, 944
　　　juvenile, 1219
　　for vasculitis, 1087–1088
　　for Wegener's granulomatosis, 1102–1103
　　in immunoregulation, 808t, 808–815, 810,
　　　811t, 812t, 814t, 823t
　　side effects of, 815–817, 816, 823t
Cytoxan. See Cyclophosphamide.

Dactylitis, in psoriatic arthritis, 1002, 1002
　　in Reiter's syndrome, with human im-
　　　munodeficiency virus infection,
　　　1269, 1269
Danazol, for thrombocytopenia, in
　　systemic lupus erythematosus, 1052
Dapsone, for lupus dermatitis, 1043, 1043t
　　for polychondritis, relapsing, 1407
　　for rheumatoid arthritis, vs. antimalarial
　　　drugs, 752t
　　in immunosuppression, 822, 823t
Dawbarn's sign, in rotator cuff
　　impingement, 423
Daypro (oxaprozin), 723t, 727, 727
　　use of, in elderly, 722
　　in renal disorders, 721
de Quervain's tenosynovitis,
　　glucocorticoid injection for, 604
　　in rheumatoid arthritis, 914
　　physical examination for, 360
Deafness, in Alport's syndrome, 1556
　　in Cogan's syndrome, 1112, 1113
　　in rheumatoid arthritis, 911
10-Deazaaminopterin, for rheumatoid
　　arthritis, 777–778
Debridement, of ankle, 1761, 1763,
　　1763–1765
　　of knee, in osteoarthritis, 1739–1740
Decadron. See Dexamethasone.
Decompression, in osteonecrosis, in
　　etiology, 1584–1585
　　in treatment, 1587–1589
Decorin, in extracellular matrix, 38, 42, 45
Defensins, in neutrophils, 147
Deglutition, disorders of, cervical spinal
　　disorders and, 403
　　in Sjögren's syndrome, 960
Delivery. See also Pregnancy.
　　peripheral nerve injury in, to mother,
　　　586
Dendritic cells, 140–141
　　in immunoregulation, 141–143, 142
Dens, of axis, anatomy of, 396, 396, 397
　　calcification of, and pain, 409
　　in juvenile rheumatoid arthritis, 1214,
　　　1214
Dense granules, in platelets, 176, 177t
Dense tubular system, in platelets, 176,
　　177t

Densitometry, of bone, in osteoporosis,
　　1565–1566, 1566, 1567t
Dental caries, in Sjögren's syndrome, 958
Dental procedures, antibiotics with, after
　　hip arthroplasty, 1730–1731
Dentinogenesis imperfecta, with osteo-
　　genesis imperfecta, 1543t, 1544, 1545
Deoxynucleosides, in purine metabolism,
　　1323, 1324
Deoxynucleotides, in purine metabolism,
　　1323, 1324
Deoxyribonucleic acid (DNA), antibodies
　　to, in systemic lupus erythematosus,
　　255t, 255–256, 1021, 1022, 1023,
　　1024, 1024t, 1031, 1031t
　　tests for, 254–255
　　in antigen-specific recognition, by B
　　　cells, 107, 109, 111
　　in genetic locus identification, 1541–1542
Depo-Medrol. See Methylprednisolone.
Dercum's disease, glucocorticoids for,
　　nonarticular injection of, 597
Dermatan sulfate, in extracellular matrix,
　　41, 43
　　in articular cartilage, 1370
Dermatitis, in Lyme disease, 1466
　　in systemic lupus erythematosus, man-
　　　agement of, conservative, 1041–
　　　1043, 1043t
　　with arthritis, after intestinal bypass,
　　　1010–1011, 1011
Dermatomes, of spinal nerves, 398, 398
Dermatomyositis, antinuclear antibodies
　　in, 259–261, 260t
　　clinical features of, 1181–1182
　　diagnosis of, criteria for, 1177–1178,
　　　1178t, 1179t
　　imaging of, 662, 663
　　in children, 1182, 1245t, 1245–1249, 1246–
　　　1249, 1249t
　　　antimalarial drugs for, 754
　　methotrexate for, 778
　　pathology of, 1182, 1182
　　D-penicillamine and, in rheumatoid ar-
　　　thritis, 943
　　skin lesions in, 504–505, 504–506, Plates
　　　5 and 6
　　treatment of, 1200–1201
　　vs. rheumatoid arthritis, 904
Dermis, constituents of, 23, 23t
Desmocollins, 304
Desmogleins, 304
Desmopressin, for hemophilia, 1489
Desmosine, in elastin metabolism, 33–34
Desmosomes, cadherins in, 303–304
Dexamethasone. See also Glucocorticoids.
　　contraindication to, in pregnancy, 1051
　　for rheumatoid arthritis, in pregnancy
　　　and lactation, 1902t
　　intra-articular injection of, 594t
　　potency of, 788t
　　structure of, 787, 788
Diabetes, 1500, 1500–1502, 1501, 1502t
　　gout with, 1318
　　neuroarthropathy in, imaging of, 670,
　　　671, 671
　　pancreatic amyloid deposits in, 1510
　　septic arthritis in, imaging of, 677, 677
　　stiff hand syndrome in, 386, 386
Diacylglycerol, in neutrophil function, 148,
　　149
Dialysis, amyloid fibril deposition with,
　　1410, 1415
　　shoulder pain with, 435
Diaminodiphenylsulfone (dapsone), for
　　lupus dermatitis, 1043t, 1943

Diaminodiphenylsulfone (dapsone)
　　(Continued)
　　for polychondritis, relapsing, 1407
　　for rheumatoid arthritis, vs. antimalarial
　　　drugs, 752t
　　in immunosuppression, 822, 823t
Diarrhea, for Whipple's disease, 1011
　　in amyloidosis, 1414, 1416t
　　in Reiter's syndrome, 990
Diarthrodial joints. See Synovial joints.
Diclofenac, 729t, 733, 733–734
　　anti-inflammatory effect of, 711
　　toxicity of, to liver, 715
Didronel (etidronate), for osteoporosis,
　　1569, 1569–1571
　　for Paget's disease of bone, 1576
Diet. See Nutrition.
Diffuse idiopathic skeletal hyperostosis,
　　and low back pain, 450
　　imaging of, 668–669, 669, 670
　　in diabetes mellitus, 1501
　　vs. ankylosing spondylitis, 655, 657
　　vs. osteoarthritis, 1391–1392
Diffuse infiltrative lymphocytosis
　　syndrome, in human immuno-
　　deficiency virus infection, 1273t,
　　1273–1277, 1274, 1276
Diflunisal, 723t, 725, 725–726
DiGeorge's syndrome, 1286t, 1292,
　　1292–1293
　　genetics of, 1284, 1284t
　　treatment of, 1301
Digestion, intracellular, in macrophages,
　　139
Digestive tract. See Gastrointestinal tract.
Digital nerves, entrapment of, in foot, 580
　　in hand, 572–573, 575, 576
Digoxin, interaction of, with nonsteroidal
　　anti-inflammatory drugs, 720, 720t
Dihydrofolate reductase, inactivation of,
　　by methotrexate, 771
Dihydropyridine receptors, in skeletal
　　muscle, 78, 79t, 81–82
1,25-Dihydroxyvitamin D₃. See Vitamin D.
Diltiazem, for Raynaud's phenomenon, in
　　scleroderma, 1153
Dipalmitoyl phosphatidylcholine, in
　　synovial joint lubrication, 18
Diphtheria toxin, interleukin-2 fused with,
　　in T cell suppression, for rheumatoid
　　arthritis, 842, 860
Disability, definition of, 1619
　　in juvenile rheumatoid arthritis, 1220
　　low back pain and, 439
Disc(s), intervertebral. See Intervertebral
　　disc(s).
Discoid lupus erythematosus, and cancer,
　　1528, 1531t
　　antimalarial drugs for, 749–750
　　complement deficiencies in, 1307, 1308,
　　　1308t
　　skin lesions in, 499–502, 501, Plate 5
Discoid rash, in systemic lupus
　　erythematosus, 1030t, 1036
Distraction test, for meniscal tears, 368
Diuretics, and hyperuricemia, 1328t, 1336
　　interactions of, with nonsteroidal anti-
　　　inflammatory drugs, 719t, 720t
Diving, decompression in, and osteo-
　　necrosis, 1584–1585
DNA, antibodies to, in systemic lupus
　　erythematosus, 255t, 255–256, 1021,
　　1022, 1023, 1024, 1024t, 1031, 1031t
　　tests for, 254–255
　　in antigen-specific recognition, by B
　　　cells, 107, 109, 111

DNA (Continued)
  in genetic locus identification, 1541–1542
Docosahexaenoic acid, anti-inflammatory
    effect of, 711
  in rheumatoid arthritis, 886–887
  synthesis of, fatty acids in, 526, 528,
    528–530
Dolobid, 723t, 725, 725–726
L-Dopa, for sleep disturbances, in
    fibromyalgia syndrome, 517
Double crush syndromes, 582
Doxycycline, for Lyme disease, 1469, 1469t
  for osteoarthritis, 1400t, 1400–1401
Drawer tests, in knee examination,
    367–368
  in sports medicine, 557
Droloxifene, for osteoporosis, 1569
Drug abuse, intravenous, and septic
    arthritis, 376, 1439, 1439t
Ductus arteriosus, patent, nonsteroidal
    anti-inflammatory drugs for, 713
Duncan's disease, 1285t, 1292
Dupuytren's contracture, 359, 1165–1166
Dwarfism, in achondroplasia, 1555
  in cartilage-hair hypoplasia, 1297
Dysbaric osteonecrosis, 1584–1585
Dysphagia, cervical spinal disorders and,
    403
  in Sjögren's syndrome, 960
Dysprosium 165, in radiation synovec-
    tomy, for rheumatoid arthritis, 947
Dystonia, 585
Dystroglycan, in extracellular matrix, 45
Dystrophin, in skeletal muscle, 79, 79t

Ear, disorders of, cervical spinal disorders
    and, 403
  in Cogan's syndrome, 1112, 1113
  external, in relapsing polychondritis,
    1404–1405, 1405, 1407
  tophi of, in gout, 1316, 1317
  ossicular erosion in, in rheumatoid ar-
    thritis, 911
Eaton-Lambert syndrome, vs. inflam-
    matory muscle disease, 1190, 1197
Ecchymosis, in familial amyloidosis, 1414,
    1414, 1416t
Echinococcosis, vertebral, and low back
    pain, 452
Echocardiography, in rheumatic fever, 1233
Echovirus infection, and arthritis, 1480
Ectopia lentis, in Marfan syndrome, 1552
Eczema, in Wiskott-Aldrich syndrome,
    1296
Edema, hemorrhagic, acute, 504
  in physical examination, 1882
  in scleroderma, 1135, 1135
  of bone marrow, magnetic resonance im-
    aging of, 639, 640
  of fingers, examination for, 360–361, 361
  of joints, in osteoarthritis, 1386
    in patient history, 354
    in physical examination, 355
  of wrist, in physical examination, 359
Ehlers-Danlos syndrome, 1546–1551,
    1547–1549, 1548t, 1551
  genetic defect in, 30–31, 31t, 33t, 1540,
    1540t, 1541
Eicosanoids, in inflammation, 296–299,
    297t
  receptors of, 294–296
  synthesis of, 287–294, 288t–290t, 289,
    292, 293, 295

Eicosanoids (Continued)
  drugs inhibiting, 708–711, 709, 710
  fatty acids in, 332, 332–335, 334, 527,
    527–530, 528, 530
Eicosapentaenoic acid, anti-inflammatory
    effect of, 711
  in rheumatoid arthritis, 886–887
  synthesis of, fatty acids in, 526, 528,
    528–530
Elafin, 329t, 329–330
Elastase, in neutrophils, 147
Elastin, biosynthesis of, 33, 34
  degradation of, by proteinases, 331
  gene for, 32–33
  defects of, and disease, 34–35
  metabolic turnover of, 33–34
Elbow, arthritis of, monarticular,
    differential diagnosis of, 373t
  post-traumatic, 1679, 1680
  arthrocentesis of, 602, 602
  arthroplasty of, 1684–1688, 1685t, 1685–
    1689, 1687t
    complications of, 1688–1690, 1690,
      1691
    distraction, 1684, 1684
    failure of, management of, 1690–1692,
      1691, 1692
    in juvenile rheumatoid arthritis, 1775,
      1780
    interposition, 1682–1684, 1683
    radiography of, 1835–1836, 1836–1838
  biomechanics of, 1675, 1676
  disorders of, glucocorticoids for, 596–
    597, 597t
    in sports medicine, 551–553, 552
  examination of, 358, 358–359
  function of, 1676, 1676–1677, 1677
  instability of, post-traumatic, 1679
  osteoarthritis of, 1679–1680, 1680, 1681
  rheumatic disease of, surgery for, 1680t,
    1680–1684, 1681–1684
    indications for, 1680–1681
    rehabilitation after, 1692, 1692–1694,
      1693
  rheumatoid arthritis of, 912
    imaging of, 649
    presentation of, 1677–1679, 1678, 1679,
      1679t
  ulnar nerve entrapment in, 573, 573–574
Elderly, bacterial arthritis in, 1441
  glucocorticoid clearance in, 793
  nonsteroidal anti-inflammatory drug use
    in, 721–722, 723t, 729t
  osteoarthritis in, 1376
    psychosocial impact of, 536
  osteoporosis in, 1563–1564
  rheumatic disease in, 541, 541–544, 543t
  rheumatoid arthritis in, onset of, 901
  rotator cuff tears in, 427
Electricity, and bony structural adaptation,
    71–72
Electrocardiography, in rheumatic fever,
    1233
Electrodiagnostic studies, in carpal tunnel
    syndrome, 568–569
  in entrapment syndromes, 566, 567t
  of cervical spinal disorders, 408
Electromyography, in carpal tunnel
    syndrome, 569
  in dermatomyositis, in children, 1247
  in entrapment syndromes, 566, 567t
  in hip pain, 469
  in inflammatory muscle disease, 1196–
    1197
  in knee pain, 462

Electromyography (Continued)
  in myopathy, 390
  in polymyositis, 1181
  in shoulder pain, 420
Electrotherapy, in osteoarthritis, 1396
  in rehabilitative medicine, 1624
ELISA (enzyme-linked immunosorbent
    assay), for antinuclear antibodies, 253
  for rheumatoid factors, 241, 242
  in evaluation of inflammation, 704
  in Lyme disease, 1467, 1467, 1873–1874
Ely test, of femoral nerve, in low back
    pain, 442
Embolism, fat, and osteonecrosis, 1584
  pulmonary, after hip arthroplasty, 1728,
    1732
    in antiphospholipid syndrome, 1061
Embryo, synovial joint development in,
    2–5, 2–5
Emphysema, α_1-antitrypsin deficiency and,
    34–35
Endocarditis, bacterial, arthritis with,
    pauciarticular, 384
    vs. rheumatoid arthritis, 904
  rheumatoid factors in, 244
  in rheumatic fever, 1229
  in rheumatoid arthritis, 921
Endocrine disorders, 1499–1510. See also
    specific disorders, e.g., Hypothyroidism.
  clinical features of, 1499–1500, 1500t
Endometriosis, and hip pain, 476
Endothelial cells, in fibroblast regulation,
    201, 203
  in inflammatory response, 183–195
    activation of, 184
    apoptosis in, 183
    desquamation of, 183
    dysfunction of, 184
    in chronic reactions, 191–194, 194t
    in vascular response, 184–186
    interaction of, with leukocytes, 186t,
      186–191, 187t, 189, 190t, 191
    lysis in, 183
    necrosis in, 183
    stimulation of, 184
  in vasculitis, pathology of, 1081, 1083,
    1085
  monocyte adhesion to, 129–130
  neutrophil adherence to, 149–150
Endothelial venules, lymphocyte
    movement in, 119–120
Endothelin-1, in synovial vasculature, 13,
    14
Endothelioma, synovial. See Synovitis,
    pigmented villonodular.
Endothelium, vascular, eosinophil
    adherence to, 157
Energy, dietary deficiency of, in
    inflammatory response, 521
English walnuts, sensitivity to, in Behçet's
    syndrome, 531
Enkephalins, in rheumatoid arthritis, 870
Entactin, in extracellular matrix, 39, 40, 42,
    47, 48
Enteritis, in Reiter's syndrome, 990
Enterobacter infection, in Reiter's
    syndrome, 993, 995
Enterocolitis, gold therapy and, 764
Enteropathic arthritis, 1006–1013
  after intestinal bypass, 1010–1011, 1011
  glucocorticoids for, intra-articular
    injection of, 596
  imaging of, 660
    in children, 653–654
  in collagenous colitis, 1011–1012, 1012

Enteropathic arthritis *(Continued)*
   in gluten-sensitive enteropathy, 1011
   in Poncet's disease, 1012–1013
   in Whipple's disease, 1011, *1012*
   monarticular, 377
   pauciarticular, 384
   physiology of, 1006, *1006*
   polyarticular, 385
   postenteritic reactive, 1008–1010, 1009t,
      1010
   vs. Reiter's syndrome, 992
   vs. rheumatoid arthritis, 903
   with inflammatory bowel disease, *1007*,
      1007–1008, 1008t
Enthesitis, in ankylosing spondylitis, 973,
   974
     physical examination for, 976
Enthesopathy, degenerative, imaging of,
   667
Entrapment syndrome(s), 564–582. See also
   specific syndromes, e.g., *Carpal tunnel*
   syndrome.
   diagnosis of, 372, 374t, 386, 566–567,
      567t, *568–570*
   double crush, 582
   nerve anatomy in, 564–565, *565, 566*
   nerve injury in, types of, 565–566
   of axillary nerve, *433*, 433–434, 578
   of femoral cutaneous nerve, lateral, 580–
      581
   of femoral nerve, 581
   of genitofemoral nerve, 581
   of ilioinguinal nerve, 581
   of median nerve, 567–573, *568, 569,* 569t,
      572
   of musculocutaneous nerve, 578
   of obturator nerve, 581
   of peroneal nerve, 579
   of pudendal nerve, 582
   of radial nerve, 575–576, *576*
   of scapular nerve, dorsal, 578
   of sciatic nerve, 578–579
   of suprascapular nerve, 434, 577–578
   of sural nerve, 580
   of thoracic nerve, long, 578
   of thoracic outlet, 577, *577*
   of tibial nerve, 579–580, *580*, 598
   of ulnar nerve, *573*, 573–575
   pseudoradicular, 582
   rectus abdominis muscle in, 582
   types of, 564, 564t
   with overuse syndromes, 585, 585t
Enzyme-linked immunosorbent assay, for
   antinuclear antibodies, 253
   for rheumatoid factors, 241, 242
   in evaluation of inflammation, 704
   in Lyme disease, 1467, *1467*, 1873–1874
Eosinophil(s), *155*, 155–158, 158t
   glucocorticoid effects on, 790t, 791
   in synovial fluid analysis, 616
   priming of, 152t, 158
Eosinophil cationic protein, 155, *155*, 156
Eosinophil peroxidase, *155*, 155–157
Eosinophil protein X, *155*, 155–156
Eosinophilia, 158, 158t
   idiopathic, vs. rheumatoid arthritis, 906
   in rheumatoid arthritis, 919
   synovial biopsy in, 623
Eosinophilia-myalgia syndrome,
   1157–1158, 1185
Eosinophilic fasciitis, 1156–1157, *1157*
   and blood disorders, 1529–1530, 1531t
   antimalarial drugs for, 754
   in children, 1253
Eosinophilic myositis, 1184–1185

Epicondylitis, examination for, 358–359
   glucocorticoids for, 596–597, 604, *605*
   in sports medicine, 552
Epidermolysis bullosa, 1556–1557
   collagen gene defect in, 31, 33t
Epiligrin, in extracellular matrix, 48
Epineurium, anatomy of, 564, *566*
Epiphyseal arteries, 68–69, *69*
Epiphyseal dysplasia, multiple, 1555
Epiphyses, in hemophilia, 680, *680*
   in juvenile chronic arthritis, *651*, 651–652
   in juvenile rheumatoid arthritis, *1213*,
      1213–1214
Episcleritis, 489t, *490*, 490–492, Plate 3
   in rheumatoid arthritis, 916–917, *917*
Epistaxis, in rheumatic fever, 1232
Epithelial neutrophil–activating peptide-78,
   in rheumatoid arthritis, 868
Epithelioma, discoid lupus erythematosus
   and, 1528, 1531t
Epstein-Barr virus, and arthritis, 1481
   and X-linked lymphoproliferative dis-
      ease, 1292
   binding of, to complement receptors, 235
   in rheumatoid arthritis, 855t855–856
   in Sjögren's syndrome, 964–965
Equilibrium, disorders of, cervical spinal
   disorders and, 403
   in Cogan's syndrome, 1112
Erythema chronicum migrans, in Lyme
   disease, 1872, *1873*
Erythema circinatum, in rheumatic fever,
   507
Erythema elevatum diutinum, 503
Erythema induratum, 504
Erythema infectiosum, with parvovirus
   arthropathy, 509
Erythema marginatum, in rheumatic fever,
   506–507, 1231
Erythema migrans, in Lyme disease, 507,
   507, 1463, 1463, 1464t, Plate 6, Plate 12
Erythema nodosum, 508, 508t
   in Reiter's syndrome, 989
   paraneoplastic, 1526
Erythema papulatum, in rheumatic fever,
   507
Erythrocyte sedimentation rate, 1884
   measurement of, in inflammation, 701–
      704, 702t
Erythromelalgia, with cancer, 1526, 1527t
Erythromycin, for Lyme disease, 1469,
   1469t
   for *Neisseria* infection, in arthritis, 1446
   for Whipple's disease, 1011
   in prevention of rheumatic fever, 1237,
      1237t, 1238, 1238t
Erythropoietin, in mononuclear phagocyte
   maturation, in bone marrow, 131t, 132
Escherichia coli infection, and arthritis,
   radiography of, 1437, *1438*
   in rheumatoid arthritis, 856, 857
E-selectin, *305*, 311–312, Plate 2
   in leukocyte–endothelial cell adhesion,
      in inflammatory response, 186t,
      187t, 188–190, *191*
   in rheumatoid arthritis, 873t, 874
   monoclonal antibodies to, in anti-inflam-
      matory treatment, 317
Esophagus, in mixed connective tissue
   disease, 1071, *1072*, 1074
   in scleroderma, 1146, *1147*, 1154
     carcinoma of, 1529, 1531t
   in Sjögren's syndrome, 960
Estrogens, and uric acid excretion, 1329
   in bone cell metabolism, 60–61

Estrogens *(Continued)*
   in contraceptives, and arthritis, 904
   in osteoporosis, 1509, 1568–1569
   in systemic lupus erythematosus, 1018–
      1019, 1054
Ethambutol, for tuberculosis, 1454
Ethanol, use of, and gout, 1319, 1346
   and osteonecrosis, 1584
10-Ethyl-10-deazaaminopterin, for
   rheumatoid arthritis, 777–778
Ethylsuccinate, in prevention of rheumatic
   fever, 1238t
Etidronate, for osteoporosis, 1569t,
   1569–1571
   for Paget's disease of bone, 1576
Etodolac, 729t, 734, *734*
Etretinate, for lupus dermatitis, 1043, 1043t
Ewald elbow prosthesis, radiography of,
   1836, *1837*
Exercise, in elderly, and muscle function,
   541
   in fibromyalgia syndrome, 517–518
   in inflammatory muscle disease, in as-
      sessment, 1199
   in neck pain, 410
   in osteoarthritis, 1395–1396
     of hip, 1851–1852
     of knee, 1856, 1856t
   in rheumatic disease, in rehabilitation,
      1621–1623, *1622*
   in rheumatoid arthritis, 934–938
     of hand, 1647
     of wrist, 1647
   muscle fiber adaptation to, 83
   range of motion, in physical examina-
      tion, of musculoskeletal disorders,
      1882
Extensor muscles, of hand, reflex testing
   of, 406t
Extensor tendons, of hand, rupture of,
   surgery for, *1648, 1649*, 1649–1650
   of toes, transfer of, 1769, *1770, 1771*
Extracellular matrix, 37–51
   at cell surface, 37–40, *38, 39*
   collagen in, synthesis of, defects of,
      1536–1539, *1537*, 1537t
     types of, 1535–1536, 1536t
   components of, *38, 39*, 44–51
     chemical structures of, 40–43, *41, 42*
     classification of, 40
   fluid phase, 37, *38, 39*
   functions of, 43–44
   in angiogenesis, in inflammatory re-
      sponse, 194
   in scleroderma, 1138–1139, 1139t
   interaction of, with fibroblasts, 202–205
   of articular cartilage, composition of,
      1369–1370, 1370t
     metabolism in, 1370–1371
   proteinases degrading, 323–327, 324t–
      327t, *328*
     enzymic mechanisms of, 330–331, *331,*
      332
     inhibitors of, endogenous, 327–330,
      329t
     regulation of, cellular, 331–334, 332t–
      335t
      extracellular, 335–338, *336, 337*, 338t
   regulators of, 44
   solid phase, 37, *38, 39*
   structural proteins of, heritable disorders
      of, 1535–1557
Eye(s), disorders of, cervical spinal
   disorders and, 403
   in ankylosing spondylitis, 494, 974

Eye(s) (Continued)
  in antiphospholipid syndrome, 1061
  in Behçet's disease, 494, 494, 1114t,
      1114–1116, Plate 4, Plate 12
  in Cogan's syndrome, 1112
  in diffuse infiltrative lymphocytosis,
      in human immunodeficiency vi-
      rus infection, 1274
  in Ehlers-Danlos syndrome, 1550
  in juvenile rheumatoid arthritis, 492,
      492, 1212, 1212, 1219–1222
  in Lyme disease, 494, 1464t
  in Marfan syndrome, 1552
  in polyarteritis, 493, 1094
  in polychondritis, relapsing, 493,
      1405–1406
  in pseudoxanthoma elasticum, 1554
  in psoriatic arthritis, 494, 1002
  in Reiter's syndrome, 494, 989–990,
      993–994
  in rheumatic diseases, 488–494, 489t,
      489–494, Plates 3 and 4
  in rheumatoid arthritis, 492, 916–917,
      917
  in sarcoidosis, 493–494, 494
  in Sjögren's syndrome, 956t, 956–957,
      957, 957t, 965
  in spondyloarthropathy, 494
  in Stickler's syndrome, 1555
  in systemic lupus erythematosus, 492–
      493, 493, 1036–1037
  in Wegener's granulomatosis, 493, 493,
      1101, Plate 4
  tear film in, 488–489, 489, 489t, Plate 3
  with myositis, localized, 1186
  protrusion of, orbital pseudotumor and,
      1166–1167
  scleritis in, 489t, 490, 490–492, 491, 916–
      917, 917, Plate 3
  toxicity to, antimalarial agents and, 747,
      755, 755t, 756
    glucocorticoids and, 796
    gold therapy and, 764
    hydroxychloroquine and, in rheuma-
        toid arthritis, 1898t, 1899–1900
  uveitis in, 489t, 489–490
  vision loss in, with optic nerve dysfunc-
      tion, in giant cell arteritis, 1126,
      1126, 1130
Eyelids, inflammation of, in Sjögren's
    syndrome, 957

Fabere test, 364, 442, 1725
Face, abnormalities of, in DiGeorge's
    syndrome, 1292, 1292
Facet blocks, in low back pain, 446–447
Facet joints, anatomy of, 397
  lumbar, computed tomography of, 631,
      632
Factor B, in complement system, 233t, 234
  gene for, 1305, 1306
Factor D, in complement system, 233t, 234
Factor increasing monocytopoiesis, 133
Fairbanks apprehension test, in knee
    examination, 367
Familial Mediterranean fever, colchicine
    for, 728
  genetic linkage analysis in, 224
  monarticular arthritis in, 378
  vs. rheumatoid arthritis, 905
Farr radioimmunoassay, for antinuclear
    antibodies, 255
Fasciitis, eosinophilic, 1156–1157, 1157

Fasciitis (Continued)
  and blood disorders, 1529–1530, 1531t
    antimalarial drugs for, 754
  in children, 1253
  palmar, in reflex sympathetic dystrophy,
      with cancer, 1525, 1527t
  plantar, 485, 486
Fat, in embolism, and osteonecrosis, 1584
  metabolism of, disorders of, glucocorti-
      coids and, 796
  presacral, herniation of, 598
  subcutaneous, inflammation of, in sys-
      temic lupus erythematosus, 1036
    paraneoplastic, 1525–1526, 1527t
    skin lesions in, 508t, 508–509
Fatigue, chronic, after sarcoidosis, 1421
  syndrome of, vs. fibromyalgia syn-
      drome, 513–514
    vs. Lyme disease, 1468
    vs. rheumatoid arthritis, 904–905
  in Lyme disease, with fibromyalgia, anti-
      biotics for, 1872–1878, 1874t–1877t
  in patient history, 354–355
  in rheumatic disease, psychosocial im-
      pact of, 537
  in Sjögren's syndrome, treatment of, 965
  in systemic lupus erythematosus, 1029,
      1043
  muscular, laboratory evaluation of, 391
  psychogenic, 392
Fatty acid acylCoA dehydrogenase
    deficiency, and myopathy, 1193
Fatty acids, in immune response, 526–531,
    527, 528, 530, 711
Fc receptors, in immune complex
    formation, 228
  on mononuclear phagocyte surfaces, 134
  on neutrophil surface, in phagocytosis,
      150, 151, 151t
Feet. See Foot (feet).
Feldene (piroxicam), 723t, 726, 726
  interaction of, with cimetidine, 720t
  use of, in elderly, 722
Felty's syndrome, 951, 951–954, 952t
  methotrexate for, 778
Femoral cutaneous nerve, lateral,
    entrapment of, 580–581
  injury to, in surgery, 586
Femoral hernia, and hip pain, 476
Femoral nerve, entrapment of, 581
  injury to, in childbirth, 586
    in surgery, 586
  testing of, in low back pain, 442
  reflexes in, 406t
Femur, bone grafting to, in hip
    replacement, 1797, 1798
  condyles of, osteonecrosis of, 1589
  fracture of, after hip arthroplasty, 1813,
      1816
  head of, aseptic necrosis of, magnetic res-
      onance imaging of, 468, 469
    avascular necrosis of, in sickle cell dis-
        ease, 1496
    in resistance to compression, 91, 91
    in knee replacement, 1743–1746, 1744,
        1746, 1747
  neck of, fracture of, 471–473, 472
    and bone marrow edema, magnetic
        resonance imaging of, 639, 640
    osteonecrosis of, 1581–1590. See also
        Osteonecrosis.
  resorption of, after hip replacement,
      1798
  prosthetic, in hip arthroplasty, fractures
      of, 1812–1813, 1815

Femur (Continued)
  osteolysis around, 1812
  positioning of, in radiography, 1788–
      1789
Fenamates, 729t, 733, 733
Fenoprofen, 729t, 731, 731–732
  toxicity of, to kidney, 716–717
Ferric hydroxide, in radiation synovec-
    tomy, for rheumatoid arthritis, 947
Ferritin. See Iron.
Fertility, drug effects on, in treatment of
    rheumatoid arthritis, 1902t, 1903
Fetus. See also Pregnancy.
  joint development in, synovial, 2–5, 2–5
  tissue transplantation from, for cellular
      immunodeficiency, 1301
Fever, in juvenile rheumatoid arthritis,
    1209, 1211
  in systemic lupus erythematosus, 1029
  nonsteroidal anti-inflammatory drugs
      for, 713
  rheumatic, 1225–1238. See also Rheumatic
      fever.
Fibrillarin, antibodies to, in inflammatory
    muscle diseases, 261
  in scleroderma, 258t, 259
Fibrillin, gene for, 32–33
  defects of, and disease, 35
  in elastic fibrils, 32
  in extracellular matrix, 42, 46–47
Fibrin, in synovial fluid, in rheumatoid
    arthritis, 887–888
Fibrinogen, in inflammation, and
    erythrocyte sedimentation rate, 701
  in acute-phase response, 699, 700
Fibrinogen A α, in amyloidosis, familial,
    1410, 1410t
Fibroblast growth factors, in acute
    inflammation, 273
  in angiogenesis, 194, 274
  in articular cartilage, 8–9
  in rheumatoid arthritis, 869
Fibroblast(s), 199–206
  activation of, 199, 199–200, 200
  cytokines of, in rheumatoid arthritis,
      866–870
  development of, cytokines in, 273
  heterogeneity of, 200, 205
  immune modulation of, 202–205, 203,
      204t
  in joint development, 3
  in response to injury, 199, 199–202, 201t,
      202t
  in rheumatic disease, interaction of, with
      mast cells, 164
  in synovial stroma, 13
Fibroblast-like cells, in synovial lining, 12
Fibroendothelioma, synovial. See Synovitis,
    pigmented villonodular.
Fibroma, of tendon sheath, 1599–1600,
    1600
Fibromodulin, in extracellular matrix, 42,
    45
Fibromyalgia, 511–518
  and polyarticular pain, 387
  causation of, 513
  clinical features of, 511, 511–512
  consequences of, 513
  diagnosis of, 512–513, 513, 513t
  epidemiology of, 512, 512
  in Lyme disease, with fatigue, antibiotics
      for, 1872–1878, 1874t–1877t
  of shoulder, 435
  pathophysiology of, 514, 514–516, 516,
      516t

Fibromyalgia (Continued)
  secondary, 514
  silicone breast implants and, 1173
  treatment of, 517–518
  vs. arthritis, monarticular, 373
    rheumatoid, 905
  vs. chronic fatigue syndrome, 513–514
  vs. multiple chemical sensitivity, 514
Fibronectin, CS1 region of, in rheumatoid
    arthritis, 874, 874
  in extracellular matrix, 37, 38, 39, 42, 44,
    47
  receptors of, on mononuclear phago-
    cytes, 134–136
Fibrosis, 199, 200
  and knee pain, 463, 464
  in chronic inflammation, cytokines in,
    276–278, 277
  in Dupuytren's contracture, 1165–1166
  in keloids, 1166
  in orbital pseudotumor, 1166–1167
  of liver, 1164–1165
  penile, in Peyronie's disease, 1166
  pulmonary, 1163–1164
    in rheumatoid arthritis, 920
  retroperitoneal, 1166
  silicone implants and, 1170
  thyroid, in Riedel's struma, 1167
  with carcinoid tumors, 1166
Fibrositis, and pain. See Fibromyalgia.
Fibroxanthoma, of tendon sheath,
    1608–1610, 1610, 1611
Fifth disease, 509
Filtration, extracellular matrix components
    in, 43
Finger(s), clubbing of, in hypertrophic
    osteoarthropathy, 1514–1516, 1515,
    1518
  elongated, in Marfan syndrome, 1552,
    1553
  flexor tendons of, biomechanics of, 88,
    89
    surgery of, 1650–1652, 1653
  in osteoarthritis, 1389, 1389, 1391, 1391
  in systemic lupus erythematosus, sur-
    gery of, 1663–1666, 1665, 1666
  interphalangeal joints of. See Interphalan-
    geal joint(s).
  necrosis of, with cancer, 1526, 1527t
  nerves of, entrapment syndromes of,
    572–573, 575, 576
  physical examination of, 360–362, 361,
    362
  psoriatic arthritis of, 1668, 1668
  rheumatoid arthritis of, 1658–1661, 1659,
    1660
  sarcoidosis of, 1670–1671
  tophi of, in gout, 1316, 1317
  trigger deformity of, 360, 604, 1650–1652
Fingernails, in clubbing, in hypertrophic
    osteoarthropathy, 1515, 1515
  in psoriasis, 498, 498
  in Reiter's syndrome, 989
    with human immunodeficiency virus
      infection, 1269, 1270
Finklestein test, for de Quervain's
    tenosynovitis, 360
Fish oil, fatty acids in, in eicosanoid
    synthesis, 332, 332–335, 334, 711
Fistulas, in rheumatoid arthritis, 918
  infection and, after hip arthroplasty,
    1809
FK-506, effect of, on cytokine production,
    105
  for rheumatoid arthritis, 945

FK-506 (Continued)
  in histamine inhibition, 163
  in immunosuppression, 820, 821, 823t
Flexor carpi radialis muscle, testing of, 360
Flexor carpi ulnaris muscle, in ulnar nerve
    entrapment, 573, 573–574
  testing of, 360
Flexor digitorum muscles, reflex testing of,
    406t
Flexor muscles, of foot, reflex testing of,
    405, 406t
Flexor pollicis longus muscle, reflex testing
    of, 406t
Flexor pollicis longus tendon, rupture of,
    surgery for, 1652, 1653
Flexor tendons, of hand, biomechanics of,
    88, 89
  surgery of, 1650–1652, 1653
  synovitis of, in rheumatoid arthritis,
    914, 1650–1652
Fluconazole, for fungal infection, 1459,
    1459t
Flufenamic acid, 733, 733
Fluid balance, maintenance of, in surgery,
    1644
Fluoride, for osteoporosis, 1570, 1572
Fluoroscopy, after hip arthroplasty, 1788
5-Fluorouracil, in immunosuppression, for
    non-neoplastic diseases, 810, 815, 823t
Flurbiprofen, 729t, 734, 734
  in cyclooxygenase pathway inhibition,
    709
Focal adhesion kinase, in fibroblast
    regulation, 202
Folic acid, structure of, 771, 772
  with methotrexate therapy, 779, 783,
    1900–1901
Folinic acid, structure of, 772
  with methotrexate therapy, 779, 780
Food. See Nutrition.
Foot (feet), arthritis in, monarticular,
    differential diagnosis of, 373t
  bursitis in, 486
  clubbing of, in sarcoidosis, 1420–1421
  disorders of, glucocorticoid injection for,
    597t, 598, 606
    surgery for, 1766–1772, 1768–1771
  in gout, 484–485
  in neuropathic osteoarthropathy, 485
  in osteoarthritis, 483, 483–484, 484
    imaging of, 665
  in psoriatic arthritis, 486, 658, 658
  in Reiter's syndrome, 486, 987, 987–988,
    988
    imaging of, 659, 659–660
    with human immunodeficiency virus
      infection, 1269, 1269, 1270
  in rheumatoid arthritis, 481–483, 482,
    915, 915–916
    imaging of, 648t, 649, 649, 650
  in scleroderma, 486–487
  in sickle cell disease, 1493–1494
  in spondyloarthropathy, 486
  in systemic lupus erythematosus, 486
  Lisfranc fracture-dislocation of, with dia-
    betic neuroarthropathy, 671, 671
  magnetic resonance imaging of, 641–642
  pain in, 479–487
    imaging in, 481
    physical examination in, 480–481, 481
  plantar fasciitis in, 485, 486
  tendinitis in, 486
Force, dissipation of, articular cartilage in,
    9–10, 10
  in joint biomechanics, 87–88, 88, 89

Force (Continued)
  frictional, minimization of, 89, 89, 90
Forearm, nodules of, needle biopsy of, 604,
    606
Forefoot. See also Foot.
  anatomy of, 479, 480
  disorders of, surgery for, 1767–1770,
    1769–1771
  squeeze test of, 481, 481
Forestier's disease (diffuse idiopathic
    skeletal hyperostosis), and low back
    pain, 450
  imaging of, 668–669, 669, 670
  in diabetes mellitus, 1501
  vs. ankylosing spondylitis, 655, 657
  vs. osteoarthritis, 1391–1392
Fosamax (alendronate), for osteoporosis,
    1569t, 1570
  for Paget's disease of bone, 1577
Fracture(s), after elbow replacement,
    1689–1690, 1836, 1838
  after knee replacement, patellar, 1752
    radiography of, 1828, 1828, 1829, 1829
  glucocorticoids and, in rheumatoid ar-
    thritis, 940
  in osteogenesis imperfecta, 1543t, 1543–
    1545
  in osteomalacia, 1573, 1573
  intra-articular loose bodies after, 1595,
    1595–1596, 1596
  Lisfranc, with diabetic neuroarthropathy,
    671, 671
  of ankle, and arthrosis, 1759–1760, 1760
    arthrodesis after, 1762
    computed tomography of, 630, 630
    in sports medicine, 560, 561
  of epiphyses, in juvenile chronic arthri-
    tis, 652
  of femoral neck, 1813, 1816
    and bone marrow edema, magnetic
      resonance imaging of, 639, 640
    and osteonecrosis, 1582–1583
  of femoral prosthetic component, after
    hip arthroplasty, 1812–1813, 1815
  of femur, after hip arthroplasty, 1813,
    1816
  of hip, 470–473, 471, 472
  of humerus, and osteonecrosis, 429
  of spine, cervical, in ankylosing spondy-
    litis, 1719–1720, 1720
  of tibia, 559–560, 1759
  pathologic, magnetic resonance imaging
    of, 637, 638, 638
Free radicals, 522–523, 523
  in ischemia, and hyperuricemia, 1320
  in synovial fluid, in rheumatoid arthri-
    tis, 886
  regulation of, trace metals in, 524–526
    vitamins in, 523–524
  release of, in uric acid formation, 1324–
    1325, 1325
Frictional force, in joint biomechanics,
    minimization of, 89, 89, 90
Fructose, intolerance to, and gout, 1331t,
    1337
Fungal infection, osteoarticular, 1450,
    1456–1459, 1457, 1459t
Fusion toxins, for rheumatoid arthritis,
    842, 860

G5 capture, in mast cell assessment, 171
Gadolinium diethylenetetraminepenta-
    acetic acid, in magnetic resonance
    imaging, of spine, 636, 637

Gait, disorders of, in osteoarthritis, 1386
  in hip examination, 363
  in rehabilitative medicine, 1629–1630
  quadriceps motion in, control of, 92, *92*
Galactose, residues of, on immunoglobulin
    G, rheumatoid factors and, 243
Galeazzi's sign, in hip examination, 364
Gallbladder, puncture of, liver biopsy and,
    1867, 1871t
Gallie atlantoaxial fusion, 1718
Gallium-67, in scintigraphy, after hip
    arthroplasty, 1811, 1811t
Gallium nitrate, for Paget's disease of
    bone, 1577
Gamma globulin, blood level of, elevated,
      in Waldenström's purpura, 1108
  reduced, cyclophosphamide and, 813
  for inflammatory muscle disease, 1201
  for polyarteritis, 1096
  for thrombocytopenia, in systemic lupus
      erythematosus, 1052
Ganglion cysts, 1593–1595, *1594, 1595*
  aspiration of, 597, 604
  physical examination for, 360
Gastrocsoleus muscle, in hindfoot motion,
    1766
Gastrointestinal tract, bypass surgery of,
      arthritis-dermatitis syndrome after,
      1010–1011, *1011*
  disorders of, and arthritis, 1006–1013.
      See also *Enteropathic arthritis.*
    and hypertrophic osteoarthropathy,
        1514t, 1516
    and low back pain, 453
    in amyloidosis, 1414, 1416t
    in Henoch-Schönlein purpura, 1258
    in mixed connective tissue disease,
        1071, *1072,* 1074
    in polyarteritis, 1094
    in Reiter's syndrome, 990
      with human immunodeficiency vi-
          rus infection, 1270
    in scleroderma, 1146–1147, *1147,* 1154
      in children, 1250, 1250t
    in Sjögren's syndrome, 960–961, 961t
    in systemic lupus erythematosus, 1036
  toxicity to, cyclophosphamide and, 813
    glucocorticoids and, 795
    gold therapy and, 764
    ketorolac and, 735
    methotrexate and, 779–780
    nonsteroidal anti-inflammatory drugs
        and, 350–351, 713–715
      in osteoarthritis, 1397, 1852–1853
      in rheumatoid arthritis, 1890–1891,
          1898, 1898t
    D-penicillamine and, 767
    sulfasalazine and, 742–743, 743t
    sulindac and, 725
Gaucher's disease, and bone loss, 1565
Gelatinases, in extracellular matrix
      degradation, 324t, 325t, 326, 327t,
      328
  with fibroblast proliferation, 204
Gelsolin, in amyloidosis, familial, 1410,
    1410t
Genetics, allele-sharing studies in, 224–225,
    225
  human leukocyte antigens in, 210–214.
      See also *Human leukocyte antigens.*
  in antigen-specific recognition, by B
      cells, 106–112, *108, 109*
  in antiphospholipid syndrome, 1058
  in calcium pyrophosphate deposition dis-
      ease, 1353–1354, 1354t

Genetics *(Continued)*
  in collagen structure, 26
  in collagen synthesis, defects of, 1538–
      1539
      and connective tissue disease, 1539–
          1542, 1540t
  in gout, 1334t, 1334–1336, 1335t, 1338
  in hemochromatosis, 1424, 1427–1428
  in immunodeficiency disorders, 1284t,
      1284–1285
  in inflammatory muscle disease, 1179,
      1187–1188
  in rheumatic disease, 209–225
    future studies in, 225
    population association studies in, 214–
        216, 217t, *220,* 220–221
  in rheumatoid arthritis, 209, 852–854,
      853t
  in rheumatoid factor synthesis, 244–245
  in Sjögren's syndrome, 964
  in susceptibility to disease, 209–210
  in systemic lupus erythematosus, 1015–
      1018, 1016t, 1018t, 1028–1029
  linkage analysis in, 221–224, *222, 223,*
      224t
  of complement system, 236, 1305–1306,
      1306
  transcription in, glucocorticoids in, 789,
      789
Genitalia, disorders of, and hip pain, 476
    in Peyronie's disease, 1166
    in Reiter's syndrome, 988, *989,* 993
Genitofemoral nerve, entrapment of, 581
    injury to, in surgery, 586
    reflex testing of, 406t
Genu recurvatum, examination for, 365
Genu valgum, examination for, 365
Genu varum, examination for, 365
German measles (rubella), in arthritis,
      1475–1477, *1476*
    rheumatoid, 856
Germline transcription, in antigen-specific
      recognition, by B cells, 110
Giant cell arteritis, 1123–1130
  clinical features of, 1125t, 1125–1127,
      1126, 1127
  definition of, 1123
  diagnosis of, 1128–1129, 1130t
  epidemiology of, 1123
  etiology of, 1123–1124
  in children, 1259–1260, *1260*
  laboratory studies in, 703–704, 1128
  pathogenesis of, 1124
  pathology of, *1124,* 1124–1125, *1125*
  polyarthritis in, vs. rheumatoid arthritis,
      908
  polymyalgia rheumatica with, 1127–1128
  skin lesions in, 503
  treatment of, 1129–1130
Giant cell myositis, 1186
Giant cell synovioma, benign, 1607–1608,
    1608–1610
Giant cell tumor, of tendon sheath,
    1608–1610, *1610, 1611*
Girdlestone-Taylor procedure, 1767–1769,
    1771
Glaucoma, glucocorticoids and, 796
Glenohumeral joint. See also *Shoulder.*
  arthritis of, and pain, 428–429, *429*
  arthroscopic surgery of, 693, *696*
  computed tomography of, 632, *632*
  disorders of, in sports medicine, 547–
      550, *548, 550*
  instability of, and pain, 432
Glenoid labrum, tears of, and pain, 431

Glenoid labrum *(Continued)*
  arthrography of, 416–417, *417*
  computed tomography of, 417, *418*
  magnetic resonance imaging of, 640–
      641, *641*
Glucocorticoids, 787–800
  adverse effects of, 793–797, 794t
  alternate-day oral administration of, 799
  and cancer, 1530
  and delayed wound healing, after foot
      surgery, 1770–1771
  and muscle wasting, vs. inflammatory
      muscle disease, 1190
  and myopathy, with weakness, 392–393
  and osteonecrosis, 1584
    of shoulder, 429–430
  and osteoporosis, 794–795, 1564
    treatment of, 1571t, 1571–1572
  anti-inflammatory effects of, 789t, 789–
      791, 790t
  continuation of, with hip arthroplasty,
      1728
  crystals of, in synovial fluid analysis,
      614, *615,* Plate 8
  effect of, on gene transcription, 789, *789*
  epidural injection of, for low back pain,
      in spinal stenosis, 450
  for Churg-Strauss syndrome, 1099
  for dermatomyositis, in children, 1247–
      1248
  for eosinophilic fasciitis, 1157
  for giant cell arteritis, 1129–1130
  for gold toxicity, 764
  for gout, with acute arthritis, 1343–1344
  for Henoch-Schönlein purpura, 1259
  for inflammatory muscle disease, 1200–
      1201
  for juvenile rheumatoid arthritis, 1219
  for mixed connective tissue disease,
      1074t, 1074–1075
  for osteoarthritis, 1399–1400
  for polyarteritis, 1096
    in children, 1254
  for polychondritis, relapsing, 1407
  for polymyalgia rheumatica, 1130
  for polymyositis, 798–800
  for rheumatic fever, 1236
  for rheumatoid arthritis. See *Rheumatoid
      arthritis, glucocorticoids for.*
  for rotator cuff impingement, 424
  for scleroderma, 1152
  for shoulder pain, in diagnosis, 420–422
  for Sjögren's syndrome, 965–966
  for spondyloarthropathy, with human
      immunodeficiency virus infection,
      1272
  for systemic lupus erythematosus, 798–
      800, 1041–1042, *1044,* 1044t, 1044–
      1046, 1047t
    in children, 1243
    in pregnancy, 1051, 1052t
    side effects of, 1049–1050, 1050t
    with central nervous system disease,
        1034, 1053
    with membranous nephritis, 1053
    with thrombocytopenia, 1052
  for Takayasu's arteritis, 1089–1090
  for vasculitis, 798–800, 1087, 1088
    cutaneous, 1104
    with rheumatoid arthritis, 1111
  globulin-binding, 791
  guidelines for use of, 800
  in Addison's disease, 1506
  in Cushing's syndrome, 1506
  in diffuse infiltrative lymphocytosis, in
      human immunodeficiency virus in-
      fection, 1276, 1277

Glucocorticoids (Continued)
　in eicosanoid pathway inhibition, for inflammatory diseases, 298
　in immunosuppression, 794, 794t, 819
　in mononuclear phagocyte regulation, 136
　interactions of, with nonsteroidal anti-inflammatory drugs, 719t
　intra-articular injection of, bacterial arthritis after, 1439, 1439t
　　contraindications to, 598t, 598–599
　　efficacy of, 593–594
　　indications for, 595t, 595–596
　　mechanism of action of, 591–592
　　precautions in, 593
　　preparations for, 594t, 594–595, 595t
　　sequelae of, 592t, 592–593
　　synovial fluid analysis after, 614, 615, Plate 8
　intramuscular injection of, 799
　metabolic effects of, non-immunomodulatory, 791
　nonarticular injection of, efficacy of, 594
　　indications for, 596–598, 597t
　　techniques of, 603–606, 604–606
　perioperative use of, 799–800
　pharmacokinetics of, 788t, 791–793, 792, 793
　pulse therapy with, 799
　receptors of, 788–789, 789
　structure of, 787, 788
　withdrawal of, joint pain in, vs. rheumatoid arthritis, 905
Glucose, in synovial fluid analysis, 617
Glutamic-oxaloacetic transaminase, serum, after methotrexate therapy, for rheumatoid arthritis, 1864t–1866t, 1864–1867, 1866
Glutamic-pyruvic transaminase, serum, after methotrexate therapy, for rheumatoid arthritis, 1864t, 1864–1866, 1865t
Glutathione, in leukotriene synthesis, 291, 294
Gluteal muscles, strengthening of, exercises for, in rehabilitation, 1622
Gluteal nerves, reflex testing of, 406t
Gluten-sensitive enteropathy, and arthritis, 1011
Gluteus maximus bursa, inflammation of, and pain, 474–475
Gluteus maximus muscle, reflex testing of, 406t
Gluteus medius muscle, reflex testing of, 406t
Glycine, in collagen fibrils, 24, 25
　in collagen gene, in mutations, 1538
　in collagen synthesis, 27, 28, 29, 30
Glycocalyx, in bacterial arthritis, 1435
Glycogen, metabolism of, disorders of, and myopathy, 1191t, 1192
Glycogen storage diseases, and hyperuricemia, 1337, 1337–1338
Glycoproteins, in articular cartilage, 7
　in extracellular matrix, 37–51. See also Extracellular matrix.
　in inflammation, in acute-phase response, 701
Glycosaminoglycans, for osteoarthritis, 1400, 1400t
　in articular cartilage, 1370
　　in aging, 10, 11
　　in resistance to compression, 91
　in bone mineralization, 64
　in extracellular matrix, 40, 41, 43

Glycosaminoglycans (Continued)
　free, 37
　in lamellar bone, 67
　in proteoglycan structure, 312, 314
Glycosylated cell adhesion molecule-1, in leukocyte homing, 315
　L-selectin binding to, 310–312
Glypican, in extracellular matrix, 38, 42, 44, 47
Gold, for rheumatoid arthritis, 759–762, 761, 940–942, 1891–1893, 1892t, 1898t, 1901
　blood tests after, for liver abnormalities, vs. methotrexate, 1864, 1864t
　in combination therapy, with antimalarial drugs, 753
　in pregnancy and lactation, 1902t
　juvenile, 1218–1219
　pharmacology of, 759, 759–760, 760
　toxicity of, 762–765, 763t
　vs. antimalarial drugs, 752, 752t
　vs. methotrexate, 776, 776, 777
Golgi complex, antimalarial drug effects in, 748, 749
Gonococcal infection, and arthritis, 1445, 1445–1447, 1446
　monarticular, 376
　polyarticular, peripheral, 383
　vs. Reiter's syndrome, 991–992, 992t
Gorlin's sign, in Ehlers-Danlos syndrome, 1547, 1547
Gottron's sign, in dermatomyositis, 504, 505, 1181
Gougerot-Sjögren syndrome. See Sjögren's syndrome.
Gout, and foot pain, 484–485
　arthritis in, acute, 1314–1315, 1338–1340
　　colchicine for, 713, 1342–1344
　　monarticular, 377
　　pauciarticular, 383–384
　arthroplasty in, evaluation for, 1636
　atherosclerosis with, 1319
　classification of, 1330, 1331t
　definition of, 1313
　diabetes with, 1318
　diagnosis of, 1885
　diclofenac for, 734
　drugs for, 829–837
　　urate destruction by, 837, 837
　　urate synthesis inhibition by, 829–831, 829–833, 832t
　　uric acid excretion enhanced by, 833–837, 834, 834t, 835, 836t
　epidemiology of, 1313–1314
　genetics of, 1338
　glucocorticoids for, intra-articular injection of, 596
　hand in, surgery of, 1671
　historical aspects of, 1313, 1314t
　hypertension with, 1318–1319
　hypertriglyceridemia with, 1318, 1346
　hypothyroidism with, 1319–1320
　imaging of, 672, 672–673
　in sickle cell disease, 1494–1495
　intercritical, 1315–1316
　leukotrienes in, 297t, 1339–1340
　meclofenamate for, 733
　negative association of, with other rheumatic diseases, 1320
　obesity with, 1318
　primary, uric acid in, overproduction of, 1332–1336, 1333, 1334t, 1335t, 1336
　　renal handling of, 1330–1332, 1332
　renal disorders with, 1320–1323, 1321
　secondary, uric acid in, overproduction of, 1337, 1337–1338

Gout (Continued)
　renal handling of, 1336
　synovial biopsy in, 622
　synovial fluid analysis in, 614, 614, 615, Plate 7
　tophaceous, chronic, 1316t, 1316–1318, 1317–1319
　　vs. osteoarthritis, 1391
　　vs. rheumatoid nodules, 918
　treatment of, 1340–1347, 1341, 1344, 1345t
　vs. rheumatoid arthritis, 905
G-protein, in neutrophil activation, 177
Grafting, of bone, in knee replacement, 1823
　to acetabulum, in hip replacement, 1797, 1797
　to femur, for osteonecrosis, 1588, 1588
　in hip replacement, 1797, 1798
Graft-versus-host disease, after bone marrow transplantation, 1525
　for cellular immunodeficiency, 1301
　in severe combined immunodeficiency, 1294
Gram's stain, in synovial fluid analysis, 616–617
Granulocyte colony–stimulating factor, in immune cell development, 271
　in mononuclear phagocyte maturation, 131, 131t, 132, 133
Granulocyte-macrophage colony–stimulating factor, 101, 103t
　in adhesion molecule expression, 269
　in dendritic cell differentiation, 141
　in immune cell development, 271, 272
　in monocyte development, in inflammation, 271, 272
　in mononuclear phagocyte maturation, 131t, 131–133, 133
　in neutrophil priming, 152, 152t
　in rheumatoid arthritis, 867, 869
Granulocytopenia, in Felty's syndrome, 951, 951–954
Granuloma annulare, vs. rheumatoid nodules, in rheumatoid arthritis, 918
Granulomas, in lymph nodes, in cancer, 1529
　in sarcoidosis, 1418, 1421
　in vasculitis, cutaneous, 1108
　in human immunodeficiency virus infection, 1278
　macrophages in, 131
Granulomatosis, lymphomatoid, 1530, 1531t
　Wegener's, 1099–1103. See also Wegener's granulomatosis.
　with allergic angiitis, 503, 1097–1099
　in children, 1261
　with chronic infection, neutrophilic metabolism in, 154
Granulomatous disease, of aorta, in rheumatoid arthritis, 921–922
Graves' disease, 1503–1505, 1504
Growth, disorders of, in achondroplasia, 1555
　in cartilage-hair hypoplasia, 1297
　in juvenile chronic arthritis, imaging in, 651, 651–652
　in juvenile rheumatoid arthritis, 1212, 1212
　in metaphyseal chondrodysplasia, 1556
　in β-thalassemia, 1497
Growth factors. See also specific factors, e.g., Platelet-derived growth factor.

Growth factors *(Continued)*
  in articular cartilage, 8–9
  in bone cell metabolism, 61, *61*
Growth hormone, in acromegaly,
    1506–1508
Guanosine triphosphatase–activating
    protein, in neutrophil function, 149
Guepar prosthesis, in knee replacement,
    1832, *1832*
Gut-associated lymphoid tissue, in
    enteropathic arthritis, 1006
Guyon's canal, ulnar nerve entrapment in,
    574

Hair, hypoplasia of, with cartilage
    hypoplasia, 1285t, 1297
  loss of, antimalarial drugs and, 754–755
    cyclophosphamide and, 812–813
    in common variable immunodefi-
      ciency, 1288, *1288*
    in lupus erythematosus, 500, 1036
Hallux rigidus, in osteoarthritis, 484, *484*,
    665
  surgery for, 1770, *1771*
Hallux valgus, in osteoarthritis, *483*,
    483–484, 665
Hamstring muscles, examination of, 458
Hamstring tendinitis, 466
Hand(s), arthritis in, monarticular,
    differential diagnosis of, 373t
  digital nerves of, entrapment syndromes
    of, 572–573, 575, 576
  disorders of, glucocorticoids for, nonar-
    ticular injection of, 597, 597t
  Dupuytren's contracture of, 359, 1165–
    1166
  examination of, 360–362, *361*, *362*
  in calcium pyrophosphate deposition dis-
    ease, 1356, *1356*
    surgery of, 1671
  in diabetes, 386, *386*, 1500
  in gout, surgery of, 1671
  in juvenile rheumatoid arthritis, surgery
    for, 1661–1662, *1662*, *1664*
  in mixed connective tissue disease, 1068,
    1069, *1069*, *1070*
  in osteoarthritis, 385, *385*
    imaging of, 664, *664*
    surgery for, 1671–1673, *1672*
  in psoriatic arthritis, clinical features of,
    1000–1002
    imaging of, 657, 657–658
    surgery of, 1667–1669, *1668*
  in Reiter's syndrome, with human im-
    munodeficiency virus infection,
    1269, *1269*
  in rheumatoid arthritis, *912*, 912–914,
    913, 913t
    imaging of, 646, 647, 648t
    nonsurgical management of, 1647–
      1648
    surgery of, in flexor tendon rupture,
      1652, *1653*
      in flexor tenosynovitis, 1650–1652
      reconstructive, 1655–1661, *1656*,
        1657, *1659*, *1660*
      synovectomy in, 1652
  in sarcoidosis, surgery of, 1670–1671
  in scleroderma, edema of, in initial pre-
    sentation, 1135, *1135*
    imaging of, 661–662, *661–663*
    surgery of, 1669–1670, *1669–1671*
  in systemic lupus erythematosus, sur-
    gery of, 1662–1667, *1665–1667*

Hand(s) *(Continued)*
  Raynaud's phenomenon in. See
    Raynaud's phenomenon.
  surgery of, 1647–1673
  swan-neck deformity of, in Parkinson's
    disease, vs. rheumatoid arthritis,
    908, *908*
Hand-arm vibration syndrome, vs. carpal
    tunnel syndrome, 570
Hand-foot syndrome, in sickle cell disease,
    1493–1494, *1494*
Haptoglobin, in inflammation, in acute-
    phase response, 699, *700*
Hashimoto's thyroiditis, 1503, 1505
Haversian remodeling, in bone, 68
Headache, cervical spinal disorders and,
    403
  Chiari malformation and, 409
  in giant cell arteritis, 1125–1126
  in mixed connective tissue disease,
    1071–1072, 1074t
  migraine, in antiphospholipid syndrome,
    1060
Hearing, loss of, in Alport's syndrome,
    1556
  in Cogan's syndrome, 1112, 1113
  in rheumatoid arthritis, 911
Heart disease, glucocorticoids and, 795
  in amyloidosis, 1412, 1413, 1416t
  in ankylosing spondylitis, 974
  in antiphospholipid syndrome, *1060*,
    1060–1061
  in giant cell arteritis, 1127
  in hypertrophic osteoarthropathy, 1514t,
    1516
  in Kawasaki disease, in children, 1256,
    1257
  in Lyme disease, 1463–1464, 1464t, *1465*,
    1469, 1469t
  in Marfan syndrome, 1552–1553
  in mixed connective tissue disease, 1070,
    1074t, 1075
  in polyarteritis, 1094
  in polychondritis, relapsing, 1406, 1407
  in pseudoxanthoma elasticum, 1554
  in Reiter's syndrome, 990
  in rheumatic fever, 1226–1227, 1229,
    1230, 1235, *1235*
  in rheumatoid arthritis, 921–922
  in scleroderma, 1141, 1142t, 1149, 1154
    in children, 1250, 1250t
  in systemic lupus erythematosus, 1034–
    1035
    in children, 1241
  omega-3 fatty acids in, 531
Heat, in rehabilitative medicine, *1623*,
    1623–1624, 1624t
  in therapy, for rheumatoid arthritis, 938–
    939
  preservation of, in surgery, 1644
Heat shock proteins, in glucocorticoid
    binding, 789, *789*
  in rheumatoid arthritis, 857
Heberden's nodes, 361, *362*
  in osteoarthritis, 385, *385*, 1389, *1389*,
    1391, *1391*
Heerfordt's disease, vs. Sjögren's
    syndrome, 960
Helicobacter pylori infection, and peptic
    ulcers, nonsteroidal anti-inflammatory
    drugs with, 714
Helix, tophi of, in gout, 1316, *1317*
Helmet deformity, in osteogenesis
    imperfecta, 1544
Hemangioma, synovial, *1598*, 1598–1599,
    1599

Hemarthrosis, acute, in hemophilia, 1485,
    1490
  bacterial arthritis with, 1439, 1439t
  synovial fluid analysis in, 610, 611t, *612*
  vs. monarticular arthritis, 377
Hematoma, after foot surgery, aspirin and,
    1771
Hematuria, D-penicillamine and, 767
Hemiarthroplasty, of knee, in juvenile
    rheumatoid arthritis, 1776
  in rheumatoid arthritis, 1739
  radiography of, 1832–1833, *1833*
Hemochromatosis. See also *Iron.*
  genetic, 1423t, 1423–1428, 1425t, *1426*,
    1427
  imaging in, 675–676, *676*
  osteoarthritis with, 385
  synovial biopsy in, 622, *623*, Plate 10
  vs. rheumatoid arthritis, 905–906
  with calcium pyrophosphate deposition
    disease, 1355
Hemodialysis, amyloid fibril deposition
    with, 1410, 1415
  shoulder pain with, 435
Hemoglobinopathy, and osteonecrosis,
    1585
  articular disorders with, imaging of, 679
  in sickle cell disease, 1493–1497, *1494*,
    1494t
Hemolytic anemia, in systemic lupus
    erythematosus, 1030t, 1035
Hemolytic complement assay, 236
Hemophilia, arthropathy in, 1485–1491
  clinical features of, 1485–1487, *1486*
  diagnosis of, 1488
  imaging of, *680*, 680–681, 1487, 1487t,
    1488
  pathology of, 1487, *1489*
  synovectomy in, arthroscopic, 690
  treatment of, 1488–1491
  vs. rheumatoid arthritis, 906
Hemophilus infection, in arthritis, synovial
    fluid examination for, 1436
Hemorrhage. See *Bleeding.*
Hemosiderin. See *Iron.*
Henoch-Schönlein purpura, 503, *1105*,
    1105–1106
  in children, 1242t, *1258*, 1258–1259
  in human immunodeficiency virus infec-
    tion, 1278
Heparan sulfate, in extracellular matrix,
    41, 50
Heparin, in antiphospholipid syndrome, in
    pregnancy, 1062
  in extracellular matrix, *41*
  in management of pregnancy, in sys-
    temic lupus erythematosus, 1051,
    1052t
  in mast cell mediation, 167–169, *168*
  in rheumatoid arthritis, 881
  with hip arthroplasty, 1732
Heparin binding growth factor, in
    rheumatoid arthritis, 869
Hepatitis, and cryoglobulinemic vasculitis,
    1109
  viral, arthritis with, vs. rheumatoid ar-
    thritis, 906–907
    in hemophilia, 1490
Hepatitis A virus infection, and arthritis,
    1482
Hepatitis B surface antigen, in poly-
    arteritis, 1094
  in vasculitis, 1080
Hepatitis B virus infection, and arthritis,
    1473–1475, *1474*

Hepatitis C, immune complex assays in, 229
Hepatocyte-stimulating factor. See *Interleukin-6.*
Hernias, and hip pain, 476
Herpes virus infection, and arthritis, 1481
 with cytotoxic drug therapy, for systemic lupus erythematosus, 1049, 1050t
5-HETE, in leukotriene synthesis, 292, *292,* 294, *527*
Heterotopic ossification, after hip arthroplasty, 1732–1733, 1733t
Hexadrol. See *Dexamethasone.*
Hexose chains, on collagen, in extracellular matrix, 40, *41*
High endothelial venules, lymphocyte movement in, 119–120
Hill-Sachs lesion, computed tomography of, *417, 418,* 432
 magnetic resonance imaging of, *422*
Hindfoot. See also *Foot.*
 anatomy of, 479, *480*
 disorders of, surgery for, 1766–1767, *1768, 1769*
Hinge prostheses, in knee replacement, radiography of, 1832, *1832*
Hip, anatomy of, 362, *363*
 arthritis of, monarticular, differential diagnosis of, 373t
  nonsurgical management of, 1726
 arthrocentesis of, 602–603, *603*
 arthrodesis of, 1727
 arthroplasty of, 1727–1737
  anesthesia for, 1729–1730
  assessment before, 1727–1728
  biologic fixation in, radiography of, 1792–1795, *1794, 1795,* 1796t
  cement fixation in, radiography of, 1789, *1790–1792*
  complications of, 1731–1733, 1733t
  contraindications to, 1727
  cost/benefit analysis of, 1633–1634
  dislocation after, 1733
   radiography of, 1798–1799, *1800*
  evaluation for, 1634–1637
  femoral component in, fractures of, 1812–1813, *1815*
  femoral fractures after, 1813, *1816*
  in protrusio acetabuli, *1725*
  indications for, 1727
  infection after, arthrography of, 1805–1807, 1807t
   para-articular cavities in, 1809
   with cement fixation, 1799–1805, 1800t, *1805*
  knee synovitis after, glucocorticoids for, 596
  loosening after, arthrography of, 1805–1809, *1806,* 1807t, *1808,* 1808t, *1809*
   with biologic fixation, 1805, *1805*
   with cement fixation, 1799–1805, 1800t, *1801–1804*
  management after, 1637–1638, 1730–1731
  mechanical interlock fixation in, 1789–1792, *1793*
  ossification after, para-articular, 1813–1816, *1817*
  osteolysis after, 1733, 1812
  prosthesis selection for, 1728–1729, *1729, 1782,* 1782–1783, *1783*
  prosthetic component disengagement after, 1812, *1814*

Hip *(Continued)*
 radiography of, 1782–1816
  acetabular positioning in, 1785–1788, *1785–1788*
  after surface replacement, 1783, *1784, 1785*
  results of, 1727, 1733–1737, 1734t–1736t
  scintigraphy after, *1810,* 1810–1812, 1811t, 1812t, *1813*
  technique of, 1730
  tumors after, 1816
  unfixed acetabular components in, 1796–1798, *1797–1799*
 arthroscopic surgery of, 1727
 avascular necrosis of, 1724
  magnetic resonance imaging of, *638*
 biomechanics of, *1723,* 1723–1724
 bursitis in, glucocorticoid injection for, 605
 compressive loads in, resistance to, 91, *91*
 computed tomography of, 632
 deformity of, osteotomy for, 1727
 dysplasia of, congenital, computed tomography of, 635
  developmental, 1724
 flexion of, with knee movement, 87, *87, 88*
 fractures of, 470–473, *471, 472*
 in ankylosing spondylitis, 974, 977
  imaging of, 656, *656*
  surgery of, 979, 980
 in calcium pyrophosphate deposition disease, *674*
 in juvenile rheumatoid arthritis, 1220, *1221*
  arthroplasty of, 1775–1781, *1777, 1778, 1780*
  contractures of, soft tissue release for, 1774
 in Paget's disease, 678, *679*
 motion of, in lifting, 92, *93*
 osteoarthritis of, 1724
  diagnosis of, 1850, 1851t
  imaging of, 664–665, *665*
  management of, drugs in, 1851t, *1852,* 1852–1853
   goals of, 1850
   occupational therapy in, 1851, 1851t
   patient education in, 1851
   physical therapy in, 1851t, 1851–1852
  surgery for, 1853
 osteonecrosis of, 1581–1590. See also *Osteonecrosis.*
 pain in, 466–476
  anatomic sources of, 466–467
  causes of, intra-articular, 470–473, *471–473*
   periarticular, 473–476
   regional, 476
  differential nerve block in, 470
  electromyography in, 469
  history in, 467, 1724–1725
  nerve conduction studies in, 469
  physical examination in, 467–468, 1725–1726
  radiography in, 468–469, *469,* 1726
 physical examination of, 362–365
 rheumatoid arthritis of, 914, 1724, *1725*
  imaging of, *646,* 648t, 650
 rotation of, force in, *88*
 snapping, 473–474
 stability of, 86, *86*

Hip *(Continued)*
 synovial cyst of, computed tomography of, *628*
Histamine, in basophil activation, 163
 in mast cell activation, 163
 in mast cell mediation, 164–166, *165, 166*
Histidine, in histamine formation, 164–165
Histiocytoma, synovial. See *Synovitis, pigmented villonodular.*
Histocompatibility complex, major, 210–214. See also *Major histocompatibility complex* and *Human leukocyte antigens.*
Histone, antibodies to, in systemic lupus erythematosus, 255t, 256
Histoplasmosis, 1459, 1459t
HIV infection, 1265–1278. See also *Human immunodeficiency virus (HIV) infection.*
HLA. See *Human leukocyte antigens.*
Hoarseness, in rheumatoid arthritis, of cricoarytenoid joints, 911
Hoffa's disease, vs. lipoma arborescens, 1598
Hormonal disorders, 1499–1510. See also specific disorders, e.g., *Acromegaly.*
 clinical features of, 1499–1500, 1500t
Howship's lacunae, in bone remodeling, 58, *58*
5-HPETE, in leukotriene synthesis, 292, *292,* 294, *295, 527,* 709, 710, *710*
HTLV-1, and arthritis, 856–857
 synovial fluid analysis in, 615–616
hUBF, antibodies to, in scleroderma, 258t, 259
Human Genome Initiative, 1541–1542
Human immunodeficiency virus (HIV) infection, 1265–1278
 acute, 1273
 arthritis with, polyarticular, 383
 arthropathy in, vs. rheumatoid arthritis, 906
 diffuse infiltrative lymphocytosis syndrome in, 1273t, 1273–1277, *1274, 1276*
 host-virus relationships in, 1265–1266
 in hemophiliacs, 1490
 mast cells in, 164
 muscle weakness in, 1191
 Mycobacterium avium infection in, 1455–1456
 myopathy in, 1277
 opportunistic infections with, and arthralgia, vs. monarticular arthritis, 376
  and arthritis, 1441
 psoriasis in, pustular, 1268–1272, *1269, 1270, 1272*
  with arthritis, 1000
 Reiter's syndrome with, 990, 1268–1272, *1269, 1270, 1272*
 renal disease in, 1273, 1273t
 rheumatic diseases with, laboratory findings in, 1266
  opportunistic infections in, 1266–1267
  types of, 1266
 spondyloarthropathy with, 1268–1272, *1272*
 tuberculosis with, 1450
 vasculitis in, 1277–1278
Human leukocyte antigens, *210–213,* 210–214, 215t, 216t, Plate 1
 alleles for, linkage disequilibrium of, 214, 220
 in ankylosing spondylitis, 971–973, *972,* 972t, 973t

Human leukocyte antigens *(Continued)*
in antiphospholipid syndrome, 1058
in autoimmune diseases, 218, 221
in diffuse infiltrative lymphocytosis, in human immunodeficiency virus infection, 1275–1276
in Felty's syndrome, 951, 952
in giant cell arteritis, 1123–1124
in immunodeficiency disorders, 1284–1285
in inflammatory muscle disease, 1179, 1187
in iron storage diseases, 1424, 1427–1428
in juvenile rheumatoid arthritis, 1207–1208, 1208t
in Lyme disease, 1466–1467
vs. rheumatoid arthritis, 855
in parvovirus infection, and rheumatoid arthritis, 856
in polymyalgia rheumatica, 1123–1124
in postenteritic reactive arthritis, 1008–1010
in psoriatic arthritis, 999
in Reiter's syndrome, 217, 217t, 983–986
with human immunodeficiency virus infection, 1270
in rheumatic disease, population association studies in, 214–216, 217t, 220, 220–221
in rheumatic fever, 1227
in rheumatoid arthritis, 218t, 218–219, 852–853, 853t
in pregnancy, 854
interferon-γ inducing, 859–862
in scleroderma, 1134
in Sjögren's syndrome, 219, 964
in spondyloarthropathy, 217t, 217–218, 218t
in systemic lupus erythematosus, 219, 1016, 1016t, 1017, 1029
in T cell recognition, 210, *210*, 859–862
in Takayasu's arteritis, 1088
in viral infection, vs. rheumatoid arthritis, 855–857
molecular polymorphism of, 214, 215t, 216t
molecular structure of, 210–212, *211, 212,* Plate 1
Human neutrophil lipocalin, 148
Human T-cell lymphotrophic virus infection, type 1, and arthritis, 856–857
synovial fluid analysis in, 615–616
Humerus, fracture of, after total elbow replacement, 1689–1690
and osteonecrosis, 429
head of, avascular necrosis of, in sickle cell disease, 1496–1497
in rheumatoid arthritis, 1700, *1701*
in traumatic arthritis, 1702, *1702*
osteonecrosis of, 1589, 1703, *1703,* 1704
prosthetic, in shoulder replacement, radiography of, 1834–1835, *1835*
surface erosion of, with rotator cuff tears, 430
Hyaluronan, in articular cartilage, 1369
in osteoarthritis, 1373–1374
in extracellular matrix, 37, *38, 39, 42,* 45–48
in joint development, 3
in synovial joints, 17, *18*
in synovial lining, 12
Hyaluronate, in extracellular matrix, *41*
in joint development, 2, 4
in streptococci, in rheumatic fever, 1226, 1227

Hyaluronidase, in joint development, 2
Hydatid disease, vertebral, and low back pain, 452
Hydeltra. See *Prednisone/prednisolone.*
Hydralazine, and lupus erythematosus, 1037
interactions of, with nonsteroidal anti-inflammatory drugs, 719t
Hydrarthrosis, intermittent, vs. rheumatoid arthritis, 907
Hydrochlorothiazide, for hypercalciuria, in osteoporosis, 1571
Hydrocortisone. See also *Glucocorticoids.*
for rheumatoid arthritis, 798
intra-articular injection of, 591–594, 594t
perioperative use of, 800
potency of, 788t
structure of, 787, *788*
Hydrogen peroxide, 523, *523*
5(S)-Hydroperoxyeicosatetraenoic acid, in leukotriene synthesis, 292, *292, 294, 295,* 709, 710, *710*
Hydrotherapy, in rehabilitative medicine, 1624, 1624t
Hydroxyapatite, in bone development, 63–64
in bone matrix, 63
in bone mineralization, 64
prosthesis coating with, with unfixed acetabular components, 1796
Hydroxyapatite crystal deposition disease, 1362t, 1362–1365, *1364*
imaging of, 674–675, *675*
with hemochromatosis, 1424
Hydroxychloroquine, adverse effects of, 754–755, 755t
for calcium pyrophosphate deposition disease, 754
for dermatomyositis, in children, 754
for eosinophilic fasciitis, 754
for inflammatory muscle disease, 1201
for juvenile rheumatoid arthritis, 1218
for osteoarthritis, erosive, 754
for rheumatoid arthritis, 750–753, 751t, 752t, 941, 946, 947, 1891–1893, 1892t, 1898t, 1899–1900
in pregnancy and lactation, 1902t
vs. gold, 761
for Sjögren's syndrome, 754, 965, 966
for systemic lupus erythematosus, 749–750, 1041, 1042, 1043t
guidelines for use of, 756
mechanisms of action of, 748t, 748–749
pharmacokinetics of, 748
structure of, 747, *747*–748
5-S-Hydroxy-eicosatetraenoic acid (5-HETE), in leukotriene synthesis, 292, *292, 294,* 527
Hydroxylysine, in collagen, 26–28
Hydroxyproline, in collagen, 24, 25, 28
5-Hydroxytryptamine, in platelet-complement interaction, 179
Hydroxyurea, in immunosuppression, for non-neoplastic diseases, 810, 815, 823t
25-Hydroxyvitamin D. See *Vitamin D.*
Hypercalcemia, with cancer, calcitonin for, 61
Hypercalciuria, in osteoporosis, 1571
Hypereosinophilia, 158, 158t
idiopathic, vs. rheumatoid arthritis, 906
synovial biopsy in, 623
Hypergammaglobulinemia, in Waldenström's purpura, 1108
Hyperimmunoglobulinemia E syndrome, 1285t, 1298

Hyperlipoproteinemia, arthropathy with, vs. rheumatoid arthritis, 906
Hypermobility, of joints, in Ehlers-Danlos syndrome, 1546–1551, *1547–1549,* 1548t, *1551*
Hyperostosis, diffuse idiopathic, imaging of, 668–669, *669, 670*
in diabetes mellitus, 1501
vs. ankylosing spondylitis, 655, 657
vs. osteoarthritis, 1391–1392
in acne-pustulosis-hyperostosis-osteitis syndrome, vs. rheumatoid arthritis, 903
with spondylosis, and low back pain, 450
Hyperparathyroidism, 1502, *1503*
with calcium pyrophosphate deposition disease, 1355
Hyperpigmentation, in iron storage disorders, 1425
Hypersensitivity, to food, and arthritis, 531
to nonsteroidal anti-inflammatory drugs, 717
Hypertension, glucocorticoids and, 795
gout with, 1318–1319
in Takayasu's arteritis, 1089, 1090
intracranial, benign, glucocorticoids and, 796
management of, in gout, 1346–1347
pulmonary, arteritis and, in rheumatoid arthritis, 921
in antiphospholipid syndrome, 1061
in mixed connective tissue disease, 1070, 1073–1074
in scleroderma, management of, 1154
in systemic lupus erythematosus, 1035
neonatal, leukotrienes in, 297t
Hyperthyroidism, 1503–1505, *1504*
and arthritis, vs. rheumatoid arthritis, 904
glucocorticoid metabolism in, 793
with hypertrophic osteoarthropathy, 1516
Hypertriglyceridemia, gout with, 1318, 1346
Hypertrophic osteoarthropathy, 1514–1519, *1515, 1517*
synovial biopsy in, 623
vs. rheumatoid arthritis, 906
Hyperuricemia. See also *Gout.*
asymptomatic, 1314
management of, 1340–1342, *1341*
classification of, 1330, 1331t
definition of, 1313
drugs for, 829–837
urate destruction by, 837, *837*
urate synthesis inhibition by, *829–831,* 829–833, 832t
uric acid excretion enhanced by, 833–837, *834,* 834t, *835,* 836t
epidemiology of, 1313
in acute illness, 1320
in pregnancy, 1320
in sickle cell disease, 1494–1495
syndrome X with, 1319
with monosodium urate deposition, management of, *1344,* 1344–1345, 1345t
Hypocomplementemia, and vasculitis, *1106,* 1106–1107
Hypofibrinolysis, and osteonecrosis, 1585
Hypogammaglobulinemia, acquired, 1285t, *1288,* 1288–1289
cyclophosphamide and, 813
transient, of infancy, 1285t, 1291

Hypogastric nerve, reflex testing of, 406t
Hypomagnesemia, with calcium pyrophosphate deposition disease, 1355
Hypoparathyroidism, 1502–1503, *1503*
Hypophosphatemia, and osteomalacia, 1503, *1504*
Hypopyon, in Behçet's disease, 1114, *1115*, Plate 12
Hypothalamus, in cortisol secretion, 787–788
    suppression of, exogenous glucocorticoids and, 796
    in inflammatory response, genetic impairment of, and rheumatoid arthritis, 854
Hypothermia, in surgery, prevention of, 1644
Hypothyroidism, *1505*, 1505–1506
    and arthritis, vs. rheumatoid arthritis, 904
    gout with, 1319–1320
    in scleroderma, 1150
    in Sjögren's syndrome, 961
    osteoarthritis with, 385
Hypoxanthine, in uric acid formation, 1324–1325, *1325*
Hypoxanthine guanine phosphoribosyltransferase deficiency, 1331t, 1332–1337, *1333*, 1334t, 1335t, *1336*
Hypoxia, and angiogenesis, in rheumatoid arthritis, 872–873

I band, in skeletal muscle, 78, 79t, *80*
Ibuprofen, 729t, 731, *731*
    adverse effects of, gastrointestinal, 714
        in systemic lupus erythematosus, 1041
    for juvenile rheumatoid arthritis, 1217
    for osteoarthritis, 1397
        of hip, *1852*
        of knee, *1857*
    in cyclooxygenase pathway inhibition, 709
    overdose of, 718
ICAM. See *Intercellular adhesion molecule entries.*
IkB, in endothelial cell gene activation, 190–191, *191*
Iliohypogastric nerve, entrapment of, and hip pain, 476
    injury to, in surgery, 586
Ilioinguinal nerve, entrapment of, 581
    injury to, in surgery, 586
    reflex testing of, 406t
Iliopsoas bursa, in snapping hip, 474
    inflammation of, and pain, 475
        examination for, 364
        glucocorticoid injection of, 597–598, 606
Iliotibial band, examination of, 364
    in snapping hip, 473–474
Iliotibial bursitis, and pain, 465–466
Imbalance, cervical spinal disorders and, 403
    in Cogan's syndrome, 1112
Immobilization, and bone remodeling, 71
Immune complexes, and complement activation, 228–229
    assays for, 229–231, 230t
        in rheumatic disease, 231t, 231–232, 232t
        in cancer, 1525, 1527t

Immune complexes (*Continued*)
    in rheumatoid arthritis, in synovial fluid, 884–885
    in systemic lupus erythematosus, 1021–1024, 1023t, 1024t
    in vasculitis, 1080–1081, *1081*
Immune globulin, for inflammatory muscle disease, 1201
    for thrombocytopenia, in systemic lupus erythematosus, 1052
Immune system, aberrant reactivity in, 807
    abnormalities of, in scleroderma, 1142–1144
        in systemic lupus erythematosus, 1019–1022, 1020t
    enhancement of, therapeutic, 808
    reaction of, to silicone, 1171–1172
    regulation of, 805–807, *806*
    suppression of, apheresis in, 817–818
        cyclosporine in, 819–821, *820*, 823t
        cytotoxic drugs in, 808t, 808–815, *810*, 811t, 812t, 814t, 823t
            side effects of, 815–817, *816*, 823t
        dapsone in, 822, 823t
        FK-506 in, *820*, 821, 823t
        for diffuse infiltrative lymphocytosis, in human immunodeficiency virus infection, 1276–1277
        for inflammatory muscle disease, 1201
        for rheumatic disease, and cancer, 1530
        for rheumatoid arthritis, 945–947
            juvenile, 1219
        for scleroderma, 1152
        glucocorticoids in, 794, 794t, 819
        levamisole in, 822, 823t
        radiation in, 818–819
        rapamycin in, 821
        therapeutic, 807–808
Immunoadhesins, in tumor necrosis factor-α binding, to soluble receptors, 281
Immunoassays, enzyme-linked, for antinuclear antibodies, 253
    for rheumatoid factors, 241, 242
    in evaluation of inflammation, 704
    in Lyme disease, 1467, *1467*, 1873–1874
    for complement, 236–237
    for mast cells, 171
Immunoblotting, of antinuclear antibodies, 254
Immunodeficiency, acquired, 1265–1278. See also *Human immunodeficiency virus (HIV) infection.*
    antibody deficiency disorders and, 1285t, 1285–1292, *1287*, *1288*
        treatment of, 1300–1301
        with near-normal immunoglobulins, 1285t, 1291–1292
    cellular, 1286t, *1292*, 1292–1296
        treatment of, *1300*, *1301*, 1301–1302
    combined, mast cells in, 164
        partial, 1286t, 1296–1299
        severed, 1286t, *1294*, 1294–1295
    common variable, 1285t, *1288*, 1288–1289
    congenital, 1282–1302
    evaluation for, with recurrent infection, 1282–1284, 1283t
    genetics of, 1284t, 1284–1285
    hypogammaglobulinemia in, transient, of infancy, 1285t, 1291
    immunoglobulin A deficiency in, selective, 1285t, 1289–1290
    immunoglobulin M deficiency in, selective, 1285t, 1290–1291
    immunoglobulin subclass deficiency in, 1285t, 1289

Immunodeficiency (*Continued*)
    in cartilage-hair hypoplasia, 1285t, 1297
    in CD8+ lymphopenia, 1285t, 1299
    in cytokine deficiency, 1285t, 1299
    in hyperimmunoglobulinemia E syndrome, 1285t, 1298
    in leukocyte adhesion deficiency, 1285t, 1298–1299
    in Nezelof's syndrome, 1286t, 1293–1294
    in T cell activation defects, 1285t, 1299
    in T cell receptor–CD3 complex defects, 1285t, 1299
    in thymic hypoplasia, 1286t, *1292*, 1292–1293
    in Wiskott-Aldrich syndrome, 1286t, 1296–1297
    in X-linked disorders, 1284, 1284t
        carrier detection in, 1300
        in lymphoproliferative disease, 1285t, 1292
        intrauterine diagnosis of, 1299–1300
    major histocompatibility complex antigen deficiency in, 1286t, 1295–1296
    nonacquired, 1282–1302
    with thymoma, 1285t, 1297–1298
Immunodiffusion testing, for antinuclear antibodies, 252–253, *253*, 253t
Immunofluorescence testing, for antinuclear antibodies, 250–252, *252*, 262
    for lupus erythematosus, 501, *502*
Immunoglobulin, *105*, 105–106, 106t
    Fc region of, receptors of, on mononuclear phagocytes, 134
    for Kawasaki disease, 1256
    for rheumatoid arthritis, 946
    in antigen-specific recognition, 107, *109*, 111
    in B cell activation, 118–119
    in immune complex formation, 228, 229
    in leukocyte-endothelial adhesion, 186t, 187t, 187–190, *189*, *191*
    in lymphocyte adhesion, in inflammatory response, 192
    receptors of, on myeloid cells, 135t
    synthesis of, in B cells, 95
    testing for, in recurrent infection, 1283, 1284
Immunoglobulin A, 106, 106t
    deficiency of, selective, 1285t, 1289–1290
Immunoglobulin D, 106, 106t
Immunoglobulin E, 106, 106t
    elevated blood level of, with immunodeficiency, 1285t, 1298
    in mast cell regulation, 161, 163, 170, *170*, 171
    rheumatoid factors reacting with, in rheumatoid arthritis, 875
Immunoglobulin G, 106, 106t
    glycosylation of, genetic defect of, in rheumatoid arthritis, 853
    in immune complexes, in synovial fluid, in rheumatoid arthritis, 884
    intravenous, for antibody deficiency disorders, 1300–1301
    replacement of, in X-linked agammaglobulinemia, 1288
    rheumatoid factors reacting with, *241*, 241–246, 242t
        in rheumatoid arthritis, 875
    subclasses of, deficiencies of, 1285t, 1289
Immunoglobulin M, 106, 106t
    deficiency of, selective, 1285t, 1290–1291
    in immune complexes, in synovial fluid, in rheumatoid arthritis, 884–885

Immunoglobulin M *(Continued)*
  rheumatoid factors reacting with, 241,
    242t, 243–246, 246t
  methotrexate inhibition of, 773
Immunoglobulin supergene family, *304,
  305,* 306, Plate 2
  in leukocyte homing, 315
Immunoprecipitation, of antinuclear
  antibodies, 253–254, *254*
Immunoregulation, drugs in, 805–824
  mononuclear phagocytes in, 141–143,
    142
Impairment, definition of, 1619
Impingement syndrome, of rotator cuff,
  422–425, *423*
Imuran. See *Azathioprine.*
Inclusion body myositis, clinical features
  of, 1183–1184
  diagnosis of, criteria for, 1178, 1178t
  pathology of, 1183–1184, *1184,* 1184t,
    1185, 1189
  treatment of, 1201
Indium-111, in scintigraphy, after hip
  arthroplasty, 1811, 1812t
Indomethacin (Indocin), 729t, *730,* 730–731
  adverse effects of, gastrointestinal, 713–
    715
  and blood disorders, 717
  contraindication to, with diflunisal, 726
  for ankylosing spondylitis, 980
  for gout, with acute arthritis, 1343, 1344
  for lupus erythematosus, with antimalar-
    ial drugs, 750
  for osteoarthritis, of knee, 1396
  for Reiter's syndrome, 993
  history of, 707
  in cyclooxygenase pathway inhibition,
    709
  in prevention of heterotopic ossification,
    after hip arthroplasty, 1733
Infants. See also *Children.*
  hypogammaglobulinemia in, transient,
    1285t, 1291
  lupus syndrome in, 1037, 1052, *1244,*
    1244–1245
  Lyme disease in, congenital, 1466
  pulmonary hypertension in, leukotrienes
    in, 297t
Infarction, of bone, in sickle cell disease,
  1496
Infertility, female, cyclophosphamide and,
  812
  in males, cyclophosphamide and, 812
  methotrexate and, 780
  sulfasalazine and, 744
Inflammation. See also specific disorders,
  e.g., *Juvenile rheumatoid arthritis.*
  acute-phase response in, 699–701, *700,*
    700t
  definition of, 699
  endothelial cells in, 183–195. See also
    Endothelial cells.
  erythrocyte sedimentation rate in, 701–
    702, 702t
  glucocorticoids in, 789t, 789–791, 790t
    endogenous, 787–788
  laboratory evaluation of, 699–704
  leukocyte homing in, cell adhesion mole-
    cules and, 314–316
  mast cells in, 161–172. See also *Mast
    cells.*
  nonsteroidal anti-inflammatory drugs
    for, 712–713
  of muscle, 1177–1201. See also *Myositis*
    and specific types, e.g., *Polymyositis.*

Inflammation *(Continued)*
  platelets in, 176–180, *177,* 177t, *178*
Inflammatory bowel disease, and arthritis,
  1007, 1007–1077, 1008t
  arthritis with, ocular disorders in, 494
    vs. Reiter's syndrome, 992
    vs. rheumatoid arthritis, 903
  leukotrienes in, 297t, 299
Infracalcaneal bursa, inflammation of, 486
Infraspinatus muscle, reflex testing of, 406t
Inguinal hernia, and hip pain, 476
Injections, intra-articular, of glucocorti-
  coids, 591–599. See also *Glucocorticoids,
  intra-articular injection of.*
Injury. See *Trauma.*
Inosinic acid, synthesis of, 1325, *1325*
Inositol 1,4,5-triphosphate, in neutrophil
  function, 148, *149*
Insoles, wedged, in osteoarthritis, 1396
Instability, of joints, in physical
  examination, 356
Insulin, in mononuclear phagocyte
  regulation, 136
Insulin-like growth factor I, in articular
  cartilage, 8, 9
  in bone cell metabolism, 61
Integrins, *304, 305,* 306–310, *307, 308,*
  Plate 2
  as fibronectin receptors, on mononuclear
    phagocytes, 134–136
  in angiogenesis, 194
  in extracellular matrix, *38, 39, 42, 43,*
    47–49
  in fibroblast regulation, 202
  in leukocyte-endothelial adhesion, 186t,
    187t, 187–189, *189*
  in leukocyte homing, 314–316
  in lymphocyte adhesion, 192
  in monocyte adhesion, to endothelial
    cells, 129
  in rheumatoid arthritis, 873, 874
Intercellular adhesion molecule-1 (CD54),
  expression of, cytokines and, 268, 269
  in diffuse infiltrative lymphocytosis, in
    human immunodeficiency virus in-
    fection, 1275
  in leukocyte-endothelial adhesion, 186t,
    187t, 187–190, *191*
  in lymphocyte migration, 120, 120t, 121,
    121t
  in rheumatoid arthritis, 873, 873t
    therapy targeting, 839, 840
  monoclonal antibodies to, in anti-inflam-
    matory treatment, 317
Intercellular adhesion molecule-2,
  expression of, cytokines and, 268, 269
  in leukocyte-endothelial adhesion, in in-
    flammatory response, 186t, 187t
Intercostal nerves, reflex testing of, 406t
Interdigital nerves, of foot, entrapment of,
  580
Interferon, in eosinophil priming, 152t, 158
  in inflammatory myopathy, 1188
Interferon-α, for polyarteritis, 1097
Interferon-γ, 101, 103t
  in immune cell development, 270, 271,
    272
  in macrophage activation, 139, 140
  in rheumatoid arthritis, 864–865
    anti-inflammatory effect of, 845
    suppression of, 861
  in scleroderma, 1139, 1152
  in Sjögren's syndrome, 964
  T cell secretion of, antigen-specific activa-
    tion and, 192–193

Interleukin, 806, *806*
  antibodies to, natural, 279–280
  antimalarial drug effects on, 749
  in B cell development, 114
  in B cell regulation, in systemic lupus
    erythematosus, 1020
  in bone cell metabolism, 61, *61*
  in bone remodeling, 59
  in eosinophil priming, 152t, 158
  in fibroblast regulation, 201, 202, 204,
    204t, 205
  in immune cell development, 270–272,
    272
  in immune system enhancement, 808
  in inflammatory response, to urate crys-
    tals, in gout, 1339, 1340
  in leukocyte-endothelial adhesion, in in-
    flammatory response, 188, 190
  in macrophage activation, 139, 140
  in macrophage development, in inflam-
    mation, 272–273
  in mast cell mediation, 162t, 170
  in monocyte development, in inflamma-
    tion, 272–273
  in neutrophil priming, 152, 152t
  in osteoporosis, 1564
  in rheumatoid arthritis, and metallopro-
    teinase synthesis, 876
  in scleroderma, 1143–1144
  in Sjögren's syndrome, 964
  in T cell stimulation, effect of, on macro-
    phages, 141–143, *142*
  receptors of, on mononuclear phago-
    cytes, 136
  secretion of, by macrophages, 137t
    by T cells, antigen-specific activation
      and, 192–193
Interleukin-1, 102t
  in adhesion molecule expression, 268
  in inflammation, chronic, 275–276
  in leukocyte homing, 315
  in Lyme disease, 1466
  in mononuclear phagocyte maturation,
    132
  in rheumatoid arthritis, 862, 866–867,
    869
    therapy targeting, 843–844
  receptor antagonist of, 281–282
    in rheumatoid arthritis, 870–871, *871*
  production of, 138, 267, 268t
  receptors of, in articular cartilage, 8, 9
    soluble, 280, 871
Interleukin-2, 101–104, 102t
  in B cell regulation, 122
  in rheumatoid arthritis, 865
    diphtheria toxin fused with, in T cell
      suppression, 842, 860
  in T cell activation, 118
  production of, deficiency of, 1285t, 1299
    replacement therapy for, *1301,* 1302
Interleukin-3, 102t
  in mononuclear phagocyte maturation,
    131t, 131–132, *133*
Interleukin-4, 102t, 104
  for arthritis, 279
  for multiple sclerosis, 279
  in B cell regulation, 122
  in rheumatoid arthritis, 845, 865
Interleukin-5, 102t, 104
Interleukin-6, 102t
  in induction of acute-phase reactants,
    273–274
  in inflammation, laboratory measure-
    ment of, 702
  in mononuclear phagocyte maturation,
    131t, 131–132, *133*

Interleukin-6 (Continued)
  in rheumatoid arthritis, 867
    therapy targeting, 845
Interleukin-8, 102t
  in rheumatoid arthritis, 867–868
Interleukin-9, 103t
Interleukin-10, 103t, 104
  in rheumatoid arthritis, 845, 871
Interleukin-11, in acute-phase reactions, 274
Interleukin-12, 103t, 104
Interleukin-13, 103t
Interleukin-14, 103t
Interleukin-15, 103t
Interosseous nerve, anterior, entrapment of, 571–572, 572
    posterior, disorders of, muscle testing for, 399t
    entrapment of, 575, 576
Interphalangeal joint(s), arthrocentesis of, 601–602, 602
  in scleroderma, 1669, 1669, 1671
  juvenile rheumatoid arthritis of, surgery for, 1662
  osteoarthritis of, imaging of, 665–666, 666
    surgery for, 1671–1672, 1672
  physical examination of, 360–362, 361, 362
  psoriatic arthritis of, surgery for, 1668, 1668
  rheumatoid arthritis of, 482, 482
    surgery for, 1658–1661, 1659, 1660
  structure of, 1
  Thiemann's disease of, vs. rheumatoid arthritis, 909
  infection of, and low back pain, 451
Intervertebral disc(s), cervical, 395–396
  degeneration of, 397–398
  degeneration of, computed tomography of, 633, 634
    magnetic resonance imaging of, 635–636, 636
  development of, 5
  in spinal stability, 86, 87
  lumbar, disorders of, and pain. See Low back pain.
  osteochondrosis of, imaging of, 667, 667
Intervertebral disc spaces, in acromegaly, imaging of, 679, 680
Interzones, in joint development, 3, 4
Intestine. See also Gastrointestinal tract.
  cancer of, Sjögren's syndrome and, 1528, 1531t
  disorders of, and arthritis. See Enteropathic arthritis.
  inflammatory disease of, leukotrienes in, 297t, 299
  small, disorders of, in scleroderma, 1147
Intra-articular injection, of glucocorticoids, 591–599. See also Glucocorticoids.
Intracellular digestion, in macrophages, 139
Invariant chain, in human leukocyte antigen molecules, 212
Iodophenylundelic acid, in myelography, 444
Iohexol, in myelography, 444–445
Iridocyclitis, 490
  in ankylosing spondylitis, 974
Iritis, 490
  in Reiter's syndrome, 990
Iron, in hemochromatosis. See Hemochromatosis.
  in immune response, 523, 526

Iron (Continued)
  in pigmented villonodular synovitis, 1606, 1607
  metabolism of, normal, 1423–1424
  storage of, diseases of, 1423t, 1423–1428, 1425t, 1426, 1427
Ischemia, and bone necrosis, in systemic lupus erythematosus, 1041
  and hyperuricemia, 1320
  cerebral, in antiphospholipid syndrome, 1059, 1060
  of bone, magnetic resonance imaging of, 637–638, 638, 639
  of retina, in Behçet's disease, 494, 494, Plate 4
Ischial (ischiogluteal) bursa, inflammation of, glucocorticoid injection for, 597–598, 606
Isoniazid, and lupus erythematosus, 1037
  for tuberculosis, 1454
Itraconazole, for fungal infection, 1459, 1459t

Jaccoud's syndrome, in systemic lupus erythematosus, surgery for, 1663–1666, 1666
Jaccoud's-type arthropathy, 1524
Jansen's metaphyseal dysplasia, 1556
Jaundice, cholestatic, gold therapy and, 764
Jaw, arthritis in, monarticular, differential diagnosis of, 373t
  articulation of, with temporal bone. See Temporomandibular joint.
  growth of, in juvenile rheumatoid arthritis, 1212, 1212
Joints. See also specific joints, e.g., Knee.
  aspiration of. See Arthrocentesis.
  biology of, 1–19
  biomechanics of, compressive stress in, resistance to, 90, 90–91, 91
    force in, 87–88, 88, 89
    in degenerative disease, 91, 92
    joint structure in, 88–90, 89, 90
    motion types in, 86–87, 87, 88
    neurologic control in, 91–92, 92, 93
    stability in, 86, 86, 87
  disorders of. See specific disorders, e.g., Osteoarthritis.
  examination of, for arthritis, 355–356
    history in, 353–355
    recording of findings in, 356, 356–357
  glucocorticoid injection into, 591–599. See also Glucocorticoids, intra-articular injection of.
  loose bodies in, 1595, 1595–1596, 1596
  pain in. See Pain.
  sepsis of, computed tomography of, 634
  synovial. See Synovial joints.
  types of, 1, 1–2
Jumper's knee, 462
Juvenile chronic arthritis, imaging of, 651–653, 651–654
Juvenile rheumatoid arthritis, 1207–1222
  antimalarial drugs for, 753, 1218
  arthroplasty in, 1635, 1775–1781, 1777–1780
  classification of, 1215, 1215t
  course of, 1220–1222, 1221, 1221t
  diagnosis of, 1215–1216
  epidemiology of, 1207, 1207–1208, 1208t
  etiology of, 1208
  extra-articular manifestations of, 1209–1212, 1211, 1212

Juvenile rheumatoid arthritis (Continued)
  fenoprofen for, 732
  interleukin-6 antibodies in, 274
  laboratory tests in, 1212–1213
  leukotrienes in, 297t
  limb angular deformities in, surgery for, 1775, 1776
  limb length discrepancy in, orthotics for, 1627
    surgery for, 1775
  methotrexate for, 778, 1218
  monarticular, 377
  nonsteroidal anti-inflammatory drugs for, 736
  nutrition in, 522, 1217
  ocular disorders with, 492, 492, 1212, 1212, 1219–1222
  of foot, 483
  of hand, surgery for, 1661–1662, 1662, 1664
  of wrist, surgery for, 1661, 1662, 1663, 1774, 1774
  onset of, types of, 1208t, 1208–1211, 1209–1211
  pathology of, 1214–1215
  radiography of, 1213, 1213–1214, 1214
  skin lesions in, 506, 506, 1209–1211, 1211, 1215, Plate 6
  soft tissue release in, 1774–1775
  surgery for, 1773–1781
  synovectomy in, 1661, 1773–1774, 1774
  tolmetin for, 733
  treatment of, 1216t, 1216–1220

Kalinin, in extracellular matrix, 48
Kallikreins, in extracellular matrix degradation, 324t, 326
Kashin-Beck disease, 1390
Kawasaki disease, 1242t, 1255t, 1255–1257, 1256, 1257
  pathogenesis of, 1081, 1084, 1084
Kelley-Seegmiller syndrome, 1332
Keloids, 1166
Kenalog (triamcinolone). See also Glucocorticoids.
  crystals of, in synovial fluid analysis, 614, 615, Plate 8
  for juvenile rheumatoid arthritis, 1219
  for rotator cuff impingement, 424
  intra-articular injection of, 591–594, 594t
Keratan sulfate, in extracellular matrix, 41
Keratitis, in Cogan's syndrome, 1112
Keratoconjunctivitis sicca, 488–489, 489, 489t, Plate 3
  in Sjögren's syndrome, 488, 956t, 956–957, 957, 957t, 965
Keratoderma blennorrhagica, in Reiter's syndrome, 498, 498, 988–989, 989, 993, Plate 4
  with human immunodeficiency virus infection, 1269, 1270
Keratopathy, band, in juvenile rheumatoid arthritis, 492, 492
Ketoprofen, 729t, 732, 732
  use in elderly, 722
Ketorolac, 729t, 734, 734–735
Kidney(s), dialysis of, amyloid fibril deposition with, 1410, 1415
  shoulder pain with, 435
  disorders of, complement deficiency and, 1306–1308, 1308t
  glucocorticoid use in, 793
  in Alport's syndrome, 1556

Kidney(s) (Continued)
in amyloidosis, 1413, 1415, 1416t
in ankylosing spondylitis, 975
in antiphospholipid syndrome, 1061
in gout, 1320–1323, 1321
management of, 829, 832, 833, 1345
in Henoch-Schönlein purpura, 1105, 1106
in human immunodeficiency virus infection, 1273, 1273t
in juvenile rheumatoid arthritis, 1211
in mixed connective tissue disease, 1070–1071, 1074, 1074t
in polychondritis, relapsing, 1406
in rhabdomyolysis, 1194
in rheumatoid arthritis, 920
in scleroderma, 1149, 1149–1150, 1154
with Raynaud's phenomenon, 1141, 1142t
in Sjögren's syndrome, 961t, 961–962
in systemic lupus erythematosus, 1032–1034. See also Systemic lupus erythematosus, renal disorders in.
in Wegener's granulomatosis, 1101–1103
naproxen use in, 724
nonsteroidal anti-inflammatory drug use in, 721–722, 723t, 729t
osteodystrophy with, in hyperparathyroidism, 1502, 1503
uric acid and, management of, 1345
toxicity to, cyclosporine and, 820, 945
gold and, 762–763, 763t, 942
methotrexate and, 780
nonsteroidal anti-inflammatory drugs and, 716–717
in rheumatoid arthritis, 1898–1899
in systemic lupus erythematosus, 1041
D-penicillamine and, 767, 942
uric acid clearance in, 1327–1329, 1328t
in gout, 1330–1332, 1332, 1336
Kienböck's disease, magnetic resonance imaging of, 639
Killer cells, in immune function, 806, 806
Kinetochore, antibodies to, in scleroderma, 258, 258t, 1143
Kinin system, in rheumatoid arthritis, 887–888
Kininogens, 329t, 330
Kinky hair syndrome, Menkes', 1551
Kirschner wire, in foot surgery, 1771
Kit, in mast cell differentiation, 164
Klebsiella infection, in ankylosing spondylitis, 971
Klinefelter's syndrome, connective tissue disease with, 1509
Klonopin, for sleep disturbances, in fibromyalgia syndrome, 517
Knee, anatomy of, 365, 365, 457, 458
angular deformities of, in juvenile rheumatoid arthritis, surgery for, 1775, 1776
arthritis in, monarticular, differential diagnosis of, 373t
arthrocentesis of, 600, 600
arthroplasty of, bone grafting in, 1823
complications of, 1751–1755, 1753
contraindications to, 1747
cost/benefit analysis of, 1633–1634
drain entrapment after, 1830
fractures after, 1828, 1828, 1829, 1829
hinge prostheses in, 1832, 1832
indications for, 1747, 1748
infection after, 1826, 1827, 1828

Knee (Continued)
loosening after, 1823–1826, 1824t, 1824–1826
MacIntosh hemiarthroplasty in, 1832–1833
management after, 1637–1638
McKeever hemiarthroplasty in, 1832–1833, 1833
metal synovitis after, 1830, 1831, 1832
patellar complications of, 1826–1830, 1828, 1829
postoperative care in, 1751
prosthesis types for, 1743–1746, 1744–1747, 1816–1818, 1818t, 1819
prosthetic wear after, 1830, 1831
radiography of, 1816–1833
alignment of, 1818–1822, 1820–1822
lucent zones in, 1822–1823, 1823
patellar component in, 1822, 1822
results of, 1755–1757, 1756, 1757
technique of, 1747–1751, 1749–1751
unicondylar, 1831, 1833
arthroscopy of, 457, 458, 460–461, 694
computed tomography of, 632–633
cysts of, 1593
development of, 4
disorders of, glucocorticoid injection for, 597, 597t, 600, 605–606
in sports medicine, 553–558, 554–557, 559
in ankylosing spondylitis, 974
in calcium pyrophosphate deposition disease, imaging of, 673, 673
in juvenile rheumatoid arthritis, arthroplasty of, 1775–1781, 1779
contractures of, soft tissue release for, 1774
synovectomy of, 1774
in Reiter's syndrome, imaging of, 660
ligaments in, 6
lipoma arborescens of, 1597, 1597–1598, 1598
magnetic resonance imaging of, 642–644, 643–645
movement of, hip flexion with, 87, 87, 88
in lifting, 92, 93
orthotic devices for, 1626
osteoarthritis of, arthrodesis for, 1739
arthroscopic lavage for, 1857–1858
arthroscopic surgery for, 691, 691, 692
cartilage transplantation for, 1740
débridement for, 1739–1740
drug treatment of, 1856t, 1856–1858, 1857t
glucocorticoids for, intra-articular injection of, 594
imaging of, 665, 666
irrigation for, 1396–1397, 1857
management of, goals of, 1855–1856
osteotomy for, 1740–1741, 1741
pathology of, 1741–1743, 1743
physical therapy for, 1856, 1856t
surgery for, 1858
wedged insoles for, 1396
osteonecrosis of, imaging of, 678, 678
pain in, 457–466
causes of, anterior, 462–464, 463
mediolateral, 464–466, 465
posterior, 466
imaging in, 458–462, 459–462
physical examination in, 457–458, 458
physical examination of, 365–369, 367
rheumatoid arthritis of, 914t, 914–915
hemiarthroplasty for, 1739

Knee (Continued)
imaging of, 648t, 650
meniscus in, synovial invasion of, 688, 689
pathology of, 1741–1743, 1742
synovectomy for, 1739, 1740
septic arthritis of, coccidioidomycosis and, 1456
swelling of, acute, quadriceps wasting with, 16
synovitis of, after hip arthroplasty, glucocorticoids for, 596
pigmented villonodular. See Synovitis, pigmented villonodular.
taping of, in osteoarthritis, 1396
Kneist's dysplasia, 1555
Koebner reaction, 498
Kohler's line, in radiography, after hip arthroplasty, 1785
Ku antigen, antibodies to, in systemic lupus erythematosus, 255t, 256
Kwashiorkor, inflammatory response in, 521

Labrum, acetabular, disorders of, and pain, 470
glenoid, tears of, and pain, 431
arthrography of, 416–417, 417
computed tomography of, 417, 418
magnetic resonance imaging of, 640–641, 641
Lachman test, in knee examination, 368, 458
in sports medicine, 553, 556
Lacrimal gland, disorders of, in sarcoidosis, 493–494, 494
Lactation, after silicone breast implantation, 1173–1174
glucocorticoid use in, 793
in rheumatoid arthritis, drug treatment in, 1902t, 1903
sulfasalazine use in, 744
Lactoferrin, in neutrophils, 148
Laminectomy, for lumbar disc herniation, with spinal stenosis, 449–450
Laminins, in extracellular matrix, 37, 39, 42, 44, 45, 48
receptors of, on mononuclear phagocytes, 134, 136
Langerhans cells, 140, 141
Lansbury articular index, in rheumatoid arthritis, 925, 925t
Large intestine. See also Gastrointestinal tract.
cancer of, Sjögren's syndrome and, 1528, 1531t
disorders of, and arthritis. See Enteropathic arthritis.
in scleroderma, 1147
inflammatory disease of, leukotrienes in, 297t, 299
Larynx, in polychondritis, relapsing, 1406
Lateral plantar nerve syndrome, 580
Lavage, arthroscopic, for osteoarthritis, of knee, 1857–1858
bronchoalveolar, in pulmonary fibrosis, 1163–1164
in sarcoidosis, 1418
Laxity testing, in shoulder examination, in sports medicine, 547–548, 548
L-Dopa, for sleep disturbances, in fibromyalgia syndrome, 517
Lead, toxicity of, and gout, 1323

Lectin domain, in selectins, 310
Leg(s), cataracts of, glucocorticoids and, 796
  length discrepancy of, correction of, in hip arthroplasty, 1730
    in juvenile rheumatoid arthritis, orthotics for, 1627
      surgery for, 1775
  lower, injuries of, in sports medicine, 558–560
  pain in, in pseudoradicular nerve entrapment syndromes, 582
  raising of, in physical examination, in low back pain, 442
Lens, ectopia of, in Marfan syndrome, 1552
  toxicity to, gold therapy and, 764
Lentivirus infection, in rheumatoid arthritis, 856
Leprosy, 1456
Lesch-Nyhan syndrome, 1331t, 1332–1337, 1333, 1334t, 1335t, 1336
Leucovorin, structure of, 772
  with methotrexate therapy, 779, 780
Leukemia, acute lymphocytic, arthritis with, vs. rheumatoid arthritis, 907
  joint involvement in, 1616
  musculoskeletal manifestations of, 1522
  vasculitis with, 1112
Leukemia inhibitory factor, in acute-phase reactions, 274
  in rheumatoid arthritis, 869
Leukocyte adhesion deficiency, 189, 1285t, 1298–1299
  genetics of, 1284, 1284t
  type 1, 130
  type 2, 130
Leukocyte antigens. See Human leukocyte antigens.
Leukocyte functional antigen–1 (CD11a/CD18), in lymphocyte migration, 120, 120t, 121, 121t
  in monocyte adhesion, to endothelial cells, 129
Leukocyte response integrin, 307, 308, 308
Leukocytes, and vascular permeability, in inflammatory response, 185–186
  homing of, in infection, cell adhesion molecules and, 314–317
  in adhesion molecule expression, 268–269
  in inflammatory response, interaction of, with endothelium, 186t, 186–191, 187t, 189, 190t, 191
  in synovial fluid, 610t, 611, 611t
  in bacterial arthritis, 1437
  interaction of, with platelets, 177–178, 178
  polymorphonuclear, development of, cytokines in, 272
    in bacterial arthritis, 1435
    in rheumatoid arthritis, 880, 884, 885
    in synovial fluid analysis, 610t, 615, 616
  radiolabeled, in scintigraphy, after hip arthroplasty, 1811–1812, 1812
  suppression of, in cytotoxic drug treatment, 815–816, 816
Leukopenia, gold therapy and, 764
  in Felty's syndrome, 951, 951–954
  in severe combined immunodeficiency, 1294, 1294, 1295
  in Sjögren's syndrome, 962
  in systemic lupus erythematosus, 1030t, 1035

Leukopenia (Continued)
  sulfasalazine and, 743, 743, 744
    in rheumatoid arthritis, 1898t, 1900
Leukoplasmapheresis, for systemic lupus erythematosus, 1053
Leukotrienes, B₄, in psoriatic arthritis, 1000
  C₄, in mast cell mediation, 169
  in inflammatory response, 296–298, 297t
  to urate crystals, in gout, 1339–1340
  in synovial fluid, in rheumatoid arthritis, 886–887
  receptors of, 295–296
  synthesis of, 291–294, 292, 293, 295, 709–711, 710
    fatty acids in, 527, 527–531, 528
Levamisole, for rheumatoid arthritis, vs. antimalarial drugs, 752t
  in immunosuppression, 822, 823t
Levodopa, for sleep disturbances, in fibromyalgia syndrome, 517
LFA–1 (lymphocyte function-associated molecule–1), in leukocyte-endothelial adhesion, 186t, 187, 187t, 188
Lidocaine, after hip arthroplasty, injection of, with arthrographic contrast agent, 1810
  before intubation, for anesthesia, 1640
  with glucocorticoid injection, for rotator cuff impingement, 424
  intra-articular, 594–595, 599
Lifting, joint motion in, control of, 92, 93
Ligaments, constitutents of, 23t, 23–24
  in joint stability, 86, 87
  in synovial joints, 6
  of ankle, injury of, in sports medicine, 560
  of knee, injury of, in sports medicine, 555–558, 556, 557, 559
  of Struthers, in median nerve entrapment, 572
Ligands, extracellular matrix components as, 43–44
Light, in therapy, for Reiter's syndrome, 993
  sensitivity to, in dermatomyositis, 504, 504, Plate 5
    in systemic lupus erythematosus, 1030t, 1036
      management of, 1041, 1042t
Linear scleroderma, 1154–1155, 1155
Link protein, in extracellular matrix, 42, 48
Linkage analysis, in complex genetic disease, 221–224, 222, 223, 224t
Linoleic acid, 527, 527
γ-Linolenic acid, 527, 527–528, 528
Lipids, elevated blood level of, arthropathy with, vs. rheumatoid arthritis, 906
  metabolism of, disorders of, and myopathy, 1191t, 1192–1194
Lipocalin, human neutrophil, 148
Lipocortins, anti-inflammatory effect of, 710, 711
  in prostaglandin inhibition, glucocorticoids and, 790
Lipoma, synovial, 1597
Lipoma arborescens, 1597, 1597–1598, 1598
Lipoxins, in inflammation, 297–298
  synthesis of, 294, 295, 710
Lipoxygenase pathways, in eicosanoid synthesis, 291–294, 292, 293, 295, 709–711, 710
  inhibition of, for inflammatory diseases, 297t, 298–299
Lisfranc fracture-dislocation, with diabetic neuroarthropathy, 671, 671

Lisfranc's arthritis, 484
Lithiasis, renal, in gout, 1322, 1345
Lithium, interactions of, with nonsteroidal anti-inflammatory drugs, 719t, 720
Livedo reticularis, in polyarteritis, 1093, 1093
Livedoid vasculitis, 504
Liver, acetaminophen toxicity to, in osteoarthritis, 1398
  complement synthesis in, 235
  disorders of, α₁-antitrypsin deficiency and, 35
    in antiphospholipid syndrome, 1061
    in polyarteritis, 1094
    in Sjögren's syndrome, 960–961
    in systemic lupus erythematosus, 1036
    nonsteroidal anti-inflammatory drug use in, 721–722, 723t, 729t
  enlargement of, in Felty's syndrome, 952
  fibrotic disease of, 1164–1165
  in glucocorticoid metabolism, 792–793, 793
  in iron storage disorders, 1423–1425, 1427, 1427
  inflammation of. See Hepatitis entries.
  methotrexate toxicity to, 781t, 781–782, 782t
    in rheumatoid arthritis, 943–944, 1898t, 1900
      monitoring for, 1860–1869, 1862t–1867t, 1866, 1869t, 1871t
        biopsy in, 1860–1863, 1862t, 1863t
        costs of, 1867, 1867t, 1871t
        risks of, 1867, 1867t, 1871t
        blood tests in, 1864t–1866t, 1864–1867, 1866
        indications for, 1860–1861
        methods of, 1861
        recommendations for, 1868–1869, 1869t
  nonsteroidal anti-inflammatory drug toxicity to, 715–716
    in rheumatoid arthritis, 1899
  transplantation of, in familial amyloidotic polyneuropathy, 1414–1415
Load, bony adaptation to, 70–72
  distribution of, articular cartilage in, 9–10, 10
Lodine (etodolac), 729t, 734, 734
Lofgren's syndrome, 1418–1419
  vs. rheumatoid arthritis, 909
Longitudinal ligaments, of spine, cervical, anatomy of, 396, 397, 397
    in diffuse idiopathic skeletal hyperostosis, 668, 669
Loose bodies, in joints, 1595, 1595–1596, 1596
Looser's zones, in osteomalacia, 1573, 1573
Low back pain, 439–454
  anatomy in, 439–440, 440
  and disability, 439
  in ankylosing spondylitis, 450, 973, 973t
  in pregnancy, 1508
  incidence of, 439
  infection and, 451–452
  nonspinal sources of, 453–454
  physical examination in, 441–443, 442t
  presentation of, 440–441, 441t
  psychologic evaluation in, 443
  radiography in, 443–447, 445–447
  research in, progress in, 439
  spinal stenosis and, 447t, 447–450, 448
  spondylolisthesis and, 452t, 452–453
  spondylolysis and, 444, 452t, 452–453
  systemic inflammatory disease and, 450

L-selectin (CD62L), 310–312
  in leukocyte-endothelial adhesion, in inflammatory response, 186t, 187t, 188–190
  in leukocyte homing, 316
  in lymphocyte homing, in inflammatory response, 192
  in lymphocyte migration, 120, 120t, 121
  in monocyte adhesion, to endothelial cells, 130
Lubricin, in minimization of frictional forces, 89
  in synovial joints, 17, 18
Ludington's sign, in bicipital tendinitis, 427
Lumbar spine. See also *Spine.*
  disorders of, and pain. See *Low back pain.*
Lumbosacral radiculopathy, and hip pain, 476
Lumican, in extracellular matrix, 45
Lunate, avascular necrosis of, magnetic resonance imaging of, *639*
  dislocation of, examination for, 361
Lung(s). See also *Pulmonary* entries.
  disorders of, and hypertrophic osteoarthropathy, 1514t, 1516
  in ankylosing spondylitis, 974–975
  in antiphospholipid syndrome, 1061
  in diffuse infiltrative lymphocytosis, in human immunodeficiency virus infection, 1274, 1276
  in mixed connective tissue disease, 1070, *1071*
  in polyarteritis, 1094
  in rheumatoid arthritis, 920–921, *922*
  in scleroderma, 1147–1149, *1148*, 1154
    in children, 1250, 1250t
    with Raynaud's phenomenon, 1142, 1142t
  in Sjögren's syndrome, 960, 961t
  in systemic lupus erythematosus, 1035
  in Wegener's granulomatosis, 1100, *1100*, 1101
  emphysema of, α$_1$-antitrypsin deficiency and, 34–35
  fibrosis of, 1163–1164
  pneumonia in, in rheumatic fever, 1232
  silicosis of, 1169
  toxicity to, methotrexate and, 781
    D-penicillamine and, 767
    sulfasalazine and, 743
Lupus erythematosus, discoid, antimalarial drugs for, 749–750
  complement deficiencies in, 1307, 1308, 1308t
  skin lesions in, 499–502, *501*, 1030t, 1036, Plate 5
  genetic susceptibility to, in twins, 209
  systemic, 1015–1054. See also *Systemic lupus erythematosus.*
Lupus erythematosus cells, in synovial fluid analysis, 615
Lupus-like syndrome, paraneoplastic, 1524, 1527t
Lyme disease, 1462–1470
  and arthritis, pauciarticular, 384
  clinical features of, 507, *507*, *1463*, 1463–1466, 1464t, *1465*, Plate 6, Plate 12
  diagnosis of, *1467*, 1467–1468, *1468*
  epidemiology of, 1462
  etiologic agent in, 1462
  fibromyalgia in, with fatigue, antibiotics for, 1872–1878, 1874t–1877t
  immune complex assays in, 229–230

Lyme disease (*Continued*)
  inflammatory response in, human leukocyte antigens in, vs. rheumatoid arthritis, 855
  monarticular symptoms in, 376
  ocular disorders in, 494, 1464t
  pathogenesis of, 1466–1467
  prevention of, 1470
  treatment of, 1468–1470, 1469t
  vs. juvenile rheumatoid arthritis, 1215
  vs. rheumatoid arthritis, 907
Lymecycline, for Reiter's syndrome, 994–995
Lymph nodes, in Kawasaki disease, 1256
  irradiation of, in immunosuppression, 818–819
Lymphadenopathy, angioimmunoblastic, vs. rheumatoid arthritis, 903
Lymphapheresis, therapeutic, 818
Lymphatic system, irradiation of, total, for rheumatoid arthritis, 947
  radiographic opacification of, after hip arthroplasty, *1806*, 1809–1810
Lymphocyte function-associated molecule-1, in inflammatory response, 186t, 187, 187t, 188
Lymphocytes. See also *B cells* and *T cells.*
  glucocorticoid effects on, 790, 790t–791
  in fibroblast regulation, 202–203, *203*
  in synovial fluid analysis, 615–616, *616*, Plate 8
  interaction of, with endothelial cells, 191–192
  large granular, in rheumatoid arthritis, 919
  suppression of, in cytotoxic drug treatment, 815–816, *816*
Lymphocytic leukemia, acute, arthritis with, vs. rheumatoid arthritis, 907
Lymphocytosis, diffuse infiltrative, in human immunodeficiency virus infection, 1273t, 1273–1277, *1274*, *1276*
Lymphoma, arthropathy with, 1524
  in Sjögren's syndrome, 962, 1528, 1531t
  in systemic lupus erythematosus, 1528, 1531t
  joint involvement in, 1616
  methotrexate and, 780, 1901
  musculoskeletal manifestations of, 1522–1523
  polyarthritis in, vs. rheumatoid arthritis, 907
  vasculitis with, 1112
  with rheumatoid arthritis, 918, 923
Lymphomatoid granulomatosis, 1530, 1531t
Lymphopenia, in systemic lupus erythematosus, 1030t, 1035
Lymphoplasmapheresis, for scleroderma, 1152
Lymphoproliferative disease, X-linked, 1285t, 1292
Lymphotoxin, 101, 103t
  in chronic inflammation, 276
Lysosomes, antimalarial drug effects on, 748, 749
  in macrophages, 130
Lysozyme, in amyloidosis, familial, 1410, 1410t
  in neutrophils, 147, 148
  secretion of, by macrophages, 138
Lysyl hydroxylase, in collagen synthesis, 1538, 1540t
Lysyl oxidase, in collagen synthesis, gene for, 1538, 1540, 1540t

MA-I, antibodies to, in Sjögren's syndrome, 261, 261t
Mac-1, in monocyte adhesion, to endothelial cells, 129
MacIntosh hemiarthroplasty, of knee, radiography of, 1832–1833
α$_2$-Macroglobulin, in proteinase inhibition, 327–328, 329t
Macroglobulinemia, Waldenström's, plasmapheresis for, 817
  rheumatoid factors in, 242, 244, 246
Macroglossia, in amyloidosis, 1412, *1413*
Macrophage(s), 128–143, 806, *806*
  activation of, 139–140
  antineoplastic function of, 140
  antiviral function of, 140
  development of, cytokines in, 272–273
  distribution of, 128, 128t
  glucocorticoid effects on, 790, 790t
  heterogeneity of, 131
  in immune response, to silicone, 1171
  in rheumatoid arthritis, cytokines of, 866–870
    therapy targeting, 842
  intracellular digestion in, 139
  phagocytosis in, 138
  pinocytosis in, 138–139
  secretory products of, 136–138, 137t
  tissue, peripheral blood monocyte differentiation into, 130–131
Macrophage colony-stimulating factor, in bone cell metabolism, 61
  in bone remodeling, 59
  in immune cell development, 271
  in mononuclear phagocyte maturation, 131, 131t, 132, *133*
MAdCAM-1 (mucosal addressin cell adhesion molecule-1), in leukocyte homing, 315–316
  in lymphocyte homing, in inflammatory response, 192
  L-selectin binding to, 310–312
Magnesium, reduced blood level of, and myopathy, 1194t
  with calcium pyrophosphate deposition disease, 1355
Magnetic resonance imaging, 635–644, 1885–1886
  in low back pain, 446
  of angiitis, of central nervous system, 1091
  of ankle, 481, 641–642
  of ankylosing spondylitis, 975, *975*, 977
  of arthritis, monarticular, 379
  of bone marrow, 637–639, *638–640*, 644
  of entrapment syndromes, 566, *568*
  of foot, 481, 641–642
  of hip, 468–469, *469*
    fractures in, *471*, 471–472
    in evaluation of pain, 1726
    osteoporosis in, transient, 473, *473*
  of knee, *461*, 461–462, *462*, 642–644, *643–645*
    in sports medicine, *555–557*, 555–558, *559*
  of liver, in iron storage disease, 1427, *1427*
  of muscle disease, 391
    inflammatory, 1198, *1198*, 1199–1200
  of osteoarthritis, 1387–1388
  of osteonecrosis, 1585, 1586, *1587*
  of rheumatoid arthritis, 924, *924*
  of sarcoidosis, 1419–1421
  of shoulder, 639–641, *641*
    in sports medicine, 549, *550*, 551

Magnetic resonance imaging *(Continued)*
  painful, 420, *421*, 422, *422*, 422t
  preoperative, 1698
  of spine, 408, 635–637, *636, 637*
    cervical, in rheumatoid arthritis, 1717
  of synovial cysts, 1593, *1594*
  of temporomandibular joint, 639, *641*
  of wrist, *639*, 641
Maisonneuve's fracture, in sports
    medicine, 560
Major basic protein, in eosinophils, 155,
    155, 157
Major histocompatibility complex, 210–214.
    See also *Human leukocyte antigens.*
  antigens of, deficiency of, in immunode-
        ficiency, 1286t, 1295–1296
      intrauterine diagnosis of, 1299–
            1300
      therapy targeting, for rheumatoid ar-
            thritis, 846
  complement genes in, 1305, *1306*
  in B cell activation, 119
  in rheumatoid arthritis, 852–853, 853t
  in T cell activation, 114–116, *115*
  in T cell–B cell collaboration, 121–122
Malar rash, in systemic lupus
    erythematosus, 1030t, 1036
Malaria, drugs used for, as antirheumatic
    agents, 747–756. See also *Antimalarial
    drugs.*
Malignancy. See *Cancer.*
Mallet finger, examination for, 361
Malnutrition. See also *Nutrition.*
  inflammatory response in, 521
Mandible, arthritis in, monoarticular,
    differential diagnosis of, 373t
  articulation of, with temporal bone. See
        Temporomandibular joint.
  growth of, retardation of, in juvenile
        rheumatoid arthritis, 1212, *1212*
Manubriosternal joint, examination of, 357
  in rheumatoid arthritis, 911
Marasmus, inflammatory response in, 521
Marble bone disease (osteopetrosis),
    carbonic anhydrase deficiency and,
    59–60
  osteoclast deficiency and, 58
Marfan syndrome, 1552–1553
  fibrillin gene defects in, 35, 46
Marrow. See *Bone marrow.*
Mast cells, 161–172
  activation of, 170, *170*
  differentiation of, 164
  immunoassays for, 171
  in arthritis, 171–172
  in rheumatic disease, *163*, 163–164
  in rheumatoid arthritis, 880–881
  in scleroderma, 163–164, 1139
  in synovial fluid analysis, 616
  mediator(s) of, 161, 162t
    histamine as, 164–166, *165, 166*
    neutral proteases as, 166–167, 167t
    newly generated lipids as, *169*, 169–
        170
    proteoglycans as, 167–169, *168*
  proteinases of, in extracellular matrix
        degradation, 324t, 325, 325t
  secretion by, 170–171
  types of, 161–164, *162*, 162t, *163*
Mastectomy, silicone breast implants after,
    and rheumatic disease, 1169t,
    1169–1174, 1172t
Matrilysin, in extracellular matrix
    degradation, 324t, 325t, 327, 327t, *328*
Matrix, extracellular, 37–51. See also
    Extracellular matrix.

Matrix metalloproteinases, 324t–327t,
    326–327, *328*
  in rheumatoid arthritis, 876t, 876–878,
        877
  inhibitors of, 329t, 330
Mayaro virus infection, and arthritis,
    1478–1479
Mayo ankle prosthesis, radiography of,
    1836, *1838*
Mayo modified Coonrad elbow prosthesis,
    1686, *1688, 1689, 1691*, 1691–1692, 1835
McArdle's disease, myopathy in, 1192
McCune-Albright syndrome, 1539
McKeever hemiarthroplasty, of knee, in
    juvenile rheumatoid arthritis, 1776
  radiography of, 1832–1833, *1833*
McKusick's metaphyseal dysplasia, 1556
McMurray's test, for meniscal tears, 368
Mechlorethamine, in immunosuppression,
    for non-neoplastic diseases, *810*, 811,
    811t
Meclofenamate (Meclomen), 729t, 733, *733*
  adverse effects of, gastrointestinal, 713–
        714
Medial plantar nerve syndrome, 580
Medial tibial stress syndrome, 466
  in sports medicine, 558–559
Median nerve, disorders of, in thoracic
    outlet syndromes, 577
  muscle testing for, 399t
  entrapment of, 567–573, *568, 569, 572*
    in carpal tunnel syndrome. See *Carpal
        tunnel syndrome.*
  reflex testing of, 406t
Medipren. See *Ibuprofen.*
Mediterranean fever, familial, colchicine
    for, 728
  genetic linkage analysis in, 224
  monarticular arthritis in, 378
  vs. rheumatoid arthritis, 905
Medroxyprogesterone, for osteoporosis,
    1568–1569
Mefenamic acid, 733, *733*
Meglumine, in myelography, in low back
    pain, 444
Melphalan, for amyloidosis, 1412–1413,
    1415, 1415t
Memory, in B cells, immune complexes
    and, 228
  in T cells, 100, 100t
Meningocele, sacral, computed
    tomography of, *629*
Meningococcal infection, and arthritis,
    1446–1447
  monarticular, 376
Meniscus (menisci), in synovial joints, 6–7
  of knee, abnormalities of, and pain, 464–
        465
    anatomy of, 457, *458*
    in osteoarthritis, arthroscopy of, *691,
        692*
    lesions of, in sports medicine, 553–
        555, *555*
    prostheses bearing, 1746
    synovial invasion of, in rheumatoid ar-
        thritis, 688, *689*
    tears of, examination for, 368
      magnetic resonance imaging of,
            642–643
Menkes' kinky hair syndrome, 1551
Menopause, and osteoporosis, 1563–1564
  collagen gene defect in, 31, 31t, 33t
Menstrual cycle, cramping in, nonsteroidal
    anti-inflammatory drugs for, 713, 731
  synovial inflammation in, in rheumatoid
        arthritis, 1509

Menstruation, in systemic lupus
    erythematosus, 1037
Meralgia paresthetica, 580–581
  after surgical injury, 586
6-Mercaptopurine, in immunosuppression,
    for non-neoplastic diseases, 810, 811t,
    813–814, 814t, 823t
Merchant's view, of patella, 459, *459*
Merosin, in extracellular matrix, 48
Mesenchyme, synovial, in joint
    development, 3–4
Mesna, with cyclophosphamide, for
    systemic lupus erythematosus,
    1048–1049
Messenger RNA, in elastin synthesis, 33
Metacarpal bones, in hemochromatosis,
    imaging of, 675–676, *676*
Metacarpophalangeal joint(s),
    arthrocentesis of, 601–602, *602*
  chondrocalcinosis in, with hemochro-
        matosis, 1426
  fourth, in Albright's hereditary osteodys-
        trophy, 1502–1503, *1503*
  in juvenile rheumatoid arthritis, surgery
        of, 1662, *1664*
    synovectomy of, 1774
  in rheumatoid arthritis, *912*, 912–914,
        913
    surgery of, 1655–1658, *1657*
  in systemic lupus erythematosus, im-
        aging of, *660*, 661, *661*
    surgery of, 1663–1666, *1665–1667*
  physical examination of, 360–362
  prostheses for, silicone rubber, radiogra-
        phy of, 1840–1841, *1841, 1842*
Metal, in knee prosthesis, and synovitis,
    1830, *1831, 1832*
Metalloproteinases, in extracellular matrix
    degradation, 204, 324t–327t,
    326–327, *328*
  in osteoarthritis, 1372–1373
  inhibitors of, 329t, 330
  in rheumatoid arthritis, 876t, 876–878,
        877, 878t, 881, 883
  regulation of, cellular, 331–334, 332t–334t
    extracellular, 335–337, *336, 337*, 338t
Metaphyses, arteries of, 68
  chondrodysplasia of, 1556
  reshaping of, in bone growth, 68
Metatarsal bones, in gout, *672*, 672–673
  in rheumatoid arthritis, 882
Metatarsophalangeal joint(s), anatomy of,
    480, *480*
  arthrocentesis of, 602
  disorders of, shoe orthotics for, 1627,
        1627
  in rheumatoid arthritis, 482, *482*–483,
        915, *915*
  of great toe, rigidity of, in osteoarthritis,
        484, *484*, 665
    surgery for, 1770, *1771*
  osteolysis of, in diabetes, 1501, *1501*
Methotrexate, and cancer, 1530
  and delayed wound healing, after foot
        surgery, 1770–1771
  continuation of, with hip arthroplasty,
        1728
  dosage of, 778–779
  for dermatomyositis, 778
  for Felty's syndrome, 778
  for inflammatory disease, as leukotriene
        inhibitor, 297t, 298
    of muscle, 1201
  for juvenile rheumatoid arthritis, 778,
        1218

Methotrexate (Continued)
  for polymyositis, 778
  for psoriatic arthritis, 778
  for Reiter's syndrome, 778, 994, 995t
  for reticulohistiocytosis, multicentric,
    1433
  for rheumatoid arthritis, 774t, 774–778,
    775–777, 943–944, 946–947, 1891–
    1893, 1892t, 1898t, 1900–1901
    in pregnancy and lactation, 1902t
    toxicity of, to liver, 1860–1869. See
      also Liver, methotrexate toxicity to.
    vs. gold, 761
    with antimalarial drugs, 753
  for spondyloarthropathy, with human
    immunodeficiency virus infection,
    1272
  for Takayasu's arteritis, 1090
  historical aspects of, 771
  interactions of, with nonsteroidal anti-in-
    flammatory drugs, 719t, 720
  patient selection for, 782–783
  pharmacology of, 771–774, 772
  structure of, 771, 772
  toxicity of, 779–782, 780, 781t, 782t,
    1898t, 1900
Methyl methacrylate, in arthroplasty, of
  hip, 1728–1730, 1729
  infection after, 1799–1805, 1800t,
    1805
  loosening after, 1799–1805, 1800t,
    1801–1804
  radiography of, 1789, 1790–1792
  results with, 1734t–1736t, 1734–1736
  of knee, 1750–1751, 1751
Methylprednisolone. See also
  Glucocorticoids.
  for giant cell arteritis, 1130
  for polychondritis, relapsing, 1407
  for rheumatoid arthritis, 940
    juvenile, 1219
  for systemic lupus erythematosus, 1045–
    1046, 1047t
  intra-articular injection of, 591, 592, 594t
  pharmacokinetics of, 788t, 792, 792
  potency of, 788t
  structure of, 787, 788
Metrizamide, in myelography, in low back
  pain, 444, 445, 445, 446
Micrognathia, in juvenile rheumatoid
  arthritis, 1212, 1212
Microsatellite markers, in genetics, 225
Midfoot. See also Foot (feet).
  anatomy of, 479, 480
  disorders of, surgery for, 1766–1767,
    1768, 1769
Midtarsal joints, anatomy of, 480, 480
Migraine, in antiphospholipid syndrome,
  1060
Milwaukee shoulder syndrome, 1379
  preoperative evaluation of, 1704
Minocycline, for rheumatoid arthritis, 947
Misoprostol, adverse effects of,
  gastrointestinal, 715
  interaction of, with nonsteroidal anti-in-
    flammatory drugs, 720t
Mithramycin, for Paget's disease of bone,
  1577
Mitochondrial myopathies, 1193
Mitral valve, in antiphospholipid
  syndrome, 1060
  in rheumatic fever, 1229, 1230
Mixed connective tissue disease, 1067–1075
  clinical features of, 1068t, 1068–1073,
    1069–1073

Mixed connective tissue disease
  (Continued)
  glucocorticoids for, intra-articular
    injection of, 596
  imaging in, 663
  in children, 1253
  juvenile, 1073
  management of, 1074t, 1074–1075
  prognosis of, 1073–1074
  skin lesions in, 502
  vs. rheumatoid arthritis, 904
Mixed cryoglobulinemia, rheumatoid
  factors in, 242, 244–246
Mobility devices, in rehabilitative
  medicine, 1628–1630, 1629
Monoclonal antibodies, in management of
  rheumatoid arthritis, 839, 841–847, 843
  to cell adhesion molecules, in anti-in-
    flammatory treatment, 317
Monocyte chemotactic and activating
  factor, 130
Monocyte chemotactic protein-1, 130
Monocytes, 128–143, 806, 806
  development of, cytokines in, 272–273
  enzyme inhibitors secreted by, 138
  glucocorticoid effects on, 790, 790t
  historical aspects of, 128
  in fibroblast regulation, 202–203, 203
  in peripheral blood, differentiation of,
    into macrophages, 130–131
    migration of, to tissue, 129–130
    morphology of, 128–129, 129
  in synovial fluid analysis, 615, 616, 616,
    Plate 8
  interleukin–1 receptor antagonist in, pro-
    duction of, 267, 268t
  therapy targeting, for rheumatoid arthri-
    tis, 842
Mononuclear phagocytes, 128–143. See
  also Macrophages and Monocytes.
  antimicrobial function of, 139
  antineoplastic function of, 140
  antiviral function of, 140
  cell surface molecules of, 134–136
  in immunoregulation, 141–143, 142
  maturation of, in bone marrow, 131t,
    131–134, 132t, 133, 135t
  secretory products of, 136–138, 137t
  types of, distribution of, 128, 128t
Monosodium urate, deposition of, in
  hyperuricemia, management of, 1344,
  1344–1345, 1345t
Morphea, 1155–1156, 1156
  in children, 1252, 1252
Morton's neuroma, 580
  glucocorticoids for, 598
Motion, limitation of, in patient history,
  354
  in physical examination, 355
Motor units, structure of, 77
  types of, 82, 83t
Motrin. See Ibuprofen.
Mouth, antigen administration through,
  tolerance after, 846
  in diffuse infiltrative lymphocytosis, in
    human immunodeficiency virus infec-
    tion, 1273t, 1273–1277, 1274
  in Sjögren's syndrome, 488, 957t, 957–
    960, 959, 962, 962, 965
  ulcers of, in Behçet's disease, 1114, 1114,
    1114t, 1116, Plate 12
M-protein, in rheumatic fever, 1226
Mseleni joint disease, 1390
Mucin clot test, in synovial fluid analysis,
  617

Mucins, 304, 312
Mucocutaneous lymph node syndrome,
  1242t, 1255t, 1255–1257, 1256, 1257
Mucosal addressin cell adhesion molecule-
  1, in leukocyte homing, 315–316
  in lymphocyte homing, 192
  L-selectin binding to, 310–312
Muller template, in radiography, after hip
  arthroplasty, 1785, 1786
Multi-colony-stimulating factor
  (interleukin-3), 102t
  in mononuclear phagocyte maturation,
    131t, 131–132, 133
Multiple chemical sensitivity, vs.
  fibromyalgia syndrome, 514
Multiple epiphyseal dysplasia, 1555
Multiple myeloma, synovial biopsy in, 622,
  622, Plate 10
Multiple sclerosis, interleukin–4 for, 279
Mumps, and arthritis, 1479–1480
Murmurs, cardiac, in rheumatic fever,
  1231, 1234
  in systemic lupus erythematosus, 1035
Murphy's sign, of lunate dislocation,
  examination for, 361
Muscle(s), claudication of, in giant cell
  arteritis, 1126
  disorders of, and polyarticular pain, 386
    glucocorticoids and, 795
    in human immunodeficiency virus in-
      fection, 1277
    in hyperthyroidism, 1504–1505
    in hypothyroidism, 1505
    in mixed connective tissue disease,
      1070, 1074t
    in rheumatologic disorders, 392–393
    in scleroderma, 1145–1146
    weakness in, 388, 390–391
  function of, in elderly, 541
  hemorrhage into, in hemophilia, 1486–
    1487
  in rheumatoid arthritis, 916
  in synovial joints, 5
  inflammatory disease of, 1177–1201. See
    also Myositis and specific types, e.g.,
    Dermatomyositis.
  pain in. See Fibromyalgia and Myalgia.
  skeletal, 76–84
    contraction of, 79–82, 82
    development of, 76, 77
    fiber types of, 82–83, 83t
    structure of, 76–79, 78, 79t, 80, 81,
      Plate 1
  strengthening of, exercises for, in rehabil-
    itation, 1621–1623, 1622
  weakness of, in acromegaly, 1507
Muscular dystrophy, vs. dermatomyositis,
  in children, 1247
  vs. inflammatory muscle disease, 1189,
    1189t
Musculocutaneous nerve, disorders of,
  muscle testing for, 399t
  entrapment of, 578
  reflex testing of, 406t
Musculoskeletal system, disorders of,
  clinical syndromes in, 1882–1884,
    1883t, 1884t
  history in, 1880–1881, 1881t, 1882t
  imaging in, 1885–1886
  laboratory studies in, 1884–1885
  psychosocial factors in, 1881
  referral criteria in, 1886
Musicians, overuse syndromes in, 585,
  585t
Myalgia. See also Fibromyalgia.

Myalgia (Continued)
  causes of, 1882–1884
  in Sjögren's syndrome, treatment of, 965
  in systemic lupus erythematosus, 1040–
    1041
  spinal nerve root irritation and, 402
  vs. arthritis, monarticular, 373
  with eosinophilia, syndrome of, 1157–
    1158, 1185
Myasthenia gravis, D-penicillamine and,
    767, 943
  vs. inflammatory muscle disease, 1190,
    1197
Mycobacterial infection, and rheumatoid
    arthritis, 855, 855t
  and tuberculosis. See Tuberculosis.
  osteoarticular, 1450, 1455t, 1455–1456
Mycobacterium avium infection, in acquired
    immunodeficiency syndrome,
    1455–1456
Mycobacterium leprae infection, 1456
Mycoplasmal infection, and rheumatoid
    arthritis, 855, 855t
Mycosis fungoides, arthritis with, vs.
    rheumatoid arthritis, 907
Myelography, in low back pain, 444–445,
    445, 446
Myeloma, joint involvement in, 1616
  multiple, synovial biopsy in, 622, 622,
    Plate 10
Myeloperoxidase, in neutrophils, 147
Myelosuppression, chlorambucil and, 813
  cyclophosphamide and, 813
  methotrexate and, 1898t, 1900
  sulfasalazine and, 1898t, 1900
Myoadenylate deaminase deficiency, and
    myopathy, 1193
Myoblasts, in skeletal muscle
    development, 76, 77
Myocardial infarction, and shoulder pain,
    435
  in antiphospholipid syndrome, 1060
  in systemic lupus erythematosus, 1035
Myocarditis, in rheumatic fever, 1229
  in rheumatoid arthritis, 921
  in systemic lupus erythematosus, 1035
Myocardium, in scleroderma, 1149, 1154
    with Raynaud's phenomenon, 1141,
      1142t
Myochrysine. See Gold.
Myofascial pain, vs. arthritis, monarticular,
    373
  vs. fibromyalgia syndrome, 514
Myofibrils, in skeletal muscle, 78, 80
Myofilaments, in skeletal muscle, 78, 80
Myoglobin, in inflammatory muscle
    disease, 1195–1196
Myophosphorylase deficiency, 1192
Myosin, in skeletal muscle, 78, 79t, 80, 81,
    Plate 1
  in contraction, 82, 82
  in fiber types, 83, 83t
Myositis. See also Dermatomyositis and
    Polymyositis.
  antinuclear antibodies in, 259–261, 260t
  biopsy in, 1197–1199, 1198
  classification of, 1177t–1179t, 1177–1178
  clinical features of, 1179–1186, 1180–1182,
    1183t, 1184t, 1184–1186
  diagnosis of, differential, 1189t–1191t,
    1189–1194, 1194t
  electromyography in, 1196–1197
  eosinophilic, 1184–1185
  epidemiology of, 1178–1179
  exercise testing in, 1199

Myositis (Continued)
  genetic markers of, 1179, 1187–1188
  giant cell, 1186
  imaging in, 1199–1200
  in juvenile rheumatoid arthritis, 1211–
    1212
  in systemic lupus erythematosus, 1032
  inclusion body, clinical features of, 1183–
    1184
    diagnosis of, criteria for, 1178, 1178t
    pathology of, 1183–1184, 1184, 1184t,
      1185, 1189
    treatment of, 1201
  laboratory tests in, 1195–1196, 1196t
  localized, 1186
  pathogenesis of, 1186–1189
  physical examination in, 1194–1195,
    1195, 1195t
  treatment of, 1200–1201
  with collagen vascular diseases, 1183
Myositis ossificans, 1185–1186, 1186
Myositis ossificans progressiva, genetic
    mutation in, 1539
Myotubes, in skeletal muscle development,
    76, 77
Myxedema, 1505, 1505

Nabumetone, 723t, 726–727, 727
NADPH oxidase, in neutrophilic
    metabolism, 152–155, 154t
Nail fold, lesions of, in dermatomyositis,
    in children, 1246, 1246
Nails, in clubbing, in hypertrophic
    osteopathy, 1515, 1515
  in psoriasis, 498, 498
  in Reiter's syndrome, 989, 989
    with human immunodeficiency virus
      infection, 1269, 1270
Nalfon (fenoprofen), 729t, 731, 731–732
  toxicity of, to kidney, 716–717
Naproxen (Naprosyn), 723t, 724, 724–725
  for juvenile rheumatoid arthritis, 1217
  in cyclooxygenase pathway inhibition,
    709
  use of, in cirrhosis, 721
    in elderly, 722
    in renal disorders, 721, 724
Natural killer cells, in immune function,
    806, 806
Nebulin, in skeletal muscle, 79, 79t
Neck, anatomy of, 394–398, 395t, 396t,
    396–398
  pain in, 394–411
    clinical examination in, 403–407, 406t
    differential diagnosis of, 409–410
    disc degeneration and, 397–398
    electrodiagnostic studies of, 408
    evaluation of, 400–403, 401
    incidence of, 394
    laboratory studies in, 408
    nerve root compression and, 397–399
    patient education in, 411
    radiography of, 407–408
    treatment of, 410–411
Necrotizing vasculitis, paraneoplastic,
    1524, 1527t
  skin lesions in, 502t, 502–504, 503, Plate
    5
Neer shoulder prosthesis, 1707, 1708, 1708,
    1709t, 1834
Neisseria infection, and arthritis, 1445,
    1445–1447, 1446
  monarticular, 376

Neisseria infection (Continued)
  polyarticular, 383
    synovial fluid examination in, 1436
    vs. Reiter's syndrome, 991–992, 992t
  recurrent, in complement deficiency,
    1308t, 1308–1310
Neonate. See also Children; Infants.
  hypogammaglobulinemia in, transient,
    1285t, 1291
  lupus syndrome in, 1037, 1052, 1244,
    1244–1245
  pulmonary hypertension in, leukotrienes
    and, 297t
Neoplasia. See Cancer and Tumor(s).
Neovascularization (angiogenesis),
    cytokines in, 274
  in inflammatory response, 184
    endothelial cells and, 183–184, 193–
      194, 194t
  in rheumatoid arthritis, 869, 872, 872–
    873
Nephritis, complement deficiency and,
    1306–1308, 1308t
  in human immunodeficiency virus infec-
    tion, 1273
  in systemic lupus erythematosus. See
    Systemic lupus erythematosus, renal
    disorders in.
Nerve blocks, differential, in knee pain,
    462
Nerve conduction studies, in hip pain, 469
  in knee pain, 462
  in shoulder pain, 420
Nerves, disorders of, and pain, vs.
    monarticular arthritis, 372
  peripheral, anatomy of, 564–565, 565,
    566
    disorders of, and weakness, 390
      laboratory evaluation of, 392
    in amyloidosis, 1414, 1416t
    in compartment syndromes, 582–584,
      583, 584
    in entrapment syndromes, 564–582.
      See also Entrapment syndrome(s)
      and specific disorders, e.g., Carpal
      tunnel syndrome.
    in polyarteritis, 1093–1094
    in repetitive strain disorders, 584–585,
      585t
    perioperative lesions of, 585–586
Nervous system, autonomic, in uric acid
    excretion, 1329
  central, angiitis of, in human immunode-
    ficiency virus infection, 1278
    isolated, 1090–1091
    in antiphospholipid syndrome, throm-
      botic disorders of, 1059, 1059–
      1060
    in ataxia, with telangiectasia, 1297
    in Behçet's disease, 1115, 1116
    in juvenile rheumatoid arthritis, 1211
    in mixed connective tissue disease,
      1071–1072
    in polychondritis, relapsing, 1406
    in psychiatric disorders, with glucocor-
      ticoid use, 796
    in systemic lupus erythematosus, 180,
      1030t, 1034, 1053
      in children, 1241–1242, 1244
    toxicity to, methotrexate and, 780–781
      nonsteroidal anti-inflammatory
        drugs and, 718
      sulfasalazine and, 744
  disorders of, and polyarticular pain, 386
    in vasculitis, in rheumatoid arthritis,
      920

Nervous system (Continued)
  vs. inflammatory muscle disease,
    1189t, 1189–1190, 1197
  in ankylosing spondylitis, 975, 975, 977
  in control of joint motion, 91–92, 92, 93
  in giant cell arteritis, 1126–1127
  in hypoxanthine guanine phosphoribo-
    syltransferase deficiency, 1334
  in Lyme disease, 1463, 1464t, 1465, 1465–
    1466, 1469, 1469t
  in Paget's disease of bone, 1574–1575
  in scleroderma, 1150
  in Sjögren's syndrome, 962–963
  in Wegener's granulomatosis, 1101
  toxicity to, gold therapy and, 764
    vinca alkaloids and, 815
  transcutaneous electrical stimulation of,
    in osteoarthritis, 1396
    in rehabilitative medicine, 1624
Neuralgia, spinal nerve root irritation and,
  402
Neurapraxia, definition of, 565
  of ulnar nerve, after total elbow replace-
    ment, 1689
Neuritis, brachial, and shoulder pain, 433
Neurocan, in extracellular matrix, 46
Neuroma, Morton's, 580
  glucocorticoids for, nonarticular
    injection of, 598
Neuromuscular junction, disorders of,
  laboratory evaluation of, 391–392
  structure of, 77
Neuromuscular syndromes, weakness in,
  388t, 388–393, 389t, 390
Neuropathic arthropathy (Charcot joint),
  bacterial arthritis with, 1439, 1439t
  imaging of, 669–672, 671
  in diabetes, 1500, 1501
  knee arthroplasty for, 1747, 1748
  monarticular, 377
Neuropathic osteoarthropathy, of ankle,
  485
  of foot, 485
Neuropeptide Y, in joint development, 4
Neuropeptides, in rheumatoid arthritis,
  870
Neurotmesis, definition of, 566
Neutropenia, monitoring for, in cytotoxic
  drug treatment, 815–816, 816
  D-penicillamine and, 943
  sulfasalazine and, 743, 744
Neutrophil elastase, in extracellular matrix
  degradation, 324t, 324–325, 325t
Neutrophilic dermatosis, acute febrile
  (Sweet's syndrome), 1112
  vs. rheumatoid arthritis, 909
Neutrophils, 146–155
  activity of, eicosanoids and, 333–335
  adherence of, to vascular endothelium,
    149–150
  biochemistry of, 146t, 146–149, 149
  degranulation in, 151
  glucocorticoid effects on, 790, 790t
  in inflammatory response, colchicine
    and, 711–712
  in phagocytosis, 150–151, 151t
  interaction of, with platelets, 176–177,
    177
  maturation of, 146, 146t
  migration of, 150, 150t
  oxidative metabolism in, 152–155, 154t
  priming of, 152, 152t, 153
Newborn. See also Children; Infants.
  hypogammaglobulinemia in, transient,
    1285t, 1291

Newborn (Continued)
  lupus syndrome in, 1037, 1052, 1244,
    1244–1245
  pulmonary hypertension in, leukotrienes
    and, 297t
Nezelof's syndrome, 1286t, 1293–1294
  carrier detection in, 1300
  intrauterine diagnosis of, 1299
NF-kB, in inhibition of intracellular
  responses, to cytokines, 282
NF-kB/IkB system, in endothelial cell gene
  activation, 190–191, 191
Nicein, in extracellular matrix, 48
Nidogen, in extracellular matrix, 39, 40, 42,
  47, 48
Nifedipine, for Raynaud's phenomenon, in
  scleroderma, 1141, 1153
Nitric oxide, in antimicrobial function, of
  mononuclear phagocytes, 139
  in neutrophilic metabolism, 155
  in synovial vasculature, 13, 14
  in vasodilatation, in inflammatory re-
    sponse, 184–185
Nitrogen mustard, in immunosuppression,
  for non-neoplastic diseases, 810, 811,
  811t, 823t
Nociception. See Pain.
Nodular synovitis, localized, 1607–1608,
  1608–1610
Nodular tenosynovitis, localized,
  1608–1610, 1610, 1611
Nodular vasculitis, 503–504
Nodules, in rheumatic fever,
  subcutaneous, 1229, 1231
  in rheumatoid arthritis, pulmonary, 921
    rheumatoid, 917–918, 923
  of forearm, needle biopsy of, technique
    of, 604, 606
Nonsteroidal anti-inflammatory drugs. See
  also specific drugs, e.g., Ibuprofen.
  adverse effects of, 350–351
    cutaneous, 717
    gastrointestinal, 713–715
    hematologic, 717–718
    hepatic, 715–716
    hypersensitivity reactions in, 717
    on central nervous system, 718
    renal, 716–717
  binding of, to plasma proteins, 712
  classification of, 712, 712t
  clinical choice of, 735–736
  for ankylosing spondylitis, 736, 980
  for arthralgia, in Sjögren's syndrome,
    965
  for arthritis, of hip, 1726
  for gout, with acute arthritis, 1342–1343
  for juvenile rheumatoid arthritis, 1216–
    1217
  for osteoarthritis, 1397–1400
    of hip, 1852, 1852–1853
    of knee, 1856–1857, 1857
  for psoriatic arthritis, 1004
  for Reiter's syndrome, 736, 993, 994
  for rheumatic disease, 707–736
  for rheumatic fever, 1236
  for rheumatoid arthritis, 735–736, 939,
    1890–1891, 1891t, 1898t, 1898–1899
    in pregnancy and lactation, 1902t
  for systemic lupus erythematosus, 1040–
    1041
  history of, 707–708
  in eicosanoid pathway inhibition, 298
  in prevention of heterotopic ossification,
    after hip arthroplasty, 1733
  interactions of, with diseases, 720–721,
    721t

Nonsteroidal anti-inflammatory drugs
    (Continued)
  with methotrexate, 773–774
  with other drugs, 718–720, 719t–720t
  mechanisms of action of, 708–711, 709,
    710
  overdoses of, 718
  package inserts with, 722
  pharmacologic activities of, 712–713
  response to, individual variability in,
    722
  use of, by elderly, 721–722
  with long half-life, 722–728, 723t, 724–
    727
  with short half-life, 728–735, 729t, 730–
    734
NOR 90, antibodies to, in scleroderma,
  258t, 259
Nose, bleeding from, in rheumatic fever,
  1232
  in polychondritis, relapsing, 1405, 1405
NSAIDs. See Nonsteroidal anti-inflammatory
  drugs.
Nuclear factor kB (NF-kB), in inhibition of
  intracellular responses, to cytokines,
  282
Nuclear factor kB/IkB system, in
  endothelial cell gene activation,
  190–191, 191
Nucleic acids, increased turnover of, and
  hyperuricemia, 1337
Nucleoside triphosphate pyrophosphohydrolase, in calcium pyrophosphate
  deposition disease, 1359
Nucleosides, in purine metabolism,
  1323–1326, 1323–1326
Nucleosomes, antibodies in, in systemic
  lupus erythematosus, 255t, 256
Nucleotides, in purine metabolism,
  1323–1326, 1323–1326
Nucleus pulposus, degeneration of,
  imaging of, 667, 667
  development of, 5
Nutrient artery, of bone, 68
Nutrition, disorders of, and weakness, 389
  food allergy in, and arthritis, 531–532
  in gout, 1346
  in juvenile rheumatoid arthritis, 522,
    1217
  in osteoarthritis, 1394
  in rheumatic disease, 521–532
  in rheumatoid arthritis, 522, 939
  in systemic lupus erythematosus, 1019
  of articular cartilage, 9

Ober's test, in hip examination, 364
Obesity, gout with, 1318, 1346
  in osteoarthritis, 385, 1379, 1385
    management of, 1394, 1852
Obturator nerve, entrapment of, 581
  injury to, in surgery, 586
  reflex testing of, 406t
Occipital neuralgia, cervical spinal
  disorders and, 403
Occupational disorder(s), cervicobrachial
  syndrome as, 394
  osteoarthritis as, 1385–1386
  overuse syndromes as, 584–585, 585t
Occupational therapy, for juvenile
  rheumatoid arthritis, 1217
  in osteoarthritis, of hip, 1851, 1851t
Ochronosis, imaging in, 676
  synovial biopsy in, 622, 622, Plate 10

Ochronosis (Continued)
 synovial fluid analysis in, 612, 613, Plate 7
Octamer motif, in immunoglobulin promotion, 110–111
Odontoid process, of axis, anatomy of, 396, 396, 397
 calcification of, and pain, 409
 in juvenile rheumatoid arthritis, 1214, 1214
Olecranon bursa, inflammation of, examination for, 358
 glucocorticoids for, 597
 in sports medicine, 552–553
 septic, 1447
 tophi of, in gout, 1316, 1317
Olecranon process, fracture of, after elbow replacement, 1836, 1838
Oligoarthralgia, causes of, 1882, 1883
Oligoarthritis, in juvenile rheumatoid arthritis, course of, 1220, 1221t
 onset of, 1208t, 1209, 1210
Oligosaccharides, in extracellular matrix, 40, 41, 43
Omeprazole, interaction of, with nonsteroidal anti-inflammatory drugs, 720t
Onychodystrophy, in Reiter's syndrome, with human immunodeficiency virus infection, 1269, 1270
Onycholysis, in Graves' disease, 1504
O'nyong-nyong virus infection, and arthritis, 1478–1479
Open canalicular system, in platelets, 176, 177t
Optic nerve, disorders of, in giant cell arteritis, 1126, 1126, 1130
Oral tolerance, of antigens, 846
Orbit, myositis of, 1186
 pseudotumor of, 1166–1167
Orotic aciduria, allopurinol and, 830, 830–831
Orthoses, for ankle disorders, 1626, 1627, 1761
 for plantar fasciitis, 485, 486
 in rehabilitative medicine, 1624–1627, 1626, 1627
 after arthroplasty, 1637
Ortolani's sign, in hip examination, 364
Orudis (ketoprofen), 729t, 732, 732
 use of, in elderly, 722
Oruvail (ketoprofen), 729t, 732, 732
 use of, in elderly, 722
Osgood-Schlatter disease, and knee pain, 462
Ossicles, intra-articular, 1596–1597, 1597
 of ear, in rheumatoid arthritis, 911
Ossification, heterotopic, after hip arthroplasty, 1732–1733, 1733t
 para-articular, after hip arthroplasty, 1813–1816, 1817
Osteitis, in acne-pustulosis-hyperostosis-osteitis syndrome, vs. rheumatoid arthritis, 903
Osteitis fibrosa cystica, in hyperparathyroidism, 1502, 1503
Osteitis pubis, and pain, 475–476
Osteoarthritis, 1369–1401
 articular cartilage changes in, etiology of, 1376–1379
  mechanisms of, 1372, 1372–1375, 1373
 bacterial arthritis with, 1439, 1439t
 classification of, 1383, 1385t
 clinical features of, 1386
 complications of, 1388

Osteoarthritis (Continued)
 costovertebral, imaging of, 668
 course of, 1388
 diagnosis of, 385, 385, 1390–1392, 1391
 diclofenac for, 734
 endemic, 1390
 epidemiology of, 1383–1386
 erosive, antimalarial drugs for, 754
 etodolac for, 734
 familial, genetic mutation in, 1540–1541
 fenamates for, 733
 fenoprofen for, 732
 glucocorticoids for, 596
 imaging of, 663–665, 664–666, 1383, 1384, 1386–1388, 1387
 in acromegaly, 1507
 inflammatory, imaging of, 665–667, 666
 laboratory tests in, 1388
 management of, 1394–1401
  diet in, 1394
  drugs in, disease-modifying, 1399–1401, 1400t
   for symptomatic relief, 1397–1399
  joint loading in, 1394
  patient compliance in, 539
  physical therapy in, 1395–1397
  psychosocial support in, 1394–1395
  sexual function in, 1395
 monarticular, in young adults, 1387, 1389
 nonsteroidal anti-inflammatory drugs for, 736
 of ankle, 483, 484, 694
 of apophyseal joints, 668
 of elbow, 1679–1680, 1680, 1681
  surgery for, 1680t, 1680–1684, 1681–1684
   arthroplastic, 1684–1692
 of foot, 483, 483–484, 484, 665
 of hand, imaging of, 664, 664
  surgery for, 1671–1673, 1672
 of hip. See Hip.
 of knee. See Knee.
 of shoulder, and pain, 429, 429
  arthroscopic surgery in, 693, 693
  Milwaukee syndrome of, 1379
  preoperative evaluation of, 1699, 1699, 1700
 osteophytes in, 1375–1376, 1376
 pauciarticular, in middle age, 1389
 polyarticular, 1389, 1389
 psychosocial aspects of, 536, 1394–1395
 rapidly progressive, 1389, 1390
 synovectomy in, arthroscopic, 691–693, 691–695
 tolmetin for, 733
 unusual sites of, 1389
 vs. rheumatoid arthritis, 907t, 907–908
 with apatite deposition, 1363, 1364
 with calcium pyrophosphate deposition, 1354, 1355
 with chondrodysplasia, genetic defects in, 31, 32, 33
 with diabetes mellitus, 1500
Osteoarthropathy, hypertrophic, 1514–1519, 1515, 1517
 synovial biopsy in, 623
 vs. rheumatoid arthritis, 906
 neuropathic, of ankle, 485
  of foot, 485
Osteoblasts, in bone remodeling, 55–57, 56, 57t
 systemic regulation of, 60–62, 61
Osteocalcin, in bone matrix, 63
 in extracellular matrix, 42, 48–49

Osteocalcin (Continued)
 in osteoporosis, 1567
Osteochondritis dissecans, of knee, and pain, 465, 465, Plate 3
 magnetic resonance imaging of, 644, 644
Osteochondromatosis, synovial, 1600–1603, 1601–1603
 imaging of, 681, 681–682
Osteochondrosis, intervertebral, imaging of, 667, 667
Osteoclasts, in bone remodeling, 58, 58–60, 59
 systemic regulation of, 60–62, 61
Osteocytes, in bone remodeling, 57, 57–58
Osteodystrophy, Albright's, 1499, 1502–1503, 1503
Osteogenesis imperfecta, 1542–1546, 1543t, 1545
 genetic defect in, 29–30, 31t, 33t, 1540, 1540t
Osteoid, in bone remodeling, 56, 57, 57t
Osteolysis, after hip arthroplasty, 1733, 1812
 after knee arthroplasty, 1753
 in scleroderma, radiography of, 662, 663
 of forefoot, in diabetes, 1501, 1501
Osteomalacia, 1572t, 1572–1574, 1573, 1574t
 hypophosphatemia and, 1503, 1504
 with cancer, 1526, 1527t
Osteomyelitis, and carcinoma, squamous cell, 1529, 1531t
 computed tomography of, 630
 in sickle cell disease, 1495
 of spine, postsurgical, magnetic resonance imaging of, 637
 pyogenic, and low back pain, 451
 tuberculous, 1453
 with human immunodeficiency virus infection, 1267
Osteonecrosis, 1581–1590
 alcohol abuse and, 1584
 and knee pain, 465
 classification of, 1586, 1586t, 1587
 corticosteroids and, 1584
 dysbaric, 1584–1585
 etiology of, 1581, 1581t, 1583
 hemoglobinopathy and, 1585
 hypofibrinolysis and, 1585
 imaging of, 678, 678, 1585, 1586, 1587, 1588, 1588
 natural history of, 1586
 of shoulder, 429–430
  preoperative evaluation of, 1703, 1703–1704
 pathogenesis of, 1581, 1582, 1583
 post-traumatic, 1582, 1582–1583
 thrombosis and, 1585
 treatment of, 1586–1589, 1588
Osteonectin, in bone matrix, 62–63
 in extracellular matrix, 49–50
Osteons, in lamellar bone, 66, 67, 67
 mineralization of, 65, 65
Osteopenia, hydroxyapatite crystallization in, 63
 in juvenile chronic arthritis, 652, 652
 in sarcoidosis, 1421
Osteopetrosis, carbonic anhydrase deficiency and, 59–60
 osteoclast deficiency and, 58
Osteophytes, in ankylosing spondylitis, 656, 656
 in osteoarthritis, 1375–1376, 1376
 in spondylosis deformans, imaging of, 667–668, 668

Osteopontin, in extracellular matrix, *42*, 49
Osteoporosis, 1563–1572
  as contraindication to glucocorticoid
    injection, 599
  calcitonin for, 61, 1569, 1571
  clinical features of, 1563
  diagnosis of, 1565–1567, *1566*, 1567t
  epidemiology of, 1563
  estrogen in, 1509
  genetic defect in, 31, 31t, 33t, 1540
  glucocorticoids and, 794–795, 1564,
    1571t, 1571–1572
    in rheumatoid arthritis, 940
    in systemic lupus erythematosus,
      1050, 1050t
  in elderly, 544
  in hemochromatosis, imaging of, 675
  in ochronosis, 676
  in rheumatoid arthritis, 645
  methotrexate and, 781
  negative association of, with osteoarthri-
    tis, 1385
  of hip, in rheumatoid arthritis, 1724,
    1725
    transient, 473, *473*
  pathogenesis of, 1563–1565, 1565t
  treatment of, 1568t, 1568–1572, 1569t,
    1571t
  with diabetes, 1500
  with iron storage disorders, 1425
Osteotomy, of ankle, with debridement,
    1763, *1763*, *1765*
  of hip, for deformity, 1727
  of knee, in osteoarthritis, 1740–1741,
    1741
  of shoulder, 1706–1707
  of tibia, in arthritis, failure of,
    arthroplasty after, 1747, *1748*
  of trochanter, in arthroplasty, 1777, 1796–
    1797
Ouchterlony technique, in antinuclear
    antibody detection, 252–253, *253*, 253t
Ovaries, disorders of, and hip pain, 476
Overlap syndromes, imaging in, 663
  mixed connective tissue disease in,
    1067–1075. See also *Mixed connective
    tissue disease.*
  polymyositis in, 1066, *1067*
  scleroderma in, 1065t, 1065–1066, *1066*
Overuse injury, 584–585, 585t
  and carpal tunnel syndrome, 571
  and medial tibial stress syndrome, 558–
    559
  of rotator cuff, in sports medicine, 550–
    551, *551*
  vs. fibromyalgia syndrome, 514
Overweight, gout with, 1318, 1346
  in osteoarthritis, 385, 1379, 1385
  management of, 1394, 1852
Oxaprozin, 723t, 727, *727*
  use of, in elderly, 722
  in renal disorders, 721
Oxipurinol, in inhibition of urate
    synthesis, *829*, 829–833, *830*
Oxygen, consumption of, by neutrophils,
    152–155, 154t
  in free radicals. See *Free radicals.*
  metabolites of, in mononuclear phago-
    cyte function, 139

Pachydermoperiostosis, 1514, *1515*, 1518
Paget's disease of bone, 1574–1577, *1575*,
    1576t

Paget's disease of bone *(Continued)*
  and sarcoma, 1529, 1531t
  calcitonin for, 61, 1576
  imaging of, 678, *679*
Pain, abdominal, in rheumatic fever, 1232
    in systemic lupus erythematosus, 1036
  in ankle, 479–487. See also *Ankle.*
  in arthritis, as indication for surgery,
    1633
  in bone, vs. arthritis, monarticular, 371
  in chest, in ankylosing spondylitis, 974
  in elbow, in rheumatic disease, as indica-
    tion for surgery, 1680
  in fibromyalgia, 511–518. See also *Fibro-
    myalgia.*
  in foot, 479–487. See also *Foot (feet).*
  in hip, 466–476. See also *Hip.*
  in knee, 457–466. See also *Knee.*
  in leg, in pseudoradicular nerve entrap-
    ment syndromes, 582
  in neck, 394–411. See also *Neck.*
  in osteoarthritis, 1386
  in patient history, 353
  in rheumatic disease, psychosocial im-
    pact of, 536–537
  in rheumatoid arthritis, assessment of,
    926, 926t
    heat for, 938–939
  in shoulder, 413–435. See also *Shoulder.*
  in Sjögren's syndrome, 965
  in synovial joints, nerves in, 16
  muscular, vs. arthritis, monarticular, 373
  musculoskeletal, clinical syndromes in,
    1880–1886, 1881t–1884t
  neuropathic, vs. arthritis, monarticular,
    372
  nonsteroidal anti-inflammatory drugs
    for, 713
  polyarticular, arthritis and, classification
    of, 382t, 382–383
    diagnosis of, 383–385, *384*, *385*
      differential, *386*, 386t, 386–387
    history in, 381
    laboratory tests in, 382, 382t
    physical examination in, 381–382
    radiography in, 382
  postoperative, analgesia for, 1644–1645
    ketorolac for, 735
Palindromic rheumatism, antimalarial
    drugs for, 754
  in onset of rheumatoid arthritis, 377,
    901, 901t
Palm, fascial thickening in, in Dupuytren's
    contracture, 1165–1166
  fasciitis of, in reflex sympathetic dystro-
    phy, with cancer, 1525, 1527t
Palmar cutaneous nerve, entrapment of,
    573
Palmar stenosing tenosynovitis (trigger
    finger), glucocorticoid injection for,
    604
  in rheumatoid arthritis, surgery for,
    1650–1652
  physical examination for, 360
Pamidronate, for osteoporosis, 1571
  for Paget's disease of bone, 1576–1577
Pancreas, disease of, arthropathy with,
    imaging of, 660
    synovial biopsy in, 623
  in diabetes, amyloid deposits in, 1510
  inflammation of, glucocorticoids and,
    795
Panniculitis, in systemic lupus
    erythematosus, 1036
  paraneoplastic, 1525–1526, 1527t

Panniculitis *(Continued)*
  skin lesions in, 508t, 508–509
Pannus-cartilage junction, destruction of,
    in rheumatoid arthritis, 881–883, *882*,
    883
Pantopaque, in myelography, in low back
    pain, 444
Para-aminobenzoic acid, for
    photosensitivity, in systemic lupus
    erythematosus, 1041, 1042t
Paraffin, in heat therapy, *1623*, 1623–1624
Paralysis, rheumatoid arthritis with, 901
Parasitosis, rheumatoid factors in, 242,
    242t
Parathyroid glands, hyperfunction of,
    1502, *1503*
  with calcium pyrophosphate deposi-
    tion disease, 1355
  hypofunction of, 1502–1503, *1503*
Parathyroid hormone, in bone cell
    metabolism, 60
  in bone remodeling, 57, 59
  in osteoporosis, 1564, 1570–1571
Paresthesia, cervical spinal disorders and,
    402
Parker-Pearson needle, for synovial biopsy,
    618, *618*
Parkinson's disease, vs. rheumatoid
    arthritis, 908, *908*
Parotid glands, in diffuse infiltrative
    lymphocytosis, in human
    immunodeficiency virus infection,
    1274, *1274*, 1276
Parry-Romberg syndrome, 505
Parvovirus infection, and arthritis, 907,
    1477–1478
  and arthropathy, skin lesions with, 509
  in rheumatoid arthritis, 855t, 856
Pasteurella multocida infection, and arthritis,
    1442
Patella, anatomy of, 457, *458*
  in arthroplasty, 1744–1745, *1745*, 1750,
    1750
    complications in, 1752
    radiography of, 1826–1830, *1828*,
      1829
  physical examination of, 367, 457–458
  prosthetic, radiography of, 1822, *1822*
  radiography of, 459, *459*
  taping of, in osteoarthritis, 1396
Patellar tendon, disorders of, and pain,
    462–463
  inflammation of, in sports medicine, 558,
    559
  magnetic resonance imaging of, *643*,
    643–644
  rupture of, with hinge knee prosthesis,
    1832, *1832*
Patellofemoral arthritis, and pain, 463–464
Patellofemoral joint, abnormality of,
    examination for, 367
  replacement of, in total knee replace-
    ment, 1816–1818, *1819*
Patent ductus arteriosus, nonsteroidal anti-
    inflammatory drugs for, 713
Pathergy, in Behçet's disease, 1114t, 1115
Patrick test, 364, 442, 1725
PCNA (proliferating cell nuclear antigen),
    antibodies to, in systemic lupus
    erythematosus, 255t, 256
p80-coilin, antibodies to, in Sjögren's
    syndrome, 261, 261t
PDGF. See *Platelet-derived growth factor.*
Pelvis, bursitis in, glucocorticoid injection
    for, 597t, 597–598, 606

Pelvis (Continued)
  fracture of, after hip arthroplasty, 1813
  tilting of, examination for, 362–363
Pemphigus, D-penicillamine and, in
    rheumatoid arthritis, 943
D-Penicillamine, 765, 765–767, 766
  for rheumatoid arthritis, 942–943, 946,
    1891, 1892, 1892t, 1898t, 1901
    in pregnancy and lactation, 1902t
  juvenile, 1219
  vs. antimalarial drugs, 752t, 752–753
  for scleroderma, 1152
Penicillin, for Lyme disease, 1469, 1469t
  for Whipple's disease, 1011
  in prevention of rheumatic fever, 1236–
    1238, 1237t, 1238t
  metabolism of, probenecid and, 836
Penis, in Reiter's syndrome, 988, 989, 993
  Peyronie's disease of, 1166
Pentamidine, contraindication to, with
    methotrexate therapy, for rheumatoid
    arthritis, 944
Pepstatin, in cathepsin D inhibition, 323
Peptic ulcers, glucocorticoids and, 795
  nonsteroidal anti-inflammatory drugs
    and, 714–715
Periaortitis, retroperitoneal fibrosis with,
    1166
Periarteritis nodosa, imaging in, 663
Periarthritis, calcific, vs. rheumatoid
    arthritis, 905
Pericarditis, in rheumatoid arthritis, 921
  in systemic lupus erythematosus, 1034–
    1035
  with juvenile rheumatoid arthritis, 1211
Perichondrium, in bone development, 64
Perineurium, anatomy of, 564–565, 566
Periodic acid–Schiff staining, in synovial
    fluid analysis, 617
Periosteum, in bone development, 64
  in hypertrophic osteoarthropathy, 1516–
    1518, 1517
Periostitis, and polyarticular pain, 387
  in juvenile chronic arthritis, imaging of,
    652
Peripheral nerves. See Nerves, peripheral.
Peritoneum, bleeding in, after liver biopsy,
    1867, 1871t
Peritonitis, after liver biopsy, 1867, 1871t
  in systemic lupus erythematosus, 1036
Perlecan, in extracellular matrix, 40–42, 42,
    49
Peroneal nerve, entrapment of, 579
  injury to, in surgery, 586
  palsy of, after knee arthroplasty, 1752
Peroneal tendon, inflammation of, and
    pain, 486
Pes anserinus bursa, inflammation of, and
    pain, 465–466
  examination for, 366
Peyer's patches, in enteropathic arthritis,
    1006
Peyronie's disease, 1166
Phagocytes, deficiency of, testing for, in
    recurrent infection, 1283
  extravasation of, L-selectin in, 311
  mononuclear. See Mononuclear phago-
    cytes.
Phagocytosis, 138
  neutrophils in, 150–151, 151t
Phalanges, arrowhead, in acromegaly, 679,
    679
Phalen's maneuver, in carpal tunnel
    syndrome, 568, 569t
Phenylbutazone, 723t, 724, 724

Phenylbutazone (Continued)
  and blood disorders, 717
  for ankylosing spondylitis, 980
  for spondyloarthropathy, with human
    immunodeficiency virus infection,
    1272
  interactions of, with other drugs, 719t,
    720
  toxicity of, to liver, 715, 716
Phenytoin, interactions of, with
    nonsteroidal anti-inflammatory drugs,
    719t, 720
Phlebitis, after knee arthroplasty, 1751
  in antiphospholipid syndrome, 1058–
    1059
Phlebotomy, for iron storage diseases, 1428
Phorbol, in mononuclear phagocyte
    regulation, 136
Phosphacan, in extracellular matrix, 46
Phosphodiesterase, inhibition of, by
    nonsteroidal anti-inflammatory drugs,
    711
Phospholipase A$_2$, in eicosanoid synthesis,
    287, 288
  in neutrophil function, 149
Phospholipase C, in neutrophil function,
    148, 149
  in T cell activation, 117
Phospholipase D, in neutrophil function,
    149, 149
  in neutrophil metabolism, 153
Phospholipids, antibodies to. See Antiphos-
    pholipid syndrome.
Phosphoribosyl pyrophosphate, in gout,
    primary, 1331t, 1336, 1336
  in purine metabolism, 1325, 1325
Phosphorus, deficiency of, and myopathy,
    1194t
Photosensitivity, in dermatomyositis, 504,
    504, Plate 5
  in systemic lupus erythematosus, 1030t,
    1036
  management of, 1041, 1042t
Phototherapy, for Reiter's syndrome, 993
Physical therapy, for ankylosing
    spondylitis, 980
  for juvenile rheumatoid arthritis, 1217
  in osteoarthritis, 1395–1397
    of hip, 1851t, 1851–1852
    of knee, 1856, 1856t
Pigmentation, disorders of, in iron storage
    disorders, 1425
Pigmented villonodular synovitis. See
    Synovitis, pigmented villonodular.
Pilon fractures, of ankle, and arthrosis,
    1759
  arthrodesis after, 1762
Pinna, in relapsing polychondritis,
    1404–1405, 1405, 1407
  tophi of, in gout, 1316, 1317
Pinocytosis, fluid-phase, 138–139
Piriformis muscle, in sciatic nerve
    entrapment, 579
Piroxicam, 723t, 726, 726
  interaction of, with cimetidine, 720t
  use of, in elderly, 722
Pituitary gland, growth hormone secretion
    by, in acromegaly, 1506–1508
  in cortisol secretion, 787–788
    suppression of, exogenous glucocorti-
    coids and, 796
Plantar fasciitis, 485, 486
Plantar nerves, entrapment of, 580
Plasmapheresis, for scleroderma, 1152
  for systemic lupus erythematosus, 1053

Plasmapheresis (Continued)
  in antiphospholipid syndrome, 1062
  therapeutic, 817–818
Plasmin, in extracellular matrix
    degradation, 324t, 325t, 325–326
  regulation of, cellular, 334, 335t
    extracellular, 335, 338t
Plasminogen activators, in extracellular
    matrix degradation, 324t, 325t,
    325–326
  inhibitors of, 328, 329t
  regulation of, cellular, 334, 335t
    extracellular, 335, 338t
Platelet(s), in scleroderma, 179
  in systemic lupus erythematosus, 179–
    180
  interaction of, with complement, 179
    with neutrophils, 176–177, 177
  structure of, 176, 177t
  transforming growth factor-β release by,
    in inflammatory response, 177–178,
    178
Platelet factor-4, 176, 177
Platelet-activating factor, 178, 178–179
  in eicosanoid synthesis, 288
Platelet-derived growth factor, 176, 177
  and fibroblast development, in inflamma-
    tion, 273
  in fibroblast activation, 200–202
  in joint development, 2
  in rheumatoid arthritis, 868–869, 880
    and metalloproteinase synthesis, 876
  in scleroderma, 1139
Pleura, disease of, in systemic lupus
    erythematosus, 1035
  inflammation of, in rheumatoid arthritis,
    920
Plicae, synovial, of knee, and pain, 463,
    463
  examination for, 367
Plicamycin, for Paget's disease of bone,
    1577
PM-Scl, antibodies to, in inflammatory
    muscle diseases, 260t, 260–261
  in scleroderma, 258t, 259
Pneumatic compression stockings, in
    prevention of thrombosis, after hip
    arthroplasty, 1732
Pneumocystis carinii infection, pentamidine
    prophylaxis against, contraindication
    to, with methotrexate therapy, 944
Pneumonia, in rheumatic fever, 1232
Pneumonitis, methotrexate and, in
    rheumatoid arthritis, 1898t, 1900
Podagra, in gout, 377, 1315
POEMS syndrome, 1499, 1525
Poikiloderma, in dermatomyositis, 504
Polyarteritis, 1091–1097, 1092, 1093, 1095
  clinical features of, 1093, 1093–1094
  cutaneous, 1107
  diagnosis of, 1095, 1095
  epidemiology of, 1091–1092
  in children, 1242t, 1254, 1254t, 1254–1255
  in human immunodeficiency virus infec-
    tion, 1278
  laboratory tests in, 1094
  microscopic, 1097
    pathogenesis of, 1081–1082, 1084
  ocular disorders in, 493, 1094
  paraneoplastic, 1525, 1527t
  pathogenesis of, 1081, 1084
  pathology of, 1092, 1092
  prognosis of, 1095, 1095
  skin lesions in, 503
  synovial biopsy in, 621

Polyarteritis (Continued)
  treatment of, 1096–1097
Polyarthralgia, causes of, 1882, 1884
Polyarthritis, causes of, 1882, 1884
  classification of, 382t, 382–383
  in juvenile rheumatoid arthritis, course
      of, 1220, 1221t
    onset of, 1208t, 1209, 1209
  in leukemia, 1522
  in reflex sympathetic dystrophy, with
      cancer, 1525, 1527t
  inflammatory, with axial involvement,
      384–385
  laboratory tests in, 382, 382t
  noninflammatory. See Osteoarthritis.
  peripheral, causes of, 383
  with carcinoma, 1523t, 1523–1524
Polychondritis, paraneoplastic, 1526, 1527t
  relapsing, 1404–1407, 1405, 1405t, 1407
    and arthritis, pauciarticular, 384
    ocular disorders in, 493, 1405–1406
    skin lesions in, 499
Polycystic kidney disease, gout in, 1322
Polymethyl methacrylate. See Methyl
    methacrylate.
Polymorphonuclear leukocytes,
    development of, cytokines in, 272
  in bacterial arthritis, 1435
  in rheumatoid arthritis, 880, 884, 885
  in synovial fluid analysis, 610t, 615, 616
Polymyalgia rheumatica, clinical features
    of, 1127
  definition of, 1123
  diagnosis of, 1129
  epidemiology of, 1123
  etiology of, 1123–1124
  giant cell arteritis with, 1127–1128
  inflammation in, laboratory evaluation
      of, 703–704
  laboratory studies in, 1128
  pain in, 386
  paraneoplastic, 1525, 1527t
  pathogenesis of, 1124
  pathology of, 1125
  treatment of, 1130
  vs. rheumatoid arthritis, 908
Polymyositis, antinuclear antibodies in,
    259–261, 260t
  clinical features of, 1179–1180
  creatine kinase in, 1180–1181
  diagnosis of, criteria for, 1177–1178,
      1178t, 1179t
    differential, 1189–1194
  glucocorticoids for, 798–800
  imaging of, 662
  in human immunodeficiency virus infec-
      tion, 1277
  in overlap syndromes, 1066, 1067
    in mixed connective tissue disease,
        1067–1075. See also Mixed connec-
        tive tissue disease.
  methotrexate for, 778
  pathology of, 1180, 1181, 1181
  D-penicillamine and, 943
  skin lesions in, 504–506
  treatment of, 1200–1201
  vs. rheumatoid arthritis, 904
Polyneuropathy, familial amyloidotic, 1410,
    1410t, 1414, 1414–1415
Polyserositis, colchicine for, 728
Poncet's disease, 1012–1013, 1455
Popeye sign, of bicipital rupture, 428
Popliteal cyst (Baker's cyst), 366, 466, 1593
  imaging of, 644, 645
  in osteoarthritis, 1388

Popliteal cyst (Baker's cyst) (Continued)
  in rheumatoid arthritis, 914t, 914–915
  ultrasonography of, 460, 460
Postcalcaneal bursa, inflammation of, 486
Postenteric reactive arthritis, 1008–1010,
    1009t, 1010
Posterior drawer test, in knee examination,
    557
Posterior interosseous nerve syndrome,
    575, 576
Posterior primary ramus, anatomy of, 440,
    440
Posterior tarsal tunnel syndrome, 579–580,
    580
Posture, in ankylosing spondylitis, in
    physical examination, 976
Posturography, dynamic, 408
Potassium, metabolism of, disorders of,
    and myopathy, 1194t
Prazosin, interactions of, with nonsteroidal
    anti-inflammatory drugs, 719t
Prednisone/prednisolone. See also
    Glucocorticoids.
  and Cushing's syndrome, 1506
  and delayed wound healing, after foot
      surgery, 1770–1771
  and hypothalamic-pituitary-adrenal sup-
      pression, 796
  and immunosuppression, 794
  and osteonecrosis, 1584
  for amyloidosis, 1412, 1415t
  for calcium pyrophosphate deposition
      disease, 1362
  for Churg-Strauss syndrome, 1099
  for dermatomyositis, in children, 1247–
      1248
  for eosinophilic fasciitis, 1157
  for giant cell arteritis, 1129–1130
  for gout, with acute arthritis, 1343
  for Henoch-Schönlein purpura, 1259
  for inflammatory muscle disease, 1200,
      1201
  for juvenile rheumatoid arthritis, 1219
  for mixed connective tissue disease,
      1074, 1074t
  for osteoarthritis, 1399–1400
  for polyarteritis, 1096, 1097
    in children, 1254
  for polychondritis, relapsing, 1407
  for polymyalgia rheumatica, 1130
  for rheumatic fever, 1236
  for rheumatoid arthritis, 797, 798, 939–
      940, 1893, 1893t
    in combination therapy, 946
    in elderly, 544
    in pregnancy and lactation, 1902t
    with gold salts, 942
    with methotrexate, 943–944
  for scleroderma, 1152
  for systemic lupus erythematosus, 1045,
      1046, 1047t
    in children, 1243
    in pregnancy, 1051, 1052t
    with central nervous system disease,
        1053
    with thrombocytopenia, 1052
  for Takayasu's arteritis, 1089–1090
  for vasculitis, cutaneous, 1104
    with rheumatoid arthritis, 1111
  in diffuse infiltrative lymphocytosis, in
      human immunodeficiency virus in-
      fection, 1276, 1277
  interaction of, with methotrexate, 774
  intra-articular injection of, 591–592, 594,
      594t

Prednisone/prednisolone (Continued)
  pharmacokinetics of, 788t, 791–793, 792,
      793
  potency of, 788t
  structure of, 787, 788
  with chlorambucil, for Behçet's disease,
      1116
  with cyclophosphamide, for Wegener's
      granulomatosis, 809
Pregnancy, antimalarial drugs in, 756
  glucocorticoid use in, 793
  hormonal changes in, 1508
  hyperuricemia in, 1320
  in antiphospholipid syndrome, 1061–
      1063
  in Ehlers-Danlos syndrome, 1550
  in mixed connective tissue disease, 1073
  in rheumatoid arthritis, drug treatment
      in, 1902t, 1903
  in scleroderma, 1150
  in systemic lupus erythematosus, 1037,
      1051–1052, 1052t
  in women with silicone breast implants,
      1173–1174
  intrauterine diagnosis in, of immunodefi-
      ciency, 1299–1300
  Lyme disease in, 1466
  methotrexate contraindicated in, 780
  D-penicillamine contraindicated in, 766
  rheumatoid arthritis in, 854
  sulfasalazine use in, 743–744
Prepatellar bursa, inflammation of, and
    pain, 462
    examination for, 366–367
    glucocorticoid injection for, 597, 605–
        606
    septic, 1447
Presacral fat pads, herniation of, 598
Pressure, changes in, and osteonecrosis,
    1584–1585
Primary biliary cirrhosis, 1165
  arthropathy with, imaging of, 660
  in scleroderma, 1147
  in Sjögren's syndrome, 960–961
Pritchard elbow prosthesis, 1686, 1686,
    1688
Probenecid, for hyperuricemia, 833–837,
    834, 836t, 1344, 1345
  interaction of, with ketoprofen, 732
    with methotrexate, 774
    with naproxen, 725
    with nonsteroidal anti-inflammatory
        drugs, 719t, 720
Procaine, intra-articular injection of, with
    glucocorticoids, 594–595, 599
Procainamide, and lupus erythematosus,
    1037
Procollagens, genes for, mutations of, and
    disease, 29–31, 30, 31t, 32, 33, 33t
  structure of, 26
  in collagen synthesis, 26–28, 27, 29, 30
Progestins, and arthritis, vs. rheumatoid
    arthritis, 904
Proliferating cell nuclear antigen,
    antibodies to, in systemic lupus
    erythematosus, 255t, 256
Proline, in collagen fibrils, 24, 25
  in collagen synthesis, 26
Promatrixin, activation of, 335, 336
Pronator teres syndrome, 572
Properdin, in complement activation, 233t,
    234
Prostacyclin, in vasodilatation, in inflam-
    matory response, 184
  synthesis of, 289, 290t, 290–291

Prostacyclin (Continued)
  inhibition of, nonsteroidal anti-inflam-
    matory drugs in, 708, 709
Prostaglandin(s), anti-inflammatory effects
    of, 710
  in inflammation, 296
  in synovial fluid, in rheumatoid arthri-
    tis, 886
  receptors of, 294–295
  synthesis of, 288–291, 289, 289t, 290t
    fatty acids in, 527, 527–529, 528
    inhibition of, glucocorticoids and, 790
      nonsteroidal anti-inflammatory
        drugs in, 708–711, 709
    and renal dysfunction, 716–717
Prostaglandin D₂, in mast cell mediation,
    169–170
Prostaglandin E, in mononuclear
    phagocyte regulation, 136
Prostaglandin E₂, in bone cell metabolism,
    61
  in inhibition of repair mechanisms, in in-
    flammation, 278
Prostaglandin I₂ (prostacyclin), in
    vasodilatation, in inflammatory
    response, 184
  synthesis of, 289, 290t, 290–291
    inhibition of, nonsteroidal anti-in-
      flammatory drugs in, 708, 709
Prosthetic joints. See also Arthroplasty and
    specific joints, e.g., Hip.
  and cancer, 1530–1532
  bacterial infection of, 1439–1440, 1440,
    1440t, 1441t
  radiography of, 1437–1438
Proteases, in neutrophils, 147
  neutral, in mast cell mediation, 166–167,
    167t
Protein, dietary deficiency of, in
    inflammatory response, 521
  metabolism of, disorders of, glucocorti-
    coids and, 796
Protein 150,95, in monocyte adhesion, to
    endothelial cells, 129
Protein kinase C, activators of, in joint
    development, 2
  in neutrophil function, 148, 149
Proteinase(s), in extracellular matrix
    degradation, 323–327, 324t–327t, 328
  enzymic mechanisms of, 330–331, 331,
    332
  inhibitors of, endogenous, 327–330,
    329t
  regulation of, cellular, 331–334, 332t–
    335t
    extracellular, 335–338, 336, 337, 338t
Proteinase 3, in extracellular matrix
    degradation, 324, 324t
  in neutrophils, 147
Proteinase nexin–1, 329, 329t
Proteinuria, gold salts and, 942
  D-penicillamine and, 943
Proteoglycans, 304, 312–314
  degradation of, by proteinases, 331, 332
  in articular cartilage, 7, 1369–1371
    in aging, 10
    in load carriage, 10
    in osteoarthritis, 1372–1375
    in resistance to compression, 91
  in bone matrix, 62
  in extracellular matrix, 37–51. See also
    Extracellular matrix.
  in mast cell mediation, 167–169, 168
  in synovial fluid analysis, 617
Protrusio acetabuli, in rheumatoid
    arthritis, 1724, 1725

Prussian blue staining, in synovial fluid
    analysis, 617
P-selectin, 304, 311
  in leukocyte-endothelial adhesion, in in-
    flammatory response, 186t, 187t,
    187–190
  monoclonal antibodies to, in anti-in-
    flammatory treatment, 317
Pseudoangina pectoris, cervical spinal
    disorders and, 403
Pseudocystic rheumatoid arthritis, imaging
    of, 646, 647
Pseudofractures, in osteomalacia, 1573,
    1573
Pseudogout. See Calcium pyrophosphate
    deposition disease.
Pseudohypoparathyroidism, 1499, 1502
  in children, 1260
Pseudolymphoma, in Sjögren's syndrome,
    962, 962
Pseudoradicular nerve entrapment
    syndromes, 582
Pseudotumor, orbital, 1166–1167
Pseudotumor cerebri, glucocorticoids and,
    796
Pseudoxanthoma elasticum, 1554
  genetic defect in, 34
Psoralen, with ultraviolet light, for Reiter's
    syndrome, 993
Psoriasis, leukotrienes in, 297t
  pustular, with human immunodeficiency
    virus infection, 1268–1272, 1269,
    1270, 1272
Psoriatic arthritis, 999–1004
  antimalarial drugs for, 753, 756
  arthroplasty in, evaluation for, 1636
  clinical features of, 1000–1002, 1000–
    1002, 1002t
  course of, 1003–1004
  diagnosis of, 1003
  digit shortening in, 361
  epidemiology of, 999
  imaging of, 657–659, 657–659, 1003, 1003
  juvenile-onset, imaging of, 653
  laboratory tests in, 1002–1003
  methotrexate for, 778
  nonsteroidal anti-inflammatory drugs
    for, 736
  ocular disorders in, 494, 1002
  of foot, 486, 658, 658
  of hand, 1000–1002
    surgery for, 1667–1669, 1668
  of wrist, surgery for, 1669
  pathogenesis of, 999–1000
  pauciarticular, 383, 384
  polyarticular, 383, 385
  skin lesions with, 498, 498–499, 499
  synovial biopsy in, 620
  treatment of, 1004
  vs. Reiter's syndrome, 992, 992t
  vs. rheumatoid arthritis, 903
Psychologic disorders, and polyarticular
    pain, 387
  and weakness, 392
  evaluation for, in low back pain, 443
  glucocorticoids and, 796
  in fibromyalgia syndrome, 512, 514, 514,
    516, 517
Psychologic support, in osteoarthritis,
    1394–1395
Psychosocial management, of rheumatic
    disease, 534–539
Pteroylglutamic acid (folic acid), structure
    of, 771, 772
  with methotrexate therapy, 771, 772, 779,
    783, 1900–1901

Pubic symphysis, inflammation of, and
    pain, 475–476
Pudendal nerve, entrapment of, 582
  reflex testing of, 405, 406t
Pulmonary. See also Lung(s).
Pulmonary arteries, in scleroderma,
    1147–1148, 1148
Pulmonary disease, chronic obstructive,
    leukotrienes in, 297t
Pulmonary embolism, after hip
    arthroplasty, 1728, 1732
  in antiphospholipid syndrome, 1061
Pulmonary hypertension. See Hypertension,
    pulmonary.
Pulseless disease (Takayasu's arteritis),
    1088–1090, 1090
  in children, 1260
  pathogenesis of, 1084, 1084
Purine nucleoside phosphorylase
    deficiency, in Nezelof's syndrome,
    1293–1294
  carrier detection in, 1300
  intrauterine diagnosis of, 1299
Purines, analogs of, in immuno-
    suppression, for non-neoplastic
    diseases, 810, 811t, 813–814, 814t, 823t
  in gout, dietary restriction of, 1346
  metabolism of, 1323–1326, 1323–1326
    inhibition of, in treatment of gout,
      829–831, 829–833, 832t
  synthesis of, methotrexate inhibition of,
    771, 772
Purpura, Henoch-Schönlein, 503, 1105,
    1105–1106
  in children, 1242t, 1258, 1258–1259
  in human immunodeficiency virus in-
    fection, 1278
  Waldenström's hypergammaglobuli-
    nemic, 1108
Pustulosis, in acne-pustulosis-hyperostosis-
    osteitis syndrome, vs. rheumatoid
    arthritis, 903
PUVA (psoralen plus ultraviolet A)
    therapy, for Reiter's syndrome, 993
Pyoderma gangrenosum, with
    inflammatory bowel disease, 1007,
    1007, 1008, 1008t
Pyomyositis, with human
    immunodeficiency virus infection,
    1267
Pyrazinamide, and uric acid excretion,
    1328–1329
  for tuberculosis, 1454
Pyridinoline, in osteoporosis, 1567
Pyrimidine, synthesis of, allopurinol
    inhibition of, 830, 830–831
Pyrophosphate, analogs of, for
    osteoporosis, 1569t, 1569–1570
  in calcium pyrophosphate deposition dis-
    ease. See also Calcium pyrophosphate
    deposition disease.
Pyrophosphate arthropathy, in calcium
    pyrophosphate deposition disease,
    1352–1362

Quadriceps muscle, active drawer test of,
    in sports medicine, 557
  motion of, control of, 92, 92
  reflex testing of, 405, 406t
  strengthening of, exercises for, in rehabil-
    itation, 1622
  wasting of, with knee swelling, 16
Quadrilateral space syndrome, 578

Quadrilateral space syndrome (Continued)
and shoulder pain, 433, 433–434
Quervain's tenosynovitis, glucocorticoid
injection for, 604
in rheumatoid arthritis, 914
physical examination for, 360
Quinacrine, for lupus erythematosus, 749,
750
with dermatitis, 1042–1043, 1043t
guidelines for use of, 756
mechanisms of action of, 748t, 748–749
structure of, 747, 748

Radial artery, cannulation of, in surgery,
1644
Radial nerve, disorders of, muscle testing
for, 399t
entrapment of, 575–576, 576
reflex testing of, 405, 406t
Radiation therapy, for ankylosing
spondylitis, 980–981
for rheumatic disease, and cancer, 1530
for rheumatoid arthritis, 860, 947
in immunosuppression, 818–819
in prevention of heterotopic ossification,
after hip arthroplasty, 1733
in thyroid ablation, and hypothyroidism,
1505
Radicals, free. See Free radicals.
Radiculopathy. See Spinal nerves.
Radiography. See also specific methods,
e.g., Computed tomography, and sites,
e.g., Spine.
plain, techniques of, 626–627, 627t
Radioimmunoassay, for antinuclear
antibodies, 253–255, 254
for rheumatoid factors, 241, 242
Radionuclide imaging, after intra-articular
glucocorticoid injection, 591–592
in arthritis, monarticular, 379
in hypertrophic osteoarthropathy, 1517,
1517–1518
in low back pain, 444
in osteoarthritis, 1387
of cervical spinal disorders, 408
of hip, 468
after arthroplasty, 1810, 1810–1812,
1811t, 1812t, 1813
fractures in, 471, 471, 472, 472
in evaluation of pain, 1726
of knee, 459, 459–460
after arthroplasty, 1824–1826, 1827
Radioulnar joint, distal, in rheumatoid
arthritis, 1655
Radius, head of, replacement of, with
synovectomy, 1681–1682, 1683
Raji cell assay, for immune complexes, 230,
230t, 231, 231t
Raloxifene, for osteoporosis, 1569
Ranawat triangle, in radiography, after hip
arthroplasty, 1785, 1787
RANTES (regulated activation, normal T
cell expressed and secreted), in
monocyte adhesion, to endothelial
cells, 130
in rheumatoid arthritis, 868
Rapamycin, in immunosuppression, 821
Rapid eye movement sleep, in
fibromyalgia syndrome, 516
Ras protein, in T cell activation, 117
Rash, allopurinol and, 833
in dermatomyositis, in children, 1245–
1246, 1246

Rash (Continued)
in juvenile rheumatoid arthritis, 1209–
1211, 1211, 1215
in rheumatic fever, 1231
in systemic lupus erythematosus, 347,
348, 1030t, 1036
in newborn, 1244, 1244
Ras-Raf kinase–mitogen activated
pathway, in neutrophil function,
148–149, 149
Raynaud's phenomenon, in mixed
connective tissue disease, 1068, 1069,
1069, 1074, 1074t
in scleroderma, 505–506, 506, 1139–1142,
1140, 1141t, 1142t
in children, 1250, 1252
in initial presentation, 1134–1135
soft tissue resorption with, imaging
of, 661, 661–662
treatment of, 1153, 1669–1670, 1670
in systemic lupus erythematosus, 1035,
1111, 1112
with polymyositis, 1066, 1067
Reactive arthritis, postenteritic, 1008–1010,
1009t, 1010
vs. rheumatoid arthritis, 903
Reactive salpingitis, in Reiter's syndrome,
988
Reconversion, marrow depletion and,
magnetic resonance imaging of,
638–639
Rectus abdominis syndrome, 582
Reflex sympathetic dystrophy, and
shoulder pain, 434–435
with cancer, 1525, 1527t
with cervical spinal disorders, 407
Reflex testing, in neck pain, 405–407, 406t
Rehabilitation, in rheumatic disease,
1619–1630
after elbow surgery, 1692, 1692–1694,
1693
assessment for, 1619–1621
assistive devices in, 1627, 1628
cold in, 1623, 1624, 1624t
electrotherapy in, 1624
environmental modifications for, 1630
exercise in, 1621–1623, 1622
heat in, 1623, 1623–1624, 1624t
independent evaluations in, 1620–1621
mobility devices in, 1628–1630, 1629
orthotics in, 1624–1627, 1626, 1627
patient education in, 1630
rest in, 1621
Reiter's syndrome, 983–995
arthritis in, pauciarticular, 383
polyarticular, 384
clinical features of, 986–990, 987–989,
Plate 11
diagnosis of, 983, 984t
differential, 991–993, 992t
epidemiology of, 986
HLA-B27 antigen in, 217, 217t, 983–986,
1270
imaging of, 659, 659–660, 987, 987, 988,
991
laboratory evaluation of, 990–991
methotrexate for, 778
nonsteroidal anti-inflammatory drugs
for, 736, 993, 994
ocular disorders in, 494, 989–990, 993–
994
of ankle, 486, 660, 1269
of foot, 486, 987, 987–988, 988
pathogenesis of, 983–986
prognosis of, 993

Reiter's syndrome (Continued)
skin lesions in, 497–498, 498, 988–989,
989, 993, Plate 4
synovial biopsy in, 621
synovial fluid analysis in, 616, 616
treatment of, 993–995, 995t
vs. Lyme disease, 1468
vs. rheumatoid arthritis, 903
with human immunodeficiency virus infection, 990, 1268–1272, 1269, 1270,
1272
Relafen, 723t, 726–727, 727
Relapsing polychondritis, 1404–1407, 1405,
1405t, 1407
and arthritis, pauciarticular, 384
ocular disorders in, 493, 1405–1406
skin lesions in, 499
Relocation test, in shoulder examination,
in sports medicine, 548
Renal. See also Kidney(s).
Renal artery, in scleroderma, 1149, 1149
Renal dialysis, amyloid fibril deposition
with, 1410, 1415
shoulder pain with, 435
Repetitive strain disorders, 584–585, 585t
and carpal tunnel syndrome, 571
and medial tibial stress syndrome, 558–
559
of rotator cuff, in sports medicine, 550–
551, 551
vs. fibromyalgia syndrome, 514
Resection arthroplasty, of shoulder, 1707
Respiration, disorders of, cervical spinal
disorders and, 403
in rheumatoid arthritis, of cricoarytenoid joints, 911
Respiratory distress, acute, gold therapy
and, 764
Respiratory distress syndrome, adult,
leukotrienes in, 297t
Respiratory tract. See also Lung(s).
disorders of, in giant cell arteritis, 1127
in polychondritis, relapsing, 1406,
1407
in Sjögren's syndrome, 960, 961t
in Wegener's granulomatosis, 1100,
1100–1101
management of, in anesthesia, 1640–
1641, 1641t, 1642
Rest, immobilization in, and bone
remodeling, 71
in rheumatic disease, in rehabilitation,
1621
in rheumatoid arthritis, 934–938
of hand, 1647
of wrist, 1647
Reticular dysgenesis, with severe
combined immunodeficiency, 1295
Reticulohistiocytosis, multicentric,
1430–1433, 1431, 1432
paraneoplastic, 1524
synovial biopsy in, 623
vs. rheumatoid arthritis, 907
Retina, disorders of, in pseudoxanthoma
elasticum, 1554
in systemic lupus erythematosus,
1036–1037
inflammation of, 490
ischemia of, in Behçet's disease, 494, 494,
Plate 4
toxicity to, antimalarial agents and, 747,
755, 755t, 756
hydroxychloroquine and, 1898t, 1899–
1900
Retinoic acid, in joint development, 2

Retrocalcaneal bursa, inflammation of, and
	pain, 486
	glucocorticoid injection for, 598, 606
Retroperitoneal fibrosis, 1166
Retroviral infection, in rheumatoid
	arthritis, 856–857
	in Sjögren's syndrome, 965
Reye's syndrome, aspirin and, in juvenile
	rheumatoid arthritis, 1217
Rhabdomyolysis, 1194, 1194t
RHAMM (receptor for hyaluronan-
	mediated motility), in extracellular
	matrix, 46
Rheumatic disease. See also specific
	disorders, e.g., *Lyme disease.*
	evaluation of, adverse drug effects in,
		350–351
		and prognosis, 348–350
		clinical disagreement in, 344–345
		diagnostic procedures in, 345–348,
			346t, *347, 348*
		history in, 343–344
		physical examination in, 343–344
	genetics in, 209–225. See also *Genetics.*
	mast cells in, *163,* 163–164
	nutrition in, 521–532. See also *Nutrition.*
	psychosocial aspects of, 534–539
	rehabilitation in, 1619–1630. See also *Re-
		habilitation.*
	skin lesions in, 497–509
	therapy for, and prognosis, 349–350
	tryptase in, 167
Rheumatic fever, 1225–1238
	arthritis in, monarticular, 378
		pauciarticular, in adults, 383
		vs. Reiter's syndrome, 992
	clinical features of, 1230–1232
	diagnosis of, 1233–1234, 1234t
	epidemiology of, 1227–1229, *1228*
	etiology of, 1225
	laboratory findings in, 1232–1233
	management of, 1235–1236
	pathogenesis of, 1225–1227
	pathology of, 1229–1230, *1230*
	prevention of, 1236–1238, 1237t, 1238t
	prognosis of, 1234–1235, *1235*
	recurrences of, 1235
	skin lesions in, 506–507
	vs. rheumatoid arthritis, 908–909
Rheumatoid arthritis, 851–966
	adhesion molecules in, 873t, 873–874,
		874
	and low back pain, 450
	and osteoporosis, 1565
	angiogenesis in, 274, 869, 872, 872–873
	antimalarial drugs for, 750–753, 751t,
		752t, 941, 946, 947
	arthroplasty in, evaluation for, 1636–
		1637
	assessment of, *924,* 924–926, 925t, 926t
	azathioprine for, 944, 946, 1898t, 1901,
		1902t
	B cells in, 875
	bacterial infection with, 855, 855t, 856,
		1438, 1439t
	biologic agents for, 839, *840,* 840t
		in antigen-specific therapy, 840t, *845,*
			845–847
		targets of, cytokines as, 839, 840t, *843,*
			843–845
			inflammatory cells as, 839–840, 840t
			lymphocyte interactions as, 840t,
				842–843
			T cell surface antigens as, 840t, 840–
				842

Rheumatoid arthritis (*Continued*)
	blood abnormalities with, 919
	bone in, 916
	bucillamine for, 767
	cancer with, 918, 923, 1528–1529, 1531t
	chlorambucil for, 944–945, 1899t, 1902t,
		1903
	classification of, 898, 899t
	course of, 902, 909–917, *912, 913,* 913t,
		914t, *915, 917*
	cyclophosphamide for, 944–946, 1899t,
		1902t, 1903
	cyclosporine for, 860, 945–947, 1899t,
		1902t, 1903
	cytokines in, and cell migration, 269,
		270t
	cytotoxic drugs for, 944–946
	diagnosis of, 898, 902
		differential, 903–909, 907t, *908*
	diclofenac for, 734
	epidemiology of, 898–899
	evaluation of, 1889–1890, 1890t
	fatty acid supplementation in, 530
	fenamates for, 733
	fenoprofen for, 732
	fistulas in, 918
	gender in, 854
	general health maintenance in, 1895
	genetics in, 209, 852–854, 853t
	glucocorticoids for, 797–800, *939,* 939–
		940, 1893, 1893t, 1899t, 1901–1903,
		1902t
		in elderly, 544
		in pregnancy and lactation, 1902t
		intra-articular injection of, 595–596
			of hand, 1648
			of wrist, 1648
			with gold, 762
	gold for. See *Gold.*
	gout with, 1320
	hearing loss in, 911
	heart disease in, 921–922
	heat shock proteins in, 857
	human leukocyte antigens in, 218t, 218–
		219, 852–854, 853t, 859–862
	hydroxychloroquine for, 750–753, 751t,
		752t, 940, 941, 946, 947, 1891–1893,
		1892t, 1898t, 1899–1900, 1902t
	imaging of, 644–651, *646, 647,* 648t, *649–
		651*
	immune complex assays in, 231, 231t,
		232t
	immunosuppressive drugs for, 945–947
	in agammaglobulinemia, 1287
	in Felty's syndrome, 951–954
	infection in, 918
	inflammation in, laboratory evaluation
		of, 703
	interleukin-1 receptor antagonist in, 282
	juvenile, 1207–1222. See also *Juvenile
		rheumatoid arthritis.*
	juvenile-onset adult-type, imaging of,
		652
	kidney disease in, 920
	leukotrienes in, 297t, 298
	lung disease in, 920–921, *922*
	lymph node irradiation for, 818–819
	manubriosternal joint in, 911
	metalloproteinases in, 876t, 876–878, *877,*
		878t, 881, 883
	methotrexate for, 753, 774t, 774–778,
		775–777, 943–944, 946–947, 1891–
		1893, 1892t, 1898t, 1900–1901, 1902t
		dosage in, 779
		patient selection for, 782–783

Rheumatoid arthritis (*Continued*)
	toxicity of, 779–782, *780,* 781t
		to liver, 1860–1869. See also *Liver,
			methotrexate toxicity to.*
	monitoring of, 1894, 1894t
	morning stiffness in, in diagnosis, 346,
		347
	muscle in, 916
	nabumetone for, 727
	naproxen for, 724–725
	nonsteroidal anti-inflammatory drugs
		for, 735–736, 939, 1890–1891, 1891t,
		1898t, 1898–1899, 1902t
	nutrition in, 522, 939
	ocular disorders in, 492, 916–917, *917*
	of ankle, 481–483, 649–650, *915,* 915–916,
		1760
	of cricoarytenoid joints, 911
	of elbow, 912
		presentation of, 1677–1679, *1678, 1679,*
			1679t
		surgery for, 1680t, 1680–1684, *1681–
			1684*
		prosthetic joint replacement in,
			1684–1692
	of foot, 481–483, *482, 915,* 915–916
	of hand. See *Hand(s), in rheumatoid arthri-
		tis.*
	of hip, 914, 1724, *1725*
		arthroplasty for. See *Hip, arthroplasty
			of.*
	of knee, 648t, 650, 914t, 914–915
		hemiarthroplasty for, 1739
		pathology of, 1741–1743, *1742*
		synovectomy for, 1739, *1740*
	of shoulder, 911–912
		preoperative evaluation of, 1699–1702,
			1701
	of spine, cervical, 1713–1718, *1714–1716*
		course of, 909–911
	of temporomandibular joint, 911
	of wrist, 912–913
		nonsurgical management of, 1647–
			1648
		surgery for, in flexor tenosynovitis,
			1650, *1651*
			reconstructive, 1653–1655
			synovectomy in, 1652
	onset of, patterns of, 899t, 899–902, 901t
	D-penicillamine for, 765–767, 942–943,
		946, 1891, 1892, 1892t, 1898t, 1901,
		1902t
	polyarticular, peripheral, 383
	prognosis in, 922–924, 923t
	refractory, 1894
	remissions in, criteria for, 923, 923t
	rheumatoid factors in, *241,* 241–247,
		242t, 246t, 858, 875, 923
	rheumatoid nodules in, 917–918
	sex hormones in, 1509
	skin lesions in, 497, 916
	sternoclavicular joint in, 911
	sulfasalazine for, 742, 777, 941, 946, 947,
		1891–1893, 1892t, 1898t, 1900, 1902t
	surgery for, 1893–1894
		anesthesia in, regional, 1643
	synovectomy in, arthroscopic, 687–688,
		689
		radiation in, 947
	synovial biopsy in, 620, *620,* Plate 9
	synovial fluid in, 883–888, *885*
	synovial pathology in, 878–883, *882, 883,*
		924
	T cells in, 858–863, *859,* 861t
	tenidap for, 728

Rheumatoid arthritis (*Continued*)
  tetracyclines for, 947
  tissue specificity of, 851
  tolmetin for, 733
  total lymphoid irradiation for, 947
  treatment of, 933–948, 1888–1895
    combination therapy in, 946–947
    diet in, 939
    drugs in, 1890–1893, 1891t–1893t
      in lactation, 1902t, 1903
      in pregnancy, 1902t, 1903
      monitoring of, 1897–1903, 1898t, 1899t, 1902t
    exercise in, 934–938
    goals of, 1888–1889, *1889*
    heat in, 938–939
    in elderly, 544
    patient education in, 934, 938
    physicians' responsibility in, 1894–1895
    principles of, 933, *934*
    rest in, 934–938
    staging and, 934, 935t–937t
  vasculitis in, 919–920, 1110–1111, *1111*
  viral infection and, 854–857, 855t
  vs. collagen-induced arthritis, 857–858
  vs. Reiter's syndrome, 992, 992t
Rheumatoid factors, 241–247
  blood testing for, 1884–1885
  detection of, 241–242, 242t
  etiology of, 243–244
  genetic basis of, 244–245
  immunochemical properties of, 243
  immunoglobulin G reacting with, *241*, 241–246, 242t
  in juvenile rheumatoid arthritis, 1213
  in rheumatoid arthritis, 245–247, 246t, 858, 875, 923
  in synovial fluid analysis, 617
  incidence of, 242t, 242–243
  monoclonal, in immune complex assays, 230t
  physiologic role of, 245, 246t
Rheumatoid nodules, in rheumatoid arthritis, 917–918
  and prognosis, 923
Rhinitis, allergic, leukotrienes in, 297t
Ribonucleic acid. See *RNA*.
Ribonucleoproteins, antibodies to, in inflammatory muscle diseases, 260, 260t
  in mixed connective tissue disease, 1067–1068, *1069*
  in Sjögren's syndrome, 261, 261t
  in systemic lupus erythematosus, 255, 255t, 257–258
Ribs, articulations of, with spine, osteoarthritis of, 668
Rickets, 1503, 1572t, 1572–1574
Ridaura. See *Gold*.
Riedel's struma, 1167
Rifampin, effect of, on glucocorticoid clearance, 793, *793*
  for tuberculosis, 1454
  metabolism of, probenecid and, 836–837
Ritchie articular index, in rheumatoid arthritis, 925, 925t
RNA, antibodies to, in systemic lupus erythematosus, 258
  in antinuclear antibodies, 250, 251t
  in collagen synthesis, in extracellular matrix, 1537, *1537*
  messenger, in elastin synthesis, 33
RNA polymerases, antibodies to, in scleroderma, 258t, 259

RNA polymerases (*Continued*)
  in systemic lupus erythematosus, 256
Rocaltrol. See *Vitamin D*.
Rodnan total skin score, in scleroderma, 1137, *1138*
Ross River virus infection, and arthritis, 1478–1479
Rotator cuff. See also *Shoulder*.
  anatomy of, 413, *415*
  arthrography of, 416, *416*
  disorders of, arthroscopic surgery for, 693, *696*
    in osteoarthritis, 1388
    in rheumatoid arthritis, 911–912
    in sports medicine, 550–551, *551*
    magnetic resonance imaging of, 639–640
  in ankylosing spondylitis, imaging of, 656, *656*
  strengthening of, exercises for, in rehabilitation, 1622
  tears of, 426–427
    arthropathy with, 430
    magnetic resonance imaging of, 420, *421*
    preoperative evaluation of, *1704*, 1704–1705
    ultrasonography of, 417–419, *419*
  tendinitis/impingement syndrome of, 422–425, *423*
  ultrasonography of, preoperative, 1697–1698
Rubefacients, for osteoarthritis, 1398–1399
Rubella, in arthritis, 1475–1477, *1476*
  rheumatoid, 856
Rufen. See *Ibuprofen*.
Running, quadriceps motion in, control of, 92, *92*
Ryanodine receptors, in skeletal muscle, 78, *78*, 79t
  in contraction, 81, 82

Sacroiliac joints, computed tomography of, 631–632
  imaging of, in ankylosing spondylitis, *654*, 654–655
    in osteoarthritis, 664
    in psoriatic arthritis, 658, *658*
    in Reiter's syndrome, 660
    in rheumatoid arthritis, 650
Sacroiliitis, bacterial infection in, 1443
  in ankylosing spondylitis, imaging of, 976, 976t, 978
    physical examination for, 976
  in psoriatic arthritis, 1001, *1001*
  in Reiter's syndrome, 988, 991
  tuberculosis and, 1452
Sacrum, meningocele of, computed tomography of, *629*
  pathologic fracture of, magnetic resonance imaging of, *638*
Sag sign, of posterior cruciate ligament injury, 557
St. Vitus' dance, in rheumatic fever, 1231
Salicylates. See also *Aspirin* and *Nonsteroidal anti-inflammatory drugs*.
  nonacetylated, for systemic lupus erythematosus, 1040–1041
Salivary glands, in diffuse infiltrative lymphocytosis, in human immunodeficiency virus infection, 1274, *1274*, 1276
  in Sjögren's syndrome, 957t, 957–960, *959*, 962, *962*, 965

Salmonella infection, gastrointestinal, and reactive arthritis, 1009, 1009t, 1010
  in Reiter's syndrome, 984, 985, 989, 993
Salpingitis, reactive, in Reiter's syndrome, 988
Saphenous nerve, entrapment of, 581
Sarcoid, skin lesions in, 508
Sarcoidosis, 1418–1421, *1419*, *1420*
  and arthritis, monarticular, 377
    pauciarticular, 384
  and cancer, 1529, 1531t
  ocular disorders in, 493–494, *494*
  of hand, surgery for, 1670–1671
  salivary gland enlargement in, vs. Sjögren's syndrome, 960
  vs. rheumatoid arthritis, 909
Sarcolemma, of skeletal muscle, 76, 77, *78*, 81
Sarcoma, of joints, primary, 1610–1615, *1611*, *1613–1615*
    secondary, 1615–1616
    Paget's disease and, 1529, 1531t
    synovial, imaging of, 682
Sarcomeres, in skeletal muscle, 78, *80*
Sarcoplasmic reticulum, structure of, 78, *78*
Satellite cells, in skeletal muscle development, 76
Scalp, tenderness of, in giant cell arteritis, 1126
Scapular nerve, dorsal, entrapment of, 578
Scapulohumeral reflex, testing of, 406t
Scars, fibrosis of, 1166
  in Ehlers-Danlos syndrome, 1547, 1549–1551
Scedosporiosis, 1459
Schirmer tests, for keratoconjunctivitis sicca, in Sjögren's syndrome, 957
Schmid's metaphyseal dysplasia, 1556
Schober test, in ankylosing spondylitis, 975–976
Schönlein-Henoch purpura, 503, *1105*, 1105–1106
  in children, 1242t, *1258*, 1258–1259
  in human immunodeficiency virus infection, 1278
Schwann cells, anatomy of, 564, *565*, *566*
Sciatic nerve, entrapment of, 578–579
  injury to, in childbirth, 586
  in surgery, 586
  reflex testing of, 406t
Sciatica, 440
  with lumbar spinal stenosis, 449, 450
Scintigraphy. See *Radionuclide imaging*.
  in Reiter's syndrome, 987, 991
  of shoulder, in pain evaluation, 416, 422t
Scl–70, antibodies to, in scleroderma, 258t, 258–259, 1143
Sclera, color of, in osteogenesis imperfecta, 1543t, 1544, 1545
Scleredema, 1156
Scleritis, 489t, *490*, 490–492, *491*, Plate 3
  in rheumatoid arthritis, 916–917, *917*
Scleroderma, 1133–1158
  antinuclear antibodies in, 258t, 258–259
  arthritis in, polyarticular, peripheral, 383
  classification of, 1133, 1134t, 1150–1151, 1151t
  definition of, 1133, 1134t
  edema in, in initial presentation, 1135, *1135*
  epidemiology of, 1133–1134
  gastrointestinal tract in, 1146–1147, *1147*
  hormonal disorders in, 1150
  imaging of, 661–662, *661–663*
  immunologic features of, 1142–1144

Scleroderma (Continued)
    in cancer, 1150, 1525, 1527t, 1529, 1531t
    in children, 1242t, 1249–1253, 1250t, *1250–1253*
    in overlap syndromes, 1065t, 1065–1066, *1066*
        in mixed connective tissue disease, 1067–1075. See also *Mixed connective tissue disease.*
    interleukin-6 antibodies in, 274
    localized, 1154–1158, *1155–1157*
    mast cells in, 163–164, 1139
    microvascular abnormalities in, *1140,* 1142
    musculoskeletal features of, 1145–1146, *1146*
    myocardial disorders in, 1141, 1142t, 1149, 1154
    myositis in, 1183
    nerve disorders in, 1150
    of foot, 486–487
    of hand, surgery for, 1669–1670, *1669–1671*
    pathogenesis of, 1144–1145, *1145*
    platelets in, 179
    pregnancy in, 1150
    pulmonary disorders in, 1142, 1142t, 1147–1149, *1148,* 1250, 1250t
    Raynaud's phenomenon in, 1139–1142, *1140,* 1141t, 1142t
        in initial presentation, 1134–1135
    renal disorders in, *1149,* 1149–1150, 1154
    silica exposure and, 1169–1170
        breast implants and, 1172–1173
    skin lesions in, 505–506, *506,* 1135–1139, *1136–1138,* 1139t
    synovial biopsy in, 621, *621,* Plate 9
    treatment of, 1150–1154, 1151t, *1153*
    vs. rheumatoid arthritis, 904
Scleromalacia, 491, *491,* Plate 3
Scleromyxedema, 1156
Sclerosing cholangitis, 1165
Scoliosis, assessment for, in low back pain, 444
    in Ehlers-Danlos syndrome, 1550, *1551*
Scurvy, synovial biopsy in, 623
Secretory leukocyte proteinase inhibitor, 329, 329t
Segond's fracture, in sports medicine, 555
Seizures, in systemic lupus erythematosus, 1030t, 1034
Selectins, *304, 305,* 310–312, Plate 2
    in leukocyte–endothelial adhesion, 186t, 187t, 187–190, *189, 191*
    in leukocyte homing, 316
    in lymphocyte homing, 192
    in monocyte adhesion, to endothelial cells, 130
    in rheumatoid arthritis, 873t, 874
        therapy targeting, 839
    monoclonal antibodies to, in anti-in-flammatory treatment, 317
Selenium, in immune response, *523,* 525–526
Semimembranosus muscle, reflex testing of, 406t
Semitendinosus muscle, reflex testing of, 406t
Sepsis, articular, computed tomography of, 634
    as contraindication to intra-articular glu-cocorticoid injection, 593, 598, 599
    in Felty's syndrome, 952
Septic arthritis, fungal infection and, 1456–1459, *1457,* 1459t

Septic arthritis (Continued)
    hemophilic, 1486
    imaging of, 676–678, *677*
    in sickle cell disease, 1495
    in systemic lupus erythematosus, 1032
    of shoulder, and pain, 430
    synovectomy in, arthroscopic, 690
    tuberculosis and, 1453–1454, *1454*
    with human immunodeficiency virus in-fection, 1266–1267
Serglycin, in extracellular matrix, *38, 42,* 49
Serine proteinases, in extracellular matrix degradation, 324t, 324–326, 325t
    inhibitors of, 328–330, 329t
        in rheumatoid arthritis, 877
Serositis, in systemic lupus erythematosus, 1043–1044
Serpins, 328–329, 329t
    extracellular regulation of, 337, *337*
    in rheumatoid arthritis, 877
Serum amyloid A, in inflammation, 699, *700,* 701
Serum glutamic-oxaloacetic transaminase, after methotrexate therapy, for rheumatoid arthritis, 1864t–1866t, 1864–1867, *1866*
Serum glutamic pyruvic transaminase, after methotrexate therapy, for rheumatoid arthritis, 1864t, 1864–1866, 1865t
Serum sickness, immune complexes in, 229
Severe combined immunodeficiency, 1286t, *1294,* 1294–1295
    carrier detection in, 1300
    intrauterine diagnosis of, 1299–1300
    treatment of, *1301,* 1301–1302
Sex hormones, and uric acid excretion, 1329
    disorders of, 1508–1510
    in bone cell metabolism, 60–61
    in contraception, and arthritis, 904
    in musculoskeletal disorders, 1509–1510
    in osteoporosis, 1509, 1568–1569
    in systemic lupus erythematosus, 1018–1019, 1054
Sexual function, disorders of, in iron storage disorders, 1425
    in osteoarthritis, 1395
    in rheumatic disease, 537
SGOT, after methotrexate therapy, for rheumatoid arthritis, 1864t–1866t, 1864–1867, *1866*
SGPT, after methotrexate therapy, for rheumatoid arthritis, 1864t, 1864–1866, 1865t
Sharp-Purser test, in rheumatoid arthritis, of cervical spine, 1715
Shier's prosthesis, in knee replacement, 1832
Shigella infection, gastrointestinal, and reactive arthritis, 1009, 1009t
    in Reiter's syndrome, 984, 989
Shin splints, 466
    in sports medicine, 558–559
Shoes, wedged insoles in, in osteoarthritis, 1396
Shoulder, adhesive capsulitis in, in hyperthyroidism, 1505
    anatomy of, 413–414, *414, 415*
    arthritis in, medical treatment of, 1705–1706
        monarticular, differential diagnosis of, 373t
    arthrocentesis of, 600, *601*
    arthrodesis of, 1707

Shoulder (Continued)
    arthroplasty of, 1707–1709, *1708,* 1709t
        imaging of, 1833–1835, *1834, 1835*
        in juvenile rheumatoid arthritis, 1775, 1780
        resection, 1707
    computed tomography of, 632, *632*
    disorders of, glucocorticoids for, 596, 597t
        in diabetes mellitus, 1500–1501
        in sports medicine, 546–551, *547–551*
    hydroxyapatite crystal deposition dis-ease in, imaging of, 675, *675*
    in ankylosing spondylitis, 974, 977
        imaging of, 656, *656*
    in rheumatoid arthritis, imaging of, 649
    magnetic resonance imaging of, 639–641, *641*
    osteoarthritis of, arthroscopic surgery in, *693, 695*
        Milwaukee syndrome of, 1379
        preoperative evaluation of, 1699, *1699, 1700*
    osteonecrosis of, preoperative evaluation of, *1703,* 1703–1704
    osteotomy of, 1706–1707
    pain in, 413–435
        adhesive capsulitis and, 425, 426, 431–432
        arthritis and, 428–429, *429,* 434
            septic, 430
        bicipital rupture and, 428
        bicipital tendinitis and, 427–428
        brachial neuritis and, 433
        calcific tendinitis and, 425–426
        cervical radiculopathy and, 433
        diagnosis of, selection of tests in, 422, 422t
        drug injection for, in diagnosis, 420–422
        electromyography in, 420
        fibrositis and, 435
        glenohumeral instability and, 432
        glenoid labral tears and, 431
        history in, 414
        imaging in, 415–420, *416–419, 421, 422*
        nerve conduction studies in, 420
        nerve entrapment syndromes and, *433,* 433–434
        physical examination in, 414–415
        referred, 435
        reflex sympathetic dystrophy and, 434–435
        rotator cuff tears and, 426–427
            with arthropathy, 430
        rotator cuff tendinitis/impingement syndrome and, 422–425, *423*
        sternoclavicular disorders and, 434
        tumors and, 435
        with neck pain, 395t
    periarthritis of, glucocorticoids for, 596
    reconstructive surgery of, 1696–1710
        evaluation for, 1696–1698, *1697, 1698*
        indications for, 1705
    rheumatoid arthritis of, 911–912
        preoperative evaluation of, 1699–1702, *1701*
    rotator cuff disorders in, arthroscopic surgery for, 693, *696*
        preoperative evaluation of, *1704,* 1704–1705
    stability of, 86, *86*
    synovectomy of, 1706
    traumatic arthritis of, preoperative evalu-ation of, *1702,* 1702–1703

Shoulder-hand syndrome, and pain, 434–435
  with cancer, 1525, 1527t
Sialography, in Sjögren's syndrome, 958
Sialoprotein, bone, in extracellular matrix, 42, 49
Sialyl-Lewis X ligand, absence of, and leukocyte adhesion deficiency, 1298–1299
  selectins binding to, 310
Sicca syndrome, 488
  in scleroderma, 1150
  in systemic lupus erythematosus, 1037
Sickle cell anemia, 1493–1497, 1494, 1494t
  and osteonecrosis, 1585
    of shoulder, 430
  articular disorders with, imaging of, 679
  synovial biopsy in, 623
  vs. rheumatoid arthritis, 906
Silicon, chemistry of, 1169, 1169t, 1170
Silicone, in breast implants, and rheumatic disease, 1169t, 1169–1174, 1172t
Silicone rubber, in prostheses, radiography of, 1840–1843, 1841, 1841t, 1842, 1843t
Silicosis, 1169–1170
Sindbis virus infection, and arthritis, 1478–1479
Sinding-Larsen-Johansson syndrome, 558
Sinemet, for sleep disturbances, in fibromyalgia syndrome, 517
Sinuvertebral nerve, anatomy of, 439–440, 440
Sjögren's syndrome, 955–966
  and cancer, 1528, 1531t
  anti-ribonucleoprotein antibodies in, 257
  autoantibodies in, 963
  blood disorders in, 961t, 962
  epidemiology of, 955–956, 956t
  fibromyalgia with, 514
  gastrointestinal tract in, 960–961, 961t
  genetics in, 964
  historical aspects of, 955
  human leukocyte antigens in, 219, 964
  hydroxychloroquine for, 754, 965, 966
  hypothyroidism in, 961
  in overlap syndromes, 1037, 1065, 1066
  keratoconjunctivitis sicca in, 488, 956t, 956–957, 957, 957t, 965
  kidneys in, 961t, 961–962
  management of, 965–966
  myositis with, 1183
  nervous system in, 962–963
  ocular disorders in, 956t, 956–957, 957, 957t, 965
  oral disorders in, 957t, 957–960, 959, 962, 962, 965
  pathogenesis of, 964–965
  respiratory tract in, 960, 961t
  rheumatoid factors in, 245–246
  skin lesions in, 497, 961, 961t
  vasculitis with, 497, 961, 1111
  vs. diffuse infiltrative lymphocytosis, in human immunodeficiency virus infection, 1273, 1273t, 1274
  vs. sarcoidosis, 1421
  with rheumatoid arthritis, gold for, 760
  with Waldenström's hypergammaglobulinemia purpura, 1108
Skin, hyperpigmentation of, in iron storage disorders, 1425
  in acromegaly, 1507
  in amyloidosis, 507–508, 508
  in antiphospholipid syndrome, 1061
  in Behçet's disease, 1114–1116
  in Churg-Strauss syndrome, 1098

Skin (Continued)
  in cutis laxa, 1553–1554
    X-linked, 1551
  in dermatomyositis, 504–505, 504–506, Plates 5 and 6
    in children, 1245–1246, 1246
  in Ehlers-Danlos syndrome, 1547, 1547, 1548t, 1549, 1549–1551, 1551
  in epidermolysis bullosa, 1556–1557
  in Graves' disease, 1504
  in Henoch-Schönlein purpura, 1105, 1105–1106, 1258, 1258
  in juvenile rheumatoid arthritis, 506, 506, 1209–1211, 1211, 1215, Plate 6
  in Lyme disease, 507, 507, 1463, 1463, 1464t, 1466, 1872, 1873, Plate 6, Plate 12
  in mixed connective tissue disease, 502, 1069
  in necrotizing vasculitis, 502t, 502–504, 503, Plate 5
  in panniculitis, 508t, 508–509
  in parvovirus arthropathy, 509
  in polyarteritis, 503, 1093, 1093, 1107
  in polychondritis, relapsing, 499, 1406
  in pseudoxanthoma elasticum, 1554
  in psoriasis, with arthritis, 1002, 1002t. See also Psoriatic arthritis.
  in Reiter's syndrome, 497–498, 498, 988–989, 989, 993, Plate 4
    with human immunodeficiency virus infection, 1268–1272, 1269, 1270, 1272
  in reticulohistiocytosis, multicentric, 1430, 1431
  in rheumatic fever, 506–507
  in rheumatoid arthritis, 497, 916
  in sarcoid, 508
  in scleroderma, 505–506, 506, 1135–1139, 1136–1138, 1139t
    in children, 1250, 1250t, 1252, 1252, 1253
    treatment of, 1151t, 1151–1154, 1153
  in Sjögren's syndrome, 497, 961, 961t
  in systemic lupus erythematosus, 499–502, 500–502, 1030t, 1036, Plates 4 and 5
    conservative management of, 1041–1043, 1042t, 1043t
  in Waldenström's hypergammaglobulinemia purpura, 1108
  in Wegener's granulomatosis, 1101
  in Wiskott-Aldrich syndrome, 1296
  inflammation of, antimalarial drug effects on, 749
  telangiectasia of, with ataxia, 1297
  toxicity to, allopurinol and, 833
    antimalarial drugs and, 754–755, 755t
    glucocorticoids and, 795–796
    gold and, 762, 763t
    methotrexate and, 780
    nonsteroidal anti-inflammatory drugs and, 717
    D-penicillamine and, 767
    sulfasalazine and, 743
  vasculitis in, 1103, 1103–1105
    granulomatous, 1108
    hypocomplementemic, 1106, 1106–1107
Skull, deformity of, in osteogenesis imperfecta, 1544
Sleep, disorders of, in fibromyalgia syndrome, 515–517, 516, 516t
Small intestine, disorders of, and arthritis. See Enteropathic arthritis.
  in scleroderma, 1147

Smith ankle prosthesis, radiography of, 1836, 1839
Smoking, and Buerger's disease, 1113–1114
  and osteoporosis, 1564
Snapping hip, 473–474
Sodium, metabolism of, disorders of, and myopathy, 1194t
Sodium pentosan polysulfate, for osteoarthritis, 1400, 1400t
Solganal. See Gold.
Somatomedin C (insulin-like growth factor I), in articular cartilage, 8, 9
  in bone cell metabolism, 61
SPARC (osteonectin), in bone matrix, 62–63
  in extracellular matrix, 49–50
Spectinomycin, for Neisseria infection, 1446
Sphincter ani externus muscle, reflex testing of, 405, 406t
Spinal cord, diseases of, and weakness, 392
  in rheumatoid arthritis, position of, in anesthesia, 1641
Spinal muscles, atrophy of, vs. inflammatory muscle disease, 1190
Spinal nerves, dermatomes of, 398, 398
  disorders of, muscle tests for, 398, 399t
  roots of, cervical, in shoulder pain, 433
    compression of, 398–399
    symptoms of, 400–403
    traction for, 410
    vs. nerve entrapment syndromes, 582
  lumbar, in low back pain, 441, 441t, 446
    in spinal stenosis, 447t, 447–450, 448
  lumbosacral, in hip pain, 476
Spindle cells, in sarcoma, synovial, 1613–1614, 1614
Spine. See also Spondyl-.
  cervical, blood supply to, 399–400
    clinical examination of, 404
    degeneration of, in double crush entrapment syndromes, 582
    disorders of, electrodiagnostic studies of, 408
      imaging of, 407–408
      laboratory studies in, 408
      patient education in, 411
      treatment of, 410–411
    pain syndromes in, 395, 395t
  computed tomography of, 629, 631–635, 632, 634
  development of, 5
  disorders of, and polyarticular pain, 386
    with inflammatory bowel disease, 1008, 1008t
  fusion of, for spondylolisthesis, 453
  in Ehlers-Danlos syndrome, 1550, 1551
  in juvenile rheumatoid arthritis, 1214, 1214
  in Marfan syndrome, 1552
  in osteogenesis imperfecta, 1544
  in psoriatic arthritis, 1001, 1001, 1002t
    imaging of, 658–659, 659
  in Reiter's syndrome, 660
  in rheumatoid arthritis, 1713–1718
    evaluation of, before reconstructive surgery, 1637
    imaging of, 648t, 650–651, 651
    subluxations in, 1713–1715, 1714–1716
  in sarcoidosis, 1419–1420
  lumbar, disorders of, and pain, 439–454
    See also Low back pain.

Spine *(Continued)*
  magnetic resonance imaging of, 635–637, *636, 637*
  motion of, in lifting, 92
  orthotic devices for, 1626
  osteochondrosis of, 667, *667*
  osteoporosis of, in ochronosis, 676
  stability of, 86, *87*
  stenosis of, in osteoarthritis, 1388
  vertebral compression in, in sickle cell disease, 1493, *1494*
Spleen, enlargement of, in Felty's syndrome, 951–954
  removal of, for thrombocytopenia, in systemic lupus erythematosus, 1052
Splinting, in rehabilitative medicine, 1625–1626, *1626*
  in rheumatoid arthritis, of hand, 1647–1648
    of wrist, 1647–1648
  of elbow, after surgery, *1693,* 1693–1694
Spondylitis, ankylosing, 969–981. See also *Ankylosing spondylitis.*
  psychosocial impact of, in adolescents, 536
  syphilitic, with low back pain, 452
  tuberculous, *1451,* 1451–1453, *1452*
Spondylitis ossificans ligamentosa (diffuse idiopathic skeletal hyperostosis), and low back pain, 450
  imaging of, 668–669, *669, 670*
  in diabetes mellitus, 1501
  vs. ankylosing spondylitis, 655, 657
  vs. osteoarthritis, 1391–1392
Spondyloarthropathy, 969–1013. See also specific disorders, e.g., *Reiter's syndrome.*
  and low back pain, 450
  classification of, 969–970, 970t
  HLA-B27 antigen in, 217t, 217–218, 218t
  in psoriatic arthritis, 1001, *1001,* 1003–1004
  inflammation in, laboratory evaluation of, 704
  leukotrienes in, 297t
  seronegative, vs. rheumatoid arthritis, 903
  synovial biopsy in, 620–621
  types of, 969, 970t
  with human immunodeficiency virus infection, 1268–1272, *1272*
Spondyloepiphyseal dysplasia, 1555–1556
  genetic mutation in, 1540–1541
Spondylolisthesis, and low back pain, 452t, 452–453
  in osteoarthritis, 1388
Spondylolysis, and low back pain, 444, 452t, 452–453
Spondylosis, hyperostotic (diffuse idiopathic skeletal hyperostosis), and low back pain, 450
  imaging of, 668–669, *669, 670*
  in diabetes mellitus, 1501
  vs. ankylosing spondylitis, 655, 657
  vs. osteoarthritis, 1391–1392
Spondylosis deformans, imaging of, 667–668, *668*
Sporotrichosis, 1458, 1459, 1459t
Sports medicine, 546–561
  ankle injuries in, 560, *561*
  elbow disorders in, 551–553, *552*
  glenohumeral instability in, 432
  historical aspects of, 546
  knee disorders in, 553–558, *554–557, 559*
  lower leg disorders in, 558–560

Sports medicine *(Continued)*
  osteoarthritis in, 1385–1386
  principles of, 546
  rotator cuff impingement in, 423
  shoulder disorders in, 546–551, *547–551*
Sprains, of ankle, 560
  of knee, 555
St. Vitus' dance, in rheumatic fever, 1231
Staining, of biopsy sample, in inflammatory muscle disease, 1198–1199
  of dried smears, in synovial fluid analysis, 615–617, *616,* Plate 8
Stance, in hip examination, 362–363
Staphylococcal binding assay, for immune complexes, 230t, 231, 231t
Staphylococcus aureus infection, and arthritis, 1441–1442
  pathophysiology of, 1435, *1436*
  with human immunodeficiency virus infection, 1267
  spinal, and low back pain, 451
Stefins, 329t, 330
Stem cell factor, in mast cell differentiation, 164
Sternoclavicular joint, bacterial arthritis in, 1443
  computed tomography of, 631, *631*
  disorders of, and pain, 434
  examination of, 357
  in rheumatoid arthritis, 911
Sternocleidomastoid muscle, examination of, 404
Sternocostal joints, examination of, 357
Steroids. See *Glucocorticoids.*
Stickler's syndrome, 1555–1556
Stiffness, in back, in ankylosing spondylitis, 973
  in joints, in patient history, 353–354
  in osteoarthritis, 1386
  in rheumatoid arthritis, in diagnosis, 346, *347*
    in disease onset, 900
Stillbirth, in systemic lupus erythematosus, 1037
Still's disease, 506, *506,* Plate 6
  adult-onset, 900–901
    imaging of, 653
    vs. malignancy, 1524
  imaging of, 652–653, *653*
  monarticular arthritis in, 378
Stockings, pneumatic compression, in prevention of thrombosis, after hip arthroplasty, 1732
Stockman's nodules, 598
Stomach. See also *Gastrointestinal tract.*
  disorders of, in scleroderma, 1146–1147
    in Sjögren's syndrome, 960
  ulcers of, glucocorticoids and, 795
    nonsteroidal anti-inflammatory drugs and, 714–715
Strain, bony adaptation to, 70–72
  repetitive, 584–585, 585t
    and carpal tunnel syndrome, 571
    and medial tibial stress syndrome, 558–559
    of rotator cuff, in sports medicine, 550–551, *551*
    vs. fibromyalgia syndrome, 514
Streptococcal cell wall injection, inflammatory response to, genetic impairment of, and rheumatoid arthritis, 854
Streptococcal infection, in arthritis, 1441–1442

Streptococcal infection *(Continued)*
  in psoriatic arthritis, 1000
  in rheumatic fever, 1225–1238. See also *Rheumatic fever.*
  in septic arthritis, with human immunodeficiency virus infection, 1267
Streptomycin, for tuberculosis, 1454
Stress fractures, of hip, *472,* 472–473
  of tibia, 466, 559–560
Stress reaction, and knee pain, 466
Stress shielding, after hip arthroplasty, 1794, 1796
  after knee arthroplasty, 1823, *1823*
Stridor, in rheumatoid arthritis, of cricoarytenoid joints, 911
Stroke, in systemic lupus erythematosus, 1034, 1053
  thrombotic, in antiphospholipid syndrome, 1059
Stromelysin, in extracellular matrix degradation, 324t, 325t, 326–327, 327t, *328*
  in rheumatoid arthritis, 876t, 876–878, *877*
Struthers ligament, in median nerve entrapment, 572
Subacromial bursa, imaging of, 417, 627
  inflammation of, glucocorticoid injection for, 604, *605*
Subchondral bone, effect of, on articular cartilage, 11
Subclavian arteries, in giant cell arteritis, 1127, *1127*
Subcostal nerves, entrapment of, and hip pain, 476
Subcutaneous nodules, in rheumatic fever, 1229, 1231
Substance P, in joint development, 4
  in rheumatoid arthritis, 870
  in synovial joint innervation, 16
Subtalar joint, anatomy of, 479
  arthritis of, 484
Sudeck's atrophy (reflex sympathetic dystrophy), and shoulder pain, 434–435
  with cancer, 1525, 1527t
  with cervical spinal disorders, 407
Sulfadiazine, in prevention of rheumatic fever, 1237, 1237t
Sulfamethoxazole, with trimethoprim, interaction of, with methotrexate, 774
Sulfapyridine, *741,* 741–742, *742*
Sulfasalazine, *741–743,* 741–744, 743t
  anti-inflammatory effect of, 711
  for ankylosing spondylitis, 980
  for Reiter's syndrome, 994, 995t
  for rheumatoid arthritis, 941, 946, 947, 1891–1893, 1892t, 1898t, 1900
    in combination therapy, with antimalarial drugs, 753
    in pregnancy and lactation, 1902t
    juvenile, 1218
    vs. antimalarial drugs, 752t, 752–753
    with methotrexate, *777*
  for spondyloarthropathy, with human immunodeficiency virus infection, 1272
Sulfinpyrazone, for hyperuricemia, *834,* 834–836, 1344, 1345
  interaction of, with salicylates, 719t
Sulfonylurea, interactions of, with nonsteroidal anti-inflammatory drugs, 719t, 720
Sulindac, 723t, 725, *725*
  adverse effects of, gastrointestinal, 713–714

Sulindac (Continued)
    in systemic lupus erythematosus, 1041
    on kidney, 716
    on liver, 715, 721
Sunscreens, for photosensitivity, in
    systemic lupus erythematosus, 1041,
    1042t
Superoxide dismutase, 523, 523
Suprascapular nerve, entrapment of,
    577–578
    and shoulder pain, 434
Supraspinatus tendon, in hydroxyapatite
    crystal deposition disease, imaging of,
    675, 675
    inflammation of, calcific, 425–426
    glucocorticoid injection for, 604, 605
    magnetic resonance imaging of, 420, 421
Supraspinatus test, in rotator cuff
    disorders, 550
Suprofen, toxicity of, to kidney, 717
Sural nerve, entrapment of, 580
Surgery, 1633–1843. See also specific sites,
    e.g., Hand(s), and indications, e.g.,
    Osteoarthritis.
    anesthesia in, 1640–1645
    evaluation for, 1634–1637
    goals of, 1633–1634
    management after, 1637–1638
    patient selection for, 1637
Swallowing, disorders of, cervical spinal
    disorders and, 403
    in Sjögren's syndrome, 960
Swan-neck deformity, of fingers,
    examination for, 361, 361
    in mixed connective tissue disease,
    1069, 1069
    in Parkinson's disease, vs. rheumatoid
    arthritis, 908, 908
    in rheumatoid arthritis, 913, 913
    surgery for, 1658–1659
Swanson metacarpophalangeal prosthesis,
    radiography of, 1840, 1841
Sweet's syndrome, 1112
    vs. rheumatoid arthritis, 909
Swelling. See Edema.
Sydenham's chorea, in rheumatic fever,
    1231
Symphysis, definition of, 1
Symphysis pubis, inflammation of, and
    pain, 475–476
Synapsin I, in skeletal muscle contraction,
    81
Synaptic cleft, in neuromuscular junction,
    77
Synaptobrevins, in skeletal muscle
    contraction, 81
Synarthroses, types of, 1
Synchondroses, definition of, 1
Syncytium, in bone formation, 64–65
Syndecans, 314
    in extracellular matrix, 37, 38, 39, 42, 50
Syndesmoses, definition of, 1
Syndrome X, hyperuricemia with, 1319
Synostoses, definition of, 1
    development of, 5
Synovectomy, arthroscopic, 687–697
    in arthritis, inflammatory, 687–688, 689
    in chondromatosis, 690–691
    in hemophilic arthropathy, 690
    in osteoarthritis, 691–693, 691–695
    in pigmented villonodular synovitis,
    691
    in septic arthritis, 690
    in hemophilic arthropathy, 1491
    in juvenile rheumatoid arthritis, 1773–
    1774, 1774

Synovectomy (Continued)
    of hand, 1661
    in rheumatoid arthritis, of hand, 1652
    of knee, 1739, 1740
    of wrist, 1652
    radiation in, 947
    of elbow, 1680t, 1681–1682, 1682, 1683
    of shoulder, 1706
Synovial cysts, 1593–1594, 1594
    of hip, computed tomography of, 628
Synovial effusion, in knee, examination
    for, 366, 367
Synovial fluid, 16–18, 17
    analysis of, 609–617, 1885
      antinuclear antibodies in, 617
      arthrocentesis for, 609–610
      blood in, 610, 611t, 612
      clarity in, 610t, 610–611, 612, Plate 7
      color in, 610, 610t, 612
      complement in, 617
      cultures in, 617
      cytokines in, 617
      dried smears in, 615–617, 616, Plate 8
      glucose in, 617
      in arthritis, monarticular, 373, 374t–
      375t, 378
      in bacterial arthritis, 1436–1437, 1437
      in hypothyroidism, 1505, 1505
      in infection, after hip arthroplasty,
      1810, 1810t
      in juvenile rheumatoid arthritis, 1213
      in rheumatoid arthritis, 883–888, 885
        in prognosis, 924
        lymphocytes in, 861–863
      leukocyte count in, 610t, 611, 611t
      microscopy in, regular, 612–613, 613,
      Plate 7
        with compensated polarized light,
        613t, 613–615, 614, 615, Plates 7
        and 8
      mucin clot test in, 617
      proteoglycans in, 617
      rheumatoid factor in, 617
      viscosity in, 610, 610t
      volume in, 610, 610t
      wet preparation in, 611–612
    in minimization of frictional forces, 89,
    90
    in nutrition of articular cartilage, 9
Synovial joints, biology of, developmental,
    2–5, 2–5
    bursae in, 6
    definition of, 1, 1
    innervation of, 15–16
    ligaments in, 6
    lubrication of, 18
    menisci in, 6–7
    muscles in, 5
    synovium of, 11–18. See also Synovium.
    tendons in, 5–6
Synovial membrane, lymphocyte
    infiltration of, in rheumatoid arthritis,
    863
Synovioma, benign, 1607–1608, 1608–1610
Synovitis, in calcium pyrophosphate
    deposition disease, 1361–1362
    in gout, urate in, 1338–1339
    in osteoarthritis, 1378–1379
    in polymyalgia rheumatica, 1127
    in rheumatoid arthritis, angiogenesis in,
    872, 872–873
      exercise in, 938
      menstrual cycle and, 1509
    localized nodular, 1607–1608, 1608–1610
    metal, after knee arthroplasty, 1830,
    1831, 1832

Synovitis (Continued)
    of elbow, in rheumatoid arthritis, 1677,
    1678
    of knee, after hip arthroplasty, glucocorti-
    coids for, 596
    of wrist, physical examination for, 359–
    360
    pigmented villonodular, 1604–1607,
    1606, 1607
      biopsy of, 623, 623, Plate 10
      imaging of, 682
      in osteoarthritis, 1390–1391
      of knee, magnetic resonance imaging
      of, 644, 645
      synovectomy in, arthroscopic, 691
      vs. localized nodular synovitis, 1607–
      1608
      vs. rheumatoid arthritis, 908
    silicone rubber prostheses and, radiogra-
    phy of, 1841t, 1841–1843, 1842, 1843t
    villonodular, 1604
    vs. juvenile rheumatoid arthritis, 1215
Synovium, 11, 11–15, 12, 14, 15
    biopsy of, 617–623
      findings in, 620–623, 620–623, Plates 9
      and 10
      tissue acquisition in, 618, 618–619
      tissue handling in, 619, 619–620, 620
    chondromatosis of, 1600–1603, 1601–1603
      imaging of, 681, 681–682
      in osteoarthritis, 1390–1391
    fatty tumors of, 1597, 1597–1598, 1598
    in hypertrophic osteoarthropathy, 1518
    in rheumatoid arthritis, pathology of,
    878–883, 882, 883, 924
    lining of, 11, 11–13, 12
    plicae of, and knee pain, 463, 463
    proteinase secretion by, 331–333, 332t
    reaction of, to bone tumors, 1523
    rheumatoid, mast cells in, 163, 163–164
      tryptase in, 167
    sarcoma of, imaging of, 682
      primary, 1612–1615, 1613–1615
    stroma of, 13
    vascular tumors of, 1598, 1598–1599,
    1599
    vasculature of, 13–15, 14, 15
Synthetase, antibodies to, in inflammatory
    muscle diseases, 259–260, 260t
Syphilis, and spondylitis, with low back
    pain, 452
Syringomyelia, neuroarthropathy in,
    imaging of, 670–671
Systemic lupus erythematosus, 1015–1054
    and cancer, 1528, 1531t
    antimalarial drugs for, 749–750, 1042–
    1043, 1043t
    antinuclear antibodies in, 254, 255t, 255–
    258, 1031t, 1031–1032
    arthritis in, polyarticular, peripheral, 383
    arthroplasty in, evaluation for, 1636
    bacterial arthritis with, 1439, 1439t
    blood disorders in, 1030t, 1035–1036,
    1052–1053
    cardiovascular disorders in, 1034–1035,
    1241
    central nervous system disorders in,
    1030t, 1034, 1053
    complement deficiencies in, 1306–1310,
    1308t
    contraception in, 1037
    cyclophosphamide for, 812, 1046–1050,
    1048t, 1050t, 1243–1244
    diagnosis of, 1029–1032, 1030t, 1031t
    likelihood ratios in, 347–348, 348

Systemic lupus erythematosus (Continued)
drug-induced, 1018t, 1019, 1037
fibromyalgia with, 514
foot in, 486
gastrointestinal tract in, 1036
glucocorticoids for, 798–800
intra-articular injection of, 596
gout with, 1320
hand in, surgery of, 1662–1667, 1665–1667
human leukocyte antigens in, 219, 1016, 1016t, 1017, 1029
imaging in, 660, 661, 661
immune complexes in, 231t, 231–232, 1021–1024, 1023t, 1024t
immune reaction in, 807
in children, 1241–1245, 1242t, 1244
in overlap syndromes, in mixed connective tissue disease, 1067–1075. See also Mixed connective tissue disease.
incidence of, 1028, 1029t
inflammation in, laboratory evaluation of, 703
interleukins in, 274, 282
liver disorders in, 1036
management of, 1040–1054
aggressive, cytotoxic drugs in, 1046–1050, 1048t, 1050t
glucocorticoids in, 1044, 1044t, 1044–1046, 1047t
side effects of, 1049–1050, 1050t
indications for, 1044, 1044t
conservative, 1040–1044, 1042t, 1043t
experimental therapies in, 1053–1054
in thrombocytopenia, 1052–1053
initial decisions in, 1040, 1040
outcome of, 1054, 1054t
menstruation in, 1037
monarticular arthritis in, 377
myositis in, 1183
neuropsychiatric disorders in, 537
ocular disorders with, 492–493, 493, 1036–1037
pathogenesis of, 1015, 1015
and organ damage, 1024, 1024t
disease mediators in, 1022t, 1022–1023, 1023, 1023t
environmental factors in, 1018t, 1018–1019
genetics in, 1015–1018, 1016t, 1018t, 1028–1029
immune response in, 1019–1022, 1020t
D-penicillamine and, in rheumatoid arthritis, 943
platelets in, 179–180
pregnancy in, 1037
management of, 1051–1052, 1052t
pulmonary disease in, 1035
renal disorders in, 1030t, 1032–1034, 1033t
and prognosis, 501–502
apheresis for, 1053–1054
cyclosporine for, 1053–1054
cytotoxic drugs for, 1046–1050, 1048t, 1050t
glucocorticoids for, 1044, 1044–1046, 1047t
in children, 1242, 1244
leukotrienes in, 297t
membranous nephritis in, 1053
sex hormones in, 1508, 1509
sicca syndrome in, 1037
skin lesions in, 499–502, 500, 502, 1030t, 1036, Plates 4 and 5
conservative management of, 1041–1043, 1042t, 1043t

Systemic lupus erythematosus (Continued)
synovial biopsy in, 621
thrombosis in, management of, 1051
vasculitis with, 1035, 1111–1112
vs. rheumatoid arthritis, 904
juvenile, 1215
wrist in, surgery of, 1662, 1663
Systemic sclerosis, 1133–1158. See also Scleroderma.

T cell(s), 97t, 97–101, 99t, 100t
activation of, 114–118, 115
defects of, and immunodeficiency, 1285t, 1299
cytokines produced by, 101–105, 102t–103t
deficiency of, in Nezelof's syndrome, 1293–1294
development of, 112–113
cytokines in, 270–272, 272
human leukocyte antigen molecules in, and autoimmune disease, 221
free radical damage to, vitamin E and, 524
in antigen-specific recognition, 112
in common variable immunodeficiency, 1289
in endothelial cell injury, in vasculitis, 1083
in human immunodeficiency virus infection, 1265–1266
in immune response, 805–806, 806
to silicone, 1171
in psoriatic arthritis, 999–1000
in Reiter's syndrome, 985
in rheumatoid arthritis, 858–863, 859, 861t
cytokines in, 863–866, 864t
in rheumatoid factor synthesis, 244
in scleroderma, dermal infiltration by, 1138, 1138, 1143
in systemic lupus erythematosus, 1020t, 1020–1024, 1023t, 1024t
in vaccination, for rheumatoid arthritis, 845, 845–846
interaction of, with B cells, 119, 119, 121–122
therapy targeting, for rheumatoid arthritis, 840t, 842–843
for systemic lupus erythematosus, 1054
with endothelial cells, in inflammatory response, 192–193
memory in, 100, 100t
migration of, to inflammatory sites, 119–121, 120t, 121t
receptors of, peptide therapy targeting, for rheumatoid arthritis, 846
recognition by, human leukocyte antigens in, 210, 210
stimulation of, mononuclear phagocytes in, 141–143, 142
subsets of, 99–101, 100t
suppression of, cyclophosphamide and, 812
purine analogs and, 814
radiation and, 818
surface antigens of, in rheumatoid arthritis, therapy targeting, 840t, 840–842
surface markers of, 97t, 97–99, 99t
testing for, in recurrent infection, 1283–1284
T cell antigen receptors, 97–98, 101

T cell antigen receptors (Continued)
in antigen-specific recognition, 107, 109, 112
in lymphocyte activation, 114–117
T cell receptor–CD3 complex, defective expression of, and immunodeficiency, 1285t, 1299
Tabes dorsalis, neuroarthropathy in, 670, 671
Tachycardia, cervical spinal disorders and, 403
Takayasu's arteritis, 1088–1090, 1090
in children, 1260
pathogenesis of, 1084, 1084
Talocalcaneal (subtalar) joint, anatomy of, 479
arthritis of, 484
Talocrural joint. See Ankle.
Talofibular ligaments, injuries of, in sports medicine, 560
Talonavicular joint, anatomy of, 480, 480
Talus, dome of, osteochondral defect of, computed tomography of, 629
fracture of, computed tomography of, 630, 630
Tamoxifen, and bone density increase, 1569
Tarsal tunnel syndrome, anterior, 579
glucocorticoids for, 598
in rheumatoid arthritis, 916
posterior, 579–580, 580
Tarsometatarsal joint, arthritis of, 484
arthrodesis of, 1769, 1770
Tarsus. See Ankle.
TASS syndrome, 1499–1500
Taste, disturbances of, D-penicillamine and, in rheumatoid arthritis, 943
TATA boxes, in immunoglobulin promotion, 110–111
Tear film, disorders of, 488–489, 489, 489t, Plate 3
in Sjögren's syndrome, 488, 956t, 956–957, 957, 957t, 965
Technetium, in imaging. See Radionuclide imaging.
Teeth, caries of, in Sjögren's syndrome, 958
in dentinogenesis imperfecta, with osteogenesis imperfecta, 1543t, 1544, 1545
Telangiectasia, with ataxia, 1286t, 1297
genetics of, 1284, 1284t
Telopeptides, in collagen fibrils, 26
in osteoporosis, 1567
Temperature, in rehabilitative medicine, 1623, 1623–1624, 1624t
in therapy, for rheumatoid arthritis, 938–939
regulation of, in surgery, 1644
synovial vasculature in, 15
sensitivity to, in Raynaud's phenomenon, in scleroderma, 1140–1142
Temporal arteritis, 1123–1130. See also Giant cell arteritis.
Temporomandibular joint, arthrocentesis of, 603, 603
computed tomography of, 630–631
development of, 4–5
examination of, 357
in rheumatoid arthritis, 911
magnetic resonance imaging of, 639, 641
Tenascin, in extracellular matrix, 38, 39, 42, 50
Tenderness, in physical examination, 355
Tendinitis, Achilles, and pain, 486
glucocorticoid injection for, 598, 606

Tendinitis (Continued)
 magnetic resonance imaging of, 642
 and polyarticular pain, 386, *386*
 apatite deposition and, 1363
 bicipital, 426–428
  glucocorticoid injection for, 603–604, *604*
 calcific, of shoulder, 425–426
 of hamstrings, and pain, 466
 patellar, and pain, 462–463
  in sports medicine, 558, *559*
 supraspinatus, glucocorticoid injection for, 604, *605*
 vs. arthritis, monarticular, 372, 373t
 with rotator cuff impingement, 422–425, *423*
Tendon sheath, chondroma of, 1603–1604
 fibroma of, 1599–1600, *1600*
 giant cell tumor of, 1608–1610, *1610, 1611*
 synovitis of. See *Tenosynovitis.*
Tendons, constituents of, 23t, 23–24
 extensor, of hand, rupture of, surgery for, *1648, 1649,* 1649–1650
 of toes, transfer of, 1769, *1770, 1771*
 in joint biomechanics, 87, *88*
 in synovial joints, 5–6
 of ankle, magnetic resonance imaging of, 641–642
 steroid injection into, sequelae of, 592
Tenidap, 723, 727, 727–728
 anti-inflammatory effect of, 711
Tennis elbow, glucocorticoid injection for, 604, *605*
 resistant, 575
Tenosynovitis, de Quervain's, glucocorticoid injection for, 604
 physical examination for, 360
 in juvenile rheumatoid arthritis, 1211
 of hand, surgery for, 1661–1662, *1662*
 in rheumatoid arthritis, 914
  surgery for, *1648,* 1648–1652, *1649, 1651*
 localized nodular, 1608–1610, *1610, 1611*
Teres minor muscle, reflex testing of, 406t
Terminal cisternae, of sarcoplasmic reticulum, 78
Terminal deoxyribonucleotidyl transferase, in recombination reaction, after antigen-specific recognition, 109
Testosterone, for osteoporosis, 1569
Tetracyclines, for osteoarthritis, 1400t, 1400–1401
 for Reiter's syndrome, 994–995
 for rheumatoid arthritis, 947
 for Whipple's disease, 1011
Th snoRNP, antibodies to, in scleroderma, 258t, 259
β-Thalassemia, 1493, 1497
Thenar muscle, in carpal tunnel syndrome, 569t, 571
Thermoplastic, in orthotics, 1625
Thermoset plastic, in orthotics, 1625
Thick filaments, in skeletal muscle, 78–79, 79t, *80*
Thiemann's disease, vs. rheumatoid arthritis, 909
Thigh, anterior, pain in, causes of, 464
Thin filaments, in skeletal muscle, 78–79, 79t, *80*
Thomas test, in hip examination, 363
Thoracic nerve, long, entrapment of, 578
Thoracic outlet syndromes, 577, *577*
Thorax, in ankylosing spondylitis, limited expansion of, 976

Thorax (Continued)
 pain in, 974
Thromboangiitis obliterans, 1113–1114
Thrombocytopenia, gold therapy and, 763–764
 in antiphospholipid syndrome, 1062, 1063
 in neonate, maternal lupus and, 1052
 in systemic lupus erythematosus, 1030t, 1035–1036
  management of, 1052–1053
 in Wiskott-Aldrich syndrome, 1296–1297
Thrombocytosis, in rheumatoid arthritis, 919
Thrombomodulin, in extracellular matrix, *42,* 50–51
Thrombophlebitis, after knee arthroplasty, 1751
Thrombosis, and osteonecrosis, 1585
 deep venous, after hip arthroplasty, 1728, 1731–1732
 in antiphospholipid syndrome, 1058–1062, *1059, 1060*
 in systemic lupus erythematosus, 1051
 in vasculitis, 1083–1085
 with complement activation, 179
Thrombospondin, in extracellular matrix, *37, 38, 42,* 51
Thromboxane A$_2$, in inflammation, 296
 inhibition of, nonsteroidal anti-inflammatory drugs in, 708, *709,* 711
 receptors of, 295
 synthesis of, 288, *289, 290,* 290t, 291
 fatty acids in, *527, 528,* 529
Throwing, and shoulder disorders, 432, 549–551, *551*
Thumb, physical examination of, 362
 surgery of, in juvenile rheumatoid arthritis, 1662
  in osteoarthritis, 1672–1673
  in psoriatic arthritis, *1668,* 1669
  in rheumatoid arthritis, 1655, *1656*
  in systemic lupus erythematosus, 1666–1667, *1667*
Thymidylate, synthesis of, methotrexate inhibition of, 771, *772*
Thymoma, with immunodeficiency, 1285t, 1297–1298
Thymus, hypoplasia of, and immunodeficiency, 1286t, *1292,* 1292–1293
 genetics of, 1284, 1284t
 treatment of, 1301
 in severe combined immunodeficiency, 1294
Thyroid gland, amyloid deposits in, 1510
 disorders of, in scleroderma, 1150
 fibrosis of, in Riedel's struma, 1167
 hyperfunction of, 1503–1505, *1504*
  and arthritis, vs. rheumatoid arthritis, 904
  glucocorticoid metabolism in, 793
  with hypertrophic osteoarthropathy, 1516
 hypofunction of, *1505,* 1505–1506
  and arthritis, vs. rheumatoid arthritis, 904
  gout with, 1319–1320
  in scleroderma, 1150
  in Sjögren's syndrome, 961
  osteoarthritis with, 385
Thyroid hormone, in muscle development, 83
Thyroiditis, Hashimoto's, 1503, 1505
Tibia, fracture of, ankle arthrosis after, 1759

Tibia (Continued)
 in knee replacement, *1743,* 1743–1746, *1744, 1746, 1747*
 injury of, in sports medicine, 558–560
 osteotomy of, in arthritis, failure of, arthroplasty after, 1747, *1748*
  in osteoarthritis, of knee, 1740–1741, *1741*
 stress fractures of, 466, 559–560
Tibial nerve, entrapment of, in tarsal tunnel syndrome, glucocorticoids for, 598
 posterior, 579–580, *580*
 reflex testing of, 406t
Tibial tendon, posterior, inflammation of, and pain, 486
 rupture of, ankle arthrosis after, 1759, 1763, *1764, 1765*
  foot surgery after, 1766–1767, *1768, 1769*
 magnetic resonance imaging of, 642
Tibialis posterior muscle, reflex testing of, 406t
Tibiofemoral arthritis, and pain, 464, 465
Tibiofibular arthritis, and pain, 466
Tietze's syndrome, glucocorticoids for, 596
Tinel's sign, in carpal tunnel syndrome, 568, 569t
Tissue inhibitor of metalloproteinases, 876t, 877–878
Tissue plasminogen activator, cellular regulation of, 334, 335t
 in extracellular matrix degradation, 324t, 325
 inhibitors of, 328, 329t
Titin, in skeletal muscle, 79, 79t
Tobacco, and Buerger's disease, 1113–1114
 and osteoporosis, 1564
α-Tocopherol, antioxidant effect of, 524
Toe(s), clubbing of, in hypertrophic osteoarthropathy, 1514–1516, 1518
 deformity of, in osteoarthritis, *483,* 483–484, *484,* 665
 elongated, in Marfan syndrome, 1552, 1553
 great, metatarsophalangeal rigidity of, surgery for, 1770, *1771*
 in gout, arthritis in, 377, 1315
 interphalangeal joints of, arthrocentesis of, 602
 necrosis of, with cancer, 1526, 1527t
 osteolysis of, in diabetes mellitus, 1501, *1501*
Toenails, in clubbing, in hypertrophic osteoarthropathy, 1515
 in psoriasis, 498
 in Reiter's syndrome, 989, *989*
 with human immunodeficiency virus infection, *1269,* 1270
Tolmetin (Tolectin), 729t, *732,* 732–733
 for juvenile rheumatoid arthritis, 1217
 side effects of, in systemic lupus erythematosus, 1041
Tomography, computed, 628–635. See also *Computed tomography.*
 conventional, indications for, 627
Tongue, enlarged, in amyloidosis, 1412, *1413*
Tooth (teeth), caries of, in Sjögren's syndrome, 958
 in dentinogenesis imperfecta, with osteogenesis imperfecta, 1543t, 1544, 1545
Tophi, in gout, chronic, 1316t, 1316–1318, *1317–1319*

Tophi (Continued)
  vs. osteoarthritis, 1391
  vs. rheumatoid nodules, 918
Topoisomerase I, antibodies to, in
    scleroderma, 258t, 258–259, 1143
Toradol, 729t, 734, 734–735
Torulosis (cryptococcosis), 1457, 1457–1458,
    1459t
  spinal, and low back pain, 451
Touraine-Solente-Golé syndrome, 1514,
    1515
Toxic oil syndrome, 1158
Toxoplasmosis, and myositis, 1191
Trachea, in relapsing polychondritis, 1406,
    1407
Traction, across joint, during radiography,
    627
  cervical spinal, for nerve root compres-
      sion, 410
    for rheumatoid arthritis, 1718
Transcutaneous electrical nerve
    stimulation, in osteoarthritis, 1396
  in rehabilitative medicine, 1624
Transcytosis, and vascular permeability,
    186
Transferrin. See also Iron.
  in inflammation, in acute-phase re-
      sponse, 700
Transforming growth factor-β, 101, 103t
  in articular cartilage, 8–9
  in bone cell metabolism, 61, 61
  in bone remodeling, 56
  in calcium pyrophosphate deposition dis-
      ease, 1360
  in fibroblast regulation, 201, 202, 204,
      205
  in inflammatory response, 177–178, 178
  in rheumatoid arthritis, 845, 868, 871,
      880
  in scleroderma, 1139
  in tissue fibrosis, in chronic inflamma-
      tion, 277, 277–278
  receptors of, in extracellular matrix, 38,
      39, 40, 44, 45, 51
    on mononuclear phagocytes, 136
Transplantation, of bone marrow, for
    cellular immunodeficiency, 1300,
    1301, 1301–1302
  graft-versus-host disease after, 1525
  in Wiskott-Aldrich syndrome, 1296–
      1297
  of cartilage, to knee, in osteoarthritis,
      1740
  of kidney, in systemic lupus erythemato-
      sus, 1034
  of organs, gout after, management of,
      1345–1346
Transthyretin, in familial amyloidotic
    polyneuropathy, 1410, 1410t, 1414,
    1414–1415
Transverse tubule network, of skeletal
    muscle, 77–78, 78, 79t, 81
Transversus abdominis muscle, reflex
    testing of, 406t
Trapezium, replacement of, in
    osteoarthritis, 1672–1673
Trapezius muscle, clinical examination of,
    404
Trauma, and osteoarthritis, 1377–1378,
    1385
  and osteonecrosis, 1582, 1582–1583
  and psoriatic arthritis, 1000
  computed tomography after, 629–630,
    630
  in surgery, and peripheral nerve lesions,
    585–586

Trauma (Continued)
  to elbow, arthritis after, 1679, 1680
    joint replacement for, 1685
  to joints, intra-articular glucocorticoid
      injection for, 596
  to shoulder, and arthritis, preoperative
      evaluation of, 1702, 1702–1703
    and rotator cuff tears, 426–427
Trendelenburg gait, in hip examination,
    363
Trendelenburg's test, in hip examination,
    363
Triadin, in skeletal muscle, 79t
Triamcinolone. See also Glucocorticoids.
  crystals of, in synovial fluid analysis,
      614, 615, Plate 8
  for juvenile rheumatoid arthritis, 1219
  for rotator cuff impingement, 424
  intra-articular injection of, 591–595, 594t
Triceps brachii muscle, dysfunction of,
    after elbow replacement, 1689
Triceps surae muscle, in hindfoot motion,
    1766
  reflex testing of, 405, 406t
Trigger finger deformity, glucocorticoid
    injection for, 604
  in rheumatoid arthritis, surgery for,
      1650–1652
  physical examination for, 360
Triglycerides, blood level of, elevated, gout
    with, 1318, 1346
Trimethoprim, with sulfamethoxazole,
    interaction of, with methotrexate, 774
Trochanter, osteotomy of, in arthroplasty,
    1777, 1796–1797
Trochanteric bursa, in snapping hip,
    474–475
  inflammation of, and pain, 474–475
    examination for, 364
    glucocorticoid injection for, 597
Troponin, in skeletal muscle, 79t
Tryptase, immunoassays for, in mast cell
    assessment, 171
  in arthritis, 171–172
  in extracellular matrix degradation, 324t,
      325, 325t
  in mast cell mediation, 166–167, 167t
L-Tryptophan, contaminated, and
    eosinophilia-myalgia syndrome, 1157,
    1185
Tuberculosis, and arthritis, synovial biopsy
    in, 621, 621, Plate 9
  and osteomyelitis, 1453
  and Poncet's disease, 1455
  and septic arthritis, 1453–1454, 1454
    imaging of, 677, 677
  and spondylitis, 1451, 1451–1453, 1452
  extrapulmonary, with arthritis, 1012–
      1013
  immunization against, bacille Calmette-
      Guérin in, and rheumatic syn-
      dromes, 1455
  osteoarticular, 1450–1451
  spinal, and low back pain, 451–452
  treatment of, 1454
  with reticulohistiocytosis, multicentric,
      1431
Tubular necrosis, acute, in
    rhabdomyolysis, 1194
Tubular system, dense, in platelets, 176,
    177t
Tumor(s), after hip arthroplasty, 1816
  and hip pain, 476
  and low back pain, 453
  and polyarticular pain, 386

Tumor(s) (Continued)
  and shoulder pain, 435
  angiogenesis with, 183–184
  computed tomography of, 630
  growth of, resistance to, macrophages
      in, 140
  macrophages in, 140
  malignant. See Cancer.
  of joints, 1597–1616
    fatty, 1597, 1597–1598, 1598
  of salivary glands, vs. Sjögren's syn-
      drome, 957t, 958–960
  of synovium, biopsy of, 622–623
    vascular, 1598, 1598–1599, 1599
  vasculitis with, skin lesions in, 503
  with scleroderma, 1150
Tumor necrosis factor(s), genes for, 213,
    213
  in autoimmune disease, in population as-
      sociation studies, 220
  in bone cell metabolism, 61, 61
  in bone remodeling, 59
  soluble receptors of, 871
Tumor necrosis factor-α, 101, 103t
  and antineoplastic function, of macro-
      phages, 140
  in chronic inflammation, 276
  in fibroblast regulation, 201, 202, 204,
      205
  in leukocyte homing, 315
  in mast cell mediation, 162t, 170
  in rheumatoid arthritis, 867, 869
    antibody to, 945
    genetic variations in, 853–854
    interaction of, with interferon-γ, 865
    therapy targeting, 844
  in scleroderma, 1139
  receptors of, soluble, 280–281
Tumor necrosis factor-β, in scleroderma,
    1139
Twins, rheumatic disease in, genetic
    susceptibility to, 209
Tyrosine, in B cell activation, 119
  in mast cell regulation, 171
  in T cell activation, 116–118
Tyrosine hydroxylase, in joint
    development, 4
Tyrosine kinase, in bone remodeling, 59,
    60
  in neutrophilic metabolism, 153
  in X-linked agammaglobulinemia, 1287

U3 snoRNP, antibodies to, in inflammatory
    muscle diseases, 261
  in scleroderma, 258t, 259
Ubiquitin C-terminal hydrolase, in joint
    development, 4
Ulcerative colitis, arthritis with, 1007,
    1007–1008, 1008t
  monarticular, 377
  vs. rheumatoid arthritis, 903
Ulcers, in Behçet's disease, 1114, 1114t,
    1114–1116, Plate 12
  in systemic lupus erythematosus, 1036
  of skin, digital, in scleroderma, treat-
      ment of, 1153, 1153
    in Reiter's syndrome, 988, 989, 989
    in vasculitis, with rheumatoid arthri-
        tis, 1110, 1111, 1111
  peptic, glucocorticoids and, 795
    nonsteroidal anti-inflammatory drugs
        and, 714–715
Ulna, articulation of, with radius, in
    rheumatoid arthritis, 1655

Ulna *(Continued)*
  subluxation of, physical examination for, 360
Ulnar nerve, disorders of, in thoracic outlet syndromes, 577
  muscle testing for, 399t
  entrapment of, *573*, 573–575
    glucocorticoids for, 597
  injury to, in surgery, 586
  neurapraxia of, after total elbow replacement, 1689
Ultrasonography, in myopathy, 390–391
  of heart, in rheumatic fever, 1233
  of knee, 460, *460*
  of rotator cuff, preoperative, 1697–1698
  of shoulder, 417–419, *419*, 422t
Ultraviolet light, sensitivity to, in systemic lupus erythematosus, 1030t, 1036
  management of, 1041, 1042t
  with psoralen, for Reiter's syndrome, 993
Uncovertebral joints, anatomy of, 397
  disorders of, imaging of, 668
Upper motor neurons, disorders of, and weakness, 392
Urate, crystals of, in gout, acute, 1338–1340
  destruction of, drugs for, 837, *837*
  in nephropathy, 1320–1321, *1321*
    familial, 1322
  synthesis of, inhibition of, drugs for, *829–831*, 829–833, 832t
Urethritis, in Reiter's syndrome, 988
Uric acid, blood level of, elevated. See *Hyperuricemia.*
  measurement of, 1885
  excretion of, enhancement of, drugs for, 833–837, *834*, 834t, *835*, 836t
  extrarenal deposition of, 1327
  formation of, 1324–1327, *1325*
  in nephropathy, 1321–1322
  overproduction of, in gout, primary, 1332–1336, *1333*, 1334t, 1335t, *1336*
    secondary, *1337*, 1337–1338
  physical properties of, 1329t, 1329–1330
  renal clearance of, 1327–1329, 1328t
  renal handling of, in gout, primary, 1330–1332, *1332*
    secondary, 1336
Uricase, for hyperuricemia, 837, *837*
Uridine diphophoglucose dehydrogenase, in joint development, 3
Urine, blood in, D-penicillamine and, 767
Urokinase-type plasminogen activator, in extracellular matrix degradation, 324t, 325t, 325–326
  inhibitors of, 328, 329t
  regulation of, cellular, 334, 335t
    extracellular, 335
Urticarial vasculitis, 503
Uterus, endometriosis of, and hip pain, 476
Uveitis, 489t, 489–490
  in ankylosing spondylitis, 974
  in Behçet's disease, 1114, *1115*, 1116, Plate 12
  in juvenile rheumatoid arthritis, 1212, *1212*, 1219–1222
  in Reiter's syndrome, 989–990, 994
  in sarcoidosis, 493
Uveoparotid fever, vs. Sjögren's syndrome, 960

Vaccination, against rubella, and arthritis, 1477

Vaccination *(Continued)*
  T cells in, for rheumatoid arthritis, *845*, 845–846
Varicella-zoster virus infection, and arthritis, 1481
Vascular adhesion protein-1, in lymphocyte migration, 121
Vascular cell adhesion molecule-1, expression of, cytokines and, 268, 269
  in leukocyte-endothelial adhesion, 186t, 187t, 188–190, *191*
  in rheumatoid arthritis, 873t, 873–874
    therapy targeting, 839–840
Vascular endothelial growth factor, in angiogenesis, 183–184, 274
  in inflammatory response, 194
  in rheumatoid arthritis, 872–873
Vascular leukocyte antigen-4, in rheumatoid arthritis, 860–861, 873t, 874
  therapy targeting, 839–840
Vasculitis, 1079–1116
  and polyarticular pain, 386
  classification of, 1079–1080, 1080t
  cryoglobulinemic, 1108–1110
  cutaneous, *1103*, 1103–1105
    granulomatous, 1108
  diagnosis of, 1085t, 1085–1087, 1086t
  glucocorticoids for, 1107
  hypocomplementemic, 1107
  immune complex in, 1080t, 1080–1085
  in Behçet's disease, 1114t, 1114–1116, *1115*, 1116
  in Buerger's disease, 1113–1114
  in children, 1242t, 1253–1261
    in giant cell arteritis, 1259–1260, *1260*
    in granulomatous arteritis, 1260–1261
    necrotizing, *1254*, 1254t, 1254–1259, 1255t, *1256–1258*
  in Cogan's syndrome, 1112–1113
  in Henoch-Schönlein purpura, *1105*, 1105–1106
  in human immunodeficiency virus infection, 1277–1278
  in polyarteritis, 1091–1097, *1092*, *1093*, *1095*, 1107
  in rheumatoid arthritis, 497, 919–920, 1110–1111, *1111*
  in sarcoidosis, 1421
  in Sjögren's syndrome, 497, 961, 1111
  in systemic lupus erythematosus, 1035, 1111–1112
  in Takayasu's arteritis, 1088–1090, *1090*
  in Waldenström's hypergammaglobulinemic purpura, 1108
  in Wegener's granulomatosis, 1099–1103, *1100*
  inflammation in, laboratory evaluation of, 703
  malignancy with, 503, 1086, 1112
  necrotizing, paraneoplastic, 1524, 1527t
  skin lesions in, 502t, 502–504, *503*, Plate 5
  of central nervous system, isolated, 1090–1091
  pathogenesis of, 1080–1085, *1081*, *1084*
  treatment of, 1087–1088
Vasodilatation, in inflammatory response, endothelium in, 184–185
Vasodilators, interactions of, with nonsteroidal anti-inflammatory drugs, 719t
Vasopressin, for hemophilia, 1489
Vaughan-Jackson lesion, surgery for, *1648*, *1649*, 1649–1650

VCAM-1. See *Vascular cell adhesion molecule-1.*
VDJ rearrangement, in antigen-specific recognition, 107–110, *108*, *109*
Venography, lumbar epidural, in low back pain, 446
Versican, in extracellular matrix, *42*, 45
Vertebrae. See *Spine.*
Vertebral arteries, anatomy of, 399–400
Vertigo, diagnosis of, dynamic posturography in, 408
  in Cogan's syndrome, 1112
Very-late-activation antigen-4, expression of, cytokines and, 269
Vestibular system, disorders of, in Cogan's syndrome, 1112, 1113
Villonodular synovitis, 1604
  pigmented. See *Synovitis, pigmented villonodular.*
Vinblastine, in immunosuppression, for non-neoplastic diseases, *810*, 814–815, 823t
Vincristine, in immunosuppression, for non-neoplastic diseases, *810*, 814–815, 823t
Viral infection. See also specific infections, e.g., *Human immunodeficiency virus (HIV) infection.*
  and antiribonucleoprotein antibody response, in mixed connective tissue disease, 1067–1068
  and arthritis, 1473–1482
    adenovirus in, 1480–1481
    alphaviruses in, 1478–1479
    coxsackievirus in, 1480
    cytomegalovirus in, 1481–1482
    echovirus in, 1480
    Epstein-Barr virus in, 1481
    hepatitis A virus in, 1482
    hepatitis B virus in, 1473–1475, *1474*
    herpes simplex virus in, 1481
    monarticular, 376
    mumps virus in, 1479–1480
    parvovirus in, 1477–1478
    polyarticular, peripheral, 383
    rubella in, 1475–1477, *1476*
    varicella-zoster virus in, 1481
    vs. rheumatoid arthritis, 906–907
  and myopathy, 1190–1191, 1191t
  and rheumatoid arthritis, 854–857, 855t
  and vasculitis, 1086, 1086t
  brachial neuritis after, and shoulder pain, 433
  immune complex assays in, 232t
  in inflammatory myopathy, 1187
  in psoriatic arthritis, 1000
  resistance to, mononuclear phagocytes in, 140
  rheumatoid factors in, 242, 242t
  with cytotoxic drug therapy, 1049, 1050, 1050t
Vision, disorders of, antimalarial agents and, 747, 755, 755t, 756
  cervical spinal disorders and, 403
  in giant cell arteritis, 1126, *1126*, 1130
Vitamin A, antioxidant effect of, 523–524
Vitamin C (ascorbic acid), antioxidant effect of, 524
  deficiency of, and scurvy, synovial biopsy in, 623
  in collagen synthesis, 26
Vitamin D, antioxidant effect of, 524
  in bone cell metabolism, 60
  in osteocalcin synthesis, 63
  in osteomalacia, 1572t, 1572–1574, 1574t

Vitamin D *(Continued)*
 resistance to, 1503
 in osteoporosis, 1564, 1565, 1570, 1571
 preventive use of, with glucocorticoids, 795
  in rheumatoid arthritis, 940
  in systemic lupus erythematosus, 1050, 1050t
Vitamin E, antioxidant effect of, 524
Vitronectin, in extracellular matrix, 37, *38*, *42*, 43, 51
VLA-4 (very-late-activation antigen-4), expression of, cytokines and, 269
Voice, disorders of, in rheumatoid arthritis, of cricoarytenoid joints, 911
Volkmann's canals, in osteal blood supply, 69
Voltaren (diclofenac), 729t, *733*, 733–734
 anti-inflammatory effect of, 711
 toxicity of, to liver, 715

Waldenström's hypergammaglobulinemic purpura, 1108
Waldenström's macroglobulinemia, plasmapheresis for, 817
 rheumatoid factors in, 242, 244, 246
Walkers, in rehabilitative medicine, *1629*, 1629–1630
Walking, disorders of, in osteoarthritis, 1386
 in hip examination, 363
 quadriceps motion in, control of, 92, *92*
Walldius prosthesis, in knee replacement, 1832
Walnuts, sensitivity to, in Behçet's syndrome, 531
Warfarin, for thrombosis, in antiphospholipid syndrome, 1062
 in systemic lupus erythematosus, 1051
 interactions of, with nonsteroidal anti-inflammatory drugs, 719t, 720
 with hip arthroplasty, 1730, 1732
 with knee arthroplasty, 1751
Wartenberg's syndrome, 576
Waugh ankle prosthesis, radiography of, 1836, *1839*
Weakness, 388–393
 classification of, 388–389, 389t, *390*
 in myopathy, 388
 in neuromuscular syndromes, 388t
 in rheumatologic disorders, 392–393
 involutional, 388
 laboratory evaluation of, 390–391
 of joints, in patient history, 354
 physical examination in, 389–390
 spinal nerve root disorders and, 402
Weber-Christian disease, 508
Wegener's granulomatosis, 1099–1103, *1100*
 antineutrophil cytoplasmic antibodies in, 1099, 1101–1102
 clinical features of, 1100–1101
 cyclophosphamide for, 809, 812, 815–816, *816*, 1102–1103
 diagnosis of, 1102
 epidemiology of, 1099
 in children, 1260–1261
 laboratory tests in, 1101
 ocular disorders in, 493, *493*, 1101, Plate 4
 pathogenesis of, 1081–1083, *1084*, 1099–1100
 pathology of, 1100, *1100*
 skin lesions in, 503

Wegener's granulomatosis *(Continued)*
 treatment of, 1102–1103
Weight, excessive, gout with, 1318, 1346
 in osteoarthritis, 385, 1379, 1385
  management of, 1394, 1852
 loss of, in systemic lupus erythematosus, 1029
Weight-bearing, articular cartilage in, 1371
 during radiography, 626–627
Werner's syndrome, and cancer, 1529
Westergren technique, in erythrocyte sedimentation measurement, 701, 704, 1884
Western blot testing, for antinuclear antibodies, 254
 in Lyme disease, 1467, *1468*, 1873
Wheelchairs, in rehabilitative medicine, 1630
Whipple's disease, 1011, *1012*
 arthritis in, monarticular, 377
  polyarticular, 385
 synovial biopsy in, 623
 vs. rheumatoid arthritis, 903
White blood cells. See *Leukocytes.*
Williams' syndrome, 1554
Wilson's disease, arthropathy in, imaging of, 676
Wiskott-Aldrich syndrome, 1286t, 1296–1297
 carrier detection in, 1300
 genetics of, 1284, 1284t
 intrauterine diagnosis of, 1299–1300
 treatment of, 1300, 1302
Wolff's law, 70
Wound healing, fibroblasts in, *199*, 199–206, *200*, 201t, 202t, *203*, 204t
Wright's stain, in synovial fluid analysis, 615, 616
Wrist, anatomy of, magnetic resonance imaging of, *568*
 arthritis in, monarticular, differential diagnosis of, 373t
 arthrocentesis of, 601, *602*
 arthroplasty of, patient selection for, 1637
 examination of, *359*, 359–360
 ganglion cyst of, 1593–1595, *1594*, *1595*
  aspiration of, 597, 604
 in calcium pyrophosphate deposition disease, imaging of, 673, *673*, 674, *675*
 in systemic lupus erythematosus, surgery of, 1662, 1663
 juvenile rheumatoid arthritis of, surgery for, 1661, 1662, *1663*
  synovectomy in, 1774, *1774*
 magnetic resonance imaging of, *639*, 641
 osteoarthritis of, imaging of, 664
  surgery for, 1673
 psoriatic arthritis of, surgery for, 1669
 rheumatoid arthritis of, 912–913
  imaging of, *647*, 647–648, 648t, *649*
  nonsurgical management of, 1647–1648
  surgery for, in flexor tenosynovitis, 1650, *1651*
   reconstructive, 1653–1655
   synovectomy in, 1652
 splints for, 1625–1626, *1626*
 surgery of, 1647–1673
  evaluation for, 1647
 ulnar nerve entrapment in, 574

Xanthine, in renal disorders, in gout, management of, 829, 832

Xanthine *(Continued)*
 in uric acid formation, 1324–1325, *1325*
Xanthine dehydrogenase, inhibition of, allopurinol in, *829*, 829–830, *830*
Xanthine oxidase, allopurinol inhibiting, 1344
 in oxidant radical production, and hyperuricemia, 1320
Xanthoma, of tendon sheath, with fibrosis, 1608–1610, *1610*, *1611*
 synovial. See *Synovitis, pigmented villonodular.*
Xanthomatosis, vs. rheumatoid nodules, 918
Xenon, in imaging, after intra-articular glucocorticoid injection, 591
Xerophthalmia, in diffuse infiltrative lymphocytosis, in human immunodeficiency virus infection, 1274
Xerosis, in Sjögren's syndrome, 497
Xerostomia, in diffuse infiltrative lymphocytosis, in human immunodeficiency virus infection, 1274
 in Sjögren's syndrome, 488, 957–958, 965
X-linked defects, and agammaglobulinemia, 1284t, 1285t, 1286–1288, *1287*
 and Alport's syndrome, 1556
 and cutis laxa, 1551
 and immunodeficiency, 1284, 1284t
  carriers of, detection of, 1300
  intrauterine diagnosis of, 1299–1300
  severe combined, 1295
 and lymphoproliferative disease, 1285t, 1292
 and rickets, 1573
 and Wiskott-Aldrich syndrome, 1284, 1284t, 1286t, 1296–1297

Yergason's supination sign, in bicipital tendinitis, 427
Yersinia infection, gastrointestinal, arthritis with, 1009, 1009t, 1010
 vs. rheumatoid arthritis, 903
 in Reiter's syndrome, 984–986, 989, 993

Z lines, in skeletal muscle, 78, 79t, *80*
ZAP-70, in T cell activation, 116
Zeta potentials, in osteopenia, 63
Zidovudine (AZT), excretion of, probenecid inhibiting, 837
 for human immunodeficiency virus infection, and myopathy, 1277
  with diffuse infiltrative lymphocytosis, 1276
  with psoriatic skin disease, 1272
Zileuton, as lipoxygenase inhibitor, for inflammatory diseases, 297t, 298–299
Zinc, in activation of metalloproteins, 335, *336*
 in immune response, *523*, 525
Zonula adherens, cadherins in, 303
Zygapophyseal joints, anatomy of, 397
 lumbar, computed tomography of, 631, *632*
Zymosan, and platelet aggregation, 179
 in neutrophil function, 149, *149*